| DRUGS WITH ILLUSTRATED MECHANISMS OF ACTION | DRUGS WITH SIM[  ] MECHANISMS OF [  ] |
|---|---|
| efalizumab | sirolimus |
| enoxacin | alatrofloxacin mesylate, cinoxacin, ciprofloxacin, gatifloxacin, levofloxacin, lomefloxacin hydrochloride, moxifloxacin hydrochloride, nalidixic acid, norfloxacin, ofloxacin, sparfloxacin, trovafloxacin mesylate |
| etanercept | infliximab |
| exenatide | none |
| ezetimibe | none |
| famotidine | cimetidine, nizatidine, ranitidine hydrochloride |
| hydrochlorothiazide | chlorothiazide, chlorothiazide sodium, chlorthalidone, indapamide, metolazone |
| ipratropium bromide | none |
| isosorbide dinitrate, isosorbide mononitrate | nitroglycerin |
| lanthanum carbonate | sevelamer hydrochloride |
| levodopa | none |
| linezolid | none |
| memantine hydrochloride | none |
| milrinone lactate | inamrinone (formerly amrinone lactate) |
| nateglinide | repaglinide |
| olmesartan medoxomil | irbesartan, losartan potassium, valsartan |
| omeprazole | esomeprazole magnesium, lansoprazole, pantoprazole sodium, rabeprazole sodium |
| orlistat | none |
| palonosetron | alosetron, dolasetron, granisetron, ondansetron |
| pegvisomant | none |
| phenelzine sulfate | isocarboxazid, tranylcypromine sulfate |
| remifentanil hydrochloride | codeine phosphate, codeine sulfate, fentanyl citrate, fentanyl transdermal, fentanyl transmucosal, hydrocodone bitartrate and acetaminophen, hydrocodone and ibuprofen, hydromorphone hydrochloride, levomethadyl acetate hydrochloride, levorphanol tartrate, meperidine hydrochloride, methadone hydrochloride, morphine |

# Mechanism of Action Illustrations (continued)

| DRUGS WITH ILLUSTRATED MECHANISMS OF ACTION | DRUGS WITH SIMILAR MECHANISMS OF ACTION |
|---|---|
| remifentanil hydrochloride | codeine phosphate, codeine sulfate, fentanyl citrate, fentanyl transdermal, fentanyl transmucosal, hydrocodone bitartrate and acetaminophen, hydrocodone and ibuprofen, hydromorphone hydrochloride, levomethadyl acetate hydrochloride, levorphanol tartrate, meperidine hydrochloride, methadone hydrochloride, morphine sulfate, oxycodone and acetaminophen, oxycodone hydrochloride, oxymorphone hydrochloride, propoxyphene hydrochloride |
| reserpine | guanadrel sulfate, guanethidine monosulfate |
| spironolactone | none |
| tacrine hydrochloride | donepezil hydrochloride, galantamine hydrobromide, rivastigmine tartrate |
| teriparatide | none |
| ticlopidine hydrochloride | clopidogrel bisulfate |
| tubocurarine chloride | atracurium besylate |
| vasopressin | desmopressin acetate, lypressin |
| ziconitide | none |

# Nurse's Drug Handbook
## 2007

# Blanchard & Loeb Publishers

Nurse's Choice for Better Care®

# Nurse's Drug Handbook 2007

Blanchard & Loeb
PUBLISHERS, LLC
*Nurse's Choice for Better Care*®

San Francisco•Philadelphia•New York

Blanchard & Loeb
PUBLISHERS, LLC
*Nurse's Choice for Better Care*®

**Publishers:** Ross Blanchard, Stanley E. Loeb
**Clinical Director:** Marlene Ciranowicz, RN, MSN, CDE
**Clinical Editors:** Patricia Fischer, RN, BSN; Nancy F. Martin, RN, MSN;
Colleen Seeber-Combs, RN, MSN
**Book Editor:** Doris Weinstock
**Editors:** Jennifer Bryant, Jane Cray, Kevin D. Dodds, Catherine E. Harold, Deborah Lyons,
Nancy Priff, Michael Shaw
**Copy Editors:** Karen Comerford, Dolores Matthews
**Indexer:** Barbara Hodgson
**Cover:** Ray Keim
**Interior Illustrations:** Rolin Graphics, Inc.
**Composition:** Matrix Publishing Services

Printed in the United States of America

Blanchard & Loeb Publishers, LLC
454 Railroad Avenue
Shiremanstown, PA 17011

# Contents

# Advisors

**Jack E. Fincham,** RPh, PhD
Dean and Professor of Pharmacy
Practice
School of Pharmacy
University of Kansas
Lawrence, KS

**Martha Mitchell Funnell,** RN, MS, CDE
Associate Director for Administration
Diabetes Research and Training Center
University of Michigan
Ann Arbor, MI

**Mary E. MacCara,** PharmD
Associate Professor
College of Pharmacy
Assistant Professor
Department of Family Medicine
Dalhousie University
Halifax, NS, Canada

**S. Edet Ohia,** PhD
Professor of Pharmaceutical Sciences
Associate Dean for Administration
School of Pharmacy and Allied Health
Professions
Creighton University
Omaha, NE

**Kristine A. Quart,** PharmD
Medical Education Consultant
Olivenhain, CA

**Ruth Stanley,** PharmD, FASHP
Consultant
Birmingham, AL

**Joseph P. Zbilut,** RN,C, DNSc, PhD, ANP
Professor
Adult Health Nursing
Rush University College of Nursing
Professor
Molecular Biophysics and Physiology
Rush Medical College
Chicago, IL

**Patti Rager Zuzelo,** RN,CS, MSN, EdD
Associate Professor
School of Nursing
La Salle University
Philadelphia, PA
Associate Director of Nursing for
Research
Albert Einstein Medical Center
Philadelphia, PA
Casual Pool Registered Nurse
Emergency Trauma Care
Abington Memorial Hospital
Abington, PA

# Reviewers and Clinical Consultants

## Reviewers

**Peter J. Ambrose, PharmD**
Associate Clinical Professor, Step III
Director
Los Angeles-Orange County Area Clerkships
University of California, San Francisco
San Francisco, CA

**Donna Barto, RN, MA, CCRN**
Nurse Educator
Helene Fuld School of Nursing
Blackwood, NJ
Staff Nurse
Virtua Memorial Hospital
Mount Holly, NJ

**Edward M. Bednarczyk, PharmD**
Clinical Assistant Professor
Pharmacy Practice and Nuclear Medicine
State University of New York at Buffalo
Buffalo, NY

**Cristina E. Bello, PharmD**
Assistant Professor of Pharmacy Practice
College of Pharmacy
Nova Southeastern University
Fort Lauderdale, FL

**Scott M. Bonnema, PharmD**
Consultant Pharmacist
Emissary Pharmacy and Infusion
Casper, WY

**Felesia R. Bowen, RN, MS, PNP,C**
Clinical Nurse Specialist
Children's Hospital at Robert Wood Johnson
University Hospital
New Brunswick, NJ

**Cynthia Burman, PharmD**
Clinical Assistant Professor
School of Pharmacy
Temple University
Philadelphia, PA

**Kimberly A. Couch, PharmD**
Clinical Pharmacy Specialist, Infectious
Diseases
Department of Pharmacy
Christiana Care Health System
Newark, DE

**Brenda S. Frymoyer, RN, MSN**
Clinical Nurse Specialist
Berks Cardiologists, Inc.
Reading, PA

**Kimberly A. Galt, PharmD, FASHP**
Associate Professor of Pharmacy Practice
Director
Drug Information Services
Co-Director
Center for Practice Improvement and Outcomes
Research
Creighton University
Omaha, NE

**Deborah L. Green, RN, MSN**
Director
Medical Telemetry-CHF Program
Moses H. Cone Health System
Greensboro, NC

**Ronald L. Greenberg, PharmD, BCPS**
Clinical Pharmacy Coordinator
Fairview Ridges Hospital
Burnsville, MN

**Jan K. Hastings, PharmD**
Assistant Professor
College of Pharmacy
University of Arkansas for Medical Science
Little Rock, AR

**Michael D. Hogue, PharmD**
Assistant Professor of Pharmacy Practice
McWhorter School of Pharmacy
Samford University
Clinical Coordinator
Walgreen Drug Store
Birmingham, AL

**Kimberly A. Hunter, PharmD**
Assistant Professor of Pharmacy Practice
Albany College of Pharmacy
Albany, NY

**William A. Kehoe, Jr., PharmD, BCPS, FCCP**
Professor of Clinical Pharmacy and Psychology
School of Pharmacy and Health Sciences
University of the Pacific
Stockton, CA

**Julienne K. Kirk, PharmD, BCPS, CDE**
Assistant Professor
Department of Family Medicine
School of Medicine
Wake Forest University
Winston-Salem, NC

**Peter G. Koval, PharmD, BCPS**
Clinical Pharmacist
Moses H. Cone Family Practice
Greensboro, NC

**Lisa M. Krupa, RN,C, CEN, FNP**
Nurse Practitioner
Medical Specialists
Munster, IN

**Amista A. Lone, PharmD**
Clinical Assistant Professor
College of Pharmacy
University of Arizona
Tucson, AZ

**Jennifer L. Lutz, PharmD**
Pharmacy Resident
Samuel S. Stratton Veterans Affairs Medical
Center
Albany, NY

**T. Donald Marsh, PharmD, FASCP, FASHP**
Director
Department of Pharmacotherapy
Mountain Area Health Education Center
Asheville, NC

**Patrick McDonnell, PharmD**
Assistant Professor of Clinical Pharmacy
School of Pharmacy
Temple University
Philadelphia, PA

**Catherine M. Oliphant, PharmD**
Assistant Professor of Pharmacy Practice
School of Pharmacy
University of Wyoming
Laramie, WY

**Michael A. Oszko, PharmD, BCPS**
Associate Professor
Dept. of Pharmacy
University of Kansas
Kansas City, KS

**Vinita B. Pai, PharmD**
Assistant Professor of Pharmacy Practice
College of Pharmacy
Idaho State University
Pocatello, ID

**David J. Quan, PharmD**
Clinical Pharmacist
University of California, San Francisco
San Francisco, CA

**Susan M. Rao, RN, MSN**
Staff Nurse
Intensive Care Unit
Saint Luke East
Fort Thomas, KY

**Susan L. Ravnan, PharmD**
Assistant Professor of Pharmacy Practice
School of Pharmacy and Health Sciences
University of the Pacific
Stockton, CA

**Brenda M. Reap-Thompson, RN, MSN**
Nurse Educator
Community College of Philadelphia
Philadelphia, PA
Nurse Consultant
Chauncey International, ETS
Princeton, NJ

**Nancy Jex Sabin, RN, MSN, CFNP**
Instructor
Hahn School of Nursing and Health Science
Family Nurse Practitioner
Student Health Center
University of San Diego
San Diego, CA

**Melissa L. Sanders, PharmD**
Assistant Professor of Clinical Pharmacy
School of Pharmacy
Temple University
Philadelphia, PA

**Regina E. Silk, PharmD, RPh, BCPS**
Assistant Clinical Professor
University of Connecticut Health Center
Farmington, CT

**Elizabeth Sloand, RN, MSN, CPNP**
Assistant Professor
School of Nursing
Johns Hopkins University
Baltimore, MD

**Thomas F. Turco, PharmD**
Clinical Pharmacist
Assistant Director of Pharmacy
Our Lady of Lourdes Medical Center
Camden, NJ

**Lili Wang, PhD**
Assistant Professor
School of Pharmacy
Memorial University of Newfoundland
St. Johns, NF, Canada

**Craig Williams, PharmD**
Clinical Specialist
Wishard Memorial Hospital
Assistant Professor of Clinical Pharmacy
School of Pharmacy
Purdue University
Indianapolis, IN

# Clinical Consultants

**Madeline Albanese, RN, MSN**
Nurse Educator
Hospital of the University of Pennsylvania
Philadelphia, PA

**Marlene Ciranowicz, RN, MSN, CDE**
Independent Consultant
Huntingdon Valley, PA

**Sheree M. Fitzgerald, RN,C, MSN, CNA**
Program Coordinator
Ancora Psychiatric Hospital
Hammonton, NJ

**Maryann Foley, RN, BSN**
Independent Consultant
Flourtown, PA

**Grace Hukushi, RN, BSN, LNC**
Critical Care Nurse
Nursing Enterprises, Inc.
Brick, NJ

**Sammie Justesen, RN, BSN**
Independent Nurse Consultant
Providence, UT

**Catherine T. Kelly, RN, PhD, CCRN, CEN, ANP**
Faculty
School of Nursing
Mount Saint Mary College
Newburgh, NY

**Sharon Kumm, RN, MN, CCRN**
Assistant Professor
School of Nursing
University of Kansas
Kansas City, KS

**Leanne McQuade, RN, BSN, CEN**
Staff Nurse
Emergency Dept.
Doylestown Hospital
Case Manager
CAB Medical Consultant
Doylestown, PA

**Pamela S. Ronning, RN, MPA**
Program Coordinator
Kirkhof School of Nursing
Grand Valley State University
Allendale, MI

**Maureen Ryan, RN,CS, MSN, FNP**
Assistant Professor
Grand Valley State University
Allendale, MI
Nurse Practitioner
Emergency Dept.
St. Mary's Hospital
Grand Rapids, MI

**Julie M. Smith, RN, BA**
Staff Nurse
Radiology-Heart Station
Rancocas Hospital
Willingboro, NJ

**Aaron J. Strehlow, RN,CS, FNP-C, NPNP**
Administrator and Director of Clinical Services
UCLA School of Nursing
Health Center at the Rescue Mission
Los Angeles, CA

**Maria Wilson, RN, MSN, CCRN**
Staff Nurse
Emergency Dept.
Chestnut Hill Hospital
Philadelphia, PA

*Blanchard & Loeb Publishers Nurse's Drug Handbook 2007*, the Nurse's Choice for Better Care®, gives you what today's nurses and nursing students need: accurate, concise, and reliable drug facts. This book emphasizes the vital information you need to know before, during, and after drug administration. And the information is presented in easy-to-understand language and organized alphabetically, so you can find what you need quickly.

## What's Special

In addition to the drug information you expect to find in each entry (see "Drug Entries" for details), *Nurse's Drug Handbook 2007* boasts these special features:

• **Practical trim size** allows the book to open flat so you can find the information you need without wrestling with a book that wants to close. You can hold the book in one hand, see complete pages at a glance, and use your other hand to document or perform other activities.

• **Introductory material** reviews essential general information you need to know to administer drugs safely and effectively, including an overview of pharmacology and the principles of drug administration. In addition, the five steps of the nursing process are explained and related specifically to drug therapy.

• **Colorful illustrations** throughout the text help you visualize selected mechanisms of action by showing how drugs work at the cellular, tissue, and organ levels. In addition, the inside front cover features a chart listing all the drugs whose mechanisms of action are illustrated as well as other drugs with the same mechanisms of action.

• **No-nonsense writing style** that speaks everyday language and uses the terms and abbreviations you typically encounter in your practice and your studies—although a few abbreviations may not be used in certain facilities. (See *Abbreviations*, pages 1126 to 1127.) And to avoid sexist language, we alternate between male and female pronouns throughout the book.

• **Up-to-date drug information,** including the latest FDA-approved drugs, new and changed indications, new warnings, and newly discovered adverse reactions.

• **Dosage adjustment,** highlighted in the text, alerts you to expected dosage changes for a patient with a specific condition or disorder, such as advanced age or renal impairment.

• **Warning,** highlighted in the text, calls attention to important facts that you need to know before, during, and after drug administration. For example, in the alatrofloxacin entry, this feature informs you that the drug usually is reserved for hospitalized patients and is given for no more than 2 weeks because of the high risk of severe liver damage.

• **Easy-to-use charts** for route, onset, peak, and duration and other charts in the appendices provide a timesaving way to track and check information. (See page xiii for details on route, onset, peak, and duration charts.) The appendices give an overview of the most important drug facts and nursing considerations for important drug groups, including insulin preparations and antihypertensive combination drugs. You'll also find handy information you can use every day in your practice and studies, such as instructions for calculating drug dosages and I.V. flow rates.

## Drug Entries

*Nurse's Drug Handbook 2007* clearly and concisely presents all the vital facts on the drugs that you'll typically administer. To help you find the information you need quickly, drug entries are organized alphabetically by generic drug name—from abciximab to zonisamide. For ease of use, every drug entry follows a consistent format. However, if specific details are unknown or don't apply, the heading isn't

## FDA pregnancy risk categories

Each drug may be placed in a pregnancy risk category based on the FDA's estimate of risk to the fetus. If the FDA hasn't provided a category, the *Drug Handbook* notes that the drug is "Not rated." The categories range from A to X, signifying least to greatest fetal risk.

**A  Controlled studies show no risk**

Adequate, well-controlled studies with pregnant women have failed to demonstrate a risk to the fetus in any trimester of pregnancy.

**B  No evidence of risk in humans**

Adequate, well-controlled studies with pregnant women haven't shown increased risk of fetal abnormalities despite adverse findings in animals, or, in the absence of adequate human studies, animal studies show no fetal risk. The chance of fetal harm is remote, but remains possible.

**C  Risk can't be ruled out**

Adequate, well-controlled human studies are lacking, and animal studies have demonstrated a risk to the fetus or are lacking as well. A chance of fetal harm exists if the drug is administered during pregnancy, but the potential benefits may outweigh the potential risk.

**D  Positive evidence of risk**

Studies in humans, or investigational or post-marketing data, have demonstrated fetal risk. Nevertheless, potential benefits from the drug's use may outweigh potential risks. For example, the drug may be acceptable if needed in a life-threatening situation or serious disease for which safer drugs can't be used or are ineffective.

**X  Contraindicated in pregnancy**

Studies in animals or humans, or investigational or post-marketing reports, have demonstrated positive evidence of fetal abnormalities or risks that clearly outweigh any possible benefit to the patient.

included so you can go right to the next section.

### GENERIC AND TRADE NAMES

First, each entry identifies the drug's main generic name as well as alternate generic names. (For drugs prescribed by trade name, you can quickly check the comprehensive index, which refers you to the appropriate generic name and page.)

Next, the entry lists the most common U.S. trade names for each drug. It also includes common trade names available *only* in Canada, marked (CAN).

### CLASS, CATEGORY, AND SCHEDULE

Each entry lists the drug's chemical and therapeutic classes. With this information, you can compare drugs in the same chemical class but in different therapeutic classes and vice versa.

The entry also lists the FDA's pregnancy risk category, which categorizes drugs based on their potential to cause birth defects. (For details, see *FDA pregnancy risk categories.*)

Where appropriate, the entry also includes the drug's controlled substance schedule. (For details, see *Controlled substance schedules,* page xiv.)

### INDICATIONS AND DOSAGES

This section lists FDA-approved therapeutic indications. For each indication, you'll find the applicable drug form or route, age-group (adults, adolescents, or children), and dosage (which includes amount per dose, timing, and duration, when known and appropriate).

### ROUTE, ONSET, PEAK, AND DURATION

Quick-reference charts show the drug's onset, peak, and duration (when known) for each administration route. The *onset of action* is the time a drug takes to be absorbed, reach a therapeutic blood level, and elicit an initial therapeutic response. The *peak therapeutic effect* occurs when a drug reaches its highest blood concen-

### MECHANISM OF ACTION

Set off by a box, this section concisely describes how a drug achieves its therapeutic effects at the cellular, tissue, and organ levels, as appropriate. Illustrations of selected mechanisms of action lend exceptional detail and clarity to sometimes complex processes.

### INCOMPATIBILITIES

You'll be alerted to drugs or solutions that are incompatible with the topic drug when mixed in a syringe or solution or infused through the same I.V. line.

### CONTRAINDICATIONS

An alphabetical list details the conditions and disorders that preclude administration of the topic drug.

### INTERACTIONS

This section presents the drugs, foods, and activities (such as alcohol use and smoking) that can cause important, problematic, or life-threatening interactions with the topic drug. For each interacting drug, food, or activity, you'll learn the effects of the interaction.

### ADVERSE REACTIONS

Organized by body system, this section highlights common, serious, and life-threatening adverse reactions in alphabetical order.

### NURSING CONSIDERATIONS

Warnings, general precautions, and key information that you must know before, during, and after drug administration are detailed in this section. Examples include whether or not a pill can be crushed and how to properly reconstitute, dilute, store, handle, or dispose of a drug.

*Patient teaching* information is also included here. You'll find important guidelines for patients, such as how and when to take each prescribed drug, how to spot and manage adverse reactions, which cautions to observe, when to call the prescriber, and more. To save you time, how-

tration and the greatest amount of drug reaches the site of action to produce the maximum therapeutic response. The *duration of action* is the amount of time that a drug remains at a blood concentration that produces a therapeutic response.

# Teaching your patient about drug therapy

Your teaching about drug therapy will vary with your patient's needs and your practice setting. To help guide your teaching, each drug entry provides key information that you must teach your patient about that drug. For all patients, however, you also should:

☑ Teach the generic and trade name for each prescribed drug that he'll take after discharge—even if he took the drug before admission.

☑ Clearly explain why each drug was prescribed, how it works, and what it's supposed to do. To help your patient understand the drug's therapeutic effects, relate its action to her disorder or condition.

☑ Review the drug form, dosage, and route with the patient. Tell him whether the drug is a tablet, suppository, spray, aerosol, or other form, and explain how to administer it correctly. Also, tell him how often to take the drug and for what length of time. Emphasize that he should take the drug exactly as prescribed.

☑ Describe the drug's appearance and explain that scored tablets can be broken in half for safe, accurate dosing. Warn the patient not to break unscored tablets because doing so may alter the drug dosage. If your patient has difficulty swallowing capsules, explain that she can open ones that contain sprinkles and take them with food or a drink but that she shouldn't do this with capsules that contain powder. Also, warn her not to crush or chew enteric-coated, extended-release, sustained-release, or similar drug forms.

☑ Teach the patient about common adverse reactions that may occur. Advise him to notify the prescriber at once if a dangerous adverse reaction, such as syncope, occurs.

☑ Warn her not to suddenly stop taking a drug if she's bothered by unpleasant adverse reactions, such as a rash and mild itching. Instead, encourage her to discuss the reactions with her prescriber, who may adjust the dosage or substitute a drug that causes fewer adverse reactions.

☑ Because many drugs cause some adverse reactions, such as dizziness and drowsiness, that can impair the patient's ability to perform activities that require alertness, help him develop a dosing schedule that prevents adverse reactions from interfering with such activities.

☑ Inform the patient which adverse reactions resolve with time.

☑ Teach the patient how to store the drug properly. Let him know if the drug is sensitive to light or temperature and how to protect it from these elements.

☑ Instruct the patient to store the drug in its original container, if possible, with the drug's name and dosage clearly printed on the label.

☑ Inform the patient which devices to use—and which ones to avoid—for drug storage or administration. For example, warn him not to take liquid cyclosporine with a plastic cup or utensils.

☑ Teach the patient what to do if she misses a dose. Generally, she should take a once-daily drug as soon as she remembers—provided that she remembers within the first 24 hours. If 24 hours have elapsed, she should take the next scheduled dose, but not double the dose. If she has questions or concerns about missed doses, tell her to contact the prescriber.

☑ Provide information that's specific to the prescribed drug. For example, if a patient takes a diuretic to manage heart failure, instruct him to weigh himself daily at the same time of day, using the same scale and wearing the same amount of clothing. Or if the patient takes digoxin or an antihypertensive drug, teach him how to measure his pulse and blood pressure and how to record the measurements. Then instruct him to bring the diary to his regular appointments so that the prescriber can monitor his response to the drug.

☑ Advise the patient to refill prescriptions promptly, unless she no longer needs the drug. Also instruct her to discard expired drugs because they may become ineffective or even dangerous over time.

☑ Warn the patient to keep all drugs out of the reach of children at all times.

ever, this section doesn't repeat basic patient-teaching points. (For a summary of those, see *Teaching your patient about drug therapy*, page xv.)

In short, *Blanchard & Loeb Publishers Nurse's Drug Handbook 2007* is designed expressly to give you more of what you need. It puts vital drug information at your fingertips and helps you remain ALWAYS CURRENT in this critical part of your practice or studies.

Safe, effective drug therapy is one of your most important responsibilities. Not infrequently, a patient's life will depend on your ability to administer drugs accurately, safely, and effectively. In addition, you must keep up with the latest drug information, including newly approved drugs and recently reported life-threatening adverse reactions, as well as those drugs withdrawn from the market after widespread use.

Despite all the drug information that is available, medication errors remain one of the greatest threats to patients' well-being and a leading cause of lawsuits against nurses, physicians, and hospitals.

## Your Responsibilities in Drug Therapy

Your basic responsibilities in drug therapy include:
- administering the right drug in the right dose by the right route at the right time to the right patient
- knowing the therapeutic use, dosage, interactions, adverse reactions, and warnings of each administered drug
- being aware of newly approved drugs that may be prescribed
- knowing about changes to existing drugs, such as new indications and dosages and recently discovered adverse reactions and interactions
- concentrating fully when preparing and administering drugs
- responding promptly and appropriately to serious or life-threatening adverse reactions, interactions, and other complications
- instructing each patient about the drug, how it's administered, which effects it causes or may cause, and which reactions to watch for and report to you or to the prescriber.

Several factors may reduce your ability to meet these basic responsibilities—and contribute to medication errors. First, hospitals and other health care facilities have budget restraints that may result in the elimination of professional nursing positions or the hiring of less qualified technicians to fill them. This forces the remaining nurses to care for more patients. Second, hospital patients are older and more acutely ill, and they typically receive more complex drug therapy than ever. Together, these factors place greater demands on you—increasing your stress level, reducing the time you have to concentrate on drug administration, and increasing your risk of making medication errors or overlooking serious adverse reactions or interactions.

The same factors reduce your time and energy for learning the latest drug facts—which you need to have at your command. You must have this information at your fingertips because your next patient may need a recently approved drug or a complex and unfamiliar drug regimen.

How can you balance your limited time, on the one hand, with your need to know the latest developments, on the other?

## Meeting Your Needs

Nurses and students need a reliable, accurate, easy-to-use, quick-reference drug book. They need a book clearly written by and for nurses that has been reviewed by experts in nursing and pharmacology. You hold such a book in your hands: *Blanchard & Loeb Publishers Nurse's Drug Handbook 2007*, the Nurse's Choice for Better Care®, with its ALWAYS CURRENT features.

The content of *Nurse's Drug Handbook 2007* was developed, written, and edited by experienced practicing nurses. Expert consultants, reviewers, and advisors—both nurses and pharmacists—help ensure the accuracy and reliability of the information covered in each entry and help target that information to your needs. What's more, every drug fact is checked against the most prominent drug references today, including the *American Hospital Formulary Service Drug Information, Drug Facts and Comparisons, The Physicians' Desk Reference,* the FDA's website of new drug approvals, and the USP DI's *Drug Information for the Health Care Professional.*

In addition, to help you quickly access much-needed information, the book is organized alphabetically by generic drug name, follows a consistent format, and is concise.

To ensure that you're always current, *Blanchard & Loeb Publishers Nurse's Drug Handbook* is updated every year. This newest edition contains:
•more than 20 new drug entries and dozens of new drugs in the appendices
•new drug facts on hundreds of existing entries, including updated information on new indications and dosages, new incompatibilities and interactions, new adverse reactions, and new nursing considerations
•hundreds of patient-teaching guidelines and suggestions
•thoroughly updated appendices on ophthalmic drugs, antihypertensive drug combinations, topical drugs, antivirals, antineoplastic drugs, and vitamins
•dozens of illustrations for important mechanisms of action
•a comprehensive new index.

Even though the book is longer than last year's, you'll find the same highly readable type size that reduces eyestrain as you speed to the information you need.

## Getting More from Your Drug Reference
Whether you work in or are preparing to work in acute care, home care, long-term care, or another health care setting, you'll want your own copy of *Nurse's Drug Handbook 2007.* That's because this book can help you:
•reduce your risk of medication errors because you'll have easy access to accurate,

reliable drug information that's relevant to your practice
•stay current on the most up-to-date drug developments of the year
•improve your drug administration skills and patient care before, during, and after drug therapy
•quickly detect and manage serious or life-threatening adverse reactions and complications or prevent them from occurring
•save time because you won't have to sift through volumes of information to find what you need, search for a book that's up-to-date, or look through several drug handbooks to get enough information
•increase your confidence about drug administration and enhance your professional interactions with other health care team members
•ensure the delivery of safe, effective care
•improve the depth and quality of your patient teaching.

## Reaping the Rewards
Your patients deserve the best and safest care possible—and you deserve to have the tools to deliver that care. Whether you're a student or an experienced clinician, *Blanchard & Loeb Publishers Nurse's Drug Handbook 2007* will help you provide safe, effective drug therapy because of its practical, easy-to-understand, accurate, and reliable information on virtually all the drugs you're likely to administer.

This handbook has aided thousands of nurses in their patient care. Take it with you to the clinical setting, share it with your peers, and use it to enhance your present and future position in the nursing profession.

Kathleen Dracup, RN, FNP, DNSc, FAAN
Dean and Professor
School of Nursing
University of California, San Francisco
San Francisco, CA

Understanding the basics of pharmacology is an essential nursing responsibility. Pharmacology is the science that deals with the physical and chemical properties, and biochemical and physiologic effects, of drugs. It includes the areas of pharmacokinetics, pharmacodynamics, pharmacotherapeutics, pharmacognosy, and toxicodynamics.

*Nurse's Drug Handbook 2007* deals primarily with pharmacokinetics, pharmacodynamics, and pharmacotherapeutics—the information you need to administer safe and effective drug therapy (discussed below). *Pharmacognosy* is the branch of pharmacology that deals with the biological, biochemical, and economic features of naturally occurring drugs. *Toxicodynamics* is the study of the harmful effects that excessive amounts of a drug produce in the body; in a drug overdose or drug poisoning, large drug doses may saturate or overwhelm normal mechanisms that control absorption, distribution, metabolism, and excretion.

### Drug Nomenclature

Most drugs are known by several names— chemical, generic, trade, and official— each of which serves a specific function. (See *How drugs are named.*) However, multiple drug names can also contribute to medication errors. You may find a familiar drug packaged with an unfamiliar name if your institution changes suppliers or if a familiar drug is newly approved in a different dose or for a new indication.

### Drug Classification

Drugs can be classified in various ways. Most pharmacology textbooks group drugs by their functional classification, such as psychotherapeutics, which is based on common characteristics. Drugs can also be classified according to their therapeutic use, such as antipanic or antiobsessional drugs. Drugs within a certain therapeutic class may be further divided into subgroups based on their mechanisms of action. For example, the therapeutic class antineoplastics can be further classified as alkylating agents, antibiotic antineoplastics, antimetabolites, antimitotics, biological response modifiers, antineoplastic enzymes, and hormonal antineoplastics.

---

## How drugs are named

A drug's chemical, generic, trade, and official names are developed at different phases of the drug development process and serve different functions. For example, the various names of the commonly prescribed anticonvulsant divalproex sodium are:
- Chemical name: Pentanoic acid, 2-propyl-, sodium salt (2:1) or ($C_{16}H_{31}O_4Na$)
- Generic name: divalproex sodium
- Trade name: Depakote
- Official name: Divalproex Sodium Delayed-Release Tablets, USP

A drug's *chemical name* describes its atomic and molecular structure. The chemical name of divalproex sodium—pentanoic acid, 2-propyl-, sodium salt (2:1), or $C_{16}H_{31}O_4Na$ (pronounced valproate semisodium)—indicates that the drug is a combination of two valproic acid compounds with a sodium molecule attached to only one side.

Once a drug successfully completes several clinical trials, it receives a *generic name,* also known as the nonproprietary name. The generic name is usually derived from but shorter than the chemical name. The United States Adopted Names Council is responsible for selecting generic names, which are intended for unrestricted public use.

Before submitting the drug for FDA approval, the manufacturer creates and registers a *trade name* (or brand name) when the drug appears ready to be marketed. Trade names are copyrighted and followed by the symbol ® to indicate that they're registered and that their use is restricted to the drug manufacturer. Once the original patent on a drug has expired, any manufacturer may produce the drug and market it with its own trade name.

A drug's *official name* is the name under which it's listed in the United States Pharmacopeia (USP) and the National Formulary (NF).

## Pharmacokinetics

Pharmacokinetics is the study of a drug's actions—or fate—as it passes through the body during absorption, distribution, metabolism, and excretion.

### ABSORPTION

Before a drug can begin working, it must be transformed from its pharmaceutical dosage form to a biologically available (bioavailable) substance that can pass through various biological cell membranes to reach its site of action. This process is known as absorption. A drug's absorption rate depends on its route of administration, its circulation through the tissue into which it's administered, and its solubility—that is, whether it's more water-soluble (*hydrophilic*) or fat-soluble (*lipophilic*).

Although drugs may penetrate cellular membranes either actively or passively, most drugs do so by *passive diffusion,* moving inertly from an area of higher concentration to an area of lower concentration. Passive diffusion may occur through water or fat. Passive diffusion through water—*aqueous diffusion*—occurs within large water-filled compartments, such as interstitial spaces, and across epithelial membrane tight junctions and pores in the epithelial lining of blood vessels. Aqueous diffusion is driven by concentration gradients. Drug molecules that are bound to large plasma proteins, such as albumin, are too large to pass through aqueous pores in this way. Passive diffusion through fat—*lipid diffusion*—plays an important role in drug metabolism because of the large number of lipid barriers that separate the aqueous compartments of the body. The ability of a drug to move through lipid layers between aqueous compartments often depends on the pH of the medium—that is, the ability of the water-soluble or fat-soluble drug to form weak acid or weak base.

Drugs whose molecules are too large to readily diffuse may rely on *active diffusion,* in which special carriers on molecules, including peptides, amino acids, and glucose, transport the drug through the membranes. However, some molecules with selective membrane carriers can expel foreign drug molecules; this is why many drugs can't cross the blood-brain barrier.

Drug absorption begins at the administration route. The three main administration route categories are enteral, parenteral, and transcutaneous. Depending on its nature or chemical makeup, a drug may be better absorbed from one site than from another.

### Enteral Administration

Enteral administration consists of the oral, nasogastric, and rectal routes.

*Oral:* Drugs administered orally are absorbed in the GI tract and then proceed by the hepatic portal vein to the liver and into the systemic circulation. Although generally considered the preferred route, oral drug administration has a number of disadvantages:

• The oral route doesn't always yield sufficiently high blood concentrations to be effective.

• Bioavailability may be less than optimal because of incomplete absorption and first-pass elimination (the part of metabolism that occurs during transit through the liver before the drug reaches the general circulation).

• Drug absorption may be incomplete if the drug is degraded by digestive enzymes or the acidic pH in the stomach or if it's excreted from the liver into the bile.

• Food in the GI tract, gastric emptying time, and intestinal motility may also impede drug absorption.

*Nasogastric:* Drugs administered through a nasogastric tube enter the stomach directly and are absorbed in the GI tract.

*Rectal:* Rectal drugs and suppositories also enter the GI tract directly after being inserted in the rectum and absorbed through the rectal mucosa. After being absorbed into the lower GI tract, rectal drugs enter the circulation through the inferior vena cava, bypassing the liver and thus avoiding first-pass metabolism. Suppositories, however, tend to travel upward into the rectum, where veins, such as the superior hemorrhoidal vein, lead to the liver. As a result, drug absorption by this route is often unreliable and difficult to predict.

### Parenteral Administration

Parenteral routes may be used whenever enteral routes are contraindicated or inadequate. These routes include intramuscular (I.M.), intravenous (I.V.), subcutaneous (S.C.) and intradermal (I.D.) administration. Drug absorption is much faster and more predictable after parenteral administration than after enteral administration.

*I.M.:* Drugs administered by the I.M. route are injected deep into the muscle, where they're absorbed relatively quickly. The rate of drug absorption depends on the vascularity of the injection site, the physiochemical properties of the drug, and the solution in which the drug is contained.

*I.V.:* I.V. drug administration involves injecting or infusing the drug directly into the blood circulation, allowing for rapid distribution throughout the body. This route usually provides the greatest bioavailability.

*S.C.:* Drugs administered by the S.C. route are injected into the alveolar connective tissue just below the skin and are absorbed by simple diffusion from the injection site. The factors that affect I.M. absorption also affect S.C. absorption. Absorption by the S.C. route may be slower than by the I.M. route.

*I.D.:* Drugs administered intradermally, such as purified protein derivative (PPD), are injected into the dermis, from which they diffuse slowly into the local microcapillary system.

### Transcutaneous Administration

Transcutaneous drug administration allows drug absorption through the skin or soft-tissue surface. Drugs may be inhaled, inserted sublingually, applied topically, or administered by the eyes, ears, nose, or vagina.

*Inhalation:* Inhaled drugs may be given as a powder and aerosolized or mixed in solution and nebulized directly into the respiratory tract, where they're absorbed through the alveoli. Inhaled drugs are usually absorbed quickly because of the abundant blood flow in the lungs.

*Sublingual:* Sublingual drug administration involves placing a tablet, troche, or lozenge under the tongue. The drug is absorbed across the epithelial lining of the mouth, usually quickly. This route avoids first-pass metabolism.

*Topical:* Topical drugs—creams, ointments, lotions, and patches—are placed on the skin and then cross the epidermis into the capillary circulation. They may also be absorbed through sweat glands, hair follicles, and other skin structures. Absorption by the skin is enhanced if the drug is in a solution.

*Ophthalmic:* Ophthalmic drugs include solutions and ointments that are instilled or applied directly to the cornea or conjunctiva as well as small, elliptical disks that are placed directly on the eyeball behind the lower eyelid. The movements of the eyeball promote distribution of these drugs over the surface of the eye. Although ophthalmic drugs produce a local effect on the conjunctiva or anterior chamber, some preparations may be absorbed systemically and therefore produce systemic effects.

*Otic:* Drops administered into the external auditory canal, otic drugs are used to treat infection or inflammation and to soften and remove ear wax. Otic solutions exert a local effect but may result in minimal systemic absorption with no adverse effects.

*Nasal:* Nasal solutions and suspensions are applied directly to the nasal mucosa by instillation or inhalation to produce local effects, such as vasoconstriction to reduce nasal congestion. Some nasal solutions, such as vasopressin, are administered by this route specifically to produce systemic effects.

*Vaginal:* Vaginal drugs include creams, suppositories, and troches that are inserted into the vagina, sometimes using a special applicator. These drugs are absorbed locally to treat such conditions as bacterial and fungal infections.

### DISTRIBUTION

Distribution is the process by which a drug is transported by the circulating fluids to various sites, including its sites of action. To ensure maximum therapeutic effectiveness, the drug must permeate all membranes that separate it from its intended site of action. Drug distribution is influenced by blood flow, tissue availability, and protein binding.

### METABOLISM

Drug metabolism is the enzymatic conversion of a drug's structure into substrate molecules or polar compounds that are either less active or inactive and are readily excreted. Drugs can also be synthesized to larger molecules. Metabolism may also convert a drug to a more toxic compound. Because the primary site of drug metabolism is the liver, children, the elderly, and patients with impaired hepatic function are at risk for altered therapeutic effects.

*Biotransformation* is the process of changing a drug into its active metabolite.

Compounds that require metabolic biotransformation for activation are known as *prodrugs*. During phase I of biotransformation, the parent drug is converted into an inactive or partially active metabolite. Much of the original drug may be eliminated during this phase. During phase II, the inactive or partially active metabolite binds with available substrates, such as acetic acid, glucuronic acid, sulfuric acid, or water, to form its active metabolite. When biotransformation leads to synthesis, larger molecules are produced to create a pharmacologic effect.

### EXCRETION

The body eliminates drugs by both metabolism and excretion. Drug metabolites—and, in some cases, the active drug itself—are eventually excreted from the body, usually through bile, feces, and urine. The primary organ for drug elimination is the kidney. Impaired renal function may cause excessive elimination of a drug, thereby reducing the drug's therapeutic effect. Other excretion routes include evaporation through the skin, exhalation from the lungs, and secretion into saliva and breast milk.

A drug's elimination *half-life* is the amount of time required for half of the drug to be eliminated from the body. The half-life roughly correlates with the drug's duration of action and is based on normal renal and hepatic function. Typically, the longer the half-life, the less often the drug has to be given and the longer it remains in the body after it's discontinued.

## Pharmacodynamics

Pharmacodynamics is the study of the biochemical and physiologic effects of drugs and their mechanisms of action. A drug's actions may be structurally specific or nonspecific. Structurally specific drugs combine with cell receptors, such as proteins or glycoproteins, to enhance or inhibit cellular enzyme actions. Drug receptors are the cellular components affected at the site of action. Many drugs form chemical bonds with drug receptors, but a drug can bond with a receptor only if it has a similar shape—much the same way that a key fits into a lock. When a drug combines with a receptor, channels are either opened or closed and cellular biochemical messengers, such as cyclic adenosine monophosphate or calcium ions, are activated. Once activated, cellular functions can be turned either on or off by these messengers. Structurally nonspecific drugs, such as biological response modifiers, don't combine with cell receptors; rather, they produce changes within the cell membrane or interior.

The mechanisms by which drugs interact with the body are not always known. Drugs may work by physical action (such as the protective effects of a topical ointment) or chemical reaction (such as an antacid's effect on the gastric mucosa), or by modifying the metabolic activity of invading pathogens (such as an antibiotic) or replacing a missing biochemical substance (such as insulin).

### AGONISTS

Agonists are drugs that interact with a receptor to stimulate a response. They alter cell physiology by binding to plasma membranes or intracellular structures. *Partial agonists* can't achieve maximal effects even though they may occupy all available receptor sites on a cell. *Strong agonists* can cause maximal effects while occupying only a small number of receptor sites on a cell. *Weak agonists* must occupy many more receptor sites than strong agonists to produce the same effect.

### ANTAGONISTS

Antagonists are drugs that attach to a receptor but don't stimulate a response; instead, they inhibit or block responses that would normally be caused by agonists. *Competitive antagonists* bind to receptor sites that are also compatible with an agonist, thus preventing the agonist from binding to the site. *Noncompetitive antagonists* bind to receptor sites that aren't occupied by an agonist; this changes the receptor site so that it's no longer recognized by the agonist. *Irreversible antagonists* work in much the same way that noncompetitive ones do, except that they permanently bind with the receptor.

Antagonism plays an important role in drug interactions. When two agonists that cause opposite therapeutic effects, such as a vasodilator and a vasoconstrictor, are combined, the effects cancel each other out. When two antagonists, such as morphine and naloxone, are combined, both drugs may become inactive.

### Pharmacotherapeutics

Pharmacotherapeutics is the study of how drugs are used to prevent or treat disease. Understanding why a drug is prescribed for a certain disease can assist you in prioritizing drug administration with other patient care activities. Knowing a drug's desired and unwanted effects may help you uncover problems not readily apparent from the admitting diagnosis. This information may also help you prevent such problems as adverse reactions and drug interactions.

A drug's *desired effect* is the intended or expected clinical response to the drug. This is the response you start to evaluate as soon as a drug is given. Dosage adjustments and the continuation of therapy often depend on your accurate evaluation and documentation of the patient's response.

An *adverse reaction* is any noxious and unintended response to a drug that occurs at therapeutic doses used for prophylaxis, diagnosis, or therapy. Adverse reactions associated with excessive amounts of a drug are considered drug overdoses. Be prepared to follow your institution's policy for reporting adverse drug reactions.

An *idiosyncratic response* is a genetically determined abnormal or excessive response to a drug that occurs in a particular patient. The unusual response may indicate that the drug has saturated or overwhelmed mechanisms that normally control absorption, distribution, metabolism, or excretion, thus altering the expected response. You may be unsure whether a reaction is adverse or idiosyncratic. Once you report the reaction, the pharmacist usually determines the appropriate course of action.

An *allergic reaction* is an adverse response that results from previous exposure to the same drug or to one that's chemically similar to it. The patient's immune system reacts to the drug as if it were a foreign invader and may produce a mild hypersensitivity reaction, characterized by localized dermatitis, urticaria, angioedema, or photosensitivity. Allergic reactions should be reported to the prescriber immediately and the drug should be discontinued. Follow-up care may include giving drugs, including antihistamines and corticosteroids, to counteract the allergic response.

An *anaphylactic reaction* involves an immediate hypersensitivity response characterized by urticaria, pruritus, and angioedema. Left untreated, an anaphylactic reaction can lead to systemic involvement, resulting in shock. It's often associated with life-threatening hypotension and respiratory distress. Be prepared to assist with emergency life support measures, especially if the reaction occurs in response to I.V. drugs, which have the fastest rate of absorption.

A *drug interaction* occurs when one drug alters the pharmacokinetics of another drug—for example, when two or more drugs are given concurrently. Such concurrent administration can increase or decrease the therapeutic or adverse effects of either drug. Some drug interactions are beneficial. For example, when taken with penicillin, probenecid decreases the excretion rate of penicillin, resulting in higher blood levels of penicillin. Drug interactions may also occur when a drug's metabolism is altered, often owing to the induction of or competition for metabolizing enzymes. For example, $H_2$-receptor agonists, which reduce secretion of the enzyme gastrin, may alter the breakdown of enteric coatings on other drugs. Drug interactions due to carrier protein competition typically occur when a drug inhibits the kidneys' ability to reduce excretion of other drugs. For example, probenecid is completely reabsorbed by the renal tubules and is metabolized very slowly. It competes with the same carrier protein as sulfonamides for active tubular secretion and so decreases the renal excretion of sulfonamides. This particular competition can lead to an increased risk of sulfonamide toxicity.

## Special Considerations

Although every drug has a usual dosage range, certain factors—such as a patient's age, weight, culture and ethnicity, gender, pregnancy status, and renal and hepatic function—may contribute to the need for dosage adjustments. When you encounter special considerations such as these, be prepared to reassess the prescribed dosage to make sure that it's safe and effective for your patient.

### CULTURE AND ETHNICITY

Certain drugs are more effective or more likely to produce adverse effects in particular ethnic groups or races. For example, blacks with hypertension respond better to thiazide diuretics than do patients of other races; on the other hand, blacks also have an increased risk of developing angioedema associated with angiotensin-converting enzyme (ACE) inhibitors. A patient's religious or cultural background may also call for special consideration. For example, a drug made from porcine products may be unacceptable to a Jewish or Muslim patient.

### ELDERLY PATIENTS

Because aging produces certain changes in body composition and organ function, elderly patients present unique therapeutic and dosing problems that require special attention. For example, the weight of the liver, the number of functioning hepatic cells, and hepatic blood flow all decrease as a person ages, resulting in slower drug metabolism. Renal function may also decrease with aging. These processes can lead to the accumulation of active drugs and metabolites as well as increased sensitivity to the effects of some drugs in elderly patients. Because they're also more likely to have multiple chronic illnesses, many elderly patients take multiple prescription drugs each day, thus increasing the risk of drug interactions.

### CHILDREN

Because their bodily functions are not fully developed, children—particularly those under age 12—may metabolize drugs differently than adults. In infants, immature renal and hepatic function delay metabolism and excretion of drugs. As a result, pediatric drug dosages are very different from adult dosages.

The FDA has provided drug manufacturers with guidelines that define pediatric age categories. Use these categories as a guide when administering drugs, unless the manufacturer provides a specific age range:
• neonates—birth up to age 1 month
• infants—ages 1 month to 2 years
• children—ages 2 to 12
• adolescents—ages 12 to 16.

### PREGNANCY

The many physiologic changes that take place in the body during pregnancy may affect a drug's pharmacokinetics and alter its effectiveness. Additionally, exposure to drugs may pose risks for the developing fetus. Before administering a drug to a pregnant patient, be sure to check its assigned FDA pregnancy risk category and intervene appropriately.

# Principles of Drug Administration

Because there are thousands of drugs and hundreds of facts about each one, taking responsibility for drug administration can seem overwhelming. One way that you can enhance your understanding of the principles of drug administration is to *associate, ask,* and *predict* during the critical thinking process. For example, *associate* each drug with general information you may already know about the drug or drug class. *Ask* yourself why a drug is administered by a certain route and why it's given multiple times throughout the day rather than only once. Learn to *predict* a drug's actions, uses, adverse effects, and possible drug interactions based on your knowledge of the drug's mechanism of action. As you apply these principles to drug administration, you'll begin to intuitively know which facts you need to make rational clinical decisions.

Prescriptions for patients in hospitals and other institutions are typically written by the physician on forms called the *physician's order sheet* or are directly input into a computerized system with an electronic signature. Drugs are prescribed based not only on their specific mechanisms of action but also on the patient's profile, which commonly includes age, ethnicity, gender, pregnancy status, smoking and drinking habits, and use of other drugs.

## "Rights" of Drug Administration

Always keep in mind the following "rights" of drug administration: the right drug, right time, right dose, right patient, right route, and right preparation and administration.

### RIGHT DRUG

Many drugs have similar spellings, different concentrations, and several generic forms. Before administering any drug, compare the exact spelling and concentration of the prescribed drug that appears on the label with the information contained in the medication administration record or drug profile. Regardless of which drug distribution system your facility uses, you should read the drug label and compare it to the medication administration record at least three times:

•before removing the drug from the dispensing unit or unit dose cart

•before preparing or measuring the prescribed dose

•before opening a unit dose package (just prior to administering the drug to the patient).

### RIGHT TIME

Various factors can affect the time that a drug is administered, such as the timing of meals and other drugs, scheduled diagnostic tests, standardized times used by the institution, and factors that may alter the consistency of blood levels and drug absorption. Before administering any p.r.n. drug, check the patient's chart to ensure that no one else has already administered it and that the specified time interval has passed. Also, document administration of a p.r.n. drug immediately.

### RIGHT DOSE

Whenever you're dispensing an unfamiliar drug or in doubt about a dosage, check the prescribed dose against the range specified in a reliable reference. Be sure to consider any reasons for a dosage adjustment that may apply to your particular patient. Also, make sure you're familiar with the standard abbreviations your institution uses for writing prescriptions.

### RIGHT PATIENT

Always compare the name of the patient on the medication record with the name on the patient's identification bracelet. When using a unit dose system, compare the name on the drug profile with that on the identification bracelet.

## RIGHT ROUTE

Each prescribed drug should specify the administration route. If the administration route is missing, consult the prescribing physician. Never substitute one route for another unless you obtain a prescription for the change.

## RIGHT PREPARATION AND ADMINISTRATION

For drugs that need to be mixed, poured, or measured, be sure to maintain aseptic technique. Follow any specific directions included by the manufacturer regarding diluent type and amount and the use of filters, if needed. Clearly label any drug that you've reconstituted with the patient's name, the strength or dose, the date and time that you prepared the drug, the amount and type of diluent that you used, the expiration date, and your initials.

## Administration Routes

Drugs may be administered by a variety of routes and dosage forms. A particular route may be chosen for convenience or to maximize drug concentration at the site of action, to minimize drug absorption elsewhere, to prolong drug absorption, or to avoid first-pass metabolism. Different dosage forms of the same drug may have different drug absorption rates, times of onset, and durations of action. For example, nitroglycerin is a coronary vasodilator that may be administered by the I.V., sublingual, oral, or buccal route, or as a topical ointment or disk. The I.V., sublingual, and buccal forms of nitroglycerin provide a rapid onset of action, whereas the oral, ointment, and disk forms have a slower onset and a prolonged duration of action.

Drug administration routes include the enteral, parenteral, and transcutaneous routes.

## ENTERAL

The enteral route consists of oral, nasogastric, and rectal administration. Drugs administered enterally enter the blood circulation by way of the GI tract. This route is considered the most natural and convenient route as well as the safest. As a result, most drugs are taken enterally, usually to provide systemic effects.

### Oral

• *Tablets:* Tablets, the most commonly used dosage form, come in a variety of colors, sizes, and shapes. Some tablets are specially coated for various purposes. Enteric coatings permit safe passage of a tablet through the stomach, where some drugs may be degraded or may produce unwanted effects, to the environment of the intestine. Some coatings protect the drug from the destructive influences of moisture, light, or air during storage; some coatings actually contain the drug, such as procainamide; still others conceal a bad taste. Coatings are also used to ensure appropriate drug release and absorption. Some tablets shouldn't be crushed or broken because doing so may alter drug release.

• *Capsules:* Capsules are solid dosage forms in which the drug and other ingredients are enclosed in a hard or soft shell of varying size and shape. Drugs are generally released faster from capsules than from tablets.

• *Solutions:* Drugs administered in solution are absorbed more rapidly than those administered in solid form; however, they don't always produce predictable drug levels in the blood. Some drugs in solution should be administered with meals or snacks to minimize their irritating effect on the gastric mucosa.

• *Suspensions:* Suspensions are preparations consisting of finely divided drugs in a suitable vehicle, usually water. Suspensions should be shaken before administration to ensure the uniformity of the preparation and administration of the proper dosage.

### Nasogastric

Drugs administered through a nasogastric or gastrostomy tube enter the stomach directly, bypassing the mouth and esophagus. They're usually administered in liquid form because an intact tablet or capsule could cause an obstruction in a gastric tube. Sometimes a tablet may be crushed or a capsule opened for nasograstic administration; however, doing so will affect the drug's release. You may need to consult a pharmacist to determine which tablets can be crushed or capsules opened.

### Rectal

Some enteral drugs are administered rectally—as suppositories, solutions, or ointments—to provide either local or systemic effects. When inserted into the rectum, suppositories soften, melt, or dissolve, releasing the drug contained inside them. The rectal route may be preferred for drugs that are destroyed or inactivated by the gastric or intestinal environment or that irritate the stomach. It may also be indicated when the oral route is contraindicated because of vomiting or difficulty swallowing. The drawbacks of rectal administration include inconvenience, noncompliance, and incomplete or irregular drug absorption.

### PARENTERAL

In parenteral drug administration, a drug enters the circulatory system through an injection rather than through GI absorption. This administration route is chosen when rapid drug action is desired; when the patient is uncooperative, unconscious, or unable to accept medication by the oral route; or when a drug is ineffective by other routes. Drugs may be injected into the joints, spinal column, arteries, veins, and muscles. However, the most common parenteral routes are the intramuscular (I.M.), intravenous (I.V.), subcutaneous (S.C.), and intradermal (I.D.) routes. Drugs administered parenterally may be mixed in either a solution or a suspension; those mixed in a solution typically act more rapidly than those mixed in a suspension. Parenteral administration has several disadvantages: The drug can't be removed or the dosage reduced once it has been injected, and injections are generally more expensive to administer than other dosage forms because they require strict sterility.

### Intramuscular

I.M. injections are administered deep into the anterolateral aspect of the thigh (vastis lateralis), the dorsogluteal muscle (gluteus maximus), the upper arm (deltoid), or the ventrogluteal muscle (gluteus medius). I.M. injections typically provide sustained drug action. This route is commonly chosen for drugs known to be irritating to subcutaneous tissue. The drug should be injected as far as possible from major nerves and blood vessels.

### Intravenous

In I.V. drug administration, an aqueous solution is injected directly into the vein—typically of the forearm. Drugs may be administered as a single, small-volume injection or as a slow, large-volume infusion. Because drugs injected I.V. don't encounter absorption barriers, this route produces the most rapid drug action, making it vital in emergency situations. Except for I.V. fat emulsions used as nutritional supplements, oleaginous preparations aren't usually administered by this route because of the risk of fat embolism.

### Subcutaneous

The S.C. route may be used to inject small volumes of medication, usually 1 ml or less. S.C. injections are generally given below the skin in the abdominal area, lateral area of the anterior thigh, posterior surface of the upper arm, or lateral lumbar area. Injection sites should be rotated to minimize tissue irritation if the patient receives frequent S.C. injections—for example, a patient who takes insulin.

### Intradermal

Common sites for I.D. injection are the arm and the back. Because only about 0.1 ml may be administered intradermally, this route is rarely used, except in diagnostic and test procedures, such as screening for allergic reactions.

#### TRANSCUTANEOUS

In transcutaneous administration, a drug crosses the skin layers, from either the outside (dermal) or the inside (mucocutaneous). This route includes sublingual (S.L.), inhalation, ophthalmic, otic, nasal, topical, and vaginal administration.

### Sublingual

In S.L. administration, tablets are placed under the tongue and allowed to dissolve. Nitroglycerin is commonly administered by this route, which allows rapid drug absorption and drug action. The S.L. route also avoids first-pass metabolism.

### Inhalation

Some drugs may be inhaled orally or nasally to produce a local effect on the respiratory tract or a systemic effect. Although drugs given by inhalation avoid first-pass hepatic metabolism, the lungs can also serve as an area of first-pass metabolism by providing respiratory conversion to more water-soluble compounds.

### Ophthalmic

Ophthalmic solutions and ointments are applied directly to the cornea or conjunctiva for enhanced local penetration and decreased systemic absorption. These drugs are usually used in eye examinations and to treat glaucoma. Ophthalmic solutions pose a greater risk of drug loss through the nasolacrimal duct into the nasopharynx than ophthalmic ointments do.

### Otic

Otic solutions are instilled directly into the external auditory canal for local penetration and decreased systemic absorption. These drugs, which include anesthetics, antibiotics, and anti-inflammatory drugs, usually require occlusion of the ear canal with cotton after instillation.

### Nasal

Nasal solutions and suspensions are applied directly to the nasal mucosa for enhanced local penetration and decreased systemic absorption. These drugs are usually used to reduce the inflammation typically associated with seasonal or perennial rhinitis.

### Topical

Topical drugs—including creams, ointments, lotions, and pastes—are applied directly to the skin. Transdermal delivery systems, usually in the form of an adhesive patch or a disk, are among the latest developments in topical drug administration. Because they provide slow drug release, these systems are typically used to avoid first-pass metabolism and ensure prolonged duration of action.

### Vaginal

Vaginal troches, suppositories, and creams are inserted into the vagina for slow, localized absorption. Body pH that differs from blood pH causes drug trapping or reabsorption, which delays drug excretion through the renal tubules. Vaginal secretions are alkaline, with a pH of 3.4 to 4.2, whereas blood has a pH of 7.35 to 7.45.

A systematic approach to nursing care, the nursing process helps guide you as you develop, implement, and evaluate your care and ensures that you'll deliver safe, consistent, and effective drug therapy to your patients. The nursing process consists of five steps, including assessment, nursing diagnosis, planning, implementation, and evaluation. Even though documentation is not a step in the nursing process, you're legally and professionally responsible for documenting all aspects of your care before, during, and after drug administration.

## Assessment

The first step in the nursing process, assessment involves gathering information that's essential to guide your patient's drug therapy. This information includes the patient's drug history, present drug use, allergies, medical history, and physical examination findings. Assessment is an ongoing process that serves as a baseline against which to compare any changes in your patient's condition; it's also the basis for developing and individualizing your patient's plan of care.

### Drug History

The patient's drug history is critical in your planning of drug-related care. Ask about his previous use of over-the-counter and prescription drugs as well as herbal remedies. For each drug, determine:
• the reason the patient took it
• the prescribed dosage
• the administration route
• the frequency of administration
• the duration of the drug therapy
• any adverse reactions the patient may have experienced and how he handled them.

Also determine if the patient has a history of drug abuse or addiction. Depending on his physical and emotional state,

you may need to obtain the drug history from other sources, such as family members, friends, other caregivers, and the medical record.

### Present Drug Use

Ask about the patient's current use of over-the-counter and prescription drugs as well as herbal remedies. As you did in the drug history, find out the specific details for each drug (dosage, route, frequency, and reason for taking). Also ask the patient if he thinks the drug has been effective and when he took the last dose.

If the patient uses herbal remedies, similarly explore the use of these products because herbs may interact with certain drugs. Also ask about the patient's use of recreational drugs, such as alcohol and tobacco, as well as illegal drugs, such as marijuana and heroin. If the patient acknowledges use of these drugs, be alert for possible drug interactions. This information may also provide you with insight about the patient's response—or lack of response—to his current drug treatment plan.

Try to find out if the patient has any other problems that might affect his compliance with the drug treatment plan, and intervene appropriately. For instance, a patient who is unemployed and has no health insurance may fail to fill a needed prescription. In such a case, contact an appropriate individual in your facility who may be able to help the patient obtain financial assistance.

Be sure to ask the patient if his drug treatment plan requires special monitoring or follow-up laboratory tests. For example, patients who take antihypertensives need to have their blood pressure checked routinely, and those who take warfarin must have their prothrombin time tested regularly. Other patients must undergo periodic blood tests to assess their hepatic and renal function. Determine whether the patient has complied with this part of his treatment plan, and ask him if he knows the results of the latest monitoring or laboratory tests.

### ALLERGIES

Find out if the patient is allergic to any drugs or foods. If he has an allergy, explore it further by determining the type of drug or food that triggers a reaction, the first time he experienced a reaction, the characteristics of the reaction, and other related information. Keep in mind that some patients consider annoying symptoms, such as indigestion, an allergic reaction. However, be sure to document a true allergy according to your facility's policy to ensure that the patient doesn't receive that drug or any related drug that may cause a similar reaction. Also, document allergies to foods because they may lead to drug interactions or adverse drug reactions. For example, sulfite is a food additive as well as a drug additive, so a patient with a known allergy to sulfite-containing foods is likely to react to sulfite-containing drugs.

### MEDICAL HISTORY

While reviewing your patient's medical history, determine if he has any acute or chronic conditions that may interfere with his drug therapy. Certain disorders involving major body systems, such as the cardiovascular, GI, hepatic, and renal systems, may affect a drug's absorption, transport, metabolism, or excretion and interfere with its action; they may also increase the incidence of adverse reactions and lead to toxicity. For each disorder identified, try to determine when the condition was diagnosed, what drugs were prescribed, and who prescribed them. This information can help you determine whether the patient is receiving incompatible drugs and whether more than one prescriber is managing his drug therapy.

Ask a female patient if she is or may be pregnant or if she's breast-feeding. Many drugs are safe to use during pregnancy, but others may harm the fetus. Also, some drugs are distributed into breast milk. If your patient is or might be pregnant, check the FDA's pregnancy risk category for the prescribed drug and notify the prescriber if the drug may pose a risk to the fetus. If the patient is breast-feeding, find out if the drug is distributed in breast milk and intervene appropriately.

### PHYSICAL EXAMINATION FINDINGS

As part of the physical examination, note the patient's age and weight. Be aware that age determines the dosage of certain drugs, such as sedatives and hypnotics, whereas weight determines the dosage of others, including some I.V. antibiotics and anticoagulants. As you perform the physical examination, note any abnormal findings that may point to body organ or system dysfunction. For example, if you detect liver enlargement and ascites, the patient may have impaired hepatic function, which can affect the metabolism of a drug he's taking and lead to harmful adverse or toxic effects. Also note whether a body organ or system appears to be responding to drug treatment. For example, if a patient has been taking an antibiotic to treat chronic bronchitis, thoroughly evaluate his respiratory status to measure his progress. And be sure to assess the patient for possible adverse reactions to the drugs he's taking.

Assess the patient's neurologic function to ensure that he can understand his drug regimen and carry out required tasks, such as performing a finger stick to obtain blood for glucose measurement. If a patient can't understand essential drug information, you'll need to identify a family member or another person who is willing to become involved in the teaching process.

## Nursing Diagnosis

Based on information derived from the assessment and physical examination findings, the nursing diagnoses are statements of actual or potential problems that a nurse is licensed to treat or manage alone or in collaboration with other members of the health care team. They're worded according to guidelines established by the North American Nursing Diagnosis Association (NANDA).

One of the most common nursing diagnoses related to drug therapy is *knowledge deficit,* which indicates that the patient doesn't have sufficient understanding of his drug regimen. However, adverse reactions are the basis for most nursing diagnoses related to drug administration. For example, a patient receiving a narcotic analgesic might have a nursing diagnosis of *constipation* related to decreased intestinal motility or *ineffective breathing pattern* related to respiratory depression. A patient receiving long-term, high-dose corticosteroids may be at *risk for impaired skin integrity* related to cortisone acetate or *self-concept disturbance* related to physical changes from prednisone therapy. Many antiarrhythmics cause orthostatic hypotension and thus may place an elderly patient at *high risk for injury* related to possible syncope. Broad-spectrum antibiotics, especially penicillin, may lead to the overgrowth of *Clostridium difficile,* a bacterium that is normally present in the intestines. This overgrowth in turn may lead to pseudomembranous enterocolitis, characterized by abdominal pain and severe diarrhea. The nursing diagnoses in such a case might include *potential for infection* related to bacterial overgrowth, *alteration in comfort* related to abdominal pain, and *fluid balance deficit* related to diarrhea.

## Planning

During the planning phase, you'll establish expected outcomes—or goals—for the patient and then develop specific nursing interventions to achieve them. Expected outcomes are observable or measurable goals that should occur as a result of nursing interventions and sometimes in conjunction with medical interventions. Developed in collaboration with the patient, the outcomes should be realistic and objective and should clearly communicate the direction of the plan of care to other nurses. They should be written as behaviors or responses for the patient, not the nurse, to achieve and should include a time frame for measuring the patient's progress. An example of a typical expected outcome is *The patient will accurately demonstrate self-administration of insulin before discharge.* Based on each outcome statement that you establish, you'd then develop appropriate nursing interventions, which might include drug administration techniques, patient teaching, monitoring of vital signs, calculation of drug dosages based on weight, and recording of intake and output.

## Implementation

As you implement the nursing interventions, be sure to stringently follow the classic rule of drug administration: administer the right dose of the right drug by the right route to the right patient at the right time. Also, keep in mind that you have a legal and professional responsibility to follow institutional policy regarding standing orders, prescription renewal, and the use of nursing judgment. During the implementation phase, you'll also begin to evaluate the patient's expected outcomes and nursing interventions and make necessary changes to the plan of care.

## Evaluation

Evaluation is an ongoing process rather than a single step in the nursing process. During this phase, you evaluate each expected outcome to determine whether or not it has been achieved and whether the original plan of care is working or needs to be modified. In evaluating a patient's drug treatment plan, you should determine whether or not the drug is controlling the signs and symptoms for which it was prescribed. You should also evaluate the patient for psychological or physiologic responses to the drug, especially adverse reactions. This constant monitoring allows you to make appropriate and timely suggestions for changes to the plan of care, such as dosage adjustments or changes in delivery routes, until each expected outcome has been achieved.

## Documentation

You're responsible for documenting all your actions related to the patient's drug therapy, from the assessment phase to evaluation. Each time you administer a drug, document the drug name, dose, time given, and your evaluation of its effect. When you administer drugs that require additional nursing judgment, such as those prescribed on an as-needed basis, document the rationale for administering the drug and follow-up assessment or interventions for each dose administered.

If you decide to withhold a prescribed drug based on your nursing judgment, document your action and the rationale for it, and notify the prescriber of your action in a timely manner. Whenever you notify a prescriber about a significant finding related to drug therapy, such as an adverse reaction, document the date and time, the person you contacted, what you discussed, and how you intervened.

# abciximab
ReoPro

## Class and Category
*Chemical:* Fab fragment of chimeric 7E3 antibody
*Therapeutic:* Platelet aggregation inhibitor
*Pregnancy category:* C

## Indications and Dosages
➤ *To prevent acute myocardial ischemic complications after percutaneous transluminal coronary angioplasty (PTCA) in patients at high risk for abrupt closure of treated coronary artery*

**I.V. INFUSION OR INJECTION**
**Adults.** 250-mcg/kg bolus 10 to 60 min before PTCA. *Maintenance:* 0.125 mcg/kg/min by continuous infusion for 12 hr. *Maximum:* 10 mcg/min.

➤ *To treat unstable angina in patients who haven't responded to conventional therapy and are scheduled for PTCA within 24 hr*

**I.V. INFUSION OR INJECTION**
**Adults.** 250-mcg/kg bolus, then 10 mcg/min by continuous infusion over 18 to 24 hr, concluding 1 hr after PTCA.

---

### Mechanism of Action
Binds to glycoprotein IIb/IIIa receptor sites on surface of activated platelets. Circulating fibrinogen can bind to these receptor sites and link platelets together, forming a clot that eventually blocks a coronary artery. By binding to receptor sites, abciximab prevents normal binding of fibrinogen and other factors and inhibits platelet aggregation.

---

| Route | Onset | Peak | Duration |
|-------|-------|------|----------|
| I.V. | Unknown | Unknown | 48 hr |

## Incompatibilities
•Don't mix abciximab with other drugs. Administer it through separate I.V. line, whenever possible.

## Contraindications
Active internal bleeding, arteriovenous malformation or aneurysm, bleeding disorders, CVA in past 2 years or that caused significant neurologic deficit at any time, GI or GU bleeding in past 6 weeks, hypersensitivity to abciximab, intracranial neoplasm, I.V. dextran therapy before or during PTCA, oral anticoagulant therapy in past 7 days unless PT is less than 1.2 times the control, severe uncontrolled hypertension, surgery in past 6 weeks, thrombocytopenia, vasculitis

## Interactions
**DRUGS**
*dipyridamole, heparin, NSAIDs, oral anticoagulants, thrombolytic drugs, ticlopidine:* Increased risk of bleeding

## Adverse Reactions
**CNS:** Confusion, dizziness, hyperesthesia
**CV:** Atrial fibrillation or flutter, bradycardia, embolism, hypotension, peripheral edema, pseudoaneurysm, supraventricular tachycardia, third-degree AV block, thrombophlebitis, weak pulse
**GI:** Dysphagia, hematemesis, nausea, vomiting
**GU:** Dysuria, hematuria, renal dysfunction, urinary frequency, urinary incontinence, urine retention
**HEME:** Anemia, bleeding, leukocytosis, thrombocytopenia
**RESP:** Bronchitis, bronchospasm, crackles, dyspnea, pleural effusion, pneumonia, pulmonary edema, pulmonary embolism, wheezing
**SKIN:** Pruritus, rash, urticaria
**Other:** Development of human antichimeric antibodies

## Nursing Considerations
•Know that abciximab may be used with heparin and aspirin therapy.
•Inspect abciximab for particles; don't use if opaque particles are present.
•For continuous I.V. infusion, withdraw 4.5 ml from 2-mg/ml solution and inject pre-

scribed amount into 250-ml bag of NS or D$_5$W, using an in-line sterile, nonpyrogenic, low–protein-binding 0.2- to 0.22-micron filter. Discard unused portion.
• Give I.V. bolus using sterile, nonpyrogenic, low–protein-binding 0.2- to 0.22-micron filter.
• Avoid I.M. injections, venipunctures, and use of indwelling urinary catheters, NG tubes, and automatic blood pressure cuffs during abciximab therapy to prevent bleeding. If appropriate, insert an intermittent I.V. access device to obtain blood samples.
• Monitor patient for GI, GU, and retroperitoneal bleeding and for bleeding at all puncture sites.
• WARNING If hemorrhage occurs, prepare to stop infusion immediately. Expect to treat severe thrombocytopenia with platelet transfusions if needed.
• Monitor patient for hypersensitivity reactions, such as rash, pruritus, wheezing, and dysphagia from laryngeal edema. If such reactions occur, stop infusion and notify prescriber immediately. If anaphylaxis occurs, give epinephrine, antihistamines, and corticosteroids, as prescribed.
• Obtain platelet count 2 to 4 hours after initial bolus and every 24 hours thereafter during abciximab therapy as ordered. Expect platelet function to return to normal within 48 hours of conclusion of therapy.
• Monitor vital signs and continuous ECG tracings during treatment.

**PATIENT TEACHING**
• Teach patient about possible adverse reactions, including bleeding and hypersensitivity reactions, such as rash, urticaria, and dyspnea.
• Tell patient to prevent injury from falls by maintaining bed rest and from bleeding by keeping limb immobile while catheter sheath is in place.

# acamprosate calcium

Campral

## Class and Category
*Chemical:* Synthetic endogenous amino acid homotaurine, gamma-aminobutyric acid (GABA) analogue

*Therapeutic:* Anti-alcoholic
*Pregnancy category:* C

## Indications and Dosages
➤ *To maintain abstinence from alcohol for alcohol-dependent patients who are abstinent at the start of treatment*
**E.R. TABLETS**
**Adults.** 666 mg t.i.d.
DOSAGE ADJUSTMENT For patients with moderate renal impairment (creatinine clearance of 30 to 50 ml/min), 333 mg t.i.d.

| Route | Onset | Peak | Duration |
|-------|-------|------|----------|
| P.O. | Unknown | 3 to 8 hr | Unknown |

## Contraindications
Hypersensitivity to acamprosate or its components, severe hepatic (Childs-Pugh class C) or renal impairment

## Interactions
**DRUGS**
*antidepressants:* Increased weight gain
*tetracyclines:* Decreased absorption of tetracyclines

## Adverse Reactions
**CNS:** Abnormal thinking, amnesia, anxiety, asthenia, chills, depression, dizziness, headache, insomnia, paresthesia, somnolence, suicidal ideation, syncope, tremor
**CV:** Chest pain, hypertension, palpitations, peripheral edema, vasodilation
**EENT:** Abnormal vision, dry mouth, pharyngitis, rhinitis, taste perversion
**GI:** Abdominal pain, anorexia, constipation, diarrhea, flatulence, increased appetite, indigestion, nausea, vomiting
**GU:** Acute renal failure, decreased libido, impotence
**HEME:** Leukopenia, lymphocytosis, thrombocytopenia
**MS:** Arthralgia, back pain, myalgia
**RESP:** Bronchitis, cough, dyspnea
**SKIN:** Diaphoresis, pruritus, rash
**Other:** Flulike symptoms, infection, weight gain

## Nursing Considerations
• Be aware that acamprosate therapy should start as soon as possible after the patient has

## Mechanism of Action

Chronic alcoholism may alter the balance between excitation and inhibition in neurons in the brain; acamprosate restores it.

When the neurotransmitter gamma-aminobutyric acid (GABA) binds to its receptors in the CNS, it *opens* the chloride ion channel and releases chloride (Cl⁻) into the cell (below left), thereby reducing neuronal excitability by inhibiting depolarization. By interacting with GABA receptor sites, acamprosate prevents GABA from binding (below right).

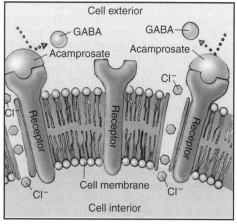

When glutamate binds to its receptors, it *closes* the chloride ion channel, increasing neuronal excitability by promoting depolarization (below left). This imbalance fosters a craving for alcohol. By interacting with glutamate receptor sites, acamprosate prevents glutamate from binding (below right).

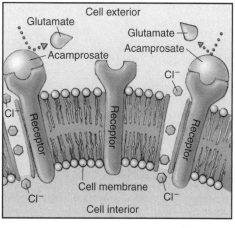

undergone alcohol withdrawal and achieved abstinence.
•Continue to administer acamprosate even during periods of alcohol relapse.

PATIENT TEACHING
•Instruct patient to take acamprosate exactly as prescribed, even if a relapse occurs, and to seek help for a relapse.
•Warn the patient that acamprosate won't reduce the symptoms of alcohol withdrawal if relapse occurs followed by cessation.
•Urge caregivers to monitor patient for signs and symptoms of depression (lack of appetite or interest in life, fatigue, excessive sleeping, difficulty concentrating) or suicidal tendencies because a small number of patients taking acamprosate have attempted suicide.
•Advise patient to use caution when performing hazardous activities until adverse CNS effects of the drug are known.
•Tell female patients to notify the prescriber if they become pregnant or intend to become pregnant while taking acamprosate; the drug may need to be stopped because fetal risks are unknown.

# acarbose

Precose

## Class and Category

*Chemical:* Alpha-glucosidase inhibitor, oligosaccharide
*Therapeutic:* Antidiabetic drug
*Pregnancy category:* B

## Mechanism of Action

Inhibits action of alpha-amylase and alpha-glucoside enzymes. Normally, alpha-amylase hydrolyzes complex starches to oligosaccharides in small intestine, and alpha-glucoside hydrolyzes oligosaccharides, trisaccharides, and disaccharides to glucose and other monosaccharides in brush border of small intestine. In diabetic patients, acarbose inhibits these actions and delays glucose absorption, which reduces the blood glucose level after meals.

## Indications and Dosages

➤ *To control blood glucose level in patients with type 2 (non–insulin-dependent) diabetes mellitus when the level can't be controlled by diet alone*

TABLETS
Adults. *Initial:* 25 mg t.i.d. with first bite of each meal. *Maintenance:* Increased to maximum at 4- to 8-wk intervals p.r.n. *Maximum:* 50 mg t.i.d. for patients who weigh 65 kg (143 lb) or less; 100 mg t.i.d. for patients who weigh more than 65 kg.

## Contraindications

Chronic intestinal disease, cirrhosis, colonic ulceration, conditions that may deteriorate because of increased gas formation in intestines, diabetic ketoacidosis, digestive or absorption disorders, history of bowel obstruction, hypersensitivity to acarbose, inflammatory bowel disease

## Interactions

DRUGS
*calcium channel blockers, digestive enzymes (such as pancreatin), diuretics, estrogen, intestinal adsorbents (such as activated charcoal), isoniazid, nicotinic acid, oral contraceptives, phenothiazines, phenytoin, sympathomimetics, thyroid hormones:* Possibly decreased therapeutic effects of acarbose
*digoxin:* Decreased serum level and therapeutic effects of digoxin
*insulin, sulfonylureas:* Decreased insulin action, possibly increased risk of hypoglycemia

## Adverse Reactions

CV: Edema
GI: Abdominal distention and pain, diarrhea, flatulence, hepatitis, hepatotoxicity, ileus, jaundice
SKIN: Erythema, exanthema, rash, urticaria

## Nursing Considerations

•WARNING Be aware that acarbose isn't recommended for patients with significant renal dysfunction and a serum creatinine level above 2 mg/dl.
•If patient is receiving acarbose and a sulfonylurea or insulin to enhance glucose control, check blood glucose level often, as appropriate.
•Store drug in sealed container in cool environment.

• Expect to decrease dosage to control GI upset.
• Monitor glycosylated hemoglobin level as ordered every 3 months for first year to evaluate glucose control and patient compliance.
• Monitor hematocrit and serum AST level every 3 months during first year of therapy and periodically thereafter, as ordered, because acarbose may decrease hematocrit and increase serum AST level.

PATIENT TEACHING
• Explain importance of self-monitoring glucose levels during acarbose therapy.
• Teach patient to recognize signs and symptoms of hypoglycemia and hyperglycemia.
• Warn patient that noncompliance with prescribed regimen can increase risk of diabetic complications, including neuropathy, retinopathy, and renal insufficiency.
• Explain that temporary insulin therapy may be needed if fever, trauma, infection, illness, surgery, or other stress alters blood glucose control.
• Warn patient not to take other drugs within 2 hours of taking acarbose unless specifically instructed by prescriber.
• Tell him to consult prescriber before taking OTC drugs during acarbose therapy.
• Advise patient who also takes another antidiabetic drug to carry glucose with him at all times in case hypoglycemia occurs.

# acebutolol hydrochloride

Monitan (CAN), Sectral

## Class and Category
*Chemical:* Beta$_1$-selective (cardioselective) adrenergic receptor blocker
*Therapeutic:* Antihypertensive, class II antiarrhythmic
*Pregnancy category:* B

## Indications and Dosages
➤ *To treat hypertension*
TABLETS
**Adults.** *Initial:* 400 mg q.d. or 200 mg b.i.d. *Usual:* 200 to 800 mg q.d. Dosage increased to 1,200 mg/day in divided doses b.i.d. for severe hypertension or hypertension that isn't well controlled with usual dosage.

➤ *To treat premature ventricular arrhythmias*

TABLETS
**Adults.** *Initial:* 200 mg b.i.d. *Usual:* 600 to 1,200 mg/day.
DOSAGE ADJUSTMENT Maximum dosage of 800 mg q.d. for elderly patients. Dosage reduced by 50% for patients with creatinine clearance of less than 50 ml/min/1.73 m$^2$. Dosage reduced by 75% for patients with creatinine clearance of less than 25 ml/min/1.73 m$^2$.

| Route | Onset | Peak | Duration |
|---|---|---|---|
| P.O. | 1 to 1.5 hr | 2 to 8 hr | 24 hr or longer |

## Mechanism of Action
Inhibits stimulation of beta$_1$ receptors in heart, decreasing cardiac excitability, heart rate, cardiac output, and myocardial oxygen demand. Acebutolol also decreases kidneys' release of renin, which helps reduce blood pressure. Drug suppresses SA node automaticity and AV node conductivity, which suppresses atrial and ventricular ectopy. By decreasing myocardial oxygen demand, acebutolol decreases myocardial ischemia. At high doses, it inhibits stimulation of beta$_2$ receptors in lungs, which may cause bronchoconstriction.

## Contraindications
Cardiogenic shock, heart failure unless caused by tachyarrhythmia, hypersensitivity to acebutolol, overt heart failure, second- and third-degree heart block, severe bradycardia

## Interactions
DRUGS
*alpha agonists, nasal decongestants:* Increased risk of hypertension
*aluminum salts, barbiturates, calcium salts, cholestyramine, colestipol, indomethacin, NSAIDs, penicillins, rifampin, salicylates, sulfinpyrazone:* Decreased antihypertensive effects
*anticholinergics, hydralazine, methyldopa, prazosin, reserpine:* Increased risk of bradycardia and hypotension
*beta$_2$ agonists, theophylline:* Decreased bronchodilation
*epinephrine:* Increased risk of blocked sympathomimetic effects
*ergot alkaloids:* Increased risk of peripheral ischemia and gangrene

*flecainide:* Possibly increased effects of both drugs
*lidocaine:* Possibly increased serum lidocaine level, causing toxicity
*oral contraceptives, quinidine:* Possibly increased serum acebutolol level
*sulfonylureas:* Possibly decreased hypoglycemic effects
*verapamil:* Increased cardiac effects, leading to bradycardia and hypotension

## Adverse Reactions
**CNS:** Abnormal dreams, anxiety, confusion, depression, dizziness, fatigue, fever, headache, insomnia
**CV:** Bradycardia, chest pain, edema, heart block, heart failure, hypotension
**EENT:** Abnormal vision, conjunctivitis, dry eyes, eye pain, pharyngitis, rhinitis
**GI:** Constipation, diarrhea, flatulence, hepatotoxicity, indigestion, nausea
**GU:** Dysuria, impotence, polyuria
**MS:** Arthralgia, myalgia
**RESP:** Bronchospasm, cough, dyspnea, wheezing
**SKIN:** Rash

## Nursing Considerations
• Before therapy begins, obtain baseline renal function tests, as ordered.
• Check apical and radial pulses before giving acebutolol. Also, frequently monitor blood pressure and pulse rate, rhythm, and quality during treatment.
• Give acebutolol with food to prevent GI upset.
• Keep in mind that acebutolol may elevate uric acid, potassium, triglyceride, lipoprotein, and ANA levels; it also may interfere with accuracy of glucose tolerance tests.
• Monitor diabetic patient's blood glucose level to spot alterations.
• Notify prescriber if you detect a heart rate below 50 beats/min or signs of heart failure, such as dyspnea, crackles, unexplained weight gain, and jugular vein distention.
• Monitor patient for peripheral edema and evaluate fluid intake and output.
**PATIENT TEACHING**
• Tell patient that tablets may be crushed or swallowed whole.
• Warn him against discontinuing acebutolol abruptly, which could cause angina or dangerously high blood pressure.

• Instruct patient to take a missed dose as soon as possible up to 6 hours before next scheduled dose but not to double the next dose.
• Advise patient to consult prescriber before taking OTC drugs that contain alpha agonists, such as nasal decongestants and cold preparations.
• Instruct patient to report dizziness, confusion, and fever immediately.
• Encourage patient to maintain diet and lifestyle changes to help control blood pressure.

# acetaminophen

Abenol (CAN), Acephen, Aceta Elixir, Acetaminophen Uniserts, Aceta Tablets, Apacet Capsules, Apacet Elixir, Apacet Extra Strength Tablets, Apacet Regular Strength Tablets, Aspirin Free Pain Relief, Exdol (CAN), Feverall, Feverall Sprinkle Caps, Genapap Infants' Drops, Genebs Extra Strength, Halenol Children's Junior Strength, Liquiprin Elixir, Liquiprin Infants' Drops, Meda Cap, Neopap, Oraphen-PD, Panadol, Panadol Infants' Drops, Redutemp, Robigesic (CAN), St. Joseph Aspirin-Free Infant Drops, Tapanol Extra Strength, Tempra, Tempra Drops, Tylenol, Tylenol Caplets, Tylenol Children's Chewable Tablets, Tylenol Extra Strength, Tylenol Gelcaps, Tylenol Infants' Drops

## Class and Category
*Chemical:* Nonsalicylate, para-aminophenol derivative
*Therapeutic:* Antipyretic, nonnarcotic analgesic
*Pregnancy category:* B

## Indications and Dosages
➤ *To relieve mild to moderate pain associated with headache, muscle ache, backache, minor arthritis, common cold, toothache, and menstrual cramps; to reduce fever*
**CAPLETS, CAPSULES, CHEWABLE TABLETS, ELIXIR, E.R. CAPLETS, GELCAPS, LIQUID, SOLUTION, SPRINKLES, SUSPENSION, TABLETS**
**Adults.** 325 to 650 mg q 4 to 6 hr, or 1,000 mg t.i.d. or q.i.d., or 2 E.R. caplets q 8 hr. *Maximum:* 4,000 mg/day.
**Children over age 14.** 650 mg q 4 hr. *Maximum:* 5 doses in 24 hr.
**Children ages 12 to 14.** 640 mg q 4 hr. *Maximum:* 5 doses in 24 hr.

**Children age 11.** 480 mg q 4 hr. *Maximum:* 5 doses in 24 hr.
**Children ages 9 to 10.** 400 mg q 4 hr. *Maximum:* 5 doses in 24 hr.
**Children ages 6 to 8.** 320 mg q 4 hr. *Maximum:* 5 doses in 24 hr.
**Children ages 4 to 5.** 240 mg q 4 hr. *Maximum:* 5 doses in 24 hr.
**Children ages 2 to 3.** 160 mg q 4 hr. *Maximum:* 5 doses in 24 hr.
**Children age 1.** 120 mg q 4 hr. *Maximum:* 5 doses in 24 hr.
**Children ages 4 to 11 months.** 80 mg q 4 hr. *Maximum:* 5 doses in 24 hr.
**Children ages 0 to 3 months.** 40 mg q 4 hr. *Maximum:* 5 doses in 24 hr.

**SUPPOSITORIES**

**Adults and adolescents.** 650 mg q 4 to 6 hr. *Maximum:* 4,000 mg/day.
**Children ages 6 to 12.** 325 mg q 4 to 6 hr. *Maximum:* 2,600 mg/day
**Children ages 3 to 6.** 120 to 125 mg q 4 to 6 hr. *Maximum:* 720 mg/day.
**Children ages 1 to 3.** 80 mg q 4 hr.
**Children ages 3 to 11 months.** 80 mg q 6 hr.

| Route | Onset | Peak | Duration |
|---|---|---|---|
| P.O., P.R. | Varies | 1 to 3 hr | 3 to 4 hr |

### Mechanism of Action

Inhibits the enzyme cyclooxygenase, thereby blocking prostaglandin production and interfering with pain impulse generation in the peripheral nervous system. Acetaminophen also acts directly on the temperature-regulating center in the hypothalamus by inhibiting synthesis of prostaglandin $E_2$.

### Contraindications

Hypersensitivity to acetaminophen or its components

### Interactions

**DRUGS**

*anticholinergics:* Decreased onset of action of acetaminophen
*barbiturates, carbamazepine, hydantoins, isoniazid, rifampin, sulfinpyrazone*: Decreased therapeutic effects and increased hepatotoxic effects of acetaminophen

*lamotrigine, loop diuretics:* Possibly decreased therapeutic effects of these drugs
*oral contraceptives:* Decreased effectiveness of acetaminophen
*probenecid:* Possibly increased therapeutic effects of acetaminophen
*propranolol:* Possibly increased action of acetaminophen
*zidovudine:* Possibly decreased effects of zidovudine

**ACTIVITIES**

*alcohol use:* Increased risk of hepatotoxicity

### Adverse Reactions

**GI:** Abdominal pain, hepatotoxicity, nausea, vomiting
**HEME:** Hemolytic anemia (with long-term use), leukopenia, neutropenia, pancytopenia, thrombocytopenia
**SKIN:** Jaundice, rash, urticaria
**Other:** Angioedema, hypoglycemic coma

### Nursing Considerations

•Before and during long-term therapy, monitor liver function test results, including AST, ALT, bilirubin, and creatinine levels, as ordered.
•Monitor renal function in patient on long-term therapy. Keep in mind that blood or albumin in urine may indicate nephritis; decreased urine output, renal failure; and dark brown urine, presence of the metabolite phenacetin.
•Expect to reduce dosage for patients with renal dysfunction.
•Store suppositories under 80° F (26.6° C).

**PATIENT TEACHING**

•Tell patient that tablets may be crushed or swallowed whole.
•Instruct patient to read manufacturer's label and follow dosage guidelines precisely. Explain that infants' and children's acetaminophen liquid aren't equal in drug concentration and aren't interchangeable.
•Advise patient to use manufacturer's dropper or dosage cup only for liquid acetaminophen.
•Advise him to contact prescriber before taking other prescription or OTC drugs; they may contain acetaminophen and lead to toxicity.
•Teach patient to recognize signs of hepatotoxicity, such as bleeding, easy bruising, and malaise, which commonly occurs with chronic overdose.

# acetazolamide

Acetazolam (CAN), Ak-Zol, Apo-Acetazo-
lamide (CAN), Dazamide, Diamox, Diamox
Sequels, Storzolamide

## Class and Category
*Chemical:* Sulfonamide derivative
*Therapeutic:* Anticonvulsant, antiglaucoma,
diuretic
*Pregnancy category:* C

## Indications and Dosages
➤ *To treat chronic simple (open-angle)*
*glaucoma*
**S.R. CAPSULES, TABLETS, I.V. OR I.M. INJECTION**
**Adults.** 250 to 1,000 mg/day (in divided
doses for dosages above 250 mg).
➤ *As short-term therapy to treat sec-*
*ondary glaucoma and preoperatively to*
*treat acute congestive (closed-angle)*
*glaucoma*
**S.R. CAPSULES, TABLETS, I.V. OR I.M. INJECTION**
**Adults.** 250 mg b.i.d. or q 4 hr; or one S.R.
capsule (500 mg) b.i.d.; or 500 mg initially,
followed by 125 to 250 mg q 4 to 6 hr for severe acute glaucoma. To initially lower intraocular pressure rapidly, 500 mg I.V.; may
repeat in 2 to 4 hr in acute cases, depending
on patient response. Oral therapy usually
initiated after initial I.V. dose.
**S.R. CAPSULES, TABLETS**
**Children.** 10 to 15 mg/kg/day in divided
doses q 6 to 8 hr.
**I.V. OR I.M. INJECTION**
**Children.** 5 to 10 mg/kg/dose q 6 hr.
➤ *To induce diuresis in heart failure*
**TABLETS, I.V. OR I.M. INJECTION**
**Adults.** *Initial:* 250 to 375 mg or 5 mg/kg q.d.
in morning. *Maintenance:* 250 to 375 mg or
5 mg/kg on alternate days or for 2 days fol-
lowed by a drug-free day.
➤ *To treat drug-induced edema*
**TABLETS, I.V. OR I.M. INJECTION**
**Adults.** 250 to 375 mg q.d. for 1 to 2 days.
**TABLETS, I.V. INJECTION**
**Children.** 5 mg/kg/dose q.d. in morning.
➤ *To treat seizures, including generalized*
*tonic-clonic, absence, and mixed*
*seizures, and myoclonic jerk patterns*
**TABLETS, I.V. OR I.M. INJECTION**
**Adults and children.** 8 to 30 mg/kg/day in
divided doses. *Optimal:* 375 to 1,000 mg/

day. When used with other anticonvulsants,
250 mg q.d.
➤ *To prevent or relieve symptoms of acute*
*mountain sickness*
**S.R. CAPSULES, TABLETS**
**Adults.** 500 to 1,000 mg/day in divided doses,
given 24 to 48 hr before ascent and continued for 48 hr or longer while at high altitude
p.r.n. to control symptoms.

| Route | Onset | Peak | Duration |
|---|---|---|---|
| P.O. | 60 to 90 min | 2 to 4 hr | 8 to 12 hr |
| P.O. (S.R.) | 2 hr | 8 to 12 hr | 18 to 24 hr |
| I.V. | 2 min | 15 min | 4 to 5 hr |

## Mechanism of Action
Inhibits the enyzme carbonic anhydrase,
which normally appears in the eyes' ciliary processes, brain's choroid plexes, and
kidneys' proximal tubule cells. In the
eyes, enzyme inhibition decreases aqueous
humor secretion, which lowers intraocular
pressure. In the brain, inhibition may
delay abnormal, intermittent, and excessive discharge from neurons that cause
seizures. In the kidneys, it increases bicarbonate excretion, which carries out
water, potassium, and sodium, thus inducing diuresis and metabolic acidosis. This
acidosis counteracts respiratory alkalosis
and reduces symptoms of mountain sickness, including headache, dizziness, nausea, and dyspnea.

## Contraindications
Chronic noncongestive closed-angle glaucoma;
cirrhosis; hyperchloremic acidosis; hypersensitivity to acetazolamide; hypokalemia; hyponatremia; severe pulmonary obstruction; severe
renal, hepatic, or adrenocortical impairment

## Interactions
**DRUGS**
*amphetamines, methenamine, phenobarbital,*
*procainamide, quinidine:* Decreased excretion
and possibly toxicity of these drugs
*corticosteroids:* Increased risk of hypokalemia
*cyclosporine:* Increased cyclosporine level,
possibly nephrotoxicity or neurotoxicity

*diflunisal:* Possibly significantly decreased intraocular pressure
*lithium:* Increased excretion and decreased effectiveness of lithium
*primidone:* Decreased serum and urine primidone levels
*salicylates:* Increased risk of salicylate toxicity

## Adverse Reactions

**CNS:** Ataxia, confusion, depression, disorientation, dizziness, drowsiness, fatigue, fever, flaccid paralysis, headache, lassitude, malaise, nervousness, paresthesia, seizures, tremor, weakness
**EENT:** Altered taste, tinnitus, transient myopia
**GI:** Anorexia, constipation, diarrhea, hepatic dysfunction, melena, nausea, vomiting
**GU:** Crystalluria, decreased libido, glycosuria, hematuria, impotence, nephrotoxicity, phosphaturia, polyuria, renal calculi, renal colic, urinary frequency
**HEME:** Agranulocytosis, hemolytic anemia, leukopenia, pancytopenia, thrombocytopenia, thrombocytopenic purpura
**SKIN:** Photosensitivity, pruritus, rash, Stevens-Johnson syndrome, urticaria
**Other:** Acidosis, hyperuricemia, hypokalemia, weight loss

## Nursing Considerations

•Use acetazolamide cautiously in patients with calcium-based renal calculi, diabetes mellitus, gout, or respiratory impairment.
•Know that acetazolamide may increase risk of hepatic encephalopathy in patients with hepatic cirrhosis.
•To avoid painful I.M. injections (caused by alkaline solution), administer acetazolamide by mouth or I.V. injection if possible.
•Reconstitute each 500-mg vial with at least 5 ml of sterile water for injection. Use within 24 hours because drug has no preservative.
•Monitor blood test results during acetazolamide therapy to detect electrolyte imbalances.
•Monitor fluid intake and output every 8 hours and body weight daily to detect excessive fluid and weight loss.

### PATIENT TEACHING

•Inform patient that acetazolamide tablets may be crushed and suspended in chocolate or another sweet syrup. Alternatively, one tablet may be dissolved in 10 ml of hot water and added to 10 ml of honey or syrup.
•Advise patient to avoid potentially hazardous activities if dizziness or drowsiness occurs.
•Instruct patient who takes high doses of salicylates to notify prescriber immediately if signs of salicylate toxicity, such as anorexia, tachypnea, and lethargy, occur.
•Advise patient who plans to mountain climb to descend mountain gradually to avoid mountain sickness and to seek immediate medical care if symptoms of mountain sickness occur.

# acetohexamide

Dimelor (CAN), Dymelor

## Class and Category

*Chemical:* Sulfonylurea
*Therapeutic:* Antidiabetic
*Pregnancy category:* C

## Indications and Dosages

➤ *To treat stable type 2 (non-insulin-dependent) diabetes mellitus*

### TABLETS

**Adults.** *Initial:* 250 to 1,500 mg/day. Dosages of 1,000 mg or more daily may be divided and given b.i.d. before morning and evening meals.

DOSAGE ADJUSTMENT For patient being switched from another antidiabetic drug, acetohexamide dosage reduced to half the usual tolbutamide dosage or twice the usual chlorpropamide dosage. For patient being switched from insulin to acetohexamide monotherapy, dosages adjusted as follows: if insulin dosage is less than 20 U/day, acetohexamide begins at 250 mg/day and insulin is discontinued; if insulin dosage exceeds 20 U/day, acetohexamide begins at 250 mg/day and insulin is tapered by 25% to 30% before being reduced further according to patient response.

| Route | Onset | Peak | Duration |
|-------|-------|------|----------|
| P.O. | 1 hr | Unknown | 12 to 24 hr |

## Mechanism of Action

Stimulates insulin release from active beta cells in the pancreas, resulting in decreased blood glucose level. Improves insulin binding to insulin receptors. Increases the number of insulin receptors (with long-term administration). May reduce basal hepatic glucose secretion.

## Contraindications

Diabetes mellitus complicated by ketoacidosis or pregnancy, hypersensitivity to acetohexamide, renal failure, sole therapy for type 1 (insulin-dependent) diabetes mellitus

## Interactions

### DRUGS

*activated charcoal:* Possibly reduced absorption and effectiveness of acetohexamide
*androgens, anticoagulants, azole antifungals, chloramphenicol, clofibrate, fluconazole, gemfibrozil, H₂-receptor antagonists, magnesium salts, MAO inhibitors, methyldopa, probenecid, salicylates, sulfinpyrazone, sulfonamides, tricyclic antidepressants, urinary acidifiers:* Enhanced hypoglycemic effect of acetohexamide
*beta blockers, calcium channel blockers, cholestyramine, corticosteroids, diazoxide, estrogens, hydantoins, isoniazid, nicotinic acid, oral contraceptives, phenothiazines, rifampin, sympathomimetics, thiazide diuretics, thyroid drugs, urinary alkalizers:* Decreased hypoglycemic effect of acetohexamide
*digitalis glycosides:* Possibly increased serum digitalis level

## Adverse Reactions

**CNS:** Anxiety, chills, confusion, depression, dizziness, drowsiness, fatigue, headache, hyperesthesia, insomnia, malaise, nervousness, paresthesia, somnolence, syncope, tremor, vertigo, weakness
**CV:** Arrhythmias, edema, hypertension, vasculitis
**EENT:** Blurred vision, conjunctivitis, eye pain, pharyngitis, retinal hemorrhage, rhinitis, tinnitus
**ENDO:** Hypoglycemia
**GI:** Abdominal pain, anorexia, constipation, diarrhea, epigastric fullness, flatulence, heartburn, hepatitis, hepatotoxicity, indigestion, nausea, proctocolitis, vomiting
**GU:** Decreased libido, dysuria, polyuria
**HEME:** Agranulocytosis, aplastic anemia, eosinophilia, hemolytic anemia, leukopenia, pancytopenia, thrombocytopenia
**MS:** Abnormal gait, arthralgia, hypertonia, leg cramps
**RESP:** Dyspnea
**SKIN:** Diaphoresis, eczema, erythema multiforme, exfoliative dermatitis, flushing, jaundice, lichenoid reaction (skin thickening and accentuated lesions), maculopapular rash, photosensitivity, pruritus, rash, urticaria
**Other:** Disulfiram-like reaction (flushing, head throbbing, hypotension, nausea, tachycardia, vomiting), hyponatremia

## Nursing Considerations

•Use acetohexamide cautiously in elderly patients and in those with cardiac, hepatic, or renal disease or thyroid dysfunction. The drug's duration of action is prolonged in patients with renal disease.
•Give acetohexamide 30 minutes before meals, crushing tablets if desired. If GI upset occurs, give in divided doses, as prescribed.
•Monitor for signs of hypoglycemia and hyperglycemia, especially after meals.
•Monitor blood glucose level frequently, as ordered. Provide additional insulin if needed during stressful periods, as prescribed.
•Monitor liver enzyme levels during therapy; acetohexamide may increase AST, ALT, and alkaline phosphatase levels.
•Store acetohexamide in tightly sealed container in a cool environment.

### PATIENT TEACHING

•Stress importance of adhering to prescribed drug regimen, diet, and exercise program.
•Advise patient to take acetohexamide with food to avoid GI upset.
•Teach patient how to self-monitor blood glucose level and check urine for glucose and ketones, as appropriate.
•Teach patient to recognize and report signs of hypoglycemia and hyperglycemia.

# acetohydroxamic acid

Lithostat

## Class and Category

*Chemical:* Synthetic hydroxylamine and ethylacetate derivative
*Therapeutic:* Urease inhibitor
*Pregnancy category:* X

## Indications and Dosages

➤ *As an adjunct to antimicrobial therapy to treat chronic UTIs caused by urea-splitting bacteria*

**TABLETS**

**Adults.** *Initial:* 12 mg/kg/day in divided doses q 6 to 8 hr. *Usual:* 250 mg t.i.d. or q.i.d. for a total daily dose of 10 to 15 mg/kg. *Maximum:* 1,500 mg/day.
**Children.** 10 mg/kg/day.
**DOSAGE ADJUSTMENT** Maximum dosage reduced to 1,000 mg/day or 500 mg q 12 hr for patients with serum creatinine level that exceeds 1.8 mg/dl.

---

### Mechanism of Action

Inhibits urease, the enzyme that catalyzes urea's hydrolysis to carbon dioxide and ammonia in urine infected with urea-splitting bacteria. This action reduces the urine ammonia level and pH, enhancing antimicrobial drug effectiveness.

---

## Contraindications

Contributing disorder that's treatable by surgery or appropriate antimicrobial therapy, hypersensitivity to acetohydroxamic acid, inadequate renal function (serum creatinine level above 2.5 mg/dl or creatinine clearance below 20 ml/min/1.73 m²), risk of pregnancy, UTI caused by non–urease-producing organisms, UTI that can be controlled by appropriate antimicrobial therapy

## Interactions

**DRUGS**

*iron:* Decreased intestinal absorption of iron, decreased effects of iron and acetohydroxamic acid

**ACTIVITIES**

*alcohol use:* Increased risk of severe rash 30 to 45 minutes after drinking alcohol

## Adverse Reactions

**CNS:** Anxiety, depression, fever, lack of coordination, malaise, headache, nervousness, slurred speech, tiredness, tremor
**CV:** Calf pain (deep vein blood clot), palpitations, sudden chest pain
**EENT:** Pharyngitis, sudden change in vision
**GI:** Anorexia, nausea, vomiting
**HEME:** Reticulocytosis, unusual bleeding
**RESP:** Dyspnea
**SKIN:** Ecchymosis, hair loss, nonpruritic macular rash

## Nursing Considerations

• Use acetohydroxamic acid cautiously in patients with severe chronic renal disease or anemia and those who've had phlebitis or thrombophlebitis.
• Be aware that risk of adverse psychomotor effects increases if patient drinks alcohol or takes drugs that affect alertness and reflexes, such as antihistamines, tranquilizers, sedatives, analgesics, and narcotics.
• Administer tablets with food or liquid, crushing them if needed.
•**WARNING** Acetohydroxamic acid chelates with dietary iron. If patient has iron deficiency anemia, expect to administer I.M. iron as needed during acetohydroxamic acid therapy.
• Monitor follow-up laboratory tests to check renal and hepatic function and urine pH, as ordered.

**PATIENT TEACHING**

• Instruct patient to take drug at same time each day, as prescribed.
• Tell patient to take a missed dose up to 2 hours after scheduled time. If more than 2 hours has passed, he should wait for next scheduled dose and shouldn't double that dose.
• Warn patient not to take drug with alcohol or iron and to consult prescriber before taking it with any other drug.
• Instruct patient to avoid hazardous activities during therapy.

# acetylcysteine

Mucomyst, Mucosil

## Class and Category

*Chemical:* N-acetyl derivative of cysteine

*Therapeutic:* Antidote (for acetaminophen overdose), mucolytic
*Pregnancy category:* B

## Indications and Dosages

➤ *To liquefy abnormal, viscid, or thickened mucus secretions in chronic pulmonary disorders (including emphysema, bronchitis, tuberculosis, bronchiectasis, and cystic fibrosis) and in pneumonia, pulmonary complications of thoracic or cardiovascular surgery, and tracheostomy care*

SOLUTION (DIRECT INSTILLATION INTO TRACHEOSTOMY)

**Adults and children.** 1 to 2 ml of 10% or 20% solution instilled q 1 to 4 hr, p.r.n.

SOLUTION (INHALATION)

**Adults and children.** 1 to 10 ml of 20% solution or 2 to 20 ml of 10% solution nebulized through face mask, mouthpiece, or tracheostomy q 2 to 6 hr. *Usual:* 3 to 5 ml of 20% solution or 6 to 10 ml of 10% solution t.i.d. or q.i.d.

➤ *To treat acetaminophen overdose*

SOLUTION (P.O.)

**Adults and children.** *Loading dose:* 140 mg/kg. *Maintenance:* 70 mg/kg 4 hr after loading dose and then q 4 hr to a total of 17 doses.

## Incompatibilities

Don't administer acetylcysteine with nebulization equipment if drug can contact iron, copper, or rubber. Don't administer drug with amphotericin B, ampicillin sodium, chlortetracycline, chymotrypsin, erythromycin, hydrogen peroxide, iodized oil, oxytetracycline, tetracycline, or trypsin.

---

### Mechanism of Action

Decreases viscosity of pulmonary secretions by breaking disulfide links that bind glycoproteins in mucus. Reduces liver damage from acetaminophen overdose. Usually, acetaminophen's toxic metabolites bind with glutathione in the liver, which detoxifies them. When acetaminophen overdose depletes glutathione stores, toxic metabolites bind with protein in liver cells, killing them. Acetylcysteine maintains or restores levels of glutathione or acts as its substitute, which reduces liver damage from acetaminophen overdose.

---

## Contraindications

Hypersensitivity to acetylcysteine, no contraindications when used as antidote

## Interactions

DRUGS

*activated charcoal:* Possibly adsorption and decreased effectiveness of acetylcysteine
*nitroglycerin:* Increased effects of nitroglycerin and possibly significant hypotension and headache

## Adverse Reactions

**CNS:** Chills, dizziness, drowsiness, fever, headache
**CV:** Hypertension, hypotension, tachycardia
**EENT:** Rhinorrhea, stomatitis, tooth damage
**GI:** Anorexia, constipation, hepatotoxicity, nausea, vomiting
**RESP:** Bronchospasm, chest tightness, hemoptysis
**SKIN:** Clammy skin, pruritus, rash, urticaria
**Other:** Angioedema

## Nursing Considerations

•Be aware that acetylcysteine should be used cautiously in patients with asthma or a history of bronchospasm because drug may adversely affect respiratory function.
•To avoid fluid overload and possibly fatal hyponatremia or seizures, adjust total administered volume, as ordered, for patients who weigh less than 40 kg (88 lb) and for those who need fluid restriction.
•If needed, dilute 20% instillation or inhalation solution with NS or sterile water if needed. The 10% solution may be used undiluted.
•To treat acetaminophen overdose, dilute 20% oral solution with cola or other soft drink to a concentration of 5% and use within 1 hour. Acetylcysteine is most effective if administered within 24 hours of acetaminophen ingestion.
•If patient vomits loading dose or any maintenance dose within 1 hour of administration, repeat dose as prescribed.
•Keep in mind that suicidal patient may not provide reliable information about vomiting. Watch such a patient to ensure that he ingests all of prescribed dosage.
•During treatment for acetaminophen overdose, monitor for signs of hepatotoxicity, such as prolonged bleeding time, altered coagulation, and easy bruising.

A

•Be aware that acetylcysteine may have a disagreeable odor, which disappears as treatment progresses.
•Because nebulization causes sticky residue on face and in mouth, have patient wash his face and rinse his mouth at the end of each treatment.
•Be aware that an open vial of solution may turn light purple but that this doesn't alter its effectiveness.
•Refrigerate opened vials and discard after 96 hours.
•Assess type, frequency, and characteristics of patient's cough. Particularly note sputum. If cough doesn't clear secretions, prepare to perform mechanical suctioning.
•Monitor patient for tachycardia.

**PATIENT TEACHING**
•Instruct patient to notify prescriber immediately about nausea, rash, or vomiting.
•Warn patient about acetylcysteine's unpleasant smell; reassure him that it subsides as treatment progresses.
•To decrease mucus viscosity, encourage patient to consume 2 to 3 L of fluid daily unless contraindicated by another condition.

# adalimumab

HUMIRA

## Class and Category
*Chemical:* Recombinant human IgG1 monoclonal antibody
*Therapeutic:* Disease-modifying antirheumatic
*Pregnancy category:* B

## Indications and Dosages
➤ *To reduce signs and symptoms, inhibit progression of structural damage, and improve physical function in patients with moderate-to-severe active rheumatoid arthritis who have had an inadequate response to other disease-modifying antirheumatics*

**S.C. INJECTION**
**Adults.** 40 mg q other wk
**DOSAGE ADJUSTMENT** Dosage may be adjusted to 40 mg q wk, as needed and prescribed, for patients not also taking methotrexate.

## Mechanism of Action
Binds to tumor necrosis factor (TNF) to block interaction with p55 and p75 cell-surface TNF receptors and lyses surface TNF-expressing cells in the presence of complement. TNF may be a major component of rheumatoid arthritis inflammation and joint destruction. Reduced TNF levels in synovial fluid improve signs and symptoms and prevent further structural damage associated with rheumatoid arthritis.

## Contraindications
Breastfeeding, hypersensitivity to adalimumab or its components

## Interactions
**DRUGS**
*anakinra:* Possibly increased risk of serious infection and neutropenia

## Adverse Reactions
**CNS:** Confusion, fever, headache, hypertensive encephalopathy, multiple sclerosis, paresthesia, subdural hematoma, syncope, tremor
**CV:** Arrhythmias, atrial fibrillation, cardiac arrest, chest pain, coronary artery disease, congestive heart failure, hypercholesterolemia, hyperlipidemia, hypertension, MI, palpitations, pericardial effusion, pericarditis, peripheral edema, tachycardia
**EENT:** Cataracts, sinusitis
**ENDO:** Ketosis, parathyroid disorder
**GI:** Abdominal pain, cholecystitis, cholelithiasis, diverticulitis, elevated alkaline phosphatase level, esophagitis, gastroenteritis, hemorrhage, hepatic necrosis, nausea, vomiting
**GU:** Hematuria, paraproteinemia, pyelonephritis, UTI
**HEME:** Agranulocytosis, aplastic anemia, granulocytopenia, leukopenia, lymphocytosis, pancytopenia, polycythemia, thrombocytopenia
**MS:** Arthritis (including pyogenic or septic arthritis); back, extremity, pelvic, or thorax pain; bone disorder, fracture, or necrosis; muscle spasms; myasthenia; prosthetic infections; synovitis
**RESP:** Asthma, bronchitis, bronchospasm, decreased pulmonary function, dyspnea, pleural effusion, pneumonia, pulmonary tuberculosis, upper respiratory tract infection

**SKIN:** Cellulitis, erysipelas, herpes zoster, rash, urticaria
**Other:** Anaphylaxis; dehydration; flare-up of disease process; flulike symptoms; healing abnormalities; injection site erythema, hemorrhage, itching, pain, or swelling; lupus-like symptoms; lymphomas; malignancies; postsurgical infections; sepsis; tuberculosis (miliary, lymphatic, or peritoneal)

## Nursing Considerations

• Use adalimumab cautiously in patients with recurrent infection or increased risk of infection, patients who live in regions where tuberculosis and histoplasmosis are endemic, and patients with a history of CNS demyelinating disorders because they occur, rarely, during adalimumab therapy.
• **WARNING** If patient has evidence of an active infection when drug is prescribed, therapy shouldn't begin until the infection has been treated. Monitor all patients for infection during therapy, especially those receiving immunosuppressants. If a serious infection develops, expect prescriber to stop drug.
• Make sure patient has a tuberculin skin test before therapy starts. If skin test is positive, treatment of latent tuberculosis will start before adalimumab, as prescribed.
• Be aware that the needle cover of the syringe contains dry rubber. Don't handle if you're allergic to latex.
• To activate the protection device on the needles of pre-filled syringes delivered to institutions, hold the syringe in one hand and, with the other hand, slide the outer protective shield over the exposed needle until it locks into place.
• **WARNING** Stop adalimumab immediately and tell prescriber if patient has an allergic reaction. Expect to provide supportive care.
• Monitor patient closely for signs and symptoms of congestive heart failure (sudden, unexplained weight gain; dyspnea; crackles; anxiety), and notify prescriber if they occur.
• Monitor patient's CBC, as ordered, because adalimumab may have adverse hematologic effects. Notify prescriber about persistent fever, bruising, bleeding, or pallor.

**PATIENT TEACHING**

• Inform patient that the first injection of adalimumab must be administered with a health care professional present.
• Teach patient or caregiver how to give adalimumab as an S.C. injection at home, if applicable. Emphasize importance of injecting the full amount in the syringe (0.8 ml) to obtain the correct dose of 40 mg.
• If patient is allergic to latex, explain that the needle cover contains rubber.
• Caution patient against reusing needles and syringes. Provide patient or caregiver with a puncture resistant container for disposal of needles and syringes at home.
• Instruct patient or caregiver to rotate injection sites and to avoid injecting in any area that is tender, bruised, red, or hard.
• Inform patient that prefilled syringes must be refrigerated (not frozen), protected from light, and stored in the original container.
• Urge patient to check expiration dates and not to use outdated drug.
• Review signs and symptoms of an allergic reaction (rash, swollen face, difficulty breathing), and tell patient to seek emergency care immediately if these occur.
• Inform patient that injection site reactions (such as redness, rash, swelling, itching, and bruising) may occur but are usually mild and transient. Instruct him to apply a towel soaked with cold water on the injection site if it hurts or remains swollen. If reaction does not disappear or seems to worsen, tell patient to call prescriber immediately.
• Inform patient that tuberculosis may occur during adalimumab therapy. Instruct him to report persistent cough, wasting or weight loss, and low-grade fever to prescriber.
• Teach patient to recognize evidence of infection and bleeding disorders and to tell prescriber if they occur; drug may need to be stopped. Advise patient to avoid people with infections and to have all prescribed laboratory tests.
• Inform patient that the risk of developing certain kinds of cancer, especially lymphomas, is higher in patients taking adalimumab but is still rare. Emphasize the importance of follow-up visits and reporting an unusual or sudden onset of signs or symptoms.
• Caution against receiving live-virus vaccines while taking adalimumab; doing so may have adverse effects on the immune system.
• Inform patient that blood samples may be required periodically, but especially around week 24 of therapy, to check for autoantibody development. Tell him that drug will need to be discontinued if autoantibodies are detected.

•Instruct patient to report lupus-like signs and symptoms that, although rare, may occur during therapy, such as chest pain that does not go away, shortness of breath, joint pain, or a rash on his cheeks or arms that's sensitive to the sun. Tell him that drug may need to be discontinued if these occur.

•Advise patient to inform all health care providers about adalimumab use and to inform prescriber about any OTC medications being taken, including herbal remedies and vitamin and mineral supplements.

# adenosine

Adenocard, Adenoscan

## Class and Category

*Chemical:* Monophosphorylated adenine riboside
*Therapeutic:* Antiarrhythmic
*Pregnancy category:* C

## Indications and Dosages

➤ *To convert paroxysmal supraventricular tachycardia (PSVT) to normal sinus rhythm*

**I.V. INJECTION**

**Adults and children who weigh 50 kg (110 lb) or more.** *Initial:* 6 mg by rapid peripheral I.V. bolus over 1 to 2 sec. If PSVT continues after 1 to 2 min, 12 mg given as rapid bolus and repeated in 1 to 2 min if needed.

**WARNING** Don't give single doses of more than 12 mg.

**Children who weigh less than 50 kg.** *Initial:* 0.05 to 0.1 mg/kg as rapid central or peripheral I.V. bolus followed by saline flush. If PSVT continues after 1 to 2 min, additional bolus injections are given, incrementally increasing dose by 0.05 to 0.1 mg/kg. Follow each bolus with saline flush. Injections continue until PSVT converts to normal sinus rhythm or until patient reaches maximum single dose of 0.3 mg/kg.

| Route | Onset | Peak | Duration |
|-------|-------|------|----------|
| I.V. | Immediate | Immediate | Unknown |

## Incompatibilities

Don't mix adenosine with other drugs.

## Mechanism of Action

Slows conduction time through the AV node and can interrupt reentry pathways through the AV node to restore normal sinus rhythm.

## Contraindications

Atrial fibrillation or flutter; hypersensitivity to adenosine; second- or third-degree heart block or sick sinus syndrome, except in patients with a functioning artificial pacemaker; ventricular tachycardia

## Interactions

**DRUGS**

*carbamazepine:* Increased heart block
*digoxin, verapamil:* Possibly increased depressant effect on SA or AV node
*dipyridamole:* Increased effects of adenosine
*methylxanthines, such as theophylline:* Antagonized effects of adenosine

**FOODS**

*caffeine:* Antagonized effects of adenosine

## Adverse Reactions

**CNS:** Apprehension, dizziness, headache, heaviness in arms, light-headedness, nervousness, paresthesia, seizures
**CV:** Atrial fibrillation, bradycardia, chest pain or pressure, heart block, hypertension, hypotension, MI, palpitations, prolonged asystole, sinus exit block or pause, torsades de pointes, transient hypertension, ventricular fibrillation, ventricular tachycardia
**EENT:** Blurred vision, metallic taste, throat tightness
**GI:** Nausea, vomiting
**MS:** Jaw, neck, and back pain
**RESP:** Bronchoconstriction, bronchospasm, dyspnea, hyperventilation, respiratory arrest
**SKIN:** Diaphoresis, facial flushing
**Other:** Injection site reaction

## Nursing Considerations

•Before use, inspect adenosine for crystals. If solution isn't clear, don't give it.

•Administer adenosine by rapid I.V. bolus over 1 to 2 seconds only. Slower administration can cause systemic vasodilation and reflex tachycardia.

•Expect prescriber to inject adenosine directly into a vein, if appropriate, to ensure that it reaches systemic circulation. If administered into an I.V. line, give as close to insertion site as possible and follow with rapid saline flush.

•Monitor heart rate and rhythm, blood pressure, and respiratory status frequently during adenosine therapy.

•Be aware that at the time of conversion to normal sinus rhythm, arrhythmias (such as PVCs, premature atrial contractions, sinus bradycardia, sinus tachycardia, and AV block) may occur for a few seconds but don't require intervention.

•WARNING Discontinue use and notify prescriber immediately if severe respiratory difficulties develop.

•Store adenosine at room temperature. Discard unused portion.

**PATIENT TEACHING**

•Instruct patient to report chest pain, palpitations, difficulty breathing, or severe headache during adenosine therapy.

•Warn patient that he may temporarily experience mild reactions, such as flushing, nausea, and dizziness.

# alatrofloxacin mesylate

Trovan I.V.

## trovafloxacin mesylate

Trovan

## Class and Category

*Chemical:* Fluoroquinolone
*Therapeutic:* Antibacterial
*Pregnancy category:* C

## Indications and Dosages

➤ *To treat life-threatening nosocomial pneumonia*

**TABLETS, I.V. INFUSION**

**Adults.** 300 mg I.V. q 24 hr followed by 200 mg P.O. q 24 hr when patient is stabilized for total of 10 to 14 days.

➤ *To treat life-threatening community-acquired pneumonia*

**TABLETS, I.V. INFUSION**

**Adults.** 200 mg I.V. q 24 hr followed by 200 mg P.O. q 24 hr when patient is stabilized for total of 7 to 14 days; or 200 mg P.O. q 24 hr for total of 7 to 14 days.

➤ *To treat complicated, life-threatening intra-abdominal infections, including*

*postsurgical, gynecologic, and pelvic infections*

**TABLETS, I.V. INFUSION**

**Adults.** 300 mg I.V. q 24 hr followed by 200 mg P.O. q 24 hr when patient is stabilized for total of 7 to 14 days.

➤ *To treat complicated, life-threatening or limb-threatening skin and soft-tissue infections, including diabetic foot infections*

**TABLETS, I.V. INFUSION**

**Adults.** 200 mg P.O. q 24 hr—or 200 mg I.V. q 24 hr followed by 200 mg P.O. q 24 hr when patient is stabilized—for total of 10 to 14 days.

DOSAGE ADJUSTMENT For patients with mild to moderate cirrhosis, 300-mg I.V. dosage reduced to 200 mg and 200-mg I.V. and P.O. dosage reduced to 100 mg.

---

### Mechanism of Action

Interferes with DNA gyrase, the enzyme needed for DNA replication in aerobic and anaerobic bacteria. May be active against pathogens resistant to such antibiotics as penicillins, cephalosporins, aminoglycosides, macrolides, and tetracyclines.

---

### Incompatibilities

Don't mix alatrofloxacin with or infuse it simultaneously through same I.V. line as other drugs. Don't dilute it with NS or LR.

### Contraindications

Hypersensitivity to alatrofloxacin, quinolone antimicrobials, trovafloxacin, or their components

### Interactions

**DRUGS**

*antacids that contain aluminum, citric acid, magnesium, or sodium citrate; iron; morphine sulfate; sucralfate:* Reduced absorption of trovafloxacin

### Adverse Reactions

**CNS:** Dizziness, headache, light-headedness, seizures
**CV:** Hypotension
**EENT:** Hoarseness, throat tightness
**GI:** Abdominal pain, acute hepatic failure (as evidenced by anorexia, dark urine, dysphagia, fatigue, jaundice, pale stool, and vomiting)
**GU:** Vaginitis
**RESP:** Dyspnea

**SKIN:** Photosensitivity, rash, urticaria or other skin reactions
**Other:** Angioedema

## Nursing Considerations
• Infuse alatrofloxacin over 60 minutes; rapid or bolus I.V. injection may cause hypotension.
• Periodically assess liver function test results. Results may be elevated for up to 21 days after alatrofloxacin administration.
• **WARNING** Be aware that alatrofloxacin may cause severe liver damage, requiring liver transplantation or leading to death. Expect therapy to last no longer than 2 weeks because more prolonged therapy increases the risk of liver damage. Alatrofloxacin is reserved for hospitalized patients with life- or limb-threatening infections.
**PATIENT TEACHING**
• Instruct patient to report rash; urticaria; difficulty swallowing; swelling of the lips, face, or tongue; hoarseness; or throat tightness.

# albuterol
## (salbutamol)
Proventil, Ventolin

## albuterol sulfate
## (salbutamol sulphate)
AccuNeb, Airet, Gen-Salbutamol (CAN), Novo-Salmol (CAN), Proventil, Proventil Repetabs, Proventil Syrup, Ventolin, Ventolin HFA, Ventolin Syrup, Volmax

## Class and Category
*Chemical:* Selective beta$_2$-adrenergic agonist, sympathomimetic
*Therapeutic:* Bronchodilator
*Pregnancy category:* C

## Indications and Dosages
➤ *To prevent exercise-induced asthma*
**INHALATION AEROSOL**
**Adults and children over age 4.** 2 inhalations 15 to 30 min before exercise.

➤ *To treat bronchospasm in patients with reversible obstructive airway disease or acute bronchospastic attack*
**E.R. TABLETS**
**Adults and children over age 12.** *Initial:* 4 or 8 mg q 12 hr. *Maximum:* 32 mg/day in divided doses q 12 hr.

**Children ages 6 to 12.** *Initial:* 4 mg q 12 hr. *Maximum:* 24 mg/day in divided doses q 12 hr.
**REPETABS**
**Adults and children over age 12.** *Initial:* 4 to 8 mg q 12 hr. *Maximum:* 32 mg/day in divided doses q 12 hr.
**Children ages 6 to 11.** *Initial:* 4 mg q 12 hr. *Maximum:* 24 mg/day in divided doses q 12 hr.
**SYRUP**
**Adults and children over age 14.** *Initial:* 2 to 4 mg (1 to 2 tsp) t.i.d. or q.i.d. *Maximum:* 32 mg/day in divided doses.
**Children ages 6 to 14.** *Initial:* 2 mg (1 tsp) t.i.d. or q.i.d. *Maximum:* 24 mg/day in divided doses.
**Children ages 2 to 6.** *Initial:* 0.1 mg/kg t.i.d. (not to exceed 2 mg t.i.d.), increased to 0.2 mg/kg t.i.d. (not to exceed 4 mg t.i.d.).
**TABLETS**
**Adults and children over age 12.** *Initial:* 2 or 4 mg t.i.d. or q.i.d. *Maximum:* 32 mg/day in divided doses.
**Children ages 6 to 12.** *Initial:* 2 mg t.i.d. or q.i.d. *Maximum:* 24 mg/day in divided doses.
**DOSAGE ADJUSTMENT** For elderly patients, initial dosage reduced to 2 mg (1 tsp) of syrup t.i.d. or q.i.d. or 2 mg of tablets t.i.d. or q.i.d. (up to 32 mg/day).
**INHALATION AEROSOL**
**Adults and children age 4 and older.** 1 inhalation q 4 hr to 2 inhalations q 4 to 6 hr.
**INHALATION CAPSULES (ROTOCAPS)**
**Adults and children age 4 and older.** 200 mcg inhaled q 4 to 6 hr using inhalation device. *Maximum:* 400 mcg q 4 to 6 hr.
**INHALATION SOLUTION**
**Adults and children age 12 and older.** 2.5 mg t.i.d. or q.i.d. by nebulization over 5 to 15 min.
**Children ages 2 to 12.** *Initial:* 0.1 to 0.15 mg/kg t.i.d. or q.i.d. *Maximum:* 2.5 mg t.i.d. or q.i.d.

| Route | Onset | Peak | Duration |
|---|---|---|---|
| P.O. (E.R. tab) | 30 min | 2 to 3 hr | 12 hr |
| P.O. (syrup) | Rapid | 2 hr | Unknown |
| P.O. (tab) | 30 min | 2 to 3 hr | 4 to 8 hr |
| Inhalation (aerosol) | 5 to 15 min | 50 to 55 min | 3 to 6 hr |
| Inhalation (rotocap) | 5 to 15 min | 0.5 to 3 hr | 2 to 6 hr |
| Inhalation (solution) | 5 to 15 min | 1 to 2 hr | 3 to 6 hr |

## Mechanism of Action

Albuterol attaches to beta₂ receptors on bronchial cell membranes, which stimulates the intracellular enzyme adenylate cyclase to convert adenosine triphosphate (ATP) to cyclic adenosine monophosphate (cAMP). This reaction decreases intracellular calcium levels. It also increases intracellular levels of cAMP, as shown. Together, these effects relax bronchial smooth-muscle cells and inhibit histamine release.

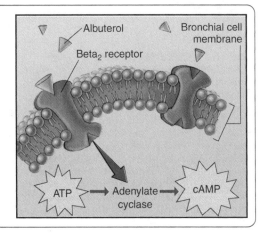

## Contraindications

Hypersensitivity to albuterol or its components

## Inteactions

### DRUGS

*beta blockers:* Inhibited effects of albuterol
*bronchodilators (sympathomimetics), such as theophylline:* Possibly adverse cardiovascular effects
*digoxin:* Decreased serum digoxin level
*MAO inhibitors, tricyclic antidepressants:* Increased vascular effects of albuterol
*methyldopa:* Increased vasopressor effect of methyldopa
*potassium-lowering drugs:* Possibly hypokalemia
*potassium-wasting diuretics:* Possibly increased hypokalemia

## Adverse Reactions

**CNS:** Anxiety, dizziness, drowsiness, headache, hyperkinesia, insomnia, irritability, nervousness, tremor, vertigo, weakness
**CV:** Angina; arrhythmias, including tachycardia; hypertension; palpitations
**EENT:** Altered taste, dry mouth and throat, taste perversion
**GI:** Anorexia, diarrhea, dysphagia, heartburn, nausea, vomiting
**RESP:** Bronchospasm, cough, dyspnea, paradoxical airway resistance (with excessive inhalation), pulmonary edema
**SKIN:** Diaphoresis, flushing, pallor, pruritus, rash, urticaria
**Other:** Hypokalemia

## Nursing Considerations

•Administer pressurized inhalations of albuterol during second half of inspiration, when airways are open wider and aerosol distribution is more effective.
•**WARNING** Use cautiously in patients with cardiac disorders, diabetes mellitus, digitalis intoxication, hypertension, hyperthyroidism, or history of seizures. Albuterol can worsen these conditions.
•Monitor serum potassium level because albuterol may cause transient hypokalemia.
•Be aware that drug tolerance can develop with prolonged use.

### PATIENT TEACHING

•Teach patient how to use inhaler properly. Tell him to shake canister well before using and to check that a new canister is working properly by spraying it once into the air while looking for a fine mist.
•Instruct patient to wash mouthpiece with water once a week and allow it to air-dry.
•Advise patient to wait at least 1 minute between inhalations.
•Tell patient to check with his prescriber before using other inhaled drugs.
•Warn patient not to exceed prescribed dose or frequency. If doses become less effective, tell him to contact his prescriber.
•Tell patient to immediately report signs and symptoms of allergic reaction, such as difficulty swallowing, itching, and rash.

# alefacept

Amevive

## Class and Category

*Chemical:* Recombinant leukocyte function-associated antigen-3 immunoglobulin GI fusion protein
*Therapeutic:* Immunosuppresant
*Pregnancy category:* B

## Indications and Dosages

➤ *To treat moderate-to-severe chronic plaque psoriasis in patients who are candidates for systemic therapy or phototherapy*

---

### Mechanism of Action

Binds to the lymphocyte antigen and CD2 and inhibits LFA-3/CD2 interaction to interfere with T-lymphocyte activation. Alefacept also reduces the subsets of CD2+ T lymphocytes. Because activation of T lymphocytes plays a role in the pathophysiology of chronic plaque psoriasis, interference with lymphocytic activity helps to prevent plaque formation.

---

**I.V. INJECTION**
**Adults.** *Initial:* 7.5 mg q wk for 12 wk. After at least 12 wk in which drug isn't given, a second 12-wk course may be given, if needed and if patient's CD4 and T-lymphocyte counts are within normal ranges.
**I.M. INJECTION**
**Adults.** 15 mg q week for 12 wk. After at least 12 wk in which drug isn't given, a second 12-wk course may be given, if needed and if patient's CD4 and T-lymphocyte counts are within normal ranges.

## Incompatibilities

Don't add other drugs to solutions containing alefacept.

## Contraindications

Breast-feeding, hypersensitivity to alefacept or its components

## Interactions

**DRUGS**
None reported

## Adverse Reactions

**CNS:** Chills, dizziness, headache
**CV:** Coronary artery disease, MI
**EENT:** Pharyngitis
**GI:** Nausea
**HEME:** Lymphopenia
**MS:** Myalgia
**RESP:** Increased cough
**SKIN:** Pruritus, urticaria
**Other:** Angioedema, injection site pain or inflammation, infection, malignancies

## Nursing Considerations

• Use alefacept cautiously in patients at high risk for malignancy because the drug increases risk of malignancy development. Know that drug isn't recommended for use in patients with a history of a systemic malignancy.
• Also use cautiously in patients with chronic infections or history of recurrent infection. Drug may increase risk of infection because of its immunosuppressive action.
• Obtain a CD4+ and T-lymphocyte count before initiating drug therapy, as ordered. If counts are below normal, be aware that therapy shouldn't be started. After therapy starts, monitor patient's CD4+ and T-lymphocyte counts weekly throughout therapy. If levels drop below 250 cells/µL, notify prescriber because drug will need to be withheld. If counts remain below 250 cells/µL for 1 month, know that drug should be discontinued.
• Reconstitute drug with 0.6 ml using only the supplied diluent (sterile water for injection) before administration. With the needle pointed at the sidewall of the vial, slowly inject the diluent into the vial of alefacept. Be aware that some foaming will occur. To prevent excessive foaming, don't shake or vigorously agitate vial. Instead, gently swirl vial during dissolution, which usually takes less than 2 minutes.
• Administer drug as soon as possible after reconstitution. Discard solution if not used within 4 hours.
• Don't filter reconstituted solution during preparation or administration.
• For I.M. administration, inject the full 0.5 ml of solution. Use a different injection site for each subsequent injection, injecting at least 1 inch away from previous sites. Never inject the drug into tender, bruised, red, or hard areas.
• For I.V. administration, prepare two syringes with 3 ml NS for pre- and post-administration flush. Then prime the winged

infusion set with 3 ml of NS and insert into the vein. Attach the filled syringe to the infusion set and administer the solution over no more than 5 seconds. Finish by flushing the set with 3 ml of NS.

•Be aware that drug therapy shouldn't be initiated in a patient with a concurrent serious infection. Monitor patient closely during and after therapy for signs and symptoms of infection. If these occur, report them to the prescriber immediately and initiate treatment, as prescribed, to reduce risk of serious infection. If infection becomes serious, expect drug to be discontinued.

•Monitor patient for allergic reactions. If these occur, discontinue drug and notify prescriber immediately.

**PATIENT TEACHING**
•Advise patient that weekly blood tests will be required to monitor his WBC during alefacept therapy.

•Teach patient the signs and symptoms of infection and common warning signs of malignancy. Emphasize the importance of complying with follow-up visits and promptly reporting to prescriber any unusual or sudden signs or symptoms suggesting malignancy or infection.

•Inform female patient to notify prescriber if she becomes pregnant while taking alefacept or within 8 weeks after discontinuing the drug.

# alendronate sodium

Fosamax

## Class and Category
*Chemical:* Aminobisphosphonate
*Therapeutic:* Bone resorption inhibitor
*Pregnancy category:* C

## Indications and Dosages
➤ *To prevent postmenopausal osteoporosis*
**TABLETS**
**Adults.** 5 mg q.d. or 35 mg once weekly in the morning with a full glass of water at least 30 min before first food, drink, or drug.
➤ *To treat postmenopausal osteoporosis*
**TABLETS**
**Adults.** 10 mg q.d. or 70 mg once weekly in the morning with a full glass of water at least 30 min before first food, drink, or drug.

➤ *To treat Paget's disease of the bone in patients whose alkaline phosphatase level is twice the upper limit of normal or higher and who are symptomatic and at risk for further complications*
**TABLETS**
**Adults.** 40 mg q.d. with a full glass of water for 6 mo.
**DOSAGE ADJUSTMENT** Dosage increased to 10 mg q.d. for postmenopausal women not receiving estrogen.
➤ *To increase bone mass in men with osteoporosis*
**TABLETS**
**Adults.** 10 mg q.d. or 70 mg once weekly in the morning with a full glass of water at least 30 min before first food, drink, or drug.
➤ *To treat glucocorticoid-induced osteoporosis in men and women who receive a daily glucocorticoid dosage equal to or greater than 7.5 mg of prednisone and who have low bone mineral density*
**TABLETS**
**Adults.** 5 mg q.d. in the morning with a full glass of water at least 30 min before first food, drink, or drug.

### Mechanism of Action
Reduces the activity of cells that cause bone loss, slows the rate of bone loss after menopause, and increases the amount of bone mass. May act by inhibiting osteoclast activity on newly formed bone resorption surfaces, which reduces the number of sites where bone is remodeled. Bone formation then exceeds bone resorption at these remodeling sites, which gradually increases bone mass. May also inhibit bone dissolution by binding to hydroxyapatite crystals, which are composed of calcium, phosphate, and hydroxide and give bone its rigid structure.

| Route | Onset | Peak | Duration |
|-------|-------|------|----------|
| P.O. | Unknown | Unknown | 6 wk* |

\* After single 5-mg dose for osteoporosis; 6 mo after single 5-mg dose for Paget's disease.

## Contraindications

Esophageal abnormalities that delay esophageal emptying, such as stricture or achalasia; hypersensitivity to alendronate; hypocalcemia; inability to stand or sit upright for at least 30 minutes

## Interactions

**DRUGS**
*antacids, calcium, iron, multivalent cations:* Decreased absorption of alendronate
*aspirin:* Increased risk of GI distress
**FOODS**
*any food:* Delayed absorption and decreased serum level of alendronate

## Adverse Reactions

**CNS:** Headache
**GI:** Abdominal distention and pain, constipation, diarrhea, dysphagia, esophageal perforation or ulceration, esophagitis, flatulence, gastritis, gastroesophageal reflux disease, heartburn, indigestion, melena, nausea, vomiting
**MS:** Arthralgia, bone pain, focal osteomalacia, muscle spasms, myalgia
**SKIN:** Photosensitivity, pruritus, rash, Stevens-Johnson syndrome, toxic epidermal necrolysis
**Other:** Hypocalcemia

## Nursing Considerations

•Monitor serum calcium level before, during, and after treatment. Expect hypocalcemia to be treated before alendronate therapy. If hypocalcemia occurs during therapy, expect prescriber to order a calcium supplement.
•Ensure adequate dietary intake of calcium and vitamin D before, during, and after treatment.
•**WARNING** Alendronate may irritate upper GI mucosa, causing such adverse reactions as esophageal ulceration. To help minimize these reactions, have patient take it with a full glass of water and remain upright for at least 30 minutes.
**PATIENT TEACHING**
•Advise patient to take alendronate in the morning with a full glass of water. Explain that such beverages as orange juice, coffee, and mineral water reduce alendronate's effects.
•To help reduce esophageal irritation, tell patient not to chew or suck on tablet.
•Instruct patient to wait at least 30 minutes after taking alendronate before eating, drinking, or taking other drugs. Teach patient to

remain upright for 30 minutes after taking alendronate *and* until she has eaten the first food of the day.
•Teach patient to consume adequate daily amounts of calcium and vitamin D.

# alfuzosin hydrochloride

Uroxatral

## Class and Category

*Chemical:* Tetrahydro-2-furancarboxamide hydrochloride
*Therapeutic:* Selective alpha$_1$-adrenergic antagonist
*Pregnancy category:* B

## Indications and Dosages

➤ *To treat signs and symptoms of benign prostatic hyperplasia*
**E.R. TABLETS**
**Adults.** 10 mg q.d. taken immediately after same meal each day.

## Contraindications

Hypersensitivity to alfuzosin or its components, moderate or severe hepatic insufficiency, use with CYP3A4 inhibitors, such as itraconazole, ketoconazole, and ritonavir

## Interactions

**DRUGS**
*alpha blockers:* May potentiate action of alfuzosin
*antihypertensives:* Possibly synergistic lowering of blood pressure
*CYP3A4 inhibitors (such as itraconazole, ketoconazole, and ritonavir):* Increased effects of alfuzosin

### Mechanism of Action

Selectively blocks alpha$_1$-adrenergic receptors in smooth muscle of the bladder neck and prostate, causing relaxation, and blocks postsynaptic alpha$_1$-adrenoreceptors in the bladder base and neck, prostate, prostatic capsule, and urethra, preventing further action at these sites. These actions improve urine flow and bladder emptying and reduce urinary hesitancy, frequency, and nocturia.

## Adverse Reactions

**CNS:** Dizziness, fatigue, headache
**CV:** Chest pain, orthostatic hypotension, tachycardia
**EENT:** Pharyngitis, sinusitis
**GI:** Abdominal pain, constipation, indigestion, nausea
**GU:** Impotence, priapism
**RESP:** Bronchitis, upper respiratory tract infection
**SKIN:** Rash
**Other:** Generalized pain

## Nursing Considerations

• Use alfuzosin cautiously in patients who have symptomatic hypotension or who have had a hypotensive response to other drugs because orthostatic hypotension (with or without symptoms such as dizziness) may occur within hours after alfuzosin administration.
• Use cautiously in patients with severe renal insufficiency because drug clearance may be hampered, increasing the risk of adverse reactions.
• Be aware that alfuzosin shouldn't be used to treat bladder symptoms in women.
• Monitor patient for chest pain. If symptoms of angina pectoris occur or worsen, notify prescriber immediately and expect drug to be discontinued.

**PATIENT TEACHING**
• Stress importance of taking alfuzosin immediately after a meal because absorption is decreased by 50% if taken on an empty stomach.
• Tell patient not to crush or chew tablets but to swallow them whole.
• Caution patient to avoid potentially hazardous activities until drug's CNS effects are known and then for several hours after taking drug because blood pressure may drop suddenly after administration

# alglucerase

Ceredase

## Class and Category

*Chemical:* Glucocerebrosidase beta-glucosidase
*Therapeutic:* Enzyme replacement
*Pregnancy category:* C

## Indications and Dosages

➤ *To treat chronic nonneuropathic Gaucher's disease in patients with moderate to severe anemia, thrombocytopenia with bleeding tendencies, bone disease, or significant hepatomegaly or splenomegaly*

**I.V. INFUSION**
**Adults.** Up to 60 U/kg infused over 1 to 2 hr, usually q 2 wk.
**DOSAGE ADJUSTMENT** Highly individualized dosage based on body size and disease severity. Some patients may need infusion once every other day; others may need it once q 4 wk. Maintenance dosage progressively reduced every 3 to 6 mo to as low as 1 U/kg.

## Contraindications

Hypersensitivity to alglucerase

| Route | Onset | Peak | Duration |
|---|---|---|---|
| I.V. | Up to 60 min | Unknown | Variable |

## Mechanism of Action

Catalyzes hydrolysis of glucocerebroside to glucose and ceramide in membrane lipids. Gaucher's disease results from deficiency of the enzyme beta-glucocerebrosidase and causes the lipid glucocerebroside to accumulate in tissue macrophages.

## Adverse Reactions

**CNS:** Chills, dizziness, fatigue, fever, headache
**CV:** Transient peripheral edema, vasomotor irritability
**EENT:** Oral ulcerations
**GI:** Abdominal discomfort, diarrhea, nausea, vomiting
**MS:** Backache
**Other:** I.V. site burning, itching, or swelling

## Nursing Considerations

• Before intitiating alglucerase therapy, expect to give antihistamines to patient who is hypersensitive to drug.
• On day of dosage, use aseptic technique to dilute alglucerase with NS to final volume of no more than 200 ml.
• Don't shake drug, which could inactivate it.
• Don't use alglucerase if it's discolored or contains precipitate.

•Be aware that drug doesn't contain preservatives. Discard unused portion.
•Infuse alglucerase with in-line I.V. particle filter.

**PATIENT TEACHING**
•Tell patient that he may experience flulike symptoms with each dose of alglucerase.
•Instruct patient to report headache, hot flashes, nausea, and other adverse reactions.
•Inform patient that alglucerase is derived from pooled human placental tissue and poses a slight risk of viral contamination.
•Advise patient to keep appointments for scheduled doses of alglucerase.

# allopurinol

Apo-Allopurinol (CAN), Lopurin, Purinol (CAN), Zyloprim

## allopurinol sodium

Aloprim

## Class and Category

*Chemical:* Hypoxanthine derivative, xanthine oxidase inhibitor
*Therapeutic:* Antigout
*Pregnancy category:* C

## Indications and Dosages

➤ *To treat gout and hyperuricemia*
**TABLETS**
**Adults.** 200 to 600 mg/day in divided doses, depending on disease severity. *Usual:* 200 to 300 mg/day. *Maximum:* 800 mg/day.
➤ *To treat secondary hyperuricemia caused by neoplastic disease*
**TABLETS**
**Children ages 6 to 10.** 300 mg/day, adjusted after 48 hr, depending on response to treatment.
**Children under age 6.** 150 mg/day, adjusted after 48 hr, depending on response to treatment.
➤ *To prevent gout attack*
**TABLETS**
**Adults.** 100 mg/day increased by 100 mg/wk until serum uric acid level is 6 mg/dl or less.
➤ *To prevent uric acid nephropathy during vigorous treatment of neoplastic disease*

**TABLETS**
**Adults.** 600 to 800 mg/day for 2 to 3 days, then adjusted to keep serum uric acid level within normal limits.

➤ *To treat recurrent calcium oxalate calculi*
**TABLETS**
**Adults.** 200 to 300 mg/day as a single dose or in divided doses, adjusted based on 24-hr urine urate level.
**DOSAGE ADJUSTMENT** For patient with impaired renal function, dosage adjusted to 200 mg/day if creatinine clearance is 10 to 20 ml/min/1.73 m$^2$, 100 mg/day if creatinine clearance is 3 to 10 ml/min/1.73 m$^2$, or 100 mg q.o.d. if creatinine clearance falls below 3 ml/min/1.73 m$^2$.

➤ *To treat increased serum and urine uric acid levels in patients with leukemia, lymphoma, and solid tumors whose cancer chemotherapy has increased those levels and who can't tolerate oral therapy*
**I.V. INFUSION**
**Adults.** 200 to 400 mg/m$^2$/day as a single infusion or in equally divided infusions q 6, 8, or 12 hr. *Maximum:* 600 mg/day.
**Children.** 200 mg/m$^2$/day as a single infusion or in equally divided infusions q 6, 8, or 12 hr.

| Route | Onset | Peak | Duration |
|-------|-------|------|----------|
| P.O. | 2 to 3 days | 1 to 3 wk* | 1 to 2 wk |

## Incompatibilities

Don't combine I.V. allopurinol in solution with amikacin, amphotericin B, carmustine, cefotaxime sodium, chlorpromazine hydrochloride, cimetidine hydrochloride, clindamycin phosphate, cytarabine, dacarbazine, daunorubicin hydrochloride, diphenhydramine hydrochloride, doxorubicin hydrochloride, doxycycline hyclate, droperidol, floxuridine, gentamicin sulfate, haloperidol lactate, hydroxyzine hydrochloride, idarubicin hydrochloride, imipenem-cilastatin sodium, mechlorethamine hydrochloride, meperidine hydrochloride, metoclopramide hydrochloride, methylprednisolone sodium succinate, minocycline hydrochloride, nalbuphine hy-

---

* For hyperuricemia; several months for gout attack prevention.

drochloride, netilmicin sulfate, ondansetron hydrochloride, prochlorperazine edisylate, promethazine hydrochloride, sodium bicarbonate, streptozocin, tobramycin sulfate, vinorelbine tartrate.

## Mechanism of Action

Inhibits uric acid production by inhibiting xanthine oxidase, the enzyme responsible for converting hypoxanthine and xanthine to uric acid. Allopurinol is metabolized to oxipurinol, which also inhibits xanthine oxidase.

## Contraindications

Hypersensitivity to allopurinol

## Interactions

**DRUGS**
*ACE inhibitors:* Increased risk of hypersensitivity reactions
*amoxicillin, ampicillin:* Increased risk of rash
*azathioprine, mercaptopurine:* Inactivation of these drugs
*chlorpropamide:* Increased risk of hypoglycemia in patients with renal insufficiency
*cyclophosphamide, other cytotoxic drugs:* Enhanced bone marrow suppression
*dicumarol:* Increased half-life and anticoagulant action of dicumarol
*thiazide diuretics:* Possibly increased risk of allopurinol toxicity
*uricosuric agents:* Increased urinary excretion of uric acid
*vitamin C (large doses):* Possibly urine acidification and increased risk of renal calculus formation

## Adverse Reactions

**CNS:** Chills, drowsiness, fever, headache, neuritis, paresthesia, peripheral neuropathy, somnolence
**CV:** Vasculitis
**EENT:** Epistaxis, loss of taste
**GI:** Abdominal pain, diarrhea, dysphagia, elevated liver function test results, gastritis, granulomatous hepatitis, hepatic necrosis, hepatomegaly, nausea, vomiting
**GU:** Exacerbation of renal calculi, renal failure
**HEME:** Agranulocytosis, aplastic anemia, bone marrow depression, eosinophilia, leukocytosis, leukopenia, thrombocytopenia

**MS:** Arthralgia, exacerbation of gout, myopathy
**SKIN:** Alopecia; ecchymosis; jaundice; maculopapular, scaly, or exfoliative rash (sometimes fatal); pruritus; urticaria

## Nursing Considerations

•As ordered, obtain baseline CBC and uric acid level and review results of renal and liver function tests before and during allopurinol therapy.
•Reconstitute and dilute I.V. preparation to a concentration of 6 mg/ml or less.
•**WARNING** Discontinue allopurinol and notify prescriber immediately at first sign of hypersensitivity reaction, such as rash, which may precede more severe reactions.
•To decrease risk of calculus formation, maintain fluid intake of up to 3 L/day and monitor patient for output of 2 L/day. Also, don't give vitamin C.
**PATIENT TEACHING**
•Advise patient to take allopurinol after meals and to drink at least 10 large glasses of water daily.
•Instruct patient to report unusual bleeding or bruising, fever, chills, gout attack, numbness, and tingling.
•Inform patient that acute gout attacks may occur more frequently early in allopurinol treatment and that results may not be noticeable for 2 weeks or longer.
•Instruct patient not to drive or perform potentially hazardous tasks if drug causes drowsiness.

# almotriptan malate

Axert

## Class and Category

*Chemical:* Selective 5-hydroxytryptamine$_1$ (5-HT$_1$) receptor agonist
*Therapeutic:* Antimigraine drug
*Pregnancy category:* C

## Indications and Dosages

➤ *To treat acute migraine*
**TABLETS**
**Adults.** *Initial:* 6.25 to 12.5 mg as a single dose, repeated in 2 hr p.r.n. *Maximum:* 2 doses/ 24 hr or 4 migraine treatments/mo.
**DOSAGE ADJUSTMENT** For patient with impaired renal or hepatic function, initial dose reduced to 6.25 mg with maximum daily dose of 12.5 mg.

## Mechanism of Action
May stimulate 5-HT$_1$ receptors on intra-cranial blood vessels and sensory nerves in the trigeminal vascular system. By activating these receptors, almotriptan selectively constricts inflamed and dilated cranial blood vessels and inhibits the production of proinflammatory neuropeptides. The drug also interrupts the transmission of pain signals to the brain.

## Contraindications
Basilar or hemiplegic migraine; cerebrovascular, peripheral vascular, or ischemic or vasospastic coronary artery disease (CAD); hypersensitivity to almotriptan or its components; hypertension (uncontrolled); use within 24 hours of other serotonin-receptor agonists or ergotamine-containing or ergot-type drugs

## Interactions
### DRUGS
*ergotamine-containing drugs:* Prolonged vasospastic reactions
*erythromycin, itraconazole, ketoconazole, ritonavir:* Possibly increased blood almotriptan level
*MAO inhibitors, verapamil:* Increased blood almotriptan level
*selective serotonin reuptake inhibitors:* Increased risk of hyperreflexia, lack of coordination, and weakness

## Adverse Reactions
**CNS:** Dizziness, headache, paresthesia, somnolence, syncope
**CV:** Coronary artery vasospasm, hypertension, ischemia, MI, palpitations, vasodilation, ventricular fibrillation, ventricular tachycardia
**EENT:** Dry mouth
**GI:** Nausea

## Nursing Considerations
•**WARNING** Because almotriptan therapy can cause coronary artery vasospasm, monitor patient with CAD for signs and symptoms of angina. Because drug also may cause peripheral vasospastic reactions, such as ischemic bowel disease, monitor patient for abdominal pain and bloody diarrhea.

•Be prepared to administer the first dose of almotriptan in a medical facility for patients who have risk factors for CAD but no known cardiovascular abnormalities.
•Obtain an ECG reading immediately after the first dose of almotriptan, as ordered, in patients who have risk factors for CAD because cardiac ischemia can occur without the patient having clinical symptoms.
•Expect to administer a lower dosage to patients with hepatic or renal dysfunction because of impaired drug metabolism or excretion.
•Monitor blood pressure regularly during therapy in patients with hypertension because almotriptan may produce a transient increase in blood pressure.

### PATIENT TEACHING
•Inform patient that almotriptan is used to treat acute migraine attacks and that he shouldn't take it to treat nonmigraine headaches.
•Advise patient to consult prescriber before taking any OTC or prescription drugs.
•Advise patient not to take more than maximum prescribed dosage during any 24-hour period.
•Caution patient that drug may cause adverse CNS reactions, and advise him to avoid potentially hazardous activities until he knows how the drug affects him.
•Instruct patient to seek emergency care immediately if he experiences cardiac symptoms—such as heaviness, pain, pressure, or tightness in the chest, jaw, neck, or throat—after taking drug.

# alosetron hydrochloride
Lotronex

## Class and Category
*Chemical:* Selective serotonin 5-HT$_3$ receptor antagonist
*Therapeutic:* Antidiarrheal
*Pregnancy category:* B

## Indications and Dosages
➤ *To treat women with severe diarrhea-predominant irritable bowel syndrome (IBS) who have failed to respond to conventional therapy*

**TABLETS**

**Adults.** *Initial:* 1 mg q.d. for 4 wk, increased to 1 mg b.i.d., if needed, or discontinued if no response seen in first 4 wk of therapy or if drug doesn't adequately control symptoms after 4 wk of b.i.d. regimen.

---

**Mechanism of Action**

Inhibits activation of $5\text{-HT}_3$ nonselective cation channels found in enteric neurons in the GI tract, thereby decreasing visceral sensations, colonic transit, and secretions in the GI tract. These changes reduce GI pain and hyperactivity, symptoms that are prominent in diarrhea-predominant IBS.

---

**Contraindications**

Administration with fluvoxamine, history of chronic or severe constipation or sequelae from constipation, Crohn's disease, diverticulitis, GI perforation or adhesions, hypercoagulable state, impaired intestinal circulation, intestinal obstruction or stricture, ischemic colitis, thrombophlebitis, toxic megacolon, or ulcerative colitis; hypersensitivity to alosetron or its components

**Interactions**

*fluvoxamine, ketoconazole:* Increased blood alosetron level
*cimetidine, clarithromycin, itraconazole, protease inhibitors, quinolones, telithromycin, voriconazole:* Possibly increased alosetron level

**Adverse Reactions**

**CNS:** Anxiety, fatigue, headache, hypnagogic effects, malaise, temperature regulation disturbances
**CV:** Tachyarrhythmias
**GI:** Abdominal or GI discomfort and pain, abdominal distention, constipation, dyspepsia, GI spasms or lesions, hemorrhoids, hyposalivation, ileus, impaction, ischemic colitis, nausea, obstruction, perforation, regurgitation and reflux, small-bowel mesenteric ischemia, ulceration
**GU:** Urinary frequency
**RESP:** Breathing disorders
**SKIN:** Diaphoresis, rash, urticaria
**Other:** Nonspecific cramps or pain

**Nursing Considerations**

• Be aware that only physicians enrolled in Glaxo-SmithKline's prescribing program for alosetron should prescribe the drug and only patients who have read and signed the patient-physician agreement can receive the drug. Confirm that the agreement has been signed before therapy starts.
• **WARNING** Monitor patient for constipation, especially if she's elderly or debilitated or she takes drugs that decrease gastrointestinal motility. Also monitor patient for signs and symptoms of ischemic colitis, such as rectal bleeding, bloody diarrhea, or new or worsening abdominal pain. If these occur, discontinue drug immediately. Be aware that once alosetron is discontinued for ischemic colitis, drug should not be resumed later; however, a patient who no longer has constipation can resume the drug, if needed.
• Ensure that program stickers required by the drug company are affixed to all prescriptions, including refills, before giving them to the patient.

**PATIENT TEACHING**

• Instruct patient to read the medication guide for alosetron, which outlines the risks and benefits of the drug.
• Instruct patient not to start alosetron if constipated and to notify prescriber.
• Advise patient to stop drug immediately and notify prescriber if signs and symptoms of ischemic colitis or constipation occur. If constipation does not resolve after drug is stopped, instruct patient to notify her prescriber.
• Inform patient that alosetron will be stopped after 4 weeks of 1 mg b.i.d. if the drug isn't effective in controlling symptoms of IBS.

# alpha₁-proteinase inhibitor (human)

Prolastin, Zemaira

## Class and Category

*Chemical:* Plasma protein
*Therapeutic:* Enzyme replacement
*Pregnancy category:* C

## Indications and Dosages

➤ *To treat congenital alpha₁-antitrypsin deficiency in patients with signs of panacinar emphysema (Prolastin); to augment and maintain patients with emphysema who are deficient in alpha₁-proteinase inhibitor*

A

### I.V. INFUSION
**Adults.** 60 mg/kg infused over 30 min for Prolastin and 15 min for Zemaira at a rate of at least 0.08 ml/kg/min once weekly.

## Mechanism of Action
Replaces the enzyme alpha₁-antitrypsin, which normally inhibits the proteolytic enzyme elastase in patients with alpha₁-antitrypsin deficiency. Without alpha₁-proteinase inhibitor, elastase attacks and destroys alveolar membranes and causes emphysema.

## Contraindications
Hypersensitivity to alpha₁-proteinase inhibitor, its components, or other alpha₁-proteinase products; selective immunoglobulin A (IgA) deficiency in patients with anti-IgA antibodies

## Interactions
### ACTIVITIES
*smoking:* Inactivation of alpha₁-proteinase inhibitor

## Adverse Reactions
**CNS:** Asthenia, dizziness, fever, headache, paresthesia
**EENT:** Sinusitis
**HEME:** Mild, transient leukocytosis
**RESP:** Exacerbation of existing COPD, upper respiratory tract infection
**SKIN:** Pruritus
**Other:** Flulike symptoms, infusion site pain

## Nursing Considerations
•Use alpha₁-proteinase inhibitor cautiously in patients at risk for circulatory overload because drug is a colloid solution that increases plasma volume.
•Before reconstituting alpha₁-proteinase inhibitor, remove drug and diluent from refrigerator and let it warm to room temperature.
•To reconstitute, remove caps from vials and cleanse rubber stoppers with antiseptic solution. After stoppers are dry, remove protective cover from diluent end of transfer device and insert into center of upright diluent vial. Then remove protective cover from drug end of transfer device, invert the diluent vial with attached transfer device, and using minimal force, insert drug end of transfer

device into center of rubber stopper of upright drug vial. Make sure flange of transfer device rests on stopper surface so that diluent flows into drug vial.
•During diluent transfer, wet lyophilized cake completely by gently tilting drug vial. Don't allow air inlet filter to face downward. (Take care not to lose the vacuum because this will prolong drug reconstitution.) Once diluent transfer is complete, pull transfer device along with attached diluent vial out of drug vial and discard. Gently swirl drug vial until powder is completely dissolved. Avoid shaking because this may cause drug to foam and degrade.
•If more than one vial of alpha₁-proteinase inhibitor is required, use aseptic technique to transfer reconstituted solution from each vial into a sterile I.V. administration container.
•Administer at room temperature within 3 hours of reconstitution as an I.V. infusion, using the large-volume 5-micron conical filter provided. Place filter between distal end of I.V. administration set and infusion set, and then infuse at a rate of 0.08 ml/kg/min or as determined by patient response and comfort. Expect the infusion to take about 15 minutes per vial.
•WARNING Alpha₁-proteinase inhibitor is made from human plasma and may contain infectious agents, such as viruses. Ensure that patient is immunized against hepatitis B before giving drug. If time doesn't allow for antibody formation, give a single dose of hepatitis B immune globulin with hepatitis B vaccine, as prescribed.
•Monitor patient for delayed fever, which may occur up to 12 hours after therapy. Fever usually resolves within 24 hours.
### PATIENT TEACHING
•Tell patient to report immediately early evidence of an allergic reaction, such as chest tightness, difficult breathing, faintness, hives, wheezing, and any other unusual symptoms.
•Advise patient to notify prescriber if signs or symptoms of viral infection (chills, drowsiness, fever, and runny nose, followed 2 weeks later by joint pain and a rash) occur after receiving drug.
•Stress the importance of receiving weekly doses to maintain an adequate antielastase barrier in the lungs. Explain that treatment must continue for life.
•Warn patient not to smoke.

# alprazolam

Apo-Alpraz (CAN), Novo-Alprazol (CAN), Nu-Alpraz, Xanax, Xanax XR

## Class, Category, and Schedule

*Chemical:* Benzodiazepine
*Therapeutic:* Antianxiety drug
*Pregnancy category:* D
*Controlled substance:* Schedule IV

## Indications and Dosages

➤ *To control anxiety disorders, relieve anxiety (short-term therapy), or treat anxiety associated with depression*

**TABLETS**

**Adults.** *Initial:* 0.25 to 0.5 mg t.i.d., adjusted to patient's needs. *Maximum:* 4 mg/day in divided doses.

**DOSAGE ADJUSTMENT** In elderly or debilitate patients or patients with advanced hepatic disease, initial dosage adjusted to 0.25 mg b.i.d. or t.i.d. and increased gradually, as needed and tolerated.

➤ *To treat panic attack*

**ORALLY DISINTEGRATING TABLETS, TABLETS**

**Adults.** *Initial:* 0.5 mg t.i.d., increased q 3 to 4 days by no more than 1 mg/day, based on patient response. *Maximum:* 10 mg/day in divided doses.

**E.R. TABLETS**

**Adults.** *Initial:* 0.5 to 1 mg q.d. in morning, increased q 3 to 4 days by no more than 1 mg/day, based on patient response. *Maximum:* 10 mg/day as single dose in morning.

## Contraindications

Acute angle-closure glaucoma; hypersensitivity to alprazolam, its components, or other benzodiazepines; itraconazole or ketoconazole therapy

---

## Mechanism of Action

May increase the effects of gamma-aminobutyric acid (GABA) and other inhibitory neurotransmitters by binding to specific benzodiazepine receptors in the limbic and cortical areas of the CNS. GABA inhibits excitatory stimulation, which helps control emotional behavior. The limbic system contains many benzodiazepine receptors, which may help explain the drug's antianxiety effects.

---

## Interactions

**DRUGS**

*antacids:* Altered rate of alprazolam absorption
*cimetidine, disulfiram, fluoxetine, isoniazid, metoprolol, oral contraceptives, propoxyphene, propranolol, valproic acid:* Decreased elimination and increased effects of alprazolam
*CNS depressants:* Possibly increased CNS effects of both drugs
*digoxin:* Possibly increased serum digoxin level, causing digitalis toxicity
*itraconazole, ketoconazole:* Possibly profoundly inhibited metabolism of alprazolam
*levodopa:* Decreased effects of levodopa
*neuromuscular blockers:* Possibly potentiated or antagonized effects of these drugs
*phenytoin:* Possibly increased serum phenytoin level, causing phenytoin toxicity
*probenecid:* Possibly faster onset or prolonged effects of alprazolam
*ranitidine:* Possibly reduced absorption of alprazolam

**ACTIVITIES**

*alcohol use:* Enhanced adverse CNS effects of alprazolam

## Adverse Reactions

**CNS:** Agitation, akathisia, confusion, depression, dizziness, drowsiness, fatigue, hallucinations, headache, insomnia, irritability, lack of coordination, light-headedness, memory loss, nervousness, paresthesia, rigidity, speech problems, syncope, tremor, weakness
**CV:** Chest pain, edema, hypotension, nonspecific ECG changes, palpitations, tachycardia
**EENT:** Blurred vision, decreased or increased salivation, dry mouth, nasal congestion, tinnitus
**ENDO:** Galactorrhea, gynecomastia, hyperprolactinemia
**GI:** Abdominal discomfort, anorexia, constipation, diarrhea, elevated liver function test results, hepatitis, hepatic failure, nausea, vomiting
**GU:** Decreased or increased libido, urinary hesitancy
**MS:** Dysarthria, muscle rigidity and spasms
**RESP:** Hyperventilation, upper respiratory tract infection
**SKIN:** Dermatitis, diaphoresis, pruritus, rash, Stevens-Johnson syndrome
**Other:** Weight gain or loss

## Nursing Considerations
•Expect to administer a higher dosage to patient with history of panic attacks that occur unexpectedly or during such situations as driving.
•Because alprazolam use can lead to dependency, expect to reduce dosage gradually when stopping the drug. To prevent withdrawal symptoms, don't stop drug abruptly.
**PATIENT TEACHING**
•Warn patient not to stop taking alprazolam abruptly because withdrawal symptoms may occur.
•Instruct patient never to increase the prescribed dosage because of the increased risk of dependency.
•Urge patient to avoid drinking alcohol during alprazolam therapy.
•Advise patient to avoid driving and activities that require alertness until alprazolam's effects are known.
•Instruct female patient of childbearing age to notify prescriber immediately if she becomes or might be pregnant because drug isn't recommended during pregnancy.


# alprostadil

Caverject, Edex, Muse

## Class and Category
*Chemical:* Prostaglandin E$_1$
*Therapeutic:* Anti-impotence drug
*Pregnancy category:* C

## Indications and Dosages
➤*To treat erectile dysfunction due to vascular or psychogenic causes or both*
**INTRACAVERNOUS INJECTION (CAVERJECT, EDEX)**
**Adults.** *Initial:* 2.5 mcg. Dosage increased to 5 mcg if partial response is apparent or 7.5 mcg if no response is apparent, followed by incremental increases of 5 to 10 mcg until erection suitable for intercourse (not exceeding 1-hr duration) is achieved. No more than 2 doses, separated by 1 hr, should be given on a single day during initial titration phase. *Maximum:* 3 doses/week; each dose separated by 24 hr.
**URETHRAL SUPPOSITORY (MUSE)**
**Adults.** *Initial:* 125 to 250 mcg. If no response, dosage increased in stepwise increments to 500 or 1,000 mcg until erection suitable for intercourse (not exceeding 1-hr duration) is achieved. *Maximum:* 2 doses/24 hr.
➤*To treat erectile dysfunction due to spinal cord injury*
**INTRACAVERNOUS INJECTION (CAVERJECT, EDEX)**
**Adults.** *Initial:* 1.25 mcg. Dosage increased to 2.5 mcg if partial response is apparent, then to 5 mcg, and increased in 5-mcg increments until erection suitable for intercourse (not exceeding 1-hr duration) is achieved. No more than 2 doses, separated by 1 hr, should be given on a single day during initial titration phase. *Maximum:* 3 doses/week; each dose separated by 24 hr.

| Route | Onset | Peak | Duration |
|-------|-------|------|----------|
| Intracavernous | 5 to 20 min | Unknown | 60 min |
| Intraurethral | 5 to 10 min | Unknown | 30 to 60 min |

## Contraindications
Anuria, balanitis (inflammation of head of penis), cavernosal fibrosis, hypersensitivity to alprostadil or its components, hyperviscosity syndrome, indwelling urethral catheter, leukemia, men for whom sexual activity is contraindicated, multiple myeloma, penile angulation, penile implants, Peyronie's disease, polycythemia, severe hypospadius (urethral opening on underside of penis), sickle cell anemia or trait, tendency to develop venous thrombosis, thrombocythemia, urethral obstruction or stricture, urethritis

## Interactions
**DRUGS**
*anticoagulants:* Possibly increased risk of bleeding
*cyclosporine:* Possibly decreased blood cyclosporine level

## Adverse Reactions
**CNS:** Dizziness, headache, syncope
**CV:** Hypertension, hypotension, tachycardia, vasodilation
**EENT:** Nasal congestion, sinusitis
**GU:** Pelvic pain; penile disorders, including edema, fibrosis, pain, and rash; priapism; prolonged erection; prostatic pain or enlargement; urethral abrasions; urethral bleeding

## Mechanism of Action

Alprostadil causes penile erection by increasing blood flow to the penis through relaxation of trabecular smooth muscles and dilation of cavernosal arteries. A naturally occurring prostaglandin, alprostadil interacts with specific membrane-bound receptors in the corpora cavernosa cells of the penis. This action activates intracellular adenyl cyclase, which in turn converts adenosine triphosphate (ATP) into cyclic adenosine monophosphate (cAMP). In-creased intracellular levels of cAMP activate protein kinase, an enzyme that activates other enzymes to initiate a cascade of chemical reactions. These chemical reactions cause the trabecular smooth muscles to relax and the cavernosal arteries to dilate. Blood flow to the penis is then increased, which distends the penile lacunar spaces and compresses the veins, trapping blood in the penis and causing it to become enlarged and rigid.

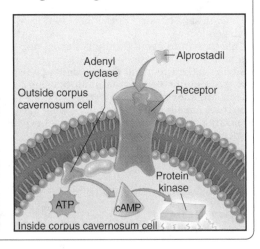

MS: Back pain
RESP: Cough, upper respiratory tract infection
Other: Flulike symptoms, injection site bruising or hematoma

## Nursing Considerations

•Reconstitute solution with 1 ml of diluent, for a concentration of 5, 10, 20, or 40 mcg/ml, depending on vial strength. Gently swirl contents of reconstituted vial. Use reconstituted solution within 24 hours when stored at room temperature. Don't use any vials that contain precipitate or discolored solution. Discard unused portion of reconstituted solution.
•Using a ½-inch 27G to 30G needle, inject drug at a 90-degree angle into the proximal third of the spongy tissue that runs the length of the dorsolateral aspect of the penis, avoiding any visible veins. Rotate injection sites by alternating sides of the penis.
•Carefully examine the penis for signs and symptoms of penile fibrosis. Expect to discontinue treatment if patient develops cavernosal fibrosis, penile angulation, or Peyronie's disease (hardening of the corpora cavernosa, which causes the penis to become distorted when erect) during therapy.
•WARNING Assess patient for prolonged erection after drug administration. Notify prescriber and be prepared to treat patient for priapism if erection lasts longer than 4 hours.
•If patient is receiving an anticoagulant, such as warfarin or heparin, monitor him for bleeding at injection site because alprostadil may inhibit platelet aggregation.

## PATIENT TEACHING

•Inform patient that initial therapy must be performed in the office setting. Teach him how to correctly administer intracavernous injections or urethral suppositories. Inform him that the goal of treatment is to produce an erection that lasts no longer than 1 hour.
•Advise patient to use alprostadil for injection no more than three times/week and to separate doses by 24 hours. Inform patient using urethral suppositories not to use more than two doses in a 24-hour period.
•Instruct patient to inform prescriber immediately of the development of nodules or hard tissue in the penis; an erection that persists for more than 4 hours; new or worsened penile pain; or persistent curvature, redness, swelling, or tenderness of the erect penis.
•Inform patient that common adverse reactions are mild to moderate pain immediately after injection, and burning after suppository insertion.
•Instruct patient using suppository form of drug to urinate just before inserting suppository and to insert suppository with the applicator supplied with drug. Tell patient to hold the penis upright after insertion and to roll it firmly between his hands to distribute drug.
•Tell patient to sit, stand, or walk for 10 minutes after inserting suppository to increase blood flow, which enhances erection.
•Inform patient that he can expect erection to occur 5 to 20 minutes after injecting drug or about 10 minutes after inserting suppository.
•Advise patient not to change drug dosage without consulting prescriber and to keep regularly scheduled follow-up appointments to monitor progress.
•Warn patient that alprostadil offers no protection from sexually transmitted diseases. Urge him to use a condom to decrease risk of blood-borne disease exposure, because injection can cause a small amount of bleeding at the injection site.
•Instruct patient not to reuse or share needles or syringes. Inform him of proper procedure for sharps disposal.
•Warn patient taking suppository form not to engage in sexual intercourse with a pregnant woman unless a condom is used because the drug's effect on pregnancy is unknown.
•Advise patient who plans to travel not to check drug with airline baggage or store it in a closed car.

# alteplase
## (tissue plasminogen activator, recombinant)

Activase, Activase rt-PA (CAN)

## Class and Category

*Chemical:* Purified glycoprotein
*Therapeutic:* Thrombolytic
*Pregnancy category:* C

## Indications and Dosages

➤ *To treat acute MI*

**ACCELERATED I.V. INFUSION**

**Adults who weigh more than 67 kg (148 lb).** 15-mg bolus followed by 50 mg infused over next 30 min and then by 35 mg infused over next 60 min.
**Adults who weigh 67 kg or less.** 15-mg bolus followed by 0.75 mg/kg (up to 50 mg) infused over next 30 min and then 0.5 mg/kg (up to 35 mg) infused over next 60 min.

**I.V. INFUSION**

**Adults who weigh more than 65 kg (143 lb).** 100 mg infused over 3 hr as follows: 6 to 10 mg by bolus over first 1 to 2 min, 50 to 54 mg over remainder of first hr, 20 mg over second hr, and 20 mg over third hr.
**Adults who weigh 65 kg or less.** 1.25 mg/kg infused over 3 hr on similar administration schedule for those weighing more than 65 kg.

➤ *To treat acute ischemic CVA*

**I.V. INFUSION**

**Adults.** 0.9 mg/kg infused over 60 min, with 10% of total dose given as bolus over first min. *Maximum:* 90 mg.

**WARNING** To avoid acute bleeding complications, treatment for acute ischemic CVA must begin within 3 hr after onset of CVA symptoms and only after computed tomography or other diagnostic imaging method excludes intracranial hemorrhage.

➤ *To treat pulmonary embolism*

**I.V. INFUSION**

**Adults.** 100 mg infused over 2 hr.

| Route | Onset | Peak | Duration |
|-------|-------|------|----------|
| I.V. | Immediate | 20 to 120 min | 4 hr |

## Mechanism of Action
Binds to fibrin in a thrombus and converts trapped plasminogen to plasmin. Plasmin breaks down fibrin, fibrinogen, and other clotting factors, which dissolves the thrombus.

## Incompatibilities
Don't add other drugs to solution that contains alteplase.

## Contraindications
*For all indications:* Active internal bleeding, arteriovenous malformation or aneurysm, bleeding diathesis, intracranial neoplasm, severe uncontrolled hypertension
*For acute MI and pulmonary embolism only:* History of CVA, intracranial or intraspinal surgery or trauma in past 2 months
*For acute ischemic CVA only:* Recent head trauma, recent intracranial surgery, recent previous CVA, seizure activity at onset of CVA, subarachnoid hemorrhage, suspicion or history of intracranial hemorrhage

## Interactions
**DRUGS**
*drugs that alter platelet function, such as abciximab, acetylsalicylic acid, and dipyridamole; heparin; vitamin K antagonists:* Increased risk of bleeding

## Adverse Reactions
**CNS:** Cerebral edema, cerebral herniation, CVA, fever, seizure
**CV:** Arrhythmias (including bradycardia and electromechanical dissociation), cardiac arrest, cardiac tamponade, cardiogenic shock, cholesterol embolism, coronary thrombolysis, heart failure, hypotension, mitral insufficiency, myocardial reinfarction or rupture, pericardial effusion, pericarditis, venous thrombosis and embolism
**EENT:** Epistaxis, gingival bleeding, laryngeal edema
**GI:** GI bleeding, nausea, retroperitoneal bleeding, vomiting
**GU:** GU bleeding
**RESP:** Pleural effusion, pulmonary edema, pulmonary reembolization
**SKIN:** Bleeding at puncture sites, ecchymosis, rash, urticaria
**Other:** Anaphylaxis

## Nursing Considerations
• Immediately before use, reconstitute alteplase with sterile water for injection only. Swirl gently to dissolve powder; don't shake.
• Monitor for bleeding, especially at arterial puncture sites.
• Monitor blood pressure and heart rate and rhythm frequently during and after therapy.
• **WARNING** Alteplase therapy may cause arrhythmias from sudden reperfusion of the myocardium. Monitor continuous ECG for arrhythmias during drug therapy.
• Minimize bleeding from noncompressible sites by avoiding internal jugular and subclavian venous puncture sites.
• Discontinue alteplase immediately if serious bleeding occurs.
• After administering alteplase, apply pressure for at least 30 minutes, followed by a pressure dressing.
• Store reconstituted solution at room temperature (about 86° F [30° C]) or refrigerated (36° to 46° F [2.2° to 7.7° C]).

**PATIENT TEACHING**
• Tell patient to immediately report bleeding, including from the nose or gums.
• Advise patient to limit physical activity during alteplase administration to reduce risk of injury and bleeding.

# aluminum carbonate
Basaljel

# aluminum hydroxide
AlternaGEL, Alu-Cap, Alugel (CAN), Alu-Tab, Amphojel, Dialume

## Class and Category
*Chemical:* Aluminum salt
*Therapeutic:* Antacid, phosphate binder
*Pregnancy category:* Not rated

## Indications and Dosages
➤ *To treat hyperacidity associated with gastric hyperacidity, gastritis, hiatal hernia, peptic esophagitis, and peptic ulcers; to prevent phosphate renal calculus formation; to reduce hyperphosphatemia in chronic renal failure*
**ALUMINUM CARBONATE CAPSULES, SUSPENSION, OR TABLETS**
**Adults.** 2 capsules or tablets or 10 ml of suspension q 2 hr up to 12 times daily p.r.n.

**ALUMINUM HYDROXIDE CAPSULES, SUSPENSION, OR TABLETS**
**Adults.** 500 to 1,500 mg as capsules or tablets in divided doses 3 to 6 times daily, taken between meals and h.s.; 5 to 30 ml as suspension p.r.n., taken between meals and h.s.

| Route | Onset | Peak | Duration |
|-------|-------|------|----------|
| P.O. | Varies | Unknown | 20 to 40 min* |

## Mechanism of Action

Neutralizes or reduces gastric acidity, resulting in increased stomach and duodenal alkalinity. Protects stomach and duodenum lining by inhibiting pepsin's proteolytic activity. Binds with phosphate ions in the intestine to form insoluble aluminum-phosphate compounds, which lower the blood phosphate level.

## Contraindications

Hypersensitivity to aluminum

## Interactions

**DRUGS**

*allopurinol, chloroquine, corticosteroids, diflunisal, digoxin, ethambutol, $H_2$-receptor blockers, iron, isoniazid, penicillamine, phenothiazines, ranitidine, tetracyclines, thyroid hormones, ticlopidine:* Decreased effects of these drugs
*benzodiazepines:* Increased effects of benzodiazepines

## Adverse Reactions

**CNS:** Encephalopathy
**GI:** Constipation, intestinal obstruction, white-speckled stool
**MS:** Osteomalacia, osteoporosis
**Other:** Aluminum accumulation in serum, bone, and CNS; aluminum intoxication; electrolyte imbalances

## Nursing Considerations

•Don't administer aluminum hydroxide within 1 to 2 hours of other oral drugs.
•Be aware that two 0.6-g aluminum hydroxide tablets can neutralize 16 mEq of acid.
•Monitor serum levels of sodium, phosphate, and other electrolytes, as appropriate.

---

* If fasting; at least 3 hr if given 1 hr after meals.

**PATIENT TEACHING**

•Instruct patient to chew tablets well before swallowing and then drink a full glass of water.
•Warn patient not to take maximum dosage for more than 2 weeks unless prescribed because this may cause stomach to secrete excess hydrochloric acid.
•Teach patient to prevent constipation with a high-fiber diet and increased fluid intake (2 to 3 L daily), if appropriate.
•If patient takes other prescription drugs, advise him to notify prescriber before taking aluminum because of risk of drug interactions.
•Advise patient to notify prescriber if symptoms worsen or don't subside.

# amantadine hydrochloride

## (adamantanamine hydrochloride)

Endantadine (CAN), Gen-Amantadine (CAN), Symmetrel

## Class and Category

*Chemical:* Adamantane derivative
*Therapeutic:* Antidyskinetic, antiviral
*Pregnancy category:* C

## Indications and Dosages

➤ *To manage symptoms of primary Parkinson's disease, postencephalitic parkinsonism, arteriosclerotic parkinsonism, and parkinsonism caused by CNS injury from carbon monoxide intoxication*
**CAPSULES, SYRUP, TABLETS**
**Adults.** *Initial:* 100 mg b.i.d. *Maximum:* 400 mg q.d. in divided doses.
➤ *To treat drug-induced extrapyramidal reactions*
**CAPSULES, SYRUP, TABLETS**
**Adults.** *Initial:* 100 mg b.i.d. *Maximum:* 300 mg q.d. in divided doses.
**DOSAGE ADJUSTMENT** For elderly patients, patients taking high doses of other antidyskinetics, and patients who have a serious medical condition (such as heart failure, epilepsy, or psychosis), initial dosage reduced to 100 mg q.d., with gradual titration to 100 mg b.i.d.

after 1 to several wk. For patients with impaired renal function, dosage adjusted to 200 mg on day 1; and then to 100 mg q.d. if creatinine clearance is 30 to 50 ml/min/1.73 m²; to 200 mg on day 1 and then to 100 mg q.o.d. if creatinine clearance is 15 to 29 ml/min/1.73 m²; and to 200 mg q wk if creatinine clearance is less than 15 ml/min/1.73 m² or if patient is receiving hemodialysis.

➤ *To prevent and treat respiratory tract infection caused by influenza A*

CAPSULES, SYRUP, TABLETS
**Adults and children age 12 and older.** *Initial:* 200 mg q.d. or 100 mg b.i.d. *Maximum:* 200 mg/day.

DOSAGE ADJUSTMENT For patients with impaired renal function, dosage adjusted to 200 mg on day 1 and then to 100 mg q.d. if creatinine clearance is 30 to 50 ml/min/1.73 m²; to 200 mg on day 1 and then to 100 mg q.o.d. if creatinine clearance is 15 to 29 ml/min/1.73 m²; and to 200 mg q wk if creatinine clearance is less than 15 ml/min/1.73 m² or if patient is receiving hemodialysis.
**Children ages 9 to 12.** 100 mg q 12 hr. *Maximum:* 200 mg/day.
**Children ages 1 to 9.** 1.5 to 3 mg/kg q 8 hr or 2.2 to 4.4 mg/kg q 12 hr. *Maximum:* 150 mg/day.

| Route | Onset | Peak | Duration |
|---|---|---|---|
| P.O. | In 48 hr* | Unknown | Unknown |

## Contraindications
Angle-closure glaucoma, hypersensitivity to amantadine or its components

## Interactions
DRUGS
*anticholinergics or other drugs with anticholinergic activity, other antidyskinetics, antihistamines, phenothiazines, tricyclic antidepressants:* Possibly increased anticholinergic effects and risk of paralytic ileus
*carbidopa-levodopa, levodopa:* Increased effectiveness of these drugs
*CNS stimulants:* Excessive CNS stimulation, possibly causing arrhythmias, insomnia, irritability, nervousness, or seizures

*hydrochlorothiazide, triamterene:* Possibly decreased amantadine clearance and increased risk of toxicity
*quinidine, quinine, trimethoprim-sulfamethoxazole:* Increased blood amantadine level

ACTIVITIES
*alcohol use:* Possibly increased risk of CNS effects—including confusion, dizziness, and light-headedness—and orthostatic hypotension

## Adverse Reactions
**CNS:** Agitation, anxiety, confusion, dizziness, drowsiness, fatigue, hallucinations, insomnia, irritability, light-headedness, mental impairment, nervousness, nightmares, suicidal ideation, syncope
**CV:** Orthostatic hypotension, peripheral edema
**EENT:** Blurred vision; dry mouth, nose, or throat
**GI:** Constipation, diarrhea, nausea
**GU:** Dysuria
**HEME:** Leukopenia, neutropenia
**SKIN:** Livedo reticularis (purplish, netlike rash)

## Mechanism of Action
Affects dopamine, a neurotransmitter that is synthesized and released by neurons leading from substantia nigra to basal ganglia and is essential for normal motor function. In Parkinson's disease, progressive degeneration of these neurons substantially reduces the supply of intrasynaptic dopamine. Amantadine may cause dopamine to accumulate in the basal ganglia by increasing dopamine release or by blocking dopamine reuptake into the presynaptic neurons of the CNS. Amantadine also may stimulate dopamine receptors or cause postsynaptic receptors to be more sensitive to dopamine. These actions help control alterations in involuntary muscle movements, such as tremors and rigidity, that are associated with Parkinson's disease.

Amantadine may inhibit influenza A viral replication by blocking the uncoating of the virus and the release of viral nucleic acid into respiratory epithelial cells. Amantadine also may interfere with early replication of viruses that have already penetrated cells.

---

* Antidyskinetic action; antiviral action unknown.

## Nursing Considerations
•Be aware that prophylactic therapy with amantadine should begin as soon as possible after exposure to persons infected with the influenza A virus and should continue for 10 days. During an influenza epidemic, expect drug to be given daily throughout the epidemic, which typically lasts 6 to 8 weeks. If patient has previously received the inactivated influenza A vaccine, prescriber may discontinue it when sure that patient has developed active immunity against the virus. If patient receives the inactivated influenza A vaccine at the same time amantadine therapy starts, expect amantadine to be given for 2 to 3 weeks.
•Expect amantadine therapy to start 24 to 48 hours after the onset of influenza A symptoms and to continue for 48 hours after their disappearance.
•Monitor patients who have a history of psychiatric illness or substance abuse because amantadine may worsen these conditions. Be aware that some patients taking amantadine have attempted suicide or had suicidal ideations.
•If patient has a history of heart failure or peripheral edema, monitor for weight gain and edema because drug may cause redistribution of body fluid.
•Be aware that amantadine may increase seizure activity in patients with a history of seizures.
•WARNING Monitor patient for signs and symptoms of neuroleptic malignant syndrome during dosage reduction or discontinuation of therapy. These include fever, hypertension or hypotension, involuntary motor activity, mental changes, muscle rigidity, tachycardia, and tachypnea. Be prepared to provide supportive treatment and additional drug therapy, as prescribed.
•Be aware that patients receiving more than 200 mg/day are more likely to experience adverse or toxic reactions.
•Monitor patient for decreased drug effectiveness over time. If therapeutic response declines, expect to increase dosage or discontinue drug therapy temporarily, as ordered.

### PATIENT TEACHING
•Instruct patient to take amantadine exactly as prescribed and not to stop taking it abruptly. Advise patient to notify prescriber if drug becomes less effective.

•Advise patient to notify prescriber if influenza symptoms don't improve after 2 to 3 days.
•WARNING Advise patient or family member to notify prescriber immediately if patient reveals thoughts of suicide.
•Encourage patient to avoid alcohol during amantadine therapy because alcohol may increase the risk of confusion, dizziness, lightheadedness, or orthostatic hypotension.
•Advise patient to avoid driving and other activities that require a high level of alertness until he knows how the drug affects him because it may cause blurred vision and mental impairment.
•Advise patient to change positions slowly to minimize effects of orthostatic hypotension.
•Tell patient to use ice chips or sugarless candy or gum to relieve dry mouth.
•Caution patient to resume physical activities gradually as signs and symptoms improve.

# ambenonium chloride
Mytelase

## Class and Category
*Chemical:* Synthetic quaternary ammonium compound
*Therapeutic:* Antimyasthenic, cholinergic
*Pregnancy category:* C

## Indications and Dosages
➤ *To improve muscle strength in patients with myasthenia gravis in whom pyridostigmine or neostigmine are contraindicated*

### TABLETS
**Adults and adolescents.** *Initial:* 5 mg t.i.d. or q.i.d., increased at 1- to 2-day intervals to optimum dosage based on patient response. *Usual:* Highly individualized but usually 5 to 50 mg t.i.d. or q.i.d.
**Children.** *Initial:* 0.3 mg/kg or 10 mg/m$^2$/day in divided doses t.i.d. or q.i.d. *Maintenance:* Up to 1.5 mg/kg or 50 mg/m$^2$/day in divided doses t.i.d. or q.i.d.

| Route | Onset | Peak | Duration |
|---|---|---|---|
| P.O. | 20 to 30 min | Unknown | 3 to 8 hr |

## Contraindications
Hypersensitivity to ambenonium, its components, or anticholinesterases; mechanical intestinal or urinary tract obstruction

## Mechanism of Action

Attaches to acetylcholinesterase and blocks acetylcholine's breakdown. This action prolongs and exaggerates acetylcholine's effects, producing cholinergic responses, such as miosis, increased intestinal and skeletal muscle tone, bronchoconstriction, bradycardia, and increased salivary and sweat gland secretions.

## Interactions

### DRUGS

*anesthetics, antiarrhythmics, corticosteroids, magnesium, methocarbamol:* Decreased effects of ambenonium
*aminoglycosides, anticholinesterase muscle stimulants, depolarizing muscle relaxants, ganglionic blockers, mecamylamine:* Increased effects of ambenonium

## Adverse Reactions

**CNS:** Dizziness, drowsiness, headache, loss of consciousness, seizures, syncope
**CV:** AV block, bradycardia, decreased cardiac output, hypotension
**EENT:** Dysphonia, increased salivation, laryngospasm
**GI:** Abdominal cramps, dysphagia, flatulence, increased gastric and intestinal secretions, increased peristalsis, mild diarrhea, nausea, vomiting
**GU:** Incontinence, urinary frequency or urgency
**MS:** Arthralgia, dysarthria, fasciculations, muscle spasms, muscle weakness
**RESP:** Bronchoconstriction, bronchospasm, dyspnea, increased tracheobronchial secretions, lung congestion, respiratory arrest or depression, respiratory muscle paralysis
**SKIN:** Diaphoresis, flushing, rash, urticaria

## Nursing Considerations

• Increase dosage gradually as prescribed to avoid ambenonium accumulation and overdose.
• When increasing dosage to optimum level, note when no further increase in muscle strength is observed. Then expect to reduce dosage to previous effective level and to use this as maintenance dosage.
• Expect prescriber to order ephedrine (25 mg per ambenonium dose) or potassium chloride (1 to 2 g per ambenonium dose) to further improve muscle strength.

• **WARNING** Drug has a narrow margin between effectiveness and overdose. If patient receives more than 200 mg/day, monitor closely for signs of overdose (cholinergic crisis), such as abdominal cramps, diarrhea, nausea, vomiting, increased salivation, diaphoresis, difficulty swallowing, blurred vision, miosis, hypertension, fasciculations, and voluntary muscle paralysis.
• Assess neuromuscular status to detect progressive or recurrent muscle weakness in patient on long-term ambenonium therapy.
• If patient develops drug resistance during long-term therapy, expect to restore drug responsiveness by decreasing dosage or briefly discontinuing ambenonium under close medical supervision.

### PATIENT TEACHING

• Instruct patient to swallow tablet with liquid or food to minimize GI irritation.
• Advise patient to consult prescriber before discontinuing drug—even if symptoms diminish or disappear.

# amikacin sulfate

Amikin

## Class and Category

*Chemical:* Aminoglycoside
*Therapeutic:* Antibiotic
*Pregnancy category:* D

## Indications and Dosages

➤ *To treat serious gram-negative bacterial infections (including septicemia; neonatal sepsis; respiratory tract, bone, joint, CNS, skin, soft-tissue, intra-abdominal, burn, and postoperative infections; and serious, complicated, and recurrent UTIs) caused by* Acinetobacter, Enterobacter, Escherichia coli, Klebsiella, Proteus, Providencia, Pseudomonas, *and* Serratia; *and staphylococcal infections when penicillin is contraindicated*

**I.V. INFUSION, I.M. INJECTION**
**Adults and children.** 15 mg/kg/day in equal doses at equally spaced intervals (7.5 mg/kg q 12 hr or 5 mg/kg q 8 hr) for 7 to 10 days. *Maximum:* 1,500 mg/day.
**DOSAGE ADJUSTMENT** For patients with impaired renal function, loading dose of 7.5 mg/

kg/day followed by maintenance dosage based on creatinine clearance and serum creatinine level and given q 12 hr. For morbidly obese patients, dosage not to exceed 1.5 g/day.
**Neonates.** *Loading dose:* 10 mg/kg. *Maintenance:* 7.5 mg/kg q 12 hr for 7 to 10 days.

➤ *To treat uncomplicated UTIs*
**I.V. INFUSION, I.M. INJECTION**
**Adults.** 250 mg b.i.d. for 7 to 10 days.

| Route | Onset | Peak | Duration |
|---|---|---|---|
| I.V. | Immediate | Unknown | Unknown |
| I.M. | Rapid | Unknown | Unknown |

### Mechanism of Action
Binds to negatively charged sites on bacteria's outer cell membrane, disrupting cell integrity. Also binds to bacterial ribosomal subunits and inhibits protein synthesis. Both actions lead to cell death.

### Incompatibilties
Don't mix or infuse amikacin with other drugs.

### Contraindications
Hypersensitivity to amikacin or other aminoglycosides

### Interactions
*cephalosporins, enflurane, methoxyflurane, vancomycin:* Increased nephrotoxic effects
*general anesthetics:* Increased risk of neuromuscular blockade
*loop diuretics:* Increased risk of ototoxicity
*neuromuscular blockers:* Possibly increased neuromuscular blockade and prolonged respiratory depression
*penicillins:* Possibly inactivation of or synergistic effects with amikacin

### Adverse Reactions
**CNS:** Drowsiness, headache, loss of balance, neuromuscular blockade, tremor, vertigo
**EENT:** Hearing loss, ototoxicity, tinnitus
**GI:** Nausea, vomiting
**GU:** Azotemia, dysuria, nephrotoxicity, oliguria or polyuria, proteinuria
**MS:** Acute muscle paralysis; arthralgia; muscle fatigue, spasms, and weakness
**RESP:** Apnea
**Other:** Hyperkalemia

### Nursing Considerations
• Expect to obtain results of culture and sensitivity testing before therapy begins.
• Prepare amikacin I.V. solution by adding contents of 500-mg vial to 100 to 200 ml of sterile diluent. Then infuse drug over 30 to 60 minutes.
• Administer I.M. injection in large muscle mass.
• Monitor for signs of ototoxicity, such as tinnitus and vertigo, especially during high-dosage or prolonged amikacin therapy.
• **WARNING** Because amikacin may produce nephrotoxic effects, assess renal function before and daily during therapy, as ordered. To minimize renal tubule irritation, maintain hydration during therapy.
• Be aware that amikacin may exacerbate muscle weakness in such conditions as myasthenia gravis and Parkinson's disease.
• Measure serum amikacin concentrations as ordered, usually 30 to 90 minutes after injection (for peak concentration) and just before administering next dose (for trough concentration).

**PATIENT TEACHING**
• Tell patient that daily laboratory tests are necessary during treatment.
• Instruct patient to report ringing in ears, hearing changes, headache, nausea, vomiting, and changes in urination.

# amiloride hydrochloride
Midamor

### Class and Category
*Chemical:* Pyrazine-carbonyl-guanidine
*Therapeutic:* Potassium-sparing diuretic
*Pregnancy category:* B

### Indications and Dosages
➤ *As adjunct to thiazide or loop diuretic in patient with heart failure or hypertension to correct diuretic-induced hypokalemia or to prevent diuretic-induced hypokalemia that increases the risk of arrhythmias or other complications*
**TABLETS**
**Adults.** 5 to 10 mg/day as single dose; if hypokalemia persists, increased to 15 mg/day and then 20 mg/day.

| Route | Onset | Peak | Duration |
|-------|-------|------|----------|
| P.O. | 2 hr | 6 to 10 hr | 24 hr |

## Mechanism of Action
Inhibits sodium reabsorption in distal convoluted tubules and cortical collecting ducts, causing sodium and water loss and enhancing potassium retention.

## Contraindications
Hypersensitivity to amiloride; impaired renal function; serum potassium level above 5.5 mEq/L; therapy with another potassium-sparing diuretic, such as spironolactone or triamterene, or a potassium supplement

## Interactions
**DRUGS**
*angiotensin II receptor antagonists, captopril, enalapril, lisinopril, potassium products, spironolactone:* Increased risk of hyperkalemia
*digoxin:* Decreased effectiveness of digoxin
*lithium:* Reduced renal clearance of lithium and increased risk of lithium toxicity
*NSAIDs:* Reduced diuretic effect of amiloride
*sympathomimetics:* Possibly reduced antihypertensive effects of amiloride
**FOODS**
*high-potassium food:* Increased risk of hyperkalemia

## Adverse Reactions
**CNS:** Confusion, depression, dizziness, drowsiness, encephalopathy, fatigue, headache, insomnia, nervousness, paresthesia, somnolence, tremor, vertigo
**CV:** Angina, arrhythmias, orthostatic hypotension, palpitations
**EENT:** Dry mouth, increased intraocular pressure, nasal congestion, tinnitus, vision disturbances
**GI:** Abdominal pain or fullness, anorexia, appetite changes, constipation, diarrhea, GI bleeding, heartburn, indigestion, nausea, thirst, vomiting
**GU:** Bladder spasms, dysuria, impotence, loss of libido, polyuria
**HEME:** Aplastic anemia, neutropenia
**MS:** Arthralgia, muscle spasms or weakness
**RESP:** Cough, dyspnea
**SKIN:** Alopecia, jaundice, pruritus, rash

**Other:** Dehydration, hyperchloremia, hyperkalemia, hypernatremia, metabolic acidosis

## Nursing Considerations
•Administer amiloride with food to reduce GI upset and early in the day to minimize sleep interference from polyuria.
•Monitor renal function test results, fluid intake and output, and weight. Also monitor serum potassium level to detect hyperkalemia.
•**WARNING** Don't administer amiloride with other potassium-sparing diuretics.
**PATIENT TEACHING**
•Warn patient to avoid high-potassium food and salt substitutes that contain potassium.
•Advise patient to consult prescriber before taking other drugs, including OTC remedies, especially sympathomimetics.
•Tell patient to report dizziness, trembling, numbness, and muscle weakness or spasms.
•Advise patient to increase fluid and fiber intake to prevent constipation.
•Warn patient to expect reversible hair loss and impotence.

# aminocaproic acid
Amicar

## Class and Category
*Chemical:* Aminohexanoic acid
*Therapeutic:* Antifibrinolytic, antihemorrhagic
*Pregnancy category:* C

## Indications and Dosages
➤ *To treat excessive bleeding caused by fibrinolysis*
**SYRUP, TABLETS**
**Adults.** *Initial:* 5 g during first hour followed by 1.0 to 1.25 g/hr to sustain drug plasma level of 0.13 mg/ml. *Maximum:* 30 g/day.
**I.V. INJECTION**
**Adults.** 4 to 5 g in 250 ml of diluent over 1 hr followed by continuous infusion of 1 g/hr in 50 ml of diluent. Continue for 8 hr or until bleeding stops.

| Route | Onset | Peak | Duration |
|-------|-------|------|----------|
| P.O. | Rapid | Unknown | Unknown |
| I.V. | Immediate | Unknown | Under 3 hr |

### Mechanism of Action
Inhibits the breakdown of blood clots by interfering with plasminogen activator substances and producing antiplasmin activity.

## Contraindications
Hypersensitivity to aminocaproic acid; signs of active intravascular clotting, as in disseminated intravascular coagulation; upper urinary tract bleeding

## Interactions
*activated prothrombin, prothrombin complex concentrates:* Increased risk of thrombosis
*estrogens, oral contraceptives:* Increased risk of hypercoagulation

## Adverse Reactions
**CNS:** CVA, delirium, dizziness, hallucinations, headache, malaise, weakness
**CV:** Bradycardia, cardiomyopathy, elevated serum CK level, hypotension, ischemia, thrombophlebitis
**EENT:** Nasal congestion, tinnitus
**GI:** Abdominal cramps and pain, diarrhea, elevated AST level, nausea, vomiting
**GU:** Elevated BUN level, intrarenal obstruction, renal failure
**HEME:** Agranulocytosis, leukopenia, thrombocytopenia
**MS:** Myopathy
**RESP:** Dyspnea, pulmonary embolism
**SKIN:** Pruritus, rash
**Other:** Elevated serum aldolase and potassium levels

## Nursing Considerations
•Be aware that patients on oral therapy may need up to 10 tablets during the first hour of treatment and tablets around the clock during continued treatment.
•Mix aminocaproic acid solution with sterile water for injection, NS, D₅W, or Ringer's solution.
•**WARNING** Avoid rapid I.V. administration because of increased risk of hypotension and bradycardia.
•Monitor neurologic status for drug-induced changes. Note that increased clotting may lead to CVA.
**PATIENT TEACHING**
•Tell patient that he'll be closely monitored during I.V. therapy and will have blood

drawn for laboratory tests before, during, and after treatment.
•Advise patient who takes aminocaproic acid at home to report adverse reactions, take drug exactly as prescribed, and keep follow-up appointments with prescriber.

# aminoglutethimide
Cytadren

## Class and Category
*Chemical:* Hormone
*Therapeutic:* Adrenal steroid inhibitor
*Pregnancy category:* D

## Indications and Dosages
➤ *To suppress adrenal function in patients with Cushing's syndrome who are waiting for surgery or for whom other treatment can't be used*
**TABLETS**
**Adults.** *Initial:* 250 mg q 6 hr. Increased as needed by 250 mg/day q 1 to 2 wk. *Maximum:* 2,000 mg/day.

| Route | Onset | Peak | Duration |
|---|---|---|---|
| P.O. | 3 to 5 days | Unknown | 72 hr |

### Mechanism of Action
Inhibits the conversion of cholesterol to delta-5-pregnenolone, which is needed to produce certain hormones, including adrenal glucocorticoids, mineralocorticoids, estrogens, and androgens.

## Contraindications
Hypersensitivity to aminoglutethimide or glutethimide

## Interactions
**DRUGS**
*antidiabetic drugs, dexamethasone, digoxin, medroxyprogesterone, synthetic glucocorticoids, theophylline, warfarin and other oral anticoagulants:* Decreased effects of these drugs

## Adverse Reactions
**CNS:** Dizziness, drowsiness, fever, headache
**CV:** Hypotension, orthostatic hypotension, tachycardia
**ENDO:** Adrenal insufficiency, hypothyroidism, masculinization
**GI:** Anorexia, nausea

**SKIN:** Hair growth, morbiliform rash, pruritus, urticaria

## Nursing Considerations

•Expect to reduce aminoglutethimide dosage or discontinue treatment if extreme drowsiness, severe rash, or excessively low cortisol level occurs.

•**WARNING** Monitor for signs of hypothyroidism, including lethargy, dry skin, and slow pulse. If prescribed, administer thyroid hormone supplement.

•Monitor blood pressure for orthostatic or persistent hypotension.

**PATIENT TEACHING**

•Teach patient to recognize signs and symptoms of orthostatic hypotension, including dizziness and weakness when moving from sitting to standing position, and how to avoid this condition, such as by rising slowly from a supine to an upright position. dizziness and weakness when moving from sitting to standing position, and how to avoid this condition, such as by rising slowly from a supine to an upright position.

•Tell patient to report dizziness, appetite loss, nausea, headache, or severe drowsiness. Warn him to avoid driving if drowsiness occurs.

•Instruct patient to take a missed dose as soon as remembered and to evenly space out the day's remaining doses.

•Advise patient that rash, sometimes accompanied by fever, may appear on day 10 of treatment and should subside by day 15 or 16. Tell him to report severe rash or one that doesn't disappear.


# aminophylline

## (theophylline ethylenediamine)

Phyllocontin, Truphylline

## Class and Category

*Chemical:* Xanthine
*Therapeutic:* Bronchodilator
*Pregnancy category:* C

## Indications and Dosages

➤ *To relieve acute bronchospasm*
**I.V. INFUSION**
**Adults (nonsmokers) not currently receiving theophylline products.** *Initial:* 6 mg/kg (equal to 4.7 mg/kg anhydrous theophylline), not to exceed 25 mg/min. *Maintenance:* 0.7 mg/kg/hr for first 12 hr, then 0.5 mg/kg/hr.

**Children ages 9 to 16 not currently receiving theophylline products.** *Initial:* 6 mg/kg (equal to 4.7 mg/kg anhydrous theophylline), not to exceed 25 mg/min. *Maintenance:* 1 mg/kg/hr for first 12 hr, then 0.8 mg/kg/hr.

**Children ages 6 months to 9 years and young adult smokers not currently receiving theophylline products.** *Initial:* 6 mg/kg (equal to 4.7 mg/kg anhydrous theophylline), not to exceed 25 mg/min. *Maintenance:* 1.2 mg/kg/hr for first 12 hr, then 1 mg/kg/hr.

**Adults and children currently receiving theophylline products.** *Initial:* If possible, determine the time, amount, administration route, and form of last dose. The loading dose is based on the principle that each 0.63 mg/kg (0.5 mg/kg anhydrous theophylline) administered as a loading dose raises the serum theophylline level by 1 mcg/ml. Defer loading dose if serum theophylline level can be readily obtained. If this isn't possible and patient isn't exhibiting obvious signs of theophylline toxicity, prescriber may order 3.1 mg/kg (2.5 mg/kg anhydrous theophylline), which may increase the serum theophylline level by about 5 mcg/ml. *Maintenance:* For adults (nonsmokers), 0.7 mg/kg/hr for first 12 hr, then 0.5 mg/kg/hr. For children ages 9 to 16, 1 mg/kg/hr for first 12 hr, then 0.8 mg/kg/hr. For children ages 6 months to 9 years and young adult smokers, 1.2 mg/kg/hr for first 12 hr, then 1 mg/kg/hr.

**DOSAGE ADJUSTMENT** For elderly patients and those with cor pulmonale, dosage reduced to 0.6 mg/kg for 12 hr, then 0.3 mg/kg. For patients with heart failure and hepatic disease, dosage reduced to 0.5 mg/kg for 12 hr, then 0.1 to 0.2 mg/kg.

➤ *To prevent or treat reversible bronchospasm from asthma, chronic bronchitis, and emphysema and to maintain patent airways*
**E.R. TABLETS, ORAL LIQUID, TABLETS, SUPPOSITORIES**
**Adults and children.** *Initial (rapidly absorbed forms):* 16 mg/kg/day or 400 mg/day (whichever is less) in divided doses q 6 to 8 hr. *Maintenance:* Daily dosage increased in increments of 25% q 3 days, as tolerated, until clinical response is achieved or maximum dose is reached. When maximum dose is

reached, dosage adjusted according to peak serum theophylline level. *Initial (E.R. forms):* 12 mg/kg/day or 400 mg/day (whichever is less) in divided doses q 8 to 12 hr. *Maintenance:* Daily dosage increased in increments of 2 to 3 mg/kg q 3 days. When maximum dose is reached, dosage adjusted according to peak serum theophylline level.

| Route | Onset | Peak | Duration |
|---|---|---|---|
| P.O. (E.R.) | Unknown | Unknown | 8 to 12 hr |
| P.O. (tab) | Unknown | Unknown | 6 to 8 hr |
| I.V. | Immediate | Unknown | 4 to 8 hr |

## Mechanism of Action
Inhibits phosphodiesterase enzymes, causing bronchodilation. Normally, these enzymes inactivate cAMP and cGMP, which are responsible for bronchial smooth-muscle relaxation. Other mechanisms of action may include translocation of calcium, prostaglandin antagonism, stimulation of catecholamines, inhibition of cGMP metabolism, and adenosine receptor antagonism.

## Incompatibilities
Don't add other drugs to prepared bag or bottle of aminophylline. Don't mix aminophylline in same syringe with doxapram. Also avoid administering amiodarone, ciprofloxacin, diltiazem, dobutamine, hydralazine, or ondansetron into the Y-port of a continuous infusion of aminophylline.

## Contraindications
Active peptic ulcer disease, hypersensitivity to aminophylline, rectal or lower intestine irritation or infection (suppository form), underlying seizure disorder

## Interactions
**DRUGS**
*activated charcoal, aminoglutethimide, barbiturates, ketoconazole, rifampin, sulfinpyrazone, sympathomimetics:* Decreased serum theophylline level
*allopurinol, calcium channel blockers, cimetidine, corticosteroids, disulfiram, ephedrine, influenza virus vaccine, interferon, macrolides, mexiletine, nonselective beta blockers, oral contraceptives, quinolones, thiabendazole:* Increased serum theophylline level

*benzodiazepines:* Antagonized sedative effects of benzodiazepines
*beta agonists:* Increased effects of aminophylline and beta agonist
*carbamazepine, isoniazid, loop diuretics:* Increased or decreased serum theophylline level
*halothane:* Increased risk of cardiotoxicity
*hydantoins:* Decreased serum hydantoin level
*ketamine:* Increased risk of seizures
*lithium:* Decreased serum lithium level
*nondepolarizing muscle relaxants:* Reversed neuromuscular blockade
*propofol:* Antagonized sedative effects of propofol
*tetracyclines:* Enhanced adverse effects of theophylline
**FOODS**
*all foods:* Altered bioavailability and absorption of E.R. aminophylline, leading to toxicity
*high-carbohydrate, low-protein diet:* Decreased theophylline elimination and prolonged aminophylline half-life
*low-carbohydrate, high-protein diet; charcoal-broiled beef:* Increased theophylline elimination and shortened aminophylline half-life
**ACTIVITIES**
*alcohol abuse:* Increased effects of aminophylline
*smoking (1 or more packs/day):* Decreased effects of aminophylline

## Adverse Reactions
**CNS:** Dizziness, fever, headache, insomnia, irritability, restlessness, seizures
**CV:** Arrhythmias (including sinus tachycardia and life-threatening ventricular arrhythmias), hypotension, palpitations
**EENT:** Bitter aftertaste
**ENDO:** Hyperglycemia, syndrome of inappropriate ADH secretion
**GI:** Anorexia, diarrhea, epigastric pain, heavy feeling in stomach, hematemesis, indigestion, nausea, rectal bleeding or irritation (suppositories), vomiting
**GU:** Diuresis, proteinuria, urine retention in men with prostate enlargement
**MS:** Muscle twitching
**RESP:** Respiratory arrest, tachypnea
**SKIN:** Alopecia, exfoliative dermatitis, flushing, rash, urticaria

## Nursing Considerations
•**WARNING** Because aminophylline has a narrow therapeutic window (10 to 20 mcg/ml), closely monitor serum theophylline level and observe for signs of toxicity, such as tachy-

cardia, tachypnea, nausea, vomiting, restlessness, and seizures. Keep in mind that acetaminophen, furosemide, phenylbutazone, probenecid, theobromine, coffee, tea, soft drinks, and chocolate can produce inaccurate serum theophylline level.
• To determine peak serum theophylline level, draw blood sample 15 to 30 minutes after administering I.V. loading dose.
• Give immediate-release and liquid forms with food to reduce GI upset. Give E.R. form 1 hour before or 2 hours after meals because food can alter drug absorption.

**PATIENT TEACHING**
• Advise patient to avoid excessive intake of caffeine (in coffee, tea, soft drinks, and chocolate), which can falsely elevate the theophylline level.
• Inform patient that blood tests may be needed to monitor aminophylline's effect.

# aminosalicylate sodium
## (para-aminosalicylate, PAS)
Nemasol Sodium (CAN), PAS

## Class and Category
*Chemical:* Para-aminobenzoic acid analogue
*Therapeutic:* Antitubercular
*Pregnancy category:* C

## Indications and Dosages
➤ *To treat tuberculosis as adjunct to isoniazid, streptomycin, or both and in patients with multidrug-resistant tuberculosis or when therapy with rifampin and isoniazid isn't possible because of resistance or intolerance*

**TABLETS**
**Adults.** 14 to 16 g/day in two or three divided doses.
**Children.** 275 to 420 mg/kg/day in three or four divided doses.

---

### Mechanism of Action
Inhibits the incorporation of para-aminobenzoic acid into folic acid and prevents the synthesis of folic acid, a compound necessary for bacterial growth. Aminosalicylate sodium is bacteriostatic against *Mycobacterium tuberculosis,* and it delays bacterial resistance to streptomycin and isoniazid.

---

## Contraindications
Hypersensitivity to aminosalicylate sodium, severe renal disease

## Interactions
**DRUGS**
*digoxin:* Decreased serum digoxin level
*probenecid:* Increased serum aminosalicylate level
*rifampin:* Decreased serum rifampin level

## Adverse Reactions
**CNS:** Encephalopathy, fever
**CV:** Vasculitis
**ENDO:** Goiter with or without myxedema
**GI:** Abdominal pain, diarrhea, hepatitis, nausea, vomiting
**HEME:** Agranulocytosis, hemolytic anemia, leukopenia, thrombocytopenia
**SKIN:** Jaundice, various types of eruptions
**Other:** Infectious mononucleosis-like syndrome, Loeffler's syndrome (anorexia, breathlessness, fever, and weight loss)

## Nursing Considerations
• Administer aminosalicylate with food to reduce GI upset.
• **WARNING** Protect drug from water, heat, and sunlight to prevent rapid deterioration. Don't administer tablets with brown or purple discoloration—a sign of deterioration.

**PATIENT TEACHING**
• Teach patient to discard aminosalicylate that appears brown or purple.
• Instruct patient to take drug with food.

# amiodarone hydrochloride
Cordarone, Pacerone

## Class and Category
*Chemical:* Iodinated benzofuran derivative
*Therapeutic:* Class III antiarrhythmic
*Pregnancy category:* D

## Indications and Dosages
➤ *To treat life-threatening, recurrent ventricular fibrillation and hemodynamically unstable ventricular tachycardia when these arrhythmias don't respond to other drugs or when patient can't tolerate other drugs*

TABLETS

**Adults.** *Loading:* 800 to 1,600 mg/day in divided doses for 1 to 3 wk. *Maintenance:* 600 to 800 mg/day in divided doses for 1 mo; then if cardiac rhythm is stable, 400 mg/day in one or two doses. Use lowest possible dose.

I.V. INFUSION

**Adults.** *Loading:* 150 mg over 10 min (15 mg/min) followed by 360 mg infused over 6 hr (1 mg/min). *Maintenance:* 540 mg infused over 18 hr (0.5 mg/min); then after the first 24 hr, 720 mg infused over 24 hr (0.5 mg/min), continued up to 96 hr or until rhythm is stable. Change to oral form as soon as possible.

| Route | Onset | Peak | Duration |
|-------|-------|------|----------|
| P.O. | 2 days to 3 wk | 1 to 5 mo | Weeks to months |
| I.V. | Hours to 3 days | 1 to 3 wk | Weeks to months |

### Mechanism of Action

Acts on cardiac cell membranes, prolonging repolarization and the refractory period and raising ventricular fibrillation threshold. Drug relaxes vascular smooth muscles, mainly in coronary circulation, and improves myocardial blood flow. It relaxes peripheral vascular smooth muscles, decreasing peripheral vascular resistance and myocardial oxygen consumption.

## Incompatibilities

Amiodarone is incompatible with heparin. To prevent precipitation, don't add amiodarone admixed with $D_5W$ to aminophylline 4 mg/ml, cefamandole nafate, cefazolin sodium, or mezlocillin sodium, and don't mix amiodarone 3 mg/ml with sodium bicarbonate.

## Contraindications

Bradycardia that causes syncope (unless pacemaker is present), cardiogenic shock, hypersensitivity to amiodarone or its components, hypokalemia, hypomagnesemia, SA node dysfunction, second- and third-degree AV block (unless pacemaker is present)

## Interactions

DRUGS

*anticoagulants:* Increased anticoagulant response, which can result in serious bleeding

*azole antifungals, fluoroquinolones, macrolide antibiotics:* Increased risk of prolonged QT interval and life-threatening arrhythmias
*beta blockers:* Increased serum levels of beta blockers with increased risk of AV block, hypotension, and bradycardia
*calcium channel blockers:* Increased serum levels of these drugs and increased risk of AV block, bradycardia, and hypotension
*cholestyramine, phenytoin, rifampin, St. John's wort:* Decreased serum amiodarone level
*cimetidine:* Increased serum amiodarone level
*cyclosporine:* Increased serum cyclosporine level
*dextromethorphan, methotrexate, phenytoin:* Increased serum levels of these drugs and increased risk of toxicity if amiodarone is taken orally for more than 2 weeks
*digoxin:* Increased serum digoxin level and risk of digitalis toxicity
*diltiazem, propranolol, verapamil:* Increased risk of hemodynamic and electrophysiologic abnormalities
*disopyramide:* Increased serum disopyramide level with QT prolongation and increased risk of arrhythmias
*fentanyl:* Increased serum fentanyl level with increased risk of bradycardia, decreased cardiac output, and hypotension
*flecainide:* Increased serum flecainide level
*hydantoins:* Increased serum hydantoin level with long-term use and reduced serum amiodarone level
*lidocaine:* Increased serum lidocaine level and increased risk of seizures and bradycardia
*potassium- and magnesium-depleting drugs:* Increased risk of hypokalemia and hypomagnesemia
*procainamide:* Increased serum procainamide or N-acetylprocainamide level
*quinidine:* Increased serum quinidine level with risk of life-threatening arrhythmias
*ritonavir:* Increased serum amiodarone level with increased risk of cardiotoxicity
*simvastatin:* Possibly increased risk of myopathy and rhabdomyolysis
*theophylline:* Increased serum theophylline level; increased risk of theophylline toxicity
*warfarin:* Increased PT and risk of bleeding

FOODS

*grapefruit juice:* Increased serum amiodarone level

## Adverse Reactions

**CNS:** Abnormal gait, ataxia, confusion, delirium, disorientation, dizziness, fatigue, hallucinations, headache, insomnia, involuntary motor activity, lack of coordination, malaise, paresthesia, peripheral neuropathy, sleep disturbances, tremor
**CV:** Arrhythmias (including bradycardia, electromechanical dissociation, torsades de pointes, and ventricular tachycardia or fibrillation), cardiac arrest, cardiogenic shock, edema, heart failure, hypotension, vasculitis
**EENT:** Abnormal salivation, abnormal taste and smell, blurred vision, corneal microdeposits, dry eyes, halo vision, lens opacities, macular degeneration, optic neuritis, optic neuropathy, papilledema, permanent blindness, photophobia, scotoma
**ENDO:** Hyperthyroidism, hypothyroidism, syndrome of inappropriate antidiuretic hormone secretion
**GI:** Abdominal pain, anorexia, cirrhosis, constipation, diarrhea, elevated liver function test results, hepatitis, nausea, pancreatitis, vomiting
**GU:** Decreased libido, epididymitis, impotence
**HEME:** Aplastic or hemolytic anemia, coagulation abnormalities, neutropenia, pancytopenia, spontaneous bruising, thrombocytopenia
**MS:** Muscle weakness, myopathy, rhabdomyolysis
**RESP:** Acute respiratory distress syndrome; bronchospasm; infiltrates that lead to dyspnea, cough, pulmonary fibrosis, pulmonary interstitial pneumonitis, crackles, and wheezing; pleuritis; pneumonia
**SKIN:** Alopecia, bluish gray pigmentation, erythema multiforme, exfoliative dermatitis, flushing, photosensitivity, pruritus, rash, Stevens-Johnson syndrome, toxic epidermal necrolysis
**Other:** Anaphylactic shock, angioedema

## Nursing Considerations

• **WARNING** Be aware that I.V. amiodarone may cause or worsen pulmonary disorders that may develop days to weeks after therapy and progress to respiratory failure or even death.
• Monitor vital signs and oxygen levels often during and after giving amiodarone. Keep emergency equipment and drugs nearby.
• **WARNING** Monitor continuous ECG; check for increased PR and QRS intervals, arrhythmias, and heart rate below 60 beats/min because amiodarone toxicity may cause or worsen arrhythmias.

• Monitor serum amiodarone level, which normally ranges from 1.0 to 2.5 mcg/ml.
• Assess liver enzyme and thyroid hormone levels; drug inhibits conversion of $T_4$ to $T_3$.
**PATIENT TEACHING**
• Explain that frequent monitoring and laboratory tests will be needed during treatment.
• Advise patient to report swollen hands and feet, wheezing, dyspnea, cough, nausea, vomiting, dark urine, fatigue, yellow skin or sclerae, stomach pain, light-headedness, fainting, or a rapid, slow, pounding, or irregular heartbeat.
• Instruct patient to report abnormal bleeding or bruising.

# amitriptyline hydrochloride

Apo-amitriptyline (CAN), Endep, Levate (CAN), Novotriptyn (CAN)

## Class and Category

*Chemical:* Tertiary amine
*Therapeutic:* Tricyclic antidepressant
*Pregnancy category:* D

## Indications and Dosages

➤ *To relieve depression, especially when accompanied by anxiety and insomnia*
**TABLETS**
**Adults and children over age 12.** *Outpatient:* 75 mg/day in divided doses, increased to 150 mg/day, if needed. *Inpatient:* 100 mg/day, gradually increased to 300 mg/day, if needed. *Maintenance:* 40 to 100 mg/day h.s.
**DOSAGE ADJUSTMENT** Maintenance dosage reduced to 10 mg t.i.d. plus 20 mg h.s. for adolescent and elderly patients.

| Route | Onset | Peak | Duration |
|-------|-------|------|----------|
| P.O. | 14 to 21 days | Unknown | Unknown |

## Contraindications

During acute recovery phase after MI, hypersensitivity to amitriptyline, MAO inhibitor therapy within 14 days

## Interactions

**DRUGS**
*anticholinergics, epinephrine, norepinephrine:* Increased effects of these drugs

## Mechanism of Action

Normally, when an impulse reaches adrenergic nerves, the nerves release serotonin and norepinephrine from their storage sites. Some serotonin and norepinephrine reaches receptor sites on target tissues. Most is taken back into the nerves and stored by the reuptake mechanism, as shown below on the left.

Amitriptyline blocks serotonin and norepinephrine reuptake by adrenergic nerves. By doing so, it raises serotonin and norepinephrine levels at nerve synapses. This action may elevate mood and reduce depression.

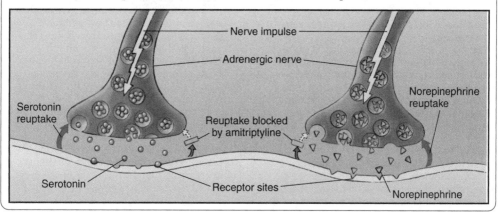

*barbiturates:* Decreased serum amitriptyline level
*carbamazepine:* Decreased serum amitriptyline level and increased serum carbamazepine level, which increases therapeutic and toxic effects of carbamazepine
*cimetidine, disulfiram, fluoxetine, fluvoxamine, haloperidol, $H_2$-receptor antagonists, methylphenidate, oral contraceptives, paroxetine, phenothiazines, sertraline:* Increased serum amitriptyline level
*cisapride:* Possibly prolonged QT interval and increased risk for arrhythmias
*clonidine, guanethidine, and other antihypertensives:* Decreased antihypertensive effects
*dicumarol:* Increased anticoagulant effect
*levodopa:* Decreased levodopa absorption; sympathetic hyperactivity, sinus tachycardia, hypertension, agitation
*MAO inhibitors:* Possibly seizures and death
*thyroid replacement drugs:* Arrhythmias and increased antidepressant effects

### ACTIVITIES

*alcohol use:* Enhanced CNS depression
*smoking:* Decreased amitriptyline effects

## Adverse Reactions

**CNS:** Anxiety, ataxia, coma, chills, delusions, disorientation, drowsiness, extrapyramidal reactions, fatigue, fever, headache, insomnia, nightmares, peripheral neuropathy, tremor
**CV:** Arrhythmias (including prolonged AV conduction, heart block, and tachycardia), cardiomyopathy, hypertension, MI, nonspecific ECG changes, orthostatic hypotension, palpitations
**EENT:** Abnormal taste, black tongue, blurred vision, dry mouth, increased salivation, nasal congestion, tinnitus
**ENDO:** Gynecomastia, increased or decreased blood glucose level, increased prolactin level, syndrome of inappropriate ADH secretion
**GI:** Abdominal cramps, constipation, diarrhea, flatulence, ileus, increased appetite, nausea, vomiting
**GU:** Impotence, libido changes, menstrual irregularities, testicular swelling, urinary hesitancy, urine retention
**HEME:** Agranulocytosis, bone marrow depression, eosinophilia, leukopenia, thrombocytopenia
**SKIN:** Alopecia, flushing, purpura
**Other:** Weight gain

## Nursing Considerations
• Because of amitriptyline's atropine-like effects, use caution if patient has a history of seizures, urine retention, or angle-closure glaucoma.
• **WARNING** Don't give an MAO inhibitor within 14 days of amitriptyline therapy because of the risk of seizures and death.
• Closely monitor patient with CV disorder because amitriptyline may cause arrhythmias, such as sinus tachycardia.
• Monitor blood pressure for hypotension or hypertension.
• Stay alert for behavior changes, such as hallucinations and decreased interest in personal appearance. Be aware that psychosis may develop in schizophrenic patients and symptoms may increase in paranoid patients.
• Abrupt withdrawal after long use may cause nausea, headache, vertigo, and nightmares.

### PATIENT TEACHING
• Instruct patient to take amitriptyline at bedtime to avoid daytime drowsiness.
• Instruct patient to avoid using alcohol or OTC drugs that contain alcohol during amitriptyline therapy because alcohol enhances CNS depressant effects.

## amlodipine besylate

Norvasc

### Class and Category
*Chemical:* Dihydropyridine
*Therapeutic:* Antianginal, antihypertensive
*Pregnancy category:* C

### Indications and Dosages
➤ *To control hypertension*
TABLETS
**Adults.** *Initial:* 5 mg/day, increased gradually over 10 to 14 days p.r.n. *Maximum:* 10 mg/day.
DOSAGE ADJUSTMENT Initial dosage of 2.5 mg/day for elderly patients or patients with impaired hepatic function. Dosage increased gradually over 7 to 14 days based on response.
➤ *To treat chronic stable angina and Prinzmetal's (variant) angina*
TABLETS
**Adults.** 5 to 10 mg/day.
DOSAGE ADJUSTMENT 5 mg/day only for elderly patients and patients with impaired hepatic function.

| Route | Onset | Peak | Duration |
|-------|-------|------|----------|
| P.O. | Unknown | 6 to 12 hr | 24 hr |

### Mechanism of Action
Binds to dihydropyridine and nondihydropyridine cell membrane receptor sites on myocardial and vascular smooth-muscle cells and inhibits the influx of extracellular calcium ions across slow calcium channels. This decreases the intracellular calcium level, inhibiting smooth-muscle cell contractions and relaxing coronary and vascular smooth muscles, decreasing peripheral vascular resistance, and reducing systolic and diastolic blood pressure. Decreased peripheral vascular resistance also decreases the workload of the myocardium and myocardial oxygen demand, which may relieve angina. Also, by inhibiting coronary artery muscle cell contractions and restoring blood flow, amlodipine may relieve Prinzmetal's angina.

### Contraindications
Hypersensitivity to amlodipine or its components

### Interactions
DRUGS
*beta blockers:* Possibly excessive hypotension
*fentanyl:* Increased risk of severe hypotension and increased fluid volume requirements during surgery

### Adverse Reactions
**CNS:** Anxiety, dizziness, fatigue, headache, lethargy, light-headedness, paresthesia, somnolence, syncope, tremor
**CV:** Arrhythmias, hot flashes, hypotension, palpitations, peripheral edema
**EENT:** Dry mouth, pharyngitis
**GI:** Abdominal cramps, abdominal pain, constipation, diarrhea, esophagitis, indigestion, nausea
**GU:** Decreased libido, impotence, urinary frequency
**MS:** Myalgia
**RESP:** Dyspnea
**SKIN:** Dermatitis, flushing, rash
**Other:** Weight loss

## Nursing Considerations
• Use amlodipine cautiously in patients with heart block, heart failure, impaired renal function, hepatic disorder, or severe aortic stenosis.
• Monitor blood pressure while adjusting dosage, especially in patients with heart failure or severe aortic stenosis.

### PATIENT TEACHING
• Tell patient to take missed dose as soon as it's remembered and next dose in 24 hours.
• Tell patient to immediately notify prescriber of dizziness, arm or leg swelling, difficulty breathing, hives, or rash.
• Suggest taking amlodipine with food to reduce GI upset.
• Advise patient to routinely have his blood pressure checked to monitor for hypotension.

# amlodipine besylate and atorvastatin calcium
Caduet

## Class and Category
*Chemical:* Dihydropyridine (amlodipine) and synthetically derived fermentation product (atorvastatin)
*Therapeutic:* Antianginal, antihypertensive (amlodipine); antihyperlipidemic, HMG-CoA reductase inhibitor (atorvastatin)
*Pregnancy category:* X

## Indications and Dosages
➤ *To continue treatment of hyperlipidemia and either hypertension or angina previously prescribed as monotherapies; to continue treatment of one component currently prescribed and start treatment with second component*

### TABLETS
**Adults.** Highly individualized. Dosage may be equivalent to monotherapy with either drug or both dosages may be higher than previously prescribed for additional effects; or dosage may be based on continuation of the component currently being prescribed and the recommended starting dose for the added monotherapy. (See monotherapy details below for usual adult dosages.)

## Monotherapy with amlodipine
➤ *To control hypertension*

### TABLETS
**Adults.** *Initial:* 5 mg/day, increased gradually over 10 to 14 days p.r.n. *Maximum:* 10 mg/day.
**DOSAGE ADJUSTMENT** Initial dosage of 2.5 mg/day for elderly patients or patients with impaired hepatic function. Increased gradually over 7 to 14 days based on response.
➤ *To treat chronic stable angina and Prinzmetal's (variant) angina*

### TABLETS
**Adults.** 5 to 10 mg/day.
**DOSAGE ADJUSTMENT** 5 mg/day only for elderly patients and patients with impaired hepatic function.

## Monotherapy with atorvastatin
➤ *To control lipid levels as an adjunct to diet in primary (heterozygous familial and nonfamilial) hypercholesterolemia and mixed dyslipidemia*

### TABLETS
**Adults.** *Initial:* 10 to 20 mg q.d., then increased according to lipid level. *Maintenance:* 10 to 80 mg q.d.
**DOSAGE ADJUSTMENT** Initial dosage may be increased to 40 mg q.d. for patients who require significant reduction (more than 45%) of cholesterol levels.
➤ *To control lipid levels in homozygous familial hypercholesterolemia*

### TABLETS
**Adults.** 10 to 80 mg/day.
➤ *To initiate treatment of hyperlipidemia and either hypertension or angina*

### TABLETS
**Adults.** *Initial:* Dosage based on appropriate combination of recommendations for monotherapies of amlodipine and atorva-statin. (See monotherapy details for usual adult dosages.) *Maximum:* 10 mg for amlodipine component; 80 mg for atorvastatin component.

| Route | Onset | Peak | Duration |
|---|---|---|---|
| P.O. (amlo-dipine) | Unknown | 6 to 12 hr | 24 hr |
| (atorva-statin) | Unknown | 1 to 2 hr | Unknown |

## Contraindications
Active liver disease; breast-feeding; hypersensitivity to atorvastatin, amlodipine, or their components; pregnancy; unexplained persistently elevated serum transaminase level

## Mechanism of Action

Amlodipine binds to dihydropyridine and nondihydropyridine cell membrane receptor sites on myocardial and vascular smooth-muscle cells and inhibits the influx of extracellular calcium ions across the slow calcium channels. This decrease in intracellular calcium level inhibits smooth-muscle cell contraction, relaxes coronary and vascular smooth muscles, and decreases peripheral vascular resistance and systolic and diastolic blood pressure. Decreased peripheral vascular resistance also reduces myocardial workload and oxygen demand, which may relieve angina. Also, by inhibiting coronary artery muscle cell contractions and restoring blood flow, amlodipine may relieve Prinzmetal's angina.

Atorvastatin reduces serum cholesterol and lipoprotein levels by inhibiting HMG-CoA reductase and cholesterol synthesis in the liver and by increasing the number of LDL receptors on liver cells, thus enhancing LDL uptake and breakdown.

## Interactions

**DRUGS**

**amlodipine component only**

*beta blockers:* Possibly excessive hypotension

*fentanyl:* Increased risk of severe hypotension and increased fluid volume requirements during surgery

**atorvastatin component only**

*antacids, colestipol:* Possibly decreased blood atorvastatin level

*cyclosporine, nicotinic acid:* Increased risk of severe myopathy or rhabdomyolysis

*digoxin:* Possibly increased blood digoxin level, causing toxicity

*erythromycin:* Increased blood atorvastatin level

*oral contraceptives (such as ethinyl estradiol and norethindrone):* Increased hormone level

## Adverse Reactions

**CNS:** Amnesia, anxiety, dizziness, emotional lability, facial paralysis, fatigue, fever, headache, hyperkinesia, lack of coordination, lethargy, light-headedness, malaise, paresthesia, peripheral neuropathy, somnolence, syncope, tremor, unusual dreams, weakness

**CV:** Arrhythmias, elevated serum CK level, hot flashes, hypotension, orthostatic hypotension, palpitations, peripheral edema, phlebitis, vasodilation

**EENT:** Amblyopia, altered refraction, cheilitis, dry eyes or mouth, epistaxis, eye hemorrhage, gingival hemorrhage, glaucoma, glossitis, hearing loss, pharyngitis, sinusitis, stomatitis, taste loss or perversion, tinnitus

**ENDO:** Hyperglycemia, hypoglycemia

**GI:** Abdominal cramps or pain, anorexia, bilary pain, colitis, constipation, diarrhea, duodenal or stomach ulcers, dysphagia, eructation, esophagitis, flatulence, gastroenteritis, hepatitis, increased appetite, indigestion, melena, nausea, pancreatitis, rectal hemorrhage, tenesmus, vomiting

**GU:** Abnormal ejaculation; cystitis; decreased libido; dysuria; epididymitis; hematuria; impotence; nephritis; nocturia; renal calculi; urinary frequency, incontinence, or urgency; urine retention; vaginal hemorrhage

**HEME:** Anemia, thrombocytopenia

**MS:** Arthralgia, back pain, bursitis, gout, leg cramps, myalgia, myasthenia gravis, myositis, neck rigidity, tendon contractures, tenosynovitis, torticollis

**RESP:** Dyspnea, pneumonia

**SKIN:** Acne, alopecia, contact dermatitis, diaphoresis, dry skin, ecchymosis, eczema, flushing, jaundice, petechiae, photosensitivity, pruritus, rash, seborrhea, ulceration, urticaria

**Other:** Allergic reaction, facial or generalized edema, flulike symptoms, infection, lymphadenopathy, weight gain or loss

## Nursing Considerations

•Use amlodipine and atorvastatin cautiously in patients with heart block, heart failure, impaired renal function, or hepatic disorder.

•Monitor blood pressure when titrating amlodipine component, especially in patients with heart failure.

•Be aware that liver function tests should be performed before initiating therapy if patient is receiving the atorvastatin component for the first time, after 6 and 12 weeks of therapy, during each dosage increase of the atorvastatin component, and every 6 months thereafter.

•Expect to measure blood levels 2 to 4 weeks after initial atorvastatin dose and adjust

dosage, as directed. Repeat this process periodically until levels are within desired range.
**PATIENT TEACHING**
• Emphasize that drug is an adjunct to—not a substitute for—a low-cholesterol diet and any other dietary restrictions prescribed before starting the drug therapy.
• Tell patient to immediately notify prescriber of dizziness, arm or leg swelling, difficulty breathing, hives, or rash. Also advise patient to notify prescriber immediately if he develops unexplained muscle pain, tenderness, or weakness, especially if accompanied by fatigue or fever.
• Suggest taking drug with food to reduce GI upset that may be caused by the amlodipine component.
• Advise patient to routinely have his blood pressure checked and his blood monitored to verify the effectiveness of therapy with amlodipine and atorvastatin.

# ammonium chloride

## Class and Category
*Chemical:* Ammonium ion
*Therapeutic:* Acidifier
*Pregnancy category:* C

## Indications and Dosages
➤ *To treat hypochloremia and metabolic alkalosis*
**I.V. INFUSION**
**Adults.** Individualized, based on serum bicarbonate level. *Usual:* 100 to 200 mEq added to 500 or 1,000 ml of NS, infused at 5 ml/min or less (about 3 hr for an infusion of 1,000 ml).

| Route | Onset | Peak | Duration |
|---|---|---|---|
| I.V. | 1 to 3 min | 3 to 6 hr | Unknown |

## Incompatibilities
Don't mix I.V. ammonium chloride with codeine, levorphanol, or methadone.

## Contraindications
Hypersensitivity to ammonium chloride or its components, markedly impaired renal or hepatic function, metabolic alkalosis caused by vomiting of hydrochloric acid and accompanied by sodium loss caused by sodium bicarbonate excretion in urine

## Mechanism of Action
Is converted to urea and hydrochloric acid in the liver. During conversion, the drug breaks into ammonium and chloride ions, and hydrogen ions are released. They enter the blood and extracellular fluid, where hydrogen reacts with bicarbonate ions to form water and carbon dioxide. This process decreases bicarbonate ions and increases chloride ions in blood and extracellular fluid, which decreases blood and urine pH and corrects alkalosis.

## Interactions
**DRUGS**
*amphetamines, salicylates, sulfonylureas, tricyclic antidepressants:* Decreased therapeutic blood level of ammonium
*chlorpropamide:* Increased ammonium effects

## Adverse Reactions
**CNS:** Fever, headache
**CV:** Phlebitis or thrombosis extending from injection site
**GI:** Indigestion, nausea, severe hepatic dysfunction, vomiting
**RESP:** Hyperventilation
**SKIN:** Extravasation
**Other:** Injection site infection, irritation, or pain; hypovolemia; severe metabolic acidosis (with large doses)

## Nursing Considerations
• Before use, warm ammonium chloride solution to room temperature to dissolve crystals by placing infusion in warm water.
• During I.V. use, keep sodium bicarbonate or sodium lactate nearby to treat overdose.
• Infuse ammonium chloride slowly to avoid I.V. site pain and irritation.
• **WARNING** Monitor for ammonia toxicity, including arrhythmias, such as bradycardia; coma; irregular breathing; pallor; retching; seizures; diaphoresis; and twitching.
• Monitor for signs of metabolic acidosis, such as increased respirations, increased serum pH, restlessness, and diaphoresis.
• Monitor serum bicarbonate level, the results of urinalysis, and the results of renal and liver function tests as appropriate.

# amobarbital sodium

Amytal, Novamobarb (CAN)

## Class, Category, and Schedule
*Chemical:* Barbiturate
*Therapeutic:* Anticonvulsant, sedative-hypnotic
*Pregnancy category:* D
*Controlled substance:* Schedule II

## Indications and Dosages
➤ *To produce preanesthesia sedation*
CAPSULES, ELIXIR, TABLETS
**Adults.** 200 mg 1 to 2 hr before surgery.
**Children.** 2 to 6 mg/kg up to a maximum of 100 mg/dose.

➤ *To produce sedation*
CAPSULES, ELIXIR, TABLETS, I.V. OR I.M. INJECTION
**Adults.** 30 to 50 mg (may range from 15 to 120 mg) b.i.d. or t.i.d. *Maximum I.V.:* 1,000 mg/dose. *Maximum I.M.:* 500 mg/dose.
**Children over age 6.** 2 mg/kg/day in four divided doses.

➤ *To treat insomnia*
CAPSULES, ELIXIR, TABLETS
**Adults.** 65 to 200 mg h.s. for up to 2 wk.

➤ *To induce a hypnotic state*
CAPSULES, ELIXIR, TABLETS, I.V. OR I.M. INJECTION
**Adults.** 65 to 200 mg/dose. *Maximum I.V.:* 1,000 mg/dose. *Maximum I.M.:* 500 mg/dose
**Children up to age 6.** 2 to 3 mg/kg I.M. per dose.

➤ *To manage seizures*
I.V. OR I.M. INJECTION
**Adults.** *Usual:* 65 to 500 mg up to a maximum of 1,000 mg. The dosage for acute seizures is determined by response. Doses of 200 to 500 mg are typically required to control seizures.
**Children age 6 and older.** 65 to 500 mg I.V.
**Children up to age 6.** 3 to 5 mg/kg/dose.
WARNING Use I.V. route only when other routes aren't appropriate. For I.V. injection, use I.M. dose and inject slowly at a rate of 50 mg/min or less to prevent sudden respiratory depression, apnea, laryngospasm, or hypotension.

## Mechanism of Action
Nonselectively acts on the CNS to depress the sensory cortex, decrease motor activity, alter cerebellar function, and produce drowsiness, sedation, and hypnosis. Appears to reduce wakefulness and alertness by acting in the thalamus, where it depresses the reticular activating system and interferes with impulse transmission from the periphery to the cortex. Produces CNS depressant effects ranging from mild sedation and anxiety reduction to anesthesia and coma, depending on the dose, route, and individual patient's response.

| Route | Onset | Peak | Duration |
|---|---|---|---|
| P.O.* | 60 min | Unknown | 10 to 12 hr |
| I.V. | Unknown | Unknown | 10 to 12 hr |
| I.M. | Unknown | Unknown | 10 to 12 hr |

## Incompatibilities
Don't mix amobarbital in solution with other drugs.

## Contraindications
Alcoholism, history of porphyria, history of sedative or barbiturate addiction, hypersensitivity to barbiturates, renal or hepatic disease, severe respiratory disease, sleep apnea, suicidal tendency, uncontrolled pain

## Interactions
DRUGS
*acetaminophen:* Increased blood acetaminophen level and risk of hepatotoxicity
*antihistamines, CNS depressants, phenothiazines, tranquilizers:* Increased CNS depression
*beta blockers, carbamazepine, clonazepam, corticosteroids, digitoxin, doxycycline, estrogens, griseofulvin, metronidazole, oral anticoagulants, oral contraceptives, phenylbutazones, quinidine, theophyllines, tricyclic antidepressants:* Decreased blood levels and effects of these drugs
*chloramphenicol:* Inhibited amobarbital metabolism; enhanced chloramphenicol metabolism
*MAO inhibitors:* Increased serum level and sedative effects of amobarbital

---

* For capsules, elixir, and tablets.

A

*methoxyflurane:* Increased nephrotoxicity
*phenytoin:* Altered effects of phenytoin
*rifampin:* Decreased serum level and effects
of amobarbital
*valproic acid:* Increased amobarbital effects
**ACTIVITIES**
*alcohol use:* Increased serum level of amobarbital and additive CNS depressant effects

## Adverse Reactions

**CNS:** Agitation, anxiety, ataxia, CNS depression, confusion, dizziness, hallucinations,
hangover, headache, hyperkinesia, insomnia,
nightmares, nervousness, paradoxical stimulation, permanent neurologic deficit (with injection near nerve), psychiatric disturbance,
somnolence, syncope, vertigo
**CV:** Bradycardia, hypotension, shock
**EENT:** Laryngospasm
**GI:** Constipation, diarrhea, epigastric pain,
nausea, vomiting
**RESP:** Apnea, bronchospasm, hypoventilation, respiratory depression
**SKIN:** Exfoliative dermatitis, rash, Stevens-
Johnson syndrome, urticaria
**Other:** Angioedema, gangrene of arm or leg
from accidental injection into artery, injection site tissue damage and necrosis, physical
and psychological dependence, potentially
fatal withdrawal syndrome, tolerance

## Nursing Considerations

• Use amobarbital cautiously in patients with
cardiac disease, debilitation, diabetes mellitus, fever, hyperthyroidism, severe anemia,
shock, status asthmaticus, or uremia.
• Administer by deep I.M. injection, preferably in large muscle.
• During I.V. administration, closely monitor
blood pressure, pulse, and respirations. Keep
emergency equipment and drugs nearby in
case respiratory depression occurs.
• WARNING Don't administer solution after 30
minutes of exposure to air. Solution quickly
becomes unstable because amobarbital sodium hydrolyzes in solution.
• To prevent withdrawal symptoms, such as
diaphoresis, insomnia, irritability, nightmares, and tremors, expect to taper amobarbital dosage gradually after long-term use,
especially for epileptic patients.
• WARNING To prevent tissue damage and necrosis at I.M. injection site, don't administer
more than 5 ml of this highly alkaline drug

at any one site. Know that accidental arterial injection may cause gangrene of the arm
or leg.

**PATIENT TEACHING**
• Advise patient to use caution when driving
or performing tasks that require alertness.
• Instruct patient not to use alcohol or other
CNS depressants (unless prescribed) because
they increase amobarbital's effects.
• Warn patient not to stop taking drug
abruptly because withdrawal symptoms can
occur.
• Instruct patient to report severe dizziness,
persistent drowsiness, rash, or skin lesions.
• Advise patient that amobarbital's effects,
such as drowsiness, may become less pronounced after a few days and when drug is
taken with food.

# amoxapine

Asendin

## Class and Category
*Chemical:* Dibenzoxazepine derivative
*Therapeutic:* Tricyclic antidepressant
*Pregnancy category:* C

## Indications and Dosages
➤ *To relieve depression, including endogenous (long-term) depression and depression associated with anxiety and agitation*

**TABLETS**
**Adults and children age 16 and older.** *Initial:*
50 mg b.i.d. or t.i.d., increased to 100 mg
b.i.d. or t.i.d. by end of first wk, if tolerated.
*Maintenance:* If 300-mg daily dose is ineffective after 2-wk trial period, dosage increased
to a maximum of 400 mg/day in divided
doses. Inpatients may receive up to a maximum of 600 mg/day in divided doses. When
effective dose is achieved, a single dose may
be given h.s., not to exceed 300 mg.
**DOSAGE ADJUSTMENT** For elderly patients: *Initial:* 25 mg b.i.d. or t.i.d., increased to 50 mg
b.i.d. or t.i.d. by end of first wk. *Maintenance:*
100 to 150 mg/day in divided doses, carefully
increased to 300 mg/day as tolerated. When
effective dose is achieved, a single dose may
be given h.s., not to exceed 300 mg.

| Route | Onset | Peak | Duration |
|-------|-------|------|----------|
| P.O. | 2 to 3 wk | Unknown | Unknown |

## Mechanism of Action

Blocks serotonin and norepinephrine reuptake by adrenergic nerves. By doing this, it raises serotonin and norepinephrine levels at nerve synapses. This action may elevate mood and reduce depression.

Normally, when an impulse reaches adrenergic nerves, they release serotonin and norepinephrine from their storage sites. Some serotonin and norepinephrine reach receptor sites on target tissues. The majority is taken back into the nerves and stored by the reuptake mechanism.

## Contraindications

Acute recovery phase after MI, hypersensitivity to amoxapine or its components, MAO inhibitor therapy within 14 days

## Interactions

**DRUGS**

*anticholinergics, epinephrine, norepinephrine:* Increased effects of these drugs
*barbiturates:* Decreased serum amoxapine level
*carbamazepine:* Decreased serum amoxapine level; increased serum carbamazepine level, increasing its therapeutic and toxic effects
*cimetidine, disulfiram, fluoxetine, fluvoxamine, haloperidol, $H_2$-receptor antagonists, methylphenidate, oral contraceptives, paroxetine, phenothiazines, sertraline:* Increased blood amoxapine level
*clonidine, guanethidine, other antihypertensives:* Decreased antihypertensive effects
*dicumarol:* Increased anticoagulant effect
*levodopa:* Decreased levodopa absorption; agitation, hypertension, sinus tachycardia, sympathetic hyperactivity
*MAO inhibitors:* Possibly seizures and death
*thyroid replacement drugs:* Arrhythmias and increased antidepressant effects

**ACTIVITIES**

*alcohol use:* Increased CNS depression
*smoking:* Decreased amoxapine effects

## Adverse Reactions

**CNS:** Agitation, anxiety, ataxia, chills, confusion, CVA, dizziness, drowsiness, excitement, extrapyramidal reactions, fatigue, fever, headache, insomnia, nervousness, nightmares, paresthesia, restlessness, sedation, seizures, syncope, tremor, weakness
**CV:** Atrial arrhythmias, heart block, heart failure, hypertension, hypotension, MI, palpitations, tachycardia
**EENT:** Blurred vision, dry mouth, increased salivation, nasal congestion, taste perversion, tinnitus
**ENDO:** gynecomastia, increased or decreased blood glucose level, increased prolactin level, syndrome of inappropriate ADH secretion
**GI:** Anorexia, constipation, diarrhea, elevated liver function test results, flatulence, increased appetite, nausea, vomiting
**GU:** Impotence, libido changes, menstrual irregularities, testicular swelling, urinary hesitancy, urine retention
**HEME:** Agranulocytosis, leukopenia
**SKIN:** Diaphoresis, flushing, photosensitivity, pruritus, rash
**Other:** Weight gain or loss; withdrawal symptoms, such as headache, nausea, nightmares, and vertigo

## Nursing Considerations

• **WARNING** Don't administer MAO inhibitors within 14 days of amoxapine therapy.
• To avoid withdrawal, don't stop drug abruptly.

**PATIENT TEACHING**

• Advise patient to take amoxapine at bedtime if daytime sedation occurs.
• Caution patient that stopping drug abruptly may cause withdrawal symptoms.
• Encourage patient to avoid alcohol because it can potentiate amoxapine's effects.
• Tell patient to report adverse drug effects.
• Instruct patient to take drug with food to prevent GI upset.

# amoxicillin trihydrate (amoxycillin)

Amoxil, Apo-Amoxi (CAN), DisperMox, Novamoxin (CAN), Nu-Amoxi (CAN), Polymox, Trimox, Wymox

## Class and Category

*Chemical:* Aminopenicillin
*Therapeutic:* Antibiotic
*Pregnancy category:* B

## Indications and Dosages

➤ *To treat ear, nose, throat, GU tract, skin, and soft-tissue infections caused by susceptible gram-positive and gram-negative organisms*

CAPSULES, CHEWABLE TABLETS, ORAL SUSPENSION, PEDIATRIC DROPS, POWDER OR TABLETS FOR ORAL SUSPENSION, TABLETS
**Adults and children who weigh 20 kg (44 lb) or more.** 250 mg q 8 hr; for severe infections, 500 mg q 8 hr or 875 mg q 12 hr.
**Children age 12 wk and older who weigh less than 20 kg.** 20 mg/kg/day in divided doses q 8 hr; for severe infections, 40 to 45 mg/kg/day in divided doses q 8 hr.
**Children younger than age 12 wk.** 30 mg/kg/day in divided doses q 12 hr.

➤ *To treat lower respiratory tract infections caused by susceptible gram-positive and gram-negative organisms*
CAPSULES, CHEWABLE TABLETS, ORAL SUSPENSION, PEDIATRIC DROPS, POWDER OR TABLETS FOR ORAL SUSPENSION, TABLETS
**Adults and children who weigh 20 kg or more.** 875 mg q 12 hr; for severe infections, 500 mg q 8 hr.
**Children age 12 wk and older who weigh less than 20 kg.** 40 to 45 mg/kg/day in divided doses q 8 hr.
**Children younger than age 12 wk.** 30 mg/kg/day in divided doses q 12 hr.

➤ *To treat gonorrhea and acute uncomplicated anogenital and urethral infections caused by susceptible strains of gram-positive and gram-negative organisms*
CAPSULES, CHEWABLE TABLETS, ORAL SUSPENSION, POWDER OR TABLETS FOR ORAL SUSPENSION, TABLETS
**Adults and postpubertal children.** 3 g as a single dose.
**Prepubertal children age 2 and older.** 50 mg/kg of amoxicillin plus 25 mg/kg of probenecid as a single dose.

➤ *As adjunct to eradicate* Helicobacter pylori *to reduce risk of duodenal ulcer recurrence*
CAPSULES, CHEWABLE TABLETS, ORAL SUSPENSION, POWDER OR TABLETS FOR ORAL SUSPENSION, TABLETS
**Adults.** 1 g q 12 hr with 500 mg of clarithromycin q 12 hr and 30 mg of lansoprazole q 12 hr for 14 days. Or, 1 g q 8 hr with 30 mg of lansoprazole q 8 hr for 14 days.

➤ *To prevent bacterial endocarditis before dental, oral, or upper respiratory tract procedures*
CAPSULES, CHEWABLE TABLETS, ORAL SUSPENSION, POWDER OR TABLETS FOR ORAL SUSPENSION, TABLETS
**Adults and children who weigh 20 kg or more.** 2 g 1 hr before procedure.

**Children who weigh less than 20 kg.** 50 mg/kg 1 hr before procedure.

| Route | Onset | Peak | Duration |
|-------|-------|------|----------|
| P.O. | Unknown | Unknown | 6 to 8 hr |

### Mechanism of Action
Kills bacteria by binding to and inactivating penicillin-binding proteins on the inner bacterial cell wall, weakening bacterial cell wall and causing lysis.

## Contraindications
Hypersensitivity to amoxicillin or its components

## Interactions
**DRUGS**
*allopurinol:* Increased risk of rash
*chloramphenicol, erythromycins, sulfonamides, tetracyclines:* Reduced bactericidal effect of amoxicillin
*methotrexate:* Increased risk of methotrexate toxicity
*oral contraceptives with estrogen:* Possibly reduced effectiveness of contraceptive
*probenecid:* Increased amoxicillin effects

## Adverse Reactions
**CNS:** Agitation, anxiety, behavior changes, confusion, dizziness, insomnia, reversible hyperactivity, seizures
**GI:** Diarrhea, nausea, vomiting
**GU:** Crystalluria, vaginal mycosis
**HEME:** Anemia, eosinophilia, granulocytosis, leukopenia, thrombocytopenia, thrombocytopenic purpura
**SKIN:** Erythema multiforme, erythematous maculopapular rash, generalized exanthematous pustulosis, Stevens-Johnson syndrome, toxic epidermal necrolysis, urticaria
**Other:** Allergic reaction, anaphylaxis, serum sickness–like reaction (such as arthralgia, arthritis, fever, myalgia, rash, and urticaria)

## Nursing Considerations
•Use amoxicillin cautiously in patients with hepatic impairment. Monitor hepatic and renal function and CBC, as ordered, in patients receiving prolonged therapy. Also use cautiously in patients who are breast-feeding or elderly.
•Expect to start therapy before culture and sensitivity test results are known.
•Be aware that chewable tablets and tablets for oral suspension contain phenylalanine.

•Don't confuse amoxicillin tablets with amoxicillin tablets for oral suspension (DisperMox). They're not interchangeable.
•**WARNING** If allergic reaction occurs, stop amoxicillin immediately and provide emergency care as indicated and ordered.
•Monitor closely for diarrhea, which may indicate pseudomembranous colitis. If it occurs, notify prescriber and expect to withhold amoxicillin and treat diarrhea, as ordered.
•Expect treatment to last at least 10 days for infections caused by hemolytic streptococci.

**PATIENT TEACHING**

•Tell patient to refrigerate reconstituted suspension and to shake well before each use.
•When amoxicillin suspension is prescribed for a child, instruct parents to place it directly on child's tongue for him to swallow. If this doesn't work, tell parents to mix dose of suspension with formula or cold drink (milk, fruit juice, ginger ale, water) and then have child drink all of it immediately.
•Instruct patient using DisperMox tablets to place one tablet and about 2 teaspoonfuls of water in a glass, drink entire mixture, add more water to the glass, and drink again to ensure delivery of full dose.
•Tell patient to chew or crush chewable tablets and not to swallow them whole.
•To prevent infection from recurring, urge patient to take amoxicillin for full length of time prescribed even if he feels better.
•Teach patient to report adverse reactions and notify prescriber if infection worsens or doesn't improve after 72 hours of therapy.
•Urge patient to tell prescriber about diarrhea that's severe or lasts longer than 3 days.


# amoxicillin trihydrate and clavulanate potassium

Augmentin, Augmentin ES, Augmentin XR, Clavulin (CAN)

## Class and Category

*Chemical:* Aminopenicillin, beta-lactamase inhibitor
*Therapeutic:* Antibiotic
*Pregnancy category:* B

## Indications and Dosages

➤ *To treat otitis media, sinusitis, skin and soft-tissue infections, and UTIs caused* *by susceptible strains of gram-positive and gram-negative organisms*

**ORAL SUSPENSION, TABLETS**

**Adults and children who weigh 40 kg (88 lb) or more.** 500 mg q 12 hr or 250 mg q 8 hr.
**Children age 12 wk and older who weigh less than 40 kg.** 25 mg/kg/day in divided doses q 12 hr or 20 mg/kg/day in divided doses q 8 hr.
**Children under age 12 wk.** 30 mg/kg/day q 12 hr.

➤ *To treat community-acquired pneumonia or acute bacterial sinusitis caused by beta-lactamase–producing pathogens and S. pneumoniae with reduced susceptibility to penicillin*

**E.R. TABLETS**

**Adults.** 4,000 mg in two divided doses daily at start of meals for 7 to 10 days for community-acquired pneumonia or 10 days for acute bacterial sinusitis.

➤ *To treat respiratory tract infections and severe otitis media and sinusitis caused by susceptible strains of gram-positive and gram-negative organisms*

**CHEWABLE TABLETS, ORAL SUSPENSION, TABLETS**

**Adults and children who weigh 40 kg or more.** 875 mg q 12 hr or 500 mg q 8 hr.
**Children age 12 wk and older who weigh less than 40 kg.** 45 mg/kg/day in divided doses q 12 hr or 40 mg/kg q 8 hr.
**Children under age 12 wk.** 30 mg/kg/day in divided doses q 12 hr.
**DOSAGE ADJUSTMENT** For a GFR of 10 to 30 ml/min, dosage reduced to 250 or 500 mg q 12 hr, depending on the severity of the infection. For a GFR less than 10 ml/min, dosage reduced to 250 to 500 mg q 24 hr, depending on the severity of the infection. For hemodialysis patients, dosage reduced to 250 or 500 mg q 24 hr with another dose during and at the end of dialysis.

➤ *To treat acute otitis media caused by beta-lactamase–producing strains of* Haemophilus influenzae, Moraxella catarrhalis, *and* Streptococcus pneumoniae *(including penicillin-resistant strains)*

**EXTRA-STRENGTH ORAL SUSPENSION**

**Children.** 90 mg/kg/day in divided doses b.i.d. for 10 days.

| Route | Onset | Peak | Duration |
|---|---|---|---|
| P.O. | Unknown | Unknown | 6 to 8 hr |

## Mechanism of Action
Kills bacteria by binding to and inactivating penicillin-binding proteins on the inner bacterial cell wall, weakening the cell wall and causing lysis. Clavulanic acid inactivates bacterial beta-lactamase enzymes, thus protecting amoxicillin from degradation by these enzymes and making the drug effective against many bacteria normally resistant to amoxicillin.

## Contraindications
History of amoxicillin and clavulanate–induced cholestatic jaundice or hepatic dysfunction; hypersensitivity to amoxicillin, clavulanate, penicillin, or their components; phenylketonuria (chewable tablets); severe renal impairment (E.R. tablets)

## Interactions
### DRUGS
*allopurinol:* Increased risk of rash
*aminoglycosides:* Inactivation of both drugs
*chloramphenicol, erythromycins, sulfonamides, tetracyclines:* Reduced bactericidal effect of amoxicillin
*heparin, oral anticoagulants:* Possibly increased risk of bleeding with large doses of amoxicillin and clavulanate potassium
*methotrexate:* Risk of methotrexate toxicity
*oral contraceptives with estrogen:* Possibly reduced effectiveness of contraceptive
*probenecid:* Increased amoxicillin effects

## Adverse Reactions
**CNS:** Agitation, anxiety, behavioral changes, confusion, dizziness, drowsiness, headache, insomnia, reversible hyperactivity
**EENT:** Black "hairy" tongue, glossitis, mucocutaneous candidiasis, stomatitis
**GI:** Diarrhea, enterocolitis, gastritis, hemorrhagic pseudomembranous colitis, indigestion, nausea, vomiting
**GU:** Hematuria, interstitial nephritis, vaginal candidiasis, vaginal mycosis
**HEME:** Agranulocytosis, anemia, eosinophilia, leukopenia, neutropenia, thrombocytopenia, thrombocytopenic purpura
**SKIN:** Erythema multiforme, exfoliative dermatitis, pruritus, rash, Stevens-Johnson syndrome, urticaria
**Other:** Allergic reaction, anaphylaxis, angioedema, serum sickness–like reaction (such as arthralgia, arthritis, fever, myalgia, rash, and urticaria)

## Nursing Considerations
• Use amoxicillin and clavulanate cautiously in patients with hepatic impairment. Monitor hepatic and renal function and CBC, as ordered, in patients receiving prolonged therapy. Also use cautiously in patients who are breast-feeding or elderly.
• For children younger than age 12 weeks, expect to use 125-mg/5-ml amoxicillin and clavulanate suspension because experience with 200-mg/5-ml suspension is limited.
•**WARNING** If allergic reaction occurs, stop drug immediately. Expect to give antihistamine and I.V. corticosteroid. If anaphylaxis occurs, expect to manage airway and give epinephrine, oxygen, and I.V. corticosteroid.
• Monitor patient closely for diarrhea, which may indicate pseudomembranous colitis. If diarrhea occurs, notify prescriber and expect to withhold drug. Expect to treat pseudomembranous colitis with fluids, electrolytes, protein, and an antibiotic effective against *Clostridium difficile.*
• Be aware that Augmentin 250-mg regular tablets should not be substituted for chewable or E.R. tablets because they contain different amounts of clavulanic acid.
• For a child under 40 kg, expect to use 250-mg chewable tablets because the ratio of amoxicillin to clavulanic acid differs from that of Augmentin 250-mg regular tablets.

### PATIENT TEACHING
• Tell patient to take amoxicillin and clavulanate with food to reduce GI upset.
• Instruct patient to refrigerate reconstituted suspension.
• Tell patient to chew or crush chewable tablets and not to swallow them whole.
• Teach patient to recognize and report adverse reactions and to seek emergency care if signs of anaphylaxis occur.
• Tell patient to notify prescriber if infection continues or worsens after 72 hours.
• Urge patient to tell prescriber about diarrhea that's severe or lasts longer than 3 days.

# amphetamine and dextroamphetamine
Adderall, Adderall XR

## Class, Category, and Schedule
*Chemical:* Phenylisopropylamine
*Therapeutic:* CNS stimulant

*Pregnancy category:* C
*Controlled substance:* Schedule II

## Indications and Dosages
➤ *To treat attention deficit hyperactivity disorder (ADHD)*

**E.R. CAPSULES**

**Adults.** 20 mg q.d.
**Adolescents ages 13 to 18.** *Initial:* 10 mg q.d. Dosage increased to 20 mg/day after 1 wk if needed.
**Children age 6 and older.** *Initial:* 5 or 10 mg q.d. Dosage increased by 5 or 10 mg/day q wk until desired response occurs. *Maximum:* 30 mg/day.

**TABLETS**

**Children age 6 and older.** *Initial:* 5 mg q.d. or b.i.d. Increased by 5 mg/day q wk until desired response occurs. *Maximum:* 40 mg/day.
**Children ages 3 to 6.** *Initial:* 2.5 mg q.d. Dosage increased by 2.5 mg/day q wk until desired response occurs. *Maximum:* 40 mg/day.

➤ *To treat narcolepsy*

**TABLETS**

**Adults and children age 12 and older.** *Initial:* 10 mg q.d. Dosage increased by 10 mg/day q wk until desired response occurs. *Maximum:* 60 mg/day for adults.
**Children ages 6 to 12.** *Initial:* 5 mg q.d. Dosage increased by 5 mg/day q wk until desired response occurs. *Maximum:* 40 mg/day.

---

### Mechanism of Action
May produce its CNS stimulant effects by facilitating the release of norepinephrine at adrenergic nerve terminals and blocking its reuptake and by directly stimulating alpha and beta receptors in the peripheral nervous system. The drug also causes the release and blocks the reuptake of dopamine in limbic regions of the brain. The main action of the drug appears to be in the cerebral cortex and, possibly, the reticular activating system. Also, dextroamphetamine may stimulate inhibitory autoreceptors in the brain. These actions decrease drowsiness, fatigue, and motor restlessness and increase mental alertness. Peripheral actions include increased blood pressure, mild bronchodilation, and respiratory stimulation.

---

## Contraindications
Advanced arteriosclerosis; agitation; glaucoma; history of drug abuse; hypersensitivity to amphetamine, dextroamphetamine, or any of their components; hyperthyroidism; MAO inhibitor therapy within 14 days; moderate to severe hypertension; symptomatic CV disease

## Interactions
**DRUGS**

*anesthetics (inhaled):* Increased risk of severe ventricular arrhythmias
*antacids that contain calcium or magnesium, carbonic anhydrase inhibitors, citrates, sodium bicarbonate:* Increased effects of amphetamine
*antihypertensives, diuretics:* Possibly decreased hypotensive effects
*beta blockers:* Increased risk of hypertension, excessive bradycardia, possibly heart block
*CNS stimulants:* Additive CNS stimulation
*digoxin, levodopa:* Possibly arrhythmias
*ethosuximide, phenobarbital, phenytoin:* Delayed intestinal absorption of these drugs
*glutamic acid hydrochloride, urinary acidifiers (such as ammonium chloride and sodium acid phosphate):* Increased excretion and decreased blood level and effects of amphetamine and dextroamphetamine
*haloperidol, loxapine, molindone, phenothiazines, pimozide, thioxanthenes:* Reduced antipsychotic effectiveness of these drugs, inhibited CNS stimulant effects of amphetamine and dextroamphetamine
*MAO inhibitors:* Potentiated effects of amphetamine, possibly hypertensive crisis
*meperidine:* Increased analgesia
*metrizamide:* Increased risk of seizures
*norepinephrine:* Possibly increased adrenergic effect of norepinephrine
*propoxyphene:* Increased CNS stimulation, risk of fatal seizures
*sympathomimetics:* Increased CV effects of both drugs
*thyroid replacement drugs:* Enhanced effects of both drugs
*tricyclic antidepressants:* Possibly increased CV effects

**FOODS**

*ascorbic acid, fruit juices:* Decreased absorption and effects of amphetamine and dextroamphetamine

## Adverse Reactions
**CNS:** Agitation, anxiety, CVA, depression, dizziness, drowsiness, emotional lability, fatigue, fever, headache, insomnia, irritability, light-headedness, motor tics, nervousness, psychosis, seizures, tremor

**CV:** Arrhythmias, hypertension, MI, sudden death, tachycardia
**EENT:** Blurred vision, dry mouth, taste perversion
**GI:** Abdominal pain, anorexia, constipation, diarrhea, indigestion, nausea, vomiting
**GU:** Decreased libido, UTI
**RESP:** Dyspnea
**SKIN:** Diaphoresis
**Other:** Infection, weight loss

## Nursing Considerations

•Keep in mind that, when signs and symptoms of ADHD occur with acute stress reactions or structural cardiac abnormalities, amphetamines usually aren't indicated because these conditions may worsen or sudden death may occur.
•Monitor pulse rate and blood pressure in patients who have hypertension, including even mild hypertension, because drug may increase blood pressure and cause arrhythmias, including tachycardia. Report abnormal findings to prescriber.
•**WARNING** If patient suddenly stops taking drug after long-term, high-dose therapy, watch for withdrawal signs and symptoms, such as abdominal pain, depression, fatigue, nausea, tremor, vomiting, and weakness. Anticipate restarting drug and gradually tapering dosage, as prescribed.
•Monitor growth and development in children because drug may adversely affect growth.
•Administer first dose of tablet form when patient awakens and additional doses at 4- to 6-hour intervals. Administer E.R. capsule form when patient awakens.
•If patient currently takes divided doses of tablet form, know that he may be switched to E.R. capsule form at the same daily dose to be taken once in the morning.
•Assess patient for potential drug dependence, drug-seeking behavior, or drug tolerance. Be alert for signs and symptoms of long-term amphetamine abuse characterized by hyperactivity, irritability, marked insomnia, personality changes, and severe dermatoses.
•Assess patient with history of Tourette syndrome or motor or vocal tics for exacerbation of these conditions during amphetamine therapy.

**PATIENT TEACHING**

•Advise patient to take amphetamine and dextroamphetamine with food or after a meal because anorexia may occur.
•Advise patient not to take drug with acidic fruit juice because it may decrease drug absorption.
•Tell patient or caregiver that E.R. capsules may be taken whole or opened and sprinkled on applesauce, then swallowed immediately without chewing.
•Stress the importance of taking drug exactly as prescribed because misuse may cause serious adverse cardiovascular reactions, including sudden death.
•Urge patient to avoid potentially hazardous activities until he knows how drug affects him.
•Inform patient of abuse potential of drug, and stress the importance of not altering dosage unless prescribed.
•Inform parents or caregivers that child may be placed on drug-free weekend and holiday schedule, as prescribed, if signs and symptoms of ADHD are controlled.

# amphetamine sulfate

## Class, Category, and Schedule

*Chemical:* Sympathomimetic amine
*Therapeutic:* CNS stimulant
*Pregnancy category:* C
*Controlled substance:* Schedule II

## Indications and Dosages

➤ *To treat attention deficit hyperactivity disorder (ADHD)*
**TABLETS**
**Children age 6 and older.** 5 mg q.d. or b.i.d., then increased by 5 mg/day at 1-wk intervals until desired response occurs. *Usual:* 0.1 to 0.5 mg/kg/day.
**Children ages 3 to 5.** 2.5 mg q.d., then increased by 2.5 mg/day at 1-wk intervals until desired response occurs. *Usual:* 0.1 to 0.5 mg/kg/day.

➤ *To treat narcolepsy*
**TABLETS**
**Adults and children age 12 and older.** *Initial:* 10 mg/day, then increased by 10 mg/day at 1-wk intervals until desired response occurs.
**Children ages 6 to 12.** 2.5 mg b.i.d., then increased by 5 mg/day at 1-wk intervals until desired response occurs or adult dosage is reached to a maximum of 60 mg/day.

## Mechanism of Action

May produce its CNS stimulant effects by facilitating the release and blocking the reuptake of norepinephrine at the adrenergic nerve terminals and by direct stimulation of alpha and beta receptors in the peripheral nervous system. It also releases and blocks the reuptake of dopamine in limbic regions of the brain. The drug's main action appears to be in the cerebral cortex and, possibly, the reticular activating system. These actions cause decreased motor restlessness, increased alertness, and diminished drowsiness and fatigue. Its peripheral actions include increased blood pressure and mild bronchodilation and respiratory stimulation.

## Contraindications

Advanced arteriosclerosis, agitation (for narcolepsy treatment), glaucoma, history of drug abuse, hypersensitivity or idiosyncratic reaction to sympathomimetic amines, hyperthyroidism, MAO inhibitor therapy within 14 days, moderate to severe hypertension, symptomatic cardiovascular disease

## Interactions

### Drugs

*adrenergic blockers:* Inhibited adrenergic blockade
*acetazolamide, alkalinizers (such as sodium bicarbonate), some thiazides:* Increased blood level and effects of amphetamine
*antihistamines:* Possibly reduced sedation from antihistamine
*antihypertensives:* Possibly decreased antihypertensive effects
*chlorpromazine:* Inhibited CNS stimulant effects of amphetamine
*ethosuximide:* Possibly delayed ethosuximide absorption
*GI acidifiers (such as ascorbic acid), reserpine:* Decreased amphetamine absorption
*guanethidine:* Decreased antihypertensive effect and decreased amphetamine absorption
*haloperidol:* Decreased CNS stimulation
*lithium carbonate:* Possibly decreased anorectic and stimulant effects of amphetamine
*MAO inhibitors:* Potentiated effects of amphetamine; possibly hypertensive crisis
*meperidine:* Increased analgesia

*methenamine:* Increased urine excretion and decreased effects of amphetamine
*norepinephrine:* Possibly increased adrenergic effect of norepinephrine
*phenobarbital, phenytoin:* Synergistic anticonvulsant action
*propoxyphene:* Increased CNS stimulation, potentially fatal seizures
*tricyclic antidepressants:* Possibly enhanced antidepressant effects and decreased effects of amphetamine
*urinary acidifiers (such as ammonium chloride and sodium acid phosphate):* Increased amphetamine excretion and decreased amphetamine blood level and effects
Veratrum *alkaloids:* Decreased hypotensive effect

### Foods

*acidic fruit juices:* Decreased amphetamine absorption

## Adverse Reactions

**CNS:** Anxiety, dizziness, dyskinesia, dysphoria, euphoria, exacerbation of motor and phonic tics and Tourette's syndrome, hallucinations, headache, insomnia, overstimulation, paranoia, psychotic episodes, restlessness, tremor
**CV:** Cardiomyopathy, hypertension, palpitations, tachycardia
**EENT:** Dry mouth, unpleasant taste
**GI:** Anorexia, constipation, diarrhea
**GU:** Impotence, libido changes
**SKIN:** Urticaria
**Other:** Weight loss

## Nursing Considerations

• Keep in mind that when symptoms of ADHD occur with acute stress reactions, treatment with amphetamines usually isn't indicated.
• **WARNING** To prevent hypertensive crisis, don't administer amphetamine during or for up to 14 days after MAO therapy.
• Administer first dose when patient awakens and additional doses at 4- to 6-hour intervals.
• If patient experiences bothersome adverse reactions, such as insomnia and anorexia, expect to decrease dosage. To minimize insomnia, administer drug earlier in day.
• Be alert for signs of long-term amphetamine abuse, such as severe dermatoses, marked insomnia, irritability, hyperactivity, and personality changes. If patient suddenly stops drug after long-term, high-dose regimen, watch for extreme fatigue and depression.

## PATIENT TEACHING

• Instruct breast-feeding patient to avoid breast-feeding during amphetamine therapy because drug is excreted in breast milk.
• Teach patient to take first dose on awakening and subsequent doses at 4- to 6-hour intervals. Tell him not to take last dose late in evening because insomnia may occur.
• Urge patient to avoid potentially hazardous activities until drug's effects are known.
• Advise patient not to take amphetamine with acidic fruit juice because it decreases drug absorption.
• Inform patient of drug's abuse potential and stress importance of not altering dosage unless prescribed.

# amphotericin B

Amphocin, Fungizone Intravenous

# amphotericin B cholesteryl sulfate complex

Amphotec

# amphotericin B lipid complex

Abelcet

# amphotericin B liposomal complex

AmBisome

## Class and Category

*Chemical:* Amphoteric polyene macrolide
*Therapeutic:* Antifungal
*Pregnancy category:* B (I.V.); C (oral suspension)

## Indications and Dosages

➤ *To treat severe fungal infections, using amphotericin B*

**I.V. INFUSION**

**Adults and adolescents.** *Initial:* 1-mg test dose in 20 ml of $D_5W$ infused over 20 to 30 min; if test dose is tolerated, then 0.25 to 0.3 mg/kg/day prepared as a 0.1 mg/ml infusion, given over 2 to 6 hr. Increased in 5- to 10-mg increments up to 50 mg/day, based on patient tolerance and infection severity, not to exceed a total daily dose of 1.5 mg/kg. *Maximum:* 50 mg/day infused over 2 to 6 hr.
**Children.** *Initial:* 0.25 mg/kg/day in $D_5W$ infused over 6 hr; then increased in 0.125- to 0.25-mg/kg increments daily or every other day as tolerated. *Maximum:* 1 mg/kg or 30 mg/m² of body surface daily.

➤ *To treat oral candidiasis, using amphotericin B*

**ORAL SUSPENSION**

**Adults and children.** 1 ml (100 mg) q.i.d. for 14 days.

➤ *To treat aspergillosis, using amphotericin B cholesteryl sulfate complex*

**I.V. INFUSION**

**Adults and children.** Test dose of 1.6 to 8.3 mg in 10 ml of $D_5W$ infused over 15 to 30 min; if test dose is tolerated, then 3 to 4 mg/kg once daily infused at 1 mg/kg/hr.

➤ *To treat invasive amphotericin B-resistant fungal infections, using amphotericin B lipid complex*

**I.V. INFUSION**

**Adults and children.** 5 mg/kg/day infused at 2.5 mg/kg/hr.

➤ *To treat severe aspergillosis, candidiasis, or cryptococcosis, using amphotericin B liposomal complex*

**I.V. INFUSION**

**Adults and children.** 3 to 5 mg/kg/day infused over 2 hr. Infusion time may be decreased to 1 hr if tolerated or increased if patient experiences discomfort.

➤ *To treat leishmaniasis, using amphotericin B liposomal complex*

**I.V. INFUSION**

**Immunocompetent adults and children.** 3 mg/kg/day for days 1 through 5 and on days 14 and 21 infused over 2 hr. Infusion time may be decreased to 1 hr if tolerated or increased if patient experiences discomfort.
**Immunocompromised adults and children.** 4 mg/kg/day for days 1 through 5 and on days 10, 17, 24, 31, and 38 infused over 2 hr. Infusion time may be decreased to 1 hr if tolerated or increased if patient experiences discomfort.

➤ *To treat presumed fungal infections in patients with febrile neutropenia, using amphotericin B lipid complex*

**I.V. INFUSION**

**Adults and children.** 3 mg/kg/day infused over 2 hr. Infusion time may be decreased to 1 hr if tolerated or increased if patient experiences discomfort.

| Route | Onset | Peak | Duration |
|-------|-------|------|----------|
| I.V. | Immediate | Unknown | Unknown |

## Mechanism of Action
Binds to sterols in fungal cell plasma membranes, which changes membrane permeability and allows loss of potassium and small molecules from cells. This action results in cell impairment or death.

## Incompatibilities
Don't reconstitute amphotericin B with diluents other than those recommended because solutions with sodium chloride or bacteriostatic agents (such as benzyl alcohol) may cause drug precipitation.

## Contraindications
Hypersensitivity to amphotericin B or its components

## Interactions
### DRUGS
*antineoplastics:* Increased risk of bronchospasm, hypotension, and nephrotoxicity
*corticosteroids, corticotropin:* Increased risk of hypokalemia and cardiac dysfunction
*cyclosporine, nephrotoxic drugs:* Increased risk of nephrotoxicity
*digitalis glycosides:* Possibly hypokalemia and more severe digitalis toxicity
*flucytosine:* Possibly increased flucytosine toxicity
*leukocyte transfusion:* Possibly dyspnea, hypoxemia, and pulmonary infiltrates
*skeletal muscle relaxants:* Possibly hypokalemia and increased muscle relaxation
*zidovudine:* Possibly myelotoxicity and nephrotoxicity

## Adverse Reactions
**CNS:** Fever, headache, shaking chills, tiredness, weakness
**CV:** Chest pain, hypotension, irregular heartbeat
**EENT:** Difficulty swallowing, pharyngitis
**GI:** Abdominal pain, anorexia, diarrhea, hepatic failure, indigestion, nausea, vomiting
**GU:** Decreased or increased urine output, impaired renal function
**HEME:** Anemia, leukopenia, thrombocytopenia, unusual bleeding or bruising
**MS:** Arthralgia, muscle spasms, myalgia
**RESP:** Apnea, dyspnea, hypoxia, pulmonary edema, tachypnea
**SKIN:** Flushing, jaundice, maculopapular rash, pruritus and redness especially around ears, urticaria
**Other:** Anaphylaxis, hypocalcemia, hypokalemia, hypomagnesemia, infusion site pain and thrombophlebitis

## Nursing Considerations
•To prepare amphotericin B, add 10 ml of sterile water for injection without a bacteriostatic agent to vial containing 50 mg of amphotericin B. For I.V. infusion, dilute the solution containing 5 mg/ml to 0.1 mg/ml by adding 1 ml (5 mg) of solution to 49 ml of $D_5W$ with a pH above 4.2.
•Before using $D_5W$ to dilute amphotericin B solution, determine the injection's pH aseptically. If the pH is below 4.2, follow the manufacturer's instructions for buffering it.
•Because reconstituted amphotericin B is a colloidal suspension, avoid using an in-line membrane filter or use one with a mean pore diameter of more than 1 micron to prevent significant drug removal.
•To prepare amphotericin B cholesteryl sulfate complex, reconstitute it with sterile water for injection. Using a sterile syringe and a 20G needle, rapidly add 10 or 20 ml of sterile water for injection to a 50- or 100-mg vial, respectively, to obtain a solution containing 5 mg of amphotericin B per milliliter. Shake gently by hand, rotating vial until solids are dissolved; fluid may be clear or opalescent. For infusion, further dilute reconstituted solution to about 0.6 mg/ml. Don't filter the solution or use an in-line filter. Flush existing line with $D_5W$ or use a separate line.
•To prepare amphotericin B lipid complex, shake vial gently until you see no yellow sediment. Using an 18G needle, withdraw prescribed dose from required number of vials into one or more 20-ml syringes. Replace needle with 5-micron filter needle that's supplied with each vial. Empty syringe contents into bag of $D_5W$ so that final concentration is 1 mg/ml. Expect to use a concentration of 2 mg/ml for children and patients with cardiovascular disease. Before infusion, shake bag until contents are mixed thoroughly. Flush existing line with $D_5W$ or use a separate line. Don't use an in-line filter. If infusion exceeds 2 hours, shake infusion bag every 2 hours.

•To prepare amphotericin B liposomal complex, add 12 ml sterile water for injection (without bacteriostatic agent) to each 50-mg vial to achieve a concentration of 4 mg amphotericin B per milliliter. Immediately shake vial vigorously for at least 30 seconds until all particles completely disperse. Withdraw prescribed dose of amphotericin B liposomal complex suspension. Then use a 5-micron filter to inject it into $D_5W$ to provide a final concentration of 1 to 2 mg/ml. Expect to use a lower concentration (0.2 to 0.5 mg/ml) for infants and young children. Flush existing line with $D_5W$ or use a separate line. You may use an in-line filter with a mean pore diameter of at least 1 micron.

•To help minimize fever and shaking chills, expect to administer an antipyretic, antihistamine, meperidine, or corticosteroid just before infusing amphotericin B.

•Before giving amphotericin B oral suspension, shake well. Drop suspension on tongue with calibrated dropper. Then tell patient to swish suspension in mouth for as long as possible before swallowing. If drug must be swabbed on, use a nonabsorbent swab.

•Administer amphotericin B oral suspension between meals to permit prolonged contact with oral lesions.

•Assess I.V. insertion site regularly to detect extravasation of amphotericin B, which may cause severe local irritation. To minimize local thrombophlebitis, plan to add heparin to infusion or expect to administer amphotericin on alternate days, which also may help prevent anorexia. Alternate-day dose shouldn't exceed 1.5 mg/kg.

•Monitor renal function because of the risk of renal impairment. Plan to obtain serum creatinine level every other day while amphotericin B dosage is increasing and then at least twice weekly during therapy. If serum creatinine or BUN level increases significantly, expect to stop amphotericin B until renal function improves. Know that a cumulative dose of more than 4 g may cause irreversible renal dysfunction.

•Expect to monitor CBC and platelet count weekly throughout therapy to detect adverse hematologic effects. Also monitor serum calcium, magnesium, and potassium levels twice weekly to detect abnormalities.

•Use reconstituted amphotericin B within 24 hours if stored at room temperature or within 1 week if refrigerated. Use reconstituted amphotericin B cholesteryl sulfate complex within 24 hours. Use amphotericin B lipid complex within 6 hours if stored at room temperature or within 48 hours if refrigerated. Use diluted amphotericin B liposomal complex within 24 hours if refrigerated, but begin infusion within 6 hours.

•Because reconstituted amphotericin B is a colloidal suspension, avoid using an in-line membrane filter or use one with a mean pore diameter of more than 1 micron to prevent significant drug removal.

**PATIENT TEACHING**

•Instruct patient to shake bottle of oral suspension well before each dose; to drop suspension directly on his tongue, using calibrated dropper; and then to swish suspension in his mouth for as long as possible before swallowing. If prescriber orders drug swabbing onto oral lesions, tell patient to use nonabsorbent swab. Instruct him to take drug four times a day—between meals and at bedtime.

•Tell patient to notify prescriber if he develops local irritation, if existing symptoms worsen or return, or if new symptoms arise.

# ampicillin

Apo-Ampi (CAN), Novo-Ampicillin (CAN), Nu-Ampi (CAN), Omnipen

## ampicillin sodium

Ampicin (CAN), Omnipen-N, Polycillin-N, Totacillin-N

## ampicillin trihydrate

D-Amp, Omnipen, Penbritin (CAN), Polycillin, Principen-250, Principen-500, Totacillin

## Class and Category

*Chemical:* Semisynthetic aminopenicillin
*Therapeutic:* Antibiotic
*Pregnancy category:* B

## Indications and Dosages

➤ *To treat GI infections and genitourinary infections (other than gonorrhea) caused by susceptible strains of* Shigella, Salmonella typhi *and other species,* Escherichia coli, Proteus mirabilis, *and enterococci*

CAPSULES, ORAL SUSPENSION, I.V. INFUSION, I.M. INJEC-
TION
**Adults and children who weigh 20 kg (44 lb)
or more.** 500 mg P.O. q 6 hr or 250 to 500 mg
I.V. or I.M. q 6 hr.
**Children who weigh less than 20 kg.** 50 to
100 mg/kg/day in divided doses P.O. q 6 hr
or 12.5 mg/kg I.V. or I.M. q 6 hr.

➤ *To treat gonorrhea caused by susceptible
strains of non-penicillinase-producing*
Neisseria gonorrhoeae
CAPSULES, ORAL SUSPENSION
**Adults and children.** 3.5 g as a single dose
with 1 g of probenecid.
I.V. INFUSION, I.M. INJECTION
**Adults and children who weigh 45 kg (99 lb)
or more.** 500 mg q 6 hr.
**Children who weigh less than 40 kg (88 lb).**
50 mg/kg/day in divided doses q 6 to 8 hr.

➤ *To treat respiratory tract infections
caused by susceptible strains of non-
penicillinase–producing* Haemophilus
influenzae, *staphylococci, and streptococci, including* Streptococcus pneumoniae
CAPSULES, ORAL SUSPENSION, I.V. INFUSION, I.M. INJEC-
TION
**Adults and children who weigh 40 kg or
more.** 250 to 500 mg I.V. or I.M. q 6 to 8 hr.
**Adults and children who weigh 20 kg or
more.** 250 mg P.O. q 6 hr.
**Children who weigh less than 40 kg.** 25 to 50
mg/kg/day I.V. or I.M. in divided doses q 6 to
8 hr.
**Children who weigh less than 20 kg.** 50 mg/
kg/day P.O. in divided doses q 6 or 8 hr or
12.5 mg/kg I.V. or I.M. q 6 hr.

➤ *To treat septicemia*
I.V. INFUSION, I.M. INJECTION
**Adults.** 8 to 14 g I.V. daily in divided doses q
3 to 4 hr for at least 3 days; then I.M.
**Children.** 150 to 200 mg/kg/day I.V. in divided
doses q 3 to 4 hr for at least 3 days; then I.M.

➤ *To prevent bacterial endocarditis from
dental, oral, or upper respiratory tract
procedures*
I.V. INFUSION, I.M. INJECTION
**Adults.** 2 g within 30 min of procedure
**Children.** 50 mg/kg within 30 min of procedure

➤ *To treat bacterial meningitis caused by
susceptible strains of* Neisseria meningitidis
I.V. INFUSION, I.M. INJECTION
**Adults.** 8 to 14 g/day or 150 to 200 mg/kg/day
I.V. in equally divided doses q 3 to 4 hr for at
least 3 days; then I.M. at same dosage and
schedule.
**Children.** 100 to 200 mg/kg/day I.V. in equally
divided doses q 3 to 4 hr for at least 3 days;
then I.M. at same dosage and schedule.

➤ *To treat listeriosis*
I.V. INFUSION, I.M. INJECTION
**Adults and children who weigh 20 kg or
more.** 50 mg/kg q 6 hr.
**Children who weigh less than 20 kg.** 12.5
mg/kg q 6 hr.

| Route | Onset | Peak | Duration |
|---|---|---|---|
| I.V. | Immediate | Unknown | Unknown |

## Mechanism of Action
Inhibits bacterial cell wall synthesis. The
rigid, cross-linked cell wall is assembled in
several steps. Ampicillin exerts its effects
on susceptible bacteria in the final stage of
the cross-linking process by binding with
and inactivating penicillin-binding proteins (enzymes responsible for linking the
cell wall strands). This action causes bacterial cell lysis and death.

## Incompatibilities
Don't mix ampicillin and any aminoglycoside
in the same I.V. bag, bottle, or tubing; otherwise, both drugs will be inactivated. If patient must receive both drugs, administer
them in separate sites at least 1 hour apart.

## Contraindications
Hypersensitivity to any penicillin, infection
caused by penicillinase-producing organism

## Interactions
DRUGS
*allopurinol:* Increased risk of rash, particularly in hyperuricemic patient
*aminoglycosides:* Possibly inactivated action
of aminoglycoside and ampicillin when given
together
*heparin, oral anticoagulants:* Increased risk
of bleeding

*oral contraceptives:* Possibly reduced contraceptive effectiveness and breakthrough bleeding
*probenecid:* Possibly increased serum ampicillin level and ampicillin toxicity
*tetracyclines:* Possibly impaired action of ampicillin

## Adverse Reactions

**CNS:** Chills, fatigue, fever, headache, malaise
**CV:** Chest pain, edema, thrombophlebitis
**EENT:** Epistaxis, glossitis, laryngeal stridor, mucocutaneous candidiasis, stomatitis, throat tightness
**GI:** Abdominal distention, diarrhea, enterocolitis, flatulence, gastritis, nausea, pseudomembranous colitis, vomiting
**GU:** Dysuria, urine retention, vaginal candidiasis
**HEME:** Agranulocytosis, anemia, eosinophilia, leukopenia, thrombocytopenia, thrombocytopenic purpura
**SKIN:** Erythema multiforme; erythematous, mildly pruritic maculopapular rash or other types of rash; exfoliative dermatitis; pruritus; urticaria
**Other:** Anaphylaxis, facial edema, injection site pain

## Nursing Considerations

• Avoid giving ampicillin to patients with mononucleosis because of increased risk of rash.
• Expect to give ampicillin for 48 to 72 hours after patient becomes asymptomatic. For streptococcal infection, expect to give ampicillin for at least 10 days after cultures show streptococcal eradication to reduce risk of rheumatic fever or glomerulonephritis.
• To dilute ampicillin for I.M. use, add (depending on manufacturer) 1.2 ml of sterile water or bacteriostatic water for injection to each 125-mg vial, 1 ml of diluent to each 250-mg vial, 1.8 ml of diluent to each 500-mg vial, 3.5 ml of diluent to each 1-g vial, or 6.8 ml of diluent to each 2-g vial.
• To dilute ampicillin for intermittent infusion, add 5 ml of sterile water or bacteriostatic water for injection to each 125-, 250-, or 500-mg vial or 7.4 to 10 ml of diluent to each 1- or 2-g vial. Infuse in suitable diluent at less than 30 mg/ml.
•**WARNING** Infuse I.V. solution for 3 to 5 minutes for each 125 or 500 mg or 10 to 15 minutes for each 1 or 2 g. More rapid infusion may cause seizures.

• Monitor patient closely for anaphylaxis, which may be life-threatening. Patients at greatest risk are those with a history of multiple allergies, hypersensitivity to cephalosporins, or a history of asthma, hay fever, or urticaria.
• Notify prescriber if patient has evidence of superinfection; expect to stop drug and provide appropriate treatment.
•**WARNING** In an anaphylactic reaction, stop drug, notify prescriber immediately, and provide immediate treatment with epinephrine, airway management, oxygen, and I.V. corticosteroids, as needed.
• If long-term or high-dose ampicillin therapy is required, closely monitor results of renal and liver function tests and CBCs.
**PATIENT TEACHING**
• Stress the importance of taking the full course of ampicillin exactly as prescribed.
• Tell patient to take ampicillin with 8 oz of water 30 minutes before or 2 hours after meals.
• Instruct patient to shake suspension well before each use, keep bottle tightly closed between uses, and discard unused portion after 14 days if refrigerated or 7 days if stored at room temperature.
• Review signs of allergic reaction; if they occur, tell patient to hold next ampicillin dose and contact prescriber immediately.

# ampicillin sodium and sulbactam sodium

Unasyn

## Class and Category

*Chemical:* Aminopenicillin, beta-lactamase inhibitor
*Therapeutic:* Antibiotic
*Pregnancy category:* B

## Indications and Dosages

➤ *To treat skin and soft-tissue infections caused by beta-lactamase–producing strains of* Staphylococcus aureus, Escherichia coli, Klebsiella *species (including* K. pneumoniae*),* Proteus mirabilis, Bacteroides fragilis, Enterobacter *species, and* Acinetobacter calcoaceticus; *intra-abdominal infections caused by beta-lactamase–producing strains of* E.

coli, Klebsiella *species (including* K. pneumoniae*)*, Bacteroides *species (including* B. fragilis*), and* Enterobacter *species; gynecologic infections caused by beta-lactamase–producing strains of* E. coli *and* Bacteroides *species (including* B. fragilis*)*

**I.V. INFUSION, I.M. INJECTION**

**Adults and children age 12 and older who weigh 40 kg (88 lb) or more.** 1.5 (1 g of ampicillin and 0.5 g of sulbactam) to 3 g (2 g of ampicillin and 1 g of sulbactam) q 6 hr, up to a maximum of 8 g of ampicillin and 4 g of sulbactam daily.

**Children age 1 and older who weigh less than 40 kg.** 300 mg/kg (200 mg of ampicillin and 100 mg of sulbactam) daily in divided doses q 6 hr.

**DOSAGE ADJUSTMENT** Dosing frequency reduced to q 6 to 8 hr for patients with creatinine clearance of 30 ml/min/1.73 m² or more. Dosing frequency reduced to q 12 hr for patients with creatinine clearance of 15 to 29 ml/min/1.73 m². Frequency reduced to 1.5 to 3.0 g q 24 hr for patients with creatinine clearance of 5 to 14 ml/min/1.73 m².

| Route | Onset | Peak | Duration |
|-------|-------|------|----------|
| I.V. | Immediate | Unknown | Unknown |

## Incompatibilities

Don't mix ampicillin sodium and sulbactam sodium with any aminoglycoside in the same I.V. bag, bottle, or tubing; otherwise, both drugs will be inactivated. If patient must receive both drugs, give them in separate sites at least 1 hour apart.

## Contraindications

Hypersensitivity to ampicillin sodium and sulbactam sodium, their components, or any penicillin

## Interactions

*allopurinol:* Increased risk of rash, particularly in hyperuricemic patient
*aminoglycosides:* Possibly inactivated action of aminoglycoside and ampicillin sodium and sulbactam sodium when given together
*heparin, oral anticoagulants:* Increased risk of bleeding
*oral contraceptives:* Possibly reduced contraceptive effectiveness and breakthrough bleeding

*probenecid:* Possibly increased serum ampicillin level and ampicillin toxicity
*tetracyclines:* Possibly impaired action of ampicillin sodium and sulbactam sodium

## Mechanism of Action

Inhibits bacterial cell wall synthesis. The rigid, cross-linked cell wall is assembled in several steps. The drug exerts its effects on susceptible bacteria in the final stage of the cross-linking process by binding with and inactivating penicillin-binding proteins (enzymes responsible for linking the cell wall strands). This action causes bacterial cell lysis and death. When ampicillin is given alone, beta-lactamases may degrade it, making it ineffective. When it's combined with sulbactam, degradation can't occur. So sulbactam extends ampicillin's bactericidal effects to beta-lactamase–producing bacteria.

## Adverse Reactions

**CNS:** Chills, fatigue, fever, headache, malaise
**CV:** Chest pain, edema, thrombophlebitis
**EENT:** Black "hairy" tongue, epistaxis, glossitis, laryngeal stridor, mucocutaneous candidiasis, stomatitis, throat tightness
**GI:** Abdominal distention, diarrhea, enterocolitis, flatulence, gastritis, nausea, pseudomembranous colitis, vomiting
**GU:** Dysuria, urine retention, vaginal candidiasis
**HEME:** Agranulocytosis, anemia, eosinophilia, leukopenia, thrombocytopenia, thrombocytopenic purpura
**SKIN:** Erythema multiforme; erythematous, mildly pruritic maculopapular rash or other rash; exfoliative dermatitis; mucosal bleeding; pruritus; urticaria
**Other:** Anaphylaxis, facial edema, injection site pain

## Nursing Considerations

• Avoid administering ampicillin sodium and sulbactam sodium to patients with mononucleosis because of the increased risk of rash.
• Administer I.V. dose by slow injection over 10 to 15 minutes or by infusion over 15 to 30 minutes in greater dilutions with 50 to 100 ml of a compatible diluent.

•Reconstitute drug for I.M. use with sterile water for injection or 0.5% or 2% lidocaine hydrochloride injection. For a 1.5-g vial, add 3.2 ml of diluent; for a 3.0-g vial, add 6.4 ml of diluent. Let solution stand until foaming dissipates. Inspect vial before withdrawing drug to ensure dissolution. After reconstituting solution, inject it within 1 hour.
•Administer by deep I.M. injection.
•Monitor closely for anaphylaxis, which may be life-threatening. Patients at greatest risk are those with a history of hypersensitivity to penicillin, multiple allergies, hypersensitivity to cephalosporins, or a history of asthma, hay fever, or urticaria.
•WARNING If drug triggers an anaphylactic reaction, discontinue drug, notify prescriber immediately, and provide appropriate therapy. Anaphylaxis requires immediate treatment with epinephrine as well as airway management and administration of oxygen and I.V. corticosteroids, as needed.
•Monitor closely for diarrhea, which may herald pseudomembranous colitis. If diarrhea occurs, notify prescriber. If pseudomembranous colitis is diagnosed, expect to discontinue drug and, possibly, administer fluids, electrolytes, protein, and antibiotic effective against *Clostridium difficile.*

**PATIENT TEACHING**
•Warn patient that I.M. injection of drug is likely to cause discomfort.
•Instruct patient to report sudden or unusual symptoms immediately. If diarrhea occurs, tell him to notify prescriber immediately.

# amyl nitrite

## Class and Category
*Chemical:* Nitrite ester
*Therapeutic:* Antianginal
*Pregnancy category:* C

## Indications and Dosages
➤ *To treat acute attacks of angina pectoris*
**CRUSHABLE AMPULES**
**Adults.** 1 ampule (0.18 or 0.3 ml) inhaled and repeated in 3 to 5 min, if needed.

| Route | Onset | Peak | Duration |
|-------|-------|------|----------|
| Inhalation | 10 to 30 sec | Unknown | 3 to 5 min |

## Mechanism of Action
After inhalation, is absorbed by pulmonary alveoli, which causes relaxation of vascular smooth-muscle cells, dilation of large coronary blood vessels, decreased systemic vascular resistance, decreased venous return to the heart, reduced afterload, decreased cardiac ouput, and subsequent relief of angina.

## Contraindications
Hypersensitivity to amyl nitrite, its components, or nitrates

## Interactions
**DRUGS**
*aspirin:* Increased serum level and action of amyl nitrite
*calcium channel blockers:* Possibly severe symptomatic hypotension
*sildenafil:* Increased risk of hypotension
*sympathomimetics:* Possibly decreased antianginal effects and severe hypotension and tachycardia
**ACTIVITIES**
*alcohol use:* Increased risk of severe hypotension and cardiovascular collapse

## Adverse Reactions
**CNS:** Dizziness, headache, restlessness, syncope, weakness
**CV:** Orthostatic hypotension, tachycardia
**GI:** Fecal incontinence, nausea, vomiting
**GU:** Urinary incontinence
**HEME:** Hemolytic anemia, methemoglobinemia
**SKIN:** Face and neck flushing, pallor, rash

## Nursing Considerations
•Use amyl nitrite cautiously in elderly patients and patients with cerebral hemorrhage, glaucoma, hyperthyroidism, recent head trauma or MI, or severe anemia.
•Monitor blood pressure during and after drug administration. Also monitor cardiac function periodically in patients who use amyl nitrite regularly.
•WARNING Stop drug and notify prescriber if you detect signs of overdose, such as bluish lips, fingernails, or palms; dizziness; fainting; extreme pressure in head; dyspnea; unusual tiredness or weakness; a weak or fast heartbeat; or increased methemoglobin level. Cyanosis may occur when methemoglobin

level reaches 1.5 g/dl. More pronounced signs occur at 20 to 50 g/dl.
• Expect to treat overdose with high-flow oxygen and I.V. methylene blue. If hypotension is severe, place patient head down. If he needs a vasopressor, avoid epinephrine because it may cause severe hypotension.

**PATIENT TEACHING**
• Advise patient to store amyl nitrate in a tight container, protected from light.
• Tell patient to crush ampule between finger and thumb, hold it to nostrils, and inhale one to six times.
• Instruct patient to remain seated or supine during administration and to rise slowly afterward to prevent dizziness.
• Inform patient that relief usually occurs in 1 to 5 minutes. If pain continues, he should repeat dose. If pain continues after another 5 minutes, he should seek emergency help.
• Remind patient not to use more amyl nitrite than prescribed because of possible overdose.
• **WARNING** Caution patient that drug is flammable and must be kept from flame and heat.
• Inform patient that amyl nitrite commonly causes headaches. Tell him to notify prescriber if they become severe or bothersome.

# anagrelide hydrochloride

Agrylin

## Class and Category
*Chemical:* Imidazo-quinazolinone
*Therapeutic:* Platelet count–reducing agent
*Pregnancy category:* C

## Indications and Dosages
➤ *To treat essential thrombocythemia*
**CAPSULES**
**Adults.** 0.5 mg q.i.d. or 1 mg b.i.d. for 1 wk; then adjusted to the lowest dose that keeps platelet count below 600,000/mm$^3$ or within normal range. Dosage shouldn't be increased by more than 0.5 mg/day in any 1 wk. *Maximum:* 10 mg/day or 2.5 mg in a single dose.
**DOSAGE ADJUSTMENT** For patients with moderate hepatic impairment, 0.5 mg/day for at least 1 wk, increased as needed by no more than 0.5 mg/day in any 1-wk period.

| Route | Onset | Peak | Duration |
|---|---|---|---|
| P.O. | 7 to 14 days | Unknown | Up to 4 days |

## Mechanism of Action
May decrease megakaryocyte hypermaturation (bone marrow cells from which platelets form), reducing platelet count. Higher doses may inhibit platelet aggregation.

## Contraindications
Hypersensitivity to anagrelide, severe hepatic impairment

## Interactions
**DRUGS**
*amrinone, cilostazol, enoximone, milrinone, olprinone:* Increased effects of these drugs; possible risk of increased adverse effects
*sucralfate:* Possibly interference with anagrelide absorption

## Adverse Reactions
**CNS:** Amnesia, asthenia, chills, confusion, CVA, depression, dizziness, fever, headache, insomnia, malaise, nervousness, paresthesia, seizures, somnolence, syncope, weakness
**CV:** Angina, arrhythmias, edema, heart failure, hypertension, MI, orthostatic hypotension, palpitations, tachycardia, vasodilation
**EENT:** Amoblyopia, diplopia, epistaxis, rhinitis, sinusitis, stomatitis, tinnitus, vision or visual field abnormality
**GI:** Abdominal pain, anorexia, constipation, diarrhea, elevated liver function test results, eructation, flatulence, gastric and duodenal ulceration, gastritis, GI hemorrhage, hepatotoxicity, indigestion, melena, nausea, pancreatitis, vomiting
**GU:** Dysuria, hematuria, renal failure
**HEME:** Anemia, hemorrhage, thrombocytopenia
**MS:** Arthralgia, back pain, leg cramps, myalgia, neck pain
**RESP:** Asthma, bronchitis, dyspnea, pneumonia
**SKIN:** Alopecia, ecchymosis, photosensitivity, pruritus, rash, urticaria
**Other:** Dehydration, flulike symptoms, generalized body pain, lymphadenoma

## Nursing Considerations
• Use anagrelide cautiously in patients with heart disease because it may cause cardiovascular problems, such as heart failure. Use it cautiously in patients with renal insufficiency (serum creatinine level 2 mg/dl or more) or hepatic dysfunction (liver function

tests more than 1.5 times normal) because of the risk of nephrotoxicity and hepatotoxicity.
•To assess efficacy and prevent thrombocytopenia, expect to monitor platelet count every 2 days for first week and then at least weekly until lowest effective dose is reached.
•While platelet count is declining (usually during first 2 weeks of therapy), assess WBC count and hemoglobin, AST, ALT, creatinine, and BUN levels to detect abnormalities.
•Monitor blood pressure to detect orthostatic hypotension.

**PATIENT TEACHING**
•Stress importance of returning for laboratory tests, such as platelet counts, to monitor drug effectiveness and adjust its dosage.
•Tell patient to keep bottle tightly capped between uses and to protect drug from light.

# anakinra

Kineret

## Class and Category

*Chemical:* Recombinant human interleukin-1 receptor antagonist
*Therapeutic:* Antirheumatic
*Pregnancy category:* B

## Indications and Dosages

➤ *To reduce signs and symptoms and slow structural damage in moderate to severe active rheumatoid arthritis in patients who have not responded to disease-modifying antirheumatics*

**S.C. INJECTION**
**Adults.** 100 mg/day.
DOSAGE ADJUSTMENT Dosage interval reduced to every other day in severe renal insufficiency or end-stage renal disease (creatinine clearance less than 30 ml/min/1.73 m$^2$).

---

## Mechanism of Action

Inhibits the binding of interleukin-1 (IL-1) to its type 1 receptor, blocking its activity. Inflammatory stimuli prompt T cells to release IL-1, a mediator of inflammation, pain, and stiffness in rheumatoid arthritis.

---

## Contraindications

Active infection; hypersensitivity to anakinra, its components, or *Escherichia coli*-derived proteins

## Interactions

**DRUGS**
*etanercept, infliximab, and other drugs that block tumor necrosis factor (TNF):* Increased risk of serious infection
*vaccines, live virus:* Possibly decreased antibody response to vaccine, potential for infection with live virus

## Adverse Reactions

**CNS:** Headache
**EENT:** Sinusitis
**GI:** Abdominal pain, diarrhea, nausea
**HEME:** Neutropenia
**MS:** Bone and joint infections
**RESP:** Pneumonia, upper respiratory tract infection
**Skin:** Cellulitis
**Other:** Flulike symptoms; hypersensitivity reaction; injection site ecchymosis, erythema, inflammation, pain, and pruritus; malignancies; positive results for anti-anakinra antibodies; serious infections

## Nursing Considerations

•Obtain baseline neutrophil count before administration, as ordered. Expect to monitor neutrophil count every month for 3 months and then every 3 months for up to 1 year.
•Discard solution if it contains particles or is discolored. Use prefilled syringe and needles to administer drug. Don't shake syringe; allow time for solution to clear if it's foamy.
•Give drug at about the same time each day.
•WARNING Be aware that anakinra is not recommended for patients with active infections. Monitor patient for evidence of infection, such as fever, chills, sore throat, and mouth sores, before and during therapy because drug increases the risk of infections, such as cellulitis, pneumonia, and bone and joint infections. Notify prescriber if signs are present. Patients with asthma and those receiving etanercept or infliximab are at increased risk for serious infections. Expect anakinra to be stopped if serious infection develops.
•Be aware that live virus vaccines should not be given to patients receiving anakinra because drug decreases the immune response.

• Monitor patients with impaired renal function for signs of anakinra toxicity; they're at increased risk because drug is excreted primarily by the kidneys.
• Store anakinra at 2° to 8° C (36° to 46° F). Protect from freezing and light.

#### PATIENT TEACHING
• Teach proper injection technique if patient will self-administer anakinra. Verify that patient understands the process and can correctly prepare and inject first few doses.
• Instruct patient to rotate injection sites among thigh, stomach, and upper arms and to avoid areas that are tender, hard, red, or bruised. Advise him to make sure that each site is at least 1″ away from previous site.
• Urge patient to discard used needles and syringes in a puncture-resistant container and not to reuse them. Instruct him to return container to prescriber for proper disposal.
• Review evidence of allergic reaction, including rash and shortness of breath.
• Urge patient to immediately report signs of infection, such as cough, fever, chills, dyspnea, or headache, to prescriber.

# anastrozole

Arimidex

## Class and Category
*Chemical:* Non-steroidal selective aromatase inhibitor
*Therapeutic:* Antineoplastic
*Pregnancy category:* D

## Indications and Dosages
➤ *To treat postmenopausal women with unknown or positive hormone receptor and locally advanced or metastatic breast cancer, and those with advanced breast cancer following disease progression after tamoxifen therapy; as adjunct to treat early breast cancer in postmenopausal women with positive hormone receptor*

#### TABLETS
Adult women. 1 mg q.d.

## Contraindications
None known

## Interactions
None

### Mechanism of Action
Anastrozole treats certain breast cancers in postmenopausal women by inhibiting the enzyme aromatase, which prevents production of estrone and estradiol. Thus, in women with breast tumors that contain estrogen receptors, anastrozole prevents the stimulatory effects of estrogen on tumor growth.

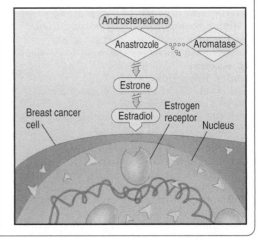

## Adverse Reactions

**CNS:** Asthenia, depression, dizziness, headache, hypertonia, insomnia, lethargy, paresthesia
**EENT:** Dry mouth, pharyngitis
**ENDO:** Hot flashes, weight gain
**CV:** Chest pain, hypertension, peripheral edema, thromboembolic disease, vasodilation
**GI:** Abdominal or pelvic pain, anorexia, increased appetite, constipation, diarrhea, nausea, vomiting
**GU:** Leukorrhea; vaginal bleeding, dryness, or hemorrhage
**MS:** Back or bone pain
**RESP:** Increased cough, dyspnea
**SKIN:** Diaphoresis, rash, urticaria
**Other:** Anaphylaxis, angioedema, flulike symptoms, pain, tumor flare

## Nursing Considerations

•Be aware that anastrozole is not recommended for premenopausal women. For these patients, obtain results of pregnancy test before giving first dose. Expect to withhold drug if results are positive.
•Assess patient for evidence of thromboembolic events during anastrozole therapy, such as shortness of breath, leg pain, and altered mental status.
•Store drug in a tightly closed container at room temperature.

**PATIENT TEACHING**

•Advise patient to notify prescriber immediately about known or suspected pregnancy because risks to the fetus will need to be evaluated.
•Inform patient about possible dizziness and lethargy, and advise her to avoid hazardous activities until drug's CNS effects are known.
•Urge patient to tell prescriber about leg pain or calf swelling, which may indicate a blood clot.
•Advise patient to consume adequate calcium and to follow an exercise program because drug may reduce bone mineral density.
•Urge patient taking anastrozole to comply with follow-up appointments.

# anisindione

Miradon

## Class and Category

*Chemical:* Indanedione derivative
*Therapeutic:* Anticoagulant
*Pregnancy category:* X

## Indications and Dosages

➤ *To prevent and treat venous thrombosis, atrial fibrillation with embolization, and pulmonary embolism; as adjunct to treat coronary artery occlusion, usually in patients who can't tolerate coumarin anticoagulants*

**TABLETS**

**Adults.** *Initial:* 300 mg on day 1; then 200 mg on day 2, and 100 mg on day 3. *Maintenance:* 25 to 250 mg q.d.

| Route | Onset | Peak | Duration |
|-------|-------|------|----------|
| P.O. | In 6 hr | 48 to 72 hr | 1 to 3 days |

## Mechanism of Action

Interferes with the liver's ability to synthesize vitamin K-dependent clotting factors, which results in the depletion of clotting factors II (prothrombin), VII, IX, and X. By depleting levels of vitamin K–dependent clotting factors that are needed to form a stable fibrin clot, anisindione interferes with the clotting cascade and prevents coagulation.

## Contraindications

Ascorbic acid deficiency; blood dyscrasias; continuous small-intestine drainage tube; diverticulitis; emaciation; GI, GU, or respiratory tract bleeding; hemophilia; hemorrhagic tendency; history of warfarin-induced necrosis; hypersensitivity to anisindione or any of its components; leukemia; major recent surgery; malnutrition; pericardial effusion; pericarditis; polyarthritis; pregnancy; prostatectomy; recent spinal puncture, percutaneous invasive procedure, diagnostic testing, or insertion of intrauterine device; recent or possible CNS or eye surgery; severe renal or hepatic disease; severe uncontrolled diabetes; severe uncontrolled malignant hypertension; subacute bacterial endocarditis; thrombocytopenic purpura; visceral carcinomas; ulcerative colitis

## Interactions

**DRUGS**

*abciximab, acetaminophen, allopurinol, alteplase, amiodarone, amitriptyline, amoxapine, androgens, aspirin, beta blockers, cephalosporins, chloral hydrate, chloramphenicol, chlorpropamide, cimetidine, cisapride, clofibrate,*

*clomipramine, corticosteroids, co-trimoxazole, cyclophosphamide, danazol, desipramine, dextrothyroxine, diclofenac, diflunisal, disulfiram, doxepin, erythromycin, etodolac, fluconazole, fluoxymesterone, fosphenytoin, gemfibrozil, glucagon, hydantoins, ifosfamide, influenza virus vaccines, imipramine, indomethacin, isoniazid, itraconazole, ketoconazole, ketolorac, lepirudin, loop diuretics, lovastatin, low–molecular-weight heparins, meclofenamate, mefenamic acid, methyltestosterone, metronidazole, miconazole, moricizine, nabumetone, naproxen, nalidixic acid, neomycin, nortriptyline, NSAIDs, omeprazole, oxandrolone, penicillins, phenylbutazones, phenytoin, piroxicam, propafenone, propoxyphene, protriptyline, quinidine, quinine, quinolones, reteplase, salicylates, stanazolol, streptokinase, sulfamethoxazole, sulfinpyrazone, sulindac, tamoxifen, testosterone, thioamines, thyroid hormones, tomentin, urokinase:* Increased anticoagulant effects
*aminoglutethimide, ascorbic acid, barbiturates, carbamazepine, cholestyramine, corticosteroids, dicloxacillin, estrogen, ethanol, ethchlorvynol, etretinate, glutethimide, griseofulvin, nafcillin, oral contraceptives, rifampin, spironolactone, sucralfate, thiazide diuretics, thiopurines, trazodone, vitamin K:* Decreased anticoagulant effects
*aminoglycosides, mineral oil, tetracycline, vitamin E:* Interference with vitamin K, leading to increased anticoagulant effects

**FOODS**
*enteral products and foods high in vitamin K, such as dark green leafy vegetables:* Interference with anticoagulant effects

**ACTIVITIES**
*alcohol use:* Possibly increased or decreased anticoagulation

## Adverse Reactions
**CNS:** Fever, headache
**EENT:** Blurred vision, mouth ulcers, pharyngitis
**GI:** Abdominal cramps, diarrhea, hepatic dysfunction, hepatitis, nausea, steatorrhea
**GU:** Albuminuria, anuria, priaprism, red-orange urine, renal tubular necrosis
**HEME:** Agranulocytosis, anemia, atypical mononuclear cells, eosinophilia, hemorrhage, leukocytosis, leukopenia, RBC aplasia, thrombocytopenia
**SKIN:** Alopecia, exfoliative dermatitis, jaundice, necrosis of the skin and tissues evidenced by gangrene and purple toes, urticaria

## Nursing Considerations
•Watch for PT to become prolonged 6 hours after anisindione administration, although maximum therapeutic effects may take 48 to 72 hours to appear.
•**WARNING** Watch for signs of overanticoagulation, such as microscopic hematuria, excessive menstrual bleeding, melena, petechiae, and bleeding from superficial trauma, such as tooth brushing or shaving.
•Monitor INR, CBC, fecal occult blood test, and urinalysis results for signs of overanticoagulation.

**PATIENT TEACHING**
•Advise patient to avoid alcohol, salicylates, and drastic changes in his intake of vitamin K–rich food.
•Instruct patient to promptly report pregnancy to prescriber.
•Provide patient with a list of vitamin K–rich food. Advise him to eat consistent daily amounts of vitamin K.
•Counsel patient to consult prescriber before undergoing dental work or elective surgery.
•Urge patient to notify prescriber immediately if he develops unusual bleeding, bruising, red or red-orange urine, red or tarry black stools, diarrhea, bleeding from gums or nose, or excessive bleeding from minor cuts or scratches.

# anistreplase
## (anisoylated plasminogen-streptokinase activator complex)
Eminase

## Class and Category
*Chemical:* p-Anisoylated derivative of the Lys-plasminogen-streptokinase activator complex
*Therapeutic:* Thrombolytic enzyme
*Pregnancy category:* C

## Indications and Dosages
➤ *To treat acute MI, lyse thrombi obstructing coronary arteries, reduce infarct size, improve ventricular function after acute MI, reduce mortality from acute MI*
**I.V. INFUSION**
**Adults.** 30 U injected over 2 to 5 min.

| Route | Onset | Peak | Duration |
|-------|-------|------|----------|
| I.V. | Immediate | 20 min to 2 hr | 4 to 6 hr |

## Mechanism of Action

Indirectly promotes the conversion of plasminogen to plasmin, an enzyme that breaks down fibrin clots, fibrinogen, and other plasma proteins, including procoagulant factors V and VIII.

## Incompatibilities

Don't add other drugs to anistreplase solution or infuse other drugs through same I.V. line.

## Contraindications

Active internal bleeding, arteriovenous malformation or aneurysm, bleeding diathesis, history of CVA, hypersensitivity to anistreplase or streptokinase, intracranial neoplasm, intracranial or intraspinal surgery or trauma within past 2 months, severe uncontrolled hypertension

## Interactions

**DRUGS**

aspirin, dipyridamole, and other drugs that alter platelet function; heparin; vitamin K antagonists: Possibly increased risk of bleeding if administered before anistreplase

## Adverse Reactions

**CNS:** Dizziness, fever, headache, intracranial hemorrhage
**CV:** Ankle edema, arrhythmias (especially accelerated idioventricular rhythm, conduction disorders, premature ventricular beats, sinus bradycardia, ventricular fibrillation, ventricular tachycardia), hypotension, vasculitis
**EENT:** Epistaxis
**GI:** Abdominal pain or swelling, constipation, GI bleeding, nausea, vomiting
**GU:** Hematuria, proteinuria, vaginal bleeding
**HEME:** Bleeding tendency, eosinophilia, mild to severe hemorrhage
**MS:** Arthralgia, back pain, joint stiffness, myalgia
**RESP:** Bronchospasm, dyspnea, hemoptysis
**SKIN:** Flushing, pruritus, rash, urticaria
**Other:** Anaphylaxis (rare), angioedema

## Nursing Considerations

•Use anistreplase cautiously in patients with acute pericarditis; cerebrovascular disease; hemorrhagic ophthalmic conditions; history of major surgery, GI or GU bleeding, or trauma within past 10 days; hypertension; mitral stenosis with atrial fibrillation; pregnancy; septic thrombophlebitis; severe hepatic or renal disease; or subacute bacterial endocarditis.
•Reconstitute anistreplase by slowly directing 5 ml of sterile water for injection USP or sodium chloride for injection against side of vial. Then gently roll vial to mix dry powder and fluid and minimize foaming. Don't shake vial. The resulting solution should be colorless to pale yellow and transparent.
•Before administering, inspect solution for particles and discoloration. If present, discard and reconstitute drug from a new vial. Then withdraw entire contents of vial. Don't dilute reconstituted solution further before administration or add it to I.V. fluid. Don't add other drugs to vial or syringe that contains anistreplase. Discard drug if it isn't administered within 30 minutes after reconstitution.
•For maximum effectiveness, expect to administer anistreplase as soon as possible after onset of MI symptoms.
•Closely monitor all puncture sites, such as catheter insertion and needle puncture sites, for bleeding.
•Don't give I.M. injections, and avoid handling patient unnecessarily during anistreplase therapy. Perform venipuncture only when necessary.
•If an arterial puncture is needed after anistreplase administration, use an arm vessel that allows easy manual compression. Apply a pressure dressing afterward and check puncture site frequently for bleeding.
•Use continuous cardiac monitoring because arrhythmias may occur during reperfusion. Keep antiarrhythmics on hand during anistreplase therapy, and manage arrhythmias according to facility policy.
•Keep epinephrine nearby to treat anaphylaxis.
•Know that anistreplase may be less effective if it's given more than 5 days after anistreplase or streptokinase administration. This occurs because patient may have developed antistreptokinase antibodies, which makes him more resistant to the drug and drug therapy less effective. Elevated serum antistreptokinase antibody levels and reduced drug effectiveness can persist for 5 days to 12 months.

•Closely monitor blood coagulation test results. The drug markedly decreases plasminogen and fibrinogen levels and increases thrombin time, APTT, and PT.

**PATIENT TEACHING**
•Instruct patient to report adverse reactions immediately, especially bleeding, dizziness, and chest pain.

# antihemophilic factor (recombinant), plasma/albumin-free method (rAHF-PFM)

Advate

## Class and Category
*Chemical:* Recombinant protein
*Therapeutic:* Antihemophilic factor
*Pregnancy category:* C

## Indications and Dosages
➤ *To prevent and control bleeding episodes in patients with hemophilia A, in patients with Factor VIII inhibitors not exceeding 10 Bethesda Units/ml*
**I.V. INJECTION**
**Adults and children.** Highly individualized. *For early hemarthrosis, muscle bleeding episode, or mild oral bleeding episode:* Dose administered to achieve peak post-infusion Factor VIII activity in blood (determined by multiplying dose administered/kg body weight by 2) between 20% and 40% of normal with infusions q 12 to 24 hr for 1 to 3 days until bleeding episode resolved. *For more extensive hemarthrosis, muscle bleeding episode, or hematoma:* Dose administered to achieve peak post-infusion Factor VIII activity in blood between 30% to 60% of normal with infusions q 12 to 24 hr for 3 or more days until pain and disability are resolved. *For life-threatening bleeding episodes:* Dose administered to achieve peak post-infusion Factor VIII activity in blood between 60% and 100% with infusions q 8 to 24 hr until bleeding episode stops.

➤ *To prevent and control perioperative bleeding in patients with hemophilia A*
**I.V. INJECTION**
**Adults and children.** Highly individualized. *For minor surgery, including tooth extrac-*

*tion:* Dose administered to achieve peak post-infusion Factor VIII activity in blood (determined by multiplying dose administered/kg body weight by 2) between 60% and 100% of normal, given as a single bolus infusion within 1 hr of operation, with optional additional dose q 12 to 24 hr, as needed. *For major surgery:* Dose administered to achieve peak post-infusion Factor VIII activity in blood between 80% to 100% pre- and postoperatively with infusions q 8 to 24 hr.

| Route | Onset | Peak | Duration |
|-------|-------|------|----------|
| I.V. | Immediate | 5 min | Unknown |

## Mechanism of Action
Provides supplemental Factor VIII, the coagulation factor required for blood to clot that is missing in patients with hemophilia A and diminished in patients with Factor VIII inhibitors. After blood clots, bleeding stops.

## Contraindications
Life-threatening, immediate hypersensitivity reactions, including anaphylaxis, experienced with prior administration of drug or exposure to mouse or hamster proteins

## Interactions
**DRUGS**
None reported.

## Adverse Reactions
**CNS:** Dizziness, fever, headache, rigidity
**CV:** Chest pain
**EENT:** Taste perversion
**GI:** Abdominal pain, diarrhea, nausea
**HEME:** Bleeding tendency, decreased coagulation factor VIII, decreased hematocrit, hematoma, hemolytic anemia
**MS:** Joint swelling, lower limb edema
**RESP:** Dyspnea
**SKIN:** Diaphoresis, pruritus
**Other:** Anaphylaxis, catheter-related infection, hot flashes

## Nursing Considerations
•Check to confirm that clotting defect is Factor VIII deficiency before administering antihemophilic factor (recombinant) because drug isn't effective in treating other coagulation factor deficiencies.

•Reconstitute drug using sterile water for injection. Bring both drug and diluent to room temperature, then clean stoppers with antiseptic solution and allow to dry. Remove protective covering from one end of double-ended needle and insert through center of diluent stopper. Remove protective covering from other end of double-ended needle. Invert diluent bottle over upright drug bottle, then rapidly insert free end of needle through drug stopper at center. The vacuum in bottle will draw in the diluent. Then disconnect the two bottles by removing needle from diluent bottle stopper and remove the needle from drug bottle. Swirl gently until all of drug is dissolved. Avoid shaking to prevent foaming and degradation of drug. Administer in a separate line within 3 hours of reconstitution.

•Take patient's pulse before and periodically during drug administration. If pulse rate increases significantly during administration, reduce administration rate or temporarily halt the injection to allow pulse rate to return to pre-administration level before resuming administration.

•To administer, use only plastic material because protein in drug will adhere to glass. Attach filter needle to syringe and draw back plunger to draw air into syringe. Insert needle into reconstituted drug vial. Inject air into bottle and then withdraw drug from vial. Remove and discard filter needle from syringe, attach a suitable needle, and inject I.V. bolus at a rate no greater than10 ml/min over no more than 5 min.

•Monitor patient's plasma Factor VIII levels during and after treatment to ensure adequate levels have been reached and are being maintained, as ordered.

•Monitor patient for anaphylaxis and have emergency equipment nearby.

•After giving drug, monitor patient for the formation of neutralizing antibodies to Factor VIII, a known complication in the treatment of hemophilia A that may be exhibited by continued bleeding. Obtain laboratory analysis to detect the neutralizing antibodies, as ordered.

•Monitor patients with blood types A, B, and AB for hemolysis when giving large doses.

**PATIENT TEACHING**

•Teach patient and caregivers how to administer drug at home in an emergency situation.

•Instruct patient to discontinue drug and seek emergency help immediately if he has an acute allergic reaction, such as hives, chest tightness, wheezing, low blood pressure, or fainting during or after drug administration.

# antithrombin III, human
## (AT-III, heparin co-factor I)
ATnativ, Thrombate III

### Class and Category
*Chemical:* Alpha$_2$-globulin
*Therapeutic:* Anticoagulant, antithrombotic
*Pregnancy category:* C

### Indications and Dosages
➤ *To treat patients with hereditary antithrombin III (AT-III) deficiency who are undergoing surgery or obstetric procedures or who have thromboembolism*

**I.V. INJECTION**
**Adults and children.** *Initial:* Individualized dosage (based on weight, degree of AT-III deficiency, and desired level of AT-III to be achieved) sufficient to increase AT-III activity to 120% of normal, administered at 50 to 100 IU/min. *Maintenance:* Individualized dosage sufficient to keep AT-III activity at 80% or more of normal, administered q 24 hr, continued for 2 to 8 days, depending on the patient's condition and history and prescriber's judgment. A pregnant, immobilized, or postsurgical patient may need more prolonged therapy.

| Route | Onset | Peak | Duration |
|-------|-------|------|----------|
| I.V. | Immediate | Unknown | 4 days |

### Mechanism of Action
Inhibits blood coagulation by inactivating thrombin; activated forms of factors IX, X, XI, and XII; and plasmin.

### Contraindications
None known

### Interactions
**DRUGS**
*heparin:* Enhanced anticoagulant effect

### Adverse Reactions
**CNS:** Chills, dizziness, fever, light-headedness

**CV:** Chest pain or tightness, hypotension, vasodilation
**EENT:** Unpleasant taste
**GI:** Abdominal cramps, bowel fullness, nausea
**GU:** Diuresis
**HEME:** Hematoma
**RESP:** Dyspnea
**SKIN:** Oozing lesions, urticaria

## Nursing Considerations
•Reconstitute AT-III with 10 ml of sterile water for injection (provided by manufacturer) or alternate solution, such as NS or $D_5W$ injection. *Don't* shake vial during reconstitution. Let solution come to room temperature before administration. If desired, dilute reconstituted solution further, using same diluent.
•WARNING Don't use diluent that contains benzyl alcohol to reconstitute AT-III for a neonate. This can cause a fatal toxic syndrome with metabolic acidosis, CNS depression, respiratory problems, renal failure, hypotension, seizures, and intracranial hemorrhage.
•Don't refrigerate reconstituted solution. Use it within 3 hours; discard unused solution.
•Administer AT-III alone. Don't mix it with other drugs or solutions.
•If after 30 minutes the initial dose doesn't increase AT-III activity to 120% of normal, expect the prescriber to increase the dosage.
•If patient requires a dosage increase, monitor AT-III activity more frequently and expect to adjust dosage accordingly.
•To avoid bleeding, anticipate a reduction in heparin dosage during AT-III therapy.
•If mild adverse reactions occur, decrease infusion rate, as prescribed. If severe reactions occur, discontinue infusion, as prescribed, until they subside.
•Evaluate serum AT-III level twice daily until dosage is stabilized. After that, evaluate level once daily, just before a dose.
PATIENT TEACHING
•Tell patient that blood will be drawn periodically to guide AT-III dosage adjustments.

# apomorphine hydrochloride

Apokyn

## Class and Category
*Chemical:* Nonergoline dopamine agonist

*Therapeutic:* Hypomobilic antiparkinsonian
*Pregnancy category:* C

## Indications and Dosages
➤ *To treat hypomobility "off" episodes (end-of-dose wearing off and unpredictable on/off episodes) in advanced Parkinson's disease*
S.C. INJECTION
**Adults.** *Initial:* 0.2 ml (2 mg) p.r.n. Dosage adjusted as needed in 0.1-ml (1-mg) increments q few days. *Maximum:* 0.6 ml (6 mg).
DOSAGE ADJUSTMENT For patients who tolerate 0.2 ml (2 mg) but have no response, a 0.4-ml (4-mg) dose may be given under medical supervision, with standing and supine blood pressure checked every 20 minutes for 1 hour at the next observed "off" period, as long as it is at least 2 hours after the initial 0.2-ml (2-mg) test dose was given. If tolerated, a dose 0.1 ml (1 mg) lower may be given p.r.n. and increased in 0.1-ml (1-mg) increments q few days as needed to a maximum dose of 0.6 ml (6 mg).
  If patient doesn't tolerate a 0.4-ml (4-mg) test dose, a 0.3-ml (3-mg) test dose may be given under medical supervision, with standing and supine blood pressure checked every 20 minutes for 1 hour at the next observed "off" period, as long as it is at least 2 hours after the initial 0.4-ml (4-mg) test dose was given. If tolerated, a 0.2-ml (2-mg) dose can be started p.r.n. and increased no higher than 0.3 ml (3 mg) if needed after a few days.
  For patients with mild to moderate renal impairment, the initial dose should be reduced to 0.1 ml (1 mg).

| Route | Onset | Peak | Duration |
|-------|-------|------|----------|
| S.C. | 10 to 60 min | Unknown | Unknown |

## Mechanism of Action
Probably stimulates postsynaptic dopamine D2 receptors in the caudate-putamen of the brain. As a result, apomorphine improves motor function and activity levels in patients with Parkinson's disease.

## Contraindications
Concurrent therapy with $5HT_3$ antagonists, such as alosetron, dolasetron, granisetron, ondansetron, and palonosetron; hypersensi-

tivity to apomorphine or its components, including sodium metabisulfite

## Interactions
**DRUGS**
*5HT₃ antagonists:* Increased risk of profound hypotension and loss of consciousness
*antihypertensives, vasodilators:* Increased risk of serious adverse reactions, such as hypotension, MI, and bone or joint injuries
*dopamine antagonists (such as butyrophenones, metoclopramide, phenothiazines, thioxanthenes):* Decreased apomorphine effectiveness
*drugs that prolong QT interval:* Increased risk of torsades de pointes
*entacapone, tolcapone:* Increased risk of tachycardia, hypertension, and arrhythmias
**ACTIVITIES**
*alcohol use:* Increased risk of hypotension

## Adverse Reactions
**CNS:** Aggravated Parkinson's disease, anxiety, confusion, depression, dizziness, drowsiness, dyskinesia, euphoria, fatigue, hallucinations, headache, insomnia, somnolence, weakness, yawning
**CV:** Angina, chest pain, congestive heart failure, edema, MI, orthostatic hypotension, prolonged QT interval
**EENT:** Rhinorrhea
**GI:** Constipation, diarrhea, nausea, vomiting
**GU:** UTI
**MS:** Arthralgia, back or limb pain
**RESP:** Dyspnea, pneumonia, tachypnea
**SKIN:** Contact dermatitis, diaphoresis, ecchymosis, flushing, pallor
**Other:** Dehydration; injection site bruising, granuloma, or pruritus

## Nursing Considerations
• Use apomorphine cautiously in patients with hepatic or renal insufficiency.
• Be aware that an antiemetic, such as trimethobenzamide 300 mg t.i.d., should be started 3 days before apomorphine therapy starts and continue for at least the first 2 months of therapy. Apomorphine may cause severe nausea and vomiting, even with an antiemetic.
• Monitor patient's blood pressure closely because apomorphine can cause severe orthostatic hypotension.
• Administer a 0.2-ml (2-mg) test dose of apomorphine, as prescribed, and then monitor patient's supine and standing blood pressure 20, 40, and 60 minutes later.
• Monitor patient closely if he has an increased risk of prolonged QT interval, as from hypokalemia, hypomagnesemia, bradycardia, use of certain drugs, or genetic predisposition. QT prolongation may lead to torsades de pointes.
• Monitor patient for evidence of abuse. Although rare, drug may cause psychosexual stimulation and increased libido, which may cause patient to use it more often than needed for Parkinson's disease symptoms.
**PATIENT TEACHING**
• Tell patient that an antiemetic will be prescribed starting three days before first apomorphine dose. Instruct patient to take the antiemetic exactly as prescribed. Explain that it will be needed for 2 months or longer during apomorphine therapy.
• Explain that a test dose will be needed to determine response and drug's effects on blood pressure before patient can go home with drug.
• Teach patient how to use dosing pen and how to give drug subcutaneously.
• Emphasize that apomorphine doses are expressed as milliliters, not milligrams. Tell patient to draw up each dose carefully to reduce the chance of dosage error.
• Instruct patient to rotate injection sites in a systematic manner.
• Stress importance of taking apomorphine only as prescribed because serious adverse reactions may occur.
• Advise patient to avoid potentially hazardous activities until drug's CNS effects are known. In particular, caution patient that apomorphine increases the risk of falling asleep suddenly, without feeling sleepy.

# aprepitant
Emend

## Class and Category
*Chemical:* Substance P/neurokinin 1 (NK1) receptor antagonist
*Therapeutic:* Antiemetic
*Pregnancy category:* B

## Indications and Dosages
➤ *To prevent acute and delayed nausea and vomiting associated with highly emetogenic chemotherapy, including high-dose cisplatin*

CAPSULES

**Adults.** 125 mg 1 hr before chemotherapy treatment, followed by 80 mg q.d. in morning on next 2 days.

| Route | Onset | Peak | Duration |
|-------|-------|------|----------|
| P.O. | Unknown | 4 hr | Unknown |

**Mechanism of Action**

Crosses the blood–brain barrier to occupy brain NK1 receptors, which prevents nerve transmission of signals that cause nausea and vomiting.

**Contraindications**

Hypersensitivity to aprepitant or its components; use of astemizole, cisapride, pimozide, or terfenadine

**Interactions**

DRUGS

*carbamazepine, phenytoin, rifampin:* Possibly decreased blood aprepitant level
*corticosteroids:* Increased blood corticosteroid level
*CYP2C9 metabolizers (such as phenytoin, tolbutamide, and warfarin):* Decreased blood level and effectiveness of CYP2C9 metabolizers
*CYP3A4 inhibitors (such as clarithromycin, diltiazem, itraconazole, ketoconazole, nefazodone, nelfinavir, and troleandomycin):* Increased blood aprepitant level
*CYP3A4 substrates (such as astemizole, benzodiazepines, cisapride, docetaxel, etoposide, ifosfamide, imatinib, irinotecan, paclitaxel, pimozide, terfenadine, vinblastine, vincristine, and vinorelbine):* Increased blood level of CYP3A4 substrates, resulting in possibly serious or life-threatening adverse reactions
*oral contraceptives:* Possibly decreased effectiveness of oral contraceptives
*paroxetine:* Possibly decreased blood level of both drugs

**Adverse Reactions**

**CNS:** Anxiety, asthenia, confusion, depression, dizziness, fatigue, fever, headache, insomnia, malaise, peripheral or sensory neuropathy, somnolence
**CV:** Deep vein thrombosis, edema, hypertension, hypotension, tachycardia

**EENT:** Increased salivation, mucous membrane alteration, nasal discharge, pharyngitis, taste perversion, tinnitus, vocal disturbance
**ENDO:** Hyperglycemia
**GI:** Abdominal pain, anorexia, constipation, diarrhea, dysphagia, elevated liver function test results, epigastric discomfort, flatulence, gastritis, gastroesophageal reflux, heartburn, hiccups, nausea, obstipation, vomiting
**GU:** Dysuria, elevated BUN and serum creatinine levels, hematuria, leukocyturia, renal insufficiency
**HEME:** Anemia, febrile neutropenia, leukocytosis, thrombocytopenia
**MS:** Muscle weakness, myalgia, pelvic pain
**RESP:** Cough, dyspnea, non–small-cell lung carcinoma, pneumonitis, pulmonary embolism, respiratory insufficiency, respiratory tract infection
**SKIN:** Alopecia, diaphoresis, flushing, rash
**Other:** Dehydration, hypokalemia, hyponatremia, malignant neoplasm, septic shock, weight loss

**Nursing Considerations**

•Use caution when giving aprepitant to patients with severe hepatic insufficiency because drug's effects on such patients aren't known.
•For maximum antiemetic effects, expect to administer aprepitant with dexamethasone and a 5-HT₃ antagonist, such as dolasetron, granisetron, or ondansetron.

PATIENT TEACHING

•Instruct patient to take 125-mg dose of aprepitant 1 hour before chemotherapy and 80-mg dose in the morning for 2 days after chemotherapy.
•Inform female patients taking oral contraceptives to use alternative or backup method of contraception because drug reduces effectiveness of oral contraceptives.
•Tell patient taking warfarin regularly to have his clotting status monitored closely for 2 weeks after the first dose of aprepitant, especially every 7 to 10 days during each chemotherapy cycle in which the drug is used.
•Caution patient to inform prescriber of any drugs he's taking, including OTC drugs and herbal preparations, because they may interact with aprepitant.

# aprotinin

Trasylol

## Class and Category

*Chemical:* Protease inhibitor
*Therapeutic:* Antifibrinolytic
*Pregnancy category:* B

## Indications and Dosages

➤ *To reduce blood loss and the need for blood transfusion in patients undergoing repeat coronary artery bypass graft surgery and for those undergoing first-time surgery who are at high risk for bleeding or when blood transfusion is unavailable or unacceptable*

**I.V. INFUSION**

**Adults.** *High-dose regimen:* Test dose of 10,000 KIU (kallikrein inactivator units, 1 ml) 10 min before initial dose. If test dose is tolerated, 2,000,000 KIU (200 ml) given over 20 to 30 min followed by maintenance dosage of 500,000 KIU/hr (50 ml/hr). To the priming fluid of the cardiopulmonary bypass circuit (pump prime dose), 2,000,000 KIU (200 ml) is added. *Low-dose regimen:* Test dose of 10,000 KIU (1 ml) 10 min before initial dose. If test dose is tolerated, 1,000,000 KIU (100 ml) given over 20 to 30 min followed by maintenance dosage of 250,000 KIU/hr (25 ml/hr). Pump prime dose of 1,000,000 KIU (100 ml) is added to priming fluid.

## Incompatibilities

Don't administer aprotinin with corticosteroids, heparin, tetracyclines, or nutrient solutions that contain amino acids or fat emulsions. Don't administer I.V. aprotinin through same I.V. line as any other drug; use a different I.V. line or catheter.

---

### Mechanism of Action

Reduces bleeding, possibly by affecting plasmin and kallikrein, which prevents fibrinolysis and may inhibit the early phase of the intrinsic clotting cascade. Aprotinin also increases the resistance of platelets to damage from elevated plasmin levels and mechanical injury during cardiopulmonary bypass.

---

## Contraindications

Hypersensitivity to aprotinin

## Interactions

**DRUGS**

*captopril:* Reduced antihypertensive effect
*fibrinolytics (such as anistreplase and streptokinase):* Inhibited fibrinolysis
*heparin:* Prolonged activated clotting time

## Adverse Reactions

**CNS:** Confusion, fever
**CV:** Arrhythmias, cardiac arrest, heart failure, hypertension, hypotension, increased CK level, MI, pericarditis, peripheral edema, shock
**ENDO:** Hyperglycemia
**GI:** Diarrhea, elevated liver function test results, nausea, vomiting
**GU:** Renal failure, UTI
**HEME:** Leukocytosis, thrombocytopenia
**RESP:** Apnea, asthma, dyspnea, pleural effusion, pneumonia, pneumothorax
**Other:** Anaphylaxis, infection, sepsis

## Nursing Considerations

• Administer aprotinin cautiously to patient with multiple allergies or history of previous aprotinin treatments. Also use drug cautiously in patient undergoing deep hypothermic circulatory arrest, especially one older than age 65.
• If aprotinin is cloudy or contains precipitate or particles, discard it and obtain a new vial.
• Use aprotinin immediately after opening vial. Discard unused portion.
• To reduce risk of anaphylaxis, expect to administer an $H_1$-receptor antagonist, such as diphenhydramine, shortly before giving a loading dose of aprotinin to patient who has received aprotinin previously.
• Give aprotinin through a central line.
• After anesthesia induction and before sternotomy, expect the initial aprotinin dose to be given with patient in supine position. Maintenance dosage is given by constant infusion until patient leaves operating room. Before cardiopulmonary bypass begins, the pump prime dose is added to priming fluid of cardiopulmonary bypass circuit by replacing an aliquot of priming fluid with aprotinin.
• If anaphylaxis occurs, discontinue aprotinin immediately and notify prescriber. Then administer oxygen and I.V. epinephrine, antihistamine, and corticosteroid, as prescribed, and maintain a patent airway.

**PATIENT TEACHING**

• Inform patient that he'll receive aprotinin during surgery and explain its purpose.

# argatroban

Acova

## Class and Category
*Chemical:* N2-substituted derivative of arginine
*Therapeutic:* Anticoagulant
*Pregnancy category:* B

## Indications and Dosages
➤ *To prevent or treat thrombosis in patients with heparin-induced thrombocytopenia (HIT)*

**I.V. INFUSION**
**Adults.** 2 mcg/kg/min as a continuous infusion. *Maximum:* 10 mcg/kg/min.
**DOSAGE ADJUSTMENT** Dosage adjusted as prescribed to maintain patient's APTT at 1.5 to 3 times the initial baseline value, not to exceed 100 sec. Initial dosage reduced to 0.5 mcg/kg/min for patients with moderate hepatic impairment.

➤ *To prevent or treat thrombosis in patients with or at risk for HIT when undergoing percutaneous coronary interventions (PCI)*

**I.V. INFUSION**
**Adults.** *Initial:* 350 mcg/kg over 3 to 5 min followed by a continuous infusion of 25 mcg/kg/min.
**DOSAGE ADJUSTMENT** Dosage adjusted as prescribed to maintain therapeutic activated clotting time (ACT) between 300 and 450 sec. If ACT is less than 300 sec, give additional I.V. bolus dose of 150 mcg/kg and increase infusion to 30 mcg/kg/min; if ACT is greater than 450 sec, reduce dosage to 15 mcg/kg/min. For dissection, impending abrupt closure, thrombus formation during PCI, or inability to achieve or maintain ACT greater than 300 sec, administer additional bolus dose of 150 mcg/kg and increase infusion to 40 mcg/kg/min.

| Route | Onset | Peak | Duration |
|-------|-------|------|----------|
| I.V. | Immediate | 3 to 4 hr | Unknown |

## Mechanism of Action
Forms a tight bond with thrombin, neutralizing this enzyme's actions, even when the enzyme is trapped within clots. Thrombin causes fibrinogen to convert to fibrin, which is essential for clot formation.

## Contraindications
Active major bleeding, hypersensitivity to argatroban or its components

## Interactions
**DRUGS**
*alteplase, antineoplastic drugs, antiplatelets, antithymocyte globulin, heparin, NSAIDs, reteplase, salicylates, streptokinase, strontium chloride Sr 89, warfarin:* Increased risk of bleeding
*porfimer:* Possibly decreased efficacy of porfimer photodynamic therapy

## Adverse Reactions
**CNS:** Cerebrovascular bleeding, fever, headache
**CV:** Atrial fibrillation, cardiac arrest, hypotension, unstable angina, ventricular tachycardia
**GI:** Abdominal pain, anorexia, diarrhea, elevated liver function test results, GI bleeding, melena, nausea, vomiting
**GU:** Elevated BUN and serum creatinine levels, hematuria (microscopic), UTI
**HEME:** Hypoprothrombinemia, unusual bleeding or bruising
**RESP:** Cough, dyspnea, hemoptysis, pneumonia
**SKIN:** Bleeding at puncture site, rash
**Other:** Sepsis

## Nursing Considerations
•**WARNING** Be aware that argatroban isn't recommended for PCI patients with significant hepatic disease or AST/ALT levels greater than or equal to three times the upper limits of normal.
•Reconstitute drug to 1 mg/ml before giving.
•Protect solution from direct sunlight.
•**WARNING** Monitor patients with thrombocytopenia or those receiving daily doses of salicylates greater than 6 g for signs and symptoms of bleeding because they're at increased risk of bleeding from hypoprothrombinemia.
•**WARNING** Expect to perform blood coagulation tests before and 2 hours after start of therapy because of the major risk of bleeding associated with argatroban. Be aware that coagulopathy must be ruled out before therapy is initiated. When giving drug to a patient undergoing PCI, expect to check ACT 5 to 10 minutes after each bolus and each infusion rate change and every 20 to 30 minutes during the PCI.
•Monitor the following patients for signs and symptoms of bleeding because they're at increased risk during argatroban therapy:

females with active menstruation; patients with vascular or organ abnormalities, such as severe uncontrolled hypertension, advanced renal disease, infective endocarditis, dissecting aortic aneurysm, diverticulitis, hemophilia, hepatic disease (especially if associated with a deficiency of vitamin K–dependent clotting factors), inflammatory bowel disease, or peptic ulcer disease; and those who have recently had a CVA, major surgery (including eye, brain, or spinal cord surgery), large vessel puncture or organ biopsy, lumbar puncture, spinal anesthesia, or major bleeding (including intracranial, GI, intraocular, retroperitoneal, or pulmonary bleeding).

• Whenever possible, avoid I.M. injections in patients receiving argatroban to decrease the risk of bleeding.

• Be aware that thrombin times may not be helpful for monitoring argatroban activity because the drug affects all thrombin-dependent coagulation tests.

• Expect drug dosage to be tapered before discontinuation to prevent the risk of rebound hypercoagulopathy; drug's effects last for only a short time once drug is discontinued.

**PATIENT TEACHING**

• Inform patient that argatroban is a blood thinner that's administered in the hospital by infusion into a vein. If he requires long-term anticoagulation, he'll be switched to another drug before discharge.

• Advise patient to immediately report unusual or unexplained bleeding, such as blood in urine, easy bruising, nosebleeds, tarry stools, and vaginal bleeding.

• Instruct patient to avoid injury while receiving argatroban. For example, suggest that he brush his teeth gently, using a soft-bristled toothbrush, and take special care when flossing.

# aripiprazole

Abilify

## Class and Category

*Chemical:* Dihydrocarbostyril
*Therapeutic:* Atypical antipsychotic
*Pregnancy category:* C

## Indications and Dosages

➤ *To treat schizophrenia*

**ORAL SOLUTION, TABLETS**

**Adults.** *Initial:* 10 or 15 mg q.d. Increased to 30 mg q.d., as needed, with dosage adjustments at 2-wk intervals.

➤ *To treat acute manic and mixed episodes associated with bipolar disorder; to maintain stability in patients with bipolar I disorder who have had a recent manic or mixed episode and who have been stabilized and then maintained for at least 6 weeks*

**ORAL SOLUTION, TABLETS**

**Adults.** *Initial:* 30 mg q.d. Decreased to 15 mg q.d., as prescribed.

**DOSAGE ADJUSTMENT** Dosage reduced to half of normal dose when administered with fluoxetine, itraconazole, ketoconazole, paroxetine, or quinidine. Dosage doubled when administered with carbamazepine.

---

### Mechanism of Action

May produce antipsychotic effects through partial agonist and antagonist actions. Aripiprazole acts as a partial agonist at dopamine—especially $D_2$—receptors and serotonin—especially $5\text{-HT}_{1A}$—receptors. The drug acts as an antagonist at $5\text{-HT}_{2A}$ serotonin receptor sites.

---

## Contraindications

Breast-feeding, hypersensitivity to aripiprazole or its components

## Interactions

**DRUGS**

*anticholinergics:* Increased risk for potentially fatal elevation of body temperature
*carbamazepine and other CYP3A4 inducers:* Possibly increased clearance and decreased blood level of aripiprazole
*CNS depressants:* Increased CNS depression
*fluoxetine, paroxetine, quinidine, and other CYP2D6 inhibitors; ketoconazole and other CYP3A4 inhibitors:* Possibly inhibited elimination and increased blood aripiprazole level

**ACTIVITIES**

*alcohol use:* Increased CNS depression

## Adverse Reactions

**CNS:** Abnormal gait, agitation, akathisia, anxiety, asthenia, cognitive and motor impairment, confusion, CVA (elderly), delusions, depression, dizziness, dream disturbances, extrapyramidal reactions, fever, hallucinations,

headache, hostility, insomnia, intracranial hemorrhage, light-headedness, mania, nervousness, neuroleptic malignant syndrome, paranoia, schizophrenic reaction, seizures, somnolence, suicidal ideation, tardive dyskinesia, transient ischemic attack (elderly), tremor
**CV:** Arrhythmias, bradycardia, cardiopulmonary arrest, chest pain, deep vein thrombosis, elevated serum CK levels, heart failure, hypertension, MI, orthostatic hypotension, peripheral edema, prolonged QT interval, tachycardia
**EENT:** Blurred vision, conjunctivitis, increased salivation, laryngospasm, pharyngitis, rhinitis, sinusitis
**ENDO:** Hyperglycemia
**GI:** Constipation, difficulty swallowing, GI bleeding, indigestion, nausea, vomiting
**GU:** Renal failure, urinary incontinence
**HEME:** Anemia, leukopenia, thrombocytopenia
**MS:** Muscle spasms, myalgia, neck and pelvic pain, neck and limb rigidity
**RESP:** Apnea, aspiration, asthma, cough, dyspnea, pneumonia, pulmonary edema or embolism, respiratory failure
**SKIN:** Diaphoresis, dry skin, ecchymosis, pruritus, rash, ulceration, urticaria
**Other:** Anaphylaxis, angioedema, dehydration, flulike symptoms, heat stroke, weight gain

## Nursing Considerations
•Use cautiously in patients with cardiovascular disease, cerebrovascular disease, or conditions that would predispose them to hypotension. Also use cautiously in those with a history of seizures or with conditions that lower seizure threshold, such as Alzheimer's disease.
•Also use cautiously in elderly patients because of increased risk of serious adverse cerebrovascular effects, such as CVA and transient ischemic attack.
•Be aware that oral solution may be given on a milligram-per-milligram basis in place of tablets up to 25 mg. For example, if patient needs 30 mg of tablet and is switched to oral solution, expect to give 25 mg of solution.
•Monitor patient for difficulty swallowing or excessive somnolence, which could predispose him to accidental injury or aspiration.
•WARNING Be aware that aripiprazole rarely may cause neuroleptic malignant syndrome, tardive dyskinesia, and seizures. Monitor patient closely throughout therapy, and take safety precautions as needed.

•Monitor patient's blood glucose level routinely because aripiprazole may increase risk of hyperglycemia.
**PATIENT TEACHING**
•Advise patient to get up slowly from a lying or sitting position to minimize orthostatic hypotension during aripiprazole therapy.
•Urge patient to avoid alcohol during aripiprazole therapy.
•Instruct patient to avoid hazardous activities until drug's effects are known.
•Caution patient to avoid activities that may suddenly increase his body temperature, such as strenuous exercise or exposure to extreme heat, and to compensate for situations that may lead to dehydration, such as vomiting or diarrhea.
•Instruct patient to inform all prescribers of any drugs he's taking, including OTC drugs, because of a potential for interactions.
•Advise female patient of childbearing age to notify prescriber if she intends to become or suspects that she is pregnant during therapy.
•Instruct diabetic patient taking the oral solution to monitor blood glucose levels closely because each milliliter of solution contains 400 mg of sucrose and 200 mg of fructose.

# aspirin
## (acetylsalicylic acid, ASA)

Ancasal (CAN), Apo-As (CAN), Apo-ASEN (CAN), Arthrinol (CAN), Arthrisin (CAN), Aspergum, Aspirin, Atria S.R. (CAN), Bayer, Easprin, Ecotrin, Ecotrin Maximum Strength, 8-Hour Bayer Time Release, Empirin, Genprin, Maximum Bayer, Norwich Extra-Strength, Novasen (CAN), Sal-Adult (CAN), Sal-Infant (CAN), St. Joseph Children's, Supasa (CAN), Therapy Bayer, ZORprin

## Class and Category
*Chemical:* Salicylate
*Therapeutic:* Anti-inflammatory, antiplatelet, antipyretic, nonopioid analgesic
*Pregnancy category:* D

## Indications and Dosages
➤ *To relieve mild pain or fever*
**CHEWABLE TABLETS, CHEWING GUM, CONTROLLED-RELEASE TABLETS, ENTERIC-COATED TABLETS, SOLUTION, TABLETS, TIMED-RELEASE TABLETS, SUPPOSITORIES**
**Adults and adolescents.** 325 to 650 mg q 4 hr, p.r.n., or 500 mg q 3 hr, p.r.n., or 1,000 mg q 6 hr, p.r.n.

**Children ages 2 to 14.** 10 to 15 mg/kg/dose q 4 hr, p.r.n., up to 80 mg/kg/day.

➤ *To relieve mild to moderate pain from inflammation, as in rheumatoid arthritis and osteoarthritis*

CHEWABLE TABLETS, CHEWING GUM, CONTROLLED-RELEASE TABLETS, ENTERIC-COATED TABLETS, SOLUTION, TABLETS, TIMED-RELEASE TABLETS, SUPPOSITORIES

**Adults and adolescents.** 3.2 to 6 g/day in divided doses. *Maximum:* 6 g/day.
**Children.** 10 to 15 mg/kg/day, up to 80 mg/kg/day, in divided doses q 4 to 6 hr.

➤ *To treat juvenile rheumatoid arthritis*

CHEWABLE TABLETS, CHEWING GUM, CONTROLLED-RELEASE TABLETS, ENTERIC-COATED TABLETS, SOLUTION, TABLETS, TIMED-RELEASE TABLETS, SUPPOSITORIES

**Children.** 60 to 110 mg/kg/day in divided doses q 6 to 8 hr.

➤ *To treat acute rheumatic fever*

CHEWABLE TABLETS, CHEWING GUM, CONTROLLED-RELEASE TABLETS, ENTERIC-COATED TABLETS, SOLUTION, TABLETS, TIMED-RELEASE TABLETS, SUPPOSITORIES

**Adults and adolescents.** 5 to 8 g/day in divided doses.
**Children.** *Initial:* 100 mg/kg/day in divided doses for first 2 wk. *Maintenance:* 75 mg/kg/day in divided doses for next 4 to 6 wk.

➤ *To reduce the risk of recurrent transient ischemic attacks or CVA in men*

CHEWABLE TABLETS, CHEWING GUM, CONTROLLED-RELEASE TABLETS, ENTERIC-COATED TABLETS, SOLUTION, TABLETS, TIMED-RELEASE TABLETS, SUPPOSITORIES

**Adults.** 650 mg b.i.d. or 325 mg q.i.d.

➤ *To reduce severity of or prevent acute MI*

CHEWABLE TABLETS, CHEWING GUM, CONTROLLED-RELEASE TABLETS, ENTERIC-COATED TABLETS, SOLUTION, TABLETS, TIMED-RELEASE TABLETS, SUPPOSITORIES

**Adults.** *Initial:* 160 to 162.5 mg (one-half of a 325-mg tablet or two 80- or 81-mg tablets) as soon as MI is suspected. *Maintenance:* 160 to 162.5 mg/day for 30 days.

➤ *To reduce risk of MI in patients with previous MI or unstable angina*

CHEWABLE TABLETS, CHEWING GUM, CONTROLLED-RELEASE TABLETS, ENTERIC-COATED TABLETS, SOLUTION, TABLETS, TIMED-RELEASE TABLETS, SUPPOSITORIES

**Adults.** 325 mg/day.

## Contraindications

Allergy to tartrazine dye, asthma, bleeding problems (such as hemophilia), hypersensitivity to aspirin or its components, peptic ulcer disease

| Route | Peak | Onset | Duration |
|---|---|---|---|
| P.O. (chewable tablets) | Rapid | Unknown | 1 to 4 hr |
| P.O. (controlled-release) | 5 to 30 min | 1 to 4 hr | 4 to 6 hr |
| P.O. (enteric-coated) | 5 to 30 min | Unknown | 1 to 4 hr |
| P.O. (solution) | 5 to 30 min | 15 to 40 min | 1 to 4 hr |
| P.O. (tablets) | 15 to 30 min | 1 to 2 hr | 4 to 6 hr |
| P.O. (timed-release) | 5 to 30 min | 1 to 4 hr | 4 to 6 hr |
| P.R. | Unknown | Unknown | 4 to 6 hr |

## Mechanism of Action

Blocks the activity of cyclooxygenase, the enzyme necessary for prostaglandin synthesis. Prostaglandins, important mediators in the inflammatory response, cause local vasodilation with swelling and pain. With the blocking of cyclooxygenase and the inhibition of prostaglandins, inflammatory symptoms subside. Pain relief is also achieved by inhibiting prostaglandins because they play a role in pain transmission from the periphery to the spinal cord. Aspirin inhibits platelet aggregation by interfering with the production of thromboxane $A_2$, a substance that stimulates platelet aggregation. Aspirin acts on the heat-regulating center in the hypothalamus and causes peripheral vasodilation, diaphoresis, and heat loss.

## Interactions
**DRUGS**
*ACE inhibitors:* Decreased antihypertensive effect
*activated charcoal:* Decreased aspirin absorption
*antacids, urine alkalinizers:* Decreased aspirin effectiveness
*anticoagulants:* Increased risk of bleeding; prolonged bleeding time
*carbonic anhydrase inhibitors:* Salicylism

*corticosteroids:* Increased excretion and decreased blood level of aspirin
*heparin:* Increased risk of bleeding
*methotrexate:* Increased blood level and decreased excretion of methotrexate, causing toxicity
*nizatidine:* Increased blood aspirin level
*NSAIDs:* Possibly decreased blood NSAID level and increased risk of adverse GI effects
*sulfonylureas:* Possibly enhanced effect of sulfonylureas with large doses of aspirin
*urine acidifiers, such as ammonium chloride and ascorbic acid:* Decreased aspirin excretion
*vancomycin:* Increased risk of ototoxicity
**ACTIVITIES**
*alcohol use:* Increased risk of ulcers

## Adverse Reactions
**CNS:** Confusion, CNS depression
**EENT:** Hearing loss, tinnitus
**GI:** Diarrhea, GI bleeding, heartburn, hepatotoxicity, nausea, stomach pain, vomiting
**HEME:** Decreased blood iron level, leukopenia, prolonged bleeding time, shortened life span of RBCs, thrombocytopenia
**SKIN:** Ecchymosis, rash, urticaria
**Other:** Angioedema, Reye's syndrome, salicylism (dizziness, tinnitus, difficulty hearing, vomiting, diarrhea, confusion, CNS depression, diaphoresis, headache, hyperventilation, and lassitude) with regular use of large doses

## Nursing Considerations
•Don't crush timed-release or controlled-release aspirin tablets unless directed.
•Ask about tinnitus. This reaction usually occurs when blood aspirin level reaches or exceeds maximum for therapeutic effect.
**PATIENT TEACHING**
•**WARNING** Advise parents not to give aspirin to a child or adolescent with chickenpox or flu symptoms because of risk of Reye's syndrome (rare life-threatening reaction characterized by vomiting, lethargy, belligerence, delirium, and coma). Tell them to consult prescriber about alternative drugs.
•Instruct patient to take aspirin with food or after meals because it may cause GI upset if taken on an empty stomach.
•Advise patient with tartrazine allergy not to take aspirin.
•Tell patient to consult prescriber before taking aspirin with any prescription drug for blood disorder, diabetes, gout, or arthritis.
•Tell patient not to use aspirin if it has a strong vinegar-like odor.

# aspirin and dipyridamole
Aggrenox

## Class and Category
*Chemical:* Salicylate (aspirin), pyrimidine (dipyridamole)
*Therapeutic:* Platelet aggregation inhibitor
*Pregnancy category:* Not rated (aspirin D, dipyridamole B)

## Indications and Dosages
➤ *To prevent the recurrence of thromboembolic CVA*
**CAPSULES**
**Adults.** *Initial:* One capsule (25 mg aspirin and 200 mg extended-release dipyridamole) b.i.d.

| Route | Onset | Peak | Duration |
|---|---|---|---|
| P.O. | 1 to 7.5 min* | Unknown | 2 to 2.5 hr* |

### Mechanism of Action
Aspirin inhibits platelet aggregation by interfering with production of thromboxane $A_2$, a substance that stimulates platelet aggregation. Dipyridamole inhibits platelet uptake of adenosine, thus increasing the amount of adenosine in surrounding blood. The increased adenosine acts on platelet $A_2$ receptors, which stimulates the activity of intraplatelet adenylate cyclase. This action in turn increases the level of cyclic adenosine monophosphate in platelets, which decreases platelet activation and aggregation.

## Contraindications
Allergy to NSAIDs or tartrazine dye; hypersensitivity to aspirin, dipyridamole, or their components

## Interactions
**DRUGS (ASPIRIN)**
*ACE inhibitors, beta blockers:* Decreased antihypertensive effect
*acetazolamide:* Increased blood acetazolamide level and risk of toxicity
*activated charcoal:* Decreased aspirin absorption
*antacids, urinary alkalinizers:* Decreased aspirin effectiveness
*carbonic anhydrase inhibitors:* Salicylism
*corticosteroids:* Increased excretion and decreased blood level of aspirin

---

* For aspirin; unknown for dipyridamole.

A

*heparin:* Increased risk of bleeding
*methotrexate:* Increased blood level and decreased excretion rate of methotrexate, causing toxicity
*nizatidine:* Increased blood aspirin level
*NSAIDs:* Possibly decreased blood NSAID level and increased risk of bleeding
*oral anticoagulants:* Increased risk of bleeding; prolonged bleeding time
*phenytoin:* Decreased blood phenytoin level
*sulfonylureas:* Possibly enhanced effect of sulfonylureas with large doses of aspirin
*urinary acidifiers, such as ammonium chloride and ascorbic acid:* Decreased aspirin excretion
*valproic acid:* Increased blood valproic acid level
*vancomycin:* Increased risk of ototoxicity
**DRUGS (DIPYRIDAMOLE)**
*adenosine:* Increased blood adenosine level; potentiated effects of adenosine
*cefamandole, cefoperazone, cefotetan, plicamyin, valproic acid:* Possibly hypoprothrombinemia and increased risk of bleeding
*cholinesterase inhibitors:* Possibly counteracted effects of these drugs and aggravation of myasthenia gravis
*heparin, NSAIDs, thrombolytics:* Possibly increased risk of bleeding
**ACTIVITIES (ASPIRIN)**
*alcohol use:* Increased risk of GI bleeding

## Adverse Reactions
**CNS:** Amnesia, asthenia, headache, seizures, somnolence, syncope
**EENT:** Epistaxis
**GI:** Abdominal pain, anorexia, diarrhea, dyspepsia, esophageal irritation, GI bleeding, hemorrhoids, hepatic impairment, nausea, vomiting
**HEME:** Anemia
**MS:** Arthralgia, arthritis, back pain
**SKIN:** Purpura

## Nursing Considerations
•Be aware that combination drug aspirin and dipyridamole isn't interchangeable with individual aspirin or dipyridamole tablets.
•**WARNING** Monitor patients with severe hepatic impairment for evidence of bleeding, such as easy bruising, tarry stools, and epistaxis. Monitor coagulation test results as appropriate, and notify prescriber immediately about significant changes. These patients already have an increased risk of bleeding, and platelet inhibition increases the risk further.

•Monitor liver function test results as appropriate if patient has hepatic impairment because dipyridamole may increase hepatic enzyme levels and cause hepatic failure.
•Monitor renal function test results, such as GFR, if patient has renal impairment. Because aspirin is excreted by the kidneys, it should be avoided in patients with a GFR below 10 ml/min. Otherwise, patient may develop aspirin toxicity.
•If patient consumes three or more alcoholic beverages daily or has hypoprothrombinemia, peptic ulcer disease, or vitamin K deficiency, monitor him for signs and symptoms of bleeding.
•If patient has coronary artery disease, assess him for chest pain and hypotension because of dipyridamole's vasodilatory effect.
**PATIENT TEACHING**
•Advise patient to swallow capsule whole and not to break, chew, or crush it.
•Instruct patient to take drug with a full glass of water and to not lie down for 15 to 30 minutes to prevent esophageal irritation.
•Warn patient to consult prescriber before taking any drug to treat pain, fever, or arthritis.
•Urge patient not to discontinue drug for any reason without first consulting prescriber.
•Advise patient to notify other health care providers that he takes aspirin and dipyridamole.

# atenolol

Apo-Atenol (CAN), Novo-Atenol (CAN), Tenormin

## Class and Category
*Chemical:* Beta-adrenergic blocker (beta$_1$ and at high doses beta$_2$)
*Therapeutic:* Antianginal, antihypertensive
*Pregnancy category:* D

## Indications and Dosages
➤ *To treat angina pectoris and control hypertension*
**TABLETS**
**Adults.** 50 mg q.d. increased, p.r.n., after 1 to 2 wk to 100 mg/day.

➤ *To treat acute MI*
**TABLETS, I.V. INFUSION**
**Adults.** *Initial:* 5 mg I.V. over 5 min followed by 5 mg I.V. 10 min later. After an additional 10 min, 50 mg given and followed by another 50 mg in 12 hr. *Maintenance:* 50 mg P.O. b.i.d. or 100 mg P.O. q.d. for 6 to 9 days or until discharged from hospital.

**DOSAGE ADJUSTMENT** Dosage reduced to 50 mg/day P.O. for renally impaired patients and elderly, renally impaired patients with creatinine clearance of 15 to 35 ml/min/1.73 m². Dosage reduced to 25 mg/day P.O. for renally impaired patients and elderly, renally impaired patients with creatinine clearance of less than 15 ml/min/1.73 m².

| Route | Onset | Peak | Duration |
|-------|-------|------|----------|
| P.O. | 1 hr | 2 to 4 hr | 24 hr |
| I.V. | Immediate | 5 min | 12 hr |

## Mechanism of Action
Inhibits stimulation of beta$_1$-receptor sites, located primarily in the heart, causing a decrease in cardiac excitability, cardiac output, and myocardial oxygen demand. Atenolol also acts to decrease the release of renin from the kidneys, aiding in reducing blood pressure. At high doses, it inhibits stimulation of beta$_2$ receptors in the lungs, which may cause bronchoconstriction.

## Contraindications
Cardiogenic shock, heart block greater than first degree, hypersensitivity to beta blockers, overt heart failure, sinus bradycardia

## Interactions
**DRUGS**
*calcium channel blockers, such as verapamil and diltiazem:* Possibly symptomatic bradycardia and conduction abnormalities
*catecholamine-depleting drugs, such as reserpine:* Additive antihypertensive effect
*clonidine:* Rebound hypertension

## Adverse Reactions
**CNS:** Depression, disorientation, dizziness, drowsiness, emotional lability, fatigue, fever, lethargy, light-headedness, short-term memory loss, vertigo
**CV:** Arrhythmias, including bradycardia and heart block; cardiogenic shock; cold arms and legs; heart failure; mesenteric artery thrombosis; mitral insufficiency; myocardial reinfarction; orthostatic hypotension; Raynaud's phenomenon
**EENT:** Dry eyes, laryngospasm, pharyngitis
**GI:** Diarrhea, ischemic colitis, nausea
**GU:** Renal failure
**HEME:** Agranulocytosis
**MS:** Leg pain

**RESP:** Bronchospasm, dyspnea, pulmonary emboli, respiratory distress, wheezing
**SKIN:** Erythematous rash
**Other:** Allergic reaction

## Nursing Considerations
•Use atenolol cautiously in patients with heart failure controlled by digitalis glycosides or diuretics. Use it cautiously in patients with conduction abnormalities or left ventricular dysfunction who are receiving verapamil or diltiazem, in those with arterial circulatory disorders, and in those with impaired renal function.
•Use atenolol cautiously in diabetic patients because it may mask tachycardia caused by hypoglycemia. Unlike other beta-adrenergic blockers, it doesn't mask other signs of hypoglycemia, cause hypoglycemia, or delay the return of blood glucose to a normal level.
•At first sign of heart failure, expect patient to receive a digitalis glycoside, a diuretic, or both and to be monitored closely. If failure continues, expect to discontinue atenolol.
•Closely monitor patient with hyperthyroidism because atenolol may mask some signs of thyrotoxicosis. Avoid abrupt withdrawal of atenolol, which may precipitate thyrotoxicosis.
•If patient also receives clonidine, expect to discontinue atenolol several days before gradually withdrawing clonidine. Then expect to restart atenolol therapy several days after clonidine has been discontinued.
•During I.V. atenolol therapy, monitor vital signs and cardiac rhythm closely.
•Discard parenteral mixture with atenolol if it isn't used within 48 hours.
•Stop atenolol therapy and notify prescriber if patient develops bradycardia, hypotension, or other serious adverse reaction.

**PATIENT TEACHING**
•Instruct patient *not* to stop taking atenolol abruptly. Otherwise, angina may worsen and an MI or arrhythmia may occur.
•While patient is being weaned from atenolol, tell him to perform minimal physical activity to prevent chest pain.
•Instruct patient to take a missed dose as soon as possible. However, if it's within 8 hours of the next scheduled dose, tell him to skip the missed dose and return to his regular schedule.
•Inform patient that atenolol may alter his serum glucose level and mask symptoms of hypoglycemia.

A

•Inform the patient that he may experience fatigue and reduced tolerance to exercise and that he should notify his prescriber if this interferes with his normal lifestyle.

# atomoxetine hydrochloride

Strattera

## Class and Catgegory

*Chemical:* Selective norepinephrine reuptake inhibitor
*Therapeutic:* Anti–attention deficit hyperactivity agent
*Pregnancy category:* C

## Indications and Dosages

➤ *To treat attention deficit hyperactivity disorder (ADHD)*

CAPSULES

**Adults and children who weigh 70 kg (154 lb) or less.** *Initial:* 0.5 mg/kg/day, increased after at least 3 days to 1.2 mg/kg/day given either as a single dose in the morning or in evenly divided doses in the morning and late afternoon or early evening, as needed. *Maximum:* 1.4 mg/kg or 100 mg/day, whichever is less.

**Adults and children who weigh more than 70 kg.** *Initial:* 40 mg/day, increased after a minimum of 3 days to 80 mg/day given either as a single dose in the morning or in evenly divided doses in the morning and late afternoon or early evening. After 2 to 4 additional wk, dosage may be increased to 100 mg/day if optimal response hasn't been achieved. *Maximum:* 100 mg/day.

DOSAGE ADJUSTMENT For patients with moderate (Child-Pugh Class B) hepatic impairment, dosage reduced by 50%. For patients with severe (Child-Pugh Class C) impairment, dosage reduced by 75%. For patients weighing 70 kg or less and taking strong CYP2D6 inhibitors, such as paroxetine, fluoxetine, or quinidine, initial dosage of 0.5 mg/kg/day should be increased to 1.2 mg/kg/day only if symptoms fail to improve after 4 wk. For patients weighing more than 70 kg and taking strong CYP2D6 inhibitors, initial dosage of 40 mg/day should be increased to 80 mg/day only if symptoms fail to improve after 4 wk.

## Mechanism of Action

Selectively inhibits presynaptic norepinephrine transport in the nervous system to increase attention span and produce a calming effect.

## Contraindications

Angle-closure glaucoma, hypersensitivity to atomoxetine or its components, use within 14 days of MAO inhibitor therapy

## Interactions

DRUGS

*albuterol and other beta$_2$ agonists:* May potentiate action of albuterol and other beta$_2$ agonists on cardiovascular system
*CYP2D6 inhibitors (such as fluoxetine, paroxetine, and quinidine):* Increased blood atomoxetine level
*MAO inhibitors:* Possibly induced hypertensive crisis
*pressor agents:* Possibly altered blood pressure

## Adverse Reactions

**CNS:** Aggressiveness, crying, depression, dizziness, early morning awakening, fatigue, headache, insomnia, irritability, lethargy, mood changes, paresthesia, peripheral coldness, pyrexia, rigors, sedation, sleep disturbance, somnolence, suicidal ideation (children and adolescents), tremor, unusual dreams
**CV:** Chest pain, hypertension, orthostatic hypotension, palpitations, tachycardia
**EENT:** Dry mouth, ear infection, mydriasis, nasal congestion, nasopharyngitis, pharyngitis, rhinorrhea, sinus congestion
**GI:** Abdominal pain (upper), anorexia, constipation, diarrhea, elevated liver function test results, flatulence, gastroenteritis (viral), indigestion, nausea, severe hepatic dysfunction, vomiting
**GU:** Decreased libido, dysmenorrhea, ejaculation disorders, erectile dysfunction, impotence, menstrual irregularities, orgasm abnormality, prostatitis, urinary hesitancy, urine retention
**MS:** Arthralgia, back pain, myalgia
**RESP:** Cough, upper respiratory tract infection
**SKIN:** Dermatitis, diaphoresis, pruritus, rash, urticaria
**Other:** Angioedema, hot flashes, influenza, weight loss

## Nursing Considerations
- Use atomoxetine cautiously in patients with cerebrovascular or CV disease (especially hypertension or tachycardia) because drug may cause an increase in blood pressure and heart rate. Also use cautiously in those who are prone to orthostatic hypotension.
- **WARNING** Monitor children and adolescents closely for evidence of suicidal thinking and suicidal behavior because atomoxetine increases the risk of suicidal ideation in these age-groups.
- Obtain baseline blood pressure and heart rate before starting therapy. Monitor patient's vital signs after dosage increases and periodically during therapy.
- Monitor patient closely for allergic reactions. If these occur, notify prescriber.
- Monitor child's or adolescent's growth and weight. Expect to interrupt therapy, as prescribed, if patient isn't growing or gaining weight appropriately.
- Monitor patient's liver function studies, as ordered. Notify prescriber immediately if enzyme levels are elevated or patient has signs or symptoms of hepatic dysfunction, such as jaundice, dark urine, pruritus, right-upper-quadrant tenderness, or unexplained flulike symptoms. Expect atomoxetine to be stopped permanently.

**PATIENT TEACHING**
- Instruct patient or parent to immediately report to prescriber any adverse reactions to atomoxetine therapy, such as facial swelling, itching, or rash.
- **WARNING** Urge parents to watch their child or adolescent closely for evidence of abnormal thinking, abnormal behavior, or increased aggression or hostility. If unusual changes occur, stress need to notify prescriber.
- Urge patient to tell prescriber immediately about yellowing of his skin or eyes, itchiness, right upper abdominal pain, dark urine, or flulike symptoms.
- Caution patient to assume sitting or standing position slowly because of drug's potential effect on blood pressure.
- Advise patient to report urinary hesitancy or urine retention to prescriber.
- Remind patient of the importance of alerting all prescribers to any OTC drugs, dietary supplements, or herbal remedies he's taking.
- Caution patient to avoid potentially hazardous activities until drug's CNS effects are known.
- Reassure patient or parent that drug doesn't cause physical or psychological dependence.
- Instruct patient or parent to monitor weight during therapy.

# atorvastatin calcium

Lipitor

## Class and Category
*Chemical:* Synthetically derived fermentation product
*Therapeutic:* Antihyperlipidemic, HMG-CoA reductase inhibitor
*Pregnancy category:* X

## Indications and Dosages
➤ *To control lipid levels as adjunct to diet in primary (heterozygous familial and nonfamilial) hypercholesterolemia and mixed dyslipidemia*

**TABLETS**
**Adults.** *Initial:* 10 or 20 mg once daily, then increased according to lipid level. *Maintenance:* 10 to 80 mg once daily.
**DOSAGE ADJUSTMENT** Initial dose may be increased to 40 mg once daily for patients who need cholesterol level reduced more than 45%.

➤ *To control lipid levels in homozygous familial hypercholesterolemia*

**TABLETS**
**Adults.** 10 to 80 mg/day.

➤ *To control lipid levels in pediatric heterozygous familial hypercholesterolemia*

**TABLETS**
**Adolescents and children ages 10 to 17.** *Initial:* 10 mg/day, adjusted at intervals of 4 wk or more, as needed. *Maximum:* 20 mg/day.

## Contraindications
Active hepatic disease, hypersensitivity to atorvastatin or its components, unexplained persistent rise in serum transaminase level

---

### Mechanism of Action
Reduces plasma cholesterol and lipoprotein levels by inhibiting HMG-CoA reductase and cholesterol synthesis in the liver and by increasing the number of LDL receptors on liver cells to enhance LDL uptake and breakdown.

# Interactions

## DRUGS

*antacid, colestipol:* Possibly decreased blood atorvastatin level

*cyclosporine:* Increased risk of severe myopathy or rhabdomyolysis

*digoxin:* Possibly increased blood digoxin level, causing toxicity

*erythromycin:* Increased blood atorvastatin level

*nicotinic acid:* Increased risk of severe myopathy or rhabdomyolysis

*oral contraceptives (such as ethinyl estradiol and norethindrone):* Increased hormone level

# Adverse Reactions

**CNS:** Abnormal dreams, amnesia, asthenia, emotional lability, facial paralysis, fever, headache, hyperkinesia, lack of coordination, malaise, paresthesia, peripheral neuropathy, somnolence, syncope, weakness

**CV:** Arrhythmias, elevated serum CK level, orthostatic hypotension, palpitations, phlebitis, vasodilation

**EENT:** Amblyopia, altered refraction, dry eyes, dry mouth, epistaxis, eye hemorrhage, gingival hemorrhage, glaucoma, glossitis, hearing loss, lip swelling, loss of taste, pharyngitis, sinusitis, stomatitis, taste perversion, tinnitus

**ENDO:** Hyperglycemia or hypoglycemia

**GI:** Abdominal or biliary pain, anorexia, colitis, constipation, diarrhea, duodenal or stomach ulcers, dysphagia, eructation, esophagitis, flatulence, gastroenteritis, hepatitis, increased appetite, indigestion, melena, pancreatitis, rectal hemorrhage, tenesmus, vomiting

**GU:** Abnormal ejaculation; cystitis; decreased libido; dysuria; epididymitis; hematuria; impotence; nephritis; nocturia; renal calculi; urinary frequency, incontinence, or urgency; urine retention; vaginal hemorrhage

**HEME:** Anemia, thrombocytopenia

**MS:** Arthralgia, back pain, bursitis, gout, leg cramps, myalgia, myasthenia gravis, myositis, neck rigidity, tendon contracture, tenosynovitis, torticollis

**RESP:** Dyspnea, pneumonia

**SKIN:** Acne, alopecia, contact dermatitis, diaphoresis, dry skin, ecchymosis, eczema, jaundice, petechiae, photosensitivity, pruritus, rash, seborrhea, ulceration, urticaria

**Other:** Allergic reaction, facial or generalized edema, flulike symptoms, infection, lymphadenopathy, weight gain

# Nursing Considerations

•Be aware that atorvastatin is used in patients with homozygous familial hypercholesterolemia as an adjunct to other lipid-lowering treatments or alone only if other treatments aren't available.

•Atorvastatin may be used with colestipol or cholestyramine for additive antihyperlipidemic effects.

•Expect atorvastatin to be used in patients without obvious coronary artery disease (CAD) but with multiple risk factors (such as age 55 or older, smoker, history of hypertension or low HDL level, or family history of early CAD). Drug is used to reduce risk of MI, angina, and adverse effects of revascularization procedures.

•Also expect drug to be used in patients with type 2 diabetes who have no obvious CAD but multiple risk factors, such as retinopathy, albuminuria, smoking, or hypertension. Drug is used in these patients to reduce the risk of MI and stroke.

•Expect liver function tests to be performed before atorvastatin therapy starts, after 6 and 12 weeks of therapy, with each dosage increase, and every 6 months thereafter.

•Expect to measure lipid levels 2 to 4 weeks after atorvastatin starts, and adjust dosage as directed. Repeat this process periodically until lipid levels are within desired range.

## PATIENT TEACHING

•Stress that atorvastatin is an adjunct to—not a substitute for—a low-cholesterol diet.

•Tell patient to take drug at the same time each day to maintain its effects.

•Instruct patient to take a missed dose as soon as possible. If it's almost time for his next dose, he should skip the missed dose. Tell him not to double the dose.

•Instruct patient to consult prescriber before taking OTC niacin preparations because of increased risk of rhabdomyolysis.

•Advise patient to notify prescriber immediately if he develops unexplained muscle pain, tenderness, or weakness, especially if accompanied by fatigue or fever.

•Be aware that atorvastatin therapy is expensive. Reinforce the benefits of therapy, and encourage patient to comply if possible.

# atovaquone

Mepron

## Class and Category
*Chemical:* Hydroxy-1,4-naphthoquinone
*Therapeutic:* Antiprotozoal
*Pregnancy category:* C

## Indications and Dosages
➤ *To prevent* Pneumocystis carinii *pneumonia in patients who can't tolerate co-trimoxazole*

**SUSPENSION, TABLETS**
**Adults and adolescents.** 750 mg (5 ml) b.i.d. with meals for 21 days.

➤ *To treat mild to moderate* P. carinii *pneumonia in patients who can't tolerate co-trimoxazole*

**SUSPENSION, TABLETS**
**Adults and adolescents.** 750 mg (5 ml) b.i.d. with meals for 21 days. *Maximum:* 1,500 mg/day.

---

### Mechanism of Action
May destroy *P. carinii* organisms by inhibiting the enzymes needed to synthesize nucleic acid and adenosine triphosphate.

---

## Contraindications
Hypersensitivity to atovaquone or its components

## Interactions
**DRUGS**
*rifabutin, rifampin:* Possibly decreased blood atovaquone level

## Adverse Reactions
**CNS:** Fever, headache, insomnia
**EENT:** Rhinitis
**GI:** Abdominal pain, diarrhea, nausea, vomiting
**HEME:** Anemia
**RESP:** Cough, dyspnea
**SKIN:** Rash
**Other:** Allergic reaction

## Nursing Considerations
•Monitor blood test results because atovaquone may decrease serum sodium and hemoglobin levels and neutrophil count and may increase AST, ALT, alkaline phosphatase, and serum amylase levels.
•Crush atovaquone tablets, if needed.
•Don't use atovaquone tablets and oral suspension interchangeably; they aren't bioequivalent.

**PATIENT TEACHING**
•Instruct patient to take atovaquone with meals for maximum effectiveness.
•Instruct patient to take a missed dose as soon as possible. If it's almost time for the next dose, tell him to skip the missed dose. Tell him not to double the dose.
•Tell patient to notify prescriber if his condition doesn't improve in a few days or if he develops signs of an allergic reaction, such as fever or rash.

# atracurium besylate

Tracrium

## Class and Category
*Chemical:* Biquaternary ammonium ester
*Therapeutic:* Skeletal muscle relaxant
*Pregnancy category:* C

## Indications and Dosages
➤ *To facilitate endotracheal intubation and induce skeletal muscle relaxation for surgery or mechanical ventilation as adjunct to anesthesia*

**I.V. INFUSION OR INJECTION**
**Adults and children age 2 or older.** *Initial:* 0.4 to 0.5 mg/kg by I.V. bolus for nearly complete neuromuscular blockade. *Maintenance:* 0.08 to 0.10 mg/kg 20 to 45 min after initial dose during prolonged surgery. Maintenance doses may be given q 15 to 25 min for patients under balanced anesthesia. For patients undergoing extended surgical procedures, after an initial I.V. bolus, an infusion of 9 to 10 mcg/kg/min may be required to counteract the spontaneous return of neuromuscular function and thereafter 5 to 10 mcg/kg/min as a constant infusion.
**Children ages 1 month to 2 years who are undergoing halothane anesthesia.** *Initial:* 0.3 to 0.4 mg/kg. Frequent maintenance doses may be required.

| Route | Onset | Peak | Duration |
|---|---|---|---|
| I.V. | 2 to 2.5 min | 3 to 5 min | 35 to 70 min |

## Mechanism of Action
Inhibits nerve impulse transmission by competing with acetylcholine for cholinergic receptors on motor end plate.

## Incompatibilities
Don't mix atracurium in same syringe or administer it through same I.V. needle as an alkaline solution, such as a barbiturate injection. Don't mix atracurium with lactated Ringer's injection.

## Contraindications
Hypersensitivity to atracurium, its components, or benzyl alcohol

## Interactions
*aminoglycosides, enflurane, furosemide, halothane, isoflurane, lithium, magnesium salts, polymyxin antibiotics, procainamide, quinidine, thiazide diuretics:* Possibly enhanced or prolonged atracurium effects
*opioid analgesics:* Possibly additive histamine release and increased risk and severity of bradycardia and hypotension

## Adverse Reactions
**CNS:** Seizures
**CV:** Bradycardia, hypertension, hypotension, tachycardia
**MS:** Inadequate or prolonged neuromuscular blockade
**RESP:** Apnea, bronchospasm, dyspnea, laryngospasm, wheezing
**SKIN:** Flushing, rash, urticaria
**Other:** Anaphylaxis, injection site reaction

## Nursing Considerations
•Use atracurium cautiously in patients with hypotension, and monitor blood pressure closely.
•Monitor closely for adverse reactions, especially those associated with histamine release. Be aware that atracurium is more likely than other neuromuscular blockers to cause skin flushing.
•Anticipate using lower doses for patients with neuromuscular disease, severe electrolyte disorders, or carcinomatosis because of risk of enhanced neuromuscular blockade and difficulties with reversal.
•Keep atropine nearby to treat atracurium-induced bradycardia.

•For I.V. infusion, dilute atracurium with NS, D$_5$W, or D$_5$NS. To prepare a solution that yields 200 mcg of atracurium per milliliter, add 2 ml of atracurium to 98 ml of diluent. To prepare a solution that yields 500 mcg per milliliter, add 5 ml of atracurium to 95 ml of diluent.
•Refrigerate solution or store at room temperature for up to 24 hours.
**PATIENT TEACHING**
•Explain atracurium's purpose and administration during anesthesia. Keep in mind that the patient can still hear.

# atropine
AtroPen

# atropine sulfate

## Class and Category
*Chemical:* Belladonna alkaloid
*Therapeutic:* Anticholinergic, antimuscarinic
*Pregnancy category:* C

## Indications and Dosages
➤ *To reduce respiratory tract secretions related to anesthesia*
**TABLETS (ATROPINE SULFATE)**
**Adults.** 0.4 to 0.6 mg preoperatively.
**Children.** 0.01 mg/kg up to total of 0.4 mg preoperatively and repeated q 4 to 6 hr, p.r.n.
**I.V., I.M., OR S.C. INJECTION**
**Adults.** 0.4 to 0.6 mg preoperatively.
**Children.** 0.01 mg/kg up to total of 0.4 mg preoperatively and repeated q 4 to 6 hr, p.r.n.
➤ *To correct bradycardia*
**I.V. INJECTION (ATROPINE SULFATE)**
**Adults.** 0.4 to 1 mg. If no response to first dose, repeat once after 5 min.
**Children.** 0.01 to 0.02 mg/kg with a minimum dose of 0.1 mg and a maximum dose of 0.5 mg. If no response to first dose, repeat once after 5 min.
➤ *To treat cholinesterase inhibitor (such as neostigmine, pilocarpine, and methacholine) toxicity*
**I.V. INJECTION (ATROPINE SULFATE)**
**Adults.** 2 to 4 mg. Then 2 mg q 5 to 10 min until muscarinic signs (bradycardia, vasodilation, and pupil dilation) disappear or signs of atropine intoxication develop.

**I.V. OR I.M. INJECTION (ATROPINE SULFATE)**
**Children.** 1 mg. Then 0.5 to 1.0 mg q 5 to 10 min until muscarinic signs disappear or signs of atropine intoxication develop.

➤ *To treat mushroom (muscarine) toxicity*
**I.V. OR I.M. INJECTION (ATROPINE SULFATE)**
**Adults.** 1 to 2 mg q hr until respiratory signs and symptoms subside.

➤ *To treat pesticide (organophosphate) toxicity*
**I.V. OR I.M. INJECTION (ATROPINE SULFATE)**
**Adults.** 1 to 2 mg, repeated in 20 to 30 min as soon as cyanosis has cleared. Then dosage continued until definite improvement is maintained, possibly for 2 or more days.

➤ *To treat known or suspected exposure to chemical nerve agent or insecticide*
**I.M. INJECTION (ATROPEN)**
**Adults and children weighing over 90 lb (41 kg) with two or more mild symptoms.**
2 mg. If severe symptoms develop afterward, two or more 2-mg injections given in rapid succession 10 min after initial injection.
**Adults and children weighing over 90 lb who are unconscious or have other severe symptoms.** 2 mg given immediately 3 times in rapid succession.
**Children weighing 40 to 90 lb (18 to 41 kg) with two or more mild symptoms.** 1 mg. If severe symptoms develop after injection, two more 1-mg injections given in rapid succession 10 min after initial injection.
**Children weighing 40 to 90 lb who are unconscious or exhibit any other severe symptoms.** 1 mg given immediately 3 times in rapid succession.
**Children weighing 15 to 40 lb (7 to 18 kg) with two or more mild symptoms.** 0.5 mg. If severe symptoms develop after injection, two more 0.5-mg injections given in rapid succession 10 min after initial injection.
**Children weighing 15 to 40 lb who are unconscious or exhibit any other severe symptoms.** 0.5 mg given immediately 3 times in rapid succession.

| Route | Onset | Peak | Duration |
|-------|-------|------|----------|
| P.O. | 30 to 120 min | 1 to 2 hr | 4 to 6 hr |
| I.V. | Immediate | 2 to 4 min | Brief |
| I.M. | 5 to 40 min | 20 to 60 min | Brief Brief |
| S.C. | Unknown | Unknown | Brief |

## Contraindications
Angle-closure glaucoma, asthma, GI obstructive disease (achalasia, pyloric obstruction, pyloroduodenal stenosis), hepatic disease, hypersensitivity to atropine or its components, ileus, intestinal atony, myasthenia gravis, myocardial ischemia, obstructive uropathy, renal disease, severe ulcerative colitis, tachycardia, toxic megacolon, unstable cardiovascular status in acute hemorrhage

## Interactions
**DRUGS**
*adsorbent antidiarrheals, antacids:* Decreased atropine absorption
*amantadine, anticholinergics, antidyskinetics, glutethimide, meperidine, muscle relaxants, phenothiazines, tricyclic antidepressants and other drugs with anticholinergic properties, including antiarrhythmics (disopyramide, procainamide, quinidine), antihistamines, buclizine, meclizine:* Increased atropine effects
*antimyasthenics:* Reduced intestinal motility
*cyclopropane:* Risk of ventricular arrhythmias
*haloperidol:* Decreased antipsychotic effect
*ketoconazole:* Decreased ketoconazole absorption
*metoclopramide:* Decreased effect on GI motility
*opioid analgesics:* Increased risk of ileus, severe constipation, and urine retention
*potassium chloride, especially wax-matrix forms:* Possibly GI ulcers
*urinary alkalizers (calcium or magnesium antacids, carbonic anhydrase inhibitors, citrates, sodium bicarbonate):* Delayed excretion and increased risk of adverse atropine effects

## Mechanism of Action
Inhibits acetylcholine's muscarinic action at the neuroeffector junctions of smooth muscles, cardiac muscles, exocrine glands, SA and AV nodes, and the urinary bladder. In small doses, atropine inhibits salivary and bronchial secretions and diaphoresis. In moderate doses, it increases impulse conduction through the AV node and increases heart rate. In large doses, it decreases GI and urinary tract motility and gastric acid secretion.

A

## Adverse Reactions

**CNS:** Agitation, amnesia, anxiety, ataxia, Babinski's or Chaddock's reflex, behavioral changes, CNS stimulation (with high doses), coma, confusion, decreased concentration, decreased tendon reflexes, delirium, dizziness, drowsiness, fever, hallucinations, headache, hyperreflexia, insomnia, lethargy, mania, mental disorders, nervousness, paranoia, restlessness, seizures, somnolence, stupor, syncope, vertigo, weakness
**CV:** Arrhythmias, bradycardia (with low doses), cardiac dilation, chest pain, hypertension, hypotension, left ventricular failure, MI, palpitations, tachycardia (with high doses), weak or impalpable peripheral pulses
**EENT:** Acute angle-closure glaucoma, altered taste, blepharitis, blindness, blurred vision, conjunctivitis, cyclophoria, cycloplegia, decreased visual acuity or accommodation, dry eyes or conjunctiva, dry mucous membranes, dry mouth, eye irritation, eyelid crusting, heterophoria, increased intraocular pressure, keratoconjunctivitis, lacrimation, laryngitis, laryngospasm, mydriasis, nasal congestion, oral lesions, photophobia, pupils poorly reactive to light, strabismus, tongue chewing
**GI:** Abdominal distention, abdominal pain, bloating, constipation, decreased bowel sounds or food absorption, delayed gastric emptying, dysphagia, heartburn, ileus, nausea, vomiting
**GU:** Bladder distention, enuresis, impotence, urinary hesitancy, urinary urgency, urine retention
**MS:** Dysarthria, hypertonia, muscle twitching
**RESP:** Bradypnea, dyspnea, inspiratory stridor, pulmonary edema, respiratory failure, shallow breathing, subcostal recession, tachypnea
**SKIN:** Cold skin, cyanosis, decreased sweating, dermatitis, flushing, rash, urticaria
**Other:** Anaphylaxis, dehydration, injection site reaction, polydipsia, sensations of warmth

## Nursing Considerations

•**WARNING** For patient prescribed AtroPen for suspected nerve gas or insecticide exposure, dosage is determined by severity of symptoms. Mild symptoms include blurred vision, miosis, excessive unexplained teary eyes or runny nose, increased salivation, chest tightness, difficulty breathing, tremors, muscle twitching, nausea, vomiting, unexplained wheezing or coughing, acute onset of stomach cramps, tachycardia, and bradycardia. Severe symptoms include confusion or other strange behavior, severe difficulty breathing, extreme secretions from airway or lungs, severe muscle twitching and general weakness, involuntary urination and defecation, seizures, and unconsciousness.
•Avoid using high-dose atropine sulfate therapy in patients with ulcerative colitis because of risk of toxic megacolon or in patients with hiatal hernia and reflux esophagitis because of risk of esophagitis
•Be aware that AtroPen has no absolute contraindications when used to treat life-threatening nerve gas or insecticide exposure.
•**WARNING** Assess for symptoms of toxic doses of atropine, such as excitement, agitation, drowsiness, and confusion, which are likely to affect elderly patients even with low doses. If these symptoms occur, take safety precautions to prevent patient injury.
•Assess bowel and bladder elimination. Notify prescriber if diarrhea, constipation, urinary hesitancy, or urine retention develop.

**PATIENT TEACHING**

•Instruct patient at increased risk for exposure to nerve gas or insecticides who is prescribed to carry AtroPen when and how to self-administer the drug.
•Instruct patient to take atropine sulfate 30 to 60 minutes before meals.
•Advise patient to notify prescriber if he has persistent or severe diarrhea, constipation, or difficulty urinating.

# auranofin

Ridaura

## Class and Category

*Chemical:* Gold salt
*Therapeutic:* Anti-inflammatory
*Pregnancy category:* C

## Indications and Dosages

➤ *To treat active rheumatoid arthritis that's unresponsive to NSAIDs*

**CAPSULES**

**Adults.** *Initial:* 6 mg q.d. or 3 mg b.i.d. *Maintenance:* Up to 9 mg/day after 3 mo of treatment, if needed.

**Children age 6 and older.** *Initial:* 0.1 mg/kg/day. *Maintenance:* 0.15 mg/kg/day. *Maximum:* 0.2 mg/kg/day.

DOSAGE ADJUSTMENT Drug discontinued if therapeutic response isn't adequate after 3 mo at 9 mg/day.

| Route | Onset | Peak | Duration |
|-------|-------|------|----------|
| P.O. | 3 to 6 mo | 1 to 2 hr | Up to 26 days |

## Mechanism of Action
Decreases rheumatoid factor and humoral antibody (immunoglobulin) levels. Although its exact anti-inflammatory action is unknown, the drug is believed to suppress the increased phagocytic activity of macrophages and polymorphonuclear leukocytes that occurs with rheumatoid arthritis and thereby inhibits the release of the destructive enzymes that cause inflammation in joints.

## Contraindications
Agranulocytosis, blood dyscrasias, bone marrow aplasia, colitis, eczema, exfoliative dermatitis, hepatic disease, history of gold or heavy metal toxicity, hypersensitivity to auranofin, marked hypertension, necrotizing enterocolitis, pulmonary fibrosis, recent radiation therapy, renal disease, severe debilitation, systemic lupus erythematosus, uncontrolled diabetes mellitus, uncontrolled heart failure, urticaria, youth (under age 6)

## Interactions
**DRUGS**
*phenytoin:* Possibly increased phenytoin level

## Adverse Reactions
**CNS:** Confusion, dizziness, EEG abnormalities, hallucinations, seizures
**EENT:** Gingivitis, glossitis, iritis or corneal ulcers from gold deposits in ocular tissue, metallic taste, stomatitis
**GI:** Abdominal cramps, anorexia, constipation, diarrhea, enterocolitis, flatulence, indigestion, melena, nausea, vomiting
**GU:** Hematuria, elevated BUN and serum creatinine levels, proteinuria, vaginitis
**HEME:** Agranulocytosis, aplastic anemia, eosinophilia, leukopenia, neutropenia, thrombocytopenia

**RESP:** Cough, dyspnea, fibrosis, interstitial pneumonitis
**SKIN:** Alopecia, dermatitis, exfoliative dermatitis, jaundice, photosensitivity, pruritus, rash, urticaria

## Nursing Considerations
•Monitor blood and urine tests for signs of gold toxicity during auranofin therapy.
•WARNING Gold toxicity may occur during treatment or several months after its discontinuation. Toxicity, which usually occurs with a cumulative dose of 400 to 800 mg, may cause a decreased hemoglobin level, WBC count of less than 4,000/mm$^3$, granulocyte count of less than 1,500/mm$^3$, platelet count of less than 150,000/mm$^3$, severe diarrhea, stomatitis, hematuria, proteinuria, rash, and pruritus.
•Monitor fluid intake and output for signs of imbalance. If urine output decreases, assess BUN and serum creatinine levels for signs of renal impairment.
•Notify prescriber if you detect signs of allergic reaction, such as dermatitis, rash, and pruritus. The drug may need to be discontinued.

**PATIENT TEACHING**
•Advise patient that diarrhea commonly occurs, but that he should notify prescriber immediately if diarrhea becomes severe.
•Instruct patient to take drug exactly as prescribed and to return monthly for blood tests.
•Inform patient that drug may take 3 to 4 months to reach a therapeutic level.
•Advise patient to report skin problems, fatigue, or stomatitis, which may signal blood dyscrasias.
•Tell patient to notify prescriber if he sees blood in his stool or urine, he bruises easily, or his gums bleed.

# azathioprine
Imuran

# azathioprine sodium
Imuran

## Class and Category
*Chemical:* Purine analogue
*Therapeutic:* Antimetabolite, immunosuppressant
*Pregnancy category:* D

## Indications and Dosages
➤ *To prevent kidney transplant rejection*
TABLETS, I.V. INFUSION
**Adults and children.** *Initial:* 3 to 5 mg/kg/day P.O. or I.V. as a single dose on, or 1 to 3 days before, day of transplantation, followed by 3 to 5 mg/kg/day I.V. after surgery until P.O. dose is tolerated. *Maintenance:* 1 to 3 mg/kg/day P.O.
DOSAGE ADJUSTMENT Dosage reduced for patients with oliguria (such as from tubular necrosis) after transplantation because their drug or metabolite excretion may be delayed.
➤ *To treat refractory rheumatoid arthritis*
TABLETS
**Adults.** *Initial:* 1 mg/kg (50 to 100 mg) daily as a single dose or b.i.d. for 6 to 8 wk. *Maintenance:* If initial therapy doesn't produce therapeutic effects or serious adverse effects, dosage increased q 4 wk by 0.5 mg/kg up to 2.5 mg/kg. Optimal dosage is 2 to 2.5 mg/kg/day.
DOSAGE ADJUSTMENT Dosage reduced to 25% to 33% of usual dosage for patients who also take allopurinol.

| Route | Onset | Peak | Duration |
|-------|-------|------|----------|
| P.O., I.V. | 4 to 8 wk | Unknown | Several days |

## Mechanism of Action
May prevent proliferation and differentiation of activated B and T cells by interfering with purine (protein) and nucleic acid (DNA and RNA) synthesis.

## Contraindications
Hypersensitivity to azathioprine

## Interactions
DRUGS
*ACE inhibitors and drugs that affect bone marrow and cell development in bone marrow, such as co-trimoxazole:* Possibly severe leukopenia
*allopurinol:* Possibly increased therapeutic and adverse effects of azathioprine
*anticoagulants:* Possibly decreased anticoagulant action
*cyclosporine:* Possibly decreased plasma cyclosporine level
*methotrexate:* Possibly increased plasma level of azathioprine's metabolite, 6-mercaptopurine, which can lead to cell death

*nondepolarizing neuromuscular blockers:* Possibly decreased or reversed action of neuromuscular blocker

## Adverse Reactions
**CNS:** Fever, malaise
**GI:** Abdominal pain, diarrhea, hepatoxicity (elevated liver function test results), nausea, pancreatitis, steatorrhea, vomiting
**HEME:** Leukopenia, macrocytic anemia, pancytopenia, thrombocytopenia
**MS:** Arthralgia, myalgia
**SKIN:** Alopecia, rash
**Other:** Infection, lymphomas and other neoplasms

## Nursing Considerations
•Before I.V. administration, add 20 ml of sterile water for injection to azathioprine vial and swirl it until clear solution forms. The resulting drug concentration is 100 mg and can be diluted further as prescribed. Calculate infusion rate based on final volume to be infused. Then administer over 30 to 60 minutes or as prescribed (from 5 minutes to 8 hours).
•Obtain results of baseline laboratory tests, including WBC, RBC, and platelet counts. Then expect to monitor results once a week during first month of therapy, twice a month during second and third months of therapy, and once a month or more frequently thereafter.
•Be aware that hematologic reactions typically are dose related and may occur late in therapy, especially in patients with transplant rejection.
•WARNING If WBC count decreases rapidly or remains significantly and consistently low, expect to reduce dosage or discontinue use of azathioprine.
•Periodically monitor liver function test results to detect early signs of hepatotoxicity.
•If patient develops thrombocytopenia, take bleeding precautions, such as avoiding I.M. injections and venipunctures, applying ice to areas of trauma, and checking I.V. infusion sites every 2 hours for bleeding.
•If patient also receives an oral anticoagulant, monitor his PT.
•Know that azathioprine therapy increases risk of viral, fungal, bacterial, and protozoal infections. Monitor for signs of infection, such as fever, chills, sore throat, and mouth sores. Expect to administer aggressive antibiotic, antiviral, or other drug therapy and reduce azathioprine dosage.

•Minimize the risk of infection. If patient has severe leukopenia, take neutropenic precautions, such as placing him in a private room and limiting visitors.

•Be aware that rheumatoid arthritis requires at least 12 weeks of azathioprine therapy. During this time, continue other pain-relief measures, such as rest, physical therapy, and other drugs, such as salicylates and corticosteroids.

•If oral azathioprine causes GI upset, administer it in divided doses or with meals.

•Plan to use lowest possible maintenance dosage for patient with rheumatoid arthritis. Expect to reduce dosage gradually in 0.5-mg/kg (about 25-mg) increments at 4-week intervals. Know that drug can be discontinued abruptly, but its effects may persist for several days.

**PATIENT TEACHING**

•Advise patient to take oral drug with food or meals to minimize GI upset.

•**WARNING** Teach patient to recognize and report signs of infection, such as sore throat and fever.

•Teach patient how to reduce the risk of bleeding and falling.

# azelastine hydrochloride

Astelin

## Class and Category

*Chemical:* Phthalazinone derivative
*Therapeutic:* Antihistamine, H₁-receptor antagonist
*Pregnancy category:* C

## Indications and Dosages

➤ *To treat symptoms of seasonal rhinitis (rhinorrhea, sneezing, and nasal itching)*

**NASAL SPRAY**

**Adults and children age 12 and older.**
2 sprays in each nostril b.i.d.

| Route | Onset | Peak | Duration |
|-------|-------|------|----------|
| Nasal | In 3 hr | Unknown | 12 hr |

## Contraindications

Hypersensitivity to azelastine or its components

## Interactions

**DRUGS**

*cimetidine, ketoconazole:* Possibly increased blood azelastine level

*CNS depressants:* Possibly increased sedative effects and reduced mental alertness

**ACTIVITIES**

*alcohol use:* Possibly increased sedative effects and reduced mental alertness

## Mechanism of Action

Binds nonselectively to central and peripheral H₁ receptors, preventing histamine from reaching its site of action, which reduces or prevents most of histamine's physiologic effects. By blocking histamine at its site of action, azelastine inhibits respiratory, vascular, and GI smooth-muscle contraction; decreases capillary permeability, which reduces wheals, flares, and itching; and decreases salivary and lacrimal gland secretions.

## Adverse Reactions

**CNS:** Dizziness, fatigue, headache, somnolence
**EENT:** Bitter taste, dry mouth, epistaxis, nasal burning, paroxysmal sneezing, pharyngitis, rhinitis
**GI:** Nausea
**Other:** Weight gain

## Nursing Considerations

•Assess for changes in alertness and take safety precautions, if needed.

**PATIENT TEACHING**

•Teach patient how to use azelastine nasal spray properly to achieve maximum therapeutic effects.

•Before patient's first use of nasal spray, instruct him to prime pump by placing his thumb on base and his index and middle fingers on shoulder area of bottle and then pressing thumb firmly and quickly against bottle four times or until fine mist appears.

•If patient hasn't used spray in more than 3 days, instruct him to reprime pump with two sprays or until fine mist appears.

•Advise patient to clear nostrils gently, if needed, before using spray.

•Teach patient to inhale deeply after each spray and then exhale through his mouth and tilt his head back so drug can spread over nasopharynx.

•Advise patient to store bottle upright and tightly closed.

•**WARNING** Emphasize that patient must check with prescriber before taking any OTC

drug, such as a cough syrup or cold remedy, because of risk of extreme CNS depression.
•Inform patient that decreased alertness may occur. Advise him to avoid activities that require alertness, such as driving or operating machinery, until drug's effects are known.

# azithromycin

Zithromax, Zmax

## Class and Category

*Chemical:* Azalide (subclass of macrolide)
*Therapeutic:* Antibiotic
*Pregnancy category:* B

## Indications and Dosages

➤ *To treat mild community-acquired pneumonia, otitis media, pharyngitis, tonsillitis, and uncomplicated skin and soft-tissue infections*

CAPSULES, ORAL SUSPENSION, TABLETS

**Adults.** 500 mg as a single dose on day 1, followed by 250 mg q.d. on days 2 through 5.
**Children age 6 months or older with acute otitis media or community-acquired pneumonia.** 10 mg/kg as a single dose (not to exceed 500 mg/day) on day 1, followed by 5 mg/kg (not to exceed 250 mg/day) q.d. on days 2 through 5. Alternatively for acute otitis media, 30 mg/kg of oral suspension as a single dose or 10 mg/kg q.d. for 3 days.
**Children age 12 or older with pharyngitis or tonsillitis.** 12 mg/kg (not to exceed 500 mg/day) as a single dose daily for 5 days.

➤ *To treat mild to moderate acute bacterial exacerbations of COPD*

CAPSULES, ORAL SUSPENSION, TABLETS

**Adults.** 500 mg q.d. for 3 days. Alternatively, 500 mg as single dose on day 1, followed by 250 mg q.d. on days 2 through 5.

➤ *To treat community-acquired pneumonia*

CAPSULES, ORAL SUSPENSION, TABLETS, I.V. INFUSION

**Adults and adolescents age 16 or older.** 500 mg I.V. as a single dose daily for at least 2 days, followed by 500 mg P.O. as a single dose daily until patient completes 7 to 10 days of therapy.

➤ *To treat community-acquired pneumonia caused by* Chlamydophila pneumoniae, Haemophilus influenzae, Mycoplasma pneumoniae, *or* Streptococcus pneumoniae

E.R. ORAL SOLUTION (ZMAX)

**Adults.** 2 g as a single dose on an empty stomach.

➤ *To treat chancroid caused by* Haemophilus ducreyi; *gonococcal pharyngitis; urethritis, cervicitis, or other infections caused by* Chlamydia trachomatis

CAPSULES, ORAL SUSPENSION, TABLETS

**Adults.** 1 g as a one-time dose.
**Children age 8 or older and children younger than age 8 who weigh 45 kg (99 lb) or more (with infections caused by *C. trachomatis*).** 1 g as a one-time dose.

➤ *To treat urethritis or cervicitis caused by* Neisseria gonorrhoeae

CAPSULES, ORAL SUSPENSION, TABLETS

**Adults.** 2 g as a one-time dose.

➤ *To prevent* Mycobacterium avium *complex in patients with advanced HIV infection*

CAPSULES, ORAL SUSPENSION, TABLETS, I.V. INFUSION

**Adults.** 1.2 g once weekly, as indicated.

➤ *To treat pelvic inflammatory disease*

CAPSULES, ORAL SUSPENSION, TABLETS, I.V. INFUSION

**Adults.** 500 mg I.V. as a single dose daily for 1 to 2 days, followed by 250 mg P.O. as a single dose daily until patient completes 7 days of therapy.

➤ *To treat acute bacterial sinusitis*

ORAL SUSPENSION, TABLETS

**Adults.** 500 mg q.d. for 3 days.
**Children.** 10 mg/kg q.d. for 3 days.

➤ *To treat acute bacterial sinusitis caused by* Haemophilus influenzae, Moraxella catarrhalis, *or* Streptococcus pneumoniae

E.R. ORAL SOLUTION (ZMAX)

**Adults.** 2 g as a single dose on an empty stomach.

| Route | Onset | Peak | Duration |
|---|---|---|---|
| P.O. | Varies | Unknown | Unknown |

## Mechanism of Action

Binds to a ribosomal subunit of susceptible bacteria, blocking peptide translocation and inhibiting RNA-dependent protein synthesis. Drug concentrates in phagocytes, macrophages, and fibroblasts, which release it slowly and may help move it to infection sites.

## Incompatibilities
Don't add I.V. substances, additives, or drugs to azithromycin I.V. solution, and don't infuse them through the same I.V. line as azithromycin.

## Contraindications
Hypersensitivity to azithromycin, erythromycin, or other macrolide antibiotics

## Interactions
**DRUGS**
*antacids that contain aluminum or magnesium:* Possibly decreased peak blood azithromycin level, but extent of absorption is unchanged
*carbamazepine, cyclosporine, phenytoin, terfenadine (drugs metabolized by P-450 cytochrome system):* Possibly increased blood levels of these drugs
*digoxin:* Possibly increased blood digoxin level
*dihydroergotamine, ergotamine:* Possibly severe peripheral vasospasm and abnormal sensations (acute ergot toxicity)
*HMG-CoA reductase inhibitors:* Increased risk of severe myopathy or rhabdomyolysis
*pimozide:* Possibly sudden death
*theophylline:* Possibly increased blood theophylline level
*triazolam:* Possibly decreased excretion and increased therapeutic effects of triazolam
*warfarin:* Possibly increased anticoagulation
**FOODS**
*food:* Dramatically increased absorption rate of azithromycin

## Adverse Reactions
**CNS:** Dizziness, fatigue, headache, somnolence, vertigo
**CV:** Chest pain, elevated serum CK level, palpitations, prolonged QT interval, torsades de pointes
**EENT:** Hearing loss, mucocutaneous candidiasis, tinnitus
**ENDO:** Hyperglycemia
**GI:** Abdominal pain, diarrhea, elevated liver function test results, nausea, pseudomembranous colitis, vomiting
**GU:** Elevated BUN and serum creatinine levels, nephritis, vaginal candidiasis
**HEME:** Leukopenia, neutropenia, thrombocytopenia
**SKIN:** Jaundice, photosensitivity, rash, Stevens-Johnson syndrome, toxic epidermal necrolysis, urticaria
**Other:** Allergic reaction, angioedema, elevated serum phosphorus level, hyperkalemia, infusion site reaction (such as pain and redness), superinfection

## Nursing Considerations
• Obtain culture and sensitivity test results, if possible, before starting therapy.
• Use drug cautiously in patients with hepatic dysfunction (because drug is metabolize in the liver) or renal dysfunction (because effects are unknown in this group).
• Administer azithromycin capsules 1 hour before or 2 to 3 hours after food. Give tablets or suspension without regard to food.
• **WARNING** Don't give azithromycin by I.V. bolus or I.M. injection because it may cause erythema, pain, swelling, tenderness, or other reaction at the site. Infuse it over 60 minutes or longer, as prescribed (typically 1 mg/ml over 3 hours or 2 mg/ml over 1 hour.)
• If hepatic function is impaired, monitor liver function studies because azithromycin is eliminated mainly by the liver.
• Assess patient for bacterial or fungal superinfection, which may occur with prolonged or repeated therapy. If it occurs, expect to give another antibiotic or antifungal.
• Monitor bowel elimination; if needed, obtain stool culture to rule out pseudomembranous colitis. If it occurs, expect to stop azithromycin and give fluid, electrolytes, and antibiotics effective against *Clostridium difficile*.
**PATIENT TEACHING**
• Tell patient to take azithromycin capsules 1 hour before or 2 to 3 hours after food. Instruct patient to take tablets or suspension without regard to food.
• **WARNING** Urge patient to ask prescriber before taking OTC drugs, including antacids. If they're prescribed, tell patient to take drug 1 hour before or 2 to 3 hours after taking antacids.
• Tell patient to immediately report evidence of allergic reactions, such as rash, itching, hives, chest tightness, and trouble breathing.
• Warn patient that abdominal pain and loose, watery stools may occur. If diarrhea persists or becomes severe, urge him to contact prescriber and replace fluids.
• Because azithromycin may destroy normal flora, teach patient to watch for and immediately report signs of superinfection, such as white patches in the mouth.

# aztreonam

Azactam

## Class and Category

*Chemical:* Monobactam
*Therapeutic:* Antibiotic
*Pregnancy category:* B

## Indications and Dosages

➤ *To treat infections of the urinary tract, lower respiratory tract, skin, soft tissue, female reproductive tract; intra-abdominal infections; septicemia; and surgical abscesses caused by susceptible strains of gram-negative bacteria*

**I.V. INFUSION, I.V. OR I.M. INJECTION**

**Adults.** 0.5 to 2.0 g q 8 to 12 hr up to a maximum of 8 g/day. For life-threatening systemic infection, 2 g q 6 to 8 hr up to a maximum of 8 g/day.

**Children ages 9 months to 16 years.** 30 mg/kg q 6 to 8 hr up to 120 mg/kg/day; 50 mg/kg q 4 to 6 hr (for *Pseudomonas aeruginosa*).

**DOSAGE ADJUSTMENT** If creatinine clearance is 10 to 30 ml/min/1.73 $m^2$, initial dose is 1 to 2 g; then 50% of usual dose at usual interval. If creatinine clearance less than 10 ml/min/1.73 $m^2$, initial dose is 500 mg to 2 g; then 25% of the usual dose q 6, 8, or 12 hr.

| Route | Onset | Peak | Duration |
|---|---|---|---|
| I.V. infusion | Immediate | Immediate | Unknown |
| I.V. injection | Immediate | Immediate | Unknown |
| I.M. | Variable | 60 min | Unknown |

### Mechanism of Action

Inhibits bacterial cell wall synthesis in susceptible aerobic gram-negative bacteria. These bacteria assemble rigid, cross-linked cell walls in several steps. Aztreonam affects the final cross-linking stage by inactivating penicillin-binding protein 3 (the enzyme that links cell wall strands), which causes cell lysis and death.

## Incompatibilities

Don't mix aztreonam in same I.V. solution as cephradine, metronidazole, or nafcillin sodium. Don't mix it in same I.M. injection solution as local anesthetic.

## Contraindications

Hypersensitivity to aztreonam or its components

## Interactions

**DRUGS**

*aminoglycosides (prolonged or high-dose therapy):* Increased risk of nephrotoxicity and ototoxicity
*cefoxitin, imipenem:* Possibly antagonized action of aztreonam
*furosemide, probenecid:* Possibly increased blood aztreonam level

## Adverse Reactions

**CNS:** Confusion, dizziness, fever, headache, insomnia, malaise, paresthesia, seizures, vertigo
**CV:** Chest pain, hypotension, transient ECG changes
**EENT:** Altered taste, diplopia, halitosis, mouth ulcers, mucocutaneous candidiasis, nasal congestion, sneezing, tinnitus, tongue numbness
**GI:** Abdominal cramps, diarrhea, elevated liver function test results, GI bleeding, hepatitis, nausea, pseudomembranous colitis, vomiting
**GU:** Breast tenderness, elevated serum creatinine level, vaginal candidiasis
**HEME:** Anemia, eosinophilia, leukocytosis, neutropenia, pancytopenia, positive Coombs' test, prolonged PT and APTT, thrombocytopenia, thrombocytosis
**MS:** Myalgia
**RESP:** Bronchospasm, dyspnea, wheezing
**SKIN:** Diaphoresis, erythema multiforme, exfoliative dermatitis, flushing, jaundice, petechiae, pruritus, purpura, rash, toxic epidermal necrolysis, urticaria
**Other:** Allergic reaction; injection site pain, phlebitis, swelling, or thrombophlebitis

## Nursing Considerations

•Obtain culture and sensitivity test results, if possible, before initiating therapy. If patient is acutely ill, expect to begin therapy before results are available.

•Keep in mind that other antimicrobials may be used with aztreonam in seriously ill patients at risk for gram-positive infection.

•Expect to use I.V. route for patients who need single doses over 1 g and those with life-threatening systemic infections, such as septicemia or peritonitis.

•To reconstitute aztreonam for I.V. bolus injection, use sterile water for injection.

•Immediately after adding diluent to vial, shake it vigorously to mix. After obtaining correct dose, discard unused solution.

•Be aware that reconstituted solution may turn light pink on standing at room temperature. This doesn't affect drug potency.

•Administer I.V. bolus injection directly into I.V. tubing over 3 to 5 minutes.

•**WARNING** When preparing aztreonam for I.V. infusion, use at least 50 ml of appropriate infusion solution per gram of aztreonam. Further dilute drug in I.V. solution, such as NS, D$_5$W, D$_5$NS, LR, or Ringer's solution.

•Know that I.V. infusion may be administered over 20 to 60 minutes.

•Flush I.V. tubing with solution, such as NS, before and after administering I.V. infusion to reduce risk of incompatibilities.

•If prescribed, mix aztreonam in same I.V. solution with other antibiotics (such as ampicillin sodium, cefazolin sodium, clindamycin phosphate, gentamicin sulfate, or tobramycin sulfate), or mix it with cloxacillin sodium and vancomycin hydrochloride in peritoneal dialysis solution.

•Prepare solution for I.M. injection using sterile or bacteriostatic water or sodium chloride for injection. Administer injection deep into large muscle, such as in dorsogluteal or ventrogluteal area.

•Assess for signs of bacterial or fungal superinfection, which may occur with prolonged or repeated therapy. If superinfection occurs, treat it as prescribed.

•Monitor bowel elimination; if needed, obtain stool culture to rule out pseudomembranous colitis. If this adverse reaction occurs, expect to discontinue aztreonam and administer fluid, electrolytes, and antibiotics that are effective against *Clostridium difficile.*

•Evaluate patient's renal and liver function test results, as ordered, if the patient has renal or hepatic impairment.

•Monitor renal function if patient is receiving an aminoglycoside because of the increased risk of nephrotoxicity.

**PATIENT TEACHING**

•Stress the importance of taking the full course of aztreonam exactly as prescribed, even if the patient feels better before finishing it.

•Teach patient to recognize and immediately report signs and symptoms of allergic reactions, such as chest tightness, difficulty breathing, hives, itching, and rash.

•Warn patient that abdominal pain and loose, watery stools may occur. If diarrhea persists or becomes severe, urge him to contact prescriber and replace fluids.

•Because aztreonam may destroy normal flora, teach patient to watch for and immediately report signs of superinfection, such as white patches in mouth.

# B

## bacampicillin hydrochloride

Penglobe (CAN), Spectrobid

### Class and Category
*Chemical:* Aminopenicillin
*Therapeutic:* Antibiotic
*Pregnancy category:* B

### Indications and Dosages
➤ *To treat upper respiratory tract infections (including otitis media) caused by* streptococci, pneumococci, non-penicillinase-producing staphylococci, *and* Haemophilus influenzae; *UTIs caused by* Escherichia coli, Proteus mirabilis, *and* Streptococcus faecalis; *skin and soft-tissue infections caused by streptococci and susceptible staphylococci*

TABLETS
**Adults.** 400 mg q 12 hr; 800 mg q 12 hr for severe infections and those caused by less susceptible organisms.
**Children who weigh 25 kg (55 lb) or more.** 25 mg/kg/day in divided doses q 12 hr; 50 mg/kg/day in divided doses q 12 hr for severe infections and those caused by less susceptible organisms.
➤ *To treat lower respiratory tract infections caused by streptococci, pneumococci, non-penicillinase-producing staphylococci, and* H. influenzae

TABLETS
**Adults.** 800 mg q 12 hr.
**Children who weigh 25 kg or more.** 50 mg/kg/day in divided doses q 12 hr.
➤ *To treat uncomplicated gonorrhea caused by* Neisseria gonorrhoeae

TABLETS
**Adults.** 1.6 g plus 1 g of probenecid as a single dose.

| Route | Onset | Peak | Duration |
|-------|-------|------|----------|
| P.O. | Variable | Unknown | 12 hr |

### Contraindications
Cholestatic jaundice and hepatic dysfunction associated with amoxicillin and clavulanate potassium; hypersensitivity to penicillins, cephalosporins, imipenem and cilastatin, or beta-lactamase inhibitors, such as piperacillin and tazobactam

### Mechanism of Action
Inhibits bacterial cell wall synthesis in susceptible bacteria. These bacteria assemble rigid, cross-linked cell walls in several steps. Bacampicillin, which undergoes hydrolysis to ampicillin, affects final stage of cross-linking by binding with and inactivating penicillin-binding protein (enzyme responsible for linking cell wall strands). This action inhibits bacterial cell wall synthesis and causes cell lysis and death.

### Interactions
DRUGS
*allopurinol:* Increased risk of rash from bacampicillin use
*beta-adrenergic blockers:* Increased risk of anaphylaxis
*disulfiram:* Possibly disulfiram reaction when administered together
*oral contraceptives:* Possibly reduced effectiveness of oral contraceptives, contraceptive failure, and breakthrough bleeding
*tetracyclines:* Possibly impaired bactericidal effects of bacampicillin

### Adverse Reactions
**CNS:** Anxiety, confusion, CVA, depression, fatigue, fever, hallucinations, lethargy, malaise, neuromuscular irritability, seizures, syncope
**CV:** Hypotension, palpitations, periarteritis nodosa, pulmonary hypertension, tachycardia, vascular collapse
**EENT:** Altered taste, black "hairy" tongue, blurred vision, glossitis, laryngospasm, mouth soreness, mucocutaneous candidiasis, stomatitis, taste disorders
**GI:** Abdominal cramps or pain, anorexia, diarrhea, enterocolitis, epigastric distress, elevated liver function test results, gastritis, nausea, pseudomembranous colitis, vomiting
**GU:** Elevated BUN and serum creatinine levels, hematuria, impotence, interstitial nephritis, neurogenic bladder, priapism, renal failure, vaginal candidiasis
**HEME:** Agranulocytosis, anemia, bone marrow depression, decreased hemoglobin level and hematocrit, eosinophilia, leukopenia, neutropenia, prolonged PT, thrombocytopenia, thrombocytopenic purpura

**MS:** Arthralgia, arthritis exacerbation
**RESP:** Bronchospasm
**SKIN:** Exfoliative dermatitis, rash, urticaria
**Other:** Allergic reaction, lymphadenopathy, serum sickness

## Nursing Considerations
• Obtain culture and sensitivity test results, if possible, before initiating therapy. Be prepared to start bacampicillin therapy before results are available.
• Expect to continue treatment for at least 48 hours after symptoms resolve or culture detects no signs of infection.
• **WARNING** Expect to administer bacampicillin for 10 days to treat infection caused by group A beta-hemolytic streptococci to prevent development of acute rheumatic fever or acute glomerulonephritis.
• Assess for signs of bacterial or fungal superinfection, which may occur with prolonged or repeated therapy. If superinfection occurs, expect to administer another antibiotic or antifungal drug.
• Monitor bowel elimination; if needed, obtain stool culture to rule out pseudomembranous colitis. If this adverse reaction occurs, expect to discontinue bacampicillin and administer fluid, electrolytes, and antibiotics that are effective against *Clostridium difficile*.
**PATIENT TEACHING**
• Teach patient to recognize and immediately report signs of allergic reaction, including rash, itching, hives, chest tightness, and difficulty breathing.
• Warn patient that abdominal pain and loose, watery stools may occur. If diarrhea persists or becomes severe, urge him to contact prescriber and drink plenty of fluids.
• Because bacampicillin may destroy normal flora, teach patient to watch for and immediately report signs of superinfection, such as white patches in mouth and vaginal itching and discharge.

# bacitracin
Baci-IM

## Class and Category
*Chemical:* Bacillus subtilis derivative (polypeptide)
*Therapeutic:* Antibiotic
*Pregnancy category:* C

## Indications and Dosages
➤ *To treat pneumonia and empyema caused by susceptible staphylococci*
**I.M. INJECTION**
**Infants who weigh more than 2.5 kg (5.5 lb).** 1,000 U/kg/day in two or three divided doses.
**Infants who weigh less than 2.5 kg.** 900 U/kg/day in two or three divided doses.

| Route | Onset | Peak | Duration |
|---|---|---|---|
| I.M. | Rapid | Unknown | About 6 hr |

### Mechanism of Action
Interferes with bacterial cell wall synthesis by binding with isoprenyl pyrophosphate (a lipid-carrying molecule that transports substances out of bacterial cells to help build new cell walls), forming an unusable complex in bacterial cells. This weakens cell walls and causes lysis and death. Bacitracin is considered a bacteriostatic and bactericidal drug.

## Incompatibilities
Don't dilute bacitracin with a solution that contains parabens.

## Contraindications
Hypersensitivity or toxic reaction to bacitracin

## Interactions
**DRUGS**
*aminoglycosides:* Increased risk of respiratory paralysis and renal dysfunction
*nondepolarizing neuromuscular blockers:* Possibly increased neuromuscular blockade

## Adverse Reactions
**GI:** Nausea, vomiting
**GU:** Albuminuria, azotemia, cylindrical mucus casts in urine, nephrotoxicity
**SKIN:** Rash
**Other:** Injection site pain, superinfection

## Nursing Considerations
• Obtain culture and sensitivity test results before therapy begins, if possible. However, be prepared to start bacitracin therapy before results are available.
• **WARNING** Use parenteral bacitracin for I.M. injection only.
• For an I.M. solution of 5,000 U/ml, reconstitute 50,000 U of bacitracin powder with

9.8 ml of sodium chloride for injection that contains 2% procaine hydrochloride.
• Administer I.M. injection into upper outer quadrant of buttocks, alternating right and left sides. To prevent pain at injection site, avoid multiple injections in same site.
• During therapy, compare daily results of renal function tests with baseline results, as appropriate.
• Assess urine output frequently (even hourly, if indicated), and replace fluids orally and parenterally to maintain adequate renal function.
• **WARNING** Because of increased risk of nephrotoxicity, avoid concurrent use of other nephrotoxic drugs, such as streptomycin, kanamycin, polymyxin B, and neomycin.
• Assess infant for signs of superinfection, especially white patches in mouth and perineal area. If superinfection develops, plan to treat it with appropriate antibiotics.

**PATIENT TEACHING**
• Advise parents that daily blood tests are needed to assess infant's renal function.
• Encourage parents to provide oral fluids to promote renal function. Teach them how to record infant's fluid intake.
• Instruct parents to report signs of superinfection, such as white patches in mouth or perineal area and bright red diaper rash.

# baclofen

Apo-Baclofen (CAN), Lioresal, Lioresal Intrathecal, Novo-Baclofen (CAN)

## Class and Category

*Chemical:* Gamma-aminobutyric acid (GABA) chlorophenyl derivative
*Therapeutic:* Skeletal muscle relaxant, spasmolytic
*Pregnancy category:* C

## Indications and Dosages

➤ *To relieve symptoms of spasticity caused by multiple sclerosis (particularly flexor spasms and pain, clonus, and muscle rigidity) and spasticity from spinal cord injury or disease and brain injury*

**TABLETS**
**Adults and children age 12 and older.** 5 mg t.i.d. for 3 days, then 10 mg t.i.d. for 3 days, then 15 mg t.i.d. for 3 days, then 20 mg t.i.d. for 3 days, then increased if needed up to 80 mg/day. Usual dosage ranges from 40 to 80 mg/day.

➤ *To relieve severe symptoms of spasticity of spinal cord origin when symptoms don't respond to oral drug or when oral drug causes severe adverse CNS effects*

**INTRATHECAL BOLUS, INTRATHECAL INFUSION**
**Adults.** *For screening before implantable pump insertion:* 50 mcg in 1 ml of sterile preservative-free sodium chloride for injection as bolus injection into intrathecal space over 1 min or more. After 4 to 8 hr, if symptoms don't improve as much as desired, second bolus of 75 mcg in 1.5 ml of sterile preservative-free sodium chloride for injection injected after 24 hr followed by third bolus of 100-mcg/2 ml dilution injected after another 24 hr, if needed.
*After implantable pump insertion:* Effective screening dose doubled and infused over 24 hr. Or effective screening dose (if it provided desired effects for more than 12 hr) infused over 24 hr.
*For spasticity of spinal cord origin after implantable pump insertion:* After first 24 hr, daily dose increased by 10% to 30% once every 24 hr until desired effects achieved.
*For spasticity of cerebral origin after implantable pump insertion:* Daily dose increased by 5% to 15% once every 24 hr until desired effects achieved.
*For long-term maintenance therapy in spasticity of spinal cord origin:* 12 to 2,003 mcg/day (usual dose 300 to 800 mcg/day). Lowest possible therapeutic dose should be used. If adverse effects occur, daily dose may be decreased by 10% to 20%. During periodic pump refills, daily dose may be increased by 10% up to 40% to control symptoms adequately.
*For long-term maintenance therapy in spasticity of cerebral origin:* 90 to 703 mcg/day (usual) but ranging from 22 to 1,400 mcg/day. If adverse effects occur, daily dose may be decreased by 10% to 20%. During periodic pump refills, daily dose may be increased by 5% to 20% to control symptoms adequately.
**Children.** *For screening before implantable pump insertion:* 1 ml of a 50-mcg/ml dilution or 1 ml of a 25-mcg/ml dilution (if child is very young) as bolus injection into intrathe-

B

cal space over 1 min or more. After 4 to 8 hr, if symptoms don't improve as desired, second bolus of 75 mcg in 1.5 ml of sterile preservative-free sodium chloride for injection injected after 24 hr followed by third bolus of 100-mcg/2 ml dilution injected after another 24 hr, if needed.

*After implantable pump insertion:* Daily dose increased by 5% to 15% once every 24 hr until the desired effect is achieved.

*For maintenance therapy:* In children over age 12: 90 to 703 mcg/day (usual) but ranging from 22 to 1,400 mcg/day. In children under age 12: 274 mcg/day (average) but ranging from 24 to 1,199 mcg/day.

DOSAGE ADJUSTMENT Dosage reduced for patients with renal impairment because drug is excreted primarily unchanged by kidneys.

| Route | Onset | Peak | Duration |
|---|---|---|---|
| P.O. | Hours to weeks | Unknown | Unknown |
| Intrathecal bolus injection | 30 to 60 min | About 4 hr | 4 to 8 hr |
| Intrathecal infusion | 6 to 8 hr | 24 to 48 hr | Unknown |

## Mechanism of Action

May inhibit transmission of monosynaptic and polysynaptic impulses, similar to effects of GABA. Baclofen may work in the spinal cord at the afferent spinal end of upper motor neurons, where it hyperpolarizes nerve fibers and inhibits impulse transmission. This reduces excess muscle activity caused by muscle hypertonia, spasms, and spasticity.

## Contraindications

Hypersensitivity to baclofen; treatment of skeletal muscle spasm resulting from rheumatic disorders, CVA, cerebral palsy, or Parkinson's disease (oral form only)

## Interactions

**DRUGS**

*CNS depressants:* Possibly increased CNS depression

*epidural morphine:* Possibly hypotension and dyspnea

**ACTIVITIES**

*alcohol use:* Possibly increased CNS depression

## Adverse Reactions

**CNS:** Abnormal gait, anxiety, ataxia, chills, coma, confusion, CVA, depression, dizziness, drowsiness, dystonia, emotional lability, euphoria, excitement, fatigue, fever, hallucinations, headache, hypertonia, hypothermia, hypotonia, impaired concentration, insomnia, lack of coordination, lethargy, memory loss, paresthesia, personality disorder, seizures, somnolence, syncope, tremor, weakness

**CV:** Bradycardia, chest pain, chest tightness, deep vein thrombosis, hypertension, orthostatic hypotension, palpitations, peripheral edema

**EENT:** Amblyopia, blurred vision, diplopia, dry mouth, miosis, mydriasis, nasal congestion, nystagmus, photophobia, ptosis, rhinitis, slurred speech, strabismus, taste loss, tinnitus

**ENDO:** Hyperglycemia

**GI:** Abdominal pain, anorexia, constipation, dysphagia, elevated liver function test results, flatulence, ileus, indigestion, nausea, vomiting

**GU:** Albuminuria, bladder spasms, dysuria, enuresis, hematuria, impotence, renal failure, sexual dysfunction, urinary frequency, urinary incontinence, urine retention

**HEME:** Anemia

**MS:** Muscle twitching

**RESP:** Aspiration pneumonia, pulmonary embolism, respiratory depression

**SKIN:** Alopecia, diaphoresis, facial edema, flushing, pruritus, rash, urticaria, wound dehiscence

**Other:** Dehydration, infection at pump implantation site, weight loss

## Nursing Considerations

• Expect to initiate baclofen therapy at a low dose and gradually increase it until desired effects are achieved.

• WARNING Before screening dose is administered, expect prescriber to ensure that patient is free of infection to prevent systemic infection from interfering with patient's response. Before implantable pump insertion, also expect prescriber to ensure that patient is free of infection to reduce risk of complications and interference with determining most appropriate dose.

• Use baclofen cautiously in patients with history of autonomic dysreflexia. Nociceptor stimulation may precipitate autonomic dysreflexia. Be aware that abrupt withdrawal of intrathecal infusion may produce symptoms similar to autonomic dysreflexia, high fever,

life-threatening complications such as multiple organ-system failure, and death.
•**WARNING** Never administer intrathecal form of baclofen by I.V., I.M., or S.C. route.
•Assess for signs of effectiveness, such as relief of spasms, pain, and muscle rigidity.
•Because CNS depression can occur, take safety precautions to help prevent injury. Also take precautions for patients who use spasticity to maintain locomotion or upright posture and balance. Relief of spasticity may increase risk of falls and injury.
•**WARNING** Because continuous intrathecal infusion increases risk of life-threatening CNS depression, keep emergency equipment nearby.
•Expect baclofen to be discontinued slowly; hallucinations and seizures may occur with abrupt withdrawal.
**PATIENT TEACHING**
•Teach patient how to care for and operate programmable implanted pump. Have her demonstrate all procedures.
•Advise patient not to stop taking baclofen abruptly. Stress the importance of keeping refill visits for intrathecal infusion.
•Instruct patient to avoid driving and other activities that require mental alertness, coordination, or physical dexterity until baclofen's effects are known.
•Urge patient to contact prescriber before taking OTC drugs, such as cough syrups and cold remedies, which may increase risk of sedation.
•Advise patient to notify prescriber if spasticity increases or baclofen is no longer effective.

# balsalazide disodium

Colazal

## Class and Category

*Chemical:* Prodrug of 5-aminosalicylic acid (5-ASA)
*Therapeutic:* Anti-inflammatory
*Pregnancy category:* B

## Indications and Dosages

➤ *To treat mildly to moderately active ulcerative colitis*
**CAPSULES**
**Adults.** 2.25 g t.i.d. for 8 wk. *Maximum:* 6.75 g/day for 12 wk.

## Contraindications

Hypersensitivity to balsalazide, salicylates, or their components

## Mechanism of Action

After it has been metabolized to 5-ASA, balsalazide may reduce inflammation by inhibiting the enzyme cyclooxygenase and decreasing the production of arachidonic acid metabolites, which may be increased in patients with inflammatory bowel disease. Cyclooxygenase is needed to form prostaglandin from arachidonic acid. Prostaglandin mediates inflammatory activity and produces signs and symptoms of inflammation. By inhibiting prostaglandin synthesis, balsalazide may reduce signs and symptoms of inflammation in inflammatory bowel disease. Balsalazide also may reduce inflammation by interfering with leukotrine synthesis and by inhibiting the enzyme lipoxygenase. These substances also are involved in the inflammatory response.

## Adverse Reactions

**CNS:** Headache
**GI:** Abdominal pain, diarrhea, nausea, vomiting
**MS:** Arthralgia
**RESP:** Respiratory tract infection

## Nursing Considerations

•**WARNING** Monitor patients who are sensitive to sulfasalazine or olsalazine for possible cross-sensitivity to balsalazide.
•Monitor patients with pyloric stenosis for decreased or delayed drug effects due to prolonged gastric retention of balsalazide capsules.
•Monitor patient for possible exacerbation of colitis symptoms.
**PATIENT TEACHING**
•Inform patient that balsalazide is used to reduce bowel inflammation and pain associated with ulcerative colitis and to minimize recurring inflammation.
•Instruct patient to swallow capsules whole, with a full glass of water, and not to crush or chew them.
•Advise patient to notify prescriber of any other drugs she may be taking, including OTC drugs, nutritional supplements, and herbal products, because they may interact with balsalazide.
•Instruct patient to notify prescriber immediately if her colitis symptoms worsen.
•Inform patient that she can expect some im-

B

provement in symptoms in 3 to 21 days but that she may need up to 6 weeks of treatment before she achieves optimal results.

# basiliximab

Simulect

## Class and Category

*Chemical:* Chimeric (murine or human) monoclonal antibody
*Therapeutic:* Immunosuppressant
*Pregnancy category:* B

## Indications and Dosages

➤ *To prevent acute kidney transplant rejection*

**I.V. INFUSION OR INJECTION**

**Adults and adolescents over age 15.** 20 mg within 2 hr before transplant, then 20 mg 4 days after transplant.
**Children and adolescents ages 2 to 15.** 12 mg/m$^2$ within 2 hr before transplant, then 12 mg/m$^2$ 4 days after transplant. *Maximum:* 20 mg/dose.

| Route | Onset | Peak | Duration |
|---|---|---|---|
| I.V. | Unknown | Unknown | 22 to 50 days |

## Mechanism of Action

Initiates immunosuppression by blocking interleukin-2 receptors located on the surface of activated T cells. Normally, interleukin-2 is released by stimulated T lymphocytes, causing activation and differentiation of other T lymphocytes responsible for cell-mediated immunity.

## Incompatibilities

Don't add or infuse any other drugs simultaneously through same I.V. line.

## Contraindications

Hypersensitivity to basiliximab or its components

## Adverse Reactions

**CNS:** Asthenia, dizziness, fever, headache, insomnia, tremor
**CV:** Hypertension, peripheral edema
**EENT:** Oral candidiasis, pharyngitis, rhinitis
**ENDO:** Hyperglycemia
**GI:** Abdominal pain, constipation, diarrhea, indigestion, nausea, vomiting

**GU:** Dysuria, increased urinary nitrogen level, UTI
**HEME:** Anemia
**MS:** Back pain, leg pain
**RESP:** Cough, dyspnea, upper respiratory tract infection
**SKIN:** Acne
**Other:** Hypercholesterolemia, hyperkalemia, hyperuricemia, hypocalcemia, hypokalemia, hypophosphatemia, impaired wound healing, injection site reaction, metabolic acidosis, weight gain

## Nursing Considerations

• To reconstitute basiliximab, add 5 ml of sterile water for injection to powder and shake vial gently to dissolve. Further dilute with NS or D$_5$W for infusion to a volume of 50 ml. Gently invert infusion bag to avoid foaming; don't shake. Drug should appear clear to opalescent and colorless.
• Administer reconstituted drug I.V. over 20 to 30 minutes or as a bolus dose directly through a central or peripheral I.V. line. Be aware that bolus dose may cause nausea, vomiting, and a localized injection site reaction, including pain.
• Expect drug to be given as adjunct to cyclosporine and corticosteroids.
• Don't store drug at room temperature for longer than 4 hours; don't refrigerate for longer than 24 hours.
• **WARNING** Be aware that patient may develop hypersensitivity reactions, including anaphylaxis, bronchospasm, dyspnea, hypotension, pruritus, rash, respiratory failure, sneezing, tachycardia, urticaria, and wheezing, on initial exposure or following reexposure after several months. Notify prescriber immediately if such reactions occur.
**PATIENT TEACHING**
• Inform patient that second dose of basiliximab will be given 4 days after transplant and that she may also receive cyclosporine and corticosteroid therapy.
• Inform patient that because of drug's immunosuppressant effects, she may experience slower wound healing and be more susceptible to upper respiratory tract infections.

# beclomethasone dipropionate

Beclodisk (CAN), Beclovent Rotacaps (CAN), Beconase, Beconase AQ, QVAR, Vancenase, Vanceril

## Class and Category

*Chemical:* Synthetic glucocorticoid
*Therapeutic:* Antiasthmatic, anti-inflammatory
*Pregnancy category:* C

## Indications and Dosages

➤ *To control and prevent symptoms in patients with chronic asthma and those who also require oral corticosteroids*

INHALATION AEROSOL (84 MCG)

**Adults and children age 12 and older.** *Initial:* 2 inhalations (168 mcg) b.i.d. For patients with severe asthma, 6 to 8 inhalations (504 to 672 mcg) daily with dosage reduced based on patient response. *Maximum:* 10 inhalations (840 mcg) daily.

**Children ages 6 to 12.** *Initial:* 2 inhalations (168 mcg) b.i.d. *Maximum:* 5 inhalations (420 mcg) daily.

INHALATION AEROSOL (42 MCG)

**Adults and children age 12 and older.** *Initial:* 2 inhalations (84 mcg) t.i.d. or q.i.d. or 4 inhalations (168 mcg) b.i.d. For patients with severe asthma, 12 to 16 (504 to 672 mcg) inhalations daily with dosage reduced based on patient response. *Maximum:* 20 inhalations (840 mcg) daily.

**Children ages 6 to 12.** *Initial:* 1 or 2 inhalations (42 mcg or 84 mcg) t.i.d. or q.i.d. or 4 inhalations (168 mcg) b.i.d. with dosage reduced based on patient response. *Maximum:* 10 inhalations (420 mcg) daily.

INHALATION AEROSOL (40 MCG, 80 MCG [QVAR])

**Adults and adolescents.** *Initial for patients previously taking bronchodilators alone:* 1 to 2 inhalations (40 to 80 mcg) b.i.d., depending on strength used. *Maximum:* 4 to 8 inhalations (320 mcg) b.i.d., depending on strength used. *Initial for patients previously taking inhaled corticosteroids:* 1 to 4 inhalations (160 mcg) b.i.d., depending on strength used. *Maximum:* 4 to 8 inhalations (320 mcg) b.i.d., depending on strength used.

**Children ages 5 to 11.** 1 inhalation (40 mcg) b.i.d. *Maximum:* 1 to 2 inhalations (80 mcg) b.i.d., depending on strength used.

➤ *To relieve symptoms of seasonal or perennial allergic and nonallergic (vasomotor) rhinitis and prevent nasal polyps from recurring after surgical removal*

NASAL INHALATION AEROSOL

**Adults and children age 12 and older.** *Initial:* 1 inhalation (42 mcg) in each nostril b.i.d. to q.i.d. for total dose of 168 to 336 mcg/day.

*Maintenance:* 1 inhalation (42 mcg) in each nostril t.i.d. for total dose of 252 mcg/day.
**Children ages 6 to 12.** 1 inhalation (42 mcg) in each nostril t.i.d. for total dose of 252 mcg/day.

NASAL SPRAY

**Adults and children age 12 and older.** 1 or 2 inhalations (42 or 84 mcg) in each nostril b.i.d. for total dose of 168 or 336 mcg/day.

**B**

---

## Mechanism of Action

May decrease number and activity of cells involved in the inflammatory response of asthma, allergies, and rhinitis, such as mast cells, eosinophils, basophils, lymphocytes, macrophages, and neutrophils. Also may inhibit production or secretion of chemical mediators, such as histamine, eicosanoids, leukotrienes, and cytokines. May produce direct smooth-muscle cell relaxation and decrease airway hyperresponsiveness.

---

## Contraindications

Hypersensitivity to beclomethasone's ingredients, infrequent oral corticosteroid treatment, primary treatment of status asthmaticus or other acute asthma attack, relief of acute bronchospasm or of asthma controlled by bronchodilators or other nonsteroidal drugs, treatment of nonasthmatic bronchitis

## Adverse Reactions

**CNS:** Depression, fatigue, fever, headache, insomnia, light-headedness
**CV:** Chest pain, tachycardia
**EENT:** Cataracts, dry mouth, dysphonia, earache, epistaxis, glaucoma, hoarseness, lacrimation, nasal congestion, nose and throat dryness and irritation, oral candidiasis, pharyngitis, rhinorrhea, sinusitis, sneezing, unpleasant smell and taste
**ENDO:** Adrenal insufficiency, cushingoid symptoms
**GI:** Diarrhea, indigestion, nausea, rectal hemorrhage
**GU:** Dysmenorrhea, UTI
**MS:** Arthralgia, growth suppression in children (nasal aerosol)
**RESP:** Bronchitis, bronchospasm, chest congestion, cough, pulmonary infiltrates, upper respiratory tract infection, wheezing
**SKIN:** Acne, eczema, pruritus, rash, skin discoloration, urticaria

**Other:** Angioedema, flulike symptoms, lymphadenopathy, weight gain

## Nursing Considerations
•If patient also receives an oral corticosteroid, expect to taper its dosage slowly (by decreasing the daily dosage or using the drug every other day) about 1 week after beclomethasone therapy begins. Expect dosage reductions of more than 2.5 mg/day.
•WARNING When gradually switching patient from an oral corticosteroid to inhaled beclomethasone, assess her for signs of life-threatening adrenal insufficiency, such as fatigue, lassitude, weakness, nausea, vomiting, and hypotension, during transition period and when exposed to trauma, surgery, infection, or other stressor. If signs occur, notify prescriber immediately.
•Expect to resume oral corticosteroid during a stressful period or severe asthma attack.
•Because beclomethasone may be absorbed systemically, monitor for signs of adrenal insufficiency during periods of stress.
•If patient experiences an acute asthma attack or increased wheezing after administering beclomethasone, administer a fast-acting bronchodilator, as prescribed. Expect to discontinue beclomethasone.
•Assess for signs of candidiasis, such as thick white plaques or coating on tongue and sides of mouth. If present, notify prescriber and expect to reduce drug dose or frequency or discontinue beclomethasone. Also anticipate treatment with antifungal drug.
•When administering beclomethasone nasal spray, periodically assess nasal discharge for color or consistency changes, which may indicate infection.
•Monitor the growth of children receiving beclomethasone nasally.
PATIENT TEACHING
•Advise patient not to abruptly stop taking beclomethasone because adrenal insufficiency may occur. Urge her to notify prescriber if she develops signs of adrenal insufficiency, such as nausea, fatigue, anorexia, dyspnea, hypotension, fever, malaise, dizziness, and fainting.
•Before patient uses nasal spray for first time, instruct her to prime the pump by placing her thumb on its base and index and middle fingers on its shoulder area and then pressing her thumb firmly and quickly against bottle several times or until fine mist appears. Before patient uses nasal inhalation canister for first time, instruct her to shake it and check that it's working properly by spraying it once in the air while looking for fine mist.
•Teach patient to inhale deeply after each nasal spray or inhalation, exhaling through mouth and tilting head back to let drug spread over the nasopharynx.
•Teach patient how to properly use oral inhalation aerosol, shaking canister well before using. If patient has difficulty using device and coordinating inhalation with it, suggest using a spacer device.
•If two inhalations are prescribed, advise patient to wait at minute between inhalations.
•If patient uses an inhaled bronchodilator with beclomethasone oral inhalation, instruct her to use bronchodilator first, wait 5 minutes, and then use beclomethasone.
•WARNING Warn patient that beclomethasone isn't intended to relieve acute bronchospasm. Urge patient to notify prescriber if asthma symptoms don't respond to drug.
•Advise patient to wear medical identification that states need for supplemental oral corticosteroids during stress or severe asthma attack. Inform patient that prescriber may order high-dose oral corticosteroid therapy.
•WARNING Caution patient to avoid exposure to chickenpox and measles because beclomethasone may cause immunosuppression. If she's exposed to these disorders, urge her to notify prescriber immediately.

# belladonna alkaloids

## Class and Category
*Chemical:* Tertiary amine
*Therapeutic:* GI anticholinergic
*Pregnancy category:* C

## Indications and Dosages
➤ *To treat peptic ulcer disease, functional digestive disorders (including spastic, mucous, and ulcerative colitis), diarrhea, diverticulitis, pancreatitis, dysmenorrhea, nocturnal enuresis, idiopathic and postencephalitic parkinsonism, motion sickness, and nausea and vomiting of pregnancy*
TABLETS
**Adults.** 0.25 to 0.5 mg t.i.d.
**Children over age 6.** 0.125 to 0.25 mg t.i.d.

TINCTURE
**Adults.** 0.6 to 1 ml t.i.d. or q.i.d.
**Children.** 0.03 ml/kg (0.8 ml/m$^2$) t.i.d.

| Route | Onset | Peak | Duration |
|-------|-------|------|----------|
| P.O. | 1 to 2 hr | Unknown | 4 hr |

## Mechanism of Action

Inhibits acetylcholine's muscarinic actions at postganglionic parasympathetic receptor sites, including smooth muscles, secretory glands, and CNS. These actions relax smooth muscles and diminish GI, GU, and biliary tract secretions.

## Contraindications

Hepatic disease, hypersensitivity to anticholinergic drugs or scopolamine, ileus, myasthenia gravis, myocardial ischemia, narrow-angle glaucoma, obstructive condition of GI or GU tract, renal disease, severe ulcerative colitis, tachycardia, toxic megacolon, unstable cardiovascular status in acute hemorrhage

## Interactions

DRUGS
*amantadine:* Increased adverse anticholinergic effects
*atenolol, digoxin:* Possibly increased therapeutic and adverse effects of these drugs
*phenothiazines:* Possibly decreased phenothiazine effectiveness and increased adverse effects of belladonna alkaloids
*tricyclic antidepressants:* Possibly increased adverse anticholinergic effects

## Adverse Reactions

**CNS:** CNS stimulation (with high doses), confusion, dizziness, drowsiness, headache, insomnia, nervousness, weakness
**CV:** Bradycardia, palpitations, tachycardia
**EENT:** Altered taste, blurred vision, dry mouth, increased intraocular pressure, mydriasis, nasal congestion, photophobia
**GI:** Bloating, constipation, dysphagia, heartburn, ileus, nausea, vomiting
**GU:** Impotence, urinary hesitancy, urine retention
**SKIN:** Decreased sweating, flushing, urticaria
**Other:** Anaphylaxis

## Nursing Considerations

• Avoid using high doses of belladonna alkaloids in patients with ulcerative colitis because they may inhibit intestinal motility

and precipitate or aggravate toxic megacolon. Also avoid using high doses in patients with hiatal hernia and reflux esophagitis because they may aggravate esophagitis.
• Use belladonna alkaloids cautiously in patients with allergies, arrhythmias, asthma, autonomic neuropathy, coronary artery disease, debilitating chronic lung disease, heart failure, hypertension, hyperthyroidism, and prostatic hypertrophy.
• Give drug 30 to 60 minutes before a meal.
• WARNING Monitor patient for excitement, agitation, drowsiness, and confusion. Elderly patients are more sensitive to the effects of the drug even with small doses and are more likely to develop these adverse reactions. Dosage may need to be decreased.
• Take safety precautions to protect patient from injury from falling.

PATIENT TEACHING
• Instruct patient to take belladonna alkaloids 30 to 60 minutes before eating.
• Tell patient to notify prescriber if she has persistent or severe diarrhea, constipation, or difficulty urinating.
• Caution patient to avoid driving and similar activities until the effects of belladonna alkaloids are known.
• WARNING Urge patient to avoid extreme heat and humidity because heatstroke may occur.

# benazepril hydrochloride

Lotensin

## Class and Category

*Chemical:* Ethylester of benazeprilat
*Therapeutic:* Antihypertensive
*Pregnancy category:* C (D in second and third trimesters)

## Indications and Dosages

➤ *To control hypertension alone or with a thiazide diuretic*

TABLETS
**Adults who don't receive a diuretic.** *Initial:* 10 mg/day. *Maintenance:* 20 to 40 mg/day as a single dose or in two divided doses.
**Adults who receive a diuretic.** 5 mg/day.
DOSAGE ADJUSTMENT Initial dosage of 5 mg/day for patients with impaired renal function and creatinine clearance of less than 30

ml/min/1.73 m², then increased gradually until blood pressure is controlled or dosage reaches maximum of 40 mg/day.

TABLETS, SUSPENSION

**Children age 6 and older with glomerular filtration rate of 30 ml/min/1.73 m² or higher.** *Initial:* 0.2 mg/kg/day. *Maximum:* 0.6 mg/kg q.d. or 40 mg/day.

| Route | Onset | Peak | Duration |
|-------|-------|------|----------|
| P.O. | 1 hr | 2 to 4 hr | 24 hr |

## Mechanism of Action

May reduce blood pressure by affecting renin-angiotensin-aldosterone system. By inhibiting ACE, benazepril:
• prevents conversion of angiotensin I to angiotensin II, a potent vasoconstrictor that also stimulates aldosterone release.
• may inhibit renal and vascular production of angiotensin II.
• decreases serum angiotensin II level and increases serum renin activity. This decreases aldosterone secretion, slightly increasing serum potassium level and fluid loss.
• decreases vascular tone and blood pressure.
• inhibits aldosterone release, which reduces sodium and water resorption, increases their excretion, and reduces blood pressure.

## Contraindications

Hypersensitivity to benazepril or other ACE inhibitor

## Interactions

DRUGS

*antacids:* Possibly decreased bioavailability of benazepril, requiring administration of drugs separated by 2 hours
*capsaicin:* Possibly induction or exacerbation of ACE cough caused by benazepril
*digoxin:* Increased serum digoxin level
*diuretics:* Possibly excessive hypotension
*indomethacin:* Reduced hypotensive effects of benazepril
*lithium:* Increased serum lithium level and risk of lithium toxicity
*phenothiazines:* Possibly increased therapeutic and adverse effects of benazepril
*potassium preparations, potassium-sparing diuretics:* Possibly increased serum potassium level

## Adverse Reactions

**CNS:** Anxiety, asthenia, dizziness, drowsiness, fatigue, headache, hypertonia, insomnia, nervousness, paresthesia, sleep disturbance, somnolence, syncope, weakness
**CV:** Angina, ECG changes, hypotension, orthostatic hypotension, palpitations, peripheral edema
**EENT:** Sinusitis
**ENDO:** Hyperglycemia
**GI:** Abdominal pain, constipation, elevated liver function test results, gastritis, melena, nausea, pancreatitis, vomiting
**GU:** Decreased libido, elevated BUN and serum creatinine levels, impotence, nephrotic syndrome, proteinuria, renal insufficiency, UTI
**HEME:** Agranulocytosis, decreased hemoglobin level, leukopenia, neutropenia, thrombocytopenia
**MS:** Arthralgia, arthritis, myalgia
**RESP:** ACE cough, asthma, bronchitis, bronchospasm, dyspnea
**SKIN:** Dermatitis, diaphoresis, flushing, photosensitivity, pruritus, rash
**Other:** Angioedema, hyperkalemia, hyponatremia

## Nursing Considerations

• Evaluate blood pressure with patient lying down, sitting, and standing before initiating benazepril and then every 4 to 8 hours, as appropriate, to monitor drug's effectiveness.
• Monitor urine output and BUN and serum creatinine levels, as needed, before therapy.
• **WARNING** Be alert for angioedema, especially after first dose. If angioedema extends to larynx and patient exhibits laryngeal stridor or signs of airway obstruction, prepare to give epinephrine S.C. immediately, as prescribed, and discontinue benazepril.
• Monitor WBC count periodically to detect neutropenia and agranulocytosis.
• Monitor serum potassium and other electrolyte levels to detect electrolyte imbalances.
• To prevent injury caused by orthostatic hypotension, take safety precautions, such as having patient change position slowly and sit on edge of bed before arising.

PATIENT TEACHING

• Teach patient how to monitor blood pressure, if appropriate, and how to recognize signs of hypertension and hypotension.
• **WARNING** Strongly urge patient to contact prescriber before using any OTC salt sub-

stitutes, which may contain potassium, or potassium supplements. These substances increase the risk of hyperkalemia.
•Inform patient that a persistent dry cough may develop and may not subside unless benazepril is discontinued. If cough becomes bothersome or interferes with her sleep or activities, instruct her to notify prescriber.
•**WARNING** Instruct patient to contact prescriber immediately if she experiences signs of angioedema, such as swelling of the face, eyes, lips, or tongue.
•Caution patient to avoid sudden position changes and to rise slowly from a seated or reclining position to minimize orthostatic hypotension.
•**WARNING** Advise patient to stop benazepril and notify prescriber as soon as possible if she experiences syncope.

# benzonatate

Benzonatate Softgels, Tessalon Perles

## Class and Category
*Chemical:* Para-aminobenzoic acid (tetracaine-like)
*Therapeutic:* Nonnarcotic antitussive
*Pregnancy category:* C

## Indications and Dosages
➤ *To relieve cough*
CAPSULES
**Adults and children over age 10.** 100 mg t.i.d. up to 600 mg/day.

| Route | Onset | Peak | Duration |
|-------|-------|------|----------|
| P.O. | 15 to 20 min | Unknown | 3 to 8 hr |

### Mechanism of Action
Anesthetizes stretch receptors in respiratory tract, lung tissue, and pleura, interfering with their activity and reducing cough reflex at its source. In usual doses, benzonatate doesn't inhibit respiratory center.

## Contraindications
Hypersensitivity to benzonatate or related compounds

## Adverse Reactions
**CNS:** Confusion, hallucinations, headache, mild dizziness, sedation
**CV:** Cardiogenic shock, chest numbness
**EENT:** Burning eyes, laryngospasm, nasal congestion
**GI:** Constipation, GI upset, nausea
**RESP:** Bronchospasm
**SKIN:** Pruritus, rash

## Nursing Considerations
•Assess type and frequency of cough. Don't attempt to suppress cough with benzonatate if cough has therapeutic benefit, such as to move secretions and improve airflow.
•**WARNING** Don't break or crush capsules or let patient chew or dissolve them in her mouth. This may cause benzonatate's release in patient's mouth, which can anesthetize her mouth and throat, placing her at risk for choking. Also don't let patient suck or chew the capsule to prevent severe hypersensitivity reaction.
PATIENT TEACHING
•Instruct patient to swallow capsules whole and not to chew, suck, or open them.
•Warn patient that mild dizziness and sedation may occur. Teach her to take safety measures, and encourage her to avoid activities that require mental alertness until benzonatate's effects are known.

# benzquinamide hydrochloride

Emete-Con

## Class and Category
*Chemical:* Benzoquinolizine amide
*Therapeutic:* Antiemetic
*Pregnancy category:* Not rated

## Indications and Dosages
➤ *To treat nausea and vomiting related to anesthesia or surgery*
I.V. OR I.M. INJECTION
**Adults.** 50 mg or 0.5 to 1 mg/kg I.M., repeated in 1 hr, then q 3 to 4 hr, p.r.n. Or 25 mg or 0.2 to 0.4 mg/kg by slow infusion (1 ml every 0.5 to 1 min) as a single dose. Then, I.M. doses begin.

➤ *To prevent nausea and vomiting related to anesthesia and surgery*

**I.M. INJECTION**
**Adults.** 50 mg or 0.5 to 1 mg/kg 15 min before emergence from anesthesia.

| Route | Onset | Peak | Duration |
|---|---|---|---|
| I.V., I.M. | 15 min | Unknown | Unknown |

## Mechanism of Action
Exhibits antiemetic, antihistaminic, mild cholinergic, and sedative effects by unknown mechanism.

## Contraindications
Hypersensitivity to benzquinamide or its components

## Interactions
**DRUGS**
*vasopressors:* Increased hypertensive effects

## Adverse Reactions
**CNS:** Chills, dizziness, drowsiness, excitement, fatigue, fever, headache, insomnia, nervousness, restlessness, tremor, weakness
**CV:** Atrial fibrillation, hypertension, hypotension, premature atrial or ventricular contractions
**EENT:** Blurred vision, dry mouth, increased salivation
**GI:** Anorexia, hiccups, nausea
**MS:** Muscle twitching
**SKIN:** Diaphoresis, flushing, rash, urticaria

## Nursing Considerations
•**WARNING** Avoid I.V. route in patients with cardiovascular disease because sudden blood pressure increases and transient arrhythmias may occur. Use I.V. route only for patients without cardiovascular disease who aren't receiving a preanesthetic or cardiovascular drug.
•Administer benzquinamide I.M. into large, well-developed muscle. Avoid using deltoid muscle unless it's well developed.
•Take safety precautions to reduce the risk of injury from CNS depression.
**PATIENT TEACHING**
•Advise patient to stay in bed and call for assistance to reduce risk of injury.
•Tell patient to report whether nausea and vomiting have been relieved.

# benztropine mesylate
Apo-Benztropine (CAN), Cogentin, PMS Benztropine (CAN)

## Class and Category
*Chemical:* Tertiary amine
*Therapeutic:* Antiparkinsonian, central-acting anticholinergic
*Pregnancy category:* C

## Indications and Dosages
➤ *As adjunct, to treat all forms of Parkinson's disease*
**TABLETS, I.M. OR I.V. INJECTION**
**Adults with Parkinson's disease.** 1 to 2 mg/day (usual dose) with a range of 0.5 to 6.0 mg/day.
**Adults with idiopathic Parkinson's disease.**
*Initial:* 0.5 to 1.0 mg h.s. *Maximum:* 4 to 6 mg/day.
**Adults with postencephalitic Parkinson's disease.** 2 mg/day in one or more doses; may begin with 0.5 mg h.s. and increase as needed.
➤ *To control extrapyramidal symptoms (except tardive dyskinesia) caused by phenothiazines and other neuroleptic drugs*
**TABLETS, I.M. OR I.V. INJECTION**
**Adults.** 1 to 4 mg q.d. or b.i.d.
➤ *To treat acute dystonic reactions*
**TABLETS, I.M. OR I.V. INJECTION**
**Adults.** *Initial:* 1 to 2 ml (1 to 2 mg total dose) I.V. or I.M. *Maintenance:* 1 to 2 mg P.O. b.i.d. to prevent recurrence.

| Route | Onset | Peak | Duration |
|---|---|---|---|
| P.O. | 1 to 2 hr | Unknown | 24 hr |
| I.V., I.M | 15 min | Unknown | 24 hr |

## Mechanism of Action
Blocks acetylcholine's action at cholinergic receptor sites. This restores the brain's normal dopamine and acetylcholine balance, which relaxes muscle movement and decreases drooling, rigidity, and tremor. Benztropine also may inhibit dopamine reuptake and storage, which prolongs dopamine's action.

## Contraindications
Achalasia, bladder neck obstruction, glaucoma, hypersensitivity to benztropine mesylate or its components, megacolon, myasthenia gravis, prostatic hypertrophy, pyloric or duodenal obstruction, stenosing peptic ulcer

## Interactions
**DRUGS**
*amantadine:* Possibly increased adverse anticholinergic effects
*digoxin:* Possibly increased serum digoxin level
*haloperidol:* Possibly increased schizophrenic symptoms, decreased serum haloperidol level, and development of tardive dyskinesia
*levodopa:* Possibly decreased levodopa effectiveness
*phenothiazines:* Possibly reduced phenothiazine effects and increased psychiatric symptoms

## Adverse Reactions
**CNS:** Agitation, confusion, delirium, delusions, depression, disorientation, dizziness, drowsiness, euphoria, excitement, fever, hallucinations, headache, light-headedness, listlessness, memory loss, nervousness, paranoia, psychosis, weakness
**CV:** Hypotension, mild bradycardia, orthostatic hypotension, palpitations, tachycardia
**EENT:** Blurred vision, diplopia, dry mouth, increased intraocular pressure, mydriasis, narrow-angle glaucoma, suppurative parotitis
**GI:** Constipation, duodenal ulcer, epigastric distress, ileus, nausea, vomiting
**GU:** Dysuria, urinary hesitancy, urine retention
**MS:** Muscle spasms, muscle weakness
**SKIN:** Decreased sweating, dermatoses, flushing, rash, urticaria

## Nursing Considerations
• Expect to administer I.V. or I.M. benztropine when patient needs more rapid response than oral drug can provide. Be aware that I.M. route is commonly used because it provides effects in about the same time as I.V. route. Watch for improvement a few minutes after administration. If Parkinsonian symptoms reappear, expect to repeat dose.
• Know that therapy generally begins with a low dose followed by gradual increases of 0.5 mg every 5 or 6 days because benztropine has a cumulative action.
• Assess muscle rigidity and tremor as a baseline. Then monitor them frequently for improvement, which indicates benztropine's effectiveness.
• Administer drug before or after meals based on patient's need and response. If patient has increased salivary secretions, expect to administer benztropine after meals. If patient has dry mouth, plan to give drug before meals unless nausea develops.
• **WARNING** When administering benztropine to patient with drug-induced extrapyramidal reactions, be alert for exacerbation of psychiatric symptoms.
• Know that high-dose benztropine therapy may cause weakness and inability to move specific muscle groups. If this occurs, expect to reduce benztropine dosage.

**PATIENT TEACHING**
• Warn patient that benztropine has a cumulative effect, increasing risk of adverse reactions and overdose.
• Caution patient to avoid driving and similar activities until benztropine's effects are known because drug may cause blurred vision, dizziness, or drowsiness.
• **WARNING** Because benztropine decreases sweating, urge patient to avoid extremely hot or humid conditions to reduce risk of heatstroke and severe hyperthermia. This is especially important for elderly patients and those who abuse alcohol or have chronic illness or CNS disease.
• Stress need for periodic eye examinations and intraocular pressure measurements because benztropine may cause narrow-angle glaucoma and increase intraocular pressure.

# bepridil hydrochloride
Vascor

## Class and Category
*Chemical:* Calcium channel blocker, diarylammopropylamine derivative
*Therapeutic:* Antianginal
*Pregnancy category:* C

## Indications and Dosages
➤ *To treat chronic stable angina in patients who don't respond to or can't tolerate other antianginal drugs*
**TABLETS**
**Adults.** *Initial:* 200 mg/day for 10 days followed by dosage increases, depending on patient's response (ability to perform daily activities, length of QT interval, heart rate, and frequency and severity of angina attacks). *Maintenance:* 300 to 400 mg/day (maximum).

| Route | Onset | Peak | Duration |
|-------|-------|------|----------|
| P.O. | Unknown | 8 days | Unknown |

## Mechanism of Action

Inhibits calcium movement into coronary and vascular smooth-muscle cells by blocking slow calcium channels in their membranes. This decreases intracellular calcium level, which inhibits smooth-muscle cell contractions and causes:
• relaxation of coronary and vascular smooth muscles, decreased peripheral vascular resistance, and reduced systolic and diastolic blood pressure, which decrease myocardial oxygen demand
• depression of impulse formation (automaticity) and conduction velocity.

Bepridil also inhibits fast inward sodium channels, reducing speed and degree of action potential and increasing its duration in cardiac muscle.

## Contraindications

Congenital prolonged QT interval, history of serious ventricular arrhythmias, hypersensitivity to bepridil, hypotension (systolic pressure below 90 mm Hg), sick sinus syndrome and second- or third-degree AV block unless artificial pacemaker in place, uncompensated cardiac insufficiency, use of other drugs that prolong QT interval

## Interactions

**DRUGS**

*antiarrhythmics, such as quinidine and procainamide, with actions similar to bepridil's:* Exaggerated and prolonged QT interval
*beta blockers:* Possibly increased depression of myocardial contractility and AV conduction
*digoxin:* Possibly increased serum digoxin level
*fentanyl:* Severe hypotension and increased need for fluid
*nitrates:* Additive hypotensive effect
*tricyclic antidepressants:* Exaggerated and prolonged QT interval

## Adverse Reactions

**CNS:** Amnesia, anxiety, asthenia, depression, dizziness, drowsiness, fever, hallucinations, headache, insomnia, nervousness, paranoia, paresthesia, psychosis, syncope, tremor, vertigo
**CV:** Edema, hypertension, palpitations, premature ventricular contractions, prolonged QT interval, sinus bradycardia or tachycardia, torsades de pointes, vasodila-
tion, ventricular fibrillation, ventricular tachycardia
**EENT:** Altered taste, blurred vision, dry mouth, pharyngitis, rhinitis, tinnitus
**GI:** Abdominal cramps or discomfort, anorexia, appetite increase, constipation, diarrhea, flatulence, gastritis, nausea
**GU:** Decreased libido, impotence
**HEME:** Agranulocytosis, leukopenia, neutropenia
**MS:** Arthritis, myalgia
**RESP:** Cough, dyspnea, respiratory tract infection
**SKIN:** Dermatitis, diaphoresis, rash
**Other:** Flulike symptoms

## Nursing Considerations

• Use bepridil cautiously in patients with heart failure because it can induce new arrhythmias and may worsen heart failure.
• Because bepridil is metabolized by the liver and its metabolites are excreted in urine, monitor results of liver function studies as well as BUN and serum electrolyte and creatinine levels as appropriate.
• Assess heart rate and rhythm to obtain baseline. Then monitor frequently during therapy. Also, monitor serial 12-lead ECG tracings. Be aware that bepridil can induce new arrhythmias, including ventricular tachycardia and fibrillation (which are more difficult to convert), torsades de pointes, and prolonged QT intervals.
• WARNING Be alert for QT intervals that exceed 0.52 second. If this occurs, expect to reduce bepridil dose or discontinue drug.
• Monitor WBC count to detect agranulocytosis, which may require drug discontinuation.
• WARNING Be aware that bepridil shouldn't be discontinued abruptly. Instead, gradually taper its dosage as prescribed to prevent increased frequency and duration of chest pain as increased calcium moves into cells, causing coronary artery spasm.
• Monitor blood pressure frequently if patient also receives nitrates or beta blockers. Assess for hypotension.
• Monitor serum electrolyte levels. Especially note decreased potassium level, which may exacerbate existing arrhythmias or induce new ones.

**PATIENT TEACHING**

• Advise patient to avoid driving and other activities that require alertness and coordination until bepridil's CNS effects are known.

# betamethasone
Celestone

## betamethasone acetate-betamethasone sodium phosphate
Celestone Soluspan

## betamethasone sodium phosphate
Betnesol (CAN), Celestone Phosphate, Selestoject

### Class and Category
*Chemical:* Synthetic glucocorticoid
*Therapeutic:* Anti-inflammatory
*Pregnancy category:* C

### Indications and Dosages
➤ *To treat conditions with severe inflammation and conditions requiring immunosuppression*
SYRUP, TABLETS (BETAMETHASONE)
**Adults.** 0.6 to 7.2 mg/day.
I.M. INJECTION (BETAMETHASONE ACETATE-BETAMETHASONE SODIUM PHOSPHATE)
**Adults.** 0.5 to 9 mg I.M. daily, or ⅓ to ½ of P.O. dose q 12 hr.
I.M OR I.V. INJECTION (BETAMETHASONE SODIUM PHOSPHATE)
**Adults.** *Initial:* Variable (given in emergency situations or when oral therapy isn't possible). *Maximum:* 9 mg/day.
➤ *To treat bursitis, gouty arthritis, osteoarthritis, periostitis of cuboid, peritendinitis, rheumatoid arthritis, skin lesions, tenosynovitis*
INTRA-ARTICULAR, INTRABURSAL, OR INTRADERMAL INJECTION (BETAMETHASONE ACETATE-BETAMETHASONE SODIUM PHOSPHATE)
**Adults with bursitis, peritendinitis, or tenosynovitis.** 1 ml by intrabursal or intra-articular injection. Three or four injections given q 1 to 2 wk.
**Adults with osteoarthritis or rheumatoid arthritis.** 0.5 to 2 ml, depending on joint size.
**Adults with foot bursitis.** 0.25 to 0.5 ml q 3 to 7 days.
**Adults with foot tenosynovitis or periostitis of cuboid.** 0.5 ml q 3 to 7 days.
**Adults with acute gouty arthritis.** 0.5 to 1 ml q 3 to 7 days.
**Adults with skin lesions.** 0.2 ml/cm² intradermally, up to 1 ml weekly.

DOSAGE ADJUSTMENT Dosage reduced for elderly patients and accompanied by periodic monitoring of blood pressure and blood glucose and electrolyte levels.

### Contraindications
Idiopathic thrombocytopenic purpura (I.M. injection), live virus vaccination, systemic fungal infection

| Route | Onset | Peak | Duration |
|---|---|---|---|
| P.O. | Unknown | 1 to 2 hr | 3.25 days |
| I.V., I.M. (sodium phosphate) | Rapid | Unknown | Unknown |
| I.M. (acetate-sodium phosphate) | 1 to 3 hr | Unknown | 1 wk |
| Other (acetate-sodium phosphate) | Unknown | Unknown | 1 to 2 wk* |

### Mechanism of Action
Binds to intracellular glucocorticoid receptors and suppresses inflammatory and immune responses by:
•inhibiting neutrophil and monocyte accumulation at inflammation site and suppressing their phagocytic and bactericidal activity
•stabilizing lysosomal membranes
•suppressing antigen response of macrophages and helper T cells
•inhibiting synthesis of inflammatory response mediators, such as cytokines, interleukins, and prostaglandins.

### Interactions
DRUGS
*anticholinesterase drugs:* Possibly antagonized anticholinesterase effects in myasthenia gravis
*barbiturates:* Possibly decreased effects of betamethasone
*cyclosporine:* Possibly increased risk of cyclosporine toxicity

---

*For intra-arterial or intrasynovial injection; 1 week for intralesional injection in soft tissue.

*digitalis glycosides:* Possibly increased risk of digitalis toxicity
*estrogens:* Possibly decreased excretion of betamethasone
*hydantoins, rifampin:* Possibly increased excretion and decreased therapeutic effects of betamethasone
*isoniazid:* Possibly decreased serum isoniazid level
*ketoconazole:* Possibly decreased excretion of betamethasone
*oral anticoagulants:* Possibly increased or decreased action of anticoagulants, requiring adjusted anticoagulant dosage
*oral contraceptives:* Possibly increased half-life and concentration and decreased excretion of betamethasone
*potassium-wasting diuretics:* Increased risk of hypokalemia
*salicylates:* Possibly decreased serum level and therapeutic effects of salicylates
*somatrem:* Possibly inhibition of somatrem's growth-promoting effects
*theophyllines:* Possibly changes in both drugs' effects

## Adverse Reactions

**CNS:** Fatigue, headache, increased intracranial pressure with papilledema, insomnia, malaise, neuritis, paresthesia, seizures, steroid psychosis, syncope, vertigo
**CV:** Arrhythmias, ECG changes, fat embolism, heart failure, hypertension, thromboembolism, thrombophlebitis
**EENT:** Cataracts, exophthalmos, glaucoma, increased intraocular pressure
**ENDO:** Cushingoid symptoms (buffalo hump, central obesity, decreased carbohydrate tolerance, fat pad enlargement, moon face), fluid retention, growth suppression in children, hyperglycemia, masked signs of infection, negative nitrogen balance, secondary adrenocortical and pituitary unresponsiveness (in times of stress)
**GI:** Abdominal distention, increased appetite, nausea, pancreatitis, peptic ulcer possibly with perforation, ulcerative esophagitis, vomiting
**GU:** Amenorrhea, glycosuria, menstrual irregularities
**HEME:** Leukocytosis
**MS:** Aseptic necrosis of femoral and humeral heads, loss of muscle mass, muscle weakness, osteoporosis, spontaneous pathologic and vertebral compression fractures, tendon rupture
**SKIN:** Acneiform lesions, allergic dermatitis,

ecchymosis, facial erythema, hirsutism, impaired wound healing, increased sweating, petechiae, lupuslike lesions, purpura, subcutaneous fat atrophy, thin and fragile skin, urticaria
**Other:** Angioedema, hypocalcemia, hypokalemia, sodium retention, suppressed reaction to skin tests, weight gain

## Nursing Considerations

• Expect prescriber to order baseline ophthalmologic examination before initiating therapy because prolonged betamethasone use may lead to increased intraocular pressure, glaucoma, and subsequent optic nerve damage. Use betamethasone cautiously in patients with ocular herpes simplex because corneal perforation may occur.
• Assess for signs of infection before administering betamethasone because drug may mask those signs. Because drug may cause immunosuppression, new infection may develop during therapy. If so, expect to administer appropriate antibiotic.
• Review serum electrolyte levels, as ordered, before initiating therapy. Monitor these levels frequently during therapy to detect imbalances. Sodium and water retention and potassium and calcium depletion may occur with high-dose betamethasone therapy. If so, expect to restrict sodium intake and provide potassium and calcium supplements.
• Because betamethasone is linked to peptic ulcer formation, expect to administer it with an antacid or H₂-receptor blocker.
• **WARNING** Monitor ECG tracings for arrhythmias, and evaluate patient for anaphylactic reactions, such as angioedema and seizures, which have been associated with rapid I.V. administration of high-dose corticosteroids.
• **WARNING** During long-term betamethasone therapy, assess for signs of adrenal suppression and insufficiency (fatigue, hypotension, lassitude, nausea, vomiting, and weakness) when patient is exposed to stress. If she exhibits these signs, notify prescriber at once.
• Watch for signs of steroid psychosis, such as delirium, clouded sensorium, euphoria, insomnia, mood swings, personality changes, and severe depression, which may develop 15 to 30 days after therapy begins. Be prepared to discontinue therapy. If this isn't possible, expect to administer psychotropic drugs.
• Rotate I.M. injection sites. To prevent muscle atrophy, avoid S.C. injection, injection in deltoid

site, and repeated I.M. injections into same site.
•Administer oral betamethasone before 9 a.m.,
if appropriate, to mimic body's natural release
of corticosteroids.
•After intra-articular injection, assess joint
for marked increase in pain, local swelling,
and more restricted movement. If patient
also develops fever and malaise, suspect septic arthritis and notify prescriber immediately. Expect to assist with joint fluid aspiration to confirm septic arthritis.
•Monitor patient for cushingoid signs and
symptoms, such as moon face, buffalo hump,
central obesity, striae, acne, ecchymosis, and
weight gain. Notify prescriber if you detect
these symptoms.
•Expect to slowly taper oral betamethasone
dosage to prevent adrenal insufficiency.

**PATIENT TEACHING**
•Instruct patient to take betamethasone with
food if GI upset occurs.
•Reinforce signs of adrenal insufficiency and
possible need for dosage increases during
stress. Advise patient to notify prescriber immediately if signs of insufficiency occur or if
she's exposed to stress.
•Instruct patient to avoid exposure to infections because drug can cause immunosuppression. Also teach patient to recognize and
immediately report signs of infection.
•After intra-articular injection, advise patient not to overuse joint and to continue
other treatments such as physical therapy.

# betaxolol hydrochloride

Kerlone

## Class and Category
*Chemical:* Selective beta$_1$-adrenergic blocker
*Therapeutic:* Antihypertensive
*Pregnancy category:* C

## Indications and Dosages
➤ *To treat hypertension alone or with
other antihypertensives*
**TABLETS**
**Adults.** *Initial:* 10 mg/day. If no response in 7
to 14 days, then 20 mg/day.
**DOSAGE ADJUSTMENT** For elderly patients
and patients who have renal failure or are
undergoing hemodialysis, initial dosage reduced to 5 mg/day. If desired response isn't
achieved, dosage increased by 5-mg increments q 2 wk up to 20 mg/day.

| Route | Onset | Peak | Duration |
|---|---|---|---|
| P.O. | Unknown | 3 to 4 hr | Unknown |

## Mechanism of Action
Inhibits stimulation of beta$_1$-adrenergic
receptor sites, primarily in the heart. This
decreases myocardial excitability, cardiac
output, and myocardial oxygen demand. It
also decreases renin release from the kidneys, which helps reduce blood pressure.

## Contraindications
Cardiogenic shock, heart failure unless caused
by tachyarrhythmia or overt heart failure, hypersensitivity to betaxolol, second- or third-
degree heart block, sinus bradycardia

## Interactions
**DRUGS**
*aluminum salts, barbiturates, calcium salts,
cholestyramine, colestipol, NSAIDs, penicillins, rifampin, salicylates, sulfinpyrazone:*
Decreased therapeutic and adverse effects of
betaxolol
*beta blockers:* Increased risk of additive systemic beta blockade
*calcium channel blockers:* Possibly increased
therapeutic and adverse effects of betaxolol
*ciprofloxacin, other quinolones:* Possibly increased bioavailability of betaxolol, increasing the drug's pharmacologic effect
*clonidine:* Possibly severe hypertension when
both drugs (or just clonidine) are simultaneously withdrawn
*epinephrine:* Possibly severe hypertension
followed by bradycardia
*ergot alkaloids:* Possibly peripheral ischemia
and gangrene
*flecainide:* Possibly increased therapeutic
and adverse effects of both drugs
*lidocaine:* Possibly increased risk of lidocaine
toxicity
*nondepolarizing neuromuscular blockers:*
Possibly increased or decreased neuromuscular blockade
*oral contraceptives:* Possibly increased
bioavailability and plasma level of betaxolol,
increasing the drug's pharmacologic effect
*prazosin:* Possibly increased orthostatic hypotension
*quinidine:* Possibly increased effects of betaxolol

*sulfonylureas:* Possibly masking of hypo-glycemic symptoms

## Adverse Reactions

**CNS:** Amnesia, anxiety, behavior changes, confusion, CVA, depression, dizziness, emotional lability, fatigue, fever, hallucinations, headache, insomnia, lethargy, malaise, mood changes, nightmares, paresthesia, peripheral neuropathy, sedation, syncope, tremor, vertigo

**CV:** Arrhythmias, including asystole, bradycardia, heart block, and torsades de pointes; cardiogenic shock; chest pain; claudication; heart failure; hypercholesterolemia; hyperlipidemia; hypotension; mitral insufficiency; MI; orthostatic hypotension; peripheral vascular insufficiency; Raynaud's phenomenon; renal and mesenteric artery thrombosis

**EENT:** Altered taste, blurred vision, burning eyes, conjunctivitis, dry eyes, dry mouth, earache, eye irritation, eye pain or pressure, increased salivation, laryngospasm, mouth ulcers, nasal stuffiness, pharyngitis, ptosis, rhinitis, sinusitis, tinnitus

**ENDO:** Breast pain (in women), hyperglycemia, hypoglycemia

**GI:** Acute pancreatitis, anorexia, bloating, constipation, diarrhea, elevated liver function test results, epigastric pain, flatulence, gastritis, heartburn, hepatomegaly, increased appetite, indigestion, nausea, vomiting

**GU:** Decreased libido, dysuria, impotence, nocturia, Peyronie's disease, prostatitis, renal colic, renal failure, urinary frequency, urine retention, UTI

**HEME:** Agranulocytosis, eosinophilia, leukopenia, thrombocytopenia

**MS:** Arthralgia, arthritis, gout, muscle spasms or twitching, myalgia, neck pain, tendinitis

**RESP:** Bronchial obstruction, bronchitis, bronchospasm, cough, pulmonary embolus, respiratory distress, upper respiratory tract infection, wheezing

**SKIN:** Acne, diaphoresis, dry skin, eczema, erythema, exfoliative dermatitis, flushing, increased pigmentation, pallor, photophobia, pruritus, rash

**Other:** Acidosis, facial edema, hyperkalemia, hyperuricemia, lymphadenopathy, positive ANA titer, weight gain

## Nursing Considerations

•Use betaxolol cautiously in patients with peripheral vascular disease. Assess color, temperature, and pulses of patient's arms and legs and ask about numbness or tingling and pain.

•Check blood pressure with patient lying, sitting, and standing before starting betaxolol therapy and periodically throughout day to detect changes.

•Review renal function test results before and during therapy.

•Closely monitor diabetic patient's blood glucose level for hypoglycemia because betaxolol may mask tachycardia, but not dizziness and diaphoresis. Be aware that betaxolol may mask tachycardia and blood pressure changes associated with hyperthyroidism.

•**WARNING** Avoid abrupt withdrawal of betaxolol, which can exacerbate or precipitate thyroid storm. Instead, expect to withdraw drug gradually and monitor patient closely.

•Expect to discontinue betaxolol over 2 weeks to prevent MI, ventricular arrhythmias, and, possibly, death from catecholamine hypersensitivity caused by beta blocker therapy.

•If systolic pressure falls below 90 mm Hg, expect to discontinue drug and prepare for hemodynamic monitoring.

•Take safety precautions to prevent injury from falls caused by orthostatic hypotension.

**PATIENT TEACHING**

•Teach patient how to check her blood pressure, if appropriate. Also discuss signs and symptoms of hypertension and hypotension.

•Advise patient to avoid sudden position changes and to rise slowly from a sitting or lying position to minimize the effects of orthostatic hypotension.

•Advise patient to avoid driving and activities that require mental alertness until drug's CNS effects are known.

•Counsel patient to consult prescriber before using an OTC product, such as a cold remedy or nasal decongestant.

# bethanechol chloride

Duvoid, PMS-Bethanechol chloride (CAN), Urabeth, Urecholine

## Class and Category

*Chemical:* Synthetic choline ester
*Therapeutic:* Cholinergic, parasympathomimetic
*Pregnancy category:* C

## Indications and Dosages

➤ *To treat postoperative and postpartal urine retention and retention caused by neurogenic atony of bladder*

B

TABLETS
**Adults.** 10 to 50 mg t.i.d. or q.i.d. *To determine minimum effective dose:* 5 to 10 mg repeated q hr until response is obtained or maximum of 50 mg is reached.

S.C. INJECTION
**Adults.** 2.5 to 5.0 mg t.i.d. or q.i.d. *To determine minimum effective dose:* 2.5 mg repeated q 15 to 30 min until response is obtained or maximum of four doses is reached. Minimum effective dose may be repeated t.i.d. or q.i.d., p.r.n.

| Route | Onset | Peak | Duration |
|-------|-------|------|----------|
| P.O. | 30 to 90 min | 60 min | 6 hr |
| S.C. | 5 to 15 min | 15 to 30 min | 2 hr |

### Mechanism of Action
Acts directly on muscarinic receptors of parasympathetic nervous system, increasing detrusor muscle tone in bladder and allowing contraction of sufficient strength to initiate voiding. Similar to natural neurotransmitter acetylcholine, bethanechol also stimulates gastric motility, increases gastric tone, and enhances peristalsis.

### Contraindications
Acute inflammatory lesions of GI tract, AV conduction defects, bronchial asthma, coronary artery disease, epilepsy, hypersensitivity to bethanecol or its components, hypertension, hyperthyroidism, hypotension, marked vagotonia, mechanical obstruction of GI or GU tract, Parkinson's disease, peptic ulcer disease, peritonitis, pronounced bradycardia, questionable integrity of GI or GU mucosa, spastic GI disorders, vasomotor instability

### Interactions
DRUGS
*cholinergic drugs:* Possibly increased effects of bethanechol
*ganglionic blockers:* Possibly severe hypotension, usually first manifested by severe adverse GI reactions
*procainamide, quinidine:* Possibly decreased effects of bethanechol

### Adverse Reactions
**CNS:** Headache, malaise
**CV:** Hypotension with reflex tachycardia, vasomotor response
**EENT:** Excessive salivation, lacrimation, miosis

**GI:** Abdominal cramps, colicky pain, diarrhea, eructation, nausea, vomiting
**GU:** Urinary urgency
**RESP:** Asthma attack, bronchoconstriction

### Nursing Considerations
• Assess urine elimination before initiating bethanechol therapy.
• WARNING Be aware that patient must have functioning urinary sphincter because a sphincter that doesn't relax when bladder contracts can push urine up into renal pelvis and cause reflux infection.
• Administer oral bethanechol 1 hour before or 2 hours after meals to reduce risk of nausea and vomiting.
• WARNING Don't administer bethanechol I.M. or I.V. because of risk of cholinergic overstimulation, which can cause abdominal cramps, bloody diarrhea, hypotension, shock, or sudden cardiac arrest. Always keep atropine nearby during S.C. administration.
PATIENT TEACHING
• Advise patient to take bethanechol on an empty stomach 1 hour before or 2 hours after meals to reduce risk of nausea and vomiting.

# biperiden hydrochloride
Akineton

## biperiden lactate
Akineton Lactate

### Class and Category
*Chemical:* Tertiary amine
*Therapeutic:* Anticholinergic, antidyskinetic
*Pregnancy category:* C

### Indications and Dosages
➤ *As adjunct to treat all forms of Parkinson's disease*
TABLETS
**Adults.** 2 mg t.i.d. or q.i.d up to 16 mg/day.
➤ *To control extrapyramidal symptoms (except tardive dyskinesia) caused by phenothiazines and other neuroleptic drugs*
TABLETS
**Adults.** 2 mg q.d. to t.i.d.
I.V. OR I.M. INJECTION
**Adults.** 2 mg repeated q 30 min until symptoms resolve or maximum of four consecutive doses in 24 hr is reached.

| Route | Onset | Peak | Duration |
|-------|-------|------|----------|
| I.V. | 15 min | Unknown | 1 to 8 hr |
| I.M. | 10 to 30 min | Unknown | Unknown |

### Mechanism of Action
Blocks acetylcholine's action at cholinergic receptor sites. This action restores the brain's normal dopamine and acetylcholine balance, which relaxes muscle movement and decreases rigidity and tremors. Biperiden also may inhibit dopamine reuptake and storage, which prolongs dopamine's action.

### Contraindications
Achalasia, bladder neck obstruction, hypersensitivity to biperiden, myasthenia gravis, narrow-angle glaucoma, prostatic hypertrophy, pyloric or duodenal obstruction, stenosing peptic ulcer, toxic megacolon

### Interactions
**DRUGS**
*amantadine:* Possibly increased adverse anticholinergic effects
*digoxin:* Possibly increased serum digoxin level
*haloperidol:* Possibly increased schizophrenic symptoms, decreased serum haloperidol level, and development of tardive dyskinesia
*levodopa:* Possibly decreased levodopa effectiveness
*phenothiazines:* Possibly reduced phenothiazine effects and increased psychiatric symptoms

### Adverse Reactions
**CNS:** Agitation, confusion, delirium, delusions, depression, disorientation, dizziness, drowsiness, euphoria, excitement, fever, hallucinations, headache, light-headedness, listlessness, memory loss, nervousness, paranoia, psychosis, weakness
**CV:** Hypotension, mild bradycardia, orthostatic hypotension, palpitations, tachycardia
**EENT:** Blurred vision, diplopia, dry mouth, increased intraocular pressure, mydriasis, narrow-angle glaucoma, suppurative parotitis
**GI:** Constipation, duodenal ulcer, epigastric distress, ileus, nausea, vomiting
**GU:** Dysuria, urinary hesitancy, urine retention
**MS:** Muscle spasms, muscle weakness
**SKIN:** Decreased sweating, dermatosis, flushing, rash, urticaria

### Nursing Considerations
•Expect to administer I.V. or I.M. biperiden when patient needs more rapid response than oral drug can provide.
•Assess muscle rigidity and tremor as baseline. Then monitor them frequently for improvement, which indicates biperiden's effectiveness.
•**WARNING** When administering biperiden to patient with drug-induced extrapyramidal reactions, be alert for exacerbation of psychiatric symptoms.
**PATIENT TEACHING**
•Caution patient to avoid driving and other activities that require alertness until biperiden's CNS effects are known.
•**WARNING** Because biperiden decreases sweating, urge patient to avoid extremely hot and humid conditions to reduce risk of heatstroke and severe hyperthermia. This is especially important for elderly patients and those who abuse alcohol or have chronic illness or CNS disease.
•Stress need for periodic eye examinations and intraocular pressure measurements because biperiden may cause narrow-angle glaucoma and increase intraocular pressure.

# bisoprolol fumarate
Zebeta

### Class and Category
*Chemical:* Selective beta₁-adrenergic blocker
*Therapeutic:* Antihypertensive
*Pregnancy category:* C

### Indications and Dosages
➤ *To treat hypertension, alone or with other antihypertensives*
**TABLETS**
**Adults.** 5 mg q.d., increased to 10 to 20 mg q.d. if blood pressure doesn't respond to lower dosage.
**DOSAGE ADJUSTMENT** Dosage reduced to 2.5 mg q.d. initially and increased gradually for patients with impaired renal function and creatinine clearance of less than 40 ml/min/ 1.73 m$^2$ or with impaired hepatic function, such as from cirrhosis or hepatitis.

### Contraindications
Cardiogenic shock, heart failure unless caused by tachyarrhythmia, overt heart failure, second- or third-degree heart block, sinus bradycardia

## Mechanism of Action

Inhibits stimulation of beta$_1$-receptors primarily in the heart, which decreases cardiac excitability, cardiac output, and myocardial oxygen demand. Bisoprolol also decreases renin release from kidneys, which helps reduce blood pressure.

## Interactions

**DRUGS**

*aluminum salts, barbiturates, calcium salts, cholestyramine, colestipol, NSAIDs, penicillins, rifampin, salicylates, sulfinpyrazone:* Possibly decreased therapeutic and adverse effects of bisoprolol
*calcium channel blockers:* Possibly increased therapeutic and adverse effects of bisoprolol
*ciprofloxacin, quinolones:* Possibly increased bioavailability of bisoprolol
*clonidine:* Possibly severe hypertension caused by withdrawal of clonidine or both drugs
*epinephrine:* Possibly hypertension followed by bradycardia
*ergot alkaloids:* Possibly peripheral ischemia and gangrene
*flecainide:* Possibly increased therapeutic and adverse effects of either drug
*lidocaine:* Possibly increased risk of lidocaine toxicity
*oral contraceptives:* Possibly increased bioavailability and plasma level of bisoprolol
*prazosin:* Possibly increased orthostatic hypotension
*quinidine:* Possibly increased effects of bisoprolol
*sulfonylureas:* Possibly masking of hypoglycemic symptoms

## Adverse Reactions

**CNS:** Anxiety, confusion, depression, dizziness, emotional lability, fatigue, fever, hallucinations, headache, insomnia, malaise, nightmares, paresthesia, sleep disturbances, syncope, tremor, unsteadiness, vertigo
**CV:** Bradycardia, heart block, and other arrhythmias; chest pain; claudication; cold arms and legs; edema; heart failure; hypercholesterolemia; hyperlipidemia; hypotension; MI; orthostatic hypotension; palpitations; peripheral vascular insufficiency; renal and mesenteric artery thrombosis
**EENT:** Altered taste, blurred vision, dry mouth, eye pain or pressure, hearing loss, increased salivation, laryngospasm, pharyngitis, rhinitis, sinusitis, tinnitus
**GI:** Constipation, diarrhea, epigastric pain, gastritis, indigestion, ischemic colitis, nausea, vomiting
**GU:** Cystitis, decreased libido, impotence, Peyronie's disease, renal colic
**HEME:** Agranulocytosis, eosinophilia, leukopenia, thrombocytopenia, thrombocytopenic purpura
**MS:** Arthralgia, gout, muscle twitching, neck pain
**RESP:** Asthma, bronchitis, bronchospasm, cough, dyspnea, respiratory distress, upper respiratory tract infection
**SKIN:** Alopecia, dermatitis, diaphoresis, eczema, exfoliative dermatitis, flushing, pruritus, psoriasis, rash
**Other:** Angioedema, hyperkalemia, hyperuricemia, weight gain

## Nursing Considerations

• Use bisoprolol cautiously in patients with peripheral vascular disease because reduced cardiac output can precipitate or aggravate symptoms of arterial insufficiency. Assess arms and legs for changes in color, temperature, and pulses; ask about numbness, tingling, and pain.
• Measure blood pressure with patient lying, sitting, and standing before initiating bisoprolol therapy and then every 4 to 8 hours, as appropriate, to evaluate effectiveness.
• If patient has diabetes, monitor closely for signs of hypoglycemia, which drug may mask.
• If patient has hyperthyroidism, monitor for tachycardia and hypertension, which may be masked by bisoprolol.
• **WARNING** Keep in mind that abrupt withdrawal of bisoprolol may exacerbate or precipitate thyroid storm. During drug withdrawal, monitor patient closely.
• Expect to discontinue bisoprolol over 1 to 2 weeks to prevent MI, ventricular arrhythmias, and, possibly, death from catecholamine hypersensitivity caused by beta blocker therapy.
• If systolic blood pressure falls below 90 mm Hg, expect to discontinue drug. Prepare for hemodynamic monitoring, if needed.
• **WARNING** If patient is scheduled for surgery with general anesthesia, expect to discontinue bisoprolol about 48 hours beforehand to reduce risk of excessive myocardial depression during anesthesia.

B

•Teach patient how to monitor her blood pressure, if appropriate, and to recognize signs of hypertension and hypotension.
•Instruct patient to avoid sudden position changes and to rise slowly from a sitting or lying position to minimize the effects of orthostatic hypotension.
•Advise patient to avoid driving and other activities that require mental alertness until bisoprolol's CNS effects are known.
•Instruct patient to contact prescriber before using any OTC product, such as a cold remedy or nasal decongestant.

# bitolterol mesylate

Tornalate

## Class and Category

*Chemical:* Acid ester of colterol
*Therapeutic:* Bronchodilator, sympathomimetic
*Pregnancy category:* C

## Indications and Dosages

➤ *To prevent and treat asthma and other conditions associated with reversible bronchospasm, such as emphysema and chronic bronchitis*

INTERMITTENT AEROSOL SOLUTION

**Adults and children age 12 and older.** 1 mg of bitolterol diluted in 0.5 ml of NS and inhaled over 10 to 15 min t.i.d. *Maximum:* 8 mg/day.

CONTINUOUS AEROSOL SOLUTION

**Adults and children age 12 and older.** 2.5 mg of bitolterol diluted in 1.25 ml of NS and inhaled over 10 to 15 min t.i.d. *Maximum:* 14 mg/day.

METERED-DOSE INHALER

**Adults and children age 12 and older.** *To treat acute bronchospasm:* 2 inhalations over 1 to 3 min followed by a third inhalation, if needed.
*To prevent bronchospasm:* 2 inhalations q 8 hr not to exceed 3 inhalations q 6 hr or 2 inhalations q 4 hr.

| Route | Onset | Peak | Duration |
|---|---|---|---|
| Aerosol, inhalation | In 2 to 3 min | 30 to 60 min | 6 to 8 hr |
| Metered-dose inhalation | 3 to 5 min | 30 min to 2 hr | 4 to 8 hr |

## Mechanism of Action

Is hydrolyzed to active agent colterol (a long-acting agent that primarily affects $beta_2$-adrenergic receptors). Then it attaches to $beta_2$ receptors on bronchial cell membranes. This action stimulates the intracellular enzyme adenylate cyclase to convert adenosine triphosphate to cyclic adenosine monophosphate (cAMP). An increased intracellular level of cAMP relaxes bronchial smooth-muscle cells, stabilizes mast cells, and inhibits histamine release.

## Incompatibilities

Don't mix bitolterol in inhalation solution with cromolyn sodium or acetylcysteine.

## Contraindications

Hypersensitivity to bitolterol or its ingredients

## Interactions

DRUGS

*beta blockers:* Possibly inhibition of bronchodilating effect of bitolterol
*epinephrine, other sympathomimetic drugs:* Possibly additive effects of either drug
*MAO inhibitors, tricyclic antidepressants:* Possibly potentiation of bitolterol's action on cardiovascular system

## Adverse Reactions

**CNS:** Dizziness, fatigue, headache, hyperkinesia, insomnia, light-headedness, nervousness, paresthesia, somnolence, tremor, vertigo
**CV:** Chest pain, hypertension, irregular pulse, palpitations, tachycardia, transient ECG changes
**EENT:** Mouth and throat irritation, rhinitis
**GI:** Elevated liver function test results, nausea
**HEME:** Decreased hemoglobin level, hematocrit, and WBC count
**RESP:** Bronchospasm, cough

## Nursing Considerations

•Assess respiratory rate, rhythm, and depth and breath sounds before, during, and after bitolterol therapy. Expect improved air movement and improvement in abnormal breath sounds.
•Because beta-adrenergic bronchodilators can significantly increase blood pressure and pulse rate, monitor blood pressure and pulse rate frequently.
•Expect therapy to begin with lowest effective dose because higher doses or more fre-

quent use may reduce drug effectiveness and cause paradoxical reactions or overdose.

**PATIENT TEACHING**

•Teach patient how to properly use and care for aerosol nebulizer or metered-dose inhaler. Before patient uses aerosol nebulizer, advise her to look for slight bubbling in solution-filled chamber and fine mist when nebulizer is turned on. Before patient uses inhaler for first time, instruct her to check that it's working properly by spraying it once in the air and looking for fine mist.

•Teach patient to mix nebulizer solution immediately before use. Afterward, he should clean nebulizer and solution chamber according to manufacturer's recommendations.

•**WARNING** Advise patient not to use more than the recommended dosage; excessive use of sympathomimetic drugs may be fatal.

•Tell patient to wait 1 to 3 minutes between metered-dose inhalations.

# bivalirudin

Angiomax

## Class and Category

*Chemical:* Hirudin analogue
*Therapeutic:* Anticoagulant
*Pregnancy category:* B

## Indications and Dosages

➤ *As adjunct to provide anticoagulation and prevent thrombosis in patients with unstable angina who are having PTCA or percutaneous coronary intervention*

**I.V. INFUSION**

**Adults.** *Initial:* Immediately before angioplasty, 0.75-mg/kg bolus followed by 1.75 mg/kg/hr as a continuous infusion for duration of procedure. Five minutes after bolus dose and while continuous infusion is running, additional 0.3-mg/kg dose may be given if needed. After procedure, 1.75 mg/kg/hr may be given for 4 hr by continuous infusion, followed by 0.2 mg/kg/hr for up to 20 hr if needed.

**DOSAGE ADJUSTMENT** Infusion dosage possibly reduced to 1 mg/kg/hr for patients with severe renal impairment (glomerular filtration rate of 10 to 29 ml/min) and to 0.25 mg/kg/hr for patients undergoing dialysis.

| Route | Onset | Peak | Duration |
|-------|-------|------|----------|
| I.V. | Immediate | Unknown | 1 hr after end of infusion |

## Mechanism of Action

Selectively binds to thrombin, including thrombin trapped in established clots. Without thrombin, fibrinogen can't convert to fibrin and clots can't form.

B

## Incompatibilities

Don't mix other drugs in same I.V. line before or during bivalirudin administration. Mixing with alteplase, amiodarone, amphotericin B, chlorpromazine HCL, diazepam, prochlorperazine edisylate, reteplase, streptokinase, or vancomycin HCL can result in haze, particulate formation, or precipitation.

## Contraindications

Active major bleeding, hypersensitivity to bivalirudin or its components

## Interactions

**DRUGS**

*alteplase, antineoplastics, antithymocyte globulin, heparin, NSAIDs, platelet inhibitors, reteplase, streptokinase, strontium chloride Sr 89, warfarin:* Risk of bleeding
*porfimer:* Possibly decreased efficacy of porfimer photodynamic therapy
*salicylates:* Increased risk of hypoprothrombinemia and bleeding

## Adverse Reactions

**CNS:** Headache, intracranial hemorrhage
**CV:** Hypotension, thrombosis (with gamma brachytherapy)
**EENT:** Epistaxis, gingival bleeding
**GI:** Abdominal cramps, diarrhea, GI or retroperitoneal bleeding, nausea, vomiting
**GU:** Hematuria, vaginal bleeding
**MS:** Back pain
**RESP:** Hemoptysis, hemothorax
**SKIN:** Ecchymosis
**Other:** Injection site bleeding, hematoma, or pain

## Nursing Considerations

•To reconstitute bivalirudin, add 5 ml of sterile water for injection to each 250-mg vial and swirl gently until dissolved. For initial infusion, dilute each reconstituted vial in 50 ml of $D_5W$ or NS to yield 5 mg/ml.

•For subsequent low-rate infusion, further dilute reconstituted drug in 500 ml of $D_5W$ or NS to a final concentration of 0.5 mg/ml.

•Expect to give patient 300 to 325 mg of aspirin P.O. daily, as prescribed, during bivalirudin therapy.

•**WARNING** Expect to monitor blood coagulation tests before and regularly during therapy because bleeding is a major risk of bivalirudin therapy.

•**WARNING** Monitor patient often for evidence of bleeding because no antidote for bivalirudin is available. If life-threatening bleeding occurs, notify prescriber immediately, stop drug, and prepare to monitor APTT and other coagulation tests as ordered. Be aware that blood transfusions may be needed. Patients with an increased risk of bleeding include females with active menstruation; patients with vascular or organ abnormalities, such as severe uncontrolled hypertension, advanced renal disease, infective endocarditis, dissecting aortic aneurysm, diverticulitis, hemophilia, hepatic disease (especially from a deficiency in vitamin K–dependent clotting factors), inflammatory bowel disease, or peptic ulcer disease; and those who have recently had a CVA, major surgery (including eye, brain, or spinal cord surgery), large vessel or lumbar puncture, organ biopsy, spinal anesthesia, or major bleeding (including intracranial, GI, intraocular, retroperitoneal, or pulmonary bleeding).

•If patient is receiving gamma brachytherapy, watch closely for evidence of thrombosis (weak or absent pulse, pallor, pain) because drug may increase the risk of thrombosis in these patients.

•If possible, avoid I.M. injections of any kind to decrease the risk of bleeding.

•Discard any unused portion of drug.

**PATIENT TEACHING**

•Inform patient that bivalirudin is a blood thinner used only in the hospital setting.

•Instruct patient to check her skin for bruising or red spots and to immediately report back or stomach pain, difficulty breathing, dizziness or fainting, and unusual bleeding, such as black or tarry stools, blood in urine, coughing up blood, heavy menstrual bleeding, or nosebleeds. Drug may need to be discontinued.

•Urge patient to avoid injury while receiving bivalirudin—for example, by brushing her teeth gently, using a soft-bristled toothbrush.

•Caution patient not to take anti-inflammatories, such as ibuprofen, naproxen, ketoprofen, aspirin, and aspirin-like products, or other blood thinners, such as warfarin, while receiving bivalirudin unless prescriber instructs her to do so.

# bosentan

Tracleer

## Class and Category

*Chemical:* Endothelin receptor antagonist, pyrimidine derivative
*Therapeutic:* Antihypertensive
*Pregnancy category:* X

## Indications and Dosages

➤ *To treat pulmonary arterial hypertension in patients with World Health Organization class III or IV symptoms, to improve exercise ability, and to slow worsening of clinical condition*

**TABLETS**

**Adults.** *Initial:* 62.5 mg b.i.d. in the morning and evening for 4 wk. *Maintenance:* 125 mg b.i.d. in the morning and evening.

**DOSAGE ADJUSTMENT** For adults who weigh less than 40 kg (88 lb), maintenance dosage is 62.5 mg b.i.d. morning and evening.

## Contraindications

Hypersensitivity to bosentan or its components, concurrent use of cyclosporine or glyburide, pregnancy

## Interactions

**DRUGS**

*atorvastatin, lovastatin, simvastatin:* Decreased blood level and efficacy of these drugs
*cyclosporine:* Markedly increased blood bosentan level
*glyburide:* Increased liver enzyme and possibly glucose levels; possibly decreased blood level of both drugs (and of other oral antidiabetics metabolized by CYP2C9 or CYP3A4)
*hormonal contraceptives (oral, injected, implanted):* Possibly decreased effects of these drugs
*ketoconazole and other CYP3A4 inhibitors:* Increased blood level and effects of bosentan
*tacrolimus:* Possibly marked increase in blood bosentan level
*warfarin:* Increased elimination and decreased blood level of warfarin

## Adverse Reactions

**CNS:** Fatigue, headache
**CV:** Edema, hypotension, palpitations
**EENT:** Nasopharyngitis
**GI:** Elevated liver function test results, hepatic injury, indigestion

## Mechanism of Action

Bosentan is an endothelin receptor antagonist that inhibits the effects of endothelin (ET), a potent vasoconstrictor. ET, a neurohormone produced by endothelial cells that line blood vessels, normally increases during times of cardiovascular stress. Patients with pulmonary arterial hypertension have an abnormal increase in serum ET level.

ET binds with its receptors, $ET_A$ and $ET_B$, which are located on endothelial and vascular smooth-muscle cells. When ET binds with these receptors, it causes vasoconstriction, as shown below left, and such long-term effects as fibrosis and hypertrophy. By binding to $ET_A$ and $ET_B$ receptors, as shown below right, bosentan blocks the vasoconstrictive effects of ET, causing pulmonary artery vasodilation and decreased pulmonary artery pressure. As a result, the patient experiences increased exercise tolerance and decreased breathlessness.

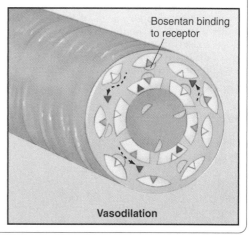

**HEME:** Decreased hemoglobin level and hematocrit
**SKIN:** Flushing, pruritus, rash
**Other:** Hypersensitivity

## Nursing Considerations

•Before giving bosentan, obtain baseline hemoglobin level and liver function test results, as ordered.
•WARNING Because bosentan use may cause major birth defects, make sure that female patient of childbearing age has had a negative pregnancy test before giving drug.
•WARNING Be aware that bosentan may put patient at risk for serious hepatic injury. Assess patient for signs and symptoms of hepatic dysfunction, including abdominal pain, fatigue, fever, jaundice, nausea, and vomiting. Monitor liver function test results every month, as ordered.
•Expect dosage to be adjusted or drug stopped if liver function test results become elevated. Expect treatment to be stopped if bilirubin level increases to twice the upper limit of normal (or higher) or if clinical symptoms occur in conjunction with liver function test elevations. Bosentan probably won't be prescribed for patients with moderate to severe hepatic dysfunction or for those with liver function test levels higher than three times the upper limit of normal.
•Monitor hemoglobin level 1 and 3 months after initiation of therapy and every 3 months thereafter, as ordered.
•Monitor patient's response to drug, and evaluate her activity tolerance.
**PATIENT TEACHING**
•WARNING Because major birth defects are associated with bosentan, caution female patient of childbearing age to have a urine or serum pregnancy test monthly during bosentan therapy to verify that she isn't pregnant. Advise her to notify prescriber immediately if she experiences a late or missed menstrual

period. Instruct patient to use a reliable non-hormonal method of contraception because bosentan may decrease the effectiveness of hormonal contraceptives.

•Urge patient to immediately report signs or symptoms of hepatic dysfunction, including yellow skin or eyes, fever, nausea, vomiting, fatigue, and abdominal pain.

•Stress the importance of keeping appointments for follow-up testing so that drug's effects can be evaluated.

•Inform patient that bosentan is dispensed only by a special access program set up by the drug's manufacturer and isn't available from commercial pharmacies. Advise patient to allow for adequate delivery time when refilling prescription so that she doesn't run out of drug. Instruct her to review the medication guide that comes with each renewed prescription.

# bretylium tosylate

Bretylate (CAN), Bretylol

## Class and Category

*Chemical:* Bromobenzyl quaternary ammonium compound
*Therapeutic:* Class III antiarrhythmic
*Pregnancy category:* C

## Indications and Dosages

➤ *To prevent and treat ventricular fibrillation and treat life-threatening ventricular arrhythmias that don't respond to first-line antiarrhythmics, such as lidocaine*

**I.V. INFUSION, I.V. OR I.M. INJECTION**

**Adults with immediate life-threatening ventricular arrhythmias.** *Initial:* 5 mg/kg undiluted by rapid I.V. injection; if ventricular fibrillation persists, 10 mg/kg repeated as often as needed. *Continuous suppression:* 1 to 2 mg/min or 5 to 10 mg/kg of diluted I.V. solution infused over at least 8 min q 6 hr.

**Adults with other ventricular arrhythmias.** *Initial:* 5 to 10 mg/kg of diluted I.V. solution infused over at least 8 min, repeated q 1 to 2 hr if arrhythmia continues; or 5 to 10 mg/kg undiluted I.M. injection, repeated q 1 to 2 hr if arrhythmia continues. *Maintenance:* 5 to 10 mg/kg diluted I.V. solution infused over at least 8 min q 6 hours, 1 to 2 mg/min infused continuously, or 5 to 10 mg/kg undiluted I.M. injection q 6 to 8 hr.

**DOSAGE ADJUSTMENT** Interval between dosages increased for patients with impaired renal function because bretylium is excreted primarily by kidneys.

**Children with acute ventricular fibrillation.** 5 mg/kg I.V. given over 8 to 10 min, followed by 10 mg/kg q 15 to 30 min up to total dose of 30 mg/kg. *Maintenance:* 5 to 10 mg/kg q 6 hr.

**Children with other ventricular arrhythmias.** 5 to 10 mg/kg q 6 hr.

| Route | Onset | Peak | Duration |
|---|---|---|---|
| I.V. | 5 to 10 min* | 6 to 9 hr | 6 to 24 hr |
| I.M. | 20 to 60 min* | 6 to 9 hr | 6 to 24 hr |

## Contraindications

Digitalis toxicity, hypersensitivity to bretylium

## Interactions

**DRUGS**
*catecholamines (such as dopamine and norepinephrine):* Increased vasopressor effects of catecholamines
*digoxin:* Possibly worsening of digitalis toxicity

## Adverse Reactions

**CNS:** Anxiety, confusion, dizziness, emotional lability, fever, lethargy, light-headedness, paranoia, psychosis, syncope, vertigo
**CV:** Angina, arrhythmias (including bradycardia and more frequent PVCs), hypotension, orthostatic hypotension, transient hypertension
**EENT:** Mild conjunctivitis, nasal stuffiness
**GI:** Abdominal pain, diarrhea, hiccups, nausea, vomiting
**GU:** Renal impairment
**RESP:** Dyspnea
**SKIN:** Diaphoresis, erythematous macular rash, flushing
**Other:** Injection site pain

## Nursing Considerations

•**WARNING** Use bretylium cautiously in patients with severe aortic stenosis or pulmonary hypertension because hypotension may occur.

---

* For suppression of ventricular fibrillation; 20 to 120 min for suppression of ventricular tachycardia.

## Mechanism of Action

Bretylium prolongs the repolarization phase of the action potential and lengthens the effective refractory period, which helps terminate reentry arrhythmias. The drug also acts on adrenergic nerve terminals. Initially, it causes early release of norepinephrine, which increases the heart rate and blood pressure. Then it blocks the release of norepinephrine, as shown here. This reduces the heart rate and blood pressure. Bretylium also increases the ventricular threshold, making the ventricular myocardium less responsive to ectopic impulses and preventing ventricular fibrillation.

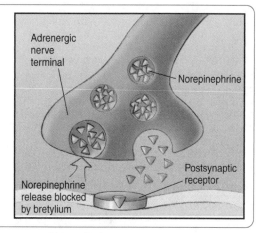

- For I.V. infusion, dilute bretylium and administer at 1 to 2 mg/min.
- Dilute bretylium in compatible I.V. solution, such as $D_5W$, $D_5NS$, $D_5LR$, NS, 5% sodium bicarbonate, 20% mannitol, 1/6 molar sodium lactate, LR, calcium chloride in $D_5W$, and potassium chloride in $D_5W$.
- **WARNING** Be aware that patient may experience hypotension while supine. Have patient remain supine until tolerance develops. If her supine systolic blood pressure falls below 75 mm Hg, expect to give dopamine or norepinephrine and monitor her blood pressure closely because vasopressor effects are increased when these drugs are given together.
- Be alert for transient hypertension and increased frequency of arrhythmias because bretylium initially triggers release of norepinephrine. Monitor patient's ECG tracings and blood pressure continuously, and notify prescriber of changes.
- Monitor blood bretylium level. Notify prescriber if level falls outside therapeutic range of 0.5 to 1.5 mcg/ml.

**PATIENT TEACHING**
- Advise patient to immediately report chest pain or pressure, pain at I.V. site, or rash.
- Warn patient that she may feel dizzy or lightheaded even when lying down. Instruct her to remain supine and ask for assistance when attempting to move or sit up. Tell her that this sensation usually subsides in a few days.

# bromocriptine mesylate

Alti-Bromocriptine (CAN), Apo-Bromocriptine (CAN), Parlodel, Parlodel SnapTabs

## Class and Category

*Chemical:* Ergot alkaloid derivative
*Therapeutic:* Antidyskinetic, antihyperprolactinemic, dopamine-receptor agonist, growth hormone suppressant, infertility therapy adjunct
*Pregnancy category:* B

## Indications and Dosages

➤ *To treat amenorrhea, galactorrhea, male hypogonadism, and infertility from hyperprolactinemia*

**CAPSULES, TABLETS**
**Adults.** *Initial:* 1.25 to 2.5 mg q h.s. with snack. Increased by 2.5 mg q 3 to 7 days as needed to a total daily dose of 5 to 7.5 mg given in divided doses with snacks. *Maintenance:* 2.5 mg b.i.d. or t.i.d. with meals.

➤ *To treat prolactin-secreting adenoma*

**CAPSULES, TABLETS**
**Adults and adolescents age 15 and older.** *Initial:* 1.25 mg b.i.d. or t.i.d. with meals. Increased gradually over several weeks, if needed, to 10 to 20 mg/day in divided doses with meals. Some patients may need higher doses. *Maintenance:* 2.5 to 20 mg/day in divided doses with meals.

➤ *To treat Parkinson's disease*

CAPSULES, TABLETS
**Adults.** *Initial:* 1.25 mg q h.s. with snack or b.i.d. with meals. Increased by 2.5 mg q 14 to 28 days, if needed. *Maintenance:* 2.5 to 40 mg/day in divided doses with meals.

➤ *To treat acromegaly*

CAPSULES, TABLETS
**Adults and children age 15 and older.** *Initial:* 1.25 to 2.5 mg q h.s. with snack for 3 days. Then increased by 1.25 to 2.5 mg q 3 to 7 days, if needed, up to 30 mg/day. *Maintenance:* Usually 10 to 30 mg/day h.s. with snack or in divided doses with meals.

| Route | Onset | Peak | Duration |
|-------|-------|------|----------|
| P.O.* | 2 hr | 8 hr | 24 hr |
| P.O.† | 30 to 90 min | 2 hr | Unknown |
| P.O.‡ | 1 to 2 hr | 4 to 8 wk | 4 to 8 hr |

**Mechanism of Action**

Inhibits release of prolactin and growth hormone from anterior pituitary gland, thus restoring testicular or ovarian function and suppressing lactation. The drug decreases dopamine turnover in the CNS, depleting dopamine or blocking its receptors in the brain, alleviating dyskinesia.

**Contraindications**

Hypersensitivity to bromocriptine, other ergot alkaloids, or their components; severe ischemic heart disease or peripheral vascular disease

**Interactions**

DRUGS
*antihypertensives:* Increased hypotensive effects
*clarithromycin, erythromycin, troleandomycin:* Increased risk of bromocriptine toxicity
*ergot alkaloids or derivatives:* Increased risk of hypertension
*haloperidol, loxapine, MAO inhibitors, methyldopa, metoclopramide, molindone, phenothiazines, pimozide, reserpine, risperidone,*

*thioxanthenes:* Increased serum prolactin level, decreased bromocriptine effectiveness
*levodopa:* Additive effects requiring reduced levodopa dose
*ritonavir:* Increased blood bromocriptine level

ACTIVITIES
*alcohol use:* Possibly disulfiram-like reaction

**Adverse Reactions**

**CNS:** Dizziness, drowsiness, fatigue, headache, light-headedness, syncope
**CV:** Hypertension, hypotension, orthostatic hypotension, Raynaud's phenomenon
**EENT:** Dry mouth, nasal congestion
**GI:** Abdominal cramps, anorexia, constipation, diarrhea, GI bleeding, indigestion, nausea, vomiting

**Nursing Considerations**

• Use bromocriptine cautiously if patient has a history of psychosis or cardiovascular disease, especially after MI with residual arrhythmia.
• Expect to perform a pregnancy test every 4 weeks during the amenorrheic period. Once menses resume, test whenever a period is missed, as ordered.
• Plan to withhold bromocriptine if patient becomes pregnant.
• If a rapidly expanding adenoma needs continued therapy, watch closely for hypertensive crisis.
• Be aware that bromocriptine shouldn't be given postpartum if patient has a history of coronary artery disease or other severe cardiovascular problem unless risk of withdrawing drug is greater than risk of use. If so, monitor closely for signs and symptoms of CV dysfunction, such as chest pain.
• Expect to give bromocriptine with levodopa if patient is being treated for Parkinson's disease.
• Assess for hypotension when therapy starts and hypertension (typically during second week). Monitor blood pressure often if patient takes other antihypertensives.
• If patient has a history of peptic ulcer or GI bleeding, watch for new bleeding.
• Take safety precautions, such as keeping the bed in low position with side rails up, because bromocriptine can cause dizziness, drowsiness, light-headedness, and syncope.

PATIENT TEACHING
• Tell patient to take each dose with a meal, milk, or a snack to minimize nausea.
• Caution patient about possible dizziness, drowsiness, and light-headedness.

---

* For amenorrhea, galactorrhea, male hypogonadism, infertility from hyperprolactinemia, and prolactin-secreting adenoma.
† For Parkinson's disease.
‡ For acromegaly.

• Advise patient to avoid sudden position changes to minimize orthostatic hypotension.
• Warn patient to avoid alcohol while taking bromocriptine because it may cause disulfiram-like reactions, such as chest pain, confusion, a fast or pounding heartbeat, facial flushing, diaphoresis, nausea, vomiting, a throbbing headache, blurred vision, and severe weakness.
• Tell patient to take a missed dose as soon as she remembers it, unless it's almost time for the next dose. In that case, tell her to wait until the next scheduled dose. Warn her not to double the dose. Advise her to contact prescriber if she misses more than one dose.
• Urge patient to report adverse reactions, such as an unremitting headache, nausea, vomiting, or other signs of CNS toxicity.
• Tell patient who takes large doses of bromocriptine to schedule regular dental checkups because the drug can decrease salivary flow, which may encourage dental caries, periodontal disease, oral candidiasis, and discomfort.
• Tell patient with acromegaly to keep her fingers warm to prevent cold-sensitive digital vasospasm.

# budesonide

Entocort EC, Pulmicort Respules, Pulmicort Turbuhaler, Rhinocort, Rhinocort Aqua, Rhinocort Turbuhaler (CAN)

### Class and Category
*Chemical:* Glucocorticoid
*Therapeutic:* Antiasthmatic, anti-inflammatory
*Pregnancy category:* B

### Indications and Dosages
➤ *To manage symptoms of seasonal or perennial allergic rhinitis*
NASAL AEROSOL
**Adults and children over age 6.** 64 mcg in each nostril b.i.d. or 128 mcg in each nostril q.d. *Maximum:* 256 mcg/day. *Maintenance:* Lowest dosage that controls symptoms.
NASAL POWDER
**Adults and children over age 6.** 200 mcg in each nostril q.d. *Maximum:* 800 mcg/day (adults and adolescents); 400 mcg/day (children). *Maintenance:* Lowest dosage that controls symptoms.
NASAL SUSPENSION
**Adults and children over age 6.** 32 mcg in each nostril q.d. *Maximum:* 256 mcg/day (adults and adolescents); 128 mcg/day (chil-

dren). *Maintenance:* Lowest dosage that controls symptoms.
➤ *To manage symptoms of perennial nonallergic rhinitis*
NASAL AEROSOL
**Adults and adolescents.** 64 mcg in each nostril b.i.d. or 128 mcg in each nostril q.d. *Maximum:* 256 mcg/day. *Maintenance:* Lowest dosage that controls symptoms.
NASAL POWDER
**Adults and adolescents.** 200 mcg in each nostril q.d. *Maximum:* 800 mcg/day. *Maintenance:* Lowest dosage that controls symptoms.
➤ *To provide maintenance therapy in chronic bronchial asthma*
ORAL INHALATION
**Adults previously on bronchodilators alone.** 1 or 2 inhalations (200 to 400 mcg) b.i.d. *Maximum:* 800 mcg/day.
**Adults previously on inhaled corticosteroids.** 1 or 2 inhalations (200 to 400 mcg) b.i.d. *Maximum:* 800 mcg b.i.d. as needed and tolerated.
**Adults previously on systemic corticosteroids.** 2 to 4 inhalations (400 to 800 mcg) b.i.d. *Maximum:* 1,600 mcg/day.
**Children age 6 and older.** 1 inhalation (200 mcg) b.i.d. *Maximum:* 400 mcg b.i.d. as needed and tolerated.
➤ *To prevent or provide maintenance therapy in chronic bronchial asthma*
NEBULIZED INHALATION (PULMICORT RESPULES)
**Children ages 1 to 8 previously on bronchodilators alone.** 0.25 mg b.i.d. or 0.5 mg q.d. inhaled by jet nebulizer. *Maximum:* 0.5 mg/day.
**Children ages 1 to 8 previously on inhaled steroids.** 0.25 mg b.i.d. or 0.5 mg q.d. inhaled by jet nebulizer. *Maximum:* 1 mg/day.
**Children ages 1 to 8 previously on systemic corticosteroids.** 0.5 mg b.i.d. or 1 mg q.d. inhaled by jet nebulizer. *Maximum:* 1 mg/day.
➤ *To treat mild to moderate active Crohn's disease involving the ileum, the ascending colon, or both*
CAPSULES
**Adults.** 9 mg q.d. in the morning for 8 weeks.
➤ *To maintain clinical remission of mild to moderate Crohn's disease involving the ileum, the ascending colon, or both*
CAPSULES
**Adults.** 6 mg q.d. in the morning for up to 3 months.
DOSAGE ADJUSTMENT Dosage reduced for patients with heptic insufficiency and those taking ketoconazole or other CYP3A4 inhibitor.

| Route | Onset | Peak | Duration |
|---|---|---|---|
| Nasal aerosol | 10 hr to 3 days | 3 days to 3 wk | Unknown |
| Nasal powder or suspension, oral inhalation | In 4 wk | Unknown | Unknown |
| Nebulized inhalation | 2 to 8 days | 4 to 6 wk | Unknown |
| Oral capsules | Unknown | 30 min to 10 hr | Unknown |

## Mechanism of Action

Inhibits inflammatory cells and mediators, possibly by decreasing their influx into nasal passages or bronchial walls. As a result, nasal or airway inflammation decreases. Oral inhalation form also inhibits mucus secretion in airways, decreasing the amount and viscosity of sputum.

## Contraindications

Hypersensitivity to budesonide or its components, recent septal ulcers or nasal surgery or trauma (nasal spray); status asthmaticus or other acute asthma episodes (oral inhalation)

## Interactions

**DRUGS**

*clarithromycin, erythromycin, itraconazole, ketoconazole, other CYP3A4 inhibitors:* Possibly increased blood budesonide level

## Adverse Reactions

**CNS:** Amnesia, asthenia, dizziness, fatigue, fever, headache
**EENT:** Bad taste, dry mouth, epistaxis, nasal irritation, oral candidiasis, pharyngitis, rhinitis, sinusitis
**ENDO:** Growth suppression in children
**GI:** Abdominal pain, diarrhea, dyspepsia, flatulence, indigestion, nausea, vomiting
**GU:** UTI
**MS:** Arthralgia, back pain
**RESP:** Increased cough, respiratory tract infection
**SKIN:** Purpura

## Nursing Considerations

•Use budesonide cautiously if patient has tubercular infection; untreated fungal, bacterial, or systemic viral infection; or ocular herpes simplex.
•Closely monitor a child's growth pattern; budesonide may stunt growth.
•**WARNING** Assess patient who switches from a systemic corticosteroid to inhaled budesonide for adrenal insufficiency (fatigue, hypotension, lassitude, nausea, vomiting, weakness), which may be life-threatening. Hypothalamic-pituitary-adrenal axis function may take several months to recover after systemic corticosteroids stop. Stopping budesonide abruptly may cause adrenal insufficiency.
•Administer Respules by a jet nebulizer connected to an air compressor.
•Patient exposed to chickenpox may receive varicella zoster immune globulin or pooled I.V. immunoglobulin. If chickenpox develops, give antiviral as ordered. Patient exposed to measles may need pooled I.M. immunoglobulin.

**PATIENT TEACHING**

•Urge patient taking oral capsules to swallow them whole and not to chew or break them.
•Instruct patient who uses nasal spray to shake container before each use. Instruct her to blow her nose, tilt her head slightly forward, and insert tube into a nostril, pointing toward inner corner of eye, away from nasal septum. Tell her to hold the other nostril closed and spray while inhaling gently. Then have her repeat the procedure in the other nostril.
•Instruct patient to prime oral inhaler before using it for first time by holding canister upright with mouthpiece on top and then twisting base of device fully to the right and then fully to the left until it clicks. Teach patient to load each subsequent dose just before use in the same manner. After loading a dose, caution patient not to shake device or blow into it. Instruct patient to turn her head away from device and exhale. Then have her hold device upright, place her lips around mouthpiece, and inhale deeply. The device will discharge a dose. Tell patient to remove her lips from mouthpiece to exhale.
•Caution patient not to use an oral inhaler with a spacer device.
•Instruct patient not to use budesonide as a rescue inhaler.
•Instruct patient to contact prescriber if symptoms persist or have worsened after 3 weeks.

•Inform parents of small children using nebulized Respules that improvement may begin within 2 to 8 days but that full effect may not be evident for 4 to 6 weeks.
•Caution patient to avoid exposure to chickenpox and measles and, if exposed, to contact prescriber immediately.

# bumetanide

Bumex

## Class and Category

*Chemical:* Sulfonamide derivative
*Therapeutic:* Loop diuretic
*Pregnancy category:* C

## Indications and Dosages

➤ *To treat edema caused by heart failure, hepatic disease, and renal disease, including nephrotic syndrome*

TABLETS

**Adults.** 0.5 to 2 mg q.d., increased as needed, with a second or third dose q 4 to 5 hr or 0.5 to 2 mg q.o.d. or q.d. for 3 or 4 days each week. *Maximum:* 10 mg/day.

I.V. INFUSION, I.V. OR I.M. INJECTION

**Adults.** 0.5 to 1 mg over 1 to 2 min q.d., increased p.r.n. with a second or third dose q 2 to 3 hr. *Maximum:* 10 mg/day.

DOSAGE ADJUSTMENT Continuous infusion (12 mg over 12 hr) may be more effective and less toxic than intermittent infusion in patients with severe chronic renal insufficiency.

| Route | Onset | Peak | Duration |
|-------|-------|------|----------|
| P.O. | 30 to 60 min | 1 to 2 hr | 4 to 6 hr |
| I.V. | In min | 15 to 30 min | 3.5 to 4 hr |

## Mechanism of Action

Inhibits the reabsorption of sodium, chloride, and water in the ascending limb of the loop of Henle, which promotes their excretion and reduces fluid volume.

## Contraindications

Anuria, hepatic coma, hypersensitivity to bumetanide or its components, severe electrolyte depletion

## Interactions

DRUGS

*aminoglycosides:* Increased risk of ototoxicity
*antihypertensives:* Increased antihypertensive effect
*indomethacin:* Slowed increase in urine and sodium excretion, inhibited plasma renin activity
*lithium:* Reduced lithium renal clearance, increased risk of lithium toxicity
*probenecid:* Reduced sodium excretion

## Adverse Reactions

**CNS:** Dizziness, encephalopathy, headache
**CV:** Hypotension
**EENT:** Ototoxicity
**ENDO:** Hyperglycemia
**GI:** Nausea
**GU:** Azotemia, elevated serum creatinine level
**MS:** Muscle spasms
**Other:** Hyperuricemia, hypocalcemia, hypochloremia, hypokalemia, hyponatremia, hypovolemia

## Nursing Considerations

•WARNING Know that a patient who is hypersensitive to sulfonamides may be hypersensitive to bumetanide. Monitor such a patient closely when starting therapy.
•Expect to use the parenteral route for patients with impaired GI absorption or in whom the oral route isn't practical. Switch to the oral route, as prescribed, as soon as possible.
•Discard unused parenteral solution 24 hours after preparation.
•Assess fluid and electrolyte balance closely because bumetanide is a potent diuretic (40 to 60 times more potent than furosemide). Monitor fluid intake and output once every 8 hours, evaluate serum electrolyte levels when ordered, and assess for imbalances.
•WARNING Be aware that high-dose or too-frequent administration can cause profound diuresis and water and electrolyte depletion, especially in elderly patients.
•Monitor serum potassium level regularly to check for hypokalemia, especially if patient takes a digitalis glycoside for heart failure or has hepatic cirrhosis, ascites, aldosteronism, potassium-losing nephropathy, diarrhea, or a history of ventricular arrhythmias.
•Assess for signs of ototoxicity, such as tinnitus, daily. Rarely, bumetanide may cause ototoxicity, especially with I.V. administra-

tion, high doses, and increased frequency of dosing in a patient with renal impairment.
•Monitor results of renal function tests during therapy to detect adverse reactions.

**PATIENT TEACHING**
•Advise patient to avoid potentially hazardous activities until drug's CNS effects are known.
•Stress the importance of monitoring fluid intake and output and watching for signs and symptoms of electrolyte imbalances, such as dizziness, headache, and muscle spasms.
•Review adverse reactions, and tell patient to notify prescriber about severe or persistent reactions.
•Review potassium-rich foods, and encourage patient to include them in her daily diet.
•Encourage patient to return for appropriate follow-up care, especially if she's receiving bumetanide for a chronic condition.
•Tell diabetic patient to monitor blood glucose level regularly and to notify prescriber if hyperglycemia persistently occurs.

# buprenorphine hydrochloride

Buprenex, Subutex

## Class, Category, and Schedule
*Chemical:* Opioid, thebaine derivative
*Therapeutic:* Narcotic analgesic
*Pregnancy category:* C
*Controlled substance:* Schedule V

## Indications and Dosages
➤ *To control moderate to severe pain*
**I.V OR I.M. INJECTION**
**Adults and children age 12 and older.** 0.3 mg q 6 hr or more, p.r.n. A second 0.3-mg dose given 30 to 60 min after first dose, if needed.
**DOSAGE ADJUSTMENT** In patients not at high risk for opioid toxicity, I.M. dose increased to 0.6 mg or frequency increased to q 4 hr, if needed, depending on pain severity and patient response. I.V. or I.M. dose reduced by half in elderly or debilitated patients and in those who have respiratory disease or also use another CNS depressant.
**Children ages 2 to 12.** 0.002 to 0.006 mg/kg q 4 to 6 hr, p.r.n.
➤ *To treat opioid dependence*
**S.L. TABLETS**
**Adults.** 12 to 16 mg q.d.

| Route | Onset | Peak | Duration |
|-------|-------|------|----------|
| I.V. | Under 15 min | Under 1 hr | 6 to 10 hr* |
| I.M. | 15 min | 1 hr | 6 to 10 hr* |

## Mechanism of Action
May bind with CNS receptors to alter the perception of and emotional response to pain. Buprenorphine may act by displacing narcotic agonists from their binding sites and competitively inhibiting their actions.

## Incompatibilities
Don't administer I.V. buprenorphine through the same I.V. line as diazepam or lorazepam.

## Contraindications
Hypersensitivity to buprenorphine or its components

## Interactions
**DRUGS**
*CNS depressants, MAO inhibitors:* Additive hypotensive and respiratory and CNS depressant effects of these drugs
*narcotic analgesics:* Reduced therapeutic effects if buprenorphine is given before another narcotic analgesic

## Adverse Reactions
**CNS:** Dizziness, headache, sedation, vertigo
**CV:** Bradycardia, hypertension, hypotension
**EENT:** Miosis
**GI:** Nausea, vomiting
**RESP:** Bronchospasm, hypoventilation
**SKIN:** Diaphoresis, pruritus, rash, urticaria
**Other:** Anaphylaxis; angioedema; injection site pain, redness, and swelling

## Nursing Considerations
•Use buprenorphine cautiously in patients with severe hepatic or renal impairment, myxedema, hypothyroidism, adrenal insufficiency, CNS depression, coma, toxic psychosis, prostatic hypertrophy, urethral stricture, acute alcoholism, alcohol withdrawal syndrome, kyphoscoliosis, or biliary tract dysfunction. Also use cautiously in patients who receive a drug that decreases hepatic clearance, are known drug abusers, or have been addicted to narcotics.

---

* 4 to 5 hr in children ages 2 to 12.

• Use drug cautiously in patients with head injury, intracranial lesions, or other conditions that could increase CSF pressure.
• To avoid causing withdrawal, buprenorphine shouldn't be given for opioid dependence until signs of withdrawal are evident.
• Administer I.V. form over at least 2 minutes.
• Inspect injection site for local reactions; don't use the same site twice.
• Monitor vital signs and response to drug often, especially after giving first dose.

**PATIENT TEACHING**
• Instruct patient taking S.L. form to place tablets under her tongue until they dissolve. If patient takes more than two tablets per dose, tell her to place all tablets under her tongue at the same time. If they won't fit, tell her to place two at a time under her tongue until full dose has dissolved. Caution her not to swallow the tablets.

# bupropion hydrochloride

Wellbutrin, Wellbutrin SR, Wellbutrin XL, Zyban

## Class and Category
*Chemical:* Aminoketone derivative
*Therapeutic:* Antidepressant, smoking cessation adjunct
*Pregnancy category:* B

## Indications and Dosages
➤ *To treat depression*
**E.R. TABLETS (WELLBUTRIN SR)**
**Adults.** *Initial:* 150 mg q.d. in the morning for 3 days; then 150 mg b.i.d. and, after several weeks, 200 mg b.i.d., as needed and tolerated. *Maximum:* 400 mg/day or 200 mg/dose.
**E.R. TABLETS (WELLBUTRIN XL)**
**Adults.** *Initial:* 150 mg q.d. in the morning for at least 3 days; then 300 mg q.d. and, after 4 wk, 450 mg q.d., as needed and tolerated. *Maximum:* 450 mg q.d.
**TABLETS**
**Adults.** *Initial:* 100 mg b.i.d., increased after 3 or more days to 100 mg t.i.d., as needed. *Maximum:* 450 mg/day or 150 mg/dose.
➤ *To aid in smoking cessation*
**E.R. TABLETS**
**Adults.** *Initial:* 150 mg q.d. for 3 days and then 150 mg b.i.d. for 7 to 12 wk. *Maximum:* 300 mg/day or 150 mg/dose.

**DOSAGE ADJUSTMENT** For patients with severe hepatic cirrhosis, no more than 75 mg/day of Wellbutrin, 100 mg/day or 150 mg q.o.d. of Wellbutrin SR, or 150 mg q.o.d. of Wellbutrin XL and Zyban. In renal impairment, frequency decreased on an individual basis.

| Route | Onset | Peak | Duration |
|---|---|---|---|
| P.O. | 1 to 3 wk | Unknown | Unknown |

## Mechanism of Action
May inhibit norepinephrine, serotonin, and dopamine uptake by neurons, which significantly relieves evidence of depression.

## Contraindications
Anorexia, bulimia, use of another form of bupropion, hypersensitivity to bupropion or its components, seizure disorder, treatment requiring abrupt discontinuation of alcohol or sedatives (including benzodiazepines), use within 14 days of an MAO inhibitor

## Interactions
**DRUGS**
*amantadine, levodopa:* Increased adverse reactions to bupropion
*carbamazepine, cimetidine, phenobarbital, phenytoin:* Increased bupropion metabolism
*clozapine, fluoxetine, haloperidol, lithium, loxapine, maprotiline, molindone, phenothiazines, thioxanthenes, trazodone, tricyclic antidepressants:* Increased risk of major motor seizures
*levodopa:* Increased adverse bupropion effects
*MAO inhibitors:* Increased risk of acute bupropion toxicity
*nicotine:* Possibly increased blood pressure
*warfarin:* Possibly altered PT and INR; risk of hemorrhagic or thrombotic complications
**ACTIVITIES**
*alcohol use, recreational drug abuse:* Lowered seizure threshold

## Adverse Reactions
**CNS:** Agitation, anxiety, asthenia, CNS stimulation, coma, confusion, CVA, decreased concentration or memory, delusions, dizziness, euphoria, fever, general or migraine headache, hallucinations, insomnia, irritability, nervousness, paranoia, paresthesia, seizures, somnolence, suicidal ideation, syncope, tremor, vertigo

**CV:** Chest pain, complete AV block, hypertension, MI, orthostatic hypotension, palpitations, phlebitis, tachycardia, vasodilation
**EENT:** Altered taste, amblyopia, blurred vision, dry mouth, hearing loss, pharyngitis, sinusitis, tinnitus
**ENDO:** Hyperglycemia, hypoglycemia, syndrome of inappropriate ADH secretion
**GI:** Abdominal pain, anorexia, constipation, diarrhea, dysphagia, GI hemorrhage, GI ulceration, hepatitis, intestinal perforation, nausea, pancreatitis, vomiting
**GU:** Urinary frequency and urgency, UTI, vaginal hemorrhage
**HEME:** Anemia, leukocytosis, leukopenia, lymphadenopathy, pancytopenia, thrombocytopenia
**MS:** Arthralgia, arthritis, muscle twitching, myalgia, rhabdomyolysis
**RESP:** Bronchospasm, cough, pulmonary embolism
**SKIN:** Diaphoresis, exfoliative dermatitis, flushing, pruritus, rash, urticaria
**Other:** Angioedema, generalized pain, hot flashes, infection, serum sickness–like reaction, weight loss

## Nursing Considerations

•Monitor depressed patient closely for worsened depression and suicide risk, especially when therapy starts and dosage is adjusted.
•To reduce the risk of seizures, allow at least 4 hours between doses of bupropion tablets and 8 hours between doses of E.R. tablets.
•Use seizure precautions, especially in patients who take OTC stimulants or anorectics; use excessive alcohol or sedatives; are addicted to opioids, cocaine, or stimulants; take drugs that lower the seizure threshold; have a history of seizures, head trauma, or CNS tumors; have severe hepatic cirrhosis; or take insulin or an oral antidiabetic.
•Using transdermal nicotine with bupropion may cause hypertension. Watch closely.
**PATIENT TEACHING**
•Advise patient to take bupropion for 7 or more days before stopping smoking.
•Tell patient to swallow E.R. tablets whole.
•Tell patient to take bupropion with food.
•Urge patient to avoid or minimize alcohol and sedatives during therapy and not to stop drug abruptly because seizures may occur.
•Urge caregivers to monitor depressed patient closely for worsened depression, especially when therapy starts or dosage increases.

# buspirone hydrochloride
BuSpar, BuSpar DIVIDOSE, Bustab (CAN)

## Class and Category
*Chemical:* Azaspirodecanedione
*Therapeutic:* Antianxiety
*Pregnancy category:* B

## Indications and Dosages
➤ *To manage anxiety*
**TABLETS**
**Adults.** *Initial:* 5 mg t.i.d. or 7.5 mg b.i.d. increased by 5 mg/day at 2- to 3-day intervals until desired response occurs. *Maintenance:* 20 to 30 mg/day (usual therapeutic range). *Maximum:* 60 mg/day.
**DOSAGE ADJUSTMENT** When used with nefazodone, dosage as little as 2.5 mg q.d.

| Route | Onset | Peak | Duration |
|-------|-------|------|----------|
| P.O. | 1 to 4 wk | 3 to 6 wk | Unknown |

## Mechanism of Action
May act as a partial agonist at serotonin 5-hydroxytryptamine$_{1A}$ receptors in the brain, producing antianxiety effects.

## Contraindications
Hypersensitivity to buspirone or its components

## Interactions
**DRUGS**
*diltiazem, erythromycin, itraconazole, nefazodone, verapamil:* Increased blood level and adverse effects of buspirone
*haloperidol:* Increased blood haloperidol level
*hepatic enzyme CYP3A4 inducers, such as dexamethasone and certain anticonvulsants (phenytoin, phenobarbital, carbamazepine):* Possibly increased rate of buspirone metabolism
*hepatic enzyme CYP3A4 inhibitors, such as ketoconazole and ritonavir:* Possibly inhibited buspirone metabolism and increased blood level
*MAO inhibitors:* Increased risk of hypertension
*nefazadone:* Increased risk of adverse CNS effects
*rifampin:* Decreased blood buspirone level and pharmacodynamic effects
**FOODS**
*food:* Possibly decreased buspirone clearance
*grapefruit juice:* Increased blood buspirone level

## Adverse Reactions

**CNS:** Anger, confusion, decreased concentration, depression, dizziness, dream disturbances, drowsiness, excitement, fatigue, headache, hostility, insomnia, lack of coordination, light-headedness, nervousness, paresthesia, tremor, weakness
**CV:** Chest pain, palpitations, tachycardia
**EENT:** Blurred vision, dry mouth, nasal congestion, pharyngitis, tinnitus
**GI:** Abdominal or gastric distress, constipation, diarrhea, nausea, vomiting
**MS:** Myalgia
**SKIN:** Diaphoresis, rash

## Nursing Considerations

• Use buspirone cautiously in patients with hepatic or renal impairment.
• Institute safety precautions because of possible adverse CNS reactions.

**PATIENT TEACHING**
• Advise patient to take buspirone consistently, either always with or always without food.
• Caution patient to avoid drinking large amounts of grapefruit juice.
• Inform patient that 1 to 2 weeks of therapy may be needed before she notices drug's antianxiety effect.
• Stress the importance of not taking more buspirone than prescribed.
• Advise patient to avoid potentially hazardous activities until drug's CNS effects are known.

# butabarbital sodium

Busodium, Butalan, Butisol, Sarisol No. 2

## Class, Category, and Schedule

*Chemical:* Barbiturate
*Therapeutic:* Sedative-hypnotic
*Pregnancy category:* D
*Controlled substance:* Schedule III

## Indications and Dosages

➤ *To provide daytime sedation*
**ELIXIR, TABLETS**
**Adults.** 15 to 30 mg t.i.d. or q.i.d.
➤ *To treat insomnia*
**ELIXIR, TABLETS**
**Adults.** 50 to 100 mg q h.s.
➤ *To provide preoperative sedation*
**ELIXIR, TABLETS**
**Adults.** 50 to 100 mg 60 to 90 min before surgery.
**Children.** 2 to 6 mg/kg. *Maximum:* 100 mg/dose.

**DOSAGE ADJUSTMENT** Dosage reduced in patients with impaired renal or hepatic function and in elderly or debilitated patients because they may be more sensitive to drug.

| Route | Onset | Peak | Duration |
|-------|-------|------|----------|
| P.O. | 45 to 60 min | Unknown | 6 to 8 hr |

## Mechanism of Action

Inhibits the upward conduction of nerve impulses in the brain's reticular formation, which disrupts impulse transmission to the cortex. As a result, butabarbital depresses the CNS and produces drowsiness, sedation, and hypnosis.

## Contraindications

History of addiction to sedative or hypnotic drug, hypersensitivity to butabarbital or its components, porphyria, severe hepatic or respiratory disease

## Interactions

**DRUGS**
*acetaminophen:* Increased risk of hepatotoxicity (with large doses of or long-term therapy with butabarbital)
*activated charcoal:* Reduced butabarbital absorption
*carbamazepine:* Decreased blood carbamazepine level
*chloramphenicol, corticosteroids, digitalis glycosides:* Increased metabolism and decreased effects of these drugs
*clonazepam:* Increased clearance and reduced efficacy of clonazepam
*CNS depressants, including OTC sedatives and hypnotics:* Additive CNS depression
*doxycycline:* Shortened half-life and decreased effects of doxycycline
*fenoprofen:* Reduced bioavailability and effects of fenoprofen
*griseofulvin:* Reduced griseofulvin absorption
*hydantoins, such as phenytoin:* Unpredictable effects on barbiturate metabolism
*MAO inhibitors:* Prolonged barbiturate effects
*meperidine:* Prolonged CNS depressant effects of meperidine
*methadone:* Reduced methadone actions
*methoxyflurane:* Increased risk of nephrotoxicity

*metronidazole:* Decreased antimicrobial effect of metronidazole
*oral anticoagulants:* Decreased anticoagulant effect
*oral contraceptives with estrogen:* Decreased contraceptive effect
*phenylbutazone:* Reduced elimination half-life of phenylbutazone
*rifampin:* Decreased butabarbital effectiveness
*sodium valproate, valproic acid:* Decreased butabarbital metabolism and increased adverse CNS effects
*theophylline:* Decreased blood level and effects of theophylline
**ACTIVITIES**
*alcohol use:* Additive CNS depression

## Adverse Reactions

**CNS:** Agitation, anxiety, ataxia, clumsiness, CNS depression, confusion, depression, dizziness, drowsiness, fever, hallucinations, headache, hyperkinesia, insomnia, irritability, nervousness, nightmares, psychiatric disturbance, somnolence, syncope
**CV:** Hypertension
**EENT:** Laryngospasm
**GI:** Constipation, hepatic dysfunction, nausea, vomiting
**MS:** Rickets
**RESP:** Apnea, bronchospasm, respiratory depression
**SKIN:** Exfoliative dermatitis, Stevens-Johnson syndrome
**Other:** Drug tolerance, physical and psychological dependence

## Nursing Considerations

• Use butabarbital cautiously, if at all, in patients with depression, suicidal tendency, history of drug abuse, or hepatic dysfunction. Don't administer drug to patients with premonitory signs of hepatic coma.
• Expect to give drug for no more than 2 weeks to treat insomnia because, like all barbiturates, it loses effectiveness for sleep induction and sleep maintenance after 2 weeks.
• Monitor butabarbital intake closely during long-term use because tolerance and psychological and physical dependence may develop.
• Avoid abrupt withdrawal of butabarbital to prevent withdrawal symptoms.
• Monitor elderly and debilitated patients closely because drug may cause marked excitement, depression, and confusion in these patients.
• If patient in pain receives butabarbital, monitor closely for paradoxical excitement.
• If pregnant woman took butabarbital during last trimester, monitor infant for withdrawal symptoms.
**PATIENT TEACHING**
• Stress the importance of taking butabarbital exactly as prescribed because it can be addictive. Warn against increasing the dose or decreasing the dosage interval without consulting prescriber.
• Tell patient to avoid alcohol and OTC sedatives and hypnotics during butabarbital therapy because of additive CNS effects.
• Advise patient to avoid potentially hazardous activities until drug's CNS effects are known.
• Advise female patient not to rely on oral contraceptives during butabarbital therapy.

# butorphanol tartrate

Stadol, Stadol NS

## Class, Category, and Schedule

*Chemical:* Opioid
*Therapeutic:* Anesthesia adjunct, narcotic analgesic
*Pregnancy category:* C
*Controlled substance:* Schedule II

## Indications and Dosages

➤ *To manage pain*
**I.V. INJECTION**
**Adults.** 0.5 to 2 mg (usually 1 mg) q 3 to 4 hr, p.r.n.
**I.M. INJECTION**
**Adults.** 1 to 4 mg (usually 2 mg) q 3 to 4 hr, p.r.n. *Maximum:* 4 mg/single dose.
**NASAL INHALATION**
**Adults.** 1 spray (1 mg) in one nostril. Dose repeated after 60 to 90 min; two-dose sequence repeated q 3 to 4 hr, p.r.n. For severe pain, 2 sprays (one in each nostril) q 3 to 4 hr, p.r.n.

**DOSAGE ADJUSTMENT** Dose reduced to 1 spray in one nostril for elderly patients and those with impaired hepatic or renal function; dose repeated after 90 to 120 min; two-dose sequence repeated q 6 hr or more, p.r.n.

➤ *As adjunct to provide preoperative anesthesia*
**I.V. OR I.M. INJECTION**
**Adults.** Individualized. *Average:* 2 mg 60 to 90 min before surgery.
➤ *As adjunct to provide anesthesia*
**I.V. INJECTION**
**Adults.** Individualized. *Average:* 1 to 4 mg and then supplemental doses of 0.5 to 1 mg, p.r.n. Total usually required during surgery is 60 to 180 mcg/kg.

**DOSAGE ADJUSTMENT** Parenteral doses reduced by half for elderly patients and those with impaired hepatic or renal function.

| Route | Onset | Peak | Duration |
|---|---|---|---|
| I.V. | 2 to 3 min | 30 min | 2 to 4 hr |
| I.M. | 10 to 30 min | 30 to 60 min | 3 to 4 hr |
| Inhalation | In 15 min | 1 to 2 hr | 4 to 5 hr |

**Mechanism of Action**
Binds with specific CNS receptors to alter the perception of and emotional response to pain.

**Contraindications**
Hypersensitivity to butorphanol or its components (including the preservative benzethonium chloride)

**Interactions**
**DRUGS**
*CNS depressants:* Additive CNS depression
*nasal vasoconstrictors, such as oxymetazoline:* Decreased absorption rate and delayed onset of butorphanol
**ACTIVITIES**
*alcohol use:* Additive CNS depression

**Adverse Reactions**
**CNS:** Anxiety, confusion, difficulty performing purposeful movements, difficulty speaking, dizziness, euphoria, floating feeling, headache, insomnia (with nasal form), lethargy, nervousness, paresthesia, sensation of heat, somnolence, syncope, tremor, vertigo
**CV:** Chest pain, hypotension, palpitations, tachycardia, vasodilation
**EENT:** Blurred vision, dry mouth, ear pain, epistaxis, nasal congestion or irritation (with

nasal form), pharyngitis, rhinitis, sinus congestion, sinusitis, tinnitus, unpleasant taste
**GI:** Anorexia, constipation, epigastric pain, nausea, vomiting
**RESP:** Apnea, bronchitis, cough, dyspnea, respiratory depression, shallow breathing, upper respiratory tract infection
**SKIN:** Clammy skin, pruritus

**Nursing Considerations**
•Use butorphanol cautiously, if at all, in patients with depression, suicidal tendency, history of drug abuse, or hepatic or renal dysfunction.
•Because drug can raise CSF pressure, use it cautiously, if at all, in patients with head injury. Because it can increase cardiac workload, use with extreme caution in patients with acute MI, ventricular dysfunction, or coronary insufficiency.
•Be aware that butorphanol has a high potential for abuse.
•Monitor patient after first dose of nasal form because hypotension and syncope may occur.
•Take safety precautions because butorphanol causes CNS depression.
•Assess respiratory status closely because drug causes respiratory depression.
•Frequently monitor blood pressure after giving drug. If severe hypertension develops (rare), stop drug at once and notify prescriber. If patient isn't narcotic-dependent, expect to administer naloxone to reverse butorphanol's effects.
**PATIENT TEACHING**
•Stress the importance of taking butorphanol exactly as prescribed because it can be addictive. Warn patient not to increase the dose or decrease the dosage interval without consulting prescriber.
•Advise patient to avoid potentially hazardous activities until drug's CNS effects are known.
•Tell patient to avoid alcohol and other CNS depressants, including OTC drugs, while taking butorphanol because of additive adverse CNS reactions.
•Teach patient how to use nasal form properly. After blowing the nose to clear the nostrils, pull the clear cover from the pump unit and remove the protective clip from its neck. Prime the pump unit by placing the nozzle between the first and second fingers with the

thumb on the bottom of the bottle. Then pump the sprayer unit firmly and quickly until a fine spray appears (7 or 8 strokes). Insert the spray tip about 1 cm ($\frac{1}{3}''$) into one nostril, pointing the tip toward the back of the nose. Close the other nostril with one finger and tilt the head slightly forward. Then pump the sprayer firmly and quickly by pushing down on the pump unit's finger grips and against the thumb at the bottom of the bottle. Sniff gently with the mouth closed. After spraying, remove the pump from the nose, tilt the head back, and sniff gently for a few more seconds. Then replace the protective clip and clear cover.

# C

# cabergoline

Dostinex

## Class and Category

*Chemical:* Ergot alkaloid derivative
*Therapeutic:* Antihyperprolactinemic
*Pregnancy category:* B

## Indications and Dosages

➤ *To treat idiopathic or adenoma-induced hyperprolactinemic disorders*

**TABLETS**

**Adults.** 0.25 mg twice a week. Increased by 0.25 mg/wk at 4-wk intervals, if needed, up to 1 mg twice a week.

| Route | Onset | Peak | Duration |
|-------|-------|------|----------|
| P.O. | Unknown | 48 hr | Up to 14 days |

## Mechanism of Action

Binds with dopamine$_2$ receptors to block prolactin synthesis and secretion by the anterior pituitary gland, thereby reducing the serum prolactin level.

## Contraindications

Hypersensitivity to cabergoline, ergot derivatives, or their components; uncontrolled hypertension

## Interactions

**DRUGS**

*antihypertensives:* Increased risk of hypotension
*dopamine antagonists (butyrophenones, metoclopramide, phenothiazines, or thioxanthenes):* Decreased cabergoline effectiveness

## Adverse Reactions

**CNS:** Asthenia, depression, fatigue, headache, nervousness, paresthesia, somnolence, vertigo
**CV:** Orthostatic hypotension
**EENT:** Dry mouth
**ENDO:** Breast pain
**GI:** Abdominal pain, constipation, diarrhea, flatulence, indigestion, nausea, vomiting
**GU:** Dysmenorrhea, increased libido

## Nursing Considerations

•Before each dose increase, check serum prolactin level to assess cabergoline's effectiveness.
•If patient has moderate to severe hepatic impairment, monitor closely for adverse reactions because of decreased cabergoline metabolism.
•**WARNING** If you detect signs of overdose, such as syncope, hallucinations, light-headedness, tachycardia, and nasal congestion, notify prescriber and treat as ordered.

**PATIENT TEACHING**

•Urge patient to read and follow printed information that explains how to use cabergoline for maximum therapeutic results.
•Advise patient to take drug with meals to help decrease GI distress.
•Tell patient to take a missed dose as soon as possible within 1 to 2 days. If the missed dose isn't remembered until it's time for the next dose, instruct him to double the dose if the drug is generally well tolerated and doesn't cause nausea. If the drug isn't well tolerated, instruct him to consult prescriber before taking the missed dose.
•Instruct patient to change positions slowly to avoid the effects of orthostatic hypotension. Tell him to notify prescriber if such effects occur.
•Encourage patient to keep regular appointments to monitor drug effectiveness.
•Advise patient that drug therapy will end when serum prolactin level is normal for 6 months. Explain that he'll need periodic monitoring of the level to determine whether therapy should resume.
•Tell female patient to notify prescriber and discuss possible drug discontinuation if pregnancy occurs or is suspected during therapy or if she plans to become pregnant during therapy.

# calcifediol

Calderol

## Class and Category

*Chemical:* Sterol derivative, vitamin D analogue
*Therapeutic:* Antihypocalcemic
*Pregnancy category:* C

## Indications and Dosages

➤ *To treat metabolic bone disease or hypocalcemia in patients receiving renal dialysis*

**CAPSULES**

**Adults and children age 10 and older.** 300 to 350 mcg/wk given in divided doses q.d. or q.o.d. Increased at 4-wk intervals, p.r.n. Most patients respond to 50 to 100 mcg q.d. or 100 to 200 mcg q.o.d.

**Children ages 2 to 10.** 0.05 mg q.d.

**Children up to age 2.** 0.02 to 0.05 mg q.d.

DOSAGE ADJUSTMENT Dosage decreased as low as 20 mcg q.o.d. in patients with normal serum calcium level.

| Route | Onset | Peak | Duration |
|-------|-------|------|----------|
| **P.O.** | Unknown | Unknown | 15 to 20 days |

### Mechanism of Action

Is converted to calcitriol in the kidneys and then binds to specific receptors in the intestinal mucosa to increase calcium absorption from the intestines. Calcifediol may also regulate calcium ion transfer from bone to blood and stimulate calcium reabsorption in the distal renal tubules, making more calcium available in the body.

## Contraindications

Abnormal sensitivity to vitamin D's effects, decreased renal function, hypercalcemia, hyperphosphatemia, hypervitaminosis, malabsorption syndrome, vitamin D toxicity

## Interactions

**DRUGS**

*aluminum-containing antacids:* Increased blood aluminum level, especially in patients with chronic renal failure

*barbiturates, corticosteroids, hydantoin anticonvulsants, primidone:* Decreased effects of vitamin D

*calcitonin, etidronate, gallium nitrate, pamidronate, plicamycin:* Decreased effects of these drugs

*calcium (high doses), thiazide diuretics:* Increased risk of hypercalcemia

*cholestyramine, colestipol, mineral oil:* Decreased vitamin D absorption

*digitalis glycosides:* Increased risk of arrhythmias from hypercalcemia

*magnesium-containing antacids:* Hypermagnesemia, especially in chronic renal failure

*phosphorous-containing drugs:* Increased risk of hyperphosphatemia

*verapamil:* Increased risk of atrial fibrillation

*vitamin D derivatives, such as calcitriol, dihydrotachysterol, ergocalciferol:* Increased risk of vitamin D toxicity

## Adverse Reactions

None with usual dosages

## Nursing Considerations

•Use calcifediol cautiously in patients with sarcoidosis or other granulomatous disease because of increased sensitivity to effects of vitamin D.

•If hypercalcemia develops, expect to discontinue therapy. Calcium level usually returns to normal in 2 to 4 weeks. To manage acute hypercalcemia, administer I.V. NS and, possibly, a loop diuretic as prescribed to enhance diuresis or prepare for dialysis with a calcium-free dialysate if needed. Be aware that chronic hypercalcemia may lead to diffuse vascular calcification, nephrocalcinosis, and other soft-tissue calcification.

•If patient receives high-dose or long-term calcifediol therapy, be alert for vitamin D toxicity. Early signs and symptoms include bone pain, constipation, dry mouth, headache, metallic taste, myalgia, nausea, somnolence, vomiting, and weakness. Late signs and symptoms include albuminuria, anorexia, arrhythmias, azotemia, conjunctivitis (calcific), decreased libido, elevated AST and ALT levels, elevated BUN level, generalized vascular calcification, hypercholesterolemia, hypertension, hyperthermia, irritability, mild acidosis, nephrocalcinosis, nocturia, pancreatitis, photophobia, polydipsia, polyuria, pruritus, rhinorrhea, and weight loss.

**PATIENT TEACHING**

•Instruct patient to swallow capsule whole and not to crush or chew it.

•Advise patient to consult prescriber before taking OTC drugs.

•Instruct patient to store drug tightly capped in a cool, dry place away from direct light.

•Encourage patient to eat a balanced diet that includes foods high in vitamin D and calcium. Calcifediol is most effective when patient follows a high-calcium diet.

•If patient takes vitamin supplements, warn him not to exceed recommended daily allowances.

•Tell patient to avoid calcium-, magnesium-, and phosphate-containing laxatives and antacids; mineral oil; and vitamin D preparations because they may increase the risk of calcifediol's toxic effects.
•Advise patient to notify prescriber immediately if signs of toxicity, such as headache, irritability, nausea, photophobia, vomiting, weakness, and weight loss, develop.
•Stress the importance of follow-up care, including laboratory tests to evaluate progress and identify signs of toxicity early.

# calcitonin, human

Cibacalcin

## calcitonin, salmon

Calcimar, Miacalcin

## Class and Category

*Chemical:* Polypeptide hormone
*Therapeutic:* Antihypercalcemic, bone resorption inhibitor, osteoporosis therapy adjunct
*Pregnancy category:* C

## Indications and Dosages

➤ *To treat hypercalcemic emergency*
**I.M. OR S.C. INJECTION**
**Adults.** *Initial:* 4 IU/kg q 12 hr. Increased after 1 or 2 days, if needed, to 8 IU/kg q 12 hr. *Maximum:* 8 IU/kg q 6 hr.

➤ *To treat postmenopausal osteoporosis*
**I.M. OR S.C. INJECTION (CALCITONIN, SALMON)**
**Adults.** *Initial:* 100 IU q.d., q.o.d., or 3 times/wk. *Maximum:* 100 IU q.d.
**NASAL SPRAY**
**Adults.** 200 IU (1 spray) q.d., alternating nostrils.

➤ *To treat Paget's disease of the bone*
**I.M. OR S.C INJECTION (CALCITONIN, SALMON)**
**Adults.** *Initial:* 100 IU q.d. *Maintenance:* 50 to 100 IU q.d. or q.o.d. *Maximum:* 100 IU q.d.
**S.C. INJECTION (CALCITONIN, HUMAN)**
**Adults.** 0.5 mg/day, 0.5 mg 2 or 3 times/wk, or 0.25 mg/day.

| Route | Onset | Peak | Duration |
|---|---|---|---|
| I.M., S.C. | In 15 min* | 2 hr† | 6 to 8 hr† |

* For hypercalcemia; 6 to 24 mo for Paget's disease.
† For hypercalcemia; unknown for other indications.

## Mechanism of Action

Directly inhibits bone resorption. Besides reducing the serum calcium level, this action slows bone metabolism (a major factor in the development of Paget's disease) and calcium loss from the bone (a major factor in the development of osteoporosis).

## Contraindications

Hypersensitivity to calcitonin, human; calcitonin, salmon; or their components

## Adverse Reactions

**CNS:** Agitation, anxiety, CVA, dizziness, headache, insomnia, neuralgia, paresthesia, vertigo
**CV:** Bundle-branch block, hypertension, MI, palpitations, peripheral edema, tachycardia, thrombophlebitis
**EENT:** Blurred vision; dry mouth; earache; epistaxis; eye pain; hearing loss; nasal irritation, lesions, or redness; pharyngitis; rhinitis; salty taste; sinusitis; taste perversion; tinnitus; vitreous floaters
**ENDO:** Goiter, hyperthyroidism
**GI:** Anorexia, cholelithiasis, epigastric discomfort, flatulence, gastritis, hepatitis, increased appetite, nausea, thirst, vomiting
**GU:** Hematuria, nocturia, pyelonephritis, renal calculi
**HEME:** Anemia
**MS:** Arthritis, arthrosis, back pain, joint stiffness, polymyalgia rheumatica
**RESP:** Bronchitis, cough, dyspnea, pneumonia, upper respiratory tract infection
**SKIN:** Alopecia, diaphoresis, eczema, flushing of face or hands, pruritus of earlobes, rash, ulceration
**Other:** Antibody formation, feverish sensation, injection site inflammation, lymphadenopathy, mild tetanic symptoms

## Nursing Considerations

•If sensitivity to calcitonin, human; calcitonin, salmon; or their components is suspected, expect to perform a skin test before administration. Prepare a mixture of 10 IU/ml by withdrawing 0.05 ml of 200-IU solution in a tuberculin syringe and filling the syringe to 1 ml with sodium chloride for injection. Mix well, discard 0.9 ml, and inject 0.1 ml intradermally on the inner forearm. Observe the site for 15 minutes after injection. If you detect signs of sensitivity, such as more than mild erythema or a wheal, notify prescriber.

•If patient receives calcitonin for hypercalcemia, monitor serum calcium level. During first several doses, keep parenteral calcium available in case the calcium level is inadvertently overcorrected.

•If the calcitonin dose exceeds 2 ml, expect to use I.M. route and multiple injection sites.

•For patient receiving calcitonin for postmenopausal osteoporosis, also expect to administer 1.5 g of supplemental calcium carbonate and at least 400 U of vitamin D daily. Plan to provide a balanced diet that includes foods high in calcium and vitamin D.

•Assess for nausea, especially with the first dose. Nausea tends to decrease or disappear with continued use.

•If patient with Paget's disease relapses after treatment, check for antibody formation, as ordered.

**PATIENT TEACHING**

•Tell patient to refrigerate injection or unopened nasal spray container.

•Teach patient how to self-administer injections.

•If patient has postmenopausal osteoporosis, teach her about dietary needs, including foods rich in calcium and vitamin D.

•For a nasal spray user, explain how to activate the nasal pump by holding the bottle upright and depressing two white side arms toward the bottle six times. When the bottle emits a faint spray, the pump is activated. Tell patient to store the activated nasal pump upright at room temperature and to discard it after 30 days.

•Tell patient to place the nozzle firmly into a nostril while holding the head upright and then to depress the pump toward the bottle.

•Remind patient that he doesn't need to reactivate the pump before each daily dose.

•Instruct patient to report nasal symptoms, such as redness, lesions, sinusitis, and rhinitis, to prescriber.

# calcitriol

## (1,25-dihydroxycholecalciferol)

Calcijex, Rocaltrol

## Class and Category

*Chemical:* Sterol derivative, vitamin D analogue

*Therapeutic:* Antihypocalcemic, antihypoparathyroid
*Pregnancy category:* C

## Indications and Dosages

➤ *To treat hypocalcemia in dialysis patients*

**CAPSULES, ORAL SOLUTION**

**Adults.** *Initial:* 0.25 mcg q.d. Increased by 0.25 mcg/day q 4 to 8 wk, if needed to achieve normal serum calcium level. *Maintenance:* 0.5 to 3 mcg q.d.

➤ *To treat hypocalcemia in predialysis patients*

**CAPSULES, ORAL SOLUTION**

**Adults and children age 3 and older.** *Initial:* 0.25 mcg q.d. Increased after 4 to 8 wk, if needed, to 0.5 mcg q.d.

**ORAL SOLUTION**

**Children up to age 3.** 10 to 15 ng/kg/day.

➤ *To treat hypoparathyroidism*

**TABLETS**

**Adults and children age 6 and older.** *Initial:* 0.25 mcg q.d. in the morning. Increased q 2 to 4 wk, if needed to achieve normal serum calcium level. *Usual:* 0.5 to 2 mcg q.d.

**Children ages 1 to 5.** 0.25 to 0.75 mcg q.d in the morning.

**I.V. INJECTION**

**Adults.** *Initial:* 1 to 2 mcg 3 times/wk given q.o.d. Each dose increased 0.5 to 1 mcg at 2- to 4-wk intervals, if needed.

| Route | Onset | Peak | Duration |
|-------|-------|------|----------|
| P.O. | 2 to 6 hr | 10 hr | 3 to 5 days |

## Mechanism of Action

Binds to specific receptors of the intestinal mucosa to increase calcium absorption from the intestines. It also may regulate calcium ion transfer from bone to blood and stimulate calcium reabsorption in the distal renal tubules, making more calcium available in the body.

## Contraindications

Hypercalcemia, vitamin D toxicity

## Interactions

**DRUGS**

*cholestyramine:* Decreased calcitriol absorption

*digitalis glycosides:* Possibly arrhythmias

*ketoconazole:* Decreased blood calcitriol level
*magnesium-containing antacids (I.V. form):*
Hypermagnesemia
*mineral oil:* Decreased blood calcitriol level
(with prolonged use of mineral oil)
*phenobarbital, phenytoin:* Decreased synthesis and blood level of calcitriol
*thiazide diuretics:* Hypercalcemia

## Adverse Reactions
**SKIN:** Erythema multiforme, lip swelling, pruritus, rash, urticaria

## Nursing Considerations
• Make sure patient has adequate calcium intake.
• Store drug at room temperature and protect from heat and direct light.
• In high-dose or long-term calcitriol therapy, be alert for vitamin D toxicity. Early evidence includes abdominal or bone pain, constipation, dry mouth, headache, metallic taste, myalgia, nausea, somnolence, vomiting, and weakness. Late evidence includes albuminuria, anorexia, arrhythmias, azotemia, conjunctivitis (calcific), decreased libido, elevated AST and ALT levels, elevated BUN level, vascular calcification, hypercholesterolemia, hypertension, hyperthermia, irritability, mild acidosis, nephrocalcinosis, nocturia, pancreatitis, photophobia, polydipsia, polyuria, pruritus, rhinorrhea, and weight loss.
**PATIENT TEACHING**
• Warn patient not to take other forms of vitamin D while taking calcitriol.
• Instruct patient to take a missed dose as soon as possible.
• Advise patient to notify prescriber immediately if signs of toxicity, such as headache, irritability, nausea, photophobia, vomiting, weakness, and weight loss, develop.

# calcium acetate
PhosLo

## calcium carbonate
Apo-Cal (CAN), Calci-Mix, Calsan (CAN), Liqui-Cal, Liquid Cal-600, Titralac

## calcium chloride
Calciject (CAN)

## calcium citrate
Citracal, Citracal Liquitabs

## calcium glubionate
Calcionate, Calcium-Sandoz (CAN), Neo-Calglucon

## calcium gluceptate
Calcium Stanley (CAN)

## calcium gluconate

## calcium lactate

## Class and Category
*Chemical:* Elemental cation
*Therapeutic:* Antacid, antihypermagnesemic, antihyperphosphatemic, antihypocalcemic, calcium replacement, cardiotonic
*Pregnancy category:* C (Not rated for calcium carbonate, citrate, and lactate)

## Indications and Dosages
➤ *To treat hyperphosphatemia*
**TABLETS (CALCIUM ACETATE)**
**Adults.** *Initial:* 2 tabs (338 mg elemental calcium, 1,334 mg calcium acetate) t.i.d. with meals. Dosage increased to reduce serum phosphorous level below 6 mg/dl as long as hypercalcemia doesn't develop. *Maintenance:* 3 or 4 tabs t.i.d. with each meal.

➤ *To prevent hypocalcemia*
**CAPSULES, ORAL SUSPENSION, TABLETS (CALCIUM CARBONATE); EFFERVESCENT TABLETS, TABLETS (CALCIUM CITRATE); SYRUP (CALCIUM GLUBIONATE); TABLETS (CALCIUM GLUCONATE OR LACTATE)**
**Adults and children over age 10.** 800 to 1,200 mg/day.
**Pregnant and breast-feeding women.** 1,200 mg/day.
**Children ages 4 to 10.** 800 mg/day.
**Children up to age 4.** 400 to 800 mg/day.

➤ *To provide antacid effects*
**CHEWABLE TABLETS, ORAL SUSPENSION, TABLETS (CALCIUM CARBONATE)**
**Adults and children age 12 and older.** 350 to 1,500 mg 1 hr p.c. and h.s., p.r.n.

➤ *To replace calcium in hypocalcemia*
**I.V. INFUSION (CALCIUM CHLORIDE)**
**Adults.** 0.5 to 1 g q 1 to 3 days, infused at less than 1 ml/min.
**Children.** 25 mg/kg given over several minutes.
**I.V. OR I.M. INJECTION (CALCIUM GLUCEPTATE)**
**Adults and children.** 0.44 to 1.1 g I.M. or 1.1 to 4.4 g I.V. at a rate not to exceed 2 ml (36 mg)/min.

**I.V. INJECTION (CALCIUM GLUCONATE)**

**Adults.** 970 mg given slowly, repeated if needed until tetany is controlled.

**Children.** 200 to 500 mg as a single dose given slowly, repeated if needed until tetany is controlled.

➤ *As adjunct to treat magnesium intoxication*

**I.V. INJECTION (CALCIUM CHLORIDE)**

**Adults.** 500 mg promptly and repeated p.r.n., based on response.

➤ *As adjunct in cardiac resuscitation*

**I.V. INJECTION (CALCIUM CHLORIDE)**

**Adults.** 0.5 to 1 g.
**Children.** 0.2 ml/kg.

➤ *As adjunct in exchange transfusion*

**I.V. INJECTION (CALCIUM GLUCONATE)**

**Adults.** 1.35 mEq with each 100 ml of citrated blood exchanged.
**Neonates.** 0.45 mEq after each 100 ml of citrated blood exchanged.

**I.V. INJECTION (CALCIUM GLUCEPTATE)**

**Neonates.** 110 mg after each 100 ml of citrated blood exchanged.

### Mechanism of Action

Increases levels of intracellular and extracellular calcium, which is needed to maintain homeostasis, especially in the nervous and musculoskeletal systems. Also plays a role in normal cardiac and renal function, respiration, coagulation, and cell membrane and capillary permeability. Helps regulate the release and storage of neurotransmitters and hormones. Oral forms also neutralize or buffer stomach acid to relieve discomfort cause by hyperacidity.

### Incompatibilities

To avoid precipitation, don't administer I.V. calcium chloride, gluceptate, or gluconate through the same I.V. line as bicarbonates, carbonates, phosphates, sulfates, or tartrates.

### Contraindications

Hypercalcemia, hypersensitivity to calcium salts or their components, hypophosphatemia, renal calculi

## Interactions

**DRUGS**

*aluminum-containing antacids:* Enhanced aluminum absorption with use of calcium citrate
*atenolol:* Decreased blood atenolol level and beta blockade
*calcitonin:* Possibly antagonized effects of calcitonin in hypercalcemia treatment
*calcium supplements, magnesium-containing preparations:* Increased serum calcium or magnesium level, especially in patients with impaired renal function
*cellulose sodium phosphate:* Decreased effectiveness of cellulose sodium phosphate in preventing hypercalciuria
*digitalis glycosides:* Increased risk of arrhythmias
*estrogens, oral contraceptives (estrogen-containing):* Increased calcium absorption
*etidronate:* Decreased etidronate absorption
*fluoroquinolones:* Reduced fluoroquinolone absorption by calcium carbonate
*gallium nitrate:* Antagonized effects of gallium nitrate
*iron salts:* Decreased gastric absorption of iron
*magnesium sulfate (parenteral):* Neutralized effects of magnesium by parenteral calcium salts
*neuromuscular blockers (except succinylcholine):* Possibly reversal of neuromuscular blockade by parenteral calcium salts; enhanced or prolonged neuromuscular blockade induced by tubocurarine
*norfloxacin:* Decreased norfloxacin bioavailability
*phenytoin:* Decreased bioavailability of phenytoin and calcium
*potassium phosphates, potassium and sodium phosphates:* Increased risk of calcium deposition in soft tissue
*sodium bicarbonate:* Possibly milk-alkali syndrome
*sodium fluoride:* Reduced fluoride and calcium absorption
*sodium polystyrene sulfonate:* Possibly metabolic alkalosis if patient has renal impairment
*tetracyclines:* Decreased tetracycline absorption and blood level, leading to decreased anti-infective response
*thiazide diuretics:* Possibly hypercalcemia
*verapamil:* Reversed verapamil effects
*vitamin A (more than 25,000 U/day):* Possibly stimulation of bone loss, decreased ef-

fects of calcium supplementation, and hypercalcemia

*vitamin D (high doses):* Excessively increased calcium absorption

**FOODS**

*caffeine, high-fiber food:* Possibly decreased calcium absorption

**ACTIVITIES**

*alcohol use (excessive), smoking:* Possibly decreased calcium absorption

### Adverse Reactions

**CNS:** Paresthesia (parenteral form)

**CV:** Hypotension, irregular heartbeat (parenteral form)

**GI:** Nausea or vomiting (parenteral form)

**SKIN:** Diaphoresis, flushing, or sensation of warmth (parenteral form)

**Other:** Hypercalcemia; injection site burning, pain, rash, or redness (parenteral form)

### Nursing Considerations

•Store at room temperature and protect from heat, moisture, and direct light. Don't freeze.

•Warm solution to room temperature before parenteral administration.

•Maintain patient in a recumbent position for 30 minutes after parenteral administration to prevent dizziness from hypotension.

•Administer I.V. calcium through an infusing I.V. solution, using a small-bore needle inserted into a large vein to minimize irritation. Give calcium slowly to prevent excess calcium from reaching the heart and causing adverse cardiovascular reactions. Adverse reactions often result from too-rapid administration. If ECG tracings are abnormal or patient reports injection site discomfort, expect to temporarily discontinue administration.

•Check regularly for infiltration because calcium causes necrosis. If infiltration occurs, stop infusion and tell prescriber immediately.

•Divide I.M. calcium gluceptate dose of 5 ml or more in half and inject in gluteal region.

•Regularly monitor serum calcium level and evaluate therapeutic response by assessing for Chvostek's and Trousseau's signs, which shouldn't appear.

•Be aware that calcium chloride injection contains three times as much calcium per milliliter as calcium gluconate injection.

**PATIENT TEACHING**

•If chewable tablets are prescribed, urge patient to chew them thoroughly before swallowing and to drink a glass of water afterward.

•If suspension is prescribed, tell patient to shake bottle well before each use.

•If calcium citrate effervescent tablets are prescribed, tell patient to dissolve them in water and drink immediately.

•Instruct patient to take calcium carbonate tablets 1 to 2 hours after meals, calcium glubionate syrup before meals (diluted in water or fruit juice, if desired, for an infant or a child), and other calcium supplements with meals.

•Advise storing calcium at room temperature away from heat, moisture, and direct light. Warn against freezing suspension or syrup.

•Instruct patient to avoid taking calcium within 2 hours of taking another oral drug because of risk of interactions.

•Urge patient to see prescriber before taking OTC drugs because of risk of interactions.

•Tell patient to avoid excessive use of tobacco and excessive consumption of alcoholic beverages, caffeine-containing products, and high-fiber foods because these substances may decrease calcium absorption.

# candesartan cilexetil

Atacand

### Class and Category

*Chemical:* Angiotensin II receptor antagonist

*Therapeutic:* Antihypertensive

*Pregnancy category:* C (first trimester), D (later trimesters)

### Indications and Dosages

➤ *To manage, or as adjunct in managing, hypertension*

**TABLETS**

**Adults.** *Initial:* 16 mg q.d. Maintenance: 8 to 32 mg q.d. or 4 to 16 mg q 12 hr. *Maximum:* 32 mg/day.

**DOSAGE ADJUSTMENT** Initial dosage decreased to 2 mg for patients with moderate to severe hepatic impairment and to 4 mg for those with renal impairment, need for hemodialysis, or possibly a risk of hypotension.

➤ *To treat heart failure in patients with an ejection fraction of 40% or less and NYHA class II–IV to reduce the risk of death from cardiovascular causes and reduce hospitalizations for heart failure*

**TABLETS**

**Adults.** *Initial:* 4 mg q.d. for 2 wk; then doubled q 2 wk as tolerated until reaching target dose of 32 mg q.d.

| Route | Onset | Peak | Duration |
|-------|-------|------|----------|
| P.O. | In 2 wk | In 4 to 5 wk | Unknown |

## Mechanism of Action

Selectively blocks binding of angiotensin (AT) II to $AT_1$ receptor sites in many tissues, including vascular smooth muscle and adrenal glands. This inhibits vasoconstrictive and aldosterone-secreting effects of AT II, which reduces blood pressure.

## Contraindications

Hypersensitivity to candesartan or components

## Interactions

**DRUGS**
*diuretics, other antihypertensives:* Possibly increased risk of hypotension
*heparin, potassium-sparing diuretics, potassium supplements, potassium-containing salt substitutes:* Possibly increased risk of hyperkalemia
*lithium:* Increased blood lithium level

## Adverse Reactions

**CNS:** Dizziness, headache
**CV:** Hypotension
**EENT:** Pharyngitis, rhinitis
**GI:** Elevated liver function test results, hepatitis
**GU:** Elevated BUN and serum creatinine levels
**HEME:** Agranulocytosis, leukopenia, neutropenia
**MS:** Back pain, rhabdomyolysis
**RESP:** Upper respiratory tract infection
**Other:** Hyperkalemia, hyponatremia

## Nursing Considerations

•If patient has known or suspected hypovolemia, expect to provide treatment, such as I.V. normal saline solution, as prescribed, to correct it before starting candesartan.
•Watch for elevated BUN and serum creatinine levels, especially if patient has heart failure or impaired renal function; drug may cause acute renal failure. Report significant or persistent increases immediately.
•If blood pressure isn't controlled with candesartan alone, expect to give a diuretic, such as hydrochlorothiazide, as prescribed.
•WARNING If patient receives a diuretic or antihypertensive with candesartan, has heart failure, or is elderly, assess blood pressure often because of added risk of hypotension.
•If patient develops hypotension, expect to stop drug temporarily. Immediately place patient in supine position and prepare to give I.V. normal saline solution, as prescribed. Expect to resume therapy after blood pressure stabilizes.
•If patient also receives a diuretic, provide hydration, as appropriate, to help prevent hypovolemia. Watch for evidence of hypovolemia, such as hypotension with dizziness and fainting. If patient has heart failure and develops hypotension, dosage of diuretic, candesartan, or both may be reduced when blood pressure stablizes and therapy resumes.
•Check patient's CBC for decreases in hemoglobin and hematocrit. If they're significant or persistent, notify prescriber immediately.

**PATIENT TEACHING**
•Advise patient that full effects of candesartan may not occur for 4 to 5 weeks.
•Explain the importance of lifestyle choices in controlling hypertension.
•Advise female patient to immediately report known or suspected pregnancy. Explain that if she becomes pregnant, prescriber may replace candesartan with another antihypertensive that is safe to use during pregnancy.

# capreomycin sulfate

Capastat

## Class and Category

*Chemical:* Polypeptide antibiotic isolated from *Streptomyces capreolus*
*Therapeutic:* Antitubercular
*Pregnancy category:* C

## Indications and Dosages

➤ *As adjunct to treat pulmonary tuberculosis caused by* Mycobacterium tuberculosis *in which primary drugs are ineffective or can't be used because of toxicity*

**I.V. INFUSION, I.M. INJECTION**
**Adults.** 1 g q.d. for 60 to 120 days followed by 1 g 2 or 3 times/wk for 12 to 24 mo. *Maximum:* 20 mg/kg/day.

## Contraindications

Hypersensitivity to capreomycin or its components

## Mechanism of Action
May interfere with lipid and nucleic acid biosynthesis in actively growing tubercle bacilli.

## Interactions
### DRUGS
*aminoglycosides (parenteral):* Increased risk of ototoxicity, nephrotoxicity, and neuromuscular blockade
*nephrotoxic drugs, such as amphotericin B:* Increased risk of nephrotoxicity
*nondepolarizing neuromuscular blockers:* Enhanced neuromuscular blockade
*ototoxic drugs, such as quinidine:* Increased risk of ototoxicity
*polymyxins (parenteral):* Increased risk of nephrotoxicity and neuromuscular blockade

## Adverse Reactions
**CNS:** Dizziness, vertigo
**EENT:** Ototoxicity
**GI:** Elevated liver function test results
**GU:** Nephrotoxicity
**HEME:** Leukocytosis, leukopenia
**SKIN:** Maculopapular rash, sterile abscess, urticaria
**Other:** Injection site pain, induration, and bleeding

## Nursing Considerations
• Use capreomycin cautiously in patients with renal insufficiency, impaired hearing, or a history of hypersensitivity, especially to other drugs.
• To reconstitute drug for I.V. injection, add 100 ml of NS. Administer over 60 minutes.
• To reconstitute drug for I.M. injection, add 2 ml of sodium chloride for injection or sterile water for injection to each 1-g vial. Allow 2 to 3 minutes for complete dissolution.
• Give I.M. injection deep into a large muscle mass, such as the gluteus maximus.
• Observe injection site for excessive bleeding or sterile abscess.
• Monitor results of renal function tests to detect nephrotoxicity.
• Make sure patient receives audiometric tests and vestibular function assessment regularly.
• Closely monitor for urticaria and maculopapular rash.
### PATIENT TEACHING
• Advise patient to alert nurse or prescriber if injection site bleeds excessively.

• Warn patient to contact prescriber immediately about hearing loss or tinnitus.
• Explain the need for frequent laboratory tests to monitor renal function.
• Tell patient that tuberculosis therapy lasts for 12 to 24 months.
• Explain that noncompliance may decrease effectiveness and lengthen treatment.

# captopril
Capoten

## Class and Category
*Chemical:* ACE inhibitor
*Therapeutic:* Antihypertensive
*Pregnancy category:* C (first trimester), D (later trimesters)

## Indications and Dosages
➤ *To control hypertension*
### TABLETS
**Adults and adolescents.** *Initial:* 25 mg b.i.d. or t.i.d. Increased to 50 mg b.i.d. or t.i.d. after 1 to 2 wk, if needed. If blood pressure isn't well controlled at this dosage and with the addition of a diuretic, dosage increased to 100 mg b.i.d. or t.i.d. and then, if needed, to 150 mg b.i.d. or t.i.d. while continuing diuretic. *Maximum:* 450 mg/day.
➤ *To control accelerated or malignant hypertension when temporary discontinuation of current antihypertensive therapy isn't practical or when prompt titration of blood pressure is needed*
### TABLETS
**Adults and adolescents.** *Initial:* 25 mg b.i.d. or t.i.d while continuing diuretic but discontinuing current antihypertensive drug. Increased q 24 hr as needed until satisfactory response is obtained or maximum dosage is reached. *Maximum:* 450 mg/day.
➤ *To treat heart failure that's unresponsive to conventional therapy*
### TABLETS
**Adults and adolescents.** *Initial:* 25 mg b.i.d. or t.i.d. Increased to 50 mg b.i.d. or t.i.d., as needed. After 14 days, increased to 100 mg t.i.d. and then to 150 mg t.i.d, if needed. *Maximum:* 450 mg/day.
➤ *To treat left-sided heart failure after MI*
### TABLETS
**Adults and adolescents.** *Initial:* 6.25 mg as a single dose starting 3 days after MI and then

C

12.5 mg t.i.d. Increased to 25 mg t.i.d. for several days and then increased again to maintenance dosage. *Maintenance:* 50 mg t.i.d.

➤ *To treat diabetic nephropathy*

**TABLETS**

**Adults and adolescents.** 25 mg t.i.d.

DOSAGE ADJUSTMENT Starting dosage reduced to 6.25 mg b.i.d. or t.i.d. if patient with hypertension also has heart failure, is undergoing dialysis, or is being vigorously treated with diuretics that result in hyponatremia or hypovolemia.

| Route | Onset | Peak | Duration |
|---|---|---|---|
| P.O. | 15 to 60 min | 60 to 90 min | 6 to 12 hr |

**Mechanism of Action**

May reduce blood pressure by affecting the renin-angiotensin-aldosterone system. By inhibiting ACE, captopril:

• prevents conversion of angiotensin I to angiotensin II, a potent vasoconstrictor that also stimulates the adrenal cortex to secrete aldosterone. Inhibiting aldosterone increases sodium and water excretion, reducing blood pressure.

• may inhibit renal and vascular production of angiotensin II.

• decreases serum angiotensin II level and increases renin activity. This decreases aldosterone secretion, slightly increasing serum potassium level and fluid loss.

• decreases vascular tone and blood pressure.

**Contraindications**

Hypersensitivity to captopril, other ACE inhibitors, or their components

**Interactions**

**DRUGS**

*allopurinol:* Increased risk of hypersensitivity reactions, including Stevens-Johnson syndrome, skin eruptions, fever, arthralgia

*antacids:* Possibly impaired captopril absorption

*capsaicin:* Possibly initiation or worsening of cough caused by ACE inhibitor

*cyclosporine, potassium-containing drugs, potassium-sparing diuretics, potassium supplements:* Increased risk of hyperkalemia

*digoxin:* Increased blood digoxin level

*diuretics; hypotension-producing drugs, such as hydralazine:* Additive hypotensive effects

*lithium:* Increased risk of lithium toxicity

*NSAIDs:* Decreased antihypertensive response to ACE inhibition

*probenecid:* Increased blood level and decreased total clearance of captopril

**ACTIVITIES**

*alcohol use:* Additive hypotensive effects

**Adverse Reactions**

**CNS:** Fever

**CV:** Chest pain, hypotension, orthostatic hypotension, palpitations, tachycardia

**EENT:** Loss of taste

**GU:** Dysuria, impotence, nephrotic syndrome, nocturia, oliguria, polyuria, proteinuria, urinary frequency

**HEME:** Eosinophilia

**MS:** Arthralgia

**RESP:** Cough

**SKIN:** Photosensitivity, pruritus, rash

**Other:** Angioedema, hyperkalemia, hyponatremia, positive ANA titer

**Nursing Considerations**

• Closely monitor blood pressure, especially when therapy starts and dosage increases. Keep patient supine if hypotension occurs.

• Monitor renal function tests for signs of nephrotic syndrome, such as proteinuria and increased BUN and serum creatinine levels. Also watch for renal symptoms, such as oliguria, polyuria, and urinary frequency.

• Monitor WBC regularly, as ordered, especially if patient has collagen vascular disease or renal disease.

**PATIENT TEACHING**

• Instruct patient to take captopril 1 hour before meals.

• Tell patient to rise slowly from sitting or lying down to minimize orthostatic hypotension.

• Tell patient to avoid sunlight or to wear sunscreen in direct sunlight because photosensitivity may occur.

• Warn patient not to stop taking drug abruptly.

• Advise patient not to use salt substitutes that contain potassium and to consult prescriber before increasing dietary potassium intake to avoid increasing the risk of hyperkalemia.

• Urge patient to tell prescriber about signs of infection, such as sore throat or fever.

# carbamazepine

Apo-Carbamazepine (CAN), Atretol, Carbatrol, Epitol, Equetro, Novo-Carbamaz (CAN), Tegretol, Tegretol-XR

## Class and Category

*Chemical:* Tricyclic iminostilbene derivative
*Therapeutic:* Analgesic, anticonvulsant
*Pregnancy category:* C

## Indications and Dosages

➤ *To treat epilepsy*

**E.R. CAPSULES (CARBATROL), E.R. TABLETS (TEGRETOL-XR)**

**Adults and children age 12 and older.** *Initial:* 200 mg b.i.d. Increased weekly by 200 mg/day, if needed. *Maximum:* 1,600 mg/day in adults, 1,200 mg/day in children age 16 and older, and 1,000 mg/day in children ages 12 to 16.
**Children ages 6 to 12.** *Initial:* 100 mg b.i.d. Increased weekly by 100 mg/day, if needed. *Maximum:* 1,000 mg/day.

**ORAL SUSPENSION**

**Adults and children age 12 and older.** *Initial:* 100 mg q.i.d. Increased weekly by 200 mg/day, if needed, given in divided doses t.i.d or q.i.d. *Maximum:* 1,600 mg/day in adults, 1,200 mg/day in children age 16 and older, and 1,000 mg/day in children ages 12 to 16.
**Children ages 6 to 12.** *Initial:* 50 mg q.i.d. Increased weekly by 100 mg/day, if needed, given in divided doses t.i.d or q.i.d. *Maximum:* 1,000 mg/day.
**Children up to age 6.** *Initial:* 10 to 20 mg/kg/day in divided doses q.i.d. *Maximum:* 35 mg/kg/day.

**TABLETS**

**Adults and children age 12 and older.** *Initial:* 200 mg b.i.d. Increased weekly by 200 mg/day, if needed, given in divided doses t.i.d. or q.i.d. *Maximum:* 1,600 mg/day in adults, 1,200 mg/day in children age 16 and older, and 1,000 mg/day in children ages 12 to 16.
**Children ages 6 to 12.** *Initial:* 100 mg b.i.d. Increased weekly by 100 mg/day, if needed, given in divided doses t.i.d. or q.i.d. *Maximum:* 1,000 mg/day.
**Children up to age 6.** *Initial:* 10 to 20 mg/kg/day in divided doses b.i.d. or t.i.d. Increased weekly, if needed, divided and given t.i.d. or q.i.d. *Maximum:* 35/kg/day.

➤ *To relieve pain in trigeminal neuralgia*

**E.R. CAPSULES (CARBATROL), E.R. TABLETS (TEGRETOL-XR), TABLETS**

**Adults.** *Initial:* 100 mg b.i.d. Increased by up to 200 mg/day, if needed, in increments of 100 mg q 12 hr. *Maintenance:* 400 to 800 mg/day. *Maximum:* 1,200 mg/day.

**ORAL SUSPENSION (100 MG/5 ML)**

**Adults.** 50 mg q.i.d. Increased by up to 200 mg/day, if needed, in increments of 50 mg q.i.d. *Maintenance:* 400 to 800 mg/day. *Maximum:* 1,200 mg/day.

➤ *To treat acute manic and mixed episodes in bipolar disorder*

**E.R. CAPSULES (EQUETRO)**

**Adults.** *Initial:* 200 mg b.i.d., increased as needed in 200-mg increments. *Maximum:* 1,600 mg/day.

| Route | Onset | Peak | Duration |
|---|---|---|---|
| P.O. (all forms) | In 1 mo* | Unknown | Unknown |

## Contraindications

History of bone marrow depression; hypersensitivity to carbamazepine, tricyclic compounds, or their components; MAO inhibitor therapy

## Interactions

**DRUGS**

*acetaminophen (long-term use):* Increased metabolism, leading to acetaminophen-induced hepatotoxicity or decreased acetaminophen effectiveness
*bupropion, cyclosporine, haloperidol:* Decreased blood levels of these drugs
*cimetidine, clarithromycin, danazol, diltiazem, erythromycin, fluoxetine, fluvoxamine, itraconazole, ketoconazole, niacinamide, nicotinamide, propoxyphene, troleandomycin, verapamil:* Increased blood carbamazepine level
*cisplatin, doxorubicin, phenytoin, rifampin, theophylline:* Decreased blood carbamazepine level
*doxycycline:* Decreased doxycycline half-life
*felbamate:* Decreased blood level of felbamate or carbamazepine
*felodipine:* Decreased felodipine effects
*isoniazid:* Increased risk of carbamazepine toxicity and isoniazid hepatotoxicity
*lamotrigine, phenobarbital, primidone, tricyclic antidepressants, valproic acid:* De-

---

\* For anticonvulsant use; 8 to 72 hr for use in trigeminal neuralgia.

## Mechanism of Action

Normally, sodium moves into a neuronal cell by passing through a gated sodium channel in the cell membrane. Carbamazepine may prevent or halt seizures by closing or blocking sodium channels, as shown, thus preventing sodium from entering the cell. Keeping sodium out of the cell may slow nerve impulse transmission, thus slowing the rate at which neurons fire.

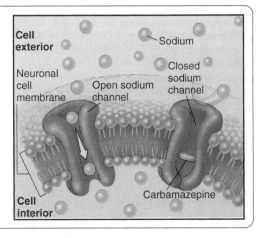

creased blood levels of these drugs, increased blood level of carbamazepine
*lithium:* Increased risk of CNS toxicity
*oral anticoagulants:* Increased metabolism and decreased effectiveness of anticoagulant
*oral contraceptives:* Decreased contraceptive effectiveness
*nondepolarizing neuromuscular blockers:* Possibly reduced duration or decreased effectiveness of neuromuscular blocker

### Adverse Reactions

**CNS:** Chills, confusion, dizziness, drowsiness, fatigue, fever, headache, syncope, talkativeness, unsteadiness, visual hallucinations
**CV:** Arrhythmias, including AV block; edema; heart failure; hypertension; hypotension; thromboembolism; thrombophlebitis; worsened coronary artery disease
**EENT:** Blurred vision, conjunctivitis, dry mouth, glossitis, nystagmus, oculomotor disturbances, stomatitis, tinnitus, transient diplopia
**ENDO:** Syndrome of inappropriate ADH secretion, water intoxication
**GI:** Abdominal pain, anorexia, constipation, diarrhea, dyspepsia, elevated liver function test results, hepatitis, nausea, pancreatitis, vomiting
**GU:** Acute urine retention, albuminuria, azotemia, glycosuria, impotence, oliguria, renal failure, urinary frequency
**HEME:** Acute intermittent porphyria, agranulocytosis, aplastic anemia, bone marrow depression, eosinophilia, leukocytosis, leukopenia, pancytopenia, thrombocytopenia

**MS:** Arthralgia, leg cramps, myalgia
**RESP:** Pulmonary hypersensitivity (dyspnea, fever, pneumonia, or pneumonitis)
**SKIN:** Aggravation of disseminated lupus erythematosus, alopecia, altered skin pigmentation, diaphoresis, erythema multiforme, erythema nodosum, exfoliative dermatitis, jaundice, Lyell's syndrome, photosensitivity reactions, pruritic and erythematous rash, purpura, Stevens-Johnson syndrome, urticaria
**Other:** Adenopathy, lymphadenopathy

### Nursing Considerations

• Use carbamazepine cautiously in patients with impaired hepatic function because it's mainly metabolized in the liver. Monitor results of liver function tests, as directed.
• Monitor patient closely for adverse reactions because many are serious.
• Periodically monitor blood carbamazepine level to assess for therapeutic and toxic levels; a blood level of 6 to 12 mcg/ml is optimal for anticonvulsant effects.
• **WARNING** Monitor WBC and platelet counts monthly for first 2 months. Decreased counts may indicate bone marrow depression.

**PATIENT TEACHING**
• Tell patient to take carbamazepine with food (except oral suspension, which shouldn't be taken with other liquid drugs or diluents).
• Warn patient about possible dizziness, blurred vision, and unsteadiness.
• Inform patient that the coating of E.R. tablets isn't absorbed and may appear in stool.
• Advise patient not to crush or chew E.R. capsules or tablets. If he can't swallow cap-

sules whole, have him open them and sprinkle contents on food.
• Urge patient to wear sunscreen and protective clothing to prevent photosensitivity.
• Tell patient to report unusual bleeding or bruising, fever, rash, or mouth ulcers.
• Warn woman that drug decreases oral contraceptive effectiveness and urge her to use another form of contraception. Because drug may cause fetal harm, urge her to notify prescriber if pregnancy is suspected or occurs.

# carbenicillin indanyl sodium

Geocillin, Geopen, Pyopen (CAN)

## Class and Category
*Chemical:* Carboxypenicillin
*Therapeutic:* Antibiotic
*Pregnancy category:* B

## Indications and Dosages
➤ *To treat acute and chronic infections of the upper and lower urinary tract and asymptomatic bacteriuria caused by susceptible strains of* Escherichia coli, Morganella morganii, Proteus mirabilis, Proteus vulgaris, *and* Providencia rettgeri
**TABLETS**
**Adults.** 382 or 764 mg (1 or 2 tabs) q.i.d.
➤ *To treat acute and chronic infections of the upper and lower urinary tract and asymptomatic bacteriuria caused by susceptible strains of* Enterobacter *sp.,* Enterococcus *sp., and* Pseudomonas *sp.*
**TABLETS**
**Adults**: 764 mg (2 tabs) q.i.d.
➤ *To treat prostatitis caused by susceptible strains of* E. coli, Enterobacter *sp.,* Enterococcus *sp., and* P. mirabilis
**TABLETS**
**Adults:** 764 mg (2 tabs) q.i.d.

## Contraindications
Hypersensitivity to carbenicillin, penicillin, or their components

## Mechanism of Action
Is bactericidal to susceptible organisms by inhibiting the biosynthesis of cell wall mucopeptides, especially when target cells are actively multiplying.

## Interactions
**DRUGS**
*probenecid:* Increased and prolonged blood level of carbenicillin indanyl sodium and increased risk of toxicity

## Adverse Reactions
**EENT:** Altered taste, glossitis
**GI:** Diarrhea, flatulence, mildly elevated AST level, nausea, vomiting
**SKIN:** Pruritus, rash, urticaria
**Other:** Anaphylaxis

## Nursing Considerations
• **WARNING** If anaphylaxis occurs, stop drug, tell prescriber immediately, and provide care, including epinephrine, airway management, oxygen, and I.V. corticosteroids.
• Watch closely for evidence of superinfection, and tell prescriber if it develops. Expect to stop drug and give appropriate care.
**PATIENT TEACHING**
• Urge patient to take full course of drug exactly as prescribed, even if feeling better.
• Tell patient to take carbenicillin on empty stomach 1 hour before or 2 hours after meals.
• Instruct patient to space doses evenly around the clock, if possible.
• Encourage patient to drink plenty of fluids unless he's on fluid restriction.
• Tell patient to notify prescriber immediately if a rash, itching, or difficulty breathing develops, especially if he hasn't taken a penicillin product before.

# carbidopa-levodopa

Apo-Levocarb (CAN), Atamet, Parcopa, Sinemet, Sinemet CR

## Class and Category
*Chemical:* Hydralazine analogue of levodopa (carbidopa), levorotatory isomer of dihydroxyphenylalanine (levodopa)
*Therapeutic:* Antidyskinetic
*Pregnancy category:* C

## Indications and Dosages
➤ *To relieve symptoms of Parkinson's disease*
**E.R. TABLETS**
**Adults not currently taking levodopa.** *Initial:* 1 tab of 25 mg carbidopa/100 mg levodopa b.i.d. or 1 tab of 50 mg carbidopa/200 mg levodopa b.i.d. with doses spaced at least 6 hr apart. Dose increased or decreased q 3 days or more, if needed, based on response.

*Maintenance:* 400 to 1,600 mg levodopa/day in divided doses q 4 to 8 hr. *Maximum:* 2,400 mg levodopa/day.

**Adults currently taking levodopa regardless of dose.** 1 tab of 25 mg carbidopa/100 mg levodopa b.i.d. or 1 tab of 50 mg carbidopa/ 200 mg levodopa b.i.d. at least 12 hr after levodopa is stopped. *Maximum:* 2,400 mg levodopa/day.

**Adults currently taking conventional carbidopa-levodopa.** If patient takes 300 to 400 mg of levodopa in combination product, regimen switched to 1 E.R. tab (200 mg levodopa) b.i.d. given 4 to 8 hr apart; if patient takes 500 to 600 mg of levodopa in combination product, regimen switched to 1 E.R. tab (300 mg levodopa) b.i.d. or t.i.d. given 4 to 8 hr apart; if patient takes 700 to 800 mg of levodopa in combination product, regimen switched to 4 E.R. tabs (800 mg levodopa)/ day divided into three doses and given 4 to 8 hr apart. *Maximum:* 2,400 mg levodopa/day.

TABLETS

**Adults not currently taking levodopa.** *Initial:* 1 tab of 25 mg carbidopa/100 mg levodopa t.i.d., or 1 tab of 10 mg carbidopa/100 mg levodopa t.i.d. or q.i.d. Increased by 1 tab q.d. or q.o.d., if needed, up to maximum. *Maximum:* 200 mg carbidopa/2,000 mg levodopa daily.

**Adults currently taking more than 1,500 mg of levodopa.** 1 tab of 25 mg carbidopa/ 250 mg levodopa t.i.d. or q.i.d. at least 12 hr after levodopa stops. *Maximum:* 200 mg carbidopa/2,000 mg levodopa daily.

**Adults currently taking less than 1,500 mg of levodopa.** 1 tab of 25 mg carbidopa/100 mg levodopa t.i.d. or q.i.d. or 1 tab of 10 mg carbidopa/100 mg levodopa t.i.d. or q.i.d. at least 12 hr after levodopa stops. *Maximum:* 200 mg carbidopa/2,000 mg levodopa daily.

ORALLY DISINTEGRATING TABLETS

**Adults.** *Initial:* 1 tab of 25 mg carbidopa/100 mg levodopa t.i.d., increased as needed by 1 tab q.d. or q.o.d. Or 1 tab of 10 mg carbidopa/ 100 mg levodopa t.i.d. or q.i.d., increased as needed by 1 tab q.d. or q.o.d. *Maximum:* 8 tabs of 25 mg carbidopa/100 mg levodopa or 10 mg carbidopa/100 mg levodopa daily.

## Contraindications

Concurrent MAO inhibitor therapy; history of melanoma; hypersensitivity to carbidopa, levodopa, or their components; narrow-angle glaucoma; suspicious undiagnosed skin lesions

## Mechanism of Action

Carbidopa inhibits peripheral distribution of levodopa, making more levodopa available to the brain. In extracerebral tissues, levodopa is converted to dopamine and moves to the CNS, where it replenishes dopamine, thus helping to improve muscle control and normalize body movements.

## Interactions

DRUGS

*antihypertensives:* Increased risk of symptomatic orthostatic hypotension
*benzodiazepines, droperidol, haloperidol, hydantoin anticonvulsants, loxapine, metoclopramide, metyrosine, molindone, papaverine, phenothiazines, rauwolfia alkaloids, thioxanthenes:* Decreased carbidopa-levodopa effects
*bromocriptine:* Additive carbidopa-levodopa effects
*iron salts:* Decreased absorption, blood level, and effectiveness of levodopa
*MAO inhibitors:* Increased risk of severe orthostatic hypotension
*methyldopa:* Altered antiparkinsonian effects of levodopa, additive toxic CNS effects
*pyridoxine:* Reversed levodopa effects
*tricyclic antidepressants:* Increased risk of adverse reactions to carbidopa-levodopa

FOODS

*high-protein food:* Possibly delayed or reduced drug absorption

## Adverse Reactions

**CNS:** Anxiety, confusion, depression, headache, insomnia, mood or mental changes, nervousness, neuroleptic malignant syndrome, nightmares, tiredness, uncontrolled movements, weakness
**CV:** Arrhythmias, orthostatic hypotension
**EENT:** Blurred vision, darkened saliva, dry mouth, eyelid spasm, ptosis
**GI:** Anorexia, constipation, diarrhea, nausea, vomiting
**GU:** Darkened urine, dysuria
**MS:** Muscle twitching
**SKIN:** Darkened sweat, flushing

## Nursing Considerations

• Use drug cautiously in patients with history of psychosis. Monitor all patients for depression and suicidal tendencies.
• Administer cautiously to patients with severe CV or pulmonary disease; bronchial

asthma; renal, hepatic, or endocrine disease; history of MI and residual atrial, nodal, or en- ventricular arrhythmias; or history of peptic ulcer. Monitor closely, especially when ther- apy begins and dosage is adjusted.

•**WARNING** Avoid giving carbidopa-levodopa within 2 weeks of an MAO inhibitor because sudden, extreme hypertension may occur.

•Assess patient for neuroleptic malignant syndrome if drug is stopped or dose reduced, especially if patient also takes a neuroleptic drug. Rare but life-threatening, the syndrome causes altered level of consciousness, auto- nomic dysfunction, diaphoresis, fever, altered blood pressure, involuntary movement, muscle rigidity, tachycardia, and tachypnea. If these changes occur, notify prescriber immediately.

**PATIENT TEACHING**

•If patient can't swallow E.R. tablet whole, tell him to break it in half for swallowing but not to crush or chew it.

•If patient takes orally disintegrating form, tell him to gently remove tab from bottle with dry hands, place it on top of his tongue, let it dissolve (which takes seconds), and swallow it with saliva. Explain that no other liquids are needed.

•Remind patient that it may take several weeks or months to feel full drug effects.

•Stress importance of taking carbidopa- levodopa regularly and in exact dose pre- scribed. Altering the dose or dosing interval may increase the risk of adverse reactions or decrease drug effectiveness.

•Tell patient to notify prescriber if involun- tary movements appear or worsen during therapy; dose may need to be adjusted.

•Inform patient being switched from regular to E.R. tablets that effect may be delayed for up to 1 hour after the first morning dose, compared with the effect usually obtained from the regular tablet. If this delay poses a problem, tell patient to notify prescriber.

# carbidopa, levodopa, and entacapone

Stalevo

## Class and Category

*Chemical:* Hydralazine analogue of levodopa (carbidopa), levorotatory isomer of dihy- droxyphenylalanine (levodopa), catechol-*O*- methyltransferase (COMT) inhibitor (enta- capone)

*Therapeutic:* Antidyskinetic
*Pregnancy category:* C

## Indications and Dosages

➤ *To treat idiopathic Parkinson's disease*

**TABLETS**

**Adults.** Highly individualized and used only as a substitute for patients already stabilized on equivalent doses of carbidopa-levodopa and entacapone. *Maintenance:* Highly indi- vidualized. When less levodopa is required, strength or frequency of dosage can be de- creased; when more levodopa is required, dosage frequency can be increased or next higher strength can be administered. *Maxi- mum:* One tablet of equivalent strength (12.5 mg carbidopa/50 mg levodopa/200 mg enta- capone; 25 mg carbidopa/100 mg levo- dopa/200 mg entacapone; or 37.5 mg car- bidopa/150 mg levodopa/200 mg entacapone) per dosing interval; 8 tablets/day.

## Contraindications

Angle-closure glaucoma; history of mela- noma; hypersensitivity to carbidopa, levo- dopa, entacapone, or their components; sus- picious, undiagnosed skin lesions; use within 14 days of an MAO inhibitor

---

### Mechanism of Action

Carbidopa inhibits peripheral distribution of levodopa, making more levodopa avail- able in the brain. Entacapone inhibits pe- ripheral COMT, the major metabolizing enzyme for levodopa. During levodopa metabolism, COMT produces a levodopa metabolite that reduces levodopa effec- tiveness. By inhibiting COMT, entacapone increases blood levels of levodopa, making more available for diffusion into the CNS. Levodopa is transported to the CNS, where it replenishes depleted dopamine, which is thought to cause Parkinson's dis- ease, thus helping to improve muscle con- trol and normalize body movements.

---

## Interactions

**DRUGS**

**Carbidopa, levodopa, and entacapone**
*alpha-methyldopa, apomorphine, bitolterol, dobutamine, dopamine, epinephrine, isoetharine, isoproterenol, norepinephrine, other COMT metabolizers:* Possibly increased

heart rate, arrhythmias, and extreme changes in blood pressure

*anti-hypertensives:* Possibly symptomatic orthostatic hypotension

*iron salts:* Possibly reduced bioavailability of carbidopa, levodopa, and entacapone

*MAO inhibitors:* Possibly inhibited catecholamine metabolism

*selegiline:* Possibly severe orthostatic hypotension

*tricyclic antidepressants:* Possibly hypertension and dyskinesia

**Levodopa component only**

*dopamine D₂-receptor antagonists (such as butyrophenones, isoniazid, phenothiazines, and risperidone):* Possible reduced effectiveness of levodopa

*metoclopramide:* Increased bioavailability but decreased effectiveness of levodopa

*papaverine, phenytoin:* Possible reversed effects of levodopa in Parkinson's disease

**Entacapone component only**

*ampicillin, cholestyramine, erythromycin, probenecid, rifampin:* Possible interference with biliary excretion of entacapone

**FOODS**

*high-protein food:* Possibly delayed or reduced drug absorption

## Adverse Reactions

**CNS:** Activation of latent Horner's syndrome, aggravation of Parkinson's disease symptoms, agitation, anxiety, asthenia, ataxia, bradykinetic episodes, confusion, decreased mental acuity, delusions, dementia, depression, disorientation, dizziness, dyskinesia, euphoria, fatigue, gait abnormalities, hallucinations, headache, hyperkinesia, hypokinesia, insomnia, malaise, memory loss, nervousness, neuroleptic malignant syndrome, nightmares, paranoia, paresthesia, peripheral neuropathy, sense of stimulation, somnolence, syncope, tremor increase, trismus

**CV:** Arrhythmias; chest pain; edema; hypotension, including orthostatic; hypertension; MI; palpitations; phlebitis

**EENT:** Blepharospasm, blurred vision, darkened saliva, dilated pupils, diplopia, dry mouth, excessive salivation, hoarseness, oculogyric crisis, taste disturbance, tongue burning

**ENDO:** Hyperglycemia

**GI:** Abdominal pain, elevated function test results, anorexia, bruxism, constipation, diarrhea, duodenal ulcer, dysphagia, flatulence, gastritis, GI bleeding, GI pain, hiccups, indigestion, nausea, vomiting

**GU:** Bacteria, blood, glucose, or protein in urine, darkened urine; elevated BUN and serum creatinine levels; elevated uric acid levels; elevated WBC count in urine; increased libido; urinary frequency, incontinence, or retention; UTI

**HEME:** Agranulocytosis, decreased hemoglobin and hematocrit, hemolytic and nonhemolytic anemia, leukopenia, positive Coombs' test, thrombocytopenia

**MS:** Back, leg, and shoulder pain; muscle cramps or twitching; rhabdomyolysis

**RESP:** Abnormal breathing patterns, dyspnea, upper respiratory tract infection

**SKIN:** Alopecia, bullous lesions, darkened sweat, diaphoresis, flushing, malignant melanoma, pruritus, purpura, rash, urticaria

**Other:** Angioedema, hot flashes, hypokalemia, weight gain or loss

## Nursing Considerations

• Use drug cautiously in patients with past or current psychosis because drug may cause depression and suicidal tendencies.

• Use cautiously in patients with severe CV or pulmonary disease; biliary obstruction; bronchial asthma; or renal, hepatic, or endocrine disease.

• If patient has chronic open-angle glaucoma, make sure intraocular pressure is well controlled because drug may lead to increased intraocular pressure.

• If patient has a history of MI with residual atrial, nodal, or ventricular arrhythmias, expect to make initial dosage adjustment in a facility with intensive cardiac care.

• Monitor patient closely for adverse CNS effects. Such adverse effects as dyskinesia may occur at lower dosages and more quickly with the use of carbidopa, levodopa, and entacapone tablets than when levodopa is used alone. If dyskinesia occurs, notify prescriber and expect to decrease dosage.

• Closely monitor patient with a history of peptic ulcer because drug may increase risk of GI hemorrhage.

• If drug must be stopped, taper it slowly to prevent high fever or severe rigidity.

• Assess for neuroleptic malignant syndrome during dosage reduction or drug discontinuation, especially in a patient who also receives a neuroleptic drug. This uncommon syndrome is life-threatening and causes altered level of consciousness, autonomic dysfunction, diaphoresis, fever, high or low blood pressure, involuntary movement, muscle rigidity, tachycardia, and tachypnea. If these occur, notify prescriber immediately.

**PATIENT TEACHING**
•To provide uniform drug effect, stress importance of taking carbidopa, levodopa, and entacapone at regular intervals according to the prescribed schedule.
•Advise patient to avoid a high-protein diet and iron salts (such as those found in many multi-vitamin tablets) because protein and iron may delay absorption of the levodopa component of drug and reduce the amount available for the body to use to control the symptoms of Parkinson's disease.
•Alert patient to the possibility of nausea, especially at the beginning of therapy. Tell him that this adverse reaction usually resolves with continued therapy.
•Tell patient to notify prescriber if he's taking any other medication, including OTC and herbal preparations, because of potential drug interactions.
•Inform patient that drug's effect may sometimes appear to wear off at the end of a dosing interval. If this occurs, instruct him to notify his prescriber to determine if a dosage adjustment is needed.
•Caution patient that hallucinations may occur and advise him to avoid potentially hazardous activities until drug's CNS effects are known.
•Advise patient to rise slowly after sitting or lying down to avoid a sudden drop in blood pressure.
•Instruct patient to notify prescriber if dyskinesia occurs.
•Tell patient that body fluids, such as saliva, urine and sweat, may turn a dark color, such as red, brown, or black. Reassure him that this effect is harmless but that fluids may stain clothing.
•Advise female patients of child-bearing age to notify prescriber immediately about known or suspected pregnancy because changes to drug therapy may be required.
•Inform patient with diabetes that drug may cause a false-positive result for urinary ketones when a test tape product is used to check for ketonuria and a false-negative result for urine glucose when a glucose-

oxidase method is used. Encourage patient to monitor blood glucose levels and seek medical attention if he suspects ketonuria.

# carisoprodol

Soma, Vanadom

## Class and Category
*Chemical:* Dicarbamate
*Therapeutic:* Skeletal muscle relaxant
*Pregnancy category:* Not rated

## Indications and Dosages
➤ *As adjunct to relieve acute musculo-skeletal pain and stiffness*
**TABLETS**
**Adults and children over age 12.** 350 mg t.i.d. and h.s.
**Children ages 5 to 12.** 6.25 mg/kg t.i.d. and h.s.

| Route | Onset | Peak | Duration |
|-------|-------|------|----------|
| P.O. | 30 min | Unknown | 4 to 6 hr |

### Mechanism of Action
Blocks interneuronal activity in the descending reticular formation and spinal cord, producing muscle relaxation and sedation.

## Contraindications
Hypersensitivity to carisoprodol or its components, intermittent porphyria

## Interactions
**DRUGS**
*CNS depressants, psychotropic drugs:* Additive CNS depression
**ACTIVITIES**
*alcohol use:* Additive CNS depression

## Adverse Reactions
**CNS:** Agitation, ataxia, depression, dizziness, drowsiness, fever, headache, insomnia, irritability, syncope, tremor, vertigo
**CV:** Orthostatic hypotension, tachycardia
**EENT:** Diplopia, transient vision loss
**GI:** Epigastric discomfort, hiccups, nausea, vomiting
**HEME:** Eosinophilia
**SKIN:** Erythema multiforme, facial flushing, pruritus, rash

## Nursing Considerations
• Use carisoprodol cautiously in patients with history of drug addiction.
• Closely monitor for hypersensitivity or idiosyncratic reactions, which usually occur before the fourth dose in patients who have had no previous contact with drug.
• Provide rest and other pain-relief measures.
• To avoid mild withdrawal symptoms, expect to taper therapy as prescribed, rather than stopping it abruptly.

**PATIENT TEACHING**
• Tell patient to take carisoprodol with meals if GI distress occurs.
• Warn patient about possible dizziness, drowsiness, syncope, and vertigo.
• Inform patient that abruptly stopping drug can cause headache, insomnia, nausea, and other adverse reactions.
• Instruct patient to avoid alcohol and other CNS depressants while taking drug.
• Inform patient that saliva, urine, and sweat may appear darker (red, brown, or black). Reassure him that this discoloration is harmless but may stain garments.
• Tell patient to store drug in a tightly capped container at room temperature.
• Tell patient not to store drug in the bathroom, near the kitchen sink, or in other damp places to avoid heat and moisture.

# carteolol hydrochloride

Cartrol

## Class and Category
*Chemical:* Beta-adrenergic blocker
*Therapeutic:* Antihypertensive
*Pregnancy category:* C

## Indications and Dosages
➤ *To control hypertension*

**TABLETS**
**Adults.** *Initial:* 2.5 mg q.d. If response is inadequate, dosage increased to 5 mg and then 10 mg q.d., p.r.n. *Maintenance:* 2.5 or 5 mg q.d.

**DOSAGE ADJUSTMENT** Dosage interval increased to q 48 hr for patients with creatinine clearance of 20 to 60 ml/min/1.73 $m^2$ or to q 72 hr for patients with creatinine clearance below 20 ml/min/1.73 $m^2$.

| Route | Onset | Peak | Duration |
|-------|-------|------|----------|
| P.O. | Unknown | 1 to 3 hr | Unknown |

## Mechanism of Action
May reduce blood pressure by competing with beta-adrenergic receptor agonists, which helps reduce cardiac output, decrease sympathetic outflow to peripheral blood vessels, and inhibit renin.

## Contraindications
Asthma, bradycardia (less than 45 beats/min), cardiogenic shock, hypersensitivity to carteolol or its components, second- or third-degree heart block

## Interactions
**DRUGS**
*allergen immunotherapy, allergenic extracts for skin testing:* Increased risk of serious systemic reaction or anaphylaxis
*catecholamine-depleting drugs, such as reserpine:* Additive effects, increased risk of hypotension and bradycardia
*clonidine:* Increased risk of tachycardia and hypertension after clonidine discontinuation
*diltiazem, nifedipine, verapamil:* Potentiated effects of carteolol
*general anesthetics:* Exaggeration of hypotension
*NSAIDs:* Reduced antihypertensive effect of carteolol
*oral antidiabetic drugs:* Reduced symptomatic responses to hypoglycemia
*sympathomimetics with alpha- and beta-adrenergic effects, such as pseudoephedrine:* Possibly hypertension and excessive bradycardia or heart block

## Adverse Reactions
**CNS:** Fatigue, insomnia, lassitude, paresthesia, tiredness, weakness
**CV:** Chest pain, heart failure, peripheral edema
**EENT:** Dry mouth, nasal congestion, pharyngitis
**GI:** Abdominal pain, diarrhea, flatulence, nausea
**MS:** Arthralgia, back pain, leg pain, muscle spasms
**SKIN:** Rash

## Nursing Considerations
• **WARNING** Be aware that abrupt cessation of carteolol in patients with angina may cause angina exacerbation or MI; abrupt cessation in patients with hyperthyroidism may cause thyroid storm.

• Carefully monitor blood glucose level in diabetic patient because carteolol can mask hypoglycemic symptoms. It also can interfere with endogenous insulin release in response to hyperglycemia, requiring dosage adjustment of oral antidiabetic drug.

### PATIENT TEACHING
• Advise patient to follow dosing schedule even if he feels better and not to discontinue therapy abruptly.
• Instruct patient to report signs of heart failure, such as fatigue, difficulty breathing, cough, and unusually fast heartbeat.
• Tell diabetic patient to frequently monitor his blood glucose level.
• Advise patient to consult prescriber before taking OTC preparations, such as nasal decongestants and cold preparations that contain sympathomimetics, because of the risk of serious drug interactions.

# carvedilol

Coreg

## Class and Category
*Chemical:* Nonselective beta-adrenergic blocker with alpha$_1$-adrenergic blocking activity
*Therapeutic:* Antihypertensive, heart failure treatment adjunct
*Pregnancy category:* C

## Indications and Dosages
➤ *To control hypertension*
### TABLETS
**Adults.** 6.25 mg b.i.d. for 7 to 14 days, if tolerated. Then dosage increased to 12.5 mg b.i.d. for 7 to 14 days, and up to 25 mg, if tolerated and needed. *Maximum:* 50 mg/day.
➤ *As adjunct to treat mild to severe heart failure of ischemic or cardiomyopathic origin*
### TABLETS
**Adults.** 3.125 mg b.i.d. for 2 wk, then increased to 6.25, 12.5, and 25 mg b.i.d. at successive 2-wk intervals, as tolerated. *Maximum (for patients with mild to moderate heart failure):* 50 mg b.i.d. if patient weighs more than 85 kg (187 lb).
➤ *To reduce CV mortality after acute phase of MI in patients with left ventricular ejection fraction of 40% or less*

### TABLETS
**Adults.** 6.25 mg b.i.d. for 3 to 10 days, if tolerated. Then dosage increased to 12.5 mg b.i.d. for 3 to 10 days and up to 25 mg b.i.d., if needed and tolerated.
DOSAGE ADJUSTMENT For patient with fluid retention or low blood pressure or heart rate, starting dosage may be decreased to 3.125 mg b.i.d., increase may be slowed, or both.

| Route | Onset | Peak | Duration |
|-------|-------|------|----------|
| P.O. | In 30 min | 1.5 to 7 hr | Unknown |

### Mechanism of Action
Reduces cardiac output and tachycardia, causes vasodilation, and decreases peripheral vascular resistance, which reduces blood pressure and cardiac workload. When administered for at least 4 weeks, carvedilol reduces plasma renin activity.

## Contraindications
Asthma or related bronchospastic conditions; cardiogenic shock; decompensated heart failure that requires I.V. inotropics; hypersensitivity to car-vedilol or its components; and second- or third-degree AV block, severe bradycardia, or sick sinus syndrome unless pacemaker is in place

## Interactions
### DRUGS
*calcium channel blockers (especially diltiazem and verapamil):* Abnormal cardiac conduction and, possibly, increased adverse effects of calcium channel blockers
*catecholamine-depleting drugs (such as reserpine and MAO inhibitors):* Additive effects, increased risk of hypotension and bradycardia
*cimetidine:* Increased blood carvedilol level
*clonidine:* Risk of tachycardia and hypertension when clonidine is discontinued
*cyclosporine, digoxin:* Increased blood levels of these drugs
*digoxin:* Possibly increased blood digoxin level
*oral antidiabetic drugs:* Increased risk of hypoglycemia
*rifampin:* Decreased blood carvedilol level

## Adverse Reactions
**CNS:** Asthenia, CVA, depression, dizziness, fatigue, fever, headache, hypesthesia, hypotonia, insomnia, light-headedness, malaise, paresthesia, somnolence, syncope, vertigo

**CV:** Angina, AV block, bradycardia, edema, heart failure, hypertension, hypertriglyceridemia, orthostatic hypotension, palpitations, peripheral vascular disorder
**EENT:** Blurred vision, dry eyes, periodontitis, pharyngitis, rhinitis
**ENDO:** Hyperglycemia, hypoglycemia
**GI:** Abdominal pain, diarrhea, elevated liver function test results, melena, nausea, vomiting
**GU:** Albuminuria, hematuria, elevated BUN and creatinine levels, impotence, renal insufficiency, UTI
**HEME:** Aplastic anemia, decreased PT, thrombocytopenia, unusual bleeding or bruising
**MS:** Arthralgia, arthritis, back pain, muscle cramps
**RESP:** Dyspnea, increased cough
**SKIN:** Jaundice, pruritus, purpura
**Other:** Anaphylaxis, fluid overload, gout, hyperkalemia, hyperuricemia, hyponatremia, hypovolemia, viral infection, weight gain or loss

## Nursing Considerations

• Use carvedilol cautiously in patients with peripheral vascular disease because it may aggravate symptoms of arterial insufficiency; in patients with diabetes mellitus it may mask signs of hypoglycemia, such as tachycardia, and may delay recovery.
• **WARNING** Avoid stopping drug abruptly in patients with hyperthyroidism because thyroid storm may occur and in patients with angina because it may worsen or MI may occur.

• If patient has heart failure, expect to also give digoxin, a diuretic, and an ACE inhibitor.
**PATIENT TEACHING**
• Warn patient that drug may cause orthostatic hypotension, light-headedness, and dizziness; advise him to take safety precautions.
• Tell patient with heart failure to notify prescriber if he gains 5 lb or more in 2 days or if shortness of breath increases. These changes may signal worsening heart failure.

# caspofungin acetate

Cancidas

## Class and Category

*Chemical:* Echinocandins
*Therapeutic:* Antifungal
*Pregnancy category:* C

## Indications and Dosages

➤ *To treat invasive aspergillosis in patients refractory to or intolerant of other therapies; to treat candidemia and candidal infections in intra-abdominal abscesses, peritonitis, and pleural space infections*
**I.V. INFUSION**
**Adults.** *Initial:* 70 mg on day 1, followed by 50 mg q.d. *Maximum:* 70 mg/day.
➤ *To treat presumed fungal infections in febrile, neutropenic patients*
**I.V. INFUSION**
**Adults.** *Initial:* 70 mg on day 1, followed by 50 mg q.d. for at least 14 days, including at

## Mechanism of Action

Caspofungin acetate interferes with fungal cell membrane synthesis by inhibiting the synthesis of $\beta$ (1,3)-D-glucan. A polypeptide, $\beta$ (1,3)-D-glucan is the essential component of the fungal cell membrane that makes it rigid and protective. Without it, fungal cells rupture and die. This mechanism of action is most effective against susceptible filamentous fungi, such as *Aspergillus*.

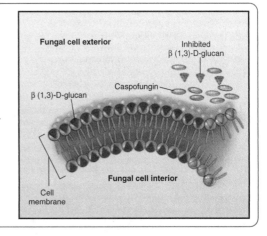

Fungal cell exterior

Inhibited
$\beta$ (1,3)-D-glucan

$\beta$ (1,3)-D-glucan

Caspofungin

Fungal cell interior

Cell membrane

least 7 days after neutropenia and symptoms have resolved. Increased to 70 mg/day as needed. *Maximum:* 70 mg/day.

**DOSAGE ADJUSTMENT** Dosage reduced to 35 mg q.d. after initial 70-mg loading dose in moderate hepatic insufficiency.

➤ *To treat esophageal candidiasis*

**I.V. INFUSION**

**Adults.** 50 mg q.d.

**DOSAGE ADJUSTMENT** Dosage reduced to 35 mg q.d. in moderate hepatic insufficiency.

## Incompatibilities

Don't mix or infuse with other drugs. Don't admix with diluents that contain dextrose.

## Contraindications

Hypersensitivity to caspofungin acetate or its components

## Interactions

**DRUGS**

*carbamazepine, dexamethasone, efavirenz, nelfinavir, nevirapine, phenytoin, rifampin:* Possibly decreased blood caspofungin level

*cyclosporine:* Transient increases in ALT and AST levels

*tacrolimus:* Possibly decreased blood tacrolimus level

## Adverse Reactions

**CNS:** Chills, dizziness, fever, headache, insomnia, paresthesia, tremor

**CV:** Edema, hypertension, hypotension, phlebitis, tachycardia, thrombophlebitis

**GI:** Abdominal pain, diarrhea, elevated liver function test results, hepatic dysfunction, jaundice, nausea, vomiting

**GU:** Elevated BUN or serum creatinine level, proteinuria, renal insufficiency

**HEME:** Decreased hemoglobin and hematocrit

**MS:** Back pain, myalgia

**RESP:** Bronchospasm, dyspnea, stridor, tachypnea

**SKIN:** Diaphoresis, erythema, flushing, pruritus, rash, sensation of warmth

**Other:** Decreased serum bicarbonate level, facial edema, hypercalcemia, hyperkalemia, hyperphosphatemia, hypokalemia, hypomagnesemia, infusion site reaction

## Nursing Considerations

•To prepare 70-mg loading dose, let vial reach room temperature. Reconstitute by adding 10.5 ml of NS to vial. Dilute for administration by transferring 10 ml of reconstituted drug to 250 ml of NS.

•To prepare 70-mg loading dose from two 50-mg vials, add 10.5 ml of NS to each vial; then transfer 14 ml of prepared solution to 250 ml of NS.

•To prepare daily 50-mg infusion, let vial reach room temperature. Reconstitute by adding 10.5 ml of NS to vial. Dilute for administration by transferring only 10 ml of reconstituted drug to 250 ml of NS.

•To prepare daily 50-mg infusion at reduced volume, add 10 ml of reconstituted drug to 100 ml of NS.

•To prepare 35-mg daily dose for patient with moderate hepatic insufficiency, reconstitute 50-mg vial with 10.5 ml of NS. To dilute, transfer only 7 ml of reconstituted drug to 250 ml of NS or, if needed, to 100 ml of NS.

•When preparing powder for reconstitution, mix gently to obtain a clear solution. Don't use if solution is cloudy or contains precipitate. Discard unused solution after 24 hours.

•Infuse drug slowly over approximately 1 hour.

•Expect to increase daily dose to 70 mg, as prescribed, for patients not responding to carbamazepine, dexamethasone, efavirenz, nelfinavir, nevirapine, phenytoin, or rifampin.

•Watch for flushed skin, and assess patient often for unexplained temperature elevation.

•Assess for airway patency if patient develops excessive facial edema or respiratory stridor. Provide emergency airway management if complete obstruction occurs.

•Monitor patient's liver function test results, as ordered, and report abnormalities.

**PATIENT TEACHING**

•Urge patient to notify prescriber immediately if he has difficulty talking, swallowing, or breathing during drug administration.

# cefaclor

Apo-Cefaclor (CAN), Ceclor, Ceclor CD, Raniclor

## Class and Category

*Chemical:* Second-generation cephalosporin, 7-aminocephalosporanic acid

*Therapeutic:* Antibiotic

*Pregnancy category:* B

## Indications and Dosages

➤ *To treat otitis media caused by* Haemophilus influenzae, *staphylococci,* Streptococcus pneumoniae, *and* Streptococcus pyogenes; *lower respiratory tract infections, including pneumonia caused by* H. influenzae, S. pneumoniae, *and* S. pyogenes; *pharyngitis and tonsillitis caused by* S. pyogenes; *UTIs, including cystitis and pyelonephritis, caused by* Escherichia coli, Klebsiella *sp.,* Proteus mirabilis, *and coagulase-negative staphylococci; and skin and soft-tissue infections caused by* S. pyogenes *and* Staphylococcus aureus

**CAPSULES**

**Adults and adolescents.** 250 mg q 8 hr. For severe infections, such as pneumonia, or those caused by less susceptible organisms, 500 mg q 8 hr. *Maximum:* 4 g/day.

**CHEWABLE TABLETS, ORAL SUSPENSION**

**Adults and adolescents.** 250 mg q 8 hr. For severe infections, such as pneumonia, or those caused by less susceptible organisms, 500 mg q 8 hr. *Maximum:* 4 g/day.

**Children.** 20 mg/kg/day in divided doses q 8 hr. For serious infections, such as otitis media, and infections caused by less susceptible organisms, 40 mg/kg/day in divided doses q 8 hr. For otitis media and pharyngitis, total daily dosage divided and given q 12 hr, if needed. *Maximum:* 1 g/day.

➤ *To treat acute bacterial infection in chronic bronchitis or secondary bacterial infection in acute bronchitis (not caused by* H. influenzae*)*

**E.R. TABLETS**

**Adults and adolescents age 16 and older.** 500 mg q 12 hr for 7 days.

➤ *To treat pharyngitis and tonsillitis (not caused by* H. influenzae*)*

**E.R. TABLETS**

**Adults and adolescents age 16 and older.** 375 mg q 12 hr for 10 days.

➤ *To treat uncomplicated skin and soft-tissue infections caused by* S. aureus

**E.R. TABLETS**

**Adults and adolescents age 16 and older.** 375 mg q 12 hr for 7 to 10 days.

---

## Mechanism of Action

Interferes with bacterial cell wall synthesis by inhibiting cross-linking of peptidoglycan strands, which stiffen cell membranes. As a result, bacterial cells rupture.

---

## Contraindications

Hypersensitivity to cephalosporins or their components

## Interactions

**DRUGS**

*aminoglycosides, loop diuretics:* Increased risk of nephrotoxicity

*antacids:* Decreased blood cefaclor level (E.R. tablets)

*oral anticoagulants:* Increased anticoagulation

## Adverse Reactions

**CNS:** Chills, fever, headache, seizures

**CV:** Edema

**EENT:** Hearing loss

**GI:** Abdominal cramps, diarrhea, elevated liver function test results, hepatic failure, hepatomegaly, nausea, oral candidiasis, pseudomembranous colitis, vomiting

**GU:** Elevated BUN level, nephrotoxicity, renal failure, vaginal candidiasis

**HEME:** Eosinophilia, hemolytic anemia, hypoprothrombinemia, neutropenia, thrombocytopenia, unusual bleeding

**MS:** Arthralgia

**RESP:** Dyspnea

**SKIN:** Ecchymosis, erythema, erythema multiforme, pruritus, rash, Stevens-Johnson syndrome

**Other:** Anaphylaxis, superinfection

## Nursing Considerations

• Use cefaclor cautiously in patients with impaired renal function or a history of GI disease, particularly colitis. Also use cautiously in patients hypersensitive to penicillin; about 10% of such patients have cross-sensitivity.

• If possible, obtain culture and sensitivity test results, as ordered, before giving drug.

• Monitor BUN and serum creatinine levels for early signs of nephrotoxicity. Also monitor fluid intake and output; decreasing urine output may indicate nephrotoxicity.

• Be aware that an allergic reaction may occur a few days after therapy starts.

• Assess bowel pattern daily; severe diarrhea may indicate pseudomembranous colitis.

• Assess for superinfection: perineal itching, fever, malaise, redness, pain, swelling, rash, drainage, diarrhea, cough, sputum changes.

**PATIENT TEACHING**

• Instruct patient to complete the prescribed course of therapy, even if he feels better.

• Tell patient to swallow E.R. tablets whole and not to crush, break, or chew them.

- Advise patient to take E.R. tablets with food to enhance absorption.
- Instruct patient to take capsules or E.R. tablets with a full glass of water.
- Tell patient to shake oral suspension well before measuring and to use a liquid-measuring device to ensure accurate dose.
- Instruct patient to refrigerate oral suspension and to discard unused portion after 14 days.
- Tell patient to immediately report severe diarrhea to prescriber.
- Explain that yogurt and buttermilk protect intestinal flora and decrease diarrhea.
- Tell patient to report signs of superinfection.

# cefadroxil

Duricef

## Class and Category

*Chemical:* First-generation cephalosporin, 7-aminocephalosporanic acid
*Therapeutic:* Antibiotic
*Pregnancy category:* B

## Indications and Dosages

➤ *To treat UTIs caused by* Escherichia coli, Klebsiella *sp., and* Proteus mirabilis

CAPSULES, TABLETS

**Adults.** For uncomplicated lower UTIs, 1 to 2 g q.d. or in divided doses q 12 hr. For all other UTIs, 2 g q 12 hr.

ORAL SUSPENSION

**Adults.** For uncomplicated lower UTIs, 1 to 2 g q.d. or in divided doses q 12 hr. For all other UTIs, 2 g q 12 hr.

**Children.** 30 mg/kg/day in divided doses q 12 hr. *Maximum:* Adult dosage.

➤ *To treat skin and soft-tissue infections caused by staphylococci or streptococci*

CAPSULES, TABLETS

**Adults.** 1 g q.d. or 500 mg q 12 hr.

ORAL SUSPENSION

**Adults.** 1 g q.d. or 500 mg q 12 hr.

**Children.** 30 mg/kg/day in divided doses q 12 hr. *Maximum:* Adult dosage.

➤ *To treat pharyngitis and tonsillitis caused by group A beta-hemolytic streptococci*

CAPSULES, TABLETS

**Adults.** 1 g q.d. or 500 mg b.i.d for 10 days.

ORAL SUSPENSION

**Adults.** 1 g q.d. or 500 mg b.i.d. for 10 days.

**Children.** 30 mg/kg/day in divided doses q 12 hr for 10 days. *Maximum:* 1 g q.d. or 500 mg b.i.d. for 10 days.

DOSAGE ADJUSTMENT Initial dose of 1 g followed by maintenance dosage of 0.5 g q 12 hr for patients with creatinine clearance of 25 to 50 ml/min/1.73 m$^2$; 0.5 g q 24 hr for patients with creatinine clearance of 10 to 25 ml/min/1.73 m$^2$; and 0.5 g q 36 hr for those with creatinine clearance of 0 to 10 ml/min/1.73 m$^2$.

### Mechanism of Action

Interferes with bacterial cell wall synthesis by inhibiting the final step in the cross-linking of peptidoglycan strands. Peptidoglycan makes cell membranes rigid and protective. Without it, bacterial cells rupture and die.

## Contraindications

Hypersensitivity to cephalosporins or their components

## Interactions

DRUGS

*aminoglycosides, loop diuretics:* Increased toxicity of these drugs

## Adverse Reactions

**CNS:** Chills, fever, headache, seizures
**CV:** Edema
**EENT:** Hearing loss
**GI:** Abdominal cramps, diarrhea, elevated liver function test results, hepatic failure, hepatomegaly, nausea, oral candidiasis, pseudomembranous colitis, vomiting
**GU:** Elevated BUN level, nephrotoxicity, renal failure, vaginal candidiasis
**HEME:** Eosinophilia, hemolytic anemia, hypoprothrombinemia, neutropenia, thrombocytopenia, unusual bleeding
**MS:** Arthralgia
**RESP:** Dyspnea
**SKIN:** Ecchymosis, erythema, erythema multiforme, pruritus, rash, Stevens-Johnson syndrome
**Other:** Anaphylaxis, superinfection

## Nursing Considerations

- Use cefadroxil cautiously in patients with impaired renal function or a history of GI disease, particularly colitis. Also use drug cautiously in patients who are hypersensitive to penicillin because cross-sensitivity has occurred in about 10% of such patients.
- If possible, obtain culture and sensitivity test results, as ordered, before giving drug.

• Be aware that an allergic reaction may occur a few days after therapy starts.
• Monitor BUN and serum creatinine levels for early signs of nephrotoxicity. Also monitor fluid intake and output; decreasing urine output may indicate nephrotoxicity.
• Assess bowel pattern daily; severe diarrhea may indicate pseudomembranous colitis.
• Assess for signs of superinfection, such as perineal itching, fever, malaise, redness, pain, swelling, drainage, rash, diarrhea, and cough or sputum changes.

**PATIENT TEACHING**
• Instruct patient to complete the prescribed course of therapy.
• Tell patient to shake oral suspension well before measuring and to use a liquid-measuring device to ensure accurate dosage.
• Instruct patient to refrigerate oral suspension and to discard unused portion after 14 days.
• Urge patient to immediately report severe diarrhea to prescriber.
• Inform patient that yogurt and buttermilk can help maintain intestinal flora and decrease diarrhea.
• Teach patient to recognize and report signs of superinfection, such as furry tongue, perineal itching, and loose, foul-smelling stools.

# cefazolin sodium

Ancef

## Class and Category
*Chemical:* First-generation cephalosporin, 7-aminocephalosporanic acid
*Therapeutic:* Antibiotic
*Pregnancy category:* B

## Indications and Dosages
➤ *To treat respiratory tract infections caused by group A beta-hemolytic streptococci,* Haemophilus influenzae, *Klebsiella sp.,* Staphylococcus aureus, *and* Streptococcus pneumoniae; *skin and soft-tissue infections caused by* S. aureus, *group A beta-hemolytic and other strains of streptococci; biliary tract infections caused by* Escherichia coli, Klebsiella sp., *Proteus mirabilis,* S. aureus, *and various strains of streptococci; bone and joint infections caused by* S. aureus; *genital infections, such as epididymitis and prosta-*

*titis, caused by* E. coli, Klebsiella sp., P. mirabilis, *and some strains of enterococci; septicemia caused by* E. coli, Klebsiella sp., P. mirabilis, S. aureus, *and* S. pneumoniae; *and endocarditis caused by group A beta-hemolytic streptococci and* S. aureus

**I.V. INFUSION, I.V. OR I.M. INJECTION**
**Adults.** For mild infections, 250 to 500 mg q 8 hr; for moderate to severe infections, 500 to 1,000 mg q 6 to 8 hr; and for severe life-threatening infections, 1,000 to 1,500 mg q 6 hr. *Maximum:* 6 g/day.
**Children**: For mild to moderate infections, 25 to 50 mg/kg/day divided equally and given t.i.d. or q.i.d.; for severe infections, 100 mg/kg/day divided equally and given t.i.d. or q.i.d.
➤ *To treat pneumococcal pneumonia*
**I.V. INFUSION, I.V. OR I.M. INJECTION**
**Adults.** 500 mg q 12 hr.
➤ *To treat acute uncomplicated UTIs caused by* E. coli, Klebsiella sp., *P. mirabilis, and some strains of* Enterobacter *and* Enterococcus
**I.V. INFUSION, I.V. OR I.M. INJECTION**
**Adults.** 1 g q 12 hr.
➤ *To provide surgical prophylaxis*
**I.V. INFUSION, I.V. OR I.M. INJECTION**
**Adults.** 1 g 30 to 60 min before surgery; 0.5 to 1 g during surgery if it lasts 2 hr or longer; 0.5 to 1 g q 6 to 8 hr for 24 hr after surgery.
**DOSAGE ADJUSTMENT** After initial loading dose appropriate to infection's severity, dosage interval restricted to at least 8 hr for adults with creatinine clearance of 35 to 54 ml/min/1.73 m$^2$; dosage reduced by 50% and given q 12 hr for adults with creatinine clearance of 11 to 34 ml/min/1.73 m$^2$; and dosage reduced by 50% and given q 18 to 24 hr for adults with creatinine clearance of 10 ml/min/1.73 m$^2$ or less. Dosage reduced to 60% and given q 12 hr for children with creatinine clearance of 40 to 70 ml/min/1.73 m$^2$; dosage reduced to 25% and given q 12 hr for children with creatinine clearance of 20 to 40 ml/min/1.73 m$^2$; and dosage reduced to 10% and given q 24 hr for children with creatinine clearance of 5 to 20 ml/min/1.73 m$^2$.

## Incompatibilities
To prevent mutual inactivation, don't mix cefazolin with aminoglycosides. Also avoid mixing cefazolin with other drugs, including pentamidine isethionate.

## Contraindications

Hypersensitivity to cephalosporins or their components

---

### Mechanism of Action

Interferes with bacterial cell wall synthesis by inhibiting the final step in the cross-linking of peptidoglycan strands. Peptidoglycan makes cell membranes rigid and protective. Without it, bacterial cells rupture and die.

---

## Interactions

**DRUGS**

*aminoglycosides, loop diuretics:* Additive nephrotoxicity

*probenecid:* Increased and prolonged blood cefazolin level

## Adverse Reactions

**CNS:** Chills, fever, headache, seizures
**CV:** Edema
**EENT:** Hearing loss
**GI:** Abdominal cramps, diarrhea, elevated liver function test results, hepatic failure, hepatitis, hepatomegaly, nausea, oral candidiasis, pseudomembranous colitis, vomiting
**GU:** Elevated BUN and serum creatinine levels, nephrotoxicity, renal failure, vaginal candidiasis
**HEME:** Eosinophilia, hemolytic anemia, hypoprothrombinemia, neutropenia, thrombocytopenia, unusual bleeding
**MS:** Arthralgia
**RESP:** Dyspnea
**SKIN:** Ecchymosis, erythema, erythema multiforme, pruritus, rash, Stevens-Johnson syndrome
**Other:** Anaphylaxis; injection site pain, redness, and swelling; superinfection

## Nursing Considerations

• Use cefazolin cautiously in patients with impaired renal function or a history of GI disease, particularly colitis. Also use drug cautiously in patients who are hypersensitive to penicillin because cross-sensitivity has occurred in 10% of such patients.
• If possible, obtain culture and sensitivity test results, as ordered, before giving drug.
• **WARNING** To prevent unintentional overdose, cefazolin for injection USP and dextrose injection USP shouldn't be used in children who require less than the full adult dose.

• Reconstitute 500-mg vial of drug with 2 ml of sterile water for injection (or 1-g vial with 2.5 ml). Shake well until dissolved.
• For direct I.V. injection, further dilute reconstituted solution with at least 5 ml of sterile water for injection. Inject slowly over 3 to 5 minutes through tubing of a flowing compatible I.V. solution.
• For intermittent I.V. infusion, reconstitute 500 to 1,000 mg in 50 to 100 ml of NS, $D_5W$, $D_{10}W$, $D_5LR$, $D_50.2NS$, $D_50.45NS$, $D_5NS$, LR injection, 5% or 10% invert sugar in sterile water for injection, 5% sodium bicarbonate (Ancef), or Ringer's injection.
• Administer I.M injection deep into large muscle mass, such as the gluteus maximus.
• Store reconstituted cefazolin up to 24 hours at room temperature or 10 days under refrigeration.
• Monitor I.V. site for irritation, phlebitis, and extravasation.
• Monitor BUN and serum creatinine levels for early signs of nephrotoxicity. Also monitor fluid intake and output; decreasing urine output may indicate nephrotoxicity.
• Be aware that an allergic reaction may occur a few days after therapy starts.
• Assess bowel pattern daily; severe diarrhea may indicate pseudomembranous colitis.
• Watch for evidence of superinfection: cough, diarrhea, drainage, fever, malaise, pain, perineal itching, rash, redness, swelling.
• Assess for pharyngitis, ecchymosis, bleeding, and arthralgia; they may indicate a blood dyscrasia.

**PATIENT TEACHING**

• Instruct patient to complete the prescribed course of therapy.
• Reassure patient that I.M. injection doesn't typically cause pain.
• Tell patient to immediately report severe diarrhea to prescriber.

# cefdinir

Omnicef

## Class and Category

*Chemical:* Cephalosporin
*Therapeutic:* Antibiotic
*Pregnancy category:* B

## Indications and Dosages

➤ *To treat community-acquired pneumonia caused by* Haemophilus influenzae *(including beta-lactamase–producing strains),* Haemophilus parainfluenzae *(including beta-lactamase–producing strains),* Streptococcus pneumoniae *(penicillin-susceptible strains only), and* Moraxella catarrhalis *(including beta-lactamase–producing strains)*

**CAPSULES**

**Adults and adolescents.** 300 mg q 12 hr for 10 days. *Maximum:* 600 mg/day.

➤ *To treat pharyngitis or tonsillitis caused by* Streptococcus pyogenes *and acute exacerbations of chronic bronchitis caused by* H. influenzae *(including beta-lactamase–producing strains),* H. parainfluenzae *(including beta-lactamase–producing strains),* S. pneumoniae *(penicillin-susceptible strains only), and* M. catarrhalis *(including beta-lactamase–producing strains)*

**CAPSULES**

**Adults and adolescents.** 300 mg q 12 hr for 5 to 10 days or 600 mg q 24 hr for 10 days. *Maximum:* 600 mg/day.

**ORAL SUSPENSION**

**Children ages 6 months to 12 years.** 7 mg/kg q 12 hr for 5 to 10 days or 14 mg/kg q 24 hr for 10 days (for pharyngitis or tonsillitis).

➤ *To treat acute maxillary sinusitis caused by* H. influenzae *(including beta-lactamase–producing strains),* S. pneumoniae *(penicillin-susceptible strains only), and* M. catarrhalis *(including beta-lactamase–producing strains)*

**CAPSULES**

**Adults and adolescents.** 300 mg q 12 hr or 600 mg q 24 hr for 10 days. *Maximum:* 600 mg/day.

**ORAL SUSPENSION**

**Children ages 6 months to 12 years.** 7 mg/kg q 12 hr or 14 mg/kg q 24 hr for 10 days.

➤ *To treat uncomplicated skin and soft-tissue infections caused by* Staphylococcus aureus *(including beta-lactamase–producing strains) and* Streptococcus pyogenes

**CAPSULES**

**Adults and adolescents.** 300 mg q 12 hr for 10 days. *Maximum:* 600 mg/day.

**ORAL SUSPENSION**

**Children ages 6 months to 12 years.** 7 mg/kg q 12 hr for 10 days.

➤ *To treat acute bacterial otitis media caused by* H. influenzae *(including beta-lactamase–producing strains),* S. pneumoniae *(penicillin-susceptible strains only), and* M. catarrhalis *(including beta-lactamase–producing strains)*

**ORAL SUSPENSION**

**Children ages 6 months to 12 years.** 7 mg/kg q 12 hr for 5 to 10 days or 14 mg/kg q 24 hr for 10 days.

**DOSAGE ADJUSTMENT** For adults with creatinine clearance of less than 30 ml/min/1.73 m$^2$, expect to reduce dosage to 300 mg q.d.; for children with creatinine clearance of less than 30 ml/min/1.73 m$^2$, dosage is 7 mg/kg (up to 300 mg) q.d. For patients undergoing intermittent hemodialysis, dosage is 300 mg or 7 mg/kg q.o.d., beginning at the end of each hemodialysis session, as prescribed.

## Mechanism of Action

Interferes with bacterial cell wall synthesis by inhibiting the final step in the cross-linking of peptidoglycan strands. Peptidoglycan makes cell membranes rigid and protective. Without it, bacterial cells rupture and die. Because cefdinir is not degraded by some bacterial beta-lactamase enzymes, it's effective against many organisms that are resistant to both penicillins and some cephalosporins.

## Contraindications

Hypersensitivity to cefdinir, other cephalosporins, or their components

## Interactions

**DRUGS**

*antacids that contain aluminum or magnesium:* Decreased cefdinir absorption if given within 2 hours of antacid
*iron salts:* Reduced cefdinir absorption if given within 2 hours of iron
*probenecid:* Increased blood level and prolonged half-life of cefdinir

## Adverse Reactions

**CNS:** Asthenia, dizziness, drowsiness, headache, insomnia, somnolence
**EENT:** Dry mouth, pharyngitis, rhinitis
**GI:** Abdominal pain, anorexia, constipation, diarrhea, flatulence, indigestion, nausea,

pseudomembranous colitis, stool discoloration, vomiting
**GU:** Leukorrhea, vaginal candidiasis, vaginitis
**HEME:** Leukopenia
**SKIN:** Pruritus, rash
**Other:** Serum sickness–like reaction

## Nursing Considerations

• To reconstitute powder for oral suspension, tap bottle to loosen powder. Dilute with water to 125 mg/5 ml. Shake well before each use. Discard any unused portion after 10 days. Keep suspension bottle tightly closed and store it at room temperature.
• Administer antacids that contain aluminum or magnesium and iron salts at least 2 hours before or after cefdinir because they may interfere with cefdinir absorption.
• Monitor patient who is allergic to penicillin for signs and symptoms of a hypersensitivity reaction, ranging from a mild rash to fatal anaphylaxis, because cross-sensitivity can occur.
• Monitor patient with a chronic GI condition, such as colitis, for signs and symptoms of a drug-related exacerbation.
• Because all cephalosporins have the potential to cause bleeding, monitor elderly patients and patients with a preexisting coagulopathy, including vitamin K deficiency, for elevated PT or APTT.
• Assess bowel pattern daily; severe diarrhea may indicate pseudomembranous colitis. Notify prescriber immediately if you detect signs or symptoms of this adverse reaction.
• Assess for other evidence of superinfection, including perineal itching; loose, foul-smelling stools; and vaginal drainage.

### PATIENT TEACHING

• Advise patient taking cefdinir oral suspension to shake bottle well before use and to use a liquid-measuring device to ensure accurate dose.
• Inform patient that tablet coating may cause stools to become a reddish color.
• Instruct patient to complete entire course of therapy, even if he feels better.
• Advise patient to take iron salts and aluminum- or magnesium-containing antacids at least 2 hours before or after taking cefdinir.
• Inform patient with history of colitis that cefdinir may worsen the condition; urge him to notify prescriber immediately if symptoms develop.
• Inform patient with diabetes mellitus that oral suspension contains 2.86 g of sucrose

per teaspoon; advise him to monitor his blood glucose levels as appropriate.
• Teach patient to recognize and report signs of superinfection, such as perineal itching; loose, foul-smelling stools; and vaginal drainage.
• Inform patient that yogurt and buttermilk can help prevent superinfection and may decrease diarrhea.

# cefditoren pivoxil

Spectracef

## Class and Category

*Chemical:* Cephalosporin
*Therapeutic:* Antibiotic
*Pregnancy category:* B

## Indications and Dosages

➤ *To treat mild to moderate acute bacterial exacerbation of chronic bronchitis or community-acquired pneumonia caused by* Haemophilus influenzae *(including beta-lactamase–producing strains),* H. parainfluenzae *(including beta-lactamase–producing strains),* Streptococcus pneumoniae *(penicillin-susceptible strains), or* Moraxella catarrhalis *(including beta-lactamase–producing strains)*

**TABLETS**

**Adults and children age 12 and older.** 400 mg b.i.d. for 10 days or for 14 days for community-acquired pneumonia.

➤ *To treat mild to moderate pharyngitis and tonsillitis caused by* Streptococcus pyogenes

**TABLETS**

**Adults and children age 12 and older.** 200 mg b.i.d. for 10 days.

➤ *To treat mild to moderate uncomplicated skin and soft-tissue infections caused by* Staphylococcus aureus *(including beta-lactamase–producing strains) or* S. pyogenes

**TABLETS**

**Adults and children age 12 and older.** 200 mg b.i.d. for 10 days.

**DOSAGE ADJUSTMENT** For patients with moderate renal impairment (creatinine clearance of 30 to 49 ml/min/1.73 m²), maximum dosage reduced to 200 mg b.i.d. For patients with severe renal impairment (creatinine clearance less than 30 ml/min/1.73 m²), maximum dosage reduced to 200 mg q.d.

## Mechanism of Action
Interferes with bacterial cell wall synthesis by inhibiting the final step in the cross-linking of peptidoglycan strands. Peptidoglycan makes the cell membrane rigid and protective. Without it, bacterial cells rupture and die. This mechanism of action is most effective against bacteria that divide rapidly, including many gram-positive and gram-negative bacteria. Cefditoren isn't inactivated by beta lactamase produced by some bacteria.

## Contraindications
Carnitine deficiency or inborn metabolic disorder that causes carnitine deficiency; hypersensitivity to cephalosporins or their components

## Interactions
**DRUGS**
*aluminum- and magnesium-containing antacids, H₂-receptor antagonists:* Reduced cefditoren absorption
*probenecid:* Increased and prolonged blood cefditoren level
**FOODS**
*food:* Increased cefditoren absorption

## Adverse Reactions
**CNS:** Headache, hyperactivity, hypertonia, seizures
**GI:** Abdominal pain, diarrhea, dyspepsia, hepatic dysfunction, nausea, pseudomembranous colitis, vomiting
**GU:** Acute renal failure, renal dysfunction, toxic nephropathy
**HEME:** Aplastic anemia, hemolytic anemia, hemorrhage, thrombocytopenia
**MS:** Arthralgia
**RESP:** Pneumonia
**SKIN:** Erythema multiforme, Stevens-Johnson syndrome, toxic epidermal necrolysis
**Other:** Allergic reaction, anaphylaxis, carnitine deficiency, drug fever, serum sickness–like reaction, superinfection

## Nursing Considerations
•**WARNING** Before instituting cefditoren therapy, determine if patient is hypersensitive to milk protein because cefditoren contains sodium caseinate, a milk protein. Be aware that drug should not be given to patient with this hypersensitivity. Also determine if patient has had a hypersensitivity reaction to cefditoren or other cephalosporins (because drug is contraindicated in these patients) or to penicillin (because cross-sensitivity has occurred in about 10% of patients).
•Cefditoren shouldn't be used for prolonged treatment because of the risk of carnitine deficiency.
•If possible, obtain culture and sensitivity test results, as ordered, before giving cefditoren.
•Assess patient for evidence of *Clostridium difficile* infection and pseudomembranous colitis, such as profuse, watery diarrhea. For mild cases, expect to discontinue cefditoren. For moderate to severe cases, expect to also administer fluids and electrolytes, protein supplementation, and an antibacterial drug effective against *C. difficile* colitis, as prescribed.
•If an allergic reaction occurs, expect to discontinue drug, as prescribed. For serious acute hypersensitivity reactions, expect to also administer epinephrine, oxygen, I.V. fluids, I.V. antihistamines, I.V. corticosteroids, and I.V. vasopressors, as prescribed.
•Monitor BUN and serum creatinine levels to detect early signs of renal dysfunction. Also monitor fluid intake and output.
•Watch for a decreased PT, as ordered, in at-risk patients, such as those with renal or hepatic impairment, those with a poor nutritional state, and those receiving anticoagulant or prolonged antibiotic therapy. Notify prescriber if a decrease occurs, and give vitamin K as ordered.
**PATIENT TEACHING**
•Urge patient to complete prescribed course of therapy.
•Instruct patient to take cefditoren with meals to enhance drug absorption.
•Advise patient not to take cefditoren with aluminum- or magnesium-containing antacids or other drugs used to reduce stomach acids because these drugs may interfere with cefditoren absorption.
•Explain that yogurt and buttermilk help maintain normal intestinal flora and can decrease diarrhea during therapy.
•Instruct patient to immediately report severe diarrhea to prescriber.

# cefepime hydrochloride

Maxipime

## Class and Category

*Chemical:* Fourth-generation cephalosporin, 7-aminocephalosporanic acid
*Therapeutic:* Antibiotic
*Pregnancy category:* B

## Indications and Dosages

➤ *To treat mild to moderate UTIs caused by* Escherichia coli, Klebsiella pneumoniae, *and* Proteus mirabilis

I.V. INFUSION, I.M. INJECTION (ONLY FOR UTI CAUSED BY
E. COLI)

**Adults and children age 12 and older.** 500 to 1,000 mg q 12 hr for 7 to 10 days.

➤ *To treat severe UTIs caused by* E. coli *or* K. pneumoniae, *moderate to severe skin and soft-tissue infections caused by* Staphylococcus aureus *or* Streptococcus pyogenes

I.V. INFUSION

**Adults and children age 12 and older.** 2 g q 12 hr for 10 days.

➤ *To treat moderate to severe pneumonia caused by* Enterobacter *sp.,* K. pneumoniae, Pseudomonas aeruginosa, *or* Streptococcus pneumoniae

I.V. INFUSION

**Adults and children age 12 and older.** 1 to 2 g q 12 hr for 10 days.

➤ *To treat febrile neutropenia*

I.V. INFUSION

**Adults and children age 12 and older.** 2 g q 8 hr for 7 days or until neutropenia resolves.

➤ *To treat complicated intra-abdominal infections (together with metronidazole) caused by* alpha-hemolytic streptococci, Bacteroides fragilis, E. coli, Enterobacter *sp.,* K. pneumoniae, *or* P. aeruginosa

I.V. INFUSION

**Adults and children age 12 and older.** 2 g q 12 hr for 7 to 10 days.

DOSAGE ADJUSTMENT Dosing interval increased from 12 to 24 hr and from 8 to 12 hr for patients with creatinine clearance of 30 to 60 ml/min/1.73 m$^2$; dosing interval increased from 8 or 12 hr to 24 hr and dose decreased from 2 g q 12 hr to 1 g q 24 hr (all other doses remain unchanged) for patients with creatinine clearance of 11 to 29 ml/min/

1.73 m$^2$; dosage decreased from 500 mg q 12 hr to 250 mg q 24 hr, from 1,000 mg q 12 hr to 250 mg q 24 hr, from 2,000 mg q 12 hr to 500 mg q 24 hr, and from 2 g q 8 hr to 1 g q 24 hr if creatinine clearance is less than 11 ml/min/1.73 m$^2$.

## Incompatibilities

Don't add cefepime to solutions that contain ampicillin in a concentration of more than 40 mg/ml. Don't add drug to solutions that contain aminophylline, gentamycin, metronidazole, netilmicin sulfate, tobramycin, or vancomycin.

## Mechanism of Action

Interferes with bacterial cell wall synthesis by inhibiting the final step in the cross-linking of peptidoglycan strands. Peptidoglycan makes cell membranes rigid and protective. Without it, bacterial cells rupture and die.

## Contraindications

Hypersensitivity to cephalosporins or their components

## Interactions

DRUGS

*aminoglycosides, loop diuretics:* Increased risk of renal failure in patients with renal disease

## Adverse Reactions

**CNS:** Chills, fever, headache, seizures
**CV:** Edema
**EENT:** Hearing loss
**GI:** Abdominal cramps, diarrhea, elevated liver function test results, hepatic failure, hepatomegaly, nausea, oral candidiasis, pseudomembranous colitis, vomiting
**GU:** Elevated BUN level, nephrotoxicity, renal failure, vaginal candidiasis
**HEME:** Eosinophilia, hemolytic anemia, hypoprothrombinemia, neutropenia, thrombocytopenia, unusual bleeding
**MS:** Arthralgia
**RESP:** Dyspnea
**SKIN:** Ecchymosis, erythema, erythema multiforme, pruritus, rash, Stevens-Johnson syndrome
**Other:** Anaphylaxis; injection site pain, redness, and swelling; superinfection

## Nursing Considerations
• Use cefepime cautiously in patients with impaired renal function or a history of GI disease, particularly colitis. Also use drug cautiously in patients who are hypersensitive to penicillin because cross-sensitivity has occurred in about 10% of such patients.
• If possible, obtain culture and sensitivity test results, as ordered, before giving drug.
• For I.V. infusion, reconstitute according to manufacturer's guidelines. Administer over 30 minutes.
• For I.M. injection, reconstitute 500-mg vial of drug with 1.3 ml of diluent, such as sterile water for injection (or 1-g vial with 2.4 ml of diluent). See manufacturer's guidelines for complete list of appropriate diluents.
• Be aware that an allergic reaction may occur a few days after therapy starts.
• Monitor BUN and serum creatinine levels for early signs of nephrotoxicity. Also monitor fluid intake and output; decreasing urine output may indicate nephrotoxicity. Be aware that unadjusted dosages of cefepime in renally impaired patients may cause myoclonus and seizures.
• Assess bowel pattern daily; severe diarrhea may indicate pseudomembranous colitis.
• Assess for signs of superinfection, such as perineal itching, fever, malaise, redness, pain, swelling, drainage, rash, diarrhea, and cough or sputum changes.
• Assess for pharyngitis, ecchymosis, bleeding, and arthralgia; they may indicate a blood dyscrasia.

**PATIENT TEACHING**
• Tell patient to immediately report severe diarrhea to prescriber.


# cefixime

Suprax

## Class and Category
*Chemical:* Third-generation cephalosporin, 7-aminocephalosporanic acid
*Therapeutic:* Antibiotic
*Pregnancy category:* B

## Indications and Dosages
➤ *To treat uncomplicated UTIs caused by* Escherichia coli *and* Proteus mirabilis; *otitis media caused by* Haemophilus influenzae, Moraxella catarrhalis, *and* Streptococcus pyogenes; *pharyngitis and tonsillitis caused by* S. pyogenes; *acute bronchitis and acute exacerbations of chronic bronchitis caused by* H. influenzae *and* Streptococcus pneumoniae

**ORAL SUSPENSION**
**Children.** 8 mg/kg q.d. or 4 mg/kg q 12 hr.
**TABLETS**
**Adults and children over 50 kg (110 lb) or age 12.** 400 mg q.d. or 200 mg q 12 hr.

➤ *To treat uncomplicated gonorrhea caused by* Neisseria gonorrhoeae
**TABLETS**
**Adults and children over 50 kg or age 12.** 400 mg q.d.

**DOSAGE ADJUSTMENT** Dosage reduced to 75% for patients who have creatinine clearance of 21 to 60 ml/min/1.73 m² or receive hemodialysis. Dosage reduced to 50% for patients who have creatinine clearance of 20 ml/min/1.73 m² or less.

---

### Mechanism of Action
Interferes with bacterial cell wall synthesis by inhibiting the final step in the cross-linking of peptidoglycan strands. Peptidoglycan makes cell membranes rigid and protective. Without it, bacterial cells rupture and die.

---

## Contraindications
Hypersensitivity to cephalosporins or their components

## Interactions
**DRUGS**
*aminoglycosides, loop diuretics:* Increased risk of nephrotoxicity
*carbamazepine:* Increased blood carbamazepine level

## Adverse Reactions
**CNS:** Chills, fever, headache, seizures
**CV:** Edema
**EENT:** Hearing loss
**GI:** Abdominal cramps, diarrhea, elevated liver function test results, hepatic failure, hepatitis, hepatomegaly, jaundice, nausea, oral candidiasis, pseudomembranous colitis, vomiting
**GU:** Elevated BUN level, nephrotoxicity, renal failure, vaginal candidiasis
**HEME:** Eosinophilia, hemolytic anemia, hypoprothrombinemia, neutropenia, thrombocytopenia, unusual bleeding

**MS:** Arthralgia
**RESP:** Dyspnea
**SKIN:** Ecchymosis, erythema, erythema multiforme, pruritus, rash, Stevens-Johnson syndrome, toxic epidermal necrolysis
**Other:** Anaphylaxis, angioedema, facial edema, superinfection

## Nursing Considerations

•Use cefixime cautiously in patients with impaired renal function or a history of GI disease, especially colitis. Also use drug cautiously in patients who are hypersensitive to penicillin because cross-sensitivity has occurred in 10% of such patients.
•If possible, obtain culture and sensitivity test results, as ordered, before giving drug.
•Be aware that tablets shouldn't be substituted for oral suspension to treat otitis media because cefixime suspension produces a higher peak blood level than do tablets when administered at the same dose.
•Monitor BUN and serum creatinine levels to detect early signs of nephrotoxicity. Also monitor fluid intake and output; decreasing urine output may indicate nephrotoxicity.
•Be aware that an allergic reaction may occur a few days after therapy starts.
•Assess bowel pattern daily; severe diarrhea may indicate pseudomembranous colitis.
•Assess for signs of superinfection, such as perineal itching, fever, malaise, redness, pain, swelling, drainage, rash, diarrhea, and cough or sputum changes.
•Assess for pharyngitis, ecchymosis, bleeding, and arthralgia; they may indicate a blood dyscrasia.

**PATIENT TEACHING**
•Instruct patient to complete the prescribed course of therapy.
•Advise patient to shake oral suspension well before pouring dose and to use a liquid-measuring device to obtain an accurate dose.
•Instruct patient to store oral suspension at room temperature and to discard unused portion after 14 days.
•Tell patient to immediately report severe diarrhea to prescriber.
•Inform patient that yogurt and buttermilk can help maintain intestinal flora and decrease diarrhea.
•Teach patient to recognize and report signs of superinfection, such as furry tongue, perineal itching, and loose, foul-smelling stools.

# cefmetazole sodium

Zefazone

## Class and Category

*Chemical:* Second-generation cephalosporin, 7-aminocephalosporanic acid
*Therapeutic:* Antibiotic
*Pregnancy category:* B

## Indications and Dosages

➤ *To treat UTIs caused by* Escherichia coli; *lower respiratory tract infections, such as bronchitis and pneumonia, caused by* E. coli, Haemophilus influenzae, Staphylococcus aureus, *and* Streptococcus pneumoniae; *skin and soft-tissue infections caused by* Bacteroides fragilis, Bacteroides melaninogenicus, E. coli, Klebsiella oxytoca, Klebsiella pneumoniae, Morganella morganii, Proteus mirabilis, Proteus vulgaris, S. aureus, Staphylococcus epidermidis, Streptococcus agalactiae, *and* Streptococcus pyogenes; *intra-abdominal infections caused by* B. fragilis, Clostridium perfringens, E. coli, K. oxytoca, *and* K. pneumoniae

**I.V. INFUSION**
**Adults.** 2 g q 6 to 12 hr for 5 to 14 days.
**DOSAGE ADJUSTMENT** Dosage reduced to 1 to 2 g q 12 hr if creatinine clearance is 50 to 90 ml/min/1.73 m$^2$; 1 to 2 g q 16 hr if creatinine clearance is 30 to 49 ml/min/1.73 m$^2$; 1 to 2 g q 24 hr if creatinine clearance is 10 to 29 ml/min/1.73 m$^2$; and 1 to 2 g q 48 hr if creatinine clearance is less than 10 ml/min/1.73 m$^2$.

➤ *To provide surgical prophylaxis for vaginal hysterectomy*

**I.V. INFUSION**
**Adults.** 2 g as a single dose 30 to 90 min before surgery or 1 g 30 to 90 min before surgery and repeated 8 and 16 hr later.

➤ *To provide surgical prophylaxis for abdominal hysterectomy and for high-risk cholecystectomy*

**I.V. INFUSION**
**Adults.** 1 g 30 to 90 min before surgery and repeated 8 and 16 hr later.

➤ *To provide surgical prophylaxis for cesarean section*

**I.V. INFUSION**
**Adults.** 2 g as a single dose after cord is clamped or 1 g after cord is clamped and then repeated 8 and 16 hr later.
➤ *To provide surgical prophylaxis for colorectal surgery*
**I.V. INFUSION**
**Adults.** 2 g as a single dose 30 to 90 min before surgery or 2 g 30 to 90 min before surgery and repeated 8 and 16 hr later.

## Mechanism of Action
Interferes with bacterial cell wall synthesis by inhibiting the final step in the cross-linking of peptidoglycan strands. Peptidoglycan makes cell membranes rigid and protective. Without it, bacterial cells rupture and die.

## Contraindications
Hypersensitivity to cephalosporins or their components

## Interactions
**DRUGS**
*aminoglycosides, loop diuretics:* Increased risk of nephrotoxicity
*anticoagulants:* Possibly increased anticoagulant effect
*probenecid:* Increased and prolonged blood cefmetazole level
**ACTIVITIES**
*alcohol use:* Possibly disulfiram-like reaction

## Adverse Reactions
**CNS:** Chills, fever, headache, seizures
**CV:** Edema
**EENT:** Hearing loss
**GI:** Abdominal cramps, diarrhea, elevated liver function test results, hepatic failure, hepatomegaly, nausea, oral candidiasis, pseudomembranous colitis, vomiting
**GU:** Elevated BUN level, nephrotoxicity, renal failure, vaginal candidiasis
**HEME:** Eosinophilia, hemolytic anemia, hypoprothrombinemia, neutropenia, thrombocytopenia, unusual bleeding
**MS:** Arthralgia
**RESP:** Dyspnea
**SKIN:** Ecchymosis, erythema, erythema multiforme, pruritus, rash, Stevens-Johnson syndrome
**Other:** Anaphylaxis; injection site pain, redness, and swelling; superinfection

## Nursing Considerations
•Use cefmetazole cautiously in patients who are hypersensitive to penicillin; cross-sensitivity has occurred in 10% of such patients.
•If possible, obtain culture and sensitivity test results, as ordered, before giving drug.
•Reconstitute drug with sterile or bacteriostatic water for injection or sodium chloride for injection.
•Dilute primary solution as needed to 1 to 20 mg/ml in $D_5W$, NS, LR, or 1% lidocaine solution without epinephrine.
•Store reconstituted solution for up to 24 hours at room temperature or 7 days under refrigeration.
•Monitor BUN and serum creatinine levels and fluid intake and output to detect early signs of nephrotoxicity.
•Assess bowel pattern daily; severe diarrhea may indicate pseudomembranous colitis.
•Assess for signs of superinfection, such as perineal itching, fever, malaise, redness, rash, diarrhea, and cough or sputum changes.
•Assess for pharyngitis, bleeding, and arthralgia, which may indicate blood dyscrasia. Monitor PT and bleeding time, as ordered.
**PATIENT TEACHING**
•Advise patient to immediately report severe diarrhea to prescriber.
•Instruct patient to avoid alcohol during therapy and for at least 3 days after last dose.

# cefonicid sodium

Monocid

## Class and Category
*Chemical:* Second-generation cephalosporin, 7-aminocephalosporanic acid
*Therapeutic:* Antibiotic
*Pregnancy category:* B

## Indications and Dosages
➤ *To treat lower respiratory tract infections caused by* Escherichia coli, Haemophilus influenzae, Klebsiella pneumoniae, *and* Streptococcus pneumoniae; *UTIs caused by* E. coli, K. pneumoniae, Morganella morganii, Proteus mirabilis, Proteus vulgaris, *and* Providencia rettgeri; *skin and soft-tissue infections caused by* Staphylococcus aureus, Staphylococcus epidermidis, Streptococcus agalactiae, *and* Streptococcus pyogenes; *septicemia caused by* E. coli *and*

S. pneumoniae; *and bone and joint in-fections caused* by S. aureus

**I.V. INFUSION, I.V. OR I.M. INJECTION**

**Adults.** For mild to moderate infections, 1 g q 24 hr. For severe or life-threatening infections, 2 g q 24 hr.

➤ *To treat uncomplicated UTIs*

**I.V. INFUSION, I.V. OR I.M. INJECTION**

**Adults.** 500 mg q 24 hr.

**DOSAGE ADJUSTMENT** Initial dose reduced to 75 mg/kg I.V. or I.M. in patients with impaired renal function. Then dosage reduced to 10 to 25 mg/kg q 24 hr if creatinine clearance ranges from 60 to 79 ml/min/1.73 m²; 8 to 20 mg/kg q 24 hr if creatinine clearance ranges from 40 to 59 ml/min/1.73 m²; 4 to 15 mg/kg q 24 hr if creatinine clearance ranges from 20 to 39 ml/min/1.73 m²; 4 to 15 mg/kg q 48 hr if creatinine clearance ranges from 10 to 19 ml/min/1.73 m²; 4 to 15 mg/kg q 3 to 5 days if creatinine clearance ranges from 5 to 9 ml/minute/1.73 m²; and 3 to 4 mg/kg q 3 to 5 days if creatinine clearance is less than 5 ml/min/1.73 m².

➤ *To provide surgical prophylaxis*

**I.V. INFUSION, I.V. OR I.M. INJECTION**

**Adults.** 1 g 60 min before surgery. Dose repeated once daily, if needed, for 2 days after prosthetic arthroplasty or open-heart surgery.

**Mechanism of Action**

Interferes with bacterial cell wall synthesis by inhibiting the final step in the cross-linking of peptidoglycan strands. Peptidoglycan makes cell membranes rigid and protective. Without it, bacterial cells rupture and die.

**Incompatibilities**

To prevent mutual inactivation, don't mix cefonicid with aminoglycosides.

**Contraindications**

Hypersensitivity to cephalosporins or their components

**Interactions**

**DRUGS**

*aminoglycosides, loop diuretics:* Increased risk of nephrotoxicity

**Adverse Reactions**

**CNS:** Chills, fever, headache, seizures
**CV:** Edema

**EENT:** Hearing loss
**GI:** Abdominal cramps, diarrhea, elevated liver function test results, hepatic failure, hepatomegaly, nausea, oral candidiasis, pseudomembranous colitis, vomiting
**GU:** Elevated BUN level, nephrotoxicity, renal failure, vaginal candidiasis
**HEME:** Eosinophilia, hemolytic anemia, hypoprothrombinemia, neutropenia, thrombocytopenia, unusual bleeding
**MS:** Arthralgia
**RESP:** Dyspnea
**SKIN:** Ecchymosis, erythema, erythema multiforme, pruritus, rash, Stevens-Johnson syndrome
**Other:** Anaphylaxis; injection site pain, redness, and swelling; superinfection

**Nursing Considerations**

•Use cefonicid cautiously in patients with impaired renal function. Also use drug cautiously in patients who are hypersensitive to penicillin because cross-sensitivity has occurred in about 10% of such patients.
•If possible, obtain culture and sensitivity test results, as ordered, before giving drug.
•Reconstitute each 500-mg vial of drug with 2 ml of sterile water for injection (or each 1-g vial with 2.5 ml).
•For I.V. infusion, dilute further in 50 to 100 ml of compatible solution, such as D₅W, D₁₀W, D₅/0.2NS, D₅/0.45NS, or D₅NS.
•Administer I.V. injection slowly over 3 to 5 minutes through tubing of a flowing compatible I.V. solution.
•For I.M. dose larger than 1 g, divide dose in half and give into large muscle mass, such as the gluteus maximus, at two different sites.
•Store reconstituted solution at room temperature for 24 hours or under refrigeration for 72 hours.
•Monitor BUN and serum creatinine levels to detect early signs of nephrotoxicity. Also monitor fluid intake and output; decreasing urine output may indicate nephrotoxicity.
•Assess bowel pattern daily; severe diarrhea may indicate pseudomembranous colitis.
•Assess for signs of superinfection, such as perineal itching, fever, malaise, redness, pain, swelling, drainage, rash, diarrhea, and cough or sputum changes.
•Assess for pharyngitis, ecchymosis, bleeding, and arthralgia; they may indicate a blood dyscrasia.

•Warn patient that I.M. injection may be painful.
•Tell patient to immediately report severe diarrhea to prescriber.

# cefoperazone sodium

Cefobid

## Class and Category

*Chemical:* Third-generation cephalosporin, 7-aminocephalosporanic acid
*Therapeutic:* Antibiotic
*Pregnancy category:* B

## Indications and Dosages

➤ *To treat respiratory tract infections caused by* Enterobacter *sp.,* Escherichia coli, Haemophilus influenzae, Klebsiella pneumoniae, Proteus mirabilis, Pseudomonas aeruginosa, Staphylococcus aureus, Streptococcus pneumoniae, Streptococcus pyogenes, *and other streptococci (excluding enterococci); UTIs caused by* E. coli *and* P. aeruginosa; *uncomplicated gonorrhea caused by* Neisseria gonorrhoeae; *gynecologic infections caused by anaerobic gram-positive cocci,* Bacteroides *sp.,* Clostridium *sp.,* E. coli, Staphylococcus epidermidis, *and* Streptococcus agalactiae; *bacterial septicemia caused by* E. coli, Klebsiella *sp.,* S. aureus, Serratia marcescens, *and streptococci; skin and soft-tissue infections caused by* P. aeruginosa, S. aureus, *and* S. pyogenes; *and intra-abdominal infections caused by anaerobic gram-negative bacilli,* E. coli, *and* P. aeruginosa

**I.V. INFUSION, I.M. INJECTION**

**Adults.** 1 to 2 g q 12 hr. For severe infections or those caused by less sensitive organisms, 6 to 12 g/day divided into equal doses and given b.i.d., t.i.d., or q.i.d. *Maximum:* 12 g/day.

## Mechanism of Action

Interferes with bacterial cell wall synthesis by inhibiting the final step in the cross-linking of peptidoglycan strands. Peptidoglycan makes cell membranes rigid and protective. Without it, bacterial cells rupture and die.

## Incompatibilities

To prevent mutual inactivation, don't mix cefoperazone with aminoglycosides. Also avoid mixing cefoperazone with other drugs, including pentamidine isethionate.

## Contraindications

Hypersensitivity to cephalosporins or their components

## Interactions

**DRUGS**

*aminoglycosides, loop diuretics:* Increased risk of nephrotoxicity
*oral anticoagulants, other drugs that affect blood clotting:* Increased anticoagulant effect

**ACTIVITIES**

*alcohol use:* Disulfiram-like reaction

## Adverse Reactions

**CNS:** Chills, fever, headache, seizures
**CV:** Edema
**EENT:** Hearing loss
**GI:** Abdominal cramps, diarrhea, elevated liver function test results, hepatic failure, hepatomegaly, nausea, oral candidiasis, pseudomembranous colitis, vomiting
**GU:** Elevated BUN level, nephrotoxicity, renal failure, vaginal candidiasis
**HEME:** Eosinophilia, hemolytic anemia, hypoprothrombinemia, neutropenia, thrombocytopenia, unusual bleeding
**MS:** Arthralgia
**RESP:** Dyspnea
**SKIN:** Ecchymosis, erythema, erythema multiforme, pruritus, rash, Stevens-Johnson syndrome
**Other:** Anaphylaxis; injection site pain, redness, and swelling; superinfection

## Nursing Considerations

•Use cefoperazone cautiously in patients with a history of bleeding problems, GI disease (especially colitis), or severely impaired hepatic or renal function. Also use drug cautiously in patients who are hypersensitive to penicillin because cross-sensitivity has occurred in 10% of such patients.
•If possible, obtain culture and sensitivity test results, as ordered, before giving drug.
•For I.V. use, reconstitute drug with required amount of diluent, and then further dilute in compatible solution, such as $D_5W$, $D_5LR$, $D_5.2NS$, $D_5NS$, $D_{10}W$, LR injection, NS, Normosol M and $D_5W$, or Normosol R. (See manufacturer's guidelines for details.)

• Administer I.V. drug as intermittent infusion over 15 to 30 minutes or as continuous infusion. Direct bolus injection isn't recommended.
• For I.M. injection, reconstitute drug with bacteriostatic water for injection (that contains benzyl alcohol or parabens) or sterile water for injection.
• After reconstitution, let foam dissipate and inspect the solution to ensure complete dissolution.
• Store reconstituted solution at room temperature for 24 hours.
• Monitor BUN and serum creatinine levels to detect early signs of nephrotoxicity. Also monitor fluid intake and output; decreasing urine output may indicate nephrotoxicity.
• Assess bowel pattern daily; severe diarrhea may indicate pseudomembranous colitis.
• Assess for pharyngitis, ecchymosis, bleeding, and arthralgia; they may indicate a blood dyscrasia.
• Assess for signs of superinfection, such as perineal itching, fever, malaise, redness, pain, swelling, drainage, rash, diarrhea, and cough or sputum changes.

**PATIENT TEACHING**
• Advise patient to avoid alcohol during therapy and for at least 3 days after taking the last dose.
• Warn patient that I.M. injection may cause pain.
• Tell patient to immediately report severe diarrhea to prescriber.

# cefotaxime sodium

Claforan

## Class and Category
*Chemical*: Third-generation cephalosporin, 7-aminocephalosporanic acid
*Therapeutic*: Antibiotic
*Pregnancy category:* B

## Indications and Dosages
➤ *To provide perioperative prophylaxis*
**I.V. INFUSION, I.V. OR I.M. INJECTION**
**Adults and children who weigh more than 50 kg (110 lb).** 1 g 30 to 90 min before surgery.
➤ *To provide perioperative prophylaxis related to cesarean section*
**I.V. INFUSION, I.V. OR I.M. INJECTION**
**Adults.** 1 g as soon as cord is clamped, then 1 g q 6 hr for up to two doses.

➤ *To treat gonococcal urethritis and cervicitis in men and women*
**I.M. INJECTION**
**Adults who weigh more than 50 kg.** 500 mg as a single dose.
➤ *To treat rectal gonorrhea in women*
**I.M. INJECTION**
**Adults who weigh more than 50 kg.** 500 mg as a single dose.
➤ *To treat rectal gonorrhea in men*
**I.M. INJECTION**
**Adults who weigh more than 50 kg.** 1 g as a single dose.
➤ *To treat disseminated gonorrhea*
**I.V. INFUSION OR INJECTION**
**Adults and children who weigh more than 50 kg.** 1 g q 8 hr.
➤ *To treat uncomplicated infections caused by susceptible organisms*
**I.V. INFUSION, I.V. OR I.M. INJECTION**
**Adults and children who weigh more than 50 kg.** 1 g q 12 hr.
**Children ages 1 month to 12 years who weigh less than 50 kg.** 50 to 180 mg/kg/day in four to six divided doses.
**Children ages 1 to 4 weeks.** 50 mg/kg I.V. q 8 hr.
**Children age 1 week and younger.** 50 mg/kg I.V. q 12 hr.
➤ *To treat moderate to severe infections caused by susceptible organisms*
**I.V. INFUSION, I.V. OR I.M. INJECTION**
**Adults and children who weigh more than 50 kg.** 1 to 2 g q 8 hr.
**Children ages 1 month to 12 years who weigh less than 50 kg.** 50 to 180 mg/kg/day in four to six divided doses. For more serious infections, including meningitis, higher dosages are used.
**Children ages 1 to 4 weeks.** 50 mg/kg I.V. q 8 hr.
**Children age 1 week and younger.** 50 mg/kg I.V. q 12 hr.
➤ *To treat septicemia and other infections that commonly require antibiotics in higher doses than those used to treat moderate to severe infections*
**I.V. INFUSION OR INJECTION**
**Adults and children who weigh more than 50 kg.** 2 g q 6 to 8 hr.
➤ *To treat life-threatening infections caused by susceptible organisms*
**I.V. INFUSION OR INJECTION**
**Adults and children who weigh more than 50 kg.** 2 g q 4 hr. *Maximum:* 12 g/day.

**Children ages 1 month to 12 years who weigh less than 50 kg.** 50 to 180 mg/kg/day in four to six divided doses.

**Children ages 1 to 4 weeks.** 50 mg/kg q 8 hr.

**Children age 1 week and younger.** 50 mg/kg q 12 hr.

**DOSAGE ADJUSTMENT** Dosage reduced by 50% for patients with estimated creatinine clearance below 20 ml/min/1.73 m².

## Incompatibilities
To prevent mutual inactivation, don't mix cefotaxime with aminoglycosides. Also avoid mixing cefotaxime with other drugs, including pentamidine isethionate.

## Mechanism of Action
Interferes with bacterial cell wall synthesis by inhibiting the cross-linking of peptidoglycan strands. Peptidoglycan makes cell membranes rigid and protective. Without it, bacterial cells rupture and die.

## Contraindications
Hypersensitivity to cephalosporins or their components

## Interactions
**DRUGS**
*aminoglycosides, loop diuretics:* Increased risk of nephrotoxicity
*probenecid:* Increased and prolonged blood cefotaxime level

## Adverse Reactions
**CNS:** Chills, fever, headache, seizures
**CV:** Edema
**EENT:** Hearing loss
**GI:** Abdominal cramps, diarrhea, elevated liver function test results, hepatic failure, hepatomegaly, nausea, oral candidiasis, pseudomembranous colitis, vomiting
**GU:** Elevated BUN level, nephrotoxicity, renal failure, vaginal candidiasis
**HEME:** Eosinophilia, hemolytic anemia, hypoprothrombinemia, neutropenia, thrombocytopenia, unusual bleeding
**MS:** Arthralgia
**RESP:** Dyspnea
**SKIN:** Ecchymosis, erythema, erythema multiforme, pruritus, rash, Stevens-Johnson syndrome, toxic epidermal necrolysis

**Other:** Anaphylaxis; injection site pain, redness, and swelling; superinfection

## Nursing Considerations
• Use cefotaxime cautiously in patients with impaired renal function, a history of GI disease (especially colitis), or hypersensitivity to penicillin because cross-sensitivity has occurred in 10% of such patients.
• If possible, obtain culture and sensitivity test results, as ordered, before giving drug.
• For I.V. use, reconstitute each 0.5-, 1-, or 2-g vial with 10 ml of sterile water for injection. Shake to dissolve.
• For intermittent I.V. infusion, further dilute in 50 to 100 ml of D₅W or NS.
• For I.M. use, reconstitute each 500-mg vial with 2 ml of sterile water for injection or bacteriostatic water for injection; each 1-g vial with 3 ml of diluent; and each 2-g vial with 5 ml of diluent. Shake to dissolve.
• **WARNING** When preparing drug for a neonate, don't use diluent that contains benzyl alcohol; it could cause a fatal toxic syndrome.
• Give cefotaxime by I.V. injection over 3 to 5 minutes through tubing of a flowing compatible I.V. solution. Temporarily stop other solutions being given through same I.V. site.
• Discard unused drug after 24 hours if stored at room temperature, 5 days if refrigerated.
• Protect cefotaxime powder and solution from light and heat.
• Monitor I.V. sites for signs of phlebitis or extravasation. Rotate I.V. sites every 72 hours.
• Monitor BUN and serum creatinine levels and fluid intake and output for signs of nephrotoxicity.
• Be aware that an allergic reaction may occur a few days after therapy starts.
• Assess bowel pattern daily; severe diarrhea may indicate pseudomembranous colitis.
• Assess patient for pharyngitis, ecchymosis, bleeding, and arthralgia, which may indicate a blood dyscrasia. Monitor CBC, PT, and bleeding time, as ordered.
• Monitor patient closely for superinfection. If signs appear, notify prescriber and expect to stop drug and give appropriate care.
**PATIENT TEACHING**
• Caution patient that I.M. injection may be painful.
• Instruct patient to immediately report severe diarrhea to prescriber.

# cefotetan disodium

Cefotan

## Class and Category

*Chemical:* Second-generation cephalosporin, 7-aminocephalosporanic acid
*Therapeutic:* Antibiotic
*Pregnancy category:* B

## Indications and Dosages

➤ *To provide surgical prophylaxis*

**I.V. INJECTION**

**Adults.** 1 to 2 g 30 to 60 min before surgery or, in cesarean section, as soon as cord is clamped.

➤ *To treat lower respiratory tract infections caused by* Escherichia coli, Haemophilus influenzae, Klebsiella *sp.,* Proteus mirabilis, Serratia marcescens, Staphylococcus aureus, *and* Streptococcus pneumoniae; *gynecologic infections caused by* Bacteroides sp. (excluding B. distasonis, B. ovatus, *and* B. thetaiotaomicron), E. coli, Fusobacterium *sp., gram-positive anaerobic cocci,* Neisseria gonorrhoeae, P. mirabilis, S. aureus, Staphylococcus epidermidis, *and* Streptococcus sp. (excluding enterococci); intra-abdominal infections caused by* Bacteroides sp. (excluding B. distasonis, B. ovatus, *and* B. thetaiotaomicron), Clostridium *sp.,* E. coli, Klebsiella *sp., and* Streptococcus sp. (excluding enterococci); and bone and joint infections caused by* S. aureus

**I.V. INFUSION, I.V. OR I.M. INJECTION**

**Adults.** For mild to moderate infections, 1 to 2 g q 12 hr.

**I.V. INFUSION OR INJECTION**

**Adults.** For severe infections, 2 g q 12 hr; for life-threatening infections, 3 g q 12 hr.

➤ *To treat UTIs caused by* E. coli, Klebsiella *sp., and* Proteus sp.

**I.V. INFUSION, I.V. OR I.M. INJECTION**

**Adults.** 0.5 to 2 g q 12 hr or 1 to 2 g q 24 hr.

➤ *To treat skin and soft-tissue infections caused by* E. coli, Klebsiella pneumoniae, Peptostreptococcus *sp.,* S. aureus, S. epidermidis, Streptococcus pyogenes, *and* Streptococcus sp. (excluding enterococci)

**I.V. INFUSION, I.V. OR I.M. INJECTION**

**Adults.** For mild to moderate infections due to *K. pneumoniae,* 1 or 2 g q 12 hr. For mild to moderate infections caused by other organisms, 1 g I.M. or I.V. q 12 hr or 2 g I.V. q 24 hr; for severe infections, 2 g I.V. q 12 hr.

**DOSAGE ADJUSTMENT** Dosing interval reduced to 24 hr in patients with creatinine clearance of 10 to 30 ml/min/1.73 $m^2$ and to 48 hr in patients with creatinine clearance below 10 ml/min/1.73 $m^2$.

---

### Mechanism of Action

Interferes with bacterial cell wall synthesis by inhibiting the final step in the cross-linking of peptidoglycan strands. Peptidoglycan makes cell membranes rigid and protective. Without it, bacterial cells rupture and die.

---

## Incompatibilities

To prevent mutual inactivation, don't mix cefotetan with aminoglycosides.

## Contraindications

Hypersensitivity to cephalosporins or their components

## Interactions

**DRUGS**

*aminoglycosides, loop diuretics:* Increased risk of nephrotoxicity
*oral anticoagulants, other drugs that affect blood clotting:* Enhanced anticoagulant effect
*probenecid:* Increased and prolonged blood cefotetan level

**ACTIVITIES**

*alcohol use:* Disulfiram-like reaction

## Adverse Reactions

**CNS:** Chills, fever, headache, seizures
**CV:** Edema
**EENT:** Hearing loss
**GI:** Abdominal cramps, diarrhea, elevated liver function test results, hepatic failure, hepatomegaly, nausea, oral candidiasis, pseudomembranous colitis, vomiting
**GU:** Elevated BUN level, nephrotoxicity, renal failure, vaginal candidiasis
**HEME:** Eosinophilia, hemolytic anemia, hypoprothrombinemia, neutropenia, thrombocytopenia, unusual bleeding
**MS:** Arthralgia
**RESP:** Dyspnea
**SKIN:** Ecchymosis, erythema, erythema multiforme, pruritus, rash, Stevens-Johnson syndrome
**Other:** Anaphylaxis; injection site pain, redness, and swelling; superinfection

## Nursing Considerations

•Use cefotetan cautiously in patients with impaired renal function or a history of GI disease, especially colitis. Also use drug cautiously in patients who are hypersensitive to penicillin because cross-sensitivity has occurred in 10% of such patients.

•If possible, obtain culture and sensitivity test results, as ordered, before giving drug.

•For I.V. use, reconstitute each 1-g vial of drug with 10 ml of sterile water for injection. For each 2-g vial, use 10 to 20 ml of diluent. For I.V. infusion, further dilute solution in 50 to 100 ml of D$_5$W or NS.

•For direct I.V. injection, administer drug slowly over 3 to 5 minutes through tubing of a flowing compatible I.V. solution.

•For I.M. use, reconstitute each 1-g vial of drug with 2 ml of sterile or bacteriostatic water for injection, or sodium chloride for injection. For a 2-g vial, use 3 ml of diluent.

•Monitor I.V. site for signs of phlebitis and extravasation; rotate sites every 72 hours.

•Protect reconstituted solution from light and store for up to 24 hours at room temperature or 96 hours under refrigeration.

•Be aware than an allergic reaction may occur a few days after therapy starts.

•Monitor BUN and serum creatinine levels and fluid intake and output for signs of nephrotoxicity.

•Monitor patient receiving even short-term cefotetan therapy for evidence of hemolytic anemia, such as marked pallor and fatigue.

•If patient receives long-term therapy, monitor CBC and serum AST, ALT, bilirubin, LD, and alkaline phosphatase levels.

•Assess bowel pattern daily; severe diarrhea may indicate pseudomembranous colitis.

•Watch for pharyngitis, ecchymosis, bleeding, and arthralgia, which may indicate a blood dyscrasia. Monitor PT and bleeding time, as ordered. Be prepared to give vitamin K, if ordered, to treat hypoprothrombinemia.

**PATIENT TEACHING**

•Explain that I.M. injection may be painful.

•Tell patient to immediately report severe diarrhea to prescriber.

•Urge patient to avoid alcohol during and for at least 3 days after cefotetan therapy.

# cefoxitin sodium

Mefoxin

## Class and Category

*Chemical:* Second-generation cephalosporin, 7-aminocephalosporanic acid
*Therapeutic:* Antibiotic
*Pregnancy category:* B

## Indications and Dosages

➤ *To provide surgical prophylaxis*

**I.V. INFUSION OR INJECTION**

**Adults.** 2 g 30 to 60 min before surgery and then 2 g q 6 hr after first dose for up to 24 hr.
**Children age 3 months or older.** 30 to 40 mg/kg 30 to 60 min before surgery and then q 6 hr after first dose for up to 24 hr.

➤ *To provide surgical prophylaxis for cesarean section*

**I.V. INFUSION OR INJECTION**

**Adults.** 2 g as a single dose as soon as cord is clamped or 2 g as soon as cord is clamped followed by 2 g 4 and 8 hr after initial dose.

➤ *To provide surgical prophylaxis for transurethral prostatectomy*

**I.V. INFUSION OR INJECTION**

**Adults.** 1 g 30 to 60 min before surgery and then 1 g q 8 hr for up to 5 days.

➤ *To treat infections, including septicemia, gynecologic infections, intra-abdominal infections, UTIs, and infections of the lower respiratory tract, skin, soft tissue, bones, and joints caused by anaerobes (including* Bacteroides *sp.,* Clostridium *sp.,* Fusobacterium *sp.,* Peptococcus niger, *and* Peptostreptococcus *sp.), gram-negative organisms (including* Escherichia coli, Haemophilus influenzae *[also ampicillin-resistant strains],* Klebsiella, *and* Proteus *sp.), and gram-positive organisms (including* Staphylococcus aureus *[penicillinase- and non-penicillinase-producing strains],* Staphylococcus epidermidis, Streptococcus agalactiae, Streptococcus pneumoniae, *and* Streptococcus pyogenes)*

**I.V. INFUSION OR INJECTION**

**Adults.** For uncomplicated infections, 1 g q 6 to 8 hr; for moderate to severe infections, 1 g q 4 hr or 2 g q 6 to 8 hr; for infections that commonly require high-dose antibiotics (such as gas gangrene), 2 g q 4 hr or 3 g q 6 hr.
**Children age 3 months or older.** 80 to 160 mg/kg/day in equal doses and given q 4 to 6 hr (with higher dosages used for more severe infections). *Maximum:* 12 g/day.

➤ *To treat uncomplicated gonorrhea*

**I.M. INJECTION**

**Adults.** 2 g as a single dose along with 1 g oral probenecid concurrently or within 30 min of cefoxitin.

**DOSAGE ADJUSTMENT** Dosage reduced to 1 to 2 g q 8 to 12 hr if creatinine clearance is 30 to 50 ml/min/1.73 m$^2$; 1 to 2 g q 12 to 24 hr if clearance is 10 to 29 ml/ min/1.73 m$^2$; 0.5 to 1 g q 12 to 24 hr if clearance is 5 to 9 ml/min/1.73 m$^2$; and 0.5 to 1 g q 24 to 48 hr if clearance is less than 5 ml/min/1.73 m$^2$.

## Mechanism of Action
Interferes with bacterial cell wall synthesis by inhibiting the final step in the cross-linking of peptidoglycan strands. Peptidoglycan makes cell membranes rigid and protective. Without it, bacterial cells rupture and die.

## Incompatibilities
To prevent mutual inactivation, don't mix cefoxitin with aminoglycosides. Also avoid mixing cefoxitin with other drugs, including pentamidine isethionate.

## Contraindications
Hypersensitivity to cephalosporins or their components

## Interactions
**DRUGS**
*aminoglycosides, loop diuretics:* Increased risk of nephrotoxicity

## Adverse Reactions
**CNS:** Chills, fever, headache, seizures
**CV:** Edema
**EENT:** Hearing loss
**GI:** Abdominal cramps, diarrhea, elevated liver function test results, hepatic failure, hepatomegaly, nausea, oral candidiasis, pseudomembranous colitis, vomiting
**GU:** Elevated BUN level, nephrotoxicity, renal failure, vaginal candidiasis
**HEME:** Eosinophilia, hemolytic anemia, hypoprothrombinemia, neutropenia, thrombocytopenia, unusual bleeding
**MS:** Arthralgia
**RESP:** Dyspnea
**SKIN:** Ecchymosis, erythema, erythema multiforme, flushing, pruritus, rash, Stevens-Johnson syndrome, urticaria
**Other:** Anaphylaxis; injection site pain, redness, and swelling; superinfection

## Nursing Considerations
•Use cefoxitin cautiously in patients hypersensitive to penicillin; cross-sensitivity has occurred in 10% of such patients. Also use cautiously in patients with a history of GI disease, particularly colitis, because of an increased risk of pseudomembranous colitis.
•If possible, obtain culture and sensitivity test results, as ordered, before giving drug.
•For I.V. use, reconstitute 1 g with 10 ml of sterile water for injection or 2 g with 10 to 20 ml of diluent.
•For I.V. injection, administer slowly over 3 to 5 minutes through tubing of a flowing compatible I.V. solution.
•For intermittent infusion, further dilute with 50 to 100 ml of D$_5$W or NS.
•For continuous high-dose infusion, add cefoxitin to I.V. solutions of D$_5$W, NS, or D$_5$NS.
•For I.M. use, reconstitute each 1 g with 2 ml of sterile water for injection.
•Discard unused drug after 24 hours if stored at room temperature or after 1 week if refrigerated.
•Be aware that powder or solution may darken during storage, a change that doesn't reflect altered potency.
•Be aware that an allergic reaction may occur a few days after therapy starts.
•Monitor BUN and serum creatinine levels for early signs of nephrotoxicity. Also monitor fluid intake and output; decreasing urine output may indicate nephrotoxicity.
•Assess bowel pattern daily; severe diarrhea may indicate pseudomembranous colitis.
•Assess for pharyngitis, ecchymosis, bleeding, and arthralgia; they may indicate a blood dyscrasia.

**PATIENT TEACHING**
•Tell patient to immediately report severe diarrhea to prescriber.
•Instruct patient to complete the course of therapy as prescribed.

# cefpodoxime proxetil
Vantin

## Class and Category
*Chemical:* Third-generation cephalosporin, 7-aminocephalosporanic acid
*Therapeutic:* Antibiotic
*Pregnancy category:* B

## Indications and Dosages
➤ *To treat acute community-acquired pneumonia caused by* Haemophilus influenzae *or* Streptococcus pneumoniae

ORAL SUSPENSION, TABLETS
**Adults and adolescents over age 13.** 200 mg q 12 hr for 14 days.

➤ *To treat acute bacterial exacerbation of chronic bronchitis caused by* H. influenzae, Moraxella catarrhalis, *or* S. pneumoniae

TABLETS
**Adults and adolescents over age 13.** 200 mg q 12 hr for 10 days.

➤ *To treat uncomplicated gonorrhea in men and women and rectal gonococcal infections in women caused by* Neisseria gonorrhoeae

ORAL SUSPENSION, TABLETS
**Adults.** 200 mg as a single dose.

➤ *To treat uncomplicated UTIs caused by* Escherichia coli, Klebsiella pneumoniae, Proteus mirabilis, *or* Staphylococcus saprophyticus

ORAL SUSPENSION, TABLETS
**Adults.** 100 mg q 12 hr for 7 days.

➤ *To treat skin and soft-tissue infections caused by* Staphylococcus aureus *or* Staphylococcus pyogenes

ORAL SUSPENSION, TABLETS
**Adults and adolescents over age 13.** 400 mg q 12 hr for 7 to 14 days.

➤ *To treat acute otitis media caused by* H. influenzae, M. catarrhalis, *or* S. pneumoniae

ORAL SUSPENSION, TABLETS
**Children ages 5 months through 12 years.** 5 mg/kg q 12 hr (*Maximum:* 200 mg/dose) or 10 mg/kg q 24 hr (*Maximum:* 400 mg/dose) for 10 days.

➤ *To treat pharyngitis and tonsillitis caused by* S. pyogenes

ORAL SUSPENSION, TABLETS
**Adults and adolescents over age 13.** 100 mg q 12 hr for 5 to 10 days.
**Children ages 2 months through 12 years.** 5 mg/kg q 12 hr for 5 to 10 days. *Maximum:* 100 mg/dose.

DOSAGE ADJUSTMENT Dosing interval increased to 24 hr in patients with creatinine clearance of less than 30 ml/min/1.73 m$^2$.

## Contraindications
Hypersensitivity to cephalosporins or their components

## Mechanism of Action
Interferes with bacterial cell wall synthesis by inhibiting the final step in the cross-linking of peptidoglycan strands. Peptidoglycan makes cell membranes rigid and protective. Without it, bacterial cells rupture and die.

## Interactions
DRUGS
*aminoglycosides, loop diuretics:* Increased risk of nephrotoxicity
*antacids, H$_2$-receptor antagonists:* Reduced bioavailability and blood level of cefpodoxime
*oral anticholinergics:* Delayed peak blood level of cefpodoxime
*probenecid:* Possibly increased and prolonged blood cefpodoxime level

## Adverse Reactions
**CNS:** Chills, fever, headache, seizures
**CV:** Edema
**EENT:** Hearing loss
**GI:** Abdominal cramps, diarrhea, elevated liver function test results, hepatic failure, hepatomegaly, nausea, oral candidiasis, pseudomembranous colitis, vomiting
**GU:** Elevated BUN level, nephrotoxicity, renal failure, vaginal candidiasis
**HEME:** Eosinophilia, hemolytic anemia, hypoprothrombinemia, neutropenia, thrombocytopenia, unusual bleeding
**MS:** Arthralgia
**RESP:** Dyspnea
**SKIN:** Ecchymosis, erythema, erythema multiforme, pruritus, rash, Stevens-Johnson syndrome
**Other:** Anaphylaxis, superinfection

## Nursing Considerations
• Use cefpodoxime cautiously in patients who have impaired renal function or are receiving potent diuretics. Also use drug cautiously in patients who are hypersensitive to penicillin because cross-sensitivity has occurred in 10% of such patients.
• If possible, obtain culture and sensitivity test results, as ordered, before giving drug.
• Assess bowel pattern daily; severe diarrhea may indicate pseudomembranous colitis.
• Be aware that an allergic reaction may occur a few days after therapy starts.

PATIENT TEACHING
• Urge patient to complete the prescribed course of therapy.

- Tell patient to take tablets with food to enhance absorption.
- Advise patient to refrigerate oral suspension and discard after 14 days.
- Instruct patient to shake oral suspension bottle well before pouring dose and to use a liquid-measuring device to ensure accurate doses.
- Inform patient that yogurt and buttermilk can help maintain intestinal flora and decrease diarrhea.
- Warn patient not to take an antacid within 2 hours before or after taking cefpodoxime.
- Tell patient to immediately report severe diarrhea to prescriber.

# cefprozil

Cefzil

## Class and Category

*Chemical*: Second-generation cephalosporin, 7-aminocephalosporanic acid
*Therapeutic*: Antibiotic
*Pregnancy category:* B

## Indications and Dosages

➤ *To treat secondary bacterial infections in patients with acute bronchitis and acute bacterial exacerbations of acute bronchitis caused by* Haemophilus influenzae, Moraxella catarrhalis, *and* Streptococcus pneumoniae

ORAL SUSPENSION, TABLETS
**Adults and adolescents.** 500 mg q 12 hr for 10 days.

➤ *To treat uncomplicated skin and soft-tissue infections caused by* Staphylococcus aureus *and* Streptococcus pyogenes

ORAL SUSPENSION, TABLETS
**Adults and adolescents.** 250 mg q 12 hr or 500 mg q 12 to 24 hr for 10 days.
**Children ages 2 to 12.** 20 mg/kg q 24 hr for 10 days.

➤ *To treat pharyngitis and tonsillitis caused by* S. pyogenes

ORAL SUSPENSION, TABLETS
**Adults and adolescents.** 500 mg q 24 hr for 10 days.
**Children ages 2 to 12.** 7.5 mg/kg q 12 hr for 10 days.

➤ *To treat otitis media caused by* H. influenzae, M. catarrhalis, *and* S. pneumoniae

ORAL SUSPENSION, TABLETS
**Children ages 6 months to 12 years.** 15 mg/kg q 12 hr for 10 days.

➤ *To treat acute sinusitis caused by* H. influenzae, M. catarrhalis, *and* S. pneumoniae

ORAL SUSPENSION, TABLETS
**Adults and adolescents.** 250 to 500 mg q 12 hr for 10 days.
**Children ages 6 months to 12 years.** 7.5 or 15 mg/kg q 12 hr for 10 days.
DOSAGE ADJUSTMENT Dosage reduced by half and given at usual intervals in patients with creatinine clearance of less than 30 ml/min/ 1.73 m².

## Contraindications

Hypersensitivity to cephalosporins or their components

## Mechanism of Action

Interferes with bacterial cell wall synthesis by inhibiting the final step in the cross-linking of peptidoglycan strands. Peptidoglycan makes the cell membrane rigid and protective. Without it, bacterial cells rupture and die.

## Interactions

DRUGS
*aminoglycosides, loop diuretics:* Increased risk of nephrotoxicity
*probenecid:* Increased blood cefprozil level

## Adverse Reactions

**CNS:** Chills, fever, headache, seizures
**CV:** Edema
**EENT:** Hearing loss
**GI:** Abdominal cramps, diarrhea, elevated liver function test results, hepatic failure, hepatomegaly, nausea, oral candidiasis, pseudomembranous colitis, vomiting
**GU:** Elevated BUN level, nephrotoxicity, renal failure, vaginal candidiasis
**HEME:** Eosinophilia, hemolytic anemia, hypoprothrombinemia, neutropenia, thrombocytopenia, unusual bleeding
**MS:** Arthralgia
**RESP:** Dyspnea
**SKIN:** Ecchymosis, erythema, erythema multiforme, pruritus, rash, Stevens-Johnson syndrome
**Other:** Anaphylaxis, superinfection

## Nursing Considerations

• Use cefprozil cautiously in patients with impaired renal function or a history of GI disease, especially colitis. Also use drug cautiously in patients who are hypersensitive to penicillin because cross-sensitivity has occurred in 10% of such patients.

• If possible, obtain culture and sensitivity test results, as ordered, before giving drug.

• **WARNING** Don't administer oral suspension to patients with phenylketonuria because it contains phenylalanine 28 mg/5 ml.

• Monitor BUN and serum creatinine levels to detect early signs of nephrotoxicity. Also monitor fluid intake and output; decreasing urine output may indicate nephrotoxicity.

• Be aware that an allergic reaction may occur a few days after therapy starts.

• Assess bowel pattern daily; severe diarrhea may indicate pseudomembranous colitis.

### PATIENT TEACHING

• Urge patient to complete the prescribed course of therapy.

• Tell patient to refrigerate oral suspension and discard after 14 days.

• Instruct patient to shake oral suspension bottle well before pouring and to use a liquid-measuring device to ensure accurate doses.

• Inform patient that yogurt and buttermilk can help maintain intestinal flora and decrease diarrhea.

• Tell patient to immediately report severe diarrhea to prescriber.

# ceftazidime

Ceptaz, Fortaz, Tazicef, Tazidime

## Class and Category

*Chemical*: Third-generation cephalosporin, 7-aminocephalosporanic acid
*Therapeutic*: Antibiotic
*Pregnancy category*: B

## Indications and Dosages

➤ *To treat infections caused by gram-negative organisms (including* Acinetobacter, Citrobacter, Enterobacter, Escherichia coli, Haemophilus influenzae, Klebsiella, Neisseria, Proteus mirabilis, Proteus vulgaris, Pseudomonas aeruginosa, Salmonella, Serratia, *and* Shigella*), gram-positive organisms (including* Streptococcus agalactiae, Streptococcus pneu-

moniae, *and* Streptococcus pyogenes *[group B streptococci]), as well as* Staphylococcus aureus *(penicillinase- and non-penicillinase-producing strains)*

**I.V. INFUSION, I.M. INJECTION**
**Adults and children age 12 and older.** 1 g q 8 to 12 hr.

**I.V. INFUSION**
**Children ages 1 month to 12 years.** 30 to 50 mg/kg q 8 hr.
**Neonates up to age 1 month.** 30 mg/kg q 12 hr. *Maximum:* 6 g/day.

➤ *To treat uncomplicated UTIs*

**I.V. INFUSION, I.M. INJECTION**
**Adults and children age 12 and older.** 250 mg q 12 hr.

➤ *To treat complicated UTIs*

**I.V. INFUSION, I.M. INJECTION**
**Adults and children age 12 and older.** 500 mg q 8 to 12 hr.

➤ *To treat uncomplicated pneumonia and mild skin and soft-tissue infections*

**I.V. INFUSION, I.M. INJECTION**
**Adults and children age 12 and older.** 0.5 to 1 g q 8 hr.

➤ *To treat bone and joint infections*

**I.V. INFUSION**
**Adults and children age 12 and older.** 2 g q 12 hr.

➤ *To treat serious gynecologic and intra-abdominal infections, meningitis, and life-threatening infections, especially in immunocompromised patients*

**I.V. INFUSION**
**Adults and children age 12 and older.** 2 g q 8 hr.

➤ *To treat pseudomonal lung infection in patients with cystic fibrosis and normal renal function*

**I.V. INFUSION**
**Adults and children age 1 month and older.** 30 to 50 mg/kg q 8 hr. *Maximum:* 6 g/day.
**Neonates up to age 1 month.** 30 mg/kg q 12 hr.

**DOSAGE ADJUSTMENT** Dosage reduced to 1 g q 12 hr if creatinine clearance is 31 to 50 ml/min/1.73 m$^2$; to 1 g q 24 hr if 16 to 30 ml/min/1.73 m$^2$; to 0.5 g q 24 hr if 6 to 15 ml/min/1.73 m$^2$; and to 0.5 g q 48 hr if less than 6 ml/min/1.73 m$^2$.

## Incompatibilities

Don't mix ceftazidime with aminoglycosides to prevent mutual inactivation. Vancomycin is physically incompatible with ceftazidime (precipitate may form); flush I.V. line between these drugs if given through same tubing. Avoid mixing ceftazidime with other drugs, including pentamidine isethionate.

## Mechanism of Action

Interferes with bacterial cell wall synthesis by inhibiting the cross-linking of peptidoglycan strands. Peptidoglycan makes the cell membrane rigid and protective. Without it, bacterial cells rupture and die.

## Contraindications

Hypersensitivity to cephalosporins or their components

## Interactions

**DRUGS**
*aminoglycosides, loop diuretics:* Increased risk of nephrotoxicity

## Adverse Reactions

**CNS:** Chills, fever, headache, seizures
**CV:** Edema
**EENT:** Hearing loss
**GI:** Abdominal cramps, diarrhea, elevated liver function test results, hepatic failure, hepatomegaly, nausea, oral candidiasis, pseudomembranous colitis, vomiting
**GU:** Elevated BUN level, nephrotoxicity, renal failure, vaginal candidiasis
**HEME:** Eosinophilia, hemolytic anemia, hypoprothrombinemia, neutropenia, thrombocytopenia, unusual bleeding
**MS:** Arthralgia
**RESP:** Dyspnea
**SKIN:** Ecchymosis, erythema, erythema multiforme, pruritus, rash, Stevens-Johnson syndrome
**Other:** Anaphylaxis; injection site pain, redness, and swelling; superinfection

## Nursing Considerations

• Use ceftazidime cautiously in patients hypersensitive to penicillin because cross-sensitivity occurs in 10% of them. Watch for allergic reactions a few days after therapy starts.
• Use cautiously in patients with a history of GI disease, particularly colitis, because risk of pseudomembranous colitis is increased.
• Know that ceftazidime L-arginine (Ceptaz) is not recommended for children under age 12.
• If possible, obtain culture and sensitivity test results, as ordered, before giving drug.

• Protect ceftazidime powder and reconstituted drug from heat and light; both tend to darken during storage.
• If pharmacy delivers frozen solution, thaw it at room temperature, not in water bath or microwave. Store thawed solution for up to 12 hours at room temperature or 7 days in refrigerator; don't refreeze.
• **WARNING** When preparing drug for neonates or immature infants, don't use diluents containing benzyl alcohol because they are linked to a fatal toxic syndrome.
• For I.V. bolus, reconstitute 1 to 2 g with 10 ml sterile water for injection, $D_5W$, or sodium chloride for injection. Shake to dissolve. Administer I.V. injection slowly over 3 to 5 minutes through tubing of a flowing compatible I.V. fluid.
• For intermittent infusion, further dilute in 50 to 100 ml of $D_5W$ or NS. Avoid using sodium bicarbonate injection as a diluent because drug is least stable in it. During ceftazidime administration, temporarily stop other solutions being given at the same I.V. site.
• For I.M. use, reconstitute each gram with 3 ml sterile water for injection or bacteriostatic water for injection.
• Give I.M. injection deep into large muscle mass, such as gluteus maximus.
• Rotate I.V. sites every 72 hours. Assess for phlebitis and extravasation.
• Assess bowel pattern daily; severe diarrhea may indicate pseudomembranous colitis.
• Monitor CBC, hematocrit, and serum AST, ALT, bilirubin, LD, and alkaline phosphatase levels during long-term therapy.
• Monitor PT, as ordered, in at-risk patients, such as those with renal or hepatic impairment or poor nutritional state and those receiving anticoagulant or prolonged antibiotic therapy. Notify prescriber if PT decreases, and expect to give vitamin K.
• Assess for perineal itching, fever, malaise, redness, swelling, rash, and change in cough or sputum; they may indicate a superinfection.
• Watch for pharyngitis, ecchymosis, bleeding, and arthralgia (possible blood dyscrasia). Monitor PT and bleeding time.

**PATIENT TEACHING**
• Tell patient to take ceftazidine exactly as prescribed.
• Urge patient to report severe diarrhea or signs of blood dyscrasia or superinfection.

# ceftibuten

Cedax

## Class and Category

*Chemical*: Third-generation cephalosporin, 7-aminocephalosporanic acid
*Therapeutic*: Antibiotic
*Pregnancy category:* B

## Indications and Dosages

➤ *To treat acute bacterial exacerbations of chronic bronchitis caused by* Haemophilus influenzae, Moraxella catarrhalis, *or* Streptococcus pneumoniae; *pharyngitis and tonsillitis caused by* Streptococcus pyogenes; *and acute bacterial otitis media caused* by H. influenzae, M. catarrhalis, *or* S. pneumoniae

**CAPSULES, ORAL SUSPENSION**

**Adults and children age 12 and older.** 400 mg q.d. for 10 days.

➤ *To treat pharyngitis and tonsillitis caused by* S. pyogenes *and acute bacterial otitis media caused* by H. influenzae, M. catarrhalis, *or* S. pneumoniae

**ORAL SUSPENSION**

**Children under age 12.** 9 mg/kg q.d. for 10 days. *Maximum:* 400 mg/day.

**DOSAGE ADJUSTMENT** Dosage reduced to 4.5 mg/kg or 200 mg q 24 hr if creatinine clearance is 30 to 49 ml/min/1.73 m$^2$; to 2.25 mg/kg or 100 mg q 24 hr if it's 5 to 29 ml/min/1.73 m$^2$.

---

### Mechanism of Action

Interferes with bacterial cell wall synthesis by inhibiting the cross-linking of peptidoglycan strands. Peptidoglycan makes the cell membrane rigid and protective. Without it, bacterial cells rupture and die.

---

## Contraindications

Hypersensitivity to cephalosporins or their components

## Interactions

**DRUGS**

*aminoglycosides, loop diuretics:* Increased risk of nephrotoxicity

## Adverse Reactions

**CNS:** Chills, fever, headache, seizures
**CV:** Edema
**EENT:** Hearing loss

**GI:** Abdominal cramps, diarrhea, elevated liver function test results, hepatic failure, hepatomegaly, nausea, oral candidiasis, pseudomembranous colitis, vomiting
**GU:** Elevated BUN level, nephrotoxicity, renal failure, vaginal candidiasis
**HEME:** Eosinophilia, hemolytic anemia, hypoprothrombinemia, neutropenia, thrombocytopenia, unusual bleeding
**MS:** Arthralgia
**RESP:** Dyspnea
**SKIN:** Ecchymosis, erythema, erythema multiforme, pruritus, rash, Stevens-Johnson syndrome
**Other:** Anaphylaxis, superinfection

## Nursing Considerations

• Use ceftibuten cautiously in patients hypersensitive to penicillins because cross-sensitivity occurs in up to 10% of such patients.
• If possible, obtain culture and sensitivity test results, as ordered, before giving drug.
• Refrigerate oral suspension; shake well before using. Discard after 14 days.
• Monitor BUN and serum creatinine levels to detect early signs of nephrotoxicity. Also, monitor fluid intake and output; decreasing urine output may indicate nephrotoxicity.
• Be aware that an allergic reaction may occur a few days after therapy starts.
• Assess bowel pattern daily; severe diarrhea may indicate pseudomembranous colitis.
• Assess for perineal itching, fever, malaise, redness, swelling, rash, and change in cough or sputum; they may indicate a superinfection.
• Assess for pharyngitis, ecchymosis, bleeding, and arthralgia; they may indicate a blood dyscrasia.

**PATIENT TEACHING**

• Urge patient to complete the drug therapy.
• Instruct patient to take drug on an empty stomach at least 2 hours before or 1 hour after meals.
• Inform patient that unflavored oral suspension has a bitter taste. Suggest that he ask that a flavor be added when prescription is filled.
• Advise patient that yogurt and buttermilk can help maintain intestinal flora and decrease diarrhea during therapy.
• Tell patient to immediately report hypersensitivity reactions, severe diarrhea, and evidence of blood dyscrasia or superinfection to prescriber.

# ceftizoxime sodium

Cefizox

## Class and Category

*Chemical:* Third-generation cephalosporin,
7-aminocephalosporanic acid
*Therapeutic:* Antibiotic
*Pregnancy category:* B

## Indications and Dosages

➤ *To treat mild to moderate infections of the*
*lower respiratory tract, skin, soft tissue,*
*bones, and joints; septicemia; meningitis;*
*and intra-abdominal infections caused by*
*anaerobes (such as* Bacteroides *sp.,* Peptococcus, *and* Peptostreptococcus*), gram-*
*negative organisms (including* Escherichia
coli, Haemophilus influenzae, Klebsiella,
*and* Proteus mirabilis*), and gram-positive*
*organisms (including* Enterobacter *sp.,*
Serratia *sp.,* Staphylococcus aureus,
Staphylococcus epidermidis, Streptococcus agalactiae, Streptococcus pneumoniae,
*and* Streptococcus pyogenes*)*

**I.V. INFUSION, I.V. OR I.M. INJECTION**

**Adults and children age 12 and older.** 1 to
2 g q 8 to 12 hr.

➤ *To treat severe or refractory infections*
*of the type listed above*

**I.V. INFUSION OR INJECTION**

**Adults and children age 12 and older.** 1 g q
8 hr or 2 g q 8 to 12 hr.

➤ *To treat life-threatening infections of the*
*type listed above*

**I.V. INFUSION OR INJECTION**

**Adults and children age 12 and older.** 3 to 4 g
q 8 hr or, if required, up to 2 g q 4 hr.

➤ *To treat bacterial infections in children*

**I.V. INFUSION, I.V. OR I.M. INJECTION**

**Children age 6 months and older.** 50 mg/kg q
6 to 8 hr.

➤ *To treat uncomplicated UTIs*

**I.V. INFUSION, I.V. OR I.M. INJECTION**

**Adults.** 500 mg q 12 hr.

➤ *To treat pelvic inflammatory disease*

**I.V. INFUSION OR INJECTION**

**Adults.** 2 g q 8 hr.

➤ *To treat uncomplicated gonococcal infec-*
*tions*

**I.M. INJECTION**

**Adults.** 1 g as a single dose.

**DOSAGE ADJUSTMENT** Dosage reduced to 0.5 g
q 8 hr for less severe infections and 0.75 to
1.5 g q 8 hr for life-threatening infections if
creatinine clearance is 50 to 79 ml/min/1.73 m$^2$;
to 0.25 to 0.5 g q 12 hr for less severe infections and 0.5 to 1 g q 12 for life-threatening
infections if creatinine clearance is 5 to
49 ml/min/1.73 m$^2$; and to 0.5 g q 48 hr or
0.25 g q 24 hr for less severe infections and
0.5 to 1 g q 48 hr or 0.5 g q 24 hr for life-
threatening infections if creatinine clearance
is 4 ml/min/1.73 m$^2$ or less.

## Mechanism of Action

Interferes with bacterial cell wall synthesis by inhibiting the final step in the
cross-linking of peptidoglycan strands.
Peptidoglycan makes the cell membrane
rigid and protective. Without it, bacterial
cells rupture and die.

## Contraindications

Hypersensitivity to cephalosporins or their
components

## Interactions

**DRUGS**

*aminoglycosides, loop diuretics:* Increased
risk of nephrotoxicity

## Adverse Reactions

**CNS:** Chills, fever, headache, seizures
**CV:** Edema
**EENT:** Hearing loss
**GI:** Abdominal cramps, diarrhea, elevated
liver function test results, hepatic failure, hepatomegaly, nausea, oral candidiasis, pseudomembranous colitis, vomiting
**GU:** Elevated BUN level, nephrotoxicity,
renal failure, vaginal candidiasis
**HEME:** Eosinophilia, hemolytic anemia, hypoprothrombinemia, neutropenia, thrombocytopenia, unusual bleeding
**MS:** Arthralgia
**RESP:** Dyspnea
**SKIN:** Ecchymosis, erythema, erythema multiforme, pruritus, rash, Stevens-Johnson syndrome
**Other:** Anaphylaxis; injection site pain, redness, and swelling; superinfection

## Nursing Considerations

•Use ceftizoxime cautiously in patients who are
hypersensitive to penicillin because cross-sensitivity has occurred in 10% of such patients.

•If possible, obtain culture and sensitivity test results, as ordered, before giving drug.
•For I.V. administration, reconstitute with sterile water for injection as follows: for 500-mg vial, add 5 ml; for 1-g vial, add 10 ml; and for 2-g vial, add 20 ml. Shake well. Dilute reconstituted solution further with 50 to 100 ml of a compatible solution, such as NS or $D_5W$, before administration. Administer I.V. injection slowly over 3 to 5 minutes through tubing of a flowing compatible I.V. fluid.
•For I.M. administration, reconstitute with sterile water for injection as follows: for 500-mg vial, add 1.5 ml; for 1-g vial, add 3 ml; and for 2-g vial, add 6 ml. Shake well. Divide 2-g doses and administer in different sites. Inject deeply in large muscle mass, such as the gluteus maximus.
•Reconstituted drug may be stored for 24 hours at room temperature or 96 hours if refrigerated.
•Assess I.V. site for extravasation and phlebitis.
•Monitor BUN and serum creatinine levels to detect early signs of nephrotoxicity. Also, monitor fluid intake and output; decreasing urine output may indicate nephrotoxicity.
•Assess bowel pattern daily; severe diarrhea may indicate pseudomembranous colitis.
•Monitor for allergic reactions a few days after therapy starts.
•Assess CBC, hematocrit, and serum AST, ALT, bilirubin, LD, and alkaline phosphatase levels during long-term therapy.
•Assess for pharyngitis, ecchymosis, bleeding, and arthralgia; they may indicate a blood dyscrasia.

**PATIENT TEACHING**
•Advise patient to immediately report severe diarrhea or evidence of blood dyscrasia to prescriber.

# ceftriaxone sodium

Rocephin

## Class and Category

*Chemical*: Third-generation cephalosporin, 7-aminocephalosporanic acid
*Therapeutic*: Antibiotic
*Pregnancy category*: B

## Indications and Dosages

➤ *To treat infections of the lower respiratory tract, skin, soft tissue, urinary tract, bones, and joints; sinusitis; intra-abdominal infections; and septicemia caused by anaerobes (including* Bacteroides bivius,

Bacteroides fragilis, Bacteroides melaninogenicus, *and* Peptostreptococcus *sp.), gram-negative organisms (including* Citrobacter *sp.,* Enterobacter aerogenes, Escherichia coli, Haemophilus influenzae, Klebsiella *sp.,* Neisseria *sp.,* Proteus mirabilis, Proteus vulgaris, Providencia *sp.,* Salmonella *sp.,* Serratia marcescens, Shigella, *and some strains of* Pseudomonas aeruginosa*), and gram-positive organisms (including* Staphylococcus aureus, Streptococcus pneumoniae, *and* Streptococcus pyogenes*)*

**I.V. INFUSION, I.M. INJECTION**
**Adults.** 1 to 2 g q.d. or in equally divided doses b.i.d. *Maximum:* 4 g/day.
**Children.** 50 to 75 mg/kg/day in divided doses q 12 hr. *Maximum:* 2 g/day.
➤ *To treat meningitis*
**I.V. INFUSION**
**Children.** *Initial:* 100 mg/kg on first day, then 100 mg/kg q.d. or in divided doses q 12 hr for 7 to 14 days. *Maximum:* 4 g/day.
➤ *To treat acute bacterial otitis media*
**I.M. INJECTION**
**Children.** 50 mg/kg as a single dose. *Maximum:* 1 g.
➤ *To treat chancroid (Haemophilus ducreyi infection) and uncomplicated gonorrhea*
**I.M. INJECTION**
**Adults.** 250 mg as a single dose.
➤ *To treat gonococcal conjunctivitis*
**I.M. INJECTION**
**Adults.** 1 g as a single dose.
➤ *To treat disseminated gonoccocal infection and pelvic inflammatory disease*
**I.V. INFUSION, I.M. INJECTION**
**Adults:** 1 g q 24 hr.
➤ *To treat gonococcal meningitis and endocarditis*
**I.V. INFUSION**
**Adults.** 1 to 2 g q 12 hr for 10 to 14 days (meningitis) or for 4 wk or longer (endocarditis).
➤ *To provide surgical prophylaxis*
**I.V. INFUSION**
**Adults.** 1 g 30 min to 2 hr before surgery.

## Incompatibilities

Don't admix ceftriaxone with pentamidine isethionate, labetalol, or other antibiotics, such as aminoglycosides, because of potential for incompatibility, such as substantial mutual inactivation.

> *To treat acute otitis media*

**ORAL SUSPENSION**

**Children ages 3 months to 12 years.** 30 mg/kg/day in equally divided doses b.i.d. for 10 days. *Maximum:* 1,000 mg/day.

**TABLETS**

**Children under age 13 who can swallow tablets.** 250 mg b.i.d. for 10 days.

> *To treat impetigo*

**ORAL SUSPENSION**

**Children ages 3 months to 12 years.** 30 mg/kg/day in equally divided doses b.i.d. for 10 days. *Maximum:* 1,000 mg/day.

> *To treat acute bacterial maxillary sinusitis*

**ORAL SUSPENSION**

**Children ages 3 months to 12 years.** 30 mg/kg/day in equally divided doses b.i.d. for 10 days. *Maximum:* 1,000 mg/day.

**TABLETS**

**Adults and children age 13 and older and children under age 13 who can swallow tablets.** 250 mg b.i.d. for 10 days.

> *To treat acute bacterial exacerbations of chronic bronchitis and uncomplicated skin and soft-tissue infections*

**TABLETS**

**Adults and children age 13 and older.** 250 to 500 mg b.i.d. for 10 days.

**I.V. INFUSION, I.V. OR I.M. INJECTION**

**Adults.** 750 mg q 8 hr.

> *To treat secondary bacterial infection in patients with acute bronchitis*

**Adults and children age 13 and older.** 250 to 500 mg b.i.d. for 5 to 10 days.

> *To treat early Lyme disease*

**TABLETS**

**Adults and children age 13 and older.** 500 mg b.i.d. for 20 days.

> *To treat uncomplicated UTIs*

**TABLETS**

**Adults.** 125 to 250 mg b.i.d. for 7 to 10 days.

**I.V. INFUSION, I.V. OR I.M. INJECTION**

**Adults.** 750 mg q 8 hr.

> *To treat uncomplicated gonorrhea*

**TABLETS**

**Adults.** 1 g as a single dose.

**I.M. INJECTION**

**Adults.** 1.5 g as a single dose divided equally and injected into two different sites; given with oral probenecid 1 g.

> *To treat disseminated gonococcal infection and uncomplicated pneumonia*

**I.V. INFUSION, I.V. OR I.M. INJECTION**

**Adults.** 750 mg q 8 hr.

> *To treat bone and joint infections*

**I.V. INFUSION, I.V. OR I.M. INJECTION**

**Adults.** 1.5 g q 8 hr.

**Children over age 3 months.** 50 to 150 mg/kg/day in divided doses q 8 hr. *Maximum:* Adult dose.

> *To treat bacterial meningitis*

**I.V. INFUSION**

**Adults.** 1.5 to 3 g q 8 hr..

**Children over age 1 month.** 50 to 80 mg/kg q 6 to 8 hr.

**Neonates up to age 1 month.** 33.3 to 50 mg/kg q 8 to 12 hr.

> *To treat moderate infections other than those listed above*

**I.V. INFUSION, I.V. OR I.M. INJECTION**

**Adults.** 750 mg q 8 hr for 5 to 10 days.

**I.V. INFUSION OR INJECTION**

**Children over age 3 months.** 50 mg/kg/day in equally divided doses q 6 to 8 hr.

> *To treat severe or complicated infections other than those listed above*

**I.V. INFUSION OR INJECTION**

**Adults.** 1.5 g q 8 hr.

**Children over age 3 months.** 100 mg/kg/day in equally divided doses q 6 to 8 hr.

> *To treat life-threatening infections other than those listed above*

**I.V. INFUSION OR INJECTION**

**Adults.** 1.5 g q 6 hr.

> *To provide perioperative prophylaxis*

**I.V. INFUSION OR INJECTION**

**Adults.** 1.5 g 30 to 60 min before surgery (at induction of anesthesia for open-heart surgery), and then 0.75 g q 8 hr thereafter (1.5 g q 12 hr for total of 6 g with open-heart surgery).

**DOSAGE ADJUSTMENT** Parenteral dosage reduced to 0.75 g q 12 hr if creatinine clearance is 10 to 20 ml/min/1.73 m$^2$ or to 0.75 g q 24 hr if less than 10 ml/min/1.73 m$^2$.

## Incompatibilities

Don't admix parenteral cefuroxime with other antibiotics, such as aminoglycosides, because of potential for incompatibility, such as substantial mutual inactivation. If they're administered concurrently, don't mix them in the same I.V. bag or bottle.

## Contraindications

Hypersensitivity to cephalosporins or their components

## Mechanism of Action
Interferes with bacterial cell wall synthesis by inhibiting the final step in the cross-linking of peptidoglycan strands. Peptidoglycan makes the cell membrane rigid and protective. Without it, bacterial cells rupture and die.

## Interactions
**DRUGS**
*aminoglycosides, loop diuretics:* Increased risk of nephrotoxicity
*antacids, H₂-receptor antagonists, omeprazole:* Decreased cefuroxime axetil absorption
*probenecid:* Increased and prolonged blood cefuroxime level

## Adverse Reactions
**CNS:** Chills, fever, headache, seizures
**CV:** Edema
**EENT:** Hearing loss, oral candidiasis
**GI:** Abdominal cramps, diarrhea, elevated liver function test results, hepatic failure, hepatomegaly, nausea, pseudomembranous colitis, vomiting
**GU:** Elevated BUN level, nephrotoxicity, renal failure, vaginal candidiasis
**HEME:** Eosinophilia, hemolytic anemia, hypoprothrombinemia, neutropenia, thrombocytopenia, unusual bleeding
**MS:** Arthralgia
**RESP:** Dyspnea
**SKIN:** Ecchymosis, erythema, erythema multiforme, pruritus, rash, Stevens-Johnson syndrome
**Other:** Anaphylaxis; injection site edema, pain, and redness; superinfection

## Nursing Considerations
• Use cefuroxime cautiously in patients hypersensitive to penicillin because cross-sensitivity has occurred in 10% of such patients.
• If possible, obtain culture and sensitivity results, as ordered, before giving drug.
• Give oral form with food to decrease GI distress, as needed.
• Remember that oral forms—tablets and suspension—aren't bioequi1valent.
• For I.V. use, reconstitute following manufacturer's instructions according to type of preparation available. Solution ranges in color from light yellow to amber.
• For I.M. use, add 3 or 3.6 ml of sterile water for injection to each 750-mg vial to yield 220 mg/ml.

• If using a container of frozen parenteral solution, thaw at room temperature or under refrigeration before administration; make sure all ice crystals have melted. Don't force thawing by microwave irradiation.
• Store reconstituted parenteral drug for up to 24 hours at room temperature or 96 hours in refrigerator. (Thawed solutions may be stable for 24 hours at room temperature or 28 days if refrigerated.) Store reconstituted oral suspension in refrigerator or at room temperature for up to 10 days.
• Administer I.V. injection over 3 to 5 minutes through tubing of a flowing compatible I.V. fluid.
• Monitor I.V. site for extravasation and phlebitis.
• Monitor patient's BUN and serum creatinine levels and fluid intake and output to detect signs of nephrotoxicity. Monitor patients with renal impairment closely because they may have greater toxic reactions to cefuroxime.
• Monitor patient for allergic reactions continuing up to a few days after therapy starts. Patients with a history of some form of allergy, especially to drugs, are at increased risk for an allergic reaction.
• Assess bowel pattern daily; severe diarrhea may indicate pseudomembranous colitis. If it's suspected, stop drug, as ordered, and provide treatment as prescribed.
• Assess patient for pharyngitis, ecchymosis, bleeding, and arthralgia, which may indicate a blood dyscrasia.
• Monitor PT and bleeding time, as ordered. Be prepared to administer vitamin K, if ordered, to treat hypothrombinemia.

**PATIENT TEACHING**
• Instruct patient to shake oral suspension well before measuring each dose and to use an accurate liquid-measuring device for each dose.
• Advise patient using single-dose packets of oral suspension to empty the contents of one packet into a glass and add at least 10 ml (2 tsp) of cold water; apple, grape, or orange juice; or lemonade. Tell him to stir well and consume entire mixture at once.
• Inform patient that yogurt and buttermilk help maintain intestinal flora and can decrease diarrhea during therapy.
• Instruct patient to immediately report to prescriber severe diarrhea or evidence of blood dyscrasia.

# celecoxib

Celebrex

## Class and Category

*Chemical:* Diaryl-substituted pyrazole derivative
*Therapeutic:* Anti-inflammatory, antirheumatic
*Pregnancy category:* C

## Indications and Dosages

➤ *To relieve pain from osteoarthritis*
**CAPSULES**
**Adults.** 200 mg q.d. or 100 mg b.i.d.
➤ *To relieve pain from rheumatoid arthritis*
**CAPSULES**
**Adults.** 100 to 200 mg b.i.d.
➤ *To relieve pain from ankylosing spondylitis*
**CAPSULES**
**Adults.** 200 mg q.d. or 100 mg b.i.d. Dosage increased to 400 mg q.d. or 200 mg b.i.d. after 6 weeks if needed.
➤ *As adjunct to reduce adenomatous colorectal polyps in patients with familial adenomatous polyposis*
**CAPSULES**
**Adults.** 400 mg b.i.d.
➤ *To manage acute pain, to treat primary dysmenorrhea*
**CAPSULES**
**Adults.** 400 mg, followed by 200 mg if needed, on 1st day. On subsequent days, 200 mg b.i.d. as needed.
**DOSAGE ADJUSTMENT** Daily dosage reduced for patients with hepatic impairment. For patients weighing less than 50 kg (110 lb), expect to begin therapy with lowest recommended dose.

## Contraindications

Allergic reaction (such as anaphylaxis or angioedema) to aspirin, other NSAIDs, or sulfonamide derivatives or history of aspirin-induced nasal polyps with bronchospasm; hypersensitivity to celecoxib or its components; treatment of perioperative pain after coronary artery bypass graft surgery

## Interactions

**DRUGS**
*ACE inhibitors:* Decreased antihypertensive effect of ACE inhibitors, increased risk of renal failure
*aspirin:* Increased risk of GI ulceration and other GI complications
*fluconazole:* Increased blood celecoxib level
*furosemide, thiazide diuretics:* Reduced diuretic effects of these drugs, increased risk of renal failure
*lithium:* Possibly elevated blood lithium level
*warfarin:* Possibly increased PT and risk of bleeding

## Mechanism of Action

Selectively inhibits the enzymatic activity of cyclooxygenase-2 (COX-2), the enzyme needed to convert arachidonic acid to prostaglandin. Prostaglandins are responsible for mediating the inflammatory response and causing local vasodilation, swelling, and pain. Prostaglandins also play a role in peripheral pain transmission to the spinal cord. By inhibiting COX-2 activity and prostaglandin production, this NSAID reduces inflammatory symptoms and relieves pain. Celecoxib's mechanism of action in reducing the number of colorectal polyps is unknown.

## Adverse Reactions

**CNS:** Asceptic meningitis, cerebral hemorrhage, dizziness, headache, insomnia, ischemic CVA, transient ischemic attacks
**CV:** Deep vein thrombosis, fluid retention, hypertension, MI, peripheral edema, unstable angina, vasculitis
**EENT:** Pharyngitis, rhinitis, sinusitis
**ENDO:** Hypoglycemia
**GI:** Abdominal pain, bleeding or ulceration, diarrhea, elevated liver function test results, flatulence, hepatic failure, indigestion, jaundice, nausea, perforation of stomach or intestine, vomiting
**GU:** Acute renal failure, interstitial nephritis
**HEME:** Agranulocytosis, aplastic anemia, leukopenia, pancytopenia, thrombocytopenia
**MS:** Back pain
**RESP:** Pulmonary embolism, upper respiratory tract infection
**SKIN:** Erythema multiforme, exfoliative dermatitis, rash, Stevens-Johnson syndrome, toxic epidermal necrolysis
**Other:** Anaphylaxis, angioedema, hyponatremia

## Nursing Considerations

•Use celecoxib with extreme caution in patients who have a history of ulcer disease or GI bleeding because NSAIDs, such as celecoxib, increase the risk of GI bleeding and ulceration. In these patients, drug should be used for the shortest time possible.

•Be aware that serious GI tract ulceration and bleeding as well as perforation of the stomach or intestine can occur without warning or symptoms. Elderly patients are at greatest risk. To minimize this risk, give celecoxib with food. If patient develops GI distress, withhold celecoxib and notify prescriber immediately.

•Use celecoxib cautiously in patients with hypertension, and monitor blood pressure closely throughout therapy because drug can start or worsen hypertension.

•WARNING Monitor patient closely for thrombotic events, including MI and CVA, because use of NSAIDs, such as celecoxib, increases the risk.

•WARNING In patient who has bone marrow suppression or is receiving antineoplastic drug therapy, monitor laboratory results (including WBC) and assess for signs and symptoms of infection because celecoxib has anti-inflammatory and antipyretic actions that may mask signs and symptoms, such as fever and pain.

•Monitor patient—especially if he's elderly or receiving long-term celecoxib therapy— for less common but serious adverse GI reactions, including anorexia, constipation, diverticulitis, dysphagia, esophagitis, gastritis, gastroenteritis, gastroesophageal reflux disease, hemorrhoids, hiatal hernia, melena, stomatitis, and vomiting.

•Monitor liver function test results because, in rare cases, elevations may progress to severe hepatic reactions, including fatal hepatitis, hepatic necrosis, and hepatic failure.

•Monitor BUN and serum creatinine levels in elderly patients, patients taking diuretics or ACE inhibitors, and patients with heart failure, impaired renal function, or hepatic dysfunction because drug may cause renal failure.

•Monitor CBC for decreased hemoglobin level and hematocrit because drug may worsen anemia.

•Assess patient's skin regularly for signs of rash or other hypersensitivity reaction because celecoxib is a sulfur drug and may cause serious skin reactions without warning, even in patients with no history of sensivity to sulfur. At first sign of reaction, stop drug and notify prescriber.

**PATIENT TEACHING**

•Instruct patient to swallow celecoxib capsules whole with a full glass of water and with food or milk to prevent stomach upset.

•Advise patient to notify prescriber if pain continues or is poorly controlled.

•Explain that celecoxib may increase the risk of serious adverse CV events; urge patient to seek immediate medical attention if signs or symptoms arise, such as chest pain, shortness of breath, slurred speech, and weakness.

•Tell patient that celecoxib may also increase the risk of serious adverse GI reactions. Stress the need to seek immediate medical attention if signs or symptoms develop, such as epigastric or abdominal pain, indigestion, black or tarry stools, and vomiting blood or material that resembles coffee grounds.

•Alert patient that celecoxib may cause serious skin reactions. Advise seeking immediate medical attention if signs or symptoms develop, such as rash, blisters, fever, itching, or other evidence of hypersensitivity.

•Urge patient to avoid smoking and alcohol during celecoxib therapy because they may increase the risk of adverse GI reactions.

# cephalexin hydrochloride

Keftab

## cephalexin monohydrate

Apo-Cephalex (CAN), Keflex, Novo-Lexin (CAN), Nu-Cephalex (CAN), PMS-Cephalexin (CAN)

## Class and Category

*Chemical:* First-generation cephalosporin, 7-aminocephalosporanic acid
*Therapeutic:* Antibiotic
*Pregnancy category:* B

## Indications and Dosages

➤ *To treat streptococcal tonsillitis, pharyngitis, and skin and soft-tissue infections*

**CAPSULES, ORAL SUSPENSION, TABLETS**

**Adults and adolescents age 15 and older.**
500 mg q 12 hr. *Maximum:* 4 g/day.

**Children and adolescents ages 2 to 15.** 25 to 50 mg/kg/day divided into two equal doses and given q 12 hr. If infection is severe, dose may be doubled.

➤ *To treat mild to moderate respiratory tract, skin, soft-tissue, bone, and GU infections caused by susceptible organisms other than streptococci*

**CAPSULES, ORAL SUSPENSION, TABLETS**

**Adults.** 250 mg q 6 hr.

## Mechanism of Action

Like all cephalosporins, cephalexin interferes with bacterial cell wall synthesis by inhibiting the final step in the cross-linking of peptidoglycan strands. Peptidoglycan makes the cell membrane rigid and protective. Without it, bacterial cells rupture and die. This mechanism of action is most effective against bacteria that divide rapidly, including many gram-positive and gram-negative bacteria.

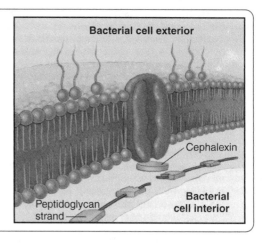

Bacterial cell exterior

Cephalexin

Peptidoglycan strand

Bacterial cell interior

ORAL SUSPENSION

**Children.** 25 to 50 mg/kg/day in equally divided doses b.i.d. or q.i.d.

➤ *To treat severe respiratory tract, skin, soft-tissue, bone, and GU infections*

CAPSULES, ORAL SUSPENSION, TABLETS

**Adults.** 0.5 to 1 g q 6 hr. *Maximum:* 4 g/day.
**Children.** 50 to 100 mg/kg/day in equally divided doses q.i.d.z

➤ *To treat otitis media*

ORAL SUSPENSION

**Children.** 75 to 100 mg/kg/day in equally divided doses q.i.d.

➤ *To treat uncomplicated cystitis*

CAPSULES, ORAL SUSPENSION, TABLETS

**Adults and adolescents age 15 and older.**
500 mg q 12 hr.

## Contraindications

Hypersensitivity to cephalosporins or their components

## Interactions

DRUGS

*aminoglycosides, loop diuretics:* Increased risk of nephrotoxicity
*probenecid:* Increased and prolonged blood cephalexin level

## Adverse Reactions

**CNS:** Chills, fever, headache, seizures
**CV:** Edema
**EENT:** Hearing loss
**GI:** Abdominal cramps, diarrhea, elevated liver function test results, hepatic failure, hepatomegaly, nausea, oral candidiasis, pseudomembranous colitis, vomiting
**GU:** Elevated BUN level, nephrotoxicity, renal failure, vaginal candidiasis
**HEME:** Eosinophilia, hemolytic anemia, hypoprothrombinemia, neutropenia, thrombocytopenia, unusual bleeding
**MS:** Arthralgia
**RESP:** Dyspnea
**SKIN:** Ecchymosis, erythema, erythema multiforme, pruritus, rash, Stevens-Johnson syndrome
**Other:** Anaphylaxis, superinfection

## Nursing Considerations

•Use cephalexin cautiously in patients who are hypersensitive to penicillin because cross-sensitivity has occurred in about 10% of such patients.
•If possible, obtain culture and sensitivity test results, as ordered, before giving drug.
•Monitor BUN and serum creatinine levels to detect early signs of nephrotoxicity. Also, monitor fluid intake and output; decreasing urine output may indicate nephrotoxicity.
•Monitor for allergic reactions a few days after therapy starts.
•Assess CBC, hematocrit, and serum AST, ALT, bilirubin, LD, and alkaline phosphatase levels during long-term therapy.
•Assess patient's bowel pattern daily; severe diarrhea may indicate pseudomembranous colitis.
•Assess patient for pharyngitis, ecchymosis, bleeding, and arthralgia; they may indicate a blood dyscrasia.

C

PATIENT TEACHING
•Advise patient to complete prescribed course of therapy.
•Instruct patient to shake oral suspension well before measuring each dose and to use a liquid-measuring device to ensure an accurate dose.
•Tell patient that yogurt and buttermilk can help maintain intestinal flora and decrease diarrhea during therapy.
•Instruct patient to immediately report severe diarrhea to prescriber.

# cephapirin sodium

Cefadyl

## Class and Category

*Chemical*: First-generation cephalosporin, 7-aminocephalosporanic acid
*Therapeutic*: Antibiotic
*Pregnancy category*: B

## Indications and Dosages

➤ *To treat respiratory tract infections, skin and soft-tissue infections, UTIs, septicemia, endocarditis, and osteomyelitis caused by gram-negative organisms (including* Escherichia coli, Haemophilus influenzae, Klebsiella *sp., and* Proteus mirabilis) *and gram-positive organisms (including group A beta-hemolytic streptococci,* Streptococcus pneumoniae, *and staphylococci, including coagulase-positive, coagulase-negative, and penicillinase-producing strains but not methicillin-resistant* Staphylococcus aureus)

I.V. INFUSION, I.V. OR I.M. INJECTION
**Adults.** 0.5 to 1 g q 4 to 6 hr. *Maximum:* 12 g/day. For serious infections, higher doses are given by I.V. route.
**Children older than age 3 months.** 40 to 80 mg/kg/day divided into four equal doses and given q 6 hr. *Maximum:* 12 g/day.

➤ *To provide surgical prophylaxis*
I.V. INFUSION, I.V. OR I.M. INJECTION
**Adults.** 1 to 2 g 30 to 60 min before surgery, 1 to 2 g during long procedure, and 1 to 2 g q 6 hr after surgery for 24 hr.
DOSAGE ADJUSTMENT For open-heart surgery or prosthetic arthroplasty, prophylaxis continued 3 to 5 days after procedure, if needed.

## Contraindications

Hypersensitivity to cephalosporins or their components

## Mechanism of Action

Interferes with bacterial cell wall synthesis by inhibiting the final step in the cross-linking of peptidoglycan strands. Peptidoglycan makes the cell membrane rigid and protective. Without it, bacterial cells rupture and die.

## Interactions
DRUGS
*aminoglycosides, loop diuretics:* Increased risk of nephrotoxicity
*probenecid:* Increased and prolonged blood cephapirin level

## Adverse Reactions

**CNS:** Chills, fever, headache, seizures
**CV:** Edema
**EENT:** Hearing loss
**GI:** Abdominal cramps, diarrhea, elevated liver function test results, hepatic failure, hepatomegaly, nausea, oral candidiasis, pseudomembranous colitis, vomiting
**GU:** Elevated BUN level, nephrotoxicity, renal failure, vaginal candidiasis
**HEME:** Eosinophilia, hemolytic anemia, hypoprothrombinemia, neutropenia, thrombocytopenia, unusual bleeding
**MS:** Arthralgia
**RESP:** Dyspnea
**SKIN:** Ecchymosis, erythema, erythema multiforme, pruritus, rash, Stevens-Johnson syndrome
**Other:** Anaphylaxis; injection site pain, redness, and swelling; superinfection

## Nursing Considerations

•Use cephapirin cautiously in patients who are hypersensitive to penicillins because cross-sensitivity has occurred in about 10% of such patients.
•If possible, obtain culture and sensitivity test results, as ordered, before giving drug.
•For I.V. injection, reconstitute 1 g with 10 ml or more of appropriate diluent, such as sterile water for injection. Administer I.V. injection slowly over 3 to 5 minutes through tubing of a flowing compatible I.V. fluid.
•For I.V. infusion, dilute further in 50 ml of D₅W or NS and infuse over 15 to 30 minutes. Stop primary I.V. solution during cephapirin administration.
•For I.M. injection, reconstitute 1-g vial with 2 ml of sterile water for injection or bacteriosta-

tic water for injection. Inject deeply into large muscle mass, such as the gluteus maximus.
•Store reconstituted drug for up to 24 hours at room temperature or 10 days in refrigerator.
•Don't give a cloudy solution.
•Assess I.V. site for extravasation and phlebitis.
•Monitor BUN and serum creatinine levels to detect early signs of nephrotoxicity. Also, monitor fluid intake and output; decreasing urine output may indicate nephrotoxicity.
•Monitor for allergic reactions a few days after therapy starts.
•Assess CBC, hematocrit, and serum AST, ALT, bilirubin, LD, and alkaline phosphatase levels during long-term therapy.
•Assess bowel pattern daily; severe diarrhea may indicate pseudomembranous colitis.
•Assess for pharyngitis, ecchymosis, bleeding, and arthralgia; they may indicate a blood dyscrasia.
•Assess for furry tongue, perineal itching, and loose, foul-smelling stool; they may indicate superinfection.

**PATIENT TEACHING**
•Instruct patient to immediately report severe diarrhea or evidence of blood dyscrasia or superinfection to prescriber.

# cephradine

Velosef

## Class and Category

*Chemical:* First-generation cephalosporin, 7-aminocephalosporanic acid
*Therapeutic:* Antibiotic
*Pregnancy category:* B

## Indications and Dosages

➤ *To treat respiratory tract infections (other than lobar pneumonia) and skin and soft-tissue infections*
**CAPSULES, ORAL SUSPENSION**
**Adults.** 250 mg q 6 hr or 500 mg q 12 hr. *Maximum:* 4 g/day.
**ORAL SUSPENSION**
**Children age 9 months and older.** 25 to 50 mg/kg/day in equally divided doses q 6 or 12 hr. *Maximum:* 4 g/day.
➤ *To treat lobar pneumonia*
**CAPSULES, ORAL SUSPENSION**
**Adults.** 0.5 g q 6 hr or 1 g q 12 hr. *Maximum:* 4 g/day.
**ORAL SUSPENSION**
**Children age 9 months and older.** 25 to 50 mg/

kg/day in equally divided doses q 6 or 12 hr. *Maximum:* 4 g/day.
➤ *To treat uncomplicated UTIs*
**CAPSULES, ORAL SUSPENSION**
**Adults.** 500 mg q 12 hr. For more serious infections, 500 mg q 6 hr or 1,000 mg q 12 hr. *Maximum:* 4 g/day.
➤ *To treat otitis media caused by* Haemophilus influenzae
**ORAL SUSPENSION**
**Children.** 75 to 100 mg/kg/day in equally divided doses q 6 to 12 hr. *Maximum:* 4 g/day.
**DOSAGE ADJUSTMENT** Dosage reduced to 500 mg q 6 hr if creatinine clearance exceeds 20 ml/min/1.73 m$^2$; 250 mg q 6 hr if creatinine clearance is 5 to 20 ml/min/1.73 m$^2$; and 250 mg q 12 hr if creatinine clearance is less than 5 ml/min/1.73 m$^2$.

## Contraindications
Hypersensitivity to cephalosporins or their components

---

### Mechanism of Action
Interferes with bacterial cell wall synthesis by inhibiting the final step in the cross-linking of peptidoglycan strands. Peptidoglycan makes the cell membrane rigid and protective. Without it, bacterial cells rupture and die.

---

## Interactions
**DRUGS**
*aminoglycosides, loop diuretics:* Increased risk of nephrotoxicity
*probenecid:* Increased and prolonged blood cephradine level

## Adverse Reactions
**CNS:** Chills, fever, headache, seizures
**CV:** Edema
**EENT:** Hearing loss, oral candidiasis
**GI:** Abdominal cramps, diarrhea, elevated liver function test results, hepatic failure, hepatomegaly, nausea, pseudomembranous colitis, vomiting
**GU:** Elevated BUN level, nephrotoxicity, renal failure, vaginal candidiasis
**HEME:** Eosinophilia, hemolytic anemia, hypoprothrombinemia, neutropenia, thrombocytopenia, unusual bleeding
**MS:** Arthralgia
**RESP:** Dyspnea

SKIN: Ecchymosis, erythema, erythema multiforme, pruritus, rash, Stevens-Johnson syndrome
Other: Anaphylaxis, superinfection

## Nursing Considerations
•If possible, obtain culture and sensitivity test results, as ordered, before giving drug.
•Monitor patients who are hypersensitive to penicillin for signs and symptoms of a hypersensitivity reaction because cross-sensitivity has occurred in 10% of such patients.
•Store oral suspension for 7 days at room temperature or for 14 days if refrigerated.
•Monitor BUN and serum creatinine levels to detect early signs of nephrotoxicity. Also monitor fluid intake and output; decreasing urine output may indicate nephrotoxicity.
•Monitor patient for allergic reactions a few days after therapy starts. If patient develops hypersensitivity, be prepared to discontinue the drug and administer antihistamines, corticosteroids, and vasopressors, as ordered. Also prepare to administer oxygen, maintain an open airway, and assist with endotracheal intubation, as appropriate.
•Assess CBC, hematocrit, and serum AST, ALT, bilirubin, LD, and alkaline phosphatase levels during long-term therapy.
•Assess bowel pattern daily; severe diarrhea may indicate pseudomembranous colitis. Obtain a stool specimen to test for *Clostridium difficile*. Keep in mind that this serious adverse reaction can occur during therapy or up to several weeks after therapy is discontinued. Also avoid giving antiperistaltic antidiarrheals, such as atropine and diphenoxylate or loperamide, because they may delay elimination of toxins from the bowel and cause damage to the colon from toxin retention. Mild cases may respond after drug is discontinued. For moderate or severe cases, be prepared to administer fluid, electrolyte, and protein replacement as ordered.
•If patient has a history of GI disease, especially ulcerative colitis, regional enteritis, or antibiotic-associated colitis, assess him frequently for diarrhea because he is at risk for pseudomembranous colitis.
•Assess for pharyngitis, ecchymosis, bleeding, and arthralgia; these may indicate a blood dyscrasia.
•If patient has a seizure, notify prescriber immediately and expect to discontinue drug.

Institute seizure precautions according to facility policy.

PATIENT TEACHING
•If patient develops GI distress, advise him to take cephradine with food.
•Advise patient to complete prescribed course of therapy.
•Explain that patient should avoid missing doses and that he should take the drug at evenly spaced intervals. If patient misses a dose, instruct him to take the dose as soon as possible unless it's almost time for the next dose. Emphasize that he shouldn't double the dose.
•Tell patient that yogurt and buttermilk help maintain intestinal flora and can decrease diarrhea during therapy.
•Instruct patient to immediately report to prescriber severe diarrhea or evidence of blood dyscrasia or superinfection. Warn patient not to take any OTC antidiarrheals before consulting prescriber.
•Advise patient to notify prescriber if symptoms don't improve within a few days.

# cevimeline hydrochloride
Evoxac

## Class and Category
*Chemical:* Quinuclidine derivative of acetylcholine
*Therapeutic:* Cholinergic enhancer, dry mouth reliever
*Pregnancy category:* C

## Indications and Dosages
➤ *To treat dry mouth associated with Sjögren's syndrome*
CAPSULES
Adults. 30 mg t.i.d. *Maximum:* 90 mg/day.

## Contraindications
Acute iritis, angle-closure glaucoma, hypersensitivity to cevimeline or its components, uncontrolled asthma

## Mechanism of Action
As a cholinergic agonist, binds to and activates muscarinic receptors of the parasympathetic nervous system and increases secretions of the exocrine glands, such as salivary glands.

## Interactions

**DRUGS**

*amiodarone, cimetidine, clarithromycin, diltiazem, erythromycin, fluconazole, haloperidol, itraconazole, ketoconazole, metoclopramide, mibefradil, nefazodone, propafenone, quinidine, ritonavir, selective serotonin reuptake inhibitors, thioridazine, tricyclic antidepressants, troleandomycin, verapamil:* Possibly inhibited metabolism and increased blood level of cevimeline
*anticholinergics:* Decreased effectiveness of anticholinergics
*antimuscarinics:* Altered effects of antimuscarinics and decreased therapeutic action of cevimeline
*beta blockers:* Possibly cardiac conduction disturbances
*parasympathomimetics:* Additive effects of either drug

## Adverse Reactions

**CNS:** Depression, fatigue, fever, hypoesthesia, insomnia, migraine headache, tremor
**CV:** Edema, palpitations
**EENT:** Abnormal vision, conjunctivitis, dry mouth, earache, epistaxis, excessive salivation, eye pain, rhinitis, salivary gland pain
**GI:** Abdominal pain, anorexia, constipation, eructation, heartburn, hiccups, nausea, vomiting
**HEME:** Anemia
**MS:** Arthralgia, leg cramps, myalgia
**RESP:** Cough, dyspnea
**SKIN:** Diaphoresis, pruritus
**Other:** Flulike symptoms, hot flashes

## Nursing Considerations

• Administer cevimeline on an empty stomach because food may decrease rate and extent of drug absorption and thus delay peak blood concentrations.
• Assess patient with a pulmonary disorder for wheezing and increased respiratory secretions because drug may cause increased bronchiolar smooth-muscle contractions, airway resistance, and respiratory secretions.
• Monitor patient with known or suspected gallbladder disease for abdominal pain or other signs and symptoms that may indicate biliary obstruction, cholecystitis, or cholangitis; each of these conditions may be precipitated by cevimeline.

**PATIENT TEACHING**

• Instruct patient to take cevimeline on an empty stomach.
• Inform patient that drug may cause vision changes; advise him to avoid driving at night or performing potentially hazardous activities until drug's adverse effects are known.
• Urge patient to drink plenty of fluids during hot weather and while exercising because drug may cause excessive sweating and dehydration.

# chloral hydrate

Aquachloral Supprettes, Novo-Chlorhydrate (CAN), PMS-Chloral Hydrate (CAN)

## Class, Category, and Schedule

*Chemical:* Chloral derivative
*Therapeutic:* Sedative-hypnotic
*Pregnancy category:* C
*Controlled substance:* Schedule IV

## Indications and Dosages

➤ *To prevent or suppress alcohol withdrawal symptoms, act as an adjunct to opioids and analgesics to control postoperative pain*

**CAPSULES, SYRUP, SUPPOSITORIES**

**Adults.** 250 mg t.i.d. p.c. *Maximum:* 2,000 mg.

➤ *To produce nocturnal sedation*

**CAPSULES, SYRUP, SUPPOSITORIES**

**Adults.** 0.5 to 1 g 30 min before bedtime. *Maximum:* 2 g.

➤ *To produce preoperative sedation*

**CAPSULES, SYRUP, SUPPOSITORIES**

**Adults.** 0.5 to 1 g 30 min before surgery.

➤ *To provide sedation before dental or medical procedure*

**SYRUP, SUPPOSITORIES**

**Children.** 25 mg/kg up to 500 mg/single dose; up to 75 mg/kg for dental procedure supplemented by nitrous oxide.

| Route | Onset | Peak | Duration |
|-------|-------|------|----------|
| P.O. | 30 min to 1 hr | Unknown | 4 to 8 hr |
| P.R. | Unknown | Unknown | 4 to 8 hr |

## Contraindications

Gastritis; hypersensitivity or idiosyncrasy to chloral hydrate or its components; severe cardiac, hepatic, or renal disease

## Mechanism of Action
Produces CNS depression by an unknown mechanism involving trichloroethanol, the drug's active metabolite.

## Interactions
**DRUGS**
*CNS depressants:* Increased CNS effects of chloral hydrate
*furosemide (I.V.):* Increased incidence of adverse effects when administered after chloral hydrate
*phenytoin:* Increased excretion and subsequent decreased effectiveness of phenytoin
*warfarin:* Transient increase in anticoagulant effect
**ACTIVITIES**
*alcohol use:* Increased CNS effects of chloral hydrate

## Adverse Reactions
**CNS:** Ataxia, disorientation, hangover, incoherence, paranoia, somnolence
**GI:** Gastric irritation, nausea, vomiting
**SKIN:** Rash, urticaria
**Other:** Drug dependence

## Nursing Considerations
•Administer with full glass of water or juice to minimize GI distress from chloral hydrate capsules. Dilute syrup in a half-glass of water, ginger ale, or fruit juice.
•**WARNING** Monitor carefully for hypersensitivity reaction in patients with a history of tartrazine sensitivity.
•Suspect physical or psychological dependence if withdrawal of chloral hydrate produces confusion, hallucinations, nausea, nervousness, restlessness, stomach pain, tremor, unusual excitement, or vomiting.
**PATIENT TEACHING**
•Advise patient to take capsules with a full glass of water or juice or to mix syrup in a half-glass of water, ginger ale, or fruit juice.
•Advise patient to avoid hazardous activities until drug's CNS effects are known.
•Caution patient that drug may be habit-forming. Advise taking it exactly as prescribed and not to stop taking it abruptly because withdrawal symptoms could occur.
•Instruct patient to notify prescriber at once about stomach pains or tarry stools.

# chloramphenicol
Chloromycetin, Novochlorocap (CAN)

# chloramphenicol palmitate
Chloromycetin

# chloramphenicol sodium succinate
Chloromycetin

## Class and Category
*Chemical*: Dichloroacetic acid derivative
*Therapeutic*: Antibiotic
*Pregnancy category:* Not rated

## Indications and Dosages
➤ *To treat serious infections for which less potentially dangerous drugs are ineffective or contraindicated*
**I.V. INFUSION**
**Adults.** 12.5 mg/kg q 6 hr. *Maximum:* 4 g/day.
**Children.** 50 to 75 mg/kg/day in divided doses q 6 hr.
**Full-term infants age 2 weeks and older.** 12.5 mg/kg q 6 hr or 25 mg/kg q 12 hr.
**Preterm and full-term infants up to age 2 weeks.** 6.25 mg/kg q 6 hr.
➤ *To treat bacteremia or meningitis*
**I.V. INFUSION**
**Children.** 50 to 100 mg/kg/day in divided doses q 6 hr.
**DOSAGE ADJUSTMENT** Dosage limited to 25 mg/kg/day for infants and children with immature metabolic processes.

## Contraindications
Hypersensitivity to chloramphenicol or its components

## Mechanism of Action
Produces a bacteriostatic effect on susceptible organisms by inhibiting protein synthesis, thereby preventing amino acids from being transferred to growing polypetide chains.

## Interactions
**DRUGS**
*alfentanil:* Prolonged alfentanil effect
*barbiturates:* Increased blood barbiturate

level; decreased blood chloramphenicol level

*blood-dyscrasia–causing drugs (such as captopril and cephalosporins), bone marrow depressants (including colchicine and methotrexate):* Increased bone marrow depression
*chlorpropamide, tolbutamide:* Increased hypoglycemic effects
*clindamycin, erythromycin, lincomycin:* Decreased antibacterial effects of these drugs
*cyclophosphamide:* Decreased or delayed activation of cyclophosphamide, increased bone marrow depression
*hepatic enzyme inducers (including rifampin):* Decreased blood chloramphenicol level
*hydantoins:* Increased blood hydantoin level, possibly resulting in toxicity; increased or decreased blood chloramphenicol level
*iron salts:* Increased serum iron level
*oral anticoagulants:* Enhanced anticoagulant action
*oral contraceptives containing estrogen:* Decreased contraceptive effect with prolonged chloramphenicol use
*penicillins:* Decreased penicillin activity; synergistic effects with treatment of certain microorganisms
*vitamin B$_{12}$:* Antagonized hematopoietic response to vitamin B$_{12}$

### Adverse Reactions

**CNS:** Confusion, delirium, depression, fever, headache, peripheral neuropathy
**CV:** Gray syndrome in neonates
**EENT:** Optic neuritis
**GI:** Diarrhea, nausea, vomiting
**HEME:** Aplastic anemia, bone marrow depression, granulocytopenia, hypoplastic anemia, leukopenia, reticulocytopenia, thrombocytopenia
**SKIN:** Rash
**Other:** Anaphylaxis, angioedema

### Nursing Considerations

• As appropriate and ordered, obtain specimen for culture and sensitivity testing before beginning chloramphenicol therapy.
• Keep in mind that chloramphenicol should never be used to treat minor infections or for prophylaxis because of the many serious toxicities associated with its use.
• Be aware that repeated courses of therapy should be avoided because of the risk of serious adverse reactions.

• For I.V. use, prepare a 10% solution by adding 10 ml of sterile water for injection or D$_5$W to each 1-g vial. Administer over at least 1 minute.
• Know that diluted I.V. solution is stable for 24 to 48 hours when stored at room temperature or refrigerated. Don't use if cloudy.
• Assess patient for fever, sore throat, tiredness, unusual bleeding, or ecchymosis; these may indicate a blood dyscrasia.
• Perform neurologic assessments regularly, looking for signs and symptoms of peripheral neuropathy.
• **WARNING** If early signs of gray syndrome appear (failure to eat, pallor, cyanosis, abdominal distention, irregular respirations, and vasomotor collapse), notify prescriber and be prepared to stop drug immediately.
• Monitor blood chloramphenicol level as appropriate. Keep in mind that therapeutic peak levels are 10 to 20 mcg/ml and trough levels are 5 to 10 mcg/ml.
• Monitor CBC and platelet and reticulocyte counts as ordered to detect signs of blood dyscrasia. Notify prescriber immediately about abnormal results.

**PATIENT TEACHING**
• Instruct patient to immediately report to prescriber signs of blood dyscrasia.
• **WARNING** Tell patient to stay alert for signs of potentially fatal, irreversible bone marrow depression that leads to aplastic anemia and is characterized by fever, pallor, pharyngitis, severe fatigue and weakness, and unusual bleeding or bruising. Bone marrow depression may occur weeks to months after therapy stops. Stress the importance of follow-up care.

# chlordiazepoxide hydrochloride

Apo-Chlordiazepoxide (CAN), Librium, Novo-Poxide (CAN)

### Class, Category, and Schedule
*Chemical:* Benzodiazepine
*Therapeutic:* Antianxiety
*Pregnancy category:* Not rated
*Controlled substance:* Schedule IV

### Indications and Dosages
➤ *To provide short-term management of mild anxiety*
**CAPSULES, TABLETS**
**Adults.** 5 to 10 mg t.i.d. or q.i.d.

**Children over age 6.** 5 mg b.i.d. to q.i.d. increased as needed to 10 mg b.i.d. or t.i.d., or 0.5 mg/kg/day in equally divided doses q 6 to 8 hr.

➤ *To provide short-term management of severe anxiety*

**CAPSULES, TABLETS**

**Adults.** 20 to 25 mg t.i.d. or q.i.d.

**I.V. OR I.M. INJECTION**

**Adults.** *Initial:* 50 to 100 mg. Then, 25 to 50 mg t.i.d. or q.i.d., p.r.n. *Maximum:* 300 mg/day.

**I.M. INJECTION**

**Children age 12 and older.** 0.5 mg/kg/day in equally divided doses q 6 to 8 hr.

➤ *To provide short-term treatment of acute alcohol withdrawal*

**CAPSULES, TABLETS, I.V. OR I.M. INJECTION**

**Adults.** *Initial:* 50 to 100 mg, usually given I.V. or I.M. Repeated in 2 to 4 hr followed by individualized oral dosage if needed to control symptoms. *Maximum:* 300 mg/day.

➤ *To provide perioperative relaxation and reduce apprehension and anxiety*

**CAPSULES, TABLETS, I.M. INJECTION**

**Adults.** 5 to 10 mg P.O. t.i.d. or q.i.d. several days before surgery; 50 to 100 mg I.M. 1 hr before surgery.

DOSAGE ADJUSTMENT Dosage reduced to 5 mg P.O. b.i.d. to q.i.d., p.r.n., for elderly or debilitated patients.

---

## Mechanism of Action

May potentiate the effects of gamma-aminobutyric acid (GABA) and other inhibitory neurotransmitters by binding to specific benzodiazepine receptors in the limbic and cortical areas of the CNS. By binding to these receptors, chlordiazepoxide increases GABA's inhibitory effects and blocks cortical and limbic arousal, which helps control emotional behavior. It also helps relieve symptoms of alcohol withdrawal by causing CNS depression.

---

## Contraindications

Hypersensitivity to chlordiazepoxide or its components

## Interactions

**DRUGS**

*antacids:* Altered rate of chlordiazepoxide absorption

*cimetidine, disulfiram, fluoxetine, isoniazid,* *ketoconazole, metoprolol, oral contraceptives, propoxyphene, propranolol, valproic acid:* Increased blood chlordiazepoxide level

*CNS depressants:* Increased CNS effects

*digoxin:* Increased blood digoxin level and risk of digitalis toxicity

*levodopa:* Decreased efficacy of levodopa's antiparkinsonian effects

*neuromuscular blockers:* Potentiated, counteracted, or diminished effects of neuromuscular blockers

*phenytoin:* Possibly increased phenytoin toxicity

*probenecid:* Shortened onset of action or prolonged effect of chlordiazepoxide

*rifampin:* Decreased chlordiazepoxide effect

*theophyllines:* Antagonized sedative effects of chlordiazepoxide

**ACTIVITIES**

*alcohol use:* Increased CNS effects

## Adverse Reactions

**CNS:** Ataxia, confusion, depression, drowsiness

**CV:** ECG changes, hypotension, tachycardia

**GI:** Hepatic dysfunction

**HEME:** Agranulocytosis

**SKIN:** Jaundice

**Other:** Injection site pain, redness, and swelling

## Nursing Considerations

•Use chlordiazepoxide cautiously in patients with renal or hepatic impairment or porphyria.

•WARNING Be aware that prolonged use of therapeutic doses can lead to dependence.

•For I.V. use, reconstitute ampule contents with 5 ml of sterile water for injection or sodium chloride for injection. Agitate gently until completely dissolved. Give slowly over 1 minute.

•For I.M. use, reconstitute only with diluent provided by manufacturer.

•WARNING Don't use supplied diluent to prepare drug for I.V. use because air bubbles form on the surface.

•Don't give opalescent or hazy solution.

•Observe for signs of phlebitis or thrombophlebitis after I.V. administration.

•Monitor liver function test results during therapy.

•If patient is a hyperactive, aggressive child or has a history of psychiatric disorders, monitor for paradoxical reactions, such as excitement, stimulation, and acute rage, during first 2 weeks of therapy.

**PATIENT TEACHING**

•Warn patient about possible drowsiness.

• Advise patient to avoid other CNS depressants during therapy.
• Warn patient not to take antacids with drug.

# chlorothiazide
Diuril

# chlorothiazide sodium
Diuril

## Class and Category
*Chemical*: Sulfonamide derivative
*Therapeutic*: Antihypertensive, diuretic
*Pregnancy category:* B

## Indications and Dosages
➤ *To treat hypertension*
**ORAL SUSPENSION, TABLETS**
**Adults.** 250 to 1,000 mg/day in a single dose or divided doses b.i.d. *Maximum:* 2,000 mg/day in divided doses.
**Children age 6 months and older.** 10 to 20 mg/kg/day in a single dose or divided doses b.i.d. *Maximum:* 1,000 mg/day for ages 2 to 12; 375 mg/day for ages 6 months to 2 years.
**Children under age 6 months.** Up to 30 mg/kg/day in divided doses given b.i.d.
➤ *To produce diuresis*
**ORAL SUSPENSION, TABLETS**
**Adults.** 250 mg q 6 to 12 hr. Administered on an intermittent schedule, if needed, such as alternate days or 3 to 5 days/wk.
**Children age 6 months and older.** 10 to 20 mg/kg/day in a single dose or divided doses b.i.d. *Maximum:* 1,000 mg/day for children ages 2 to 12; 375 mg/day for children ages 6 months to 2 years.
**Children under age 6 months.** Up to 33 mg/kg/day in divided doses b.i.d.
**I.V. INFUSION OR INJECTION**
**Adults.** 250 mg q 6 to 12 hr.

| Route | Onset | Peak | Duration |
|-------|-------|------|----------|
| P.O. | 2 hr | 4 hr | 6 to 12 hr |
| I.V. | 15 min | 4 hr | 6 to 12 hr |

## Contraindications
Anuria; hepatic coma; hypersensitivity to chlorothiazide or its components, sulfonamides, or related thiazide diuretics; renal failure

## Mechanism of Action
May promote sodium, chloride, and water excretion by inhibiting sodium reabsorption in the kidneys' distal tubules. Initially, chlorothiazide may reduce blood pressure by decreasing extracellular fluid volume, plasma volume, and cardiac output. It also may dilate arteries directly, reducing peripheral vascular resistance. After several weeks, extracellular fluid and plasma volume and cardiac output return to normal, but peripheral vascular resistance remains decreased.

## Interactions
**DRUGS**
*allopurinol:* Increased risk of allopurinol hypersensitivity
*amiodarone:* Increased risk of arrhythmias from hypokalemia
*amphotericin B, glucocorticoids:* Intensified electrolyte depletion
*anesthetics:* Potentiated effects of anesthetics
*anticholinergics:* Increased chlorothiazide absorption
*anticoagulants, methenamines, sulfonylureas:* Decreased effects of these drugs
*antihypertensives:* Increased antihypertensive effect
*antineoplastics:* Prolonged antineoplastic-induced leukopenia
*calcium:* Possibly increased blood calcium level
*cholestyramine, colestipol:* Decreased chlorothiazide absorption
*diazoxide:* Hyperglycemia, hypotension
*digitalis glycosides:* Increased risk of digitalis-induced arrhythmias
*dopamine:* Increased diuretic effect of both drugs
*lithium:* Increased risk of lithium toxicity
*loop diuretics:* Synergistic effects, resulting in profound diuresis and serious electrolyte imbalances
*methyldopa:* Potential development of hemolytic anemia
*neuromuscular blockers:* Increased neuromuscular blockade
*NSAIDs:* Possibly reduced diuretic effect of chlorothiazide
*sympathomimetics:* Possibly inhibited antihypertensive effect of chlorothiazide
*vitamin D:* Enhanced vitamin D action

## Adverse Reactions
**CNS:** Dizziness, headache, paresthesia, restlessness, vertigo, weakness
**CV:** Orthostatic hypotension
**ENDO:** Hyperglycemia
**GI:** Abdominal cramps, anorexia, constipation, diarrhea, gastric irritation, nausea, pancreatitis, vomiting
**GU:** Glycosuria, hematuria (I.V. form), impotence, interstitial nephritis, renal dysfunction or failure
**HEME:** Agranulocytosis, aplastic anemia, hemolytic anemia, leukopenia, thrombocytopenia
**MS:** Muscle spasms
**SKIN:** Jaundice, photosensitivity, purpura, rash, urticaria
**Other:** Anaphylactic reactions, hypercalcemia, hyperuricemia, hypochloremic alkalosis, hypokalemia, hypomagnesemia, hyponatremia, hypovolemia

## Nursing Considerations
•Don't give parenteral form of chlorothiazide by I.M. or S.C. route.
•For I.V. use, reconstitute with at least 18 ml of sterile water for injection. Discard unused solution after 24 hours. Reconstituted solution is compatible with dextrose solution or NS for infusion.
•Watch I.V. site closely. If extravasation occurs, stop infusion and tell prescriber at once.
•Weigh patient daily to assess fluid loss and drug effectiveness. Also, check blood pressure often if used to treat hypertension; antihypertensive effect may not appear for days.
•Assess patient for electrolyte imbalances.
•Monitor renal function closely, especially in elderly patients, because the risk of toxicity increases with renal impairment.

**PATIENT TEACHING**
•Tell patient to take chlorothiazide early in the day to avoid nocturia and to take it with food or milk if GI distress occurs.
•Encourage patient to eat a high-potassium diet.
•Instruct patient to rise slowly to minimize effects of orthostatic hypotension.
•Urge patient to weigh himself at least weekly and to notify prescriber if weight rises or falls by 5 lb (2.25 kg) or more in 2 days.
•Tell patient to immediately notify prescriber about weakness, cramps, nausea, vomiting, restlessness, excessive thirst, drowsiness, tiredness, increased heart rate, diarrhea, sudden joint pain, or dizziness.

•If patient has diabetes mellitus, tell him to monitor his blood glucose level often. Oral antidiabetic dosage may need to be increased.
•Tell patient to avoid prolonged exposure to sun, use sunscreen, and wear protective clothing.
•Advise patient to consult prescriber or pharmacist before using alcohol and such OTC drugs as those used for appetite control, colds, cough, hay fever, and sinus problems.

# chlorphenesin carbamate
Maolate

## Class and Category
*Chemical:* Chemically related to mephenesin
*Therapeutic:* Skeletal muscle relaxant
*Pregnancy category:* Not rated

## Indications and Dosages
➤ *As adjunct to relieve pain in acute musculoskeletal conditions*
**TABLETS**
**Adults:** 800 mg t.i.d. until desired effect occurs. *Maintenance:* 400 mg q.i.d or less, p.r.n.

> ### Mechanism of Action
> May act on the CNS, rather than directly on skeletal muscle, producing a sedative effect that aids in muscle relaxation.

## Contraindications
Hypersensitivity to chlorphenesin or its components

## Interactions
**DRUGS**
*CNS depressants:* Increased adverse CNS effects
**ACTIVITIES**
*alcohol use:* Increased adverse CNS effects

## Adverse Reactions
**CNS:** Confusion, dizziness, drowsiness, headache, insomnia, nervousness, paradoxical stimulation
**EENT:** Diplopia, transient vision loss
**GI:** Epigastric discomfort, nausea
**Other**: Anaphylaxis, drug-induced fever

## Nursing Considerations
•**WARNING** Use chlorphenesin cautiously in patients hypersensitive to aspirin; it contains tartrazine, which may cause hypersensitivity.

•Expect drug therapy to last for no more than 8 weeks because safety beyond this point is unknown.

•Provide rest and other pain-relief measures.

**PATIENT TEACHING**

•Because of possible reduced alertness, advise patient to avoid potentially hazardous activities until drug's CNS effects are known.

•Instruct patient to notify prescriber if these symptoms occur: confusion, dizziness, drowsiness, insomnia, nervousness, or paradoxical stimulation.

•Tell patient to immediately notify prescriber if he develops a fever or any signs or symptoms of an allergic reaction, such as rash, hives, itching, facial swelling, or difficulty breathing.

# chlorpromazine

Largactil (CAN), Thorazine

## chlorpromazine hydrochloride

Chlorpromanyl (CAN), Novo-Chlorpromazine (CAN), Thorazine, Thorazine Spansule

## Class and Category

*Chemical*: Propylamine derivative of phenothiazine
*Therapeutic*: Antiemetic, antipsychotic, tranquilizer
*Pregnancy category:* Not rated

## Indications and Dosages

➤ *To manage symptoms of psychotic disorders or control manic manifestations of manic-depression in outpatients*

**E.R. CAPSULES**

**Adults.** 30 to 300 mg q.d. to t.i.d. with dosage adjusted as needed. *Maximum:* 1 g/day.

**ORAL CONCENTRATE, SYRUP, TABLETS**

**Adults.** 10 mg t.i.d. or q.i.d., or 25 mg b.i.d. or t.i.d. After 1 or 2 days, dose increased by 20 to 50 mg semiweekly until patient is calm. After 2 wk of calmness, dosage gradually reduced to maintenance level of 200 to 800 mg/day in equally divided doses.

➤ *To control acutely disturbed or manic hospitalized patients*

**I.M. INJECTION**

**Adults.** 25 mg. Repeated 25 to 50 mg in 1 hr, if needed. Increased gradually over several days up to 400 mg q 4 to 6 hr for severe cases until behavior is controlled. Then, regi-

men switched to oral form and outpatient dosage.

➤ *To treat severe behavioral problems in children*

**ORAL CONCENTRATE, SYRUP, TABLETS**

**Children ages 6 months to 12 years.** 0.55 mg/kg q 4 to 6 hr, p.r.n.

**SUPPOSITORIES**

**Children ages 6 months to 12 years.** 1 mg/kg q 6 to 8 hr, p.r.n.

**I.M. INJECTION**

**Children ages 6 months to 12 years.** 0.55 mg/kg q 6 to 8 hr. *Maximum:* 75 mg/day for children ages 5 to 12 years or weighing 50 to 100 lb (23 to 45 kg), except in unmanageable cases; 40 mg/day for children up to age 5 years or weighing up to 50 lb.

➤ *To treat nausea and vomiting*

**ORAL CONCENTRATE, SYRUP, TABLETS**

**Adults and adolescents.** 10 to 25 mg q 4 to 6 hr, p.r.n.

**Children ages 6 months to 12 years.** 0.55 mg/kg q 4 to 6 hr, p.r.n.

**I.M. INJECTION**

**Adults.** 25 mg. If no hypotension occurs, 25 to 50 mg q 3 to 4 hr, p.r.n., until vomiting stops; then drug switched to oral form.

**Children age 6 months and older.** 0.55 mg/kg q 6 to 8 hr, p.r.n. *Maximum:* 75 mg/day for children ages 5 to 12 years or weighing 50 to 100 lb; 40 mg/day for children up to age 5 years or weighing up to 50 lb.

**SUPPOSITORIES**

**Adults and adolescents.** 50 to 100 mg q 6 to 8 hr, p.r.n.

**Children ages 6 months to 12 years.** 1 mg/kg q 6 to 8 hr, p.r.n.

➤ *To provide intraoperative control of nausea and vomiting*

**I.V. INJECTION**

**Adults.** 25 mg diluted to 1 mg/ml with sodium chloride for injection and given at a rate not to exceed 2 mg q 2 min. *Maximum:* 25 mg.

**Children age 6 months and older.** 0.275 mg/kg diluted to at least 1 mg/ml with sodium chloride for injection and given at a rate not to exceed 1 mg q 2 min. *Maximum:* 75 mg/day for children ages 5 to 12 years or weighing 50 to 100 lb; 40 mg/day for children up to age 5 years or weighing up to 50 lb.

**I.M. INJECTION**

**Adults.** 12.5 mg. Repeated in 30 min if needed and no hypotension occurs.

**Children age 6 months and older.** 0.275 mg/kg. Repeated in 30 min if needed and tolerated.

> *To treat intractable hiccups*

**TABLETS**

**Adults.** 25 to 50 mg t.i.d. or q.i.d. If hiccups last longer than 2 days, route switched to I.M., as prescribed.

**I.V. INFUSION**

**Adults.** 25 to 50 mg diluted in 500 to 1,000 ml of NS and administered at a rate of 1 mg/min with patient in supine position.

**I.M. INJECTION**

**Adults.** 25 to 50 mg given only if oral route is ineffective. If symptoms persist, route switched to I.V., as prescribed.

> *To provide preoperative relaxation*

**ORAL CONCENTRATE, SYRUP, TABLETS**

**Adults and adolescents.** 25 to 50 mg 2 to 3 hr before surgery.

**Children ages 6 months to 12 years.** 0.55 mg/kg 2 to 3 hr before surgery.

**I.M. INJECTION**

**Adults.** 12.5 to 25 mg 1 to 2 hr before surgery.

**Children age 6 months and older.** 0.55 mg/kg 1 to 2 hr before surgery.

> *To treat acute intermittent porphyria*

**ORAL CONCENTRATE, SYRUP, TABLETS**

**Adults and adolescents.** 25 to 50 mg t.i.d. or q.i.d.

**I.M. INJECTION**

**Adults.** 25 mg t.i.d. or q.i.d. until oral route is possible.

> *To treat tetanus (usually as adjunct with barbiturates)*

**I.V. INFUSION**

**Adults.** 25 to 50 mg diluted to at least 1 mg/ml and given at a rate not to exceed 1 mg/min.

**Children age 6 months and older.** 0.55 mg/kg q 6 to 8 hr, diluted to at least 1 mg/ml and given at a rate not to exceed 1 mg/2 min. *Maximum:* 75 mg/day for children ages 5 to 12 years or weighing 50 to 100 lb; 40 mg/day for children up to age 5 years or weighing up to 50 lb.

**I.M. INJECTION**

**Adults.** 25 to 50 mg t.i.d. or q.i.d.

**Children age 6 months and older.** 0.55 mg/kg q 6 to 8 hr. *Maximum:* 75 mg/day for children ages 5 to 12 years or weighing 50 to 100 lb; 40 mg/day for children up to age 5 years or weighing up to 50 lb.

**DOSAGE ADJUSTMENT** Dosage possibly reduced for patients with hepatic dysfunction. Dosage reduced to one-third to one-half the normal adult dosage for elderly or debilitated patients.

## Mechanism of Action

Depresses areas of the brain that control activity and aggression, including the cerebral cortex, hypothalamus, and limbic system, by an unknown mechanism. Drug prevents nausea and vomiting by inhibiting or blocking dopamine receptors in the medullary chemoreceptor trigger zone and peripherally by blocking the vagus nerve in the GI tract. It may relieve anxiety by causing indirect reduction in arousal and increased filtering of internal stimuli to the reticular activating system in the brain stem.

## Incompatibilities

Don't mix chlorpromazine with thiopental, atropine, or solutions that don't have a pH of 4 to 5 because a precipitate will form. Don't mix chlorpromazine injection with other drugs in a syringe.

## Contraindications

Comatose states; hypersensitivity to chlorpromazine, phenothiazines, or their components; use of large amounts of CNS depressants

## Interactions

**DRUGS**

*amphetamines:* Decreased amphetamine effectiveness, decreased antipsychotic effectiveness of chlorpromazine
*antacids (aluminum hydroxide or magnesium trisilicate gel):* Decreased chlorpromazine absorption and effectiveness
*barbiturates:* Decreased plasma level and, possibly, effectiveness of chlorpromazine
*CNS depressants:* Prolonged and intensified CNS depression
*metrizamide:* Possibly lowered seizure threshold
*oral anticoagulants:* Decreased anticoagulant effect
*phenytoin:* Interference with phenytoin metabolism, increased risk of phenytoin toxicity
*propranolol:* Increased plasma levels of both drugs
*thiazide diuretics:* Possibly increased orthostatic hypotension

**ACTIVITIES**

*alcohol use:* Prolonged and intensified CNS depression

## Adverse Reactions

**CNS:** Drowsiness, extrapyramidal reactions (such as dystonia, fever, motor restlessness,

pseudoparkinsonism, and tardive dyskinesia), neuroleptic malignant syndrome, seizures
**CV:** ECG changes, such as nonspecific, usually reversible Q- and T-wave changes; orthostatic hypotension; tachycardia
**EENT:** Blurred vision, dry mouth, nasal congestion, ocular changes (fine particle deposits in lens and cornea) with long-term therapy
**ENDO:** Gynecomastia, hyperglycemia, hypoglycemia, lactation, moderate breast engorgement
**GI:** Constipation, ileus, nausea
**GU:** Amenorrhea, ejaculation disorders, impotence, priapism, urine retention
**HEME:** Agranulocytosis, aplastic anemia, eosinophilia, hemolytic anemia, leukopenia, pancytopenia, thrombocytopenic purpura
**SKIN:** Exfoliative dermatitis, jaundice, photosensitivity, tissue necrosis, urticaria

## Nursing Considerations
•Don't open or crush E.R. capsules.
•Use chlorpromazine cautiously in patients (especially children) with chronic respiratory disorders (such as severe asthma or emphysema) or acute respiratory tract infections because drug has CNS depressant effect. Also use cautiously in patients with cardiovascular, hepatic, or renal disease because of increased risk of developing hypotension, heart failure, and arrhythmias.
•Because of chlorpromazine's anticholinergic effects, use it cautiously in patients with glaucoma. Also use it cautiously in those who are exposed to extreme heat or organophosphorus insecticides and those receiving atropine or related drugs.
•Protect concentrate from light. Refrigeration isn't required.
•Dilute concentrate in at least 60 ml of diluent just before giving it. Use tomato or fruit juice, milk, simple syrup, orange syrup, a carbonated beverage, coffee, tea, water, or semisolid food, such as pudding and soup.
•Protect parenteral solution from light. Solution should be clear and colorless to pale yellow. Discard markedly discolored solution.
•Don't inject drug by S.C. route because it can cause severe tissue necrosis.
•Wear gloves when working with liquid or injectable form because parenteral solution may cause contact dermatitis.
•For I.V. injection, dilute chlorpromazine with sodium chloride to a concentration of 1 mg/ml.
•Give I.M. injection slowly and deep into upper outer quadrant of buttocks, such as in

the gluteus maximus. To minimize hypotensive effects, keep patient lying flat and monitor blood pressure for 30 minutes after injection.
•**WARNING** Stay alert for possible suppressed cough reflex, which increases the risk of the patient's aspirating vomitus.
•Monitor for increased sensitivity to drug's CNS effects if patient has a history of hepatic encephalopathy from cirrhosis.
•**WARNING** If neuroleptic malignant syndrome (hyperpyrexia, muscle rigidity, altered mental status, autonomic instability) develops, notify prescriber immediately and expect to stop drug and start intensive treatment. Watch for recurrence if patient resumes antipsychotic therapy.

**PATIENT TEACHING**
•Instruct patient to swallow E.R. capsules whole and not to crush, break, or chew them.
•Tell patient not to take drug within 2 hours of taking an antacid. Allow him to take drug with food or a full glass of milk or water.
•If patient uses suppository form, tell him to chill the suppository, moisten it with cold water, and insert it well inside the rectum.
•Tell patient to store oral concentrate at room temperature, away from light. Instruct him to measure it with the dropper provided and to dilute it in 4 oz of fluid just before use.
•Because of possible drowsiness, dizziness, and blurred vision (especially during the first few days of therapy), advise the patient to avoid potentially hazardous activities until drug's CNS effects are known.
•Tell patient to avoid alcohol because of possible additive effects and hypotension.
•Advise patient, especially if elderly, to rise slowly from a supine or seated position to avoid dizziness, light-headedness, and fainting.
•Tell patient to inform doctors and dentists that he's taking chlorpromazine before he undergoes surgery, medical tests, or dental work.
•Explain that drug may reduce the body's response to heat and cold; tell patient to avoid temperature extremes, as in a sauna, hot tub, or very cold or hot shower. Remind patient to dress warmly in cold weather.
•Warn patient not to take OTC drugs for a cold or an allergy; they can increase the risk of heatstroke and other unwanted effects.
•Inform patient that drug increases sensitivity to sunlight; tell him to stay out of the sun as much as possible and to protect his skin.

•If patient reports dry mouth, suggest sugarless chewing gum, hard candy, and fluids.
•Urge patient to report sudden sore throat or other signs of infection.

# chlorpropamide

Apo-Chlorpropamide (CAN), Diabinese, Novo-Propamide (CAN)

## Class and Category
*Chemical:* Sulfonylurea
*Therapeutic:* Antidiabetic
*Pregnancy category:* C

## Indications and Dosages
➤ *As adjunct to manage non–insulin-dependent diabetes when diet alone fails to lower blood glucose level*

**TABLETS**
**Adults.** *Initial:* 250 mg q.d. for 5 to 7 days. After therapy begins, dosage may be adjusted up or down by increments of 50 to 125 mg at intervals of 3 to 5 days to obtain optimal control. *Maintenance:* 100 to 500 mg q.d. *Maximum:* 750 mg q.d.

DOSAGE ADJUSTMENT Dosage reduced to half usual insulin dose during first few days of chlorpropamide therapy if patient takes more than 40 U of insulin daily. Insulin dose can be reduced, depending on response. If patient takes oral antidiabetic drug or less than 40 U of insulin daily, it may be stopped abruptly when chlorpropamide starts.

Dosage reduced to half usual dose if patient has mild renal failure because metabolites and unchanged drug are excreted in urine. To avoid hypoglycemic reactions, initial dosage reduced to 100 to 125 mg q.d. for elderly, debilitated, or malnourished patients and patients with impaired hepatic function.

| Route | Onset | Peak | Duration |
|-------|-------|------|----------|
| P.O. | 1 hr | 3 to 6 hr | 24 to 72 hr |

## Mechanism of Action
Lowers blood glucose level by stimulating release of insulin from the pancreas in patients who have functioning beta cells. It also may increase insulin sensitivity in target tissues, which may result in a decrease in liver breakdown of glycogen to glucose or the liver's production of new glucose.

## Contraindications
Diabetic ketoacidosis (with or without coma), hypersensitivity to chlorpropamide or its components, type I diabetes mellitus

## Interactions
**DRUGS**
*androgens, anticoagulants, azole antifungals, chloramphenicol, clofibrate, fenfluramine, fluconazole, gemfibrozil, H₂-receptor antagonists, magnesium salts, MAO inhibitors, methyldopa, probenecid, salicylates, sulfinpyrazone, sulfonamides, tricyclic antidepressants, urinary acidifiers:* Increased hypoglycemic effect
*barbiturates:* Prolonged barbiturate action
*beta blockers, calcium channel blockers, cholestyramine, corticosteroids, diazoxide, estrogens, hydantoins, isoniazid, nicotinic acid, oral contraceptives, phenothiazines, rifampin, sympathomimetics, thiazide diuretics, thyroid drugs, urinary alkalinizers:* Decreased hypoglycemic effect
*digitalis glycosides:* Increased blood digitalis level
*oral miconazole:* Risk of severe hypoglycemia
**ACTIVITIES**
*alcohol use:* Disulfiram-like reaction

## Adverse Reactions
**ENDO:** Hypoglycemia
**GI:** Anorexia, diarrhea, hunger, nausea, vomiting
**SKIN:** Maculopapular eruptions, photosensitivity, pruritus, urticaria
**Other:** Disulfiram-like reaction

## Nursing Considerations
•Use chlorpropamide cautiously in patients with renal or hepatic dysfunction; in elderly, debilitated, or malnourished patients; and in those with adrenal or pituitary insufficiency because of increased susceptibility to drug's hypoglycemic action.
•Monitor patient's blood glucose level frequently at start of therapy and during dosage adjustments or changes in patient's life, such as stress and illness. Hypoglycemia may be difficult to recognize in elderly patients and those who take beta-adrenergic blockers.
•Assess patient for hypoglycemia—the most common adverse reaction to chlorpropamide—especially in patients whose caloric intake is deficient, who have just engaged in strenuous or prolonged exercise, who have ingested alcohol, or who receive more than one glucose-lowering drug.

•Treat hypoglycemia promptly by giving 15 g of simple carbohydrate, such as 4 oz of orange juice or soda or 8 oz of milk. Repeat in 15 minutes, if needed. Because of drug's long half-life, careful monitoring and frequent feedings are required for 3 to 5 days after a hypoglycemic episode. Hospitalization and I.V. glucose may be needed.

•Monitor patients receiving long-term chlorpropamide therapy for secondary failure, which causes loss of blood glucose control despite adherence to prescribed drug therapy and diet and exercise guidelines. If it occurs, therapy should be discontinued and a different antidiabetic drug substituted.

**PATIENT TEACHING**

•Instruct patient to store chlorpropamide in a sealed container, away from heat and light.

•Tell patient to take chlorpropamide with breakfast.

•Stress that drug works with diet and exercise to help control blood glucose level and isn't a substitute for them.

•Tell patient to monitor blood glucose level as instructed.

•Instruct patient not to skip meals or exercise excessively.

•Teach patient how to recognize and treat hypoglycemia. Tell him to report frequent or severe hypoglycemia to prescriber.

•Caution patient with confirmed or suspected hypoglycemia not to drive or operate machinery until blood glucose levels return to normal.

•Tell patient to take a missed dose as soon as he remembers it unless it's almost time for the next scheduled dose.

•Urge patient to wear or carry medical identification showing that he has diabetes and listing his drugs.

•Advise the patient to protect his skin from the sun.

•Instruct the patient to report a fever, sore throat, dark yellow or brown urine, yellow skin and eyes, bleeding, and bruising.

# chlorthalidone

Apo-Chlorthalidone (CAN), Hygroton, Novo-Thalidone (CAN), Thalitone, Uridon (CAN)

## Class and Category

*Chemical:* Phthalimidine derivative of benzenesulfonamide (thiazide-like diuretic)

*Therapeutic:* Antihypertensive, diuretic
*Pregnancy category:* B

## Indications and Dosages

➤ *To reduce edema caused by heart failure, hepatic cirrhosis, corticosteroid or estrogen therapy, or renal dysfunction*

**TABLETS**

**Adults.** *Initial:* 50 to 100 mg (Thalitone, 30 to 60 mg) q.d., 100 mg (Thalitone, 60 mg) q.o.d., or 150 to 200 mg (Thalitone, 90 to 120 mg) q.d. or q.o.d. *Maintenance:* Individualized; may be lower than initial dosage.

➤ *To treat hypertension*

**TABLETS**

**Adults.** *Initial:* 25 mg q.d. (Thalitone, 15 mg q.d.). If response is insufficient, dosage increased to 50 mg q.d. (Thalitone, 30 to 50 mg q.d.). If additional control is required, dosage increased to 100 mg q.d. (except Thalitone) or a second antihypertensive added. *Maintenance:* Individualized; may be lower than initial dosage.

| Route | Onset | Peak | Duration |
|-------|-------|------|----------|
| P.O. | 2 to 3 hr | 2 to 6 hr | 24 to 72 hr |

## Mechanism of Action

May promote sodium, chloride, and water excretion by inhibiting sodium reabsorption in the distal tubules of the kidneys. Initially, chlorthalidone may decrease extracellular fluid volume, plasma volume, and cardiac output, which helps explain how it reduces blood pressure. It also may dilate arteries directly, which helps reduce peripheral vascular resistance and blood pressure. After several weeks, extracellular fluid and plasma volume and cardiac output return to normal, but peripheral vascular resistance remains decreased.

## Contraindications

Anuria; hypersensitivity to chlorthalidone, other sulfonamides, or their components; renal decompensation

## Interactions

**DRUGS**

*allopurinol:* Increased risk of allopurinol hypersensitivity
*amphotericin B, glucocorticoids:* Intensified electrolyte depletion

*anesthetics:* Potentiated effects of anesthetics
*anticholinergics:* Increased chlorthalidone absorption
*antidiabetics, methenamines, oral anticoagulants, sulfonylureas:* Decreased effects of these drugs
*antihypertensives:* Potentiated action of antihypertensives and chlorthalidone
*antineoplastics:* Prolonged antineoplastic-induced leukopenia
*cholestyramine, colestipol:* Decreased chlorthalidone absorption
*diazoxide:* Increased risk of hyperglycemia and hypotension
*digitalis glycosides:* Increased risk of digitalis-induced arrhythmias
*lithium:* Decreased renal lithium clearance and increased risk of lithium toxicity
*loop diuretics:* Increased synergistic effects, resulting in profound diuresis and serious electrolyte imbalances
*methyldopa:* Potential development of hemolytic anemia
*neuromuscular blockers:* Increased neuromuscular blockade
*NSAIDs:* Possibly reduced diuretic effect of chlorthalidone
*vitamin D:* Enhanced vitamin D action

### Adverse Reactions
**CNS:** Dizziness, headache, insomnia, lightheadedness, paresthesia, restlessness, vertigo, weakness
**CV:** Orthostatic hypotension, vasculitis
**EENT:** Yellow vision
**ENDO:** Hyperglycemia
**GI:** Abdominal cramps or pain, anorexia, bloating, constipation, diarrhea, gastric irritation, nausea, pancreatitis, vomiting
**GU:** Decreased libido, impotence
**HEME:** Agranulocytosis, aplastic anemia, hypoplastic anemia, leukopenia, thrombocytopenia
**MS:** Gout attacks, muscle spasms
**SKIN:** Cutaneous vasculitis, exfoliative dermatitis, jaundice, necrotizing vasculitis, photosensitivity, purpura, rash, urticaria
**Other:** Hyperuricemia

### Nursing Considerations
• Use chlorthalidone cautiously in patients with impaired hepatic function or progressive hepatic disease because minor changes in fluid and electrolyte balance may cause hepatic coma.

• Assess BUN, serum electrolyte, uric acid, and blood glucose levels before therapy and periodically throughout therapy. Monitor patient for signs of fluid and electrolyte imbalance.
•**WARNING** Monitor renal function periodically to detect cumulative drug effects, which may cause azotemia in patients with impaired renal function.
**PATIENT TEACHING**
• Stress the importance of taking chlorthalidone even when feeling well.
• Tell patient to store drug at room temperature in tightly closed container.
• Tell patient to take drug in the morning with food or milk.
• To minimize effects of orthostatic hypotension, instruct patient to rise slowly from a seated or lying position.
• Advise patient to check blood pressure regularly.
• Instruct patient to report signs of low potassium level, such as muscle weakness and fatigue.
• Advise patient to protect his skin from the sun.
• Urge patient to immediately report sudden joint pain to prescriber because drug can cause sudden gout attacks.
• Instruct patient to take a missed dose as soon as he remembers it. If he misses one day in an every-other-day schedule, tell him to take the dose on the off day and then resume usual dosing schedule. Warn against taking double or extra doses.

## chlorzoxazone

EZE-DS, Paraflex, Parafon Forte DSC, Relaxazone, Remular, Remular-S, Strifon Forte DSC

### Class and Category
*Chemical:* Benzoxazole derivative
*Therapeutic:* Skeletal muscle relaxant
*Pregnancy category:* C (Parafon Forte DSC, not rated)

### Indications and Dosages
➤ *As adjunct to relieve acute musculoskeletal pain and stiffness*
**TABLETS**
**Adults.** 250 to 750 mg t.i.d. or q.i.d., usually 500 mg t.i.d. or q.i.d., increased or decreased according to patient response.

| Route | Onset | Peak | Duration |
|---|---|---|---|
| P.O. | In 1 hr | Unknown | 3 to 4 hr |

## Mechanism of Action
Reduces muscle spasm by inhibiting multisynaptic reflex arcs at the level of the spinal cord and subcortical areas of the brain that are active in producing and maintaining skeletal muscle spasm.

## Contraindications
Hypersensitivity or known intolerance to chlorzoxazone or any of its components

## Interactions
**DRUGS**
*CNS depressants:* Additive CNS depression
**ACTIVITIES**
*alcohol use:* Additive CNS depression

## Adverse Reactions
**CNS:** Dizziness, drowsiness, headache, lightheadedness, malaise, paradoxical stimulation
**GI:** Abdominal cramps or pain, constipation, diarrhea, GI bleeding, heartburn, hepatotoxicity, nausea, vomiting
**GU:** Urine discoloration
**HEME:** Agranulocytosis, anemia
**SKIN:** Allergic dermatitis, ecchymosis, petechiae
**Other:** Anaphylaxis, angioedema

## Nursing Considerations
•If necessary, crush chlorzoxazone tablets and mix with food or liquid for easier swallowing.
•Assess patients, especially those with a history of allergies, for signs and symptoms of hypersensitivity, such as rash, hives, and itching.
•WARNING Monitor patient for signs of hepatotoxicity, including fever, rash, jaundice, and darkened urine. Notify prescriber immediately and expect to discontinue drug if any of these signs or symptoms occur. Monitor patient for abnormal liver function test results, such as elevated AST, ALT, alkaline phosphatase, and bilirubin levels, and expect to discontinue drug, as ordered, if any of these occurs.
•Provide rest and other pain-relief measures.
•Institute safety measures to prevent falls or injury (such as raising bed rails and assisting with ambulation) until drug's full CNS effects are known.

**PATIENT TEACHING**
•Advise patient to take a missed dose of chlorzoxazone as soon as possible unless it's almost time for the next dose.
•Advise patient to avoid potentially hazardous activities until drug's CNS effects are known.
•Instruct patient to avoid alcohol and other CNS depressants during chlorzoxazone therapy.
•Inform patient that, in rare instances, urine may turn orange or reddish purple during therapy.
•Advise patient to store drug in a tightly capped container at room temperature.

# cholestyramine

Questran, Questran Light

## Class and Category
*Chemical:* Quaternary ammonium anion exchange resin
*Therapeutic:* Antihyperlipidemic, antipruritic (cholestasis)
*Pregnancy category:* Not rated

## Indications and Dosages
➤ *As adjunct to reduce serum cholesterol level in patients with primary hypercholesterolemia, to relieve pruritus associated with partial biliary obstruction*

**ORAL SUSPENSION**
**Adults.** *Initial:* 4 g q.d. or b.i.d. before meals. *Maintenance:* 8 to 24 g equally divided and given 2 to 6 times a day. *Maximum:* 24 g/day when used as antihyperlipidemic drug and 16 g/day when used as antipruritic drug.

| Route | Onset | Peak | Duration |
|---|---|---|---|
| P.O. | In 1 to 2 wk* | Unknown | 2 to 4 wk† |

## Contraindications
Complete biliary obstruction (when bile isn't excreted into intestine), hypersensitivity to cholestyramine or its components

---

\* For hypercholesterolemia; in 1 to 3 wk for pruritus.
† For hypercholesterolemia; 1 to 2 wk for pruritus.

## Mechanism of Action
Increases bile acid excretion in the feces. The resulting decreased bile acid level increases the activity of the enzyme that regulates cholesterol synthesis in the liver. As a result, the liver increases its cholesterol synthesis to produce more bile acids. However, the liver's synthesis of cholesterol typically can't match the amount needed to synthesize bile acids, which reduces the cholesterol level. Also, a decreased cholesterol level causes liver cells to increase their uptake of LDLs, which further reduces the cholesterol level. Cholestyramine may relieve pruritus by decreasing the body's bile acid level. This reduces the amount of excess bile acids that are deposited in the dermis and that typically cause pruritus in patients with cholestasis.

## Interactions
**DRUGS**
*chenodiol, digitalis glycosides, fat-soluble vitamins, folic acid, gemfibrozil, penicillin G (oral), phenylbutazone, propranolol (oral), tetracyclines (oral), thiazide diuretics (oral), thyroid hormones, ursodiol, vancomycin (oral):* Decreased absorption and effects of these drugs
*oral anticoagulants:* Decreased or increased anticoagulant effect

## Adverse Reactions
**CNS:** Headache, dizziness
**GI:** Bloating, constipation, diarrhea, epigastric pain, eructation, fecal impaction, flatulence, indigestion, nausea, vomiting

## Nursing Considerations
•Store cholestyramine at room temperature.
•Don't administer dry powder without mixing it in a beverage because it may cause esophageal distress.
•**WARNING** Be aware that long-term use may increase bleeding tendency from hyperprothrombinemia caused by vitamin K deficiency. If this occurs, patient will require treatment with vitamin $K_1$.
•Monitor for deficiencies of fat-soluble vitamins, such as A and D. If long-term therapy prevents absorption of these vitamins, expect to provide supplementation.

**PATIENT TEACHING**
•Urge patient to follow a low-fat, low-cholesterol diet and regular exercise program.
•Tell patient to take drug before meals.
•Instruct patient to mix dry powder as follows: Place the amount of powder equal to his dosage in any beverage and stir vigorously. Then, vigorously stir an additional 2 to 4 oz of beverage into the mixture. After drinking the mixture, rinse the glass with more liquid, and swallow that liquid to make sure all the drug is taken. Explain that the drug also can be mixed in thin soups or moist, pulpy fruits, such applesauce and crushed pineapple.
•Tell patient to drink plenty of fluids and increase bulk in his diet to minimize constipation; remind him to notify prescriber if constipation, nausea, or other adverse GI reactions develop.
•Explain that the serum cholesterol level will need to be measured frequently during the first few months of therapy and periodically thereafter.
•Advise patient to take other drugs at least 1 hour before or 4 to 6 hours after cholestyramine to avoid interference with their absorption.
•Tell patient to take a missed dose as soon as he remembers but not to take double or extra doses.

# choline and magnesium salicylates
Tricosal, Trilisate

## Class and Category
*Chemical:* Salicylate
*Therapeutic:* Analgesic, anti-inflammatory, antipyretic
*Pregnancy category:* C (first trimester), Not rated (later trimesters)

## Indications and Dosages
➤ *To treat osteoarthritis, rheumatoid arthritis, and acute painful shoulder*
**LIQUID, TABLETS**
**Adults.** 1,500 mg b.i.d. or 3,000 mg h.s.
**Children who weigh more than 37 kg (81 lb).** 2,250 mg/day in equally divided doses b.i.d.
**Children who weigh 37 kg or less.** 50 mg/kg/day in equally divided doses b.i.d.

➤ *To treat mild to moderate pain, to reduce fever*

**LIQUID, TABLETS**

**Adults.** 2,000 to 3,000 mg/day in equally divided doses b.i.d.

**DOSAGE ADJUSTMENT** Dosage reduced to 750 mg t.i.d. for elderly patients.

| Route | Onset | Peak | Duration |
|-------|-------|------|----------|
| P.O. | Unknown | Several wk* | Unknown |

### Mechanism of Action

Block the activity of cyclooxygenase, the enzyme needed for prostaglandin synthesis. As mediators in the inflammatory process, prostaglandins cause local vasodilation with swelling and pain. They also play a role in pain transmission from the periphery to the spinal cord. By blocking cyclooxygenase and inhibiting prostaglandins, this NSAID decreases inflammatory symptoms and relieves pain. It acts on the heat-regulating center in the hypothalamus and causes peripheral vasodilation, sweating, and heat loss.

### Contraindications

Hypersensitivity to nonacetylated salicylates

### Interactions

**DRUGS**

*antacids:* Increased clearance and decreased blood level of salicylate
*carbonic anhydrase inhibitors, phenytoin, valproic acid:* Decreased blood levels and therapeutic effects of these drugs
*corticosteroids:* Decreased blood salicylate level, increased salicylate dosage requirements
*insulin, sulfonylureas:* Increased hypoglycemic response
*methotrexate:* Increased therapeutic and toxic effects of methotrexate, especially when given in chemotherapeutic doses
*oral anticoagulants:* Increased blood level of unbound anticoagulant and risk of bleeding
*salicylate-containing products:* Increased plasma salicylate level, possibly to toxic level
*uricosuric drugs:* Decreased uricosuric drug efficacy

### Adverse Reactions

**CNS:** Dizziness, drowsiness, headache, lethargy, light-headedness

---

* For rheumatoid arthritis.

**EENT:** Hearing loss, tinnitus
**GI:** Constipation, diarrhea, epigastric pain, heartburn, indigestion, nausea, vomiting
**HEME:** Easy bruising, unusual bleeding

### Nursing Considerations

• Use choline and magnesium salicylates cautiously in patients with gastritis, hepatic or renal dysfunction, or peptic ulcer disease.
• Don't give salicylates to children and adolescents with chickenpox or influenza symptoms because of the risk of Reye's syndrome.
• **WARNING** During high-dose or long-term therapy, monitor for signs of salicylate intoxication, such as headache, dizziness, tinnitus, hearing loss, confusion, drowsiness, diaphoresis, vomiting, diarrhea, and hyperventilation. CNS disturbance, electrolyte imbalance, respiratory acidosis, hyperthermia, and dehydration also may occur. If intoxication occurs, prepare to induce vomiting, administer gastric lavage, and give activated charcoal, as ordered. In extreme cases, prepare patient for peritoneal dialysis or hemodialysis.

**PATIENT TEACHING**

• Tell patient to store drug at room temperature, away from heat, light, and moisture.
• Instruct patient to take drug with food or after meals with a full glass of water.
• Tell patient to take a missed dose as soon as he remembers but to avoid double-dosing.
• Advise patient that optimal effects may not occur for 2 to 3 weeks.
• Teach patient to recognize and immediately report signs of salicylate toxicity.
• Explain that drug is closely related to aspirin. Advise against taking aspirin-containing OTC remedies during therapy.

## choline salicylate

Arthropan

### Class and Category

*Chemical:* Salicylate
*Therapeutic:* Analgesic, anti-inflammatory, antipyretic
*Pregnancy category:* C (first trimester), Not rated (later trimesters)

### Indications and Dosages

➤ *To treat mild to moderate pain, reduce fever*

**LIQUID**

**Adults and adolescents.** 435 to 870 mg q 4 hr, p.r.n. *Maximum:* 5,325 mg/day.

**Children ages 11 to 12.** 435 to 652.5 mg q 4 hr, p.r.n. *Maximum:* Five doses/day.
**Children ages 9 to 11.** 435 to 543.8 mg q 4 hr, p.r.n. *Maximum:* Five doses/day.
**Children ages 6 to 9.** 435 mg q 4 hr, p.r.n. *Maximum:* Five doses/day.
**Children ages 4 to 6.** 326.5 mg q 4 hr, p.r.n. *Maximum:* Five doses/day.
**Children ages 2 to 4.** 217.5 mg q 4 hr, p.r.n. *Maximum:* Five doses/day.
**Children up to age 2.** Individualized dosage. *Maximum:* Five doses/day.

➤ *To treat rheumatoid arthritis*
LIQUID
**Adults and adolescents.** 870 to 1,740 mg up to four times/day.
**Children age 12 and younger.** 107 to 133 mg/kg/day in divided doses.

| Route | Onset | Peak | Duration |
|-------|-------|------|----------|
| P.O. | Unknown | Several wk* | Unknown |

---

**Mechanism of Action**

Blocks cyclooxygenase, an enzyme needed for prostaglandin synthesis. As mediators in the inflammatory process, prostaglandins cause local vasodilation, swelling, and pain. They also influence pain transmission from the periphery to the spinal cord. By blocking cyclooxygenase and inhibiting prostaglandins, this NSAID decreases inflammatory symptoms and relieves pain. It also acts on the heat-regulating center in the hypothalamus and causes peripheral vasodilation, sweating, and heat loss.

---

**Contraindications**

Hypersensitivity to nonacetylated salicylates

**Interactions**
DRUGS
*antacids:* Increased clearance and decreased blood level of salicylate
*carbonic anhydrase inhibitors, phenytoin, valproic acid:* Decreased blood levels and therapeutic effects of these drugs
*corticosteroids:* Decreased blood salicylate level, increased salicylate dosage requirements
*insulin, sulfonylureas:* Increased hypoglycemic response

---

*For rheumatoid arthritis.

*methotrexate:* Increased therapeutic and toxic effects of methotrexate, especially when given in chemotherapeutic doses
*oral anticoagulants:* Increased blood level of unbound anticoagulant and risk of bleeding
*salicylate-containing products:* Increased plasma salicylate level, possibly to toxic level
*uricosuric drugs:* Decreased uricosuric drug efficacy

**Adverse Reactions**

**CNS:** Confusion, dizziness, drowsiness, hallucinations, headache, light-headedness
**CV:** Tachycardia
**EENT:** Hearing loss, tinnitus
**GI:** Constipation, diarrhea, epigastric pain, heartburn, indigestion, nausea, vomiting
**HEME:** Easy bruising, unusual bleeding

**Nursing Considerations**

•Use choline salicylate cautiously in patients with renal impairment.
•Don't give salicylates to children and adolescents with chickenpox or influenza symptoms because of the risk of Reye's syndrome.
•WARNING During high-dose or long-term therapy, watch for salicylate intoxication, (headache, dizziness, tinnitus, hearing loss, confusion, drowsiness, diaphoresis, vomiting, diarrhea, hyperventilation, and possibly CNS disturbance, electrolyte imbalance, respiratory acidosis, hyperthermia, and dehydration). Prepare for induced vomiting, gastric lavage, activated charcoal, and peritoneal dialysis or hemodialysis, as ordered.
PATIENT TEACHING
•Tell patient to store drug at room temperature, away from heat, light, and moisture.
•Instruct patient to take drug with full glass of water or with food.
•Tell patient to take a missed dose as soon as he remembers but to avoid double-dosing.
•If patient has arthritis, explain that optimal drug effects may not occur for 2 to 3 weeks.
•Teach patient to recognize and immediately report signs of salicylate toxicity.
•Because drug is closely related to aspirin, advise against taking aspirin-containing OTC products during therapy.

# cilostazol

Pletal

**Class and Category**
*Chemical:* Quinolinone derivative

*Therapeutic:* Phosphodiesterase III inhibitor, platelet aggregation inhibitor
*Pregnancy category:* C

## Indications and Dosages

➤ *To reduce symptoms of intermittent claudication*

**TABLETS**

**Adults.** 100 mg b.i.d. taken at least 30 min before or 2 hr after breakfast and dinner.

## Contraindications

Heart failure, hypersensitivity to cilostazol or its components

---

### Mechanism of Action

May inhibit phosphodiesterase, decreasing phosphodiesterase activity and suppressing cAMP degradation. This action increases cAMP in platelets and blood vessels, which inhibits platelet aggregation and causes vasodilation. This in turn relieves symptoms of claudication.

---

## Interactions

**DRUGS**

*diltiazem, erythromycin, itraconazole, ketoconazole, omeprazole:* Increased plasma cilostazol level

**FOODS**

*grapefruit:* Increased risk of adverse reactions
*high-fat foods:* Faster cilostazol absorption and increased risk of adverse reactions

**ACTIVITIES**

*smoking:* Decreased cilostazol effects by about 20%

## Adverse Reactions

**CNS:** Cerebral hemorrhage, dizziness, headache, paresthesia
**CV:** Angina, chest pain, hypotension, palpitations, peripheral edema, tachycardia
**EENT:** Pharyngitis, rhinitis
**ENDO:** Diabetes mellitus, hot flashes, hyperglycemia
**GI:** Abdominal pain, abnormal stool, diarrhea, elevated liver function test results, flatulence, hepatic dysfunction, indigestion, jaundice, vomiting
**GU:** Elevated BUN level, hematuria
**HEME:** Bleeding tendency, leukopenia, thrombocytopenia
**MS:** Back pain, myalgia
**RESP:** Cough, interstitial pneumonia, pulmonary hemorrhage
**SKIN:** Eruptions, pruritus, rash, Stevens-Johnson syndrome
**Other:** Hot flashes, infection

## Nursing Considerations

• Monitor vital signs and cardiovascular status closely because cilostazol may cause cardiovascular lesions, which could lead to problems, such as endocardial hemorrhage.
• Monitor blood glucose level to detect hyperglycemia. Also assess for signs of type 2 diabetes mellitus, such as polyuria, polydipsia, polyphagia, and fatigue.

**PATIENT TEACHING**

• Instruct patient to take cilostazol on an empty stomach because high-fat foods can increase the risk of adverse reactions.
• Warn patent to avoid grapefruit juice during therapy because it can increase the risk of adverse reactions.
• Urge patient not to smoke because it decreases drug's effects.
• Explain that assessment of drug effectiveness is based on ability to walk increased distances. Stress that drug effects won't appear until 2 to 4 weeks after therapy starts and that full effects may take up to 12 weeks.

# cimetidine

Apo-Cimetidine (CAN), Gen-Cimetidine (CAN), Novo-Cimetine (CAN), Nu-Cimet (CAN), PMS-Cimetidine (CAN), Tagamet, Tagamet HB

## cimetidine hydrochloride

Novo-Cimetine (CAN), Tagamet

## Class and Category

*Chemical:* Imidazole derivative
*Therapeutic:* Antiulcer agent, gastric acid secretion inhibitor, $H_2$-receptor antagonist
*Pregnancy category:* B

## Indications and Dosages

➤ *To treat and prevent recurrence of duodenal ulcer*

**ORAL SOLUTION, TABLETS**

**Adults and adolescents.** *Initial:* 800 mg h.s., 300 mg q.i.d. with meals and h.s., or 400 to 600 mg in morning and h.s. for 4 to 6 wk. *Maintenance:* 400 mg h.s.
**Children.** 20 to 40 mg/kg/day in divided doses q.i.d. with meals and h.s.

**I.V. OR I.M. INJECTION**

**Adults.** *Initial:* 300 mg q 6 to 8 hr. Dosage increased, if needed, by increasing frequency. *Maximum:* 2,400 mg/day.

➤ *To treat active, benign gastric ulcer*

**ORAL SOLUTION, TABLETS**

**Adults and adolescents.** 800 mg h.s., 300 mg q.i.d. with meals and h.s., or 600 mg b.i.d. in morning and h.s., or 800 mg h.s. for up to 8 wk.

**Children.** 20 to 40 mg/kg/day in divided doses q.i.d. with meals and h.s.

**I.V. OR I.M. INJECTION**

**Adults and adolescents.** *Initial:* 300 mg q 6 to 8 hr. Dosage increased, if needed, by increasing frequency. *Maximum:* 2,400 mg/day.

➤ *To manage gastroesophageal reflux disease*

**ORAL SOLUTION, TABLETS**

**Adults and adolescents.** 1,600 mg/day in divided doses (800 mg b.i.d or 400 mg q.i.d.) for up to 12 wk.

**Children.** 40 to 80 mg/kg/day in divided doses q.i.d.

➤ *To treat pathological hypersecretory conditions, such as Zollinger-Ellison syndrome*

**ORAL SOLUTION, TABLETS**

**Adults and adolescents.** 300 mg q.i.d. with meals and h.s. Given more often, if needed. *Maximum:* 2,400 mg/day.

**I.V. OR I.M. INJECTION**

**Adults and adolescents.** *Initial:* 300 mg q 6 to 8 hr. Dosage increased, if needed, by increasing frequency. *Maximum:* 2,400 mg/day.

➤ *To treat heartburn and acid indigestion*

**ORAL SOLUTION, TABLETS**

**Adults and adolescents.** *Initial:* 200 mg with water at onset of symptoms. *Maximum:* 400 mg q 24 hr for no more than 2 wk unless prescribed.

**DOSAGE ADJUSTMENT** Oral dosage for all indications reduced to 300 mg q 12 hr (and increased to q 8 hr with caution, if needed) for patients with renal impairment.

➤ *To prevent stress-related upper GI bleeding during hospitalization*

**I.V. INFUSION**

**Adults.** 50 mg/hr by continuous infusion for 7 days.

| Route | Onset | Peak | Duration |
|---|---|---|---|
| P.O. | Unknown | 1 to 2 hr | 4 to 5 hr |
| I.V., I.M. | Unknown | Unknown | 4 to 5 hr |

## Mechanism of Action

Blocks histamine's action at $H_2$-receptor sites on the stomach's parietal cells. This action reduces gastric fluid volume and acidity. Cimetidine also decreases the amount of gastric acid that's secreted in response to food, caffeine, insulin, betazole, or pentagastrin.

## Incompatibilities

Don't mix cimetidine with aminophylline or barbiturates in I.V. solution. Don't mix drug with pentobarbital sodium in the same syringe.

## Contraindications

Hypersensitivity to cimetidine or its components

## Interactions

**DRUGS**

*antacids, anticholinergics, metoclopramide:* Decreased cimetidine absorption

*benzodiazepines, calcium channel blockers, carbamazepine, chloroquine, labetalol, lidocaine, metoprolol, metronidazole, moricizine, pentoxifylline, phenytoin, propafenone, propranolol, quinidine, quinine, sulfonylureas, tacrine, theophyllines, triamterene, tricyclic antidepressants, valproic acid, warfarin:* Reduced metabolism and increased blood levels and effects of these drugs, possibly toxicity from these drugs

*carmustine:* Increased carmustine myelotoxicity

*digoxin, fluconazole:* Possibly decreased blood levels of these drugs

*ferrous salts, indomethacin, ketoconazole, tetracyclines:* Decreased effects of these drugs

*flecainide:* Increased flecainide effects

*fluorouracil:* Increased blood fluorouracil level after long-term cimetidine use

*ketoconazole:* Decreased blood ketoconazole level

*narcotic analgesics:* Increased toxic effects of narcotic analgesics

*oral anticoagulants:* Increased anticoagulant effect

*procainamide:* Increased blood procainamide level

*succinylcholine:* Increased neuromuscular blockade

*tocainide:* Decreased tocainide effects

**FOODS**
*caffeine:* Reduced metabolism and increased blood level and effects of caffeine
**ACTIVITIES**
*alcohol use:* Possibly increased blood alcohol level

## Adverse Reactions

**CNS:** Confusion, dizziness, hallucinations, headache, peripheral neuropathy, somnolence
**ENDO:** Mild gynecomastia if used longer than 1 month
**GI:** Mild and transient diarrhea
**GU:** Impotence, transiently elevated serum creatinine level
**SKIN:** Rash
**Other:** Pain at I.M. injection site

## Nursing Considerations

•**WARNING** Be aware that rapid administration of cimetidine can increase patient's risk of developing arrhythmias and hypotension.
•For I.V. injection, dilute cimetidine in NS to a total volume of 20 ml. Inject drug over 5 minutes or more.
•For intermittent I.V. infusion, dilute drug in at least 50 ml of $D_5W$ or other compatible I.V. solution. Infuse over 15 to 20 minutes.
•For I.M. injection, don't dilute drug.
•Be especially alert for confusion in elderly or debilitated patients who receive cimetidine.
**PATIENT TEACHING**
•Tell patient to use a liquid-measuring device to ensure accurate measurement of oral solution.
•Advise patient to avoid alcohol while taking cimetidine to prevent interactions.
•Instruct patient to avoid taking antacids within 1 hour of taking cimetidine.
•Warn patient that cigarette smoking increases gastric acid secretion and can worsen gastric disease.
•Caution patient not to take drug for more than 14 days, unless prescribed.

# cinacalcet hydrochloride

Sensipar

## Class and Category

Chemical: Calcimimetic
Therapeutic: Calcium reducer
Pregnancy category: C

## Indications and Dosages

➤ *To treat secondary hyperparathyroidism in patients with chronic renal disease who are on dialysis*

**TABLETS**
**Adults.** Initial: 30 mg q.d. P.O., increased q 2 to 4 wk in sequential doses of 60, 90, 120, and 180 mg q.d., as needed.
➤ *To treat hypercalcemia in patients with parathyroid carcinoma*
**TABLETS**
**Adults.** Initial: 30 mg q.d. P.O., increased q 2 to 4 wk in sequential doses of 30 mg b.i.d., 60 mg b.i.d., 90 mg b.i.d., and then 90 mg t.i.d. or q.i.d., as needed to normalize serum calcium level.

| Route | Onset | Peak | Duration |
|---|---|---|---|
| P.O. | Unknown | 2 to 6 hr | Unknown |

## Mechanism of Action

Increases the sensitivity of calcium-sensing receptors on the surface of parathyroid cells to extracellular calcium. This sensitivity directly reduces parathyroid hormone (PTH) level, which in turn decreases serum calcium level.

## Contraindications

Hypersensitivity to cinacalcet or its components

## Interactions

**DRUGS**
*amitriptyline, flecainide, thioridazine, tricyclic antidepressants (most), vinblastine:* Possibly increased blood level of these drugs
*erythromycin, itraconazole, ketoconazole:* Possibly increased blood cinacalcet level

## Adverse Reactions

**CNS:** Asthenia, dizziness
**CV:** Hypertension
**ENDO:** Hypocalcemia
**GI:** Anorexia, diarrhea, nausea, vomiting
**MS:** Myalgia
**Other:** Noncardiac chest pain

## Nursing Considerations

•Use cinacalcet cautiously in patients with a history of seizures because reduced blood calcium level may lower seizure threshold. Also use cautiously in patients with hepatic insufficiency because cinacalcet metabolism may be reduced.
•Monitor patient for hypocalcemia exhibited by cramping, myalgia, paresthesia, seizures, and tetany. Also monitor patient's blood cal-

cium and phosphorus levels within 1 week after starting therapy or adjusting dosage, and every month or two once the maintenance dose is established, as ordered. If hypocalcemia develops, notify prescriber immediately because treatment to raise calcium level will be needed. Treatment may include supplemental calcium, initiating or increasing dosage of calcium-based phosphate binder or vitamin D sterols, or temporarily withholding cinacalcet.
• Be aware that if patient begins or stops therapy with a strong CYP3A4 inhibitor, such as erythromycin, itraconazole, or ketoconazole, cinacalcet dosage may need to be adjusted.
• Monitor dialysis patient's intact PTH levels 1 to 4 weeks after therapy starts or dose is adjusted and then every 1 to 3 months thereafter, as ordered. Expect to reduce dosage or discontinue cinacalcet therapy, as ordered, in a patient whose intact PTH level falls below the target range of 150 to 300 pg/ml.

**PATIENT TEACHING**
• Instruct patient to take cinacalcet with food or shortly after a meal.
• Caution patient to take tablet whole and not divide it or crush it.
• Review signs and symptoms of hypocalcemia with patient and urge him to notify prescriber of changes.

# cinoxacin

Cinobac

## Class and Category

*Chemical:* Quinolone derivative
*Therapeutic:* Antibiotic
*Pregnancy category:* B

## Indications and Dosages

➤ *To treat UTIs caused by* Enterobacter *sp.,* Escherichia coli, Klebsiella *sp.,* Proteus mirabilis, *and* Proteus vulgaris

**CAPSULES**
**Adults.** 1 g/day in divided doses b.i.d. to q.i.d. for 7 to 14 days.

**DOSAGE ADJUSTMENT** After initial dose of 500 mg, dosage reduced to 250 mg t.i.d. if creatinine clearance is 50 to 80 ml/min/ 1.73 $m^2$, 250 mg b.i.d. if creatinine clearance is 20 to 50 ml/min/1.73 $m^2$, and 250 mg q.d. if creatinine clearance is less than 20 ml/min/ 1.73 $m^2$.

➤ *To prevent UTIs in women with a history of chronic UTIs*

**CAPSULES**
**Adults.** 250 mg h.s. for up to 5 mo.

## Contraindications

Hypersensitivity to cinoxacin, other quinolones, or their components

> **Mechanism of Action**
> Inhibits the enzyme DNA gyrase, which is responsible for the unwinding and supercoiling of bacterial DNA before it replicates. By inhibiting this enzyme, cinoxacin causes bacterial cells to die.

## Interactions

**DRUGS**
*antacids that contain aluminum or magnesium, didanosine (chewable tablets, buffered tablets, pediatric powder for oral solution), metal cations (such as iron), multivitamins that contain zinc, sucralfate:* Possibly interference with cinoxacin absorption
*probenecid:* Increased blood cinoxacin level
*theophylline:* Possibly increased blood theophylline level

**FOODS**
*caffeine:* Decreased metabolism of caffeine, resulting in increased blood caffeine level

## Adverse Reactions

**CNS:** Dizziness, headache
**CV:** Edema
**EENT:** Altered taste
**GI:** Abdominal cramps, anorexia, diarrhea, elevated liver function test results, nausea, vomiting
**GU:** Perineal burning
**HEME:** Eosinophilia
**SKIN:** Angioedema, photosensitivity, pruritus, rash, urticaria

## Nursing Considerations

• Obtain results of urine culture and sensitivity test before administering first dose of cinoxacin.
• Review results of liver function tests, as indicated, during treatment.
• Administer drug with food, if needed; food decreases peak blood level but doesn't change total absorption.

**PATIENT TEACHING**
• Tell patient to take cinoxacin with food, if needed, to avoid GI distress.

•Instruct patient to drink 2 to 3 L of fluid daily unless contraindicated.

•Inform patient not to take antacids that contain aluminum or magnesium; didanosine chewable tablets, buffered tablets, or pediatric powder for oral solution; sucralfate; metal cations such as iron; or multivitamins that contain zinc for at least 2 hours before or after taking cinoxacin because they can interfere with absorption of the drug.

•Advise patient to limit caffeine intake while taking cinoxacin because the drug may cause caffeine to accumulate in the body.

•Advise patient to immediately report edema, rash, or severe adverse GI reactions.

•Tell patient to immediately report tendon inflammation, pain, or rupture to prescriber because other drugs in the same class as cinoxacin have been known to cause tendon rupture, requiring drug therapy to be discontinued.

•Warn patient about the potential for seizures, which have occurred with other drugs in the same class as cinoxacin.

# ciprofloxacin

Cipro, Cipro I.V., Cipro XR, Proquin XR

## Class and Category

*Chemical:* Fluoroquinolone derivative
*Therapeutic:* Antibiotic
*Pregnancy category:* C

## Indications and Dosages

➤ *To prevent inhalation anthrax after exposure or to treat inhalation anthrax*

**ORAL SUSPENSION, TABLETS**

**Adults and adolescents.** 500 mg q 12 hr for 60 days.

**Children.** 15 mg/kg q 12 hr for 60 days. *Maximum:* 500 mg/dose.

**I.V. INFUSION**

**Adults and adolescents.** 400 mg q 12 hr for 60 days.

**Children.** 10 mg/kg q 12 hr for 60 days. *Maximum:* 400 mg/dose or 800 mg/day.

➤ *To treat acute sinusitis caused by gram-negative organisms (including* Campylobacter jejuni, Citrobacter diversus, Citrobacter freundii, Enterobacter cloacae, Escherichia coli, Haemophilus influenzae, Haemophilus parainfluenzae, Klebsiella pneumoniae, Morganella morganii, Neisseria gonorrhoeae, Proteus

mirabilis, Proteus vulgaris, Providencia rettgeri, Providencia stuartii, Pseudomonas aeruginosa, Serratia marcescens, Shigella flexneri, *and* Shigella sonnei) *and gram-positive organisms (including* Enterococcus faecalis, Staphylococcus aureus, Staphylococcus epidermidis, *and* Streptococcus pneumoniae)

**ORAL SUSPENSION, TABLETS**

**Adults.** 500 mg q 12 hr for 10 days.

**I.V. INFUSION**

**Adults.** For mild to moderate infections, 400 mg q 12 hr.

➤ *To treat bone and joint infections caused by susceptible organisms listed above*

**ORAL SUSPENSION, TABLETS**

**Adults.** For mild to moderate infections, 500 mg q 12 hr for 4 to 6 wk. For severe or complicated infections, 750 mg q 12 hr for 4 to 6 wk.

**I.V. INFUSION**

**Adults.** For mild to moderate infections, 400 mg q 12 hr for 4 to 6 wk. For severe or complicated infections, 400 mg q 8 hr.

➤ *To treat skin and soft-tissue infections caused by susceptible organisms listed above*

**ORAL SUSPENSION, TABLETS**

**Adults.** For mild to moderate infections, 500 mg q 12 hr for 7 to 14 days. For severe or complicated infections, 750 mg q 12 hr for 7 to 14 days.

**I.V. INFUSION**

**Adults.** For mild to moderate infections, 400 mg q 12 hr. For severe or complicated infections, 400 mg q 8 hr.

➤ *To treat chronic bacterial prostatitis caused by susceptible organisms listed above*

**ORAL SUSPENSION, TABLETS**

**Adults.** 500 mg q 12 hr for 28 days.

**I.V. INFUSION**

**Adults.** 400 mg q 12 hr.

➤ *To treat infectious diarrhea caused by susceptible organisms listed above*

**ORAL SUSPENSION, TABLETS**

**Adults.** 500 mg q 12 hr for 5 to 7 days.

➤ *To treat UTIs caused by susceptible organisms listed above*

**ORAL SUSPENSION, TABLETS**

**Adults.** For acute uncomplicated infections, 100 mg q 12 hr for 3 days. For mild to moderate infections, 250 mg q 12 hr for 7 to 14 days. For severe or complicated infections, 500 mg q 12 hr for 7 to 14 days.

**I.V. INFUSION**

**Adults.** For mild to moderate infections, 200 mg q 12 hr. For severe or complicated infections, 400 mg q 12 hr.

➤ *To treat complicated UTIs caused by* E. coli, K. pneumoniae, Enterococcus faecalis, P. mirabilis, *or* P. aeruginosa *or acute uncomplicated pyelonephritis caused by* E. coli

**E.R. TABLETS**

**Adults.** 1,000 mg q.d. for 7 to 14 days.

➤ *To treat acute cystitis caused by* E. coli, P. mirabilis, E. faecalis, *or* Staphylococcus saprophyticus

**E.R. TABLETS**

**Adults.** 500 mg q.d. for 3 days.

➤ *To treat lower respiratory tract infections caused by susceptible organisms listed above*

**ORAL SUSPENSION, TABLETS**

**Adults.** For mild to moderate infections, 500 mg q 12 hr for 7 to 14 days. For severe or complicated infections, 750 mg q 12 hr for 7 to 14 days.

**I.V. INFUSION**

**Adults.** For mild to moderate infections, 400 mg q 12 hr. For severe or complicated infections, 400 mg q 8 hr.

➤ *To treat intra-abdominal infections caused by susceptible organisms listed above*

**I.V. INFUSION**

**Adults.** 400 mg q 8 hr along with parenteral metronidazole.

➤ *To treat mild to severe nosocomial pneumonia caused by susceptible organisms listed above*

**I.V. INFUSION**

**Adults.** 400 mg q 8 hr.

➤ *To treat typhoid fever caused by* Salmonella typhi *or infectious diarrhea caused by* C. jejuni, E. coli, S. flexneri, *or* S. sonnei

**ORAL SUSPENSION, TABLETS**

**Adults.** 500 mg q 12 hr for 10 days.

➤ *To treat uncomplicated urethral or cervical gonococcal infections caused by* N. gonorrhoeae

**ORAL SUSPENSION, TABLETS**

**Adults.** 250 mg as a single dose.

**DOSAGE ADJUSTMENT** Dosage reduced to 250 to 500 mg q 12 hr in patients with creatinine clearance of 30 to 50 ml/min/1.73 $m^2$; and to 250 to 500 mg P.O. or 200 to 400 mg I.V. q 18 hr in patients with creatinine clearance of 5 to 29 ml/min/1.73 $m^2$.

➤ *To treat acute cystitis caused by* E. coli *or* K. pneumoniae

**E.R. TABLETS (PROQUIN XR)**

**Adults.** 500 mg q.d. for 3 days with evening meal.

## Incompatibilities

Don't administer parenteral ciprofloxacin with aminophylline, amoxicillin, cefepime, clindamycin, dexamethasone, floxacillin, furosemide, heparin, or phenytoin.

### Mechanism of Action

Inhibits the enzyme DNA gyrase, which is responsible for the unwinding and supercoiling of bacterial DNA before it replicates. By inhibiting this enzyme, ciprofloxacin causes bacterial cells to die.

## Contraindications

Hypersensitivity to ciprofloxacin, quinolones, or their components

## Interactions

**DRUGS**

*antacids, didanosine, iron supplements, sucralfate, multivitamins that contain iron or zinc:* Decreased ciprofloxacin absorption

*cyclosporine:* Elevated serum creatinine and blood cyclosporine levels

*glyburide:* Severe hypoglycemia

*methotrexate:* Increased blood methotrexate level and increased risk of methotrexate toxicity

*NSAIDs (except acetylsalicylic acid):* Increased risk of seizures with high doses of ciprofloxacin

*oral anticoagulants:* Enhanced anticoagulant effects

*phenytoin:* Increased or decreased blood phenytoin level

*probenecid:* Increased blood ciprofloxacin level and, possibly, toxicity

*theophylline:* Increased blood level, half-life, and risk of adverse effects of theophylline

**FOODS**

*caffeine:* Increased caffeine effects

*dairy products:* Delayed drug absorption

## Adverse Reactions

**CNS:** Agitation, anxiety, cerebral thrombosis, confusion, dizziness, headache, insomnia, light-headedness, migraine, nightmares,

paranoia, peripheral neuropathy, restlessness, seizures, syncope, toxic psychosis
**CV:** Angina, atrial flutter, cardiopulmonary arrest, cardiovascular collapse, hypertension, MI, orthostatic hypotension, palpitations, phlebitis, tachycardia, torsades de pointes, vasculitis, ventricular ectopy
**EENT:** Oral candidiasis
**GI:** Abdominal pain, constipation, diarrhea, elevated liver function test results, flatulence, GI bleeding, hepatic failure or necrosis, hepatitis, indigestion, intestinal perforation, jaundice, nausea, pancreatitis, pseudomembranous colitis, vomiting
**GU:** Crystalluria, hematuria, increased serum creatinine level, interstitial nephritis, nephrotoxicity, renal calculi, renal failure, urine retention, vaginal candidiasis
**HEME:** Agranulocytosis, bone marrow depression, hemolytic anemia, lymphadenopathy, pancytopenia
**MS:** Tendon rupture
**SKIN:** Erythema multiforme, exfoliative dermatitis, photosensitivity, rash, Stevens-Johnson syndrome, toxic epidermal necrolysis, urticaria
**RESP:** Bronchospasm, pulmonary embolism, respiratory arrest
**Other:** Acidosis, anaphylaxis, angioedema, serum sickness–like reaction

## Nursing Considerations
•Obtain culture and sensitivity test results, as ordered, before giving ciprofloxacin.
•Use drug cautiously in patients with CNS disorders.
•Dilute I.V. ciprofloxacin concentrate to 1 to 2 mg/ml using $D_5W$ or sodium chloride for injection. Don't dilute solutions that come from the manufacturer in $D_5W$ before I.V. infusion. Infuse slowly over 1 hour.
•Store reconstituted solution for up to 14 days at room temperature or refrigerated.
•Don't give oral suspension by feeding tube.
•Be aware that E.R. and immediate-release tablets aren't interchangeable and that Proquin XR and Cipro XR aren't interchangeable.
•Be aware that patient should be well hydrated during therapy to help prevent alkaline urine, which may lead to crystalluria and nephrotoxicity.
•Assess patient's hepatic, renal, and hematologic functions periodically, as ordered, if

he's receiving prolonged therapy.
•Monitor patient closely for diarrhea, which may reflect pseudomembranous colitis. If it occurs, notify prescriber and expect to withhold ciprofloxacin and treat diarrhea.
•Assess patient for evidence of peripheral neuropathy. Notify prescriber and expect to stop drug if patient complains of burning, numbness, pain, tingling, or weakness in extremities or if physical examination reveals deficits in light touch, pain, temperature, position sense, vibratory sensation, or motor strength.
•Monitor patients (especially children, elderly patients, and patients receiving corticosteroids) for evidence of tendon rupture, such as inflammation, pain, and swelling at the site. Be aware that tendon rupture may occur during or after ciprofloxacin therapy. Notify prescriber about suspected tendon rupture, and have patient rest and refrain from exercise until tendon rupture has been ruled out. If present, expect to provide supportive care as ordered.
•Assess patient's skin routinely for signs of rash or other hypersensitivity reactions because ciprofloxacin may cause serious skin reactions. Stop drug at first sign of reaction and notify prescriber.

PATIENT TEACHING
•Urge patient to complete the prescribed course of therapy, even if he feels better before it's finished.
•Tell patient not to take drug with dairy products or calcium-fortified juices alone.
•Advise patient to take ciprofloxacin 2 hours before or 6 hours after antacids, iron supplements, or multivitamins that contain iron or zinc. Tell him to shake oral suspension for 15 seconds, not to chew microcapsules, and not to split, crush, or chew E.R. tablets.
•Encourage patient to drink plenty of fluids during therapy to help prevent crystalluria.
•Urge patient to avoid caffeinated products because caffeine may accumulate in the body during ciprofloxacin therapy and cause excessive stimulation.
•Instruct patient to notify prescriber at first sign of allergy, such as rash.
•Caution patient to avoid excessive exposure to sunlight or artificial ultraviolet light because severe sunburn may result. Tell patient to notify prescriber if sunburn develops because ciprofloxacin will need to be stopped.

•Urge patient to avoid hazardous activities until CNS effects of drug are known.

•Advise patient to notify prescriber about severe or prolonged diarrhea, changes in limb sensation or movement, and inflammation, pain, or swelling over a joint.

•Tell patient to stop taking drug and to notify prescriber at first sign of rash or other hypersensitivity reaction.

# citalopram hydrobromide

Celexa

## Class and Category

*Chemical:* Racemic, bicyclic phthalate derivative

*Therapeutic:* Antidepressant

*Pregnancy category:* C

## Indications and Dosages

➤ *To treat depression*

ORAL SOLUTION, TABLETS

**Adults.** *Initial:* 20 mg q.d. Daily dosage increased by 20 mg at weekly intervals, as prescribed. *Usual:* 40 mg q.d. *Maximum:* 60 mg/day.

DOSAGE ADJUSTMENT For elderly patients, maximum dosage is 40 mg/day.

| Route | Onset | Peak | Duration |
|-------|-------|------|----------|
| P.O. | 1 to 4 wk | Unknown | Unknown |

### Mechanism of Action

Blocks serotonin reuptake by adrenergic nerves, which normally release this neurotransmitter from their storage sites when activated by a nerve impulse. This blocked reuptake increases serotonin levels at nerve synapses, which may elevate mood and reduce depression.

## Contraindications

Hypersensitivity to citalopram or its components, use within 14 days of MAO inhibitor therapy

## Interactions

DRUGS

*amitriptyline, bromocriptine, buspirone, clomipramine, dextromethorphan, fluoxetine, fluvoxamine, furazolidone, imipramine, levodopa, lithium, meperidine, naratriptan, nefa-* *zodone, paroxetine, pentazocine, phenelzine, procarbazine, selegiline, sertraline, sibutramine, sumatriptan, tramadol, tranylcypromine, trazodone, venlafaxine, zolmitriptan:* Possibly enhanced serotonergic effects of citalopram, resulting in agitation, chills, confusion, diaphoresis, diarrhea, fever, hyperreflexia, hypomania, incoordination, myoclonus, or tremor

*aspirin, NSAIDs, warfarin:* Increased risk of upper GI bleeding

*carbamazepine:* Possibly increased clearance of citalopram

*cimetidine:* Possibly increased blood citalopram level

*desipramine, metoprolol:* Increased blood levels of these drugs

*furazolidone, procarbazine, selegiline:* Possibly hyperthermia, rigidity, myoclonus, and extreme agitation progressing to delirium and coma

*itraconazole, ketoconazole, macrolide antibiotics, omeprazole:* Possibly decreased clearance of citalopram

*warfarin:* Possibly increased PT

## Adverse Reactions

**CNS:** Agitation, akathisia, anxiety, asthenia, delirium, dizziness, drowsiness, dyskinesia, fatigue, fever, insomnia, myoclonus, neuroleptic malignant syndrome, seizures, serotonin syndrome, tremor

**CV:** Chest pain, prolonged QT interval, thrombosis, ventricular arrhythmias

**EENT:** Blurred vision, dry mouth, rhinitis, sinusitis

**GI:** Abdominal pain, anorexia, diarrhea, GI bleeding, hepatic necrosis, indigestion, nausea, pancreatitis, vomiting

**GU:** Acute renal failure, anorgasmia, decreased libido, dysmenorrhea, ejaculation disorders, impotence, priapism

**HEME:** Abnormal bleeding, decreased PT, hemolytic anemia, thrombocytopenia

**MS:** Arthralgia, myalgia, rhabdomyolysis

**RESP:** Upper respiratory tract infection

**SKIN:** Diaphoresis, ecchymosis, erythema multiforme

**Other:** Anaphylaxis, angioedema, weight gain or loss

## Nursing Considerations

•WARNING Whenever citalopram dosage is increased, monitor patient for possible serotonin syndrome, characterized by agitation,

chills, confusion, diaphoresis, diarrhea, fever, hyperactive reflexes, poor coordination, restlessness, shaking, talking or acting with uncontrolled excitement, tremor, and twitching.
•Be aware that effective antidepressant therapy may transform depression into mania in predisposed individuals. If your patient develops symptoms of mania, notify prescriber immediately and expect to discontinue citalopram.
•Monitor patient with hepatic disease for increased adverse reactions because drug is extensively metabolized in the liver.
•Assess elderly patients and those taking diuretics for signs suggesting syndrome of inappropriate secretion of antidiuretic hormone, including hyponatremia and increased serum and urine osmolarity.
•If patient takes citalopram for depression, monitor him closely for suicidal tendencies, especially when therapy starts or dosage changes, because depression may worsen at these times.
•If drug will be stopped, expect to reduce the dosage gradually to avoid serious adverse reactions.

**PATIENT TEACHING**
•Inform patient that citalopram's full effects may take up to 4 weeks to occur.
•Advise patient not to self-medicate for coughs, colds, or allergies without consulting prescriber because some ingredients in these preparations can increase the risk of adverse reactions.
•Caution patient not to stop citalopram abruptly because doing so may lead to serious adverse reactions.
•If patient takes citalopram for depression, urge caregivers to monitor him closely for suicidal tendencies, especially when therapy starts or dosage changes.
•Caution against taking OTC NSAIDs, aspirin, or other remedies (including herbal products, such as St. John's wort) while taking citalopram because they may increase the risk of bleeding.

# clarithromycin

Biaxin, Biaxin XL, Biaxin XL-PAK

## Class and Category
*Chemical:* Macrolide derivative

*Therapeutic:* Antibiotic
*Pregnancy category:* C

## Indications and Dosages
➤ *To treat pharyngitis and tonsillitis caused by* Streptococcus pyogenes
**ORAL SUSPENSION, TABLETS**
**Adults and adolescents.** 250 mg q 12 hr for 10 days.
**Children.** 15 mg/kg/day in divided doses q 12 hr for 10 days.
➤ *To treat acute maxillary sinusitis caused by* Haemophilus influenzae, Moraxella catarrhalis, *or* Streptococcus pneumoniae
**ORAL SUSPENSION, TABLETS**
**Adults and adolescents.** 500 mg q 12 hr for 14 days.
**Children.** 15 mg/kg/day in divided doses q 12 hr for 10 days.
**EXTENDED-RELEASE TABLETS**
**Adults and adolescents.** 1,000 mg q 24 hr for 14 days.
➤ *To treat acute exacerbations of chronic bronchitis caused by* H. influenzae, M. catarrhalis, *or* S. pneumoniae
**ORAL SUSPENSION, TABLETS**
**Adults and adolescents.** 250 to 500 mg q 12 hr for 7 to 14 days.
**Children.** 15 mg/kg/day in divided doses q 12 hr for 10 days.
**EXTENDED-RELEASE TABLETS**
**Adults and adolescents.** 1,000 mg q 24 hr for 7 days.
➤ *To treat uncomplicated skin and soft-tissue infections caused by* Staphylococcus aureus *or* S. pyogenes
**ORAL SUSPENSION, TABLETS**
**Adults and adolescents.** 250 mg q 12 hr for 7 to 14 days.
**Children.** 15 mg/kg/day in divided doses q 12 hr for 10 days.
➤ *To treat pneumonia caused by* Chlamydia pneumoniae, Mycoplasma pneumoniae, *or* S. pneumoniae
**ORAL SUSPENSION, TABLETS**
**Adults and adolescents.** 250 mg q 12 hr for 7 to 14 days.
**Children.** 15 mg/kg/day in divided doses q 12 hr for 10 days.
➤ *To treat pneumonia caused by* H. influenzae
**ORAL SUSPENSION, TABLETS**
**Adults and adolescents.** 250 mg q 12 hr for 7 days.

**Children.** 15 mg/kg/day in divided doses q 12 hr for 10 days.

➤ *To treat acute otitis media caused by* H. influenzae, M. catarrhalis, *or* S. pneumoniae

ORAL SUSPENSION, TABLETS

**Children.** 15 mg/kg/day in divided doses q 12 hr for 10 days.

➤ *To treat active duodenal ulcer caused by* Helicobacter pylori

ORAL SUSPENSION, TABLETS

**Adults and adolescents.** 500 mg q 8 hr for 14 days with omeprazole 40 mg q.d. in the morning. Then, omeprazole continued at 20 mg q.d. in the morning for days 15 through 28. Alternatively, 500 mg q 12 hr for 14 days with lansoprazole 30 mg and amoxicillin 1 g q 12 hr for 14 days.

➤ *To prevent or treat* Mycobacterium avium *complex in patients with HIV infection*

ORAL SUSPENSION, TABLETS

**Adults and adolescents.** 500 mg q 12 hr for 7 to 14 days.

**Children.** 7.5 mg/kg q 12 hr. *Maximum:* 500 mg b.i.d.

---

## Mechanism of Action

Inhibits RNA-dependent protein synthesis in many types of aerobic, anaerobic, gram-positive, and gram-negative bacteria. By binding with the 50S ribosomal subunit of the bacterial 70S ribosome, clarithromycin causes bacterial cells to die.

---

## Contraindications

Concurrent therapy with astemizole, cisapride, pimozide, or terfenadine; hypersensitivity to clarithromycin, erythromycin, or any macrolide antibiotic

## Interactions

DRUGS

*astemizole, disopyramide, quinidine:* Possibly prolonged QT interval or torsades de pointes

*carbamazepine, other drugs metabolized by cytochrome P450 enzyme system:* Increased blood levels of these drugs

*cisapride, disopyramide, pimozide, quinidine, terfenadine:* Increased risk of arrhythmias

*digoxin:* Increased serum digoxin level

*dihydroergotamine, ergotamine:* Risk of acute ergot toxicity

*lovastatin, simvastatin:* Risk of rhabdomyolysis

*oral anticoagulants:* Potentiated anticoagulant effects

*rifabutin, rifampin:* Decreased blood clarithromycin level by more than 50%

*sildenafil:* Possibly prolonged blood sildenafil level

*theophylline:* Increased blood theophylline level

*triazolam:* Possibly increased CNS effects

*zidovudine:* Decreased blood zidovudine level

## Adverse Reactions

**CNS:** Anxiety, confusion, dizziness, fatigue, hallucinations, headache, insomnia, mania, nightmares, seizures, somnolence, tremor, vertigo

**CV:** Prolonged QT interval, ventricular arrhythmias

**EENT:** Altered smell, altered taste, glossitis, hearing loss, oral moniliasis, stomatitis, tinnitus, tongue or tooth discoloration

**ENDO:** Hypoglycemia

**GI:** Abdominal pain, diarrhea, indigestion, nausea, pancreatitis, pseudomembranous colitis

**GU:** Anorexia, elevated BUN level, hepatic dysfunction, vomiting

**HEME:** Leukopenia, neutropenia, increased prothrombin time, thrombocytopenia

**SKIN:** Pruritus, rash, Stevens-Johnson syndrome, toxic epidermal necrolysis, urticaria

**Other:** Anaphylaxis, superinfection

## Nursing Considerations

•Expect to obtain a specimen for culture and sensitivity tests before giving first dose of clarithromycin.

•Use clarithromycin cautiously in patients with renal impairment. Be aware that patients with severe renal impairment may need decreased dosage or prolonged dosage interval and that clarithromycin is not recommended in combination with ranitidine bismuth citrate therapy if patient has a creatinine clearance less than 2.5 ml/min/1.73 m$^2$ or a history of acute porphyria.

PATIENT TEACHING

•Stress the importance of taking the full course of clarithromycin exactly as prescribed, even after feeling better.

•Caution patient not to crush or chew E.R. tablets.

•Advise patient to take clarithromycin with food if he takes E.R. tablets or experiences GI distress.

•If patient takes suspension form, instruct him not to refrigerate it.

•Tell patient to report severe or watery diarrhea, severe nausea, rash, or itching.

•Instruct patient not to take OTC or prescription drugs without consulting prescriber of clarithromycin.

# clidinium bromide

Quarzan

## Class and Category

*Chemical:* Synthetic quaternary ammonium derivative

*Therapeutic:* Anticholinergic

*Pregnancy category:* Not rated

## Indications and Dosages

➤ *As adjunct to treat peptic ulcers*

CAPSULES

**Adults.** 2.5 to 5 mg t.i.d. or q.i.d. 30 to 60 min before meals and h.s.

DOSAGE ADJUSTMENT Dosage limited to 2.5 mg t.i.d. before meals for elderly or debilitated patients.

| Route | Onset | Peak | Duration |
|-------|-------|------|----------|
| P.O. | 1 hr | Unknown | Up to 3 hr |

### Mechanism of Action

Inhibits acetylcholine's muscarinic actions at postganglionic parasympathetic receptor sites, including smooth muscles, secretory glands, and the CNS. These actions relax smooth muscles and diminish GI, GU, and biliary tract secretions.

## Contraindications

Angle-closure glaucoma, benign bladder neck obstruction, hypersensitivity to clidinium bromide or its components, ileus, intestinal atony (elderly or debilitated patients), intestinal obstruction, myasthenia gravis, myocardial ischemia, ocular adhesions between lens and iris, prostatic hypertrophy, renal disease, severe ulcerative colitis, tachycardia, toxic megacolon, unstable cardiovascular status in acute hemorrhage

## Interactions

DRUGS

*amantadine*: Increased risk of clidinium adverse effects

*atenolol*: Increased atenolol effects

*CNS depressants:* Increased clidinium effects

*phenothiazines*: Decreased antipsychotic effectiveness

*tricyclic antidepressants*: Increased clidinium adverse effects

ACTIVITIES

*alcohol use:* Increased clidinium effects

## Adverse Reactions

**CNS:** Confusion, dizziness, drowsiness, excitement, fever, headache, insomnia, memory loss, nervousness, weakness

**CV:** Palpitations, tachycardia

**EENT:** Blurred vision, cycloplegia, dry mouth, increased intraocular pressure, loss of taste, mydriasis, nasal congestion, pharyngitis, photophobia

**GI:** Bloating, constipation, dysphagia, heartburn, ileus, nausea, vomiting

**GU:** Impotence, urinary hesitancy, urine retention

**SKIN:** Decreased sweating, flushing, rash, urticaria

## Nursing Considerations

•Avoid high doses of clidinium in patients with ulcerative colitis because drug may inhibit intestinal motility and precipitate or aggravate toxic megacolon. Also avoid high doses in patients with hiatal hernia or reflux esophagitis because drug may aggravate esophagitis.

•Use clidinium cautiously in patients with heart failure, arrhythmias, hypertension, autonomic neuropathy, hyperthyroidism, allergies, asthma, and debilitating chronic lung disease.

•WARNING Monitor for excitement, agitation, drowsiness, and confusion in elderly patients, even with small doses, because they're more sensitive to clidinium's effects. If these reactions occur, notify prescriber and expect to decrease dosage.

•Take safety precautions to protect patient from injury from falling.

PATIENT TEACHING

•Instruct patient to take clidinium exactly as prescribed and not to stop taking it suddenly because it can cause withdrawal symptoms, such as vomiting, diaphoresis, and dizziness.

•Advise patient to take drug 30 to 60 minutes before meals.

•Tell patient not to store capsules in the bathroom, near the kitchen sink, or in other damp places.

•Teach patient how to prevent or relieve constipation and dry mouth.

•Instruct patient to avoid alcohol and other CNS depressants because they increase the drug's effects.

•Instruct patient to report constipation, vision changes, sore throat, difficulty urinating, and palpitations.

# clindamycin hydrochloride

Cleocin, Dalacin C

## clindamycin palmitate hydrochloride

Cleocin Pediatric, Dalacin C Flavored Granules (CAN)

## clindamycin phosphate

Cleocin, Clindesse, Dalacin C Phosphate (CAN), Evoclin

## Class and Category

*Chemical:* Lincosamide
*Therapeutic:* Antibacterial and antiprotozoal antibiotic
*Pregnancy category:* B

## Indications and Dosages

➤ *To treat serious respiratory tract infections caused by anaerobes such as occur with anaerobic pneumonitis, empyema, and lung abscess and those caused by pneumococci, staphylococci, and streptococci; serious skin and soft-tissue infections caused by anaerobes, staphylococci, and streptococci; septicemia caused by anaerobes; intra-abdominal infections caused by anaerobes such as occur with intra-abdominal abscess and peritonitis; infections of the female pelvis and genital tract caused by anaerobes such as occur with endometritis, nongonococcal tubo-ovarian abscess, pelvic cellulitis, and postsurgical vaginal cuff infection; bone and joint infections caused by* Staphylococcus aureus; *as adjunct therapy in chronic bone and joint infections*

CAPSULES, ORAL SOLUTION

**Adults and adolescents.** For serious infections, 150 to 300 mg q 6 hr; for severe infections, 300 to 450 mg q 6 hr.

**Children.** For serious infections, 8 to 16 mg/kg/day in equally divided doses t.i.d. or q.i.d.; for severe infections, 16 to 20 mg/kg/day in equally divided doses t.i.d. or q.i.d.

I.V. INFUSION, I.M. INJECTION

**Adults and adolescents age 16 and older.** For serious infections, 600 to 1,200 mg/day in equally divided doses b.i.d. to q.i.d.; for severe infections, 1,200 to 2,700 mg/day in equally divided doses b.i.d. to q.i.d.; for life-threatening infections, 4,800 mg/day in equally divided doses b.i.d. to q.i.d.

**Children ages 1 month to 16 years.** 20 to 40 mg/kg/day in equally divided doses t.i.d. or q.i.d., depending on severity of infection.

**Neonates less than age 1 month.** 15 to 20 mg/kg/day in equally divided doses t.i.d. or q.i.d., depending on severity of infection.

➤ *To treat vaginal infections caused by* Gardnerella *or* Haemophilus

VAGINAL CREAM

**Nonpregnant adults.** 100 mg (1 applicatorful) into vagina q.d., preferably h.s., for 3 to 7 consecutive days.

**Pregnant adults in second or third trimester.** 100 mg (1 applicatorful) into vagina q.d., preferably h.s., for 7 consecutive days.

➤ *To treat acne vulgaris*

FOAM

**Adults and adolescents.** Apply to affected area q.d.

## Incompatibilities

To prevent physical incompatibility, don't administer with aminophylline, ampicillin, barbiturates, calcium gluconate, magnesium sulfate, or phenytoin.

> ### Mechanism of Action
> Inhibits protein synthesis in susceptible bacteria by binding to the 50S subunits of bacterial ribosomes and preventing peptide bond formation, which causes bacterial cells to die.

## Contraindications

Hypersensitivity to clindamycin or lincomycin

## Interactions

DRUGS

*erythromycin:* Possibly blocked access of clindamycin to its site of action

*kaolin-pectin antidiarrheals:* Decreased absorption of oral clindamycin
*neuromuscular blockers:* Increased neuromuscular blockade

## Adverse Reactions

**CNS:** Fatigue, headache
**CV:** Hypotension, thrombophlebitis (after I.V. injection)
**EENT:** Glossitis, metallic or unpleasant taste (with high I.V. doses), stomatitis
**GI:** Abdominal pain, diarrhea, esophagitis, nausea, pseudomembranous colitis, vomiting
**GU:** Cervicitis, vaginitis, and vulvar irritation (with vaginal form)
**HEME:** Agranulocytosis, eosinophilia, leukopenia, neutropenia, thrombocytopenic purpura
**SKIN:** Pruritus, rash, urticaria
**Other:** Anaphylaxis; induration, pain, or sterile abscess after injection; superinfection

## Nursing Considerations

• Expect to obtain a specimen for culture and sensitivity testing before giving first dose.
• Use clindamycin cautiously in patients who have a history of asthma, significant allergies, or GI disease; in those with renal or hepatic dysfunction; and in elderly or atopic patients.
• **WARNING** Don't give 75- and 150-mg capsules to tartrazine-sensitive patients.
• Store oral solution for up to 2 weeks at room temperature or reconstituted parenteral solution for up to 24 hours at room temperature.
• Administer I.V. dose by infusion only; don't give bolus dose. Dilute 300 mg of clindamycin in 50 ml of diluent and administer over 10 minutes. Dilute 600 mg of clindamycin in 100 ml of diluent and administer over 20 minutes. Dilute 900 mg of clindamycin in 100 ml of diluent and administer over 30 minutes.
• **WARNING** Don't use diluents that contain benzyl alcohol when clindamycin is to be administered to neonates because a fatal toxic syndrome may occur.
• Give I.M. injection deep into large muscle mass, such as the gluteus maximus. Rotate injection sites, and avoid giving more than 600 mg by I.M. injection.
• Check I.V. site frequently for phlebitis and irritation.
• For topical foam, wash the affected area with mild soap, let it dry fully, and then apply foam to entire affected area.

• Monitor results of liver function tests, CBC, and platelet counts during prolonged therapy.
• Observe patient for signs and symptoms of superinfection, such as vaginal itching and sore mouth, and signs of pseudomembranous colitis, which may occur 2 to 9 days after therapy begins.

### PATIENT TEACHING

• Tell patient to complete the prescribed course of therapy, even if he feels better before it's finished.
• Instruct patient to take oral clindamycin with at least 8 oz of water to prevent esophageal irritation.
• Advise patient to take oral drug with food, if needed, to reduce GI distress.
• Tell patient not to refrigerate reconstituted oral solution because it may become thick and difficult to pour and to discard unused drug after 14 days.
• If patient will use topical foam, tell him to wash affected area with mild soap, let it dry fully, and then apply foam to entire area. Caution against dispensing foam directly onto hands or face because foam will melt when it contacts warm skin. Instead, patient should dispense amount to be used into the cap or onto a cool surface. Tell patient to pick up a small amount with fingertips and gently massage into affected area until foam disappears. If foam feels warm or looks runny, tell patient to run the can under cold water before dispensing.
• Warn patient not to rely on latex or rubber condoms and diaphragms for 72 hours after vaginal treatment because mineral oil in the vaginal cream may weaken these items.
• Explain that engaging in sexual intercourse after using vaginal cream can increase irritation.
• Inform patient that I.M. injection may be painful.
• Tell patient to immediately report symptoms of colitis (severe diarrhea and abdominal cramps), an inflamed mouth or vagina, and rash or lesions.

# clofibrate

Abitrate, Atromid-S, Claripex (CAN), Novofibrate (CAN)

## Class and Category

*Chemical:* Aryloxyisobutyric acid derivative

*Therapeutic:* Antihyperlipidemic
*Pregnancy category:* C

## Indications and Dosages

➤ *To treat primary hyperlipidemia (type III) that doesn't respond to diet and type IV and type V hyperlipidemia that don't respond to diet in patients at risk for abdominal pain and pancreatitis*

**CAPSULES**

**Adults.** 1.5 to 2 g/day in divided doses b.i.d. to q.i.d.

| Route | Onset | Peak | Duration |
|-------|-------|------|----------|
| P.O.  | 2 to 5 days | 3 wk | 3 wk |

### Mechanism of Action

Increases the amount of cholesterol that's secreted into bile and of bile that's excreted in the feces. Clofibrate also may increase the activity of lipoprotein lipase, which degrades VLDLs.

## Contraindications

Hepatic dysfunction, hypersensitivity to clofibrate, lactation, peptic ulcer, pregnancy, primary biliary cirrhosis, renal dysfunction

## Interactions

**DRUGS**

*chenodiol, ursodiol:* Counteracted effectiveness of these drugs
*dantrolene:* Decreased plasma protein binding of dantrolene
*furosemide:* Increased furosemide and clofibrate effects
*insulin, sulfonylureas:* Increased antidiabetic effect
*oral anticoagulants:* Increased bleeding tendency
*oral contraceptives:* Decreased effectiveness of clofibrate
*phenytoin*: Displacement of phenytoin from binding site
*probenecid:* Increased clofibrate effects
*rifampin:* Decreased clofibrate effects

## Adverse Reactions

**CNS:** Dizziness, drowsiness, fatigue, headache, weakness
**CV:** Angina, edema, phlebitis
**EENT:** Stomatitis
**GI:** Abdominal pain, bloating, diarrhea, flatulence, nausea, vomiting

**GU:** Decreased libido, decreased urine output, impotence, proteinuria
**HEME:** Eosinophilia
**MS:** Arthralgia, myalgia
**SKIN:** Alopecia, dry skin and hair, pruritus, rash, urticaria
**Other:** Weight gain

## Nursing Considerations

•Obtain baseline CBC, liver and renal function studies, and cholesterol profile, as ordered.
•Use clofibrate cautiously in patients with a history of hepatic disease or jaundice and in those with peptic ulcer disease.

**PATIENT TEACHING**

•Tell patient to take clofibrate with milk or food to reduce GI distress.
•Tell patient that repeated laboratory tests will be needed to evaluate serum cholesterol and triglyceride levels.
•Stress the importance of diet, exercise, and weight loss to control cholesterol.
•Tell patient to report ankle or leg swelling, chest pain, decreased urine output, severe GI reactions, and unusual weight gain.
•If patient takes an anticoagulant, instruct him to watch carefully for abnormal bleeding.
•If patient takes antidiabetic drugs, instruct him to stay alert for signs of hypoglycemia from interactions with these drugs.
•Advise women of childbearing age to use contraception during and for several months after therapy because of teratogenic effects.

# clomipramine hydrochloride

Anafranil

## Class and Category

*Chemical:* Dibenzazepine derivative
*Therapeutic:* Antiobsessional tricyclic antidepressant
*Pregnancy category:* C

## Indications and Dosages

➤ *To treat obsessive-compulsive disorder*

**CAPSULES, TABLETS**

**Adults.** *Initial:* 25 mg q.d. Gradually increased to 100 mg/day in divided doses over 2 wk, then to maximum of 250 mg/day in divided doses over next few weeks. At maximum dose, total daily amount may be given h.s.
**Children age 10 and older.** *Initial:* 25 mg q.d. Gradually increased to the lesser of 3 mg/kg/

day or 100 mg/day in divided doses over 2 wk, then to maximum of 3 mg/kg/day or 200 mg/day, whichever is less. At maximum dose, total daily amount may be given h.s.

| Route | Onset | Peak | Duration |
|-------|-------|------|----------|
| P.O. | Unknown | 2 to 4 wk | Unknown |

## Mechanism of Action

May inhibit neuronal reuptake of norepinephrine and serotonin, which may be a factor in normalizing neurotransmission in obsessive-compulsive behavior.

## Contraindications

Acute recovery period after MI, hypersensitivity to clomipramine or its components, use of an MAO inhibitor within 14 days

## Interactions

### DRUGS

*anticholinergics:* Increased anticholinergic effects
*barbiturates:* Decreased level and effects of clomipramine; additive CNS depression
*bupropion, cimetidine, haloperidol, $H_2$-receptor antagonists, selective serotonin reuptake inhibitors, valproic acid:* Increased blood level and therapeutic and adverse effects of clomipramine
*carbamazepine:* Decreased blood clomipramine level; increased carbamazepine level
*clonidine:* Severely increased blood pressure and risk of hypertensive crisis
*CNS depressants:* Increased CNS depression
*dicumarol:* Increased anticoagulant effect
*grepafloxacin, quinolones, sparfloxacin:* Increased risk of life-threatening arrhythmias
*guanethidine:* Antagonized antihypertensive effect of guanethidine
*levodopa:* Delayed absorption and decreased bioavailability of levodopa
*MAO inhibitors:* Increased risk of seizures, coma, or death
*rifamycins:* Decreased clomipramine level
*sympathomimetics:* Possibly potentiated cardiovascular effects
*thyroid drugs:* Increased effects of thyroid drugs and clomipramine

### ACTIVITIES

*alcohol use:* Increased CNS depression

## Adverse Reactions

**CNS:** Anxiety, confusion, depersonalization, depression, dizziness, drowsiness, emotional lability, fatigue, headache, insomnia, panic reaction, paresthesia, somnolence, suicidal ideation (children and teens), syncope, tremor, unusual dreams, yawning
**CV:** Orthostatic hypotension, palpitations, tachycardia
**EENT:** Blurred vision, dry mouth, epistaxis, pharyngitis, rhinitis, sinusitis, unpleasant taste
**GI:** Abdominal pain, anorexia, constipation, diarrhea, flatulence, increased appetite, indigestion, nausea, vomiting
**GU:** Dysmenorrhea, ejaculation failure, impotence, urinary hesitancy, urine retention
**RESP:** Bronchospasm
**SKIN:** Abnormal skin odor, acne, dermatitis, dry skin, photosensitivity, rash, urticaria
**Other:** Weight gain

## Nursing Considerations

• Be aware that stopping clomipramine abruptly may cause withdrawal symptoms and worsen disorder.

• **WARNING** Don't give drug within 14 days of an MAO inhibitor to avoid possible seizures, coma, or death.

• **WARNING** Monitor children and teens closely for evidence of suicidal ideation; clomipramine increases the risk in these groups.

### PATIENT TEACHING

• Tell patient not to use alcohol, barbiturates, or other CNS depressants; clomipramine increases their effects.

• **WARNING** Urge parents to watch their child or teen closely for abnormal thinking or behavior or increased aggression or hostility. Stress need to notify prescriber if they occur.

• Inform male patients about risk of sexual dysfunction while taking drug.

• Caution patient about possible drowsiness, especially during initial dosage adjustment.

• Warn patient not to stop drug abruptly.

• Instruct patient to take a missed dose as soon as he remembers unless it's almost time for the next scheduled dose, in which case he should skip the missed dose. Warn against doubling the next dose.

• Teach patient how to prevent photosensitivity reactions.

• Tell patient to report difficulty urinating, dizziness, dry mouth, sedation, and mental changes.

• Caution patient to avoid hazardous activities until CNS effects of drug are known.

# clonazepam

Apo-Clonazepam (CAN), Clonapam (CAN), Gen-Clonazepam (CAN), Klonopin, Rivotril (CAN)

## Class, Category, and Schedule

*Chemical:* Benzodiazepine
*Therapeutic:* Anticonvulsant
*Pregnancy category:* D
*Controlled substance:* Schedule IV

## Indications and Dosages

➤ *To treat Lennox-Gastaut syndrome (type of absence seizure disorder) and akinetic and myoclonic seizures*

TABLETS

**Adults and children over age 10.** 1.5 mg/day in divided doses t.i.d. Increased by 0.5 to 1 mg q 3 days, if needed, until seizures are controlled. *Maximum:* 20 mg/day.
**Children age 10 and under or weighing less than 30 kg (66 lb).** 0.01 to 0.03 mg/kg/day in divided doses b.i.d. or t.i.d. Increased by 0.25 to 0.5 mg every third day up to maintenance dosage. *Maintenance:* 0.1 to 0.2 mg/kg/day, preferably in three equal doses, or if unequal, with largest dose given h.s. *Maximum:* 0.05 mg/kg/day.

➤ *To treat panic disorder*

TABLETS

**Adults.** *Initial:* 0.25 mg b.i.d. Increased, if needed, to 1 mg/day after 3 days. If more than 1 mg/day is required, dosage increased in increments of 0.125 to 0.25 mg b.i.d. q 3 days until panic disorder is controlled or adverse reactions make further increases undesirable. This maintenance dosage may be given as a single dose h.s. *Maximum:* 4 mg/day.

---

### Mechanism of Action

Prevents seizures by potentiating the effects of gamma-aminobutyric acid, which is an inhibitory neurotransmitter. Suppresses the spread of seizure activity caused by seizure-producing foci in the cortex, thalamus, and limbic structures.

---

## Contraindications

Acute angle-closure glaucoma, hepatic disease, hypersensitivity to benzodiazepines or their components

## Interactions

DRUGS

*antianxiety drugs, barbiturates, MAO inhibitors, narcotics, phenothiazines, tricyclic antidepressants:* Increased CNS depression

ACTIVITIES

*alcohol use:* Increased CNS depression

## Adverse Reactions

**CNS:** Ataxia, confusion, depression, dizziness, drowsiness, emotional lability, fatigue, headache, memory loss, nervousness, reduced intellectual ability
**CV:** Palpitations
**EENT:** Blurred vision, eyelid spasm, increased salivation, loss of taste, pharyngitis, rhinitis, sinusitis
**GI:** Abdominal pain, anorexia, constipation
**GU:** Difficult ejaculation, dysmenorrhea, dysuria, enuresis, impotence, nocturia, urine retention, UTI
**HEME:** Anemia, eosinophilia, leukopenia, thrombocytopenia
**MS:** Dysarthria, myalgia
**RESP:** Bronchitis, cough
**Other:** Allergic reaction

## Nursing Considerations

•Use clonazepam cautiously in patients with renal failure, mixed seizure disorder (because drug can increase the risk of generalized tonic-clonic seizures), or respiratory disease and troublesome secretions (because clonazepam increases salivation) and in elderly patients (because they're more sensitive to drug's CNS effects).
•Monitor blood drug level, CBC, and liver function test results during long-term or high-dose therapy, as ordered.
•**WARNING** Don't stop drug abruptly; expect to taper dosage gradually to avoid withdrawal symptoms and seizures.

PATIENT TEACHING

•Instruct patient to take drug exactly as prescribed. Explain that stopping drug abruptly can cause seizures and withdrawal symptoms.
•Advise patient to avoid alcohol and sleep-inducing drugs during therapy. Instruct him to consult prescriber before taking any OTC drugs.
•Urge patient to carry medical identification indicating his seizure disorder and drug therapy.
•Warn patient about possible drowsiness.
•Instruct patient to report severe dizziness, persistent drowsiness, palpitations, difficulty

urinating, seizure activity, and other disruptive adverse reactions.

• Suggest that parents monitor child's performance in school because clonazepam can cause drowsiness or inattentiveness.

# clonidine

Catapres-TTS

## clonidine hydrochloride

Catapres, Dixarit (CAN), Duraclon

## Class and Category

*Chemical:* Imidazoline derivative
*Therapeutic:* Analgesic, antihypertensive
*Pregnancy category:* C

## Indications and Dosages

➤ *To manage hypertension*

TABLETS

**Adults.** *Initial:* 0.1 mg b.i.d. Dosage increased by 0.1 mg/wk to produce desired response. *Maintenance:* 0.2 to 0.6 mg/day in divided doses b.i.d. or t.i.d. *Maximum:* 2.4 mg/day.

TRANSDERMAL PATCH

**Adults.** *Initial:* 0.1-mg patch applied to hairless area of intact skin on upper arm or torso q 7 days. After 1 to 2 wk, if blood pressure isn't controlled, two 0.1-mg patches or one 0.2-mg patch applied to skin. Dosage adjusted, as needed, q 7 days. *Maximum:* Two 0.3-mg patches worn at same time.

➤ *To treat severe hypertension*

TABLETS

**Adults.** 0.2 mg, then 0.1 mg q 1 hr until diastolic blood pressure reaches acceptable range or 0.8 mg have been administered.

DOSAGE ADJUSTMENT Dosage individualized for patients with renal failure.

➤ *As adjunct to relieve severe pain (in cancer patients) that isn't adequately relieved by opioid analgesics alone*

CONTINUOUS EPIDURAL INFUSION

**Adults.** *Initial:* 30 mcg/hr. Titrated up or down, if needed, depending on comfort. *Maximum:* 40 mcg/hr.

**Children old enough to tolerate placement and management of epidural catheter.** *Initial:* 0.5 mcg/kg/hr. Then, titrated to achieve comfort.

| Route | Onset | Peak | Duration |
|---|---|---|---|
| P.O. | 30 to 60 min | 2 to 4 hr | 8 hr |
| Transdermal | 2 to 3 days | Unknown | 7 days |

## Mechanism of Action

Stimulates peripheral alpha-adrenergic receptors in the CNS to produce transient vasoconstriction and then stimulates central alpha-adrenergic receptors in the brain stem to reduce peripheral vascular resistance, heart rate, and systolic and diastolic blood pressure. May produce analgesia by preventing transmission of pain signals to the brain at presynaptic and postjunctional $alpha_2$-adrenoreceptors in the spinal cord. With epidural administration, clonidine produces analgesia in body areas innervated by the spinal cord segments in which the drug concentrates.

## Contraindications

Anticoagulant therapy (epidural infusion); bleeding diathesis; hypersensitivity to clonidine or its components, including components of the transdermal patch adhesive; injection site infection (epidural infusion)

## Interactions

DRUGS

*barbiturates, other CNS depressants:* Increased depressant effects of these drugs
*beta blockers, calcium channel blockers, digoxin:* Additive effects, such as bradycardia and AV block; increased risk of exacerbated hypertensive response when clonidine is withdrawn (beta blockers only)
*diuretics, other antihypertensive drugs:* Increased hypotensive effect
*epidural local anesthetics:* Prolonged effects of epidural local anesthetics when used with epidural clonidine
*levodopa:* Decreased levodopa effectiveness
*prazosin, tricyclic antidepressants:* Decreased antihypertensive effect of clonidine

ACTIVITIES

*alcohol use:* Enhanced CNS depressant effects of alcohol

## Adverse Reactions

**CNS:** Agitation, depression, dizziness, drowsiness, fatigue, headache, malaise, nervousness, sedation, weakness

**CV:** Chest pain, orthostatic hypotension
**EENT:** Blurred vision, burning eyes, dry eyes and mouth
**GI:** Constipation, mildly elevated liver function test results, nausea, vomiting
**GU:** Decreased libido, impotence, nocturia
**SKIN:** Rash
**Other:** Weight gain, withdrawal symptoms

## Nursing Considerations
• Use clonidine cautiously in elderly patients, who may be more sensitive to its hypotensive effect.
• Monitor blood pressure and heart rate frequently during clonidine therapy.
• Expect transdermal clonidine to take 2 to 3 days to lower blood pressure.
• Be aware that stopping drug abruptly can elevate serum catecholamine levels and cause such withdrawal symptoms as nervousness, agitation, headache, confusion, tremor, and rebound hypertension.
• Expect hypertension to return within 48 hours after drug is discontinued.

**PATIENT TEACHING**
• Advise patient to take drug exactly as prescribed and not to stop taking it abruptly because withdrawal symptoms and severe hypertension may occur.
• Instruct patient to consult prescriber if dry mouth or drowsiness becomes a problem during oral clonidine therapy. To minimize these effects, prescriber may suggest taking most of dosage at bedtime.
• If a transdermal patch loosens during the 7-day application period, tell patient to place the adhesive overlay directly over the patch to ensure adhesion.
• Tell patient to rotate transdermal application sites.
• Instruct patient to remove the patch and place a fresh patch on another site if skin irritation, redness, or rash develops at the patch site.
• Advise patient to fold used transdermal patch in half with the adhesive sides together and discard it out of the reach of children.
• Because of possible sedation, advise patient to avoid potentially hazardous activities until drug's CNS effects are known.
• Advise male patients about possibly decreased libido.
• Instruct patient to report chest pain, dizziness with position changes, excessive drowsiness, rash, urine retention, and vision changes. As needed, tell patient to rise slowly to avoid hypotensive effects.

# clopidogrel bisulfate
Plavix

## Class and Category
*Chemical:* Thienopyridine derivative
*Therapeutic:* Platelet aggregation inhibitor
*Pregnancy category:* B

## Indications and Dosages
➤ *To reduce atherosclerotic events, such as CVA and MI, in patients with atherosclerosis documented by recent CVA, MI, or peripheral artery disease*
**TABLETS**
**Adults.** 75 mg q.d.

➤ *To reduce atherosclerotic events, such as CVA and MI, in patients with acute coronary syndrome (unstable angina or non-Q-wave MI)*
**TABLETS**
**Adults.** *Loading dose:* 300 mg. *Maintenance:* 75 mg q.d.

| Route | Onset | Peak | Duration |
|-------|-------|------|----------|
| P.O. | 2 hr | 3 to 7 days* | 5 days |

### Mechanism of Action
Binds to adenosine diphosphate (ADP) receptors on the surface of activated platelets. This action blocks ADP, which deactivates nearby glycoprotein IIb/IIIa receptors and prevents fibrinogen from attaching to receptors. Without fibrinogen, platelets can't aggregate and form thrombi.

## Contraindications
Active pathological bleeding, including peptic ulcer and intracranial hemorrhage; hypersensitivity to clopidogrel or its components

## Interactions
**DRUGS**
*fluvastatin, phenytoin, tamoxifen, tolbutamide, torsemide:* Interference with metabolism of these drugs

___
* With repeated doses.

*NSAIDs:* Increased risk of GI bleeding, interference with NSAID metabolism
*warfarin:* Prolonged bleeding time, interference with warfarin metabolism

## Adverse Reactions
**CNS:** Confusion, depression, dizziness, fatigue, hallucinations, headache
**CV:** Chest pain, edema, hypercholesterolemia, hypertension, hypotension
**EENT:** Altered taste; conjunctival, ocular, or retinal bleeding; epistaxis; rhinitis
**GI:** Abdominal pain, diarrhea, elevated liver function test results, indigestion, nausea, noninfectious hepatitis, pancreatitis
**GU:** Elevated serum creatinine level, glomerulopathy, UTI
**HEME:** Agranulocytosis, aplastic anemia, neutropenia, pancytopenia, prolonged bleeding time, thrombocytopenic purpura, thrombotic thrombocytopenic purpura, unusual bleeding or bruising
**MS:** Arthralgia, back pain, myalgia
**RESP:** Bronchitis, bronchospasm, cough, dyspnea, upper respiratory tract infection
**SKIN:** Erythema multiforme, lichen planus, pruritus, purpura, rash, Stevens-Johnson syndrome
**Other:** Anaphylaxis, angioedema, flulike symptoms

## Nursing Considerations
• Use clopidogrel cautiously in patients with severe hepatic disease; risk of bleeding from trauma or surgery; or conditions that predispose to bleeding (such as peptic ulcer disease or thrombotic thrombocytopenic purpura).
• In patient with acute coronary syndrome, expect to give aspirin with clopidogrel.
• ◆WARNING Drug prolongs bleeding time; expect to stop it 5 days before elective surgery.
**PATIENT TEACHING**
• Discourage the use of NSAIDs, including OTC preparations, during clopidogrel therapy because of potential for bleeding.
• Caution patient that bleeding may continue for longer than usual. Instruct him to notify prescriber about unusual bleeding or bruising.
• Instruct patient to inform his health care providers about his clopidogrel therapy.

# clorazepate dipotassium
Apo-Clorazepate (CAN), Novo-Clopate (CAN), Tranxene (CAN), Tranxene-SD, Tranxene-SD Half Strength

## Class, Category, and Schedule
*Chemical:* Benzodiazepine
*Therapeutic:* Alcohol withdrawal adjunct, antianxiety drug, anticonvulsant
*Pregnancy category:* Not rated
*Controlled substance:* Schedule IV

## Indications and Dosages
➤ *To relieve anxiety*
**CAPSULES, TABLETS**
**Adults and adolescents.** *Initial:* 15 mg h.s. or 7.5 to 15 mg b.i.d. Dosage adjusted, as needed, to 15 to 60 mg/day in divided doses b.i.d. to q.i.d. *Maximum:* 90 mg/day.
**E.R. TABLETS**
**Adults and adolescents.** 11.25 mg q.d. as substitute for capsules or tablets in patients who were stabilized on 3.75 mg t.i.d. of those forms; 22.5 mg q.d. as substitute for capsules or tablets in patients who were stabilized on 7.5 mg t.i.d. of those forms.
➤ *To relieve symptoms of acute alcohol withdrawal*
**CAPSULES, TABLETS**
**Adults.** *Initial:* 30 mg followed by 15 mg b.i.d. to q.i.d. on day 1 of therapy; 15 mg three to six times on day 2; 7.5 to 15 mg t.i.d. on day 3; 7.5 mg b.i.d. to q.i.d. on day 4; and thereafter, 3.75 mg b.i.d. to q.i.d. *Maximum:* 90 mg/day.
➤ *As adjunct to treat partial seizure disorder*
**CAPSULES, TABLETS**
**Adults and adolescents.** *Initial:* Up to 7.5 mg t.i.d. Increased, if needed, by up to 7.5 mg/wk. *Maximum:* 90 mg/day.
**Children ages 9 to 12.** *Initial:* 7.5 mg b.i.d. Increased, if needed, by up to 7.5 mg/wk. *Maximum:* 60 mg/day.
**E.R. TABLETS**
**Adults and adolescents.** 11.25 mg q.d. as substitute for capsules or tablets in patients who were stabilized on 3.75 mg t.i.d. of those forms; 22.5 mg q.d. as substitute for capsules or tablets in patients who were stabilized on 7.5 mg t.i.d. of those forms.
**DOSAGE ADJUSTMENT** Initial dosage reduced to 3.75 to 15 mg/day to treat anxiety in elderly patients.

## Mechanism of Action
Potentiates the action of gamma-amino-butyric acid (GABA) and other inhibitory neurotransmitters by binding to specific benzodiazepine receptor sites in the limbic and cortical areas of the CNS, which helps control emotional behavior and suppresses the spread of seizure activity. The drug also helps relieve symptoms of alcohol withdrawal by depressing the CNS.

## Contraindications
Angle-closure glaucoma, hypersensitivity to chlorazepate dipotassium or its components

## Interactions
**DRUGS**
*barbiturates, MAO inhibitors, narcotics, other antidepressants, phenothiazines:* Potentiated effects of clorazepate
*cimetidine, disulfiram, fluoxetine, isoniazid, ketoconazole, metoprolol, oral contraceptives, propoxyphene, propranolol, valproic acid:* Increased blood clorazepate level
*clozapine:* Possibly increased risk of shock
**ACTIVITIES**
*alcohol use:* Potentiated effects of clorazepate

## Adverse Reactions
**CNS:** Anxiety, ataxia, confusion, depression, dizziness, drowsiness, fatigue, headache, insomnia, irritability, nervousness, psychosis, slurred speech, tremor
**CV:** Hypotension
**EENT:** Blurred vision, diplopia, dry mouth
**GI:** Anorexia, constipation, diarrhea, elevated liver function test results, nausea, vomiting
**GU:** Elevated BUN and serum creatinine levels, incontinence, libido changes, menstrual irregularities, urine retention
**HEME:** Decreased hematocrit
**SKIN:** Rash
**Other:** Drug dependence

## Nursing Considerations
•**WARNING** Be aware that prolonged use of therapeutic doses can lead to dependence.
•Monitor liver function test results during therapy.
**PATIENT TEACHING**
•Tell patient to take clorazepate with food if GI distress occurs.

•Advise patient to avoid alcohol and other CNS depressants while taking drug.
•Urge patient to avoid potentially hazardous activities until drug's CNS effects are known.

# cloxacillin sodium
Apo-Cloxi (CAN), Cloxapen, Novo-Cloxin (CAN), Nu-Cloxi (CAN), Orbenin (CAN), Tegopen

## Class and Category
*Chemical:* Penicillinase-resistant isoxazolyl penicillin derivative
*Therapeutic:* Antibiotic
*Pregnancy category:* B

## Indications and Dosages
➤ *To treat mild to moderate upper respiratory tract infections or localized skin and soft-tissue infections caused by penicillinase-producing staphylococci*
**CAPSULES, ORAL SOLUTION, I.V. INFUSION, I.V. OR I.M. INJECTION**
**Adults and children who weigh 20 kg (44 lb) or more.** 250 mg q 6 hr. *Maximum:* 6 g/day.
**Children and infants who weigh less than 20 kg.** 50 mg/kg/day in equally divided doses q 6 hr.

➤ *To treat severe lower respiratory tract infections or disseminated infections caused by penicillinase-producing staphylococci*
**CAPSULES, ORAL SOLUTION, I.V. INFUSION, I.V. OR I.M. INJECTION**
**Adults and children who weigh 20 kg or more.** 500 mg q 6 hr. *Maximum:* 6 g/day.
**Infants and children who weigh less than 20 kg.** 100 mg/kg/day in divided doses q 6 hr.

## Mechanism of Action
Inhibits cell wall synthesis and causes cell lysis and death in bacteria that make rigid, cross-linked cell walls in several steps. Cloxacillin affects the final stage of cross-linking by binding with and inactivating penicillin-binding protein, the enzyme that causes linkage in cell wall strands.

## Incompatibilities
Don't mix cloxacillin with aminoglycosides because of risk of mutual inactivation.

## Contraindications
Hypersensitivity to cloxacillin, penicillin, or their components

## Interactions
**DRUGS**
*chloramphenicol, erythromycins, sulfonamides, tetracyclines:* Decreased cloxacillin effects
*hepatotoxic drugs, such as fluconazole:* Increased risk of hepatotoxicity
*methotrexate:* Increased blood methotrexate level and risk of toxicity
*probenecid:* Increased and prolonged blood cloxacillin level

## Adverse Reactions
**CNS:** Headache
**EENT:** Glossitis, oral candidiasis
**GI:** Abdominal pain, diarrhea, elevated liver function test results, nausea, pseudomembranous colitis, vomiting
**GU:** Hematuria, vaginal candidiasis
**MS:** Muscle twitching
**SKIN:** Pruritus, rash, urticaria
**Other:** Anaphylaxis

## Nursing Considerations
•Use cloxacillin cautiously in patients hypersensitive to cephalosporins (allergic reaction may be delayed) and those with hypertension (drug is relatively high in sodium).
•For I.V. injection, reconstitute 250-mg vial with 4.9 ml of sterile water for injection, 500-mg vial with 4.8 ml, and 2,000-mg vial with 6.8 ml. Shake to dissolve.
•For direct I.V. injection, give over 2 to 4 minutes through the tubing of a compatible infusing I.V. solution. If giving by intermittent I.V. infusion, further dilute with a suitable diluent (see manufacturer's package insert) and administer over 30 to 40 minutes.
•For I.M. injection, reconstitute 250-mg vial with 1.9 ml of sterile water for injection and 500-mg vial with 1.7 ml of sterile water. Shake to dissolve.
•Be aware that parenteral solutions are stable for 24 hours at room temperature and for 72 hours if refrigerated.
**PATIENT TEACHING**
•Tell patient to finish the course of therapy, even if he feels better before drug is gone.
•Instruct patient to take oral cloxacillin 1 to 2 hours before meals.
•Tell patient to take oral form with a full glass of water only, not with fruit juice or a carbonated beverage.
•Instruct patient taking oral solution to refrigerate container and to discard unused portion after 14 days. Also instruct him to use a calibrated device to measure the dose.
•Advise patient to report allergic reaction.

# clozapine
Clozaril, Fazaclo

## Class and Category
*Chemical:* Dibenzodiazepine derivative
*Therapeutic:* Antipsychotic
*Pregnancy category:* B

## Indications and Dosages
➤ *To treat severe schizophrenia unresponsive to standard drugs; to reduce risk of recurrent suicidal behavior in schizophrenia or schizoaffective disorders*
**ORALLY DISINTEGRATING TABLETS, TABLETS**
**Adults.** *Initial:* 12.5 mg q.d. or b.i.d. Increased by 25 to 50 mg/day to 300 to 450 mg/day by the end of 2 wk. Subsequent dosage adjustments shouldn't exceed 100 mg once or twice per wk. *Maximum:* 900 mg/day.

| Route | Onset | Peak | Duration |
|---|---|---|---|
| P.O. | 1 to 6 hr | Unknown | 4 to 12 hr |

## Mechanism of Action
May produce antipsychotic effects by interfering with dopamine binding to dopamine—especially $D_4$—receptors in the limbic region of the brain and by antagonizing adrenergic, cholinergic, histaminic, and serotoninergic receptors.

## Contraindications
Angle-closure glaucoma, coma, history of clozapine-induced agranulocytosis or severe granulocytopenia, hypersensitivity to clozapine or its components, myeloproliferative disorders, severe CNS depression, uncontrolled epilepsy, WBC count below 3,500/mm$^3$

## Interactions

**DRUGS**

*anticholinergics:* Potentiated anticholinergic effects

*benzodiazepines, psychotropics:* Additive hypotensive effects; increased risk of cardiopulmonary collapse

*bone marrow depressants:* Potentiated myelosuppressive effects

*carbamazepine, phenytoin:* Decreased blood clozapine level

*cimetidine, erythromycin:* Increased blood clozapine level

*CNS depressants:* Increased CNS depression

*digoxin, warfarin:* Increased blood level of digoxin and warfarin; displacement of clozapine from its binding site

*lithium:* Increased risk of confusion, dyskinesia, neuroleptic malignant syndrome, and seizures

*selective serotonin reuptake inhibitors:* Markedly increased blood clozapine level; increased risk of adverse effects and leukocytosis

**ACTIVITIES**

*alcohol use:* Increased CNS depression

## Adverse Reactions

**CNS:** Agitation, akinesia, anxiety, ataxia, confusion, depression, dizziness, drowsiness, fatigue, fever, headache, hyperkinesia, hypokinesia, insomnia, lethargy, myoclonic jerks, neuroleptic malignant syndrome, nightmares, restlessness, rigidity, sedation, seizures, sleep disturbance, slurred speech, syncope, tardive dyskinesia, tremor, vertigo, weakness

**CV:** Cardiac arrest, cardiomyopathy, chest pain, deep vein thrombosis, ECG changes, hypertension, hypotension, myocarditis, orthostatic hypotension, tachycardia

**EENT:** Blurred vision, dry mouth, increased nasal congestion, increased salivation, pharyngitis, tongue numbness or soreness

**ENDO:** Ketoacidosis, severe hyperglycemia

**GI:** Abdominal discomfort, anorexia, constipation, diarrhea, elevated liver function test results, heartburn, nausea, vomiting

**GU:** Abnormal ejaculation; urinary frequency, urgency, and incontinence; urine retention

**HEME:** Agranulocytosis, eosinophilia, leukopenia, neutropenia

**MS:** Back or leg pain, muscle spasm or weakness, myalgia

**RESP:** Dyspnea, respiratory arrest

**SKIN:** Rash

**Other:** Weight gain

## Nursing Considerations

• Use clozapine cautiously in patients with hepatic, renal, or cardiovascular disease and in elderly patients with dementia-related psychosis because they have increased risk of serious or fatal adverse reactions.

• **WARNING** Rarely, clozapine causes severe or life-threatening adverse reactions, such as agranulocytosis, cardiac or respiratory arrest, deep vein thrombosis, myocarditis (especially in first month), neuroleptic malignant syndrome, and severe hyperglycemia with ketoacidosis in nondiabetic patients. It also may cause seizures and tardive dyskinesia. Monitor patient closely.

• **WARNING** Check baseline WBC count and absolute neutrophil count (ANC) before therapy and weekly for first 6 months. If WBC count is at least 3,500/mm$^3$ and ANC at least 2,000/mm$^3$, check every 2 weeks for next 6 months. If counts remain stable, expect to continue checking every 4 weeks thereafter.

• If patient develops mild leukopenia (WBCs 3,000 to 3,500/mm$^3$) or granulocytopenia (ANC 1,500 to 2,000/mm$^3$), expect to check counts twice weekly until normal. In moderate leukopenia (WBCs 2,000 to 3,000/mm$^3$) or granulocytopenia (ANC 1,000 to 1,500/mm$^3$), expect to stop drug temporarily and check counts daily until improved. Follow manufacturer's direction for resuming drug and monitoring. In severe leukopenia (WBCs less than 2,000/mm$^3$) or granulocytopenia (ANC less than 1,000/mm$^3$), expect to stop drug permanently and monitor counts daily, then as specified by manufacturer.

• Monitor temperature. A transient increase above 100.4° F (38° C) may occur, most often within the first 3 weeks of therapy.

• When therapy ends, expect to check WBC count and ANC weekly for at least 4 weeks or until WBC count is 3,500/mm$^3$ or more and ANC is 2,000/mm$^3$ or more.

**PATIENT TEACHING**

• Tell patient that he'll receive only a 1-week supply at a time.

•Tell patient taking orally disintegrating tablets (Fazaclo) to leave tablet in blister pack until ready to take it. Tell him to peel foil back to remove tablet (rather than pushing tablet through foil) and then to immediately place tablet in mouth and let it dissolve before swallowing. Explain that no water is needed.
•Inform patient that he'll need weekly blood tests. Review evidence of dyscrasias (fatigue, fever, sore throat, weakness); urge patient to report them to prescriber if they occur.
•Instruct patient to avoid hazardous activities until clozapine's CNS effects are known.
•Advise patient to rise slowly from lying or sitting to minimize orthostatic hypotension.
•If patient stops drug for more than 2 days, stress need to contact prescriber for instructions; dosage will need to be changed.
•Tell patient to consult prescriber before using alcohol or taking OTC drugs.
•Advise female patients to notify prescriber if pregnancy occurs or is suspected.

# codeine phosphate

## codeine sulfate

### Class, Category, and Schedule
*Chemical:* Phenanthrene derivative
*Therapeutic:* Antitussive, narcotic analgesic
*Pregnancy category:* C
*Controlled substance:* Schedule II

### Indications and Dosages
➤ *To treat mild to moderate pain*
ORAL SOLUTION, TABLETS, I.M. OR S.C. INJECTION
**Adults.** 15 to 60 mg (usual, 30 mg) q 4 hr, p.r.n.
**Children age 1 year or older.** 0.5 mg/kg q 4 to 6 hr, p.r.n.
I.V. INJECTION
**Adults.** 15 to 60 mg (usual, 30 mg) q 4 hr.
➤ *To treat cough from chemical or mechanical irritation of respiratory system*
ORAL SOLUTION, TABLETS
**Adults and adolescents.** 10 to 20 mg q 4 to 6 hr. *Maximum:* 120 mg/day.
**Children ages 6 to 12.** 5 to 10 mg q 4 to 6 hr. *Maximum:* 60 mg/day.
**Children ages 2 to 6.** 2.5 to 5 mg q 4 to 6 hr. *Maximum:* 30 mg/day.

| Route | Onset | Peak | Duration |
|---|---|---|---|
| P.O. | 30 to 45 min | 1 to 2 hr | 4 hr* |
| I.M. | 10 to 30 min | 30 to 60 min | 4 hr* |
| S.C. | 10 to 30 min | Unknown | 4 hr* |

### Mechanism of Action
May produce analgesia through partial metabolism to morphine. Drug binds with mu, delta, and kappa receptors in the spinal cord and with mu$_1$ and kappa$_3$ receptors higher in the CNS, decreasing intracellular cAMP, which inhibits adenylate cyclase activity and prevents release of pain neurotransmitters, such as substance P and dopamine, and altering perception of and emotional response to pain. Drug also suppresses cough by acting on opiate receptors in the cough center.

### Contraindications
Hypersensitivity to codeine, other opioids, or their components; significant respiratory depression

### Interactions
DRUGS
*anticholinergics, paregoric:* Increased risk of severe constipation
*antihypertensives, diuretics:* Potentiated hypotensive effects
*buprenorphine:* Decreased codeine effectiveness
*CNS depressants:* Additive CNS effects
*hydroxyzine:* Increased analgesia; increased CNS depressant and hypotensive effects
*MAO inhibitors:* Increased risk of unpredictable, severe, and sometimes fatal reactions
*metoclopramide:* Antagonized effect of metoclopramide on GI motility
*naloxone:* Antagonized codeine effect
*naltrexone:* Precipitated withdrawal symptoms in codeine-dependent patients
*neuromuscular blockers:* Additive respiratory depressant effects
*other opioids:* Additive CNS, respiratory depressant, and hypotensive effects

* For pain; 4 to 6 hr for cough.

ACTIVITIES
*alcohol use:* Additive CNS effects

## Adverse Reactions
**CNS:** Coma, delirium, depression, disorientation, dizziness, drowsiness, euphoria, hallucinations, headache, lack of coordination, lethargy, light-headedness, mental and physical impairment, mood changes, restlessness, sedation, seizures, tremor
**CV:** Bradycardia, heart block, hypertension, orthostatic hypotension, palpitations, tachycardia
**EENT:** Altered taste, blurred vision, diplopia, dry mouth, laryngeal edema, laryngospasm, miosis
**GI:** Abdominal cramps and pain, anorexia, constipation, flatulence, gastroesophageal reflux, ileus, indigestion, nausea, vomiting
**GU:** Decreased libido, difficult ejaculation, dysuria, impotence, oliguria, ureteral spasm, urinary incontinence, urine retention
**MS:** Muscle rigidity
**RESP:** Apnea, bronchoconstriction, bronchospasm, depressed cough reflex, respiratory depression
**SKIN:** Diaphoresis, flushing, pallor, pruritus, rash, urticaria
**Other:** Anaphylaxis, facial edema, physical and psychological dependence

## Nursing Considerations
•Evaluate for therapeutic response, including decreased pain, cough, and facial grimacing.
•Take safety precautions, if needed.
•Monitor respiratory depth, effort, and rate. Notify prescriber immediately if respiratory rate drops below 10 breaths/min.
•Assess urine output to detect retention.
•WARNING Assess patient for evidence of physical and psychological dependence.
•Rotate sites when giving codeine S.C. Tissue irritation, pain, and induration may occur with repeated injection into same site.
PATIENT TEACHING
•Advise patient to avoid alcohol or other CNS depressants while taking codeine.
•To minimize nausea, suggest that patient take drug with food.
•Advise patient to avoid potentially hazardous activities until drug's CNS effects are known.
•Caution patient to get up slowly from a sitting or lying position.

•To prevent constipation, encourage patient to consume plenty of fluids and high-fiber foods, if not contraindicated by another condition.
•Instruct patient to take codeine exactly as prescribed and not to adjust dose or frequency without consulting prescriber.
•Advise patient to report shortness of breath or difficulty breathing.

# colchicine

## Class and Category
*Chemical:* Colchicum alkaloid derivative
*Therapeutic:* Antigout, anti-inflammatory
*Pregnancy category:* C (oral form), D (parenteral forms)

## Indications and Dosages
➤ *To prevent gouty arthritis attacks*
TABLETS
**Adults.** 0.5 to 0.6 mg q.d. Dosage increased to 0.5 to 0.6 mg b.i.d. or t.i.d., if needed.
I.V. INFUSION OR INJECTION
**Adults.** 0.5 to 1 mg q.d. or b.i.d. *Maximum:* 4 mg/day.

➤ *To prevent gouty arthritis attacks before, during, and after surgery*
TABLETS
**Adults.** 0.5 to 0.6 mg t.i.d. for 3 days before and 3 days after surgery.
➤ *To treat acute gouty arthritis*
TABLETS
**Adults.** *Initial:* 0.5 to 1.2 mg; then 0.5 to 0.6 mg q 1 to 2 hr, or 1 to 1.2 mg q 2 hr until pain decreases or adverse reactions occur. *Maximum:* 6 mg/day.
I.V. INFUSION OR INJECTION
**Adults.** 2 mg over 2 to 5 min; then 0.5 mg q 6 hr or 1 mg q 6 to 12 hr until pain decreases. *Maximum:* 4 mg/day.
DOSAGE ADJUSTMENT For elderly patients, maximum I.V. dosage reduced to 2 mg/24 hr; maximum oral dosage reduced to 2 mg/24 hr. After initial course of I.V. therapy, elderly patient should receive no form of colchicine for 21 days.

| Route | Onset | Peak | Duration |
|-------|-------|------|----------|
| P.O. | In 12 hr | In 24 to 48 hr | Unknown |
| I.V. | In 6 to 12 hr | Unknown | Unknown |

## Mechanism of Action

In gouty arthritis, leukocytes phagocytose urate crystals in affected joints, a process that releases chemotactic factors, degradation enzymes, and other inflammatory substances. Colchicine helps stop this process, probably by disrupting microtubules within leukocytes. Normally, microtubules contribute to cell structure and movement. When colchicine binds to tubulin (the protein from which microtubules are made), the microtubule falls apart, as shown. This process disrupts cell function and prevents leukocytes from invading joints and producing inflammation.

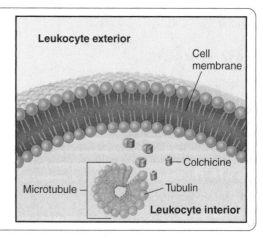

## Contraindications

Blood dyscrasias; hypersensitivity to colchicine or its components; serious cardiac, GI, hepatic, or renal disorders

## Incompatibilities

Don't combine colchicine with bacteriostatic agents, any solution or injection that contains $D_5W$, and any other solution that may change colchicine's pH because precipitation may occur.

## Interactions

### DRUGS

*anticoagulants, such as heparin; platelet aggregation inhibitors, such as aspirin; thrombolytics, such as alteplase:* Possibly significantly increased risk of GI ulceration or hemorrhage
*antineoplastics:* Possibly increased serum uric acid level and decreased therapeutic effectiveness of colchicine
*cyclosporine:* Increased blood cyclosporine level
*NSAIDs, such as phenylbutazone:* Possibly increased risk of bone marrow depression, GI bleeding, leukopenia, or thrombocytopenia
*vitamin $B_{12}$:* Possibly impaired absorption of and increased dosage requirements for vitamin $B_{12}$

### ACTIVITIES

*alcohol use:* Increased risk of adverse GI effects

## Adverse Reactions

**CNS:** Peripheral neuropathy
**CV:** Arrhythmias (I.V. form)
**GI:** Abdominal pain, anorexia, diarrhea, nausea, vomiting
**HEME:** Agranulocytosis, aplastic anemia, thrombocytopenia
**MS:** Myopathy
**SKIN:** Alopecia, rash
**Other:** Injection site pain and tenderness, median nerve neuritis in affected arm, and skin and soft-tissue necrosis if extravasation occurs (I.V. form)

## Nursing Considerations

•WARNING Avoid S.C. or I.M. administration of colchicine because these routes may cause tissue necrosis and sloughing. To prevent extravasation, ensure that the I.V. catheter is patent and correctly positioned before administering drug. Throughout therapy, check I.V. injection site frequently for pain, tenderness, and skin peeling. Consult prescriber about switching to oral form as soon as necessary.

•WARNING To reduce the risk of toxicity, avoid giving colchicine by any route within 7 days after a full I.V. course (4 mg). Expect to wait 3 days after oral therapy before beginning second oral course. Be aware that elderly or debilitated patients and those with a history of cardiac disease or impaired renal or hepatic function are at increased risk for cumulative toxicity.

•Dilute I.V. form with 10 to 20 ml of NS. Alternatively, administer colchicine into a large vein through an I.V. line with NS infusion.
•Administer I.V. form over 2 to 5 minutes.
•Expect to monitor CBC and platelet and reticulocyte counts at baseline and every 3 months after therapy starts.
•Notify prescriber immediately and expect to stop therapy if patient develops signs or symptoms of colchicine toxicity, such as abdominal pain, diarrhea, nausea, or vomiting.

PATIENT TEACHING
•Instruct patient to return for blood tests every 3 months, as ordered, while taking colchicine.
•Explain that gouty arthritis pain and swelling typically subside in 24 to 48 hours after therapy begins.
•Advise patient to notify prescriber immediately if abdominal pain, diarrhea, nausea, or vomiting occurs.

# colesevelam hydrochloride

Welchol

## Class and Category
*Chemical:* Nonabsorbed hydrogel polymer
*Therapeutic:* Bile acid sequestrant
*Pregnancy category:* B

## Indications and Dosages
➤ *As adjunct to diet and exercise to reduce elevated low-density-lipoprotein (LDL) cholesterol levels in patients with primary hypercholesterolemia*

TABLETS
**Adults.** *Initial:* 1.9 g b.i.d. *Usual:* 3.8 g/day. *Maximum:* 4.5 g/day.

## Contraindications
Bowel obstruction, cholelithiasis or complete biliary obstruction, hypersensitivity to colesevelam or its components

## Interactions
DRUGS
*sustained-release verapamil:* Possibly decreased blood level of sustained-release verapamil

## Adverse Reactions
**CNS:** Asthenia
**EENT:** Pharyngitis

**GI:** Constipation, indigestion
**MS:** Myalgia

## Nursing Considerations
•Because colesevelam may decrease or delay absorption of other drugs, administer it separately if possible.
•Ensure that patient drinks enough fluids when taking drug.
•**WARNING** Monitor patients with preexisting constipation, who are at increased risk for developing fecal impaction.
•Monitor frequency of bowel movements and consistency of stools in patients with coronary artery disease or hemorrhoids because constipation may aggravate these conditions.

PATIENT TEACHING
•Instruct patient to take colesevelam with meals and to drink plenty of liquids when taking drug.
•Advise patient to protect tablets from moisture.
•Caution patient not to change prescribed dosage or stop taking drug abruptly because significant increases in serum lipid levels may result.
•Remind patient that drug therapy doesn't reduce the importance of making dietary changes.
•Encourage patient to keep regularly scheduled appointments for follow-up blood tests.

## Mechanism of Action
Binds with bile acids in the intestines, preventing their absorption and forming an insoluble complex that's excreted in feces. This action decreases the amount of bile acids returning through the enterohepatic circulation to the liver. As a result, the liver must convert more cholesterol to bile acids, which increases the liver's demand for cholesterol. This, in turn, causes an increase in the production and activity of the hepatic enzyme hydroxymethyl-glutaryl-coenzyme A (HMG-CoA) reductase, which is necessary for cholesterol production. However, the liver's synthesis of cholesterol typically can't match the amount needed to synthesize bile acids. Because the cholesterol levels can't be sustained, LDLs, lipoproteins composed mostly of cholesterol, are increasingly removed from the blood, thereby decreasing the blood LDL level.

# colestipol hydrochloride

Colestid

## Class and Category

*Chemical*: Diethylenetriamine and 1-chloro-2,3-epoxypropane copolymer, high-molecular-weight anion exchange resin
*Therapeutic*: Antihyperlipidemic
*Pregnancy category*: Not rated

## Indications and Dosages

➤ *To treat primary hypercholesterolemia*

**GRANULES**

**Adults.** 15 to 30 g/day in divided doses b.i.d. to q.i.d., a.c. and h.s.

**TABLETS**

**Adults.** *Initial:* 2 g q.d. or in divided doses b.i.d., increased q 1 to 2 mo in 2-g increments q.d. or b.i.d. *Maximum:* 16 g/day.

---

### Mechanism of Action

Combines with bile acids in the intestine, preventing their absorption and forming an insoluble complex that's excreted in feces. Loss of bile acids increases hepatic production of cholesterol to form new bile acids and increases oxidation of cholesterol to bile acids. The depletion of cholesterol increases hepatic LDL receptor activity, which removes LDLs from the blood.

---

## Contraindications

Complete biliary obstruction, hypersensitivity to colestipol or its components

## Interactions

**DRUGS**

*chenodiol, ursodiol:* Possibly reduced therapeutic effects of colestipol
*digitalis glycosides:* Possibly increased risk of digitalis toxicity when colestipol is discontinued
*furosemide, sulfonylureas, thyroid hormones:* Decreased absorption and therapeutic effects of these drugs
*oral anticoagulants:* Possibly increased or decreased anticoagulant effect
*penicillin G, propranolol, tetracyclines (oral), thiazide diuretics:* Decreased absorption of these drugs

*vancomycin (oral):* Possibly markedly decreased antibacterial action of vancomycin
*vitamins (fat-soluble):* Possibly interference with vitamin absorption

## Adverse Reactions

**CNS:** Headache
**GI:** Abdominal distention and pain, constipation, diarrhea, eructation, esophageal reaction, fecal impaction, heartburn, nausea, vomiting

## Nursing Considerations

•Mix colestipol granules with at least 90 ml of fluid before administration to prevent accidental inhalation or esophageal distress.
•Because colestipol may interact with various drugs, administer it on a separate schedule from other drugs when possible.
•Ensure that patient has adequate fluid intake, and obtain an order for a stool softener or laxative to prevent constipation. To prevent impaction, expect to decrease dosage or discontinue drug if constipation occurs or worsens.
•Expect to discontinue drug if no response occurs after 3 months.
•Monitor serum cholesterol level as appropriate, usually at baseline, 4 to 6 weeks after starting therapy, and then every 3 months. Expect to reduce monitoring frequency to every 4 months if response is adequate.
•Be aware that HDL and serum triglyceride levels may increase or remain unchanged during colestipol therapy.
•Keep in mind that adverse GI reactions are more common in patients older than age 60.

**PATIENT TEACHING**

•To help minimize adverse GI reactions, advise patient to mix granules thoroughly in fluid so that they're completely wet before drinking.
•Remind patient that drug therapy doesn't reduce the importance of dietary changes.
•Caution patient not to increase or decrease the prescribed dosage or to suddenly stop taking drug. Inform him that abrupt discontinuation may significantly increase serum lipid levels.
•Instruct patient to keep appointments for follow-up blood tests.
•Teach patient how to prevent constipation, and advise him to contact prescriber if constipation occurs or worsens.

# conivaptan hydrochloride

Vaprisol

## Class and Category

*Chemical:* Arginine vasopressin antagonist (antidiuretic hormone)
*Therapeutic:* Aquaretic (sodium/water stabilizer)
*Pregnancy category:* C

## Indications and Dosages

➤ To *treat euvolemic hyponatremia in hospitalized patients such as may occur in the syndrome of inappropriate antidiuretic hormone, hypothyroidism, adrenal insufficiency, or pulmonary disorders*

**I.V. INFUSION**

**Adults.** *Loading dose:* 20 mg over 30 minutes followed by 20 mg as a continuous infusion over 24 hours. An additional 20 mg/day may be given by continuous infusion for 1 to 3 days, as needed. *Maximum:* 40 mg/day with total duration of therapy, including loading dose, not to exceed 4 days.

| Route | Onset | Peak | Duration |
|-------|-------|------|----------|
| I.V. | Unknown | 24 hr | Unknown |

## Mechanism of Action

Conivaptan binds with arginine vasopressin V2 receptor sites in the collecting ducts of the kidneys. By doing so, it blocks the action of arginine vasopressin on the V2 receptor, decreasing water resorption in the collecting ducts. This increases excretion of free water (urine output) and increases serum sodium concentration, thereby correcting the water and sodium imbalance.

## Incompatibilities

Don't mix conivaptan with LR, NS, or other drugs.

## Contraindications

Hypersensitivity to conivaptan or its components; patients with hypovolemic hyponatremia; use with potent CYP3A4 inhibitors such as clarithromycin, indinavir, itraconazole, ketoconazole, and ritonavir

## Interactions

**DRUGS**

*amphotericin B, cisplatin, corticosteroids:* Possibly additive hypokalemic effects
*clarithromycin, indinavir, itraconazole, ketoconazole, ritonavir, and other strong CYP3A4 inhibitors:* Increased blood conivaptan level
*digoxin:* Possibly increased digoxin level and risk of digoxin toxicity
*drugs metabolized by CYP3A4, such as HMG-CoA reductase inhibitors:* Possibly increased risk of rhabdomyolysis

## Adverse Reactions

**CNS:** Confusion, fever, headache, insomnia
**CV:** Atrial fibrillation, hypertension, hypotension, orthostatic hypotension, peripheral edema
**EENT:** Dry mouth, oral candidiasis
**ENDO:** Hyperglycemia, hypoglycemia
**GI:** Constipation, diarrhea, nausea, thirst, vomiting
**GU:** Hematuria, pollakiuria, polyuria, UTI
**HEME:** Anemia
**RESP:** Pneumonia
**SKIN:** Erythema
**Other:** Dehydration, hypokalemia, hypomagnesemia, hyponatremia, infusion site reactions (erythema, pain, phlebitis, swelling)

## Nursing Considerations

• Be aware that conivaptan shouldn't be used to treat patients with heart failure.
• Use conivaptan cautiously in patients with hepatic or renal dysfunction because conivaptan levels remain elevated longer in these patients, resulting in increased exposure to the drug.
• Administer conivaptan only through large veins, and change the infusion site every 24 hours. This drug may cause serious infusion site reactions even when diluted and infused correctly. Inspect the site regularly; change it immediately if reactions occur, such as erythema, pain, phlebitis, or swelling.
• Dilute 20-mg (4-ml) loading dose with 100 ml of 5% dextrose injection before administration. Gently invert the bag several times to mix thoroughly. Use mixture within 24 hours, infusing over 30 minutes.
• Dilute 20-mg (4-ml) or 40-mg (8-ml) continuous infusion dose with 250 ml of $D_5W$ before administration. Gently invert the bag several times to mix thoroughly. Infuse im-

mediately over 24 hours. If infusion is interrupted for any reason, discard any remaining solution 24 hours after mixing.
•Monitor patient's neurologic status and serum sodium level closely throughout conivaptan administration because a rapid increase in serum sodium level (more than 12 mEq/L/24 hr) may result in serious neurologic impairment. If serum sodium level rises faster than expected, stop infusion temporarily and notify prescriber. If it continues to rise, expect conivaptan to be discontinued. If hyponatremia persists or recurs and the patient has no neurologic abnormalities, conivaptan may be resumed at a reduced rate.
•Monitor patient's vital signs, and assess patient regularly for evidence of hypovolemia. If patient develops hypovolemia or hypotension while receiving conivaptan, stop infusion, notify prescriber, and provide supportive care, as prescribed. After hypovolemia and hypotension have been corrected, drug may be resumed at a reduced rate.
•Store ampules in cardboard container, protected from light, until ready for use.

**PATIENT TEACHING**
•Instruct patient to report any infusion site discomfort immediately.
•Tell patient that frequent laboratory tests will be performed to monitor his serum sodium level and volume status.

# cortisone acetate

Cortisone Acetate-ICN (CAN), Cortone (CAN), Cortone Acetate

## Class and Category
*Chemical*: Glucocorticoid
*Therapeutic*: Anti-inflammatory, corticosteroid replacement, immunosuppressant
*Pregnancy category*: Not rated

## Indications and Dosages
➤ *To treat allergic and inflammatory disorders, collagen disorders, congenital adrenal hyperplasia, dermatologic disorders, edema (from systemic lupus erythematosus or nephrotic syndrome), GI disorders, hematologic disorders, multiple sclerosis (acute exacerbations), neoplastic diseases, primary or secondary*

*adrenocortical insufficiency, respiratory disorders, rheumatic disorders, trichinosis with myocardial or neurologic involvement, and tuberculous meningitis*

**TABLETS**
**Adults and adolescents.** *Initial:* 25 to 300 mg before 9 a.m. q.d. *Maintenance:* Dosage adjusted based on patient response.
**Children.** 2.5 to 10 mg/kg/day before 9 a.m. For adrenocortical insufficiency, 0.7 mg/kg/day before 9 a.m.

**I.M. INJECTION**
**Adults and adolescents.** *Initial:* 25 to 300 mg q.d. *Maintenance:* Dosage adjusted based on patient response.
**Children.** 0.83 to 5 mg/kg q 12 to 24 hr. For adrenocortical insufficiency, 0.7 mg/kg q.d. or q third day, or 0.23 to 0.35 mg/kg q.d.

| Route | Onset | Peak | Duration |
|-------|-------|------|----------|
| P.O. | Rapid | 2 hr | 1.25 to 1.5 days |
| I.M. | Slow | 20 to 48 hr | 1.25 to 1.5 days |

## Mechanism of Action
Binds to intracellular glucocorticoid receptors and suppresses the inflammatory and immune responses by:
•inhibiting neutrophil and monocyte accumulation at the inflammation site and suppressing their phagocytic and bactericidal activity
•stabilizing lysosomal membranes
•suppressing the antigen response of macrophages and helper T cells
•inhibiting the synthesis of cellular mediators of the inflammatory response, such as cytokines, interleukins, and prostaglandins.

## Contraindications
Hypersensitivity to cortisone or its components, idiopathic thrombocytopenic purpura (parenteral form), live-virus vaccine administration, systemic fungal infection

## Interactions
**DRUGS**
*anticholinesterases:* Possibly antagonized anticholinesterase effects in myasthenia gravis
*barbiturates:* Decreased cortisone effectiveness, increased cortisol clearance

*digitalis glycosides:* Increased risk of digitalis toxicity
*estrogens, oral contraceptives:* Increased cortisone effects and risk of toxicity
*hydantoins, rifampin:* Increased metabolism and decreased effects of cortisone
*isoniazid:* Decreased blood isoniazid level
*neuromuscular blockers:* Possibly enhanced blockade of neuromuscular blockers, leading to increased or prolonged respiratory depression or apnea
*oral anticoagulants:* Possibly obstructed anticoagulant effects
*potassium-wasting diuretics:* Possibly hypokalemia
*salicylates:* Decreased effectiveness and blood level of salicylates
*somatrem:* Decreased growth-promoting effect

## Adverse Reactions

**CNS:** Ataxia, behavior changes, depression, dizziness, euphoria, fatigue, headache, increased ICP with papilledema, insomnia, lassitude, malaise, mood swings, paresthesia, seizures, steroid psychosis, syncope, vertigo
**CV:** Arrhythmias (from hypokalemia), fat embolism, heart failure, hypertension, hypotension, thromboembolism, thrombophlebitis
**EENT:** Exophthalmos, glaucoma, increased intraocular pressure, nystagmus, posterior subcapsular cataracts
**ENDO:** Adrenal insufficiency during stress, Cushing's syndrome, diabetes mellitus, growth uppression in children, hyperglycemia, negative nitrogen balance from protein catabolism
**GI:** Abdominal distention, hiccups, increased appetite, nausea, pancreatitis, peptic ulcer, ulcerative esophagitis, vomiting
**GU:** Glycosuria, menstrual irregularities, perineal burning or tingling
**HEME:** Leukocytosis
**MS:** Arthralgia; aseptic necrosis of femoral and humeral heads; compression fractures; muscle atrophy, weakness, and twitching; myalgia; osteoporosis; spontaneous fractures; steroid myopathy; tendon rupture
**SKIN:** Acne; diaphoresis; ecchymosis; erythema; hirsutism; hyperpigmentation; hypopigmentation; necrotizing vasculitis; petechiae; purpura; rash; scarring; sterile abscesses; striae; subcutaneous fat atrophy; thin, fragile skin; urticaria
**Other:** Anaphylaxis, hypocalcemia, hypokalemia, hypokalemic alkalosis, impaired wound healing, masking of infection, metabolic alkalosis, suppressed skin test reaction, weight gain

## Nursing Considerations

•Use cortisone cautiously in patients with ocular herpes simplex because corneal perforation may occur.
•Expect prescriber to order baseline ophthalmologic examination before beginning therapy because prolonged use of cortisone may result in glaucoma, increased intraocular pressure, and damage to optic nerve.
•Assess for signs and symptoms of infection before giving cortisone because drug may mask them. Be aware that new infections may develop during therapy because of risk of immunosuppression. If a new infection develops, expect to administer appropriate antibiotics.
•Obtain serum electrolyte levels before beginning therapy, as ordered, and monitor results frequently during therapy to detect electrolyte imbalances. Increased calcium excretion, potassium depletion, and sodium and water retention may occur with large doses of cortisone. Anticipate the need for potassium and calcium supplementation and sodium restriction, if indicated.
•Keep in mind that prescriber will order lowest effective dose.
•To avoid peptic ulcer formation from cortisone, expect patient to receive concurrent antacid or antihistamine therapy.
•**WARNING** Be aware that live-virus vaccines shouldn't be given during cortisone therapy because patient may become immunosuppressed and develop the viral infection.
•**WARNING** Assess for adrenal suppression or insufficiency (fatigue, hypotension, lassitude, nausea, vomiting, and weakness) in patient exposed to stress or receiving prolonged cortisone therapy. Notify prescriber immediately if patient exhibits signs or symptoms of this life-threatening adverse reaction.
•Watch for signs of steroid psychosis (confusion, delirium, euphoria, insomnia, mood swings, personality changes, severe depression), which may develop 15 to 30 days after starting drug. Be prepared to stop drug if such signs occur. If stopping isn't possible, expect to administer a psychotropic drug.
•Watch for cushingoid signs, such as acne, buffalo hump, central obesity, ecchymosis, moon face, striae, and weight gain. Notify prescriber at once if they occur.

•Expect to taper oral cortisone dosage slowly to prevent withdrawal syndrome (abdominal or back pain, anorexia, dizziness, fever, headache, and syncope).

**PATIENT TEACHING**

•Instruct patient to take oral cortisone exactly as prescribed, every morning before 9 a.m. Advise him to take it with food if GI distress occurs.

•Caution patient not to stop drug abruptly because doing so may lead to adrenal insufficiency, withdrawal symptoms, or both.

•Inform patient about adrenal insufficiency and need for possible dosage increases during stress. Advise him to notify prescriber immediately if signs or symptoms develop or if he's exposed to stress.

•Caution patient to avoid exposure to people with infections because cortisone can cause immunosuppression. Also, teach him to recognize and immediately report signs and symptoms of infection.

•Teach patient to recognize and report adverse reactions to cortisone, including Cushing's syndrome.

•Urge patient receiving long-term cortisone therapy to carry medical identification.

•Advise patient to have regular eye examinations.

•Urge him to keep follow-up appointments with prescriber, which may include laboratory tests, to evaluate effects of therapy.

# co-trimoxazole

## (sulfamethoxazole and trimethoprim)

Apo-Sulfatrim (CAN), Bactrim, Bactrim-DS, Bactrim Pediatric, Cofatrim Forte, Cotrim, Cotrim DS, Cotrim Pediatric, Novo-Trimel (CAN), Nu-Cotrimox (CAN), Roubac (CAN), Septra, Septra DS, Septra Pediatric, Sulfatrim, Sulfatrim DS, Sulfatrim S/S, Sulfatrim Suspension

## Class and Category

*Chemical:* Sulfonamide derivative (sulfamethoxazole), dihydrofolic acid analogue (trimethoprim)
*Therapeutic:* Antibiotic
*Pregnancy category:* C

## Indications and Dosages

➤ *To treat acute otitis media, shigellosis, UTIs, and other infections caused by gram-negative organisms (including* Enterobacter *sp.,* Escherichia coli, Haemophilus ducreyi, Haemophilus influenzae, *indole-positive* Proteus *sp.,* Klebsiella pneumoniae, Neisseria gonorrhoeae, Proteus mirabilis, Providencia *sp.,* Salmonella *sp.,* Serratia *sp., and* Shigella *sp.) and gram-positive organisms (including group A beta-hemolytic streptococci, No-cardia *sp.,* Staphylococcus aureus, and Streptococcus pneumoniae)*

**ORAL SUSPENSION, TABLETS**

**Adults.** 800 mg of sulfamethoxazole (SMZ) and 160 mg of trimethoprim (TMP) q 12 hr for 10 to 14 days (5 days for shigellosis).

**Children age 2 months and older.** 40 mg/kg of SMZ and 8 mg/kg of TMP daily in two divided doses q 12 hr for 10 days (5 days for shigellosis).

**DOSAGE ADJUSTMENT** Dosage reduced by one-half if creatinine clearance is 15 to 30 ml/min/1.73 m². Drug avoided if creatinine clearance is less than 15 ml/min/1.73 m².

**I.V. INFUSION**

**Adults and children over age 2 months.** 40 to 50 mg/kg of SMZ and 8 to 10 mg/kg of TMP daily in divided doses q 6, 8, or 12 hr for up to 5 days for shigellosis, 14 days for UTIs.

➤ *To treat acute exacerbation of chronic bronchitis*

**ORAL SUSPENSION, TABLETS**

**Adults.** 800 mg of SMZ and 160 mg of TMP q 12 hr for 14 days.

➤ *To treat traveler's diarrhea*

**ORAL SUSPENSION, TABLETS**

**Adults.** 800 mg of SMZ and 160 mg of TMP q 12 hr for 5 days.

➤ *To prevent* Pneumocystis carinii *pneumonia*

**ORAL SUSPENSION, TABLETS**

**Adults.** 800 mg of SMZ and 160 mg of TMP q 24 hr.

**Children.** 750 mg/m² of SMZ and 150 mg/m² of TMP daily in two divided doses on 3 consecutive days weekly. *Maximum:* 1,600 mg of SMZ and 320 mg of TMP daily.

➤ *To treat* P. carinii *pneumonia*

**ORAL SUSPENSION, TABLETS**

**Adults.** 100 mg/kg of SMZ and 15 to 20 mg/kg

of TMP daily in divided doses q 6 hr for 14 to 21 days.

**I.V. INFUSION**

**Adults and children over age 2 months.** 75 to 100 mg/kg of SMZ and 15 to 20 mg/kg of TMP daily in three or four divided doses q 6 to 8 hr for up to 14 days.

## Incompatibilities
Don't mix co-trimoxazole with other drugs or solutions.

## Contraindications
Age younger than 2 months; hypersensitivity to sulfamethoxazole, sulfonamides, trimethoprim, or their components; megaloblastic anemia caused by folate deficiency

## Mechanism of Action
Blocks two consecutive steps in the formation of essential nucleic acids and proteins in susceptible organisms. Sulfamethoxazole inhibits synthesis of dehydrofolic acid (a nucleic acid) by competing with para-aminobenzoic acid. Trimethoprim inhibits the action of the enzyme dihydrofolate reductase, thus blocking production of tetrahydrofolic acid.

## Interactions
**DRUGS**

*ACE inhibitors:* Possibly increased risk of hyperkalemia in elderly patients

*cyclosporine:* Decreased blood level and therapeutic effectiveness of cyclosporine, increased risk of nephrotoxicity

*digoxin:* Possibly increased blood digoxin level resulting in increased risk of digoxin toxicity

*diuretics:* Increased risk of thrombocytopenic purpura in elderly patients

*indomethacin:* Possibly increased blood co-trimoxazole level

*methotrexate:* Increased blood methotrexate level and risk of methotrexate toxicity

*phenytoin:* Possibly decreased hepatic clearance and prolonged half-life of phenytoin

*pyrimethamine (dosage greater than 25 mg/wk):* Increased risk of megaloblastic anemia

*sulfonylureas:* Possibly increased hypoglycemic effects of sulfonylureas

*tricyclic antidepressants:* Decreased effectiveness of tricyclic antidepressant

*warfarin:* Increased anticoagulant effects

## Adverse Reactions
**CNS:** Anxiety, aseptic meningitis, ataxia, chills, depression, fatigue, hallucinations, headache, insomnia, seizures, vertigo

**EENT:** Glossitis, stomatitis

**GI:** Abdominal pain, anorexia, diarrhea, hepatitis, nausea, pancreatitis, pseudomembranous enterocolitis, vomiting

**GU:** Crystalluria, renal failure, toxic nephrosis

**HEME:** Agranulocytosis, eosinophilia, hemolytic anemia, leukopenia, methemoglobinemia, neutropenia, thrombocytopenia

**RESP:** Cough, dyspnea

**SKIN:** Dermatitis, erythema, photosensitivity, rash, Stevens-Johnson syndrome, toxic epidermal necrolysis, urticaria

**Other:** Anaphylaxis, hyperkalemia, injection site inflammation and pain

## Nursing Considerations
•Use cautiously in patients with impaired hepatic or renal function, severe allergy or bronchial asthma, or possible folate deficiency (the elderly, long-term alcoholics, patients taking anticonvulsants, patients who are malnourished or have malabsorption).

•Expect to obtain culture and sensitivity test results before beginning co-trimoxazole.

•For I.V. infusion, dilute each 5 ml of co-trimoxazole with 75 to 125 ml of $D_5W$ before administration.

•When giving drug to neonates, don't mix with solutions that contain benzyl alcohol because this preservative has been linked to a fatal toxic syndrome involving circulatory, CNS, renal, and respiratory impairment and metabolic acidosis.

•Infuse slowly over 60 to 90 minutes.

•Assess for evidence of blood dyscrasia, including bleeding, ecchymosis, and joint pain, especially in elderly patients who are also taking a thiazide diuretic.

•Monitor elderly patients closely because they have an increased risk of bone marrow suppression, hyperkalemia, and severe skin reactions.

**PATIENT TEACHING**

•To minimize photosensitivity, advise patient to avoid direct sunlight and to use sunscreen.

•Instruct patient to notify prescriber immediately if rash, severe diarrhea, or other serious adverse reactions occur.

# cromolyn sodium
## (disodium cromoglycate, sodium cromoglycate)

Apo-Cromolyn (CAN), Gastrocrom, Intal, Intal Syncroner (CAN), Nalcrom (CAN), Nasalcrom, Novo-cromolyn (CAN)

## Class and Category
*Chemical*: Disodium chromoglycate
*Therapeutic*: Antiasthmatic, anti-inflammatory
*Pregnancy category*: B

## Indications and Dosages
➤ *To prevent bronchial asthma attacks*

**AEROSOL (METERED-DOSE INHALER)**
**Adults and children over age 5.** 2 metered sprays (1.6 to 2 mg) q 4 to 6 hr. *Maximum:* 16 sprays (12.8 to 16 mg)/day.

**CAPSULES FOR INHALATION**
**Adults and children over age 2.** 1 capsule (20 mg) q 4 to 6 hr. *Maximum:* 8 capsules (160 mg)/day.

**SOLUTION FOR NEBULIZATION**
**Adults and children over age 2.** 20 mg q 4 to 6 hr. *Maximum:* 160 mg/day.

➤ *To prevent bronchospasm caused by environmental exposure or exercise*

**AEROSOL (METERED-DOSE INHALER)**
**Adults and children over age 5.** 2 metered sprays (1.6 to 2 mg) as a single dose at least 10 to 15 min (no longer than 1 hr) before exposure or exercise. *Maximum:* 16 sprays (12.8 to 16 mg)/day.

**CAPSULES FOR INHALATION**
**Adults and children over age 2.** 1 capsule (20 mg) as a single dose inhaled at least 10 to 15 min (no longer than 1 hr) before exposure or exercise. *Maximum:* 8 capsules (160 mg)/day.

**SOLUTION FOR NEBULIZATION**
**Adults and children over age 2.** *Initial:* 20 mg inhaled 10 to 15 min (no longer than 1 hr) before exposure or exercise. Repeated p.r.n. during prolonged exercise. *Maximum:* 160 mg/day.

➤ *To treat allergic rhinitis*

**NASAL SOLUTION**
**Adults and children over age 2.** 1 spray (5.2 mg) in each nostril at regular intervals t.i.d. or q.i.d. *Maximum:* 1 spray (5.2 mg) in each nostril 6 times/day.

➤ *To prevent systemic mastocytosis*

**CAPSULES, ORAL CONCENTRATE**
**Adults and adolescents.** 200 mg q.i.d., 30 min before meals and h.s.
**Children ages 2 to 12.** 100 mg q.i.d., 30 min before meals and h.s. *Maximum:* 40 mg/kg/ day.
**Children under age 2.** 5 mg/kg q.i.d. *Maximum:* 40 mg/kg/day.

| Route | Onset | Peak | Duration |
|---|---|---|---|
| Aerosol | In minutes | Unknown | Up to 2 hr |
| Nasal solution | In 1 wk | 1 to 4 wk | Unknown |
| Nebulizer solution | In minutes | Unknown | 3 to 6 hr |

## Mechanism of Action
In asthma, inflammation results when antigen reexposure causes mast cells to degranulate and release histamine and chemical mediators. Cromolyn helps reduce inflammation by preventing mast cells from degranulating. After exposure to an antigen, mast cells become sensitized to it, and immunoglobulin E (IgE) antibodies appear on their surfaces. When the antigen returns, it attaches to IgE antibodies (1) and triggers events that lead to degranulation (2). By preventing granules from opening on the cells' surfaces (3), cromolyn blocks the release of histamine and chemical mediators.

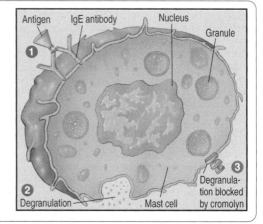

## Contraindications
Arrhythmias, coronary artery disease (aerosol); hypersensitivity to cromolyn or its components, status asthmaticus (all forms); nasal polyps (nasal solution)

## Adverse Reactions
**CNS:** Dizziness, headache, neuritis
**EENT:** Burning eyes, hoarseness, laryngeal edema, nasal congestion, and swollen parotid glands (all forms); increased sneezing, nasal stinging, and throat irritation (nasal solution); taste perversion (aerosol)
**GI:** Anorexia, diarrhea (capsules and oral concentrate), nausea, vomiting
**GU:** Dysuria, urinary frequency
**MS:** Arthralgia, joint swelling
**RESP:** Cough, wheezing
**SKIN:** Rash, urticaria

## Nursing Considerations
•**WARNING** Be aware that cromolyn sodium shouldn't be used to relieve acute asthma attack or severe bronchospasm; it should be used only for prevention.
•Don't give drug through handheld nebulizer. Instead, administer via power-operated nebulizer with a face mask or mouthpiece.
•Evaluate patient for effective inhalation; patient must be able to inhale adequately for nebulizer solution to be effective.
•Thoroughly mix oral concentrate or capsule contents into half a glass of hot water (not fruit juice, milk, or food), and let cool before administering.
•Give drug at regular intervals to maximize effectiveness.

**PATIENT TEACHING**
•Teach patient how to use power-operated nebulizer; warn against using handheld nebulizer.
•Advise patient to use cromolyn sodium 10 to 15 minutes before exercising or exposing himself to precipitating factors.
•Instruct patient to thoroughly mix oral concentrate with hot water (not fruit juice, milk, or food) and let it cool before drinking.
•Inform patient that nasal spray may cause minor nasal irritation.
•Explain that cromolyn may take up to 1 month to achieve its full therapeutic effects.

# crotamiton
Eurax

## Class and Category
*Chemical:* Synthetic chloroformate salt
*Therapeutic:* Antipruritic, scabicide
*Pregnancy category:* C

## Indications and Dosages
➤ *To treat scabies*
**CREAM, LOTION**
**Adults.** 30 to 60 g (thin layer) massaged into skin from chin down and repeated in 24 hr. Applied p.r.n. to skin folds, creases, and areas of intense pruritus for up to 48 hr.
➤ *To relieve pruritus caused by scabies*
**CREAM, LOTION**
**Adults.** 30 to 60 g (thin layer) massaged gently into affected areas until drug is completely absorbed. Repeated p.r.n.

> ## Mechanism of Action
> Exerts a toxic effect on *Sarcoptes scabiei* by an unknown mechanism.

## Contraindications
Abrasions, application to mucous membranes, breaks in skin, hypersensitivity to crotamiton or its components, inflammation

## Adverse Reactions
**SKIN:** Contact dermatitis, irritation, pruritus, rash

## Nursing Considerations
•Expect pruritus to continue for 4 to 6 weeks after treatment.
**PATIENT TEACHING**
•Advise patient to shake lotion bottle well before applying.
•Warn him to keep drug away from eyes, nose, mouth, and inflamed skin.
•Advise patient to use a topical corticosteroid for dermatitis and an antihistamine for pruritus, as prescribed.
•Instruct patient to change clothing and bed linens the morning after final application and to take a cleansing bath 48 hours after final application.
•Inform patient that pruritus may continue for 4 to 6 weeks after treatment.
•Advise patient to notify prescriber if skin irritation or rash occurs.

# cyclizine hydrochloride

Marezine

## cyclizine lactate

Marzine (CAN)

## Class and Category

*Chemical*: Piperazine derivative
*Therapeutic*: Anticholinergic, antiemetic
*Pregnancy category:* B

## Indications and Dosages

➤ *To prevent postoperative vomiting*

**I.M. INJECTION**

**Adults and adolescents.** 50 mg 15 to 30 min before surgery ends, then q 4 to 6 hr, p.r.n., during first few postoperative days.
**Children ages 6 to 12.** 25 mg 15 to 30 min before surgery ends, then t.i.d., p.r.n., during first few postoperative days.
**Children up to age 6.** 12.5 mg 15 to 30 min before surgery ends, then t.i.d., p.r.n., during first few postoperative days.

➤ *To prevent and treat motion sickness*

**TABLETS**

**Adults and adolescents.** 50 mg 30 min before travel, then q 4 to 6 hr, p.r.n. *Maximum:* 200 mg/day.
**Children ages 6 to 12.** 25 mg 30 min before travel, then q 6 to 8 hr, p.r.n. *Maximum:* 75 mg/day.

**I.M. INJECTION**

**Adults and adolescents.** 50 mg q 4 to 6 hr, p.r.n.
**Children.** 1 mg/kg t.i.d., p.r.n.

| Route | Onset | Peak | Duration |
|---|---|---|---|
| P.O., I.M. | 30 to 60 min | Unknown | 4 to 6 hr |

## Mechanism of Action

May act centrally on the vomiting center by blocking chemoreceptor trigger zones. Cyclizine also may reduce the sensitivity of the labyrinthine apparatus in the inner ear.

## Contraindications

Hypersensitivity to cyclizine or its components, shock

## Interactions

**DRUGS**

*anticholinergics:* Possibly potentiated anticholinergic effects

*apomorphine:* Possibly decreased emetic response of apomorphine
*CNS depressants:* Possibly potentiated CNS depression

**ACTIVITIES**

*alcohol use:* Possibly potentiated CNS depression

## Adverse Reactions

**CNS:** Dizziness, drowsiness, euphoria, excitation, hallucinations, insomnia, nervousness, restlessness, seizures (in children), vertigo
**CV:** Hypotension, palpitations, tachycardia
**EENT:** Blurred vision; diplopia; dry mouth, nose, and throat; tinnitus
**GI:** Anorexia, constipation, diarrhea, nausea, vomiting
**GU:** Urinary frequency and hesitancy, urine retention
**SKIN:** Jaundice, rash, urticaria

## Nursing Considerations

•Help patient with ambulation and take safety precautions to prevent injury from falls if drowsiness or dizziness occurs.
•Don't schedule skin tests using allergens until at least 5 days after cyclizine therapy stops because drug may interfere with test results.

**PATIENT TEACHING**

•Urge patient to avoid alcohol and other CNS depressants during cyclizine therapy.
•Advise patient to ask for help with ambulation if he feels drowsy or dizzy.

# cyclobenzaprine hydrochloride

Flexeril

## Class and Category

*Chemical:* Tricyclic amine salt
*Therapeutic:* Skeletal muscle relaxant
*Pregnancy category:* B

## Indications and Dosages

➤ *As adjunct to rest and physical therapy for relief of muscle spasm associated with acute, painful musculoskeletal conditions*

**TABLETS**

**Adults and adolescents.** 5 mg t.i.d., increased as needed to 10 mg t.i.d. *Maximum:* 30 mg/day for 3 wk.

**DOSAGE ADJUSTMENT** Dosage frequency reduced in elderly patients and those with hepatic impairment.

| Route | Onset | Peak | Duration |
|-------|-------|------|----------|
| P.O. | 1 hr | 1 to 2 wk | 12 to 24 hr |

### Mechanism of Action
Acts in the brain stem to reduce or abolish tonic muscle hyperactivity. Because cyclobenzaprine doesn't act at the neuromuscular junction or directly on skeletal muscle, it relieves muscle spasm without disrupting muscle function.

### Contraindications
Acute recovery phase of MI; age less than 12; arrhythmias, including heart block and other conduction disturbances; heart failure; hypersensitivity to cyclobenzaprine or its components; hyperthyroidism; MAO inhibitor use within 14 days

### Interactions
**DRUGS**
*anticholinergics, antidyskinetics:* Possibly potentiated anticholinergic effects of these drugs
*CNS depressants, tricyclic antidepressants:* Possibly additive CNS depressant effects of these drugs, increased risk of adverse effects of antidepressants and cyclobenzaprine
*guanadrel, guanethidine:* Possibly decreased or blocked antihypertensive effects of these drugs
*MAO inhibitors:* Possibly hyperpyretic crisis, severe seizures, and death
**ACTIVITIES**
*alcohol use:* Possibly additive CNS depression

### Adverse Reactions
**CNS:** Asthenia, confusion, depression, dizziness, drowsiness, fatigue, fever, headache, insomnia, irritability, nervousness, paresthesia, seizures, tremor, weakness
**CV:** Arrhythmias, including tachycardia; orthostatic hypotension; palpitations; vasodilation
**EENT:** Blurred vision, diplopia, dry mouth, transient vision loss, unpleasant taste
**GI:** Constipation, hiccups, indigestion, nausea, vomiting
**GU:** Libido changes, urinary frequency, urine retention
**SKIN:** Diaphoresis, facial flushing, pruritus, rash

### Nursing Considerations
• Use cyclobenzaprine cautiously in patients with history of low seizure threshold.
• Keep in mind that elderly patients shouldn't receive drug, if possible, because of its anticholinergic effects.
• To prevent injury from falls, take safety precautions if patient experiences confusion, dizziness, or weakness.
**PATIENT TEACHING**
• Urge patient to avoid alcohol and other CNS depressants during therapy.
• Inform patient about possible lack of alertness and dexterity.
• Advise patient to ask for assistance with walking, driving, or potentially hazardous activities if he experiences dizziness or weakness.

# cycloserine
Seromycin

### Class and Category
*Chemical*: D-alanine analogue, *Streptomyces garyphalus* or *Streptomyces orchidaceus* derivative
*Therapeutic*: Antitubercular
*Pregnancy category: C*

### Indications and Dosages
➤ *To treat tuberculosis along with other antitubercular drugs after failure of primary drugs, including ethambutol, isoniazid, pyrazinamide, rifampin, and streptomycin*
**CAPSULES**
**Adults and adolescents.** 250 mg q 12 hr for 2 wk, then q 6 to 8 hr for 2 wk. Dosage increased gradually to maintain blood cycloserine level below 30 mcg/ml. *Maximum:* 1 g/day.
**Children.** 10 to 20 mg/kg/day in divided doses q 12 hr. *Maximum:* 1 g/day.

### Mechanism of Action
Inhibits bacterial cell wall synthesis in gram-positive organisms, including *Mycobacterium tuberculosis.* In the early stages of bacterial cell wall synthesis, cycloserine inhibits two enzymes that help form peptidoglycan, which is needed to make the cell membrane rigid and protective.

## Contraindications

Chronic alcoholism, depression, hypersensitivity to cycloserine or its components, psychosis, renal disease, seizure disorder, severe anxiety

## Interactions

### DRUGS

*ethionamide*: Possibly increased risk of seizures
*isoniazid*: Possibly increased risk of adverse CNS effects
*phenytoin*: Possibly increased blood phenytoin level
*pyridoxine*: Possibly anemia or peripheral neuritis

### ACTIVITIES

*alcohol use:* Possibly increased risk of seizures

## Adverse Reactions

**CNS:** Aggression, anxiety, coma, confusion, depression, dizziness, drowsiness, headache, irritability, lethargy, memory loss, nervousness, nightmares, psychosis, restlessness, seizures, suicidal tendencies, tremor, vertigo
**CV:** Heart failure
**HEME:** Leukocytosis, megaloblastic anemia
**MS:** Dysarthria, hyperreflexia
**SKIN:** Dermatitis, photosensitivity
**Other:** Folic acid deficiency, vitamin $B_{12}$ deficiency

## Nursing Considerations

• Monitor blood cycloserine level, as appropriate. Blood level should be maintained at 25 to 30 mcg/ml.
• Monitor mental status, mood, and affect for aggression or depression.
• Monitor CBC to detect blood dyscrasias.
• To prevent injury from falls, take safety precautions if adverse CNS reactions, such as dizziness or drowsiness, develop.

### PATIENT TEACHING

• Urge patient to avoid alcohol while taking cycloserine.
• Instruct patient to seek help immediately if he has suicidal thoughts.
• Advise patient to avoid driving and to ask for assistance with walking or hazardous activities if he develops adverse CNS reactions, such as dizziness and drowsiness.
• Advise patient to contact prescriber if he notices no improvement after 2 to 3 weeks.
• Emphasize the importance of complying with drug therapy because effective treatment may take years to complete.

# cyclosporine

## (cyclosporin A)

Neoral, Sandimmune, SangCya

## Class and Category

*Chemical:* Tolypocladium inflatum Gams- or Cylindrocarpon lucidum Booth-derived polypeptide
*Therapeutic:* Antipsoriatic, antirheumatic,
*Therapeutic:* Antipsoriatic, antirheumatic, immunosuppressant
*Pregnancy category:* C

## Indications and Dosages

➤ *To prevent or treat organ rejection in kidney, liver, and heart allogenic transplantation*

CAPSULES, MODIFIED CAPSULES, MODIFIED ORAL SOLUTION, ORAL SOLUTION

**Adults and children.** *Initial:* 12 to 15 mg/kg/day in divided doses q 12 hr beginning 4 to 12 hr before surgery and continuing for 1 to 2 wk postoperatively. Then, dosage reduced by 5%/wk to maintenance dose. *Maintenance:* 5 to 10 mg/kg/day in divided doses q 12 hr.

I.V. INFUSION

**Adults.** 2 to 6 mg/kg/day beginning 4 to 12 hr before surgery and continuing postoperatively until patient can tolerate oral form.

➤ *To treat severe rheumatoid arthritis*

MODIFIED CAPSULES, MODIFIED ORAL SOLUTION

**Adults.** 2.5 mg/kg/day in divided doses q 12 hr, increased by 0.5 to 0.75 mg/kg/day after 8 wk and again after 12 wk. *Maximum:* 4 mg/kg/day.

➤ *To treat psoriasis*

MODIFIED CAPSULES, MODIFIED ORAL SOLUTION

**Adults.** *Initial:* 2.5 mg/kg/day in divided doses b.i.d., increased by 0.5 mg/kg/day after 4 wk. Then dosage increased q 2 wk, if needed. *Maximum:* 4 mg/kg/day.

---

### Mechanism of Action

Causes immunosuppression by inhibiting the proliferation of T lymphocytes, the production and release of lymphokines, and the release of interleukin-2.

---

## Contraindications

Abnormal renal function, neoplastic diseases, and uncontrolled hypertension in patients with psoriasis or rheumatoid arthritis (modified capsules and oral solution); hypersensitivity to cyclosporine, its components, or polyoxyethylated castor oil (I.V. infusion)

## Interactions

### DRUGS

*ACE inhibitors, angiotensin II receptor antagonists, potassium-sparing diuretics, potassium supplements:* Increased risk of hyperkalemia
*amiodarone, azithromycin, bromocriptine, clarithromycin, colchicine, danazol, diltiazem, erythromycin, fluconazole, hormonal contraceptives, imatinib, itraconazole, ketoconazole, methylprednisolone, metoclopramide, nicardipine, quinupristin and dalfopristin, verapamil:* Increased blood cyclosporine level
*amphotericin B, azapropazon, cimetidine, ciprofloxacin, colchicine, co-trimoxazole, fibric acid derivatives (such as bezafibrate and fenofibrate), gentamicin, ketoconazole, melphalan, NSAIDs, ranitidine, tacrolimus, tobramycin, vancomycin:* Increased risk of nephrotoxicity
*atorvastatin, fluvastatin, lovastatin, pravastatin, simvastatin:* Increased risk of myotoxicity
*carbamazepine, nafcillin, octreotide, orlistat, phenobarbital, phenytoin, rifampin, St. John's wort, sulfinpyrazone, terbinafine, ticlopidine:* Decreased blood cyclosporine level and therapeutic response
*digoxin:* Increased blood digoxin level and risk of digitalis toxicity
*indinavir, nelfinavir, ritonavir, saquinavir:* Possibly increased blood cyclosporine level
*methotrexate:* Increased blood methotrexate level
*methylprednisolone (high dose):* Increased risk of seizures
*other immunosuppressants:* Possibly excessive immunosuppression
*prednisolone:* Increased blood prednisolone level
*sirolimus:* Increased blood sirolimus level
*vaccines (killed or live virus):* Possibly suppressed immune response and increased adverse effects of vaccine

### FOODS

*Grapefruit, grapefruit juice:* Increased risk of nephrotoxicity
*Potassium-rich foods:* Increased risk of hyperkalemia

## Adverse Reactions

**CNS:** Altered level of consciousness, confusion, headache, intracranial hypertension, loss of motor function, paresthesia, psychiatric disturbances, seizures, tremor
**CV:** Chest pain, hypertension
**EENT:** Gingival hyperplasia, optic disc edema, oral candidiasis, visual impairment
**ENDO:** Gynecomastia
**GI:** Diarrhea, nausea, pancreatitis, vomiting
**GU:** Albuminuria, hematuria, proteinuria, renal failure
**HEME:** Anemia, leukopenia, thrombocytopenia
**SKIN:** Acne, flushing, hirsutism, rash
**Other:** Anaphylaxis, hyperkalemia, hypomagnesemia, lymphoma

## Nursing Considerations

•Be aware that capsules and oral solution aren't interchangeable with modified capsules and modified oral solution. Modified forms have greater bioavailability.
•Prepare I.V. infusion by diluting each milliliter of concentrate in 20 to 100 ml of NS or $D_5W$. Use glass containers because of possible leaching of diethylhexyphthalate from polyvinyl chloride bags into cyclosporine solution.
•Administer I.V. infusion over 2 to 6 hr. If needed, the drug may be infused over 24 hr.
•WARNING Closely monitor for anaphylaxis at least during first 30 minutes of I.V. administration. Make sure emergency equipment and drugs are immediately available.
•WARNING Be aware that rapid I.V. infusion may cause acute nephrotoxicity.
•Don't draw blood to measure cyclosporine level through same I.V. tubing used to administer drug, even if line was flushed after administration. Blood level may be falsely elevated.
•Discard diluted solution after 24 hours.
•Be aware that oral solution contains alcohol and shouldn't be administered to patient who drinks heavily or has a history of alcohol dependence.
•Don't add water to oral solution because it will alter drug's effectiveness.
•Avoid giving oral forms of cyclosporine with grapefruit juice, which may raise trough level, increasing risk of nephrotoxicity.

•Monitor blood pressure, especially in patients with a history of hypertension, because drug can worsen this condition. Expect to decrease cyclosporine dosage if hypertension develops.

•Monitor results of liver and renal function tests, as ordered, to detect signs of decreased function.

•Although uncommon, cyclosporine may cause neurotoxicity, especially after liver transplantation. Watch for evidence of encephalopathy, such as impaired consciousness, loss of motor function, psychiatric disurbance, seizures, and visual disturbance.

•Be aware that cyclosporine use may result in increased serum cholesterol levels.

•Be aware that St. John's wort may decrease blood cyclosporine level.

•Store capsules at 77° F (25° C) and in prepackaged foil wrap to protect them from light.

•Expect about 50% of patients treated for psoriasis to relapse about 4 months after therapy stops.

**PATIENT TEACHING**

•Instruct patient to take drug at same time each day and in same relation to type and timing of food intake to help increase compliance and maintain steady blood level.

•Advise patient to mix oral solution in a glass—not plastic—container with room-temperature orange or apple juice to improve flavor. Also advise him to avoid grapefruit juice because it alters drug metabolism.

•Instruct patient to use accompanying syringe supplied by manufacturer to ensure accurate measurement of oral solution dose and to wipe syringe—not rinse it—after use to prevent cloudiness.

•Advise patient not to stop taking drug without consulting prescriber.

•Instruct patient not to receive virus vaccines during therapy. Urge him to avoid people who have received such vaccines or to wear a protective mask when he's around them.

•Caution patient to avoid contact with people who have infections during therapy because cyclosporine causes immunosuppression.

•Urge patient to maintain good dental hygiene because of risk of gingival hyperplasia.

•Advise patient to discard oral solution after it has been opened for 2 months.

•Inform patient with rheumatoid arthritis that drug effects may not appear for 4 to 6 weeks.

# daclizumab

## (dacliximab)

Zenapax

## Class and Category

*Chemical:* Monoclonal antibody
*Therapeutic:* Immunosuppressant
*Pregnancy category:* C

## Indications and Dosages

➤ *To prevent acute organ rejection after kidney transplantation*

**I.V. INFUSION**

**Adults and children.** 1 mg/kg given in five doses: dose 1 given no more than 24 hr before transplantation; doses 2 through 5, at 14-day intervals.

---

### Mechanism of Action

Inhibits interleukin-2–mediated activation of lymphocytes, which prevents WBCs from attacking the transplanted kidney. Daclizumab also reduces the body's infection-fighting ability.

---

## Contraindications

Hypersensitivity to daclizumab or its components

## Adverse Reactions

**CNS:** Anxiety, chills, depression, dizziness, fatigue, fever, headache, insomnia, prickly sensation, tremor, weakness
**CV:** Chest pain, edema, hypertension, hypotension, tachycardia, thrombosis
**EENT:** Blurred vision, pharyngitis, rhinitis
**ENDO:** Hyperglycemia
**GI:** Abdominal distention and pain, constipation, diarrhea, flatulence, gastritis, heartburn, hemorrhoids, indigestion, nausea, vomiting
**GU:** Dysuria, hematuria, hydronephrosis, oliguria, renal insufficiency, renal tubular necrosis, urine retention
**HEME:** Bleeding
**MS:** Arthralgia, back pain, leg cramps, myalgia

**RESP:** Atelectasis, cough, crackles, dyspnea, hypoxia, lung congestion, pleural effusion, pulmonary edema
**SKIN:** Acne, diaphoresis, hirsutism, impaired wound healing, night sweats, pruritus, rash
**Other:** Dehydration, fluid overload, injection site pain and redness, lymphocele

## Nursing Considerations

•Dilute calculated dose of daclizumab in 50 ml of NS. Gently invert bag to mix; to prevent foaming, don't shake it.
•Use room temperature solution within 4 hours or refrigerate it for up to 24 hours. Discard unused solution.
•Because daclizumab's compatibility with other drugs isn't known, don't add or simultaneously infuse other drugs through same I.V. line.
•Monitor blood glucose level for increases during therapy.
•**WARNING** Although daclizumab seldom causes severe hypersensitivity reactions, keep drugs to treat such a reaction nearby for immediate use.

**PATIENT TEACHING**

•Urge patient to complete the course of therapy and return for follow-up visits.

# dalteparin sodium

## (tedelparin)

Fragmin

## Class and Category

*Chemical:* Low-molecular-weight heparin
*Therapeutic:* Anticoagulant, antithrombotic
*Pregnancy category:* B

## Indications and Dosages

➤ *To prevent ischemic complications in patients who receive aspirin as part of treatment for unstable angina and non-Q wave MI*

**S.C. INJECTION**

**Adults.** 120 IU/kg q 12 hr with aspirin (75 to 165 mg/day) until patient is stable, usually 5 to 8 days. *Maximum:* 10,000 IU/dose.

➤ *To prevent blood clots in patients undergoing hip replacement surgery*

**S.C. INJECTION**

**Adults.** *Initial:* 2,500 IU 1 to 2 hr before surgery, repeated in 8 to 12 hr and again 8 to

12 hr later. *Maintenance:* 5,000 IU q morning for 5 to 10 days postoperatively or until patient is fully ambulatory. *Alternate:* 5,000 IU the evening before surgery followed by 5,000 IU q.d. (starting the next evening) for 5 to 10 days or until patient is fully ambulatory.

➤ *To prevent blood clots in patients undergoing abdominal surgery who are at risk for thromboembolic complications*

**S.C. INJECTION**

**Adults.** 2,500 IU q.d., starting 1 to 2 hr before surgery and repeated for 5 to 10 days. For patients at high risk (those with cancer), 5,000 IU the evening before surgery, repeated q.d. for 5 to 10 days; or 2,500 IU 1 to 2 hr before surgery followed by 2,500 IU 12 hr later and then 5,000 IU q.d. for 5 to 10 days.

➤ *To prevent blood clots in patients with severe mobility restrictions during acute illness*

**S.C. INJECTION**

**Adults.** 5,000 IU q.d.

---

## Mechanism of Action

Binds to and accelerates the activity of antithrombin III, thus inhibiting thrombin and blocking the formation of fibrin clots.

---

## Incompatibilities

Don't mix dalteparin with other drugs.

## Contraindications

Active major bleeding; hypersensitivity to low-molecular-weight heparins, heparin, or pork products; thrombocytopenia associated with positive laboratory tests for antiplatelet antibodies in the presence of dalteparin

## Interactions

**DRUGS**

*NSAIDs, oral anticoagulants, platelet aggregation inhibitors, thrombolytics:* Possibly increased risk of hemorrhage

## Adverse Reactions

**HEME:** Hemorrhage, thrombocytopenia
**SKIN:** Bullous eruption, necrosis, pruritus, rash
**Other:** Anaphylaxis, injection site hematoma and pain

## Nursing Considerations

•Use dalteparin with extreme caution in patients with a history of heparin-induced

thrombocytopenia; those at increased risk for hemorrhage (such as those who use a platelet inhibitor or have bacterial endocarditis, bleeding disorders, active ulcerative GI disease, uncontrolled hypertension, or hemorrhagic CVA); and those who have recently had brain, eye, or spinal surgery.

•Use drug cautiously in patients with bleeding diathesis, diabetic retinopathy, platelet defects, recent GI bleeding, severe hepatic or renal insufficiency, or thrombocytopenia.

•Before giving first dose, tell Jewish patients that drug comes from porcine intestine.

•Be aware that risk factors for thromboembolic events include age over 40, cancer, history of deep vein thrombosis or pulmonary embolism, obesity, and planned use of anesthesia for more than 30 minutes.

•Don't give drug by I.M. or I.V. injection.

•With the patient seated or supine, administer drug deep into S.C. tissue in U-shaped area around navel, upper outer thigh, or upper outer quadrant of buttocks. If using area around navel or on thigh, lift skin fold with thumb and forefinger while giving injection. Insert entire length of needle at a 45- to 90-degree angle. Rotate sites daily.

•Be aware that routine coagulation tests and dosage adjustments usually aren't required.

**PATIENT TEACHING**

•If therapy will continue at home, teach patient or caregiver how to give S.C. injections, select injection sites, and rotate sites daily. Tell patient to discard drug if it's discolored or contains particles. Review safe handling and disposal of syringes and needles.

•Teach patient to store drug at room temperature, away from moisture and heat.

•Urge patient to report adverse reactions, especially bleeding, and to seek help immediately if signs of thromboembolism develop, such as severe dyspnea (pulmonary embolism) or neurologic deficits (cerebral embolism).

•Stress the importance of follow-up visits.

# danaparoid sodium

Orgaran

## Class and Category

*Chemical*: Glycosaminoglycan heparinoid, low-molecular-weight heparin
*Therapeutic*: Anticoagulant, antithrombotic
*Pregnancy category*: B

## Indications and Dosages

➤ *To prevent deep vein thrombosis after hip replacement surgery*

**S.C. INJECTION**

**Adults.** 750 anti-factor Xa U b.i.d. (first dose 1 to 4 hr preoperatively; second dose no sooner than 2 hr after surgery) for 7 to 14 days, as indicated.

---

### Mechanism of Action

Inhibits thrombin generation in coagulation pathway, thus preventing fibrin formation and clotting.

---

## Contraindications

Active major bleeding (including hemorrhagic CVA); hypersensitivity to low-molecular-weight heparins, heparin, or pork products; severe hemorrhagic disorders, such as hemophilia and thrombocytopenic purpura; sulfite sensitivity; type II thrombocytopenia associated with positive laboratory tests for antiplatelet antibodies in the presence of danaparoid

## Interactions

**DRUGS**

*NSAIDs, oral anticoagulants, platelet aggregation inhibitors:* Possibly increased risk of bleeding

## Adverse Reactions

**CNS:** Asthenia, dizziness, fever, headache, insomnia
**CV:** Chest pain, edema
**GI:** Abdominal pain, constipation, nausea, vomiting
**GU:** Urine retention, UTI
**HEME:** Anemia, excessive bleeding
**MS:** Arthralgia, myalgia
**SKIN:** Pruritus, rash
**Other:** Anaphylaxis, injection site pain

## Nursing Considerations

• Use danaparoid with extreme caution in patients who are at increased risk for hemorrhage (such as those with severe uncontrolled hypertension, acute bacterial endocarditis, bleeding disorders, active ulcerative GI disease, severe renal dysfunction, or nonhemorrhagic CVA); those with a postoperative indwelling epidural catheter; and those who have recently had brain, eye, or spinal surgery.
• Don't give drug by I.M. or I.V. injection.

• Administer drug with patient lying down. Use a 25G or 26G needle to minimize tissue trauma. Select site on left or right anterolateral or posterolateral abdominal wall. Hold skin fold gently between thumb and forefinger, and insert entire length of needle deep into S.C. tissue at a 45- to 90-degree angle. Don't pinch or rub site afterward. Rotate sites.
• Expect to monitor results of CBCs and fecal occult blood tests during therapy. Typical coagulation tests, such as PT, APTT, clotting time, whole blood clotting time, and thrombin time, aren't useful for monitoring danaparoid's anticoagulant effect.

**PATIENT TEACHING**

• Before administering first dose, inform Jewish patients that drug comes from porcine intestinal mucosa.
• If therapy must continue at home, teach patient or caregiver how to administer S.C. injections. Review appropriate injection sites, and instruct her to rotate them daily. Also instruct her to discard drug if it's discolored or contains particles. Review safe handling and disposal of syringes and needles.
• Teach patient to store drug at room temperature, away from moisture and heat.
• Instruct patient to consult prescriber before using aspirin, ibuprofen, indomethacin, ketoprofen, naproxen, and other NSAIDs because they may increase the risk of bleeding.
• Advise patient to stop taking drug and seek help immediately if she experiences severe dizziness, fever, rash, wheezing, or prolonged or unexplained bleeding and pain at the injection site.

# dantrolene sodium

Dantrium, Dantrium Intravenous

## Class and Category

*Chemical:* Hydantoin derivative, imidazolidinedione sodium salt
*Therapeutic:* Antispastic, malignant hyperthermia therapy adjunct
*Pregnancy category:* C (parenteral), Not rated (oral)

## Indications and Dosages

➤ *To treat chronic spastic conditions caused by severe chronic disorders, such as cerebral palsy, CVA, multiple sclerosis, and spinal cord injury*

D

CAPSULES

**Adults and adolescents.** *Initial:* 25 mg q.d. for 7 days. Then dosage increased to 25 mg/day q 4 to 7 days until desired response occurs or dosage reaches 100 mg q.i.d. *Maximum:* 400 mg/day.

**Children.** *Initial:* 0.5 mg/kg b.i.d. for 7 days. Then increased by 0.5 mg/kg/day q 4 to 7 days until desired response occurs or dosage reaches 3 mg/kg q.i.d. *Maximum:* 400 mg/day.

➤ *To prevent malignant hyperthermia before surgery*

CAPSULES

**Adults and children.** 4 to 8 mg/kg/day in divided doses t.i.d. or q.i.d. 1 or 2 days before surgery, with last dose given 3 to 4 hr before surgery.

**I.V. INFUSION**

**Adults and children.** *Initial:* 2.5 mg/kg 60 to 75 min before anesthesia and infused over 1 hr. Additional individualized doses given as needed during surgery.

➤ *To treat malignant hyperthermic crisis*

**I.V. INJECTION**

**Adults and adolescents.** *Initial:* 1 mg/kg by rapid bolus repeated as needed until symptoms subside or cumulative dose of 10 mg/kg has been reached. Dose repeated if symptoms reappear.

➤ *To treat postmalignant hyperthermic crisis*

CAPSULES

**Adults and children.** 4 to 8 mg/kg/day in divided doses q.i.d. for 1 to 3 days.

**I.V. INJECTION**

**Adults and children**: *Initial:* Individualized dosage beginning with 1 mg/kg or more as needed if oral therapy can't be used. *Maximum:* 10 mg/kg total dose.

| Route | Onset | Peak | Duration |
|-------|-------|------|----------|
| P.O. | 1 wk* | Unknown | Unknown |

## Incompatibilities

Don't administer parenteral dantrolene with acidic solutions, including $D_5W$ and NS.

## Contraindications

*For oral drug only:* Active hepatic disease (such as cirrhosis and hepatitis), conditions in which spasticity helps maintain upright posture and improve balance or function, skeletal muscle spasms caused by rheumatic disorders

---

* For spasticity; unknown for malignant hyperthermia.

## Mechanism of Action

Acts directly on skeletal muscle to reduce the force of reflex muscle contraction. This in turn reduces hyperreflexia, spasticity, involuntary movements, and clonus, probably by preventing calcium release from the sarcoplasmic reticulum of skeletal muscle cells. Blocked calcium release also inhibits the activation of acute catabolism associated with malignant hyperthermic crisis syndrome.

## Interactions

DRUGS

*calcium channel blockers (especially verapamil):* Possibly hyperkalemia, life-threatening arrhythmias, shock
*hepatotoxic drugs:* Increased risk of hepatotoxicity with long-term oral dantrolene use
*sedatives:* Possibly profound sedation

ACTIVITIES

*alcohol use:* Possibly increased CNS depression

## Adverse Reactions

**CNS:** Chills, confusion, depression, dizziness, drowsiness, fatigue, fever, headache, insomnia, light-headedness, malaise, nervousness, seizures, slurred speech or other speech problems, weakness
**CV:** Heart failure (I.V.), labile blood pressure, pericarditis, phlebitis, tachycardia
**EENT:** Abnormal vision, altered taste, diplopia, lacrimation
**GI:** Abdominal cramps, anorexia, constipation, diarrhea, dysphagia, gastric irritation, GI bleeding, hepatitis, hepatotoxicity
**GU:** Crystalluria, dysuria, erectile dysfunction, hematuria, nocturia, urinary frequency, urinary incontinence, urine retention
**MS:** Backache, myalgia
**RESP:** Feeling of suffocation, pleural effusion
**SKIN:** Acne, diaphoresis, eczematoid eruption, erythema (I.V.), extravasation with tissue damage, hirsutism, pruritus, rash, urticaria

## Nursing Considerations

• Use dantrolene cautiously in patients with impaired pulmonary function, especially those with COPD, and in those with severe cardiac or hepatic dysfunction.
• Reconstitute drug with 60 ml of sterile water for injection. Shake vial until clear. Store reconstituted solution at room temperature, protected from direct sunlight. Discard after 6 hours.
• To prevent precipitation, transfer reconsti-

tuted drug to a plastic I.V. bag, rather than a glass bottle, for infusion.
•Because drug has a high pH, infuse into a central vein, if possible, to avoid tissue damage from extravasation.
•Monitor blood pressure and heart rate frequently during drug administration to detect tachycardia and blood pressure changes.
•Notify prescriber if persistent diarrhea develops with oral therapy; drug may need to be stopped.
•Monitor results of liver function tests—especially ALT, AST, alkaline phosphatase, and total bilirubin levels—to detect hepatotoxicity. Expect to stop drug after 45 days if benefits aren't sufficient because the risk of hepatotoxicity increases with dose and time, especially for women and patients over age 35.

**PATIENT TEACHING**
•Advise patient to take dantrolene with food if gastric irritation develops.
•Inform patient that drug may weaken muscles used for walking and climbing stairs.
•Warn patient about drug's sedating effects. Caution her to avoid sedatives, unless prescribed, and other sedating substances, such as alcohol.
•Advise patient to notify prescriber if yellow skin or sclerae, itching, anorexia, or fatigue develop.
•Advise patient that if she misses a dose, she should wait until the next scheduled dose if more than 2 hours have passed since the missed dose. Instruct her not to double-dose.
•Caution patient not to stop taking drug without consulting prescriber. Gradual dosage reduction may be required, especially after long-term use.

# darbepoetin alfa

Aranesp

## Class and Category

*Chemical:* 165-amino acid glycoprotein identical to human erythropoietin
*Therapeutic:* Antianemic
*Pregnancy category:* C

## Indications and Dosages

➤ *To treat anemia from chronic renal failure*
**I.V. OR S.C. INJECTION**
**Adults.** *Initial:* 0.45 mcg/kg as a single dose q wk. *Maintenance:* Dosage individualized and increased once a month to maintain a hemoglobin level not to exceed 12 g/dl.

DOSAGE ADJUSTMENT Dosage reduced by about 25% if hemoglobin level increases and approaches 12 g/dl. If hemoglobin level continues to increase, doses temporarily withheld until hemoglobin level begins to decrease; then therapy is restarted at a dose about 25% below previous dose. Dosage reduced by about 25% if hemoglobin level increases by more than 1.0 g/dl in a 2-week period. Dosage increased by about 25% of previous dose if hemoglobin level increases less than 1 g/dl over 4 weeks but only if serum ferritin level is 100 mcg/L or greater and serum transferrin saturation is 20% or greater. Further increases made at 4-week intervals until specified hemoglobin level is obtained.

DOSAGE ADJUSTMENT For conversion from epoetin alfa to darbepoetin alfa, dosage administered q wk for patient who previously received epoetin alfa 2 to 3 times/wk and once every 2 wk for patient who previously received epoetin alfa once/wk. For patients being converted from epoetin alfa, 6.25 mcg/wk darbepoetin alfa given q wk for patients who received < 2,500 units/wk of epoetin alfa; 12.5 mcg/wk darbepoetin alfa given q wk for patients who received 2,500 to 4,999 units/wk of epoetin alfa; 25 mcg/wk darbepoetin alfa given q wk for patients who received 5,000 to 10,999 units/wk of epoetin alfa; 40 mcg/wk darbepoetin alfa given q wk for patients who received 11,000 to 17,999 units/wk of epoetin alfa; 60 mcg/wk darbepoetin alfa given q wk for patients who received 18,000 to 33,999 units/wk of epoetin alfa; 100 mcg/wk darbepoetin alfa given q wk for patients who received 34,000 to 89,999 units/wk of epoetin alfa; 200 mcg/wk darbepoetin alfa given q wk for patients who received 90,000 or more units/wk of epoetin alfa.

➤ *To treat chemotherapy-induced anemia in patients with nonmyeloid malignancies*
**S.C. INJECTION**
**Adults.** *Initial:* 2.25 mcg/kg as a single dose q wk. *Maintenance:* Dosage individualized to maintain a target hemoglobin level.

DOSAGE ADJUSTMENT Dosage increased up to 4.5 mcg/kg if there is less than 1.0 g/dl increase in hemoglobin after 6 wk of therapy. If hemoglobin level increases by more than 1.0 g/dl over 2 wk or if hemoglobin exceeds 12 g/dl, dosage reduced by approximately 25%. If hemoglobin exceeds 13 g/dl, doses temporarily withheld until hemoglobin falls to 12 g/dl. Then therapy is restarted at a dose about 25% less than last dose given.

| Route | Onset | Peak | Duration |
|-------|-------|------|----------|
| I.V., S.C. | In 2 to 6 wk | Unknown | Unknown |

## Mechanism of Action
Stimulates the release of reticulocytes from the bone marrow into the bloodstream, where they develop into mature RBCs.

## Incompatibilities
Don't mix darbepoetin alfa with any other drug.

## Contraindications
Hypersensitivity to human albumin or products made from mammal cells; uncontrolled hypertension

## Interactions
**DRUGS**
None known

## Adverse Reactions
**CNS:** Asthenia, dizziness, fatigue, fever, headache, seizures
**CV:** Arrhythmias, cardiac arrest, chest pain, congestive heart failure, hypertension, hypotension, peripheral edema, vascular access hemorrhage, vascular access thrombosis
**GI:** Abdominal pain, constipation, diarrhea, nausea, vomiting
**MS:** Arthralgia, back pain, limb pain, myalgia
**RESP:** Bronchitis, cough, dyspnea, upper respiratory tract infection
**SKIN:** Rash, urticaria
**Other:** Fluid overload, infection, flulike symptoms, injection site pain, sepsis

## Nursing Considerations
• Before starting therapy, expect to correct folic acid or vitamin $B_{12}$ deficiencies because these conditions may interfere with drug's effectiveness.
• To ensure effective drug response, expect to obtain serum ferritin level and serum transferrin saturation before beginning and during therapy, as ordered. If serum ferritin level is less than 100 mcg/l or serum transferrin saturation is less than 20%, expect to begin supplemental iron therapy.
• Don't shake vial during preparation to avoid denaturing drug and rendering it biologically inactive.
• Discard drug if you see particulate matter or discoloration.

• Don't dilute drug before giving it.
• Discard unused portion of drug because it contains no preservatives.
• Monitor blood pressure frequently during therapy for hypertension. Expect to reduce dosage or withhold drug if blood pressure is poorly controlled with antihypertensive and dietary measures.
• Monitor hemoglobin level weekly, as ordered, until hemoglobin stabilizes and maintenance dosage has been achieved. Thereafter, monitor hemoglobin level regularly, as ordered. After each dosage adjustment, expect to monitor hemoglobin level weekly for 4 weeks until hemoglobin level stabilizes in response to dosage change.
• **WARNING** Be aware that the risk of cardiac arrest, seizures, CVA, exacerbations of hypertension, congestive heart failure, vascular thrombosis, vascular ischemia, vascular infarction, acute myocardial infarction, and fluid overload with peripheral edema increases if hemoglobin level increases more than about 1 g/dl during any 2-week period. Expect to decrease darbepoetin dosage if this occurs.
• Institute seizure precautions according to facility policy.
• For patients with chronic renal failure who aren't receiving dialysis, expect to administer doses lower than those given to patients receiving dialysis. Also, monitor renal function test results and fluid and electrolyte balance in these patients for signs of deteriorating renal function.
• Store drug at 2° to 8° C (36° to 46° F). Don't freeze, and do protect from light.

**PATIENT TEACHING**
• Advise patient that the risk of seizures is highest during the first 90 days of drug therapy. Discourage her from engaging in hazardous activities during this time.
• Stress the importance of complying with the dosage regimen and keeping follow-up medical and laboratory appointments.
• Advise patient to follow up with her prescriber for blood pressure monitoring.
• Encourage patient to eat adequate quantities of iron-rich foods.
• If patient will self-administer darbepoetin, teach her and her caregiver the proper administration technique.
• Caution patient and her caregiver not to reuse needles, syringes, or drug product. Thoroughly instruct them in proper needle

and syringe disposal using a puncture-resistant container.
•Review possible adverse reactions, and urge patient to notify prescriber if she experiences chest pain, headache, rash, seizures, shortness of breath, or swelling.

# darifenacin

Enablex

## Class and Category
*Chemical:* Muscarinic receptor antagonist
*Therapeutic:* Bladder antispasmodic
*Pregnancy category:* C

## Indications and Dosages
➤ *To treat overactive urinary bladder with symptoms of urge incontinence, including urgency and frequency*
**E.R. TABLETS**
**Adults.** *Initial:* 7.5 mg q.d., increased to 15 mg q.d. after 2 wk as needed.
DOSAGE ADJUSTMENT For patients with moderate hepatic impairment and patients taking potent CYP3A4 inhibitors (such as clarithromycin, itraconazole, ketoconazole, nefazodone, nelfinavir, and ritonavir) daily dosage should not exceed 7.5 mg.

| Route | Onset | Peak | Duration |
|-------|-------|------|----------|
| P.O. | Unknown | 7 hr | Unknown |

## Contraindications
Gastric retention, hypersensitivity to darifenacin or its components, uncontrolled narrow-angle glaucoma, urine retention, and patients at risk for these conditions

## Interactions
**DRUGS**
*anticholinergics:* Increased frequency and severity of anticholinergic adverse reactions
*flecainide, thioridazine, tricyclic antidepressants:* Increased risk of toxicity of these drugs
*potent CYP3A4 inhibitors (such as clarithromycin, itraconazole, ketoconazole, nefazodone, nelfinavir, and ritonavir):* Decreased metabolism and increased effects of darifenacin, possibly increasing the risk of adverse reactions

## Adverse Reactions
**CNS:** Asthenia, dizziness
**CV:** Hypertension, peripheral edema
**EENT:** Abnormal vision, dry eyes or mouth, pharyngitis, rhinitis, sinusitis
**GI:** Abdominal pain, constipation, diarrhea, indigestion, nausea, vomiting
**GU:** Urine retention, UTI, vaginitis
**MS:** Arthralgia, back pain
**RESP:** Bronchitis
**SKIN:** Dry skin, pruritus, rash
**Other:** Flulike symptoms, weight gain

## Mechanism of Action
Antagonizes the effect of acetylcholine on muscarinic receptors in the detrusor muscle, decreasing the muscle spasms that cause inappropriate bladder emptying. This action increases bladder capacity and volume, which relieves the sensations of urgency and frequency and enhances bladder control.

## Nursing Considerations
•Administer darifenacin cautiously to patients with significant bladder outflow obstruction because they have an increased risk of urine retention.
•Use darifenacin cautiously in patients with severe constipation, ulcerative colitis, or myasthenia gravis because darifenacin may decrease GI motility. Also use it cautiously in patients with obstructive GI disorders because drug increases the risk of gastric retention.
**PATIENT TEACHING**
•Tell the patient to swallow darifenacin tablets with liquid and not to crush, split, or break them.
•Advise patient to avoid exercising in hot weather because darifenacin decreases sweating, which can increase the risk of heatstroke.
•Caution patient to avoid potentially hazardous activities until drug's CNS effects are known.

# demeclocycline hydrochloride

Declomycin

## Class and Category
*Chemical:* Tetracycline derivative
*Therapeutic:* Antibiotic
*Pregnancy category:* D

## Indications and Dosages

➤ *To treat Rocky Mountain spotted fever, typhus infections, Q fever, and rickettsialpox and tick fevers caused by Rickettsieae; psittacosis (ornithosis), lymphogranuloma venereum, granuloma inguinale, and* Mycoplasma pneumoniae *or* Borrelia recurrentis *infections; infections caused by gram-negative organisms, such as* Bacteroides *sp.,* Bartonella bacilliformis, Brucella *sp.,* Campylobacter fetus, Francisella tularensis, Haemophilus ducreyi, Vibrio cholerae, *and* Yersinia pestis*; infections caused by susceptible strains of* Acinetobacter calcoaceticus, Enterobacter aerogenes, Escherichia coli, Haemophilus influenzae *(respiratory tract infections),* Herellea *sp.,* Klebsiella *sp. (respiratory tract infections and UTIs), and* Shigella *sp.; infections caused by susceptible strains of* Staphylococcus aureus *(skin and soft-tissue infections) and* Streptococcus *sp.; infections caused by* Actinomyces *sp.,* Bacillus anthracis, Clostridium *sp.,* Fusobacterium fusiforme, Listeria monocytogenes, Treponema pallidum, *and* Treponema pertenue*; and acute intestinal amebiasis*

CAPSULES, TABLETS

**Adults and adolescents.** 150 mg q 6 hr or 300 mg q 12 hr.

**Children ages 8 to 12.** 6 to 12 mg/kg/day in divided doses q 6 to 12 hr.

➤ *To treat gonorrhea*

CAPSULES, TABLETS

**Adults and adolescents.** 600 mg followed by 300 mg q 12 hr for 4 days for total dose of 3,000 mg.

---

### Mechanism of Action

Binds with ribosomal subunits of susceptible bacteria and alters the cytoplasmic membrane, inhibiting bacterial protein synthesis and rendering the organism ineffective.

---

## Contraindications

Hypersensitivity to demeclocycline or other tetracyclines

## Interactions

DRUGS

*antacids, calcium supplements, cholestyramine, choline, colestipol, iron supplements, magnesium-containing laxatives, magnesium salicylate, sodium bicarbonate:* Decreased demeclocycline absorption

*digoxin:* Possibly increased blood digoxin level and risk of digitalis toxicity

*methoxyflurane:* Increased nephrotoxic effect

*oral anticoagulants:* Increased anticoagulant effects

*oral contraceptives:* Decreased contraceptive effectiveness

*penicillins:* Decreased bactericidal action of penicillins

*vitamin A:* Possibly benign intracranial hypertension

FOODS

*milk, other dairy products:* Decreased drug absorption

## Adverse Reactions

**CNS:** Dizziness, headache, light-headedness, vertigo

**EENT:** Tinnitus, vision changes

**GI:** Abdominal cramps, diarrhea, nausea, pseudomembranous colitis, vomiting

**GU:** Elevated BUN level, nephrogenic diabetes insipidus

**HEME:** Eosinophilia, hemolytic anemia, neutropenia, thrombocytopenia

**SKIN:** Photosensitivity, pruritus, rash, urticaria

**Other:** Anaphylaxis, angioedema

## Nursing Considerations

•Monitor results of renal and liver function tests during demeclocycline therapy, as indicated.

•**WARNING** Watch for development of nephrogenic diabetes insipidus during long-term therapy.

PATIENT TEACHING

•Stress the importance of completing therapy as prescribed, even if symptoms improve.

•Advise patient not to take demeclocycline within 3 hours of taking other drugs or dairy products because they may decrease its absorption.

•Instruct patient to avoid taking antacids while taking demeclocycline because of impaired absorption.

•Advise patient to avoid direct sunlight, use sunscreen, and wear protective clothing out-

doors; among tetracyclines, demeclocycline causes the most photosensitivity.
• Urge patient to notify prescriber immediately if edema, rash, or severe GI problems develop.
• Advise patient to avoid potentially hazardous activities if light-headedness, dizziness, or vertigo occurs.
• Instruct female patient of childbearing age to notify prescriber if she may be pregnant because demeclocycline may need to be discontinued.

# desipramine hydrochloride

Norpramin, Pertofrane (CAN)

## Class and Category
*Chemical*: Dibenzazepine derivative
*Therapeutic*: Antidepressant
*Pregnancy category*: C

## Indications and Dosages
➤ *To treat depression*
**TABLETS**
**Adults.** *Initial:* 100 to 200 mg/day as a single dose or in divided doses. Increased gradually to 300 mg/day, if needed. *Maximum:* 300 mg/day.
**Adolescents.** *Initial:* 25 to 50 mg/day in divided doses. Increased gradually, if needed. *Maximum:* 100 mg/day.
**Children ages 6 to 12.** *Initial:* 10 to 30 mg/day, or 1 to 5 mg/kg, in divided doses.
**DOSAGE ADJUSTMENT** Initial dosage decreased to 25 to 50 mg/day and given in divided doses for elderly patients; then increased gradually if needed to maximum of 150 mg/day.

| Route | Onset | Peak | Duration |
|-------|-------|------|----------|
| P.O. | 2 to 3 wk | Unknown | Unknown |

## Contraindications
Acute recovery phase of MI; hypersensitivity to desipramine, other tricyclic antidepressants, or their components; MAO inhibitor therapy within 14 days

## Interactions
**DRUGS**
*activated charcoal:* Prevention of desipramine absorption, reduced therapeutic effects

*barbiturates:* Decreased blood desipramine level, increased CNS depression
*bupropion, haloperidol, H2-receptor antagonists, valproic acid*: Increased blood level and adverse effects of desipramine
*carbamazepine:* Increased blood carbamazepine level, decreased blood desipramine level
*cimetidine:* Increased blood desipramine level and anticholinergic effects (dry mouth, urine retention, blurred vision)
*clonidine:* Increased risk of hypertensive crisis
*dicumarol:* Increased anticoagulant effect
*grepafloxacin, quinolones, sparfloxacin:* Increased risk of arrhythmias, including torsades de pointes
*guanethidine:* Antagonized antihypertensive effect of guanethidine
*levodopa:* Delayed levodopa absorption, increased risk of hypotension
*MAO inhibitors:* Increased risk of life-threatening adverse effects, such as hyperpyretic or hypertensive crisis and severe seizures
*phenothiazines:* Increased desipramine level, risk of inhibited phenothiazine metabolism and neuroleptic malignant syndrome
*quinidine:* Increased blood quinidine level
*rifamycins:* Decreased desipramine effects
*selective serotonin reuptake inhibitors:* Increased desipramine effects
*sympathomimetics:* Possibly arrhythmias, possibly increased or decreased vasopressor effects of sympathomimetics
**ACTIVITIES**
*alcohol use:* Possibly increased CNS or respiratory depression, hypotension, alcohol effects

## Mechanism of Action
Blocks serotonin and norepinephrine reuptake by adrenergic nerves, which normally release these neurotransmitters from their storage sites when activated by a nerve impulse. By blocking reuptake, this tricyclic antidepressant increases serotonin and norepinephrine levels at nerve synapses, which may elevate mood and reduce depression.

## Adverse Reactions
**CNS:** Agitation, akathisia, anxiety, ataxia, confusion, CVA, delusions, disorientation, dizziness, drowsiness, exacerbation of psychosis, extrapyramidal reactions, fatigue, headache, hypomania, insomnia, lack of co-

ordination, nervousness, nightmares, paresthesia, peripheral neuropathy, restlessness, seizures, sleep disturbance, suicidal ideation (children and teens), tremor, weakness
**CV:** Arrhythmias, including heart block; hypertension; hypotension; palpitations
**EENT:** Black tongue, blurred vision, dry mouth, mydriasis, stomatitis, taste perversion, tinnitus
**ENDO:** Breast enlargement and galactorrhea (in women), gynecomastia (in men), hyperglycemia, hypoglycemia, syndrome of inappropriate ADH secretion
**GI:** Abdominal cramps, anorexia, constipation, diarrhea, elevated liver function test results, elevated pancreatic enzyme levels, epigastric distress, hepatitis, ileus, increased appetite, nausea, vomiting
**GU:** Acute renal failure, impotence, libido changes, nocturia, painful ejaculation, testicular swelling, urinary frequency and hesitancy, urine retention
**HEME:** Agranulocytosis, eosinophilia, thrombocytopenia
**SKIN:** Acne, alopecia, dermatitis, diaphoresis, dry skin, flushing, petechiae, photosensitivity, pruritus, purpura, rash, urticaria
**Other:** Angioedema, drug fever, weight gain

## Nursing Considerations

•Use desipramine with extreme caution in patients with cardiovascular disease, glaucoma, seizure disorder, thyroid disease, or urine retention.
•**WARNING** Desipramine increases the risk of suicidal ideation in children and teens; monitor them closely for evidence.
•**WARNING** Expect drug to produce sedation and possibly to lower seizure threshold. Take safety and seizure precautions.
•Monitor blood glucose level frequently.
•Be prepared to obtain blood sample for leukocyte and differential counts from patients in whom fever develops during therapy.
•Expect to discontinue drug as soon as possible before elective surgery because of its possible adverse cardiovascular effects.
**PATIENT TEACHING**
•**WARNING** Urge parents to watch their child or teen closely and report abnormal thinking or behavior, aggression, and hostility.
•Advise patient to use sunscreen when outdoors and to avoid sunlamps and tanning beds.
•Instruct patient to notify prescriber immediately about a fast and pounding heart-

beat, fainting, severe agitation or restlessness, and strange behavior or thoughts.
•Caution patient not to stop drug abruptly; doing so may cause dizziness, headache, hyperthermia, irritability, malaise, nausea, sleep disturbances, and vomiting.
•Advise against drinking alcohol because of increased risk of adverse CNS reactions.
•Advise patient to avoid potentially hazardous activities until drug's CNS effects are known.
•Urge diabetic patient to monitor blood glucose level often.

# desmopressin acetate

DDAVP Injection, DDAVP Nasal Spray, DDAVP Rhinal Tube, DDAVP Rhinyle Nasal Solution (CAN), DDAVP Tablets, Octostim (CAN), Stimate, Stimate Nasal Spray

## Class and Category

*Chemical:* Synthetic ADH analogue
*Therapeutic:* Antidiuretic, antihemorrhagic
*Pregnancy category:* B

## Indications and Dosages

➤ *To manage primary nocturnal enuresis*
**TABLETS**
**Adults and children age 6 and older.** *Initial:* 0.2 mg h.s., increased as needed. *Maximum:* 0.6 mg/day.
**NASAL SOLUTION**
**Adults and children age 6 and older.** 10 mcg in each nostril h.s. for 4 to 8 wk. Reduced to 10 mcg in only one nostril h.s. if response is adequate to 10 mcg in each nostril, or increased to 20 mcg in each nostril h.s. if response is inadequate to 10 mcg in each nostril daily.

➤ *To control symptoms of central diabetes insipidus*
**TABLETS**
**Adults and children age 6 and older.** *Initial:* 0.05 mg b.i.d., increased as needed. *Usual:* 0.1 to 0.8 mg in divided doses b.i.d. or t.i.d. *Maximum:* 1.2 mg/day.
**I.V. INFUSION, I.M. OR S.C. INJECTION**
**Adults.** 2 to 4 mcg/day in divided doses b.i.d. Dosage adjusted as needed.
**NASAL SOLUTION**
**Adults and adolescents.** 0.1 to 0.4 ml/day (10 to 40 mcg/day) as a single dose or in divided doses b.i.d. or t.i.d. Dosage adjusted as need-

ed. If daily dose is divided, each dose adjusted separately.

**Children ages 3 months to 12 years.** 0.25 mcg/kg/day as a single dose or in divided doses b.i.d. Dosage adjusted as needed. If daily dose is divided, each dose adjusted separately.

➤ *To prevent or manage bleeding episodes in hemophilia A or mild to moderate type I von Willebrand's disease*

**I.V. INFUSION**

**Adults and children who weigh more than 10 kg (22 lb).** 0.3 mcg/kg diluted in 50 ml of NS and infused over 15 to 30 min. If used preoperatively, give 30 min before procedure.

**Children who weigh 10 kg or less.** 0.3 mcg/kg diluted in 10 ml of NS and infused over 15 to 30 min. If used preoperatively, dose is given 30 min before procedure.

**NASAL SOLUTION (STIMATE NASAL SPRAY)**

**Adults and children who weigh more than 50 kg (110 lb).** 150 mcg in each nostril. If used preoperatively, dose is given 2 hr before procedure.

**Adults and children who weigh 50 kg or less.** 150 mcg in one nostril. If used preoperatively, dose is given 2 hr before procedure.

| Route | Onset | Peak | Duration |
|-------|-------|------|----------|
| P.O. | 1 hr* | 4 to 7 hr* | 8 to 12 hr* |
| I.V. | 15 to 30 min† | 30 to 60 min† | 3 hr‡ |
| Nasal | In 1 hr* | 1 to 5 hr* | 8 to 20 hr* |

## Contraindications

Hypersensitivity to desmopressin or its components

## Interactions

**DRUGS**

*carbamazepine, chlorpropamide, clofibrate:* Possibly potentiated antidiuretic effect of desmopressin

*demeclocycline, lithium:* Possibly decreased antidiuretic effect of desmopressin

*vasopressor drugs:* Possibly potentiated vasopressor effect of desmopressin

---

\* For antidiuretic effect.

† For antihemorrhagic effect.

‡ For von Willebrand's disease; 4 to 20 hr for mild hemophilia A.

## Mechanism of Action

Exerts an antidiuretic effect similar to that of vasopressin by increasing cellular permeability of renal collecting ducts and distal tubules, thus enhancing water reabsorption, reducing urine flow, and increasing osmolality. As an antihemorrhagic, drug increases blood level of clotting factor VIII (antihemophilic factor) and activity of von Willebrand's factor (factor VII$_{VWF}$). It also may increase platelet aggregation and adhesion at injury sites by directly affecting blood vessel walls.

**D**

## Adverse Reactions

**CNS:** Asthenia, chills, dizziness, headache

**CV:** Hypertension (with high doses), transient hypotension

**EENT:** Conjunctivitis, epistaxis, lacrimation, nasal congestion (nasal form), ocular edema, pharyngitis, rhinitis

**GI:** Nausea

**GU:** Vulvar pain (parenteral form)

**SKIN:** Flushing

**Other:** Anaphylaxis, injection site pain and redness; water intoxication

## Nursing Considerations

• Use desmopressin cautiously in patients with conditions associated with fluid and electrolyte imbalance, such as cystic fibrosis; such patients are prone to hyponatremia.

• Be aware that nasal cavity scarring, edema, and other abnormalities may cause erratic absorption and require the use of a different administration route.

• Monitor blood pressure frequently during therapy.

**PATIENT TEACHING**

• To prevent hyponatremia and water intoxication in a child or an elderly patient, instruct family to restrict fluids as prescribed.

• Instruct patient to refrigerate nasal solution.

• Teach patient to prime nasal spray pump (only once) and spray dose into one or both nostrils, as prescribed, while inhaling briskly. Instruct her to clean tip of sprayer with hot water and dry it with clean tissue. Advise her to keep track of doses given and to discard bottle after 50 doses.

• Instruct patient who uses Stimate Nasal Spray to prime pump before first use by pressing down four times. Advise her to discard pump after 25 or 50 doses, depending on bottle, because delivery of an accurate dose can't be assured.

• Teach patient who uses nasal tube delivery system to draw prescribed amount of solution into calibrated flexible plastic tube, insert one end of tube into a nostril and the other end into her mouth, and gently blow into tube to deposit solution deep into nasal cavity. Caution her not to let drug drain into her mouth.

• Teach patient or caregiver how to administer S.C. injection, if appropriate.

• Urge patient to notify prescriber if adverse reactions occur.

# dexamethasone

Decadron, Decadron Elixir, Deronil (CAN), Dexamethasone Intensol, Dexasone (CAN), Dexone, Hexadrol, Oradexon (CAN)

## dexamethasone acetate

Cortastat LA, Dalalone D.P., Dalalone L.A., Decadron-LA, Decaject L.A., Dexacen LA-8, Dexacorten-LA, Dexasone L.A., Dexone LA, Solurex LA

## dexamethasone sodium phosphate

Cortastat, Dalalone, Decadrol, Decadron Respihaler, Decaject, Dexacen-4, Dexacorten, Dexacort Turbinaire, Dexasone, Dexone, Hexadrol Phosphate, Primethasone, Solurex

## Class and Category

*Chemical:* Synthetic adrenocortical steroid
*Therapeutic:* Anti-inflammatory, diagnostic aid, immunosuppressant
*Pregnancy category:* C

## Indications and Dosages

➤ *To treat endocrine disorders, such as congenital adrenal hyperplasia, hypercalcemia associated with cancer, and non-suppurative thyroiditis; acute episodes or exacerbations of rheumatic disorders; collagen diseases, such as systemic lupus erythematosus and acute rheumatic carditis; severe dermatologic diseases; se-vere allergic conditions, such as seasonal or perennial allergic rhinitis, bronchial asthma, serum sickness, and drug hypersensitivity reactions; respiratory diseases, such as symptomatic sarcoidosis, Löffler's syndrome, berylliosis, fulminating or dis-seminated pulmonary tuberculosis, and aspiration pneumonitis; hematologic disorders, such as idiopathic thrombocyto-penic purpura and secondary thrombocy-topenia in adults, autoimmune hemolytic anemia, aplastic crisis, and congenital hypoplastic anemia; tuberculous menin-gitis and trichinosis with neurologic or myocardial involvement*

➤ *To manage leukemias and lymphomas in adults and acute leukemia in children; to induce diuresis or remission of pro-teinuria in idiopathic nephrotic syn-drome without uremia or nephrotic syn-drome caused by systemic lupus erythe-matosus*

➤ *To provide palliative therapy during acute exacerbations of GI diseases, such as ulcerative colitis and regional enteritis*

ELIXIR, ORAL SOLUTION, TABLETS, I.V. OR I.M. INJECTION
**Adults.** Highly individualized dosage based on severity of disorder. *Usual:* 0.75 to 9 mg/ day as a single dose or in divided doses.

ELIXIR, ORAL SOLUTION, TABLETS
**Children.** Highly individualized dosage based on severity of disorder. *Usual:* 83.3 to 333.3 mcg/kg/day in divided doses t.i.d. or q.i.d.

I.M. INJECTION
**Children.** Highly individualized dosage based on severity of disorder. *Usual:* 27.76 to 166.65 mcg/kg q 12 to 24 hr.

➤ *To manage adrenocortical insufficiency*
ELIXIR, ORAL SOLUTION, TABLETS, I.V. OR I.M. INJECTION
**Adults.** 0.5 to 9 mg/day as a single dose or in divided doses.

ELIXIR, ORAL SOLUTION, TABLETS
**Children.** 23.3 mcg/kg/day in divided doses t.i.d.

I.M. INJECTION
**Children.** 23.3 mcg/kg/day in divided doses t.i.d. given q third day; alternatively, 7.76 to 11.65 mcg/kg/day.

➤ *To test for Cushing's syndrome*
ELIXIR, ORAL SOLUTION, TABLETS
**Adults.** 0.5 mg q 6 hr for 48 hr followed by collection of 24-hr urine specimen to deter-mine 17-hydroxycorticosteroid level. Alterna-

tively, 1 mg at 11 p.m. followed by plasma cortisol test performed at 8 a.m. the next day.

➤ *To distinguish Cushing's syndrome related to pituitary corticotropin excess from Cushing's syndrome related to other causes*

ELIXIR, ORAL SOLUTION, TABLETS

**Adults.** 2 mg q 6 hr for 48 hr followed by collection of 24-hr urine specimen to determine 17-hydroxycorticosteroid level.

➤ *To decrease cerebral edema*

ELIXIR, ORAL SOLUTION, TABLETS

**Adults.** 2 mg q 8 to 12 hr as maintenance after parenteral form has controlled initial symptoms.

I.V. OR I.M. INJECTION

**Adults.** 10 mg I.V. followed by 4 mg I.M. q 6 hr. Decreased after 2 to 4 days, if needed, gradually tapering off over 5 to 7 days unless inoperable or recurring brain tumor is present. If such a tumor is present, dosage gradually decreased after 2 to 4 days to maintenance dosage of 2 mg I.M. q 8 to 12 hr and switched to P.O. regimen as soon as possible.

➤ *To treat unresponsive shock*

I.V. INFUSION AND INJECTION

**Adults.** 20 mg as a single dose followed by 3 mg/kg over 24 hr as a continuous infusion; 40 mg as a single dose followed by 40 mg q 2 to 6 hr, as needed; or 1 mg/kg as a single dose. All regimens used for no more than 3 days.

➤ *To decrease localized inflammation*

INTRA-ARTICULAR INJECTION

**Adults.** 2 to 4 mg for large joint; 0.8 to 1 mg for small joint; 2 to 3 mg for bursae; 0.4 to 1 mg for tendon sheaths.

SOFT-TISSUE INJECTION

**Adults.** 2 to 6 mg; 1 to 2 mg for ganglia.

INTRALESIONAL INJECTION

**Adults.** 0.8 to 1.6 mg/injection site.

➤ *To decrease inflammation in allergic conditions or nasal polyps (except in sinuses)*

NASAL AEROSOL

**Adults and children age 12 and older.** 2 sprays (0.2 mg) in each nostril b.i.d. or t.i.d. *Maximum:* 12 sprays (1.2 mg)/day.
**Children ages 6 to 12.** 1 or 2 sprays (0.1 to 0.2 mg) in each nostril b.i.d. *Maximum:* 8 sprays (0.8 mg)/day.

## Mechanism of Action

Binds to intracellular glucocorticoid receptors and suppresses inflammatory and immune responses by:
• inhibiting neutrophil and monocyte accumulation at inflammation site and suppressing their phagocytic and bactericidal activity
• stabilizing lysosomal membranes
• suppressing antigen response of macrophages and helper T cells
• inhibiting synthesis of inflammatory response mediators, such as cytokines, interleukins, and prostaglandins.

## Contraindications

Administration of live virus vaccine to patient or family member, hypersensitivity to dexamethasone or its components (including sulfites), idiopathic thrombocytopenic purpura (I.M. use), systemic fungal infections

## Interactions

DRUGS

*aminoglutethimide, antacids, barbiturates, carbamazepine, hydantoins, mitotane, rifampin:* Decreased dexamethasone effectiveness
*amphotericin B (parenteral), carbonic anhydrase inhibitors:* Risk of hypokalemia
*anticholinesterases:* Decreased anticholinesterase effectiveness in myasthenia gravis
*aspirin, NSAIDs:* Increased risk of adverse GI effects
*cholestyramine:* Increased dexamethasone clearance
*cyclosporine:* Increased activity of both drugs, possibly resulting in seizures
*digoxin:* Increased risk of digitalis toxicity related to hypokalemia
*ephedrine:* Decreased half-life and increased clearance of dexamethasone
*erythromycin, indinavir:* Increased clearance and decreased plasma concentrations of these drugs
*estrogens, ketoconazole, macrolide antibiotics:* Decreased dexamethasone clearance
*isoniazid:* Decreased blood isoniazid level
*neuromuscular blockers:* Possibly potentiated or counteracted neuromuscular blockade
*oral anticoagulants:* Altered coagulation times, requiring reduced anticoagulant dosage

*oral contraceptives:* Increased half-life and concentration of dexamethasone
*phenytoin:* Increased risk of seizures
*potassium-wasting diuretics:* Increased potassium loss and risk of hypokalemia
*salicylates:* Decreased blood level and effectiveness of salicylates
*somatrem:* Possibly inhibition of somatrem's growth-promoting effect
*thalidomide:* Increased risk of toxic epidermal necrolysis
*theophyllines:* Altered effects of either drug
*toxoids, vaccines:* Decreased antibody response

**ACTIVITIES**
*alcohol use:* Increased risk of GI bleeding

## Adverse Reactions

**CNS:** Depression, emotional lability, euphoria, fever, headache, increased ICP with papilledema, insomnia, light-headedness, malaise, neuritis, neuropathy, paresthesia, psychosis, seizures, syncope, tiredness, vertigo, weakness
**CV:** Arrhythmias, bradycardia, edema, fat embolism, heart failure, hypercholesterolemia, hyperlipidemia, hypertension, myocardial rupture, tachycardia, thromboembolism, thrombophlebitis, vasculitis
**EENT:** Cataracts, glaucoma, vision changes (all forms); epistaxis, loss of smell and taste, nasal burning and dryness, oral candidiasis, perforated nasal septum, pharyngitis, rebound nasal congestion, rhinorrhea, sneezing (nasal aerosol)
**ENDO:** Cushingoid symptoms, decreased iodine uptake, growth suppression in children, hyperglycemia, menstrual irregularities, secondary adrenocortical and pituitary unresponsiveness
**GI:** Abdominal distention, bloody stools, elevated liver function test results, heartburn, hepato-megaly, increased appetite, indigestion, intestinal perforation, melena, nausea, pancreatitis, peptic ulcer with possible perforation, ulcerative esophagitis, vomiting
**GU:** Glycosuria, increased or decreased number and motility of spermatozoa, perineal irritation, urinary frequency
**HEME:** Leukocytosis, leukopenia
**MS:** Aseptic necrosis of femoral and humeral heads; muscle atrophy, spasms, or weakness; myalgia; osteoporosis; pathologic fracture of long bones; tendon rupture (intra-articular injection); vertebral compression fracture
**RESP:** Bronchospasm

**SKIN:** Acne, allergic dermatitis, diaphoresis, ecchymosis, erythema, hirsutism, necrotizing vasculitis, petechiae, subcutaneous fat atrophy, striae, thin and fragile skin, urticaria
**Other:** Aggravated or masked signs of infection, anaphylaxis, angioedema, hypernatremia, hypocalcemia, hypokalemia, hypokalemic alkalosis, impaired wound healing, metabolic acidosis, sodium and fluid retention, suppressed skin test reaction, weight gain

## Nursing Considerations

• Use dexamethasone cautiously in patients with congestive heart failure, hypertension, or renal insufficiency because drug can cause sodium retention, which may lead to edema and hypokalemia.
• Also use cautiously in patients who have had intestinal sugery and in those with peptic ulcer, diverticulitis, or ulcerative colitis because of the risk of perforation.
• Give once-daily dose of dexamethasone in the morning to coincide with the body's natural cortisol secretion.
• Give oral drug with food to decrease GI distress.
• Be aware that dosage forms with a concentration of 24 mg/ml are for I.V. use only.
• Shake I.M. solution before injecting deep into large muscle mass.
• **WARNING** Avoid S.C. injection; it may cause atrophy and sterile abscess.
• Inject undiluted I.V. dose directly into I.V. tubing of infusing compatible solution over 30 seconds or less, as prescribed.
• **WARNING** Don't give acetate form by I.V. injection.
• Shake nasal aerosol container well, and hold it upright about 6″ (15 cm) from area being treated. Keep spray out of patient's eyes, and advise her not to inhale it.
• Expect to taper drug rather than stopping it abruptly; prolonged use can cause adrenal suppression.
• Monitor fluid intake and output and daily weight, and assess patient for crackles, dyspnea, peripheral edema, and steady weight gain.
• Periodically evaluate growth if patient is a child.
• Test stool for occult blood.
• Monitor results of hematology studies as well as blood glucose and serum electrolyte, cholesterol, and lipid levels. Dexamethasone may

cause hyperglycemia, hypernatremia, hypocalcemia, hypokalemia, or leukopenia. It also may increase serum cholesterol and lipid levels, and it may decrease iodine uptake by the thyroid.
•Assess for evidence of osteoporosis, Cushing's syndrome, and other systemic effects during long-term use.
•Monitor neonate for signs of hypoadrenocorticism if mother received dexamethasone during pregnancy. Be aware that some preparations also contain benzyl alcohol, which may cause a fatal toxic syndrome in neonates and immature infants.
•Assess for hypersensitivity reactions after giving acetate or sodium phosphate form; both may contain bisulfites or parabens, inactive ingredients to which some people are allergic.

**PATIENT TEACHING**
•Instruct patient not to store drug in damp or hot places and to protect liquid form from freezing.
•Instruct patient to take once-daily oral dose in the morning with food to help prevent GI distress.
•Caution patient to avoid alcoholic beverages during therapy because they increase the risk of GI bleeding.
•Advise patient to follow a low-sodium, high-potassium, high-protein diet, if prescribed, to help minimize weight gain (common with this drug). Instruct her to inform prescriber if she's on a special diet.
•Instruct patient not to stop using drug abruptly.
•Advise patient to notify prescriber if condition recurs or worsens after dosage is reduced or therapy stops.
•Urge patient to have regular eye examinations during long-term use.
•Advise patient receiving long-term therapy to carry medical identification and to notify all health care providers that she takes dexamethasone.
•Instruct patient (especially a child) to avoid close contact with anyone who has chickenpox or measles and to notify prescriber immediately if exposure occurs.
•Advise patient and family members to avoid live virus vaccinations, such as oral polio vaccine, during therapy unless prescriber approves.

•Inform diabetic patient that drug may affect her blood glucose level.
•If drug is injected into a joint, instruct patient not to put excessive pressure on joint and to notify prescriber if it becomes red or swollen.
•Advise patient to notify prescriber about anorexia, depression, light-headedness, malaise, muscle pain, nausea, vomiting, and signs of early hyperadrenocorticism (abdominal distention, amenorrhea, easy bruising, extreme weakness, facial hair, increased appetite, moon face, weight gain). Inform patient and family about possible changes in appearance.
•Encourage patient to notify prescriber about illness, surgery, or changes in stress level.

# dexchlorpheniramine maleate

Dexchlor, Polaramine, Polaramine Repetabs

## Class and Category
*Chemical:* Propylamine derivative
*Therapeutic:* Antihistamine
*Pregnancy category:* B

## Indications and Dosages
➤ *To treat allergic conjunctivitis; transfusion reaction; dermographism; mild, uncomplicated allergic skin reactions, such as urticaria and angioedema; perennial and seasonal allergic rhinitis; and vasomotor rhinitis and as adjunct to treat anaphylaxis*
**E.R. TABLETS**
**Adults and adolescents.** 4 to 6 mg/day h.s. or q 8 to 10 hr, p.r.n.
**SYRUP, TABLETS**
**Adults and adolescents.** 2 mg q 4 to 6 hr, p.r.n.
**Children ages 6 to 12.** 1 mg q 4 to 6 hr or 150 mcg/kg in divided doses q.i.d., p.r.n.
**Children ages 2 to 6.** 0.5 mg q 4 to 6 hr, p.r.n.

| Route | Onset | Peak | Duration |
|---|---|---|---|
| P.O. | 15 to 60 min* | Unknown* | 4 to 8 hr* |

* For syrup and tablets; unknown for E.R. tablets.

## Mechanism of Action

Binds to central and peripheral $H_1$ receptors, competing with histamine for these sites and preventing histamine from reaching its site of action. By blocking histamine, dexchlorpheniramine:
• inhibits respiratory, vascular, and GI smooth-muscle contraction, which prevents wheezing
• decreases capillary permeability, which reduces itching, flares, and wheals
• decreases lacrimal and salivary gland secretions, which prevents increased nasal secretions, itching, sneezing, and watery eyes.

## Contraindications

Angle-closure glaucoma; benign prostatic hyperplasia; bladder neck obstruction; hypersensitivity to dexchlorpheniramine or other antihistamines; lower respiratory tract disorders, such as asthma; MAO inhibitor therapy within 14 days; pyloroduodenal obstruction; stenosing peptic ulcer

## Interactions

**DRUGS**
*anticholinergics:* Potentiated anticholinergic effects
*CNS depressants:* Increased CNS depression
*MAO inhibitors:* Possibly severe hypotension and prolonged and intensified anticholinergic and sedative effects of dexchlorpheniramine
**ACTIVITIES**
*alcohol use:* Increased CNS depression

## Adverse Reactions

**CNS:** Ataxia, confusion, dizziness, drowsiness, euphoria, excitement, headache, insomnia, irritability, nervousness, neuritis, nightmares, paresthesia, restlessness, vertigo, weakness
**CV:** Hypotension, palpitations, tachycardia
**EENT:** Acute labyrinthitis, blurred vision, dry mouth, tinnitus, vision changes
**GI:** Anorexia, constipation, diarrhea, indigestion, nausea, vomiting
**GU:** Urinary hesitancy, urine retention
**RESP:** Tenacious bronchial secretions
**SKIN:** Diaphoresis, photosensitivity, rash

## Nursing Considerations

• Use dexchlorpheniramine cautiously in elderly patients and those with cardiovascular disease, hyperthyroidism, increased intraocular pressure, prostatic hypertrophy, or renal disease.
• Monitor for adverse reactions, especially in elderly patients and children.
• Assess for signs of overdose, including clumsiness; drowsiness; dry mouth, nose, or throat; dyspnea; flushed or red face; hallucinations; insomnia; light-headedness; seizures; and unsteadiness.
**PATIENT TEACHING**
• Inform patient that drug provides temporary relief of symptoms.
• Advise patient to take drug with food, water, or milk to reduce GI irritation. Inform her that she can crush regular (not E.R.) tablets and mix with food or fluid.
• If patient takes E.R. tablets, tell her not to break, crush, or chew them before swallowing.
• Advise patient to take missed dose as soon as possible unless it's almost time for next dose.
• Because drug may cause drowsiness, caution patient to avoid potentially hazardous activities until its CNS effects are known.
• Instruct her to avoid prolonged sun exposure and to use a sunscreen.
• Suggest that patient use sugarless candy or gum, ice chips, or saliva substitute to relieve dry mouth. If dryness lasts longer than 2 weeks, advise her to notify prescriber.
• Caution patient to avoid alcohol and CNS depressants, such as sedatives, sleepng pills, and tranquilizers, while taking dexchlorpheniramine.
• If patient takes high doses of aspirin, urge her to inform prescriber because antihistamines may mask adverse reactions to aspirin overdose, such as tinnitus.
• Inform patient that drug needs to be discontinued 3 to 4 days before skin tests for allergies are performed.

# dexmethylphenidate hydrochloride

Focalin, Focalin XR

## Class, Category, and Schedule

*Chemical:* d-*threo*-enantiomer of methylphenidate
*Therapeutic:* CNS stimulant
*Pregnancy category:* C
*Controlled substance:* Schedule II

## Indications and Dosages

➤ *To treat attention deficit hyperactivity disorder (ADHD)*

**TABLETS**

**Adults and children age 6 and older who are new to methylphenidate.** 2.5 mg b.i.d. at least 4 hr apart, increased in weekly increments of 2.5 to 5 mg. *Maximum:* 10 mg b.i.d.

**Adults and children age 6 and older who are currently using methylphenidate.** One-half of racemic methylphenidate dosage. *Maximum:* 10 mg b.i.d. at least 4 hr apart.

DOSAGE ADJUSTMENT Drug stopped if no improvement within 1 month after appropriate dosage adjustments. Dosage decreased or drug stopped for paradoxical aggravation of symptoms or adverse reactions.

**E.R. CAPSULES, E.R. TABLETS**

**Adults who are new to methylphenidate.** 10 mg q.d., increased after 1 wk as needed to 20 mg q.d.

**Children age 6 and older who are new to methylphenidate.** 5 mg q.d., increased as needed in weekly intervals by 5-mg increments. *Maximum:* 20 mg/day.

**Adults and children age 6 and older who are currently using methylphenidate.** One-half of racemic methylphenidate dosage. *Maximum:* 20 mg/day.

## Mechanism of Action

May block the reuptake of norepinephrine and dopamine into presynaptic neurons in the cerebral cortex, which increases the availability of norepinephrine and dopamine in the extraneuronal space.

## Contraindications

Diagnosis or family history of Tourette syndrome; glaucoma; hypersensitivity to dexmethylphenidate, methylphenidate, or their components; marked anxiety, tension, and agitation; motor tics; use within 14 days of MAO inhibitor therapy

## Interactions

**DRUGS**

*anticoagulants (oral), anticonvulsants, antidepressants (tricyclic and selective serotonin reuptake inhibitors):* Possibly decreased metabolism of these drugs

*antihypertensives:* Decreased therapeutic effect of these drugs

*dopamine and other vasopressors:* Increased therapeutic effect of these drugs

*MAO inhibitors:* Increased adverse effects, risk of hypertensive crisis

## Adverse Reactions

**CNS:** Cerebral arteritis or occlusion, dizziness, drowsiness, dyskinesia, fever, headache, insomnia, motor or vocal tics, nervousness, seizures, Tourette syndrome, toxic psychosis

**CV:** Angina, arrhythmias, hypertension, hypotension, increased or decreased pulse rate, palpitations, tachycardia

**GI:** Abdominal pain, anorexia, nausea

**HEME:** Thrombocytopenic purpura

**MS:** Arthralgia

**SKIN:** Erythema multiforme, exfoliative dermatitis, necrotizing vasculitis, rash, urticaria

**Other:** Weight loss (with prolonged dexmethylphenidate therapy)

## Nursing Considerations

•WARNING Be aware that dexmethylphenidate may induce CNS stimulation and psychosis and may worsen behavior disturbances and thought disorders. Use drug cautiously in children with psychosis. Be aware that withdrawal symptoms may occur with long-term use.

•Monitor patient's blood pressure and pulse rate to detect hypertension and signs of excessive stimulation. Notify prescriber if you detect such signs.

•Be aware that dexmethylphenidate shouldn't be used to treat severe depression or to prevent or treat normal fatigue.

•WARNING Monitor patient for signs of physical or psychological dependence. Use drug cautiously in patients with a history of drug abuse, including alcoholism.

•Monitor CBC and differential and platelet counts, as ordered, during prolonged therapy.

•Expect to stop drug if seizures occur. Drug may lower seizure threshold, especially in patients with a history of seizures or EEG abnormalities.

•Monitor children on long-term therapy for signs of growth suppression, which has been noted during long-term use of stimulants.

•Be aware that the dosages of drugs affected by dexmethylphenidate, such as anticoagulants and antihypertensives, may need adjustment.

D

•Tell patient that extended-release capsules should either be taken whole, without being chewed, crushed, or divided, or capsule contents should be sprinkled on a small amount of applesauce.
•Encourage patient to notify her prescriber if she experiences excessive nervousness, fever, insomnia, nausea, palpitations, or rash while undergoing dexmethylphenidate therapy.
•Caution patient with seizure disorder that drug may cause seizures.
•Advise patient to protect drug from light and moisture.
•Teach patient (or parent) to watch for improvement in signs and symptoms of ADHD, such as decreased impulsiveness and increased attention. Stress the need for continued follow-up care, and suggest participation in an ADHD program.

# dexrazoxane

Zinecard

## Class and Category

*Chemical:* Piperazinedione
*Therapeutic:* Cardioprotective agent, chelating agent
*Pregnancy category:* C

## Indications and Dosages

➤ *To prevent or reduce severity of cardiomyopathy associated with doxorubicin therapy in women with metastatic breast cancer*

**I.V. INJECTION**
**Adults.** *Initial:* 500 mg/m$^2$ for every 50 mg/m$^2$ of doxorubicin q 3 wk.
DOSAGE ADJUSTMENT In patients with hyperbilirubinemia, dosage proportionately reduced (depending on severity) to maintain a dexrazoxane-to-doxorubicin ratio of 10:1. In patients with creatinine clearance of less than 40 ml/min, dosage decreased 50%.

## Incompatibilities

Don't mix dexrazoxane in same I.V. line with other drugs.

## Contraindications

Hypersensitivity to dexrazoxane or its components; use with chemotherapy regimens that do not contain an anthracycline, such as daunorubicin, doxorubicin, epirubicin, idarubicin, or mitoxantrone

## Mechanism of Action

Rapidly enters cardiac cells and acts as an intracellular heavy metal chelator. In cardiac tissues, anthracyclines, such as doxorubicin, form complexes with iron or copper, resulting in damage to cardiac cell membranes and mitochondria. Dexrazoxane combines with intracellular iron and protects against anthracycline-induced free radical damage to the myocardium. It also prevents the conversion of ferrous ions back to ferric ions for use by free radicals.

## Interactions

*bone marrow depressants:* Possibly enhanced bone marrow depression

## Adverse Reactions

**HEME:** Myelosuppression including granulocytopenia, leukopenia, or thrombocytopenia
**Other:** Injection site pain

## Nursing Considerations

•WARNING Use gloves when preparing reconstituted solution. If dexrazoxane powder or solution comes in contact with your skin or mucosa, immediately and thoroughly wash with soap and water.
•Reconstitute drug by mixing with 25 or 50 ml of 0.167 molar sodium lactate, supplied by the manufacturer, to produce a final concentration of 10 mg/ml. Administer reconstituted solution by slow I.V. push, or further dilute with either NS or D$_5$W to a concentration of 1.3 to 5 mg/ml, as prescribed, for rapid I.V. infusion.
•Be aware that dexrazoxane may interfere with tumor response to doxorubicin, especially in patients receiving drug at start of fluorouracil-doxorubicin-cyclophosphamide therapy.
•Monitor patient with immunosuppression or decreased bone marrow reserves resulting from prior chemotherapy or radiation therapy to prevent worsening of her condition. Notify prescriber if condition deteriorates.
•Inform patient that dexrazoxane is used to protect the heart from damage caused by myelosuppression and that she'll be given the drug by a health care professional in the hospital or clinic before receiving chemotherapy.

•Inform patient that dexrazoxane and chemotherapy may make her feel generally unwell, but urge her to continue treatment unless prescriber tells her to stop.

•Instruct patient to report chills, fever, mouth sores, pain at injection site, sore throat, unusual bleeding or bruising, unusual tiredness or weakness, and vomiting. Dosage may need to be changed or therapy stopped.

•Inform patient that drug may exacerbate symptoms of bone marrow suppression caused by anthracycline chemotherapy, including increased risk of infection.

•Teach patient importance of avoiding injury and infection during dexrazoxane therapy. For example, advise her to use a soft-bristled toothbrush to prevent damage to teeth and gums; to avoid people with colds, the flu, or bronchitis; and to avoid anyone who has recently had oral polio vaccine because of the increased risk of infection from live virus.

# dextrose

## (d-glucose)

B-D Glucose, Glutose, Insta-Glucose, Insulin Reaction

## glucose

2.5% Dextrose Injection, 5% Dextrose Injection, 10% Dextrose Injection, 20% Dextrose Injection, 25% Dextrose Injection, 50% Dextrose Injection, 60% Dextrose Injection, 70% Dextrose Injection

### Class and Category

*Chemical:* Monosaccharide
*Therapeutic:* Antidiabetic, nutritional supplement
*Pregnancy category:* C

### Indications and Dosages

➤ *To treat insulin-induced hypoglycemia*
CHEWABLE TABLETS, ORAL GEL
**Adults and children.** *Initial:* 10 to 20 g. Repeated in 10 to 20 min, if needed, based on serum glucose level.
I.V. INFUSION OR INJECTION
**Adults and children.** *Initial:* 20 to 50 ml of 50% solution given at 3 ml/min. *Maintenance:* 10% to 15% solution by continuous infusion until blood glucose level reaches therapeutic range.

**Infants and neonates.** 2 ml/kg of 10% to 25% solution until blood glucose level reaches therapeutic range.
➤ *To replace calories*
I.V. INFUSION
**Adults and children.** Individualized dosage of 2.5%, 5%, or 10% solution, based on need for fluids or calories and given through peripheral I.V. line. Or a 10% to 70% solution given through a large central vein, if needed, typically mixed with amino acids or other solutions.

| Route | Onset | Peak | Duration |
|---|---|---|---|
| P.O. | 10 to 20 min | 40 min | Unknown |
| I.V. | 2 to 3 min | Unknown | Unknown |

### Mechanism of Action
Prevents protein and nitrogen loss, promotes glycogen deposition, prevents or decreases ketosis, and, in large amounts, acts as an osmotic diuretic. Dextrose is readily metabolized and undergoes oxidation to carbon dioxide and water. The oral form—glucose—is absorbed directly into the bloodstream from the intestines and is distributed, used, or stored in the liver.

### Incompatibilities
Don't give dextrose through same infusion set as blood or blood products because pseudoagglutination of RBCs may occur.

### Contraindications
*For all solutions:* Diabetic coma with excessively elevated blood glucose level
*For concentrated solutions:* Anuria, alcohol withdrawal syndrome in dehydrated patient, glucose-galactose malabsorption syndrome, hepatic coma, hypersensitivity to corn or corn products, intracranial or intraspinal hemorrhage, overhydration

### Interactions
DRUGS
*corticosteroids, corticotropin:* Increased risk of fluid and electrolyte imbalance if dextrose solution contains sodium ions

### Adverse Reactions
**CNS:** Confusion, fever
**GU:** Glycosuria

**Other:** Dehydration; hyperosmolar coma; hypervolemia; hypovolemia; injection site extravasation with tissue necrosis, infection, phlebitis, and venous thrombosis

### Nursing Considerations
•Use dextrose cautiously in patients with renal impairment because dextrose solutions contain aluminum, which may reach toxic levels when these patients receive prolonged parenteral therapy.
•Give highly concentrated dextrose solution by central venous catheter—not by S.C. or I.M. route.
•**WARNING** Avoid rapid or excessive administration of dextrose solution in a very low–birth-weight infant because it can increase serum osmolality and possibly cause intracerebral hemorrhage.
•Assess infusion site regularly for signs of infiltration, such as pain or swelling.
•Assess for glucosuria by using a urine reagent strip or collecting a urine sample and reviewing urinalysis results.
•When discontinuing a concentrated solution, expect to give a 5% to 10% dextrose infusion to avoid rebound hypoglycemia.
•Monitor for signs of hypervolemia, such as jugular vein distention and crackles.
**PATIENT TEACHING**
•Advise patient to swallow oral dextrose, which isn't absorbed from the buccal cavity.
•Instruct patient to monitor her blood glucose level as directed.
•Stress the importance of reporting discomfort, pain, or signs of infection at I.V. site.

# dezocine

Dalgan

## Class and Category
*Chemical:* Aminotetralin, synthetic opioid
*Therapeutic:* Analgesic
*Pregnancy category:* C

## Indications and Dosages
➤ *To relieve pain*
**I.V. INJECTION**
**Adult.** *Initial:* 5 mg followed by 2.5 to 10 mg q 2 to 4 hr, p.r.n. *Maximum:* 120 mg/day.
**I.M. INJECTION**
**Adult.** *Initial:* 10 mg followed by 5 to 20 mg q 3 to 6 hr, p.r.n. *Maximum:* 20 mg/dose, 120 mg/day.

| Route | Onset | Peak | Duration |
|-------|-------|------|----------|
| I.V. | In 15 min | 30 min | 2 to 4 hr |
| I.M. | In 30 min | 1 to 2 hr | 2 to 4 hr |

### Mechanism of Action
Binds with opioid receptors at many CNS sites. This affects the perception of and emotional response to pain.

## Contraindications
Hypersensitivity to dezocine or its components

## Interactions
**DRUGS**
*CNS depressants, general anesthetics, hypnotics, sedatives, tranquilizers:* Increased CNS depressant effects
*opioids:* Possibly decreased therapeutic effects of opioid and withdrawal symptoms in patient receiving long-term opioid therapy
**ACTIVITIES**
*alcohol use:* Increased CNS depressant effects

## Adverse Reactions
**CNS:** Dizziness, sedation, vertigo
**GI:** Nausea, vomiting
**Other:** Injection site redness and swelling

## Nursing Considerations
•Use dezocine cautiously and in low doses in elderly patients and those who have common bile duct, hepatic, renal, or respiratory disease.
•Discard solution if it contains precipitate.
•Frequently monitor blood pressure and pulse and respiratory rates after giving first dose, especially if given by I.V. route.
•**WARNING** Avoid administering dezocine to a patient who is opioid-dependent. Doing so may precipitate withdrawal symptoms because drug can antagonize opioid effects.
•Assess for pain relief and document findings frequently.
**PATIENT TEACHING**
•Instruct patient to notify prescriber if pain isn't relieved within 1 hour.
•Advise patient to avoid potentially hazardous activities until drug's CNS effects are known.

# diazepam

Apo-Diazepam (CAN), Diastat, Diazepam
Intensol, Dizac, Novo-Dipam (CAN), Valium,
Vivol (CAN)

## Class, Category, and Schedule
*Chemical*: Benzodiazepine
*Therapeutic*: Anticonvulsant, anxiolytic,
sedative-hypnotic, skeletal muscle relaxant
*Pregnancy category:* D
*Controlled substance:* Schedule IV

## Indications and Dosages
➤ *To relieve anxiety*
ORAL SOLUTION, TABLETS
**Adults.** 2 to 10 mg b.i.d. to q.i.d.
DOSAGE ADJUSTMENT Dosage reduced to 2 to
2.5 mg q.d. or b.i.d. and increased gradually
as needed and tolerated for elderly or debilitated patients.
**Children age 6 months and older.** *Initial:* 1 to
2.5 mg t.i.d. or q.i.d. Increased gradually as
needed and tolerated.
I.V. OR I.M. INJECTION
**Adults.** 2 to 5 mg q 3 to 4 hr, p.r.n., for mod-
erate anxiety; 5 to 10 mg q 3 to 4 hr, p.r.n.,
for severe anxiety.
**Children.** Individualized dosage. *Maximum:*
0.25 mg/kg given over 3 min and repeated
after 15 to 30 min if needed and after another 15 to 30 min if needed.
➤ *To treat symptoms of acute alcohol
withdrawal*
ORAL SOLUTION, TABLETS
**Adults.** 10 mg t.i.d. or q.i.d. during first 24 hr.
Then 5 mg t.i.d. or q.i.d., if needed.
I.V. OR I.M. INJECTION
**Adults.** 10 mg and then 5 to 10 mg in 3 to
4 hr, if needed.
➤ *To provide muscle relaxation, to provide
sedation*
ORAL SOLUTION, TABLETS
**Adults.** 2 to 10 mg t.i.d. or q.i.d.
DOSAGE ADJUSTMENT Dosage reduced to 2 to
2.5 mg q.d. or b.i.d. and increased gradually
as needed and tolerated for elderly or debili-
tated patients.
**Children age 6 months and older.** *Initial:* 1 to
2.5 mg t.i.d. or q.i.d. Increased gradually as
needed and tolerated.
I.V. OR I.M. INJECTION
**Adults.** 2 to 5 mg q 3 to 4 hr, p.r.n., for moderate anxiety; 5 to 10 mg q 3 to 4 hr, p.r.n.,
for severe anxiety.

**Children.** Individualized dosage. *Maximum:*
0.25 mg/kg given over 3 min and repeated
after 15 to 30 min if needed and after an-
other 15 to 30 min if needed.
➤ *To treat symptoms of acute alcohol
withdrawal*
ORAL SOLUTION, TABLETS
**Adults.** 10 mg t.i.d. or q.i.d. during first 24 hr.
Then 5 mg t.i.d. or q.i.d., if needed.
I.V. OR I.M. INJECTION
**Adults.** 10 mg and then 5 to 10 mg in 3 to
4 hr, if needed.
➤ *To provide muscle relaxation, to provide
sedation*
ORAL SOLUTION, TABLETS
**Adults.** 2 to 10 mg t.i.d. or q.i.d.
DOSAGE ADJUSTMENT Dosage reduced to 2 to
5 mg/dose and increased as needed and tol-
erated for debilitated patients.
➤ *To treat seizures*
ORAL SOLUTION, TABLETS
**Adults.** 2 to 10 mg b.i.d. to q.i.d.
DOSAGE ADJUSTMENT Dosage reduced to 2 to
2.5 mg q.d. or b.i.d. and increased gradually
as needed and tolerated for elderly or debili-
tated patients.
**Children age 6 months and older.** *Initial:* 1 to
2.5 mg t.i.d. or q.i.d. Increased gradually as
needed and tolerated.
➤ *To treat status epilepticus and severe recurrent seizures*
I.V. INJECTION
**Adults.** 5 to 10 mg repeated q 10 to 15 min,
as needed, up to a cumulative dose of 30 mg.
Regimen repeated, if needed, in 2 to 4 hr.
(Use I.M. route if I.V. access is impossible.)
**Children age 5 and older.** 1 mg repeated q 2
to 5 min, as needed, up to a cumulative dose
of 10 mg. Regimen repeated, if needed, in 2
to 4 hr.
**Children ages 1 month to 5 years.** 0.2 to
0.5 mg repeated q 2 to 5 min, as needed, up

D

to a cumulative dose of 5 mg. Regimen repeated, if needed, in 2 to 4 hr.

**RECTAL GEL**

**Adults and adolescents.** 0.2 mg/kg rounded up to next available unit dose (or rounded down for elderly or debilitated patient). Repeated in 4 to 12 hr, if needed.

**Children ages 6 to 12.** 0.3 mg/kg rounded up to next available unit dose. Repeated in 4 to 12 hr, if needed.

**Children ages 2 to 6.** 0.5 mg/kg rounded up to next available unit dose. Repeated in 4 to 12 hr, if needed.

➤ *To provide preoperative sedation*

**I.V. OR I.M. INJECTION**

**Adults.** 5 to 10 mg 30 min before surgery.

➤ *To reduce anxiety before cardioversion*

**I.V. INJECTION**

**Adults.** 5 to 15 mg 5 to 10 min before procedure.

➤ *To reduce anxiety before endoscopic procedures*

**I.V. INJECTION**

**Adults.** Up to 20 mg titrated to desired sedation and administered immediately before procedure.

**I.M. INJECTION**

**Adults.** 5 to 10 mg 30 min before procedure.

➤ *To treat tetanus*

**I.V. OR I.M. INJECTION**

**Adults and children age 5 and older.** *Initial:* 5 to 10 mg repeated q 3 to 4 hr, if needed. Sometimes larger doses are needed for adults.

**DOSAGE ADJUSTMENT** Initial dose reduced to 2 to 5 mg and increased gradually as needed and tolerated for debilitated patients.

**Children ages 1 month to 5 years.** 1 to 2 mg repeated q 3 to 4 hr, as needed.

## Mechanism of Action

May potentiate the effects of gamma-aminobutyric acid (GABA) and other inhibitory neurotransmitters by binding to specific benzodiazepine receptors in the limbic and cortical areas of the CNS. GABA inhibits excitatory stimulation, which helps control emotional behavior. The limbic system contains a highly dense area of benzodiazepine receptors, which may explain the drug's antianxiety effects. Diazepam suppresses the spread of seizure activity caused by seizure-producing foci in the cortex, thalamus, and limbic structures.

## Incompatibilities

Don't mix diazepam injection with aqueous solutions. Don't mix diazepam emulsion for I.M. injection with morphine or glycopyrrolate or administer it through an infusion set that contains polyvinyl chloride.

## Contraindications

Acute angle-closure glaucoma, hypersensitivity to diazepam or its components, untreated open-angle glaucoma

## Interactions

**DRUGS**

*antacids:* Altered rate of diazepam absorption
*cimetidine, disulfiram, fluoxetine, isoniazid, itraconazole, ketoconazole, metoprolol, oral contraceptives, propoxyphene, propranolol, valproic acid:* Decreased diazepam metabolism, increased blood level and risk of adverse effects of diazepam
*CNS depressants:* Increased CNS depression
*digoxin:* Increased serum digoxin level and risk of digitalis toxicity
*levodopa:* Decreased antidyskinetic effect of levodopa
*probenecid:* Faster onset or more prolonged effects of diazepam
*ranitidine:* Delayed elimination and increased blood level of diazepam
*rifampin:* Decreased blood diazepam level
*theophyllines:* Antagonized sedative effect of diazepam

**ACTIVITIES**

*alcohol use:* Increased CNS depression

## Adverse Reactions

**CNS:** Anterograde amnesia, anxiety, ataxia, confusion, depression, dizziness, drowsiness, fatigue, headache, insomnia, lethargy, lightheadedness, sedation, sleepiness, slurred speech, tremor, vertigo
**CV:** Hypotension, palpitations, tachycardia
**EENT:** Blurred vision, diplopia, increased salivation
**GI:** Anorexia, constipation, diarrhea, nausea, vomiting
**GU:** Libido changes, urinary incontinence, urine retention
**RESP:** Respiratory depression
**SKIN:** Dermatitis
**Other:** Physical and psychological dependence

## Nursing Considerations

•Use diazepam cautiously in patients with hepatic or renal impairment.

•Mix concentrated oral solution (Intensol) with liquid or semisolid food for administration. Use supplied calibrated dropper for accurate dosing.

•Protect diazepam injection from light. Don't use solution that's more than slightly yellow or that contains precipitate.

•Administer I.M. injection into deltoid muscle for rapid and complete absorption. Administration into other sites may cause slow, erratic absorption.

•Before administering emulsion form, ask if patient is allergic to soybeans because this form contains soybean oil.

•For an infant or a child, administer I.V. injection slowly over 3 minutes in a dose not to exceed 0.25 mg/kg.

•Administer emulsion form within 6 hours of opening ampule because this form contains no preservatives and allows rapid microbial growth. Use polyethylene-lined or glass infusion sets and polyethylene or polypropylene plastic syringes for administration. Don't use a filter with a pore size of less than 5 microns because it may break down the emulsion.

•Don't mix emulsion form with anything other than its emulsion base. Otherwise, it may become unstable and increase the risk of serious adverse reactions.

•Monitor patient for adverse reactions, especially if she has hypoalbuminemia, which increases the risk of sedation.

•**WARNING** Observe for signs of physical and psychological dependence: a strong desire or need to continue taking diazepam, a need to increase the dose to maintain drug effects, and posttherapy withdrawal symptoms, such as abdominal cramps, insomnia, irritability, nervousness, and tremor.

**PATIENT TEACHING**

•Instruct patient not to take more drug than prescribed, more often, or for a longer time. Warn her that physical and psychological dependence can occur, and teach her to recognize signs of dependence.

•Advise patient not to take drug to relieve everyday stress.

•Advise patient to avoid potentially hazardous activities until drug's CNS effects are known.

•Advise patient to avoid CNS depressants and alcohol during therapy.

•Instruct patient not to abruptly stop taking drug without prescriber supervision. If patient has a history of seizures, warn her that abrupt drug withdrawal may trigger them.

•Instruct patient to mix Diazepam Intensol with water, soda, or a similar beverage; applesauce; or pudding just before taking it. Caution her not to save the mixture for later. Also tell patient to use calibrated dropper that's provided to measure each dose.

•Teach patient how to self-administer a rectal form, if prescribed.

# diazoxide

Hyperstat, Proglycem

## Class and Category

*Chemical:* Benzothiadiazine derivative
*Therapeutic:* Antihypertensive, antihypoglycemic
*Pregnancy category:* C

## Indications and Dosages

➤ *To manage hypoglycemia caused by hyperinsulinism*

**CAPSULES, ORAL SUSPENSION**

**Adults and children.** *Initial:* 1 mg/kg q 8 hr. *Maintenance:* 3 to 8 mg/kg/day in 2 or 3 equal doses given q 8 or 12 hr. *Maximum:* 15 mg/kg/day.

**Infants and neonates.** *Initial:* 3.3 mg/kg q 8 hr. *Maintenance:* 8 to 15 mg/kg/day in 2 or 3 equal doses given q 8 or 12 hr.

➤ *To treat severe hypertension in hospitalized patients*

**I.V. INJECTION**

**Adults and children.** *Initial:* 1 to 3 mg/kg by rapid bolus, repeated q 5 to 15 min until diastolic pressure falls below 100 mm Hg. Repeated in 4 hr and again in 24 hr, if needed, until oral antihypertensive therapy begins. *Maximum:* 150 mg/dose, 1.2 g/day.

| Route | Onset | Peak | Duration |
|-------|-------|------|----------|
| P.O. | In 1 hr | Unknown | 8 hr |
| I.V. | 1 min | 2 to 5 min | 2 to 12 hr |

## Mechanism of Action

Directly affects smooth muscle cells of peripheral arteries and arterioles, causing them to dilate. This action decreases peripheral resistance, which helps reduce blood pressure. Diazoxide also inhibits insulin release from the pancreas, stimulates catecholamine release, and increases hepatic glucose release.

## Contraindications

Acute aortic dissection; hypersensitivity to diazoxide, thiazides, other sulfonamide derivatives, or their components; treatment of compensatory hypertension, as occurs with aortic coarctation

## Interactions

### DRUGS

*allopurinol, colchicine, probenecid, sulfinpyrazone:* Increased serum uric acid level
*antihypertensives:* Additive hypotensive effects
*beta blockers:* Increased hypotensive effects of diazoxide
*diuretics, especially thiazides:* Potentiated hyperglycemic, hyperuricemic, and antihypertensive effects of diazoxide
*estrogens, NSAIDs, sympathomimetics:* Antagonized hypotensive effects of diazoxide
*insulin, oral antidiabetic drugs:* Possibly decreased effectiveness of these drugs
*oral anticoagulants:* Increased anticoagulant effects
*peripheral vasodilators, ritodrine (I.V.):* Additive, possibly severe, hypotensive effects

## Adverse Reactions

**CNS:** Anxiety, apprehension, cerebral ischemia, dizziness, euphoria, headache, insomnia, light-headedness, malaise, somnolence, weakness
**CV:** Bradycardia, chest pain, hypotension, palpitations, tachycardia, transient hypertension
**EENT:** Blurred vision, dry mouth, increased salivation, taste perversion, tinnitus, transient hearing loss
**ENDO:** Transient hyperglycemia
**GI:** Abdominal pain, anorexia, constipation, diarrhea, ileus, nausea, vomiting
**MS:** Gout
**SKIN:** Diaphoresis, flushing, pruritus, rash, sensation of warmth
**Other:** Extravasation with injection site cellulitis and pain; fluid and sodium retention

## Nursing Considerations

• Use diazoxide cautiously in patients with uncompensated heart failure (because it can cause fluid retention and heart failure) and in patients with impaired cardiac or cerebral circulation in whom abrupt blood pressure reduction, mild tachycardia, and decreased blood perfusion may be harmful.

• Administer I.V. drug undiluted over 10 to 30 seconds. Don't give drug by I.M. or S.C. route.
• Keep patient supine during I.V. injection and for 1 hour afterward.
• Monitor blood pressure throughout treatment to check for hypertension. Before ending surveillance, measure patient's standing blood pressure if she's ambulatory.
• Frequently assess I.V. site for extravasation because the alkaline drug can irritate tissue.
• Expect to adjust dosage as prescribed if patient switches from oral suspension to capsules; suspension produces a higher blood diazoxide level.
• If diabetic patient receives I.V. diazoxide to treat hypertension, monitor for signs and symptoms of hyperglycemia because parenteral form commonly causes transient hyperglycemia.
• Monitor the blood glucose level of all patients who receive oral diazoxide to determine if drug has raised the blood glucose level to normal.

### PATIENT TEACHING

• For patient receiving I.V. diazoxide, explain that she'll be on bed rest until oral therapy starts.
• Advise patient to protect oral suspension from light.
• Instruct patient to take oral drug on a regular schedule and not to skip or double doses.
• Instruct patient to check her blood glucose level regularly if she takes oral diazoxide to treat hypoglycemia.
• Caution patient not to take antidiabetic drugs unless prescribed.
• Advise patient to notify prescriber if she experiences signs of hyperglycemia, such as increased urinary frequency, increased thirst, and fruity breath.

# dichloralphenazone

*(all contain 325 mg of acetaminophen, 100 mg of dichloralphenazone, and 65 mg of isometheptene mucate)*

Amidrine, I.D.A., Iso-Acetozone, Isocom, Midchlor, Midrin, Migquin, Migragap, Migratine, Migrazone, Migrend, Migrex, Mitride

## Class and Category

*Chemical:* Sympathomimetic amine
*Therapeutic:* Analgesic
*Pregnancy category:* Not rated

## Indications and Dosages
➤ *To relieve tension headache*
**CAPSULES**
**Adults.** 1 to 2 caps q 4 hr. *Maximum:* 8 caps/day.
➤ *To relieve migraine headache*
**CAPSULES**
**Adults.** 2 caps followed by 1 cap q hr until relief occurs. *Maximum:* 5 caps/12 hr.

| Route | Onset | Peak | Duration |
|---|---|---|---|
| P.O. | 30 to 60 min | 1 to 3 hr | 3 to 4 hr |

### Mechanism of Action
Acetaminophen raises the pain threshold by acting on the hypothalamus. Dichloralphenazone reduces the patient's emotional reaction to pain through its mild sedative effect. Isometheptene constricts dilated cranial and cerebral arterioles through sympathomimetic action, which reduces stimuli that lead to vascular headaches.

### Contraindications
Heart disease, hepatic disease, hypersensitivity to acetaminophen or isometheptene, MAO inhibitor therapy within 14 days, severe renal disease, uncontrolled glaucoma, uncontrolled hypertension

### Interactions
**DRUGS**
*CNS depressants:* Additive sedative effects
*hepatic enzyme inducers, other hepatotoxic drugs:* Increased risk of hepatotoxicity
*MAO inhibitors:* Increased risk of severe hypertension and hyperpyrexia
**ACTIVITIES**
*alcohol use:* Additive sedative effects, increased risk of hepatotoxicity

### Adverse Reactions
**CNS:** Dizziness, drowsiness
**SKIN:** Rash

### Nursing Considerations
• Because dichloralphenazone has vasoconstrictive and sympathomimetic actions, assess patients with peripheral vascular disease or recent angina pectoris or MI for signs and symptoms indicating aggravation or deterioration of these conditions.
• Institute safety precautions to prevent injury from falls.

**PATIENT TEACHING**
• **WARNING** Caution patient not to take dichloralphenazone if she has taken an MAO inhibitor within the past 14 days; doing so can cause severe hypertension or hyperpyrexia.
• Advise patient to take drug only after a headache or migraine warning sign occurs. Too-frequent use may make drug less effective and may worsen headaches.
• Instruct patient to lie down in a quiet, dark room after taking drug.
• Because of possible dizziness or drowsiness, advise patient to avoid potentially hazardous activities until drug's CNS effects are known.
• Caution patient to avoid alcohol and CNS depressants during therapy because they increase dizziness, drowsiness, and the risk of hepatotoxicity.
• Advise patient to notify prescriber if drug becomes less effective or if headaches occur more frequently.
• Teach patient how to read drug labels, and stress the need to avoid taking too much acetaminophen, which can cause hepatic or renal damage.
• Inform patient that decreasing the dichloralphenazone dose may prevent transient dizziness or rash.
• Instruct patient to store drug away from heat, moisture, and direct light.

# dichlorphenamide
Daranide

### Class and Category
*Chemical:* Sulfonamide derivative
*Therapeutic:* Antiglaucoma drug
*Pregnancy category:* C

### Indications and Dosages
➤ *To manage chronic open-angle glaucoma, secondary glaucoma, and acute angle-closure glaucoma (preoperatively)*
**TABLETS**
**Adults.** *Initial:* 100 to 200 mg followed by 100 mg q 12 hr. *Maintenance:* 25 to 50 mg q.d. to t.i.d.

| Route | Onset | Peak | Duration |
|---|---|---|---|
| P.O. | 30 to 60 min | 2 to 4 hr | 6 to 12 hr |

## Mechanism of Action

Inhibits the enzyme carbonic anhydrase, which normally exists in renal proximal tubule cells, choroid plexes of the brain, and ciliary processes of the eyes. In the eyes, enzyme inhibition decreases aqueous humor secretion, which reduces intraocular pressure.

## Contraindications

Adrenocortical insufficiency, hepatic insufficiency, hyperchloremic acidosis, hypersensitivity to dichlorphenamide or sulfa drugs, hypokalemia, hyponatremia, renal failure, severe obstructive pulmonary disease

## Interactions

### DRUGS

*diflunisal:* Increased adverse effects of dichlorphenamide, significantly decreased intraocular pressure
*salicylates:* Increased risk of dichlorphenamide toxicity, including CNS depression and metabolic acidosis

## Adverse Reactions

**CNS:** Depression, disorientation, dizziness, drowsiness, lassitude, paresthesia
**CV:** Arrhythmias
**EENT:** Metallic taste, pharyngitis
**ENDO:** Hyperglycemia
**GI:** Anorexia, diarrhea, hepatic dysfunction, nausea, vomiting
**GU:** Phosphaturia, renal calculi, renal colic, urinary frequency
**HEME:** Hemolytic anemia, leukopenia, pancytopenia, thrombocytopenia
**SKIN:** Photosensitivity
**Other:** Hyperchloremia, hyperuricemia, weight loss

## Nursing Considerations

• Use dichlorphenamide cautiously in patients who have emphysema, pulmonary obstruction, or severe respiratory acidosis.
• Frequently monitor serum potassium level (especially in elderly patients and those taking digoxin) because diuresis may cause hypokalemia.

### PATIENT TEACHING

• Instruct patient to take dichlorphenamide with food or full glass of water to decrease GI distress.

• Advise patient to avoid potentially hazardous activities until drug's CNS effects are known.
• **WARNING** Urge patient to immediately report signs and symptoms of blood dyscrasias, such as fever, numbness or tingling, rash, sore throat, and unusual bleeding or bruising.
• Advise patient to avoid prolonged exposure to sunlight, to apply sunscreen, and to wear protective clothing outdoors.
• Instruct patient to take a missed dose as soon as she remembers it, unless it's almost time for the next dose.
• Advise patient to store drug at room temperature and to protect it from moisture and heat.

# diclofenac potassium

Cataflam, Voltaren Rapide (CAN)

## diclofenac sodium

Apo-Diclo (CAN), Novo-Difenac (CAN), Nu-Diclo (CAN), Voltaren, Voltaren SR (CAN)

## Class and Category

*Chemical:* Phenylacetic acid derivative
*Therapeutic:* Analgesic, anti-inflammatory
*Pregnancy category:* B

## Indications and Dosages

➤ *To relieve pain and inflammation in rheumatoid arthritis*

### DELAYED-RELEASE TABLETS, TABLETS

**Adults.** *Initial:* 150 to 200 mg/day in divided doses t.i.d. or q.i.d. *Maintenance:* 75 to 100 mg/day, divided, t.i.d. *Maximum:* 225 mg/day.

### E.R. TABLETS

**Adults.** *Initial:* 75 or 100 mg q.d. in the morning or evening, or 75 mg b.i.d. in the morning and evening.

### RECTAL SUPPOSITORIES

**Adults.** 50 or 100 mg as substitute for last P.O. dose of day.

➤ *To relieve pain and inflammation in osteoarthritis*

### DELAYED-RELEASE TABLETS, TABLETS

**Adults.** 100 to 150 mg/day in divided doses b.i.d. or t.i.d. *Maximum:* 150 mg/day.

➤ *To relieve pain in ankylosing spondylitis*

### DELAYED-RELEASE TABLETS, TABLETS

**Adults.** 100 to 125 mg/day in 4 or 5 divided doses.

➤ *To relieve pain and dysmenorrhea*
**TABLETS**
**Adults.** 50 mg t.i.d., p.r.n.; if needed, 100 mg for first dose only.
**DOSAGE ADJUSTMENT** Dosage reduced, if needed, for elderly patients and those with serious renal dysfunction.

| Route | Onset | Peak | Duration |
|-------|-------|------|----------|
| P.O.* | 30 min | Unknown | 8 hr |

### Mechanism of Action
Blocks the activity of cyclooxygenase, the enzyme needed to synthesize prostaglandins, which mediate the inflammatory response and cause local pain, swelling, and vasodilation. By blocking cyclooxygenase and inhibiting prostaglandins, diclofenac reduces inflammatory symptoms. This mechanism also relieves pain because prostaglandins promote pain transmission from the periphery to the spinal cord.

### Contraindications
Active GI bleeding or ulcers; asthma attacks, rhinitis, or urticaria precipitated by aspirin or other NSAIDs; hypersensitivity to diclofenac or NSAIDs; treatment of perioperative pain after coronary artery bypass grafting

### Interactions
**DRUGS**
*acetaminophen:* Increased risk of adverse renal effects with long-term concurrent use
*anticoagulants, thrombolytics:* Prolonged PT, increased risk of bleeding
*antihypertensives:* Decreased antihypertensive effectiveness
*aspirin, other NSAIDs, salicylates:* Increased GI irritability and bleeding, decreased diclofenac effectiveness
*beta blockers*: Impaired antihypertensive effect
*cefamandole, cefoperazone, cefotetan, plicamycin, valproic acid*: Increased risk of hypoprothrombinemia
*cimetidine*: Altered blood diclofenac level
*colchicine, corticotropin (long-term use), glucocorticoids, potassium supplements:* Increased GI irritability and bleeding

---

*For tablets; unknown for delayed-release and E.R. tablets.

*cyclosporine, gold compounds, nephrotoxic drugs:* Increased risk of nephrotoxicity
*digoxin:* Increased blood digoxin level
*insulin, oral antidiabetic drugs:* Decreased effects of these drugs
*lithium:* Increased risk of lithium toxicity
*loop diuretics:* Decreased loop diuretic effectiveness
*methotrexate:* Increased risk of methotrexate toxicity
*phenytoin:* Increased blood phenytoin level
*potassium-sparing diuretics:* Increased risk of hyperkalemia
*probenecid:* Increased diclofenac toxicity
**FOODS**
*food:* Delayed absorption of delayed-release tablets
**ACTIVITIES**
*alcohol use:* Increased risk of GI irritability and bleeding

### Adverse Reactions
**CNS:** Aseptic meningitis, cerebral hemorrhage, dizziness, drowsiness, headache
**CV:** Bradycardia and other arrhythmias, hypotension, vasculitis
**EENT:** Glaucoma, hearing loss, tinnitus
**ENDO:** Hypoglycemia
**GI:** Abdominal pain, constipation, diarrhea, dysphagia, elevated liver function test results, esophageal ulceration, flatulence, GI bleeding or ulceration, hepatic failure, hepatitis, indigestion, jaundice, nausea, perforation of stomach or intestine
**GU:** Acute renal failure, interstitial nephritis
**HEME:** Agranulocytosis, aplastic anemia, eosinophilia, leukocytosis, leukopenia, pancytopenia, porphyria, thrombocytopenia
**SKIN:** Erythema multiforme, exfoliative dermatitis, pruritus, rash, Stevens-Johnson syndrome, toxic epidermal necrolysis
**Other:** Anaphylaxis, angioedema, fluid retention, hyperkalemia, hyperuricemia, hyponatremia, lymphadenopathy

### Nursing Considerations
•Use diclofenac with extreme caution in patients with a history of GI bleeding or ulcer disease because NSAIDs increase the risk of GI bleeding and ulceration. Use diclofenac for shortest possible time in these patients.
•Be aware that serious GI tract ulceration and bleeding, as well as perforation of stomach or intestine, can occur without warning

or symptoms. Elderly patients are at greater risk. Monitor patient for signs of GI irritation and ulceration, especially if patient has a predisposing condition (such as a history of GI bleeding); takes an oral corticosteroid, anticoagulant, or NSAID (long-term); smokes; is an alcoholic; is over age 60; has poor general health; or tests positive for *Helicobacter pylori*. To minimize risk, give diclofenac with food. If patient develops GI distress, withhold diclofenac and notify prescriber immediately.

•Use diclofenac cautiously in patients with hypertension, and monitor blood pressure closely during therapy; drug can cause or worsen hypertension.

•Assess for hypotension. If patient takes a potassium-sparing diuretic, check for elevated serum potassium level.

•WARNING Monitor patient closely for thrombotic events, including MI and CVA, because NSAIDs such as diclofenac increase the risk.

•Report signs of bleeding, such as bleeding gums, bloody or cloudy urine, ecchymoses, melena, and petechiae.

•Monitor BUN and serum creatinine levels in elderly patients, patients taking ACE inhibitors or diuretics, and patients with heart failure or impaired renal or hepatic function. These patients may have an increased risk of renal failure.

•Assess patient's skin routinely for rash or other signs of hypersensitivity reaction; drug may cause serious skin reactions without warning. At first sign of reaction, stop drug and notify prescriber.

•Monitor liver function test results and serum uric acid level. Liver enzyme elevations usually occur within 2 months of starting diclofenac therapy.

•Report weight gain of more than 1 kg (2 lb) in 24 hours because it suggests fluid retention.

**PATIENT TEACHING**

•Advise patient not to chew, crush, or dissolve diclofenac tablet, but to swallow it whole.

•Instruct patient to take drug with food to minimize GI distress.

•To decrease risk of esophageal ulceration, instruct patient not to lie down for 15 to 30 minutes after taking drug.

•Warn patient to avoid potentially hazardous activities until drug's CNS effects are known.

•Instruct patient to notify prescriber if she experiences ringing or buzzing in the ears, impaired hearing, dizziness, or GI distress or bleeding.

•Advise patient to consult prescriber before taking aspirin or other OTC analgesics or drinking alcohol.

•Explain that diclofenac may increase the risk of serious adverse cardiovascular reactions; urge patient to seek immediate medical attention for signs and symptoms such as chest pain, shortness of breath, weakness, and slurred speech.

•Tell patient that diclofenac also may increase the risk of serious adverse GI reactions; stress the need to seek immediate medical attention for signs and symptoms such as epigastric or abdominal pain, indigestion, black or tarry stools, and vomiting blood or material that resembles coffee grounds.

•Alert patient about possibly serious skin reactions and the need to seek immediate medial attention for such as problems as blisters, fever, itching, rash, and other signs of hypersensitivity.

# dicloxacillin sodium

Dycill, Dynapen, Pathocil

## Class and Category

*Chemical:* Isoxazolyl penicillin derivative
*Therapeutic:* Antibiotic
*Pregnancy category:* B

## Indications and Dosages

➤ *To treat mild to moderate upper respiratory tract and localized skin and soft-tissue infections caused by penicillinase-producing staphylococci*

**CAPSULES, ORAL SOLUTION**

**Adults and children who weigh 40 kg (88 lb) or more.** 125 mg q 6 hr.

**Children who weigh less than 40 kg.** 12.5 mg/kg/day divided into four equal doses and given q 6 hr.

➤ *To treat severe infections, such as lower respiratory tract or disseminated infections, caused by penicillinase-producing staphylococci*

**CAPSULES, ORAL SOLUTION**

**Adults and children who weigh 40 kg or more.** 250 mg q 6 hr, or higher doses, if needed. *Maximum:* 6 g/day.

**Children over age 1 month who weigh less than 40 kg.** 25 mg/kg/day divided into four equal doses and given q 6 hr, or higher doses if needed.

---

### Mechanism of Action
Inhibits cell wall synthesis in susceptible bacteria. These bacteria assemble rigid, cross-linked cell walls in several steps. Dicloxacillin affects the final stage of cross-linking by binding with and inactivating penicillin-binding protein (the enzyme responsible for linking cell wall strands). This action inhibits cell wall synthesis and causes cell lysis and death.

---

### Contraindications
Hypersensitivity to dicloxacillin, other penicillins, beta-lactamase inhibitors (such as piperacillin/tazobactam), cephalosporins, imipenem, or their components

### Interactions
**DRUGS**
*hepatotoxic drugs:* Increased risk of hepatotoxicity
*methotrexate:* Decreased methotrexate clearance and increased risk of methotrexate toxicity
*oral contraceptives:* Decreased contraceptive action
*probenecid:* Increased and prolonged blood dicloxacillin level
*tetracyclines:* Decreased dicloxacillin effectiveness
**FOODS**
*All foods:* Possibly delayed absorption

### Adverse Reactions
**CNS:** Dizziness, fatigue, fever, insomnia
**EENT:** Black "hairy" tongue, dry mouth, glossitis, laryngeal edema, laryngospasm, stomatitis, taste perversion
**GI:** Abdominal pain, anorexia, diarrhea, flatulence, nausea, pseudomembranous colitis, transient hepatitis, vomiting
**GU:** Nephropathy, vaginitis
**MS:** Prolonged muscle relaxation
**SKIN:** Dermatitis, erythema multiforme, pruritus, rash, urticaria, vesicular eruptions
**Other:** Anaphylaxis, serum sickness–like reaction, superinfection

### Nursing Considerations
•Before dicloxacillin therapy begins, expect to obtain body fluid and tissue samples for culture and sensitivity tests, as ordered, and review the results, if possible. Also check for history of sensitivity to cephalosporins, penicillins, and other substances.
•If diarrhea develops, notify prescriber because of possibility of pseudomembranous colitis.
**PATIENT TEACHING**
•Instruct patient to take dicloxacillin 1 hour before or 2 hours after meals.
•Instruct patient to take drug around the clock, not to miss a dose, and to complete the entire prescription unless directed otherwise by prescriber.
•Advise patient to take oral solution with a cold beverage but not acidic juice, such as orange juice. Explain that solution is effective for 7 days at room temperature and for 14 days if refrigerated.
•Caution patient not to open capsules and mix contents with food or liquids because an unpleasant taste and decreased drug absorption will result.
•Instruct parent to shake oral solution thoroughly and measure doses with a calibrated device for accuracy.
•Advise patient to notify prescriber if she experiences adverse GI reactions or signs of hypersensitivity or superinfection.
•If patient takes an oral contraceptive, advise her to use an additional form of contraception during therapy.
•Instruct patient to store drug away from heat, moisture, and direct light and to refrigerate—but not freeze—oral solution.

# dicumarol

### Class and Category
*Chemical:* Coumarin derivative
*Therapeutic:* Anticoagulant
*Pregnancy category:* X

### Indications and Dosages
➤ *To prevent and treat pulmonary embolus, thromboembolus, and venous thrombus; to prevent thromboembolism related to atrial fibrillation and mechanical heart valves*

**Adults.** *Initial:* 200 to 300 mg on the first day. *Maintenance:* 25 to 200 mg q.d.
DOSAGE ADJUSTMENT Dosage reduced for elderly patients and those with hepatic or renal impairment.

| Route | Onset | Peak | Duration |
|-------|-------|------|----------|
| P.O. | 1 to 5 days | Unknown | 5 to 6 days |

### Mechanism of Action
Prevents coagulation by interfering with the liver's ability to synthesize vitamin K–dependent clotting factors. This in turn depletes clotting factors II (prothrombin), VII, IX, and X. Normally, clots result from a cascade of proteolytic reactions that involve several clotting factors, including vitamin K–dependent factors. These clotting factors must be converted to an activated form before the clotting cascade can continue. By depleting vitamin K–dependent clotting factors, dicumarol interferes with the clotting cascade and prevents coagulation.

### Contraindications
Active bleeding; aneurysm; ascorbic acid deficiency; bacterial endocarditis; blood dyscrasia; continuous tube drainage of small intestine; CVA; diverticulitis; eclampsia or preclampsia; emaciation; hemophilia; hemorrhagic tendency; history of bleeding diathesis or warfarin-induced necrosis; leukemia; major regional lumbar block anesthesia; malnutrition; pericardial effusion; pericarditis; polyarthritis; pregnancy; prostatectomy; recent surgery on brain, eye, GI tract, or prostate; recovery from spinal puncture; severe hepatic or renal impairment; surgery resulting in large, open surfaces; threatened abortion; thrombocytopenic purpura; uncontrolled or malignant hypertension; visceral cancer; vitamin K deficiency

### Interactions
DRUGS
*acetaminophen, androgens, beta blockers, chlorpropamide, clofibrate, corticosteroids, cyclophosphamide, dextrothyroxine, disulfiram, erythromycin, fluconazole, gemfibrozil, glucagon, hydantoins, influenza virus vaccine, isoniazid, ketoconazole, miconazole, moricizine, propoxyphene, quinolones, streptokinase, sulfonamides, tamoxifen, thio-*

*amines, thyroid drugs, urokinase:* Increased effects of dicumarol and risk of bleeding

### Adverse Reactions
**CNS:** Fever, malaise
**ENDO:** Adrenal hemorrhage
**GI:** Abdominal cramps and distention, anorexia, diarrhea, flatulence, nausea, vomiting
**GU:** Menorrhagia, priapism
**HEME:** Hemorrhage, leukopenia
**SKIN:** Alopecia, pruritus, rash, urticaria
**Other:** Allergic reaction, purple toes syndrome

### Nursing Considerations
• Use dicumarol cautiously in elderly patients and in those with hepatic or renal impairment.
• Monitor results of serial tests for PT and INR and expect to adjust dosage accordingly.
• If patient also receives heparin, expect heparin therapy to continue until INR reaches desired level: 2 to 3 times the control value for pulmonary embolus, thromboembolus, or venous thrombus; or 3 to 4.5 times the control value for thromboembolism related to atrial fibrillation or mechanical valves.
• If PT or INR are prolonged, withhold one dose of dicumarol, as prescribed. To reverse anticoagulation immediately, administer vitamin K, as prescribed. If patient has severe bleeding, expect to administer blood to offset vitamin K's delayed onset.
• Assess for signs of hemorrhage, such as ecchymosis, epistaxis, gingival bleeding, hematuria, and melena.
• To avoid excessive bleeding, apply pressure to I.M. or venipuncture sites for up to 5 minutes.

PATIENT TEACHING
• Instruct patient to take dicumarol at the same time every day.
• Inform patient that drug's full effects may not occur for 2 to 7 days.
• Instruct patient to have frequent coagulation tests, as prescribed.
• Advise patient to stabilize her intake of foods high in vitamin K. Urge her to consult prescriber before starting a weight-loss diet, altering eating habits, or taking new vitamins or other nutritional supplements; these activities may alter her vitamin K intake.
• Caution patient to avoid activities that may cause bleeding. Advise the use of a soft toothbrush and an electric razor.

•Encourage patient to consult prescriber before taking OTC drugs, including herbs, which may affect dicumarol's anticoagulant effect.

•Instruct patient to take a missed dose as soon as she remembers unless it's nearly time for the next dose. Urge her to report missed doses to prescriber.

•Caution patient to immediately notify prescriber if signs of bleeding occur, such as abdominal pain or swelling; back pain; bloody or black stools; bloody urine; coughing up blood; joint pain, swelling, or stiffness; severe or continuing headache; and vomiting blood or material that looks like coffee grounds.

•Urge patient to carry medical identification and tell all health care providers that she takes dicumarol.

•Explain that coagulation will gradually return to normal after therapy stops. Remind her to continue watching for signs of bleeding.

# dicyclomine hydrochloride

Bentyl, Bentylol (CAN), Formulex (CAN), Spasmoban (CAN)

## Class and Category

*Chemical:* Tertiary amine
*Therapeutic:* Anticholinergic, antispasmodic
*Pregnancy category:* Not rated

## Indications and Dosages

➤ *To control diarrhea and GI tract spasms*
**CAPSULES, TABLETS**
**Adults and adolescents.** 10 to 20 mg t.i.d. or q.i.d., increased as needed and tolerated. *Maximum:* 160 mg/day.
**Children ages 6 to 12.** 10 mg t.i.d. or q.i.d.
**E.R. TABLETS**
**Adults and adolescents.** 30 mg b.i.d.
**SYRUP**
**Adults and adolescents.** 10 to 20 mg t.i.d. or q.i.d., increased as needed and tolerated. *Maximum:* 60 mg/day.
**Children ages 2 to 13.** 10 mg t.i.d. or q.i.d.
**Children ages 6 months to 2 years.** 5 to 10 mg t.i.d. or q.i.d.
**I.M. INJECTION**
**Adults.** 20 mg q 4 to 6 hr. Dosage adjusted as needed and tolerated.

## Mechanism of Action

Inhibits acetylcholine's muscarinic actions at postganglionic parasympathetic receptors in smooth muscles, secretory glands, and the CNS. These actions relax smooth muscles and diminish GI, GU, and biliary tract secretions.

## Contraindications

Adhesions between iris and lens, angle-closure glaucoma, GI obstruction, hemorrhagic shock, hepatic disease, hiatal hernia, hypersensitivity to any anticholinergic, ileus, intestinal atony in elderly or debilitated patients, myasthenia gravis, myocardial ischemia, obstructive uropathy, renal disease, severe ulcerative colitis, tachycardia, toxic megacolon

## Interactions

**DRUGS**
*adsorbent antidiarrheals, antacids:* Decreased dicyclomine absorption
*amantadine, anticholinergics, phenothiazines, tricyclic antidepressants:* Increased dicyclomine effects
*antimyasthenics:* Reduced intestinal motil-ity
*atenolol:* Increased atenolol effects
*cyclopropane:* Risk of ventricular arrhythmias
*haloperidol:* Decreased antipsychotic effect of haloperidol
*ketoconazole:* Decreased ketoconazole absorption
*metoclopramide:* Decreased effect of metoclopramide on GI motility
*opioid analgesics:* Increased risk of ileus, severe constipation, and urine retention
*potassium chloride, especially wax-matrix preparations:* Possibly GI ulceration
*urinary alkalinizers (antacids that contain calcium or magnesium, carbonic anhydrase inhibitors, citrates, sodium bicarbonate):* Delayed excretion and increased risk of adverse effects of dicyclomine

## Adverse Reactions

**CNS:** Agitation, dizziness, drowsiness, dyskinesia, excitement, fever, insomnia, lethargy, light-headedness (with I.M. use), nervousness, paresthesia, syncope
**CV:** Palpitations, tachycardia

**EENT:** Blurred vision, cycloplegia, dry mouth, loss of taste, mydriasis, nasal congestion, photophobia
**GI:** Constipation, dysphagia, heartburn, ileus, vomiting
**GU:** Impotence, urine retention
**SKIN:** Decreased sweating, flushing, pruritus
**Other:** Heatstroke; injection site pain, redness, and swelling

## Nursing Considerations
• Assess for tachycardia before giving dicyclomine because drug may increase heart rate.
• Don't give drug by I.V. route.
• Monitor for symptoms of hypersensitivity, such as agitation and pruritus. They usually resolve within 48 hours after stopping drug.
• During long-term use, assess patient for chronic constipation and fecal impaction, and take apropriate corrective measures, as prescribed.

### PATIENT TEACHING
• Instruct patient to store dicyclomine in a tightly sealed container at room temperature, protected from moisture and direct light. Advise her not to refrigerate syrup.
• Inform patient that dicyclomine relieves symptoms but doesn't cure the underlying disorder.
• For best results, instruct patient to take drug 30 to 60 minutes before eating.
• Advise patient not to take an antacid or antidiarrheal within 2 hours of taking dicyclomine.
• Inform patient that blurred vision, dizziness, or drowsiness may occur.
• To prevent constipation, advise patient to eat high-fiber foods and drink at least 8 glasses of water daily.
• WARNING Urge patient to avoid getting overheated during exercise or in hot weather because heatstroke may result. Inform patient that hot baths or saunas may cause dizziness or fainting.
• Instruct patient to change position slowly to avoid light-headedness.
• Inform patient that stopping drug abruptly may cause dizziness and vomiting.
• Advise patient to take a missed dose as soon as she remembers unless it's nearly time for the next dose. Caution her not to double-dose.

# difenoxin hydrochloride and atropine sulfate
Motofen

## Class, Category, and Schedule
*Chemical:* Meperidine analogue (difenoxin), tertiary amine belladonna alkaloid (atropine)
*Therapeutic:* Antidiarrheal
*Pregnancy category:* C
*Controlled substance:* Schedule IV

## Indications and Dosages
➤ *To treat acute and chronic diarrhea*
TABLETS
**Adults and adolescents.** 2 mg (difenoxin) immediately and then 1 mg (difenoxin) after each loose stool or q 3 to 4 hr, p.r.n. *Maximum:* 8 mg (difenoxin)/day.
DOSAGE ADJUSTMENT Dosage reduced for patients with hepatic or renal dysfunction.

> ### Mechanism of Action
> Directly affects circular smooth muscles of the GI tract, reducing intestinal motility. Subtherapeutic doses of atropine help prevent drug abuse.

## Contraindications
Diarrhea caused by pseudomembranous enterocolitis or enterotoxin-producing bacteria, such as *Escherichia coli, Salmonella* sp., or *Shigella* sp.; hypersensitivity to atropine, difenoxin, diphenoxylate, or their components; angle-closure glaucoma; obstructive jaundice

## Interactions
DRUGS
*barbiturates, narcotics, tranquilizers:* Possibly potentiated effects of these drugs
*MAO inhibitors:* Possibly hypertensive crisis
*naltrexone:* Possibly precipitated withdrawal symptoms (in patient physically dependent on difenoxin) and interference with difenoxin's therapeutic effects
ACTIVITIES
*alcohol use:* Possibly potentiated effects of difenoxin

## Adverse Reactions
**CNS:** Confusion, dizziness, drowsiness, euphoria, fatigue, headache, insomnia, lethargy, light-headedness, nervousness, sedation

**EENT:** Dry mouth
**GI:** Abdominal distention and pain, anorexia, constipation, nausea, pancreatitis, vomiting
**SKIN:** Pruritus, urticaria
**Other:** Physical and psychological dependence

## Nursing Considerations
• Closely monitor patients who are elderly or very ill or who have respiratory problems; they're more sensitive to drug's effects and may require a lower dosage.

**PATIENT TEACHING**
• Inform patient that diarrhea may not be controlled for 12 to 24 hours but that abdominal cramps usually subside in 30 to 90 minutes. Advise patient to consult prescriber if diarrhea doesn't improve within 2 days.
• Instruct patient to continue taking drug until diarrhea has stopped for 24 to 36 hours.
• Urge patient to consult prescriber before consuming alcohol or CNS depressants.
• Advise patient to avoid potentially hazardous activities until drug's CNS effects are known.
• Instruct patient to protect drug from heat, moisture, and direct light.

# diflunisal

Apo-Diflunisal (CAN), Dolobid, Novo-Diflunisal (CAN)

## Class and Category
*Chemical:* Difluorophenyl, salicylic acid derivative
*Therapeutic:* Analgesic, anti-inflammatory
*Pregnancy category:* C (first trimester), Not rated (later trimesters)

## Indications and Dosages
➤ *To relieve mild to moderate pain*
**TABLETS**
**Adults.** 1 g followed by 0.5 g q 8 to 12 hr. *Maximum:* 1.5 g/day.
➤ *To reduce inflammation in osteoarthritis or rheumatoid arthritis*
**TABLETS**
**Adults.** 0.5 to 1 g/day in divided doses b.i.d. *Maximum:* 1.5 g/day.
**DOSAGE ADJUSTMENT** Dosage reduced for elderly patients and those who use diuretics; who could be harmed by prolonged bleeding time; or who have compromised cardiac function, conditions that cause fluid retention, hepatic or renal impairment, hypertension, or upper GI disease.

| Route | Onset | Peak | Duration |
|-------|-------|------|----------|
| P.O.* | 1 hr | 2 to 3 hr | 8 to 12 hr |

## Mechanism of Action
Blocks the activity of cyclooxygenase, the enzyme needed to synthesize prostaglandins, which mediate the inflammatory response and cause local vasodilation, swelling, and pain. By blocking cyclooxygenase and inhibiting prostaglandins, this NSAID reduces inflammatory symptoms. This mechanism also relieves pain because prostaglandins promote pain transmission from the periphery to the spinal cord.

## Contraindications
Asthma attacks, rhinitis, or urticaria precipitated by aspirin or other NSAIDs; hypersensitivity to diflunisal; treatment of perioperative pain after coronary artery bypass graft surgery

## Interactions
**DRUGS**
*acetaminophen:* Increased risk of adverse renal effects with long-term use of both drugs
*antacids:* Decreased blood diflunisal level
*antihypertensives:* Decreased antihypertensive effects
*aspirin, other NSAIDs, salicylates:* Increased GI irritability and bleeding, decreased diflunisal effectiveness
*beta blockers:* Impaired antihypertensive effects of beta blocker
*cefamandole, cefoperazone, cefotetan, plicamycin, valproic acid:* Increased risk of hypoprothrombinemia
*colchicine, corticotropin (long-term use), glucocorticoids, potassium supplements:* Increased GI irritability and bleeding
*cyclosporine, gold compounds, nephrotoxic drugs:* Increased risk of nephrotoxicity
*digoxin:* Increased blood digoxin level
*heparin, oral anticoagulants, thrombolytics:* Prolonged PT, increased risk of bleeding
*hydrochlorothiazide:* Increased blood hydrochlorothiazide level
*insulin, oral antidiabetic drugs:* Increased hypoglycemic effects

* For analgesia; unknown for anti-inflammatory effects.

*loop diuretics:* Decreased loop diuretic effectiveness
*methotrexate:* Increased risk of methotrexate toxicity
*phenytoin:* Increased blood phenytoin level
*probenecid:* Increased diflunisal toxicity
**ACTIVITIES**
*alcohol use:* Increased GI irritability and bleeding

## Adverse Reactions

**CNS:** Aseptic meningitis, cerebral hemorrhage, dizziness, drowsiness, headache, insomnia
**CV:** Vasculitis
**EENT:** Tinnitus
**ENDO:** Hypoglycemia
**GI:** Abdominal pain, constipation, diarrhea, esophageal irritation, GI bleeding or ulceration, hepatic failure, hepatitis, indigestion, jaundice, nausea, perforation of stomach or intestine, vomiting
**GU:** Acute renal failure, interstitial nephritis
**HEME:** Agranulocytosis, aplastic anemia, leukopenia, pancytopenia, thrombocytopenia
**SKIN:** Erythema multiforme, exfoliative dermatitis, rash, Stevens-Johnson syndrome, toxic epidermal necrolysis
**Other:** Anaphylaxis, angioedema, hyponatremia

## Nursing Considerations

•Use diflunisal with extreme caution in patients with a history of GI bleeding or ulcer disease because NSAIDs such as diflunisal increase the risk. Use drug for the shortest time possible in these patients.
•Be aware that serious GI tract ulceration and bleeding, as well as perforation of stomach or intestine, can occur without warning or symptoms. Elderly patients are at greater risk. To minimize risk, give diflunisal with food. If patient develops GI distress, withhold diflunisal and notify prescriber immediately.
•Use diflunisal cautiously in patients with hypertension, and monitor blood pressure closely during therapy; drug can cause or worsen hypertension.
•Use diflunisal cautiously in elderly patients, those with renal dysfunction, and those who should avoid a prolonged bleeding time.
•**WARNING** Monitor patient closely for thrombotic events, including CVA and MI, because NSAIDs such as diflunisal increase the risk of these events.

•Monitor BUN and serum creatinine levels in elderly patients, patients taking ACE inhibitors or diuretics, and patients with heart falure or impaired hepatic or renal function. These patients may have an increased risk of renal failure.
•Assess patient's skin routinely for rash or other signs of hypersensitivity reaction; drug may cause serious skin reactions without warning. At first sign of reaction, stop drug and notify prescriber.
•Assess type, location, and intensity of pain before and 1 to 2 hours after giving drug.
•Assess patient carefully because long-term or high-dose therapy may mask fever.

**PATIENT TEACHING**
•Teach patient not to crush or chew diflunisal tablets.
•Instruct patient to take tablet with a full glass of water and not to lie down for 30 minutes afterward to avoid esophageal irritation.
•Inform patient that drug will start working in about 1 week but that full effects may not occur for several weeks.
•Explain that diflunisal may increase the risk of serious adverse cardiovascular reactions; urge patient to seek immediate medical attention for such signs and symptoms as chest pain, shortness of breath, slurred speech, and weakness.
•Tell patient that diflunisal also may increase the risk of serious adverse GI reactions; stress the need to seek immediate medical attention for signs and symptoms such as abdominal or epigastric pain, black or tarry stools, indigestion, and vomiting blood or material that resembles coffee grounds.
•Alert patient about possibly serious skin reactions and the need to seek immediate medial attention for such as problems as blisters, fever, itching, rash, and other signs of hypersensitivity.
•Caution patient to avoid acetaminophen, alcohol, aspirin, and other salicylates during diflunisal therapy, unless directed otherwise by prescriber.
•Advise patient to avoid potentially hazardous activities until drug's CNS effects are known.
•Advise patient to tell health care providers about diflunisal therapy before surgery, including dental surgery. Therapy should stop for 1 week before procedure.

# digoxin

Lanoxicaps, Lanoxin, Lanoxin Elixir Pediatric, Lanoxin Injection, Lanoxin Injection Pediatric, Novo-Digoxin (CAN)

## Class and Category

*Chemical:* Digitalis glycoside
*Therapeutic:* Antiarrhythmic, cardiotonic
*Pregnancy category:* C

## Indications and Dosages

➤ *To treat heart failure, atrial flutter, atrial fibrillation, and paroxysmal atrial tachycardia with rapid digitalization*

CAPSULES, I.V. INJECTION

**Adults.** *Loading:* 10 to 15 mcg/kg in 3 divided doses q 6 to 8 hr, with first dose equal to 50% of total dose. *Maintenance:* 125 to 350 mcg/day q.d. or b.i.d.
**Children over age 10.** *Loading:* 8 to 12 mcg/kg in 3 or more divided doses, with first dose equal to 50% of total dose. Subsequent doses given q 6 to 8 hr. *Maintenance:* 2 to 3 mcg/kg/day q.d.
**Children ages 6 to 10.** *Loading:* 15 to 30 mcg/kg in 3 or more divided doses, with first dose equal to 50% of total dose. Subsequent doses given q 6 to 8 hr. *Maintenance:* 4 to 8 mcg/kg/day in 2 divided doses.
**Children ages 2 to 5.** *Loading:* 25 to 35 mcg/kg in 3 or more divided doses, with first dose equal to 50% of total dose. Subsequent doses given q 6 to 8 hr. *Maintenance:* 6 to 9 mcg/kg/day in 2 divided doses.
**Infants ages 1 to 24 months.** *Loading:* 30 to 50 mcg/kg in 3 or more divided doses, with first dose equal to 50% of total dose. Subsequent doses given q 6 to 8 hr. *Maintenance:* 7.5 to 12 mcg/kg/day in 2 divided doses.
**Full-term neonates.** *Loading:* 20 to 30 mcg/kg in 3 or more divided doses, with first dose equal to 50% of total dose. Subsequent doses given q 6 to 8 hr. *Maintenance:* 5 to 8 mcg/kg/day in 2 divided doses.
**Premature neonates.** *Loading:* 15 to 25 mcg/kg in 3 or more divided doses, with first dose equal to 50% of total dose. Subsequent doses given q 6 to 8 hr. *Maintenance:* 4 to 6 mcg/kg/day in 2 divided doses.

ELIXIR, TABLETS

**Adults.** *Loading:* 10 to 15 mcg/kg total dose given in 3 divided doses q 6 to 8 hr, with first dose equal to 50% of total dose. *Maintenance:* 125 to 500 mcg/day.

**Children over age 10.** *Loading:* 10 to 15 mcg/kg total dose given in 3 divided doses q 6 to 8 hr, with first dose equal to 50% of total dose. *Maintenance:* 2.5 to 5 mcg/kg/day.
**Children ages 5 to 10.** *Loading:* 20 to 35 mcg/kg in 3 divided doses q 6 to 8 hr. *Maintenance:* 5 to 10 mcg/kg/day in 2 divided doses.
**Children ages 2 to 5.** *Loading:* 30 to 40 mcg/kg in 3 divided doses q 6 to 8 hr. *Maintenance:* 7.5 to 10 mcg/kg/day in 2 divided doses.
**Infants ages 1 to 24 months.** *Loading:* 35 to 60 mcg/kg in 3 divided doses q 6 to 8 hr. *Maintenance:* 10 to 15 mcg/kg/day in 2 divided doses.
**Full-term neonates.** *Loading:* 25 to 35 mcg/kg in 3 divided doses q 6 to 8 hr. *Maintenance:* 6 to 10 mcg/kg/day in 2 divided doses.
**Premature neonates.** *Loading:* 20 to 30 mcg/kg in 3 divided doses q 6 to 8 hr. *Maintenance:* 5 to 7.5 mcg/kg/day in 2 divided doses.

DOSAGE ADJUSTMENT Dosage carefully adjusted for patients who are elderly or debilitated or have implanted pacemakers because toxicity may develop at doses tolerated by most patients.

| Route | Onset | Peak | Duration |
|-------|-------|------|----------|
| P.O. | 30 to 120 min | 6 to 8 hr | 3 to 4 days |
| I.V. | 5 to 30 min | 1 to 5 hr | 3 to 4 days |

## Mechanism of Action

Increases the force and velocity of myocardial contraction, resulting in positive inotropic effects. Digoxin produces antiarrhythmic effects by decreasing the conduction rate and increasing the effective refractory period of the AV node.

## Contraindications

Hypersensitive carotid sinus syndrome, hypersensitivity to digoxin, presence or history of digitalis toxicity or idiosyncratic reaction to digoxin, ventricular fibrillation, ventricular tachycardia unless heart failure occurs unrelated to digoxin therapy

## Interactions

DRUGS

*adsorbent antidiarrheals, such as kaolin and pectin; bulk laxatives; cholestyramine; colestipol; oral neomycin; sulfasalazine:* Inhibited digoxin absorption

*amiodarone, propafenone:* Elevated blood digoxin level, possibly to toxic level
*antacids:* Inhibited digoxin absorption
*antiarrhythmics, pancuronium, parenteral calcium salts, rauwolfia alkaloids, sympathomimetics:* Possibly increased risk of arrhythmias
*diltiazem, verapamil:* Increased blood digoxin level, possibly excessive bradycardia
*edrophonium:* Excessive slowing of heart rate
*erythromycin, neomycin, tetracycline:* Possibly increased blood digoxin level
*hypokalemia-causing drugs, potassium-wasting diuretics:* Increased risk of digitalis toxicity from hypokalemia
*indomethacin:* Decreased renal clearance and increased blood level of digoxin
*magnesium sulfate (parenteral):* Possibly cardiac conduction changes and heart block
*quinidine, quinine:* Increased blood digoxin level
*spironolactone:* Increased half-life and risk of adverse effects of digoxin
*succinylcholine:* Increased risk of digoxin-induced arrhythmias
*sucralfate:* Decreased digoxin absorption
**Foods**
*high-fiber food:* Inhibited digoxin absorption

## Adverse Reactions

**CNS:** Confusion, depression, drowsiness, extreme weakness, headache, syncope
**CV:** Arrhythmias, heart block
**EENT:** Blurred vision, colored halos around objects
**GI:** Abdominal discomfort or pain, anorexia, diarrhea, nausea, vomiting
**Other:** Electrolyte imbalances

## Nursing Considerations

•Administer parenteral digoxin undiluted, or dilute with a fourfold or greater volume of sterile water for injection, NS, or D₅W for I.V. administration. Once diluted, administer immediately. Discard if solution is markedly discolored or contains precipitate.
•Before giving each dose, take patient's apical pulse and notify prescriber if pulse is below 60 beats/minute (or other specified level).
•Monitor closely for signs of digitalis toxicity: altered mental status, arrhythmias, heart block, nausea, vision disturbances, and vomiting. If they appear, notify prescriber,

check serum digoxin level as ordered, and expect to withhold drug until level is known. Monitor ECG tracing continuously.
•If patient has acute or unstable chronic atrial fibrillation, assess for drug effectiveness. Ventricular rate may not normalize even when serum drug level falls within therapeutic range; raising the dosage probably won't produce a therapeutic effect and may lead to toxicity.
•Frequently obtain ECG tracings as ordered in elderly patients because of their smaller body mass and reduced renal clearance. Elderly patients, especially those with coronary insufficiency, are more susceptible to arrhythmias—particularly ventricular fibrillation—if digitalis toxicity occurs.
•Monitor serum potassium level regularly because hypokalemia predisposes to digitalis toxicity and serious arrhythmias. Also monitor potassium level frequently when giving potassium salts because hyperkalemia in patients receiving digoxin can be fatal.

**PATIENT TEACHING**
•Stress the importance of taking digoxin exactly as prescribed. Warn patient about possible toxicity from taking too much and decreased effectiveness from taking too little.
•Instruct patient to take drug at the same time each day to help increase compliance.
•Teach patient how to take her pulse, and instruct her to do so before each dose. Urge her to notify prescriber if pulse falls below 60 beats/minute or suddenly increases.
•Inform patient that small, white 0.25-mg tablets can easily be confused with other drugs. Caution against carrying drug in anything other than original labeled container.
•Emphasize the need to use the special dropper supplied with elixir to ensure accurate dose measurement.
•Instruct patient to take a missed dose as soon as she remembers if within 12 hours of scheduled dose. If not, urge her to notify prescriber immediately.
•Urge patient to notify prescriber if she experiences adverse reactions, such as GI distress or pulse changes.
•Instruct patient to carry medical identification that indicates her need for digoxin.
•Advise patient to consult prescriber before using other drugs, including OTC preparations.

# digoxin immune Fab (ovine)

Digibind

## Class and Category

*Chemical:* Digoxin-specific antigen-binding fragments
*Therapeutic:* Digitalis glycoside antidote
*Pregnancy category:* C

## Indications and Dosages

➤ *To treat acute toxicity from a known amount of digoxin elixir or tablets*

**I.V. INJECTION**

**Adults and children.** Individualized dosage based on amount ingested. Dose (mg) = dose ingested (mg) multiplied by 0.8 and then divided by 0.5, multiplied by 38, and rounded up to next whole vial.

➤ *To treat acute toxicity from a known amount of digoxin capsules, digitoxin tablets, or I.V. injection of digoxin or digitoxin*

**I.V. INJECTION**

**Adults and children.** Individualized dosage based on amount ingested. Dose (mg) = dose ingested (mg) divided by 0.5, then multiplied by 38 and rounded up to next whole vial.

➤ *To treat acute toxicity from an unknown amount of digoxin or digitoxin during long-term therapy*

**I.V. INJECTION**

**Adults and children.** Individualized dosage for digoxin toxicity: dose (mg) = serum digoxin level (ng/ml) multiplied by body weight (kg), then divided by 100, and then multiplied by 38. Individualized dosage for digitoxin toxicity: dose (mg) = serum digitoxin level (ng/ml) multiplied by body weight (kg) and then divided by 1,000, multiplied by 38, and rounded up to next whole vial.

**DOSAGE ADJUSTMENT** Higher dose delivered, as prescribed, if the dose based on ingested amount differs substantially from the dose based on serum digoxin or digitoxin level. Dose repeated after several hours, if needed.

| Route | Onset | Peak | Duration |
|-------|-------|------|----------|
| I.V. | 15 to 30 min | Unknown | 8 to 12 hr |

## Mechanism of Action

Binds with digoxin or digitoxin molecules. The resulting complex is excreted through the kidneys. As the free serum digoxin level declines, tissue-bound digoxin enters the serum and also is bound and excreted.

## Contraindications

Hypersensitivity to digoxin immune Fab

## Adverse Reactions

**CV:** Increased ventricular rate (in atrial fibrillation), worsening of heart failure or low cardiac output
**Other:** Allergic reaction (difficulty breathing, urticaria), febrile reaction, hypokalemia

## Nursing Considerations

• Expect each 38-mg vial of purified digoxin immune Fab to bind about 0.5 mg of digoxin or digitoxin.

• Reconstitute for I.V. use by dissolving 38 mg in 4 ml of sterile water for injection to yield 9.5 mg/ml. Mix gently. Further dilute with NS to a convenient volume for I.V. infusion. For very small doses, reconstituted 38-mg vial may be diluted with 34 ml of NS to yield 1 mg/ml.

• **WARNING** Before administering digoxin immune Fab to high-risk patient, test for allergic reaction as prescribed by diluting 0.1 ml of reconstituted drug in 9.9 ml of sodium chloride for injection and then injecting 0.1 ml (9.5 mcg/0.1 ml) intradermally. After 20 minutes, observe for an urticarial wheal surrounded by erythema. Alternatively, perform a scratch test by placing one drop of 9.5 mcg/0.1 ml dilution on patient's skin and making a ¼″ scratch through the drop with a sterile needle. Inspect site in 20 minutes. Test is considered positive if it produces a wheal surrounded by erythema. If test causes a systemic reaction, apply tourniquet above test site, notify prescriber, and prepare to respond to anaphylaxis. Be aware that if a skin or systemic reaction occurs, additional drug shouldn't be given unless essential; if more of the drug must be given, expect prescriber to pretreat patient with corticosteroids and diphenhydramine. Prescriber should be on standby to treat anaphylaxis.

D

•For an infant, reconstitute digoxin immune Fab as ordered and administer with a tuberculin syringe.
•When administering to a child, monitor for fluid volume overload.
•When giving a large dose, expect a faster onset but watch closely for febrile reaction.
•Administer I.V. infusion through a 0.22-micron membrane filter over 30 minutes. Keep in mind that drug may be given by rapid I.V. injection if cardiac arrest is imminent.
•Monitor serum potassium level frequently, especially during first few hours of therapy. The potassium level may drop rapidly.

**PATIENT TEACHING**
•Inform patient of the purpose of digoxin immune Fab and how it will be administered.
•Advise patient to notify you immediately if she experiences adverse reactions, especially difficulty breathing and urticaria.

# dihydroergotamine mesylate

D.H.E. 45, Dihydroergotamine-Sandoz (CAN), Migranal

## Class and Category
*Chemical:* Semisynthetic ergot alkaloid
*Therapeutic:* Antimigraine
*Pregnancy category:* X

## Indications and Dosages
➤ *To treat acute migraine with or without aura*
**I.V. INJECTION**
**Adults.** 1 mg, repeated in 1 hr, if needed. *Maximum:* 6 mg/wk.
**I.M. INJECTION**
**Adults.** 1 mg at first sign of headache, repeated q hr up to 3 mg, if needed. *Maximum:* 3 mg/24 hr, 6 mg/wk.
**NASAL SPRAY**
**Adults.** 1 spray (0.5 mg) in each nostril, repeated in 15 min for a total dose of 2 sprays in each nostril or 2 mg. *Maximum:* 3 mg/ 24 hr, 4 mg/wk.

| Route | Onset | Peak | Duration |
|-------|-------|------|----------|
| I.V. | In 5 min | 15 min to 2 hr | About 8 hr |
| I.M. | 15 to 30 min | 15 min to 2 hr | 3 to 4 hr |
| Nasal | In 30 min | 30 to 60 min | Unknown |

## Mechanism of Action
Produces intracranial and peripheral vasoconstriction by binding to all known 5-hydroxytryptamine$_1$ (5-HT$_1$) receptors, alpha$_1$- and alpha$_2$-adrenergic receptors, and dopaminergic receptors. Activation of 5-HT$_1$ receptors on intracranial blood vessels probably constricts large intracranial arteries and closes arteriovenous anastomoses to relieve migraine headache. Activation of 5-HT$_1$ receptors on sensory nerves in the trigeminal system also may inhibit the release of pro-inflammatory neuropeptides.

Peripherally, dihydroergotamine causes vasoconstriction by stimulating alpha-adrenergic receptors. At therapeutic doses, it inhibits norepinephrine reuptake, increasing vasoconstriction. The drug constricts veins more than arteries, increasing venous return while decreasing venous stasis and pooling.

## Contraindications
Coronary artery disease, including vasospasm; hemiplegic or basilar migraine; hypersensitivity to dihydroergotamine or other ergot alkaloids; malnutrition; peripheral vascular disease or after vascular surgery; pregnancy; sepsis; severe hepatic or renal impairment; severe pruritus; uncontrolled hypertension; use of macrolide antibiotics or protease inhibitors; use within 24 hours of 5-HT$_1$ agonist, ergotamine-containing or ergot-type drug, or methysergide

## Interactions
**DRUGS**
*beta blockers:* Possibly peripheral vasoconstriction and peripheral ischemia, increased risk of gangrene
*macrolides, protease inhibitors:* Possibly increased risk of vasospasm, acute ergotism with peripheral ischemia
*nitrates:* Decreased antianginal effects of nitrates
*other ergot drugs, including ergoloid mesylates, ergonovine, methylergonovine, methysergide, and sumatriptan:* Increased risk of serious adverse effects from nasal dihydroergotamine
*systemic vasoconstrictors:* Risk of severe hypertension
**ACTIVITIES**
*smoking:* Possibly increased ischemic response to ergot therapy

## Adverse Reactions
**CNS:** Anxiety, confusion, dizziness, fatigue, headache, paresthesia, somnolence, weakness
**CV:** Bradycardia, chest pain, peripheral vasospasm (calf or heel pain with exertion, cool and cyanotic hands and feet, leg weakness, weak or absent pulses), tachycardia
**EENT:** Abnormal vision; dry mouth; epistaxis, nasal congestion or rhinitis, and sore nose (nasal spray); miosis; pharyngitis; sinusitis; taste perversion
**GI:** Diarrhea, nausea, vomiting
**MS:** Muscle stiffness
**SKIN:** Localized edema of face, feet, fingers, and lower legs; sensation of heat or warmth; sudden diaphoresis

## Nursing Considerations
•**WARNING** Monitor for signs of dihydroergotamine overdose, such as abdominal pain, confusion, delirium, dizziness, dyspnea, headache, nausea, pain in legs or arms, paresthesia, seizures, and vomiting.
•Assess peripheral pulses, skin sensation, warmth, and capillary refill. After giving nasal dihydroergotamine, monitor for signs of widespread blood vessel constriction and adverse reactions caused by decreased circulation to many body areas.
**PATIENT TEACHING**
•Instruct patient to use nasal spray when headache pain—not aura—begins.
•Teach her to prime spray pump by squeezing it four times.
•Advise patient to wait 15 minutes between each set of nasal sprays.
•Encourage patient to lie down in a quiet, dark room after using drug.
•Instruct patient to use more drug if headache returns or worsens but not to exceed maximum prescribed amount or dosing schedule.
•Remind patient to take drug only as needed, not on a daily basis.
•Instruct patient to discard residual nasal spray in an open ampule after 8 hours.
•If patient experiences a headache different from her usual migraines, caution her not to use dihydroergotamine and to notify prescriber.
•Inform patient that nasal form of drug won't relieve pain other than throbbing headaches.
•Advise patient to avoid alcohol, which can exacerbate or cause headaches, and to avoid smoking, which may cause an ischemic response.

•Warn patient about possible dizziness during or after a migraine for which she took dihydroergotamine.

# dihydrotachysterol
DHT, DHT Intensol, Hytakerol

## Class and Category
*Chemical:* Sterol derivative, vitamin D analogue
*Therapeutic:* Antihypocalcemic, antihypoparathyroid
*Pregnancy category:* C

## Indications and Dosages
➤ *To treat hypocalcemic and idiopathic tetany*
**CAPSULES, ORAL SOLUTION, TABLETS**
**Adults and adolescents.** *Initial:* 0.75 to 2.5 mg q.d. for 3 days for acute cases; 0.25 to 0.5 mg q.d. for 3 days for less acute cases. *Maintenance:* 0.25 mg/wk to 1 mg q.d., as needed to maintain normal serum calcium level.
➤ *To treat hypoparathyroidism*
**CAPSULES, ORAL SOLUTION, TABLETS**
**Adults and adolescents.** *Initial:* 0.75 to 2.5 mg q.d. for several days. *Maintenance:* 0.2 to 1 mg q.d.
**Children.** *Initial:* 1 to 5 mg q.d. for 4 days and then continued or decreased to one-quarter the dose. *Maintenance:* 0.5 to 1.5 mg q.d.

| Route | Onset | Peak | Duration |
|-------|-------|------|----------|
| P.O. | Several hr | Unknown | Up to 9 wk |

### Mechanism of Action
Stimulates intestinal calcium absorption and mobilizes bone calcium when parathyroid hormone and renal tissue fail to raise the serum calcium level.

## Contraindications
Hypercalcemia, hypersensitivity to vitamin D, hypervitaminosis D, malabsorption syndrome, renal dysfunction

## Interactions
**DRUGS**
*aluminum-containing antacids:* Possibly increased serum aluminum level, leading to toxicity
*barbiturates, phenytoin:* Decreased half-life and therapeutic effects of vitamin D

*calcium-containing drugs, thiazide diuretics:* Risk of hypercalcemia in patients with hypoparathyroidism
*cholestyramine, colestipol, mineral oil:* Decreased vitamin D absorption
*digitalis glycosides:* Possibly hypercalcemia; possibly potentiated effects of digitalis glycosides, resulting in arrhythmias
*magnesium-containing antacids:* Risk of hypermagnesemia, especially in patients with chronic renal failure
*phosphorus-containing drugs:* Increased risk of hyperphosphatemia
*vitamin D analogues:* Increased risk of vitamin D toxicity

## Adverse Reactions
**Other:** Vitamin D toxicity (long-term, high-dose therapy)

## Nursing Considerations
•After thyroid surgery, expect to give 0.25 mg once daily with 6 g of oral calcium lactate until danger of tetany has passed.
•Monitor serum calcium level regularly to determine dosage schedule and to detect or prevent hypercalcemia. Be aware that the difference between therapeutic and toxic doses may be small.
•Monitor closely for signs of vitamin D toxicity: abdominal cramps, amnesia, anorexia, ataxia, coma, constipation, depression, diarrhea, disorientation, hallucinations, headache, hypotonia, lethargy, nausea, syncope, tinnitus, vertigo, vomiting, and weakness. Renal impairment may cause albuminuria, polydipsia, and polyuria. Delayed treatment can result in death from cardiac and renal failure caused by widespread calcification of soft tissues, including the heart, blood vessels, kidneys, and lungs.
•If toxicity occurs, notify prescriber and expect to stop dihydrotachysterol immediately. Place patient on bed rest, administer fluids and a laxative, and place her on a low-calcium diet as ordered. For hypercalcemic crisis with dehydration, prepare to give I.V. NS and a loop diuretic (such as furosemide or ethacrynic acid) to increase urinary calcium excretion.
**PATIENT TEACHING**
•Stress the importance of not exceeding prescribed dihydrotachysterol dosage because of the risk of vitamin D toxicity.

•If patient detects signs of toxicity, caution her not to take the next dose and to notify prescriber immediately.
•Advise patient to drop solution directly into her mouth or to mix it with fruit juice, cereal, or other food.
•Instruct patient to take a missed dose as soon as she remembers unless it's nearly time for the next dose. Warn her not to double the dose.
•Advise patient to avoid OTC drugs and dietary supplements that contain aluminum, calcium, phosphorus, or vitamin D, unless directed by prescriber. Also advise her to avoid antacids that contain magnesium.
•Urge patient to keep follow-up appointments and to have her serum calcium level measured periodically.

# diltiazem hydrochloride
Apo-Diltiaz (CAN), Cardizem, Cardizem CD, Cardizem LA, Cardizem SR, Dilacor XR, Novo-Diltiazem (CAN), Nu-Diltiaz (CAN)

## Class and Category
*Chemical:* Benzothiazepine derivative
*Therapeutic:* Antianginal, antiarrhythmic, antihypertensive
*Pregnancy category:* C

## Indications and Dosages
➤ *To treat Prinzmetal's (variant) angina and chronic stable angina*
**TABLETS**
**Adults and adolescents.** *Initial:* 30 mg t.i.d. or q.i.d. a.c. and h.s., increased q 1 or 2 days as appropriate. *Maximum:* 360 mg/day in divided doses t.i.d. or q.i.d.
**E.R. TABLETS**
**Adults and adolescents.** *Initial:* 180 mg q.d., increased q 7 to 14 days as needed. *Maximum:* 360 mg/day.
➤ *To control hypertension*
**E.R. CAPSULES**
**Adults and adolescents.** *Initial:* 180 to 240 mg q.d., adjusted after 14 days as appropriate. *Maximum:* 360 mg/day.
**S.R. CAPSULES**
**Adults and adolescents.** *Initial:* 60 to 120 mg b.i.d., adjusted after 14 days as appropriate. *Maximum:* 360 mg/day.

## Mechanism of Action

Diltiazem inhibits calcium movement into coronary and vascular smooth-muscle cells by blocking slow calcium channels in cell membranes, as shown. This action decreases intracellular calcium, which:
• inhibits smooth-muscle cell contractions
• decreases myocardial oxygen demand by relaxing coronary and vascular smooth muscle, reducing peripheral vascular resistance and systolic and diastolic blood pressures
• slows AV conduction time and prolongs AV nodal refractoriness
• interrupts the reentry circuit in AV nodal reentrant tachycardias.

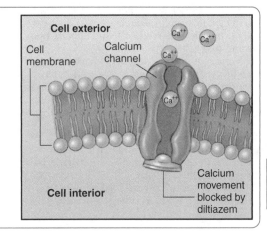

**TABLETS**
**Adults and adolescents.** *Initial:* 30 mg t.i.d. or q.i.d. a.c. and h.s., increased q 1 or 2 days as appropriate. *Maximum:* 360 mg/day in divided doses t.i.d. or q.i.d.
**E.R. TABLETS**
**Adults.** *Initial:* 180 to 240 mg q.d., adjusted after 14 days, as needed. *Maximum:* 540 mg/day.

➤ *To treat atrial fibrillation, atrial flutter, and paroxysmal supraventricular tachycardia*
**I.V. INFUSION OR INJECTION**
**Adults and adolescents.** 0.25 mg/kg given by bolus over 2 min. If response is inadequate after 15 min, 0.35 mg/kg given by bolus over 2 min. Then 10 mg/hr for continued reduction of heart rate after bolus, increased by 5 mg/hr, as needed. *Maximum:* 15 mg/hr for up to 24 hr.

## Incompatibilities

Don't give diltiazem through same I.V. line as acetazolamide, acyclovir, aminophylline, ampicillin sodium/sulbactam sodium, cefamandole, cefoperazone, diazepam, furosemide, heparin, hydrocortisone sodium succinate, methylprednisolone sodium succinate, mezlocillin, nafcillin, phenytoin, rifampin, or sodium bicarbonate.

| Route | Onset | Peak | Duration |
|---|---|---|---|
| P.O. | 30 to 60 min | In 2 wk | Unknown |
| P.O. (E.R.) | 2 to 3 hr | In 2 wk | Unknown |
| P.O. (S.R.) | Unknown | In 2 wk | Unknown |
| I.V. | In 3 min | 2 to 7 min | 30 min to 10 hr* |

## Contraindications

Acute MI; cardiogenic shock; Lown-Ganong-Levine or Wolff-Parkinson-White syndrome, second- or third-degree AV block, and sick sinus syndrome, unless artificial pacemaker is in place; pulmonary edema; systolic blood pressure below 90 mm Hg; ventricular tachycardia (wide complex)

## Interactions

**DRUGS**
*anesthetic:* Additive hypotension; possibly decreased cardiac contractility, conductivity, and automaticity
*benzodiazepines:* Increased risk of prolonged sedation

---

*For infusion; 1 to 3 hr for injection.

*beta blockers:* Possibly increased risk of adverse cardiovascular effects
*buspirone:* Increased effects and risk of buspirone toxicity
*carbamazepine, cyclosporine, lovastatin, quinidine, theophyllines:* Decreased hepatic clearance and increased serum levels of these drugs, leading to toxicity
*cimetidine:* Decreased diltiazem metabolism, increased blood diltiazem level
*digoxin:* Increased blood digoxin level
*lithium:* Possibly neurotoxicity
*NSAIDs:* Possibly antagonized antihypertensive effect of diltiazem
*prazocin:* Possibly increased risk of hypotension
*procainamide:* Possibly increased risk of prolonged QT interval
*quinidine:* Increased risk of adverse quinidine effects
*rifampin:* Decreased blood diltiazem level to undetectable amounts

## Adverse Reactions

**CNS:** Abnormal gait, amnesia, asthenia, depression, dizziness, dream disturbances, extrapyramidal reactions, fatigue, hallucinations, headache, insomnia, nervousness, paresthesia, personality change, somnolence, syncope, tremor, weakness
**CV:** Angina, atrial flutter, AV block (first-, second-, and third-degree), bradycardia, bundle-branch block, heart failure, hypotension, palpitations, peripheral edema, PVCs, sinus arrest, sinus tachycardia, 12-lead ECG abnormalities, ventricular fibrillation, ventricular tachycardia
**EENT:** Amblyopia, dry mouth, epistaxis, eye irritation, gingival bleeding and hyperplasia, gingivitis, nasal congestion, retinopathy, taste perversion, tinnitus
**ENDO:** Hyperglycemia
**GI:** Anorexia, constipation, diarrhea, elevated liver function test results, indigestion, nausea, thirst, vomiting
**GU:** Acute renal failure, impotence, nocturia, polyuria, sexual dysfunction
**HEME:** Hemolytic anemia, leukopenia, prolonged bleeding time, thrombocytopenia
**MS:** Arthralgia, muscle spasms, myalgia
**RESP:** Cough, dyspnea
**SKIN:** Alopecia, diaphoresis, erythema multiforme, exfoliative dermatitis, flushing, leukocytoclastic vasculitis, petechiae, photosensitivity, pruritus, purpura, rash, Stevens-Johnson syndrome, toxic epidermal necrolysis, urticaria
**Other:** Angioedema, hyperuricemia, weight gain

## Nursing Considerations

•Use diltiazem cautiously in patients with impaired hepatic or renal function, and monitor liver and renal function test results, as appropriate; diltiazem is metabolized mainly in the liver and excreted by the kidneys.
•**WARNING** Monitor blood pressure, pulse rate, and heart rate and rhythm by continuous ECG as appropriate during therapy. Keep emergency equipment and drugs available.
•Assess patient for signs of heart failure.
•If patient takes digoxin, watch for signs of digitalis toxicity, such as nausea, vomiting, halo vision, and elevated serum digoxin level.
•Administer sublingual nitroglycerin, as prescribed, during diltiazem therapy.
•Expect to discontinue drug if adverse skin reactions, usually transient, persist.

### PATIENT TEACHING

•Explain that regular tablets can be crushed but that capsules and E.R. tablets must be swallowed whole.
•**WARNING** Tell patient that stopping drug suddenly may cause life-threatening effects.
•Advise patient to monitor blood pressure and pulse rate regularly and to report significant changes to prescriber.
•Urge patient to report chest pain, difficulty breathing, dizziness, fainting, irregular heartbeat, rash, or swollen ankles.
•Instruct patient to maintain good oral hygiene, perform gum massage, and see a dentist every 6 months to prevent gingival bleeding and hyperplasia and gingivitis.

# dimenhydrinate

Dinate, Dramanate, Gravol (CAN), Hydrate

## Class and Category

*Chemical:* Ethanolamine derivative
*Therapeutic:* Antiemetic, antivertigo
*Pregnancy category:* B

## Indications and Dosages

➤ *To treat nausea, vomiting, dizziness, or vertigo associated with motion sickness*
**CHEWABLE TABLETS, ORAL SOLUTION, SYRUP, TABLETS**
**Adults and adolescents.** 50 to 100 mg q 4 to 6 hr, p.r.n. *Maximum:* 400 mg/24 hr.

**Children ages 6 to 12.** 25 to 50 mg q 6 to 8 hr, p.r.n. *Maximum:* 150 mg/24 hr.
**Children ages 2 to 6.** 12.5 to 25 mg q 6 to 8 hr, p.r.n. *Maximum:* 75 mg/24 hr.

**I.M. INJECTION**
**Adults and adolescents.** 50 mg q 4 hr, p.r.n.
**Children.** 1.25 mg/kg or 37.5 mg/m² q 6 hr, p.r.n. *Maximum:* 300 mg/day.

**I.V. INFUSION OR INJECTION**
**Adults and adolescents.** 50 mg in 10 ml of NS administered slowly, over at least 2 min, q 4 hr, p.r.n.
**Children.** 1.25 mg/kg or 37.5 mg/m² in 10 ml of NS administered slowly, over at least 2 min, q 6 hr, p.r.n. *Maximum:* 300 mg/day.

| Route | Onset | Peak | Duration |
|---|---|---|---|
| P.O. | Unknown | Unknown | 3 to 6 hr |
| I.M. | 20 to 30 min | Unknown | 3 to 6 hr |
| I.V. | Immediate | Unknown | 3 to 6 hr |

**Mechanism of Action**
May inhibit vestibular stimulation and labyrinthine stimulation and function by acting on the otolith system and, with larger doses, on the semicircular canals.

**Contraindications**
Age less than 1 month, hypersensitivity to dimenhydrinate or its components

**Interactions**
**DRUGS**
*aminoglycosides, other ototoxic drugs:* Masked symptoms of ototoxicity
*anticholinergics, drugs with anticholinergic activity:* Potentiated anticholinergic effects of dimenhydrinate
*apomorphine:* Possibly decreased emetic response to apomorphine in treatment of poisoning
*barbiturates, other CNS depressants:* Possibly increased CNS depression
*MAO inhibitors:* Increased anticholinergic and CNS depressant effects of dimenhydrinate
**ACTIVITIES**
*alcohol use:* Possibly increased CNS depression

**Adverse Reactions**
**CNS:** Confusion, drowsiness, hallucinations, nervousness, paradoxical stimulation
**CV:** Hypotension, palpitations, tachycardia

**EENT:** Blurred vision, diplopia, dry eyes, dry mouth, nasal congestion
**GI:** Anorexia, constipation, diarrhea, epigastric discomfort, nausea, vomiting
**GU:** Dysuria
**HEME:** Hemolytic anemia
**RESP:** Thickening of bronchial secretions, wheezing
**SKIN:** Photosensitivity, rash, urticaria
**Other:** Anaphylaxis

**Nursing Considerations**
•**WARNING** Be aware that I.V. dimenhydrinate shouldn't be administered to premature or full-term neonates. Some I.V. preparations may contain benzyl alcohol, which can cause a fatal toxic syndrome characterized by CNS, respiratory, circulatory, and renal impairment and metabolic acidosis.
•**WARNING** Be aware that 50-mg/ml concentration of dimenhydrinate is intended for I.M. use. For I.V. use, the solution must be diluted further with at least 10 ml of diluent, such as D₅W or NS, for each milliliter of dimenhydrinate.
•Monitor patients with prostatic hyperplasia, stenosing peptic ulcer, pyloroduodenal obstruction, bladder neck obstruction, angle-closure glaucoma, bronchial asthma, or cardiac arrhythmias for worsening of these conditions caused by anticholinergic effects.
•Monitor elderly patients for signs of increased sensitivity to dimenhydrinate, such as excessive drowsiness, confusion, and restlessness.
•Assess patients, especially children and elderly patients, for evidence of paradoxical stimulation, such as nightmares, unusual excitement, nervousness, restlessness, or irritability.
•Store parenteral drug at 15° to 30° C (59° to 86° F); don't freeze.
**PATIENT TEACHING**
•Because dimenhydrinate may cause drowsiness, instruct patient to avoid potentially hazardous activities until drug's CNS effects are known.
•Advise patient to inform health care providers about dimenhydrinate therapy, especially if she's being evaluated for medical conditions that are affected by this drug, such as appendicitis.
•Instruct patient to avoid alcohol, sedatives, and tranquilizers while receiving this drug.
•Encourage patient to use sunscreen to prevent photosensitivity reactions.

# diphenhydramine hydrochloride

Allerdryl (CAN), Banophen, Benadryl, Benadryl Allergy, Diphenhist CapTabs, Genahist, Hyrexin, Nytol QuickCaps, Siladryl, Sleep-Eze D Extra Strength, Unisom SleepGels Maximum Strength

## Class and Category

*Chemical:* Ethanolamine derivative
*Therapeutic:* Antianaphylactic adjunct, antidyskinetic, antiemetic, antihistamine, antitussive (syrup), antivertigo, sedative-hypnotic
*Pregnancy category:* B

## Indications and Dosages

➤ *To treat hypersensitivity reactions, such as perennial and seasonal allergic rhinitis, vasomotor rhinitis, allergic conjunctivitis, uncomplicated allergic skin eruptions, and transfusion reactions*

CAPSULES, TABLETS
**Adults and adolescents.** 25 to 50 mg q 4 to 6 hr, p.r.n. *Maximum:* 300 mg/day.
**Children ages 6 to 12.** 12.5 to 25 mg q 4 to 6 hr. *Maximum:* 150 mg/day.
**Children up to age 6.** 6.25 to 12.5 mg q 4 to 6 hr.

ELIXIR
**Adults and adolescents.** 25 to 50 mg q 4 to 6 hr, p.r.n. *Maximum:* 300 mg/day.
**Children.** 1.25 mg/kg q 4 to 6 hr. *Maximum:* 300 mg/day.

I.V. OR I.M. INJECTION
**Adults and adolescents.** 10 to 50 mg q 4 to 6 hr up to 100 mg/dose, if needed. *Maximum:* 400 mg/day.
**Children.** 1.25 mg/kg q 4 to 6 hr. *Maximum:* 300 mg/day.

➤ *To treat sleep disorders*

CAPSULES, TABLETS
**Adults and adolescents.** 50 mg 20 to 30 min before bedtime.

➤ *To provide antitussive effects*

ELIXIR
**Adults and adolescents.** 25 mg q 4 hr. *Maximum:* 100 mg/24 hr.
**Children ages 6 to 12.** 12.5 mg q 4 to 6 hr. *Maximum:* 75 mg/day.
**Children ages 2 to 6.** 6.25 mg q 4 to 6 hr. *Maximum:* 25 mg/day.

➤ *To prevent motion sickness or treat vertigo*

CAPSULES, ELIXIR, TABLETS
**Adults and adolescents.** 25 to 50 mg q 4 to 6 hr, p.r.n. *Maximum:* 300 mg/day.
**Children.** 1 to 1.5 mg/kg q 4 to 6 hr, p.r.n. *Maximum:* 300 mg/day.

I.V. OR I.M. INJECTION
**Adults and adolescents.** *Initial:* 10 mg. Increased to 20 to 50 mg q 2 to 3 hr, if needed. *Maximum:* 100 mg/dose, 400 mg/day.
**Children.** 1 to 1.5 mg/kg I.M. q 4 to 6 hr, p.r.n. *Maximum:* 300 mg/day.

➤ *To treat symptoms of Parkinson's disease and drug-induced extrapyramidal reactions in elderly patients who can't tolerate more potent antidyskinetic drugs*

CAPSULES, ELIXIR, TABLETS
**Adults.** 25 mg t.i.d. increased gradually to 50 mg q.i.d., if needed. *Maximum:* 300 mg/day.

I.V. OR I.M. INJECTION
**Adults and adolescents.** 10 to 50 mg q.i.d., as needed. *Maximum:* 100 mg/dose, 400 mg/day.

| Route | Onset | Peak | Duration |
|-------|-------|------|----------|
| P.O. | 15 to 60 min | 1 to 3 hr | 6 to 8 hr |
| I.V. | Immediate | 1 to 3 hr | 6 to 8 hr |
| I.M. | 30 min | 1 to 3 hr | 6 to 8 hr |

## Mechanism of Action

Binds to central and peripheral $H_1$ receptors, competing with histamine for these sites and preventing it from reaching its site of action. By blocking histamine, diphenhydramine produces antihistamine effects, inhibiting respiratory, vascular, and GI smooth-muscle contraction; decreasing capillary permeability, which reduces wheals, flares, and itching; and decreasing salivary and lacrimal gland secretions.

Diphenhydramine produces antidyskinetic effects, possibly by inhibiting acetylcholine in the CNS. It also produces antitussive effects by directly suppressing the cough center in the medulla oblongata. Diphenhydramine's antiemetic and antivertigo effects may be related to its ability to bind to CNS muscarinic receptors and depress vestibular stimulation and labyrinthine function. Its sedative effects are related to its CNS depressant action.

## Contraindications

Bladder neck obstruction, hypersensitivity to diphenhydramine or its components, lower respiratory tract symptoms (including asthma), MAO inhibitor therapy, narrow-angle glaucoma, pyloroduodenal obstruction, stenosing peptic ulcer, symptomatic benign prostatic hyperplasia

## Interactions

**DRUGS**

*apomorphine:* Possibly decreased emetic response to apomorphine in treatment of poisoning
*barbiturates, other CNS depressants:* Possibly increased CNS depression
*MAO inhibitors:* Increased anticholinergic and CNS depressant effects of diphenhydramine

**ACTIVITIES**

*alcohol use:* Possibly increased CNS depression

## Adverse Reactions

**CNS:** Confusion, dizziness, drowsiness
**CV:** Arrhythmias, palpitations, tachycardia
**EENT:** Blurred vision, diplopia
**GI:** Epigastric distress, nausea
**HEME:** Agranulocytosis, hemolytic anemia, thrombocytopenia
**RESP:** Thickened bronchial secretions
**SKIN:** Photosensitivity

## Nursing Considerations

•Expect to give parenteral form of diphenhydramine only when oral ingestion isn't possible.
•Keep elixir container tightly closed. Protect elixir and parenteral forms from light.
•Expect to discontinue drug at least 72 hours before skin tests for allergies because drug may inhibit cutaneous histamine response, thus producing false-negative results.

**PATIENT TEACHING**

•Instruct patient to take diphenhydramine at least 30 minutes before exposure to situations that may cause motion sickness.
•Advise her to take drug with food to minimize GI distress.
•Urge patient to avoid alcohol while taking diphenhydramine.
•Instruct her to use sunscreen to prevent photosensitivity reactions.
•Advise patient to avoid taking other OTC drugs that contain diphenhydramine to prevent additive effects.

# diphenoxylate hydrochloride and atropine sulfate

Lofene, Logen, Lomocot, Lomotil, Lonox, Vi-Atro

## Class, Category, and Schedule

*Chemical:* Belladonna alkaloid, tertiary amine (atropine), phenylpiperidine derivative opioid (diphenoxylate)
*Therapeutic:* Antidiarrheal
*Pregnancy category:* C
*Controlled substance:* Schedule V

## Indications and Dosages

➤ *To treat acute and chronic diarrhea*

**ORAL SOLUTION, TABLETS**

**Adults and adolescents.** *Initial:* 5 mg of diphenoxylate and 0.05 mg of atropine t.i.d. or q.i.d. *Maintenance:* 5 mg of diphenoxylate and 0.05 mg of atropine q.d., p.r.n. *Maximum:* 20 mg of diphenoxylate daily.

**DOSAGE ADJUSTMENT** Dosage reduced as soon as symptoms are controlled. Expect prescriber to consider alternative treatment if no improvement occurs after 10 days at maximum dosage. Dosage also reduced in elderly or very ill patients and in those with respiratory problems.

| Route | Onset | Peak | Duration |
|---|---|---|---|
| P.O. | 45 to 60 min | Unknown | 3 to 4 hr |

### Mechanism of Action

Directly affects circular smooth muscles of the GI tract, reducing intestinal motility. Subtherapeutic doses of atropine are added to diphenoxylate to reduce its potential for abuse.

## Contraindications

Diarrhea caused by pseudomembranous enterocolitis or enterotoxin-producing bacteria; hypersensitivity to atropine, diphenoxylate, or their components; obstructive jaundice; ulcerative colitis

## Interactions

**DRUGS**

*anticholinergics:* Possibly enhanced effects of atropine
*barbiturates, tranquilizers, and other habit-forming CNS depressants:* Potentiated CNS

depression, possibly increased risk of drug dependence
*MAO inhibitors*: Possibly hypertensive crisis
*naltrexone*: Withdrawal symptoms if patient is physically dependent on diphenoxylate
*opioid analgesics*: Increased risk of severe constipation, additive CNS depression
**ACTIVITIES**
*alcohol use:* Possibly potentiated CNS depression

## Adverse Reactions
**CNS:** Confusion, depression, dizziness, drowsiness, euphoria, fever, headache, hyperthermia, lethargy, malaise, paresthesia, restlessness, sedation
**CV:** Tachycardia
**EENT:** Gingival hyperplasia
**GI:** Abdominal cramps or pain, anorexia, ileus, nausea, pancreatitis, toxic megacolon, vomiting
**GU:** Urine retention
**RESP:** Respiratory depression
**SKIN:** Dry skin and mucous membranes, flushing, pruritus, urticaria
**Other:** Anaphylaxis, physical and psychological dependence

## Nursing Considerations
•**WARNING** Use diphenoxylate-atropine combination with extreme caution in patients with abnormal hepatic or renal function because drug can cause hepatic coma. Monitor liver function test results as appropriate during long-term therapy.
•**WARNING** Monitor for respiratory depression, especially in elderly or very ill patients and in those with respiratory problems; expect to give lower doses as prescribed.
•If severe fluid or electrolyte imbalance develops, expect to withhold drug as ordered until imbalance is corrected. Drug-induced ileus or toxic megacolon may cause fluid retention in the intestine, aggravating dehydration and electrolyte imbalance.
•Closely monitor patient with ulcerative colitis because drug has caused toxic megacolon. Notify prescriber immediately about unexpected adverse reactions, especially abdominal distention and hypoactive or absent bowel sounds.
•During long-term therapy, assess for tolerance to drug's antidiarrheal effects.
**PATIENT TEACHING**
•Caution patient not to exceed the prescribed dosage because of the risk of adverse

reactions, including drug dependence.
•Stress the importance of keeping drug away from children because overdose can cause permanent brain damage in them.
•Instruct patient to take drug with food if GI distress occurs.
•Advise patient to avoid potentially hazardous activities until drug's CNS effects are known.
•Urge patient to avoid alcohol and CNS depressants because of additive effects.
•Instruct patient to notify prescriber if diarrhea isn't improved or controlled within 48 hours or if a fever develops.

# dipyridamole

Apo-Dipyridamole FC (CAN), Apo-Dipyridamole SC (CAN), Novo-Dipiradol (CAN), Persantine

## Class and Category
*Chemical:* Pyrimidine
*Therapeutic:* Coronary vasodilator, diagnostic aid, platelet aggregation inhibitor
*Pregnancy category:* B

## Indications and Dosages
➤ *To prevent thromboembolic complications of cardiac valve replacement*
**TABLETS**
**Adults.** 75 to 100 mg q.i.d. with coumarin or indanedione derivative anticoagulant.
➤ *To aid diagnosis during thallium perfusion imaging of myocardium*
**I.V. INFUSION**
**Adults.** 0.57 mg/kg in 50 ml of $D_5W$ infused over 4 min. *Maximum:* 60 mg.

| Route | Onset | Peak | Duration |
|-------|-------|------|----------|
| I.V. | Unknown | 3.8 to 8.7 min* | Unknown |

## Contraindications
Asthma (I.V.), hypersensitivity to dipyridamole or its components, hypotension, unstable angina pectoris

## Interactions
**DRUGS**
*adenosine:* Potentiated effects of adenosine
*cefamandole, cefoperazone, cefotetan, pli-*

---

* After start of infusion, for increased velocity of coronary artery blood flow.

*camycin, valproic acid*: Possibly hypoprothrombinemia and increased risk of bleeding
*heparin, NSAIDs, thrombolytics*: Possibly increased risk of bleeding
*theophylline*: Reversal of coronary vasodilation caused by dipyridamole, possibly false-negative thallium imaging result

## Mechanism of Action
May increase the intraplatelet level of adenosine, which causes coronary vasodilation and inhibits platelet aggregation. Dipyridamole also may increase the intraplatelet level of cAMP and may inhibit formation of the potent platelet activator stimulant thromboxane $A_2$, which decreases platelet activation. Vasodilation and increased blood flow occur preferentially in nondiseased coronary vessels, which results in redistribution of blood away from significantly diseased vessels. These changes in perfusion are observed during thallium imaging studies.

## Adverse Reactions
**CNS:** Dizziness, headache
**CV:** Angina, arrhythmias, ECG changes (specifically ST-segment and T-wave changes)
**GI:** Abdominal pain, diarrhea, nausea, vomiting
**RESP:** Dyspnea
**SKIN:** Flushing, pruritus, rash

## Nursing Considerations
• Protect I.V. form of dipyridamole from direct light and freezing.
• Monitor blood pressure, pulse rate and rhythm, and breath sounds every 10 to 15 minutes during I.V. infusion.
• Keep parenteral aminophylline available to relieve adverse reactions to dipyridamole infusion.
• At therapeutic doses, expect adverse reactions to be minimal and transient. They typically resolve with long-term use.
**PATIENT TEACHING**
• Urge patient to take drug at least 1 hour before or 2 hours after meals for faster absorption. If she experiences GI distress, advise her to take drug with meals or milk.
• Advise patient to take drug at evenly spaced intervals.
• Inform patient that drug commonly is taken with other anticoagulants.
• Urge her to keep appointments for coagulation tests.

• Instruct patient to seek immediate emergency treatment if chest pain occurs.
• Caution patient to consult prescriber before taking aspirin and other OTC NSAIDs because of increased risk of bleeding.
• Advise patient to notify all health care providers about dipyridamole use.

# dirithromycin

Dynabac

## Class and Category
*Chemical:* Semisynthetic macrolide
*Therapeutic:* Antibiotic
*Pregnancy category:* C

## Indications and Dosages
➤ *To treat acute bacterial exacerbations and secondary bacterial infections in patients with bronchitis caused by* Moraxella catarrhalis *or* Streptococcus pneumoniae, *and uncomplicated skin and soft-tissue infections caused by methicillin-susceptible* Staphylococcus aureus
**TABLETS**
**Adults and adolescents.** 500 mg q.d. for 7 days.
➤ *To treat streptococcal pharyngitis*
**TABLETS**
**Adults and adolescents.** 500 mg q.d. for 10 days.

➤ *To treat community-acquired pneumonia caused by* Legionella pneumophila, Mycoplasma pneumoniae, *or* S. pneumoniae
**TABLETS**
**Adults and adolescents.** 500 mg q.d. for 14 days.

## Mechanism of Action
Binds with the 50S ribosomal subunit of the 70S ribosome in susceptible bacteria. This action inhibits RNA-dependent protein synthesis in bacterial cells, causing them to die.

## Contraindications
Concurrent use of astemizole, cisapride, or pimozide; hypersensitivity to dirithromycin, erythromycin, other macrolide antibiotics, or their components; known, potential, or suspected bacteremia

## Interactions
**DRUGS**
*antacids, H₂-receptor antagonists:* Increased dirithromycin absorption
*astemizol, terfenadine:* Possibly life-threatening arrhythmias
*theophylline:* Possibly increased serum theophylline level

## Adverse Reactions
**CNS:** Dizziness, headache, weakness
**GI:** Abdominal pain, diarrhea, nausea, pseudomembranous colitis, vomiting
**SKIN:** Pruritus, rash, urticaria

## Nursing Considerations
•Use dirithromycin cautiously in patients with impaired hepatic function. Monitor liver function test results as indicated because drug is metabolized in liver.
**PATIENT TEACHING**
•Instruct patient to take dirithromycin at the same time each day with food or within 1 hour of eating.
•Caution patient not to cut, chew, or crush tablets.
•Advise patient to store drug at room temperature in a dry place.
•Instruct patient to complete the full course of therapy, even if she feels better before it's finished.
•Advise patient to notify prescriber immediately if GI problems persist.

# disopyramide

Rythmodan (CAN)

## disopyramide phosphate

Norpace, Norpace CR, Rythmodan-LA (CAN)

## Class and Category
*Chemical:* Substituted pyramide derivative
*Therapeutic:* Class IA antiarrhythmic
*Pregnancy category:* C

## Indications and Dosages
➤ *To rapidly control ventricular arrhythmias*
**CAPSULES**
**Adults.** *Loading:* 300 mg (200 mg if patient weighs less than 50 kg [110 lb]). If no response to loading dose within 6 hr, 200 mg given q 6 hr. If no response within 48 hr, drug discontinued or dosage carefully increased to 250 to 300 mg q 6 hr.

➤ *To treat ventricular arrhythmias*
**CAPSULES**
**Adults.** 400 to 800 mg/day in divided doses q 6 hr, limited to 400 mg/day if patient weighs less than 50 kg. *Maximum:* 800 mg/day.
**Children ages 12 to 18.** 6 to 15 mg/kg/day in divided doses q 6 hr.
**Children ages 4 to 12.** 10 to 15 mg/kg/day in divided doses q 6 hr.
**Children ages 1 to 4.** 10 to 20 mg/kg/day in divided doses q 6 hr.
**Children younger than age 1.** 10 to 30 mg/kg/day in divided doses q 6 hr.
**DOSAGE ADJUSTMENT** Initial dosage reduced to 100 mg q 6 to 8 hr for adults with cardiomyopathy or possible cardiac decompensation. In patients with renal insufficiency, dosage reduced to 100 mg q 6 hr if creatinine clearance exceeds 40 ml/min/1.73 m² or hepatic function is impaired; 100 mg q 8 hr if creatinine clearance is 30 to 40 ml/min/1.73 m²; 100 mg q 12 hr if creatinine clearance is 15 to 29 ml/min/1.73 m²; and 100 mg q 24 hr if creatinine clearance is less than 15 ml/min/1.73 m².
**E.R. CAPSULES, E.R. TABLETS**
**Adults.** 400 to 800 mg/day in divided doses q 12 hr, limited to 200 mg q 12 hr if patient weighs less than 50 kg. *Maximum:* 800 mg/day.

## Mechanism of Action
Inhibits sodium influx through fast channels of myocardial cell membranes, thus increasing the recovery period after repolarization. Disopyramide decreases automaticity in the His-Purkinje system and conduction velocity in the atria, ventricles, and accessory pathways. It prolongs the QRS and QT intervals in normal sinus rhythm and atrial arrhythmias. The drug has a potent negative inotropic effect. It also acts as an anticholinergic and increases peripheral vascular resistance.

## Contraindications
Cardiogenic shock, congenital QT-interval prolongation, hypersensitivity to disopyramide or its components, second- or third-degree AV block (without pacemaker), sick sinus syndrome

## Interactions
**DRUGS**
*antiarrhythmics:* Widened QRS complex, prolonged QT interval, risk of arrhythmias,

serious negative inotropic effects
*anticholinergics:* Possibly additive anticholinergic effects
*cisapride:* Possibly increased risk of prolonged QT interval
*clarithromycin, erythromycin:* Increased blood disopyramide level
*digoxin:* Increased serum digoxin level
*hydantoins, rifampin:* Decreased blood disopyramide level
*insulin, oral antidiabetic drugs:* Possibly intensified antidiabetic effects
*quinidine:* Increased blood disopyramide level, decreased blood quinidine level, or both
*verapamil:* Widened QRS complex, prolonged QT interval, possibly death

### Adverse Reactions

**CNS:** Depression, dizziness, fatigue, fever, headache, insomnia, nervousness, syncope
**CV:** Chest pain; conduction disturbances; edema; heart failure (new or worsened); hypercholesterolemia; hypertriglyceridemia; hypotension; palpitations; proarrhythmias, including torsades de pointes; ventricular fibrillation; ventricular tachycardia
**EENT:** Blurred vision; dry eyes, mouth, nose, and throat
**ENDO:** Gynecomastia, hypoglycemia
**GI:** Abdominal distention, anorexia, constipation, diarrhea, vomiting
**GU:** Impotence, urinary frequency and urgency, urine retention
**HEME:** Reversible agranulocytosis (rare), thrombocytopenia
**MS:** Muscle weakness
**RESP:** Dyspnea
**SKIN:** Decreased sweating, pruritus, rash, reversible cholestatic jaundice
**Other:** Hypokalemia, lupus erythematosus–like symptoms

### Nursing Considerations

•**WARNING** Because of disopyramide's anticholinergic activity, avoid using drug in patients with glaucoma, myasthenia gravis, or urine retention.
•Use disopyramide cautiously and expect to reduce dosage in patients with impaired hepatic or renal function. Monitor hepatic and renal function, as ordered. Be aware that E.R. form shouldn't be given to patients with severe renal insufficiency.
•When changing from immediate-release to E.R. form, expect to start maintenance schedule 6 hours after last immediate-release dose.
•At therapeutic doses in hemodynamically uncompromised patients, expect drug to reduce cardiac output without decreasing resting sinus rate or affecting blood pressure. Keep in mind, however, that 2 mg/kg given I.V. over 3 minutes can increase heart rate and total peripheral resistance.
•Monitor heart rate and rhythm by continuous ECG.
•Assess serum electrolyte levels, especially the potassium level, because drug may be ineffective in hypokalemia and its toxic effects enhanced in hyperkalemia.
•If patient takes quinidine, expect to start disopyramide 6 to 12 hours after the last dose of quinidine. If patient takes procainamide, expect to start disopyramide 3 to 6 hours after the last dose of procainamide. A loading dose may not be required in either case.

**PATIENT TEACHING**
•Warn patient not to stop taking disopyramide abruptly; doing so may cause life-threatening cardiac problems.
•Advise patient to take a missed dose as soon as possible after she remembers, unless it's nearly time for the next dose. Caution her against doubling the dose. Urge her to notify prescriber if she misses more than one dose.
•Instruct patient to store drug at room temperature in a dry place.
•Instruct patient to check her pulse rate regularly and report significant changes to prescriber.
•Urge patient to notify prescriber about blurred vision, constipation, difficulty urinating, dizziness, dry mouth, and trouble breathing.
•Advise patient to avoid potentially hazardous activities until drug's CNS effects are known.
•Instruct patient to rise slowly from a lying or sitting position to reduce dizziness.
•Urge patient to avoid becoming overheated during hot weather or exercise because of risk of heatstroke.

# disulfiram

Antabuse

### Class and Category

*Chemical:* Thiuram derivative
*Therapeutic:* Alcohol abuse deterrent
*Pregnancy category:* Not rated

## Indications and Dosages

➤ *As adjunct to maintain sobriety in treatment of chronic alcoholism*

**TABLETS**

**Adults.** *Initial:* Up to 500 mg q.d. for 1 to 2 wk. *Maintenance:* 125 to 500 mg q.d. *Maximum:* 500 mg q.d.

| Route | Onset | Peak | Duration |
|-------|-------|------|----------|
| P.O. | In 1 to 2 hr | Unknown | Up to 14 days |

## Mechanism of Action

Interferes with the enzyme responsible for hepatic oxidation of acetaldehyde to acetate, which occurs during alcohol catabolism. Ingestion of even a small amount of alcohol after taking disulfiram raises the blood acetaldehyde level to 5 to 10 times normal. Disulfiram doesn't alter the rate at which alcohol is eliminated. Its major metabolite, diethyldithiocarbamate, inhibits norepinephrine synthesis and may be responsible for the drug's hypotensive effect.

## Contraindications

Alcohol intoxication; coronary artery occlusion; hypersensitivity to disulfiram, its components, rubber, pesticides, or fungicides; psychosis; recent use of alcohol, alcohol-containing preparations, metronidazole, or paraldehyde; severe myocardial disease

## Interactions

**DRUGS**

*alfentanil:* Decreased plasma clearance and prolonged duration of action of alfentanil
*amoxicillin-clavulanate, bacampicillin:* Possibly disulfiram-alcohol reaction
*ascorbic acid:* Possibly interference with disulfiram-alcohol reaction
*CNS depressants:* Possibly increased CNS depressant effects of either drug
*isoniazid:* Increased risk of additive neurotoxic effect of disulfiram; possibly increased adverse CNS effects
*metronidazole:* Risk of CNS toxicity, resulting in confusion and psychosis
*oral anticoagulants:* Possibly increased anticoagulant effects
*paraldehyde*: Decreased paraldehyde metabolism, increased blood paraldehyde level
*phenytoin*: Possibly increased blood phenytoin level and risk of phenytoin toxicity

*tricyclic antidepressants:* Possibly temporary delirium

**FOODS**

*caffeine:* Possibly increased cardiovascular and CNS effects of caffeine

**ACTIVITIES**

*alcohol use:* Disulfiram-alcohol reaction (if used within 14 days of disulfiram therapy)

## Adverse Reactions

**CNS:** Drowsiness, headache, peripheral neuropathy, psychotic reaction, tiredness
**EENT:** Blurred vision, garlic or metallic taste, optic atrophy, optic neuritis
**GU:** Impotence
**SKIN:** Rash

## Nursing Considerations

•Know that disulfiram is given only to patients who are highly motivated to stop drinking and who are receiving psychotherapy or substance abuse counseling.
•Be aware that alcohol content of patient's other drugs should be checked before starting therapy.
•**WARNING** Never give drug to patient without her knowledge or who is intoxicated.
•If needed, crush tablet and mix with fluids before administration.
•Don't give drug within 14 days of patient's ingestion of a substance that contains alcohol.
•Expect alcohol ingestion during disulfiram therapy to produce a severe reaction that lasts from 30 minutes to several hours. Symptoms may include angina, anxiety, blurred vision, confusion, diaphoresis, dyspnea, heart failure, hypotension, nausea, palpitations, sinus tachycardia, syncope, thirst, throbbing headache, throbbing in neck, vertigo, vomiting, and weakness. A deep sleep usually follows.
•**WARNING** Be aware that ingestion of three or more alcoholic beverages with a disulfiram dose greater than 500 mg/day may cause respiratory depression, arrhythmias, and cardiac arrest.
•If patient takes phenytoin, monitor blood phenytoin level before and during disulfiram therapy, and adjust dosage of either drug as prescribed. Drug interactions may not occur if disulfiram therapy starts before phenytoin therapy. Be aware that a subtherapeutic phenytoin level may result if disulfiram therapy stops.
•If patient takes an oral anticoagulant, monitor PT before and during disulfiram therapy, and adjust anticoagulant dosage as

prescribed. Drug interactions may not occur if disulfiram therapy starts before warfarin therapy. If disulfiram therapy stops, be prepared to adjust warfarin dosage to avoid loss of hypoprothrombinemic effects.
•Expect some adverse reactions, such as drowsiness, headache, and impotence, to subside over time or with a brief dosage reduction.
•Because one-fifth of a disulfiram dose may stay in the body for 1 week or longer, know that alcohol ingestion may continue to produce unpleasant symptoms for up to 2 weeks after therapy stops.
•Expect therapy to last months to years, depending on patient's ability to abstain from alcohol.

**PATIENT TEACHING**
•Teach patient's household and family members about precautions needed and risks associated with disulfiram therapy.
•Inform patient that drug doesn't cure alcoholism but does help deter alcohol consumption.
•If patient reports daytime drowsiness, advise her to take drug in the evening.
•Warn patient to avoid alcohol-containing substances, such as vinegar, cough syrup, and sauces, during therapy because a disulfiram-alcohol reaction may occur after ingesting as little as 15 ml of 100-proof alcohol. Encourage patient to avoid alcohol-containing liniments and lotions as well.
•Teach patient what to expect if a disulfiram-alcohol reaction occurs. Inform her that a deep sleep usually follows the reaction.
•Advise patient that a reaction can occur up to 14 days after therapy stops and that a severe reaction may cause respiratory depression, arrhythmias, and cardiac arrest.
•Instruct patient to carry medical identification that indicates drug, describes possible reactions, and lists someone to notify in case of emergency.

# dobutamine hydrochloride

Dobutrex

## Class and Category
*Chemical*: Synthetic catecholamine
*Therapeutic*: Cardiac stimulant
*Pregnancy category:* Not rated

## Indications and Dosages
➤ *To treat low cardiac output and heart failure*

**I.V. INFUSION**
**Adults.** 2.5 to 10 mcg/kg/min as continuous infusion adjusted according to hemodynamic response.
**Children.** 5 to 20 mcg/kg/min as continuous infusion adjusted according to hemodynamic response.

| Route | Onset | Peak | Duration |
|---|---|---|---|
| I.V. | 1 to 2 min | Unknown | Under 5 min |

## Mechanism of Action
Primarily stimulates beta$_1$-adrenergic receptors, and mildly stimulates beta$_2$- and alpha$_1$-adrenergic receptors. Beta$_1$-receptor stimulation produces a positive inotropic effect on the myocardium. This increases cardiac output by boosting myocardial contractility and stroke volume. Increased myocardial contractility raises coronary blood flow and myocardial oxygen consumption. Systolic blood pressure typically rises as a result of increased stroke volume. Other hemodynamic effects include decreased systemic vascular resistance, which reduces afterload, and decreased ventricular filling pressure, which reduces preload.

## Incompatibilities
Don't combine dobutamine with cefamandole, cefazolin, hydrocortisone sodium succinate, cephalothin, penicillin, sodium ethycrynate, and sodium heparin because of incompatibility. Don't mix dobutamine with alkaline solutions, such as sodium bicarbonate, because of possible physical incompatibility. Don't use diluents that contain sodium bisulfite or ethanol.

## Contraindications
Hypersensitivity to dobutamine or its components, idiopathic hypertrophic subaortic stenosis

## Interactions
**DRUGS**
*beta blockers:* Possibly increased alpha-adrenergic activity and peripheral resistance
*bretylium:* Potentiated vasopressor activity, possibly arrhythmias
*cyclopropane, halothane:* Possibly serious arrhythmias

*guanethidine:* Decreased hypotensive effect of guanethidine, possibly resulting in severe hypertension

*thyroid hormones:* Increased cardiovascular effects of thyroid hormones or dobutamine

*tricyclic antidepressants:* Possibly potentiated cardiovascular and vasopressor effects of dobutamine, resulting in arrhythmias, hyperpyrexia, or severe hypertension

## Adverse Reactions

**CNS:** Fever, headache, nervousness, restlessness
**CV:** Angina, bradycardia, hypertension, hypotension, palpitations, PVCs, tachycardia
**GI:** Nausea, vomiting
**RESP:** Dyspnea
**SKIN:** Extravasation with tissue necrosis and sloughing, rash
**Other:** Hypokalemia

## Nursing Considerations

• Avoid giving dobutamine to patients with uncorrected hypovolemia. Expect prescriber to order whole blood or plasma volume expanders to correct hypovolemia. Also avoid giving dobutamine to patients with acute MI because it can intensify or extend myocardial ischemia.

• Use drug cautiously in patients who are allergic to sulfites because drug may cause anaphylactic-like signs and symptoms; commercially available dobutamine injections contain sodium bisulfite. Also use drug cautiously in patients with atrial fibrillation because drug increases AV conduction. Keep in mind that patient should be adequately digitalized before administration.

• Dilute concentrate with at least 50 ml of compatible I.V. solution. A common dilution is 500 mg (40 ml from 250-ml bag) in 210 ml of D$_5$W or NS to yield 2,000 mcg/ml. Or dilute 1,000 mg (80 ml from 250-ml bag) in 170 ml of D$_5$W or NS to yield 4,000 mcg/ml. Adjust maximum concentration according to patient's fluid requirements as prescribed. Don't exceed a concentration of 5,000 mcg/ml. Discard solution after 24 hours.

• Inspect parenteral solution for particles and discoloration before administering it.

• Administer I.V. drug using an infusion pump.

• Monitor blood pressure frequently during therapy, preferably by continuous intra-arterial monitoring; a systolic pressure increase of 10 to 20 mm Hg may indicate a dobuta-

mine-induced increase in cardiac output.

• If hypotension develops, expect to reduce dosage or discontinue drug.

• Monitor heart rate and rhythm continuously for PVCs, which may result from drug's stimulatory effect on the heart's conduction system, and sinus tachycardia, which results from positive chronotropic effect of beta stimulation and may increase the heart rate by 5 to 15 beats/minute.

• Monitor hemodynamic parameters, such as central venous pressure, pulmonary artery wedge pressure, and cardiac output, as indicated, to assess drug's effectiveness.

• **WARNING** Monitor serum potassium level to check for hypokalemia, a rare result of beta$_2$ stimulation that causes electrolyte imbalance.

• Monitor urine output hourly, as appropriate, to assess for improved renal blood flow.

• Be aware that dobutamine isn't indicated for long-term treatment of heart failure because it may not be effective and may increase the risk of hospitalization and death.

**PATIENT TEACHING**

• Explain the need for frequent hemodynamic monitoring.

# docusate calcium

## (dioctyl calcium sulfosuccinate)

Albert Docusate (CAN), DC Softgels, Docucal-P, Doxidan (CAN), Pro-Cal-Sof, Sulfolax, Surfak

## docusate potassium (dioctyl potassium sulfosuccinate)

Diocto-K, Kasof

## docusate sodium (dioctyl sodium sulfosuccinate)

Afko-Lube, Afko-Lube Lax, Bilax, Colace, Colax, Correctol Stool Softener Soft Gels, Dialose, Diocto, Dioeze, DOK, D.O.S. Softgels, Ex-Lax Light Formula (CAN), Modane Soft, Regulax SS, Silace

## Class and Category

*Chemical:* Anionic surfactant
*Therapeutic:* Laxative, stool softener
*Pregnancy category:* C

## Indications and Dosages

➤ *To treat constipation*

CAPSULES (DOCUSATE CALCIUM)

**Adults and adolescents.** 240 mg h.s. until bowel movements are normal.

**Children age 6 and older.** 50 to 150 mg h.s.

CAPSULES, LIQUID, SYRUP, TABLETS (DOCUSATE SODIUM)

**Adults and adolescents.** 50 to 500 mg h.s.

**Children ages 6 to 12.** 40 to 120 mg h.s.

**Children ages 3 to 6.** 20 to 60 mg h.s.

**Children under age 3.** 10 to 40 mg h.s.

CAPSULES, TABLETS (DOCUSATE POTASSIUM)

**Adults and adolescents.** 100 mg t.i.d. until bowel movements are normal.

**Children age 6 and older.** 100 mg h.s.

| Route | Onset | Peak | Duration |
|-------|-------|------|----------|
| P.O. | 24 to 72 hr | Unknown | Unknown |

### Mechanism of Action

Acts as a surfactant that softens stool by decreasing the surface tension between the oil and water in fecal matter. This action lets more fluid penetrate the stool, thus forming a softer fecal mass.

## Contraindications

Fecal impaction; hypersensitivity to docusate salts or their components; intestinal obstruction; nausea, vomiting, or other symptoms of appendicitis; undiagnosed abdominal pain

## Interactions

DRUGS

*mineral oil:* Increased mineral oil absorption, increased risk of toxicity

*tetracycline:* Decreased tetracycline absorption

## Adverse Reactions

**CNS:** Dizziness, syncope

**CV:** Palpitations

**GI:** Abdominal cramps and distention, diarrhea, nausea, perianal irritation, vomiting

**MS:** Muscle weakness

## Nursing Considerations

•WARNING Expect long-term or excessive use of docusate to cause dependence on laxatives for bowel movements, electrolyte imbalances, osteomalacia, steatorrhea, and vitamin and mineral deficiencies.

•Assess for laxative abuse syndrome, especially in women with depression, personality disorders, or anorexia nervosa.

PATIENT TEACHING

•Instruct patient not to use docusate when she's experiencing abdominal pain, nausea, or vomiting.

•Advise patient to take docusate with a full glass of water or milk.

•To help prevent constipation, encourage patient to increase her fiber intake, exercise regularly, and drink 6 to 8 glasses (240 ml/glass) of water daily.

•Instruct patient to notify prescriber about rectal bleeding; symptoms of electrolyte imbalances, such as dizziness, light-headedness, muscle cramping, and weakness; and unrelieved constipation.

# dofetilide

Tikosyn

## Class and Category

*Chemical:* Methanesulfonanilide derivative

*Therapeutic:* Class III antiarrhythmic

*Pregnancy category:* C

## Indications and Dosages

➤ *To convert symptomatic atrial fibrillation or flutter to normal sinus rhythm or to maintain normal sinus rhythm in patients converted from symptomatic atrial fibrillation or flutter*

CAPSULES

**Adults.** *Initial:* 500 mcg b.i.d. for patients with creatinine clearance greater than 60 ml/min/1.73 m$^2$. *Maintenance:* Dosage based on QTc interval. If, 2 to 3 hr after initial dose, QTc interval increase is 15% of baseline or less, initial dose given b.i.d. *Maximum:* 500 mcg b.i.d.

DOSAGE ADJUSTMENT Initial dose reduced to 250 mcg b.i.d. for patients with creatinine clearance of 40 to 60 ml/min/1.73 m$^2$ and to 125 mcg b.i.d. for creatinine clearance of 20 to 39 ml/min/1.73 m$^2$, as prescribed. If, 2 to 3 hr after initial dose, QTc interval has increased by at least 15% or is more than 500 msec (more than 550 msec in patients with ventricular conduction abnormalities), dosage is decreased by 50%, as prescribed; however, for patients receiving lowest initial dose of 125 mcg b.i.d., dosage is reduced to 125 mcg q.d., as prescribed. During next four doses (given q 2 to 3 hr, as prescribed), if QTc interval increases to more than 500 msec (more than 550 msec in patients with ventricular conduction abnormalities), expect to discontinue therapy, as prescribed.

| Route | Onset | Peak | Duration |
|-------|-------|------|----------|
| P.O. | Unknown | 2 hr | 4 hr |

## Mechanism of Action

Selectively blocks potassium channels in myocardial cell membranes involved in cardiac repolarization. By blocking potassium channels, dofetilide prolongs ventricular refractoriness (widens QT interval), effective refractory period, and action potential duration. These actions terminate or prevent reentrant tachyarrhythmias, such as atrial fibrillation, atrial flutter, and ventricular tachycardia.

## Contraindications

Cardiac conduction disturbances without an artificial pacemaker; congenital or acquired QT prolongation syndrome; concurrent therapy with cimetidine, hydrochlorothiazide, ketoconazole, trimethoprim, or verapamil; hypersensitivity to dofetilide or its components; severe renal impairment (creatinine clearance less than 20 ml/min/1.73 m$^2$)

## Interactions

### DRUGS

*amiloride, cimetidine, co-trimoxazole, ketoconazole, megestrol, metformin, triamterene, trimethoprim:* Possibly increased blood dofetilide level
*azole antifungals, diltiazem, nefazodone, norfloxacin, protease inhibitors, quinine, selective serotonin reuptake inhibitors, zafirlukast:* Possibly increased blood dofetilide level and risk of dofetilide toxicity
*bepridil, cisapride, macrolide antibiotics, phenothiazines, tricyclic antidepressants:* Possibly prolonged QT interval
*class I and III antiarrhythmics, especially amiodarone:* Possibly prolonged QT interval and increased risk of dofetilide-induced proarrhythmias
*diuretics (potassium-depleting):* Increased risk of torsades de pointes in patients with hypokalemia or hypomagnesemia
*hydrochlorothiazide, verapamil:* Possibly increased blood dofetilide level and increased risk of torsades de pointes

### FOODS

*grapefruit juice:* Increased blood dofetilide level

### ACTIVITIES

*marijuana use:* Increased blood dofetilide level

## Adverse Reactions

**CNS:** Cerebral ischemia, CVA, dizziness, facial or flaccid paralysis, headache, insomnia, paresthesia, slurred speech, syncope
**CV:** AV block, bradycardia, cardiac arrest, chest pain, edema, MI, tachycardia, ventricular arrhythmias (including torsades de pointes and ventricular tachycardia)
**GI:** Abdominal pain, diarrhea, hepatic dysfunction, nausea
**MS:** Back pain, muscle weakness
**RESP:** Cough, dyspnea, respiratory tract infection
**SKIN:** Jaundice, rash
**Other:** Angioedema, flulike symptoms, weight gain

## Nursing Considerations

•**WARNING** If patient has previously received amiodarone drug therapy, be aware that dofetilide therapy should not be initiated until blood amiodarone level is less than 0.3 mcg/ml or until amiodarone has been withdrawn for at least 3 months.
•Evaluate and document QTc interval before and during dofetilide therapy.
•Place patient on continuous ECG monitoring for at least 3 days, as ordered, during dofetilide therapy.
•**WARNING** If patient does not convert to normal sinus rhythm within 24 hours of starting dofetilide, expect to prepare her for possible synchronized electrical cardioversion.
•Be prepared to reevaluate renal function and QTc every 3 months, as ordered, during dofetilide therapy.
•When switching to dofetilide from class I or class III antiarrhythmics, or after withdrawing antiarrhythmic treatment, monitor continuous ECG for at least 30 hours, as ordered.
•If patient requires a drug that may interact with dofetilide, expect to discontinue dofetilide, as prescribed, for 2 or more days before starting the other drug.
•**WARNING** Monitor laboratory test results for hypokalemia or hypomagnesemia, especially in patients who are taking diuretics, because of the increased risk of dofetilide-induced torsades de pointes.
•Frequently monitor female patients for adverse reactions, including prolonged QTc in-

terval and torsades de pointes, because women have approximately 12% to 18% lower renal clearance of drug than men and therefore a greater risk of experiencing adverse drug reactions.

**PATIENT TEACHING**
• Advise patient to swallow dofetilide capsules with water.
• Instruct patient to avoid drinking grapefruit juice while taking this drug.
• Inform patient that she may be hospitalized for at least 3 days if dosage is increased.
• Teach patient how to measure pulse rate and blood pressure during dofetilide therapy.
• Urge patient to report chest discomfort immediately, including fluttering or palpitations.
• Advise patient to consult prescriber before using any OTC drugs, nutritional supplements, or herbal products.
• Instruct patient to keep follow-up appointments to monitor heart rhythm.

# dolasetron mesylate

Anzemet

## Class and Category

*Chemical:* Carboxylate monomethanesulfonate
*Therapeutic:* Antiemetic
*Pregnancy category:* B

## Indications and Dosages

➤ *To prevent nausea and vomiting due to chemotherapy*

**ORAL SOLUTION, TABLETS**
**Adults and children over age 16.** 100 mg within 1 hr before chemotherapy.
**Children ages 2 to 16.** 1.8 mg/kg within 1 hr before chemotherapy. *Maximum:* 100 mg.

**I.V. INJECTION**
**Adults and children over age 16.** 1.8 mg/kg or 100 mg as a single dose within 30 min before chemotherapy.
**Children ages 2 to 16.** 1.8 mg/kg as a single dose within 30 min before chemotherapy. *Maximum:* 100 mg.

➤ *To prevent postoperative nausea and vomiting*

**ORAL SOLUTION, TABLETS**
**Adults and children over age 16.** 100 mg within 2 hr before surgery.
**Children ages 2 to 16.** 1.2 mg/kg within 2 hr before surgery. *Maximum:* 100 mg.

**I.V. INJECTION**
**Adults and children over age 16.** 12.5 mg 15 min before end of anesthesia.
**Children ages 2 to 16.** 0.35 mg/kg 15 min before end of anesthesia. *Maximum:* 12.5 mg/ dose.

➤ *To treat postoperative nausea and vomiting*

**I.V. INJECTION**
**Adults and children over age 16.** 12.5 mg as a single dose as soon as symptoms develop.
**Children ages 2 to 16.** 0.35 mg/kg as a single dose as soon as symptoms develop. *Maximum:* 12.5 mg/dose.

**D**

---

## Mechanism of Action

With its active metabolite hydrodolasetron, prevents activation of the serotonin 5-HT$_3$ receptors located peripherally on the vagal nerve terminals and centrally in the chemoreceptor trigger zone, thereby decreasing the vomiting reflex.

---

## Contraindications

Hypersensitivity to dolasetron or its components

## Interactions

**DRUGS**
*atenolol:* Possibly decreased clearance of dolasetron
*cimetidine:* Possibly increased blood dolasetron level
*rifampin:* Possibly decreased blood dolasetron level

## Adverse Reactions

**CNS:** Headache
**CV:** Hypertension, hypotension
**GI:** Diarrhea
**SKIN:** Rash
**Other:** Injection site pain

## Nursing Considerations

• Expect to administer up to 100 mg of dolasetron I.V. in 30 seconds or to dilute drug in NS, D$_5$W, D$_5$.45NS, or lactated Ringer's solution and infuse for up to 15 minutes, as prescribed.
• Flush I.V. line with compatible solution before and after drug administration.
• Expect to prepare an oral solution of dolasetron for patients unable to swallow tablets by diluting injection solution with apple or apple-grape juice.

•**WARNING** Monitor patients receiving dolasetron for ECG changes, including prolonged PR, QTc, and QT intervals and widened QRS complex.

**PATIENT TEACHING**
•Advise parents of pediatric patients and patients who have difficulty swallowing that oral solution can be prepared by diluting injection form of drug with apple or apple-grape juice.
•Inform the patient that oral solution may be refrigerated for up to 48 hours but should be discarded after 2 hours at room temperature.

# donepezil hydrochloride

Aricept

## Class and Category
*Chemical:* Piperidine derivative
*Therapeutic:* Antidementia
*Pregnancy category:* C

## Indications and Dosages
➤ *To treat mild to moderate dementia of the Alzheimer type*

**TABLETS**
**Adults.** *Initial:* 5 mg h.s. After 4 to 6 wk, dosage increased to 10 mg h.s., as indicated. *Maximum:* 10 mg/day.

---

### Mechanism of Action
Reversibly inhibits acetylcholinesterase and improves acetylcholine's concentration at cholinergic synapses. Raising the acetylcholine level in the cerebral cortex may improve cognition. Donepezil becomes less effective as Alzheimer's disease progresses and the number of intact cholinergic neurons declines.

---

## Contraindications
Hypersensitivity to donepezil, piperidine derivatives, or their components

## Interactions
**DRUGS**
*anticholinergics:* Possibly interference with activity of these drugs
*carbamazepine, dexamethasone, phenobarbital, phenytoin, rifampin:* Increased donepezil elimination rate

*cholinergic agonists, neuromuscular blockers:* Possibly synergistic effects of these drugs
*ketoconazole, quinidine:* Inhibited donepezil metabolism
*NSAIDs:* Possibly increased gastric acid secretion and increased risk of GI bleeding

## Adverse Reactions
**CNS:** Depression, dizziness, dream disturbances, fatigue, headache, insomnia, somnolence, syncope
**GI:** Anorexia, constipation, diarrhea, nausea, vomiting
**GU:** Urinary frequency
**MS:** Arthralgia, muscle spasms
**SKIN:** Ecchymosis

## Nursing Considerations
•Use donepezil cautiously in patients with bladder obstruction because drug's weak peripheral cholinergic effect could obstruct outflow.
•Use drug cautiously in patients with asthma, COPD, or other pulmonary disorders because drug has a weak affinity for peripheral cholinesterase, which may increase bronchoconstriction and bronchial secretions.
•If patient has cardiac disease, monitor heart rate and rhythm for bradycardia, which may result from increased vagal tone caused by drug's inhibition of peripheral cholinesterase. Reduced heart rate may be especially significant if patient has sick sinus syndrome, bradycardia, or other supraventricular arrhythmia.
•Take safety precautions if patient experiences dizziness or other adverse CNS reactions.

**PATIENT TEACHING**
•Advise patient to take donepezil just before going to bed.
•Inform her that drug may be taken with or without food.
•Instruct patient to avoid potentially hazardous activities, such as driving, until drug's CNS effects are known. Encourage her to take safety precautions to prevent falling if she experiences adverse reactions, such as dizziness.
•Inform patient with history of peptic ulcer disease or gastric irritation that drug may aggravate these conditions by increasing gastric acid secretion.
•Caution patient to avoid NSAIDs during therapy because of risk of GI bleeding. Urge her to notify prescriber immediately if she notices black, tarry stools.

# dopamine hydrochloride

Intropin, Revimine (CAN)

## Class and Category

*Chemical*: Catecholamine
*Therapeutic*: Cardiac stimulant, vasopressor
*Pregnancy category*: C

## Indications and Dosages

▶ *To correct hypotension that is unrespon-sive to adequate fluid volume replace-ment or occurs as part of shock syn-drome caused by bacteremia, chronic cardiac decompensation, drug overdose, MI, open-heart surgery, renal failure, trauma, or other major systemic ill-nesses; to improve low cardiac output*

**I.V. INFUSION**

**Adults.** 0.5 to 3 mcg/kg/min for vasodilation of renal arteries; 2 to 10 mcg/kg/min for pos-itive inotropic effects and increased cardiac output; 10 mcg/kg/min, increased gradually according to patient's response, for increased systolic and diastolic blood pressures.

**DOSAGE ADJUSTMENT** Initial dosage reduced to 10% of usual amount if patient has re-ceived MAO inhibitor in previous 2 to 3 wk.

**Children.** 1 to 5 mcg/kg/min increased grad-ually in increments of 2.5 to 5 mcg/kg/min to achieve desired results. *Maximum:* 20 mcg/kg/min.

| Route | Onset | Peak | Duration |
|-------|-------|------|----------|
| I.V. | In 5 min | Unknown | Up to 10 min |

## Incompatibilities

Don't add dopamine to 5% sodium bicarbon-ate, alkaline I.V. solutions, oxidizing agents, or iron salts.

## Contraindications

Pheochromocytoma, uncorrected ventricular fibrillation, ventricular tachycardia, and other tachyarrhythmias

## Interactions

**DRUGS**

*alpha blockers, haloperidol, loxapine, pheno-thiazines, thioxanthenes:* Antagonized peripheral vasoconstriction with high doses of dopamine
*anesthetics, such as chloroform, enflurane, halothane, isoflurane, and methoxyflurane:* Increased risk of severe atrial and ventricu-lar arrhythmias

*antihypertensives, diuretics used as antihy-pertensives:* Possibly decreased antihyperten-sive effects of these drugs
*beta blockers:* Antagonized beta receptor-mediated inotropic effects of dopamine
*digitalis glycosides:* Possibly increased risk of arrhythmias and additive inotropic ef-fects
*diuretics:* Possibly increased diuretic effects of dopamine or diuretic
*doxapram:* Possibly increased vasopressor ef-fects of dopamine or doxapram
*ergot alkaloids:* Enhanced peripheral vaso-constriction
*guanadrel, guanethidine:* Possibly decreased hypotensive effects of these drugs and poten-tiated vasopressor response to dopamine, re-sulting in hypertension and arrhythmias
*levodopa:* Possibly increased risk of arrhyth-mias
*MAO inhibitors:* Prolonged and intensified cardiac stimulation and vasopressor effect of dopamine
*maprotiline, tricyclic antidepressants:* Possi-bly potentiated cardiovascular and vasopres-sor effects of dopamine, resulting in arrhyth-mias, hyperpyrexia, or severe hypertension
*mecamylamine, methyldopa:* Possibly de-creased hypotensive effects of these drugs and enhanced vasopressor effect of dopamine
*methylphenidate:* Possibly potentiated vaso-pressor effect of dopamine
*nitrates:* Possibly decreased antianginal ef-fects of nitrates; possibly decreased vaso-pressor effect of dopamine, resulting in hy-potension
*oxytocic drugs:* Possibly severe hypertension
*phenoxybenzamine:* Possibly antagonized pe-ripheral vasoconstriction of dopamine, caus-ing hypotension and tachycardia
*phenytoin:* Possibly sudden bradycardia and hypotension
*rauwolfia alkaloids:* Possibly decreased hy-potensive effects of these drugs
*sympathomimetics:* Possibly increased ad-verse cardiovascular and other effects
*thyroid hormones:* Increased risk of coronary insufficiency

## Adverse Reactions

**CNS:** Headache
**CV:** Angina, bradycardia, hypertension, hypo-tension, palpitations, peripheral vasoconstric-tion, sinus tachycardia, ventricular arrhythmias
**GI:** Nausea, vomiting

D

**RESP:** Dyspnea
**SKIN:** Extravasation with tissue necrosis

## Mechanism of Action

Stimulates dopamine$_1$ (D$_1$) and dopamine$_2$ (D$_2$) postsynaptic receptors. D$_1$ receptors mediate vasodilation in renal, mesenteric, coronary, and cerebral blood vessels. D$_2$ receptors, when stimulated, inhibit norepinephrine release. In higher doses, dopamine also stimulates alpha$_1$ and alpha$_2$ receptors, causing vascular smooth-muscle contraction.

At doses of 0.5 to 3 mcg/kg/min, this naturally occurring catecholamine mainly affects dopaminergic receptors in renal, mesenteric, coronary, and cerebral vessels, resulting in vasodilation, increased renal blood flow, improved GFR, and increased urine output. At doses of 2 to 10 mcg/kg/min, dopamine stimulates beta$_1$-adrenergic receptors, increasing cardiac output while maintaining dopaminergic-induced vasodilation. At doses of 10 mcg/kg/min or more, alpha-adrenergic agonism takes over, causing increased peripheral vascular resistance and renal vasoconstriction.

## Nursing Considerations

•If possible, avoid giving dopamine to patients with occlusive vascular disease, such as atherosclerosis, Buerger's disease, diabetic endarteritis, or Raynaud's disease, because of the risk of decreased peripheral circulation.
•Use drug cautiously in patients with cardiac disease, particularly coronary artery disease, because dopamine increases myocardial oxygen demand. Also use drug cautiously in patients who are allergic to sulfites, which are contained in some forms of dopamine.
•Inspect parenteral solution for particles and discoloration before administration.
•Dilute dopamine concentrate with a compatible I.V. solution before administering. Typical dilution is 400 mg in 250 ml to yield 1.6 mg/ml. Don't exceed 3.2 mg/ml.
•If patient has hypovolemia, ensure adequate fluid resuscitation before giving drug.
•Give drug by I.V. infusion using an infusion pump.
•**WARNING** When the infusion rate exceeds 20 mcg/kg/min, monitor patient for excessive vasoconstriction and loss of renal vasodilating effects. Avoid using an infusion rate above 50 mcg/kg/min.
•If you must infuse more than 20 mcg/kg/min of dopamine to maintain blood pressure, expect to infuse norepinephrine as prescribed.
•To avoid extravasation and tissue necrosis, administer infusion through a central catheter. If you must administer drug through a peripheral line, inspect site frequently for signs of extravasation and necrosis. If you detect such signs, start a new I.V. line for dopamine infusion, discontinue previous I.V. line, and notify prescriber immediately.
•If drug extravasates, expect prescriber to give 5 to 10 mg of phentolamine diluted in 10 to 15 ml of NS, as prescribed. Phentolamine infiltrates directly into area to antagonize vasoconstriction and minimize sloughing and tissue necrosis.
•Titrate dopamine gradually to minimize hypotension, especially after a high infusion rate.
•Monitor blood pressure continuously with an intra-arterial line, as indicated.
•Place patient on continuous ECG monitoring, and assess heart rate and rhythm for arrhythmias.
•Monitor hemodynamic parameters, such as central venous pressure, pulmonary artery wedge pressure, and cardiac output, as indicated, to assess drug's effectiveness.
•Monitor urine output hourly as appropriate to assess patient for improved renal blood flow.

**PATIENT TEACHING**
•Explain the need for frequent hemodynamic monitoring.

# doxapram hydrochloride

Dopram

## Class and Category

*Chemical:* Pyrrolidinone derivative
*Therapeutic:* Respiratory stimulant
*Pregnancy category:* B

## Indications and Dosages

➤ *To stimulate respiration in COPD-related acute respiratory insufficiency*

**I.V. INFUSION**

**Adults and adolescents.** 1 to 2 mg/min titrated according to respiratory response. *Maximum:* 3 mg/min for up to 2 hr.

➤ *To treat respiratory depression after anesthesia*

**I.V. INFUSION**

**Adults and adolescents.** 5 mg/min until desired response occurs and then reduced to 1 to 3 mg/min. *Maximum:* Cumulative dose of 4 mg/kg or 300 mg.

**I.V. INJECTION**

**Adults and adolescents.** 0.5 to 1 mg/kg, repeated q 5 min, if needed. *Maximum:* 1.5 mg/kg as a single dose or 2 mg/kg q 5 min.

| Route | Onset | Peak | Duration |
|---|---|---|---|
| I.V. | 20 to 40 sec | 1 to 2 min | 5 to 12 min |

**Mechanism of Action**

Activates peripheral carotid, aortic, and other chemoreceptors to stimulate respiration, resulting in increased tidal volume and respiratory rate. Doxapram also may increase respiratory rate and tidal volume by directly stimulating the respiratory center in the medulla oblongata.

**Incompatibilities**

To avoid precipitation and gas formation, don't mix doxapram with alkaline solutions, such as aminophylline, sodium bicarbonate, or 2.5% thiopental.

**Contraindications**

Age less than 1 month; cerebral edema; CVA; head injury; hypersensitivity to doxapram or its components; mechanical disorders of ventilation, including acute bronchial asthma, flail chest, muscle paresis, obstruction, pneumothorax, and pulmonary fibrosis; pulmonary embolism; seizure disorder; severe cardiovascular disorder; severe hypertension; uncompensated heart failure

**Interactions**

**DRUGS**

*chloroform, cyclopropane, enflurane, halothane, isoflurane, methoxyflurane, trichloroethylene:* Possibly adverse myocardial effects if doxapram given within 10 minutes of these drugs

*CNS stimulants:* Possibly excessive CNS stimulation, resulting in arrhythmias, insomnia, irritability, nervousness, or seizures

*MAO inhibitors, sympathomimetics:* Additive vasopressor effects

*skeletal muscle relaxants:* Masked residual effects of muscle relaxants

**Adverse Reactions**

**CNS:** Disorientation, dizziness, headache

**CV:** Arrhythmias, including sinus tachycardia; hypertension

**GI:** Diarrhea, hiccups, nausea, vomiting

**GU:** Urine retention

**RESP:** Bronchospasm, cough, dyspnea

**SKIN:** Diaphoresis

**Other:** Injection site pain, redness, swelling, and thrombophlebitis

**Nursing Considerations**

• Avoid giving doxapram to patients receiving mechanical ventilation.

• Maintain a patent airway, and assess for optimal oxygenation before administering drug.

• Monitor I.V. insertion site for extravasation and signs of thrombophlebitis or local skin irritation.

• If hypertension or dyspnea develops suddenly, stop infusion as directed.

• Assess for early signs of overdose, including enhanced deep tendon reflexes, skeletal muscle hyperactivity, and tachycardia.

**PATIENT TEACHING**

• Explain the need for frequent pulse and blood pressure monitoring.

# doxazosin mesylate

Cardura, Cardura-1 (CAN), Cardura-2 (CAN), Cardura-4 (CAN)

**Class and Category**

*Chemical:* Quinazoline derivative

*Therapeutic:* Antihypertensive, benign prostatic hyperplasia therapeutic agent

*Pregnancy category:* C

**Indications and Dosages**

➤ *To manage hypertension*

**TABLETS**

**Adults.** *Initial:* 1 mg q.d. Doubled q 1 to 2 wk, if needed to achieve desired blood pressure. *Maximum:* 16 mg/day.

➤ *To treat benign prostatic hyperplasia (BPH)*

**TABLETS**

**Adults.** *Initial:* 1 mg q.d. Doubled q 1 to 2 wk, if needed, based on signs and symptoms. *Maximum:* 8 mg/day.

| Route | Onset | Peak | Duration |
|-------|-------|------|----------|
| P.O. | 1 to 2 hr* | 2 to 6 hr† | 24 hr† |

## Mechanism of Action
Competitively inhibits alpha$_1$-adrenergic receptors in the sympathetic nervous system, causing peripheral vasodilation and reduced peripheral vascular resistance. This action increases heart rate and decreases blood pressure, especially in a standing position. Doxazosin also relaxes smooth muscle of the bladder neck, prostate, and prostate capsule, which reduces urethral resistance and pressure and urinary outflow resistance, which helps treat BPH.

## Contraindications
Hypersensitivity to doxazosin, prazosin, terazosin, or their components

## Interactions
**DRUGS**
*antihypertensives, diuretics:* Enhanced hypotensive effects
*cimetidine:* Possibly increased blood doxazosin level
*dopamine:* Antagonized vasopressor effect of high-dose dopamine
*ephedrine, metaraminol, methoxamine, phenylephrine:* Possibly decreased vasopressor effects of these drugs
*epinephrine:* Possibly severe hypotension and tachycardia
*NSAIDs:* Possibly loss of hypotensive activity from sodium or fluid accumulation

## Adverse Reactions
**CNS:** Dizziness, drowsiness, headache, nervousness, restlessness, vertigo
**CV:** Arrhythmias, including sinus tachycardia; first-dose orthostatic hypotension; palpitations; peripheral edema
**EENT:** Rhinitis
**GI:** Nausea
**RESP:** Dyspnea

## Nursing Considerations
• Don't give doxazosin to hypotensive patients.

---

*For hypertension; in 2 wk for BPH.
† For hypertension; unknown for BPH.

• Use drug cautiously in patients with hepatic disease (because normal dosage may cause exaggerated effects) and in elderly patients (because hypotensive response may be more pronounced).
• **WARNING** Monitor for orthostatic hypotension (which may cause syncope) early in therapy, especially after exercise and in patients with hypovolemia.
• Monitor blood pressure for 2 to 6 hours after first dose and with each dose increase because orthostatic hypotension commonly occurs during this time. Adjust dose as prescribed, based on standing blood pressure.
• Carefully monitor patients with renal disease for exaggerated effects, such as first-dose orthostatic hypotension.
• Monitor urination, checking for difficulty urinating and urine retention, to assess drug's effects on BPH.

**PATIENT TEACHING**
• Inform patient that she may take doxazosin in the morning or evening and with food, if desired.
• Instruct patient to change position slowly to minimize effects of orthostatic hypotension.
• Advise patient to avoid standing for long periods, exercising, using alcohol, and going outside in hot weather; these activities may exacerbate orthostatic hypotension.
• Advise patient to avoid potentially hazardous activities until drug's CNS effects are known.

# doxepin hydrochloride
Novo-Doxepin (CAN), Sinequan, Triadapin (CAN)

## Class and Category
*Chemical*: Dibenzoxepin derivative
*Therapeutic*: Antidepressant
*Pregnancy category:* Not rated

## Indications and Dosages
➤ *To treat mild to moderate depression or anxiety*
**CAPSULES, ORAL SOLUTION**
**Adults and adolescents.** 75 to 150 mg q.d. h.s. *Maximum:* 150 mg q.d.

➤ *To treat mild to moderate depression or anxiety with organic disease*
**CAPSULES, ORAL SOLUTION**
**Adults and adolescents.** 25 to 50 mg q.d.

➤ *To treat severe depression or anxiety*
**CAPSULES, ORAL SOLUTION**
**Adults and adolescents.** 50 mg t.i.d., gradually increased to 300 mg q.d., as indicated.

| Route | Onset | Peak | Duration |
|-------|-------|------|----------|
| P.O. | 2 to 3 wk | Unknown | Unknown |

## Mechanism of Action
May block serotonin and norepinephrine reuptake by adrenergic nerves. In this way, the tricyclic antidepressant raises serotonin and norepinephrine levels at nerve synapses, which may elevate mood and reduce depression.

## Incompatibilities
Don't mix doxepin solution with carbonated beverages or grape juice.

## Contraindications
Acute recovery phase of MI; concurrent use of MAO inhibitor; glaucoma; hypersensitivity to doxepin, other tricyclic antidepressants, or their components; urine retention

## Interactions
**DRUGS**
*amantadine, anticholinergics, antidyskinetics, antihistamines:* Possibly intensified anticholinergic effects, causing confusion, hallucinations, and nightmares
*anticonvulsants:* Possibly lowered seizure threshold and decreased effects of these drugs
*antithyroid drugs:* Possibly increased risk of agranulocytosis
*barbiturates, carbamazepine:* Increased doxepin metabolism, decreased blood doxepin level, possibly lowered seizure threshold
*bupropion, clozapine, cyclobenzaprine, haloperidol, loxapine, maprotiline, molindone, phenothiazines, thioxanthenes:* Possibly prolonged and intensified sedative and anticholinergic effects of either drug, possibly increased risk of seizures
*cimetidine, flecainide, phenothiazines, propafenone, quinidine, selective serotonin reuptake inhibitors, tricyclic antidepressants:* Increased blood doxepin level from inhibited systemic clearance, resulting in increased risk of toxicity

*clonidine, guanadrel, guanethidine:* Increased risk of hypertension, especially during second week of doxepin therapy
*CNS depressants:* Possibly potentiated CNS depression, hypotension, and respiratory depression
*corticosteroids:* Possibly exacerbated depression
*direct-acting sympathomimetics, such as epinephrine and norepinephrine:* Potentiated effects of these drugs
*disulfiram:* Possibly transient delirium
*fluoxetine:* Possibly increased blood doxepin level
*MAO inhibitors:* Possibly hyperpyrexia, hypertension, seizures, and death
*oral anticoagulants:* Possibly increased anticoagulant effects of these drugs
*pimozide:* Increased risk of arrhythmias
*probucol:* Possibly prolonged QT interval and increased risk of ventricular tachycardia
*thyroid hormones:* Possibly increased therapeutic and toxic effects of both drugs
*tolazamide:* Possibly severe hypoglycemia
**ACTIVITIES**
*alcohol use:* Possibly enhanced CNS depression, hypotension, and respiratory depression

## Adverse Reactions
**CNS:** Confusion, delirium, dream disturbances, drowsiness, fatigue, hallucinations, headache, nervousness, parkinsonism, restlessness, sedation, seizures, suicidal ideation (children and teens), tremor
**CV:** ECG changes, orthostatic hypotension, palpitations
**EENT:** Blurred vision, dry mouth, taste perversion
**GI:** Constipation, diarrhea, heartburn, ileus, increased appetite, nausea, vomiting,
**GU:** Decreased libido, ejaculation disorders
**SKIN:** Diaphoresis, jaundice
**Other:** Weight gain

## Nursing Considerations
•If desired, mix oral solution in 120 ml of water; milk; or orange, grapefruit, tomato, or pineapple juice.
•Expect to observe adverse reactions within a few hours after giving drug.
•Evaluate patient for therapeutic response: decreased anxiety, apprehension, depression, fear, guilt, somatic symptoms, and worry; increased energy; and more restful sleep.

•**WARNING** Monitor children and teens closely for evidence of suicidal thinking and behavior because doxepin increases the risk in these groups.

•Keep in mind that abrupt withdrawal of doxepin after prolonged therapy can cause cholinergic rebound effects, including diarrhea, nausea, and vomiting.

•Plan to discontinue drug, as prescribed, several days before elective surgery to avoid hypertension.

•Monitor elderly patients for signs of parkinsonism, especially with high-dose therapy.

•Be alert for seizures. Patients with a seizure disorder may need an increased anticonvulsant dosage to maintain seizure control.

•For patients with asthma or sulfite sensitivity, know that doxepin tablets may aggravate asthma or cause allergic reactions because they contain sulfites.

•Follow diabetic patient's serum glucose level closely; drug may alter glucose metabolism.

•If patient takes a thyroid hormone, be alert for increased responses to both drugs and, possibly, exaggerated drug-induced effects, such as arrhythmias and CNS stimulation. Untreated hypothyroidism prevents adequate response to therapy.

**PATIENT TEACHING**

•**WARNING** Alert parents to watch their child or teen closely for abnormal thinking or behavior and increased aggression or hostility. Stress importance of notifying prescriber about unusual changes.

•Instruct patient to avoid alcohol during doxepin therapy because mental alertness may decrease.

•Advise diabetic patient to measure her serum glucose level more often than usual.

# doxercalciferol

Hectorol

## Class and Category

*Chemical:* Fat-soluble vitamin D analogue
*Therapeutic:* Antihyperparathyroid drug
*Pregnancy category:* B

## Indications and Dosages

➤ *To reduce elevated intact parathyroid hormone (iPTH) serum level when man-*
*aging secondary hyperparathyroidism in patients undergoing chronic hemodialysis*

**CAPSULES**

**Adults.** *Initial:* 10 mcg 3 times/wk (about every other day) before, during, or after dialysis. *Maintenance:* If iPTH level is decreased by 50% and above 300 picograms (pg)/ml, dosage increased by 2.5 mcg at 8-wk intervals, as needed. If iPTH level is between 150 and 300 pg/ml, initial dosage maintained. If iPTH level is less than 100 pg/ml, drug stopped for 1 wk and then restarted at a dose that's at least 2.5 mcg less than previous dose. *Maximum:* 20 mcg 3 times/wk for a total of 60 mcg/wk.

➤ *To reduce elevated iPTH blood level when managing secondary hyperparathyroidism in patients with stage 3 or 4 chronic renal disease*

**CAPSULES**

**Adults.** 1 mcg q.d. *Maintenance:* If iPTH level exceeds 70 pg/ml for stage 3 or 110 pg/ml for stage 4, dosage increased by 0.5 mcg at 2-wk intervals, as needed. If iPTH level is 35 to 70 pg/ml for stage 3 or 70 to 110 pg/ml for stage 4, dosage is maintained. If iPTH is less than 35 pg/ml for stage 3 or less than 70 pg/ml for stage 4, drug is stopped for 1 wk and then restarted with a dose that's at least 0.5 mcg lower than previous dose. *Maximum:* 3.5 mcg q.d.

## Contraindications

Evidence of vitamin D toxicity, hypersensitivity to doxercalciferol or its components, risk or history of hypercalcemia or hyperphosphatemia

## Interactions

**DRUGS**

*antacids that contain magnesium:* Possibly additive drug effects and increased risk of hypermagnesemia

*cholestyramine, mineral oil, orlistat, and other drugs that affect lipid absorption:* Possibly decreased doxercalciferol absorption

*glutethimide, phenobarbital:* Possibly increased doxercalciferol metabolism and risk of adverse reactions

*erythromycin, ketoconazole:* Possibly inhibited doxercalciferol metabolism and decreased effectiveness

*vitamin D and its analogues:* Possibly additive effects, resulting in increased adverse effects, such as hypercalcemia

## Mechanism of Action

Undergoes hepatic conversion to an active metabolite (1,25-dihydroxyvitamin $D_2$ [1,25-dihydroxyergocalciferol]), which increases intestinal absorption of dietary calcium and renal tubular reabsorption of urinary calcium. Together with parathyroid hormone, doxercalciferol also mobilizes calcium from bone. These effects serve to maintain the blood calcium levels in patients with chronic renal failure, which in turn prevents hyperparathyroidism.

In patients with renal failure, decreased metabolic activation of vitamin D in the kidneys leads to chronic hypocalcemia. The parathyroid gland compensates by increasing PTH secretion, but renal failure prevents it from achieving a normal serum calcium level. Thus, secondary hyperparathyroidism develops. Because doxercalciferol doesn't require renal conversion to form its active metabolite, it can regulate the serum calcium level and thus suppress PTH secretion and reduce its serum level in patients with chronic renal failure. An elevated PTH level in these patients lead to metabolic bone disease, such as renal osteodystrophy.

## Adverse Reactions

**CNS:** Depression, dizziness, headache, insomnia, malaise, paresthesia
**CV:** Bradycardia, chest pain, peripheral edema
**EENT:** Rhinitis
**ENDO:** Oversuppression of iPTH
**GI:** Anorexia, constipation, indigestion, nausea, vomiting
**HEME:** Anemia
**MS:** Hypertonia
**RESP:** Cough, dyspnea
**SKIN:** Pruritus
**Other:** Dehydration, hypercalcemia, hypercalciuria, hyperphosphatemia, weight gain

## Nursing Considerations

•**WARNING** Be aware that patients who take vitamin D also should not take doxercalciferol because they may develop severe vitamin D toxicity and hypercalcemia.
•Be alert for signs and symptoms of vitamin D toxicity and hypercalcemia in patients receiving high-dose or long-term doxercalciferol therapy. Early signs and symptoms include bone pain, constipation, dry mouth, headache, metallic taste, myalgia, nausea, somnolence, vomiting, and weakness. Late signs and symptoms include albuminuria, anorexia, arrhythmias, azotemia, conjunctivitis (calcific), decreased libido, elevated AST and ALT levels, elevated BUN level, generalized vascular calcification, hypercholesterolemia, hypertension, hyperthermia, irritability, mild metabolic acidosis, nephrocalcinosis, nocturia, pancreatitis, photophobia, polydipsia, polyuria, pruritus, rhinorrhea, and weight loss.
•Keep emergency equipment readily available in case patient develops toxicity.
•Expect to monitor blood iPTH, calcium, and phosphorus levels before starting drug therapy and weekly during early treatment.
•For patients with renal failure who are undergoing hemodialysis, be aware that oral calcium-based or other non–aluminum-containing phosphate binders and a low-phosphate diet typically are used to control the serum phosphorus level. An elevated serum phosphorus level worsens secondary hyperparathyroidism and may decrease doxercalciferol's effectiveness in reducing the blood iPTH level.
•After doxercalciferol therapy starts, expect to decrease dosage of phosphate binders to correct persistent mild hypercalcemia. Expect to increase dosage to correct persistent mild hyperphosphatemia.
•Avoid giving magnesium-containing antacids with doxercalciferol if patient receives long-term hemodialysis because doing so may lead to hypermagnesemia.

**PATIENT TEACHING**
•Urge patient who takes doxercalciferol to strictly follow a low-phosphorus diet and to take calcium supplement, as prescribed, to maintain serum calcium level. Stress that diet and calcium-based phosphate binder should provide 1.5 to 2 g of calcium daily.
•Explain the importance of periodic follow-up blood work to measure drug effectiveness. Mention that it may take several months to achieve optimal PTH suppression.
•Warn patient not to take other forms of vitamin D while taking doxercalciferol and to consult prescriber before taking any OTC drugs.

• Advise patient to contact prescriber immediately if early signs or symptoms of toxicity, such as headache or nausea, develop.

# doxycycline calcium

*(contains 50 mg of base per 5 ml of oral suspension)*

Vibramycin

## doxycycline hyclate

*(contains 50 or 100 mg of base per capsule, 100 mg of base per delayed-release capsule, 100 mg of base per tablet, and 100 or 200 mg of base per injection vial)*

Alti-Doxycycline (CAN), Apo-Doxy (CAN), Doryx, Doxycin (CAN), Vibramycin, Vibra-Tabs

## doxycycline monohydrate

*(contains 50 or 100 mg of base per capsule and 25 mg of base per 5 ml of oral suspension)*

Monodox, Vibramycin

### Class and Category
*Chemical*: Oxytetracycline derivative
*Therapeutic*: Antibiotic
*Pregnancy category*: D

### Indications and Dosages
➤ *To treat cutaneous, GI, or inhalation anthrax*
CAPSULES, DELAYED-RELEASE CAPSULES, ORAL SUSPENSION, TABLETS, I.V. INFUSION
**Adults, adolescents, and children who weigh more than 45 kg (99 lb).** 100 mg (base) q 12 hr for 60 days.
**Children who weigh less than 45 kg.** 2.2 mg/kg (base) q 12 hr for 60 days.
➤ *To treat endocervical, rectal, and urethral infections caused by* Chlamydia trachomatis
CAPSULES, DELAYED-RELEASE CAPSULES, ORAL SUSPENSION, TABLETS
**Adults and children over age 8 who weigh more than 45 kg.** 100 mg (base) b.i.d. for 7 days. *Maximum:* 300 mg (base)/day.
**Children who weigh 45 kg or less.** 2.2 mg (base)/kg b.i.d. on day 1 and then 2.2 to 4.4 mg (base)/kg q.d. or 1.1 to 2.2 mg (base)/kg b.i.d.
I.V. INFUSION
**Adults and children over age 8 who weigh more than 45 kg.** 200 mg (base) q.d. or 100 mg (base) q 12 hr on day 1 and then 100 to

200 mg (base) q.d. or 50 to 100 mg (base) q 12 hr. *Maximum:* 300 mg (base)/day.
**Children who weigh 45 kg or less.** 4.4 mg (base)/kg q.d. or 2.2 mg (base)/kg q 12 hr on day 1 and then 2.2 to 4.4 mg (base)/kg q.d. or 1.1 to 2.2 mg (base)/kg q 12 hr.
➤ *To treat epididymo-orchitis caused by* C. trachomatis *or* Neisseria gonorrhoeae *or nongonococcal urethritis caused by* C. trachomatis *or* Ureaplasma urealyticum
CAPSULES, DELAYED-RELEASE CAPSULES, ORAL SUSPENSION, TABLETS
**Adults and children over age 8 who weigh more than 45 kg.** 100 mg (base) b.i.d. for at least 10 days. *Maximum:* 300 mg (base)/day.
**Children who weigh 45 kg or less.** 2.2 mg (base)/kg b.i.d. on day 1 and then 2.2 to 4.4 mg (base)/kg q.d. or 1.1 to 2.2 mg (base)/kg b.i.d.
I.V. INFUSION
**Adults and children over age 8 who weigh more than 45 kg.** 200 mg (base) q.d. or 100 mg (base) q 12 hr on day 1 and then 100 to 200 mg (base) q.d. or 50 to 100 mg (base) q 12 hr. *Maximum:* 300 mg (base)/day.
**Children who weigh 45 kg or less.** 4.4 mg (base)/kg q.d. or 2.2 mg (base)/kg q 12 hr on day 1 and then 2.2 to 4.4 mg (base)/kg q.d. or 1.1 to 2.2 mg (base)/kg q 12 hr.
➤ *To prevent malaria*
CAPSULES, DELAYED-RELEASE CAPSULES, ORAL SUSPENSION, TABLETS
**Adults and children over age 8 who weigh more than 45 kg.** 100 mg (base) q.d. beginning 1 to 2 wk before travel, continued daily during travel, and then daily for 4 wk after travel ends. *Maximum:* 300 mg (base)/day.
**Children over age 8.** 2 mg (base)/kg q.d. beginning 1 to 2 days before travel, continued daily during travel, and then daily for 4 wk after travel ends. *Maximum:* 100 mg (base) q.d.
➤ *To treat early syphilis in penicillin-allergic patients*
CAPSULES, DELAYED-RELEASE CAPSULES, ORAL SUSPENSION, TABLETS
**Adults and children over age 8 who weigh more than 45 kg.** 100 mg (base) b.i.d. for 2 wk. *Maximum:* 600 mg (base)/day.
**Children who weigh 45 kg or less.** 2.2 mg (base)/kg b.i.d. on day 1 and then 2.2 to 4.4 mg (base)/kg q.d. or 1.1 to 2.2 mg (base)/kg b.i.d.
I.V. INFUSION
**Adults and children over age 8 who weigh more than 45 kg.** 150 mg (base) q 12 hr for at least 10 days. *Maximum:* 300 mg (base)/day.

**Children who weigh 45 kg or less.** 4.4 mg (base)/kg q.d. or 2.2 mg (base)/kg q 12 hr on day 1 and then 2.2 to 4.4 mg (base)/kg q.d. or 1.1 to 2.2 mg (base)/kg q 12 hr.

➤ *To treat syphilis of more than 1 year's duration in patients allergic to penicillin*
**CAPSULES, DELAYED-RELEASE CAPSULES, ORAL SUSPENSION, TABLETS**
**Adults and children over age 8 who weigh more than 45 kg.** 100 mg (base) b.i.d. for 4 wk. *Maximum:* 300 mg (base)/day.

**I.V. INFUSION**
**Adults and children over age 8 who weigh more than 45 kg.** 150 mg (base) q 12 hr for at least 10 days. *Maximum:* 300 mg (base)/day.
**Children who weigh 45 kg or less.** 4.4 mg (base)/kg q.d. or 2.2 mg (base)/kg q 12 hr on day 1 and then 2.2 to 4.4 mg (base)/kg q.d. or 1.1 to 2.2 mg (base)/kg q 12 hr.

➤ *To treat all other infections caused by susceptible organisms*
**CAPSULES, DELAYED-RELEASE CAPSULES, ORAL SUSPENSION, TABLETS**
**Adults and children over age 8 who weigh more than 45 kg.** 100 mg (base) q 12 hr on day 1 and then 100 mg (base) q.d. or 50 mg (base) b.i.d. For severe infections, 100 mg (base) continued q 12 hr. *Maximum:* 300 mg (base)/day.
**Children who weigh 45 kg or less.** 2.2 mg (base)/kg b.i.d. on day 1 and then 2.2 to 4.4 mg (base)/kg q.d. or 1.1 to 2.2 mg (base)/kg b.i.d.

**I.V. INFUSION**
**Adults and children over age 8 who weigh more than 45 kg.** 200 mg (base) q.d. or 100 mg (base) q 12 hr on day 1 and then 100 to 200 mg (base) q.d. or 50 to 100 mg (base) q 12 hr. *Maximum:* 300 mg (base)/day.
**Children who weigh 45 kg or less.** 4.4 mg (base)/kg q.d. or 2.2 mg (base)/kg q 12 hr on day 1 and then 2.2 to 4.4 mg (base)/kg q.d. or 1.1 to 2.2 mg (base)/kg q 12 hr.

## Mechanism of Action

Exerts a bacteriostatic effect against a wide variety of gram-positive and gram-negative organisms. Doxycycline is more lipophilic than other tetracyclines, which allows it to pass more easily through the bacterial lipid bilayer, where it binds reversibly to 30S ribosomal subunits. Bound doxycycline blocks the binding of aminoacyl transfer RNA to messenger RNA, thus inhibiting bacterial protein synthesis.

## Contraindications
Hypersensitivity to any tetracycline

## Interactions
**DRUGS**
*antacids that contain aluminum, calcium, magnesium, or zinc; calcium supplements; choline and magnesium salicylates; iron salts; laxatives that contain magnesium:* Decreased doxycycline absorption and therapeutic effects
*barbiturates, carbamazepine, phenytoin:* Increased clearance and decreased effects of doxycycline
*cholestyramine, colestipol:* Decreased doxycycline absorption
*digoxin:* Increased bioavailability of digoxin, possibly leading to digitalis toxicity
*oral anticoagulants:* Possibly increased hypoprothrombinemic effects of these drugs
*oral contraceptives:* Decreased effectiveness of estrogen-containing oral contraceptives, increased risk of breakthrough bleeding
*penicillins:* Inhibited bactericidal action
*sodium bicarbonate:* Altered doxycycline absorption from increased gastric pH
**FOODS**
*dairy products, other foods high in calcium or iron:* Decreased doxycycline absorption

## Adverse Reactions
**CNS:** Paresthesia
**CV:** Phlebitis
**EENT:** Black "hairy" tongue, glossitis, hoarseness, oral candidiasis, pharyngitis, stomatitis, tooth discoloration
**GI:** Anorexia; bulky, loose stools; diarrhea; dysphagia; enterocolitis; epigastric distress; esophageal ulceration; hepatotoxicity; nausea; rectal candidiasis; vomiting
**GU:** Anogenital lesions, dark yellow or brown urine, elevated BUN level, vaginal candidiasis
**HEME:** Eosinophilia, hemolytic anemia, neutropenia, thrombocytopenia, thrombocytopenic purpura
**SKIN:** Dermatitis, photosensitivity, rash, urticaria
**Other:** Anaphylaxis, injection site phlebitis

## Nursing Considerations
•Avoid giving doxycycline to breast-feeding women because of the risk of enamel hypoplasia, inhibited linear skeletal growth, oral and vaginal candidiasis, photosensitivity reactions, and tooth discoloration in breast-feeding infant.

•Avoid giving drug to children younger than age 8; it may cause permanent discoloration and enamel hypoplasia of developing teeth.
•Use oral suspension cautiously in patients who are allergic to sulfites because it contains sodium metabisulfite.
•Expect to adjust dosage for patients who have hepatic disease to avoid drug accumulation.
•**WARNING** Don't give doxycycline by I.M. or S.C. route.
•Give doxycycline without regard to meals. Although food and milk may delay absorption, they don't significantly reduce it.
•Observe patient frequently for injection site phlebitis, a common adverse reaction to I.V. administration.
•Monitor liver function test results as appropriate to detect hepatotoxicity.
•Expect oral or parenteral doxycycline to increase risk of oral, rectal, or vaginal candidiasis—especially in elderly or debilitated patients and those on prolonged therapy—by changing the normal balance of microbial flora.
•Monitor patient closely for diarrhea, which may indicate pseudomembranous colitis. If diarrhea occurs, notify prescriber and expect to withhold doxycycline. Expect to treat pseudomembranous colitis with fluids, electrolytes, protein, and an antibiotic effective against *Clostridium difficile*.

**PATIENT TEACHING**
•Instruct patient to avoid taking doxycycline just before bed because drug may not dissolve properly when she's recumbent and may cause esophageal burning and ulceration.
•Advise patient to avoid dairy products and other foods high in calcium or iron during therapy.
•Caution patient not to take bismuth subsalicylate while taking doxycycline because doxycycline absorption will be reduced.
•Instruct patient to drink plenty of fluids while taking doxycycline to reduce the risk of esophageal burning and ulceration.
•Inform patient that her urine may become dark yellow or brown during therapy.
•Instruct patient to avoid sun exposure and ultraviolet light as much as possible during therapy and to use a sunscreen or sunblock when exposure can't be avoided. If patient develops evidence of phototoxicity, such as skin eruption, tell her to stop drug and notify prescriber.

•Advise patients who take an oral contraceptive to use an additional contraceptive method during therapy.
•If patient is being treated for a sexually transmitted disease, explain that her partner may need treatment as well.
•Instruct patient to notify prescriber immediately if she experiences anorexia, diarrhea, epigastric distress, nausea, and vomiting during therapy.
•Alert female patients that doxycycline may increase the risk of vaginal candidiasis. Tell her to notify prescriber if she develops vaginal itching or discharge.
•Advise patient taking doxycycline for malaria prevention to start taking drug 1 to 2 days before traveling to the region and continue it for 4 weeks after leaving the area. Note that the total length of therapy shouldn't exceed 4 months.

# dronabinol

## (delta-9-tetrahydrocannabinol, THC)

Marinol

### Class, Category, and Schedule
*Chemical*: Synthetic tetrahydrocannabinol
*Therapeutic*: Antiemetic, appetite stimulant
*Pregnancy category:* C
*Controlled substance:* Schedule II

### Indications and Dosages
➤ *To prevent nausea and vomiting caused by chemotherapy and unresponsive to other antiemetics*

**CAPSULES**
**Adults.** 5 mg/m$^2$ 1 to 3 hr before and 2 to 4 hr after chemotherapy, increased by 2.5 mg/m$^2$, as needed. *Maximum:* 15 mg/m$^2$/dose or a total of 4 to 6 doses/day.

➤ *To stimulate appetite in cancer and AIDS patients*

**CAPSULES**
**Adults.** *Initial:* 2.5 mg b.i.d. before lunch and supper, increased as needed. *Maximum:* 20 mg/day in divided doses.

**DOSAGE ADJUSTMENT** Dosage reduced to 2.5 mg before supper or h.s. for patients who can't tolerate 5 mg/day.

| Route | Onset | Peak | Duration |
|-------|-------|------|----------|
| P.O. | Unknown | Unknown | 24 hr or longer* |

## Mechanism of Action

May exert antiemetic effect by inhibiting the vomiting control mechanism in the medulla oblongata. As the main psychoactive substance in marijuana (*Cannabis sativa* L.), dronabinol's effects may be mediated by cannabinoid receptors in neural tissues.

## Contraindications

Hypersensitivity to dronabinol, its components, sesame oil, or marijuana

## Interactions

**DRUGS**
*anticholinergics, antihistamines:* Possibly increased risk of tachycardia
*apomorphine:* Possibly potentiated CNS depression, possibly decreased emetic response with prior use of dronabinol
*CNS stimulants (such as amphetamines), and CNS depressants (such as benzodiazepines):* Additive CNS effects
*sympathomimetics:* Possibly enhanced hypertension, tachycardia, and other adverse cardiovascular effects
**ACTIVITIES**
*alcohol use:* Additive CNS depressant effects

## Adverse Reactions

**CNS:** Amnesia, anxiety, ataxia, confusion, delusions, depression, dizziness, drowsiness, euphoria, hallucinations, irritability, mood changes, nervousness, sleep disturbance
**CV:** Orthostatic hypotension, palpitations, sinus tachycardia
**GI:** Nausea, vomiting
**Other:** Physical and psychological dependence

## Nursing Considerations

•**WARNING** Be aware that drug shouldn't be discontinued abruptly; otherwise, withdrawal syndrome may occur.
•Know that patients under age 45 may tolerate drug better than those over age 45.
•Monitor for adverse reactions that mimic psychosis, such as hallucinations and, possi-

---

* For appetite stimulant effects; unknown for antiemetic effects.

bly, acute anxiety, especially with high doses.
•Anticipate higher risk of cardiovascular reactions, such as increased heart rate and blood pressure changes (especially orthostatic hypotension), at higher doses.
•**WARNING** Expect tolerance to drug to develop over time, especially if patient has smoked marijuana.
•Be aware that short-term, low-dose therapy doesn't typically lead to physical and psychological dependence, which may occur with long-term, high-dose therapy.
•Expect drug to alter REM sleep pattern, even after therapy stops.
**PATIENT TEACHING**
•Caution patient not to stop taking dronabinol abruptly because withdrawal symptoms may occur.
•Urge patient not to use alcohol while taking dronabinol because it may enhance CNS depression.
•Instruct patient to rise slowly to sitting or standing position to minimize effects of orthostatic hypotension.
•Advise patient to avoid potentially hazardous activities until drug's CNS effects are known.
•Inform patient that sleep pattern may be adversely affected during therapy and for sometime afterward.

# droperidol

Inapsine

## Class and Category

*Chemical:* Butyrophenone derivative
*Therapeutic:* Antiemetic
*Pregnancy category:* C

## Indications and Dosages

➤ *To reduce nausea and vomiting after surgery or diagnostic procedures when other treatments are ineffective*
**I.V. OR I.M. INJECTION**
**Adults and adolescents.** Dosage individualized up to a maximum initial dose of 2.5 mg I.M. or slow I.V. Additional 1.25 mg may be administered to achieve desired effect if potential benefit outweighs potential risk.
**Children ages 2 to 12.** Dosage individualized up to a maximum initial dose of 0.1 mg/kg. Additional dose may be administered to achieve desired effect if potential benefit outweighs potential risk.

D

DOSAGE ADJUSTMENT Initial dosage reduced for elderly, debilitated, or critically ill patients because of the increased risk of hypotension and excessive sedation.

| Route | Onset | Peak | Duration |
|-------|-------|------|----------|
| I.V., I.M. | 3 to 10 min | In 30 min | 2 to 4 hr |

## Mechanism of Action
Produces sedation by blocking postsynaptic dopamine receptors in the limbic system. Droperidol may reduce nausea by blocking dopamine receptors in the chemoreceptor trigger zone in the reticular formation of the medulla oblongata. It also may produce antiemetic effects by attaching to postsynaptic gamma-aminobutyric acid receptors in the chemoreceptor trigger zone.

## Contraindications
Hypersensitivity to droperidol or its components, known or suspected prolonged QT interval (including congenital long QT syndrome)

## Interactions
**DRUGS**
*amoxapine, haloperidol, loxapine, metoclopramide, metyrosine, molindone, olanzapine, phenothiazines, pimozide, rauwolfia alkaloids, risperidone, tacrine, thioxanthenes:* Possibly increased risk of severe extrapyramidal reactions
*anesthetics:* Possibly hypotension and peripheral vasodilation
*antiarrhythmics (class I or III), antidepressants, antimalarials, benzodiazepines, diuretics, I.V. opiates, laxatives, MAO inhibitors, volatile anesthetics, and other drugs that prolong QT interval (such as some antihistamines):* Increased risk of serious adverse effects of droperidol, such as prolonged QT interval and arrhythmias
*antihypertensives:* Possibly orthostatic hypotension
*bromocriptine, levodopa:* Possibly inhibited actions of these drugs
*CNS depressants:* Additive CNS depression
*epinephrine:* Possibly paradoxical reduction of blood pressure
*propofol:* Possibly decreased antiemetic effect of both drugs
**ACTIVITIES**
*alcohol use:* Additive CNS depression

## Adverse Reactions
**CNS:** Anxiety, drowsiness, dystonia, restlessness
**CV:** Cardiac arrest, hypertension, hypotension, potentially fatal arrhythmias (such as torsades de pointes and ventricular tachycardia), prolonged QT interval, sinus tachycardia
**EENT:** Fixed upward position of eyeballs, laryngospasm
**MS:** Spasms of tongue, face, neck, and back muscles
**RESP:** Bronchospasm

## Nursing Considerations
•WARNING Use droperidol cautiously in patients over age 65 and in patients with alcoholism, bradycardia, heart failure, hypokalemia, hypomagnesemia, parkinsonism, or preexisting QT-interval prolongation because they're at increased risk for prolonged QT interval and potentially fatal adverse reactions. Patients who take drugs that prolong the QT interval, such as some antiarrhythmics and benzodiazepines, and patients who take drugs that may cause an electrolyte imbalance, such as diuretics and laxatives, are also at increased risk.
•Expect a 12-lead ECG to be performed on all patients before droperidol administration to verify the absence of prolonged QT interval. Monitor ECG continuously for 2 to 3 hours after administering drug. Also monitor serum electrolyte levels to detect electrolyte imbalances.
•Use droperidol cautiously in patients with cardiac disease, who may not be able to compensate for drug's hypotensive effect. Monitor vital signs, including blood pressure, frequently. Be aware that hypertension and tachycardia may occur in patients with a history of pheochromocytoma.
•Expect altered level of consciousness to last up to 12 hours after drug is given. Expect dosage to be reduced if patient is taking an opioid analgesic.
•If drug causes extrapyramidal reactions, such as restlessness, dystonia, and oculogyric crisis, expect to administer an anticholinergic, such as benztropine or diphenhydramine. Be sure to maintain a patent airway and oxygenation.
•If severe hypotension develops, expect to administer phenylephrine. If hypotension is related to hypovolemia, expect to administer fluids.

## PATIENT TEACHING
•Advise patient to immediately report palpitations or faintness, which may indicate an abnormal cardiac rhythm.
•Instruct patient to ask for help with ambulation on the first postoperative day because altered consciousness may last up to 12 hours.
•Caution patient to avoid drinking alcohol, taking CNS depressants, driving, and operating machinery for 24 hours after receiving droperidol.

# drospirenone and estradiol

Angeliq

## Class and Category
*Chemical:* Synthetic progestin and spirono-lactone analog (drospirenone), estrogenic steroid hormone derivative (estradiol)
*Therapeutic:* Ovarian hormone replacement
*Pregnancy category:* X

## Indications and Dosages
➤ *To treat moderate to severe vasomotor symptoms associated with menopause; to treat moderate to severe vulvar and vaginal atrophy associated with menopause*
**TABLETS**
**Adult females.** 0.5 mg drospirenone and 1 mg estradiol (1 tablet) q.d.

## Contraindications
Active deep vein thrombosis, pulmonary embolism, or history of these conditions; adrenal insufficiency; hepatic disorders; hypersensitivity to drospirenone, estradiol, or their components; known or suspected breast cancer or history of breast cancer from estrogen use; known or suspected estrogen-dependent cancer; new or recent (within past year) CVA or MI; post hysterectomy; pregnancy; renal insufficiency; undiagnosed abnormal genital bleeding

## Interactions
**DRUGS**
**drospirenone component only**
*ACE inhibitors, angiotensin receptor blockers, heparin, NSAIDs, potassium-sparing diuretics, potassium supplements:* Increased risk of hyperkalemia

**estradiol component only**
*barbiturates, carbamazepine, hydantoins, rifabutin, rifampin:* Possibly reduced activity of estradiol
*clarithromycin, erythromycin, itraconazole, ketoconazole, ritonivir:* Decreased metabolism and possible increased adverse effects of estradiol
*corticosteroids:* Increased therapeutic and toxic effects of corticosteroids
*cyclosporine:* Increased risk of hepatotoxicity and nephrotoxicity
*didanosine, lamivudine, zalcitabine:* Possibly pancreatitis
*hepatotoxic drugs (such as isoniazid):* Increased risk of hepatitis and hepatotoxicity
*oral antidiabetic drugs:* Decreased therapeutic effects of these drugs
*warfarin:* Decreased or increased anticoagulant effect
**FOODS**
*Grapefruit juice:* Decreased metabolism and possibly increased adverse effects of estradiol
**ACTIVITIES**
*Smoking:* Increased risk of CVA, pulmonary embolism, thrombophlebitis, and transient ischemic attack

## Mechanism of Action
Drospirenone counters the estrogenic effects associated with menopause by decreasing the number of nuclear estradiol receptors and suppressing epithelial DNA synthesis in endometrial tissue. It also is an aldosterone antagonist, which increases excretion of sodium and water.

Estradiol increases the rate of DNA and RNA synthesis in cells of female reproductive organs, pituitary gland, hypothalamus, and other target organs. In the hypothalamus, estrogens reduce release of gonadotropin-releasing hormone, which decreases pituitary release of follicle-stimulating hormone and luteinizing hormone. In women, these hormones are required for normal genitourinary and other essential body functions. At the cellular level, estrogens increase cervical secretions, cause endometrial cell proliferation, and improve uterine tone. Estrogen replacement helps maintain genitourinary function and reduces vasomotor symptoms when estrogen production declines as a result of menopause, surgical removal of ovaries, or other estrogen deficiency states.

## Adverse Reactions

**CNS:** Chorea, CVA, dementia, depression, dizziness, exacerbation of epilepsy, headache, irritability, migraine, mood disturbance, nervousness, porphyria

**CV:** Hypertension, hypertriglyceridemia, MI, peripheral edema, pulmonary embolism, thromboembolism, thrombophlebitis

**EENT:** Diplopia, intolerance of contact lenses, retinal vascular thrombosis, sinusitis, vision changes or loss

**ENDO:** Breast enlargement, pain, tenderness, or tumors; endometrial hyperplasia; galactorrhea; gynecomastia; hyperglycemia; nipple discharge

**GI:** Abdominal cramps or pain, anorexia, bloating, constipation, diarrhea, elevated liver function test results, enlargement of hepatic hemangiomas, gallbladder obstruction, hepatitis, increased appetite, nausea, pancreatitis, vomiting

**GU:** Amenorrhea, breakthrough bleeding, cervical erosion, clear vaginal discharge, dysmenorrhea, endometiral or ovarian tumors, increased libido, leukorrhea, prolonged or heavy menstrual bleeding, vaginal candidiasis

**MS:** Arthralgias, back or extremity pain, leg cramps

**RESP:** Exacerbation of asthma, upper respiratory tract infection

**SKIN:** Alopecia, chloasma, erythema multiforme or nodosum, hirsutism, jaundice, melasma, pruritus, purpura, rash, urticaria

**Other:** Anaphylaxis, angioedema, flulike symptoms, folic acid deficiency, hypercalcemia (with bone metastases), hypocalcemia, hyperkalemia, hyponatremia, weight gain or loss

## Nursing Considerations

•Use drospirenone and estradiol cautiously in women with asthma, diabetes mellitus, epilepsy, migraines, porphyria, systemic lupus erythematosus, or hepatic hemangiomas because estrogens such as estradiol can worsen these conditions.

•Give drospirenone and estradiol with or immediately after food to decrease nausea.

•WARNING Assess patient for possible intolerance of contact lenses or changes in vision or visual acuity because estrogens can cause keratoconus. Be prepared to stop drug immediately, as prescribed, if patient experiences sudden partial or complete loss of vision or sudden onset of diplopia or migraine.

•If patient takes warfarin, monitor PT for loss of anticoagulant effect because estrogens increase production of clotting factors VII, VIII, IX, and X and promote platelet aggregation.

•Watch for elevated liver function test results because estrogens and progestins may worsen such conditions as acute intermittent or variegate hepatic porphyria.

•Monitor patient's electrolyte levels, especially early in therapy, as ordered, because drospirenone has antialdosterone activity, which may increase serum potassium and decrease serum sodium levels in high-risk patients.

•Closely monitor patient's blood pressure. A few patients may experience a substantial increase as an indiosyncratic reaction to estrogen. Monitor hypertensive patients for increased blood pressure because estrogens may cause fluid retention.

•If patient has diabetes mellitus, check serum glucose level often because estrogens may decrease insulin sensitivity and alter glucose tolerance.

•Expect to stop drospirenone and estradiol in any woman who develops signs or symptoms of cardiovascular disease, such as CVA, MI, pulmonary embolism, or venous thrombosis.

•Be aware that drospirenone and estradiol may worsen mood disorders, including depression. Monitor patient for depression, mood changes, anxiety, fatigue, dizziness, or insomnia.

•WARNING Be aware that severe hypercalcemia may occur in patients with bone metastasis from breast cancer because estrogens influence the metabolism of calcium and phosphorus. Monitor patient for toxic effects of increased calcium absorption in patients predisposed to hypercalcemia or nephrolithiasis.

•Assess skin for melasma (tan or brown patches), which may develop on forehead, cheeks, temples, and upper lip. These patches may persist after drug is stopped.

•Monitor thyroid function in patients with hypothyroidism; long-term use of estradiol may disrupt thyroid therapy.

•Expect to stop drospirenone and estradiol therapy several weeks before patient undergoes major surgery, as prescribed, because prolonged immobilization poses a risk of thromboembolism.

## PATIENT TEACHING

•Before therapy starts, explain risks involved in estrogen/progestin therapy, such as increased risk of breast or endometrial cancer, cardiovascular disease, dementia, gallbladder disease, and vision abnormalities.
•Inform patient that a cyclic combination regimen of drospirenone and estradiol may cause monthly withdrawal bleeding.
•Instruct patient to avoid eating large amounts of foods high in potassium, such as bananas, oranges, or spinach, or using salt substitutes that contain potassium.
•Instruct patient to report any abnormal signs and symptoms to prescriber.
•Stress importance of having follow-up visits every 3 to 6 months to determine drug's effectiveness at relieving menopausal symptoms and to test for adverse reactions.

# drotrecogin alfa (activated)

## (recombinant human activated protein C)

Xigris

## Class and Category

*Chemical:* Serine protease glycoprotein
*Therapeutic:* Anti-inflammatory, antithrombolytic
*Pregnancy category:* C

## Indications and Dosages

➤ *To reduce high risk of death in patients with severe sepsis (associated with acute organ dysfunction)*

**I.V. INFUSION**
**Adults.** 24 mcg/kg/hr for 96 hr.

## Incompatibilities

Don't infuse any other drugs or solutions, except $D_5W$, NS, LR, or dextrose and saline mixtures, through the same I.V. line as drotrecogin alfa.

## Contraindications

Active internal bleeding; evidence of cerebral herniation; hemorrhagic stroke within the past 3 months; hypersensitivity to drotrecogin alfa or its components; intracranial or intraspinal surgery or severe head trauma within the past 2 months; intracranial neoplasm or lesion; presence of epidural catheter; trauma with an increased risk of life-threatening bleeding

## Mechanism of Action

Interferes with a number of the body's responses to severe sepsis, including increased thrombin generation and fibrin formation, impaired fibrinolysis, and systemic inflammation. Drotrecogin alfa produces its antithrombotic effect by inhibiting factors Va and VIIIa and exhibits indirect profibrinolytic activity by inhibiting plasminogen activator inhibitor-1 and limiting the generation of activated thrombin-activatable-fibrinolysis-inhibitor.

Drotrecogin may produce its anti-inflammatory effect by inhibiting production of human tumor necrosis factor and other cytokines, preventing leukocyte adhesion to selectins, and limiting thrombin-induced inflammatory responses in the microvascular endothelium.

## Interactions

### DRUGS

*abciximab, eptifibatide, and other glycoprotein IIb/IIIa inhibitors; aspirin and other platelet inhibitors; heparin; oral anticoagulants; thrombolytics:* Increased risk of bleeding

## Adverse Reactions

**CNS:** Intracranial hemorrhage
**CV:** Intrathoracic bleeding
**GI:** GI, intra-abdominal, or retroperitoneal bleeding
**GU:** Genitourinary bleeding
**HEME:** Prolonged APTT
**SKIN:** Ecchymosis

## Nursing Considerations

•Be aware that drotrecogin alfa is used only for patients with severe sepsis who are at high risk for death, as determined by an APACHE II score, which is a method of assessing the risk of mortality. Patients with only single-organ dysfunction who are recovering from recent surgery may not be candidates for drotrecogin alfa despite an adequate APACHE II score.
•Reconstitute 5-mg and 20-mg vials of drotrecogin alfa by slowly adding 2.5 ml or 10 ml of sterile water for injection, respec-

tively, to yield a concentration of 2 mg/ml. Gently swirl—don't shake—vial until powder is completely dissolved. Use immediately or store for up to 3 hours at 15° to 30° C (59° to 86° F).

•Add reconstituted drug to NS by directing stream to side of bag to minimize agitation. Gently invert the bag to mix; don't shake. Dilute drug to a final concentration of 100 to 200 mg/ml if it will be administered by I.V. infusion pump and to a final concentration of 100 to 1,000 mg/ml if it will be administered by syringe pump. Be aware that infusion bag shouldn't be transported by a mechanical delivery system, such as a tube delivery system between the pharmacy and nursing unit.

•Prime infusion set for 15 minutes at a flow rate of 5 ml/hour when infusing a concentration of less than 200 mg/ml at a rate of less than 5 ml/hour. Use prepared I.V. solution within 12 hours.

•Administer drotrecogin alfa through a dedicated I.V. line or a dedicated lumen of a multilumen central venous catheter. Don't infuse any other drugs or solutions—other than $D_5W$, NS, LR, or dextrose and saline mixtures—through the same line.

•Be aware that total duration of the infusion must equal 96 hours, even if you need to interrupt it for a period. For example, if you calculate that infusion should end on 5 p.m. Friday, but then have to stop to give the patient blood for 2 hours on Thursday, add those 2 hours to your estimated completion time, which would then be 7 p.m. Friday.

•**WARNING** Monitor patient closely for signs of bleeding; if bleeding occurs, stop drotrecogin alfa infusion immediately and notify prescriber. Patients at increased risk for bleeding include those with chronic severe hepatic disease, intracranial arteriovenous malformation or aneurysm, known bleeding diathesis, recent (in the past 6 weeks) GI bleeding, or recent (in the past 3 months) ischemic stroke; those receiving concurrent therapeutic heparin (15 U/kg/hour or more); those who have recently received thrombolytic therapy (in the past 3 days), aspirin (at dosage greater than 650 mg/day) or other platelet inhibitors (in the past 7 days), or oral anticoagulants or glycoprotein IIb/IIIa inhibitors (in the past 7 days); those with any other condition in which bleeding would

constitute a significant hazard or be difficult to manage because of its location; and those with a platelet count less than 30,000 × $10^6$/L or PT (as INR) greater than 3.0.

•Expect to discontinue drotrecogin alfa 2 hours before an invasive surgical or other procedure that poses a risk of bleeding and to resume administration immediately after uncomplicated, less-invasive procedures or 12 hours after major invasive procedures or surgery at the same rate of 24 mg/kg/hour, as prescribed.

•Be aware that drotrecogin alfa may prolong APTT during administration; PT may need to be used to monitor coagulopathy status during treatment.

•Before using drotrecogin alfa, refrigerate it at 2° to 8° C (36° to 46° F); don't freeze it. Protect from heat and direct sunlight.

**PATIENT TEACHING**

•Teach patient about adverse reactions to drotrecogin alfa, including bleeding from gums or nose or increased bruising. Instruct her to immediately report any signs of bleeding.

•Reassure patient that she'll be monitored closely throughout therapy.

# duloxetine hydrochloride

Cymbalta

## Class and Category

*Chemical:* Selective serotonin and norepinephrine reuptake inhibitor
*Therapeutic:* Antidepressant, neuropathic pain reliever
*Pregnancy category:* C

## Indications and Dosages

➤ *To treat major depressive disorder*

**E.R. CAPSULES**

**Adults.** 20 mg b.i.d. Alternatively, 60 mg q.d. or 30 mg b.i.d.

➤ *To relieve neuropathic pain associated with diabetic peripheral neuropathy*

**E.R. CAPSULES**

**Adults.** 60 mg q.d.

| Route | Onset | Peak | Duration |
|-------|-------|------|----------|
| P.O. | Unknown | 6 hr | Unknown |

## Mechanism of Action
Inhibits neuronal serotonin, norepineph-rine, and dopamine reuptake to potentiate serotonergic and noradrenergic activity in the CNS. These activities may elevate mood and inhibit pain signals stemming from peripheral nerves adversely affected by chronically elevated serum glucose levels.

## Contraindications
Hypersensitivity to duloxetine or its compo-nents, uncontrolled angle-closure glaucoma, use within 14 days of MAO inhibitor therapy

## Interactions
**DRUGS**
*amiodarone, celecoxib, cimetidine, erythro-mycin, fluoxetine, fluvoxamine, haloperidol, ketoconazole, methadone, paroxetine, quini-dine, quinolones, ritonavir:* Increased blood duloxetine level
*amiodarone, amitriptyline, desipramine, fle-cainide, haloperidol, imipramine, methadone, nortriptyline, phenothiazines, propafenone, ritonavir, thioridazine:* Increased blood levels of these drugs
*CNS drugs:* Increased effect of duloxetine
*MAO inhibitors:* Serious, sometimes fatal, autonomic instability, hyperthermia, my-oclonus, rigidity
*plasma protein binders (warfarin, phenytoin):* Increased free concentration of these drugs and increased risk of adverse reactions
**ACTIVITIES**
*alcohol use:* Increased risk of hepatotoxicity

## Adverse Reactions
**CNS:** Anxiety, asthenia, dizziness, fatigue, fever, headache, insomnia, somnolence, tremor
**CV:** Hypertension, palpitations, peripheral edema
**EENT:** Blurred vision, dry mouth, naso-pharyngitis, pharyngitis
**ENDO:** Hot flashes
**GI:** Anorexia, constipation, diarrhea, indiges-tion, nausea, upper abdominal pain, vomiting
**GU:** Abnormal orgasm, decreased libido, erectile or ejaculatory dysfunction, urinary frequency
**MS:** Arthralgia, back pain, extremity pain, muscle cramp, myalgia

**RESP:** Cough, upper respiratory tract infec-tion
**SKIN:** Diaphoresis, pruritus
**Other:** Weight loss

## Nursing Considerations
• Avoid giving duloxetine to patients with se-vere renal impairment or end-stage renal disease that requires hemodialysis because blood drug levels increase significantly in these patients. Also avoid duloxetine in pa-tients with hepatic insufficiency because drug is metabolized by the liver.
• Use duloxetine cautiously in patients with delayed gastric emptying because drug has an enteric coating that resists dissolution until it reaches an area where pH exceeds 5.5.
• Give duloxetine cautiously to patients with a history of mania (which it may activate) and patients with a seizure disorder (because drug effects aren't known in these patients).
• Obtain baseline blood pressure before du-loxetine therapy starts, and assess it periodi-cally thereafter for increases.
• Monitor patient's hepatic function, as or-dered, because drug may increase the risk of hepatotoxicity.
• If patient takes duloxetine for depression, watch closely for suicidal tendencies, espe-cially when therapy starts or dosage changes.
**PATIENT TEACHING**
• Tell patient to take capsule whole and not to chew it, crush it, or sprinkle contents on food or liquids because doing so alters en-teric coating and may affect drug absorption.
• Inform patient that full effect of drug may take weeks; stress the importance of continu-ing to take drug as directed.
• Advise against excessive alcohol consump-tion while taking duloxetine because it may increase risk of hepatic dysfunction.
• Advise patient not to stop duloxetine abruptly because adverse reactions may occur. Explain that drug will be stopped gradually.
• Instruct patient to notify prescriber of any serious or troublesome adverse effects.
• Advise patient to avoid hazardous activities until drug's CNS effects are known.
• Instruct female patients of childbearing po-tential to notify prescriber if they are, could be, or wish to become pregnant during ther-apy; duloxetine may cause adverse reactions in neonates exposed to it during the third trimester.

**D**

# dutasteride

Avodart

## Class and Category

*Chemical:* Synthetic 4-azasteroid compound
*Therapeutic:* Benign prostatic hyperplasia agent
*Pregnancy category:* X

## Indications and Dosages

➤ *To treat symptomatic benign prostatic hyperplasia*

**CAPSULES**
**Adult males.** 0.5 mg q.d.

## Contraindications

Children; females; hypersensitivity to dutasteride, its components, or other 5-alpha reductase inhibitors

## Interactions

**DRUGS**
*cimetidine, ciprofloxacin, diltiazem, keto-conazole, ritonavir, verapamil, and other CYP3A4 inhibitors:* Risk of decreased metabolism and enhanced effects of dutasteride

## Adverse Reactions

**ENDO:** Gynecomastia, increased serum testosterone and thyroid-stimulating hormone levels
**GU:** Decreased ejaculatory volume, decreased libido, impotence
**SKIN:** Localized edema, pruritus, rash, urticaria

## Nursing Considerations

•**WARNING** Be aware that dutasteride is absorbed through the skin. If you are female and pregnant or of childbearing age, do *not*

## Mechanism of Action

Dutasteride reduces prostate gland enlargement by inhibiting the conversion of the male hormone testosterone to its active metabolite, 5-alpha dihydrotestosterone (DHT). DHT is the principal hormone that stimulates prostate cells to grow. As men age, they may become more sensitive to the effects of DHT, resulting in an excessive growth of prostatic cells and enlargement of the prostate. This condition, known as benign prostatic hyperplasia, may cause such signs and symptoms as urinary hesitancy, urinary urgency, and nocturia.

The intracellular enzyme 5-alpha-reductase (5α-R), which is present in the liver, prostate, and skin, converts testosterone to DHT, as shown below left. The two forms of 5α-R are type 1 and type 2. Dutasteride, a dual 5α-R inhibitor, deactivates both forms. When 5α-R is inhibited by dutasteride, the production of DHT is suppressed, as shown below right. With less circulating DHT, the prostate gland becomes smaller and the patient experiences an improvement in his symptoms.

handle the dutasteride capsule when administering it to a patient.
•Expect patient to undergo a digital rectal examination of the prostate before and periodically during dutasteride therapy.
•Anticipate the need to obtain a new baseline prostate-specific antigen (PSA) value after 3 to 6 months of treatment because dutasteride can decrease PSA concentration by 40% to 50%.

**PATIENT TEACHING**
•WARNING Urge patient and female partners to use reliable contraceptive method during dutasteride therapy because semen of men who take drug can harm male fetuses. Caution women and children against handling capsules.
•Advise patient to inform prescriber if he has liver disease.
•Explain how to take drug properly, and advise patient to follow instructions that accompany drug. Instruct him to swallow capsule whole and to notify pharmacist if capsules are cracked or leaking.
•Inform patient that drug may decrease ejaculatory volume and libido and may cause impotence.
•Instruct patient to postpone blood donations for 6 months after final dose to avoid transmitting dutasteride to a pregnant female during a blood transfusion.
•Urge patient to have periodic follow-up evaluations.

# dyphylline

Dilor, Lufyllin

## Class and Category
*Chemical*: Xanthine derivative
*Therapeutic*: Bronchodilator
*Pregnancy category*: C

## Indications and Dosages
➤ *To prevent or relieve bronchospasm from acute and chronic bronchial asthma, chronic bronchitis, and emphysema*

**ELIXIR, TABLETS**
**Adults.** Up to 15 mg/kg q 6 hr.
**I.M. INJECTION**
**Adults.** *Initial:* 500 mg. *Maintenance:* 250 to 500 mg q 2 to 6 hr, as needed.

## Contraindications
Hypersensitivity to dyphylline, xanthines, or their components; peptic ulcer disease; seizure disorder (unless controlled by anticonvulsant therapy)

## Mechanism of Action
May cause bronchodilation by inhibiting phosphodiesterase enzymes. These enzymes normally inactivate cAMP and cGMP, which are responsible for bronchial smooth-muscle relaxation. Other possible mechanisms of action include calcium translocation, prostaglandin antagonism, catecholamine stimulation, and adenosine-receptor antagonism.

## Interactions
**DRUGS**
*beta blockers:* Possibly inhibited bronchodilation by dyphylline
*ephedrine:* Possibly increased frequency of insomnia, nausea, and nervousness
*hydrocarbon inhalation anesthetics:* Possibly increased risk of ventricular arrhythmias
*probenecid:* Possibly decreased renal excretion of dyphylline
*sucralfate:* Possibly adsorption of dyphylline if drugs given within 2 hours of each other

## Adverse Reactions
**CNS:** Headache, insomnia, irritability, nervousness, seizures, tremor
**CV:** Arrhythmias, hypotension, tachycardia
**GI:** Diarrhea, gastroesophageal reflux, nausea, vomiting
**GU:** Increased diuresis

## Nursing Considerations
•Inspect I.M. form of dyphylline for precipitate. If precipitate is present, discard drug and obtain a new ampule.
•Give oral drug at least 1 hour after meals for best absorption. However, if drug causes GI distress, give it with food if prescribed.
•Don't give parenteral drug by I.V. route.
•Evaluate for therapeutic response: decreased respiratory rate and effort.
•Assess for signs of dyphylline toxicity, including seizures and ventricular tachycardia.
**PATIENT TEACHING**
•Instruct patient to take oral dyphylline with a full glass of water and on an empty stomach to promote absorption.
•Advise patient to consult prescriber about taking drug with food if she experiences GI distress.

# E·F

## efalizumab

Raptiva

### Class and Category

*Chemical:* Recombinant humanized IgG1
kappa isotype monoclonal antibody
*Therapeutic:* Immunosuppressant
*Pregnancy category:* C

### Indications and Dosages

➤ *To treat chronic, moderate-to-severe
plaque psoriasis in patients who are
candidates for systemic therapy or phototherapy*

**S.C. INJECTION**

**Adults.** *Initial:* 0.7 mg/kg S.C. as a single
dose. Maintenance: 1 mg/kg S.C. weekly, beginning 1 wk after initial dose. *Maximum:*
200 mg/injection weekly.

### Incompatibilities

Don't add any other medications to efalizumab solution, and don't reconstitute with
any other diluent except that provided by
manufacturer.

### Contraindications

Hypersensitivity to efalizumab or its components, or to murine or humanized monoclonal antibodies

### Interactions

**DRUGS**

*other immunosuppressants:* Additive effects
and increased risk of adverse reactions or infection

### Mechanism of Action

Inhibits T-cell activation and reactivation,
which may play a central role in the development of the silvery plaques of psoriasis.
The disorder begins when T cells bind to
Langerhans cells in the dermis. These cells
mediate immune responses, and protect the
skin from antigens. When T cells are activated by the psoriasis antigen, the T-cell
surface molecule, leukocyte function anti-
gen-1 (LFA-1), binds to the intracellular
adhesion molecule-1 (ICAM-1) on Langerhans cells. Then T cells move through

blood vessel walls and into the dermis and
epidermis, where they're reactivated by another exposure to the psoriasis antigen. The
T cells then bind to keratinocytes and endothelial cells, causing hyperproliferation,
cytokine secretion, dermal and epidermal
thickening, and plaque formation.

Efalizumab binds to the CD11a, a subunit of LFA-1 on T cells, blocking its interaction with ICAM-1. This action inhibits T-
cell activation and reactivation, preventing
the underlying mechanism of psoriasis.

*vaccines (killed or live virus):* Possibly suppressed immune response and increased adverse effects of vaccine

## Adverse Reactions

**CNS:** Asthenia, chills, fever, headache
**EENT:** Laryngospasm
**GI:** Nausea, vomiting
**HEME:** Hemolytic anemia, leukocytosis, lymphocytosis, thrombocytopenia
**MS:** Arthralgia, arthritis, back pain, myalgia, myositis
**RESP:** Asthma, dyspnea, eosinophilic pneumonitis
**SKIN:** Acne, erythema multiforme, maculopapular rash, photosensitivity, toxic epidermal necrolysis, urticaria, worsening psoriasis
**Other:** Alkaline phosphatase elevation; angioedema; flulike symptoms; generalized pain; serious infections, such as necrotizing fasciitis, tuberculous pneumonia, bacterial sepsis with seeding of distant sites, severe pneumonia with neutropenia, and worsening cellulitis despite treatment; malignancies; serum sickness–like reaction

## Nursing Considerations

•Be aware that efalizumab may increase infection risk and may reactivate latent, chronic infections; therefore, it shouldn't be given to patients with acute or serious infections. Also exercise caution when administering drug to a patient with a chronic infection or a history of recurrent infections.
•Administer efalizumab using the sterile disposable syringe and needle provided.
•Prepare injection by first removing the cap from the prefilled syringe containing sterile water and attaching the needle to the syringe. Remove the plastic cap protecting the rubber stopper of the vial, and wipe the top of the rubber stopper with alcohol. Inject the 1.3 ml of sterile water from the prefilled syringe into the vial and swirl gently to dissolve. Don't shake the vial because foaming will occur. Be aware that dissolution takes less than 5 minutes. Use for only one dose; administer immediately if possible, although the reconstituted solution may be stored at room temperature for up to 8 hours.
•Inject efalizumab into thigh, abdomen, buttocks, or upper arm. Rotate injection sites. After administration, discard any unused reconstituted solution.
•Monitor patient for first-dose reactions, which may include headache, fever, nausea,

and vomiting. Notify prescriber of reactions because dosage may need to be altered.
•Monitor patient throughout efalizumab therapy for signs and symptoms of serious infections, such as abscess, aseptic meningitis, bronchitis, cellulitis, gastroenteritis, Legionnaire's disease, pneumonia, sepsis, and vertebral osteomyelitis. Notify prescriber immediately if you suspect a serious infection because hospitalization may be required.
•Monitor patient's platelet count, as ordered, monthly initially and then every 3 months with continued therapy. If thrombocytopenia develops, notify prescriber, and expect to stop drug. Observe patient for such signs of bleeding as ecchymosis, epistaxis, hematemesis, hematuria, melena, and petechiae.
•Assess patient's psoriasis for improvement or worsening throughout treatment. If psoriasis worsens, notify prescriber because efalizumab may need to be discontinued.
•Monitor patient for severe arthritis pain; although uncommon, drug may cause new or recurrent arthritis, including psoriatic arthritis, that may be severe.

**PATIENT TEACHING**

•Teach patient or caregiver how to administer efalizumab as an S.C. injection.
•Alert patient to the increased risk for malignancies during efalizumab therapy. Review common warning signs, and advise patient to notify prescriber if any occur.
•Inform patient about the increased risk of bleeding; urge him to avoid injuries and to use a soft toothbrush and an electric razor.
•Instruct patient and family to watch for and report abdominal or lower-back pain, black stools, bleeding gums, bloody urine, excessive menstrual bleeding, nosebleeds, and severe headaches.
•Instruct patient not to receive acellular, live, or attenuated live-virus vaccines during therapy. Urge him to avoid people who have received such vaccines or to wear a protective mask when he's around them.
•Caution patient to avoid contact with people who have infections during therapy because efalizumab causes immunosuppression.
•Tell women of childbearing age to notify prescriber promptly if they suspect pregnancy during or within 6 weeks of discontinuing efalizumab therapy; drug effects on fetal development are unknown. Urge them to enroll in the Raptiva Pregnancy Registry by calling 1-877-RAPTIVA.

# eflornithine hydrochloride

## (alpha-difluoromethyl-ornithine, DFMO)

Ornidyl

### Class and Category

*Chemical:* Difluoromethylornithine
*Therapeutic:* Antiprotozoal
*Pregnancy category:* C

### Indications and Dosages

➤ *To treat the meningoencephalitic stage of* Trypanosoma brucei gambiense *infection (sleeping sickness)*

**I.V. INFUSION**

**Adults.** 100 mg/kg given over at least 45 min q 6 hr for 14 days.

| Route | Onset | Peak | Duration |
|-------|-------|------|----------|
| I.V. | Unknown | 4 to 6 hr | Unknown |

### Mechanism of Action

Inhibits the enzyme ornithine decarboxylase, which is needed for decarboxylation of ornithine. This process is the first step in polyamine synthesis, which is needed for protozoal cell division and differentiation.

### Incompatibilities

Don't administer eflornithine with any other drug.

### Contraindications

Hypersensitivity to eflornithine or its components

### Adverse Reactions

**CNS:** Asthenia, dizziness, headache, seizures
**EENT:** Hearing loss
**GI:** Abdominal pain, anorexia, diarrhea, vomiting
**HEME:** Anemia, eosinophilia, leukopenia, myelosuppression, thrombocytopenia
**Other:** Alopecia, facial edema

### Nursing Considerations

•Plan to reduce eflornithine dosage as prescribed, based on renal function. Monitor creatinine clearance in patients with renal dysfunction.

•Before infusion, dilute eflornithine concentrate with sterile water for injection. Using strict aseptic technique, withdraw the contents of a 100-ml vial and inject 25 ml into each of four I.V. diluent bags that contain 100 ml of sterile water. The resulting solution contains 40 mg/ml of eflornithine (5,000 mg of eflornithine in 125 ml total volume).

•Store bags of diluted eflornithine at 4° C (39° F) to reduce the risk of contamination. Use diluted drug within 24 hours.

•Expect to monitor the patient's CBC, including platelet count, before eflornithine treatment, twice weekly during treatment, and weekly after therapy stops until the patient's hematologic values return to baseline.

•Take infection-control and bleeding precautions because drug may cause myelosuppression. Adjust dosage or stop therapy as prescribed, based on severity.

•Take seizure precautions during eflornithine therapy.

•Consult prescriber about the need for serial audiography, if appropriate.

•Store undiluted vials of eflornithine at room temperature, and protect from freezing and light.

**PATIENT TEACHING**

•Stress the importance of follow-up visits because the risk of relapse lasts for 24 months after treatment.

•Teach patient how to follow infection-control and bleeding precautions if myelosuppression occurs.

•Warn patient about risk of seizures; advise against performing potentially hazardous activities during therapy.

# eletriptan hydrobromide

Relpax

### Class and Category

*Chemical:* Serotonin 5-HT$_{1D}$–receptor agonist
*Therapeutic:* Antimigraine agent
*Pregnancy category:* C

### Indications and Dosages

➤ *To relieve acute migraine attacks with or without aura*

**TABLETS**

**Adults.** *Initial:* 20 or 40 mg as a single dose. Repeated in 2 hr, as needed and ordered. *Maximum:* 40 mg as single dose, 80 mg daily.

E
F

## Mechanism of Action

May stimulate 5-HT$_1$ receptors, causing selective vasoconstriction of inflamed and dilated cranial blood vessels in carotid circulation, which decreases carotid arterial blood flow and relieves acute migraines.

## Contraindications

Bibasilar or hemiplegic migraine, cardiovascular disease (significant), cerebrovascular syndromes (CVA, transient ischemic attack), hepatic impairment (severe), hypersensitivity to eletriptan or components, ischemic bowel disease, ischemic or vasospastic coronary artery disease (CAD), peripheral vascular disease, uncontrolled hypertension, use within 24 hours of another serotonin 5-HT$_1$–receptor agonist or ergot-type drug, use within 72 hours of a potent PYP3A4 inhibitor

## Interactions

**DRUGS**

*clarithromycin, ketoconazole, itraconazole, nefazodone, nelfinavir, ritonavir, troleandomycin and other potent CYP3A4 inhibitors:* Increased metabolism of eletriptan and decreased blood eletriptan level
*ergot-containing drugs, 5-HT$_1$-receptor agonists:* Possibly additive or prolonged vasoconstrictive effects
*fluoxetine, fluvoxamine, paroxetine, sertraline:* Increased risk of weakness, hyperreflexia, and incoordination

## Adverse Reactions

**CNS:** Asthenia, dizziness, headache, paresthesia, somnolence, tiredness, weakness
**CV:** Chest tightness, pain, or pressure; coronary artery vasospasm; hypertension, MI or myocardial ischemia (transient); ventricular fibrillation or tachycardia
**EENT:** Dry mouth, throat tightness
**GI:** Abdominal pain, cramps, discomfort, or pressure; dysphagia; indigestion; nausea
**SKIN:** Flushing
**Other:** Feeling of warmth, pain, or pressure

## Nursing Considerations

•Ensure that patients who are at risk for CAD undergo a satisfactory CV evaluation before you administer the first dose of eletriptan and that they have a periodic re-evaluation of their cardiac status during intermittent long-term therapy.
•Obtain an ECG immediately after first dose of drug in patients who have CV risk factors but who have had a satisfactory CV evaluation because of the drug's potential to cause coronary vasospasm.
•Evaluate patient for CV signs and symptoms after administration of eletriptan and notify prescriber if they occur. Expect drug to be withheld, as ordered, while patient undergoes an extensive CV workup, and discontinued if abnormalities are detected.
•Monitor patient's blood pressure during therapy because of drug's potential to increase blood pressure.

**PATIENT TEACHING**

•Advise patient to take eletriptan as soon as possible after onset of migraine symptoms.
•Urge patient to contact prescriber and avoid taking drug if headache symptoms aren't typical.
•Remind patient not to exceed prescribed daily dose.
•Instruct patient to seek emergency care for chest, jaw, or neck tightness after taking drug because these may indicate adverse CV reactions; subsequent doses may require ECG monitoring.
•Urge patient to report palpitations to prescriber.
•Advise patient to avoid potentially hazardous activities until drug's CNS effects are known.
•Encourage yearly ophthalmic examinations for patients who require prolonged eletriptan therapy.
•Instruct patient to inform prescriber of all drugs he's taking, including OTC products and herbal remedies.

# enalapril maleate

Vasotec

# enalaprilat

Vasotec I.V.

## Class and Category

*Chemical:* Dicarbocyl-containing ACE inhibitor
*Therapeutic:* Antihypertensive
*Pregnancy category:* C (first trimester), D (later trimesters)

# Indications and Dosages

➤ *To control hypertension*

**TABLETS**

**Adults.** *Initial:* 5 mg q.d., increased after 1 to 2 wk, as needed. *Maintenance:* 10 to 40 mg q.d. or in divided doses b.i.d.

**Children.** 0.08 mg/kg q.d., titrated according to blood pressure response up to 5 mg q.d. *Maximum:* 0.58 mg/kg/dose or 40 mg/dose.

**I.V. INJECTION**

**Adults.** 1.25 mg q 6 hr.

**DOSAGE ADJUSTMENT** Initial dose reduced to 2.5 mg P.O. or 0.625 mg I.V. for patients who have sodium and water depletion from diuretic therapy, are receiving diuretics, or have a creatinine clearance below 30 ml/min/ 1.73 m². If response to I.V. dose is inadequate after 1 hr, I.V. dose of 0.625 mg is repeated and therapy continued at 1.25 mg q 6 hr.

➤ *To treat heart failure*

**TABLETS**

**Adults.** *Initial:* 2.5 mg q.d. or b.i.d., increased after 1 to 2 wk, as needed. *Maintenance:* 5 to 40 mg q.d. or in divided doses b.i.d.

➤ *To treat asymptomatic left ventricular dysfunction*

**TABLETS**

**Adults.** *Initial:* 2.5 mg b.i.d., increased to 20 mg/day in divided doses.

**DOSAGE ADJUSTMENT** Initial dosage reduced to 2.5 mg q.d. and, if possible, diuretic dosage reduced in patients who have a serum sodium level below 130 mEq/L or a serum creatinine level above 1.6 mg/dl.

| Route | Onset | Peak | Duration |
|---|---|---|---|
| P.O. | 1 hr | 4 to 6 hr | About 24 hr |
| I.V. | 15 min | 1 to 4 hr | About 6 hr |

# Contraindications

History of angioedema from previous ACE inhibitor; hypersensitivity to enalapril, enalaprilat, or their components

# Interactions

**DRUGS**

*allopurinol, bone marrow depressants (such as amphotericin B and methotrexate), procainamide, systemic corticosteroids:* Possibly increased risk of fatal neutropenia or agranulocytosis

*cyclosporine, potassium-sparing diuretics, potassium supplements:* Increased risk of hyperkalemia

*diuretics, other antihypertensives:* Additive hypotensive effects

*lithium:* Increased blood lithium level and lithium toxicity

*NSAIDs:* Possibly reduced antihypertensive effects of enalapril and enalaprilat

*sympathomimetics:* Possibly reduced therapeutic effects of enalapril and enalaprilat

**FOODS**

*potassium-containing salt substitutes:* Increased risk of hyperkalemia

**ACTIVITIES**

*alcohol use:* Possibly additive hypotensive effect

# Mechanism of Action

May reduce blood pressure by affecting the renin-angiotensin-aldosterone system. By inhibiting ACE, enalapril:

• prevents conversion of angiotensin I to angiotensin II, a potent vasoconstrictor that also stimulates the adrenal cortex to secrete aldosterone

• may inhibit renal and vascular production of angiotensin II

• decreases the serum angiotensin II level and increases serum renin activity, which decreases aldosterone secretion and slightly increases serum potassium level and fluid loss

• decreases vascular tone and blood pressure

• inhibits aldosterone release, which reduces sodium and water reabsorption and increases their excretion, further reducing blood pressure.

# Adverse Reactions

**CNS:** Ataxia, confusion, CVA, depression, dizziness, dream disturbances, fatigue, headache, insomnia, nervousness, peripheral neuropathy, somnolence, syncope, vertigo, weakness

**CV:** Angina, arrhythmias, cardiac arrest, hypotension, MI, orthostatic hypotension, palpitations, pulmonary embolism and infarction, Raynaud's phenomenon

**EENT:** Blurred vision, conjunctivitis, dry eyes and mouth, glossitis, hoarseness, lacrimation, loss of smell, pharyngitis, rhinorrhea, stomatitis, taste perversion, tinnitus

**ENDO:** Gynecomastia

**GI:** Abdominal pain, anorexia, constipation, diarrhea, hepatic failure, hepatitis, ileus, indigestion, melena, nausea, pancreatitis, vomiting
**GU:** Flank pain, impotence, oliguria, renal failure, UTI
**MS:** Muscle spasms
**RESP:** Asthma, bronchitis, bronchospasm, cough, dyspnea, pneumonia, pulmonary edema, pulmonary infiltrates, upper respiratory tract infection
**SKIN:** Alopecia, diaphoresis, erythema multiforme, exfoliative dermatitis, flushing, pemphigus, photosensitivity, pruritus, rash, Stevens-Johnson syndrome, toxic epidermal necrolysis, urticaria
**Other:** Anaphylaxis, angioedema, herpes zoster, hyperkalemia

## Nursing Considerations

• Use enalapril and enalaprilat cautiously in patients with impaired renal function. Be aware that drug shouldn't be given to children with a GFR of less than 30 ml/min/1.73m².
• For children who can't swallow tablets, consult with prescriber and pharmacist about preparation of an oral suspension from tablets as directed by manufacturer.
• Give each I.V. dose over at least 5 minutes.
• Measure blood pressure immediately after first dose and frequently for at least 2 hours thereafter. If hypotension requires a dosage reduction, monitor blood pressure frequently for 2 hours after reduced dosage is administered and for another hour after blood pressure has stabilized.
• Monitor blood pressure regularly during therapy. If hypotension develops, place patient in a supine position and expect to give I.V. NS or other volume expander as prescribed.
• Monitor heart rate and rhythm. Expect to obtain repeated 12-lead ECG tracings.
• Monitor laboratory test results to check hepatic and renal function, leukocyte count, and serum potassium level.
• Monitor patient closely for angioedema of the face, lips, tongue, glottis, larynx, and limbs. For angioedema of the face and lips, stop drug and give an antihistamine, as prescribed. If tongue, glottis, or larynx is involved, assess patient for airway obstruction and prepare to give epinephrine 1:1,000 (0.3 to 0.5 ml) S.C. and maintain a patent airway.

**PATIENT TEACHING**
• Advise patient to take enalapril or enalaprilat at the same time each day.
• Instruct patient not to split, crush, or chew tablets.
• Inform patient that light-headedness and fainting may occur, especially during first few days of therapy. Advise him to change position slowly and avoid potentially hazardous activities until drug's CNS effects are known.
• Inform patient that diarrhea, excessive sweating, vomiting, and other conditions may cause dehydration, which can lead to dizziness, fainting, and very low blood pressure during therapy. Urge sufficient fluid intake to prevent dehydration and related adverse reactions. If diarrhea or vomiting is severe or prolonged, instruct patient to notify prescriber.
• Urge patient to immediately notify prescriber if angioedema and other adverse reactions, including persistent dry cough, occur.
• Advise patient to consult prescriber before using salt substitutes, potassium supplements, or other drugs (including OTC drugs) while taking drug.

# enoxacin

Penetrex

## Class and Category

*Chemical:* Fluoroquinolone
*Therapeutic:* Antibiotic
*Pregnancy category:* C

## Indications and Dosages

➤ *To treat gonorrhea*
**TABLETS**
**Adults.** 400 mg as a single dose.
➤ *To treat uncomplicated UTIs*
**TABLETS**
**Adults.** 200 mg q 12 hr for 7 days.
➤ *To treat complicated UTIs*
**TABLETS**
**Adults.** 400 mg q 12 hr for 14 days.
**DOSAGE ADJUSTMENT** Dosage reduced to one-half in patients with creatinine clearance of 30 ml/min/1.73 m² or less.

## Mechanism of Action

Normally, the enzyme DNA gyrase is responsible for unwinding and supercoiling bacterial DNA before it replicates, as shown below left. Enoxacin inhibits this enzyme, as shown below right, interfering with bacterial cell replication and causing cell death.

## Contraindications

History of tendinitis or tendon rupture, hypersensitivity to enoxacin or any quinolone antibiotic

## Interactions

### DRUGS

*aluminum-, calcium-, or magnesium-containing antacids; didanosine (chewable or buffered tablets); ferrous sulfate; magnesium-containing laxatives; sucralfate; zinc:* Interference with enoxacin absorption, decreased blood enoxacin level

*bismuth:* Decreased enoxacin bioavailability (by about 25% if given with or up to 60 minutes after enoxacin)

*cyclosporine:* Possibly increased blood cyclosporine level

*digoxin:* Increased serum digoxin level and risk of digitalis toxicity

*NSAIDs:* Possibly increased risk of CNS stimulation and seizures

*theophylline:* Interference with theophylline metabolism, increased risk of theophylline toxicity

*warfarin:* Possibly increased anticoagulant effect of warfarin and increased risk of bleeding

### FOODS

*caffeine:* Decreased caffeine clearance, increased adverse effects of caffeine, increased blood enoxacin level

## Adverse Reactions

**CNS:** Dizziness, drowsiness, hallucinations, headache, insomnia, nervousness, seizures, vertigo
**EENT:** Taste perversion
**GI:** Abdominal pain, diarrhea, indigestion, nausea, pseudomembranous colitis, vomiting
**GU:** Vaginitis
**MS:** Tendinitis, tendon rupture
**SKIN:** Photosensitivity, pruritus, rash
**Other:** Anaphylaxis

## Nursing Considerations

• Be aware that enoxacin shouldn't be given to a patient under age 18 because it may cause arthropathy.
• Use drug cautiously in patients with a history of or susceptibility to seizures.
• Obtain a specimen for culture and sensitivity tests, as ordered, but expect to begin therapy before results are available.
• Monitor closely for signs and symptoms of anaphylaxis after first dose: shock, dyspnea, facial or laryngeal edema, loss of con-

sciousness, paresthesia, pruritus, and urticaria. If they occur, stop enoxacin immediately, notify prescriber, and prepare to treat symptoms.
•Ask if patient has a history of seizures. Take seizure and safety precautions because drug may induce seizures and other adverse CNS reactions after a single dose.
•Report severe or prolonged diarrhea, which may indicate pseudomembranous colitis.
•Watch for pain, inflammation, and tendon rupture, especially in shoulders, hands, and ankles.
•If patient has gonorrhea, expect to obtain a serologic test for syphilis at diagnosis and 3 months after enoxacin therapy ends.

**PATIENT TEACHING**
•Stress the importance of taking the full course of enoxacin exactly as prescribed, even if patient feels better before it's finished.
•Instruct patient to take drug at the same times each day—1 hour before or 2 hours after meals—with 8 oz of water.
•Urge patient to avoid potentially hazardous activities until drug's CNS effects are known.
•Advise patient to notify prescriber if symptoms don't improve within a few days.
•Urge patient to drink plenty of fluids but to avoid caffeine during therapy.
•Caution patient not to take aluminum-, calcium-, or magnesium-containing antacids; bismuth; didanosine (chewable or buffered tablets), if prescribed; or products that contain iron or zinc for 8 hours before or 2 hours after taking enoxacin.
•Tell patient to avoid direct sunlight and to use sunscreen and wear protective clothing outdoors. Urge him to report photosensitivity.
•Instruct patient to stop taking enoxacin and notify prescriber immediately if a rash or other allergic reaction develops.
•Instruct patient to take a missed dose as soon as he remembers, unless it's nearly time for the next. Warn against doubling the dose.
•Tell patient to report tendon pain or inflammation, to stop enoxacin, and to rest until tendinitis or tendon rupture is ruled out.

# enoxaparin sodium

Lovenox

## Class and Category
*Chemical:* Low-molecular-weight heparin
*Therapeutic:* Antithrombotic
*Pregnancy category:* B

## Indications and Dosages
➤ *To prevent deep vein thrombosis (DVT) after hip or knee replacement and for continued prophylaxis after hospitalization for hip replacement*
**S.C. INJECTION**
**Adults.** 30 mg q 12 hr, starting 12 to 24 hr after surgery and lasting up to 14 days. Alternatively, 40 mg q.d., starting 9 to 15 hr after hip replacement surgery. *Prophylaxis:* 40 mg q.d. for 3 wk.

➤ *To prevent DVT after abdominal surgery for patients with thromboembolic risk factors (over age 40, obesity, general anesthesia lasting longer than 30 minutes, cancer, or a history of DVT or pulmonary embolism)*
**S.C. INJECTION**
**Adults.** 40 mg q.d., starting 2 hr before surgery and lasting 7 to 10 days.

➤ *To prevent ischemic complications of unstable angina and non–Q-wave MI*
**S.C. INJECTION**
**Adults.** 1 mg/kg q 12 hr with 100 to 325 mg of aspirin q.d. for 2 to 8 days or until condition is stable.
**DOSAGE ADJUSTMENT** Dosage reduced to 30 mg q.d. if creatinine clearance is less than 30 ml/min and patient is receiving drug as prophylaxis in abdominal, hip, or knee replacement surgery or is acutely ill. Dosage reduced to 1 mg/kg q.d. if creatinine clearance is less than 30 ml/min and drug is given with aspirin to prevent ischemic complications of unstable angina and non–Q-wave MI, with warfarin as inpatient treatment for acute DVT with or without pulmonary embolism, or with warfarin as outpatient treatment of acute DVT without pulmonary embolism.

| Route | Onset | Peak | Duration |
|-------|-------|------|----------|
| S.C. | Unknown | 3 to 5 hr | Up to 24 hr |

## Mechanism of Action
Potentiates the action of antithrombin III, a coagulation inhibitor. By binding with antithrombin III, enoxaparin rapidly binds with and inactivates clotting factors (primarily thrombin and factor Xa). Without thrombin, fibrinogen can't convert to fibrin and clots can't form.

## Incompatibilities
Don't mix enoxaparin with other I.V. fluids or drugs.

## Contraindications
Active major bleeding; hypersensitivity to benzyl alcohol (if only the multidose vial is available), enoxaparin, heparin (including low-molecular-weight heparins), or pork products; thrombocytopenia and positive antiplatelet antibody test while taking low-molecular-weight heparins

## Interactions
### DRUGS
*cefamandole, cefoperazone, cefotetan, plicamycin, valproic acid:* Possibly increased risk of hemorrhage
*NSAIDs; oral anticoagulants; platelet aggregation inhibitors, such as aspirin, dipyridamole, sulfinpyrazone, and ticlopidine; thrombolytics, such as alteplase, anistreplase, streptokinase, and urokinase:* Possibly increased risk of bleeding

## Adverse Reactions
**CNS:** Confusion, CVA, fever, paralysis
**CV:** Atrial fibrillation, congestive heart failure, peripheral edema, pulmonary embolism
**EENT:** Epistaxis
**GI:** Bloody stools, diarrhea, elevated liver function test results, hematemesis, melena, nausea, vomiting
**GU:** Hematuria, menstrual irregularities
**HEME:** Anemia, hemorrhage, thrombocytopenia
**RESP:** Dyspnea, pneumonia, pulmonary edema
**SKIN:** Cutaneous vasculitis, ecchymosis, persistent bleeding or oozing from mucous membranes or surgical wounds, pruritus, urticaria, vesiculobullous rash
**Other:** Anaphylaxis; injection site erythema, hematoma, irritation, and pain

## Nursing Considerations
•Use enoxaparin with extreme caution in patients with a history of heparin-induced thrombocytopenia or an increased risk of hemorrhage. Use it cautiously in patients with bleeding diathesis, recent GI ulceration or hemorrhage, or uncontrolled hypertension. Expect possible delayed elimination in elderly patients and those with renal insufficiency.
•Enoxaparin is not recommended for patients with prosthetic heart valves, especially pregnant women, because of the risk of prosthetic valve thrombosis. If enoxaparin is needed, monitor peak and trough anti-Factor Xa levels often and adjust dosage as needed.
•Use multidose vials cautiously in pregnant women because benzyl alcohol may cross the placenta and cause fetal harm.
•Don't give drug by I.M. injection.
•Expect to give drug with aspirin to patient with unstable angina and non–Q-wave MI.
•Watch closely for bleeding. Notify prescriber immediately if platelet count falls below 100,000/mm$^3$. Expect to stop drug and start treatment if patient has a thromboembolic event, such as a CVA.
•Test stool for occult blood, as ordered.
•Keep protamine sulfate nearby in case of accidental overdose.
### PATIENT TEACHING
•Advise patient to notify prescriber about adverse reactions, especially bleeding.
•Instruct patient to seek immediate help for signs of thromboembolism, such as neurologic changes and severe shortness of breath.
•Stress the importance of complying with follow-up visits with prescriber.
•Teach patient or family member how to give enoxaparin at home, if needed. Show patient how to give by deep S.C. injection while lying down. Instruct him not to expel the air bubble from a prefilled syringe to avoid losing some of the drug. Tell him to insert the entire needle into a skin fold held between the thumb and forefinger. Remind him to alternate injection sites between the left and right anterolateral abdominal wall.
•To minimize bruising, caution patient not to rub the site after giving the injection.
•Review safe handling and disposal of syringes and needles.

# entacapone

Comtan

## Class and Category
*Chemical:* COMT inhibitor
*Therapeutic:* Antidyskinetic
*Pregnancy category:* C

## Indications and Dosages
➤ *As adjunct to manage symptoms of Parkinson's disease*
### TABLETS
**Adults.** 200 mg with each dose of carbidopa-levodopa. *Maximum:* 1,600 mg/day.

## Mechanism of Action

Inhibits peripheral catechol-*O*-methyl-transferase (COMT), the major metabolizing enzyme for levodopa. During levodopa metabolism, COMT causes the formation of a levodopa metabolite that reduces the effectiveness of levodopa. By inhibiting COMT, entacapone leads to higher sustained blood levels of levodopa and its increased availability for diffusion into the CNS, where it is converted to dopamine. Depleted dopamine stores are thought to cause Parkinson's disease. By replenishing dopamine stores, entacapone increases dopaminergic stimulation in the brain and reduces the symptoms of Parkinson's disease. Carbidopa is given with levodopa because it inhibits the peripheral distribution of levodopa, making more levodopa available for transport to the brain.

## Contraindications

Hypersensitivity to entacapone or its components, use within 14 days of nonselective MAO inhibitor therapy

## Interactions

### Drugs

*ampicillin, chloramphenicol, cholestyramine, erythromycin, probenecid, rifampin:* Decreased biliary excretion of entacapone
*apomorphine, bitolterol, dobutamine, dopamine, epinephrine, isoetharine, isoproterenol, methyldopa, norepinephrine:* Possibly increased heart rate, arrhythmias, and excessive changes in blood pressure
*MAO inhibitors (nonselective):* Possibly inhibited entacapone metabolism

## Adverse Reactions

**CNS:** Agitation, anxiety, asthenia, dizziness, dyskinesia, fatigue, hallucinations, hyperkinesia, hypokinesia, somnolence
**EENT:** Dry mouth
**GI:** Abdominal pain, constipation, diarrhea, indigestion, gastritis, nausea
**GU:** Brown-orange urine
**MS:** Back pain
**RESP:** Dyspnea
**SKIN:** Diaphoresis, purpura

## Nursing Considerations

•WARNING Be aware that entacapone should not be discontinued abruptly because doing so may precipitate signs and symptoms resembling those of neuroleptic malignant syndrome, such as fever, muscle rigidity, altered level of consciousness, confusion, and elevated creatine kinase level. Patients may also experience a rapid reemergence of parkinsonian symptoms.
•Monitor for drug-induced diarrhea during first 4 to 12 weeks of entacapone therapy.
•Assist patient with activities as necessary because drug may increase occurrence of orthostatic hypotension or syncope in susceptible patients.
•Monitor for worsening dyskinesia because entacapone potentiates dopaminergic adverse effects of levodopa and may exacerbate preexisting dyskinesia.
•Be aware that drug may be taken with selective MAO inhibitors, such as selegiline.

### PATIENT TEACHING

•Instruct patient to always take entacapone with carbidopa-levodopa because drug has no antidyskinetic effect of its own.
•Inform patient that dizziness and sleepiness are more common at beginning of treatment, especially in those with hypotension.
•Advise patient not to participate in potentially hazardous activities until drug's CNS effects are known, especially if he's also taking CNS depressants.
•If patient is scheduled for surgery, instruct him to inform surgeon and anesthesiologist of entacapone use beforehand because COMT inhibitors may interact with some drugs used in surgical procedures.
•Caution patient that entacapone may increase adverse effects of carbidopa-levodopa, such as nausea and uncontrolled movements. If these adverse effects do increase, advise him to contact prescriber immediately because carbidopa-levodopa dosage may need to be lowered.
•Inform patient that urine may turn brown-orange while he's taking entacapone but that this is a harmless effect.

# epinephrine

## (adrenaline)

Adrenalin, Adrenalin Chloride Solution, Ana-Guard, Bronkaid Mist, Bronkaid Mistometer (CAN), EpiPen (CAN), EpiPen Auto-

Injector, EpiPen Jr. (CAN), EpiPen Jr. Auto-Injector, Primatene Mist

## epinephrine bitartrate
Asthmahaler Mist, Bronkaid Suspension Mist

## racepinephrine
AsthmaNefrin, MicroNefrin, Nephron, Vaponefrin

## Class and Category
*Chemical:* Catecholamine
*Therapeutic:* Antianaphylactic, bronchodilator, cardiac stimulant, vasopressor
*Pregnancy category:* C

## Indications and Dosages
➤ *To treat bronchospasm*
INHALED SOLUTION (EPINEPRHINE)
**Adults and children age 4 and older.** 1 to 3 inhalations (10 drops) by hand-bulb nebulizer no more than q 3 hr.
INHALED SOLUTION (RACEPINEPHRINE)
**Adults and children age 4 and older.** 3 inhalations of 0.5 ml (10 drops) by hand-bulb nebulizer, or 0.2 to 0.5 ml (4 to 10 drops) of diluted solution given over 15 min by jet nebulizer; repeated after 3 to 4 hr, if needed.
ORAL INHALED AEROSOL (EPINEPHRINE BITARTRATE)
**Adults and children age 4 and older.** 1 inhalation (160 mcg) repeated after 1 min, if needed; then repeated after at least 3 hr.
ORAL INHALER (EPINEPHRINE)
**Adults and children age 4 and older.** 1 inhalation (200 to 275 mcg) repeated after at least 1 min, if needed; then repeated after at least 3 hr.
➤ *To treat croup*
INHALED SOLUTION (RACEPINEPHRINE)
**Children.** 0.05 ml/kg diluted to 3 ml in NS and given over 15 min q 2 hr, as needed. *Maximum:* 0.5 ml/dose.
➤ *To treat anaphylaxis*
I.V. INFUSION
**Adults and adolescents.** 100 to 250 mcg given slowly.
I.M. OR S.C. INJECTION
**Adults and adolescents.** 100 to 500 mcg repeated q 10 to 15 min, as needed. *Maximum:* 1 mg/dose; three doses.
**Children.** 10 mcg/kg repeated q 15 min for three doses. *Maximum:* 300 mcg/dose.
➤ *To treat severe anaphylactic shock*

I.V. INFUSION
**Adults.** 1 mcg/min titrated to 2 to 10 mcg/min for desired hemodynamic response.
➤ *To treat cardiac arrest*
I.V. INJECTION
**Adults.** 0.5 to 1 mg q 3 to 5 min during resuscitation.
**Children.** 10 mcg/kg followed by 100 mcg/kg q 3 to 5 min, if needed. If two doses produce no response, subsequent doses are increased to 200 mcg/kg q 5 min.
**Neonates.** 10 to 30 mcg/kg q 3 to 5 min.

| Route | Onset | Peak | Duration |
|---|---|---|---|
| I.V., I.M. | Rapid | Unknown | 1 to 2 min |
| S.C. | 5 to 10 min | In 20 min | Short |
| Oral inhalation | 1 to 5 min | In 5 to 15 min | Up to 3 hr |

### Mechanism of Action
Acts on alpha and beta receptors. This nonselective adrenergic agonist stimulates:
• alpha$_1$ receptors, which constricts arteries and may decrease bronchial secretions
• presynaptic alpha$_2$ receptors, which inhibits norepinephrine release by way of negative feedback
• postsynaptic alpha$_2$ receptors, which constricts arteries
• beta$_1$ receptors, which induces positive chronotropic and inotropic responses
• beta$_2$ receptors, which dilates arteries, relaxes bronchial smooth muscles, increases glycogenolysis, and prevents mast cells from secreting histamine and other substances, thus reversing bronchoconstriction and edema.

### Incompatibilities
Don't mix epinephrine with alkalies or oxidizing agents, including bromine, chlorine, chromates, iodine, metal salts (as from iron), nitrites, oxygen, and permanganates, because these substances can destroy epinephrine.

### Contraindications
Cerebral arteriosclerosis, coronary insufficiency, counteraction of phenothiazine-induced hypotension, dilated cardiomyopathy, general anesthesia with halogenated hydrocarbons or cyclopropane, hypersensitivity to

E
F

epinephrine or its components, labor, angle-closure glaucoma, organic brain damage, shock (nonanaphylactic)

## Interactions
### DRUGS
*alpha-adrenergic blockers, drugs with alpha-adrenergic action, rapid-acting vasodilators:* Blockage of epinephrine's alpha-adrenergic effect, possibly causing severe hypotension and tachycardia
*amyl nitrite, nitrates:* Decreased antianginal effects
*antihypertensives, diuretics used to treat hypertension:* Decreased antihypertensive effects
*beta blockers:* Mutual inhibition of therapeutic effects, possibly severe hypertension and cerebral hemorrhage
*digoxin, quinidine:* Increased risk of arrhythmias
*dihydroergotamine, ergoloid mesylates, ergonovine, ergotamine, methylergonovine, methysergide, oxytocin:* Increased risk of vasoconstriction, causing gangrene, peripheral vascular ischemia, or severe hypertension
*hydrocarbon inhalation anesthetics:* Increased risk of severe atrial and ventricular arrhythmias
*insulin, oral antidiabetic drugs:* Decreased effects of these drugs
*MAO inhibitors:* Possibly increased vasopressor effect of epinephrine and hypertensive crisis
*maprotiline, tricyclic antidepressants:* Potentiated cardiovascular effects of epinephrine, possibly causing arrhythmias, hyperpyrexia, severe hypertension, or tachycardia
*sympathomimetics:* Additive CNS stimulation, increased cardiovascular effects of either drug
*thyroid hormones:* Increased effects of either drug
*xanthines:* Increased CNS stimulation, additive toxic effects

## Adverse Reactions
**CNS:** Anxiety, chills, fever, dizziness, drowsiness, hallucinations, headache, insomnia, light-headedness, nervousness, restlessness, seizures, tremor, weakness
**CV:** Chest discomfort or pain; fast, irregular, or slow heartbeat; palpitations; severe hypertension
**EENT:** Blurred vision, dry mouth or throat, miosis
**GI:** Anorexia, heartburn, nausea, vomiting
**GU:** Dysuria

**MS:** Muscle twitching, severe muscle spasms
**RESP:** Dyspnea
**SKIN:** Cold skin, diaphoresis, ecchymosis, flushed or red face or skin, pallor, tissue necrosis
**Other:** Hyperkalemia, hypokalemia, injection site pain and stinging

## Nursing Considerations
• Use epinephrine with extreme caution in patients with angina, arrhythmias, asthma, degenerative heart disease, or emphysema. Epinephrine's inotropic effect equals that of dopamine and dobutamine; its chronotropic effect exceeds that of both.
• Use drug cautiously in elderly patients and those with cardiovascular disease (other than listed above), diabetes mellitus, hypertension, hyperthyroidism, prostatic hypertrophy, and psychoneurologic disorders.
• Be aware that some preparations contain sulfites, which may cause allergic-type reactions. However, the presence of sulfites in epinephrine should not deter its use in a patient with anaphylaxis, even if patient is sensitive to sulfites. Monitor patient closely for adverse effects.
• Dilute the 1:1,000 (1-mg/ml) solution of parenteral epinephrine before I.V. administration.
• Shake suspension thoroughly before withdrawing dose; refrigerate it between uses.
• Inspect epinephrine solution or suspension before use. If it's pink or brown, air has entered a multidose vial. If it's discolored or contains particles, discard it. Also discard unused portions of parenteral epinephrine.
• When injecting drug, rotate sites because repeated injections in the same site may cause vasoconstriction and localized necrosis.
• Be aware that drug shouldn't be given by intra-arterial injection because marked vasoconstriction may cause gangrene.
• Avoid I.M. injection into buttocks. Vasoconstriction reduces oxygen tension in tissues, which may allow anaerobic Clostridium welchii to multiply and cause gas gangrene.
• Monitor for potassium imbalances. Initially, hyperkalemia occurs when hepatocytes release potassium. Hypokalemia may quickly follow as skeletal muscles take up potassium.
• To minimize insomnia, give the last dose a few hours before bedtime.
• **WARNING** To treat cardiac arrest, at least twice the peripheral I.V. dose of epinephrine

may be given by endotracheal instillation. Two dilutions are needed for this regimen; use great caution to avoid medication errors.

**PATIENT TEACHING**
•Warn patient not to exceed recommended dosage or to shorten dosing interval because of the risk of adverse reactions and tolerance.
•Advise patient to notify prescriber if symptoms don't improve or if they improve but then worsen.
•Instruct patient to take the day's last dose a few hours before bedtime to avoid insomnia.
•Caution patient not to use inhalation solution that is pink or brown or that contains particles.
•Teach patient how to use oral inhaler or inhalation solution, as needed.
•If patient also uses an oral corticosteroid inhaler, instruct him to use epinephrine inhaler first, wait 5 minutes, and then use corticosteroid inhaler to increase its effectiveness.
•Advise patient to notify prescriber immediately if he experiences blurred vision, chest pain, difficulty breathing, a fast or irregular heartbeat, or increased sweating.

# eplerenone

Inspra

## Class and Category
*Chemical:* Methyl ester
*Therapeutic:* Antihypertensive
*Pregnancy category:* B

## Indications and Dosages
➤ *To improve survival of stable patients with left ventricular systolic dysfunction and congestive heart failure after an acute MI*
**TABLETS**
**Adults.** *Initial:* 25 mg q.d., increased to 50 mg q.d. within 4 wk, if needed.
➤ *To treat hypertension alone or with other anti-hypertensive drugs*
**TABLETS**
**Adults.** *Initial:* 50 mg/day, increased to 50 mg b.i.d. after 4 wk, if needed.
**DOSAGE ADJUSTMENT** For patients taking weak CYP450 3A4 inhibitors, such as erythromycin, saquinavir, verapamil, and fluconazole, initial dosage should be reduced to 25 mg/day.

## Mechanism of Action
Blocks the binding of aldosterone at its mineralocorticoid receptor sites located in the kidneys, heart, blood vessels, and brain. This action decreases blood pressure by preventing aldosterone from inducing sodium reabsorption and possibly other mechanisms that contribute to raising blood pressure.

## Contraindications
Hyperkalemia (serum potassium level greater than 5.5. mEq/L); hypersensitivity to eplerenone or its components; renal insufficiency (serum creatinine level greater than 2.0 mg/dl in men or 1.8 mg/dl in women or creatinine clearance less than 50 ml/min); type 2 diabetes mellitus complicated by microalbuminuria; use of potassium supplements, potassium-sparing diuretics, or strong CYP450 3A4 inhibitors, such as ketoconazole or itraconazole

## Interactions
**DRUGS**
*ACE inhibitors, angiotensin II receptor antagonists:* Increased risk of hyperkalemia
*CYP450 3A4 inhibitors:* Increased blood level and effect of eplerenone
*lithium:* Possibly lithium toxicity
*NSAIDs:* Possibly reduced antihypertensive effect of eplerenone
**FOODS**
*grapefruit:* Possibly increased blood level and effect of eplerenone

## Adverse Reactions
**CNS:** Dizziness, fatigue, headache
**CV:** Angina pectoris, hypercholesterolemia, hypertriglyceridemia, MI
**ENDO:** Gynecomastia, mastodynia
**GI:** Abdominal pain, diarrhea, increased liver enzyme levels
**GU:** Albuminuria, elevated BUN and serum creatinine levels, vaginal bleeding
**RESP:** Cough
**Other:** Flulike symptoms, hyperkalemia, hyponatremia, increased uric acid level

## Nursing Considerations
•Monitor patient's blood pressure regularly to evaluate the effectiveness of eplerenone therapy.
•Monitor patient's serum potassium level every 2 weeks for the first month or two of therapy and then monthly thereafter, as ordered.

•Be aware that patients who take an ACE inhibitor or an angiotensin II receptor antagonist during eplerenone therapy have an increased risk of hyperkalemia.

**PATIENT TEACHING**

•Caution patient not to use potassium supplements or salt substitutes containing potassium because increased potassium levels can lead to serious adverse reactions to eplerenone.

•Urge patient to tell all prescribers about eplerenone because of possible interactions.

# epoetin alfa

## (EPO, erythropoietin alfa, recombinant erythropoietin, r-HuEPO)

Epogen, Eprex (CAN), Procrit

### Class and Category

*Chemical:* 165–amino acid glycoprotein identical to human erythropoietin
*Therapeutic:* Antianemic
*Pregnancy category:* C

### Indications and Dosages

➤ *To treat anemia from renal failure*

**I.V. OR S.C. INJECTION**

**Adults and adolescents.** *Initial:* 50 to 100 U/kg 3 times/wk, increased by 25 U/kg after 8 wk if hematocrit hasn't risen by 5 or 6 points or is below desired range (30% to 36%). *Maintenance:* Dosage gradually decreased by 25 U/kg q 4 wk or more to lowest dose that keeps hematocrit at 30% to 36%. *Maximum:* 300 U/kg 3 times/wk.

**Children on dialysis.** 50 U/kg 3 times/wk; increased after 8 wk if hematocrit hasn't risen by 5 or 6 points and is still below desired range of 30% to 36%. *Maintenance:* Dosage gradually decreased to lowest dose that keeps hematocrit at 30% to 36%.

➤ *To treat anemia in HIV-infected patients who take zidovudine*

**I.V. OR S.C. INJECTION**

**Adults with serum erythropoietin level of 500 mU/ml or less who receive 4,200 mg or less of zidovudine/wk.** *Initial:* 100 U/kg 3 times/wk, increased by 50 to 100 U/kg q 4 to 8 wk after 8 wk of therapy. *Maintenance:* Dosage gradually titrated to maintain desired response, based on such factors as

variations in zidovudine dosage and occurrence of infection or inflammation. *Maximum:* 300 U/kg 3 times/wk.

➤ *To treat anemia from chemotherapy*

**S.C. INJECTION**

**Adults.** *Initial:* 150 U/kg 3 times/wk. Dosage decreased by 25% if hemoglobin level approaches 12 g/dl or increases more than 1 g/dl in any 2-wk period. Dose withheld if hemoglobin exceeds 13 g/dl and resumed at 25% less than previous dose after hemoglobin has fallen to 12 g/dl. Dosage increased to 300 U/kg 3 times/wk after 8 wk if response is inadequate. *Maximum:* 300 U/kg 3 times/wk. Alternatively, 40,000 U weekly. Dosage decreased by 25% if hemoglobin level approaches 12 g/dl or increases more than 1 g/dl in any 2-wk period. Dose withheld if hemoglobin level exceeds 13 g/dl and resumed at 25% less than previous dose after hemoglobin has fallen to 12 g/dl. Dosage increased to 60,000 U weekly after 8 wk if hemoglobin level has not increased at least 1 g/dl without RBC transfusion.

➤ *To reduce the need for blood transfusion in anemic patients having surgery*

**S.C. INJECTION**

**Adults.** 300 U/kg q.d. for 10 days before surgery, on day of surgery, and 4 days after surgery; or 600 U/kg/wk starting 3 wk before surgery for a total of 3 doses. Dose of 300 U/kg repeated on day of surgery.

**DOSAGE ADJUSTMENT** For patients with anemia from renal failure, dosage temporarily reduced or drug discontinued if hematocrit reaches or exceeds 36%; drug is resumed at a lower dose when hematocrit returns to desired range. For patients with anemia from zidovudine use, therapy temporarily discontinued if hematocrit reaches or exceeds 40% and is resumed at a 25% lower dose when hematocrit returns to desired range.

| Route | Onset | Peak | Duration |
|---|---|---|---|
| I.V., S.C. | In 2 to 6 wk | In 2 mo | About 2 wk |

### Mechanism of Action

Stimulates the release of reticulocytes from the bone marrow into the bloodstream, where they develop into mature RBCs.

### Incompatibilities

Don't mix epoetin alfa with any other drug.

## Contraindications

Hypersensitivity to human albumin or products made from mammal cells, uncontrolled hypertension

## Interactions

**DRUGS**

*antihypertensives:* Increased blood pressure (to hypertensive level), especially when hematocrit rises rapidly
*heparin:* Increased heparin requirement in hemodialysis patients
*iron supplements:* Increased iron requirement and need for increased dose

## Adverse Reactions

**CNS:** Anxiety, asthenia, CVA, dizziness, fatigue, fever, headache, insomnia, paresthesia, seizures
**CV:** Chest pain, deep vein thrombosis, edema, hypertension, MI, tachycardia
**GI:** Constipation, diarrhea, indigestion, nausea, vomiting
**GU:** UTI
**HEME:** Polycythemia
**MS:** Arthralgia, bone pain, muscle weakness
**RESP:** Cough, dyspnea, pulmonary congestion, upper respiratory tract infection
**SKIN:** Rash, pruritus, urticaria
**Other:** Flulike symptoms, hyperkalemia, injection site reaction, trunk pain

## Nursing Considerations

•Use epoetin alfa cautiously in patients who have conditions that could decrease or delay response to drug, such as aluminum intoxication, folic acid deficiency, hemolysis, infection, inflammation, iron deficiency, malignant neoplasm, osteitis (fibrosa cystica), or vitamin $B_{12}$ deficiency.
•Also use drug cautiously in patients with cardiovascular disorders caused by hypertension, a history of seizures, vascular disease, or a hematologic disorder, such as hypercoagulation, myelodysplastic syndrome, or sickle cell disease.
•**WARNING** Be aware that the multidose vial of epoetin contains benzyl alcohol, which can cause a fatal toxic syndrome in neonates and immature infants characterized by CNS, respiratory, circulatory, and renal impairment and metabolic acidosis.
•Don't shake vial during preparation to avoid denaturing glycoprotein and inactivating epoetin alfa.

•Discard unused portion of single-dose vial because it contains no preservatives. Discard unused portion of multidose vial after 21 days.
•Be aware that baseline hemoglobin level should be above 10 but below 13 g/dl if drug is given to patient scheduled for surgery.
•Expect to increase heparin dose if patient receives hemodialysis because epoetin alfa can increase the RBC volume, which could cause clots to form in the dialyzer, hemodialysis vascular access, or both.
•Expect to give an iron supplement (I.V. iron dextran, if needed) because iron requirements rise when erythropoiesis consumes existing iron stores.
•Monitor drug effectiveness by checking hematocrit, typically twice weekly until it stabilizes at 30% to 36%. After that, monitoring can be less frequent.
•Take seizure precautions.
•Be aware that the risk of hypertensive or thrombotic complications increases if the hematocrit rises more than 4 points in 2 weeks.

**PATIENT TEACHING**

•Teach patient how to dispose of needles properly, and caution him against reusing needles.
•Advise patient that the risk of seizures is highest during the first 90 days of epoetin alfa therapy. Urge him not to engage in hazardous activities during this time.
•Stress the importance of complying with the dosage regimen and keeping follow-up medical appointments and appointments for laboratory tests.
•Encourage patient to eat iron-rich foods.
•Review possible adverse reactions, and urge patient to notify prescriber if he experiences chest pain, headache, hives, rapid heartbeat, rash, seizures, shortness of breath, or swelling.

# epoprostenol sodium

## ($PGI_2$, PGX, prostacyclin)

Flolan

## Class and Category

*Chemical:* Natural prostaglandin
*Therapeutic:* Antihypertensive, vasodilator
*Pregnancy category:* B

## Indications and Dosages

➤ *To provide long-term treatment of primary pulmonary hypertension*

**I.V. INFUSION**

**Adults.** *Initial:* 2 ng/kg/min, increased by 2 ng/kg/min q 15 min or longer until dose-limiting effects occur (abdominal, chest, or musculoskeletal pain; anxiety; bradycardia; dizziness; dyspnea; flushing; headache; hypotension; nausea; tachycardia; vomiting; or other adverse reactions). *Maintenance:* Dosage reduced by at least 4 ng/kg/min by continuous infusion.

DOSAGE ADJUSTMENT Continuous infusion rate adjusted, based on persistence, recurrence, or worsening of primary pulmonary hypertension and dose-related adverse reactions.

## Mechanism of Action

Directly relaxes vascular smooth muscles through its action as a natural prostaglandin. This results in arterial dilation and inhibition of platelet aggregation. These actions decrease pulmonary vascular resistance, increase cardiac index and oxygen delivery, and limit thrombus formation.

## Incompatibilities

Don't mix epoprostenol with other parenteral solutions or drugs.

## Contraindications

Hypersensitivity to epoprostenol or its components; long-term use in patients with heart failure caused by severe left ventricular systolic dysfunction; pulmonary edema that developed while establishing epoprostenol dosage

## Interactions

**DRUGS**

*anticoagulants, antiplatelet drugs, NSAIDs:* Increased risk of bleeding

*antihypertensives, diuretics, vasodilators:* Decreased blood pressure

## Adverse Reactions

**CNS:** Anxiety, chills, confusion, dizziness, fever, headache, nervousness, paresthesia, syncope, weakness

**CV:** Bradycardia, chest pain, hypotension, tachycardia

**GI:** Abdominal pain, diarrhea, nausea, vomiting

**HEME:** Thrombocytopenia

**MS:** Arthralgia, jaw pain, myalgia

**RESP:** Dyspnea, hypoxia

**SKIN:** Flushing

**Other:** Flulike symptoms, injection site infection and pain, sepsis, weight loss or gain

## Nursing Considerations

• Use epoprostenol cautiously in elderly patients because they may have decreased hepatic, renal, or cardiac function, or other diseases or may receive other drugs that can interact with epoprostenol.

• Reconstitute drug only with sterile diluent that comes with package. Don't dilute reconstituted epoprostenol.

• To make 100 ml of reconstituted solution at 3,000 ng/ml, dissolve contents of 0.5-mg vial with 5 ml of diluent; withdraw 3 ml and add enough diluent to make 100 ml. To make 100 ml of solution at 5,000 ng/ml, dissolve contents of 0.5-mg vial with 5 ml of diluent; withdraw contents and add enough diluent to make 100 ml. To make 100 ml of solution at 10,000 ng/ml, dissolve contents of two 0.5-mg vials each with 5 ml of diluent; withdraw contents and add enough diluent to make 100 ml. To make 100 ml of solution at 15,000 ng/ml, dissolve contents of 1.5-mg vial with 5 ml of diluent; withdraw contents and add enough diluent to make 100 ml.

• Give continuous infusion through a central venous catheter. Use peripheral I.V. infusion only until central access is established.

• Use an ambulatory infusion pump that's small, lightweight, and able to deliver 2 ng/kg/min. It should have alarms for occlusion, end of infusion, and low battery. Use a polyvinyl chloride, polypropylene, or glass reservoir. Keep a backup pump and infusion set nearby to minimize disruptions in delivery of drug.

• At room temperature, administer a single container of reconstituted solution over 8 hours. For extended use at temperatures above 77° F (25° C), use a cold pouch with frozen gel packs to keep drug at 36° to 46° F (2° to 8° C) for 12 hours.

• After a new infusion rate has been established, monitor patient closely for adverse reactions. Measure each blood pressure with patient standing and supine. Also, monitor heart rate for several hours after dosage adjustment.

• During prolonged infusion, monitor patient for dose-related adverse reactions. If they develop, expect to decrease infusion rate by 2 ng/kg/min every 15 minutes, as prescribed, until dose-limiting reactions resolve.

• Avoid abrupt withdrawal or a sudden large reduction in infusion rate, which could cause rebound pulmonary hypertension (asthenia, dizziness, and dyspnea) or death.

•Protect reconstituted drug from light, and refrigerate for no more than 48 hours. Discard solution that has been frozen or that has been refrigerated for more than 48 hours.

**PATIENT TEACHING**
•Inform patient that epoprostenol is infused continuously through a permanent indwelling central venous catheter by a small infusion pump.
•Stress that patient must commit to long-term therapy, possibly for years.
•Teach patient or caregiver how to reconstitute drug, administer it, and care for the permanent central venous catheter.
•Urge patient to maintain prescribed infusion rate and to consult prescriber before altering it.
•Caution patient that even brief interruptions in drug delivery may cause rapid worsening of symptoms.
•Instruct patient to notify prescriber if adverse reactions occur.
•Make sure patient or caregiver has ready access to emergency phone numbers.

# eprosartan mesylate

Teveten

## Class and Category

*Chemical*: Monomethanesulfonate, non-biphenyl nontetrazole angiotensin II receptor antagonist
*Therapeutic*: Antihypertensive
*Pregnancy category:* Not rated

## Indications and Dosages

➤ To *control blood pressure in patients with essential hypertension*

**TABLETS**
**Adults.** *Initial:* 600 mg q.d. *Maximum:* 800 mg q.d. or in divided doses b.i.d.

---

### Mechanism of Action

Blocks the effects of angiotensin II (a potent vasoconstrictor that's part of the renin-angiotensin-aldosterone system) by blocking its binding to angiotensin I receptors in vascular smooth muscles, adrenal glands, and other tissues. This action halts angiotensin II's negative feedback on renin secretion. Thus, circulating renin and angiotensin II levels rise and vascular resistance declines.

---

## Contraindications

Hypersensitivity to eprosartan or components

## Adverse Reactions

**CNS:** Depression, dizziness, drowsiness, fatigue
**CV:** Angina pectoris, atrial fibrillation, bradycardia, extrasystole, hypertriglyceridemia, hypotension, palpitations, tachycardia
**EENT:** Pharyngitis, rhinitis
**GI:** Abdominal pain
**GU:** Oliguria, UTI
**MS:** Myalgia, rhabdomyolysis
**RESP:** Cough, upper respiratory tract infection

## Nursing Considerations

•Monitor for excessive hypotension if patient receives other cardiac drugs.
•Expect maximum blood pressure response after about 3 weeks.
•Be aware that, unlike ACE inhibitors, eprosartan doesn't affect bradykinin breakdown and cause the characteristic ACE cough.

**PATIENT TEACHING**
•Inform patient that maximum blood pressure response may not occur for 3 to 4 weeks.
•Explain that drug may cause dizziness, drowsiness, or very low blood pressure. Tell patient to rise slowly to upright positions.

# eptifibatide

Integrilin

## Class and Category

*Chemical:* Cyclic heptapeptide
*Therapeutic:* Platelet aggregation inhibitor
*Pregnancy category:* B

## Indications and Dosages

➤ *To treat unstable angina and non–Q-wave MI*

**I.V. INFUSION**
**Adults.** *Initial:* 180 mcg/kg over 1 to 2 min as soon as possible after diagnosis. *Maintenance:* 2 mcg/kg/min by continuous infusion beginning immediately after initial dose and continuing until discharge or coronary artery bypass grafting, up to 72 hr.

**DOSAGE ADJUSTMENT** For patients with serum creatinine level of 2 to 4 mg/dl, initial dosage reduced to 135 mcg/kg over 1 to 2 min and maintenance dosage to 0.5 mcg/kg/min by continuous infusion. Dosage discontinued before coronary artery bypass graft surgery or if platelet count is less than 100,000/mm³.

➤ *To prevent thrombosis related to percutaneous transluminal coronary angioplasty (PTCA)*

**I.V. INFUSION**

**Adults.** *Initial:* 135 mcg/kg over 1 to 2 min immediately before procedure. *Maintenance:* 0.5 mcg/kg/min by continuous infusion beginning immediately after initial dose and continuing for 20 to 24 hr. *Maximum:* 96 hr of therapy.

| Route | Onset | Peak | Duration |
|-------|-------|------|----------|
| I.V. | Immediate | In 15 min | 4 to 8 hr |

## Mechanism of Action

Reversibly inhibits platelet aggregation by preventing the binding of fibrinogen, von Willebrand factor, and other adhesive ligands to glycoprotein IIb/IIIa receptors on activated platelets. As a result, eptifibatide disrupts the final cross-linking stage of platelet aggregation—and thrombus formation.

## Incompatibilities

Don't administer eptifibatide through the same I.V. line as furosemide.

## Contraindications

Active bleeding or CVA during previous 30 days, bleeding diathesis, dependency on dialysis, history of hemorrhagic CVA, hypersensitivity to eptifibatide, major surgery during previous 4 weeks, serum creatinine level of 2 mg/dl or higher for 180 mcg/kg dose or 2 mcg/kg/min infusion, serum creatinine level of 4 mg/dl or higher for 135 mcg/kg dose or 0.5 mcg/kg/min infusion, severe uncontrolled hypertension (systolic pressure above 200 mm Hg, diastolic pressure above 110 mm Hg), thrombocytopenia (platelet count below 100,000/mm$^3$)

## Interactions

**DRUGS**

*anticoagulants, clopidogrel, dipyridamole, NSAIDs, thrombolytics, ticlopidine:* Additive pharmacologic effects, increased risk of bleeding
*other platelet aggregation inhibitors (especially inhibitors of platelet receptor glycoprotein IIb/IIIa, such as abciximab):* Increased risk of additive pharmacologic effects

## Adverse Reactions

**CNS:** Intracranial hemorrhage
**CV:** Hypotension

**GI:** Hematemesis
**GU:** Hematuria
**HEME:** Bleeding, decreased hemoglobin level, thrombocytopenia
**Other:** Anaphylaxis

## Nursing Considerations

•Expect to obtain APTT and PT as a baseline and hematocrit, platelet count, and hemoglobin and serum creatinine levels before eptifibatide therapy to detect abnormalities.
•Withdraw bolus dose of eptifibatide from a 10-ml (2 mg/ml) vial into a syringe.
•Using a vented I.V. infusion set, administer a continuous infusion directly from the 100-ml (0.75 mg/ml) vial. Be sure to center the spike in the circle on top of the vial stopper.
•Expect to maintain APTT between 50 and 70 seconds or according to facility protocol during therapy unless patient undergoes PTCA.
•If patient undergoes PTCA, expect to maintain his activated clotting time between 200 and 250 seconds during the procedure.
•During therapy, avoid arterial and venous punctures, I.M. injections, urinary catheter use, nasotracheal or nasogastric intubation, and use of noncompressible I.V. sites, such as subclavian and jugular veins.
•Expect to discontinue eptifibatide and heparin and monitor patient closely if platelet count falls below 100,000/mm$^3$.
•Plan to discontinue drug, as prescribed, if patient undergoes coronary artery bypass surgery.

**PATIENT TEACHING**

•Instruct patient to immediately report bleeding during eptifibatide therapy.
•Reassure patient that he'll be monitored closely throughout therapy.
•Advise patient to avoid activities that may lead to bruising and bleeding.

# ergoloid mesylates

## (dihydrogenated ergot alkaloids)

Gerimal, Hydergine, Hydergine LC

## Class and Category

*Chemical:* Dihydrogenated ergot alkaloid derivative
*Therapeutic:* Antidementia adjunct, cerebral metabolic enhancer
*Pregnancy category:* Not rated

# Indications and Dosages

➤ *To treat age-related decline in mental capacity*

CAPSULES, ORAL SOLUTION, S.L. TABLETS, TABLETS

**Adults.** 1 to 2 mg t.i.d.

| Route | Onset | Peak | Duration |
|-------|-------|------|----------|
| P.O. | 3 wk or more | Unknown | Unknown |

## Mechanism of Action

May increase cerebral metabolism, blood flow, and oxygen uptake. These actions may increase neurotransmitter levels.

## Contraindications

Acute or chronic psychosis, hypersensitivity to ergoloid mesylates or their components

## Interactions

**DRUGS**

*delavirdine, efavirenz, indinavir, nelfinavir, saquinavir:* Increased risk of ergotism (blurred vision, dizziness, and headache)
*dopamine:* Increased risk of gangrene

## Adverse Reactions

**CNS:** Dizziness, headache, light-headedness, syncope
**CV:** Bradycardia, orthostatic hypotension
**EENT:** Blurred vision, nasal congestion, tongue soreness (with S.L. tablets)
**GI:** Abdominal cramps, anorexia, nausea, vomiting
**SKIN:** Flushing, rash

## Nursing Considerations

• Expect ergoloid mesylates to be prescribed only after a pathophysiologic cause for mental decline has been ruled out.
• Measure blood pressure and pulse rate and rhythm before therapy begins and monitor them frequently during therapy.
• If bradycardia or hypotension develops, expect to discontinue drug permanently.

**PATIENT TEACHING**

• Stress the importance of adhering to prescribed dosage and schedule.
• Teach caregiver to place S.L. tablet under patient's tongue and withhold food, fluids, and cigarettes until tablet dissolves.
• Instruct patient not to swallow S.L. tablets.
• Advise caregiver to skip a missed dose and resume the regular dosing schedule. Warn against doubling the dose, and urge caregiver to notify prescriber if patient misses two or more doses in a row.
• Instruct caregiver to store drug in a tightly closed, light-resistant container.
• Inform caregiver and family that drug may take 3 to 4 weeks to produce its effects.
• Stress the importance of follow-up care.

# ergotamine tartrate

Ergomar (CAN), Ergostat, Gynergen (CAN), Medihaler Ergotamine (CAN)

## Class and Category

*Chemical:* Ergot alkaloid
*Therapeutic:* Vascular headache suppressant
*Pregnancy category:* X

## Indications and Dosages

➤ *To relieve vascular headaches, such as migraine, migraine variants, and cluster headaches*

**S.L. TABLETS**

**Adults.** *Initial:* 2 mg at first sign of attack and repeated q 30 min, p.r.n. *Maximum:* 6 mg/day and no more than two times/wk at least 5 days apart.

**TABLETS**

**Adults.** *Initial:* 1 to 2 mg at first sign of attack and repeated q 30 min, p.r.n. Dosage increased to 3 mg for subsequent attacks if needed and if lower dose was well tolerated. *Maximum:* 6 mg/day.

**ORAL INHALATION AEROSOL**

**Adults:** 1 (360-mcg) inhalation at first sign of attack and repeated q 5 min, p.r.n. *Maximum:* 2.16 mg/day and no more than two times/wk at least 5 days apart.

| Route | Onset | Peak | Duration |
|-------|-------|------|----------|
| P.O., S.L. | Unknown | 1 to 5 hr | Unknown |

## Mechanism of Action

Directly stimulates vascular smooth muscles, constricting arteries and veins and depressing vasomotor centers in the brain.

## Contraindications

Coronary artery disease, hypersensitivity to ergot alkaloids, hypertension, impaired hepatic or renal function, malnutrition, peripheral vascular disease (Raynaud's disease, severe arteriosclerosis, syphilitic arteritis,

E
F

thromboangiitis obliterans, thrombophlebitis), pregnancy or risk of pregnancy, sepsis, severe pruritus

## Interactions

**DRUGS**

*beta blockers:* Increased risk of vasoconstriction and, possibly, peripheral gangrene
*erythromycin, troleandomycin:* Increased risk of peripheral vasospasm and ischemia
*nitrates:* Increased ergotamine effects, decreased antianginal effects of nitrates, increased risk of hypertension
*sumatriptan:* Possibly additive vasoconstriction
*vasoconstrictors:* Increased risk of dangerous hypertension

**ACTIVITIES**

*smoking:* Possibly increased risk of peripheral vasoconstriction and ischemia

## Adverse Reactions

**CNS:** Anxiety, confusion, dizziness, drowsiness, paresthesia, severe headache
**CV:** Chest pain, fast or slow heart rate, heart valve fibrosis, increased or decreased blood pressure, MI, weak pulse
**EENT:** Dry mouth, miosis, vision changes
**GI:** Nausea, vomiting
**MS:** Arm, back, or leg pain; muscle weakness in legs
**SKIN:** Cold, cyanotic, or pale feet or hands; pruritus
**Other:** Edema of face, feet, fingers, or lower legs; physical dependence

## Nursing Considerations

• Use ergotamine cautiously in elderly patients.
• If patient receives long-term therapy, monitor pain control; he may need increasingly higher doses to obtain relief.
• Notify prescriber at the first sign of vasospasm and expect to discontinue drug.

**PATIENT TEACHING**

• Teach patient to take a tablet at the first sign of headache and to lie down in a quiet, dark room.
• Instruct patient not to swallow S.L. tablet but to let it dissolve under his tongue. Advise him not to drink, eat, or smoke until tablet has dissolved.
• Stress the importance of adhering to prescribed dosage and schedule because of drug's potential for dependence.
• Warn patient not to smoke while taking ergotamine (especially heavy smokers) because the combination of drug and nicotine, which

also constricts vessels, may increase the risk of peripheral vascular ischemia.
• Advise patient to notify prescriber if usual doses fail to relieve headaches or if headache frequency or severity increases.
• Urge patient to avoid alcohol because it worsens headaches. Also suggest that patient avoid excessive cold, which may increase peripheral vasoconstriction.
• Instruct patient to notify prescriber if an infection develops because severe infection may increase sensitivity to drug.
• Advise patient to notify prescriber if he experiences chest pain; numbness, pain, or tingling in fingers or toes; pulse rate changes; swelling of face, feet, fingers, or lower legs; or vision changes.

# ertapenem sodium

Invanz

## Class and Category

*Chemical:* Synthetic 1-β methyl-carbapenem
*Therapeutic:* Antibiotic
*Pregnancy category:* B

## Indications and Dosages

➤ *To treat moderate to severe infections, such as complicated intra-abdominal infections due to* Escherichia coli, Clostridium clostridioforme, Eubacterium lentum, Peptostreptococcus *sp.,* Bacteroides fragilis, B. distasonis, B. ovatus, B. thetaiotaomicron, *or* B. uniformis; *complicated skin and skin-structure infections due to* Staphylococcus aureus *(methicillin-susceptible strains only),* Streptococcus pyogenes, E. coli, *or* Peptostreptococcus *sp.; community-acquired pneumonia due to* Streptococcus pneumoniae *(penicillin-susceptible strains only, including cases with concurrent bacteremia),* Haemophilus influenzae *(beta-lactamase–negative strains only), or* Moraxella catarrhalis; *complicated UTIs (including pyelonephritis) due to* E. coli *(including cases with concurrent bacteremia) or* Klebsiella pneumoniae; *and acute pelvic infections (including postpartum endomyometritis, septic abortion, and postsurgical gynecologic infections) due to* Streptococcus agalactiae, E. coli,

B. fragilis, Porphyromonas asaccharolytica, Peptostreptococcus *sp., or* Prevotella bivia

**I.V. INFUSION**
**Adults and adolescents.** 1 g q.d., infused over 30 min, for up to 14 days.
**Children ages 3 months to 13 years.** 15 mg/kg b.i.d., infused over 30 min, for up to 14 days. *Maximum:* 1 g/day.

**I.M. INJECTION**
**Adults and adolescents.** 1 g q.d. for up to 7 days.
**Children ages 3 months to 13 years.** 15 mg/kg b.i.d. for up to 7 days. *Maximum:* 1 g/day.
**DOSAGE ADJUSTMENT** Dosage decreased to 500 mg q.d. for patients with advanced renal insufficiency (creatinine clearance less than or equal to 30 ml/min/1.73 m$^2$) or end-stage renal insufficiency (creatinine clearance less than or equal to 10 ml/min/1.73 m$^2$). For patients on hemodialysis who have received 500 mg of ertapenem within 6 hr of hemodialysis, supplemental dose of 150 mg given after hemodialysis.

---

### Mechanism of Action
Inhibits bacterial cell wall synthesis by binding to specific penicillin-binding proteins inside the cell wall. Penicillin-binding proteins are responsible for various steps in bacterial cell wall synthesis. By binding to these proteins, ertapenem leads to bacterial cell wall lysis.

---

### Incompatibilities
Don't mix ertapenem with other drugs. Don't dilute it with solutions containing dextrose.

### Contraindications
Hypersensitivity to ertapenem, its components, or other drugs in the same class; hypersensitivity to local anesthetics (I.M. form only, because lidocaine hydrochloride 1% is used as a diluent); patients who have experienced anaphylactic reactions to beta-lactam drugs

### Interactions
**DRUGS**
*probenecid:* Increased ertapenem half-life, increased and prolonged blood ertapenem level

### Adverse Reactions
**CNS:** Agitation, anxiety, asthenia, confusion, disorientation, dizziness, fatigue, fever, hallucinations, headache, hypothermia, insomnia, mental changes, seizures, somnolence, stupor
**CV:** Chest pain, edema, hypertension, hypotension, tachycardia, thrombophlebitis
**EENT:** Nasopharyngitis, oral candidiasis, viral pharyngitis
**ENDO:** Hyperglycemia
**GI:** Abdominal pain, acid regurgitation, constipation, diarrhea, elevated liver function test results, indigestion, nausea, vomiting
**GU:** Elevated serum creatinine level, RBCs and WBCs in urine, vaginitis
**HEME:** Anemia, decreased hematocrit, decreased WBC count, eosinophilia, neutropenia, prolonged PT, thrombocytopenia, thrombocytosis
**MS:** Leg pain
**RESP:** Cough, crackles, dyspnea, respiratory distress, upper respiratory tract infection, wheezing
**SKIN:** Dermatitis, erythema, extravasation, pruritus, rash
**Other:** Anaphylaxis; death; hyperkalemia; hypokalemia; infusion site induration, pain, phlebitis, redness, swelling, or warmth

### Nursing Considerations
•Obtain sputum, urine, or other specimens for culture and sensitivity testing, as ordered, before giving ertapenem. Expect to begin therapy before results are available.
•When preparing drug for I.V. use, reconstitute 1 g of drug with 10 ml of sterile water for injection, 0.9% sodium chloride injection, or bacteriostatic water for injection. Don't use solutions that contain dextrose. Shake well to dissolve. Immediately transfer reconstituted drug to 50 ml of NS. Use within 6 hours if stored at room temperature or within 24 hours if refrigerated at 5° C (41° F). Don't freeze. Administer I.V. infusion over 30 minutes.
•Inspect drug for particles and discoloration after reconstitution.
•For I.M. injection, reconstitute 1 g of drug with 3.2 ml of 1% lidocaine hydrochloride injection (*without* epinephrine). Shake thoroughly to form solution. Use within 1 hour after preparation. Withdraw contents of vial and inject deep into a large muscle mass such as the gluteal muscle.
•**WARNING** Don't administer reconstituted I.M. solution by I.V. route because of the potential for adverse reactions from the lidocaine hydrochloride injection used to reconstitute drug.

E
F

• Monitor patient closely for a life-threatening anaphylactic reaction. Patients with a history of hypersensitivity to penicillin, cephalosporins, other beta-lactams, or other allergens are at increased risk.

• **WARNING** If ertapenem triggers an anaphylactic reaction, stop drug, notify prescriber immediately, and provide appropriate therapy. Anaphylaxis requires immediate treatment with epinephrine as well as airway management and administration of oxygen and I.V. corticosteroids, as needed.

• Be aware that patients with a history of seizures, other CNS disorders that predispose them to seizures (such as brain lesions), or compromised renal function may be at increased risk for seizures. Administer anticonvulsant, as ordered.

• Monitor patient for diarrhea during or shortly after drug therapy; diarrhea may signal pseudomembranous colitis.

• Be aware that because ertapenem is excreted in breast milk, its use by nursing mothers is carefully evaluated.

**PATIENT TEACHING**

• Instruct patient receiving ertapenem to immediately report signs of an anaphylaxis, such as rash, itching, or shortness of breath; or signs of superinfection, such as severe diarrhea or white patches on tongue or in mouth.

# erythromycin

*(contains 250, 333, or 500 mg of base per delayed-release capsule, delayed-release tablet, or tablet)*

Apo-Erythro (CAN), E-Mycin, Erybid (CAN), ERYC, Ery-Tab, Ilotycin, Novo-Rythro Encap (CAN), PCE

## erythromycin estolate

*(contains 250 mg of base per capsule or tablet, or 125 or 250 mg of base per 5 ml of oral suspension)*

Ilosone, Novo-Rythro (CAN)

## erythromycin ethylsuccinate

*(contains 1 g of base per 1.6 g of oral suspension or tablet)*

Apo-Erythro-ES (CAN), E.E.S., EryPed, Erythro, Novo-Rythro (CAN)

## erythromycin gluceptate

*(contains 500 or 1,000 mg of base per vial)*

Ilotycin

## erythromycin lactobionate

*(contains 500 or 1,000 mg of base per vial)*

Erythrocin

## erythromycin stearate

*(contains 125 or 250 mg of base per 5 ml of oral suspension, or 250 or 500 mg of base per tablet)*

Apo-Erythro-S (CAN), Erythrocin, Erythrocot, My-E, Novo-Rythro (CAN), Wintrocin

## Class and Category

*Chemical:* Macrolide
*Therapeutic:* Antiacne agent, antibiotic
*Pregnancy category:* B

## Indications and Dosages

➤ *To treat mild to moderate upper respiratory tract infections caused by* Haemophilus influenzae, Streptococcus pneumoniae, *or* Streptococcus pyogenes *(group A beta-hemolytic streptococcus)*

**CAPSULES, CHEWABLE TABLETS, DELAYED-RELEASE CAPSULES, DELAYED-RELEASE TABLETS, ORAL SUSPENSION, TABLETS, I.V. INFUSION**

**Adults.** 250 to 500 mg (base) q 6 hr for 10 days.
**Children.** 250 to 500 mg (base) q.i.d. or 20 to 50 mg (base)/kg/day in divided doses for 10 days. For *H. influenzae* infections, erythromycin ethylsuccinate is administered with 150 mg/kg/day of sulfisoxazole. *Maximum:* Adult dosage, or 6 g/day for erythromycin ethylsuccinate.

➤ *To treat lower respiratory tract infections caused by* S. pneumoniae *or* S. pyogenes *(group A beta-hemolytic streptococcus)*

**CAPSULES, CHEWABLE TABLETS, DELAYED-RELEASE CAPSULES, DELAYED-RELEASE TABLETS, ORAL SUSPENSION, TABLETS, I.V. INFUSION**

**Adults.** 250 to 500 mg (base) q 6 hr for 10 days.
**Children.** 250 to 500 mg (base) q.i.d. or 20 to 50 mg (base)/kg/day in divided doses for 10 days. *Maximum:* Adult dosage.

➤ *To treat respiratory tract infections caused by* Mycoplasma pneumoniae

**CAPSULES, CHEWABLE TABLETS, DELAYED-RELEASE CAPSULES, DELAYED-RELEASE TABLETS, ORAL SUSPENSION, TABLETS, I.V. INFUSION**

**Adults.** 500 mg (base) q 6 hr for 5 to 10 days or up to 3 wk for severe infections.

➤ *To treat mild to moderate skin and soft-tissue infections caused by* S. pyogenes *or* Staphylococcus aureus

CAPSULES, CHEWABLE TABLETS, DELAYED-RELEASE
CAPSULES, DELAYED-RELEASE TABLETS, ORAL SUSPENSION,
TABLETS, **I.V.** INFUSION
**Adults.** 250 mg (base) q 6 hr or 500 mg (base) q 12 hr for 10 days. *Maximum:* 4 g (base)/day.
**Children.** 250 to 500 mg (base) q.i.d. or 20 to 50 mg (base)/kg/day in divided doses for 10 days. *Maximum:* Adult dosage.

➤ *To treat acne vulgaris*
DELAYED-RELEASE CAPSULES, DELAYED-RELEASE TABLETS,
TABLETS
**Adults and adolescents.** *Initial:* 250 mg (base) q 6 hr, 333 mg (base) q 8 hr, or 500 mg (base) q 12 hr for 4 wk. *Maintenance:* 333 to 500 mg (base) q.d.

➤ *To treat pertussis (whooping cough) caused by* Bordetella pertussis
CAPSULES, CHEWABLE TABLETS, DELAYED-RELEASE CAP-
SULES, DELAYED-RELEASE TABLETS, ORAL SUSPENSION,
TABLETS, **I.V.** INFUSION
**Children.** 500 mg (base) q.i.d. or 40 to 50 mg (base)/kg/day in divided doses for 5 to 14 days.

➤ *To treat diphtheria*
CAPSULES, CHEWABLE TABLETS, DELAYED-RELEASE
CAPSULES, DELAYED-RELEASE TABLETS, ORAL SUSPENSION,
TABLETS, **I.V.** INFUSION
**Adults and children.** 500 mg (base) q 6 hr for 10 days.

➤ *To treat erythrasma*
CAPSULES, CHEWABLE TABLETS, DELAYED-RELEASE CAP-
SULES, DELAYED-RELEASE TABLETS, ORAL SUSPENSION,
TABLETS, **I.V.** INFUSION
**Adults and children.** 250 mg (base) t.i.d. for 21 days.

➤ *To treat intestinal amebiasis*
CAPSULES, CHEWABLE TABLETS, DELAYED-RELEASE
CAPSULES, DELAYED-RELEASE TABLETS, ORAL SUSPENSION,
TABLETS, **I.V.** INFUSION
**Adults.** 250 mg (base) q 6 hr for 10 to 14 days.
**Children.** 30 to 50 mg (base)/kg/day in divided doses for 10 to 14 days

➤ *To treat pelvic inflammatory disease caused by* Neisseria gonorrhoeae
CAPSULES, CHEWABLE TABLETS, DELAYED-RELEASE CAP-
SULES, DELAYED-RELEASE TABLETS, ORAL SUSPENSION,
TABLETS, **I.V.** INFUSION
**Adults.** 500 mg (base) I.V. q 6 hr for 3 days and then 250 mg (base) P.O. or I.V. q 6 hr for 7 days.

➤ *To treat newborn conjunctivitis*
**I.V.** INFUSION
**Neonates.** 50 mg (base)/kg/day in four divided doses for 14 days.

➤ *To treat pneumonia in neonates*
**I.V.** INFUSION
**Neonates.** 50 mg (base)/kg/day in divided doses for 21 days.

➤ *To treat urogenital infections caused by* Chlamydia trachomatis *during pregnancy*
CAPSULES, CHEWABLE TABLETS, DELAYED-RELEASE CAPSULES,
DELAYED-RELEASE TABLETS, ORAL SUSPENSION, TABLETS
**Adults.** 500 mg (base) on an empty stomach q 6 hr for 7 days; or 250 mg (base) on an empty stomach q 6 hr for at least 14 days.

➤ *To treat nongonococcal urethritis or uncomplicated urethral, endocervical, or rectal infections caused by* C. trachomatis
CAPSULES, CHEWABLE TABLETS, DELAYED-RELEASE
CAPSULES, DELAYED-RELEASE TABLETS, ORAL SUSPENSION,
TABLETS
**Adults.** 500 mg (base) q 6 hr for 7 days. If patient can't tolerate high doses, 250 mg (base) q 6 hr for 14 days.

➤ *To treat primary syphilis*
CAPSULES, CHEWABLE TABLETS, DELAYED-RELEASE CAPSULES,
DELAYED-RELEASE TABLETS, ORAL SUSPENSION, TABLETS
**Adults.** 20 to 40 g (base) in divided doses over 10 to 15 days.

➤ *To treat Legionnaire's disease*
CAPSULES, CHEWABLE TABLETS, DELAYED-RELEASE CAP-
SULES, DELAYED-RELEASE TABLETS, ORAL SUSPENSION,
TABLETS, **I.V.** INFUSION
**Adults.** 1 to 4 g (base)/day in divided doses for 10 to 14 days.

➤ *To treat rheumatic fever*
CAPSULES, CHEWABLE TABLETS, DELAYED-RELEASE
CAPSULES, DELAYED-RELEASE TABLETS, ORAL SUSPENSION,
TABLETS, **I.V.** INFUSION
**Adults.** 250 mg (base) q 12 hr.

➤ *To prevent bacterial endocarditis in patients with penicillin allergy who plan dental or upper respiratory tract surgery*
CAPSULES, CHEWABLE TABLETS, DELAYED-RELEASE
CAPSULES, DELAYED-RELEASE TABLETS, ORAL SUSPENSION,
TABLETS, **I.V.** INFUSION
**Adults.** 1 g (base) given 1 to 2 hr before procedure and then 500 mg (base) 6 hr after initial dose.
**Children.** 20 mg (base)/kg given 2 hr before procedure and then 10 mg (base)/kg 6 hr after initial dose.

➤ *To treat listeriosis*
CAPSULES, CHEWABLE TABLETS, DELAYED-RELEASE
CAPSULES, DELAYED-RELEASE TABLETS, ORAL SUSPENSION,
TABLETS, **I.V.** INFUSION
**Adults.** 250 mg (base) q 6 hr or 500 mg (base) q 12 hr. *Maximum:* 4 g (base)/day.

E
F

## Mechanism of Action
Binds with the 50S ribosomal subunit of the 70S ribosome in many types of aerobic, anaerobic, gram-positive, and gram-negative bacteria. This action inhibits RNA-dependent protein synthesis in bacterial cells, causing them to die.

## Contraindications
Astemizole, cisapride, pimozide, or terfenadine therapy; hypersensitivity to erythromycin, macrolide antibiotics, or their components; hepatic disease (erythromycin estolate)

## Interactions
### DRUGS
*alfentanil*: Decreased alfentanil clearance, prolonged alfentanil action
*astemizole, cisapride, terfenadine*: Increased risk of cardiotoxicity, torsades de pointes, ventricular tachycardia, and death
*atorvastatin, lovastatin, pravastatin, simvastatin*: Increased risk of rhabdomyolysis
*carbamazepine, valproic acid:* Possibly inhibited metabolism of these drugs, increasing their blood levels and risk of toxicity
*chloramphenicol, lincomycins*: Antagonized effects of these drugs
*cyclosporine*: Increased risk of nephrotoxicity
*digoxin*: Increased serum digoxin level and risk of digitalis toxicity
*diltiazem, verapamil:* Increased risk of life-threatening cardiac events
*ergotamine*: Decreased ergotamine metabolism, increased risk of vasospasm from ergotamine use
*hepatotoxic drugs*: Increased risk of hepatotoxicity
*midazolam, triazolam*: Increased pharmacologic effects of these drugs
*oral contraceptives:* Failed contraception, hepatotoxicity
*ototoxic drugs*: Increased risk of ototoxicity if patient with impaired renal function receives high doses of erythromycin
*penicillins*: Interference with bactericidal effects of penicillins
*sildenafil*: Increased effects of sildenafil
*warfarin:* Prolonged PT and risk of hemorrhage, especially in elderly patients
*xanthines (except dyphylline)*: Increased serum theophylline level and risk of theophylline toxicity

### ACTIVITIES
*alcohol use*: Increased alcohol level (by 40%) with I.V. erythromycin

## Adverse Reactions
**CNS:** Fatigue, fever, malaise, weakness
**CV:** Prolonged QT interval, torsades de pointes, ventricular arrhythmias
**EENT:** Hearing loss, oral candidiasis
**GI:** Abdominal cramps and pain, diarrhea, hepatotoxicity, nausea, vomiting
**GU:** Vaginal candidiasis
**SKIN:** Erythema, jaundice, pruritus, rash
**Other:** Fluid overload (from I.V. infusion), injection site inflammation and phlebitis

## Nursing Considerations
•Use erythromycin cautiously in patients with impaired hepatic function because drug is metabolized by the liver.
•Before administering the first erythromycin dose, expect to obtain body fluid or tissue sample for culture and sensitivity testing.
•Reconstitute parenteral form before administration. Add at least 10 ml of preservative-free sterile water for injection to each 500-mg vial or at least 20 ml of diluent to each 1-g vial.
•For prolonged infusion, expect to infuse a buffered solution up to 24 hours after dilution.
•For intermittent infusion, dilute the dose if needed in 100 to 250 ml of NS or D$_5$W and administer slowly over 20 to 60 minutes.
•When giving I.V. erythromycin gluceptate, dilute the solution if needed to 1 g/L in NS or D$_5$W injection for slow, continuous infusion. Diluted solution remains potent for 7 days if refrigerated.
•When giving I.V. erythromycin lactobionate, dilute the solution if needed to 1 to 5 mg/ml in NS, LR, or other electrolyte solution for slow, continuous infusion. Diluted solution remains potent for 14 days if refrigerated and for 24 hours at room temperature.
•Be aware that infusions prepared in piggyback infusion bottles remain potent for 30 days if frozen, 24 hours if refrigerated, or 8 hours at room temperature. Don't store infusions prepared in the ADD-vantage system.
•Don't use diluent with benzyl alcohol if parenteral erythromycin is for a neonate. It may cause a fatal toxic syndrome of CNS depression, hypotension, metabolic acidosis, renal failure, respiratory problems, and, possibly, seizures and intracranial hemorrhage.
•Periodically monitor liver function test results to detect hepatotoxicity, which is most

common with erythromycin estolate. Signs typically appear within 2 weeks after continuous therapy starts and resolve when it stops.
•Assess hearing regularly, especially in elderly patients and those who receive 4 g or more/day or have hepatic or renal disease. Hearing impairment begins 36 hours to 8 days after treatment starts and usually begins to improve 1 to 14 days after it stops.
•During I.V. therapy, watch for signs of fluid overload, such as acute dyspnea and crackles.
•Monitor infants for vomiting or irritability with feeding because infantile hypertrophic pyloric stenosis has been reported.
•Monitor myasthenia gravis patients for weakness because drug may aggravate it.
•Monitor patient closely for signs and symptoms of superinfection. If they occur, notify prescriber and expect to stop drug and provide appropriate therapy.
•If patient receives an order for urine catecholamine analysis, notify prescriber; erythromycin interferes with fluorometric measurement of urine catecholamines.

**PATIENT TEACHING**
•Urge patient to complete prescribed therapy, even if he feels better before it's finished.
•Tell patient to notify prescriber if symptoms worsen or don't improve after a few days.
•Teach patient how to administer prescribed drug form. Instruct him to swallow capsules or tablets whole. For an oral suspension, teach him to use the measuring device provided to ensure accurate doses. Remind him to shake the suspension before measuring a dose.
•Advise patient to take any oral form with a full glass of water on an empty stomach (except erythromycin ethylsuccinate, which is better absorbed with food).
•If GI distress occurs, instruct patient to take oral form with food.
•Instruct patient to promptly notify prescriber about allergic reactions, hearing changes, or signs of hepatic dysfunction.


# escitalopram oxalate

Lexapro

## Class and Category
*Chemical:* Pure S+ enantiomer of racemic bicyclic phthalane derivative citalopram
*Therapeutic:* Antidepressant
*Pregnancy category:* C

## Indications and Dosages
➤ *To treat generalized anxiety disorder or major depression*
**ORAL SOLUTION, TABLETS**
**Adults.** *Initial:* 10 mg q.d. in morning or evening, increased to 20 mg q.d. after one or more wk, as needed.
**DOSAGE ADJUSTMENT** Dosage shouldn't exceed 10 mg q.d. for elderly patients and those with hepatic impairment.

### Mechanism of Action
Inhibits reuptake of the neurotransmitter serotonin by CNS neurons, thereby increasing the amount of serotonin available in nerve synapses. An elevated serotonin level may result in elevated mood and reduced depression.

## Contraindications
Hypersensitivity to escitalopram, citalopram or its components; use within 14 days of MAO inhibitor therapy

## Interactions
**DRUGS**
*aspirin, NSAIDs, warfarin:* Possibly increased risk of bleeding
*carbamazepine:* Possibly increased clearance of escitalopram
*cimetidine:* Possibly increased plasma escitalopram level
*CNS drugs:* Additive CNS effects
*lithium:* Possible enhancement of the serotonergic effects of escitalopram
*MAO inhibitors:* Possibly hyperpyretic episodes, hypertensive crisis, serotonin syndrome, and severe seizures
*metoprolol:* Increased plasma metoprolol levels with decreased cardioselectivity of metoprolol
*naratriptan, sumatriptan, zolmitriptan:* Possibly weakness, hyperreflexia, and incoordination
*St. John's wort:* Increased risk of serotonin syndrome
*sibutramine:* Increased risk of serotonin syndrome
**ACTIVITIES**
*alcohol use:* Possibly increased cognitive and motor effects of alcohol

## Adverse Reactions
**CNS:** Abnormal gait, aggression, akathisia, delirium, dizziness, dyskinesia, dystonia, ex-

trapyramidal effects, fatigue, headache, hypomania, insomnia, lethargy, mania, myoclonus, neuroleptic malignant syndrome, paresthesia, seizures, serotonin syndrome, somnolence

**CV:** Atrial fibrillation, hypotension, MI, prolonged QT interval, thrombosis, torsades de pointes, ventricular arrhythmias

**EENT:** Diplopia, dry mouth, nystagmus, rhinitis, sinusitis, toothache, visual hallucinations

**ENDO:** Syndrome of inappropriate ADH secretion

**GI:** Abdominal pain, constipation, decreased appetite, diarrhea, flatulence, GI bleeding or hemorrhage, hepatic necrosis, hepatitis, indigestion, nausea, pancreatitis, vomiting

**GU:** Acute renal failure, anorgasmia, decreased libido, ejaculation disorders, impotence, priapism

**HEME:** Bleeding, decreased prothrombin time, hemolytic anemia, thrombocytopenia

**MS:** Neck or shoulder pain, rhabdomyolysis

**RESP:** Pulmonary embolism

**SKIN:** Ecchymosis, erythema multiforme, increased sweating, toxic epidermal necrolysis

**Other:** Anaphylaxis, angioedema, flulike symptoms

## Nursing Considerations

•Use escitalopram cautiously in patients with history of mania or seizures, patients with severe renal impairment, or those with diseases or conditions that produce altered metabolism or hemodynamic responses.

•Monitor patient for hypo-osmolarity of serum and urine and for hyponatremia, which may indicate escitalopram-induced syndrome of inappropriate ADH secretion.

•Observe patient for signs of misuse or abuse, such as development of tolerance, increasing dosage without approval, and drug-seeking behavior, because escitalopram's potential for physical and psychological dependence is unknown.

•Expect prescriber to reassess patient periodically to determine the continued need for therapy and confirm the appropriate dosage.

•If patient takes escitalopram to treat depression, watch closely for suicidal tendencies, especially when therapy starts or dosage changes, because depression may worsen temporarily.

•If drug will be stopped, expect to taper dosage to avoid serious adverse reactions.

**PATIENT TEACHING**

•Inform patient that alcohol use isn't recommended during escitalopram therapy because it may decrease his ability to think clearly and perform motor skills.

•Advise patient to avoid potentially hazardous activities until drug's CNS effects are known.

•Instruct patient that drug shouldn't be taken with citalopram hydrobromide because of potentially additive effects.

•Tell patient that improvement may not be noticed for 1 to 4 weeks after therapy begins. Emphasize the importance of continuing therapy as prescribed.

•Warn patient not to stop taking drug abruptly. Explain that gradual tapering helps to avoid withdrawal symptoms.

•Urge patient to inform prescriber of any OTC drugs he takes because of potential for interactions.

# esmolol hydrochloride

Brevibloc

## Class and Category

*Chemical:* Beta blocker
*Therapeutic:* Antiarrhythmic, antihypertensive
*Pregnancy category:* C

## Indications and Dosages

➤ *To treat supraventricular tachycardia*

**I.V. INFUSION**

**Adults.** *Loading:* 500 mcg/kg over 1 min. *Maintenance:* If response to loading dose is adequate after 5 min, 50 mcg/kg/min infused for 4 min. If response is inadequate after 5 min, another 500 mcg/kg may be given over 1 min followed by 100 mcg/kg/min for 4 min. Sequence repeated, as needed, until adequate response occurs, increasing maintenance dosage by 50 mcg/kg/min at each step. *Maximum:* 200 mcg/kg/min for 48 hr.

**Children.** 50 mcg/kg/min titrated q 10 min up to 300 mcg/kg/min.

➤ *To treat intraoperative and postoperative tachycardia and hypertension*

**I.V. INFUSION**

**Adults.** *Initial:* 250 to 500 mcg/kg over 1 min. *Maintenance:* 50 mcg/kg/min infused

over 4 min. If response is inadequate after 5 min, another 250 to 500 mcg/kg may be given over 1 min followed by 100 mcg/kg/ min for 4 min. Sequence repeated, as needed, up to 4 times, increasing by 50 mcg/kg/min each time. *Maximum:* 200 mcg/kg/min for 48 hr.
DOSAGE ADJUSTMENT Loading doses omitted, increments decreased to 25 mcg/kg/min, and titration intervals increased to 10 min as heart rate approaches desired level or if blood pressure decreases too much.

| Route | Onset | Peak | Duration |
|-------|-------|------|----------|
| I.V. | Immediate | Unknown | 10 to 20 min |

## Mechanism of Action

Inhibits stimulation of beta$_1$ receptors primarily in the heart, which decreases cardiac excitability, cardiac output, and myocardial oxygen demand. Esmolol also decreases renin release from the kidneys, which helps reduce blood pressure.

## Incompatibilities

Don't mix esmolol with 5% sodium bicarbonate injection.

## Contraindications

Cardiogenic shock, hypersensitivity to beta blockers, overt heart failure, second- or third-degree heart block, sinus bradycardia

## Interactions

**DRUGS**
*antihypertensives:* Possibly hypotension
*insulin, oral antidiabetic drugs:* Possibly masking of signs and symptoms of hypoglycemia caused by these drugs
*MAO inhibitors:* Possibly severe hypertension if esmolol is administered within 14 days of discontinuing MAO inhibitor therapy
*neuromuscular blockers:* Possibly potentiated and prolonged action of these drugs
*phenytoin:* Possibly increased cardiac depression
*reserpine:* Possibly bradycardia and hypotension
*sympathomimetics, xanthine derivatives:* Possibly inhibited therapeutic effects of both drugs

## Adverse Reactions

**CNS:** Anxiety, confusion, depression, dizziness, fatigue, fever, headache, syncope
**CV:** Bradycardia, chest pain, decreased peripheral circulation, heart block, hypotension

**GI:** Nausea, vomiting
**RESP:** Dyspnea, wheezing
**SKIN:** Diaphoresis, flushing, pallor
**Other:** Infusion site pain, redness, and swelling

## Nursing Considerations

•Use esmolol cautiously if patient has supraventricular arrhythmias with decreased cardiac output, hypotension, or other hemodynamic compromise or is taking drugs that decrease peripheral resistance or myocardial filling, contractility, or impulse generation.
•Also use drug cautiously in patients with impaired renal function because drug is excreted by the kidneys. Patients with end-stage renal disease have an increased risk of adverse reactions.
•Avoid giving esmolol for intraoperative or postoperative hypertension caused by hypothermia-induced vasoconstriction.
•Expect to give lowest possible dose to patients with allergies, asthma, bronchitis, or emphysema. If patient develops bronchospasm, expect to discontinue infusion immediately and give a beta$_2$ stimulating drug, as ordered.
•Don't give 250 mg/ml (2,500 mg/10 ml) dosage strength by direct I.V. push. Dilute it to a 10-mg/ml infusion by first removing 20 ml from 500 ml of a compatible I.V. solution, such as D$_5$W or D$_5$NS, and then adding 5 g of esmolol to the solution.
•Use diluted solution within 24 hours if stored at room temperature.
•Use 100-mg vial (prediluted to 10 mg/ml) for loading dose. For 70-kg (154-lb) patient, loading dose for 500 mcg/kg/min is 3.5 ml.
•Monitor blood pressure and heart rate frequently during therapy. Keep in mind that hypotension can occur at any dose but usually is dose related. Hypotension typically reverses within 30 minutes after dose is decreased or infusion is stopped.
•Inspect site often for thrombophlebitis (pain, redness, swelling at site). Infusion of 20 mg/ml is more likely to cause serious vein irritation than 10 mg/ml. Extravasation of 20 mg/ml may cause a serious local reaction and skin necrosis. Don't give more than 10 mg/ml into a small vein or using a butterfly catheter.

**PATIENT TEACHING**
•Urge patient to report adverse reactions immediately.

E
F

•Reassure patient that his blood pressure, heart rate, and response to therapy will be monitored throughout esmolol therapy.

# esomeprazole magnesium

Nexium, Nexium I.V.

## Class and Category

*Chemical:* Substituted benzimidazole
*Therapeutic:* Antiulcerative
*Pregnancy category:* B

## Indications and Dosages

➤ *To treat gastroesophageal reflux disease (GERD)*

**DELAYED-RELEASE CAPSULES**

**Adults.** 20 to 40 mg q.d. for 4 to 8 wk; may be repeated for another 4 to 8 wk if ulcer hasn't healed. *Maintenance:* 20 mg q.d. for up to 6 mo.

➤ *To treat GERD in a patient with a history of erosive esophagitis who can't take the drug by mouth*

**I.V. INFUSION, I.V. INJECTION**

**Adults.** 20 to 40 mg q.d. infused for no less than 3 min (I.V. injection) or 10 to 30 min (I.V. infusion).

➤ *As adjunct to treat duodenal or gastric ulcer associated with* Helicobacter pylori

**DELAYED-RELEASE CAPSULES**

**Adults.** 40 mg q.d. in combination with amoxicillin 1,000 mg b.i.d. and clarithromycin 500 mg b.i.d. for 10 days.

➤ *To reduce the risk of gastric ulcer formation in patients who are receiving continuous NSAID therapy and who either are older than age 60 or have a history of gastric ulcer*

**DELAYED-RELEASE CAPSULES**

**Adults.** 20 to 40 mg q.d. for up to 6 mo.

**DOSAGE ADJUSTMENT** Maximum, 20 mg q.d. for patients who have severe hepatic insufficiency.

## Incompatibilities

Don't give esomeprazole with any other drug through the same I.V. site or tubing.

## Contraindications

Hypersensitivity to esomeprazole or its components

## Mechanism of Action

Interferes with gastric acid secretion by inhibiting the hydrogen-potassium-adenosine triphosphatase ($H^+$-$K^+$-ATPase) enzyme system, or proton pump, in gastric parietal cells. Normally, the proton pump uses energy from the hydrolysis of ATPase to drive $H^+$ and chloride ($Cl^-$) out of parietal cells and into the stomach lumen in exchange for potassium ($K^+$), which leaves the stomach lumen and enters parietal cells. After this exchange, $H^+$ and $Cl^-$ combine in the stomach to form hydrochloric acid (HCl). Esomeprazole irreversibly inhibits the final step in gastric acid production by blocking the exchange of intracellular $H^+$ and extracellular $K^+$, thus preventing $H^+$ from entering the stomach and additional HCl from forming.

## Interactions

**DRUGS**

*Antimicrobials:* Increased blood esomeprazole levels

*diazepam:* Possibly increased blood diazepam level

*digoxin, iron salts, ketoconazole:* Possibly decreased absorption of these drugs

*warfarin:* Possibly increased INR and PT, leading to abnormal bleeding

**FOODS**

*all foods:* Decreased bioavailability of esomeprazole

## Adverse Reactions

**CNS:** Dizziness, headache
**EENT:** Dry mouth, sinusitis
**GI:** Abdominal pain, constipation, diarrhea, dyspepsia, flatulence, hepatitis, jaundice, nausea, pancreatitis
**MS:** Myalgia
**RESP:** Respiratory tract infection
**SKIN:** Erythema multiforme, pruritus, Stevens-Johnson syndrome, toxic epidermal necrolysis
**Other:** Anaphylaxis, infusion site redness or pruritus

## Nursing Considerations

•Give oral esomeprazole at least 1 hour before meals because food decreases bioavailability.

•**WARNING** If patient takes drug with amoxicillin or clarithromycin for *H. pylori*–related ulcer, severe diarrhea may indicate pseudomembranous colitis. Obtain stool cultures, as ordered.
•Always flush I.V. line with NS injection, LR injection, or 5% dextrose injection before and after giving esomeprazole intravenously.
•For I.V. injection, reconstitute powder with 5 ml of NS injection and give as a bolus dose over 3 or more minutes. Once reconstituted, drug may be stored at room temperature for up to 12 hours.
•For I.V. infusion, reconstitute powder with 5 ml of NS injection, LR injection, or 5% dextrose injection. Further dilute reconstituted solution to make a final volume of 50 ml, and infuse over 10 to 30 minutes. Reconstituted drug may be stored at room temperature up to 6 hours if mixed with 5% dextrose injection or up to 12 hours if mixed with NS or LR injection.
•Be aware that patient receiving I.V. esomeprazole should be switched to oral form as soon as possible.
**PATIENT TEACHING**
•If patient has trouble swallowing esomeprazole capsules, tell him to open capsule and sprinkle pellets into a tablespoon of cool applesauce. Tell him not to chew pellets and to discard any unused pellets.
•Urge patient to tell prescriber if he takes antacids.

# estazolam

ProSom

## Class, Category, and Schedule
*Chemical:* Benzodiazepine
*Therapeutic:* Sedative-hypnotic
*Pregnancy category:* X
*Controlled substance:* Schedule IV

## Indications and Dosages
➤ *To treat insomnia*
**TABLETS**
**Adults.** 1 to 2 mg h.s.
**DOSAGE ADJUSTMENT** Starting dose 0.5 mg for small or debilitated elderly patients.

| Route | Onset | Peak | Duration |
|-------|-------|------|----------|
| P.O. | Unknown | Unknown | 6 to 8 hr |

## Mechanism of Action
May potentiate the effects of gamma-aminobutyric acid (GABA) and other inhibitory neurotransmitters by binding to specific benzodiazepine receptors in the limbic and cortical areas of the CNS. By binding to these receptors, estazolam increases GABA's inhibitory effects and blocks cortical and limbic arousal.

## Contraindications
Acute angle-closure glaucoma; hypersensitivity to estazolam, other benzodiazepines, or their components; pregnancy; psychosis

## Interactions
**DRUGS**
*barbiturates, carbamazepine, phenytoin, rifampin:* Possibly decreased estazolam levels
*carbamazepine:* Possibly increased blood carbamazepine level
*cimetidine, diltiazem, disulfiram, erythromycin, fluoxetine, fluvoxamine, isoniazid, itraconazole, ketoconazole, nefazodone, oral contraceptives, propoxyphene, ranitidine, verapamil:* Possibly increased blood level and impaired hepatic metabolism of estazolam
*clozapine:* Possibly cardiac arrest or respiratory depression
*CNS depressants:* Possibly potentiated CNS depression
*levodopa:* Possibly decreased therapeutic effects of levodopa
**FOODS**
*grapefruit juice:* Possibly increased blood level and impaired hepatic metabolism of drug
**ACTIVITIES**
*alcohol use:* Possibly potentiated CNS depression

## Adverse Reactions
**CNS:** Amnesia, anxiety, ataxia, confusion, delusions, depression, dizziness, drowsiness, euphoria, headache, hypokinesia, irritability, malaise, nervousness, slurred speech, tremor
**CV:** Chest pain, palpitations, tachycardia
**EENT:** Blurred vision, dry mouth, increased salivation, photophobia
**GI:** Abdominal pain, constipation, diarrhea, nausea, thirst, vomiting
**GU:** Libido changes
**RESP:** Respiratory depression
**SKIN:** Diaphoresis
**Other:** Physical or psychological dependence

E
F

## Nursing Considerations
•Use estazolam with extreme caution in patients with a history of drug or alcohol abuse because of the risk of addiction. Expect to give drug for no more than 12 weeks.
•Use drug cautiously in elderly or debilitated patients and those with depression or impaired hepatic, renal, or respiratory function.
•Expect to stop estazolam gradually to prevent withdrawal symptoms. Avoid stopping it abruptly if patient has a history of seizures.
•Monitor respiratory status, especially in patients with respiratory compromise, who are at increased risk for respiratory depression.
•If patient takes estazolam for depression, watch for suicidal tendencies, especially when therapy starts or dosage changes.
**PATIENT TEACHING**
•Warn patient not to exceed prescribed amount of time because of risk of addiction.
•Because estazolam can reduce alertness, advise patient to avoid hazardous activities until CNS effects of the drug are known.
•Advise patient not to drink alcohol or take other CNS depressants during estazolam therapy because of the risk of additive effects.
•Warn elderly and debilitated patients and those with impaired hepatic or renal function about the risk of excessive sedation or mental impairment and the need to report them.
•If patient takes 2-mg dosage for a long time, warn against stopping drug abruptly.

## estradiol
Estrace, Estrasorb, Estring, Estrogel

### estradiol acetate
Femtrace, Femring

### estradiol cypionate
depGynogen, Depo-Estradiol, Depogen, Dura-Estrin, E-Cypionate, Estragyn LA 5, Estro-Cyp, Estrofem, Estro-L.A.

### estradiol transdermal system
Alora, Climara, Esclim, Estraderm, Estrasorb, Estrogel, FemPatch, Menostar, Vivelle, Vivelle-Dot

### estradiol valerate
Clinagen LA 40, Delestrogen, Dioval 40, Dioval XX, Duragen-20, Estra-L 40, Estro-Span, Femogex (CAN), Gynogen L.A. 20, Gynogen

L.A. 40, Menaval-20, Valergen 10, Valergen 20, Valergen 40

## ethinyl estradiol
Estinyl

## Class and Category
*Chemical:* Estrogen derivative, steroid hormone
*Therapeutic:* Antineoplastic, antiosteoporotic agent, ovarian hormone replacement
*Pregnancy category:* X

## Indications and Dosages
➤ *To treat menopausal symptoms*
**TABLETS (ESTRADIOL)**
**Adult menopausal and postmenopausal females.** Starting on day 5 of a cycle, 0.5 to 2 mg q.d. in cycles of 3 wk on, 1 wk off.
**Adult postmenopausal females with intact uterus receiving progestin.** 0.5 to 2 mg q.d. with daily progestin; or 0.5 to 2 mg q.d. on days 1 through 25 of a 28-day cycle, with progestin starting day 12 or 16 and continuing through day 25 of the cycle; then no drugs on days 26 through 28, as prescribed.
**VAGINAL RING (ESTRADIOL ACETATE [FEMRING])**
**Adult females.** One ring (0.05 mg or 0.1 mg of estradiol/24 hr) inserted into upper third of vaginal vault and replaced q 3 mo.
**TABLETS (ESTRADIOL ACETATE [FEMTRACE])**
**Adult menopausal and postmenopausal females.** *Initial:* 0.45 mg q.d. May be increased to 0.9 mg q.d. and then 1.8 mg q.d. as needed.
**TABLETS (ETHINYL ESTRADIOL)**
**Adult menopausal and postmenopausal females.** 0.02 to 0.05 mg q.d. in cycles of 3 wk on, 1 wk off.
**Adult postmenopausal females with intact uterus receiving progestin.** 0.02 to 0.05 mg q.d. with daily progestin; or 0.02 to 0.05 mg q.d. on days 1 through 25 of a 28-day cycle, with progestin starting day 12 or 16 and continuing through day 25; then no drugs on days 26 through 28, as prescribed.
**DOSAGE ADJUSTMENT** Dosage may be reduced to less than 1 mg/day (estradiol) or 0.05 mg/day (ethinyl estradiol) for patients with only vaginal or vulvar symptoms.
**I.M. INJECTION (ESTRADIOL CYPIONATE IN OIL)**
**Adult females.** 1 to 5 mg as a single dose q 3 to 4 wk as needed.
**I.M. INJECTION (ESTRADIOL VALERATE IN OIL)**
**Adult females.** 10 to 20 mg q 4 wk as needed.

**TRANSDERMAL (ALORA, ESTRADERM, VIVELLE, VIVELLE-DOT)**

**Adult menopausal and postmenopausal females.** *Initial:* 0.025 to 0.05 mg/day in cycles of 3 wk on, 1 wk off. One patch applied to trunk or buttocks and replaced twice/wk (q 3 to 4 days). Adjust dosage to control symptoms, as prescribed.

**TRANSDERMAL (CLIMARA)**

**Adult females.** *Initial:* 0.025 mg/day. One patch applied to trunk or buttocks and replaced q wk. Titrate dosage to control symptoms, as prescribed. Schedule will be cyclic unless patient has had a hysterectomy.

**TRANSDERMAL (ESCLIM)**

**Adult females.** *Initial:* 0.025 mg/day. One patch applied to upper arm, upper thigh, or buttocks and replaced twice/wk (q 3 to 4 days). Adjust dosage to control symptoms, as prescribed. Use a cyclic schedule, as prescribed, unless patient has had a hysterectomy.

**TRANSDERMAL (ESTRASORB)**

**Adult females.** 3.48 g q.d. in morning. Half of dose (one pouchful) applied to one thigh and rubbed over entire thigh and calf for 3 min, and then repeated on other thigh and calf.

**TRANSDERMAL (ESTROGEL)**

**Adult females.** 1.25 g q.d. applied in thin layer from wrist to shoulder on inside and outside of one arm.

**TRANSDERMAL (FEMPATCH)**

**Adult females.** *Initial:* 0.025 mg/day. One patch applied to buttocks and replaced q wk. If symptoms aren't relieved after 4 to 6 wk, increased to two patches q wk, as prescribed. Follow a cyclic schedule, as prescribed, unless patient has had a hysterectomy.

➤ *To treat menopausal symptoms as combination therapy in patients with an intact uterus*

**TRANSDERMAL ESTRADIOL (ALORA, ESTRADERM, VIVELLE, VIVELLE-DOT) IN COMBINATION WITH ESTRADIOL AND NORETHINDRONE ACETATE (COMBIPATCH)**

**Adult females.** 0.05 mg/day estradiol-only transdermal system applied for first 14 days of a 28-day cycle and replaced twice/wk, according to product directions. Estradiol and norethindrone acetate transdermal system applied for remaining 14 days of 28-day cycle and replaced twice/wk during this period.

➤ *To treat postmenopausal vaginal and urogenital symptoms*

**VAGINAL CREAM (ESTRACE)**

**Adult females.** *Initial:* 2 to 4 g (200 to 400 mcg) q.d. for 1 to 2 wk. Then, dosage gradually reduced to one-half of initial dose, as prescribed, for 1 to 2 wk. *Maintenance:* 1 g (100 mcg) q.d. 1 to 3 times/wk for 3 wk, followed by 1 wk of no drugs. Repeat cyclically as needed.

**VAGINAL RING (ESTRING)**

**Adult females.** One ring (7.5 mcg of estradiol/24 hr) inserted into upper third of vaginal vault and replaced q 3 mo.

**VAGINAL RING (FEMRING)**

**Adult females.** One ring (0.05 or 0.1 mg of estradiol/24 hr) inserted into upper third of vaginal vault and replaced q 3 mo.

➤ *To prevent osteoporosis secondary to estrogen deficiency due to either natural or surgical menopause*

**TABLETS (ESTRADIOL)**

**Adult females.** At least 0.5 mg q.d. cyclically or continuously, adjusted as needed to control concurrent menopausal symptoms, as prescribed.

**TABLETS (ETHINYL ESTRADIOL)**

**Adult females.** At least 0.02 mg q.d. cyclically or continuously, as prescribed.

**TRANSDERMAL (ALORA, VIVELLE-DOT)**

**Adult females.** *Initial:* 0.025 mg/day continuously. One patch applied to lower abdomen or buttocks and replaced twice/wk. Adjust dosage to control symptoms and maintain bone density, as prescribed.

**TRANSDERMAL (CLIMARA)**

**Adult females.** *Initial:* 0.025 mg/day. One patch applied to trunk or buttocks and replaced q wk. Adjust dosage to control symptoms, as prescribed. Follow a cyclic schedule, as prescribed, unless patient has had a hysterectomy.

**TRANSDERMAL (ESTRADERM)**

**Adult females.** *Initial:* 0.05 mg/day. One patch applied to trunk or buttocks and replaced twice/wk. Adjust dosage to control symptoms, as prescribed. Follow a cyclic schedule, as prescribed, unless patient has had a hysterectomy.

**TRANSDERMAL (MENOSTAR)**

**Adult females.** *Initial:* 0.014 mg/day. One patch applied to lower abdomen and replaced q wk. Follow a cyclic schedule, as prescribed, unless patient has had a hysterectomy.

➤ *To treat estrogen deficiency due to oophorectomy, primary ovarian failure, or female hypogonadism*

**TABLETS (ESTRADIOL)**

**Adult females.** 0.5 to 2 mg q.d. continuously or in cycles of 3 wk on, 1 wk off.

E
F

TABLETS (ETHINYL ESTRADIOL)
**Adult females.** For primary ovarian failure or oophorectomy, 0.05 mg t.i.d. initially, then 0.05 mg q.d. after a few weeks, cyclically or continuously. For female hypogonadism, 0.05 mg q.d. to t.i.d. for first 2 wk of a theoretical menstrual cycle. A progestin may be added, as prescribed, during last half of cycle to help induce menses.

I.M. INJECTION (ESTRADIOL CYPIONATE IN OIL)
**Adult females.** 1.5 to 2 mg q mo (for female hypogonadism only).

I.M. INJECTION (ESTRADIOL VALERATE IN OIL)
**Adult females.** 10 to 20 mg q mo as needed.

TRANSDERMAL (ALORA, ESTRADERM, VIVELLE)
**Adult females.** *Initial:* 0.05 mg/day. One patch applied to trunk or buttocks and replaced twice/wk. Titrate dosage to control symptoms, as prescribed. Follow a cyclic schedule, as prescribed, unless patient has had a hysterectomy.

TRANSDERMAL (CLIMARA)
**Adult females.** *Initial:* 0.05 mg/day. One patch applied to trunk or buttocks and replaced q wk. Adjust dosage to control symptoms, as prescribed. Follow a cyclic schedule, as prescribed, unless patient has had a hysterectomy.

TRANSDERMAL (ESCLIM)
**Adult females.** *Initial:* 0.025 mg/day. One patch applied to upper arm, upper thigh, or buttocks and replaced twice/wk (q 3 to 4 days). Adjust dosage to control symptoms, as prescribed. Follow a cyclic schedule, as prescribed, unless patient has had a hysterectomy.

TRANSDERMAL (FEMPATCH)
**Adult females.** *Initial:* 0.025 mg. One patch applied to buttocks and replaced q wk. If symptoms aren't relieved after 4 to 6 wk, increased to two patches q wk, as prescribed. Follow a cyclic schedule, as prescribed, unless patient has had a hysterectomy.

➤ *To treat dysfunctional uterine bleeding caused by hormonal imbalance in patients with a hypoplastic or atrophic endometrium and without uterine disease*

TRANSDERMAL (CLIMARA)
**Adult females.** *Initial:* 0.05 mg/day. One patch applied to trunk or buttocks and replaced q wk. Adjust dosage to control symptoms, as prescribed. Follow a cyclic schedule, as prescribed.

TRANSDERMAL (FEMPATCH)
**Adult females.** *Initial:* 0.025 mg/day. One patch applied to buttocks and replaced q wk. If symptoms aren't relieved after 4 to 6 wk, increased to two patches q wk, as prescribed. Follow a cyclic schedule, as prescribed.

➤ *To provide palliative treatment for inoperable, progressive breast cancer in selected men and postmenopausal women*

TABLETS (ESTRADIOL)
**Adults.** 10 mg t.i.d. for at least 3 mo.

TABLETS (ETHINYL ESTRADIOL)
**Adults.** 1 mg t.i.d. for at least 3 mo.

➤ *To treat advancing inoperable prostate cancer*

TABLETS (ESTRADIOL)
**Adult males.** 1 to 2 mg b.i.d. or t.i.d., adjusted or continued, as prescribed, according to patient response.

TABLETS (ETHINYL ESTRADIOL)
**Adult males.** 0.15 to 3 mg q.d., adjusted or continued, as prescribed, according to patient response.

I.M. INJECTION (ESTRADIOL VALERATE)
**Adult males.** 30 mg q 1 to 2 wk, adjusted or continued, as prescribed, according to patient response.

## Contraindications
Active deep vein thrombosis, pulmonary embolism, or history of these conditions; active or recent (within past year) arterial thromboembolic disease, such as CVA or MI; hepatic dysfunction or disease; hypersensitivity to estradiol, ethinyl estradiol, or their components; hypersensitivity to tartrazine dye (contained in 0.02-mg estradiol and ethinyl estradiol tablets); known or suspected breast cancer or history of breast cancer except in appropriately selected patients being treated for metastatic disease; known or suspected estrogen-dependent cancer; pregnancy; undiagnosed abnormal genital bleeding

## Interactions
DRUGS
*aminocaproic acid:* Possibly increased hypercoagulability caused by aminocaproic acid
*barbiturates, carbamazepine, hydantoins, rifabutin, rifampin:* Possibly reduced activity of estradiol
*bromocriptine:* Possibly decreased therapeutic effects of bromocriptine
*calcium:* Possibly increased calcium absorption

## Mechanism of Action

Increases the rate of DNA and RNA synthesis in the cells of female reproductive organs, pituitary gland, hypothalamus, and other target organs. In the hypothalamus, estrogens reduce the release of gonadotropin-releasing hormone, which decreases pituitary release of follicle-stimulating hormone and luteinizing hormone. In women, these hormones are required for normal genitourinary and other essential body functions. At the cellular level, estrogens increase cervical secretions, cause endometrial cell proliferation, and improve uterine tone. Estrogen replacement helps maintain genitourinary function and reduces vasomotor symptoms when estrogen production declines as a result of menopause, surgical removal of ovaries, or other estrogen deficiency states. Estrogen replacement also helps prevent osteoporosis by inhibiting bone resorption.

In men, estrogens inhibit pituitary secretion of luteinizing hormone and decrease testicular secretion of testosterone. These actions may decrease prostate tumor growth and lower the level of prostate-specific antigen (PSA).

**E**
**F**

*corticosteroids:* Increased therapeutic and toxic effects of corticosteroids
*cyclosporine:* Increased risk of hepatotoxicity and nephrotoxicity
*didanosine, lamivudine, zalcitabine:* Possibly pancreatitis
*hepatotoxic drugs, such as isoniazid:* Increased risk of hepatitis and hepatotoxicity
*oral antidiabetic drugs:* Decreased therapeutic effects of these drugs
*somatrem, somatropin:* Possibly accelerated epiphyseal maturation
*tamoxifen:* Possibly decreased therapeutic effects of tamoxifen
*vitamin C:* Decreased metabolism and possibly increased adverse effects of estradiol
*warfarin:* Decreased anticoagulant effect

**FOODS**
*grapefruit juice:* Decreased metabolism and possibly increased adverse effects of estradiol

**ACTIVITIES**
*smoking:* Increased risk of CVA, pulmonary embolism, thrombophlebitis, and transient ischemic attack

### Adverse Reactions

**CNS:** CVA, dementia, depression, dizziness, headache, migraine headache
**CV:** Hypertension, MI, peripheral edema, pulmonary embolism, thromboembolism, thrombophlebitis
**EENT:** Intolerance of contact lenses, retinal vascular thrombosis, vision changes
**ENDO:** Breast enlargement, pain, tenderness, or tumors; gynecomastia; hyperglycemia
**GI:** Abdominal cramps or pain, anorexia, constipation, diarrhea, elevated liver function test results, enlargement of hepatic hemangiomas, gallbladder obstruction, hepatitis, increased appetite, nausea, pancreatitis, vomiting
**GU:** Amenorrhea, breakthrough bleeding, cervical erosion, clear vaginal discharge, decreased libido (males), dysmenorrhea, endometrial cancer, impotence, increased libido (females), ovarian cancer, prolonged or heavy menstrual bleeding, testicular atrophy, vaginal candidiasis
**SKIN:** Acne, alopecia, hirsutism, jaundice, melasma, oily skin, purpura, rash, seborrhea, urticaria
**Other:** Folic acid deficiency, hypercalcemia (in metastatic bone disease), weight gain

### Nursing Considerations

• **WARNING** Be aware that estradiol (Estrace) and ethinyl estradiol (Estinyl) are distinct and separate products and that their dosing isn't equivalent.
• Administer oral preparations with or immediately after food to decrease nausea.
• For I.M. injection of estradiol cypionate or estradiol valerate, roll vial and syringe between palms to evenly disperse drug. Use at least a 21-gauge needle because of viscosity of oil-based solution. Use a dry, sterile syringe. Inject deep into upper outer quadrant of gluteal muscle. Aspirate before injection to avoid injection into a blood vessel.
• Be aware that, in patients who are converting from oral estrogen to transdermal system, oral estrogen should be stopped 1 week before skin patches are applied.
• Expect to begin prophylaxis treatment against osteoporosis at the start of menopause.

•Be aware that estrogen therapy should be given cyclically or combined with a progestin for 10 to 14 days per month in women with an intact uterus to minimize the risk of endometrial hyperplasia.

•**WARNING** Be aware that severe hypercalcemia may occur in patients with bone metastasis due to breast cancer because estrogens influence the metabolism of calcium and phosphorus. Monitor for toxic effects of increased calcium absorption in patients who are predisposed to hypercalcemia or nephrolithiasis.

•**WARNING** Assess patient for possible contact lens intolerance or changes in vision or visual acuity because estrogens can cause keratoconus, leading to increased curvature of the cornea. Be prepared to discontinue drug immediately, as prescribed, if patient experiences sudden partial or complete loss of vision or sudden onset of diplopia, migraine, or proptosis.

•Monitor PT test results of patients receiving warfarin for loss of anticoagulant effect because estrogens increase production of clotting factors VII, VIII, IX, and X and promote platelet aggregation.

•Watch for elevated liver function test results because estrogens may worsen such conditions as acute intermittent or variegate hepatic porphyria.

•Closely monitor patient's blood pressure. A few patients may experience a substantial increase in blood pressure as an indiosyncratic reaction to estrogen. Monitor patients who already have hypertension for increases in blood pressure because estrogens may cause fluid retention. Also monitor patients with asthma, heart disease, migraines, renal disease, or seizure disorder for exacerbation of these conditions.

•Watch for peripheral edema or mild weight gain because estrogens can cause sodium and fluid retention.

•Frequently monitor serum glucose level in patients who have diabetes mellitus because estrogens may decrease insulin sensitivity and alter glucose tolerance.

•**WARNING** Expect to stop estrogen therapy in any woman who develops signs or symptoms of cancer; cardiovascular disease, such as CVA, MI, pulmonary embolism, or venous thrombosis; or dementia.

•Be aware that exogenous estradiol and progestins may worsen mood disorders, including depression. Monitor patient for anxiety, depression, dizziness, fatigue, insomnia, or mood changes.

•Assess skin for melasma (tan or brown patches), which may develop on forehead, cheeks, temples, and upper lip. These patches may persist after drug is stopped.

•Check patient's triglyceride level routinely because, in patients with hypertriglyceridemia, estrogen therapy may increase serum triglyceride level enough to cause pancreatitis and other complications.

•Monitor serum PSA level in patients with inoperable prostate cancer to determine if patient is responding to hormone therapy. If patient responds (usually within 3 months), expect therapy to continue until disease is significantly advanced.

•Monitor thyroid function test results in patients with hypothyroidism because long-term use of ethinyl estradiol may decrease effectiveness of thyroid therapy.

•Expect to stop estrogen therapy several weeks before patient undergoes major surgery, as prescribed, because certain procedures are associated with prolonged immobilization and therefore pose a risk of thromboembolism.

**PATIENT TEACHING**

•Before therapy starts, inform patient of risks involved in estrogen therapy, such as increased risk of breast, endometrial, or ovarian cancer; cardiovascular disease; dementia (if age 65 or older); gallbladder disease; and vision abnormalities.

•Advise patient to remain recumbent for at least 30 minutes after applying estradiol vaginal cream. Inform her that she may use a sanitary napkin (but not a tampon) to protect clothing after application.

•Teach patient proper application and use of transdermal patch. Instruct her not to apply patch to breasts, waistline, or other areas where it may not adhere properly. Advise her to rotate application sites at least weekly and to remove old patch before applying new one. If patch falls off, instruct her to reapply it to another area or to apply a new patch and continue the original treatment schedule. Caution her not to expose patch to sun for long periods. Explain that she may bathe while wearing the patch.

•Teach patient to apply Estrogel to clean, dry skin of one arm, using applicator. Stress importance of transferring all of the gel from applicator to arm. Tell patient to spread gel as thinly as possible over entire inside and outside of arm from wrist to shoulder. Advise her to wash her hands with soap and water afterward and to avoid fire and smoking until gel has dried because it's flammable. Tell patient never to apply gel to breasts.

•Inform patient that each pouch of Estrasorb contains half of daily dose. Instruct her to apply emulsion to clean, dry skin on top of thigh and to rub it into entire thigh and calf for 3 minutes. Tell her to rub any excess emulsion onto her buttocks. Then, advise her to repeat procedure on her other thigh and calf using the second pouch. Tell her to wash her hands with soap and water after the application and to dress only after affected areas are dry.

•Teach patient proper use of estradiol vaginal ring. Instruct her to insert ring in upper third of vagina, to keep it there for 90 days, and then to remove it and insert a new ring. Or she may remove it during the 90-day dosage period, rinse it with lukewarm (not hot or boiling) water, and reinsert it as needed for personal hygiene. Remind patient that she shouldn't be able to feel the ring when it's in place. If she does, she should use a finger to push the ring farther into her vagina.

•Inform patient receiving estradiol treatment that she should have an annual pelvic examination to screen for cervical dysplasia.

•Tell patient who has an intact uterus and is prescribed transdermal Menostar that she will need to receive progestin for 14 days every 6 to 12 months and have an endometrial biopsy yearly.

# estradiol and norethindrone acetate

Activella, CombiPatch

## Class and Category

*Chemical:* Estrogen derivative, steroid hormone
*Therapeutic:* Antiosteoporotic agent, ovarian hormone replacement
*Pregnancy category:* X

## Indications and Dosages

➤ *To treat estrogen deficiency due to hypogonadism, oophorectomy, or primary ovarian failure in patients with an intact uterus*

TRANSDERMAL (COMBIPATCH)
**Adult females.** Continuous combined regimen for women who don't want to resume menses: 0.05-mg estradiol/0.14-mg norethindrone acetate/day transdermal system (9-cm$^2$ CombiPatch) is worn continuously on lower abdomen; may be increased to 0.05-mg estradiol/0.25-mg norethindrone acetate/day system (16-cm$^2$ CombiPatch), as prescribed, if a greater progestin dose is desired. New system is applied twice/wk (q 3 to 4 days) during a 28-day cycle.

**Adult females.** Continuous sequential regimen in combination with an estradiol-only transdermal delivery system: 0.05-mg/day estradiol transdermal system (Vivelle) is worn for the first 14 days of a 28-day cycle and is replaced twice/wk according to product directions. For the remaining 14 days of the 28-day cycle, 0.05-mg estradiol/0.14-mg norethindrone acetate/day transdermal system (9-cm$^2$ CombiPatch) is worn on the lower abdomen; may be increased to 0.05-mg estradiol/0.25-mg norethindrone acetate/day system (16-cm$^2$ CombiPatch), as prescribed, if a greater progestin dose is desired. CombiPatch system should be replaced twice/wk (q 3 to 4 days) during this period in the cycle.

➤ *To treat menopausal symptoms and to prevent osteoporosis due to estrogen deficiency in postmenopausal women with an intact uterus*

TABLETS (ACTIVELLA)
**Adult females.** 1 tablet (1 mg estradiol and 0.5 mg norethindrone acetate) q.d.

TRANSDERMAL (COMBIPATCH)
**Adult females.** Continuous combined regimen for women who don't want to resume menses: 0.05-mg estradiol/0.14-mg norethindrone acetate/day transdermal system (9-cm$^2$ CombiPatch) is worn continuously on lower abdomen; may be increased to 0.05-mg estradiol/0.25-mg norethindrone acetate/day system (16-cm$^2$ CombiPatch), as prescribed, if a greater progestin dose is desired. New system is applied twice/wk (q 3 to 4 days) during a 28-day cycle.

**Adult females.** Continuous sequential regimen in combination with an estradiol-only transdermal delivery system: 0.05-mg/day estradiol transdermal system (Vivelle) is worn for the first 14 days of a 28-day cycle and is replaced twice/wk according to product directions. For remaining 14 days of 28-

day cycle, 0.05-mg estradiol/0.14-mg norethindrone acetate/day transdermal system (9-cm² CombiPatch) is worn on lower abdomen; may be increased to 0.05-mg estradiol/0.25-mg norethindrone acetate/day system (16-cm² CombiPatch), as prescribed, if a greater progestin dose is desired. CombiPatch system is replaced twice/wk (q 3 to 4 days) during this period in the cycle.

| Route | Onset | Peak | Duration |
|-------|-------|------|----------|
| Transdermal | Unknown | In 24 hr | Unknown |

## Mechanism of Action

Estradiol increases the rate of DNA and RNA synthesis in the cells of female reproductive organs, pituitary gland, hypothalamus, and other target organs. In the hypothalamus, estrogens decrease the release of gonadotropin-releasing hormone, which reduces pituitary release of follicle-stimulating hormone and luteinizing hormone. In women, these hormones are required for normal genitourinary and other essential body functions. At the cellular level, estrogens increase cervical secretions, cause endometrial cell proliferation, and improve uterine tone. Estrogen replacement helps maintain genitourinary function and reduces vasomotor symptoms when estrogen production declines as a result of menopause, surgical removal of ovaries, or other estrogen deficiency states. Estrogen replacement also helps prevent osteoporosis by inhibiting bone resorption.

Norethindrone is a progestin. Progestins prolong some of the positive effects of estrogens on HDL cholesterol. Norethindrone diffuses freely into target cells of the female reproductive tract, mammary glands, hypothalamus, and pituitary gland and binds to the progesterone cell receptor. It converts a proliferative endometrium into a secretory one in women with adequate estrogen replacement, reducing endometrial growth and the risk of endometrial cancer compared with women who have an intact uterus and take unopposed estrogens. Norethindrone also decreases nuclear estradiol receptors and suppresses epithelial DNA synthesis in endometrial tissues.

## Contraindications

Active deep vein thrombosis, pulmonary embolism, or history of these conditions; endometrial hyperplasia; hepatic disorders; hypersensitivity to estradiol, norethindrone, or their components; jaundice; known or suspected breast cancer or history of breast cancer from estrogen use; known or suspected estrogen-dependent cancer; new or recent (within past year) CVA or MI; pregnancy; undiagnosed abnormal genital bleeding; vaginal disorders

## Interactions

### DRUGS

*aminocaproic acid:* Possibly an increase in hypercoagulability caused by aminocaproic acid

*barbiturates, carbamazepine, hydantoins, rifabutin, rifampin:* Possibly reduced activity of estradiol and norethindrone

*bromocriptine:* Possibly decreased therapeutic effects of bromocriptine

*calcium:* Possibly increased calcium absorption

*corticosteroids:* Increased therapeutic and toxic effects of corticosteroids

*cyclosporine:* Increased risk of hepatotoxicity and nephrotoxicity

*didanosine, lamivudine, zalcitabine:* Possibly pancreatitis

*hepatotoxic drugs (such as isoniazid):* Increased risk of hepatitis and hepatotoxicity

*oral antidiabetic drugs:* Decreased therapeutic effects of these drugs

*somatrem, somatropin:* Possibly accelerated epiphyseal maturation

*tamoxifen:* Possibly decreased therapeutic effects of tamoxifen

*vitamin C:* Decreased metabolism and possibly increased adverse effects of estradiol and norethindrone

*warfarin:* Decreased anticoagulant effect

### FOODS

*grapefruit juice:* Decreased metabolism and possibly increased adverse effects of estradiol and norethindrone

### ACTIVITIES

*smoking:* Increased risk of CVA, pulmonary embolism, thrombophlebitis, and transient ischemic attack

## Adverse Reactions

**CNS:** CVA, dementia, depression, dizziness, headache, irritability, migraine headache, mood swings, worsening of epilepsy

**CV:** Deep and superficial venous thrombosis, hypertension, hypertriglyceridemia, MI, peripheral edema, pulmonary embolism, thromboembolism, thrombophlebitis
**EENT:** Intolerance of contact lenses, retinal vascular thrombosis, vision changes
**ENDO:** Breast enlargement, pain, tenderness, or tumors; gynecomastia; hyperglycemia; nipple discharge
**GI:** Abdominal cramps or pain, anorexia, constipation, diarrhea, elevated liver function test results, enlargement of hepatic hemangiomas, gallbladder obstruction, hepatitis, increased appetite, nausea, pancreatitis, vomiting
**GU:** Amenorrhea, breakthrough bleeding, cervical erosion, clear vaginal discharge, decreased libido (males), dysmenorrhea, endometrial hyperplasia or cancer, impotence, increased libido (females), ovarian cancer, prolonged or heavy menstrual bleeding, testicular atrophy, vaginal candidiasis
**MS:** Leg cramps
**SKIN:** Acne, alopecia, hirsutism, jaundice, melasma, oily skin, purpura, rash, seborrhea, urticaria
**Other:** Anaphylaxis, folic acid deficiency, hypercalcemia (in metastatic bone disease), hypocalcemia, weight gain

## Nursing Considerations

•**WARNING** Be aware that severe hypercalcemia may occur in patients with bone metastasis due to breast cancer because estrogens influence the metabolism of calcium and phosphorus. Monitor for toxic effects of increased calcium absorption in patients who are predisposed to hypercalcemia or nephrolithiasis.

•**WARNING** Assess patient for contact-lens intolerance or changes in vision or visual acuity because estrogens can cause keratoconus, leading to increased curvature of the cornea. Be prepared to discontinue drug immediately, as prescribed, if patient experiences sudden partial or complete loss of vision or sudden onset of diplopia, migraine, or proptosis.

•Monitor PT test results of patients receiving warfarin for loss of anticoagulant effect because estrogens increase production of clotting factors VII, VIII, IX, and X and promote platelet aggregation.

•Watch for elevated liver function test results because estrogen and progestins may exacerbate such conditions as acute intermittent or variegate hepatic porphyria.

•Closely monitor patient's blood pressure. A few patients may have a substantial increase in blood pressure as an idiosyncratic reaction to estrogen. Monitor patients who already have hypertension for increases in blood pressure because estrogens may cause fluid retention. Also monitor patients with asthma, heart disease, migraines, renal disease, or seizure disorder for worsening of these conditions.

•Monitor for peripheral edema or mild weight gain because estrogens can cause sodium and fluid retention.

•Check patient's triglyceride level routinely because, in patients with hypertriglyceridemia, estrogen therapy may increase serum triglyceride level enough to cause pancreatitis and other complications.

•Observe patients, especially those with diabetes mellitus, for changes in glucose tolerance when estrogen therapy is started or stopped. Patients with diabetes mellitus may develop altered glucose tolerance secondary to decreased insulin sensitivity.

•Be aware that exogenous estradiol and norethindrone may worsen mood disorders, including depression. Monitor patient for anxiety, depression, dizziness, fatigue, insomnia, or mood changes. If significant depression occurs, expect to stop hormone replacement therapy.

•Assess skin for melasma (tan or brown patches), which may develop on forehead, cheeks, temples, and upper lip. These patches may persist after drug is stopped.

•Expect to stop estrogen combination therapy in any woman who develops evidence of dementia, cancer, or cardiovascular disease, such as CVA, MI pulmonary embolism, or venous thrombosis.

•Expect to stop estrogen therapy several weeks before major surgery, as prescribed, because certain procedures increase the risk of thromboembolism by causing prolonged immobilization.

### PATIENT TEACHING

•Before therapy starts, explain the risks of estrogen/progestin therapy, such as increased risk of breast, endometrial, or ovarian cancer; cardiovascular disease; gallbladder disease; and vision abnormalities.

•Teach patient proper application and use of CombiPatch transdermal system. Instruct her to tear pouch open, rather than cutting it open with scissors, and to remove stiff pro-

tective liner covering adhesive without touching adhesive. Tell her not to cut or trim the patch. Advise her to apply patch to a clean, dry, hairless part of lower abdomen. Caution her not to apply patch to breasts; to injured, irritated, callused, or scarred areas; or to areas where it may not adhere properly, such as waistline.
• Advise patient to rotate application sites at least weekly and to remove old patch before applying new one. If patch falls off, instruct her to reapply it to another area, or to apply a new patch and continue the original treatment schedule. Caution her not to expose patch to sun for prolonged periods. Explain that she may bathe while wearing the patch.
• Advise patient taking estradiol and norethindrone not to smoke because smoking increases the risk of deep vein thrombosis, MI, and other thromboembolic disorders.
• Explain that estradiol and norethindrone may cause monthly withdrawal bleeding.
• Advise patient receiving estradiol treatment to have an annual pelvic examination, including a Papanicolaou (Pap) smear, to screen for cervical dysplasia.

# estrogens (conjugated)

C.E.S. (CAN), Congest (CAN), Premarin

## estrogens (conjugated) and medroxyprogesterone

Premphase, Prempro

## synthetic estrogens, A (conjugated)

Cenestin

## synthetic estrogens, B (conjugated)

Enjuvia

## Class and Category

*Chemical:* Estrogen derivative, steroid hormone
*Therapeutic:* Antiosteoporotic agent, ovarian hormone replacement
*Pregnancy category:* X

## Indications and Dosages

➤ *To treat moderate to severe vasomotor menopausal symptoms*
TABLETS (CENESTIN, PREMARIN)
**Adults.** 0.3 to 1.25 mg q.d. (Cenestin, Premarin) or cyclicly 25 days on, 5 days off (Pre-

marin only). Dosage increased as needed to control symptoms.
TABLETS (ENJUVIA)
**Adults.** 0.625 mg q.d. Dosage increased as needed to control symptoms.
TABLETS (PREMPRO)
**Adults.** 0.3 mg of conjugated estrogens and 1.5 mg of medroxyprogesterone q.d. Increased up to 0.625 mg of conjugated estrogens and 5 mg of medroxyprogesterone q.d. as needed.
TABLETS (PREMPHASE)
**Adults.** 0.625 mg of conjugated estrogens q.d. on days 1 through 14 and combination product (0.625 mg of conjugated estrogens and 5 mg of medroxyprogesterone) on days 15 through 28.

➤ *To treat vaginal and vulvar atrophy*
TABLETS (CENESTIN, PREMARIN)
**Adults.** 0.3 to 1.25 mg q.d. (Cenestin, Premarin) or cyclicly 25 days on, 5 days off (Premarin only). Dosage increased as needed to control symptoms.
TABLETS (PREMPRO)
**Adults.** 0.3 mg of conjugated estrogens and 1.5 mg of medroxyprogesterone q.d. Increased up to 0.625 mg of conjugated estrogens and 5 mg of medroxyprogesterone q.d. as needed.
TABLETS (PREMPHASE)
**Adults.** 0.625 mg of conjugated estrogens q.d. on days 1 through 14 and combination product (0.625 mg of conjugated estrogens and 5 mg of medroxyprogesterone) on days 15 through 28.

➤ *To treat atrophic vaginitis and vaginal and vulvar atrophy*
VAGINAL CREAM (PREMARIN)
**Adults.** 0.5 to 2 g q.d. in cycles of 3 wk on, 1 wk off.

➤ *To prevent postmenopausal osteoporosis*
TABLETS (CENESTIN, PREMARIN)
**Adults.** 0.625 mg q.d. continuously or cyclicly 25 days on, 5 days off.
TABLETS (PREMPRO)
**Adults.** 0.3 mg of conjugated estrogens and 1.5 mg of medroxyprogesterone q.d. Increased to 0.625 mg conjugated estrogens and 5 mg medroxyprogesterone q.d. as needed.
TABLETS (PREMPHASE)
**Adults.** 0.625 mg of conjugated estrogens q.d. on days 1 through 14 and combination product (0.625 mg of conjugated estrogens and 5 mg of medroxyprogesterone) on days 15 through 28.

➤ *To provide palliative treatment for advanced androgen-dependent prostate cancer*
TABLETS (PREMARIN)
**Adults.** 1.25 to 2.5 mg t.i.d.

➤ *To provide palliative treatment for metastatic breast cancer*
TABLETS (PREMARIN)
**Adults.** 10 mg t.i.d. for 3 mo or longer.

➤ *To treat dysfunctional uterine bleeding*
I.V. INFUSION, I.M. INJECTION (PREMARIN)
**Adults.** 25 mg, repeated in 6 to 12 hr if needed.

➤ *To treat estrogen deficiency from oophorectomy or primary ovarian failure*
TABLETS (PREMARIN)
**Adults.** 1.25 mg q.d. in cycles of 3 wk on, 1 wk off.

➤ *To treat female hypogonadism*
TABLETS (PREMARIN)
**Adults.** 0.3 to 0.625 mg q.d. in cycles of 3 wk on, 1 wk off. Increased as needed q 6 to 12 mo.

## Mechanism of Action

Increase the rate of DNA and RNA synthesis in the cells of female reproductive organs, hypothalamus, pituitary glands, and other target organs. In the hypothalamus, estrogens reduce the release of gonadotropin-releasing hormone, which decreases pituitary release of follicle-stimulating hormone and luteinizing hormone. In women, these hormones are required for normal genitourinary and other essential body functions. At the cellular level, estrogens increase cervical secretions, cause endometrial cell proliferation, and increase uterine tone. Estrogen replacement helps maintain genitourinary function and reduce vasomotor symptoms when estrogen production declines from menopause, surgical removal of ovaries, or other estrogen deficiency. It also helps prevent osteoporosis by keeping bone resorption from exceeding bone formation.

In men, estrogens inhibit pituitary secretion of luteinizing hormone and decrease testicular secretion of testosterone. These actions may decrease prostate tumor growth and lower the level of prostate-specific antigen.

## Contraindications

Active deep vein thrombosis, pulmonary embolism, or history of these conditions; active or recent (within past year) arterial thromboembolic disease such as CVA or MI; hepatic dysfunction or disease; hypersensitivity to estrogens or their components; known or suspected breast cancer or history of breast cancer; known or suspected estrogen-dependent cancer; pregnancy; undiagnosed abnormal genital bleeding

## Incompatibilities

Don't combine I.V. estrogens with acid solutions, ascorbic acid, and protein hydrolysate because they're incompatible.

## Interactions
DRUGS
*aminocaproic acid:* Possibly increased level of hypercoagulability caused by aminocaproic acid
*barbiturates, carbamazepine, hydantoins, rifabutin, rifampin:* Possibly reduced activity of estrogen and medroxyprogesterone
*bromocriptine:* Possibly interference with bromocriptine's therapeutic effects
*calcium:* Possibly increased calcium absorption
*corticosteroids:* Increased therapeutic and toxic effects of corticosteroids
*cyclosporine:* Increased risk of hepatotoxicity and nephrotoxicity
*didanosine, lamivudine, zalcitabine:* Possibly pancreatitis
*hepatotoxic drugs (such as isoniazid):* Increased risk of hepatitis and hepatotoxicity
*oral antidiabetic drugs:* Decreased therapeutic effects of these drugs
*somatrem, somatropin:* Possibly accelerated epiphyseal maturation
*tamoxifen:* Possibly interference with tamoxifen's therapeutic effects
*warfarin:* Decreased anticoagulant effect
ACTIVITIES
*smoking:* Increased risk of CVA, pulmonary embolism, thrombophlebitis, and transient ischemic attack

## Adverse Reactions
**CNS:** CVA, dementia, depression, dizziness, headache, migraine headache
**CV:** MI, peripheral edema, pulmonary embolism, thromboembolism, thrombo-phlebitis
**EENT:** Intolerance of contact lenses, retinal vascular thrombosis

E
F

**ENDO:** Breast enlargement, pain, tenderness, or tumors; gynecomastia; hyperglycemia
**GI:** Abdominal cramps or pain, anorexia, constipation, diarrhea, gallbladder obstruction, hepatitis, increased appetite, nausea, pancreatitis, vomiting
**GU:** Amenorrhea, breakthrough bleeding, cervical erosion, clear vaginal discharge, decreased libido (males), dysmenorrhea, endometrial cancer, impotence, increased libido (females), ovarian cancer, prolonged or heavy menstrual bleeding, testicular atrophy, vaginal candidiasis
**SKIN:** Acne, alopecia, hirsutism, jaundice, melasma, oily skin, purpura, rash, seborrhea, urticaria
**Other:** Folic acid deficiency, hypercalcemia (in metastatic bone disease), weight gain

## Nursing Considerations

•Use conjugated estrogens cautiously in patients with severe hypocalcemia because a sudden increase in serum calcium level may cause adverse reactions.
•Reconstitute conjugated estrogens with NS, dextrose, or invert sugar solution and use within a few hours. Discard solution that contains precipitate.
•Monitor serum calcium level to detect severe hypercalcemia in patients with bone metastasis from breast cancer.
•Watch for elevated liver function test results because estrogen and progestins may worsen such conditions as acute intermittent or variegate hepatic porphyria.
•Assess hypertensive patients for increases in blood pressure because estrogens may cause fluid retention.
•Monitor patients with asthma, diabetes mellitus, endometriosis, heart disease, lupus erythematosus, migraine headaches, renal disease, or seizure disorder for worsening of these conditions.
•If patient takes warfarin, assess PT test results as prescribed for loss of anticoagulant effects because estrogens increase production of clotting factors and promote platelet aggregation.
•Expect to stop drug during periods of immobilization, 4 weeks before elective surgery, and if jaundice develops.
•Expect to stop estrogen combination therapy in any woman who develops signs or symptoms of cancer; cardiovascular disease,

such as CVA, MI, pulmonary embolism, or venous thrombosis; or dementia.
**PATIENT TEACHING**
•Explain the risks of estrogen therapy, including increased risk of breast, endometrial, or ovarian cancer; cardiovascular disease; dementia; and gallbladder disease.
•Urge patient to immediately report breakthrough bleeding to prescriber.
•Instruct patient to perform a monthly breast self-examination and to comply with all prescribed follow-up examinations.
•Warn female patient that long-term use may increase risk of dementia, heart disease, CVA, gallbladder disease, and breast or endometrial cancer.

# eszopiclone

Lunesta

## Class, Category, and Schedule

*Chemical:* Pyrrolopyrazine derivative of cyclopyrrolone class
*Therapeutic:* Sedative-hypnotic
*Pregnancy category:* C
*Controlled substance:* Schedule IV

## Indications and Dosages

➤ *To treat insomnia*
**TABLETS**
**Adults.** *Initial:* 2 mg immediately h.s. May be increased to 3 mg h.s., as needed. *Maintenance:* 3 mg h.s.
**DOSAGE ADJUSTMENT** For elderly patients who have trouble falling asleep or patients with severe hepatic impairment, dosage decreased to 1 mg immediately h.s. For elderly patients who have trouble staying asleep, dosage may be increased to 2 mg h.s.

| Route | Onset | Peak | Duration |
|-------|-------|------|----------|
| P.O. | Unknown | 1 hr | Unknown |

## Contraindications

Hypersensitivity to eszopiclone or its components

## Interactions

**DRUGS**
*clarithromycin, itraconazole, ketoconazole, nefazodone, nelfinavir, ritonavir, troleandomycin:* Increased blood level of eszopiclone
*rifampin:* Decreased blood level of eszopiclone

ACTIVITIES
*alcohol use:* Additive effect on psychomotor performance

---

### Mechanism of Action
May potentiate the effects of the inhibitory neurotransmitter gamma-aminobutyric acid (GABA) by binding close to or with benzodiazepine receptors in the limbic and cortical areas of the CNS. By binding to these receptor sites and areas, eszopiclone increases GABA's inhibitory effects and blocks cortical and limbic arousal, thereby inducing and maintaining sleep.

---

## Adverse Reactions
**CNS:** Anxiety, confusion, depression, dizziness, hallucinations, headache (including migraine), nervousness, neuralgia, somnolence, unusual dreams
**CV:** Chest pain, peripheral edema
**EENT:** Dry mouth, taste perversion
**ENDO:** Gynecomastia
**GI:** Diarrhea, hepatitis, indigestion, nausea, vomiting
**GU:** Decreased libido, dysmenorrhea, UTI
**RESP:** Asthma, respiratory tract infection
**SKIN:** Pruritus, rash
**Other:** Generalized pain, heat stroke, viral infection

## Nursing Considerations
• Use eszopiclone cautiously in patients with severe mental depression or reduced respiratory function; drug may intensify depression and lead to respiratory depression.

PATIENT TEACHING
• Instruct patient not to exceed prescribed eszopiclone dosage and not to abruptly stop taking the drug because withdrawal symptoms may occur.
• Because eszopiclone can reduce alertness, advise patient to take drug immediately before bedtime and to avoid hazardous activities until drug's CNS effects are known.
• Caution patient to avoid alcohol and CNS depressants during therapy because of additive effects.
• Advise female patient of childbearing age to notify prescriber if she becomes or intends to become pregnant during therapy.

• Inform patient that sleep may be disturbed for the first few nights after he stops taking drug.

# etanercept
Enbrel

## Class and Category
*Chemical:* Dimeric recombinant human p75 tumor necrosis factor receptor (TNFR)
*Therapeutic:* Disease-modifying antirheumatoid drug
*Pregnancy category:* B

## Indications and Dosages
➤ *To reduce signs and symptoms of rheumatoid or psoriatic arthritis, slow structural damage in active arthritis, and improve physical function in patients with psoriatic arthritis, alone or in combination with methotrexate*

S.C. INJECTION
**Adults.** 50 mg once weekly on the same day each week.

➤ *To reduce signs and symptoms of active ankylosing spondylitis*

S.C. INJECTION
**Adults.** 50 mg once weekly on the same day each week.

➤ *To reduce signs and symptoms of juvenile rheumatoid arthritis*

S.C. INJECTION
**Children ages 4 to 17.** 0.4 mg/kg twice/wk 3 to 4 days apart for 3 to 7 mo; or 0.8 mg/kg once weekly on the same day each week for 3 to 7 mo. *Maximum:* 25 mg twice/wk or 50 mg weekly.

➤ *To treat chronic moderate to severe plaque psoriasis in candidates for systemic therapy or phototherapy*

S.C. INJECTION
**Adults.** *Initial:* 50 mg twice/wk 3 to 4 days apart for 3 mo; then reduced to 50 mg/wk.

## Incompatibilities
Don't combine etanercept with other drugs.

## Contraindications
Hypersensitivity to etanercept, hamster protein, or their components, sepsis or risk of it

E
F

## Mechanism of Action

Etanercept reduces joint inflammation from rheumatoid arthritis by binding with tumor necrosis factor (TNF), a cytokine, or protein, that plays an important role in normal inflammatory and immune responses.

In rheumatoid arthritis, the immune and inflammatory process triggers release of TNF, mainly from macrophages. TNF then binds to TNF receptors on cell membranes, as shown below left. This action renders TNF biologically active and triggers a cas-

cade of inflammatory events that results in increased inflammation of the synovial membrane, release of destructive lysosomal enzymes, and further joint destruction.

Etanercept binds specifically to TNF and prevents it from binding with TNF receptors on the cell membranes, as shown below right. This action renders the bound TNF biologically inactive, prevents TNF-mediated cellular responses, and results in significant reduction in inflammatory activity.

## Interactions

**DRUGS**

*sulfasalazine:* Possibly decreased neutrophil count

## Adverse Reactions

**CNS:** Asthenia, chills, dizziness, fever, headache

**CV:** Hypertension, hypotension, peripheral edema

**EENT:** Pharyngitis, rhinitis, sinusitis

**GI:** Abdominal abscess, abdominal pain, cholecystitis, diarrhea, gastroenteritis, indigestion, nausea, noninfectious hepatitis, vomiting

**GU:** Pyelonephritis

**HEME:** Lymphoma

**MS:** Osteomyelitis, septic arthritis

**RESP:** Bronchitis, cough, pneumonia, upper respiratory tract infection

**SKIN:** Cellulitis, foot abscess, leg ulceration, pruritus, rash, urticaria

**Other:** Angioedema; injection site edema, erythema, itching, and pain; sepsis; varicella infection

## Nursing Considerations

•**WARNING** Don't use the diluent provided with etanercept (bacteriostatic water for injection, USP, with 0.9% benzyl alcohol) for patients with benzyl alcohol hypersensitivity. Use sterile water for injection instead.

•**WARNING** If you have a latex allergy, don't handle needle cover of diluent syringe because it contains dry natural rubber (latex).

•**WARNING** Expect to stop etanercept if patient develops sepsis.

•Avoid giving live virus vaccines to patients taking etanercept because the drug decreases immune response and increases the risk of secondary transmission of vaccine virus.

•Monitor patients with immunosuppression for evidence of acute or chronic infection, including chills, fever, and tachycardia, be-

cause etanercept decreases patient's defenses against infection. It also increases patient's risk of developing malignant tumors.
•Continue giving corticosteroids, NSAIDs, and other analgesics, as prescribed, during etanercept therapy.

**PATIENT TEACHING**
•Inform patient that etanercept is given by a small injection under the skin, and teach him proper injection technique if needed.
•If patient will be taking a 50-mg dose, explain that a prefilled syringe is available to eliminate the need to mix or draw up drug.
•If patient will be taking less than a 50-mg dose or prefers not to use prefilled syringe, advise him to use drug as soon as possible after dissolving powder. Dissolved powder may be kept in refrigerator for up to 6 hours after mixing and then should be discarded.
•Instruct patient to rotate injection sites among the thigh, stomach, and upper arms and to avoid areas that are tender, red, bruised, or hard. Advise him to keep each site at least 1″ away from a previous site.
•Urge patient to use needles and syringes once and discard in puncture-proof container.
•Caution patient that the risk of lymphoma may be higher in those who take etanercept; tell him to seek medical attention promptly for any suspicious signs and symptoms.
•Urge patient to consult prescriber immediately if he develops an infection because drug may decrease infection-fighting ability.
•Caution patient who hasn't had chickenpox to contact prescriber right away if he's exposed because he may develop a more serious infection.

# ethacrynic acid
Edecrin

# ethacrynate sodium
Edecrin

## Class and Category
*Chemical:* Ketone derivative of anyloxyacetic acid
*Therapeutic:* Diuretic
*Pregnancy category:* B

## Indications and Dosages
➤ *To promote diuresis in heart failure; hepatic cirrhosis; renal disease; ascites of short duration caused by cancer, idio-*pathic edema, or lymphedema; and edema in children (excluding infants with congenital heart disease or nephrotic syndrome)*

**ORAL SOLUTION, TABLETS**
**Adults.** *Initial:* 50 to 100 mg/day as a single dose or in divided doses. Dosage increased by 25 to 50 mg/day, if needed. *Maintenance:* 50 to 200 mg/day. *Maximum:* 400 mg/day.
**Children (except infants).** *Initial:* 25 mg q.d. Dosage increased in 25-mg increments daily, if needed.

**I.V. INFUSION**
**Adults.** *Initial:* 50 mg or 0.5 to 1 mg/kg. Dose repeated in 2 to 4 hr, if needed, then q 4 to 6 hr based on patient response. In an emergency, dose repeated q 1 hr, if needed. *Maximum:* 100 mg as a single dose.

| Route | Onset | Peak | Duration |
|-------|-------|------|----------|
| P.O. | 30 min | 2 hr | 6 to 8 hr |
| I.V. | 5 min | 15 to 30 min | 2 hr |

## Mechanism of Action
Probably inhibits the sulfhydryl-catalyzed enzyme systems that cause sodium and chloride resorption in the proximal and distal tubules and the ascending limb of the loop of Henle. These inhibitory effects increase urinary excretion of sodium, chloride, and water, causing profound diuresis. The drug also increases the excretion of potassium, hydrogen, calcium, magnesium, bicarbonate, ammonium, and phosphate.

## Contraindications
Anuria; hypersensitivity to ethacrynic acid, ethacrynate sodium, sulfonylureas, or their components; infancy; severe diarrhea

## Interactions
**DRUGS**
*ACE inhibitors, antihypertensives:* Possibly hypotension
*aminoglycosides:* Increased risk of ototoxicity
*amiodarone:* Increased risk of arrhythmias
*amphotericin B:* Increased risk of electrolyte imbalances, nephrotoxicity, and ototoxicity
*anticoagulants, thrombolytics:* Possibly potentiated anticoagulation and risk of hemorrhage
*corticosteroids:* Increased risk of gastric hemorrhage

*digoxin*: Increased risk of digitalis toxicity
*insulin, oral antidiabetic drugs*: Possibly increased serum glucose level and decreased therapeutic effects of these drugs
*lithium:* Increased risk of lithium toxicity
*neuromuscular blockers*: Possibly increased neuromuscular blockade
*NSAIDs:* Possibly decreased effects of ethacrynic acid
*sympathomimetics*: Possibly interference with hypotensive effects of ethacrynic acid and ethacrynate sodium

**ACTIVITIES**
*alcohol use:* Possibly potentiated hypotensive and diuretic effects of ethacrynic acid and ethacrynate sodium

## Adverse Reactions

**CNS:** Confusion, fatigue, headache, malaise, nervousness
**CV:** Orthostatic hypotension
**EENT:** Blurred vision, hearing loss, ototoxicity (ringing or buzzing in ears), sensation of fullness in ears, yellow vision
**ENDO:** Hyperglycemia, hypoglycemia
**GI:** Abdominal pain, anorexia, diarrhea, dysphagia, GI bleeding (I.V. form), nausea, vomiting
**GU:** Hematuria (I.V. form), interstitial nephritis, polyuria
**HEME:** Agranulocytosis, severe neutropenia, thrombocytopenia
**SKIN:** Rash
**Other:** Hyperuricemia, hypochloremic alkalosis, hypokalemia, hypomagnesemia, hyponatremia, hypovolemia, infusion site irritation and pain

## Nursing Considerations

•**WARNING** Administer ethacrynic acid and ethacrynate sodium cautiously in patients with advanced hepatic cirrhosis, especially those who also have a history of electrolyte imbalance or hepatic encephalopathy; both forms of drug may lead to lethal hepatic coma.
•Dilute ethacrynate sodium with $D_5W$ or NS for I.V. infusion. Discard unused portion after 24 hours.
•Don't use diluted ethacrynate sodium that's cloudy or opalescent.
•Infuse I.V. ethacrynate sodium slowly over 30 minutes.
•Weigh patient daily and assess for signs of electrolyte imbalances and dehydration. Monitor blood pressure and fluid intake and

output, and check laboratory test results. Notify prescriber about significant changes. Prescriber may reduce dosage or temporarily discontinue drug.
•If hypokalemia develops, administer replacement potassium, as ordered.
•Monitor serum glucose level frequently, especially if patient has diabetes mellitus; both forms of drug may cause hyperglycemia or hypoglycemia.
•Notify prescriber if patient experiences hearing loss, vertigo, or ringing, buzzing, or sense of fullness in his ears. Drug may need to be discontinued.

**PATIENT TEACHING**
•Instruct patient to take the last dose of ethacrynic acid several hours before bedtime to avoid sleep interruption from diuresis. If patient receives once-daily dosing, advise him to take the dose in the morning to avoid sleep disturbance caused by nocturia.
•Suggest that patient take ethacrynic acid with food or milk to reduce the likelihood of GI distress.
•Advise patient to change position slowly to minimize effects of orthostatic hypotension, especially if he also takes an antihypertensive.
•Unless contraindicated, urge patient to eat more high-potassium foods and to take a potassium supplement, if prescribed, to prevent hypokalemia.
•Caution patient not to drink alcohol, stand for prolonged periods, or exercise during hot weather because these activities may exacerbate orthostatic hypotension.
•Instruct patient to notify prescriber if he experiences diarrhea; buzzing, fullness, or ringing in his ears; hearing loss; severe nausea; vertigo; or vomiting. Drug may need to be discontinued.
•Remind diabetic patients to check their serum glucose levels frequently to detect alterations.

# ethambutol hydrochloride

Etibi (CAN), Myambutol

## Class and Category

*Chemical:* Diisopropylethylene diamide derivative
*Therapeutic:* Antitubercular
*Pregnancy category:* C

## Indications and Dosages

➤ *As adjunct to treat tuberculosis and atypical mycobacterial infections caused by* Mycobacterium tuberculosis

**TABLETS**

**Adults and adolescents who haven't received previous antituberculotic therapy.** 15 mg/kg q.d.

**Adults and adolescents who have received previous antituberculotic therapy.** 25 mg/kg q.d.; after 60 days, decreased to 15 mg/kg q.d.

---

**Mechanism of Action**

May suppress bacterial multiplication by interfering with RNA synthesis in susceptible bacteria that are actively dividing.

---

## Contraindications

Hypersensitivity to ethambutol or its components, inability to report changes in vision, optic neuritis

## Interactions

**DRUGS**

*antacids that contain aluminum hydroxide:* Decreased absorption of ethambutol
*other neurotoxic drugs:* Increased risk of neurotoxicity, such as optic and peripheral neuritis

## Adverse Reactions

**CNS:** Burning sensation or weakness in arms and legs, confusion, disorientation, dizziness, fever, headache, malaise, paresthesia, peripheral neuritis

**EENT:** Blurred vision, decreased visual acuity, eye pain, optic neuritis, red-green color blindness

**GI:** Abdominal pain, anorexia, hepatic dysfunction, nausea, vomiting

**HEME:** Leukopenia, neutropenia, thrombocytopenia

**MS:** Arthralgia, gouty arthritis

**RESP:** Pulmonary infiltrates

**SKIN:** Dermatitis, pruritus, rash

**Other:** Anaphylaxis, hypersensitivity syndrome (rash or exfoliative dermatitis, eosinophilia, and one of the following: hepatitis, pneumonitis, nephritis, myocarditis, pericarditis), lymphadenopathy

## Nursing Considerations

• Expect prescriber to refer patient for an ophthalmologic examination that includes tests for visual fields, acuity, and red-green color blindness before taking ethambutol and monthly thereafter. This is especially likely if therapy is prolonged or dosage exceeds 15 mg/kg/day.

• **WARNING** Notify prescriber immediately if the patient develops vision changes; expect ethambutol therapy to be discontinued if they occur.

• Expect to give the patient at least one other antituberculotic with ethambutol, as prescribed, because bacteria may become resistant quickly when therapy includes a single drug.

• Monitor laboratory test results for changes in liver function or for increased serum uric acid level if patient has gouty arthritis or impaired renal function. Notify prescriber of any abnormalities.

• Obtain a monthly sputum specimen, as ordered, to check bacteriologic response in sputum-positive patient.

• Keep in mind that successful drug therapy typically takes 6 to 12 months but may take years.

**PATIENT TEACHING**

• Teach patient to recognize possible adverse reactions to ethambutol.

• Advise patient to take drug with food if he experiences adverse GI reactions.

• Instruct patient to take a missed dose as soon as he remembers, unless it's nearly time for the next dose, but not to double-dose.

• Inform patient that therapy may last months or years and that compliance is essential.

• Advise patient to notify prescriber if no improvement occurs within 3 weeks of taking drug; if bothersome or severe adverse reactions occur; if his vision changes; or if a rash, fever, or joint pain (signs of hypersensitivity) develops.

# ethchlorvynol

Placidyl

## Class, Category, and Schedule

*Chemical:* Chlorinated tertiary acetylenic carbinol
*Therapeutic:* Sedative-hypnotic
*Pregnancy category:* C
*Controlled substance:* Schedule IV

## Indications and Dosages

➤ *To provide short-term relief from insomnia*

CAPSULES

Adults. 0.5 to 1 g h.s. for no longer than 1 wk.

| Route | Onset | Peak | Duration |
|-------|-------|------|----------|
| P.O. | 15 to 60 min | Unknown | 5 hr |

## Mechanism of Action

Exerts sedative-hypnotic, muscle relaxant, and anticonvulsant effects possibly by depressing the reticular activating system.

## Contraindications

Hypersensitivity to ethchlorvynol or its components, porphyria

## Interactions

DRUGS

*CNS depressants, tricyclic antidepressants:* Increased CNS depression
*oral anticoagulants:* Decreased anticoagulant effects

ACTIVITIES

*alcohol use:* Increased CNS depression

## Adverse Reactions

**CNS:** Ataxia, dizziness, facial numbness, fatigue, light-headedness, syncope, unsteadiness, weakness
**CV:** Hypotension
**EENT:** Blurred vision, unpleasant aftertaste
**GI:** Epigastric pain, indigestion, nausea, vomiting
**HEME:** Thrombocytopenia
**SKIN:** Jaundice, rash, urticaria
**Other:** Physical and psychological dependence

## Nursing Considerations

•If patient awakens too early after taking 0.5 or 0.75 g of ethchlorvynol at bedtime, ask prescriber if he may take a single supplemental dose of 200 mg.
•Assess for signs of addiction if patient has taken drug for 2 weeks or longer.
•Be aware that ethchlorvynol shouldn't be given for longer than 1 week. If patient has received prolonged therapy, expect to discontinue drug gradually to prevent withdrawal symptoms. Notify prescriber if you detect ev-

idence of withdrawal: diaphoresis, hallucinations, irritability, muscle twitching, nausea, nervousness, restlessness, seizures, sleep disturbance, tremor, vomiting, and weakness.

PATIENT TEACHING

•Caution patient not to exceed prescribed dosage or dosing frequency because of ethchlorvynol's habit-forming potential. Instruct him not to use drug for more than 1 week.
•Advise patient to take drug with food or milk to minimize adverse GI reactions.
•If patient has taken long-term ethchlorvynol therapy, warn against stopping drug abruptly; advise him to contact prescriber for guidelines to reduce dosage.
•Direct patient to avoid alcohol and other CNS depressants during therapy because they increase the risk of adverse reactions.
•Advise patient to avoid potentially hazardous activities until drug's CNS effects are known.

# ethinyl estradiol and norethindrone

Femhrt

## Class and Category

*Chemical:* Estrogen steroid hormone derivative (ethinyl estradiol), progesterone derivative (norethindrone)
*Therapeutic:* Antiosteoporotic agent, ovarian hormone replacement
*Pregnancy category:* X

## Indications and Dosages

➤ *To treat moderate to severe vasomotor symptoms associated with menopause; to prevent osteoporosis due to estrogen deficiency in postmenopausal women with an intact uterus*

TABLETS

Adult females. 0.05 mg ethinyl estradiol and 1 mg norethindrone (1 tablet) q.d.

## Contraindications

Current or previous thrombophlebitis or thromboembolic disorders; hypersensitivity to ethinyl estradiol, norethindrone, or their components; known or suspected breast cancer or history of breast cancer from estrogen use; known or suspected estrogen-dependent cancer; pregnancy; undiagnosed abnormal genital bleeding

## Mechanism of Action

An estrogen, ethinyl estradiol increases DNA and RNA synthesis in cells of the female reproductive organs, pituitary gland, hypothalamus, and other target organs. In the hypothalamus, estrogens decrease release of gonadotropin-releasing hormone, which decreases pituitary release of follicle-stimulating and luteinizing hormones needed for genitourinary and other essential body functions in women. Estrogens also increase cervical secretions, cause endometrial cell proliferation, and improve uterine tone. Estrogen replacement helps maintain genitourinary function and reduces vasomotor symptoms when estrogen production declines from menopause, surgical removal of ovaries, or other estrogen deficiency. It also helps prevent osteoporosis by inhibiting bone resorption.

A progestin, norethindrone prolongs some positive effects of estrogens on HDL cholesterol. Norethindrone diffuses freely into target cells of the female reproductive tract, mammary glands, hypothalamus, and pituitary gland and binds to progesterone cell receptor. It converts a proliferative endometrium into a secretory one in women with adequate estrogen replacement, reducing endometrial growth and the risk of endometrial cancer compared with women who have an intact uterus and take unopposed estrogens. Norethindrone also decreases nuclear estradiol receptors and suppresses epithelial DNA synthesis in endometrial tissues.

## Interactions

**Drugs**

**ethinyl estradiol and norethindrone**
*corticosteroids:* Increased therapeutic and toxic effects of corticosteroids
*cyclosporine:* Increased risk of hepatotoxicity and nephrotoxicity
*hepatotoxic drugs, such as isoniazid:* Increased risk of hepatitis and hepatotoxicity
*oral antidiabetic drugs:* Decreased therapeutic effects of these drugs
*thyroid hormones:* Decreased effectiveness of thyroid hormones
*warfarin:* Altered anticoagulant effect
**ethinyl estradiol component only**

*vitamin C:* Decreased metabolism and possibly increased adverse effects of ethinyl estradiol

**Foods**
*grapefruit juice:* Decreased metabolism and possibly increased adverse effects of ethinyl estradiol

**Activities**
*smoking:* Increased risk of CVA, pulmonary embolism, thrombophlebitis, and transient ischemic attack

## Adverse Reactions

**CNS:** Chorea, CVA, dementia, depression, dizziness, exacerbation of epilepsy, headache, irritability, migraine headache, mood disturbances, nervousness, porphyria
**CV:** Hypertension, hypertriglyceridemia, MI, peripheral edema, pulmonary embolism, thromboembolism, thrombophlebitis
**EENT:** Diplopia, intolerance of contact lenses, retinal vascular thrombosis, sinusitis, vision changes or loss
**ENDO:** Breast enlargement, pain, tenderness, or tumors; endometrial hyperplasia; galactorrhea; hyperglycemia; nipple discharge
**GI:** Abdominal cramps or pain, aggravation of hepatic porphyria, anorexia, bloating, constipation, diarrhea, elevated liver function test results, enlargement of hepatic hemangiomas, flatulence, gallbladder obstruction, hepatitis, increased appetite, nausea, pancreatitis, vomiting
**GU:** Amenorrhea, breakthrough bleeding, cervical erosion, clear vaginal discharge, dysmenorrhea, endometrial or ovarian tumors, increased libido, increased size of uterine leiomyomata, leukorrhea, prolonged or heavy menstrual bleeding, urinary tract infection, vaginitis including vaginal candidiasis
**MS:** Arthralgias, back or extremity pain, leg cramps
**RESP:** Bronchitis, exacerbation of asthma, upper respiratory tract infection
**SKIN:** Alopecia, application site irritation, erythema multiforme or nodosum, hirsutism, jaundice, melasma, pruritus, purpura, rash, urticaria
**Other:** Anaphylaxis, angioedema, flulike symptoms, folic acid deficiency, hypercalcemia (with bone metastases), hyperkalemia, hypocalcemia, hyponatremia, weight gain or loss

E
F

## Nursing Considerations
•Use ethinyl estradiol and norethindrone cautiously in women with asthma, diabetes mellitus, epilepsy, hepatic hemangiomas, migraine headaches, porphyria, or systemic lupus erythematosus because ethinyl estradiol may worsen these conditions.
•Make sure patient has an intact uterus before starting ethinyl estradiol and norethindrone; if she has no uterus, she doesn't need the progestin.
•WARNING Assess patient for contact-lens intolerance or changes in vision or visual acuity because estrogens can cause increased curvature of the cornea. Be prepared to stop drug immediately, as prescribed, if patient has sudden partial or complete loss of vision or sudden onset of diplopia or migraine.
•If patient takes warfarin, monitor PT test results for loss of anticoagulant effect because ethinyl estradiol increases production of clotting factors VII, VIII, IX, and X and promotes platelet aggregation.
•Watch for elevated liver function test results because ethinyl estradiol and norethindrone may worsen such conditions as acute intermittent or variegate hepatic porphyria.
•Closely monitor patient's blood pressure. A few patients may experience a substantial increase in blood pressure as an indiosyncratic reaction to estrogens. If patient has hypertension, watch for increases in blood pressure because estrogens may cause fluid retention. Also monitor patients with asthma, heart disease, migraines, renal disease, or seizure disorder for worsening of these conditions.
•Frequently monitor serum glucose levels in patients who have diabetes mellitus because estrogens may decrease insulin sensitivity and alter glucose tolerance.
•WARNING Expect to stop ethinyl estradiol and norethindrone therapy in any woman who develops signs or symptoms of dementia or cardiovascular disease, such as CVA, MI, pulmonary embolism, or venous thrombosis.
•Be aware that ethinyl estradiol and norethindrone may worsen mood disorders, including depression. Monitor patient for anxiety, depression, dizziness, fatigue, insomnia, or mood changes.
•WARNING Be aware that severe hypercalcemia may occur in patients with bone metastasis from breast cancer because estrogens

influence the metabolism of calcium and phosphorus. Watch for toxic reactions to increased calcium absorption in patients wh oare predisposed to hypercalcemia or nephrolithiasis.
•Assess skin for melasma (tan or brown patches) on forehead, cheeks, temples, and upper lip. These patches may persist after combination drug is stopped.
•Monitor thyroid function test results in patients with hypothyroidism because long-term use of ethinyl estradiol may decrease effectiveness of thyroid therapy.
•Expect to stop ethinyl estradiol and norethindrone several weeks before patient undergoes major surgery because prolonged immobilization poses a risk of thromboembolism.

PATIENT TEACHING
•Before therapy starts, inform patient of risks involved with taking ethinyl estradiol and norethindrone, such as increased risk of breast or endometrial cancer, cardiovascular disease, dementia, gallbladder disease, and vision abnormalities.
•Tell patient to notify prescriber immediately if vaginal bleeding or any other abnormal signs and symptoms occur while using ethinyl estradiol and norethindrone.
•Advise patient to avoid smoking while using ethinyl estradiol and norethindrone.
•Stress the importance of complying with follow-up visits every 3 to 6 months to the determine effectiveness of ethinyl estradiol and norethindrone at relieving menopausal symptoms and osteoporosis. Also urge compliance with scheduled diagnostic tests to detect adverse reactions.
•Emphasize the importance of good dental hygiene and regular dental checkups because an elevated serum progestin (norethindrone) level increases the growth of normal oral flora, which may lead to gum tenderness, bleeding, or swelling.

# ethinyl estradiol and norgestimate
Ortho-Cyclen, Ortho Tri-Cyclen

## Class and Category
Chemical: Estrogenic steroid hormone derivative (ethinyl estradiol), progesterone steroid hormone derivative (norgestimate)

*Therapeutic:* Ovarian hormone replacement
*Pregnancy category:* X

## Indications and Dosages

➤ *To treat moderate acne vulgaris in patients who desire contraception, who have achieved menarche, and who also are unresponsive to topical antiacne medication*

TABLETS

**Adult and adolescent females age 15 and older.** 0.035 mg ethinyl estradiol and 0.180 mg, 0.215 mg, or 0.250 mg norgestimate (1 active tablet) daily for 21 days starting first day of monthly menstruation followed by 1 inactive tablet daily for 7 days; cycle repeated q 28 days. Alternatively, 0.035 mg ethinyl estradiol and 0.180 mg, 0.215 mg, or 0.250 mg norgestimate 1 active tablet daily for 21 days starting first Sunday after onset of monthly menstruation, followed by 1 inactive tablet daily for 7 days; cycle repeated q 28 days.

## Contraindications

Cerebrovascular or coronary artery disease; deep vein thrombosis, pulmonary embolism, or history of these conditions; hepatic disorders, including cholestatic jaundice with previous pregnancy or oral contraceptive use; hypersensitivity to ethinyl estradiol, norgestimate, or their components; known or suspected breast cancer or history of breast cancer from estrogen use; known or suspected estrogen-dependent cancer; migraine with focal aura; new or recent (within past year) CVA or MI; pregnancy; undiagnosed abnormal genital bleeding

## Interactions

DRUGS

**ethinyl estradiol and norgestimate**

*ampicillin, barbiturates, carbamazepine, griseofulvin, phenylbutazone, phenytoin, rifabutin, rifampin, St. John's wort, tetracyclines, topiramate:* Possibly reduced effectiveness of ethinyl estradiol and norgestimate; increased risk of breakthrough bleeding and menstrual irregularities

**ethinyl estradiol component only**

*corticosteroids:* Increased therapeutic and toxic effects of corticosteroids
*cyclosporine:* Increased risk of hepatotoxicity and nephrotoxicity

*hepatotoxic drugs (such as isoniazid):* Increased risk of hepatitis and hepatotoxicity
*oral antidiabetic drugs:* Decreased therapeutic effects of these drugs
*warfarin:* Decreased anticoagulant effect

FOODS

*grapefruit juice:* Decreased metabolism and possibly increased adverse effects of ethinyl estradiol

ACTIVITIES

*smoking:* Increased risk of CVA, pulmonary embolism, thrombophlebitis, and transient ischemic attack

## Mechanism of Action

An estrogen, ethinyl estradiol increases DNA and RNA synthesis in cells of the female reproductive organs, pituitary gland, hypothalamus, and other target organs. In the hypothalamus, estrogens decrease release of gonadotropin-releasing hormone, which decreases pituitary release of follicle-stimulating and luteinizing hormones, needed for ovulation and follicular maturation. Estrogens also increase cervical secretions.

A progestin, norgestimate prevents ovulation and follicular maturation by inhibiting secretion of gonadotropins from the anterior pituitary. It also thickens cervical secretions, disrupting the passage of sperm, and alters the endometrial lining, reducing the likelihood of implantation.

Together, these actions interfere with the normal mechanisms of reproduction to prevent pregnancy. They also may increase sex hormone–binding globulin and decrease free testosterone, which in turn decreases the severity of facial acne.

## Adverse Reactions

**CNS:** Chorea, CVA, dementia, depression, dizziness, exacerbation of epilepsy, headache, irritability, migraine headache, mood disturbances, nervousness, porphyria
**CV:** Hypertension, hypertriglyceridemia, MI, peripheral edema, pulmonary embolism, thromboembolism, thrombophlebitis
**EENT:** Diplopia, intolerance of contact lenses, retinal vascular thrombosis, sinusitis, vision changes or loss
**ENDO:** Breast enlargement, pain, tenderness, or tumors; endometrial hyperplasia, galac-

torrhea; gynecomastia; hyperglycemia; nipple discharge

**GI:** Abdominal cramps or pain, aggravation of porphyria, anorexia, bloating, constipation, diarrhea, elevated liver function test results, enlargement of hepatic hemangiomas, flatulence, gallbladder obstruction, hepatitis, increased appetite, nausea, pancreatitis, vomiting

**GU:** Amenorrhea, breakthrough bleeding, cervical erosion, clear vaginal discharge, dysmenorrhea, endometrial or ovarian tumors, increased libido, increased size of uterine leiomyomata, leukorrhea, prolonged or heavy menstrual bleeding, urinary tract infection, vaginitis including vaginal candidiasis

**MS:** Arthralgias, back or extremity pain, leg cramps

**RESP:** Bronchitis, exacerbation of asthma, upper respiratory tract infection

**SKIN:** Alopecia, application site irritation, erythema multiforme or nodosum, hirsutism, jaundice, melasma, pruritus, purpura, rash, urticaria

**Other:** Anaphylaxis, angioedema, flulike symptoms, folic acid deficiency, hypercalcemia (with bone metastases), hyperkalemia, hypocalcemia, hyponatremia, weight gain or loss

## Nursing Considerations

•Use ethinyl estradiol and norgestimate cautiously in women with asthma, diabetes mellitus, epilepsy, hepatic hemangiomas, migraine headaches, porphyria, and systemic lupus erythematosus because ethinyl estradiol may worsen these conditions.

•**WARNING** Assess patient for possible contact lens intolerance or changes in vision or visual acuity because estrogens may cause increased curvature of the cornea. Be prepared to stop drug immediately, as prescribed, if patient has sudden partial or complete loss of vision or sudden onset of diplopia or migraine.

•If patient takes warfarin, monitor PT test results for loss of anticoagulant effect because ethinyl estradiol increases production of clotting factors VII, VIII, IX, and X and promotes platelet aggregation.

•Watch for elevated liver function test results because progestins and estrogens may worsen such conditions as acute intermittent or variegate hepatic porphyria.

•Closely monitor patient's blood pressure. A few patients may experience a substantial increase in blood pressure as an indiosyncratic reaction to ethinyl estradiol. Monitor patients who already have hypertension for increases in blood pressure because estrogens may cause fluid retention. Also monitor patients with asthma, heart disease, migraines, renal disease, or seizure disorder for exacerbation of these conditions.

•Frequently monitor serum glucose levels in patients who have diabetes mellitus because ethinyl estradiol may decrease insulin sensitivity and alter glucose tolerance.

•Expect to stop drug in any woman who develops dementia or signs or symptoms of cardiovascular disease, such as CVA, MI, pulmonary embolism, or venous thrombosis.

•Be aware that ethinyl estradiol and norgestimate may worsen mood disorders, including depression. Monitor patient for depression, mood changes, anxiety, fatigue, dizziness, or insomnia.

•**WARNING** Be aware that severe hypercalcemia may occur in patients with bone metastasis from breast cancer because estrogens influence the metabolism of calcium and phosphorus. Watch for toxic reactions to increased calcium absorption in patients who are predisposed to hypercalcemia or nephrolithiasis.

•Assess skin for melasma (tan or brown patches), which may develop on forehead, cheeks, temples, and upper lip. These patches may persist after drug is stopped.

•Monitor thyroid function test results in patients with hypothyroidism because long-term use of the ethinyl estradiol may decrease effectiveness of thyroid therapy.

•Expect to stop ethinyl estradiol and norgestimate several weeks before patient undergoes major surgery, as prescribed, because prolonged immobilization poses a risk of thromboembolism.

### PATIENT TEACHING

•Before therapy starts, explain the risks involved in taking ethinyl estradiol and norgestimate, such as increased risk of breast or endometrial cancer, cardiovascular disease, dementia, gallbladder disease, and vision abnormalities.

•Tell patient to notify prescriber immediately if vaginal bleeding or any other abnormal signs and symptoms occur while taking this drug.

•Advise patient to avoid smoking during therapy.

•Stress importance attending follow-up visits.

•Emphasize the need for good dental hygiene and regular dental checkups because an elevated serum progestin level increases the growth of normal oral flora, which may lead to gum tenderness, bleeding, or swelling.

# ethionamide

Trecator-SC

## Class and Category

*Chemical:* Thiamide analogue of isonicotinic acid
*Therapeutic:* Antituberculotic
*Pregnancy category:* Not rated

## Indications and Dosages

➤ *As adjunct to treat tuberculosis*

**TABLETS**

**Adults.** 0.5 to 1 g/day in divided doses q 8 to 12 hr, together with other antituberculotics. *Maximum:* 1 g/day.
**Children.** 15 to 20 mg/kg/day in divided doses q 8 to 12 hr, together with other antituberculotics. *Maximum:* 750 mg/day.

---

### Mechanism of Action

May inhibit peptide synthesis, resulting in bacteriostatic action against *Mycobacterium tuberculosis*.

---

## Contraindications

Hypersensitivity to ethionamide or its components, severe hepatic damage

## Interactions

**DRUGS**

*cycloserine:* Increased risk of adverse CNS effects, especially seizures
*other neurotoxic drugs:* Increased risk of neurotoxicity, such as optic and peripheral neuritis

## Adverse Reactions

**CNS:** Burning or pain in arms and legs, clumsiness, confusion, depression, mental or mood changes, paresthesia, unsteadiness
**CV:** Orthostatic hypotension
**EENT:** Blurred vision, eye pain, increased salivation, metallic taste, optic neuritis, stomatitis, vision loss

**ENDO:** Goiter, hypoglycemia, hypothyroidism
**GI:** Anorexia, hepatitis, nausea, vomiting
**SKIN:** Jaundice, rash

## Nursing Considerations

•Use ethionamide cautiously in patients with a history of hypersensitivity to isoniazid, niacin, pyrazinamide, or chemically related drugs; these ptients also may be hypersensitive to ethionamide.

•Expect to give another antituberculotic with ethionamide to decrease the risk of development of bacterial resistance.

•Also plan to give pyridoxine to prevent or minimize peripheral neuritis (burning, numbness, pain, or tingling in hands and feet), especially if patient has already had isoniazid-induced peripheral neuritis.

•Monitor liver function test results, and assess for signs of impaired function, such as hepatitis and jaundice.

•Question patient regularly about vision changes. Notify prescriber about blurred vision, eye pain, or loss of vision or acuity.

•Monitor compliance; treatment may need to continue for 1 to 2 years or indefinitely.

**PATIENT TEACHING**

•Advise patient to take ethionamide with food if adverse GI reactions occur.

•Instruct patient to take a missed dose as soon as he remembers unless it's nearly time for the next dose. Caution him not to double the dose.

•Advise patient to notify prescriber if no improvement occurs within 3 weeks; if bothersome or severe adverse reactions occur; if his vision changes; or if he has burning, numbness, pain, or tingling in his hands and feet.

•Inform patient that therapy may have to continue for months or years and that compliance is essential.

# ethosuximide

Zarontin

## Class and Category

*Chemical:* Succinimide derivative
*Therapeutic:* Anticonvulsant
*Pregnancy category:* Not rated

## Indications and Dosages

➤ *To manage absence seizures in a patient who also has generalized tonic-clonic seizures*

**Adults and children age 6 and older.** *Initial:* 500 mg q.d. *Maintenance:* Increased by 250 mg q 4 to 7 days until control is achieved with minimal adverse reactions.
**Children ages 3 to 6.** *Initial:* 250 mg q.d. *Maintenance:* Increased by 250 mg q 4 to 7 days until control is achieved with minimal adverse reactions.

## Mechanism of Action
Elevates the seizure threshold and reduces the frequency of attacks by depressing the motor cortex and elevating the threshold of CNS response to convulsive stimuli.

## Contraindications
Hypersensitivity to ethosuximide, succinimides, or their components

## Interactions
DRUGS
*carbamazepine, phenobarbital, phenytoin, primidone:* Possibly decreased blood ethosuximide level
*CNS depressants:* Possibly increased CNS depression
*haloperidol:* Possibly decreased blood haloperidol level
*loxapine, MAO inhibitors, maprotiline, molindone, phenothiazines, pimozide, tricyclic antidepressants:* Possibly lowered seizure threshold and reduced therapeutic effect of ethosuximide
*valproic acid:* Increased or decreased blood ethosuximide level
ACTIVITIES
*alcohol use:* Possibly increased CNS depression

## Adverse Reactions
**CNS:** Aggressiveness, ataxia, decreased concentration, dizziness, drowsiness, euphoria, fatigue, headache, hyperactivity, irritability, lethargy, nightmares, sleep disturbance
**EENT:** Gingival hypertrophy, myopia, tongue swelling
**GI:** Abdominal and epigastric pain, abdominal cramps, anorexia, diarrhea, hiccups, indigestion, nausea, vomiting
**GU:** Increased libido, microscopic hematuria, vaginal bleeding
**HEME:** Agranulocytosis, aplastic anemia, eosinophilia, leukopenia, pancytopenia

**SKIN:** Erythematous and pruritic rash, hirsutism, Stevens-Johnson syndrome, systemic lupus erythematosus, urticaria
**Other:** Weight loss

## Nursing Considerations
•Use ethosuximide with extreme caution in patients with hepatic or renal disease.
•Give other anticonvulsants concurrently, as prescribed, to control generalized tonic-clonic seizures.
•Monitor CBC and platelet count and assess for signs of infection, such as cough, fever, and pharyngitis. Also routinely evaluate liver and renal function test results.
•Take safety precautions because drug may cause adverse CNS reactions, such as dizziness and drowsiness.
PATIENT TEACHING
•Stress the importance of complying with ethosuximide regimen.
•Advise patient to take a missed dose as soon as he remembers unless it's nearly time for the next dose. Warn him not to double the dose.
•Instruct patient not to engage in potentially hazardous activities until drug's CNS effects are known.
•Caution patient not to stop taking drug abruptly; doing so increases the risk of absence seizures.

# ethotoin

Peganone

## Class and Category
*Chemical:* Hydantoin derivative
*Therapeutic:* Anticonvulsant
*Pregnancy category:* D

## Indications and Dosages
➤ *To treat tonic-clonic and simple or complex partial seizures as initial or adjunct therapy, or when other drugs are ineffective*
TABLETS
**Adults and adolescents.** *Initial:* 0.5 to 1 g on the first day in four to six divided doses, increased over several days until desired response is reached. *Maintenance:* 2 to 3 g/day in four to six divided doses. *Maximum:* 3 g/day.
**Children.** *Initial:* Up to 750 mg/day, based on weight and age, in four to six divided doses,

adjusted as needed and tolerated. *Maintenance:* 0.5 to 1 g/day in four to six divided doses. *Maximum:* 3 g/day.

DOSAGE ADJUSTMENT For debilitated patients, initial dosage lowered to reduce the risk of adverse reactions.

## Mechanism of Action

Limits the spread of seizure activity and the start of new seizures by:
• regulating voltage-dependent sodium and calcium channels in neurons
• inhibiting calcium movement across neuronal membranes
• enhancing sodium-potassium adenosine triphosphatase activity in neurons and glial cells.

These actions may result from ethotoin's ability to slow the recovery rate of inactivated sodium channels.

## Contraindications

Hematologic disorders; hepatic dysfunction; hypersensitivity to ethotoin, phenytoin, other hydantoins, or their components

## Interactions

### DRUGS

*acetaminophen:* Increased risk of hepatotoxicity with long-term acetaminophen use
*amiodarone:* Possibly increased blood ethotoin level and risk of toxicity
*antacids:* Possibly decreased ethotoin effectiveness
*bupropion, clozapine, loxapine, MAO inhibitors, maprotiline, phenothiazines, pimozide, thioxanthenes:* Possibly lowered seizure threshold and decreased therapeutic effects of ethotoin; possibly intensified CNS depressant effects of these drugs
*chloramphenicol, cimetidine, disulfiram, fluconazole, isoniazid, methylphenidate, metronidazole, omeprazole, phenylbutazone, ranitidine, salicylates, sulfonamides, trimethoprim:* Possibly impaired metabolism of these drugs and increased risk of ethotoin toxicity
*corticosteroids, cyclosporine, digoxin, disopyramide, doxycycline, furosemide, levodopa, mexiletine, quinidine:* Decreased therapeutic effects of these drugs
*diazoxide:* Possibly decreased therapeutic effects of both drugs

*estrogens, progestins:* Decreased therapeutic effects of these drugs, increased blood ethotoin level
*folic acid, leucovorin:* Increased ethotoin metabolism, decreased seizure control
*haloperidol:* Possibly lowered seizure threshold and decreased therapeutic effects of ethotoin; possibly decreased blood haloperidol level
*insulin, oral antidiabetic drugs:* Possibly increased blood glucose level and decreased therapeutic effects of these drugs
*lidocaine:* Increased lidocaine metabolism, leading to reduced concentration
*methadone:* Possibly increased methadone metabolism, leading to withdrawal symptoms
*molindone:* Possibly lowered seizure threshold and impaired absorption and decreased therapeutic effects of ethotoin
*oral anticoagulants:* Possibly impaired metabolism of these drugs and increased risk of ethotoin toxicity; possibly increased anticoagulant effect initially, but decreased effect with prolonged therapy
*oral contraceptives that contain estrogen and progestin:* Possibly breakthrough bleeding and decreased contraceptive effectiveness
*rifampin:* Possibly decreased therapeutic effects of ethotoin
*streptozocin:* Possibly decreased therapeutic effects of streptozocin
*sucralfate:* Possibly decreased ethotoin absorption
*tricyclic antidepressants:* Possibly lowered seizure threshold and decreased therapeutic effects of ethotoin; possibly decreased blood level of tricyclic antidepressants
*valproic acid:* Possibly decreased blood ethotoin level, increased blood valproic acid level
*vitamin D analogues:* Decreased vitamin D analogue activity; risk of anticonvulsant-induced rickets and osteomalacia
*xanthines:* Possibly inhibited ethotoin absorption and increased clearance of xanthines

### ACTIVITIES

*alcohol use:* Possibly decreased ethotoin effectiveness, enhanced CNS depressant effects

## Adverse Reactions

**CNS:** Clumsiness, confusion, drowsiness, excitement, peripheral neuropathy, sedation, slurred speech, stuttering, tremor
**EENT:** Nystagmus

**GI:** Constipation, diarrhea, nausea, vomiting
**HEME:** Agranulocytosis, leukopenia, thrombocytopenia
**SKIN:** Rash, Stevens-Johnson syndrome, toxic epidermal necrolysis
**Other:** Lymphadenopathy, systemic lupus erythematosus

## Nursing Considerations

•Obtain CBC and differential before treatment and at monthly intervals for the first few months of ethotoin therapy, as ordered.
•**WARNING** Be aware that ethotoin shouldn't be discontinued abruptly because of a risk of causing status epilepticus. Plan to reduce dosage gradually or substitute another drug, as prescribed.
•Monitor patient for signs and symptoms of infection or unusual bleeding because ethotoin may cause hematologic toxicity.
•Because of ethotoin's potential for hepatotoxicity, monitor liver function test results and expect drug to be discontinued if test results are abnormal.
•Notify prescriber immediately and expect ethotoin to be discontinued and substituted with another drug if patient develops decreased blood counts, enlarged lymph nodes, or rash.
•Be aware that ethotoin may be substituted for phenytoin without loss of seizure control if patient develops severe gingival hyperplasia or other adverse reactions. Expect ethotoin dosage to be four to six times greater than phenytoin dosage.
•Institute and maintain seizure precautions according to facility protocol.

### PATIENT TEACHING

•Instruct patient to take ethotoin exactly as prescribed and not to discontinue drug abruptly.
•Advise patient to take drug with food to enhance absorption and reduce adverse GI effects.
•Advise patient to report easy bruising, epistaxis, fever, malaise, petechiae, or sore throat to prescriber immediately.
•Instruct patient to keep medical appointments to monitor drug effectiveness and check for adverse reactions. Explain the need for periodic laboratory tests.
•Urge patient to avoid alcohol during therapy.
•Caution patient to avoid hazardous activities until drug's adverse effects are known.

•Encourage patient to wear or carry medical identification indicating his diagnosis and drug therapy.

# etidronate disodium

Didronel

## Class and Category

*Chemical:* Bisphosphonate
*Therapeutic:* Antihypercalcemic agent, bone resorption inhibitor
*Pregnancy category:* B (oral), C (parenteral)

## Indications and Dosages

➤ *To treat Paget's disease of bone (osteitis deformans)*

### TABLETS

**Adults.** 5 to 10 mg/kg/day for up to 6 mo, or 11 to 20 mg/kg/day for up to 3 mo.

➤ *To prevent and treat heterotopic ossification after total hip replacement*

### TABLETS

**Adults.** 20 mg/kg/day for 1 mo before surgery and then 20 mg/kg/day for 3 mo after surgery for a total of 4 mo of treatment.

➤ *To prevent and treat heterotopic ossification after spinal cord injury*

### TABLETS

**Adults.** 20 mg/kg/day for 2 wk and then 10 mg/kg/day for 10 wk for a total of 12 wk of treatment.

➤ *To treat moderate to severe hypercalcemia caused by cancer*

### I.V. INFUSION

**Adults.** *Initial:* 7.5 mg/kg/day infused over at least 2 hr for 3 to 7 successive days. Oral etidronate therapy may begin at 20 mg/kg/day for 30 days on the day after last infusion.
**DOSAGE ADJUSTMENT** Dosage reduced if patient has renal impairment. Drug not given if serum creatinine level exceeds 5 mg/dl.

## Contraindications

Hypersensitivity to etidronate, bisphosphonates, or their components; severe renal impairment

## Interactions

### DRUGS

*antacids that contain aluminum, calcium, or magnesium; vitamin and mineral supplements that contain aluminum, calcium, iron, or magnesium:* Decreased etidronate absorption

## Foods
*high-calcium food (such as milk and other dairy products):* Decreased etidronate absorption

### Mechanism of Action
Inhibits normal and abnormal bone resorption by reducing bone turnover and slowing the remodeling of pagetic or heterotopic bone. Etidronate also decreases the elevated cardiac output that's seen in Paget's disease of bone and reduces local increases in skin temperature. It also inhibits the abnormal bone resorption that may occur with cancer and reduces the amount of calcium that enters the blood from resorbed bone.

## Adverse Reactions
**EENT:** Altered taste, metallic taste
**GI:** Diarrhea, elevated liver function test results, nausea
**GU:** Nephrotoxicity
**MS:** Bone fractures, bone pain
**Other:** Hypocalcemia

## Nursing Considerations
•Anticipate beginning etidronate therapy as soon as possible after spinal cord injury, preferably before evidence of heterotopic ossification exists.
•Expect etidronate not to inhibit healing of spinal fractures, affect prosthesis, or disrupt trochanter attachment when used after total hip replacement.
•Give oral form 2 hours before meals to prevent decreased absorption.
•Dilute parenteral form in at least 250 ml of NS.
•Give parenteral form slowly over at least 2 hours.
•Store diluted parenteral solution at room temperature for up to 48 hours.
•**WARNING** Monitor for hypocalcemia if patient receives parenteral form for more than 3 days.
•When treating hypercalcemia, expect to continue drug for up to 90 days if serum calcium level remains within acceptable range.
### Patient Teaching
•Instruct patient to take etidronate tablets on an empty stomach—2 hours before meals, antacids, or calcium supplements. Urge him to drink a full glass of water with tablets

and to avoid taking drug with milk or other high-calcium foods.
•Tell patient to take a missed dose as soon as he remembers as long as 2 hours have elapsed since his last meal. Instruct him not to eat for another 2 hours. Warn against doubling the dose.
•Inform patient with Paget's disease that his response to etidronate may be slow and may continue for months after treatment.

# etodolac
Lodine, Lodine XL

## Class and Category
*Chemical:* Pyranoindoleacetic acid derivative
*Therapeutic:* Analgesic, anti-inflammatory
*Pregnancy category:* C

## Indications and Dosages
➤ *To manage osteoarthritis*
**Capsules, tablets**
**Adults.** *Initial:* 800 to 1,200 mg/day in divided doses. *Maintenance:* 600 to 1,200 mg/day in divided doses. *Maximum:* 1,200 mg/day for patients who weigh 60 kg (132 lb) or more; 20 mg/kg/day for those less than 60 kg.
**E.R. tablets**
**Adults.** 400 to 1,000 mg/day.
➤ *To relieve mild to moderate pain*
**Capsules, tablets**
**Adults.** *Initial:* 400 mg and then 200 to 400 mg q 6 to 8 hr. *Maximum:* 1,200 mg/day for patients who weigh 60 kg or more; 20 mg/kg/day for patients who weigh less than 60 kg.

| Route | Onset | Peak | Duration |
|-------|-------|------|----------|
| P.O. | 30 min | 1 to 2 hr | 4 to 12 hr |

### Mechanism of Action
Blocks the activity of cyclooxygenase, the enzyme needed for prostaglandin synthesis. Prostaglandins, important mediators of the inflammatory response, cause local vasodilation with swelling and pain. By inhibiting cyclooxygenase and prostaglandins, this NSAID causes inflammatory symptoms and pain to subside.

## Contraindications
Angioedema, asthma, bronchospasm, nasal polyps, rhinitis, or urticaria induced by as-

pirin, iodides, or NSAIDs; hypersensitivity to etodolac or its components

## Interactions

**DRUGS**

*ACE inhibitors:* Possibly decreased hypotensive effects of these drugs
*acetaminophen (long-term use):* Increased risk of adverse renal effects
*antacids:* Decreased blood etodolac level
*antiplatelets, oral anticoagulants, thrombolytics:* Prolonged PT (with warfarin), increased risk of bleeding
*cidofovir:* Possibly nephrotoxicity
*corticosteroids:* Increased risk of adverse GI effects
*cyclosporine:* Increased nephrotoxic effects
*digoxin:* Increased blood digoxin level and risk of digitalis toxicity
*insulin, oral antidiabetic drugs:* Increased risk of hypoglycemia
*lithium:* Increased blood lithium level and, possibly, toxicity
*loop diuretics:* Possibly decreased effects of loop diuretics
*methotrexate:* Increased risk of methotrexate toxicity
*phenylbutazone:* Possibly altered etodolac clearance
*salicylates:* Decreased blood etodolac level, increased risk of adverse GI effects

**ACTIVITIES**

*alcohol use, smoking:* Increased risk of adverse GI effects

## Adverse Reactions

**CNS:** Chills, CVA, dizziness, drowsiness, fever, malaise, seizures
**CV:** Edema, heart failure, hypertension, MI, tachycardia
**EENT:** Tinnitus
**GI:** Abdominal pain, anorexia, constipation, diarrhea, diverticulitis, dyspepsia, dysphagia, elevated liver function test results, esophagitis, flatulence, gastritis, gastroenteritis, gastroesophageal reflux disease, GI bleeding and ulceration, GI perforation, hemorrhoids, hepatic failure, hepatitis, hiatal hernia, indigestion, melena, nausea, perforation of stomach or intestines, stomatitis, vomiting
**GU:** Dysuria, elevated serum creatinine level, hematuria, renal failure or insufficiency
**HEME:** Agranulocytosis, anemia, easy bruising, hemolytic anemia, leukopenia, neutropenia, pancytopenia, thrombocytopenia

**RESP:** Asthma, respiratory depression
**SKIN:** Erythema multiforme, pruritus, Stevens-Johnson syndrome, toxic epidermal necrolysis, urticaria, vesiculobullous or other rash
**Other:** Anaphylaxis, angioedema, lymphadenopathy

## Nursing Considerations

•Use etodolac with extreme caution in patients with a history of ulcer disease or GI bleeding because NSAIDs such as etodolac increase the risk of GI bleeding and ulceration. Expect to use etodolac for the shortest time possible in these patients.
•Be aware that serious GI tract ulceration, bleeding, and perforation may occur without warning symptoms. Elderly patents are at greater risk. To minimize risk, give drug with food. If GI distress occurs, withhold drug and notify prescriber immediately.
•Use etodolac cautiously in patients with hypertension, and monitor blood pressure closely throughout therapy. Drug may cause hypertension or worsen it.
•**WARNING** Monitor patient closely for thrombotic events, including CVA and MI, because NSAIDs increase the risk.
•Especially if patient is elderly or taking etodolac long-term, watch for less common but serious adverse GI reactions, including anorexia, constipation, diverticulitis, dysphagia, esophagitis, gastritis, gastroenteritis, gastroesophageal reflux disease, hemorrhoids, hiatal hernia, melena, stomatitis, and vomiting.
•Monitor liver function test results because, in rare cases, elevated levels may progress to severe hepatic reactions, including fatal hep-atitis, hepatic necrosis, and hepatic failure.
•Monitor BUN and serum creatinine levels in patients with heart failure, hepatic dysfunction, or impaired renal function; those taking diuretics or ACE inhibitors; and elderly patients because drug may cause renal failure.
•Monitor CBC for decreased hemoglobin level and hematocrit because drug may worsen anemia.
•**WARNING** If patient has bone marrow suppression or is receiving antineoplastic drug therapy, monitor laboratory results (including WBC count), and watch for evidence of

infection because anti-inflammatory and antipyretic actions of etodolac may mask signs and symptoms, such as fever and pain.

•Assess patient's skin routinely for rash or other signs of hypersensitivity reaction because etodolac and other NSAIDs may cause serious skin reactions without warning, even in patients with no history of NSAID hypersensitivity Stop drug at first sign of reaction and notify prescriber.

•If patient also takes acetaminophen, monitor fluid intake and output and BUN and serum creatinine levels for signs of adverse renal reactions.

### PATIENT TEACHING

•Instruct patient to take etodolac with food or after meals if adverse GI reactions occur.

•Caution him to avoid aspirin or aspirin-containing products while taking drug.

•Advise patient not to smoke or drink alcoholic beverages during therapy because these activities increase the risk of adverse GI reactions.

•Inform patient that he may experience dizziness or drowsiness.

•Instruct him to notify prescriber immediately if he experiences blood in urine, easy bruising, itching, rash, swelling, or yellow eyes or skin.

•Caution pregnant patient not to take etodolac or other NSAIDs during the third trimester because drug may cause premature closure of the ductus arteriosus.

•Explain that etodolac may increase the risk of serious adverse cardiovascular reactions; urge patient to seek immediate medical attention if signs or symptoms arise, such as chest pain, shortness of breath, weakness, and slurring of speech.

•Tell patient that etodolac also may increase the risk of serious adverse GI reactions; stress the importance of seeking immediate medical attention for such signs and symptoms as epigastric or abdominal pain, indigestion, black or tarry stools, or vomiting blood or material that looks like coffee grounds.

•Alert patient to the possibility of rare but serious skin reactions. Urge him to seek immediate medical attention for rash, blisters, itching, fever, or other indications of hypersensitivity.

# exenatide

Byetta

## Class and Category

*Chemical:* Amino acid peptide amide
*Therapeutic:* Antidiabetic drug
*Pregnancy category:* C

## Indications and Dosages

➤ *Adjunct treatment to improve blood glucose levels in patients with type 2 diabetes mellitus who are taking metformin, a sulfonylurea, or a combination of metformin and a sulfonylurea but have not achieved adequate glucose control*

### S.C. INJECTION

**Adults.** *Initial:* 5 mcg b.i.d. within 60 min before morning and evening meals. After 1 mo, increased as needed to 10 mcg b.i.d. within 60 min before morning and evening meals.

| Route | Onset | Peak | Duration |
|-------|-------|------|----------|
| S.C. | Immediate | 2.1 hr | Unknown |

## Contraindications

Hypersensitivity to exenatide or its components, ketoacidosis, type 1 diabetes mellitus

## Interactions

### DRUGS

*oral antidiabetics:* Increased risk of hypoglycemia
*oral drugs:* May decrease rate and extent of absorption of these drugs

## Adverse Reactions

**CNS:** Asthenia, dizziness, headache, jitteriness
**GI:** Anorexia, diarrhea, gastroesophageal reflux, indigestion, nausea, vomiting
**SKIN:** Diaphoresis
**Other:** Elevated antiexenatide antibody level, weight loss

## Nursing Considerations

•Know that exenatide is not recommended for patients with severe GI disease, patients with creatinine clearance less than 30 ml/min/1.73 $m^3$, or patients undergoing dialysis because of drug's adverse GI effects.

•Be aware that when exenatide is given to a patient also receiving a sulfonylurea, the sul-

E
F

## Mechanism of Action

Normally, when serum glucose level rises, insulin is secreted within 10 minutes. This first-phase insulin response is absent in patients with type 2 diabetes.

Exenatide, an incretin mimetic, restores the first-phase insulin response and improves the second-phase insulin response that immediately follows. It does so by promoting incretins that spur insulin synthesis and release from beta cells by binding and activating human GLP-1 receptors to reduce fasting and postprandial serum glucose levels.

The drug also suppresses inappropriately elevated glucagon secretion. Lower serum glucagon level leads to decreased hepatic glucose output and decreased insulin demand. Exenatide also slows gastric emptying, which slows the rise of serum glucose levels.

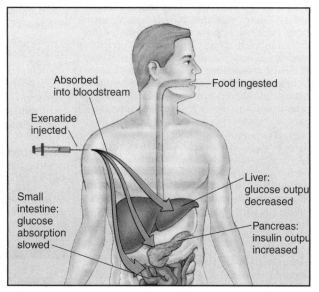

Absorbed into bloodstream

Food ingested

Exenatide injected

Liver: glucose outpu decreased

Small intestine: glucose absorption slowed

Pancreas: insulin outpu increased

fonylurea dosage may need to be decreased to reduce the risk of hypoglycemia. Usually, no dosage adjustment is needed for a patient taking metformin.

•If patient is also receiving a sulfonylurea, monitor him for hypoglycemia and treat as needed.

•Administer drug into the patient's thigh, abdomen, or upper arm.

**PATIENT TEACHING**

•Teach patient how to administer an S.C. injection and how to use the pen injection device.

•Inform patient that the drug may be administered in the thigh, abdomen, or upper arm. Stress the importance of rotating injection sites.

•Stress the importance of administering drug within 60 minutes before morning and evening meals, never after a meal.

•If patient misses a dose, tell him to resume treatment with the next scheduled dose.

•Advise patient that drug should look clear and colorless. Caution against using any pre-filled pen device in which the solution looks cloudy or colored or contains particles.

•Instruct patient to be aware of expiration date on vial and not to use drug if date has passed.

•Advise patient to keep drug refrigerated and protected from light.

•Advise patient to discard pen injection device 30 days after initial use, even if some of drug is left in the pen.

•Alert patient that pen doesn't come already equipped with needles and that he'll need to buy them separately.

•Warn patient that nausea may occur at the beginning of therapy.

•Inform patient taking a sulfonylurea to be alert for hypoglycemic reactions because risk increases when both drugs are taken. Review ways to treat such reactions, and tell patient to alert prescriber if they occur frequently or become severe.

•Instruct female patients of childbearing potential to tell their prescriber if they are, could be, or are planning to become pregnant.

# ezetimibe

Zetia

## Class and Category

*Chemical:* Azetidinone
*Therapeutic:* Antihypercholesterolemic
*Pregnancy category:* C

## Indications and Dosages

➤ *To treat heterozygous familial and non-familial hypercholesterolemia, homozygous familial hypercholesterolemia, and homozygous sitosterolemia*

**TABLETS**
**Adults.** 10 mg q.d.

## Contraindications

Active hepatic dysfunction, hypersensitivity to ezetimibe or its components

## Interactions

**DRUGS**
*cholestyramine:* Reduced effects of ezetimibe
*cyclosporine:* Increased blood cyclosporine and ezetimibe levels
*fenofibrate, gemfibrozil:* Increased blood ezetimibe level

## Adverse Reactions

**CNS:** Dizziness, fatigue, headache
**CV:** Chest pain
**EENT:** Pharyngitis, sinusitis
**GI:** Abdominal pain, cholelithiasis, cholecystitis, diarrhea, elevated liver function test results, hepatitis, nausea, pancreatitis
**HEME:** Thrombocytopenia
**MS:** Arthralgia, back pain, myalgia, myopathy, rhabdomyolysis
**RESP:** Cough, upper respiratory tract infection
**SKIN:** Rash
**Other:** Angioedema, viral infection

## Nursing Considerations

• Monitor liver function test results before and during ezetimibe therapy, as ordered.

E
F

## Mechanism of Action

Ezetimibe reduces blood cholesterol by inhibiting its absorption through the small intestine. Normally, within the intestinal lumen, lipids break down into cholesterol and other substances that create smaller droplets called micelles, as shown below left. The micelles enter intestinal epithelial cells called enterocytes, where they combine with triglycerides, cholesterol, and other substances to form chylomicrons.

Chylomicrons then pass through to the lymphatic system to be carried to the blood.

Ezetimibe blocks cholesterol absorption into enterocytes and prevents the movement of cholesterol through the intestinal wall, as shown below right. This reduced cholesterol absorption from the intestine decreases chylomicron and LDL cholesterol content.

• Know that you should give ezetimibe 2 hours before or 4 hours after giving bile acid sequestrant, cholestyramine, or colestipol.

PATIENT TEACHING

• Direct patient to follow a low-cholesterol diet as an adjunct to ezetimibe therapy. Recommend weight loss and exercise programs, as appropriate.

• Instruct patient who is also taking a bile acid sequestrant to take ezetimibe either 2 hours before or at least 4 hours after the bile acid sequestrant to prevent drug interactions.

• Advise patient to report unexplained muscle pain, tenderness, or weakness.

# ezetimibe and simvastatin

Vytorin

## Class and Category

*Chemical:* Azetidinone (ezetimibe), synthetically derived fermentation product of *Aspergillus terreus* (simvastatin)
*Therapeutic:* Antihyperlipidemic
*Pregnancy category:* X

## Indications and Dosages

➤ *To treat primary hypercholesterolemia*

TABLETS

**Adults.** *Initial:* 10 mg/10 mg daily for mild LDL-C level reduction, 10 mg/20 mg daily for moderate LDL-C level reduction, or 10 mg/40 mg daily for aggressive (more than 55%) LDL-C level reduction. Dosage adjusted, as needed, after 2 or more weeks. *Maximum:* 10 mg/80 mg daily.

➤ *To treat homozygous familial hypercholesterolemia*

TABLETS

**Adults.** 10 mg/40 mg daily or 10 mg/80 mg daily h.s.

DOSAGE ADJUSTMENT For patients with severe renal insufficiency, drugs are given only if patient has already received simvastatin at a dose of 5 mg or higher. For patients receiving cyclosporine, they are given only if patient has already received simvastatin at a dose of 5 mg or higher with the dosage not to exceed 10 mg/10 mg daily. For patients receiving amiodarone or verapamil, dosage should not exceed 10 mg/20 mg daily.

## Mechanism of Action

Ezetimibe and simvastatin work complementarily to decrease the blood cholesterol level. Normally, lipids in the intestinal lumen break down into cholesterol and other substances that create smaller droplets called micelles. Micelles enter intestinal epithelial cells (called enterocytes), where they combine with triglycerides, cholesterol, and other substances to form chylomicrons. Chylomicrons enter the lymphatic system and are carried to the bloodstream.

Ezetimibe blocks cholesterol absorption into enterocytes. This decreased movement of cholesterol through the intestinal wall decreases chylomicron and LDL cholesterol levels in the bloodstream.

Simvastatin interferes with the hepatic enzyme hydroxymethylglutaryl-coenzyme A reductase. This action reduces formation of mevalonic acid, a cholesterol precursor, thus interrupting cholesterol synthesis. When the cholesterol level declines in hepatic cells, LDLs are consumed, which in turn reduces the levels of circulating total cholesterol and serum triglycerides.

## Contraindications

Active liver disease; breast-feeding; hypersensitivity to ezetimibe, simvastatin, or their components; pregnancy

## Interactions

DRUGS

**Ezetimibe component**

*cholestyramine:* Reduced effectiveness of ezetimibe
*cyclosporine, fenofibrate, gemfibrozil:* Increased blood ezetimibe level

**Simvastatin component**

*amiodarone, antiretroviral protease inhibitors (amprenavir, indinavir, nelfinavir, ritonavir, saquinavir), clarithromycin, cyclosporine, danazol, erythromycin, gemfibrozil and other fibrates, itraconazole, ketoconazole, nefazodone, niacin (1 g/day or more), telithromycin, verapamil:* Increased risk of myopathy or rhabdomyolysis
*azole antifungals, cyclosporine, gemfibrozil, immunosuppressants, macrolide antibiotics*

*(including erythromycin), niacin, verapamil:* Increased risk of acute renal failure
*bile acid sequestrants, cholestyramine, colestipol:* Decreased bioavailability of simvastatin
*digoxin:* Possibly slight elevation in blood digoxin level
*diltiazem, verapamil:* Possibly increased blood simvastatin level and increased risk of myopathy
*oral anticoagulants:* Increased risk of bleeding or prolonged PT
**FOODS**
**Simvastatin component**
*grapefruit juice (1 or more quarts/day):* Possibly increased blood simvastatin level; increased risk of myopathy or rhabdomyolysis

## Adverse Reactions

**CNS:** Asthenia, dizziness, fatigue, headache
**CV:** Chest pain
**EENT:** Pharyngitis, rhinitis, sinusitis, taste alteration
**GI:** Abdominal pain, cholelithiasis, cholecystitis, constipation, diarrhea, elevated liver function test results, flatulence, heartburn, hepatitis, nausea, pancreatitis, vomiting
**HEME:** Thrombocytopenia
**MS:** Arthralgia, back pain, myalgia, myopathy, rhabdomyolysis
**RESP:** Cough, upper respiratory tract infection
**SKIN:** Eczema, pruritus, rash
**Other:** Angioedema, viral infection

## Nursing Considerations

• Use ezetimibe and simvastatin cautiously in elderly patients and those with hepatic or renal impairment.
• Monitor patient's liver function test results before ezetimibe and simvastatin therapy and every 3 to 6 months during therapy, as ordered.
• Give ezetimibe and simvastatin 2 hours before or 4 hours after giving a bile acid sequestrant (such as cholestyramine or colestipol).
• Monitor serum lipoprotein level, as ordered, to evaluate patient's response to therapy.
**PATIENT TEACHING**
• Advise patient to take ezetimibe and simvastatin in the evening.
• Encourage patient to follow a low-fat and low-cholesterol diet.

• Instruct patient who's taking a bile acid sequestrant (cholestyramine, colestipol) to take ezetimibe and simvastatin 2 hours before or 4 hours after taking the bile acid sequestrant.
• Urge patient to notify prescriber immediately if he develops symptoms of myopathy, such as muscle pain, tenderness, and weakness.
• Instruct female patient of childbearing age to use reliable contraception while taking drug. Instruct her to notify prescriber at once if she suspects pregnancy.
• Advise patient to avoid grapefruit juice to decrease risk of drug toxicity.

# famotidine

Act (CAN), Apo-Famotidine (CAN), Dyspep HB (CAN), Gen-Famotidine (CAN), Mylanta-AR, Novo-Famotidine (CAN), Nu-Famotidine (CAN), Pepcid, Pepcid AC, Pepcid RPD

## Class and Category

*Chemical:* Thiazole derivative
*Therapeutic:* Antiulcer agent, gastric acid secretion inhibitor
*Pregnancy category:* B

## Indications and Dosages

➤ *To provide short-term treatment of active duodenal ulcer*
**ORAL SUSPENSION, TABLETS (CHEWABLE, ORAL DISINTEGRATING, AND REGULAR)**
**Adults and adolescents.** 40 mg q.d. h.s. or 20 mg b.i.d.
**Children.** 0.5 mg/kg/day as a single dose h.s. or in divided doses b.i.d.
**I.V. INFUSION OR INJECTION**
**Adults and adolescents over age 16.** 20 mg q 12 hr, infused over 15 to 30 min or injected over at least 2 min.
**Children ages 1 to 16.** *Initial:* 0.25 mg/kg q 12 hr, infused over 15 to 30 min or injected over at least 2 min. *Maximum:* 40 mg/day.
➤ *To prevent recurrence of duodenal ulcer*
**ORAL SUSPENSION, TABLETS (CHEWABLE, ORAL DISINTEGRATING, AND REGULAR)**
**Adults and adolescents.** 20 mg q.d. h.s.
➤ *To provide short-term treatment for active, benign gastric ulcer*
**ORAL SUSPENSION, TABLETS (CHEWABLE, ORAL DISINTEGRATING, AND REGULAR)**
**Adults and adolescents.** 40 mg q.d. h.s.

E
F

**Children**. 0.5 mg/kg/day as a single dose h.s. or in divided doses b.i.d.

**I.V. INFUSION OR INJECTION**

**Adults and adolescents over age 16**. 20 mg q 12 hr.

**Children ages 1 to 16.** *Initial*: 0.25 mg/kg q 12 hr. *Maximum:* 40 mg/day.

➤ *To treat gastroesophageal reflux disease*

**ORAL SUSPENSION, TABLETS (CHEWABLE, ORAL DISINTE-GRATING, AND REGULAR)**

**Adults and adolescents.** 20 mg b.i.d. for up to 6 wk.

**Children who weigh more than 10 kg (22 lb).** 1 to 2 mg/kg/day in divided doses b.i.d.

**Children who weigh less than 10 kg.** 1 to 2 mg/kg/day in divided doses t.i.d.

**ORAL SUSPENSION**

**Infants age 4 months to 1 year.** 0.5 mg/kg/day in divided doses b.i.d. for up to 8 wk.

**Infants age 3 months or less.** 0.5 mg/kg q.d. for up to 8 wk.

**I.V. INFUSION OR INJECTION**

**Children ages 1 to 16.** *Initial:* 0.25 mg/kg q 12 hr. *Maximum:* 40 mg/day.

➤ *To treat esophagitis caused by gastro-esophageal reflux*

**ORAL SUSPENSION, TABLETS (CHEWABLE, ORAL DISINTE-GRATING, AND REGULAR)**

**Adults and adolescents.** 20 to 40 mg b.i.d. for up to 12 wk.

➤ *To treat gastric hypersecretory conditions, such as Zollinger-Ellison syndrome*

**ORAL SUSPENSION, TABLETS (CHEWABLE, ORAL DISINTE-GRATING, AND REGULAR)**

**Adults and adolescents.** *Initial:* 20 mg q 6 hr. Dosage adjusted, if needed, based on patient response.

**I.V. INFUSION OR INJECTION**

**Adults and adolescents.** 20 mg q 12 hr.

➤ *To prevent heartburn and indigestion*

**TABLETS (CHEWABLE, ORAL DISINTEGRATING, AND REGULAR)**

**Adults and adolescents.** 10 mg 1 hr before eating. *Maximum:* 20 mg q 24 hr.

➤ *To treat heartburn and indigestion*

**TABLETS (CHEWABLE, ORAL DISINTEGRATING, AND REGULAR)**

**Adults and adolescents.** 10 mg at onset of symptoms. *Maximum:* 20 mg q 24 hr for up to 2 wk unless prescriber advises otherwise.

**DOSAGE ADJUSTMENT** Oral or parenteral dosage reduced or dosing interval increased (to 36 to 48 hr), if needed, in patients with renal insufficiency and creatinine clearance of 49 ml/min/1.73 $m^2$ or less.

| Route | Onset | Peak | Duration |
|---|---|---|---|
| P.O. | 1 hr | 1 to 4 hr | 10 to 12 hr |
| I.V. | In 30 min | 0.5 to 3 hr | 10 to 12 hr |

## Contraindications

Hypersensitivity to famotidine, other $H_2$-receptor antagonists, or their components

## Interactions

**DRUGS**

*antacids, sucralfate:* Possibly decreased absorption of famotidine

*bone marrow depressants:* Increased risk of blood dyscrasias

*itraconazole, ketoconazole:* Possibly decreased absorption of these drugs

**ACTIVITIES**

*alcohol use:* Possibly increased blood alcohol level

## Adverse Reactions

**CNS:** Agitation (infants), dizziness, fever, headache, insomnia, mental or mood changes

**CV:** Arrhythmias, palpitations

**EENT:** Dry mouth, laryngeal edema, tinnitus

**GI:** Abdominal pain, anorexia, constipation, diarrhea, hepatitis, nausea, vomiting

**HEME:** Aplastic anemia, leukopenia, neutropenia, pancytopenia, thrombocytopenia

**RESP:** Bronchospasm, dyspnea, wheezing

**SKIN:** Alopecia, dry skin, erythema multiforme, exfoliative dermatitis, jaundice, pruritus, rash, Stevens-Johnson syndrome, toxic epidermal necrolysis, urticaria

**Other:** Anaphylaxis, angioedema, facial edema, hyperuricemia

## Nursing Considerations

•Shake famotidine oral suspension vigorously for 5 to 10 seconds before administration.

•Dilute injection form (2 ml) with NS or other solution to 5 to 10 ml; give I.V. injection over at least 2 minutes. Or dilute in 100 ml of $D_5W$ and infuse over 15 to 30 minutes. Or infuse premixed injection (20 mg/50 ml NS) over 15 to 30 minutes.

•**WARNING** Be aware that Pepcid AC chewable tablets contain aspartame, which can be dangerous for patients with phenylketonuria.

## Mechanism of Action

In normal digestion, parietal cells in the gastric epithelium secrete hydrogen (H⁺) ions, which combine with chloride ions (Cl⁻) to form hydrochloric acid (HCl), as shown below left. However, HCl can inflame, ulcerate, and perforate the gastric and intestinal mucosa that's normally protected by mucus. Famotidine, an H₂-receptor antagonist, reduces HCl formation by preventing histamine from binding with H₂ receptors on the surface of parietal cells, as shown below right. By doing so, the drug helps prevent peptic ulcers from forming and helps heal existing ones.

•Instruct patient to store famotidine oral suspension at room temperature (below 86° F [30° C]) and to protect it from freezing. Tell her to shake the bottle vigorously for 5 to 10 seconds after adding water and right before use.
•Advise patient who uses Pepcid RPD to store drug in unopened package. For each dose, instruct her to open blister pack with dry hands, place a tablet on her tongue, let it dissolve, and swallow it with saliva.
•If patient uses chewable tablets, instruct her to chew them thoroughly before swallowing.
•If patient also takes antacids, instruct her to wait 30 to 60 minutes after taking famotidine, if possible, before taking antacid.
•Caution patient to avoid alcohol and smoking during famotidine therapy because they irritate the stomach and can delay ulcer healing.
•Advise patient to notify prescriber if she develops pain or has trouble swallowing or if she has bloody vomit or black stools.

•Caution patient not to take famotidine with other acid-reducing products.

# felbamate

Felbatol

## Class and Category
*Chemical:* Dicarbamate
*Therapeutic:* Anticonvulsant
*Pregnancy category:* C

## Indications and Dosages
➤ *To treat partial seizures in patients who don't respond to other drugs*
ORAL SUSPENSION, TABLETS
**Adults and adolescents over age 14.** *Initial:* 1,200 mg/day in divided doses t.i.d. or q.i.d. Dosage increased over several weeks based on patient response. *Maximum:* 3,600 mg/day.
**Children ages 2 to 14.** *Initial:* 15 mg/kg/day in divided doses t.i.d. or q.i.d. Dosage increased over several weeks based on patient response. *Maximum:* 3,600 mg/day or 45 mg/kg/day.

➤ *As adjunct to treat generalized or partial seizures associated with Lennox-Gastaut syndrome in children*

**ORAL SUSPENSION, TABLETS**

**Children ages 2 to 14.** *Initial:* 15 mg/kg/day in divided doses t.i.d. or q.i.d. while decreasing other anticonvulsant drugs by 20% to control their blood levels. Felbamate dosage increased by 15 mg/kg/day q wk. *Maximum:* 3,600 mg/day or 45 mg/kg/day.

**DOSAGE ADJUSTMENT** Dosage reduced by 50% in patients with renal impairment.

---

## Mechanism of Action

May exert its anticonvulsant effects by antagonizing the effects of the amino acid glycine. When glycine binds to *N*-methyl-D-aspartate (NMDA) receptors in the CNS, the frequency at which receptor-gated calcium ion channels open is increased—an important factor in initiating seizures. Felbamate may raise the seizure threshold by blocking NMDA receptors so that glycine can't bind to them.

---

## Contraindications

Hepatic dysfunction; history of blood dyscrasias; hypersensitivity to felbamate, other carbamates, or their components

## Interactions

**DRUGS**

*carbamazepine:* Decreased blood carbamazepine level and increased felbamate clearance, resulting in decreased blood felbamate level

*fosphenytoin, phenytoin:* Increased blood phenytoin level and increased felbamate clearance, resulting in decreased blood felbamate level

*methsuximide:* Increased adverse effects of methsuximide

*oral contraceptives:* Possibly decreased effectiveness of oral contraceptives

*phenobarbital:* Decreased blood felbamate level, increased blood phenobarbital level and risk of adverse effects

*valproic acid:* Increased blood valproic acid level and increased risk of adverse effects

## Adverse Reactions

**CNS:** Abnormal gait, aggressiveness, agitation, anxiety, dizziness, drowsiness, fever, headache, insomnia, mood changes, tremor

**EENT:** Altered taste, diplopia, rhinitis

**GI:** Abdominal pain, anorexia, constipation, diarrhea, elevated liver function test results, hepatic failure, indigestion, nausea, vomiting

**HEME:** Aplastic anemia, leukopenia, pancytopenia, thrombocytopenia

**RESP:** Upper respiratory tract infection

**SKIN:** Photosensitivity, purpura, rash

**Other:** Anaphylaxis, lymphadenopathy, weight loss

## Nursing Considerations

• Check liver function test results before starting felbamate therapy, and expect to monitor test results every 1 to 2 weeks during treatment. Notify prescriber immediately and expect to stop drug if test results become abnormal.

• Plan to taper dosage by one-third every 4 to 5 days as prescribed. If patient receives adequate amounts of other anticonvulsant drugs, felbamate may be stopped without tapering, if needed.

• **WARNING** Assess for signs of aplastic anemia and bone marrow depression, which may occur with felbamate use. Signs may not appear until several months after therapy begins. Expect to stop felbamate therapy if bone marrow depression develops.

• If patient receives adjunctive therapy, expect adverse reactions to resolve as other anticonvulsant dosages decrease.

**PATIENT TEACHING**

• Direct patient to shake suspension before using and to use a calibrated spoon or container to measure each dose.

• Instruct patient to store felbamate oral suspension and tablets at room temperature.

• Because drug may cause photosensitivity reactions, urge patient to protect her skin from sun and to avoid sunlamps and tanning booths.

• Inform patient that dizziness and drowsiness may occur. Advise her to avoid potentially hazardous activities until drug's CNS effects are known.

• Warn patient not to stop taking felbamate abruptly.

• Advise patient to return for ordered liver function tests and to report yellow skin or eyes and dark urine to prescriber.

• Instruct patient to tell prescriber if she experiences bleeding, infection, or fatigue.

•Advise patient to carry medical identification that indicates her condition and drug therapy.
•Because felbamate decreases oral contraceptive effectiveness, discuss alternate contraceptive methods.

# felodipine

Plendil, Renedil (CAN)

## Class and Category
*Chemical:* Dihydropyridine derivative
*Therapeutic:* Antihypertensive
*Pregnancy category:* C

## Indications and Dosages
➤ *To manage essential hypertension alone or with other antihypertensives*

**E.R. TABLETS**
**Adults.** *Initial:* 5 mg q.d. Dosage adjusted q 2 wk to 2.5 to 10 mg q.d. based on patient response.
**DOSAGE ADJUSTMENT** Initial or maintenance dosage reduced, if needed, in patients who are over age 65 or have impaired hepatic function.

| Route | Onset | Peak | Duration |
|-------|-------|------|----------|
| P.O. | 2 to 5 hr | Unknown | 16 to 24 hr |

## Mechanism of Action
May slow the movement of extracellular calcium into myocardial and vascular smooth-muscle cells by deforming calcium channels in cell membranes, inhibiting ion-controlled gating mechanisms, and interfering with calcium release from the sarcoplasmic reticulum. The effect of these actions is a decrease in intracellular calcium ions, which inhibits contraction of smooth-muscle cells and dilates coronary and systemic arteries. As with other calcium channel blockers, felodipine's actions result in increased oxygen to the myocardium and reduced peripheral resistance, blood pressure, and afterload.

## Contraindications
Hypersensitivity to felodipine or its components

## Interactions
**DRUGS**
*anesthetics (hydrocarbon inhalation):* Possibly hypotension
*antihypertensives, prazocin:* Increased risk of hypotension
*beta blockers:* Increased adverse effects of beta blockers
*cimetidine:* Increased felodipine bioavailability
*digoxin:* Transiently increased blood digoxin level and risk of digitalis toxicity
*estrogens:* Possibly increased fluid retention and decreased felodipine effects
*lithium:* Increased risk of neurotoxicity
*NSAIDs, sympathomimetics:* Possibly decreased therapeutic effect of felodipine
*procainamide, quinidine:* Increased risk of prolonged Q-T interval
*tacrolimus:* Possibly increased blood tacrolimus level and risk of adverse effects
**FOODS**
*grapefruit juice:* Doubled felodipine bioavailability

## Adverse Reactions
**CNS:** Asthenia, dizziness, drowsiness, fatigue, headache, paresthesia, syncope, weakness
**CV:** Chest pain, hypotension, palpitations, peripheral edema, tachycardia
**EENT:** Gingival hyperplasia, pharyngitis, rhinitis
**GI:** Abdominal cramps, constipation, diarrhea, indigestion, nausea
**HEME:** Agranulocytosis
**MS:** Back pain
**RESP:** Cough
**SKIN:** Flushing, rash

## Nursing Considerations
•Use felodipine cautiously in patients with heart failure or reduced ventricular function.
•Monitor blood pressure during dosage titration and throughout felodipine therapy, especially in elderly patients.
•Expect drug bioavailability to increase by up to twofold when felodipine is taken with grapefruit juice.
•**WARNING** Be aware that felodipine may cause severe hypotension with syncope, which may lead to reflex tachycardia. This can precipitate angina in patients with coronary artery disease or a history of angina.
•Monitor for signs of overdose, such as excessive peripheral vasodilation, marked hy-

E
F

potension and, possibly, bradycardia. If you detect such signs, place patient in supine position with legs elevated and give I.V. fluids, as prescribed. Expect to give I.V. atropine for bradycardia.

**PATIENT TEACHING**
• Instruct patient to swallow tablets whole and not to crush or chew them.
• Caution patient not to alter her intake of grapefruit juice during therapy.
• Advise patient to store felodipine at room temperature and to protect it from light.
• Instruct patient to monitor her pulse rate and blood pressure.
• Teach patient how to minimize gingival hyperplasia.
• Advise patient to notify prescriber immediately if she experiences palpitations, pronounced dizziness, or swelling of hands or feet.

# fenofibrate

Tricor

## Class and Category

*Chemical:* Aryloxisobutyric acid derivative
*Therapeutic:* Antihyperlipidemic
*Pregnancy category:* C

## Indications and Dosages

➤ *To treat primary hypercholesterolemia or mixed hyperlipidemia*
**CAPSULES**
**Adults.** 200 mg/day.
**TABLETS**
**Adults.** 145 mg/day.
➤ *To treat hypertriglyceridemia (Fredrickson Types IV and V hyperlipidemia)*
**CAPSULES**
**Adults.** *Initial:* 67 mg/day with food, increased as needed q 4 to 8 wk. *Maximum:* 201 mg/day with meals.
**TABLETS**
**Adults.** 48 to 145 mg/day, increased as needed at 4- to 8-wk intervals. *Maximum:* 145 mg/day.
**DOSAGE ADJUSTMENT** For patients with impaired renal function, initial dosage limited to 48 mg/day (tablets) or 67 mg/day (capsules) with dosage increase only after drug's therapeutic and renal effects are known. For elderly patients, dosage limited to 48 mg/day (tablets) or 67 mg/day (capsules).

| Route | Onset | Peak | Duration |
|-------|-------|------|----------|
| P.O. | 6 to 8 wk | Unknown | Unknown |

## Mechanism of Action

May increase the lipolysis of triglyceride-rich lipoproteins and decrease the synthesis of fatty acids and triglycerides by enhancing the activation of lipoprotein lipase and acyl-coenzyme A synthetase. Fenofibrate also may:
• increase hepatic elimination of cholesterol as bile salts
• promote the catabolism of larger, less dense LDLs with a high-binding affinity for cellular LDL receptors.

## Contraindications

Gallbladder disease, hypersensitivity to fenofibrate or its components, hepatic or severe renal impairment

## Interactions

**DRUGS**
*bile acid sequestrants:* Decreased fenofibrate absorption
*cyclosporine:* Increased risk of nephrotoxicity
*HMG-CoA reductase inhibitors (atorvastatin, cerivastatin, fluvastatin, lovastatin, pravastatin, simvastatin):* Increased risk of myopathy, rhabdomyolysis, and acute renal failure
*oral anticoagulants:* Increased risk of bleeding
**FOODS**
*all foods:* Increased fenofibrate bioavailability when given in capsule form

## Adverse Reactions

**CNS:** Asthenia, headache
**EENT:** Rhinitis
**GI:** Abdominal pain, constipation, diarrhea, elevated liver function test results, nausea
**HEME:** Agranulocytosis, decreased hematocrit and hemoglobin levels, thrombocytopenia
**MS:** Back pain
**SKIN:** Rash, Stevens-Johnson syndrome, toxic epidermal necrolysis, urticaria
**Other:** Flulike symptoms

## Nursing Considerations

• As prescribed, discontinue drugs known to increase the serum triglyceride level, such as beta blockers, estrogens, and thiazides, before starting fenofibrate.

•Give capsule form with a full glass of water with meals.

•Administer drug 1 hour before or 4 hours after bile acid sequestrants.

•Monitor results of liver and renal function tests. If liver enzyme levels rise to more than three times the upper limit of normal and persist, or if the patient develops gallstones, expect to stop drug.

•Monitor serum triglyceride and cholesterol levels at 4- to 8-week intervals. If levels don't decrease after 2 months at maximum dosage, expect to stop therapy.

•WARNING Monitor patient closely for acute hypersensitivity reactions, including severe rash, and notify prescriber if they occur. Patient may need inpatient treatment with corticosteroids.

•Assess blood counts periodically, as ordered, during the first 12 months of fenofibrate therapy to detect adverse hematologic effects.

PATIENT TEACHING

•Stress that fenofibrate will be effective only if patient carefully follows prescriber's instructions about diet and exercise.

•Instruct patient to take capsule form with a full glass of water and with food.

•Advise patient to undergo laboratory tests, as directed, to determine drug's effectiveness. They typically include liver function tests after 3 to 6 months, hematocrit and hemoglobin levels, and WBC counts periodically during first year.

•Instruct patient to notify prescriber immediately if she experiences chills, fever, or sore throat. Also urge her to tell prescriber about unexplained muscle pain, tenderness, or weakness, especially if accompanied by fatigue or fever.

# fenoldopam mesylate

Corlopam

## Class and Category

*Chemical:* Dopamine agonist
*Therapeutic:* Antihypertensive
*Pregnancy category:* B

## Indications and Dosages

➤ *To treat severe hypertension when rapid, but quickly reversible, emergency reduction of blood pressure is clinically indicated, including malignant hyper-tension with deteriorating end-organ function*

I.V. INFUSION

**Adults.** *Initial:* 0.025 to 0.3 mcg/kg/min, individualized according to patient weight and desired effect. *Usual:* 0.01 to 1.6 mcg/kg/min. *Maximum:* 1.6 mcg/kg/min for up to 48 hr.

| Route | Onset | Peak | Duration |
|-------|-------|------|----------|
| I.V. | Rapid | Unknown | Unknown |

## Mechanism of Action

Stimulates dopamine-1 postsynaptic receptors, which mediate renal and mesenteric vasodilation. Vasodilation lowers blood pressure and total peripheral resistance while increasing renal blood flow.

## Contraindications

Hypersensitivity to fenoldopam or its components

## Interactions

DRUGS

*antihypertensives:* Additive hypotensive effect
*beta blockers:* Increased risk of hypotension
*dopamine antagonists, metoclopramide:* Possibly decreased effects of fenoldopam

## Adverse Reactions

**CNS:** Anxiety, headache, light-headedness
**CV:** Hypotension, ST- and T-wave changes, tachycardia
**EENT:** Increased intraocular pressure
**GI:** Abdominal pain, nausea
**SKIN:** Diaphoresis, flushing
**Other:** Hypokalemia, injection site pain

## Nursing Considerations

•Reconstitute by adding 40 mg of fenoldopam (4 ml of concentrate) to 1,000 ml of NS or D$_5$W, or 20 mg of fenoldopam (2 ml of concentrate) to 500 ml of NS or D$_5$W, or 10 mg of fenoldopam (1 ml of concentrate) to 250 ml of NS or D$_5$W to produce a final fenoldopam concentration of 40 mcg/ml.

•Infuse through a mechanical infusion pump for proper control of infusion rate.

•Expect to titrate dosage in increments of 0.05 to 0.1 mcg/kg/min, as prescribed.

•Expect to monitor heart rate and blood pressure every 15 minutes during fenoldopam therapy because most of drug's effect on blood pressure occurs within 15 minutes of any dosage change.

E
F

•Be aware that patient may be started on oral antihypertensive therapy, as prescribed, any time after blood pressure is stable during fenoldopam infusion.

•Discard any reconstituted solution not used within 24 hours.

•**WARNING** Assess patient for signs of increased myocardial oxygen demand, especially if patient has heart failure or a history of angina, because fenoldopam may produce a rapid decline in blood pressure, resulting in symptomatic hypotension and a dose-dependent increase in heart rate.

•Monitor serum potassium level because fenoldopam decreases serum potassium concentrations, which may result in hypokalemia, exacerbate arrhythmias, or precipitate conduction abnormalities, especially in patients with cardiac disease.

•Monitor patients with glaucoma or increased intraocular pressure for changes in vision because fenoldopam may cause a dose-dependent increase in intraocular pressure.

•Be alert for possible allergic- or anaphylactic-type reaction to sodium metabisulfite, a component of fenoldopam injection, especially in patients with asthma.

**PATIENT TEACHING**

•Inform patient that she'll be switched to an oral antihypertensive once her blood pressure is controlled.

•Instruct patient to expect frequent monitoring of vital signs.

# fenoprofen calcium

Nalfon

## Class and Category

*Chemical:* Propionic acid derivative
*Therapeutic:* Analgesic, anti-inflammatory, antirheumatic
*Pregnancy category:* Not rated

## Indications and Dosages

➤ *To manage mild to moderate pain*
**CAPSULES, TABLETS**
**Adults.** 200 mg q 4 to 6 hr, as needed.

➤ *To relieve pain, stiffness, and swelling from rheumatoid arthritis or osteoarthritis*
**CAPSULES, TABLETS**
**Adults.** 300 to 600 mg t.i.d. or q.i.d. *Maximum:* 3,200 mg/day.

| Route | Onset | Peak | Duration |
|-------|-------|------|----------|
| P.O. | 15 to 30 min* | Unknown† | 4 to 6 hr‡ |

## Mechanism of Action

Blocks the activity of cyclooxygenase, the enzyme needed for prostaglandin synthesis. Prostaglandins, important mediators of the inflammatory response, cause local vasodilation with swelling and pain. When cyclooxygenase is blocked and prostaglandins inhibited, inflammatory symptoms subside. Prostaglandin inhibition also relieves pain because prostaglandins play a role in pain transmission from the periphery to the spinal cord.

## Contraindications

Angioedema, asthma, bronchospasm, nasal polyps, rhinitis, or urticaria induced by aspirin, iodides, or NSAIDs; hypersensitivity to fenoprofen or its components; renal impairment; severe hepatic impairment

## Interactions

**DRUGS**
*acetaminophen:* Increased risk of renal impairment with concurrent long-term use
*antacids:* Decreased fenoprofen effectiveness
*anticoagulants, cefamandole, cefoperazone, cefotetan, heparin, plicamycin, thrombolytics, valproic acid:* Increased risk of bleeding
*antineoplastics:* Increased adverse hematologic effects
*cyclosporine:* Increased risk of nephrotoxicity
*diuretics, triamterene:* Decreased effectiveness of these drugs
*glucocorticoids, NSAIDs, potassium supplements:* Increased adverse GI effects
*insulin, oral antidiabetic drugs:* Increased risk of hypoglycemia
*lithium:* Increased risk of lithium toxicity
*methotrexate:* Increased risk of methotrexate toxicity
*phenobarbital:* Possibly decreased elimination half-life of fenoprofen
*salicylates:* Increased risk of GI bleeding

---

* For analgesia; 2 days for antirheumatic effects.
† For analgesia; 2 to 3 wk for antirheumatic effects.
‡ For analgesia; unknown for antirheumatic effects.

**ACTIVITIES**
*alcohol use, smoking:* Increased risk of GI bleeding

## Adverse Reactions

**CNS:** Agitation, confusion, dizziness, drowsiness, headache, seizures, sleep disturbance, stroke, tremor, weakness
**CV:** Hypertension, MI, palpitations, peripheral edema, tachycardia, vasodilation
**EENT:** Blurred vision, dry or sore mouth, hearing loss, tinnitus
**GI:** Abdominal cramps, distention, and pain; anorexia; constipation; diarrhea; diverticulitis; dysphagia; esophagitis; flatulence; gastritis; gastroenteritis; gastroesophageal reflux disease; GI bleeding or ulceration; hemorrhoids; hepatitis; hiatal hernia; indigestion; jaundice; liver failure; melena; nausea; perforation of stomach or intestines; vomiting
**GU:** Acute renal failure, dysuria, interstitial nephritis
**HEME:** Agranulocytosis, anemia, hemolytic anemia, leukopenia, neutropenia, pancytopenia
**MS:** Muscle spasms and twitching, myalgia
**RESP:** Dyspnea
**SKIN:** Diaphoresis, erythema, erythema multiforme, exfoliative dermatitis, pruritus, Stevens-Johnson syndrome, toxic epidermal necrolysis, urticaria
**Other:** Anaphylaxis, angioedema

## Nursing Considerations

•Use fenoprofen with extreme caution in patients with a history of ulcer disease or GI bleeding because NSAIDs such as fenoprofen increase the risk of GI bleeding and ulceration. Expect to use fenoprofen for the shortest time possible in these patients.
•Be aware that serious GI tract ulceration, bleeding, and perforation may occur without warning symptoms. Elderly patients are at greater risk. To minimize risk, give drug with food. If GI distress occurs, withhold drug and notify prescriber immediately.
•Use fenoprofen cautiously in patients with hypertension, and monitor blood pressure closely throughout therapy. Drug may cause hypertension or worsen it.
•Give drug with food, milk, or antacids to decrease adverse GI reactions.
•**WARNING** If patient receives long-term therapy, watch for signs of toxicity, such as agitation; blurred vision; coma; confusion;

drowsiness; elevated BUN and serum creatinine levels; indigestion; nausea; rash; seizures; severe headache; slow, labored breathing; tinnitus; and vomiting.
•**WARNING** Monitor patient closely for thrombotic events, including MI and stroke, because NSAIDs increase the risk.
•**WARNING** If patient has bone marrow suppression or is receiving antineoplastic drug therapy, monitor laboratory results (including WBC count), and watch for evidence of infection because anti-inflammatory and antipyretic actions of fenoprofen may mask signs and symptoms of infection, such as fever and pain.
•Monitor patient—especially if she's elderly or receiving long-term fenoprofen therapy—for less common but serious adverse GI reactions, including anorexia, constipation, diverticulitis, dysphagia, esophagitis, gastritis, gastroenteritis, gastroesophageal reflux disease, hemorrhoids, hiatal hernia, melena, stomatitis, and vomiting.
•Monitor liver function test results because, in rare cases, elevations may progress to severe hepatic reactions, including fatal hepatitis, liver necrosis, and hepatic failure.
•Monitor BUN and serum creatinine levels in elderly patients, patients taking diuretics or ACE inhibitors, and patients with heart failure, impaired renal function, or hepatic dysfunction because drug may cause renal failure.
•Monitor CBC for decreased hemoglobin and hematocrit because drug may worsen anemia.
•Assess patient's skin regularly for signs of rash or other hypersensitivity reaction because fenoprofen is an NSAID and may cause serious skin reactions without warning, even in patients with no history of NSAID sensitivity. At first sign of reaction, stop drug and notify prescriber.

**PATIENT TEACHING**
•Advise patient to take fenoprofen with food, milk, or antacids to minimize GI distress. Also instruct her to take drug with a full glass of water and to stay upright for 30 minutes afterward to decrease the risk of drug lodging in the esophagus and causing irritation.
•Instruct patient to swallow drug whole and not to crush, break, chew, or open capsules.
•Caution patient to avoid alcohol, aspirin, and other NSAIDs, unless prescribed, while taking fenoprofen.

• If patient takes an anticoagulant, urge her to immediately report bleeding, including bloody or tarry stools and bloody vomitus.
• Caution patient to avoid hazardous activities until drug's CNS effects are known.
• Explain that NSAIDs may increase the risk of serious adverse cardiovascular reactions; urge patient to seek immediate medical attention if signs or symptoms arise, such as chest pain, shortness of breath, weakness, and slurring of speech.
• Explain that fenoprofen also may increase the risk of serious adverse GI reactions; stress the importance of seeking immediate medical attention for such signs and symptoms as epigastric or abdominal pain, indigestion, black or tarry stools, or vomiting blood or material that looks like coffee grounds.
• Alert patient to the possibility of rare but serious skin reactions. Urge her to seek immediate medical attention for rash, blisters, itching, fever, or other indications of hypersensitivity.

# fentanyl citrate

Actiq, Sublimaze

## fentanyl transdermal system

Duragesic

## Class, Category, and Schedule

*Chemical:* Opioid, phenylpiperidine derivative
*Therapeutic:* Analgesic, anesthesia adjunct
*Pregnancy category:* C
*Controlled substance:* Schedule II

## Indications and Dosages

➤ *To provide surgical premedication*
**I.M. INJECTION**
**Adults.** 0.05 to 0.1 mg 30 to 60 min before surgery.
➤ *As adjunct to regional anesthesia*
**I.V. OR I.M. INJECTION**
**Adults.** 0.05 to 0.1 mg I.M. or slow I.V. over 1 to 2 min.
➤ *To manage postoperative pain in post-anesthesia care unit*
**I.M. INJECTION**
**Adults.** 0.05 to 0.1 mg. Repeated in 1 to 2 hr, if needed.
➤ *To treat breakthrough pain in cancer patients who have developed a tolerance to opioid therapy*

**TRANSMUCOSAL LOZENGE**
**Adults.** *Initial:* 200 mcg placed between cheek and gum for up to 15 min followed by second dose 15 min after first dose ends, if needed. Dosage increased according to patient's needs.
➤ *To relieve persistent moderate to severe chronic pain that doesn't respond to less potent drugs and requires around-the-clock opioid administration for an extended period of time*
**TRANSDERMAL SYSTEM**
**Adults and children age 2 and older.** *Initial:* One 25-mcg/hr patch, replaced q 72 hr (or 48 hr, if needed). Dosage increased by 12.5 mcg/hr, as needed, after first 72 hr and then q 6 days. For more than 100 mcg/hr, more than one patch is used.
**DOSAGE ADJUSTMENT** For elderly, cachectic, or debilitated patients, initial dosage should not exceed 25 mcg/hr unless patient is already receiving more than 135 mg of oral morphine/day or an equivalent dose of another opioid. For patients receiving long-term opioid therapy, dosage adjusted based on previous day's drug requirement. For cancer patients who need more than 800 mcg/day for breakthrough pain, dosage altered or another long-acting opioid given, as prescribed.

| Route | Onset | Peak | Duration |
|---|---|---|---|
| I.V. | 1 to 2 min | 3 to 5 min | 30 to 60 min |
| I.M. | 7 to 15 min | 20 to 30 min | 1 to 2 hr |
| Transdermal | 12 to 24 hr | Unknown | Over 72 hr |

## Contraindications

Age younger than 2, asthma, myasthenia gravis, opioid hypersensitivity or intolerance, significant respiratory depression, upper airway obstruction (I.V. or I.M. form); acute or chronic pain, body weight less than 10 kg (22 lb), doses above 5 mcg/kg in adults or 15 mcg/kg in children (transmucosal form); acute or postoperative pain, age less than 12 (or less than 18 if weight is less than 50 kg [110 lb]), dosage that exceeds 25 mcg/hr at the start of therapy, hypersensitivity to fentanyl (or alfentanil, sufentanil, or adhesives), treatment of mild to moderate pain responsive to nonopioid drugs (transdermal form)

## Mechanism of Action
Binds to opioid receptor sites in the CNS, altering perception of and emotional response to pain by inhibiting ascending pain pathways. Fentanyl may alter neurotransmitter release from afferent nerves responsive to painful stimuli, and it causes respiratory depression by acting directly on respiratory centers in the brain stem.

## Interactions
**DRUGS**
*anticholinergics, antidiarrheals (such as loperamide and paregoric):* Increased risk of severe constipation
*antihypertensives, diuretics:* Possibly potentiated hypotension
*benzodiazepines:* Possibly reduced fentanyl dose required for anesthesia induction
*buprenorphine:* Possibly decreased therapeutic effects of buprenorphine
*clarithromycin, erythromycin, itraconazole, ketoconazole, nefazodone, nelfinavir, ritonavir, troleandomycin:* Possibly increased opioid effect of transdermal fentanyl leading to increased or prolonged adverse effects, including severe respiratory depression
*CNS depressants:* Possibly increased CNS and respiratory depression and hypotension
*cytochrome P-450 inducers (such as rifampin, carbamazepine, and phenytoin):* Possibly induced metabolism and increased clearance of fentanyl
*hydroxyzine:* Possibly increased analgesic effect of fentanyl and increased CNS depression and hypotension
*MAO inhibitors:* Possibly unpredictable, even fatal, effects if taken within 14 days of fentanyl
*metoclopramide:* Possibly antagonized effect of metoclopramide on gastric motility
*nalbuphine, pentazocine:* Possibly antagonized analgesic, respiratory depressant, and CNS depressant effects of fentanyl; possibly additive hypotensive and CNS and respiratory depressant effects of both drugs
*naloxone:* Antagonized analgesic, hypotensive, CNS, and respiratory depressant effects of fentanyl
*naltrexone:* Possibly blocked therapeutic effects of fentanyl
*neuromuscular blockers:* Possibly prevention or reversal of muscle rigidity by fentanyl

**ACTIVITIES**
*alcohol use:* Increased CNS and respiratory depression and hypotension

## Adverse Reactions
**CNS:** Agitation, amnesia, anxiety, asthenia, ataxia, confusion, delusions, depression, dizziness, drowsiness, euphoria, fever, hallucinations, headache, lack of coordination, light-headedness, nervousness, paranoia, sedation, seizures, sleep disturbance, slurred speech, syncope, tremor, weakness, yawning
**CV:** Asystole, bradycardia, chest pain, edema, hypotension, orthostatic hypotension, tachycardia
**EENT:** Blurred vision, dental caries, dry mouth, gum line erosion, laryngospasm, rhinitis, sneezing, tooth loss
**GI:** Anorexia, constipation, ileus, indigestion, nausea, vomiting
**GU:** Anorgasmia, decreased libido, ejaculatory difficulty, urinary hesitancy, urine retention
**RESP:** Apnea, depressed cough reflex, dyspnea, hypoventilation, respiratory depression
**SKIN:** Diaphoresis, exfoliative dermatitis, localized skin redness and swelling (with transdermal form), pruritus, rash
**Other:** Drug tolerance, physical or psychological dependence with long-term use, weight loss

## Nursing Considerations
• To reduce skin irritation, spray the allergy inhaler triamcinolone on the patient's skin, as prescribed, before applying a fentanyl patch.
• Expect the blood fentanyl level to be prolonged if patient chews or swallows the transmucosal form because drug is absorbed slowly from GI tract.
• Be aware that 100 mcg of fentanyl is equivalent in potency to 10 mg of morphine.
• To achieve optimum pain control with the lowest possible fentanyl dose, also plan to give a nonopioid analgesic, such as acetaminophen, as prescribed.
• **WARNING** Monitor patient's respiratory status closely, especially during the first 24 to 72 hours after therapy starts or dosage increases, because severe hypoventilation may occur without warning at any time during therapy.
• To prevent withdrawal symptoms after long-term use, expect to taper drug dosage gradually, as prescribed.

• Assess patient for withdrawal symptoms after dosage reduction or conversion to another opioid analgesic.

• For patient with bradycardia, implement cardiac monitoring, as ordered, and assess heart rate and rhythm frequently during fentanyl therapy because drug may further slow heart rate.

• **WARNING** Expect respiratory depressant effects to last longer than analgesic effects. Also be prepared for residual drug to potentiate the effects of subsequent doses. Residual drug can be detected for at least 6 hours after I.V. dose and 17 hours after dose of other forms. Monitor patient closely for at least 24 hours after therapy ends.

• **WARNING** Assess patient for signs of overdose, such as cardiopulmonary arrest, hypoventilation, pupil constriction, respiratory and CNS depression, seizures, and shock. Give naloxone (possibly in repeated doses), as prescribed. Be prepared to assist with endotracheal intubation and mechanical ventilation and to provide fluids.

• Monitor the blood glucose level of diabetic patients who are receiving transdermal fentanyl because each unit contains about 2 g of sugar.

**PATIENT TEACHING**

• Instruct patient to avoid alcohol and other CNS depressants during fentanyl therapy unless prescribed.

• Advise patient not to stop taking drug unless directed by prescriber because withdrawal symptoms may occur. Ease the patient's fears about drug dependence.

• For transdermal form, instruct patient to choose a site with intact (not irritated or irradiated) skin on a flat surface, such as the chest, back, flank, or upper arm, and, if appropriate, to clip, not shave, hair from the site and clean it with water (no soaps, lotions, oils, or alcohol). After site preparation, instruct patient to press patch firmly in place with palm for 30 seconds, making sure edges are sealed. If patch loosens, tell her to tape edges down but not cover the entire patch. If more than one patch is needed, the edges shouldn't touch or overlap. Instruct patient to remove patch after 72 hours, fold it in half with adhesive sides together, and flush it down the toilet. Remind her not to reuse a site for at least 3 days.

• Caution patient to avoid saunas, hot tubs, heating pads, and electric blankets while wearing transdermal patch because of the risk of increased transdermal absorption and adverse reactions. Also advise patient to notify prescriber if a high fever develops during transdermal therapy; increased drug absorption could lead to an overdose.

• Urge patient not to cut or use damaged patches because the drug may be released too rapidly, which could cause a life-threatening overdose.

• For transmucosal form, instruct patient to open the package just before use and to save plastic cap for disposal of the unused portion of the lozenge. Tell her to place lozenge between her cheek and gum and to suck, not chew, it for 15 minutes. Show her how to move lozenge from one side of her mouth to the other, using the handle provided separately.

• For transmucosal form, urge patient to see a dentist regularly, to brush teeth and floss after each meal, and to avoid frequent consumption of products high in sugar because of an increased risk of dental caries.

• For transmucosal form, inform diabetic patient that each unit contains 2 g of sugar. Instruct her to monitor her blood glucose levels closely.

• Remind patient to keep used and unused dosage units out of reach of children and to dispose of drug properly.

• Caution patient that accidentally exposing others to transdermal fentanyl could cause serious adverse reactions. If accidental exposure occurs, the person should remove the patch, wash the area well with water, and seek medical attention.

• Caution patient to avoid potentially hazardous activities until drug's CNS effects are known.

• Tell patient to increase fiber and fluid intake, unless contraindicated, because drug may cause severe constipation. If it persists or becomes severe, urge patient to notify prescriber.

# ferrous fumarate

*(contains 100 mg of elemental iron per capsule or per 5 ml of oral suspension, 33 mg of elemental iron per chewable tablet or per*

5 ml of oral suspension, 106 mg of elemental iron per E.R. capsule, 15 mg of elemental iron per 0.6 ml of oral solution, and 20 to 115 mg of elemental iron per tablet)

Femiron, Feostat, Feostat Drops, Ferretts, Fumasorb, Fumerin, Hemocyte, Ircon, Neo-Fer (CAN), Nephro-Fer, Novofumar (CAN), Palafer (CAN), Span-FF

## ferrous gluconate

(contains 10 mg of elemental iron per capsule, 34 mg of elemental iron per 5 ml of elixir, 37 mg of elemental iron per E.R. tablet, 35 mg of elemental iron per 5 ml of syrup, and 34 to 38 mg of elemental iron per tablet)

Apo-Ferrous Gluconate (CAN), Fergon, Ferralet, Ferralet Slow Release, Fertinic (CAN), Novoferrogluc (CAN), Simron

## ferrous sulfate

(contains 50 mg of elemental iron per capsule, 60 mg of elemental iron per dried capsule, 30 to 50 mg of elemental iron per dried E.R. capsule, 50 mg of elemental iron per dried E.R. tablet, 65 mg of elemental iron per dried tablet, 44 mg of elemental iron per 5 ml of elixir, 60 to 65 mg of elemental iron per enteric-coated tablet, 65 to 105 mg of elemental iron per E.R. tablet, 15 mg of elemental iron per 0.6 ml of oral solution, 18 mg of elemental iron per 0.5 ml of oral solution, 25 mg of elemental iron per ml of oral solution, 30 or 60 mg of elemental iron per 5 ml of oral solution, and 39 to 65 mg of elemental iron per tablet)

Apo-Ferrous Sulfate (CAN), Feosol, Feratab, Fer-gen-sol, Fer-In-Sol Capsules, Fer-In-Sol Drops, Fer-In-Sol Syrup, Fer-Iron Drops, Fero-Grad (CAN), Fero-Gradumet, Ferospace, Ferralyn Lanacaps, Ferra-TD, Mol-Iron, Novoferrosulfa (CAN), PMS-Ferrous Sulfate (CAN), Slow-Fe

## iron, carbonyl

(contains 50 mg of elemental iron per caplet)

Feosol

## Class and Category

*Chemical:* Trace element, mineral
*Therapeutic:* Antianemic, nutritional supplement
*Pregnancy category:* Not rated

## Indications and Dosages

➤ *To prevent iron deficiency based on U.S. and Canadian recommended daily allowances*

CAPLETS, CAPSULES, CHEWABLE TABLETS, DRIED CAPSULES, DRIED E.R. CAPSULES, DRIED E.R.. TABLETS, DRIED TABLETS, ELIXIR, ENTERIC-COATED TABLETS, E.R. CAPSULES, E.R. TABLETS, ORAL SOLUTION, ORAL SUSPENSION, SYRUP, TABLETS

**Male adults and children age 11 and older.** 10 mg (8 to 10 mg Canadian) of elemental iron daily.
**Female adults and children age 11 and older.** 10 to 15 mg (8 to 13 mg Canadian) of elemental iron daily.
**Pregnant females.** 30 mg (17 to 22 mg Canadian) of elemental iron daily.
**Breast-feeding females.** 15 mg (8 to 13 mg Canadian) of elemental iron daily.
**Children ages 7 to 10.** 10 mg (8 to 10 mg Canadian) of elemental iron daily.
**Children ages 4 to 6.** 10 mg (8 mg Canadian) of elemental iron daily.
**Children from birth to age 3.** 6 to 10 mg (0.3 to 6 mg Canadian) of elemental iron daily.

➤ *To replace iron in deficiency states*

CAPLETS, CAPSULES, CHEWABLE TABLETS, DRIED CAPSULES, DRIED E.R. CAPSULES, DRIED E.R. TABLETS, DRIED TABLETS, ELIXIR, ENTERIC-COATED TABLETS, E.R. CAPSULES, E.R. TABLETS, ORAL SOLUTION, ORAL SUSPENSION, SYRUP, TABLETS

**Adults and adolescents.** 100 to 200 mg of elemental iron t.i.d. for 4 to 6 mo.
**Children ages 2 to 12 who weigh 30 to 50 kg (66 to 110 lb).** 50 to 100 mg/day of elemental iron in divided doses t.i.d. or q.i.d. for 4 to 6 mo.
**Children ages 6 months to 2 years.** Up to 6 mg/kg/day of elemental iron in divided doses t.i.d. or q.i.d. for 4 to 6 mo.
**Infants under age 6 months.** 10 to 25 mg/day of elemental iron in divided doses t.i.d. or q.i.d. for 4 to 6 mo.

➤ *To provide iron supplementation during pregnancy*

CAPLETS, CAPSULES, CHEWABLE TABLETS, DRIED CAPSULES, DRIED E.R. CAPSULES, DRIED E.R. TABLETS, DRIED TABLETS, ELIXIR, ENTERIC-COATED TABLETS, E.R. CAPSULES, E.R. TABLETS, ORAL SOLUTION, ORAL SUSPENSION, SYRUP, TABLETS

**Pregnant females.** 15 to 30 mg of elemental iron q.d. during second and third trimesters.
DOSAGE ADJUSTMENT Dosage increased if needed for elderly patients, who may not absorb iron as easily as younger adults do.

## Mechanism of Action

Acts to normalize RBC production by binding with hemoglobin or by being oxidized and stored as hemosiderin or aggregated ferritin in reticuloendothelial cells of the liver, spleen, and bone marrow. Iron is an essential component of hemoglobin, myoglobin, and several enzymes, including cytochromes, catalase, and peroxidase. Iron is needed for catecholamine metabolism and normal neutrophil function.

## Contraindications

Hemochromatosis, hemolytic anemias, hemosiderosis, hypersensitivity to iron salts or their components, other anemic conditions unless accompanied by iron deficiency

## Interactions

### DRUGS

*acetohydroxamic acid:* Reduced absorption of both drugs
*antacids, calcium supplements:* Decreased iron absorption and effectiveness
*ascorbic acid (with doses of 200 mg or more):* Increased iron absorption
*cholestyramine, cimetidine:* Decreased iron absorption
*ciprofloxacin, enoxacin, etidronate, lomefloxacin, norfloxacin, ofloxacin, oral tetracyclines:* Decreased effectiveness of these drugs
*dimercaprol:* Possibly combination with iron in body to form a harmful chemical
*levodopa:* Possibly chelation with iron, decreasing levodopa absorption and blood level
*levothyroxine:* Decreased levothyroxine effectiveness and, possibly, hypothyroidism
*methyldopa:* Decreased methyldopa absorption and efficacy
*penicillamine:* Decreased penicillamine absorption because penicillamine chelates heavy metals
*vitamin E:* Decreased vitamin E absorption

### FOODS

*coffee; eggs; foods that contain bicarbonates, carbonates, oxalates, or phosphates; milk and milk products; tea that contains tannic acid; whole-grain breads and cereals and other high-fiber foods:* Decreased iron absorption and effectiveness

### ACTIVITIES

*alcohol abuse (acute or chronic):* Increased serum iron level

## Adverse Reactions

**CNS:** Dizziness, fever, headache, paresthesia, syncope
**CV:** Chest pain, tachycardia
**EENT:** Metallic taste, tooth discoloration
**GI:** Abdominal cramps, constipation, epigastric pain, nausea, stool discoloration, vomiting
**HEME:** Hemochromatosis, hemolysis, hemosiderosis
**RESP:** Dyspnea
**SKIN:** Diaphoresis, flushing, rash, urticaria

## Nursing Considerations

• Give iron tablets and capsules with a full glass of water or juice. Don't crush enteric-coated tablets or open capsules.
• Because iron solutions may stain teeth, dilute and administer with a straw or place drops in back of patient's throat. Mix the elixir form in water. Fer-In-Sol Drops or Syrup may be mixed with water or juice.
• To maximize absorption, give iron salts 1 hour before or 2 hours after meals. If GI irritation occurs, give with or just after meals.
• Protect liquid form from freezing.
• Be aware that at usual dosages, serum hemoglobin level usually normalizes in about 2 months unless blood loss continues. Treatment lasts for 3 to 6 months to help replenish iron stores.
• **WARNING** Monitor patient for signs of iron overdose, which may include abdominal pain, diarrhea (possibly bloody), nausea, severe vomiting, and sharp abdominal cramps. In case of iron toxicity or accidental iron overdose (a leading cause of fatal poisoning in children under age 6), give deferoxamine, as prescribed. As few as 3 adult iron tablets can cause serious poisoning in young children.
• Don't give antacids, coffee, tea, dairy products, eggs, or whole-grain cereals or breads within 1 hour before or 2 hours after giving iron salts.
• Remember that unabsorbed iron turns stool green or black and can mask blood in stool. Check stool for occult blood, as ordered.

### PATIENT TEACHING

• Instruct patient not to chew any solid dosage form of iron except for chewable tablets.
• Inform patient that symptoms of iron deficiency may include decreased stamina, learning problems, shortness of breath, and tiredness.

• To improve iron absorption, encourage patient to eat lean red meat, chicken, turkey, and fish as well as foods rich in vitamin C (such as citrus fruits and fresh vegetables).
• Urge patient to avoid foods that impair iron absorption, including dairy products, eggs, spinach, and high-fiber foods, such as whole-grain breads and cereals and bran. Also advise her to avoid drinking coffee or tea within 1 hour of iron intake.
• Caution patient not to take antacids or calcium supplements within 1 hour before and 2 hours after taking iron supplement.
• Inform patient that her stool should become dark green or black during therapy. Advise her to notify prescriber if it doesn't.
• To minimize tooth stains from liquid iron, instruct patient to mix each dose with water, fruit juice, or tomato juice and to drink it with a straw. When patient must take liquid iron by dropper, direct her to place drops well back on the tongue and to follow with water or juice. Inform patient that iron stains can be removed by brushing with baking soda (sodium bicarbonate) or medicinal peroxide (hydrogen peroxide 3%).
• Advise patient to consult prescriber before taking large amounts of iron for longer than 6 months.
• Warn patient about the high risk of accidental poisoning, and urge her to keep iron preparations out of the reach of children.

# filgrastim

### (granulocyte colony-stimulating factor, rG-CSF)
Neupogen

## Class and Category
*Chemical:* Granulocyte colony-stimulating factor
*Therapeutic:* Antineutropenic, hematopoietic stimulator
*Pregnancy category:* C

## Indications and Dosages
➤ *To prevent infection after myelosuppressive chemotherapy*
**I.V. INFUSION**
**Adults.** 5 mcg/kg q.d. over 15 to 30 min. Increased, if needed, by 5 mcg/kg with each chemotherapy cycle.

**S.C. INJECTION**
**Adults.** 5 mcg/kg q.d. for up to 2 wk. Increased, if needed, by 5 mcg/kg with each chemotherapy cycle.
➤ *To reduce the duration of neutropenia after bone marrow transplantation*
**I.V. INFUSION**
**Adults.** 10 mcg/kg q.d. over 4 hr or as a continuous infusion over 24 hr.
**S.C. INFUSION**
**Adults.** 10 mcg/kg as a continuous infusion over 24 hr.
➤ *To enhance peripheral blood progenitor cell collection in autologous hematopoietic stem cell transplantation*
**S.C. INFUSION OR INJECTION**
**Adults.** 10 mcg/kg as continuous infusion over 24 hr or a single injection, beginning 4 days before first leukapheresis and continuing until last day of leukapheresis.
➤ *To reduce the occurrence and duration of neutropenia in congenital neutropenia*
**S.C. INJECTION**
**Adults.** 6 mcg/kg b.i.d.
➤ *To reduce the occurrence and duration of neutropenia in idiopathic or cyclic neutropenia*
**S.C. INJECTION**
**Adults.** 5 mcg/kg q.d.
**DOSAGE ADJUSTMENT** Dosage reduced for patients whose absolute neutrophil count remains above 10,000/mm³.

| Route | Onset | Peak | Duration |
|---|---|---|---|
| I.V. | In 5 min | Unknown | Unknown |

## Incompatibilities
Don't mix filgrastim in vial or syringe with NS because precipitate will form.

## Mechanism of Action
Is pharmacologically identical to human granulocyte colony-stimulating factor, an endogenous hormone synthesized by monocytes, endothelial cells, and fibroblasts. Filgrastim induces the formation of neutrophil progenitor cells by binding directly to receptors on the surface of granulocytes, which then divide and differentiate. It also potentiates the effects of mature neutrophils, which reduces fever and the risk of infection raised by severe neutropenia.

## Contraindications

Hypersensitivity to filgrastim, its components, or proteins derived from *Escherichia coli*

## Interactions

**DRUGS**

*lithium:* Increased neutrophil production

## Adverse Reactions

**CNS:** Fever, headache
**CV:** Transient supraventricular tachycardia
**GI:** Splenic rupture, splenomegaly
**HEME:** Leukocytosis
**MS:** Arthralgia; myalgia; pain in arms, legs, lower back, or pelvis
**SKIN:** Pruritus, rash
**Other:** Anaphylaxis, injection site pain and redness

## Nursing Considerations

• Warm filgrastim to room temperature before injection. Discard drug if stored longer than 6 hours at room temperature or 24 hours in refrigerator.
• Withdraw only one dose from a vial; don't repuncture the vial.
• Don't shake the solution.
• For continuous infusion, dilute in $D_5W$ (not NS) to produce less than 15 mcg/ml.
• For S.C. dose larger than 1 ml, give by divided doses in more than one injection site.
• After chemotherapy, give filgrastim over 15 to 30 minutes. Don't give within 24 hours before or after cytotoxic chemotherapy.
• Monitor CBC, hematocrit, and platelet count two or three times weekly, as appropriate.
• Inform prescriber and expect to stop drug if leukocytosis develops or absolute neutrophil count consistently exceeds $10,000/mm^3$.
• Anticipate decreased response to drug if patient has received extensive radiation therapy or long-term chemotherapy.

**PATIENT TEACHING**

• Teach patient how to prepare, administer, and store filgrastim. Caution her not to reuse needle, syringe, or vial.
• Provide patient with puncture-resistant container for needle and syringe disposal.
• Advise patient to promptly report left-upper-quadrant abdominal pain or shoulder-tip pain.
• Stress the importance of returning for follow-up laboratory tests.

# finasteride

Propecia, Proscar

## Class and Category

*Chemical:* 4-Azasteroid compound
*Therapeutic:* Benign prostatic hyperplasia agent, hair growth stimulant
*Pregnancy category:* X

## Indications and Dosages

➤ *To treat symptomatic benign prostatic hyperplasia; to reduce the risk of symptomatic progression of benign prostatic hyperplasia when given with doxazocin*

**TABLETS**

**Adults.** 5 mg q.d.

➤ *To treat male-pattern baldness*

**TABLETS**

**Adults.** 1 mg q.d.

| Route | Onset | Peak | Duration |
|---|---|---|---|
| P.O.* | Unknown | 8 hr | 24 hr† |
| P.O.‡ | In 3 mo | Unknown | Unknown |

---

### Mechanism of Action

Inhibits 5-alpha reductase, an intracellular enzyme that converts testosterone to its metabolite (5-alpha dihydrotestosterone) in the liver, prostate, and skin. This metabolite is a potent androgen that's partially responsible for benign prostatic hyperplasia and hair loss.

---

## Contraindications

Age (childhood), hypersensitivity to finasteride, sex (female)

## Interactions

**DRUGS**

*theophylline:* Decreased blood theophylline level

## Adverse Reactions

**CNS:** Asthenia, dizziness, headache
**CV:** Hypotension, peripheral edema
**EENT:** Lip swelling, rhinitis

---

\* For benign prostatic hyperplasia.
† With single-dose therapy; 2 wk with multiple-dose therapy.
‡ For male-pattern baldness.

**ENDO:** Gynecomastia
**GI:** Abdominal pain, diarrhea
**GU:** Decreased ejaculatory volume, decreased libido, impotence, testicular pain
**MS:** Back pain
**RESP:** Dyspnea
**SKIN:** Pruritus, rash, urticaria
**Other:** Angioedema

## Nursing Considerations
• Expect patient to have a digital rectal examination of the prostate before and periodically during finasteride therapy.

**PATIENT TEACHING**
• **WARNING** Urge patient and female partners to use reliable contraception during therapy because semen of men who take drug can harm male fetuses. Caution women and children not to handle broken tablets.
• Explain how to take drug, and urge patient to follow instructions that accompany drug.
• Inform patient that drug may cause decreased ejaculatory volume, decreased libido, and impotence.
• Urge patient to have periodic follow-up appointments to determine drug effectiveness.

# flavoxate hydrochloride

Urispas

## Class and Category
*Chemical:* Flavone derivative
*Therapeutic:* Urinary tract antispasmodic
*Pregnancy category:* B

## Indications and Dosages
➤ *To relieve dysuria, nocturia, suprapubic pain, urinary frequency and urgency, and urinary incontinence caused by cystitis, prostatitis, urethrocystitis, or urethrotrigonitis*

**TABLETS**
**Adults and adolescents.** 100 to 200 mg t.i.d. or q.i.d.

| Route | Onset | Peak | Duration |
|---|---|---|---|
| P.O. | 55 min | 112 min | Unknown |

### Mechanism of Action
Relaxes muscles by cholinergic blockade and counteracts smooth-muscle spasms in the urinary tract.

## Contraindications
Achalasia; GI hemorrhage; hypersensitivity to flavoxate or its components; obstruction of the duodenum, ileum, or pylorus; obstructive uropathies of the lower urinary tract

## Interactions
**DRUGS**
*bethanechol, metoclopramide*: Possibly antagonized GI motility effects of these drugs

## Adverse Reactions
**CNS:** Confusion, decreased concentration, dizziness, drowsiness, fever, headache, nervousness, vertigo
**CV:** Palpitations, tachycardia
**EENT:** Accommodation disturbances, blurred vision, dry mouth, eye pain, photophobia, worsening of glaucoma
**GI:** Constipation, nausea, vomiting
**GU:** Dysuria
**HEME:** Eosinophilia, leukopenia
**SKIN:** Decreased sweating, dermatoses, urticaria

## Nursing Considerations
• Monitor for eye pain if patient has glaucoma because flavoxate's anticholinergic effects may worsen glaucoma.

**PATIENT TEACHING**
• Caution patient about possible dry mouth and photophobia. Advise her to wear sunglasses outdoors, and suggest sugarless candy or gum, ice chips, sips of water, or saliva substitute for dry mouth.
• Advise patient to avoid hazardous activities until drug's CNS effects are known.
• Caution patient not to become overheated or to take hot baths or saunas because drug reduces sweating, which can lead to dizziness, fainting, or heatstroke.
• Instruct patient to notify prescriber immediately if she experiences confusion, drowsiness, dysuria, headache, high fever, hives, nausea, nervousness, palpitations, rash, tachycardia, vertigo, vision problems, vomiting, or worsening dry mouth.

# flecainide acetate

Tambocor

## Class and Category
*Chemical:* Benzamide derivative

*Therapeutic:* Class IC antiarrhythmic
*Pregnancy category:* C

## Indications and Dosages

➤ *To prevent and suppress recurrent life-threatening ventricular tachycardia*

**TABLETS**

**Adults.** *Initial:* 100 mg q 12 hr (q 8 hr for some patients). Increased by 50 mg b.i.d. q 4 days, if needed, until response occurs. *Maintenance:* Up to 150 mg q 12 hr. *Maximum:* 400 mg/day.

**DOSAGE ADJUSTMENT** Initial dose reduced to 100 mg/day or 50 mg q 12 hr for patients with creatinine clearance of less than 35 ml/min/1.73 m². 

➤ *To prevent paroxysmal atrial fibrillation or flutter or paroxysmal supraventricular tachycardia*

**TABLETS**

**Adults.** *Initial:* 50 mg q 12 hr (q 8 hr for some patients). Increased by 50 mg b.i.d. q 4 days, if needed, until response occurs. *Maintenance:* Up to 150 mg q 12 hr. *Maximum:* 300 mg/day.

### Mechanism of Action

Achieves antiarrhythmic effect by inhibiting fast sodium channels of myocardial cell membranes, which increase myocardial recovery after repolarization, and by depressing the upstroke of the action potential. Flecainide also produces its antiarrhythmic effect by:
• slowing intracardiac conduction, which slightly increases the duration of the action potential in atrial and ventricular muscle, thus prolonging the PR interval, QRS complex, and QT interval
• shortening the action potential of Purkinje fibers without affecting surrounding myocardial tissue
• inhibiting extracellular calcium influx (at high doses)
• stopping paroxysmal reentrant supraventricular tachycardias by acting on antegrade pathways of dysfunctional AV conduction
• decreasing conduction in accessory pathways in patients with Wolff-Parkinson-White syndrome.

## Contraindications

Cardiogenic shock, hypersensitivity to flecainide or its components, recent MI, right bundle-branch block associated with left hemiblock or second- or third-degree AV block unless pacemaker is present

## Interactions

**DRUGS**

*amiodarone:* Increased blood flecainide level
*beta blockers, disopyramide, verapamil:* Possibly myocardial depression and increased blood levels of both drugs
*calcium channel blockers:* Increased risk of arrhythmias
*digoxin:* Possibly increased blood digoxin level
*urinary acidifiers:* Possibly increased flecainide elimination and decreased therapeutic effects
*urinary alkalinizers:* Possibly decreased flecainide elimination and increased therapeutic effects

**FOODS**

*acidic juices, foods that decrease urine pH below 5.0:* Increased flecainide elimination and decreased therapeutic effects
*foods that increase urine pH above 7.0, strict vegetarian diet:* Decreased flecainide elimination and increased therapeutic effects

**ACTIVITIES**

*smoking:* Increased flecainide clearance

## Adverse Reactions

**CNS:** Anxiety, depression, dizziness, drowsiness, fatigue, headache, light-headedness, tremor, weakness
**CV:** Arrhythmias, chest pain, heart failure, hypotension
**EENT:** Blurred vision
**GI:** Abdominal pain, anorexia, constipation, hepatic dysfunction, nausea, vomiting
**RESP:** Dyspnea
**SKIN:** Rash

## Nursing Considerations

• Monitor urine pH at the start of flecainide therapy.
• Check blood pressure, fluid intake and output, and weight regularly during therapy.
• Monitor blood trough level of flecainide, as appropriate; therapeutic level is 0.2 to 1 mcg/ml.
• Expect drug to cause mild to moderate negative inotropic effects, minimal cardiovascular effects, and no effect on blood pressure, heart rate, and left ventricular function.

•**WARNING** Because hypokalemia or hyperkalemia may interfere with flecainide's therapeutic effects, monitor serum potassium level before and during therapy and notify prescriber immediately if potassium imbalance develops. Also monitor for and notify prescriber about prolonged PR interval, QRS complex, or QT interval; chest pain; hypotension; and signs of heart failure. Keep in mind that drug can cause fatal proarrhythmias, which is why it isn't considered a first-line antiarrhythmic.
•Expect prolonged flecainide therapy to raise blood alkaline phosphatase level.

**PATIENT TEACHING**
•Instruct patient to take flecainide at regular intervals to maintain a constant blood level.
•Advise patient to take a missed dose as soon as she remembers if it's within 6 hours of the scheduled time.
•Teach patient how to take her pulse, and instruct her to record it daily, along with her weight. Advise her to bring record to follow-up visits.
•Encourage family members to obtain instruction in basic cardiac life support.
•Advise patient to notify prescriber immediately about chest pain, difficulty breathing, and dizziness.
•Caution patient not to stop taking drug suddenly but to taper dosage gradually according to prescriber's instructions.

# fluconazole

Diflucan

## Class and Category
*Chemical:* Triazole derivative
*Therapeutic:* Antifungal
*Pregnancy category:* C

## Indications and Dosages
➤ *To treat oral and esophageal candidiasis*
ORAL SUSPENSION, TABLETS, I.V. INJECTION
**Adults and adolescents.** 200 mg on day 1 followed by 100 mg q.d. for at least 2 (oral) or 3 (esophageal) wk after symptoms resolve.
**Children.** 3 mg/kg q.d. for at least 2 (oral) or 3 (esophageal) wk and then for 2 wk after esophageal symptoms resolve.

➤ *To treat systemic candidiasis*
ORAL SUSPENSION, TABLETS, I.V. INJECTION
**Adults and adolescents.** 400 mg on day 1, followed by 200 mg q.d. for at least 4 wk and then for 2 wk after symptoms resolve.

➤ *To treat cryptococcal meningitis*
ORAL SUSPENSION, TABLETS, I.V. INJECTION
**Adults and adolescents.** 400 mg q.d. until patient responds to treatment, then 200 to 400 mg q.d. for 10 to 12 wk after CSF culture is negative. *Maintenance:* 200 mg q.d. to suppress relapse.
**Children.** 6 to 12 mg/kg/day for 10 to 12 wk after CSF culture is negative.

➤ *To prevent candidiasis after bone marrow transplantation*
ORAL SUSPENSION, TABLETS, I.V. INJECTION
**Adults and adolescents.** 400 mg q.d. starting several days before procedure if severe neutropenia is expected and continued for 7 days after absolute neutrophil count exceeds 1,000/mm$^3$.

➤ *To treat vaginal candidiasis*
CAPSULES, ORAL SUSPENSION, TABLETS
**Adults.** 150 mg as a single dose.
DOSAGE ADJUSTMENT Dosage reduced for patients with hepatic or renal impairment. Dosage reduced by 50% for patients with creatinine clearance of 11 to 50 ml/min/ 1.73 m$^2$.

### Mechanism of Action
Damages fungal cells by interfering with a cytochrome P-450 enzyme needed to convert lanosterol to ergosterol, an essential part of the fungal cell membrane. Decreased ergosterol synthesis causes increased cell permeability, which allows cell contents to leak. Fluconazole also may inhibit endogenous respiration, interact with membrane phospholipids, inhibit transformation of yeasts to mycelial forms, inhibit purine uptake, and impair biosynthesis of triglycerides and phospholipids.

## Incompatibilities
Don't add fluconazole to I.V. bag that contains any other drug.

## Contraindications
Hypersensitivity to fluconazole or its components

## Interactions
**DRUGS**
*astemizole, terfenadine:* Increased blood levels of these drugs
*benzodiazepines (short-acting):* Possibly increased blood benzodiazepine level and psychomotor effects
*cimetidine:* Decreased blood fluconazole level
*cisapride:* Possibly increased QT interval, leading to torsades de pointes
*cyclosporine:* Increased blood cyclosporine level
*glipizide, glyburide, tolbutamide:* Increased risk of hypoglycemia
*hydrochlorothiazide:* Increased blood fluconazole level from decreased excretion
*isoniazid, rifampin:* Decreased fluconazole effects
*nonsedating antihistamines:* Increased blood antihistamine level, increased risk of cardiotoxicity
*oral anticoagulants:* Increased anticoagulant effects
*phenytoin:* Increased blood phenytoin level
*rifabutin:* Increased blood rifabutin level
*theophylline:* Increased blood theophylline level
*zidovudine:* Increased blood zidovudine level

## Adverse Reactions
**CNS:** Chills, dizziness, drowsiness, fever, headache, seizures
**CV:** Prolonged QT interval, torsades de pointes
**GI:** Abdominal pain, anorexia, constipation, diarrhea, hepatic failure, nausea, vomiting
**HEME:** Agranulocytosis, leukopenia, thrombocytopenia
**SKIN:** Exfoliative dermatitis, photosensitivity, pruritus, rash
**Other:** Anaphylaxis, angioedema

## Nursing Considerations
•Use fluconazole cautiously in patients with potentially proarrhythmic conditions because drug may prolong the QT interval, which can lead to life-threatening torsades de pointes.
•Expect to obtain BUN and serum creatinine levels and culture and sensitivity and liver function test results before therapy starts.
•Refrigerate, but don't freeze, fluconazole oral suspension. Shake well before administering.
•Discard I.V. solution that's cloudy or contains precipitate. Don't infuse more than 200 mg/hr or add supplemental drugs to infusion.

•Monitor hepatic and renal function periodically during therapy, and notify prescriber if you detect signs of dysfunction.
•Assess for rash every 8 hours during therapy, and notify prescriber if rash occurs.
•If patient receives an oral anticoagulant, monitor coagulation test results and assess patient for bleeding.
•Monitor patient for symptoms of overdose, such as hallucinations and paranoia. If they occur, provide supportive treatment, gastric lavage, and, possibly, hemodialysis, which can reduce blood fluconazole level by half after about 3 hours.
**PATIENT TEACHING**
•Instruct patient to take fluconazole tablets or oral suspension 30 minutes before or 2 hours after meals. Inform her that tablets may be crushed for easier swallowing if needed.
•Advise patient to complete entire course of therapy, even if she feels better.
•If patient takes an oral antidiabetic drug, caution her to monitor blood glucose level frequently because of increased risk of hypoglycemia.
•Alert patient that fluconazole may change the taste of food.
•Advise patient to notify prescriber immediately about diarrhea, headache, nausea, rash, right-upper-quadrant abdominal pain, yellow skin or whites of eyes, or vomiting.
•Suggest that breast-feeding patient consult prescriber because breast-feeding may need to be stopped during therapy.

# fludrocortisone acetate
Florinef

## Class and Category
*Chemical:* Glucocorticoid
*Therapeutic:* Mineralocorticoid replacement
*Pregnancy category:* C

## Indications and Dosages
➤ *To treat primary and secondary chronic adrenocortical insufficiency*
**TABLETS**
**Adults and adolescents.** *Usual:* 100 mcg q.d. Dosage may range from 100 mcg 3 times/wk to 200 mcg q.d.
**Children.** 50 to 100 mcg q.d.

➤ *To treat salt-losing adrenogenital syndrome*

**TABLETS**

**Adults.** 100 to 200 mcg q.d.

**Children.** 50 to 100 mcg q.d.

DOSAGE ADJUSTMENT Dosage reduced to 50 mcg q.d. if transient hypertension develops during therapy.

| Route | Onset | Peak | Duration |
|-------|-------|------|----------|
| P.O. | Unknown | Unknown | 1 to 2 days |

## Mechanism of Action

Enhances sodium reabsorption, hydrogen and potassium excretion, and water retention by the distal renal tubules, much like aldosterone, an endogenous mineralocorticoid. In large doses, fludrocortisone can inhibit endogenous adrenocortical secretion, thymic activity, and pituitary corticotropin excretion. It also can promote glycogen deposits in the liver and induce a negative nitrogen balance when protein intake is deficient.

## Contraindications

Hypersensitivity to fludrocortisone, adrenocorticoids, or their components; systemic fungal infections

## Interactions

**DRUGS**

*digoxin:* Increased risk of digitalis toxicity and arrhythmias from hypokalemia

*phenytoin, rifampin:* Decreased fludrocortisone effects

*potassium-wasting drugs, such as loop diuretics and amphotericin B:* Increased risk of severe hypokalemia

## Adverse Reactions

**CNS:** Dizziness, headache, mental changes, seizures

**CV:** Arrhythmias, heart failure, hypertension, peripheral edema

**EENT:** Cataracts (with long-term use), increased intraocular pressure

**ENDO:** Adrenal insufficiency, growth suppression in children, hyperglycemia

**GI:** Anorexia, nausea, vomiting

**GU:** Menstrual irregularities

**HEME:** Easy bruising

**MS:** Arthralgia, muscle weakness, myalgia, osteoporosis (with long-term use), tendon contractures

**SKIN:** Acne, diaphoresis, rash, urticaria

**Other:** Hypokalemia, hypokalemic alkalosis, impaired wound healing, weight gain

## Nursing Considerations

•Monitor blood pressure, fluid status, and serum electrolyte levels periodically during fludrocortisone therapy. Assess patient for signs of heart failure, including adventitious breath sounds, peripheral edema, and weight gain.

•Monitor for signs and symptoms of overdose, such as cardiomegaly, edema, excessive weight gain, hypertension, and hypokalemia. These effects usually subside a few days after therapy stops. Potassium supplementation may be needed.

•Notify prescriber if patient experiences dizziness, headache, hypertension, hypokalemia, signs of infection, or weight gain.

**PATIENT TEACHING**

•Instruct patient to take a missed dose of fludrocortisone as soon as she remembers if it's within 12 hours of scheduled time. Warn against double-dosing. Advise her to notify prescriber if she misses more than one dose or if nausea or vomiting prevents her from taking drug.

•Instruct patient to reduce dietary sodium and to eat more potassium-rich foods during therapy.

•Direct patient to weigh herself each morning before breakfast in clothes of similar weight and to notify prescriber if she gains more than 2 lb (0.9 kg) per day or 5 lb (2.3 kg) per week. Instruct her to monitor how tightly her rings and shoes fit.

•Advise patient to notify prescriber about stressful events—such as dental extractions, emotional upset, illness, surgery, and trauma—because a dosage increase may be required.

•Instruct patient to notify prescriber about dizziness, fever, fluid retention, headache, joint pain, irregular heart rate, muscle weakness, or palpitations.

•Inform patient that drug may delay wound healing.

•Caution patient not to stop taking drug abruptly but to taper dosage gradually, as prescribed.

•Urge patient to carry medical identification that documents her corticosteroid use.

E
F

# flumazenil

Anexate (CAN), Romazicon

## Class and Category

*Chemical:* Imidazobenzodiazepine derivative
*Therapeutic:* Benzodiazepine antidote
*Pregnancy category:* C

## Indications and Dosages

➤ *To reverse sedation from benzodiazepine therapy*

**I.V. INJECTION**

**Adults.** 0.2 mg, repeated after 45 to 60 sec if response is inadequate and then repeated q 1 min, if needed. If sedation recurs, regimen is repeated q 20 min or more. *Maximum:* 1 mg over 5 min or 3 mg in 1-hr period.

➤ *To reverse benzodiazepine toxicity or suspected overdose*

**I.V. INJECTION**

**Adults.** 0.2 mg followed by 0.3 mg 30 to 60 sec later if response is inadequate and then 0.5 mg repeated q 1 min. If sedation recurs, regimen is repeated q 20 min. *Maximum:* 3 mg in 1-hr period.

| Route | Onset | Peak | Duration |
|---|---|---|---|
| I.V. | 1 to 2 min | 6 to 10 min | Variable |

### Mechanism of Action

Antagonizes the CNS effects of benzo-diazepines by competing for their binding sites.

## Contraindications

Evidence of tricyclic antidepressant overdose; hypersensitivity to flumazenil, benzodiazepines, or their components; use of benzodiazepine to control intracranial pressure, status epilepticus, or a potentially life-threatening condition

## Interactions

**DRUGS**

*benzodiazepines:* Benzodiazepine withdrawal symptoms, including seizures
*nonbenzodiazepine agonists:* Loss of effectiveness of these drugs
*tetracyclic or tricyclic antidepressant overdose:* High risk of seizures

**FOODS**

*all foods:* Increased flumazenil clearance (by half) with food ingestion during I.V. injection

## Adverse Reactions

**CNS:** Agitation, anxiety, ataxia, confusion, dizziness, drowsiness, emotional lability, fatigue, headache, hypoesthesia, insomnia, paresthesia, resedation, seizures, tremor, vertigo
**CV:** Hot flashes, hypertension, palpitations
**EENT:** Blurred vision, diplopia, dry mouth
**GI:** Nausea, vomiting
**RESP:** Dyspnea, hyperventilation, hypoventilation
**SKIN:** Diaphoresis, flushing, rash
**Other:** Injection site pain and thrombophlebitis

## Nursing Considerations

• Use flumazenil cautiously in patients with cardiac disease. Assess for increased stress or anxiety from benzodiazepine withdrawal because cardiac patient's blood pressure may rise.
• Give flumazenil undiluted or diluted in a syringe with D₅W, NS, or LR solution. Administer over 15 to 30 seconds directly into tubing of a free-flowing compatible I.V. solution. Use a large vein, if possible, to minimize pain at site. Avoid extravasation because drug may irritate tissue.
• Be aware that drug may cause signs of benzodiazepine withdrawal in drug-dependent patient. Also, abrupt awakening from benzodiazepine overdose can cause agitation, dysphoria, and increased adverse reactions.
• Be aware that benzodiazepine reversal may cause an anxiety or a panic attack for patient with a history of these episodes. Expect to adjust dosage carefully.
• Monitor for signs of resedation and hypoventilation for at least 2 hours after giving flumazenil because drug has a short half-life. Be aware that patient shouldn't be discharged until the risk of resedation has resolved.

**PATIENT TEACHING**

• Caution patient to avoid alcohol and OTC drugs for 10 to 24 hours after taking flumazenil.
• Advise patient to avoid hazardous activities for 18 to 24 hours after discharge.
• Inform patient and family that agitation, emotional lability, fear, and panic attack (if patient has a history of them) may occur. Tell them to seek medical care if patient develops depression, trouble breathing, flushing, hyperventilation, insomnia, palpitations, or tremor.

•Because drug doesn't always reverse post-procedure amnesia, provide written instructions or instructions to caregiver even if patient is alert.

# flunisolide

AeroBid, AeroBid-M, Bronalide (CAN), Nasalide, Nasarel, Rhinalar (CAN)

## Class and Category

*Chemical:* Corticosteroid
*Therapeutic:* Antiasthmatic, anti-inflammatory
*Pregnancy category:* C

## Indications and Dosages

➤ *To provide maintenance treatment of asthma, alone or with oral corticosteroids*

**INHALATION AEROSOL**

**Adults and adolescents age 15 and older.** 500 mcg (2 inhalations) b.i.d. morning and evening. *Maximum:* 2,000 mcg/day (4 inhalations b.i.d.). **Children ages 6 to 15.** 500 mcg (2 inhalations) b.i.d. *Maximum:* 1,000 mcg/day.

➤ *To relieve symptoms of seasonal or perennial rhinitis*

**NASAL SOLUTION**

**Adults.** 50 mcg (2 sprays) b.i.d. in each nostril. *Maximum:* 400 mcg/day (16 sprays). **Children.** 25 mcg (1 spray) t.i.d. in each nostril. *Maximum:* 200 mcg/day (8 sprays).

| Route | Onset | Peak | Duration |
|---|---|---|---|
| Inhalation | In 4 wk | Unknown | Unknown |
| Nasal | 3 to 7 days | Unknown | 4 to 6 hr |

---

### Mechanism of Action

Inhibits cells involved in inflammatory response, such as mast cells, eosinophils, basophils, lymphocytes, macrophages, and neutrophils. Also inhibits production of chemical mediators, such as histamine, eicosanoids, leukotrienes, and cytokines.

---

## Contraindications

Hypersensitivity to flunisolide or its components, primary treatment of status asthmaticus or other asthma episodes that require emergency care, recent nasal surgery (nasal form), untreated localized infection of nasal mucosa (nasal form)

## Adverse Reactions

**CNS:** Anxiety, chills, depression, dizziness, headache, hyperactivity, insomnia, irritability, lethargy, mood changes, nervousness, tremor, vertigo
**CV:** Hypertension
**EENT:** Candidiasis (oral and throat), dry mouth and throat, earache, eye infection, hoarseness, loss of smell or taste, mouth irritation, pharyngitis, rhinitis, sinusitis, sneezing
**GI:** Abdominal pain, anorexia, constipation, diarrhea, flatulence, heartburn, increased appetite, indigestion, nausea, vomiting
**GU:** Menstrual irregularities
**HEME:** Eosinophilia
**RESP:** Bronchitis, dyspnea, pleurisy, pneumonia
**SKIN:** Acne, eczema, pruritus, rash, urticaria
**Other:** Growth suppression (children), lymphadenopathy

## Nursing Considerations

•Use flunisolide cautiously in patients with ocular herpes simplex, pulmonary tuberculosis, or untreated systemic bacterial, fungal, parasitic, or viral infection.
•If patient receives an oral corticosteroid, expect to taper it slowly 1 week after changing to flunisolide. For patient who receives prednisone, expect to reduce it by no more than 2.5 mg/day at weekly intervals, beginning at least 1 week after flunisolide therapy starts.
•WARNING Assess patient switched from systemic corticosteroid to flunisolide for adrenal insufficiency (fatigue, hypotension, lassitude, nausea, vomiting, weakness) during initial treatment and during stress, trauma, surgery, infection, or other electrolyte-depleting conditions. Notify prescriber immediately if signs or symptoms arise.
•Monitor growth in children; corticosteroids may increase risk of growth suppression.

**PATIENT TEACHING**

•Teach patient how to use inhaler. When starting a new canister, advise spraying once into the air (avoiding her eyes) to check for mist.
•Instruct patient to gargle or rinse after each use to help prevent mouth and throat dryness, relieve throat irritation, and prevent oropharyngeal infection.
•Urge patient to contact prescriber if symptoms haven't improved after 3 weeks.
•WARNING Caution patient not to use flunisolide to relieve acute bronchospasm.

E
F

•If patient switches from an oral corticosteroid to flunisolide, advise her to carry medical identification indicating the need for supplemental systemic corticosteroids during stress or severe asthma attack. Advise her to ask prescriber how to respond to these problems.
•Caution patient to avoid exposure to chickenpox and measles and to contact prescriber immediately if exposure occurs.

# fluoxetine hydrochloride

Prozac, Prozac Weekly, Sarafem

## Class and Category
*Chemical:* Phenylpropylamine derivative
*Therapeutic:* Antibulimic, antidepressant, antiobsessive-compulsive
*Pregnancy category:* C

## Indications and Dosages
➤ *To treat depression*
CAPSULES, ORAL SOLUTION, TABLETS (PROZAC)
**Adults.** *Initial:* 20 mg q.d. in the morning. Dosage increased q 4 to 8 wk as needed. Dosage greater than 20 mg/day given b.i.d. morning and noon. *Maximum:* 80 mg/day.
**Children and adolescents.** *Initial:* 10 mg q.d. Dosage increased after 1 wk to 20 mg q.d.
DOSAGE ADJUSTMENT For lower-weight children, dosage increased to 20 mg q.d. only if improvement insufficient after several wk.
DELAYED-RELEASE CAPSULES (PROZAC WEEKLY)
**Adults.** 90 mg/wk, beginning 7 days after last 20-mg q.d. dose.

➤ *To treat obsessive-compulsive disorder*
CAPSULES, ORAL SOLUTION, TABLETS (PROZAC)
**Adults.** *Initial:* 20 mg q.d. in the morning. Dosage increased q 4 to 8 wk as needed. Dosage greater than 20 mg/day given b.i.d. morning and noon. *Maximum:* 80 mg/day.
**Children and adolescents.** *Initial:* 10 mg q.d. Dosage increased after 2 wk to 20 mg q.d. Subsequent dosage increased, as needed, at intervals of at least several wk. *Maintenance:* 20 to 60 mg q.d.
DOSAGE ADJUSTMENT For lower-weight children, dosage should be increased above 10 mg q.d. only if clinical improvement remains insufficient after several wk. Maintenance dosage for such patients should not exceed 30 mg q.d.

➤ *To treat moderate to severe bulimia nervosa*
CAPSULES, ORAL SOLUTION, TABLETS (PROZAC)
**Adults.** 60 mg q.d. in the morning. Some patients may be prescribed a lower dose, which is titrated to 60 mg/day as tolerated.

➤ *To treat panic disorder with or without agoraphobia*
CAPSULES, ORAL SOLUTION, TABLETS (PROZAC)
**Adults.** *Initial:* 10 mg q.d. Dosage increased in 1 wk to 20 mg/day, as needed. *Maximum:* 60 mg/day.

➤ *To treat premenstrual dysmorphic disorder*
CAPSULES (SARAFEM)
**Adults.** 20 mg q.d. Dosage increased as needed. *Maximum:* 80 mg/day.
DOSAGE ADJUSTMENT Dose or frequency reduced for patients with hepatic impairment or concurrent illness, those who take multiple medications, and for elderly patients.

| Route | Onset | Peak | Duration |
|---|---|---|---|
| P.O.* | 1 to 6 wk† | Unknown | Unknown |

## Mechanism of Action
Selectively inhibits reuptake of the neurotransmitter serotonin by CNS neurons and increases the amount of serotonin that's available in nerve synapses. An elevated serotonin level may result in elevated mood and, consequently, reduced depression.

## Contraindications
Hypersensitivity to selective serotonin reuptake inhibitors or their components, use within 14 days of MAO inhibitor therapy

## Interactions
DRUGS
*alprazolam, diazepam:* Possibly prolonged half-life of these drugs
*aspirin, NSAIDs, warfarin:* Increased anticoagulant activity and risk of bleeding
*astemizole:* Increased risk of serious arrhythmias

---

* Capsules, oral solution, and tablets.
† For depression and bulimia; 5 wk for obsessive-compulsive disorder.

*buspirone:* Decreased buspirone effects
*clozapine, fluphenazine, haloperidol, maprotiline, trazodone:* Increased risk of adverse effects
*lithium:* Increased or decreased blood lithium level
*MAO inhibitors:* Possibly severe and life-threatening adverse effects
*phenytoin:* Increased blood phenytoin level and risk of toxicity
*pimozide:* Possibly bradycardia
*serotonergics (such as amphetamines and other psychostimulants, antidepressants, and dopamine agonists):* Serotonin syndrome
*tricyclic antidepressants:* Increased risk of adverse effects, including seizures
*tryptophan:* Increased risk of central and peripheral toxicity

## Adverse Reactions

**CNS:** Anxiety, chills, dream disturbances, drowsiness, fatigue, fever, headache, hypomania, insomnia, mania, nervousness, restlessness, seizures, somnolence, tremor, vertigo, weakness, yawning
**CV:** Hypotension, palpitations
**EENT:** Abnormal vision, dry mouth, pharyngitis, sinusitis
**ENDO:** Galactorrhea, gynecomastia, hypoglycemia
**GI:** Anorexia, diarrhea, indigestion, nausea
**GU:** Decreased libido, ejaculation disorders, impotence
**HEME:** Altered platelet function, unusual bleeding
**MS:** Arthralgia, myalgia
**RESP:** Dyspnea
**SKIN:** Diaphoresis, pruritus, rash, urticaria
**Other:** Flulike symptoms, hyponatremia, weight loss

## Nursing Considerations

•Use fluoxetine cautiously in patients with a history of seizures.
•**WARNING** Avoid giving fluoxetine within 14 days of an MAO inhibitor or starting MAO inhibitor therapy within 5 weeks of discontinuing fluoxetine.
•If patient is taking fluoxetine for depression, watch closely for suicidal tendencies, especially when therapy starts and dosage changes, because depression may worsen temporarily during those times.

•Monitor patient closely for evidence of GI bleeding, especially if patient takes another drug known to increase the risk, such as aspirin, an NSAID, or warfarin.
•Expect to taper drug, as ordered, when no longer needed to minimnize adverse reactions.
•**WARNING** If patient receives another drug that raises serotonin level (such as dopamine agonists, MAO inhibitors and other antidepressants, tryptophan, and amphetamines and other psychostimulants), watch for serotonin syndrome, a rare but serious adverse effect of selective serotonin reuptake inhibitors. Signs and symptoms include agitation, confusion, diaphoresis, diarrhea, fever, hyperactive reflexes, poor coordination, restlessness, shaking, talking or acting with uncontrolled excitement, tremor, and twitching.
•Monitor patients with diabetes mellitus for altered blood glucose levels because drug may cause hypoglycemia during therapy and hyperglycemia when therapy stops. Expect to adjust dosage of antidiabetic drug, as prescribed.
•Expect patient to be reevaluated periodically to determine continued need for therapy.
•When stopping therapy, expect to taper drug to minimize adverse reactions.
**PATIENT TEACHING**
•**WARNING** Inform patient that fluoxetine increases the risk of serotonin syndrome, a rare but serious complication. Teach patient to recognize its signs and symptoms, and advise her to notify prescriber immediately if they occur.
•Urge family or caregiver to watch patient closely for suicidal tendencies, especially when therapy starts or dosage changes, particularly if patient is a child or teenager.
•Caution patient to avoid hazardous activities until CNS effects of drug are known.
•Caution against stopping drug abruptly because serious adverse effects may result.
•Advise patient to consult prescriber before taking OTC or prescription drugs, if a rash or hives develop, or if she becomes or intends to become pregnant during therapy.
•Inform patient that drug may take several weeks to achieve full effects.

# fluphenazine decanoate
Modecate (CAN), Modecate Concentrate (CAN), Prolixin Decanoate

# fluphenazine enanthate
Moditen Enanthate (CAN), Prolixin Enanthate

# fluphenazine hydrochloride
Apo-Fluphenazine (CAN), Moditen HCl (CAN), Permitil, Permitil Concentrate, PMS Fluphenazine (CAN), Prolixin, Prolixin Concentrate

## Class and Category
*Chemical:* Phenothiazine, propylpiperazine derivative
*Therapeutic:* Antipsychotic
*Pregnancy category:* Not rated

## Indications and Dosages
➤ *To control psychotic disorders*
ELIXIR, ORAL SOLUTION, TABLETS (FLUPHENAZINE HYDROCHLORIDE)
**Adults and adolescents.** *Initial:* 2.5 to 10 mg/day in divided doses q 6 to 8 hr. When symptoms are controlled, dosage reduced to 1 to 5 mg q.d. *Maximum:* 20 mg/dose with caution.
**Children.** 250 to 750 mcg q.d. to q.i.d.
I.M. INJECTION (FLUPHENAZINE HYDROCHLORIDE)
**Adults and adolescents.** *Initial:* 1.25 mg, increased as clinical condition tolerates up to 2.5 to 10 mg/day in divided doses q 6 to 8 hr. *Maximum:* 10 mg/day.
DOSAGE ADJUSTMENT For elderly or debilitated patients, dosage reduced to 1 to 2.5 mg/day in divided doses q 6 to 8 hr.
I.M. OR S.C. INJECTION (FLUPHENAZINE DECANOATE OR ENANTHATE)
**Adults.** *Initial:* 12.5 to 25 mg q 1 to 4 wk, as needed (decanoate). For doses over 50 mg, next dose increased cautiously by 12.5 mg. Or 25 mg q 2 wk, with dose and dosing interval adjusted based on patient response (enanthate). *Maximum:* 100 mg/dose.
**Adolescents and children age 12.** *Initial:* 6.25 to 18.75 mg/wk (decanoate), increased to 12.5 to 25 mg q 1 to 3 wk, according to condition.
**Children ages 5 to 12.** 3.125 to 12.5 mg q 1 to 3 wk (decanoate), according to condition.

| Route | Onset | Peak | Duration |
|---|---|---|---|
| P.O. | In 1 hr | Variable | 6 to 8 hr |
| I.M.* | In 1 hr | Variable | 6 to 8 hr |
| I.M., S.C.† | In 24 to 72 hr | Variable | 1 to 6 wk‡ |

## Mechanism of Action
May block postsynaptic dopamine receptor sites in the CNS. This action may depress areas of the brain that control activity and aggression, including the cerebral cortex, hypothalamus, and limbic system.

## Incompatibilities
Don't mix fluphenazine hydrochloride oral solution with beverages that contain caffeine, such as coffee and cola; tannins, such as tea; or pectins, such as apple juice. They're physically incompatible.

## Contraindications
Blood dyscrasias, bone marrow depression, cerebral arteriosclerosis, coma, concomitant use of large amounts of another CNS depressant, coronary artery disease, hepatic dysfunction, hypersensitivity to phenothiazines, myeloproliferative disorders, severe CNS depression, severe hypertension or hypotension, subcortical brain damage

## Interactions
DRUGS
*adsorbent antidiarrheals, aluminum- or magnesium-containing antacids:* Possibly inhibited absorption of fluphenazine
*amantadine, anticholinergics:* Possibly intensified adverse effects of both drugs
*amphetamines:* Possibly decreased therapeutic effects of both drugs
*antihypertensives:* Possibly severe hypotension
*antithyroid drugs:* Increased risk of agranulocytosis
*beta blockers:* Possibly increased blood levels and risk of adverse effects of both drugs
*bromocriptine:* Decreased bromocriptine effects

---

* For hydrochloride.
† For decanoate and enanthate.
‡ For decanoate; 2 wk for enanthate.

*CNS depressants:* Possibly prolonged and intensified CNS depression
*erythromycin:* Possibly inhibited fluphenazine metabolism
*guanethidine:* Decreased hypotensive effect of guanethidine
*levodopa:* Possibly decreased antidyskinetic effect of levodopa
*lithium:* Possibly neurotoxicity (disorientation, extrapyramidal reactions, unconsciousness)
*meperidine:* Excessive sedation and hypotension
*metrizamide:* Increased risk of seizures when injected in subarachnoid area during fluphenazine therapy
*oral anticoagulants:* Possibly decreased anticoagulant effects
*pimozide, other drugs that prolong QT interval:* Prolonged QT interval and risk of arrhythmias
*thiazide diuretics:* Increased risk of hyponatremia, hypotension, and water intoxication
*tricyclic antidepressants:* Possibly prolonged and intensified sedation

ACTIVITIES

*alcohol use:* Possibly increased CNS depression and increased risk of heatstroke

## Adverse Reactions

**CNS:** Ataxia, cerebral edema, dizziness, drowsiness, headache, insomnia, light-headedness, nervousness, seizures, slurred speech, syncope, worsening psychotic symptoms
**CV:** AV conduction disorders, bradycardia, cardiac arrest, hypercholesterolemia, hypertension, orthostatic hypotension, QT prolongation, shock, ST-segment depression, tachycardia
**EENT:** Blurred vision, dry mouth, glaucoma, increased salivation, laryngeal edema, laryngospasm, miosis, mydriasis, nasal congestion, papillary hypertrophy of the tongue, parotid gland enlargement, photophobia, pigmentary retinopathy, ptosis
**ENDO:** Breast engorgement (females), galactorrhea, hyperglycemia, hypoglycemia, mastalgia, syndrome of inappropriate ADH secretion
**GI:** Anorexia, constipation, diarrhea, fecal impaction, ileus, increased appetite, nausea, vomiting
**GU:** Amenorrhea, bladder paralysis, decreased libido, enuresis, menstrual irregularities, polyuria, urinary frequency, urinary incontinence, urine retention
**HEME:** Anemia, aplastic anemia, eosinophilia, leukopenia, thrombocytopenia, thrombocytopenic or nonthrombocytopenic purpura
**RESP:** Bronchospasm, dyspnea, increased respiratory depth
**SKIN:** Contact dermatitis, dry skin, eczema, erythema, jaundice, photosensitivity, pruritus, seborrhea
**Other:** Heatstroke, hyponatremia, lupuslike symptoms, weight gain

## Nursing Considerations

• Use fluphenazine cautiously in patients with a history of glaucoma or renal impairment.
• For I.M. and S.C. injection, use at least a 21G needle.
• Monitor temperature; a significant, unexplained rise can indicate intolerance and a need to discontinue drug. Notify prescriber immediately if this occurs.
• Assess for signs of hepatic failure, such as jaundice.
• Notify prescriber about worsening psychotic symptoms: agitation, catatonic state, confusion, depression, hallucinations, lethargy, paranoid reactions.

PATIENT TEACHING

• If patient takes elixir form of fluphenazine, instruct her to keep it in an amber or opaque bottle because drug is sensitive to light.
• Advise patient not to mix oral solution with beverages that contain caffeine (coffee, cola), tannins (tea), or pectins (apple juice).
• Caution patient about possible dizziness or light-headedness.
• Teach patient how to prevent heatstroke, orthostatic hypotension, and photosensitivity reactions.
• Warn patient not to stop taking fluphenazine abruptly.

# flurazepam hydrochloride

Apo-Flurazepam (CAN), Dalmane, Novo-Flupam (CAN), Somnol (CAN)

## Class, Category, and Schedule

*Chemical:* Benzodiazepine
*Therapeutic:* Sedative-hypnotic

*Pregnancy category:* Not rated
*Controlled substance:* Schedule IV

## Indications and Dosages

➤ *To treat insomnia characterized by difficulty falling asleep, frequent nocturnal awakening, or early-morning awakening*

**CAPSULES**

**Adults.** 15 to 30 mg h.s.

DOSAGE ADJUSTMENT Initial dose reduced to 15 mg for elderly or debilitated patients until individual response is known.

| Route | Onset | Peak | Duration |
|-------|-------|------|----------|
| P.O. | 15 to 45 min | Unknown | 7 to 8 hr |

### Mechanism of Action

May potentiate the effects of gamma-aminobutyric acid (GABA) and other inhibitory neurotransmitters by binding to specific benzodiazepine receptor sites in the limbic and cortical areas of the CNS. By binding to these receptor sites, flurazepam increases GABA's inhibitory effects and blocks cortical and limbic arousal.

## Contraindications

Acute angle-closure glaucoma, breast-feeding, hypersensitivity to other benzodiazepines, itraconazole or ketoconazole therapy, psychosis

## Interactions

**DRUGS**

*cimetidine, diltiazem, disulfiram, erythromycin, fluoxetine, fluvoxamine, itraconazole, nefazodone, estrogen-containing oral contraceptives, propoxyphene, ranitidine, verapamil:* Possibly increased blood level and impaired hepatic metabolism of flurazepam
*clozapine:* Possibly cardiac arrest or respiratory depression
*CNS depressants:* Possibly potentiated CNS depression
*levodopa:* Possibly decreased therapeutic effects of levodopa

**FOODS**

*grapefruit juice:* Possibly increased blood level and impaired hepatic metabolism of flurazepam

**ACTIVITIES**

*alcohol use:* Possibly potentiated CNS and respiratory depression

## Adverse Reactions

**CNS:** Amnesia, anxiety, ataxia, confusion, delusions, depression, dizziness, drowsiness, euphoria, headache, hypokinesia, irritability, malaise, nervousness, slurred speech, tremor
**CV:** Chest pain, palpitations, tachycardia
**EENT:** Blurred vision, dry mouth, increased salivation, photophobia
**GI:** Abdominal pain, constipation, diarrhea, nausea, thirst, vomiting
**GU:** Libido changes
**SKIN:** Diaphoresis
**Other:** Physical or psychological dependence

## Nursing Considerations

•Use flurazepam cautiously in patients with severe mental depression or reduced respiratory function; drug may intensify depression and lead to respiratory depression.
•Expect to use lowest effective dose in elderly or debilitated patients to minimize the risk of ataxia, confusion, dizziness, and oversedation.
•Monitor liver function test results, as appropriate.

**PATIENT TEACHING**

•Instruct patient not to exceed prescribed flurazepam dosage and not to stop drug abruptly.
•Caution patient about possible morning dizziness or drowsiness.
•Because flurazepam can reduce alertness, advise patient to avoid potentially hazardous activities until drug's CNS effects are known.
•Caution patient to avoid alcohol and CNS depressants during therapy.
•Advise patient to notify prescriber if she becomes or intends to become pregnant during therapy.
•Inform patient that her sleep may be disturbed for the first few nights after stopping drug.

# flurbiprofen

Ansaid, Froben (CAN), Froben SR (CAN), Novo-Flurprofen (CAN)

## Class and Category

*Chemical:* Propionic acid derivative
*Therapeutic:* Antiarthritis, anti-inflammatory
*Pregnancy category:* B (first trimester), Not rated (later trimesters)

## Indications and Dosages

➤ *To treat acute or chronic rheumatoid arthritis and osteoarthritis*

**E.R. CAPSULES**

**Adults.** 200 mg q.d. in the evening.

**TABLETS**

**Adults.** *Initial:* 200 to 300 mg/day in divided doses b.i.d. to q.i.d. *Maximum:* 300 mg/day (100 mg/dose).

## Mechanism of Action

Blocks the activity of cyclooxygenase, the enzyme necessary for prostaglandin synthesis. Prostaglandins, important mediators in the inflammatory response, cause local vasodilation with swelling and pain. They also play a role in pain transmission from the periphery to the spinal cord. By blocking cyclooxygenase and inhibiting prostaglandins, this NSAID causes inflammatory symptoms and pain to subside.

## Contraindications

Angioedema, asthma, bronchospasm, nasal polyps, rhinitis, or urticaria induced by aspirin, iodides, or NSAIDs; hypersensitivity to NSAIDs

## Interactions

**DRUGS**

*acetaminophen:* Increased risk of renal impairment with long-term use of both drugs
*antacids:* Decreased flurbiprofen effectiveness
*anticoagulants, cefamandole, cefoperazone, cefotetan, heparin, plicamycin, thrombolytics, valproic acid:* Increased risk of bleeding
*antineoplastics:* Increased adverse hematologic effects
*cyclosporine:* Increased risk of nephrotoxicity
*diuretics, triamterene:* Decreased effectiveness of these drugs
*glucocorticoids, other NSAIDs, potassium supplements:* Increased adverse GI effects
*insulin, oral antidiabetic drugs:* Increased risk of hypoglycemia
*lithium:* Increased risk of lithium toxicity
*methotrexate:* Increased risk of methotrexate toxicity
*salicylates:* Increased risk of GI bleeding

**ACTIVITIES**

*alcohol use, smoking:* Increased risk of GI bleeding

## Adverse Reactions

**CNS:** Anxiety, cerebral hemorrhage, depression, dizziness, drowsiness, forgetfulness, headache, insomnia, malaise, nervousness, stroke, tremor, weakness
**CV:** Arrhythmias, heart failure, hypertension, hypotension, palpitations, peripheral edema, tachycardia
**EENT:** Amblyopia, blurred vision, rhinitis, stomatitis, tinnitus, vision changes
**GI:** Abdominal cramps or distress, anorexia, constipation, diarrhea, diverticulitis, dysphagia, esophagitis, flatulence, gastritis, gastroenteritis, gastroesophageal reflux disease, GI bleeding or ulceration, hemorrhoids, hiatal hernia, hepatitis, increased appetite, indigestion, jaundice, liver failure, melena, nausea, perforation of stomach or intestines, stomatitis, vomiting
**GU:** Hematuria, interstitial nephritis, renal failure, UTI
**HEME:** Agranulocytosis, aplastic anemia, eosinophilia, leukopenia, neutropenia, pancytopenia, thrombocytopenia
**SKIN:** Erythema multiforme, exfoliative dermatitis, flushing, rash, Stevens-Johnson syndrome, toxic epidermal necrolysis
**Other:** Anaphylaxis, angioedema, hyponatremia

## Nursing Considerations

•Use flurbiprofen with extreme caution in patients with a history of ulcer disease or GI bleeding because NSAIDs such as flurbiprofen increase the risk of GI bleeding and ulceration. Expect to use flurbiprofen for the shortest time possible in these patients.
•Be aware that serious GI tract ulceration, bleeding, and perforation may occur without warning symptoms. Elderly patients are at greater risk. To minimize risk, give drug with food. If GI distress occurs, withhold drug and notify prescriber immediately.
•Use flurbiprofen cautiously in patients with hypertension, and monitor blood pressure closely throughout therapy. Drug may cause hypertension or worsen it.
•**WARNING** Monitor patient closely for thrombotic events, including MI and stroke, because NSAIDs increase the risk.
•Monitor patient—especially if she's elderly or receiving long-term flurbiprofen therapy—for less common but serious adverse GI reactions, including anorexia, constipation,

E
F

diverticulitis, dysphagia, esophagitis, gastritis, gastroenteritis, gastroesophageal reflux disease, hemorrhoids, hiatal hernia, melena, stomatitis, and vomiting.
•Monitor liver function test results because, in rare cases, elevations may progress to severe hepatic reactions, including fatal hepatitis, liver necrosis, and hepatic failure.
•Monitor BUN and serum creatinine levels in elderly patients, patients taking diuretics or ACE inhibitors, and patients with heart failure, impaired renal function, or hepatic dysfunction; drug may cause renal failure.
•Monitor CBC for decreased hemoglobin and hematocrit because drug may worsen anemia.
•WARNING If patient has bone marrow suppression or is receiving an antineoplastic drug, monitor laboratory results (including WBC count), and watch for evidence of infection because anti-inflammatory and anti-pyretic actions of flurbiprofen may mask signs and symptoms, such as fever and pain.
•Assess patient's skin regularly for signs of rash or other hypersensitivity reaction because flurbiprofen is an NSAID and may cause serious skin reactions without warning, even in patients with no history of NSAID sensitivity. At first sign of reaction, stop drug and notify prescriber.

PATIENT TEACHING
•Encourage patient to take flurbiprofen with food or milk to avoid GI distress.
•Caution patient about possible blurred vision, dizziness, and drowsiness.
•Advise patient to avoid aspirin, alcohol, and smoking during flurbiprofen therapy.
•Urge patient to notify prescriber immediately if she has blood in urine, easy bruising, itching, rash, swelling, or yellow eyes or skin.
•Caution pregnant patient not to take NSAIDs such as flurbiprofen during the last trimester because they may cause premature closure of the ductus arteriosus.
•Explain that flurbiprofen may increase the risk of serious adverse cardiovascular reactions; urge patient to seek immediate medical attention if signs or symptoms arise, such as chest pain, shortness of breath, weakness, and slurring of speech.
•Explain that flurbiprofen may increase the risk of serious adverse GI reactions; stress the importance of seeking immediate medical attention for such signs and symptoms as epigastric or abdominal pain, indigestion, black or tarry stools, or vomiting blood or material that looks like coffee grounds.
•Alert patient to rare but serious skin reactions. Urge her to seek immediate medical attention for rash, blisters, itching, fever, or other indications of hypersensitivity.

# fluticasone propionate

Flonase, Flovent

## Class and Category
*Chemical:* Trifluorinated corticosteroid
*Therapeutic:* Antiasthmatic, anti-inflammatory
*Pregnancy category:* C

## Indications and Dosages
➤ *To prevent asthma attacks, alone or with oral corticosteroids*
INHALATION AEROSOL
**Adults and children age 12 and older using bronchodilator therapy.** *Initial:* 88 mcg inhaled b.i.d. *Maximum:* 440 mcg inhaled b.i.d.
**Adults and children age 12 and older switching from another inhaled corticosteroid.** *Initial:* 88 to 220 mcg inhaled b.i.d. *Maximum:* 440 mcg inhaled b.i.d.
**Adults and children age 12 and older using oral corticosteroid therapy.** *Initial and maximum:* 880 mcg inhaled b.i.d.

➤ *To prevent or treat seasonal or perennial allergic rhinitis*
NASAL SUSPENSION
**Adults and children age 12 and older.** *Initial:* 100 mcg (2 sprays) in each nostril q.d. or 50 mcg (1 spray) in each nostril b.i.d, as needed. *Maintenance:* 50 mcg (1 spray) in each nostril q.d., as tolerated and needed. *Maximum:* 200 mcg/day (4 sprays).
**Children ages 4 to 11.** 50 or 100 mcg (1 or 2 sprays) in each nostril q.d. in the morning, as needed. *Maximum:* 200 mcg/day (4 sprays).

| Route | Onset | Peak | Duration |
|---|---|---|---|
| Inhalation | In 24 hr | 1 to 2 wk | Several days |
| Nasal | 12 hr to 3 days | 4 to 7 days | 1 to 2 wk |

## Mechanism of Action
Inhibits cells involved in the inflammatory response of asthma, such as mast cells, eosinophils, basophils, lymphocytes, macrophages, and neutrophils. Fluticasone also inhibits production or secretion of chemical mediators, such as histamine, eicosanoids, leukotrienes, and cytokines.

## Contraindications
Hypersensitivity to fluticasone or its components, primary treatment of status asthmaticus or other acute asthma episodes that require intensive measures, untreated nasal mucosal infection (nasal suspension)

## Interactions
**DRUGS**
*ketoconazole, ritonavir and other strong cytochrome P450 3A4 inhibitors (long-term use):* Possibly increased fluticasone level and increased risk of reduced serum cortisol level

## Adverse Reactions
**CNS:** Aggressiveness, agitation, depression, difficulty speaking, dizziness, fatigue, fever, headache, insomnia, malaise, restlessness
**EENT:** Allergic rhinitis, cataracts, conjunctivitis, dry mouth and throat, eye irritation, glaucoma, hoarseness, laryngitis, loss of voice, nasal congestion or discharge, nasal sinus pain, oropharyngeal candidiasis, otitis media, pharyngitis, sinusitis, throat irritation, tonsillitis
**ENDO:** Adrenal insufficiency, cushingoid symptoms, hyperglycemia, slower growth in children
**GI:** Abdominal pain, diarrhea, indigestion, nausea, vomiting
**GU:** Dysmenorrhea
**HEME:** Churg-Strauss syndrome, easy bruising, eosinophilia
**MS:** Arthralgia, myalgia, osteoporosis
**RESP:** Asthma exacerbation, bronchitis, bronchospasm, chest congestion and tightness, cough, dyspnea, pneumonia, upper respiratory tract infection, wheezing
**SKIN:** Dermatitis, ecchymosis, pruritus, rash, urticaria
**Other:** Anaphylaxis, angioedema, flulike symptoms, weight gain

## Nursing Considerations
•Use fluticasone cautiously in patients with ocular herpes simplex, pulmonary tuberculosis, or untreated systemic bacterial, fungal, parasitic, or viral infection.
•Although anaphylaxis is rare, monitor patient closely at start of therapy, especially if patient has severe allergy to milk.
•If patient takes a systemic corticosteroid, expect to taper dosage by no more than 2.5 mg/day at weekly intervals, starting 1 week after fluticasone therapy begins.
•**WARNING** If patient is switched from systemic corticosteroid to fluticasone, assess for adrenal insufficiency (fatigue, hypotension, lassitude, nausea, vomiting, weakness) early in therapy and when patient has infection, stress, trauma, surgery, or other electrolyte-depleting conditions or procedures. Notify prescriber immediately if signs or symptoms develop.
•As prescribed, administer a fast-acting inhaled bronchodilator if bronchospasm occurs immediately after fluticasone use. Expect to stop fluticasone and start another drug therapy.
•Expect to titrate fluticasone to lowest effective dosage after asthma has stabilized.

**PATIENT TEACHING**
•Urge patient to use fluticasone regularly, as prescribed, but not for acute bronchospasm.
•Teach patient how to administer drug according to the form prescribed (nasal spray or oral inhaler).
•Instruct patient to shake canister and to use inhaler according to package insert instructions. On first use, advise her to spray four times into the air (away from her eyes and shaking inhaler between each test spray) and look for a fine mist. If inhaler hasn't been used for more than 7 days or it's dropped, it will need to be primed again by shaking well and then releasing one test spray into the air (away from her face).
•If 2 inhalations are prescribed, direct patient to wait at least 1 minute between them.
•Instruct patient to gargle and rinse her mouth after each dose to help prevent dry mouth and throat, relieve throat irritation, and prevent oropharyngeal yeast infection.
•If patient uses more than one inhaler, instruct her to use fluticasone last, at least 5 minutes after previous inhaler.

E
F

•Instruct patient to clean inhaler according to manufacturer guidelines at least once a week after her evening dose.

•Explain that symptoms may improve within 2 days but that full improvement may not occur for 1 to 2 weeks or longer.

•Caution patient not to increase dosage but to contact prescriber after 1 week if symptoms continue or worsen.

•Instruct patient to notify prescriber immediately if asthma attacks don't respond to bronchodilators during fluticasone therapy.

•If patient is switching from an oral corticosteroid to fluticasone, urge her to carry medical identification indicating the need for supplemental systemic corticosteroids during stress or severe asthma attack.

•Caution patient to avoid contact with people who have infections because fluticasone suppresses the immune system, increasing the risk of infection. Instruct patient to notify prescriber about exposure to chickenpox, measles, or other infections because additional treatment may be needed.

# fluvastatin sodium

Lescol, Lescol XL

## Class and Category

*Chemical:* Heptenoic acid derivative
*Therapeutic:* Antihyperlipidemic
*Pregnancy category:* X

## Indications and Dosages

➤ *As adjunct to lower cholesterol level in primary hypercholesterolemia, to decrease progression of coronary atherosclerosis, to reduce risk in patients with coronary artery disease undergoing coronary revascularization*

**CAPSULES**

**Adults.** 20 to 40 mg q.d. in the evening or 40 mg b.i.d. *Maximum:* 40 mg b.i.d.

**E.R. TABLETS**

**Adults.** 80 mg in the evening. *Maximum:* 80 mg/day.

| Route | Onset | Peak | Duration |
|---|---|---|---|
| P.O. | In 1 to 2 wk | In 4 to 6 wk | Unknown |
| P.O. (E.R.) | In 2 wk | In 4 wk | Unknown |

## Mechanism of Action

Interferes with the hepatic enzyme hydroxymethylglutaryl-coenzyme A reductase, reducing formation of mevalonic acid (a cholesterol precursor) and interrupting the pathway by which cholesterol is synthesized. When cholesterol level declines in hepatic cells, LDLs are consumed, which reduces circulating total cholesterol and serum triglycerides.

## Contraindications

Acute hepatic disease, breast-feeding, hypersensitivity to fluvastatin or its components, pregnancy, unexplained persistently elevated liver enzyme levels

## Interactions

**DRUGS**

*bile acid sequestrants:* Possibly decreased fluvastatin bioavailability
*cimetidine, omeprazole, ranitidine:* Significantly increased blood fluvastatin level
*cyclosporine, erythromycin, gemfibrozil, niacin:* Increased risk of severe myopathy, rhabdomyolysis, and acute renal failure
*itraconazole, ketoconazole:* Increased risk of myopathy
*oral contraceptives:* Increased risk of bleeding
*rifampin:* Significantly decreased blood fluvastatin level, increased plasma clearance

**ACTIVITIES**

*alcohol use:* Increased bioavailability and blood level of fluvastatin

## Adverse Reactions

**CNS:** Dizziness, fatigue, headache, insomnia, weakness
**EENT:** Pharyngitis, rhinitis, sinusitis
**GI:** Abdominal cramps and pain, constipation, diarrhea, flatulence, indigestion, nausea, vomiting
**GU:** UTI
**MS:** Arthritis, back pain, myalgia, myositis, rhabdomyolysis
**RESP:** Bronchitis, cough, upper respiratory tract infection
**SKIN:** Pruritus, rash

## Nursing Considerations

•**WARNING** Expect to stop drug if serum CK level rises sharply or myopathy is suspected.

**PATIENT TEACHING**
- Urge patient to comply with monthly laboratory tests early in treatment.
- Tell patient to follow prescribed low-fat diet.
- Advise patient to notify prescriber promptly if muscle pain or unexplained weakness develops.

# fluvoxamine maleate

Luvox

## Class and Category

*Chemical:* Aralkylketone derivative
*Therapeutic:* Antiobsessional
*Pregnancy category:* C

## Indications and Dosages

➤ *To treat obsessive-compulsive disorder*

**TABLETS**

**Adults.** *Initial:* 50 mg h.s., increased by 50 mg q 4 to 7 days, if needed. *Maximum:* 300 mg/day.
**Children ages 8 to 17.** *Initial:* 25 mg h.s., increased by 25 mg q 4 to 7 days, if needed. *Maximum:* 200 mg/day.

**DOSAGE ADJUSTMENT** Doses divided for adults taking more than 100 mg/day and for children taking more than 50 mg/day; given in 2 equal doses b.i.d. or in 2 unequal doses with the larger dose h.s.

| Route | Onset | Peak | Duration |
|-------|-------|------|----------|
| P.O. | 3 to 10 wk | Unknown | Unknown |

---

### Mechanism of Action

May potentiate serotonin's action by blocking its reuptake at neuronal membranes. An elevated serotonin level may elevate mood and decrease depression and anxiety, which often accompany obsessive-compulsive disorder.

---

## Contraindications

Alosetron, astemizole, cisapride, pimozide, terfenadine, thioridazine, or tizanidine therapy, hypersensitivity to fluvoxamine maleate or its components, use within 14 days of MAO inhibitor

## Interactions

**DRUGS**

*alosetron:* Increased plasma alosetron level
*alprazolam:* Increased plasma alprazolam level
*antihistamines:* Increased risk of impaired mental and motor skills
*astemizole, cisapride, pimozide, terfenadine:* Possibly fatal QT prolongation
*benzodiazepines:* Decreased benzodiazepine clearance, possibly impaired memory and motor skills
*buspirone:* Decreased buspirone effects, increased blood fluvoxamine level, and paradoxical worsening of obsessive-compulsive disorder
*carbamazepine:* Increased risk of carbamazepine toxicity
*clozapine:* Increased blood clozapine level
*diltiazem:* Increased risk of bradycardia
*haloperidol:* Increased blood haloperidol level, possibly delayed recall and reduced memory and attention span
*lithium:* Possibly increased serotonin reuptake action of fluvoxamine
*MAO inhibitors:* Possibly serious or fatal reactions (such as agitation, autonomic instability, coma, delirium, fluctuating vital signs, hyperthermia, myoclonus, and rigidity)
*methadone:* Possibly significantly increased blood methadone level, increased risk of methadone toxicity
*metoprolol, propranolol:* Increased blood levels of these drugs, possibly reduced diastolic blood pressure and heart rate induced by these drugs
*serotonergics (such as amphetamines and other psychostimulants, antidepressants, and dopamine agonists):* Increased risk of serotonin syndrome
*sympathomimetics:* Possibly increased effects of sympathomimetics and increased risk of serotonin syndrome
*tacrine:* Increased blood level and therapeutic and adverse effects of tacrine
*theophylline:* Decreased theophylline clearance, increased risk of theophylline toxicity
*tizanidine:* Increased risk of serious adverse effects, such as hypotension and profound sedation
*tricyclic antidepressants:* Increased blood levels of antidepressants
*warfarin:* Increased blood warfarin level, prolonged PT

**FOODS**

*caffeine:* Possibly decreased hepatic clearance of caffeine

**ACTIVITIES**

*smoking:* Increased fluvoxamine metabolism

E
F

## Adverse Reactions

**CNS:** Agitation, anxiety, apathy, chills, confusion, depression, dizziness, drowsiness, fatigue, headache, hypomania, insomnia, malaise, mania, nervousness, sedation, tremor, vertigo, yawning
**CV:** Palpitations, tachycardia
**EENT:** Altered taste, blurred vision, dry mouth
**GI:** Anorexia, constipation, diarrhea, flatulence, indigestion, nausea, vomiting
**GU:** Decreased libido, ejaculation disorders, impotence, urinary frequency, urine retention
**MS:** Muscle twitching
**RESP:** Dyspnea, upper respiratory tract infection
**SKIN:** Diaphoresis, rash
**Other:** Flulike symptoms, weight gain

## Nursing Considerations

• Use fluvoxamine cautiously in patients with cardiovascular disease, impaired hepatic or renal function, mania, seizures, or suicidal tendencies.
• **WARNING** Fluvoxamine shouldn't be given within 14 days of an MAO inhibitor.
• **WARNING** If patient receives another drug that raises the serotonin level by a different mechanism, assess for serotonin syndrome, a rare but serious complication of certain selective serotonin reuptake inhibitors. Signs and symptoms include agitation, confusion, diaphoresis, diarrhea, fever, hyperactive reflexes, lack of coordination, muscle twitching, restlessness, shivering, talking or acting with uncontrolled excitement, and tremor. Drugs that raise the serotonin level include MAO inhibitors, tryptophan, amphetamines and other psychostimulants, antidepressants (buspirone, lithium), and dopamine agonists.
**PATIENT TEACHING**
• Caution patient not to drink alcohol during fluvoxamine therapy.
• Urge patient to avoid potentially hazardous activities until drug's CNS effects are known.
• **WARNING** Inform patient that fluvoxamine increases the risk of a rare but serious problem: serotonin syndrome. Encourage her to notify prescriber immediately if symptoms develop.
• Caution patient not to stop taking drug abruptly. Explain that gradual tapering helps avoid withdrawal symptoms.

# folic acid

## (vitamin B₉)

Apo-Folic (CAN), Folvite, Novo-Folacid (CAN)

## Class and Category

*Chemical:* Water-soluble B-complex vitamin
*Therapeutic:* Nutritional supplement
*Pregnancy category:* A

## Indications and Dosages

➤ *To prevent deficiency based on U.S. and Canadian recommended daily allowances*
**TABLETS**
**Male adults and children age 11 and older.**
150 to 400 mcg (150 to 220 mcg Canadian) daily.
**Female adults and children age 11 and older.** 150 to 400 mcg (145 to 190 mcg Canadian) daily.
**Pregnant females.** 400 to 800 mcg (445 to 475 mcg Canadian) daily.
**Breast-feeding females.** 260 to 800 mcg (245 to 275 mcg Canadian) daily.
**Children ages 7 to 10.** 100 to 400 mcg (125 to 180 mcg Canadian) daily.
**Children ages 4 to 6.** 75 to 400 mcg (90 mcg Canadian) daily.
**Children from birth to age 3.** 25 mcg (50 to 80 mcg Canadian) daily.
**I.V INFUSION**
**Adults and children age 11 and older.** Dosage individualized based on patient need and given as part of total parenteral nutrition solution.
➤ *To treat deficiency*
**TABLETS**
**Adults and children age 11 and older.** Dosage individualized based on severity of deficiency, as prescribed.
**I.V. INFUSION, I.M. OR S.C. INJECTION**
**Adults and children age 11 and older.** 0.25 to 1 mg q.d. until hematologic response occurs.

## Contraindications

Hypersensitivity to folic acid or its components

## Interactions

**DRUGS**
*analgesics, carbamazepine, estrogens (including oral contraceptives), phenobarbital, primidone:* Possibly increased folic acid requirements

antacids (aluminum- or magnesium-containing), cholestyramine, sulfasalazine: Possibly decreased folic acid absorption
hydantoin anticonvulsants: Possibly decreased effectiveness of these drugs, possibly increased folic acid requirements
methotrexate, pyrimethamine, triamterene, trimethoprim: Possibly decreased effectiveness of folic acid

### Mechanism of Action
Acts as a catalyst for normal production of red blood cells, helping to prevent megaloblastic anemia, and helps maintain normal homocysteine levels. After being converted to tetrahydrofolic acid in the intestines, folic acid promotes synthesis of several enzymes, including purine and thymidylates; metabolism of amino acids, including glycine and methionine; and metabolism of histidine, all of which are essential for normal cell structure and growth.

## Adverse Reactions
**Other:** Allergic reaction (bronchospasm, erythema, fever, malaise, rash, pruritus)

## Nursing Considerations
•**WARNING** Don't give injection form containing benzyl alcohol to neonates or immature infants because a fatal toxic syndrome may occur with CNS, respiratory, circulatory, and renal impairment and metabolic acidosis.
•To prevent decreased absorption, give folic acid supplements at least 1 hour before or 4 hours after cholestyramine or sulfasalazine and don't give antacids within 1 hour before or 2 hours after giving folic acid.
•Know that folic acid will correct hematologic disorders in pernicious anemia, but neurologic problems will progressively worsen.
**PATIENT TEACHING**
•Advise against taking folic acid supplements as a substitute for proper dietary intake. Explain that good sources of folic acid include green vegetables, potatoes, cereals, and organ meats. Recommend eating raw green vegetables because heat used during cooking destroys up to 90% of folic acid found in food.
•Explain to patients with pernicious anemia that folic acid won't affect the neurologic symptoms associated with the disease.

# fondaparinux sodium
Arixtra

## Class and Category
*Chemical:* Synthetic pentasaccharide Factor Xa inhibitor
*Therapeutic:* Antithrombolytic
*Pregnancy category:* B

## Indications and Dosages
➤ *To provide prophylaxis against deep vein thrombosis, which may lead to pulmonary embolism in patients undergoing hip fracture surgery, hip replacement surgery, knee replacement surgery, or abdominal surgery in patients at risk for thromboembolic complications*
**S.C. INJECTION**
**Adults.** *Initial:* After hemostasis has been established, 2.5 mg S.C. 6 to 8 hr after surgery, followed by 2.5 mg S.C. q.d. for 5 to 9 days. *Maximum:* 2.5 mg S.C. q.d. for 11 days for hip or knee replacement and abdominal surgery and 24 days for hip fracture surgery.
➤ *To treat acute deep vein thrombosis (with warfarin); to treat acute pulmonary embolism (with warfarin) in a hospital setting*
**S.C. INJECTION**
**Adults.** *Initial:* 5 mg if body weight is less than 50 kg (110 lb), 7.5 mg if body weight is 50 to 100 kg (110 to 220 lb), and 10 mg if body weight exceeds 100 kg q.d. for at least 5 days and until INR is between 2.0 and 3.0 (usually in 5 to 9 days)

## Incompatibilities
Don't mix fondaparinux sodium with other injections or infusions.

### Mechanism of Action
Selectively binds to antithrombin III, which enhances the inactivation of clotting Factor Xa by antithrombin III. Inactivation of Factor Xa interrupts the blood coagulation pathway, which then inhibits thrombin formation. Without thrombin, fibrinogen can't convert to fibrin and clots can't form.

## Contraindications
Active major bleeding; bacterial endocarditis; body weight less than 50 kg (110 lb) if

E
F

patient is having hip repair or replacement surgery or knee replacement surgery; fondaparinux-induced thrombocytopenia associated with a positive in vitro test for antiplatelet antibodies; hypersensitivity to fondaparinux; prophylactic fondaparinux therapy in patients weighing less than 50 kg (110 lb) undergoing hip repair or replacement, knee replacement, or abdominal surgery; severe renal impairment (creatinine clearance less than 30 ml/min/1.73 m$^2$)

## Interactions
**DRUGS**
*abciximab, thrombolytics, other drugs that enhance risk of bleeding:* Increased risk of hemorrhage

## Adverse Reactions
**CNS:** Confusion, dizziness, fever, headache, insomnia
**CV:** Edema, elevated serum aminotransferase level, hypotension
**GI:** Constipation, diarrhea, elevated liver function test results, indigestion, nausea, vomiting
**GU:** Urine retention, UTI
**HEME:** Anemia, bleeding, hematoma, postoperative hemorrhage, thrombocytopenia
**SKIN:** Bullous eruption, increased wound drainage, rash, purpura
**Other:** Generalized pain; hypokalemia; injection site bleeding, pruritus, and rash

## Nursing Considerations
• Use fondaparinux cautiously in elderly patients, especially those who weigh less than 50 kg (110 lb) and are receiving the drug for pulmomary embolism or deep vein thrombosis, because the risk of drug-induced bleeding increases with age.
• Inspect fondaparinux for particles or discoloration before administration.
• Alternate injection sites during treatment using the left and right anterolateral or left and right posterolateral abdominal wall. Don't expel air bubble from prefilled syringe before injection to prevent expelling drug from syringe. Don't give drug by I.M. injection.
• **WARNING** Closely monitor patients who have had epidural or spinal anesthesia or a spinal puncture for signs of neurologic impairment. They're at risk for epidural or spinal hema-

toma, which can put them at risk for paralysis.
• Closely monitor patient for bleeding (such as ecchymosis, epistaxis, hematemesis, hematuria, and melena), especially those at risk for decreased drug elimination (such as elderly patients and patients with mild to moderate renal impairment) and those at increased risk for bleeding (such as patients with congenital or acquired bleeding disorders; active ulcerative GI disease; hemorrhagic stroke; recent brain, spinal, or ophthalmologic surgery; diabetic retinopathy; or a history of heparin-induced thrombocytopenia; and those being treated concomitantly with platelet inhibitors).
• Perform periodic CBC, including platelet count, as ordered. Expect prescriber to discontinue drug if platelet count falls below 100,000/mm$^3$. Be aware that routine coagulation tests, such as PT and INR, are not used to monitor fondaparinux therapy; an anti-Xa assay may be used instead. Also, test stools for occult blood, as ordered.
• Monitor renal function test results, as ordered. Expect to discontinue drug if severe renal impairment or labile renal function occurs during fondaparinux therapy because the risk of hemorrhage increases as renal function decreases.
• Store drug at a controlled room temperature.
**PATIENT TEACHING**
• Inform patient that fondaparinux can't be taken orally.
• Instruct patient to seek immediate help if she experiences signs of thromboembolism, such as neurologic changes and severe shortness of breath.
• Inform patient about the increased risk of bleeding. Instruct her or family member to watch for and report abdominal or lower back pain, black stools, bleeding gums, bloody urine, or severe headaches.
• Teach patient or family member how to administer fondaparinux by S.C. injection at home, if needed. Instruct her not to expel air bubble from a prefilled syringe to avoid expelling some of the drug. Tell her to insert the entire needle into a skinfold held between thumb and forefinger, and remind her to alternate administration sites.
• To minimize bruising, caution the patient not to rub the injection site after giving the drug.

• Review safe handling and disposal of syringes and needles.
• Advise patient to keep follow-up appointments and undergo prescribed laboratory tests.

# formoterol fumarate dihydrate

Foradil Aerolizer, Oxeze Turbuhaler (CAN)

## Class and Category

*Chemical:* Racemic acid salt
*Therapeutic:* Bronchodilator
*Pregnancy category:* C

## Indications and Dosages

➤ *To prevent asthma-induced bronchospasm*

**POWDER FOR ORAL INHALATION**

**Adults and children age 5 and older.** 12 mcg q 12 hr through inhaler device. *Maximum:* 24 mcg/day.

➤ *To prevent exercise-induced bronchospasm*

**POWDER FOR ORAL INHALATION**

**Adults and adolescents age 12 and older.** 12 mcg at least 15 min before exercise q 12 hr p.r.n. *Maximum:* 24 mcg/day.

➤ *To provide long-term treatment of bronchospasm in patients with chronic bronchitis and emphysema*

**POWDER FOR ORAL INHALATION**

**Adults.** 12 mcg q 12 hr through inhaler device. *Maximum:* 24 mcg/day.

| Route | Onset | Peak | Duration |
|---|---|---|---|
| Oral inhalation | 1 to 3 min | Unknown | 12 hr |

## Mechanism of Action

Selectively attaches to beta$_2$ receptors on bronchial membranes, stimulating the intracellular enzyme adenyl cyclase to convert adenosine triphosphate to cAMP. The resulting increase in the intracellular cAMP level relaxes bronchial smooth-muscle cells, stabilizes mast cells, and inhibits histamine release.

## Contraindications

Acute asthma, hypersensitivity to formoterol fumarate or its components

## Interactions

**DRUGS**

*adrenergics:* Possibly increased sympathetic effects of formoterol
*beta blockers:* Decreased effects of formoterol, possibly severe bronchospasm
*corticosteroids, non-potassium-sparing diuretics, xanthine derivatives:* Possibly increased hypokalemic effect of formoterol
*disopyramide, MAO inhibitors, phenothiazines,*
*procainamide, quinidine, tricyclic antidepressants:* Possibly prolonged QTc interval, increasing risk of ventricular arrhythmias

## Adverse Reactions

**CNS:** Dizziness, fatigue, headache, insomnia, malaise, tremor
**CV:** Angina, arrhythmias, hypertension, hypotension, palpitations, tachycardia
**EENT:** Dry mouth; laryngeal spasm, irritation, or swelling; hoarseness; rhinitis and tonsillitis (in children)
**ENDO:** Hyperglycemia
**GI:** Abdominal pain, gastroenteritis, indigestion (in children); nausea
**MS:** Muscle spasms
**RESP:** Bronchitis, bronchospasm (paradoxical or hypersensitivity-induced), cough, upper respiratory tract infection
**SKIN:** Dermatitis, rash
**Other:** Hypokalemia, metabolic acidosis, viral infection (in children)

## Nursing Considerations

• Administer formoterol capsules only by oral inhalation.
• Store capsules in original blister pack, and open immediately before use.
• To use delivery system, place capsule in well of inhaler device. Press and release buttons on side of device to pierce capsule. Have patient inhale rapidly and deeply through mouthpiece; drug is dispersed into airways as patient inhales.
• **WARNING** Monitor patient for worsening or deteriorating asthma because drug isn't rapid-acting and shouldn't be used as a substitute for corticosteroid therapy.

•Monitor patient closely for paradoxical bronchospasm; if this occurs, discontinue drug immediately and notify prescriber.
•Monitor patients with a history of cardiovascular disorders, especially coronary insufficiency, arrhythmias, or hypertension. Notify prescriber of any significant increases in pulse rate or blood pressure or exacerbation of chronic conditions because formoterol may produce cardiovascular reactions, including angina, arrhythmias, hypertension or hypotension, palpitations, and tachycardia. Drug may need to be discontinued if such reactions occur.

**PATIENT TEACHING**
•Advise patient, especially if she has significant cardiac history, to inform prescriber of any other drugs she takes before beginning formoterol therapy to prevent harmful drug interactions.
•Instruct patient to use manufacturer's plastic device for inhaling formoterol, to always use new inhaler that comes with each refill, and not to use a spacer. Tell her never to swallow capsules.
•Teach patient how to properly store drug and inhaler. Instruct her to avoid exposing capsules to moisture and to always handle them with dry hands because powder inside capsules must be dry to be inhaled. Also advise her to keep inhaler in a dry place and *not* to wash it.
•Teach patient proper use of formoterol delivery system. Instruct her to remove capsule from blister pack just before use, to place capsule in well of inhaler device, to press and release buttons on side of device to pierce capsule, and then to inhale rapidly and deeply through mouthpiece. Emphasize that she should only inhale, *not exhale*, into device.
•Instruct patient who currently uses oral or inhaled corticosteroids to continue using them, as prescribed, even if she feels better after starting formoterol.
•Caution patient not to increase formoterol dosage or frequency without consulting prescriber because she may need a rapid-acting bronchodilator.
•Urge patient to notify prescriber if her symptoms worsen, if formoterol becomes less effective, or if she needs more inhalations of her short-acting beta$_2$-agonist than usual be-

cause this may indicate that her asthma is worsening.
•Instruct patient to notify prescriber immediately if she experiences palpitations, chest pain, rapid heart rate, tremor, or nervousness while taking formoterol because dosage may need to be adjusted.

# fosfomycin tromethamine

Monurol

## Class and Category
*Chemical:* Phosphonic acid derivative
*Therapeutic:* Antibiotic
*Pregnancy category:* B

## Indications and Dosages
➤ *To treat uncomplicated UTIs (acute cystitis) caused by* Enterococcus faecalis *or* Escherichia coli

**GRANULES FOR ORAL SOLUTION**
**Women age 18 and older.** 3 g as a single dose mixed with water.

| Route | Onset | Peak | Duration |
|-------|-------|------|----------|
| P.O. | 2 to 3 days | 48 hr | Unknown |

## Mechanism of Action
Disrupts the formation of bacterial cell walls by blocking cell wall precursors. Specifically, fosfomycin inactivates enolpyruvyl transferase, which irreversibly blocks the condensation of uridine diphosphate-*N*-acetylglucosamine with phospho *enol*pyruvate, a preliminary step in bacterial cell wall synthesis. Fosfomycin also decreases adherence of bacteria to epithelial cells of the urinary tract.

## Contraindications
Hypersensitivity to fosfomycin or its components

## Interactions
**DRUGS**
*metoclopramide:* Decreased blood level and urinary excretion of fosfomycin

## Adverse Reactions
**CNS:** Asthenia, dizziness, fever, headache, insomnia, nervousness, paresthesia, somnolence

**EENT:** Dry mouth, pharyngitis, rhinitis
**GI:** Abdominal pain, anorexia, constipation, diarrhea, flatulence, indigestion, nausea, vomiting
**GU:** Dysmenorrhea, dysuria, hematuria, menstrual irregularities, vaginitis
**MS:** Back pain
**SKIN:** Pruritus, rash
**Other:** Flulike symptoms, lymphadenopathy

## Nursing Considerations
•Use fosfomycin cautiously in patients with impaired renal function because drug clearance may be decreased.
•Expect to obtain urine specimens for culture and sensitivity tests before and after therapy.
•To reconstitute granules, pour contents of single-dose packet into 90 to 120 ml (3 to 4 oz) of water (not hot water) and stir. Administer immediately after dissolving.
•**WARNING** Expect adverse reactions to increase if more than one dose is used to treat a single episode of acute cystitis.

**PATIENT TEACHING**
•Explain how to reconstitute fosfomycin, and instruct patient to take drug immediately after it dissolves. Caution her not to take dry granules or mix with hot water.
•To treat each episode of acute cystitis, advise patient to use only a single dose, as prescribed, to avoid increasing the risk of adverse reactions.
•Urge patient to notify prescriber if symptoms don't improve in 2 to 3 days.
•Instruct patient to return to prescriber for further urine testing after taking fosfomycin.

# fosinopril sodium

Monopril

## Class and Category
*Chemical:* Phosphinic acid derivative
*Therapeutic:* Antihypertensive, vasodilator
*Pregnancy category:* C (first trimester), D (later trimesters)

## Indications and Dosages
➤ *To manage blood pressure, alone or with other antihypertensives*
**TABLETS**
**Adults.** *Initial:* 10 mg q.d. *Maintenance:* 20 to 40 mg q.d. *Maximum:* 80 mg/day.

➤ *To treat heart failure*
**TABLETS**
**Adults.** 10 mg q.d.
**DOSAGE ADJUSTMENT** Initial dosage reduced to 5 mg q.d., if needed, for patients with acute heart failure, moderate to severe renal failure, or recent aggressive diuresis. Dosage may be increased over several weeks to maximum of 40 mg q.d.

| Route | Onset | Peak | Duration |
|---|---|---|---|
| P.O. | 1 hr | 2 to 6 hr | 24 hr |

## Mechanism of Action
May reduce blood pressure by affecting renin-angiotensin-aldosterone system. By inhibiting angiotensin-converting enzyme, fosinopril:
•prevents conversion of angiotensin I to angiotensin II, a potent vasoconstrictor that also stimulates the adrenal cortex to secrete aldosterone
•may inhibit renal and vascular production of angiotensin II
•decreases serum angiotensin II level and increases serum renin activity, which decreases aldosterone secretion, slightly increasing the serum potassium level and fluid loss
•decreases vascular tone and blood pressure
•inhibits aldosterone release, which reduces sodium and water reabsorption and increases their excretion, further reducing blood pressure.

## Contraindications
Hypersensitivity to fosinopril, other ACE inhibitors, or their components

## Interactions
**DRUGS**
*allopurinol, bone marrow depressants, procainamide, systemic corticosteroids:* Increased risk of potentially fatal neutropenia or agranulocytosis
*antacids:* Impaired fosinopril absorption
*cyclosporine, potassium-sparing diuretics, potassium supplements:* Increased risk of hyperkalemia
*diuretics, other antihypertensives:* Possibly additive hypotension

*lithium:* Increased blood lithium level and risk of lithium toxicity
*NSAIDs:* Possibly decreased antihypertensive effect of fosinopril
**FOODS**
*salt substitutes:* Increased risk of hyperkalemia
**ACTIVITIES**
*alcohol use:* Possibly additive hypotension

## Adverse Reactions

**CNS:** Confusion, depression, dizziness, drowsiness, fatigue, fever, headache, insomnia, mood changes, sleep disturbance, syncope, tremor, vertigo, weakness
**CV:** Angina, arrhythmias (including AV conduction disorders, bradycardia, and tachycardia), claudication, hypotension, MI, orthostatic hypotension, palpitations
**EENT:** Dry mouth, epistaxis, eye irritation, hoarseness, rhinitis, sinus problems, taste perversion, tinnitus, vision changes
**GI:** Abdominal distention and pain, anorexia, constipation, diarrhea, flatulence, hepatic failure, hepatitis, hepatomegaly, nausea, pancreatitis, vomiting
**GU:** Decreased libido, flank pain, renal insufficiency, sexual dysfunction, urinary frequency
**MS:** Arthralgia, gout, myalgia
**RESP:** Asthma; bronchitis; bronchospasm; dry, persistent, tickling cough; dyspnea; tracheobronchitis; upper respiratory tract infection
**SKIN:** Diaphoresis, jaundice, photosensitivity, pruritus, rash, urticaria
**Other:** Anaphylaxis, angioedema, hyperkalemia, weight gain

## Nursing Considerations

•Monitor serum potassium level before and during fosinopril therapy, as appropriate.
•Observe patient being treated for heart failure for at least 2 hours after giving drug to detect hypotension or orthostatic hypotension. If either develops, notify prescriber and monitor patient until blood pressure stabilizes. Keep in mind that orthostatic hypotension is unlikely to develop in patients with a systolic blood pressure over 100 mm Hg who receive a 10-mg dose.
•If patient also receives an antacid, separate administration times by at least 2 hours.
•If patient also receives a diuretic or another antihypertensive, expect to reduce its dosage

over 2 to 3 days before starting fosinopril. If blood pressure isn't controlled with fosinopril alone, other antihypertensive therapy may resume, as prescribed. If so, observe for excessive hypotension.
•**WARNING** If angioedema affects the face, glottis, larynx, limbs, lips, mucous membranes, or tongue, notify prescriber immediately. Expect to discontinue fosinopril and start appropriate therapy at once. If airway obstruction threatens, promptly give 0.3 to 0.5 ml of epinephrine solution 1:1,000 S.C., as prescribed.
**PATIENT TEACHING**
•Instruct patient to take fosinopril at the same time each day to improve compliance and maintain drug's therapeutic effect.
•Emphasize the importance of taking fosinopril as prescribed, even if patient feels well. Caution her not to stop taking drug without consulting prescriber.
•Explain that drug helps control—but doesn't cure—hypertension and that patient may need lifelong therapy.
•**WARNING** Urge patient to seek immediate medical attention for difficulty breathing or swallowing, hoarseness, or swelling of the face, lips, tongue, or throat.
•Instruct patient to notify prescriber about persistent, severe nausea, vomiting, and diarrhea; resulting dehydration may lead to hypotension.
•Advise patient not to take other drugs or use salt substitutes without consulting prescriber.
•Encourage patient to keep scheduled appointments with prescriber to monitor blood pressure, blood test results, and progress.
•Caution patient about possible dizziness.
•To minimize effects of orthostatic hypotension, advise patient to rise slowly from a lying or sitting position and to dangle legs over bed for several minutes before standing.
•Reinforce prescriber's recommendations for lifestyle changes, such as smoking cessation, stress reduction, dietary improvements, alcohol avoidance, and regular exercise.
•If patient is a woman of childbearing age, urge her to use contraception during therapy because drug may harm fetus.
•Advise patient to use caution during exercise and hot weather because of the increased risk of dehydration from excessive sweating.

# fosphenytoin sodium

Cerebyx

## Class and Category
*Chemical:* Hydantoin derivative
*Therapeutic:* Anticonvulsant
*Pregnancy category:* D

## Indications and Dosages
➤ *To treat status epilepticus*
**I.V. INFUSION, I.M. INJECTION**
**Adults and adolescents.** *Initial:* 15 to 20 mg
of phenytoin equivalent (PE)/kg I.V. at 100
to 150 PE/min. *Maintenance:* 4 to 6 mg
PE/kg/day I.V. or I.M. in divided doses b.i.d.
to q.i.d.
*Maximum:* 30 mg PE/kg as total loading
dose.
**Children.** *Initial:* 15 to 20 mg PE/kg I.V.
given at up to 3 mg PE/kg/min. *Mainte-
nance:* 4 to 6 mg PE/kg/day I.V. or I.M. in di-
vided doses b.i.d. to q.i.d.
➤ *To prevent or treat seizures during and
after neurosurgery*
**I.V. INFUSION, I.M. INJECTION**
**Adults and adolescents.** *Initial:* 10 to 20 mg
PE/kg I.V., not to exceed 150 mg PE/min.
*Maintenance:* 4 to 6 mg PE/kg/day I.V. or
I.M. in divided doses b.i.d. to q.i.d. *Maxi-
mum:* 30 mg PE/kg as total loading dose.

### Mechanism of Action
Is converted from fosphenytoin (a prodrug) to phenytoin, which limits the
spread of seizure activity and the start
of new seizures. Phenytoin does so by
regulating voltage-dependent sodium
and calcium channels in neurons, inhibiting calcium movement across neuronal
membranes, and enhancing the sodium-
potassium-adenosine triphosphatase activity in neurons and glial cells. These actions may stem from phenytoin's ability
to slow the recovery rate of inactivated
sodium channels.

## Contraindications
Hypersensitivity to fosphenytoin, phenytoin,
other hydantoins, or their components

## Interactions
**DRUGS**
*acetaminophen (long-term use):* Increased
risk of hepatotoxicity

*acyclovir:* Decreased blood phenytoin level,
loss of seizure control
*alfentanil:* Increased clearance and decreased
effectiveness of alfentanil
*amiodarone, fluoxetine:* Possibly increased
blood phenytoin level and risk of toxicity
*antacids:* Possibly decreased phenytoin effectiveness
*antineoplastics:* Increased phenytoin metabolism
*beta blockers:* Increased myocardial depression
*bupropion, clozapine, loxapine, MAO inhibi-
tors, maprotiline, phenothiazines, pimozide,
thioxanthenes:* Possibly lowered seizure
threshold and decreased therapeutic effects
of phenytoin, possibly intensified CNS depressant effects of these drugs
*calcium:* Possibly impaired phenytoin absorption
*calcium channel blockers:* Possibly increased
blood phenytoin level
*carbamazepine:* Decreased blood carbamazepine level, possibly increased blood phenytoin level and risk of toxicity
*chloramphenicol, cimetidine, disulfiram, iso-
niazid, methylphenidate, metronidazole,
phenylbutazone, ranitidine, salicylates, sulfonamides, trimethoprim:* Possibly impaired
metabolism of these drugs, increased risk of
phenytoin toxicity
*CNS depressants:* Possibly increased CNS
depression
*corticosteroids, cyclosporine, digoxin, diso-
pyramide, doxycycline, furosemide, levodopa,
mexiletine, quinidine:* Decreased therapeutic
effects of these drugs
*diazoxide:* Possibly decreased therapeutic effects of both drugs
*dopamine:* Possibly sudden hypotension or
cardiac arrest after I.V. fosphenytoin administration
*estrogen- and progestin-containing contra-
ceptives:* Possibly breakthrough bleeding and
decreased contraceptive effectiveness
*estrogens, progestins:* Decreased therapeutic
effects, increased blood phenytoin level
*felbamate:* Possibly impaired metabolism and
increased blood level of phenytoin
*fluconazole, itraconazole, ketoconazole, mi-
conazole:* Increased blood phenytoin level
*folic acid:* Increased phenytoin metabolism,
decreased seizure control

*haloperidol:* Possibly lowered seizure threshold and decreased therapeutic effects of phenytoin; possibly decreased blood haloperidol level

*insulin, oral antidiabetic drugs:* Possibly increased blood glucose level and decreased therapeutic effects of these drugs

*lamotrigine:* Possibly decreased therapeutic effects of lamotrigine

*lidocaine:* Possibly decreased blood lidocaine level, increased myocardial depression

*lithium:* Increased risk of lithium toxicity

*methadone:* Possibly increased methadone metabolism, leading to withdrawal symptoms

*molindone:* Possibly lowered seizure threshold, impaired absorption, and decreased therapeutic effects of phenytoin

*omeprazole:* Possibly increased blood phenytoin level

*oral anticoagulants:* Possibly impaired metabolism of these drugs and increased risk of phenytoin toxicity; possibly increased anticoagulant effects initially and then decreased effects with prolonged therapy

*rifampin:* Possibly decreased therapeutic effects of phenytoin

*streptozocin:* Possibly decreased therapeutic effects of streptozocin

*sucralfate:* Possibly decreased phenytoin absorption

*tricyclic antidepressants:* Possibly lowered seizure threshold and decreased therapeutic effects of phenytoin; possibly decreased blood antidepressant level

*valproic acid:* Decreased blood phenytoin level, increased blood valproic acid level

*vitamin D analogues:* Decreased vitamin D analogue activity

*xanthines:* Possibly inhibited phenytoin absorption and increased clearance of xanthines

*zaleplon:* Increased clearance and decreased effectiveness of zaleplon

**ACTIVITIES**

*alcohol use:* Possibly decreased phenytoin effectiveness

## Adverse Reactions

**CNS:** Agitation, amnesia, asthenia, ataxia, cerebral edema, chills, coma, confusion, CVA, delusions, depression, dizziness, emotional lability, encephalitis, encephalopathy, extrapyramidal reactions, fever, headache, hemiplegia, hostility, hypoesthesia, lack of coordination, malaise, meningitis, nervousness, neurosis, paralysis, personality disorder, positive Babinski's sign, seizures, somnolence, speech disorders, stupor, subdural hematoma, syncope, transient paresthesia, tremor, vertigo

**CV:** Atrial flutter, bradycardia, bundle-branch block, cardiac arrest, cardiomegaly, edema, heart failure, hypertension, hypotension, orthostatic hypotension, palpitations, PVCs, shock, tachycardia, thrombophlebitis

**EENT:** Amblyopia, conjunctivitis, diplopia, dry mouth, earache, epistaxis, eye pain, gingival hyperplasia, hearing loss, hyperacusis, increased salivation, loss of taste, mydriasis, nystagmus, pharyngitis, photophobia, rhinitis, sinusitis, taste perversion, tinnitus, tongue swelling, visual field defects

**ENDO:** Diabetes insipidus, hyperglycemia, ketosis

**GI:** Anorexia, constipation, diarrhea, dysphagia, elevated liver function test results, flatulence, gastritis, GI bleeding, hepatic necrosis, hepatitis, ileus, indigestion, nausea, vomiting

**GU:** Albuminuria, dysuria, incontinence, oliguria, polyuria, renal failure, urine retention, vaginal candidiasis

**HEME:** Anemia, easy bruising, leukopenia, thrombocytopenia

**MS:** Arthralgia, back pain, leg cramps, muscle twitching, myalgia, myasthenia, myoclonus, myopathy

**RESP:** Apnea, asthma, atelectasis, bronchitis, dyspnea, hemoptysis, hyperventilation, hypoxia, increased cough, increased sputum production, pneumonia, pneumothorax

**SKIN:** Contact dermatitis, diaphoresis, maculopapular or pustular rash, photosensitivity, skin discoloration, skin nodule, Stevens-Johnson syndrome, transient pruritus, urticaria

**Other:** Cachexia, cryptococcosis, dehydration, facial edema, flulike symptoms, hyperkalemia, hypokalemia, hypophosphatemia, infection, injection site reaction, lymphadenopathy, sepsis

## Nursing Considerations

•Express the dosage, concentration, and infusion rate of fosphenytoin in PE units. Misreading an order or a label could result in massive overdose.

•Refrigerate unopened fosphenytoin at 2° to 8° C (36° to 46° F), but don't freeze.

•Dilute drug in $D_5W$ or NS to 1.5 to 25 mg PE/ml.

•Inspect parenteral solution before administration. Discard solution that contains particles or is discolored.

•Be aware that drug shouldn't be given I.M. for status epilepticus because I.V. route allows faster onset and peak.

•Keep in mind that I.V. fosphenytoin administration doesn't require use of a filter, as with phenytoin administration.

•Don't give fosphenytoin solution faster than 150 mg PE/minute because of the risk of hypotension. For a 50-kg (110-lb) patient, infusion typically takes 5 to 7 minutes. Fosphenytoin can be given more rapidly than I.V. phenytoin.

•Follow loading dose with maintenance dosage of oral or parenteral phenytoin or parenteral fosphenytoin, as prescribed.

•As prescribed, give I.V. benzodiazepine (such as lorazepam or diazepam) with fosphenytoin; otherwise, drug's full antiepileptic effect won't be immediate.

•Monitor ECG, blood pressure, and respiratory function for 10 to 20 minutes after infusion ends.

•Expect to obtain blood fosphenytoin (phenytoin) level 2 hours after I.V. infusion or 4 hours after I.M. injection. Therapeutic level generally ranges from 10 to 20 mcg/ml; steady-state may take several days to several weeks to reach.

•Be aware that I.V. or I.M. fosphenytoin may be substituted for oral phenytoin sodium at same total daily dose and frequency. If prescribed, give daily amount in two or more divided doses to maintain seizure control.

•When switching between phenytoin and fosphenytoin, remember that small differences in phenytoin bioavailability can lead to significant changes in blood phenytoin level and an increased risk of toxicity.

•If drug causes transient, infusion-related paresthesia and pruritus, decrease or discontinue infusion, as ordered.

•Monitor CBC for thrombocytopenia or leukopenia—signs of hematologic toxicity. Also monitor serum albumin level and results of renal and liver function tests.

•Anticipate increased frequency and severity of adverse reactions after I.V. administration in patients with hepatic or renal impairment or hypoalbuminemia.

•Discontinue drug, as ordered, if signs of hypersensitivity develop: acute hepatotoxicity (hepatic necrosis and hepatitis), fever, lymphadenopathy, and skin reactions during first 2 months of therapy.

•Monitor blood phenytoin level to detect early signs of toxicity, such as diplopia, nausea, severe confusion, slurred speech, and vomiting. Expect to reduce or stop drug if such signs develop.

•**WARNING** Monitor for seizures; at toxic levels, phenytoin is excitatory.

•**WARNING** If patient has bradycardia or heart block rhythm, notify prescriber and expect to withhold drug because severe cardiovascular reactions and death have occurred.

•Expect to provide vitamin D supplement if patient has inadequate dietary intake and is receiving long-term anticonvulsant treatment.

•Document type, onset, and characteristics of seizures as well as response to treatment.

**PATIENT TEACHING**

•Inform patient that fosphenytoin typically is used for short-term treatment.

•Instruct patient to notify prescriber immediately about bothersome symptoms, especially rash and swollen glands.

•Because gingival hyperplasia may develop during long-term therapy, emphasize the importance of good oral hygiene and gum massage.

•Urge patient to consume adequate amounts of vitamin D.

# frovatriptan succinate

Frova

## Class and Category

*Chemical:* Selective 5-hydroxytryptamine$_1$ (5-HT$_1$) receptor agonist, triptan
*Therapeutic:* Antimigraine agent
*Pregnancy category:* C

## Indications and Dosages

➤ *To treat acute migraine with or without aura*

**TABLETS**

**Adults.** 2.5 mg, repeated in 2 hr if needed. *Maximum:* 7.5 mg/day.

## Contraindications

Basilar or hemiplegic migraines; cerebrovascular, peripheral vascular, or ischemic or vasospastic coronary artery disease (CAD);

hypersensitivity to frovatriptan or its components; uncontrolled hypertension; use within 24 hours of other serotonin-receptor agonists or of ergotamine-containing or ergot-type drugs

## Mechanism of Action
Binds to selective 5-HT$_1$ receptors (5-HT$_{1B}$ and 5-HT$_{1D}$) on extracerebral and intracranial arteries to inhibit excessive dilation of these vessels. This action may decrease carotid arterial blood flow, thus relieving acute migraines. Frovatriptan may also relieve pain by inhibiting the release of proinflammatory neuropeptides and reducing transmission of trigeminal nerve impulses from sensory nerve endings during a migraine attack.

## Interactions
**DRUGS**
*dihydroergotamine mesylate, other ergotamine-containing drugs:* Possibly prolonged vasospastic reaction
*fluoxetine, other selective serotonin-reuptake inhibitors:* Possibly weakness, hyperreflexia, and incoordination
*oral contraceptives, propranolol:* Possibly increased blood frovatriptan level

## Adverse Reactions
**CNS:** Anxiety, dizziness, dysesthesia, fatigue, headache, hypoesthesia, insomnia, paresthesia
**CV:** Arrhythmias (such as bradycardia and tachycardia), chest pain, coronary artery vasospasm, ECG changes, MI, myocardial ischemia (transient), palpitations, ventricular fibrillation, ventricular tachycardia
**EENT:** Abnormal vision, dry mouth, indigestion, rhinitis, sinusitis, tinnitus
**GI:** Abdominal pain, diarrhea, indigestion, vomiting
**MS:** Skeletal pain
**SKIN:** Diaphoresis, flushing
**Other:** Generalized pain

## Nursing Considerations
•Be aware that frovatriptan is used cautiously in patients with peripheral vascular disease because drug may cause vasospastic reactions, leading to vascular and colonic ischemia with abdominal pain and bloody diarrhea. Assess patient's peripheral circulation and bowel sounds during therapy.
•Don't administer frovatriptan within 24 hours of another 5-HT$_1$ receptor agonist, such as sumatriptan or rizatriptan, or of an ergotamine-containing or ergot-type drug, such as dihydroergotamine or methysergide.
•Administer tablet with fluids.
•Assess patient for headache before administering second dose. Don't administer more than three 2.5-mg tablets a day.
•**WARNING** Be aware that some patients have experienced serious adverse cardiac reactions—including fatal ones—after using 5-HT$_1$ receptor agonists. However, these reactions are extremely rare; most were reported in patients with risk factors for CAD.
•Assess cardiovascular status and institute continuous ECG monitoring, as ordered, immediately after drug administration in patients with cardiovascular risk factors because they're at risk for asymptomatic cardiac ischemia.
•Assess for arrhythmias, chest pain, and other signs of heart disease in patients with risk factors for CAD. Expect to periodically assess cardiovascular status of patients on long-term therapy.
•Be aware that the safety of treating more than four migraine attacks in 30 days (on average) has not been established.
•Regularly monitor blood pressure of hypertensive patients during therapy because frovatriptan may produce a transient increase in blood pressure.

**PATIENT TEACHING**
•Instruct patient to read and follow manufacturer's instructions for using frovatriptan to ensure maximum therapeutic results.
•Remind patient not to exceed prescribed daily dosage.
•Encourage patient to lie down in a dark, quiet room after taking drug to help relieve migraine.
•Instruct patient to seek emergency care for chest, jaw, or neck tightness after drug use because drug may cause coronary artery vasospasm.
•Urge patient to report palpitations to prescriber.
•Caution patient about possible adverse CNS effects, and advise her to avoid hazardous activities until drug's CNS effects are known.

# furazolidone

Furoxone

## Class and Category

*Chemical:* MAO inhibitor, nitrofuran derivative
*Therapeutic:* Antibiotic, antiprotozoal
*Pregnancy category:* C

## Indications and Dosages

➤ *To treat bacterial diarrhea and cholera*
ORAL SUSPENSION, TABLETS
**Adults and adolescents.** 100 mg q 6 hr for 5 to 7 days.
**Infants and children age 1 month and older.** 1.25 mg/kg q 6 hr for 5 to 7 days. *Maximum:* 8.8 mg/kg/day.

➤ *To treat giardiasis*
ORAL SUSPENSION, TABLETS
**Adults and adolescents.** 100 mg q 6 hr for 7 to 10 days.
**Infants and children age 1 month and older.** 1.25 to 2 mg/kg q 6 hr for 7 to 10 days. *Maximum:* 8.8 mg/kg/day.

### Mechanism of Action

May interfere with several bacterial enzyme systems through DNA strand damage. Furazolidone also prevents the inactivation of tyramine by GI and hepatic MAO because it is similar in structure and actions to MAO inhibitors.

## Contraindications

Age less than 1 month; hypersensitivity to furazolidone, other nitrofurans, or their components

## Interactions

DRUGS
*levodopa:* Increased therapeutic and adverse effects (particularly hypertension) of levodopa
*meperidine:* Possibly agitation, apnea, coma, diaphoresis, fever, and seizures
*other MAO inhibitors, sedatives, sympathomimetics, tranquilizers, tricyclic antidepressants:* Possibly sudden and severe hypertensive crisis
*selective serotonin reuptake inhibitors:* Increased risk of serotonin syndrome
FOODS
*foods and beverages with high content of tyramine or other vasopressor amines:*

Possibly sudden and severe hypertensive crisis
ACTIVITIES
*alcohol use:* Possibly disulfiram-like reaction

## Adverse Reactions

**CNS:** Headache, malaise
**ENDO:** Hypoglycemia
**GI:** Abdominal pain, diarrhea, nausea, vomiting
**GU:** Darkened urine
**HEME:** Hemolytic anemia, leukopenia
**Other:** Allergic reaction (arthralgia, dyspnea, fever, hypotension, urticaria, vesicular morbilliform rash)

## Nursing Considerations

•Ask patient if she has a history of blood disorders—especially glucose-6-phosphate dehydrogenase (G6PD) deficiency—before giving furazolidone.
•As ordered, check G6PD level before giving furazolidone to whites of Mediterranean and Near Eastern origin, Asians, or blacks; G6PD deficiency may worsen drug's hemolytic effect.
•If no response occurs within 7 days, expect to discontinue drug because organism is resistant. Provide therapy with other antibiotics, as prescribed.
•If giardiasis symptoms persist, expect to obtain three stool specimens for analysis several days apart, starting 3 to 4 weeks after treatment ends.
PATIENT TEACHING
•Instruct patient to take drug at evenly spaced intervals around the clock.
•Advise patient to take drug with food if GI distress occurs.
•Direct patient to take a missed dose as soon as she remembers, unless it's nearly time for the next scheduled dose. Caution against double-dosing.
•Instruct patient to take furazolidone for the full time prescribed because stopping too soon could result in reinfection.
•Advise patient to store furazolidone between 59° and 86° F (15° and 30° C), protected from moisture and light.
•Inform patient that drug may cause dizziness and usually turns urine brown.
•Instruct patient to avoid alcohol during therapy and for 4 days afterward.
•Give patient a list of products to avoid during furazolidone therapy and for at least 2

weeks afterward, such as foods and beverages that contain tyramine and other vasopressor amines (for example, ripe cheese, beer, red and white wine, and smoked or pickled meat, poultry, or fish), OTC appetite suppressants, cough and cold medicines, and other drugs, unless prescribed.
• Instruct patient to notify prescriber if she experiences difficult breathing, fever, flushing, itching, muscle aches, or rash.

# furosemide

Apo-Furosemide (CAN), Furoside (CAN), Lasix, Lasix Special (CAN), Myrosemide, Novosemide (CAN), Uritol (CAN)

## Class and Category

*Chemical:* Sulfonamide
*Therapeutic:* Antihypertensive, diuretic
*Pregnancy category:* C

## Indications and Dosages

➤ *To reduce edema caused by cirrhosis, heart failure, and renal disease, including nephrotic syndrome*

ORAL SOLUTION, TABLETS

**Adults.** 20 to 80 mg as a single dose, increased by 20 to 40 mg q 6 to 8 hr until desired response occurs. *Maximum:* 600 mg/day.
**Children.** 2 mg/kg as a single dose, increased by 1 to 2 mg/kg q 6 to 8 hr until desired response occurs. *Maximum:* 6 mg/kg/dose.

I.V. INFUSION, I.V. OR I.M. INJECTION

**Adults.** 20 to 40 mg as a single dose, increased by 20 mg q 2 hr until desired response occurs.
**Children.** 1 mg/kg as a single dose, increased by 1 mg/kg q 2 hr until desired response occurs. *Maximum:* 6 mg/kg/dose.
DOSAGE ADJUSTMENT Initial single dose limited to 20 mg for elderly patients.

➤ *To manage mild to moderate hypertension, as adjunct to treat acute pulmonary edema and hypertensive crisis*

ORAL SOLUTION, TABLETS

**Adults.** *Initial:* 40 mg b.i.d., adjusted until desired response occurs. *Maximum:* 600 mg/day.

I.V. INFUSION OR INJECTION

**Adults with normal renal function.** 40 to 80 mg as a single dose over several minutes.
**Adults with acute renal failure or pulmonary edema.** 100 to 200 mg as a single dose over several minutes.

DOSAGE ADJUSTMENT For patients with acute pulmonary edema without hypertensive crisis, dosage reduced to 40 mg followed by 80 mg 1 hr later if therapeutic response doesn't occur.

| Route | Onset | Peak | Duration |
|-------|-------|------|----------|
| P.O. | 20 to 60 min | 1 to 2 hr | 6 to 8 hr |
| I.V. | 5 min | In 30 min | 2 hr |
| I.M. | 30 min | Unknown | 2 hr |

## Mechanism of Action

Inhibits sodium and water reabsorption in the loop of Henle and increases urine formation. As the body's plasma volume decreases, aldosterone production increases, which promotes sodium reabsorption and the loss of potassium and hydrogen ions. Furosemide also increases the excretion of calcium, magnesium, bicarbonate, ammonium, and phosphate. By reducing intracellular and extracellular fluid volume, the drug reduces blood pressure and decreases cardiac output. Over time, cardiac output returns to normal.

## Incompatibilities

Don't mix furosemide (a milky, buffered alkaline solution) with highly acidic solutions.

## Contraindications

Anuria unresponsive to furosemide; hypersensitivity to furosemide, sulfonamides, or their components

## Interactions

DRUGS

*ACE inhibitors:* Possibly first-dose hypotension
*aminoglycosides, cisplatin:* Increased risk of ototoxicity
*amiodarone:* Increased risk of arrhythmias from hypokalemia
*chloral hydrate:* Possibly diaphoresis, hot flashes, and hypertension
*digoxin:* Increased risk of digitalis toxicity related to hypokalemia
*insulin, oral antidiabetic drugs:* Increased blood glucose level
*lithium:* Increased risk of lithium toxicity
*NSAIDs:* Possibly decreased diuresis
*phenytoin, probenecid:* Possibly decreased therapeutic effects of furosemide

*propranolol*: Possibly increased blood propranolol level
*thiazide diuretics*: Possibly profound diuresis and electrolyte imbalances
**ACTIVITIES**
*alcohol use*: Possibly increased hypotensive and diuretic effects of furosemide

## Adverse Reactions
**CNS:** Dizziness, fever, headache, paresthesia, restlessness, vertigo, weakness
**CV:** Orthostatic hypotension, shock, thromboembolism, thrombophlebitis
**EENT:** Blurred vision, ototoxicity, stomatitis, tinnitus, transient hearing loss (rapid I.V. injection), yellow vision
**ENDO:** Hyperglycemia
**GI:** Abdominal cramps, anorexia, constipation, diarrhea, indigestion, nausea, pancreatitis, vomiting
**GU:** Bladder spasms, glycosuria
**HEME:** Agranulocytosis (rare), anemia, aplastic anemia (rare), azotemia, hemolytic anemia, leukopenia, thrombocytopenia
**MS:** Muscle spasms
**SKIN:** Erythema multiforme, exfoliative dermatitis, jaundice, photosensitivity, pruritus, purpura, rash, urticaria
**Other:** Allergic reaction (interstitial nephritis, necrotizing vasculitis, systemic vasculitis), dehydration, hyperuricemia, hypochloremia, hypokalemia, hyponatremia, hypovolemia

## Nursing Considerations
•**WARNING** Use furosemide cautiously in patients with advanced hepatic cirrhosis, especially those who also have a history of electrolyte imbalance or hepatic encephalopathy; drug may lead to lethal hepatic coma.
•Obtain patient's weight before and periodically during furosemide therapy to monitor fluid loss.
•For once-a-day dosing, give drug in the morning so patient's sleep won't be interrupted by increased need to urinate.
•Prepare drug for infusion with NS, LR, or D$_5$W.
•Administer drug slowly I.V. over 1 to 2 minutes to prevent ototoxicity.
•Expect patient to have periodic hearing tests during prolonged or high-dose I.V. therapy.
•Monitor blood pressure and hepatic and renal function as well as BUN, blood glucose, and serum creatinine, electrolyte, and uric acid levels, as appropriate.

•Be aware that elderly patients are more susceptible to hypotensive and electrolyte-altering effects and thus are at greater risk for shock and thromboembolism.
•If patient is at high risk for hypokalemia, give potassium supplements along with furosemide, as prescribed.
•Expect to discontinue furosemide at maximum dosage if oliguria persists for more than 24 hours.
•Be aware that furosemide may worsen left ventricular hypertrophy and adversely affect glucose tolerance and lipid metabolism.
•Notify prescriber if patient experiences hearing loss, vertigo, or ringing, buzzing, or sense of fullness in her ears. Drug may need to be discontinued.
**PATIENT TEACHING**
•Instruct patient to take furosemide at the same time each day to maintain therapeutic effects. Urge her to take it as prescribed, even if she feels well.
•Instruct patient to take the last dose of furosemide several hours before bedtime to avoid sleep interruption from diuresis. If patient receives once-daily dosing, advise her to take the dose in the morning to avoid sleep disturbance caused by nocturia.
•Advise patient to change position slowly to minimize effects of orthostatic hypotension and to take furosemide with food or milk to reduce GI distress.
•Caution patient about drinking alcoholic beverages, standing for prolonged periods, and exercising in hot weather because these actions increase the hypotensive effect of furosemide.
•Emphasize the importance of weight and diet control, especially limiting sodium intake.
•Unless contraindicated, urge patient to eat more high-potassium foods and to take a potassium supplement, if prescribed, to prevent hypokalemia.
•Instruct patient to keep follow-up appointments with prescriber to monitor progress. Urge her to notify prescriber about persistent, severe nausea, vomiting, and diarrhea because they may cause dehydration.
•Inform diabetic patient that furosemide may increase blood glucose level, and advise her to check her blood glucose level frequently.

E
F

# G·H·I

## gabapentin

Neurontin

### Class and Category

*Chemical:* Cyclohexane-acetic acid derivative
*Therapeutic:* Anticonvulsant
*Pregnancy category:* C

### Indications and Dosages

➤ *To manage postherpetic neuralgia*
**CAPSULES, ORAL SOLUTION, TABLETS**
**Adults.** *Initial:* 300 mg on day 1, increased to 300 mg b.i.d. on day 2, increased to 300 mg t.i.d. on day 3, and increased gradually thereafter according to pain response, up to 600 mg t.i.d. *Maximum:* 1,800 mg/day.
➤ *As adjunct to treat partial seizures*
**CAPSULES, ORAL SOLUTION, TABLETS**
**Adults and adolescents.** *Initial:* 300 mg t.i.d., increased gradually according to clinical response. *Maintenance:* 900 to 1,800 mg/day. *Maximum:* 3,600 mg/day.
**DOSAGE ADJUSTMENT** Dosage reduced to 300 mg b.i.d. if creatinine clearance is 30 to 60 ml/min/1.73 m$^2$; to 300 mg q.d. if it's 15 to 29 ml/min/1.73 m$^2$; and to 300 mg q.o.d. if it's less than 15 ml/min/1.73 m$^2$.

---

### Mechanism of Action

Is structurally like gamma-aminobutyric acid (GABA), the main inhibitory neurotransmitter in the brain. Although gabapentin's exact mechanism of action is unknown, GABA inhibits the rapid firing of neurons associated with seizures.

---

### Contraindications

Hypersensitivity to gabapentin or its components

### Interactions

**DRUGS**
*aluminum- and magnesium-containing antacids:* Decreased gabapentin bioavailability

*CNS depressants:* Increased CNS depression
**ACTIVITIES**
*alcohol use:* Increased CNS depression

### Adverse Reactions

**CNS:** Agitation, altered proprioception, amnesia, anxiety, apathy, aphasia, asthenia, ataxia, cerebellar dysfunction, chills, CNS tumors, decreased or absent reflexes, delusions, depersonalization, depression, dizziness, dream disturbances, dysesthesia, dystonia, emotional lability, euphoria, facial paralysis, fatigue, fever, hallucinations, headache, hemiplegia, hostility, hyperkinesia, hyperreflexia, hypoesthesia, hypotonia, intracranial hemorrhage, lack of coordination, malaise, migraine headache, nervousness, occipital neuralgia, paranoia, paresis, paresthesia, positive Babinski's sign, psychosis, sedation, seizures, somnolence, stupor, subdural hematoma, suicidal tendencies, syncope, tremor, vertigo
**CV:** Angina, hypertension, hypotension, murmur, palpitations, peripheral edema, peripheral vascular insufficiency, tachycardia, vasodilation
**EENT:** Abnormal vision, amblyopia, blepharospasm, cataracts, conjunctivitis, diplopia, dry eyes and mouth, earache, epistaxis, eye hemorrhage, eye pain, gingival bleeding, gingivitis, glossitis, hearing loss, increased salivation, inner ear infection, loss of taste, nystagmus, pharyngitis, photophobia, ptosis (bilateral or unilateral), rhinitis, sensation of fullness in ears, stomatitis, taste perversion, tinnitus, tooth discoloration, visual field defects
**GI:** Abdominal pain, anorexia, constipation, diarrhea, fecal incontinence, flatulence, gastroenteritis, hemorrhoids, hepatitis, hepatomegaly, increased appetite, indigestion, melena, nausea, thirst, vomiting
**GU:** Decreased libido, impotence
**HEME:** Anemia, coagulation defect, decreased WBC count, leukopenia, thrombocytopenia
**MS:** Arthralgia, arthritis, back pain, bone fractures, dysarthria, joint stiffness or swelling, muscle twitching, myalgia, positive Romberg test, tendinitis
**RESP:** Apnea, cough, dyspnea, pneumonia, pseudocroup
**SKIN:** Abrasion, acne, alopecia, cyst, diaphoresis, dry skin, eczema, hirsutism, pruritus, purpura, rash, seborrhea, urticaria
**Other:** Facial edema, lymphadenopathy, viral infection, weight gain or loss

G
H
I

## Nursing Considerations
- As needed, open gabapentin capsules and mix contents with water, fruit juice, applesauce, or pudding before administration.
- Administer initial dose at bedtime to minimize adverse reactions, especially ataxia, dizziness, fatigue, and somnolence.
- Give drug at least 2 hours after giving an antacid.
- Don't exceed 12 hours between doses on a 3-times-a-day schedule.
- Be aware that routine monitoring of blood gabapentin level isn't necessary.
- **WARNING** To discontinue drug or switch to an alternate anticonvulsant, expect to change gradually over at least 1 week, as prescribed, to avoid loss of seizure control.
- Monitor renal function test results, and expect to adjust dosage, if necessary.

### PATIENT TEACHING
- If patient has trouble swallowing gabapentin capsules, advise him to open them and sprinkle contents in juice or on soft food immediately before use.
- Instruct patient not to take drug within 2 hours after taking an antacid.
- Urge patient to take a missed dose as soon as he remembers. If the next dose is in less than 2 hours, tell him to wait 1 to 2 hours before taking it and then resume his regular schedule. Caution against doubling the dose.
- Caution patient not to stop drug abruptly.
- Inform patient about possible ataxia, dizziness, drowsiness, and nystagmus. Advise him to avoid potentially hazardous activities until drug's CNS effects are known.
- To prevent complications from adverse oral reactions (such as gingivitis), encourage patient to use good oral hygiene and to seek routine dental care.
- Inform patient that drug's adverse effects usually are mild to moderate and decline with continued use.
- Urge patient to keep follow-up appointments with prescriber to check progress.

# galantamine hydrobromide

Razadyne, Razadyne ER

## Class and Category
*Chemical:* Tertiary alkaloid
*Therapeutic:* Antidementia agent
*Pregnancy category:* B

## Indications and Dosages
➤ *To treat mild to moderate Alzheimer's-type dementia*
**ORAL SOLUTION, TABLETS**
**Adults.** *Initial:* 4 mg b.i.d. Dosage increased by 8 mg/day q 4 wk, if tolerated. *Maximum:* 12 mg b.i.d.
**DOSAGE ADJUSTMENT** For patients with moderately impaired hepatic or renal function, maximum dosage shouldn't exceed 16 mg/day.
**E.R. CAPSULES**
**Adults.** *Initial:* 8 mg/day. Dosage increased by 8 mg/day q 4 wk if tolerated. *Maximum:* 24 mg/day.

| Route | Onset | Peak | Duration |
|-------|-------|------|----------|
| P.O. | Unknown | About 1 hr | Unknown |

### Mechanism of Action
Reduces acetylcholine metabolism by competitively and reversibly inhibiting the brain enzyme acetylcholinesterase. Acetylcholine-producing neurons degenerate in the brains of patients with Alzheimer's disease. Inhibition of acetylcholinesterase increases the amount of acetylcholine, which is necessary for nerve impulse transmission.

## Contraindications
Hypersensitivity to galantamine hydrobromide or its components, severe hepatic or renal impairment (creatinine clearance less than 9 ml/min/1.73 m$^2$)

## Interactions
### DRUGS
*amitriptyline, fluoxetine, fluvoxamine, quinidine:* Possibly decreased galantamine clearance
*anticholinergics:* Possibly interference with cholinesterase activity
*cholinergic agonists, cholinesterase inhibitors, neuromuscular blockers:* Possibly exaggerated effects of these drugs and galantamine
*cimetidine:* Possibly increased galantamine bioavailability
*ketoconazole, paroxetine:* Increased galantamine bioavailability

## Adverse Reactions
**CNS:** Aggression, depression, dizziness, fatigue, headache, insomnia, somnolence, syncope, tremor
**CV:** Bradycardia
**EENT:** Rhinitis

**GI:** Abdominal pain, anorexia, diarrhea, GI bleeding, indigestion, nausea, vomiting
**GU:** Hematuria, renal failure or insufficiency, UTI
**HEME:** Anemia
**Other:** Dehydration, hypokalemia, weight loss

## Nursing Considerations
• Administer galantamine twice daily with morning and evening meals, and ensure adequate fluid intake to prevent GI symptoms.
• If therapy is interrupted for several days, expect to restart drug at lowest dose because drug's benefits are lost when it is discontinued.
• Monitor patient for progressive deterioration of mental status because drug is less effective as Alzheimer's disease progresses and intact cholinergic neurons decrease.

### PATIENT TEACHING
• Instruct patient or caregiver to give regular-strength drug with morning and evening meals. Extended-release capsules should be given once in the morning, with food.
• Tell patient or caregiver to notify prescriber immediately if therapy is stopped for several days. Prescriber may restart at lowest dose.
• Advise patient not to drive or perform activities requiring high levels of alertness, especially during first weeks of treatment, because drug may cause dizziness and drowsiness.
• Inform patient and family members that drug isn't a cure for Alzheimer's disease.

# gatifloxacin
Tequin

## Class and Category
*Chemical:* Fluoroquinolone
*Therapeutic:* Antibiotic
*Pregnancy category:* C

## Indications and Dosages
➤ *To treat acute bacterial exacerbations of chronic bronchitis caused by* Haemophilus influenzae, H. parainfluenzae, Moraxella catarrhalis, Staphylococcus aureus, *or* Streptococcus pneumoniae
**TABLETS, I.V. INFUSION**
**Adults.** 400 mg q.d. for 5 days.
➤ *To treat complicated UTIs caused by* Escherichia coli, Klebsiella pneumoniae, *or* Proteus mirabilis; *acute pyelonephritis caused by* E. coli; *and uncomplicated skin and skin-structure infections caused by* S. aureus *(methicillin-*

*susceptible strains only) or* Streptococcus pyogenes
**TABLETS, I.V. INFUSION**
**Adults.** 400 mg q.d. for 7 to 10 days.
➤ *To treat acute sinusitis due to* H. influenzae *or* S. pneumoniae
**TABLETS, I.V. INFUSION**
**Adults.** 400 mg q.d. for 10 days.
➤ *To treat community-acquired pneumonia caused by* Chlamydia pneumoniae, H. influenzae, H. parainfluenzae, Legionella pneumophila, M. catarrhalis, Mycoplasma pneumoniae, S. aureus, *or* S. pneumoniae
**TABLETS, I.V. INFUSION**
**Adults.** 400 mg q.d. for 7 to 14 days.
➤ *To treat uncomplicated cystitis caused by* E. coli, K. pneumoniae, *or* P. mirabilis
**TABLETS, I.V. INFUSION**
**Adults.** 400 mg as a single dose or 200 mg q.d. for 3 days.
➤ *To treat uncomplicated urethral gonorrhea in men, and cervical and acute rectal gonorrhea in women caused by* Neisseria gonorrhoeae
**TABLETS, I.V. INFUSION**
**Adults.** 400 mg as a single dose.
**DOSAGE ADJUSTMENT** For patients with creatinine clearance less than 40 ml/min/1.73 m$^2$ and those receiving hemodialysis or continuous peritoneal dialysis, initial dose of 400 mg is followed by reduced dosage of 200 mg q.d., as prescribed. No dosage adjustment is required for single-dose treatments or for treatment of uncomplicated cystitis.

## Mechanism of Action
Interferes with bacterial cell replication by inhibiting the bacterial enzyme DNA gyrase needed for replication, transcription, and repair of bacterial DNA. Gatifloxacin also inhibits topoisomerase IV, an enzyme involved in partitioning chromosomal DNA during bacterial cell division.

## Contraindications
Hypersensitivity to gatifloxacin, other fluoroquinolones, or their components

## Interactions
### DRUGS
*aluminum-, magnesium-, or zinc-containing antacids:* Reduced GI absorption and blood level of gatifloxacin

G
H
I

*antipsychotics; cisapride; class IA antiarrhythmics, such as procainamide and quinidine; class III antiarrhythmics, such as amiodarone and sotalol; erythromycin; tricyclic antidepressants:* Possibly prolonged QT interval, leading to torsades de pointes
*iron:* Possibly reduced gatifloxacin efficacy
*oral antidiabetic drugs:* Possibly altered glucose control
*probenecid:* Increased blood level and sustained half-life of gatifloxacin

### Adverse Reactions

**CNS:** Chills, dizziness, fever, headache, insomnia, nightmares, paresthesia, peripheral neuropathy, syncope, tremor, vertigo
**CV:** Chest pain, hypotension, palpitations, peripheral edema, prolonged QT interval, torsades de pointes, vasodilation
**ENDO:** Hyperglycemia, hyperosmolar nonketotic coma, hypoglycemia, hypoglycemic coma
**EENT:** Abnormal vision, glossitis, mouth ulcers, oral candidiasis, pharyngitis, stomatitis, taste perversion, tinnitus
**GI:** Abdominal pain, constipation, diarrhea, hepatitis, indigestion, nausea, pancreatitis, vomiting
**GU:** Acute renal failure, dysuria, hematuria, renal insufficiency, vaginitis
**HEME:** Thrombocytopenia
**MS:** Back pain, tendon rupture
**RESP:** Dyspnea
**SKIN:** Diaphoresis, rash, Stevens-Johnson syndrome
**Other:** Anaphylaxis, angioedema, infusion site inflammation

### Nursing Considerations

•Monitor patient's renal function during therapy, as ordered, because decreased renal function may delay drug elimination.
•Administer oral gatifloxacin at least 4 hours before or after preparations containing aluminum, magnesium, zinc, or iron.
•Reconstitute gatifloxacin concentrate for infusion with $D_5W$, NS, 0.45NS, $D_5LR$, 5% sodium bicarbonate, Plasma-Lyte 56 and $D_5W$, or M/6 sodium lactate to yield 2 mg/ml. Use 5% sodium bicarbonate solutions immediately, as prescribed. Be aware that premixed flexible bags need no further dilution.
•Don't add other drugs to gatifloxacin injection or infuse gatifloxacin through same I.V. line as other drugs. Use I.V. solution only

if clear and light yellow or greenish yellow. Discard if particulate matter is present.
•To avoid too rapid or bolus delivery, use an infusion pump to infuse I.V. solution over 60 minutes.
•**WARNING** Be aware that gatifloxacin may prolong the QTc interval, increasing the risk of ventricular arrhythmias, especially in patients with hypokalemia and those taking quinidine, procainamide, amiodarone, or sotalol.
•Assess patient for nightmares and insomnia because drug may cause excessive CNS stimulation. If these problems occur, notify prescriber immediately and expect to stop drug.
•Monitor blood glucose level in patients with diabetes to detect hypoglycemia or hyperglycemia, which may be caused by gatifloxacin.
•Be aware that use of any fluoroquinolone may increase the risk of tendon rupture.

**PATIENT TEACHING**
•Instruct patient to complete the full course of gatifloxacin therapy, as prescribed.
•Advise patient to take drug at least 4 hours before or after preparations containing aluminum, magnesium, iron, or zinc.
•Instruct patient to notify prescriber at first sign of allergic reaction, such as rash, and if palpitations or fainting spells occur.
•Urge patient to notify prescriber immediately about tendon pain, inflammation, or rupture.
•Advise diabetic patient taking oral antidiabetic drugs to monitor blood glucose level often and notify prescriber of significant changes.
•Instruct patient to inform all prescribers about gatifloxacin therapy to prevent potentially serious drug interactions.

# gemfibrozil

Apo-Gemfibrozil (CAN), Gen-Fibro (CAN), Lopid, Novo-Gemfibrozil (CAN), Nu-Gemfibrozil (CAN)

### Class and Category

*Chemical:* Fibric acid derivative, phenoxypentanoic acid
*Therapeutic:* Antihyperlipidemic
*Pregnancy category:* C

### Indications and Dosages

➤ *As adjunct (with diet) to treat hyperlipidemia types IIb, IV, and V*

CAPSULES, TABLETS
**Adults.** 600 mg a.c. b.i.d.

| Route | Onset | Peak | Duration |
|-------|-------|------|----------|
| P.O. | 2 to 5 days | 4 wk | Unknown |

## Mechanism of Action

May decrease hepatic triglyceride production by reducing VLDL synthesis, inhibiting peripheral lipolysis, and decreasing hepatic extraction of free fatty acids. Gemfibrozil also may inhibit synthesis and increase clearance of apolipoprotein B, a carrier molecule for VLDL. In addition, it may accelerate turnover and removal of total cholesterol from the liver while increasing cholesterol excretion into the feces. As a result of these actions, triglyceride, total cholesterol, and VLDL levels decrease; the HDL level increases; and the LDL level is unaffected.

## Contraindications

Gallbladder disease, hepatic or severe renal dysfunction, hypersensitivity to gemfibrozil or its components

## Interactions

**DRUGS**
*chenodiol, ursodiol:* Decreased effectiveness of gemfibrozil
*HMG-CoA reductase inhibitors:* Increased risk of rhabdomyolysis and acute renal failure
*oral anticoagulants*: Increased anticoagulation
*repaglinide:* Increased serum repaglinide level

## Adverse Reactions

**CNS:** Chills, fatigue, headache, hypoesthesia, paresthesia, seizures, somnolence, syncope, vertigo
**CV:** Vasculitis
**EENT:** Blurred vision, cataracts, hoarseness, retinal edema, taste perversion
**GI:** Abdominal or epigastric pain, cholelithiasis, colitis, diarrhea, flatulence, heartburn, hepatoma, nausea, pancreatitis, vomiting
**GU:** Decreased male fertility, dysuria, impotence
**HEME:** Anemia, bone marrow hypoplasia, eosinophilia, leukopenia, thrombocytopenia
**MS:** Arthralgia, back pain, myalgia, myasthenia, myopathy, myositis, rhabdomyolysis, synovitis
**RESP:** Cough

**SKIN:** Eczema, jaundice, pruritus, rash
**Other:** Anaphylaxis, angioedema, increased risk of bacterial and viral infections, lupus-like symptoms, weight loss

## Nursing Considerations

• Monitor serum triglyceride and cholesterol levels, as appropriate.
• Periodically review CBC and liver function test results during therapy, as ordered.
• If serum triglyceride and cholesterol levels don't improve within 3 months, expect to switch to a different drug, as prescribed.

**PATIENT TEACHING**
• Instruct patient to take gemfibrozil 30 minutes before breakfast and 30 minutes before dinner.
• Advise patient to take a missed dose as soon as he remembers, unless it's nearly time for the next dose. Caution against double-dosing.
• Stress the importance of a low-fat diet, regular exercise, alcohol avoidance, and smoking cessation, as appropriate.
• Caution patient to avoid potentially hazardous activities until drug's CNS effects are known.
• Instruct patient to notify prescriber if he experiences chills; cough; fever; hoarseness; lower back, side, or muscle pain; painful or difficult urination; severe abdominal pain with nausea and vomiting; tiredness; or weakness.
• If patient also takes an oral anticoagulant, urge him to report unusual bleeding or bruising; anticoagulant dosage may need to be reduced.
• Advise patient to keep scheduled appointments with prescriber to check progress.

# gemifloxacin mesylate

Factive

## Class and Category

*Chemical:* Fluoroquinolone
*Therapeutic:* Antibiotic
*Pregnancy category:* C

## Indications and Dosages

➤ *To treat acute bacterial exacerbation of chronic bronchitis caused by* Streptococcus pneumoniae, Haemophilus influenzae, H. parainfluenzae, *or* Moraxella catarrhalis

**TABLETS**
**Adults.** 320 mg q.d. for 5 days.

➤ *To treat mild to moderate community-acquired pneumonia caused by* S. pneumoniae, H. influenzae, M. catarrhalis, Mycoplasma pneumoniae, Chlamydia pneumoniae, *or* Klebsiella pneumoniae

**TABLETS**

**Adults.** 320 mg q.d. for 7 days.

**DOSAGE ADJUSTMENT** Dosage should be decreased to 160 mg q.d. in patients with creatinine clearance of 40 ml/min/1.73 m² or less.

| Route | Onset | Peak | Duration |
|---|---|---|---|
| P.O. | 0.5-2 hr | Unknown | Unknown |

### Mechanism of Action

Inhibits the actions of the enzymes DNA gyrase and topoisomerase IV, which are required for bacterial growth, and thereby causing bacterial cells to die.

## Contraindications

Hypersensitivity to gemifloxacin, its components, or other fluroroquinolones

## Interactions

**DRUGS**

*aluminum and magnesium antacids, didanosine as chewable or buffered tablets or pediatric powder for oral solution, ferrous sulfate, sucralfate, zinc or other metal cations:* Reduced blood gemifloxacin level

*antipsychotics; class Ia antiarrhythmics, such as procainamide and quinidine; class III antiarrhythmics, such as amiodarone and sotalol; erythromycin; tricyclic antidepressants:* Possibly prolonged QT interval

*probenecid:* Increased blood gemifloxacin level

*warfarin:* Possibly enhanced warfarin anticoagulant effects

## Adverse Reactions

**CNS:** Dizziness, headache
**CV:** Prolonged QT interval
**EENT:** Taste perversion
**GI:** Abdominal pain, diarrhea, elevated liver function test results, nausea, pseudomembranous colitis, vomiting
**SKIN:** Photosensitivity, rash, urticaria
**OTHER:** Anaphylaxis

## Nursing Considerations

•Review patient's medical history before administering gemifloxacin, which should not be used in a patient with a history of pro-longed QT interval, in patients with uncorrected electrolyte disorders, or in patients receiving class IA or III antiarrhythmics because of a heightened risk for prolonged QT interval.

•Use cautiously in patients with CNS disorders, such as epilepsy, or in those prone to seizures because other fluroquinolones have caused seizures, increased intracranial pressure, and toxic psychosis. Monitor patient closely; if CNS alterations occur, notify prescriber immediately and expect drug to be discontinued.

•Monitor patient closely for a hypersensitivity reaction that can occur as soon as the first dose. If signs of hypersensitivity, such as angioedema, bronchospasm, dyspnea, itching, rash, shortness of breath, and urticaria, occur, notify prescriber immediately.

•Monitor patients who are prone to tendinitis, such as the elderly, athletes, and those taking corticosteroids, for complaints of tendon pain, inflammation, or rupture. If present, notify prescriber; expect gemifloxacin to be discontinued, patient placed on bedrest with no exercise of the suspected limb, and diagnostic studies ordered to confirm rupture.

•Notify prescriber if severe or prolonged diarrhea develops; it may indicate pseudomembranous colitis.

•Monitor patients, especially women under age 40 and postmenopausal women who are receiving hormone replacement therapy, for rash. Rash may appear days after therapy is initiated and resolve in 7 days. Notify prescriber immediately if rash occurs because it can be severe in about 10% of patients.

**PATIENT TEACHING**

•Tell patient to swallow tablet whole and take with a full glass of liquid.

•Warn patient not to increase dose because doing so may cause life-threatening cardiac arrhythmias.

•Instruct patient to complete entire course of therapy, even if symptoms decrease before prescription is finished.

•Caution patient to avoid sun exposure as much as possible while taking gemifloxacin. Patient who can't avoid sun exposure should apply sunscreen and wear a hat, sunglasses, and long sleeves to cover as much skin as possible.

•Instruct patient to maintain adequate hydration throughout therapy to keep urine from becoming too concentrated. Tell patient to increase fluid intake if urine darkens or amount voided decreases.

• Caution patient to avoid performing hazardous activities until the CNS effects of the drug are known.

• Instruct patient to seek medical attention and notify prescriber immediately if he experiences tendon pain, tenderness, or rupture; signs and symptoms of a hypersensitivity reaction, such as rash, urticaria, difficulty breathing, or facial swelling; palpitations or fainting spells; or diarrhea. The drug may need to be stopped.

• Tell patient to consult prescriber before starting any new medications, including OTC products, because gemifloxacin may interact adversely.

• Inform patient that antacids containing magnesium and/or aluminum; products containing iron; multivitamin preparations containing zinc or other metal cations; and didanosine (Videx) chewable or buffered tablets and pediatric powder for oral solution (if prescribed) should not be taken within 3 hours before or 2 hours after taking gemifloxacin and that gemifloxacin should be taken at least 2 hours before sucralfate (if prescribed).

# gentamicin sulfate

Cidomycin (CAN), Garamycin, G-Mycin, Jenamicin

## Class and Category

*Chemical:* Aminoglycoside derived from *Micromonospora purpurea*
*Therapeutic:* Antibiotic
*Pregnancy category:* D

## Indications and Dosages

➤ *To treat serious bacterial infections caused by aerobic gram-negative organisms and some gram-positive organisms, including* Citrobacter *sp.,* Enterobacter *sp.,* Escherichia coli, Klebsiella *sp.,* Proteus *sp.,* Pseudomonas aeruginosa, Serratia *sp.,* Staphylococcus aureus, *and many strains of* Streptococcus *sp.*

I.V. INFUSION, I.M. INJECTION
**Adults and adolescents.** 1 to 1.7 mg/kg q 8 hr for 7 to 10 days.
**Children.** 2 to 2.5 mg/kg q 8 hr for 7 to 10 days.
**Infants.** 2.5 mg/kg q 8 to 16 hr for 7 to 10 days.

**Premature or full-term neonates up to age 1 week.** 2.5 mg/kg q 12 to 24 hr for 7 to 10 days.

INTRATHECAL (INTRALUMBAR OR INTRAVENTRICULAR) INJECTION
**Adults and adolescents.** 4 to 8 mg q.d.
**Infants and children age 3 months and older.** 1 to 2 mg q.d.

➤ *To treat uncomplicated UTIs*

I.V. INFUSION, I.M. INJECTION
**Adults and adolescents who weigh more than 60 kg (132 lb).** 160 mg q.d. or 80 mg q 12 hr.
**Adults and adolescents who weigh less than 60 kg.** 3 mg/kg q.d. or 1.5 mg/kg q 12 hr.

DOSAGE ADJUSTMENT Supplemental dose of 1 to 1.7 mg/kg (2 to 2.5 mg/kg for children) given by I.M. injection or I.V. infusion after hemodialysis, based on infection severity.

## Mechanism of Action

Binds to negatively charged sites on the outer cell membrane of bacteria, thereby disrupting the membrane's integrity. Gentamicin also binds to bacterial ribosomal subunits and inhibits protein synthesis. Both actions lead to cell death.

## Incompatibilities

Don't administer gentamicin through same I.V. line as other drugs, especially beta-lactam antibiotics (penicillins and cephalosporins), because substantial mutual inactivation may occur. Give drugs through separate sites.

## Contraindications

Hypersensitivity or serious toxic reaction to other aminoglycosides, hypersensitivity to gentamicin or its components

## Interactions

DRUGS
*aminoglycosides (concurrent use of two or more):* Decreased bacterial uptake of each drug, increased risk of ototoxicity and nephrotoxicity
*cephalosporins, enflurane, methoxyflurane, vancomycin:* Increased risk of nephrotoxicity
*loop diuretics:* Increased risk of ototoxicity and nephrotoxicity
*neuromuscular blockers:* Prolonged respiratory depression, increased neuromuscular blockade
*penicillins:* Inactivation of gentamicin by certain penicillins, increased risk of nephrotoxicity

## Adverse Reactions

**CNS:** Acute organic mental syndrome, confusion, depression, fever, headache, increased protein in cerebrospinal fluid, lethargy, myasthenia gravis–like syndrome, neurotoxicity (dizziness, hearing loss, tinnitus, vertigo), peripheral neuropathy or encephalopathy (muscle twitching, numbness, seizures, skin tingling), pseudotumor cerebri
**CV:** Hypertension, hypotension, palpitations
**EENT:** Blurred vision, increased salivation, laryngeal edema, ototoxicity, stomatitis, vision changes
**GI:** Anorexia, nausea, splenomegaly, transient hepatomegaly, vomiting
**GU:** Nephrotoxicity
**HEME:** Anemia, eosinophilia, granulocytopenia, increased or decreased reticulocyte count, leukopenia, thrombocytopenia
**MS:** Arthralgia, leg cramps
**RESP:** Pulmonary fibrosis, respiratory depression
**SKIN:** Alopecia, generalized burning sensation, pruritus, purpura, rash, urticaria
**Other:** Anaphylaxis, injection site pain, superinfection, weight loss

## Nursing Considerations

•Before gentamicin therapy begins, expect to obtain a body fluid or tissue specimen for culture and sensitivity testing, as ordered, or check test results, if available.
•Be aware that drug is best absorbed when administered by I.V. route. The blood level is unpredictable after I.M. administration.
•For I.V. use, dilute each dose with 50 to 200 ml of NS or $D_5W$ to yield no more than 1 mg/ml. Administer slowly over 30 to 60 minutes.
•Don't administer gentamicin through same I.V. line as other drugs without first consulting pharmacist.
•Expect to adjust dosage based on peak and trough blood drug levels drawn after third maintenance dose, as prescribed.
•Don't give gentamicin by S.C. route because it may be painful.
•When assisting with intrathecal injection, use only 2 mg/ml of preservative-free preparation. Drug may be injected directly or delivered by implanted reservoir.
•Don't give gentamicin to pregnant patient because drug can cause hearing loss in fetus.
•WARNING When giving pediatric injectable form of drug, be alert for allergic reactions—including anaphylaxis and, possibly, life-threatening asthmatic episodes—because drug contains sodium bisulfite.
•Assess for signs of other infections because gentamicin may cause overgrowth of nonsusceptible organisms.
•Be aware that premature infants, neonates, and elderly patients have an increased risk of nephrotoxicity.

**PATIENT TEACHING**
•Stress the importance of completing the full course of gentamicin therapy.
•Instruct patient to immediately report adverse reactions, such as hearing loss, to avoid permanent effects.

# glimepiride

Amaryl

## Class and Category

*Chemical:* Sulfonylurea
*Therapeutic:* Antidiabetic
*Pregnancy category:* C

## Indications and Dosages

➤ *To control blood glucose level in type 2 diabetes mellitus*

**TABLETS**

**Adults.** 1 to 2 mg q.d. with first meal of the day. *Maintenance:* 1 to 4 mg q.d., increased by 1 to 2 mg q 1 to 2 wk as needed for blood glucose control. *Maximum:* 8 mg/day.
**DOSAGE ADJUSTMENT** Initial dosage reduced to 1 mg q.d. if needed for patients with renal impairment.

➤ *As adjunct (with insulin) to control blood glucose level*

**TABLETS**

**Adults.** 8 mg q.d. with low-dose insulin.

| Route | Onset | Peak | Duration |
|---|---|---|---|
| P.O. | 2 to 3 hr | Unknown | Over 24 hr |

## Mechanism of Action

Stimulates insulin release from beta cells in the pancreas. The drug also increases peripheral tissue sensitivity to insulin, either by enhancing insulin binding to cellular receptors or by increasing the number of insulin receptors.

## Contraindications

Diabetes complicated by pregnancy; diabetic coma; hypersensitivity to glimepiride, sulfonylureas, or their components; ketoacidosis; sole therapy for type 1 diabetes mellitus

## Interactions

**DRUGS**

*ACE inhibitors, anabolic steroids, androgens, azole antifungals, bromocriptine, chloramphenicol, disopyramide, fibric acid derivatives, guanethidine, H₂-receptor antagonists, insulin, magnesium salts, MAO inhibitors, methyldopa, octreotide, oral anticoagulants, oxyphenbutazone, phenylbutazone, probenecid, quinidine, salicylates, sulfonamides, tetracycline, theophylline, tricyclic antidepressants, urinary acidifiers:* Increased risk of hypoglycemia

*asparaginase, calcium channel blockers, cholestyramine, clonidine, corticosteroids, danazol, diazoxide, estrogen, glucagon, hydantoins, isoniazid, lithium, morphine, nicotinic acid, oral contraceptives, phenothiazines, rifabutin, rifampin, sympathomimetics, thiazide diuretics, thyroid drugs, urinary alkalinizers:* Increased risk of hyperglycemia

*beta blockers:* Possibly hyperglycemia or masking of hypoglycemia signs

*digoxin:* Increased risk of digitalis toxicity

*pentamidine:* Initially hypoglycemia and then hyperglycemia if beta cell damage occurs

**ACTIVITIES**

*alcohol use:* Altered blood glucose control (usually hypoglycemia)

## Adverse Reactions

**CNS:** Abnormal gait, anxiety, asthenia, chills, depression, dizziness, fatigue, headache, hypertonia, hypoesthesia, insomnia, malaise, migraine headache, nervousness, paresthesia, somnolence, syncope, tremor, vertigo

**CV:** Arrhythmias, edema, hypertension, vasculitis

**EENT:** Blurred vision, conjunctivitis, eye pain, pharyngitis, retinal hemorrhage, rhinitis, taste perversion, tinnitus

**ENDO:** Hypoglycemia

**GI:** Anorexia, constipation, diarrhea, elevated liver function test results, epigastric discomfort or fullness, flatulence, heartburn, hunger, nausea, proctocolitis, trace blood in stool, vomiting

**GU:** Darkened urine, decreased libido, dysuria, polyuria

**HEME:** Agranulocytosis, aplastic anemia, eosinophilia, hemolytic anemia, hepatic porphyria, leukopenia, pancytopenia

**MS:** Arthralgia, leg cramps, myalgia

**RESP:** Dyspnea

**SKIN:** Allergic skin reactions, diaphoresis, eczema, erythema multiforme, exfoliative dermatitis, flushing, jaundice, lichenoid reactions, maculopapular or morbilliform rash, photosensitivity, urticaria

**Other:** Disulfiram-like reaction

## Nursing Considerations

•Monitor fasting blood glucose level to determine response to glimepiride. Expect to check glycosylated hemoglobin level every 3 to 6 months to evaluate long-term blood glucose control.

•Arrange for dietary consultation and diabetic teaching, if appropriate. Ask dietitian to discuss with patient the amount of alcohol he can consume without risking hypoglycemia.

•Expect to switch patient to insulin therapy, as prescribed, during physical stress, such as infection, surgery, and trauma.

•**WARNING** Expect a higher risk of hypoglycemia when giving glimepiride to a malnourished or debilitated patient or one with renal, hepatic, pituitary, or adrenal insufficiency.

**PATIENT TEACHING**

•Instruct patient to take glimepiride just before the first meal of the day. Caution him not to skip the meal after taking drug.

•Urge patient not to skip doses or increase dosage without consulting prescriber.

•Urge patient to report signs of hypoglycemia, such as anxiety, confusion, dizziness, excessive sweating, headache, and nausea.

•Encourage patient to carry candy or other simple sugars to treat mild hypoglycemia.

•Advise patient to consult prescriber before taking any OTC drug.

•Urge patient to carry identification indicating that he has diabetes.

•Teach patient how to monitor his blood glucose level.

•Teach patient about exercise, diet, signs of hyperglycemia and hypoglycemia, hygiene, foot care, and ways to avoid infection.

•Instruct patient to notify prescriber if he experiences darkened urine, difficulty controlling his blood glucose level, easy bruising, fever, rash, sore throat, or unusual bleeding.

•If photosensitivity is a problem, instruct patient to avoid direct sunlight and to wear sunscreen.

G
H
I

# glipizide
Glucotrol, Glucotrol XL

## Class and Category
*Chemical:* Sulfonylurea
*Therapeutic:* Antidiabetic
*Pregnancy category:* C

## Indications and Dosages
➤ *To control blood glucose level in type 2 diabetes mellitus*

**E.R. TABLETS**
**Adults.** *Initial:* 5 mg q.d. with breakfast. Dosage increased by 5 mg/day q 3 mo, if needed. *Maintenance:* 5 to 10 mg q.d. *Maximum:* 20 mg/day.

**TABLETS**
**Adults.** *Initial:* 5 mg 30 min before first meal of the day. Dosage adjusted by 2.5 to 5 mg q 2 to 3 days. For daily dose of 15 mg or less, give as a single dose. For dose above 15 mg/day, give in 2 divided doses. *Maximum:* 40 mg/day.

➤ *As adjunct to or replacement for insulin therapy in type 2 diabetes mellitus*

**CAPSULES, TABLETS**
**Adults who need more than 20 U insulin/day.** 5 mg q.d., while decreasing insulin dosage by one-half. Further insulin reductions are based on clinical response.

**DOSAGE ADJUSTMENT** Initial dosage reduced to 2.5 mg q.d. if needed for patients over age 65 and those with hepatic disease.

| Route | Onset | Peak | Duration |
|---|---|---|---|
| P.O. | 10 to 30 min | 30 min to 2 hr | 12 to 24 hr |
| P.O. (E.R.) | Unknown | Unknown | 18 to 24 hr |

### Mechanism of Action
Stimulates insulin release from beta cells in the pancreas. Glipizide also increases peripheral tissue sensitivity to insulin, either by enhancing insulin binding to cellular receptors or by increasing the number of insulin receptors.

## Contraindications
Diabetes complicated by pregnancy; diabetic coma; hypersensitivity to glipizide, sulfonylureas, or their components; ketoacidosis; sole therapy for type 1 diabetes mellitus

## Interactions
**DRUGS**
*ACE inhibitors, anabolic steroids, androgens, azole antifungals, bromocriptine, chloramphenicol, disopyramide, fibric acid derivatives, guanethidine, $H_2$-receptor antagonists, insulin, magnesium salts, MAO inhibitors, methyldopa, octreotide, oral anticoagulants, oxyphenbutazone, phenylbutazone, probenecid, quinidine, salicylates, sulfonamides, tetracycline, theophylline, tricyclic antidepressants, urinary acidifiers:* Increased risk of hypoglycemia
*asparaginase, calcium channel blockers, cholestyramine, clonidine, corticosteroids, danazol, diazoxide, estrogen, glucagon, hydantoins, isoniazid, lithium, morphine, nicotinic acid, oral contraceptives, phenothiazines, rifabutin, rifampin, sympathomimetics, thiazide diuretics, thyroid drugs, urinary alkalinizers:* Increased risk of hyperglycemia
*beta blockers:* Possibly hyperglycemia or masking of hypoglycemia signs
*digitalis glycosides:* Increased risk of digitalis toxicity
*pentamidine:* Initially hypoglycemia and then hyperglycemia if beta cell damage occurs
**FOODS**
*all foods:* Possibly delayed drug absorption of tablets if taken within 30 minutes of meal
**ACTIVITIES**
*alcohol use:* Altered blood glucose control (usually hypoglycemia)

## Adverse Reactions
**CNS:** Abnormal gait, anxiety, asthenia, chills, depression, dizziness, fatigue, headache, hypertonia, hypoesthesia, insomnia, malaise, migraine headache, nervousness, paresthesia, somnolence, syncope, tremor, vertigo
**CV:** Arrhythmias, edema, hypertension, vasculitis
**EENT:** Blurred vision, conjunctivitis, eye pain, pharyngitis, retinal hemorrhage, rhinitis, taste perversion, tinnitus
**ENDO:** Hypoglycemia
**GI:** Abdominal pain, anorexia, constipation, diarrhea, elevated liver function test results, epigastric discomfort or fullness, flatulence, heartburn, hunger, nausea, proctocolitis, trace blood in stool, vomiting
**GU:** Darkened urine, decreased libido, dysuria, polyuria

**HEME:** Agranulocytosis, aplastic anemia, eosinophilia, hemolytic anemia, hepatic porphyria, leukopenia, pancytopenia
**MS:** Arthralgia, leg cramps, myalgia
**RESP:** Dyspnea
**SKIN:** Allergic skin reactions, diaphoresis, eczema, erythema multiforme, exfoliative dermatitis, flushing, jaundice, lichenoid reactions, maculopapular or morbilliform rash, photosensitivity, urticaria
**Other:** Disulfiram-like reaction

## Nursing Considerations

• To improve blood glucose control, administer glipizide in divided doses instead of once a day, as prescribed.
• Check blood glucose level at least 3 times daily for a patient switching from insulin to glipizide. Patients who take more than 40 U of insulin daily may need hospitalization during transition.
• If patient gradually loses responsiveness to glipizide, expect to give a second antidiabetic drug to maintain blood glucose control, as prescribed.
• Monitor fasting blood glucose level to determine response to drug. Expect to check glycosylated hemoglobin level every 3 to 6 months or as ordered to evaluate long-term blood glucose control.
• Expect to switch patient to insulin therapy, as prescribed, during physical stress, such as infection, surgery, or trauma.
• WARNING Expect a higher risk of hypoglycemia when giving glipizide to a malnourished or debilitated patient or one with renal, hepatic, pituitary, or adrenal insufficiency.

### PATIENT TEACHING

• Instruct patient to take glipizide tablets 30 minutes before the first meal of the day. Caution him not to skip the meal after taking drug.
• Advise patient not to skip doses or increase dosage without consulting prescriber.
• Urge patient to report signs or symptoms of hypoglycemia, such as anxiety, confusion, dizziness, excessive sweating, headache, and nausea.
• Encourage patient to carry candy or other simple sugars to treat mild hypoglycemia.
• Caution patient to consult prescriber before taking any OTC drugs.
• Urge patient to carry identification indicating that he has diabetes.

• Teach patient how to monitor his blood glucose level.
• Teach patient about exercise, diet, signs of hyperglycemia and hypoglycemia, hygiene, foot care, and ways to avoid infection.
• Instruct patient to notify prescriber if he experiences darkened urine, easy bruising, fever, hypoglycemia or hyperglycemia, rash, sore throat, and unusual bleeding.
• If photosensitivity is a problem, instruct patient to avoid direct sunlight and to wear sunscreen.

# glipizide and metformin hydrochloride

Metaglip

## Class and Category

*Chemical:* Sulfonylurea (glipizide), dimethylbiguanide (metformin)
*Therapeutic:* Antidiabetic
*Pregnancy category:* C

## Indications and Dosages

➤ *To reduce blood glucose level as initial therapy in patients with type 2 diabetes mellitus*

**TABLETS**

**Adults.** *Initial:* 2.5 mg/250 mg q.d. with morning meal, or 2.5 mg/500 mg b.i.d. with morning and evening meals if fasting blood glucose is 280 to 320 mg/dl. Dosage increased by initial dosage strength q 2 wk, as needed. *Maximum:* 10 mg/1,000 mg, or 10 mg/2000 mg daily in divided doses if initial fasting glucose is 280 to 320 mg/dl.

➤ *To reduce blood glucose level in patients with type 2 diabetes mellitus who aren't adequately controlled with either a sulfonylurea or metformin alone*

**TABLETS**

**Adults.** *Initial:* 2.5 mg/500 mg or 5 mg/500 mg b.i.d. with morning and evening meals. Dosage increased by no more than 5 mg/500 mg, as needed. *Maximum:* 20 mg/2,000 mg/day.

DOSAGE ADJUSTMENT For patients taking glipizide or another sulfonylurea, metformin, or a combination of these drugs, expect initial dosage of combination drug to be equal to or less than that currently being taken individually.

| Route | Onset | Peak | Duration |
|-------|-------|------|----------|
| P.O. (glipizide) | 10 to 20 min | 30 min to 2 hr | 12 to 24 hr |
| P.O. (metformin) | Days to 1 wk | 2 wk | 2 wk after drug is stopped |

## Mechanism of Action

Glipizide and metformin hydrochloride work in complementary ways to improve glucose control. Glipizide stimulates insulin release from beta cells in the pancreas. It also increases peripheral tissue sensitivity to insulin, either by enhancing insulin binding to cellular receptors or by increasing the number of insulin receptors.

Metformin may promote storage of excess glucose as glycogen in the liver, thus reducing glucose production. It also may improve glucose use by skeletal muscle and adipose tissue by facilitating glucose transport, increasing insulin receptors, and making them more sensitive to insulin.

## Contraindications

Acute or chronic metabolic acidosis; diabetic coma; heart failure requiring drug treatment; hypersensitivity to glipizide, metformin, or their components; ketoacidosis; pregnancy, renal disease or dysfunction (serum creatinine level of 1.5 mg/dl or more in men or 1.4 mg/dl or more in women or abnormal creatinine clearance)

## Interactions

### DRUGS

**glipizide and metformin hydrochloride**
*calcium channel blockers, corticosteroids, diuretics, estrogens, isoniazid, nicotinic acid, oral contraceptives, phenothiazine, phenytoin, sympathomimetics, thiazide diuretics, thyroid hormones:* Possibly hyperglycemia or hypoglycemia when these drugs are withdrawn
*vitamin $B_{12}$:* Probably decreased vitamin $B_{12}$ absorption.

**glipizide component only**
*ACE inhibitors, anabolic steroids, androgens, azole antifungals, bromocriptine, chloramphenicol, disopyramide, fibric acid derivatives, guanethidine, $H_2$-receptor antagonists, insulin, magnesium salts, MAO inhibitors, methyldopa, octreotide, oral anticoagulants, oxyphenbutazone, phenylbutazone, probenecid, quinidine, salicylates, sulfonamides, tetracycline, theophylline, tricyclic antidepressants, urinary acidifiers:* Increased risk of hypoglycemia
*asparaginase, calcium channel blockers, cholestyramine, clonidine, corticosteroids, danazol, diazoxide, estrogen, glucagons, hydantoins, isoniazid, lithium, morphine, nicotinic acid, oral contraceptives, phenothiazines, rifabutin, rifampin, sympathomimetics, thiazide diuretics, thyroid drugs, urinary alkalinizers:* Increased risk of hyperglycemia
*beta blockers:* Possibly hyperglycemia or masking of hypoglycemia
*digitalis glycosides:* Increased risk of digitalis toxicity
*pentamidine:* Initially hypoglycemia and then hyperglycemia if beta cell damage occurs

**metformin component only**
*cationic drugs (such as amiloride, cimetidine, digoxin, morphine, procainamide, quinidine, quinine, ranitidine, triamterene, trimethoprim, vancomycin) nifedipine:* Increased blood metformin level
*calcium channel blockers, corticosteroids, estrogens, isoniazid, nicotinic acid, oral contraceptives, phenothiazines, phenytoin, sympathomimetics, thiazide and other diuretics, thyroid drugs:* Possibly hyperglycemia
*clofibrate, MAO inhibitors, probenecid, propranolol, rifabutin, rifampin, salicylates, sulfonamides, sulfonylureas:* Increased risk of hypoglycemia

### ACTIVITIES

*alcohol use:* Possibly increased risk of hypoglycemia; possibly potentiated lactate metabolism by metformin

## Adverse Reactions

**CNS:** Dizziness, headache
**CV:** Hypertension
**ENDO:** Hypoglycemia
**GI:** Abdominal pain, diarrhea, nausea, vomiting
**GU:** UTI
**MS:** Pain
**RESP:** Upper respiratory tract infection

## Nursing Considerations

•WARNING Monitor renal function, as ordered, before beginning glipizide and metformin therapy and at least annually thereafter because significant renal impairment can result in tissue hypoperfusion and hypoxemia, leading to lactic acidosis.

•**WARNING** Monitor patient closely for signs and symptoms of lactic acidosis or ketoacidosis (changes in level of consciousness, fruity breath, Kussmaul's respirations, restlessness), especially during new onset of illness or trauma. If acidosis or ketoacidosis is suspected, obtain blood samples to evaluate serum electrolyte, ketone, glucose, possibly blood pH, lactate, pyruvate, and metformin levels, as ordered. If acidosis is confirmed, expect to discontinue drug immediately and provide corrective care, as prescribed.

•Expect to discontinue drug, as ordered, if patient develops cardiovascular collapse, acute congestive heart failure, acute MI, or other conditions that exhibit hypoxemia, or if patient develops hepatic insufficiency, because lactic acidosis may develop in these conditions.

•**WARNING** Monitor patients—especially those who are malnourished or debilitated; those with renal, pituitary or adrenal insufficiency; and those with alcohol intoxication—for hypoglycemia because the drug increases the risk of this condition.

•Monitor vitamin $B_{12}$ levels at least every 2 to 3 years in patients with inadequate vitamin $B_{12}$ or calcium intake or absorption because prolonged drug use may result in decreased vitamin $B_{12}$ response.

•Know that drug should be temporarily withheld for any surgical procedure that requires restricted intake of food and fluids and should not be restarted until the patient is able to eat and drink and renal function is determined to be normal.

•Expect to discontinue glipizide and metformin for 48 hours before and after radiographic tests involving I.V. administration of iodinated contrast materials because iodinated media increase the risk of renal failure and lactic acidosis during drug therapy. Check patient's renal function before restarting glipizide and metform 48 hours after radiographic tests are completed, as ordered.

•Monitor patient's blood glucose level to determine response to drug. Expect to monitor glycosylated hemoglobin level every 3 to 6 months, as ordered, to evaluate long-term blood glucose control.

•Frequently monitor blood glucose level to detect hyperglycemia and to assess the need for supplemental insulin during periods of increased stress, such as infection, surgery, and trauma.

•Arrange for instruction about diabetes and consultation with a dietitian or certified diabetes educator, if possible.

**PATIENT TEACHING**

•Instruct patient to take glipizide and metformin with morning meal if taking once a day or morning and evening meals if taking twice a day. Caution him not to skip meal after taking drug.

•Advise patient not to skip doses, discontinue drug, or take OTC drugs without first consulting prescriber because of a risk of hyperglycemia.

•Advise patient to report signs of hypoglycemia (anxiety, confusion, dizziness, excessive sweating, headache, nausea) and teach him how to treat hypoglycemia if it occurs.

•Tell patient to stop drug and notify prescriber immediately if he develops increased respiratory rate that is unexplained by exercise or other usual activities, myalgia, malaise, unusual somnolence, or other nonspecific symptoms.

•Instruct patient to carry identification indicating that he has diabetes.

•Caution patient to avoid alcohol because it increases the risk of hypoglycemia.

•Tell patient to inform all prescribers that he is taking glipizide and metformin.

# glucagon

GlucaGen, Glucagon Diagnostic Kit, Glucagon Emergency Kit

## Class and Category

*Chemical:* Synthetic hormone
*Therapeutic:* Antihypoglycemic, diagnostic aid adjunct
*Pregnancy category:* B

## Indications and Dosages

➤ *To provide emergency treatment of severe hypoglycemia*

**I.V., I.M., OR S.C. INJECTION**

**Adults and children who weigh more than 20 kg (44 lb) or, with GlucaGen, more than 25 kg (55 lb).** 1 mg, repeated in 15 min if needed. **Children who weigh 20 kg or less or, when using GlucaGen, 25 kg or less.** 0.5 mg, or 0.02 to 0.03 mg/kg, repeated in 15 min, if needed.

➤ *To provide diagnostic assistance by inhibiting bowel peristalsis in radiologic examination of GI tract*

**I.V. INJECTION**

**Adults.** 0.25 to 2 mg before procedure. Dose,

route, and timing vary with segment of GI tract examined and length of procedure.

| Route | Onset | Peak | Duration |
|-------|-------|------|----------|
| I.V. | 5 to 20 min*† | Unknown | 90 min*‡ |
| I.M. | 15 to 26 min*§ | Unknown | 90 min*‖ |
| S.C. | 30 to 45 min* | Unknown | 90 min* |

---

### Mechanism of Action
Increases production of adenylate cyclase, which catalyzes the conversion of adenosine triphosphate to cAMP, a process that in turn activates phosphorylase. Phosphorylase promotes the breakdown of glycogen to glucose (glycogenolysis) in the liver. As a result, the blood glucose level increases and GI smooth muscles relax.

---

### Incompatibilities
Don't mix glucagon with sodium chloride or solutions that have a pH of 3.0 to 9.5; use with dextrose solutions instead.

### Contraindications
Hypersensitivity to glucagon or its components, pheochromocytoma

### Interactions
**DRUGS**
*oral anticoagulants:* Possibly increased anticoagulant effects

### Adverse Reactions
**CV:** Hypertension, hypotension (with hypersensitivity reaction), tachycardia
**GI:** Nausea, vomiting
**RESP:** Bronchospasm, respiratory distress
**SKIN:** Urticaria

### Nursing Considerations
• Rouse patient as quickly as possible because prolonged hypoglycemia can cause cerebral damage.

---

\* For antihypoglycemic action.
† 45 sec to 1 min for smooth-muscle relaxation.
‡ 9 to 25 min for smooth-muscle relaxation.
§ 4 to 10 min for smooth-muscle relaxation.
‖ 12 to 32 min for smooth-muscle relaxation.

• For I.V. use, reconstitute a 1-mg vial of glucagon with 1 ml of diluent or a 10-mg vial with 10 ml of diluent. Don't give more than 1 mg/ml. For large doses, dilute with sterile water for injection.
• Before injecting glucagon, place unconscious patient on his side to prevent aspiration of vomitus when he regains consciousness.
• Administer by slow I.V. injection to decrease the risk of adverse reactions, such as tachycardia and vomiting.
• If patient doesn't respond to glucagon, expect to administer I.V. dextrose.
• When patient has regained consciousness or as soon as diagnostic procedure is completed, give him oral carbohydrates to restore hepatic glycogen stores and prevent secondary hypoglycemia.
• Keep in mind that glucagon isn't effective in patients with depleted hepatic glycogen stores caused by such conditions as adrenal insufficiency, chronic hypoglycemia, and starvation.

**PATIENT TEACHING**
• Instruct patient to monitor his blood glucose level, especially when signs of hypoglycemia occur.
• Teach patient and family members how to recognize signs of hypoglycemia and when to notify prescriber.
• Advise patient to carry candy or other simple sugars with him to treat early hypoglycemia.
• Emphasize the importance of a consistent diet, regular exercise, and proper use of insulin or an oral antidiabetic drug.
• Make sure unstable diabetic patients and family members know how to give glucagon subcutaneously in case of hypoglycemia. Instruct family members to keep patient on his side and give him a carbohydrate when he awakens. Advise against giving fluids by mouth until patient is fully conscious.
• Instruct patient and family members to call for emergency medical assistance after glucagon treatment, especially if patient can't ingest oral glucose or if he's taking the sulfonylurea chlorpropamide, in case secondary hypoglycemia occurs.

25

# glyburide
## (glibenclamide)

Albert Glyburide (CAN), Apo-Glyburide (CAN), DiaBeta, Euglucon (CAN), Gen-Glybe (CAN), Glynase PresTab, Medi-Glybe (CAN), Micronase, Novo-Glyburide (CAN), Nu-Glyburide (CAN)

## Class and Category
*Chemical:* Sulfonylurea
*Therapeutic:* Antidiabetic
*Pregnancy category:* C (B for Glynase PresTab and Micronase)

## Indications and Dosages
➤ *To control blood glucose level in type 2 diabetes mellitus*

**MICRONIZED TABLETS**

**Adults.** *Initial:* 1.5 to 3 mg q.d. with first meal of the day, increased by up to 1.5 mg at weekly intervals, if needed. *Maintenance:* 0.75 to 12 mg as a single dose or in divided doses with meals.

**NONMICRONIZED TABLETS**

**Adults.** *Initial:* 2.5 to 5 mg q.d. with first meal of the day, increased by up to 2.5 mg at weekly intervals, if needed. *Maintenance:* 1.25 to 20 mg/day as a single dose or in divided doses with meals.

**DOSAGE ADJUSTMENT** During conversion from insulin to glyburide for adults who use more than 40 U insulin/day, initial dosage adjusted to 5-mg nonmicronized tablet or 3-mg micronized tablet as a single dose with 50% of usual insulin dose; glyburide dosage increased gradually, as needed. For adults who use less than 40 U insulin/day, usual glyburide dosage is used when insulin is discontinued.

For elderly patients, initial dosage possibly reduced to 1.25-mg nonmicronized tablet q.d. and gradually increased by 2.5 mg/wk, as needed; or 0.75- to 3-mg micronized tablet q.d. and gradually increased by 1.5 mg/wk, as needed.

| Route | Onset | Peak | Duration |
|-------|-------|------|----------|
| P.O.* | 1 hr | 2.3 to 3.5 hr | 12 to 24 hr |
| P.O.† | 15 to 60 min | 1 to 3 hr | 24 hr |

\* Micronized.
† Nonmicronized.

## Mechanism of Action
Stimulates insulin release from beta cells in the pancreas. Glyburide also increases peripheral tissue sensitivity to insulin either by enhancing insulin binding to cellular receptors or by increasing the number of insulin receptors.

## Contraindications
Diabetes complicated by pregnancy; diabetic coma; hypersensitivity to glyburide, sulfonylureas, or their components; ketoacidosis; sole therapy for type 1 diabetes mellitus

## Interactions
**DRUGS**
*ACE inhibitors, anabolic steroids, androgens, azole antifungals, bromocriptine, chloramphenicol, disopyramide, fibric acid derivatives, guanethidine, $H_2$-receptor antagonists, insulin, magnesium salts, MAO inhibitors, methyldopa, octreotide, oral anticoagulants, oxyphenbutazone, phenylbutazone, probenecid, quinidine, salicylates, sulfonamides, tetracycline, theophylline, tricyclic antidepressants, urinary acidifiers:* Increased risk of hypoglycemia
*asparaginase, calcium channel blockers, cholestyramine, clonidine, corticosteroids, danazol, diazoxide, estrogen, glucagon, hydantoins, isoniazid, lithium, morphine, nicotinic acid, oral contraceptives, phenothiazines, rifabutin, rifampin, sympathomimetics, thiazide diuretics, thyroid drugs, urinary alkalinizers:* Increased risk of hyperglycemia
*beta blockers:* Possibly hyperglycemia or masking of hypoglycemia signs
*digitalis glycosides:* Increased risk of digitalis toxicity
*pentamidine:* Initial hypoglycemia and then hyperglycemia if beta cell damage occurs

**FOODS**
*high-fat foods:* Reduced bioavailability of nonmicronized glyburide

**ACTIVITIES**
*alcohol use:* Altered blood glucose control (usually hypoglycemia)

## Adverse Reactions
**CNS:** Abnormal gait, anxiety, asthenia, chills, depression, dizziness, fatigue, headache, hy-

pertonia, hypoesthesia, insomnia, malaise, migraine headache, nervousness, paresthesia, somnolence, syncope, tremor, vertigo
**CV:** Arrhythmias, edema, hypertension, vasculitis
**EENT:** Blurred vision, conjunctivitis, eye pain, pharyngitis, retinal hemorrhage, rhinitis, taste perversion, tinnitus
**ENDO:** Hypoglycemia
**GI:** Anorexia, constipation, diarrhea, elevated liver function test results, epigastric discomfort or fullness, flatulence, heartburn, hunger, nausea, proctocolitis, trace blood in stool, vomiting
**GU:** Decreased libido, dysuria, polyuria
**HEME:** Agranulocytosis, aplastic anemia, eosinophilia, hemolytic anemia, hepatic porphyria, leukopenia, pancytopenia
**MS:** Arthralgia, leg cramps, myalgia
**RESP:** Dyspnea
**SKIN:** Allergic skin reactions, diaphoresis, eczema, erythema multiforme, exfoliative dermatitis, flushing, jaundice, lichenoid reactions, maculopapular or morbilliform rash, photosensitivity, urticaria
**Other:** Disulfiram-like reaction

## Nursing Considerations

• Give glyburide as a single dose before the first meal of the day. If patient takes more than 10 mg daily or if severe GI distress occurs, give in 2 divided doses before meals.
• Monitor fasting blood glucose level to determine patient's response to glyburide. Expect to check glycosylated hemoglobin level every 3 to 6 months or as ordered to evaluate long-term blood glucose control.
• When patient switches from insulin to glyburide, check blood glucose level 3 times daily before meals.
• Be aware that micronized tablets aren't equal to nonmicronized tablets; they contain smaller particles, which affects drug bioavailability.
• **WARNING** Expect a higher risk of hypoglycemia when giving drug to a malnourished or debilitated patient or one with renal, hepatic, pituitary, or adrenal insufficiency.
• Administer insulin as needed and prescribed during periods of increased stress, such as infection, surgery, and trauma.
• Arrange for diabetic teaching and consultation between patient and dietitian, if appropriate.

**PATIENT TEACHING**
• Instruct patient to take glyburide just before the day's first meal. Caution him not to skip the meal after taking drug.
• Advise patient not to take nonmicronized glyburide with a high-fat meal because doing so can reduce drug bioavailability.
• Caution patient to avoid skipping doses, discontinuing glyburide, or taking OTC drugs without first consulting prescriber.
• Teach patient how to monitor his blood glucose level and when to notify prescriber.
• Urge patient to report signs of hypoglycemia, such as anxiety, confusion, dizziness, excessive sweating, headache, and nausea.
• Suggest that patient carry candy or other simple sugars to treat mild hypoglycemia.
• Urge patient to avoid alcohol because it increases the risk of hypoglycemia.
• Advise patient to carry identification indicating that he has diabetes.
• Teach patient about exercise, diet, signs of hyperglycemia and hypoglycemia, hygiene, foot care, and ways to avoid infection.
• Instruct patient to notify prescriber if he experiences easy bruising, fever, hypoglycemia or hyperglycemia, rash, sore throat, and unusual bleeding.
• If photosensitivity is a problem, instruct patient to avoid direct sunlight and to wear sunscreen.

# glyburide and metformin hydrochloride

Glucovance

## Class and Category

*Chemical:* Sulfonylurea (glyburide), dimethylbiguanide (metformin)
*Therapeutic:* Antidiabetic
*Pregnancy category:* B

## Indications and Dosages

➤ *To reduce blood glucose level as initial therapy in patients with type 2 diabetes mellitus or in those receiving glyburide and metformin combination therapy who require the addition of a thiazolidinedione*
**TABLETS**
**Adults.** *Initial:* 1.25 mg/250 mg q.d. or b.i.d. Dosage increased by 1.25 mg/250 mg/day q 2 wk as needed.

➤ *To reduce blood glucose level in patients with type 2 diabetes mellitus who are not adequately controlled on either a sulfonylurea or metformin alone*

**TABLETS**

**Adults.** *Initial:* 2.5 mg/500 mg or 5 mg/500 mg b.i.d. Dosage increased, as prescribed, by 5 mg/500 mg/day. *Maximum:* 20 mg/2,000 mg/day.

DOSAGE ADJUSTMENT For patients currently receiving glyburide or another sulfonylurea, metformin, or a combination of these drugs, expect initial dosage prescribed to be equal to or less than that currently being taken. For patients currently receiving a combination of glyburide and metformin therapy who require the addition of a thiazolidinedione, expect dosage of glyburide and metformin combination to remain unchanged when the thiazolidinedione is added to patient's regimen.

| Route | Onset | Peak | Duration |
|---|---|---|---|
| P.O. (glyburide) | 45 to 60 min | 1.5 to 3 hr | 24 hr |
| P.O. (metformin) | Days to 1 wk | 2 wk | 2 wk after drug is discontinued |

## Mechanism of Action

Glyburide and metformin work in complementary ways to improve glucose control. Glyburide stimulates insulin release from beta cells in the pancreas. It also increases peripheral tissue sensitivity to insulin either by enhancing insulin binding to cellular receptors or by increasing the number of insulin receptors.

Metformin hydrochloride may promote the storage of excess glucose as glycogen in the liver, thus reducing glucose production. Metformin also may improve glucose use by skeletal muscle and adipose tissue by facilitating glucose transport across cell membranes. It also may increase the number of insulin receptors on cell membranes and make them more sensitive to insulin.

## Contraindications

Acute or chronic metabolic acidosis; diabetes complicated by pregnancy; diabetic coma; heart failure requiring drug treatment; hypersensitivity to glyburide, metformin, biguanides, sulfonylureas, or their components; ketoacidosis; renal disease or dysfunction (serum creatinine level of 1.5 mg/dl or more in men or 1.4 mg/dl or more in women); type 1 diabetes

## Interactions

**DRUGS**

**glyburide and metformin hydrochloride**
*calcium channel blockers, corticosteroids, diuretics, estrogens, isoniazid, nicotinic acid, oral contraceptives, phenothiazine, phenytoin, sympathomimetics, thiazide diuretics, thyroid hormones:* Possibly hyperglycemia, possibly hypoglycemia when these drugs are withdrawn
*vitamin B$_{12}$:* Probably decreased vitamin B$_{12}$ absorption

**glyburide component only**
*beta-adrenergic blockers, chloramphenicol, highly protein-bound drugs, MAO inhibitors NSAIDs, oral anticoagulants, probenecid, salicylates, sulfonamides:* Potentiated hypoglycemic action of glyburide, possibly hyperglycemia when these drugs are withdrawn
*ciprofloxacin:* Potentiated hypoglycemic action of glyburide
*miconazole (oral):* Possibly severe hypoglycemia

**metformin hydrochloride component only**
*cimetidine:* Increased blood metformin level, possibly increased risk of hypoglycemia
*furosemide:* Increased blood metformin level, decreased blood furosemide level
*nifedipine:* Enhanced absorption of metformin

**FOODS**
*all foods:* Delayed and reduced absorption of metformin

**ACTIVITIES**
*alcohol use:* Altered blood glucose control (usually hyperglycemia), possibly potentiated effect of metformin on lactate metabolism

## Adverse Reactions

**CNS:** Headache
**ENDO:** Hypoglycemia
**GI:** Abdominal pain, diarrhea, indigestion, nausea, vomiting
**HEME:** Megaloblastic anemia, thrombocytopenia
**RESP:** Upper respiratory tract infection
**Other:** Lactic acidosis

## Nursing Considerations

•Administer glyburide and metformin as a

G
H
I

single dose before first meal of the day. If patient takes more than 10 mg of the glyburide component daily or if severe GI distress occurs, expect to divide dose and give b.i.d. before morning and evening meals.

•**WARNING** Monitor renal function, as ordered, before beginning therapy and at least annually thereafter because significant renal impairment can result in tissue hypoperfusion and hypoxemia, leading to lactic acidosis.

•**WARNING** Expect to discontinue glyburide and metformin for 48 hours before and after radiographic tests involving I.V. administration of iodinated contrast materials because iodinated media increase the risk of renal failure and lactic acidosis during drug therapy.

•**WARNING** Monitor malnourished or debilitated patients; those with renal, hepatic, pituitary, or adrenal insufficiency; and those who are also prescribed a thiazolidinedione because they're at increased risk for hypoglycemia. Expect to monitor vitamin $B_{12}$ blood levels at least every 2 to 3 years in patients with inadequate vitamin $B_{12}$ or calcium intake or absorption because prolonged drug use may result in decreased vitamin $B_{12}$ absorption.

•Monitor fasting blood glucose level to determine patient's response to drug. Expect to monitor glycosylated hemoglobin ($HbA_{1c}$) level every 3 to 6 months, as ordered, to evaluate long-term blood glucose control.

•Frequently monitor blood glucose level to detect hyperglycemia and to assess the need for supplemental insulin during periods of increased stress, such as infection, surgery, and trauma.

•When patient switches from insulin to glyburide and metformin, expect to increase frequency of blood glucose monitoring to t.i.d. before meals.

•In pregnant females, expect to discontinue drug at least 2 weeks before expected delivery date, as prescribed, to avoid profound hypoglycemia in neonate.

•Arrange for diabetes teaching and consultation with a dietitian or certified diabetes educator, if possible.

**PATIENT TEACHING**

•Instruct patient to take glyburide and metformin with morning meal if taking once a day, or with morning and evening meals if taking twice a day. Caution him not to skip meal after taking drug.

•Advise patient not to skip doses, discontinue drug, or take OTC drugs without first consulting prescriber because hyperglycemia may result.

•Inform patient that most common adverse effects are minor, including diarrhea, nausea, and upset stomach, and typically occur during first few weeks of therapy; explain that taking drug with meals reduces these effects.

•Teach patient how to monitor his blood glucose level and when to notify prescriber.

•Advise patient to expect laboratory monitoring of $HbA_{1c}$ level every 3 months until blood glucose level is controlled.

•Instruct patient to report signs of hypoglycemia, such as anxiety, confusion, dizziness, excessive sweating, headache, and nausea.

•Advise patient to carry identification indicating that he has diabetes, and suggest that he carry candy to treat mild hypoglycemia.

•Teach patient about exercise, diet, signs of hyperglycemia and hypoglycemia, hygiene, foot care, and ways to avoid infection.

•Urge patient to notify prescriber if he develops easy bruising, unusual bleeding, fever, hypoglycemia or hyperglycemia, rash, or sore throat because drug may need to be stopped.

•Advise patient to avoid alcohol because it increases the risk of hypoglycemia.

•Inform pregnant patient that she may be taken off glyburide and metformin and switched to insulin therapy, as prescribed, at least 2 weeks before expected delivery date.

# glycopyrrolate

Robinul, Robinul Forte

## Class and Category

*Chemical:* Quaternary ammonium compound
*Therapeutic:* Antiarrhythmic, anticholinergic, cholinergic adjunct
*Pregnancy category:* B

## Indications and Dosages

➤ *To treat peptic ulcer disease*

**TABLETS**

**Adults and adolescents.** 1 to 2 mg b.i.d. or t.i.d. *Maximum:* 8 mg/day.

**I.V. OR I.M. INJECTION**

**Adults and adolescents.** 0.1 to 0.2 mg q 4 hr, p.r.n. *Maximum:* 4 doses/day.

➤ *To reduce gastric acid and respiratory secretions before anesthesia*

**I.M. INJECTION**

**Adults and adolescents.** 0.0044 mg/kg 30 to 60 min before anesthesia or when preanesthesia sedative or narcotic is given.

**Children over age 2.** 0.0044 to 0.0088 mg/kg 30 to 60 min before anesthesia or when preanesthesia sedative or narcotic is given.

➤ *To counteract intraoperative and anesthesia-induced arrhythmias*

**I.V. INJECTION**

**Adults and adolescents.** 0.1 mg, repeated q 2 to 3 min, if needed.

**Children over age 2.** 0.0044 mg/kg. Dose repeated q 2 to 3 min, if needed. *Maximum:* 0.1 mg as a single dose.

➤ *As cholinergic adjunct in curariform block*

**I.V. INJECTION**

**Adults and children over age 2.** 0.2 mg glycopyrrolate for each 1 mg neostigmine or 5 mg pyridostigmine when given together.

| Route | Onset | Peak | Duration |
|---|---|---|---|
| P.O. | 60 min | Unknown | 8 to 12 hr |
| I.V. | 1 min | Unknown | 2 to 3 hr* |
| I.M., S.C. | 15 to 30 min | 30 to 45 min | 2 to 3 hr* |

**Mechanism of Action**

Inhibits acetylcholine's action on postganglionic muscarinic receptors throughout the body. Depending on the receptors' location, glycopyrrolate produces various effects, such as:

• reducing the volume and acidity of gastric secretions

• controlling excessive bronchial, pharyngeal, and tracheal secretions and dilating the bronchi

• inhibiting vagal stimulation of the heart

• relaxing smooth muscle in the GI and GU tracts.

**Incompatibilities**

Don't mix glycopyrrolate with alkaline drugs or solutions that have a pH over 6.0 because drug stability may be affected. A pH over 6.0 may occur if glycopyrrolate is mixed with dexamethasone sodium phosphate or LR so-

lution. Gas or precipitate may form if glycopyrrolate is mixed in same syringe as chloramphenicol, diazepam, dimenhydrinate, methohexital sodium, pentobarbital sodium, secobarbital sodium, sodium bicarbonate, or thiopental sodium.

**Contraindications**

Angle-closure glaucoma, asthma, hemorrhage with unstable cardiovascular status, hepatic disease, hypersensitivity to anticholinergics, ileus, intestinal atony, myasthenia gravis, obstructive GI or urinary disorders, severe ulcerative colitis, toxic megacolon

**Interactions**

**DRUGS**

*anticholinergics, antiparkinsonian drugs, phenothiazines, tricyclic antidepressants:* Possibly increased anticholinergic effects

*antidiarrheals (adsorbent):* Decreased glycopyrrolate absorption, leading to decreased therapeutic effectiveness

*antimyasthenics:* Possibly reduced intestinal motility

*atenolol:* Possibly potentiated atenolol effects

*calcium- or magnesium-containing antacids, carbonic anhydrase inhibitors, citrates, sodium bicarbonate:* Possibly reduced excretion of glycopyrrolate and increased therapeutic and adverse effects

*cyclopropane:* Possibly ventricular arrhythmias

*digoxin:* Possibly potentiated digoxin effects

*haloperidol, phenothiazines:* Possibly decreased effectiveness of these drugs

*ketoconazole:* Possibly decreased ketoconazole absorption

*metoclopramide:* Possibly antagonized effects of metoclopramide

*opioids:* Possibly severe constipation and urine retention, risk of ileus

*potassium chloride:* Possibly increased severity of potassium chloride–induced gastric lesions

**Adverse Reactions**

**CNS:** Confusion, dizziness, drowsiness, headache, insomnia, nervousness, weakness

**CV:** Bradycardia (low doses), heart block, palpitations, prolonged QT interval, tachycardia (high doses)

**EENT:** Blurred vision, cycloplegia, dilated pupils, dry mouth, increased intraocular pressure, loss of taste, mydriasis, nasal congestion, photophobia, taste perversion

G
H
I

---

* For vagal blocking effect; up to 7 hr for reduction of saliva.

**GI:** Abdominal distention, constipation, dysphagia, nausea, vomiting
**GU:** Impotence, urinary hesitancy, urine retention
**RESP:** Dyspnea
**SKIN:** Decreased sweating (heat exhaustion), dry skin, flushing, pruritus, urticaria
**Other:** Anaphylaxis

## Nursing Considerations

• Use glycopyrrolate cautiously in patients with autonomic neuropathy, hepatic disease, mild to moderate ulcerative colitis, prostatic hypertrophy, or hiatal hernia because drug's anticholinergic effect can worsen these conditions; gastric ulcer because drug may delay gastric emptying; and renal disease because drug excretion may be altered.
• Give tablets 30 to 60 minutes before meals.
• As needed and prescribed, give 2-mg dose at bedtime to ensure overnight control of symptoms.
• For I.V. use, administer by direct injection without diluting. Or inject into tubing of a flowing I.V. solution unless it contains an alkaline drug or sodium bicarbonate.
• Closure system contains dry natural rubber that may cause hypersensitivity reaction if handled by or used to inject someone with latex sensitivity.
• Use continuous cardiac monitoring, as ordered, to assess patient for arrhythmias during drug administration.
• WARNING Check all doses carefully because even a slight overdose can lead to toxicity.
• To prevent overheating caused by decreased sweating, adjust the room temperature and make sure patient is well hydrated.

### PATIENT TEACHING

• Advise patient to take glycopyrrolate tablets 30 to 60 minutes before meals.
• Instruct patient to consult prescriber before taking any OTC drugs.
• Caution patient about possible drowsiness and dizziness and need to avoid hazardous activities until drug's effects are known.
• Suggest that he use sugarless hard candy, ice, or saliva substitute to relieve dry mouth.
• Instruct patient to avoid exertion and hot environments because he's prone to heat exhaustion while taking glycopyrrolate.
• Urge patient to maintain hydration by drinking at least 8 glasses of water daily, unless contraindicated.
• Tell patient to notify prescriber about abdominal distention, trouble breathing or urinating, eye pain, irregular heartbeat, sensitivity to light, or severe constipation.
• Advise patient to wear sunglasses in bright light.
• Inform male patient that reversible impotence may occur during therapy.
• If urinary hesitancy occurs, advise patient to void before taking each dose.

# granisetron hydrochloride

Kytril

## Class and Category

*Chemical:* Carbazole
*Therapeutic:* Antiemetic
*Pregnancy category:* B

## Indications and Dosages

➤ *To prevent nausea and vomiting caused by chemotherapy*

**ORAL SOLUTION, TABLETS**

**Adults and adolescents.** 1 mg up to 1 hr before chemotherapy and repeated 12 hr later; or 2 mg up to 1 hr before chemotherapy.

**I.V. INFUSION**

**Adults and adolescents.** 10 mcg/kg diluted and infused over 5 min, starting 30 min before chemotherapy; or 10 mcg/kg undiluted and infused over 30 sec, starting 30 min before chemotherapy.

➤ *To prevent nausea and vomiting caused by radiation therapy*

**ORAL SOLUTION, TABLETS**

**Adults and adolescents.** 2 mg q.d. given 1 hr before radiation therapy.

➤ *To prevent or treat postoperative nausea and vomiting*

**I.V. INJECTION**

**Adults and adolescents.** 1 mg administered over 30 sec before induction of anesthesia or immediately before reversal anesthesia for prevention. 1 mg administered over 30 sec after surgery for treatment.

---

### Mechanism of Action

Has a high affinity for serotonin receptors along vagal nerve endings in the intestines. Because of this affinity, granisetron prevents the nausea and vomiting that usually result when serotonin is released by damaged enterochromaffin cells.

## Incompatibilities
Don't mix granisetron in same solution as other drugs.

## Contraindications
Hypersensitivity to granisetron or its components

## Adverse Reactions
**CNS:** Asthenia, chills, CNS stimulation, drowsiness, fever, headache, insomnia, somnolence
**CV:** Hypertension
**EENT:** Taste perversion
**GI:** Abdominal pain, anorexia, constipation, diarrhea, elevated liver function test results, nausea, vomiting
**HEME:** Anemia, leukopenia, thrombocytopenia
**SKIN:** Alopecia

## Nursing Considerations
•For use with chemotherapy, dilute I.V. preparation of granisetron with NS or $D_5W$ to a total volume of 20 to 50 ml. Mixture may be stored for up to 24 hours. Use only on days when chemotherapy is given.
**PATIENT TEACHING**
•Inform patient that granisetron is given orally or I.V. before chemotherapy to help prevent nausea.
•Instruct patient to take tablet without food to avoid reducing drug bioavailability.
•Advise patient to report constipation, fever, severe diarrhea, or severe headache to prescriber. Also caution him about possible drowsiness.

# guaifenesin

Anti-Tuss, Balminil Expectorant (CAN), Benylin-E (CAN), Breonesin, Calmylin Expectorant (CAN), Gee-Gee, Genatuss, GG-CEN, Glycotuss, Glytuss, Guiatuss, Halotussin, Hytuss, Hytuss 2X, Mucinex, Organidin NR,Resyl (CAN), Robitussin, Scot-tussin Expectorant, Uni-tussin

## Class and Category
*Chemical:* Glyceryl guaiacolate
*Therapeutic:* Expectorant
*Pregnancy category:* C

## Indications and Dosages
➤ *To relieve cough, especially when secretions are thick*
**CAPSULES, ORAL SOLUTION, SYRUP, TABLETS**
**Adults and adolescents.** 200 to 400 mg q 4 hr. *Maximum:* 2,400 mg/day.

**CAPSULES, ORAL SOLUTION, SYRUP**
**Children ages 6 to 12.** 100 to 200 mg q 4 hr. *Maximum:* 1,200 mg/day.

➤ *To promote productive cough*
**E.R. TABLETS (MUCINEX)**
**Adults and adolescents.** 600 to 1,200 mg q 12 hr. *Maximum:* 2,400 mg/day.

| Route | Onset | Peak | Duration |
|-------|-------|------|----------|
| P.O. | 30 min | Unknown | 4 to 6 hr |

### Mechanism of Action
Increases fluid and mucus removal from the upper respiratory tract by increasing the volume of secretions and reducing their adhesiveness and surface tension.

## Contraindications
Hypersensitivity to guaifenesin

## Adverse Reactions
**CNS:** Dizziness, headache
**GI:** Nausea and vomiting (with large doses)
**SKIN:** Rash, urticaria

## Nursing Considerations
•As prescribed and as appropriate, give liquid forms of guaifenesin to children.
•Watch for signs of more serious condition, such as cough that lasts longer than 1 week, fever, persistent headache, and rash.
**PATIENT TEACHING**
•Instruct patient to take each dose with a full glass of water.
•Advise patient not to break, crush, or chew E.R. tablets but to swallow them whole.
•Instruct patient to increase fluid intake (unless contraindicated) to help thin secretions.
•Advise patient not to take drug longer than 1 week and to notify prescriber about fever, persistent headache, or rash.

# guanadrel sulfate

Hylorel

## Class and Category
*Chemical:* Guanidine derivative
*Therapeutic:* Antihypertensive
*Pregnancy category:* B

## Indications and Dosages
➤ *To manage hypertension*
**TABLETS**
**Adults.** 5 mg b.i.d., increased to 20 to 75 mg/day in divided doses t.i.d. or q.i.d., if needed.

G
H
I

DOSAGE ADJUSTMENT Initial dosage reduced to 5 mg q.d. if needed for patients with renal impairment or creatinine clearance of 30 to 60 ml/min/1.73 m$^2$. Then dosage adjusted after at least 7 days. Initial dosage reduced to 5 mg q.o.d. if needed for patients with creatinine clearance of less than 30 ml/min/1.73 m$^2$. Then dosage adjusted after at least 2 wk.

| Route | Onset | Peak | Duration |
|-------|-------|------|----------|
| P.O. | 30 min to 2 hr | 4 to 6 hr | 4 to 14 hr |

## Mechanism of Action

Exerts its antihypertensive effect at peripheral sympathetic nerve endings. Through an uptake mechanism, guanadrel is stored in adrenergic neurons, where it displaces norepinephrine from its storage sites. This action blocks the normal release of norepinephrine in response to nerve impulses, which depletes norepinephrine stores in the synapses and relaxes vessel walls, thus reducing peripheral resistance and blood pressure.

## Contraindications

Heart failure not caused by hypertension, hypersensitivity to guanadrel or its components, MAO inhibitor use within 1 week of guanadrel use, pheochromocytoma

## Interactions

**DRUGS**

*alpha blockers, beta blockers, rauwolfia alkaloids:* Possibly orthostatic hypotension or bradycardia
*amphetamines, appetite suppressants, cyclobenzaprine, haloperidol, loxapine, maprotiline, methylphenidate, phenothiazines, thioxanthenes, tricyclic antidepressants:* Decreased antihypertensive effect of guanadrel
*anticholinergics:* Possibly decreased inhibition of gastric acid secretion
*barbiturates, opioids:* Increased hypotensive effect
*MAO inhibitors:* Possibly severe blood pressure increase
*NSAIDs:* Possibly sodium and water retention and decreased antihypertensive effect of guanadrel
*sympathomimetics:* Possibly reduced antihypertensive effect of guanadrel, leading to hypertension; possibly potentiated effects of sympathomimetics
*vasodilators:* Increased orthostatic hypotension

**ACTIVITIES**

*alcohol use:* Increased hypotensive effect

## Adverse Reactions

**CNS:** Confusion, drowsiness, fatigue, headache, light-headedness, paresthesia, sleep disturbance
**CV:** Chest pain, orthostatic hypotension, palpitations, peripheral edema
**EENT:** Blurred vision, dry mouth and throat, glossitis
**GI:** Abdominal cramps or pain, anorexia, constipation, diarrhea, indigestion, nausea, vomiting
**GU:** Difficult ejaculation, hematuria, impotence, nocturia, urinary frequency or urgency
**MS:** Arthralgia, back or neck pain, joint inflammation, leg cramps, muscle weakness, myalgia
**RESP:** Cough, dyspnea
**Other:** Excessive weight gain or loss

## Nursing Considerations

• Use guanadrel cautiously in patients with asthma because drug may aggravate this condition. Monitor patient for acute dyspnea, wheezing, and other signs of asthma attack. Notify prescriber immediately if they develop.
• WARNING Assess for signs of overdose, such as blurred vision, dizziness, and syncope.
• Be aware that elderly patients have a greater risk of experiencing dizziness and syncope.
• Assess for signs of fluid retention and heart failure, including crackles, a new S$_3$ heart sound, and sudden weight gain.

**PATIENT TEACHING**

• Inform patient that guanadrel doesn't cure high blood pressure but does help control it.
• Instruct patient to take drug at the same time each day to improve compliance and blood pressure control.
• Caution patient about possible dizziness, light-headedness, and fainting, especially when getting up from a lying or sitting position. Advise him to rise slowly, especially in the morning, and to sit with his feet dangling for 1 to 2 minutes before standing up.
• Instruct patient to sit or lie down immediately if he feels dizzy.
• To prevent fainting, advise patient to avoid alcohol, standing for long periods, excessive exercise, and exposure to hot weather.
• Instruct patient to check with prescriber before taking OTC drugs during guanadrel therapy.

•Advise patient to follow a low-sodium diet to help reduce blood pressure and prevent fluid retention.

# guanethidine monosulfate

Apo-Guanethidine (CAN), Ismelin

## Class and Category
*Chemical:* Guanidine derivative
*Therapeutic:* Antihypertensive
*Pregnancy category:* C

## Indications and Dosages
➤ *To manage moderate to severe hypertension and renal hypertension*

**TABLETS**

**Adults.** *Initial:* 10 to 12.5 mg q.d., increased as needed by 10 to 12.5 mg q wk. *Maintenance:* 25 to 50 mg q.d. Some patients may need up to 300 mg q.d.

**Children.** 0.2 mg/kg q.d., increased p.r.n. by 0.2 mg/kg q 7 to 10 days. *Maximum:* 3 mg/kg q 24 hr.

**DOSAGE ADJUSTMENT** Initial dosage increased to 25 to 50 mg q.d. for adult hospitalized patients because they can be monitored more closely. Then dosage increased by 25 to 50 mg q.o.d., p.r.n.

| Route | Onset | Peak | Duration |
|-------|-------|------|----------|
| P.O. | Unknown | 8 hr* | Unknown* |

### Mechanism of Action
Exerts its antihypertensive effect at peripheral sympathetic nerve endings. Through an uptake mechanism, guanethidine is stored in adrenergic neurons, where it displaces norepinephrine from its storage sites. This action blocks the normal release of norepinephrine in response to nerve impulses, which depletes norepinephrine stores in the synapses and relaxes vessel walls, thus reducing peripheral resistance and blood pressure.

## Contraindications
Heart failure not caused by hypertension, hypersensitivity to guanethidine or its com-

---

* For single dose; 1 to 3 wk for multiple doses.

ponents, MAO inhibitor use within 1 week of guanethidine use, pheochromocytoma

## Interactions
**DRUGS**
*alpha blockers, beta blockers, rauwolfia alkaloids:* Possibly orthostatic hypotension or bradycardia
*amphetamines, appetite suppressants, cyclobenzaprine, haloperidol, loxapine, maprotiline, methylphenidate, phenothiazines, thioxanthenes, tricyclic antidepressants:* Decreased antihypertensive effect of guanethidine
*anticholinergics:* Possibly decreased inhibition of gastric acid secretion
*barbiturates, opioids:* Increased hypotensive effect
*insulin, oral antidiabetic drugs:* Possibly increased antidiabetic effect of these drugs
*MAO inhibitors:* Possibly severe blood pressure increase
*NSAIDs:* Possibly sodium and water retention and decreased antihypertensive effect of guanethidine
*sympathomimetics:* Possibly reduced antihypertensive effect of guanethidine, leading to hypertension; possibly potentiated effects of sympathomimetics
*vasodilators:* Increased orthostatic hypotension
**ACTIVITIES**
*alcohol use:* Increased hypotensive effect

## Adverse Reactions
**CNS:** Depression, dizziness, fatigue, headache, lassitude, paresthesia, syncope
**CV:** Angina, bradycardia, orthostatic hypotension, palpitations, peripheral edema
**EENT:** Blurred vision, dry mouth, glossitis, nasal congestion, parotid gland tenderness, ptosis
**GI:** Anorexia, constipation, diarrhea (severe), indigestion, nausea, vomiting
**GU:** Ejaculation disorders, elevated BUN level, impotence, nocturia, priapism, urinary frequency
**HEME:** Anemia, leukopenia, thrombocytopenia
**MS:** Leg cramps, muscle twitching, myalgia
**RESP:** Asthma exacerbation, dyspnea
**SKIN:** Alopecia, dermatitis
**Other:** Weight gain

## Nursing Considerations
•As prescribed, discontinue MAO inhibitor

G
H
I

therapy at least 1 week before starting guan-ethidine.
• Because guanethidine has cumulative effects, give a small initial dose and increase gradually, as prescribed. When blood pressure is controlled, expect to reduce dosage to lowest effective level.
• Monitor for orthostatic hypotension, which occurs most often when arising in the morning and is exacerbated by hot weather, exercise, and alcohol. Assess supine and standing blood pressures, especially after dosage adjustments.
• Measure daily weight to help detect fluid retention. Also observe for edema and other signs of heart failure. A thiazide diuretic may be prescribed to decrease sodium and fluid retention.
• Notify prescriber if severe diarrhea occurs. Drug may need to be discontinued.
• Monitor febrile patient for increased hypotension and adverse reactions because fever decreases drug requirements.
• As ordered, stop giving guanethidine 2 weeks before surgery to reduce the risk of cardiac arrest during anesthesia.

**PATIENT TEACHING**
• Teach patient how to recognize signs of orthostatic hypotension, and advise changing position slowly. Inform patient that symptoms are worse in the morning and exacerbated by exercise, hot weather, alcohol, and hot showers.
• Instruct patient to report fainting, frequent dizziness, and severe diarrhea.
• Caution patient to avoid alcohol because it may increase the risk of orthostatic hypotension.
• Instruct patient to weigh himself daily at the same time, on the same scale, and wearing the same amount of clothing. Advise him to report signs of fluid retention, such as reduced urine volume, sudden weight increase, and limb swelling.
• Urge patient to consult prescriber before taking OTC drugs during guanethidine therapy.
• If a diabetic patient takes insulin or a sulfonylurea, instruct him to monitor his blood glucose level more frequently to check for hypoglycemia.
• Advise patient to follow a low-sodium diet to help reduce blood pressure and prevent fluid retention.

# guanfacine hydrochloride

Tenex

## Class and Category
*Chemical:* Dichlorobenzine derivative
*Therapeutic:* Antihypertensive
*Pregnancy category:* B

## Indications and Dosages
➤ *To manage hypertension, alone or with other antihypertensives*

**TABLETS**
**Adults.** 1 mg q.d. h.s., increased if needed to 2 mg after 3 to 4 wk. Then increased to 3 mg if needed after another 3 to 4 wk. *Maintenance:* 2 or 3 mg q.d.
**DOSAGE ADJUSTMENT** Twice-daily dosing used if blood pressure tends to rise at the end of 24-hr period.

| Route | Onset | Peak | Duration |
|-------|-------|------|----------|
| P.O. | Unknown* | 8 to 12 hr† | 24 hr |

### Mechanism of Action
Decreases sympathetic nerve impulse outflow from the brain's vasomotor center to the heart and blood vessels by stimulating central alpha$_2$-adrenergic receptors. This action reduces peripheral vascular resistance, renovascular resistance, heart rate, and blood pressure. Prolonged use of guanfacine may reduce total peripheral vascular resistance, slightly reducing the heart rate. Guanfacine also stimulates growth hormone secretion, reduces circulating levels of plasma catecholamines, and reduces left ventricular hypertrophy.

## Contraindications
Hypersensitivity to guanfacine

## Interactions
**DRUGS**
*CNS depressants:* Possibly increased CNS depression
*NSAIDs, sympathomimetics, tricyclic anti-*

---

* For single dose; in 1 wk for multiple doses.
† For single dose; 1 to 3 mo for multiple doses.

*depressants:* Possibly decreased antihypertensive effect of guanfacine
*other antihypertensives:* Possibly increased antihypertensive effect, resulting in hypotension
**ACTIVITIES**
*alcohol use:* Possibly increased CNS depression

## Adverse Reactions
**CNS:** Anxiety, confusion, depression, dizziness, drowsiness, headache, nervousness, weakness
**CV:** Bradycardia, orthostatic hypotension
**EENT:** Conjunctivitis, dry mouth
**GI:** Constipation, nausea
**GU:** Decreased libido, impotence
**SKIN:** Dermatitis, diaphoresis, pruritus, purpura, rash

## Nursing Considerations
•Use guanfacine cautiously in patients with cerebrovascular disease, chronic renal or hepatic failure, recent MI, or severe coronary insufficiency.
•Give drug at bedtime to minimize daytime sedation.
•**WARNING** Expect to discontinue drug by decreasing dosage gradually over 2 to 4 days. Typically, if patient hasn't had drug for 2 or more days, he may experience withdrawal symptoms, including abdominal cramps, anxiety, chest pain, diaphoresis, headache, increased salivation, insomnia, irregular heart rate and rhythm, nausea, nervousness, restlessness, tremor, and vomiting.
•If you suspect that patient has drug-related depression, notify prescriber immediately and expect to discontinue drug.
**PATIENT TEACHING**
•Instruct patient to take guanfacine at bedtime to reduce daytime drowsiness.
•Caution patient about possible drowsiness, and advise him to avoid potentially hazardous activities until drug's CNS effects are known.
•Urge patient to avoid alcohol and other CNS depressants while taking guanfacine.
•Advise patient to report rash.
•Inform male patient that drug may cause impotence. Suggest that he discuss impotence with prescriber, if it occurs.
•Caution patient not to stop taking drug abruptly because doing so can cause a dangerous rise in blood pressure along with anxiety and nervousness.

# halazepam
Paxipam

## Class, Category, and Schedule
*Chemical:* Benzodiazepine
*Therapeutic:* Antianxiety
*Pregnancy category:* D
*Controlled substance:* Schedule IV

## Indications and Dosages
➤ *To manage anxiety*
**TABLETS**
**Adults.** 20 to 40 mg t.i.d. or q.i.d. *Optimal:* 80 to 160 mg/day.
**DOSAGE ADJUSTMENT** Dosage reduced to 20 mg q.d. or b.i.d. if needed for debilitated patients.

| Route | Onset | Peak | Duration |
|-------|-------|------|----------|
| P.O. | Slow | Unknown | 6 to 8 hr |

### Mechanism of Action
May potentiate the effects of gamma-aminobutyric acid (GABA) and other inhibitory neurotransmitters by binding to specific benzodiazepine receptor sites in the limbic and cortical areas of the CNS. By binding to these receptor sites, halazepam increases the inhibitory effects of GABA and blocks cortical and limbic arousal.

## Contraindications
Acute angle-closure glaucoma, hypersensitivity to halazepam or its components, itraconazole or ketoconazole therapy, psychosis

## Interactions
**DRUGS**
*antacids:* Possibly altered rate of halazepam absorption
*barbiturates, CNS depressants, narcotics:* Increased CNS depression, possibly sedation and impaired motor function
*cimetidine, diltiazem, disulfiram, erythromycin, fluoxetine, fluvoxamine, isoniazid, itraconazole, ketoconazole, metoprolol, nefazodone, oral contraceptives, propoxyphene, propranolol, ranitidine, valproic acid, verapamil:* Decreased clearance, increased blood level, and increased risk of adverse effects of halazepam
*clozapine:* Possibly respiratory depression

G
H
I

*digoxin:* Increased blood digoxin level and risk of digitalis toxicity
*levodopa:* Decreased antidyskinetic effect
*neuromuscular blockers:* Increased or blocked neuromuscular blockade
*theophyllines:* Decreased sedative effect of halazepam
**ACTIVITIES**
*alcohol use:* Increased CNS depression, possibly sedation and impaired motor function
*smoking:* Decreased halazepam effectiveness

## Adverse Reactions

**CNS:** Agitation, anxiety, ataxia, confusion, depression, dizziness, drowsiness, euphoria, headache, irritability, nervousness, slurred speech, tremor, weakness
**CV:** Angina, palpitations, sinus tachycardia
**EENT:** Diplopia, dry mouth, tinnitus
**GI:** Abdominal cramps or pain, constipation, diarrhea, increased salivation, nausea, vomiting
**GU:** Decreased libido, dysuria
**MS:** Arthralgia
**SKIN:** Pruritus, rash

## Nursing Considerations

•Use halazepam cautiously in patients with impaired hepatic or renal function, seizure disorders, or suicidal tendencies.
•Be aware that risk of halazepam addiction and abuse is relatively high.
•Monitor renal and liver function test results, as appropriate, during long-term treatment.
•Expect to withdraw drug gradually over 2 weeks to avoid withdrawal symptoms, which include anxiety, confusion, insomnia, psychosis, and seizures.
**PATIENT TEACHING**
•Instruct patient to take halazepam exactly as prescribed and not to stop taking it abruptly because withdrawal symptoms may occur.
•Caution patient to avoid alcohol and other CNS depressants during therapy. Advise patient to avoid OTC drugs, such as cough and cold remedies, because they may contain CNS depressants.
•Advise patient to avoid potentially hazardous activities until drug's CNS effects are known.
•Instruct patient to report depression, difficulty voiding, double vision, persistent drowsiness, and rash.
•Explain that drug's full effects may not occur for 6 weeks.

# haloperidol

Apo-Haloperidol (CAN), Haldol, Novo-Peridol (CAN), Peridol (CAN)

## haloperidol decanoate

Haldol Decanoate, Haldol LA (CAN)

## haloperidol lactate

Haldol Concentrate

## Class and Category

*Chemical:* Butyrophenone derivative
*Therapeutic:* Antidyskinetic, antipsychotic
*Pregnancy category:* C (haloperidol decanoate), Not rated (haloperidol, haloperidol lactate)

## Indications and Dosages

➤ *To treat psychotic disorders*
**ORAL SOLUTION, TABLETS**
**Adults and adolescents.** 0.5 to 5 mg b.i.d. or t.i.d. *Maximum:* Usually 100 mg/day.
**Children ages 3 to 12.** 0.05 mg/kg/day in divided doses b.i.d. or t.i.d. Increased by 0.5 mg q 5 to 7 days, if needed. *Maximum:* 0.15 mg/kg/day.

➤ *To treat nonpsychotic behavior disorders and Tourette's syndrome*
**ORAL SOLUTION, TABLETS**
**Adults and adolescents.** 0.5 to 5 mg b.i.d. or t.i.d. *Maximum:* Usually 100 mg/day.
**Children ages 3 to 12.** 0.05 to 0.075 mg/kg/day in divided doses b.i.d. or t.i.d. Increased by 0.5 mg q 5 to 7 days, if needed. *Maximum:* 0.075 mg/kg/day.
**DOSAGE ADJUSTMENT** Initial dosage reduced to 0.5 to 2 mg b.i.d. or t.i.d. if needed for elderly or debilitated patients.

➤ *To treat acute psychotic episodes*
**I.M. INJECTION**
**Adults and adolescents.** *Initial:* 2 to 5 mg followed by subsequent doses as frequently as q 60 min. Alternatively, if symptoms are controlled, dose may be repeated q 4 to 8 hr. *Maximum:* Usually 100 mg/day. First oral dose may be given 12 to 24 hr after last parenteral dose.

➤ *To provide long-term antipsychotic therapy for patients who require parenteral therapy*
**LONG-ACTING I.M. (DECANOATE) INJECTION**
**Adults.** *Initial:* 10 to 15 times the daily oral dose up to 100 mg. Repeated q 4 wk, if needed. *Maximum:* 300 mg/mo.

| Route | Onset | Peak | Duration |
|-------|-------|------|----------|
| I.M.* | Unknown | 3 to 4 days† | Unknown |

## Mechanism of Action

May block postsynaptic dopamine receptors in the limbic system and increase brain turnover of dopamine, producing an antipsychotic effect.

## Contraindications

Blood dyscrasias, bone marrow depression, cerebral arteriosclerosis, coma, concomitant use of large amounts of other CNS depressants, coronary artery disease, epilepsy, hepatic dysfunction, hypersensitivity to haloperidol or its components, Parkinson's disease, severe hypertension or hypotension, severe CNS depression, subcortical brain damage

## Interactions

**DRUGS**

*amphetamines:* Possibly decreased stimulant effects of amphetamines and decreased antipsychotic effect of haloperidol
*anticholinergics, antidyskinetics, antihistamines:* Increased anticholinergic effect and risk of decreased antipsychotic effect of haloperidol
*anticonvulsants:* Possibly decreased effectiveness of anticonvulsants and decreased blood haloperidol level
*bromocriptine:* Possibly decreased effectiveness of bromocriptine
*bupropion:* Lowered seizure threshold, increased risk of major motor seizure
*CNS depressants:* Increased CNS depression and risk of respiratory depression and hypotension
*diazoxide:* Possibly hypoglycemia
*dopamine (high-dose therapy):* Possibly decreased vasoconstriction
*ephedrine:* Possibly decreased vasopressor effect of ephedrine
*epinephrine:* Possibly severe hypotension and tachycardia
*fluoxetine:* Increased risk of severe and frequent extrapyramidal effects
*guanadrel, guanethidine:* Decreased hypotensive effects of these drugs

---

*\* For haloperidol decanoate and lactate.*
*† For haloperidol decanoate only; 30 to 45 min for haloperidol lactate.*

*levodopa, pergolide:* Possibly decreased therapeutic effects of these drugs
*lithium:* Increased risk of neurotoxicity
*MAO inhibitors, maprotiline, tricyclic antidepressants:* Increased sedative and anticholinergic effects of these drugs
*metaraminol:* Possibly decreased vasopressor effect of metaraminol
*methoxamine:* Decreased vasopressor effect, shortened duration of action of methoxamine
*methyldopa:* Possibly disorientation, slowed or difficult thought processes
*phenylephrine:* Decreased vasopressor response to phenylephrine
**ACTIVITIES**
*alcohol use:* Increased CNS depression and risk of respiratory depression and hypotension

## Adverse Reactions

**CNS:** Agitation, anxiety, confusion, drowsiness, euphoria, extrapyramidal reactions that may be irreversible (akathisia, pseudoparkinsonism, tardive dyskinesia), hallucinations, headache, insomnia, neuroleptic malignant syndrome, restlessness, slurred speech, tremor, vertigo
**CV:** Cardiac arrest, hypertension, orthostatic hypotension, QT prolongation, ventricular tachycardia
**EENT:** Blurred vision, dry mouth, increased salivation (all drug forms); stomatitis (oral solution)
**ENDO:** Breast engorgement, galactorrhea
**GI:** Constipation, nausea, vomiting
**GU:** Decreased libido, difficult ejaculation, impotence, menstrual irregularities, urine retention
**HEME:** Anemia, leukocytosis, leukopenia
**SKIN:** Diaphoresis, photosensitivity, rash
**Other:** Heatstroke, weight gain

## Nursing Considerations

• Before giving oral solution, dilute it with a beverage, such as cola or orange, apple, or tomato juice.
• Administer haloperidol decanoate (long-acting form prepared in sesame oil to produce slow, sustained release) by deep I.M. injection into gluteal muscle using Z-track technique and 21G needle. Don't give more than 3 ml at one site. Expect to reach a stable plasma level after third or fourth dose.
• If injection solution has a slight yellow discoloration, be aware that this change doesn't affect potency.

G
H
I

•Monitor for tardive dyskinesia (potentially irreversible involuntary movements) in patients receiving long-term therapy, especially elderly women who take large doses.
•If extrapyramidal reactions occur during the first few days of treatment, reduce dosage, as prescribed.
•Avoid stopping haloperidol abruptly unless severe adverse reactions occur.
•Monitor for signs of neuroleptic malignant syndrome, a rare but possibly fatal disorder linked to antipsychotic drugs. Signs include altered mental status, arrhythmias, fever, and muscle rigidity.

**PATIENT TEACHING**
•Advise patient to take haloperidol exactly as prescribed and not to stop taking it abruptly because withdrawal symptoms may occur.
•To prevent oral mucosal irritation, instruct patient to dilute liquid form with juice or cola before taking it.
•Caution patient to avoid skin contact with oral solution because it may cause a rash.
•Advise patient to take tablets with food or a full glass of milk or water to reduce GI distress.
•Instruct patient to maintain adequate fluid intake and to take precautions against heatstroke.
•Urge patient not to drink alcohol during therapy.
•If sedation occurs, caution patient to avoid driving and other potentially hazardous activities.
•Instruct patient to report repetitive movements, tremor, and vision changes to prescriber.

# heparin calcium

Calcilean (CAN), Calciparine

## heparin sodium

Hepalean (CAN), Heparin Leo (CAN), Heparin Lock Flush, Liquaemin

### Class and Category

*Chemical:* Glycosaminoglycan
*Therapeutic:* Anticoagulant
*Pregnancy category:* C

### Indications and Dosages

➤ *To prevent and treat deep vein thrombosis and pulmonary embolism, to treat*
*peripheral arterial embolism, and to prevent thromboembolism before and after cardioversion of chronic atrial fibrillation*

**I.V. INFUSION OR INJECTION**
**Adults.** *Loading:* 35 to 70 U/kg or 5,000 U by injection. Then 20,000 to 40,000 U infused over 24 hr.
**Children.** *Loading:* 50 U/kg by injection. Then 100 U/kg infused q 4 hr or 20,000 U/m² infused over 24 hr.

**I.V. INJECTION**
**Adults.** *Initial:* 10,000 U. *Maintenance:* 5,000 to 10,000 U q 4 to 6 hr.
**Children.** *Initial:* 50 U/kg. *Maintenance:* 100 U/kg/dose q 4 hr.

**I.V. OR S.C. INJECTION**
**Adults.** *Loading:* 5,000 U I.V., then 10,000 to 20,000 U S.C. *Maintenance:* 8,000 to 10,000 U S.C. q 8 hr or 15,000 to 20,000 U S.C. q 12 hr.

➤ *To diagnose and treat disseminated intravascular coagulation (DIC)*

**I.V. INFUSION OR INJECTION**
**Adults.** 50 to 100 U/kg q 4 hr. Drug may be discontinued if no improvement occurs in 4 to 8 hr.
**Children.** 25 to 50 U/kg q 4 hr. Drug may be discontinued if no improvement occurs in 4 to 8 hr.

➤ *To prevent postoperative thromboembolism*

**S.C. INJECTION**
**Adults.** 5,000 U 2 hr before surgery and then 5,000 U q 8 to 12 hr for 7 days or until patient is fully ambulatory.

➤ *To prevent clots in patients undergoing open-heart and vascular surgery*

**I.V. INFUSION OR INJECTION**
**Adults.** 300 U/kg for procedures that last less than 60 min; 400 U/kg for procedures that last longer than 60 min. *Minimum:* 150 U/kg.
**Children.** 300 U/kg for procedures that last less than 60 min. Then dosage is based on coagulation test results. *Minimum:* 150 U/kg.

➤ *To maintain heparin lock patency*

**I.V. INJECTION**
**Adults.** 10 to 100 U/ml heparin flush solution (enough to fill device) after each use of device.

| Route | Onset | Peak | Duration |
|-------|-------|------|----------|
| I.V. | Immediate | Minutes | Unknown |
| S.C. | In 20 to 60 min | Unknown | Unknown |

## Mechanism of Action

Binds with antithrombin III, enhancing antithrombin III's inactivation of the co-agulation enzymes thrombin (factor IIa) and factors Xa and XIa. At low doses, heparin inhibits factor Xa and prevents the conversion of prothrombin to throm-bin. Thrombin is necessary for the conver-sion of fibrinogen to fibrin; without fi-brin, clots can't form. At high doses, hep-arin inactivates thrombin, preventing fi-brin formation and existing clot extension.

## Incompatibilities

Don't mix heparin with any other drug un-less you have an order to do so and have checked with pharmacist. Heparin is incom-patible with many drugs and solutions, espe-cially ones that contain a phosphate buffer, sodium bicarbonate, or sodium oxalate.

## Contraindications

Hypersensitivity to heparin or its compo-nents; severe thrombocytopenia; uncontrolled bleeding, except in DIC

## Interactions

**DRUGS**

*antihistamines, digoxin, nicotine, tetracy-clines:* Decreased anticoagulant effect of hep-arin

*aspirin, NSAIDs, platelet aggregation inhibi-tors, sulfinpyrazone:* Increased platelet inhi-bition and risk of bleeding

*cefamandole, cefoperazone, cefotetan, methi-mazole, plicamycin, propylthiouracil, val-proic acid:* Possibly hypoprothrombinemia and increased risk of bleeding

*chloroquine, hydroxychloroquine:* Possibly thrombocytopenia and increased risk of hem-orrhage

*ethacrynic acid, glucocorticoids, salicylates:* Increased risk of bleeding and GI ulceration and hemorrhage

*nitroglycerin (I.V.):* Possibly decreased anti-coagulant effect of heparin

*probenecid:* Possibly increased anticoagulant effect of heparin

*thrombolytics:* Increased risk of hemorrhage

**ACTIVITIES**

*smoking:* Decreased anticoagulant effect of heparin

## Adverse Reactions

**CNS:** Chills, dizziness, fever, headache, pe-ripheral neuropathy

**CV:** Chest pain

**EENT:** Epistaxis, gingival bleeding, rhinitis

**GI:** Abdominal distention and pain, hema-temesis, melena, nausea, vomiting

**GU:** Hematuria, hypermenorrhea

**HEME:** Easy bruising, excessive bleeding from wounds, thrombocytopenia

**MS:** Back pain, myalgia, osteoporosis

**RESP:** Dyspnea, wheezing

**SKIN:** Alopecia, cyanosis, petechiae, pruri-tus, urticaria

**Other:** Anaphylaxis; injection site hematoma, irritation, pain, redness, and ulceration

## Nursing Considerations

•Use heparin cautiously in alcoholics; men-struating women; patients over age 60, espe-cially women; and patients with mild hepatic or renal disease or a history of allergies, asthma, or GI ulcer.

•**WARNING** Give heparin only S.C. or I.V.; I.M. use causes hematoma, irritation, and pain.

•Avoid injecting any drugs by I.M. route during heparin therapy to decrease the risk of bleeding and hematoma.

•Administer S.C. heparin into the anterior abdominal wall, above the iliac crest, and 5 cm (2″) or more away from the umbilicus. To minimize subcutaneous tissue trauma, lift adipose tissue away from deep tissues; don't aspirate for blood before injecting drug; don't move needle while injecting drug; and don't massage the injection site before or after injection. Keep in mind that you can apply gentle pressure to the site after you withdraw the needle.

•Alternate injection sites, and observe for signs of bleeding and hematoma formation.

•To prepare heparin for continuous infusion, invert container at least six times to prevent drug from pooling. Anticipate slight discol-oration of prepared solution; this doesn't in-dicate a change in potency.

•During continuous I.V. therapy, expect to obtain APTT after 8 hours of therapy. Use the arm opposite the infusion site.

•For intermittent I.V. therapy, expect to ad-just dose based on coagulation test results performed 30 minutes earlier. Therapeutic range is typically 1.5 to 2.5 times the control.

•Take safety precautions to prevent bleeding,

G
H
I

such as having patient use a soft-bristled toothbrush and an electric razor.

• Monitor blood test results and observe for signs of bleeding, such as ecchymosis, epistaxis, hematemesis, hematuria, melena, and petechiae.

• Make sure all health care providers know that patient is receiving heparin.

• Keep protamine sulfate on hand to use as an antidote for heparin. Be aware that each milligram of protamine sulfate neutralizes 100 U of heparin.

• Be aware that prescriber may order oral anticoagulants before discontinuing heparin to avoid increased coagulation caused by heparin withdrawal. Heparin may be discontinued when full therapeutic effect of oral anticoagulant is achieved.

• Know that women over age 60 have the highest risk of hemorrhage during therapy.

**PATIENT TEACHING**

• Explain that heparin can't be taken orally.

• Inform patient about the increased risk of bleeding; urge her to avoid injuries and to use a soft-bristled toothbrush and an electric razor.

• Advise patient to avoid drugs that interact with heparin, such as aspirin and ibuprofen.

• Instruct patient and family to watch for and report abdominal or lower back pain, black stools, bleeding gums, bloody urine, excessive menstrual bleeding, nosebleeds, and severe headaches.

• Inform patient that temporary hair loss may occur.

• Advise patient to wear or carry appropriate medical identification.

# hyaluronan (high-molecular-weight)

Euflexxa, Orthovisc

## Class and Category

*Chemical:* Natural complex glycosaminoglycan sugar
*Therapeutic:* Analgesic
*Pregnancy category:* Not rated

## Indications and Dosages

➤ *To relieve osteoarthritic knee pain in patients who respond inadequately to conservative nonpharmacologic therapy and to simple analgesics*

**INTRA-ARTICULAR INJECTION (ORTHOVISC)**
**Adults.** 30 mg/wk for 3 to 4 wk
**INTRA-ARTICULAR INJECTION (EUFLEXXA)**
**Adults.** 20 mg/wk for 3 wk

## Mechanism of Action

Instilling hyaluronan, a viscoelastic substance normally found in joint tissues and in the fluid that fills joints, directly into the joint relieves pain associated with osteoarthritis by lubricating the joint and absorbing shock when the joint moves.

## Contraindications

Hypersensitivity to hyaluronan avian, avian-derived products (such as eggs, feathers, or poultry) or any of their components; knee infections; skin diseases affecting the knee area

## Interactions

None reported.

## Adverse Reactions

**CNS:** Headache
**MS:** Acute arthritis, arthralgia, back pain, bursitis
**Other:** Injection site bruising, edema, erythema, pain, pruritus, or rash

## Nursing Considerations

• Prepare the patient for removal of joint effusion, if present, before hyaluronan injection.

• Assist the trained health care professional who gives the intra-articular injections, as needed, making sure that strict aseptic technique is followed throughout the procedure.

• Be aware that the prefilled syringe is for single use and that contents of the syringe should be used immediately after opening.

**PATIENT TEACHING**

• Inform patient that transient knee pain, swelling, or other localized reactions, such as itchiness or bruising, may occur after hyaluronan injection.

• Instruct patient to avoid strenuous or weight-bearing activities lasting longer than 1 hour for 48 hours after the injection.

• Inform patient that she may feel achy after the injection but that this discomfort is typically mild and brief.

• Advise patient that pain may not be relieved until after third injection.

# hydralazine hydrochloride

Apo-Hydralazine (CAN), Apresoline (CAN), Novo-Hylazin (CAN)

## Class and Category

*Chemical:* Phthalazine derivative
*Therapeutic:* Antihypertensive, vasodilator
*Pregnancy category:* C

## Indications and Dosages

➤ *To manage essential hypertension, alone or with other antihypertensives*

**TABLETS**
**Adults.** *Initial:* 40 mg/day in divided doses b.i.d. or q.i.d. for first 2 to 4 days and then increased to 100 mg/day in divided doses b.i.d. or q.i.d. for remainder of first wk. *Maximum:* Usually 200 mg/day, but sometimes 300 to 400 mg/day.
**Children.** 0.75 mg/kg/day in divided doses b.i.d. or q.i.d., increased gradually over 3 to 4 wk. *Maximum:* 7.5 mg/kg or 200 mg/day.

➤ *To manage severe essential hypertension when drug can't be taken orally or when need to reduce blood pressure is urgent*

**I.V. OR I.M. INJECTION**
**Adults.** 5 to 40 mg, repeated as needed.
**Children.** 1.7 to 3.5 mg/kg/day in divided doses q 4 to 6 hr, as needed.

## Incompatibilities

Don't mix hydralazine in I.V. infusion solutions.

| Route | Onset | Peak | Duration |
|---|---|---|---|
| P.O. | 20 to 30 min | 1 to 2 hr | 2 to 4 hr |
| I.V. | 5 to 20 min | 10 to 80 min | 2 to 6 hr |
| I.M. | 10 to 30 min | 1 hr | 2 to 6 hr |

## Contraindications

Coronary artery disease, hypersensitivity to hydralazine or its components, mitral valve disease

## Interactions

**DRUGS**
*beta blockers:* Increased effects of both drugs
*diazoxide, MAO inhibitors, other antihypertensives:* Risk of severe hypotension
*epinephrine:* Possibly decreased vasopressor effect of epinephrine
*NSAIDs:* Decreased hydralazine effects
*sympathomimetics:* Possibly decreased antihypertensive effect of hydralazine

**FOODS**
*all foods:* Possibly increased bioavailability of hydralazine

## Mechanism of Action

May act in a manner that resembles organic nitrates and sodium nitroprusside, except that hydralazine is selective for arteries. It:
• exerts a direct vasodilating effect on vascular smooth muscle
• interferes with calcium movement in vascular smooth muscle by altering cellular calcium metabolism
• dilates arteries rather than veins, which minimizes orthostatic hypotension and increases cardiac output and cerebral blood flow
• causes a reflex autonomic response that increases the heart rate, cardiac output, and left ventricular ejection fraction
• has a positive inotropic effect on the heart.

## Adverse Reactions

**CNS:** Chills, fever, headache, peripheral neuritis
**CV:** Angina, edema, orthostatic hypotension, palpitations, tachycardia
**EENT:** Lacrimation, nasal congestion
**GI:** Anorexia, constipation, diarrhea, nausea, vomiting
**RESP:** Dyspnea
**SKIN:** Blisters, flushing, pruritus, rash, urticaria
**Other:** Lupus-like symptoms, especially with high doses; lymphadenopathy

## Nursing Considerations

• Monitor CBC, lupus erythematosus cell preparation, and ANA titer before therapy and periodically as appropriate during long-term treatment.
• Anticipate that drug may change color in solution. Consult pharmacist if color change occurs.
• Be aware that hydralazine may undergo color changes when exposed to a metal filter.

G
H
I

•Give tablets with food to increase bioavailability.

•Monitor blood pressure and pulse rate regularly and weigh patient daily during therapy.

•Check blood pressure with patient in lying, sitting, and standing positions, and watch for signs of orthostatic hypotension. Expect orthostatic hypotension to be most common in the morning, during hot weather, and with exercise.

•**WARNING** Expect to discontinue drug immediately if patient experiences lupus-like symptoms, such as arthralgia, fever, myalgia, pharyngitis, and splenomegaly.

•Expect prescriber to withdraw drug gradually to avoid a rapid increase in blood pressure.

•Expect to treat peripheral neuritis with pyridoxine.

**PATIENT TEACHING**

•Instruct patient to take hydralazine tablets with food.

•Advise patient to change position slowly, especially in the morning. Caution her that hot showers may increase hypotension.

•Instruct patient to immediately notify prescriber about fever, muscle and joint aches, and sore throat.

•Urge patient to report numbness and tingling in her limbs, which may require treatment with another drug.

•Caution patient against stopping drug abruptly because doing so may cause severe hypertension.

# hydrochlorothiazide

Esidrix, Hydro-chlor, Hydro-D, Hydro-DIURIL, Microzide, Neo-Codema (CAN), Novo-Hydrazide (CAN), Oretic, Urozide (CAN)

### Class and Category
*Chemical:* Benzothiadiazide
*Therapeutic:* Antihypertensive, diuretic
*Pregnancy category:* B

### Indications and Dosages
➤ *To manage hypertension*
**CAPSULES**
**Adults.** 12.5 mg/day.
**ORAL SOLUTION, TABLETS**
**Adults.** 25 to 100 mg/day as a single dose or in divided doses b.i.d.
**Children age 6 months and older.** 1 to 2 mg/kg/

day as a single dose or in divided doses b.i.d.
**Infants under age 6 months.** Up to 3 mg/kg/day.

➤ *As adjunct to treat edema caused by cirrhosis, corticosteroids, estrogen, heart failure, or renal disorders*
**ORAL SOLUTION, TABLETS**
**Adults.** 25 to 100 mg b.i.d., q.d., or q.o.d for 3 to 5 days/wk.
**Children age 6 months and older.** 1 to 2 mg/kg/day as a single dose or in divided doses b.i.d.
**Infants under age 6 months.** Up to 3 mg/kg/day.

| Route | Onset | Peak | Duration |
|-------|-------|------|----------|
| P.O. | 2 hr | 4 hr | 6 to 12 hr |

### Contraindications
Anuria; hypersensitivity to hydrochlorothiazide, other thiazides, sulfonamide derivatives, or their components; renal failure

### Interactions
**DRUGS**
*amantadine:* Possibly increased blood level and risk of toxicity of amantadine
*amiodarone:* Increased risk of arrhythmias from hypokalemia
*amphotericin B, corticosteroids:* Increased electrolyte depletion, especially potassium
*antihypertensives:* Increased antihypertensive effects
*calcium:* Possibly increased serum calcium level
*cholestyramine, colestipol:* Reduced GI absorption of hydrochlorothiazide
*diazoxide:* Increased antihypertensive and hyperglycemic effects of hydrochlorothiazide
*diflunisal:* Possibly increased blood hydrochlorothiazide level
*digoxin:* Increased risk of digitalis toxicity from hypokalemia
*dopamine:* Possibly increased diuretic effects of both drugs
*insulin, oral antidiabetic drugs:* Possibly increased blood glucose level
*lithium:* Decreased lithium clearance, increased risk of lithium toxicity
*neuromuscular blockers:* Possibly enhanced neuromuscular blockade from hypokalemia
*NSAIDs:* Decreased diuretic effect of hydrochlorothiazide, increased risk of renal failure

## Mechanism of Action

A thiazide diuretic, hydro-chlorothiazide promotes the movement of sodium (Na⁺), chloride (Cl⁻), and water (H₂O) from blood in the peri-tubular capillaries into the nephron's distal convoluted tubule, as shown at right. Initially, hydrochlorothiazide may decrease extracellular fluid volume, plasma volume, and cardiac output, which helps explain blood pressure reduction. It also may reduce blood pressure by causing direct dilation of arteries. After several weeks, extracellular fluid volume, plasma volume, and cardiac output return to normal, and peripheral vascular resistance remains decreased.

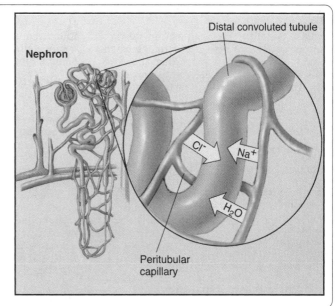

G
H
I

*oral anticoagulants:* Possibly decreased anticoagulant effects
*sympathomimetics:* Possibly decreased antihypertensive effect of hydrochlorothiazide
*vitamin D:* Increased risk of hypercalcemia

### Adverse Reactions

**CNS:** Dizziness, headache, insomnia, paresthesia, vertigo, weakness
**CV:** Hypotension, orthostatic hypotension, vasculitis
**EENT:** Blurred vision, dry mouth
**ENDO:** Hyperglycemia
**GI:** Abdominal cramps, anorexia, constipation, diarrhea, indigestion, jaundice, nausea, vomiting
**GU:** Decreased libido, impotence, interstitial nephritis, nocturia, polyuria, renal failure
**HEME:** Agranulocytosis, aplastic anemia, hemolytic anemia, leukopenia, neutropenia, thrombocytopenia
**MS:** Muscle spasms and weakness
**SKIN:** Alopecia, exfoliative dermatitis, photosensitivity, purpura, rash, urticaria
**Other:** Anaphylaxis, dehydration, hypercalcemia, hyperuricemia, hypochloremia, hypokalemia, hyponatremia, hypovolemia, metabolic alkalosis, weight loss

### Nursing Considerations

•Give hydrochlorothiazide in the morning and early in the evening to avoid nocturia.
•Monitor fluid intake and output, daily weight, blood pressure, and serum levels of electrolytes, especially potassium.
•Assess for signs of hypokalemia, such as muscle spasms and weakness.
•Monitor BUN and serum creatinine levels regularly.
•Frequently monitor blood glucose level as ordered in diabetic patients, and expect to increase antidiabetic drug dosage, as needed.
•If patient has a history of gouty arthritis, expect an increased risk of gout attacks during therapy.

**PATIENT TEACHING**

•Advise patient to take hydrochlorothiazide in the morning and early in the evening to avoid awakening during the night to urinate.
•Instruct patient to take drug with food or milk if adverse GI reactions occur.
•Direct patient to weigh herself at the same time each day wearing the same amount of clothing and to notify prescriber if she gains more than 2 lb (0.9 kg) per day or 5 lb (2.3 kg) per week.
•Instruct patient to eat a diet high in potas-

sium-rich food, including citrus fruits, bananas, tomatoes, and dates.
• Advise patient to change position slowly to minimize effects of orthostatic hypotension.
• Urge patient to notify prescriber about decreased urination, muscle cramps and weakness, and unusual bleeding or bruising.

# hydrocodone and ibuprofen

Vicoprofen

## Class, Category, and Schedule
*Chemical:* Opioid and phenanthrene derivative (hydrocodone), propionic acid derivative (ibuprofen)
*Therapeutic:* Analgesic
*Pregnancy category:* C
*Controlled substance:* Schedule III

## Indications and Dosages
➤ *To relieve acute pain*
TABLETS
**Adults.** 1 tablet (7.5 mg of hydrocodone, 200 mg of ibuprofen) q 4 to 6 hr, p.r.n., for up to 5 days. *Maximum:* 5 tablets (37.5 mg of hydrocodone, 1,000 mg of ibuprofen)/day.

| Route | Onset | Peak | Duration |
|---|---|---|---|
| P.O. | 10 to 30 min | 30 to 60 min | 4 to 6 hr |

## Mechanism of Action
Exerts a synergistic analgesic effect through two mechanisms of action. Hydrocodone, a mu opiate-receptor agonist, alters the perception of pain at the spinal cord and higher CNS levels by blocking the release of inhibitory neurotransmitters, such as gamma-aminobutyric acid and acetylcholine. It also alters the emotional response to pain.

Ibuprofen blocks the activity of cyclooxygenase, the enzyme necessary for prostaglandin synthesis. Prostaglandins, important mediators in the inflammatory response, cause local vasodilation with swelling and pain. They also play a role in pain transmission from the periphery to the spinal cord. With the inhibition of cyclooxygenase and prostaglandin synthesis, inflammatory symptoms subside.

## Contraindications
Hypersensitivity to aspirin, hydrocodone, ibuprofen, narcotics, other NSAIDs, or their components; respiratory depression; severe asthma; upper airway obstruction

## Interactions
DRUGS
*ACE inhibitors (such as benazepril, captopril, and enalapril):* Possibly decreased therapeutic effects of ACE inhibitors
*anticholinergics:* Increased risk of ileus
*aspirin, corticosteroids, NSAIDs:* Possibly increased risk of GI ulceration and hemorrhage
*CNS depressants:* Increased CNS depression
*diuretics:* Possibly decreased diuresis, increased risk of renal failure
*lithium:* Increased blood lithium level, increased risk of lithium toxicity
*methotrexate:* Increased blood methotrexate level, increased risk of methotrexate toxicity
*MAO inhibitors (such as furazolidone, phenelzine, procarbazine, selegiline, tranylcypromine):* Increased risk of adverse CNS effects
*naloxone:* Possibly withdrawal symptoms in physically dependent patients
*naltrexone:* Possibly prolonged respiratory depression and cardiac arrest
*oral anticoagulants:* Increased risk of GI bleeding
*tricyclic antidepressants:* Possibly increased adverse effects of hydrocodone or potentiated antidepressant effects
ACTIVITIES
*alcohol use:* Possibly increased CNS depression

## Adverse Reactions
**CNS:** Anxiety, confusion, depression, dizziness, euphoria, fatigue, fever, headache, insomnia, irritability, lethargy, nervousness, paresthesia, sedation, slurred speech, somnolence, tremor, weakness
**CV:** Arrhythmias, peripheral edema, hypotension, orthostatic hypotension, palpitations
**EENT:** Dry mouth, mouth ulcers, pharyngitis, rhinitis, sinusitis, tinnitus, vision changes
**GI:** Anorexia, constipation, dysphagia, esophagitis, flatulence, gastritis, gastroenteritis, indigestion, nausea, vomiting
**GU:** Impotence, urinary frequency, urine retention
**RESP:** Bronchitis, dyspnea, respiratory depression
**SKIN:** Diaphoresis, flushing, pruritus, rash, urticaria

**Other:** Physical and psychological dependence

## Nursing Considerations
•Expect to give hydrocodone and ibuprofen for short-term pain relief only (no more than 10 days).
•**WARNING** Monitor for signs of overdose, such as blurred vision; cold, clammy skin; confusion; dizziness; dyspnea; headache; hearing loss; malaise; mental or mood changes; nausea; respiratory depression; sinus bradycardia; tinnitus; and vomiting. Notify prescriber immediately if they develop.

### PATIENT TEACHING
•Inform patient that hydrocodone and ibuprofen may cause drowsiness and dizziness.
•Caution patient not to take more than prescribed dosage because of the risk of dependence.
•Urge patient to avoid using alcohol during drug therapy.
•Advise patient to change position slowly to minimize effects of orthostatic hypotension.

# hydrocodone bitartrate and acetaminophen

Allay, Anexsia, Anolor DH 5, Bancap-HC, Co-Gesic, Dolacet, Dolagesic, Duocet, Hycomed, Hyco-Pap, Hydrocet, Hydrogesic, Lorcet-HD, Lorcet Plus, Lortab, Margesic-H, Oncet, Panacet, Panlor, Polygesic, Stagesic, T-Gesic, Ugesic, Vanacet, Vendone, Vicodin, Vicodin ES, Zydone

## Class, Category, and Schedule
*Chemical:* Opioid and phenanthrene derivative (hydrocodone), para-aminophenol derivative (acetaminophen)
*Therapeutic:* Analgesic
*Pregnancy category:* C
*Controlled substance:* Schedule III

## Indications and Dosages
➤ *To treat moderate to severe back pain and pain from arthralgia, cancer, dental procedures, headache, and myalgia*
### CAPSULES
**Adults.** 1 capsule (5 mg of hydrocodone, 500 mg of acetaminophen) q 4 to 6 hr, p.r.n.; or 2 capsules (10 mg of hydrocodone, 1,000 mg of acetaminophen) q 6 hr, p.r.n. *Maximum:* 8 capsules (40 mg of hydrocodone, 4,000 mg of acetaminophen)/24 hr.

### ORAL SOLUTION
**Adults.** 5 to 15 ml (2.5 mg of hydrocodone, 167 mg of acetaminophen/5 ml) q 4 to 6 hr, p.r.n., for up to 6 days.
### TABLETS
**Adults.** 1 or 2 tablets (2.5 mg of hydrocodone, 500 mg of acetaminophen/tablet) q 4 to 6 hr, p.r.n.; or 1 tablet (5 mg of hydrocodone, 500 mg of acetaminophen) q 4 to 6 hr, p.r.n., up to 2 tablets q 6 hr, p.r.n.; or 1 tablet (7.5 mg hydrocodone, 650 mg acetaminophen) q 4 to 6 hr, p.r.n., up to 2 tablets q 6 hr, p.r.n.; or 1 tablet (7.5 mg of hydrocodone, 750 mg of acetaminophen) q 4 to 6 hr, p.r.n.; or 1 tablet (10 mg of hydrocodone, 650 mg of acetaminophen) q 4 to 6 hr, p.r.n. *Maximum:* 40 mg of hydrocodone, 4,000 mg of acetaminophen/day.

| Route | Onset | Peak | Duration |
|-------|-------|------|----------|
| P.O. | 10 to 30 min | 30 to 60 min | 4 to 6 hr |

G
H
I

## Mechanism of Action
Exerts a synergistic analgesic effect through two mechanisms of action. Hydrocodone, a mu opiate-receptor agonist, alters the perception of pain at the spinal cord and higher CNS levels by blocking the release of inhibitory neurotransmitters, such as gamma-aminobutyric acid and acetylcholine. It also alters the emotional response to pain.

Acetaminophen increases the pain threshold at the CNS level by inhibiting cyclooxygenase, an enzyme involved in prostaglandin synthesis. Prostaglandins, important mediators in the inflammatory response, cause local vasodilation with swelling and pain. They also play a role in pain transmission from the periphery to the spinal cord. With the inhibition of cyclooxygenase and prostaglandin synthesis, inflammatory symptoms subside.

## Contraindications
Acute asthma; hypersensitivity to acetaminophen, aspirin, hydrocodone, narcotics, NSAIDs, or their components; respiratory depression; upper airway obstruction

## Interactions
### DRUGS
*anticholinergics:* Increased risk of ileus, severe constipation, and urine retention

*antidiarrheals (antiperistaltic):* Increased risk of CNS depression and severe constipation
*barbiturate anesthetics:* Possibly increased respiratory and CNS depression
*chlorpromazine, thioridazine:* Increased risk of adverse and toxic effects of hydrocodone
*CNS depressants:* Increased risk of CNS and respiratory depression and hypotension
*diuretics, other antihypertensives:* Increased risk of hypotension
*MAO inhibitors (such as furazolidone, phenelzine, procarbazine, selegiline, tranylcypromine) within 14 days of receiving hydrocodone and acetaminophen:* Increased risk of adverse CNS effects
*metoclopramide:* Possibly antagonized effect of metoclopramide on GI motility
*naloxone:* Possibly withdrawal symptoms in physically dependent patients
*naltrexone:* Possibly prolonged respiratory depression or cardiac arrest
*other opioid analgesics:* Risk of increased CNS and respiratory depression and hypotension
**ACTIVITIES**
*alcohol use:* Increased risk of CNS depression

## Adverse Reactions

**CNS:** Confusion, dizziness, drowsiness, euphoria, headache, lethargy, restlessness, sedation, syncope
**CV:** Hypotension, orthostatic hypotension, tachycardia
**EENT:** Dry mouth, laryngeal edema, laryngospasm, vision changes
**GI:** Anorexia, constipation, nausea, vomiting
**GU:** Dysuria, urine retention
**RESP:** Atelectasis, bronchospasm, respiratory depression, wheezing
**SKIN:** Diaphoresis, flushing, pruritus, rash, urticaria
**Other:** Physical and psychological dependence

## Nursing Considerations

•Expect prolonged use of hydrocodone and acetaminophen to produce physical and psychological dependence; physical dependence may cause withdrawal symptoms when drug is discontinued.
•Assess carefully for adverse reactions when giving drug to elderly patients; they're especially sensitive to drug and are at increased risk for constipation.
•WARNING Monitor for signs of overdose, such as blurred vision; cold, clammy skin; confu-

sion; dizziness; dyspnea; headache; hearing loss; malaise; mental or mood changes; nausea; respiratory depression; sinus bradycardia; tinnitus; and vomiting. Notify prescriber immediately if they develop.
**PATIENT TEACHING**
•Inform patient that hydrocodone and acetaminophen may cause dizziness and drowsiness.
•Advise patient to avoid potentially hazardous activities until drug's CNS effects are known.
•Caution patient not to take more than prescribed dosage because of risk of dependence.
•Urge patient to avoid using alcohol during drug therapy.
•Advise patient to change position slowly to minimize effects of orthostatic hypotension.
•If patient reports dry mouth, suggest that she use sugarless candy or gum or ice chips.

# hydrocortisone
## (cortisol)

Cortef, Hydrocortone

# hydrocortisone acetate

Cortifoam, Hydrocortone Acetate

# hydrocortisone cypionate

Cortef

# hydrocortisone sodium phosphate

Hydrocortone Phosphate

# hydrocortisone sodium succinate

A-hydroCort, Solu-Cortef

## Class and Category

*Chemical:* Glucocorticoid
*Therapeutic:* Adrenocorticoid replacement, anti-inflammatory
*Pregnancy category:* Not rated; C (Cortifoam)

## Indications and Dosages

➤ *To treat severe inflammation or acute adrenal insufficiency*
**ORAL SUSPENSION, TABLETS (HYDROCORTISONE, HYDROCORTISONE CYPIONATE)**
**Adults.** 20 to 240 mg/day as a single dose or in divided doses.

**I.V. INFUSION OR I.V., I.M., OR S.C. INJECTION (HYDROCORTISONE SODIUM PHOSPHATE); I.M. INJECTION (HYDROCORTISONE)**

**Adults.** 15 to 240 mg/day as a single dose or in divided doses. *Usual:* ½ to ⅓ the oral dose.

**DOSAGE ADJUSTMENT** Dosage increased above 240 mg/day if needed to treat acute disease.

**I.V. INFUSION; I.V. OR I.M. INJECTION (HYDROCORTISONE SODIUM SUCCINATE)**

**Adults.** 100 to 500 mg q 2, 4, or 6 hr.

➤ *To treat joint and tissue inflammation*

**INTRA-ARTICULAR INJECTION (HYDROCORTISONE ACETATE)**

**Adults.** 25 to 37.5 mg injected into large joints or bursae as a single dose, or 10 to 25 mg injected into small joints as a single dose.

**INTRALESIONAL INJECTION (HYDROCORTISONE ACETATE)**

**Adults.** 5 to 12.5 mg injected into tendon sheaths as a single dose, or 12.5 to 25 mg injected into ganglia as a single dose.

**SOFT-TISSUE INJECTION (HYDROCORTISONE ACETATE)**

**Adults.** 25 to 50 mg as a single dose. Sometimes a dose of up to 75 mg is needed.

➤ *As adjunct to treat ulcerative proctitis of the distal portion of the rectum in patients who can't retain hydrocortisone or other corticosteroid enemas*

**RECTAL AEROSOL (HYDROCORTISONE ACETATE)**

**Adult males.** *Initial:* 1 applicatorful q.d or b.i.d. for 2 to 3 wk, then q.o.d. thereafter. *Maintenance:* Highly individualized.

| Route | Onset | Peak | Duration |
|---|---|---|---|
| P.O. (hydrocortisone) | Unknown | 1 hr | 1.25 to 1.5 days |
| P.O. (cypionate) | Unknown | 1 to 2 hr | Unknown |
| I.V. (phosphate, succinate) | Rapid | Unknown | Unknown |
| I.M. (hydrocortisone) | Unknown | 4 to 8 hr | Unknown |
| I.M. (phosphate) | Rapid | 1 hr | Unknown |
| I.M. (succinate) | Rapid | 1 hr | Variable |
| Other* (acetate) | Unknown | 24 to 48 hr | 3 days to 4 wk |

---

* Intra-articular, intralesional, and soft-tissue injection.

## Mechanism of Action

Binds to intracellular glucocorticoid receptors and suppresses the inflammatory and immune responses by:
• inhibiting neutrophil and monocyte accumulation at the inflammation site and suppressing their phagocytic and bactericidal activity
• stabilizing lysosomal membranes
• suppressing the antigen response of macrophages and helper T cells
• inhibiting the synthesis of cellular mediators of the inflammatory response, such as cytokines, interleukins, and prostaglandins.

## Contraindications

Hypersensitivity to hydrocortisone or its components, idiopathic thrombocytopenic purpura (I.M.), intestinal conditions prohibiting intrarectal steroids (P.R.), recent live-virus vaccination, systemic fungal infection

## Interactions

**DRUGS**

*acetaminophen:* Increased risk of hepatotoxicity
*amphotericin B, carbonic anhydrase inhibitors:* Possibly severe hypokalemia
*anabolic steroids, androgens:* Increased risk of edema and severe acne
*anticholinergics:* Possibly increased intraocular pressure
*anticoagulants, thrombolytics:* Increased risk of GI ulceration and hemorrhage, possibly decreased therapeutic effects of these drugs
*asparaginase:* Increased risk of hyperglycemia and toxicity
*aspirin, NSAIDs:* Increased risk of GI distress and bleeding
*cholestyramine:* Possibly increased hydrocortisone clearance
*cyclosporine:* Possibly increased action of both drugs; increased risk of seizures
*digoxin:* Possibly hypokalemia-induced arrhythmias and digitalis toxicity
*ephedrine, phenobarbital, phenytoin, rifampin:* Decreased blood hydrocortisone level
*estrogens, oral contraceptives:* Increased therapeutic and toxic effects of hydrocortisone
*insulin, oral antidiabetic drugs:* Possibly increased blood glucose level
*isoniazid:* Possibly decreased therapeutic effects of isoniazid

*macrolide antibiotics:* Possibly decreased hydrocortisone clearance
*mexiletine:* Decreased blood mexiletine level
*neuromuscular blockers:* Possibly increased neuromuscular blockade, causing respiratory depression or apnea
*potassium-depleting drugs, such as thiazide diuretics:* Possibly severe hypokalemia
*potassium supplements:* Possibly decreased effects of these supplements
*somatrem, somatropin:* Possibly decreased therapeutic effects of these drugs
*streptozocin:* Increased risk of hyperglycemia
*vaccines:* Decreased antibody response and increased risk of neurologic complications
ACTIVITIES
*alcohol use:* Increased risk of GI distress and bleeding

## Adverse Reactions

**CNS:** Ataxia, behavioral changes, depression, dizziness, euphoria, fatigue, headache, increased intracranial pressure with papilledema, insomnia, malaise, mood changes, paresthesia, seizures, steroid psychosis, syncope, vertigo
**CV:** Arrhythmias (from hypokalemia), fat embolism, heart failure, hypertension, hypotension, thromboembolism, thrombophlebitis
**EENT:** Exophthalmos, glaucoma, increased intraocular pressure, nystagmus, posterior subcapsular cataracts
**ENDO:** Adrenal insufficiency during stress, cushingoid symptoms (buffalo hump, central obesity, moon face, supraclavicular fat pad enlargement), diabetes mellitus, growth suppression in children, hyperglycemia, negative nitrogen balance from protein catabolism
**GI:** Abdominal distention, hiccups, increased appetite, nausea, pancreatitis, peptic ulcer, ulcerative esophagitis, vomiting
**GU:** Amenorrhea, glycosuria, menstrual irregularities, perineal burning or tingling
**HEME:** Easy bruising, leukocytosis
**MS:** Arthralgia; aseptic necrosis of femoral and humeral heads; compression fractures; muscle atrophy, twitching, or weakness; myalgia; osteoporosis; spontaneous fractures; steroid myopathy; tendon rupture
**SKIN:** Acne; altered skin pigmentation; diaphoresis; erythema; hirsutism; necrotizing vasculitis; petechiae; purpura; rash; scarring; sterile abscess; striae; subcutaneous fat atrophy; thin, fragile skin; urticaria
**Other:** Anaphylaxis, hypocalcemia, hypoka-lemia, hypokalemic alkalosis, impaired wound healing, masking of signs of infection, metabolic alkalosis, suppressed skin test reaction, weight gain

## Nursing Considerations

• Be aware that systemic hydrocortisone shouldn't be given to immunocompromised patients, such as those with fungal and other infections, including amebiasis, hepatitis B, tuberculosis, vaccinia, and varicella.
• Give daily dose of hydrocortisone in the morning to mimic the normal peak in adrenocortical secretion of corticosteroids.
• When possible, give oral dose with food or milk to avoid GI distress.
• Don't give acetate injectable suspension by I.V.
• Give hydrocortisone sodium succinate as a direct I.V. injection over 30 seconds to several minutes, or as an intermittent or a continuous infusion. For infusion, dilute to 1 mg/ml or less with $D_5W$, NS, or $D_5NS$.
• Inject I.M. form deep into gluteal muscle, and rotate injection sites to prevent muscle atrophy. S.C. injection may cause atrophy and sterile abscess.
• Shake foam container vigorously for 5 to 10 seconds before each use. Gently withdraw applicator plunger past the fill-line on the applicator barrel while container is upright on a level surface. Administer rectal foam only with provided applicator. After each use, wash applicator, container cap, and underlying tip with warm water.
• Be aware that high-dose therapy shouldn't be given for longer than 48 hours. Be alert for depression and psychotic episodes.
• Regularly monitor weight, blood pressure, and serum electrolyte levels during therapy.
• Expect hydrocortisone to exacerbate infections or mask their signs and symptoms.
• Monitor blood glucose level in diabetic patients, and increase insulin or oral antidiabetic drug dosage, as prescribed.
• Know that elderly patients are at high risk for osteoporosis during long-term therapy.
• Anticipate the possibility of acute adrenal insufficiency with stress, such as emotional upset, fever, surgery, and trauma. Increase hydrocortisone dosage, as prescribed.
• WARNING Avoid withdrawing drug suddenly after long-term therapy because adrenal crisis can result. Expect to reduce dosage gradually as prescribed and monitor response.

## PATIENT TEACHING

•Advise patient to take daily dose of hydrocortisone at 9 a.m.
•Instruct patient to take tablets or oral suspension with milk or food.
•Teach patient how to use foam form, if prescribed.
•Caution patient not to stop taking drug abruptly without first consulting prescriber.
•Instruct patient to report early signs of adrenal insufficiency: anorexia, difficulty breathing, dizziness, fainting, fatigue, joint pain, muscle weakness, and nausea.
•Inform patient that easy bruising may occur.
•Advise patient on long-term therapy to have periodic eye examinations.
•If patient receives long-term therapy, urge her to carry or wear medical identification.

# hydromorphone hydrochloride

## (dihydromorphinone)

Dilaudid, Dilaudid-5, Dilaudid-HP, Hydrostat IR, PMS-Hydromorphone (CAN), Palladone, PMS-Hydromorphone Syrup (CAN)

## Class, Category, and Schedule

*Chemical:* Phenanthrene derivative, semisynthetic opioid derivative
*Therapeutic:* Analgesic
*Pregnancy category:* C
*Controlled substance:* Schedule II

## Indications and Dosages

➤ *To relieve moderate to severe pain*
ORAL SOLUTION
**Adults.** 2.5 to 10 mg q 3 to 6 hr, p.r.n.
TABLETS
**Adults.** 2 mg q 3 to 6 hr, p.r.n. Increased to 4 mg or more q 4 to 6 hr, if indicated.
E.R. CAPSULES
**Adults.** Highly individualized and dependent on patient's previous total daily 24-hour opioid use. Once dosage is determined, drug is given q.d.
I.V. INJECTION
**Adults.** 1 mg q 3 hr, p.r.n.
I.M. OR S.C. INJECTION
**Adults.** 1 or 2 mg q 3 to 6 hr, p.r.n. Increased to 3 or 4 mg q 4 to 6 hr, if needed for severe pain.
SUPPOSITORIES
**Adults.** 3 mg q 4 to 8 hr, p.r.n.

| Route | Onset | Peak | Duration |
|---|---|---|---|
| P.O. | 30 min | 1.5 to 2 hr | 4 hr |
| I.V. | 10 to 15 min | 15 to 30 min | 2 to 3 hr |
| I.M. | 15 min | 30 to 60 min | 4 to 5 hr |
| S.C. | 15 min | 30 to 90 min | 4 hr |
| P.R. | 30 min | Unknown | 4 hr |

### Mechanism of Action

May bind with opioid receptors in the spinal cord and higher levels in the CNS. In this way, hydromorphone is believed to stimulate mu and kappa receptors, thus altering the perception of and emotional response to pain.

## Contraindications

Acute asthma; hypersensitivity to hydromorphone, other narcotics, or their components; increased intracranial pressure; severe respiratory depression; upper respiratory tract obstruction

## Interactions

DRUGS
*anticholinergics:* Increased risk of ileus, severe constipation, or urine retention
*antihypertensives, diuretics, guanadrel, guanethidine, mecamylamine:* Increased risk of orthostatic hypotension
*barbiturate anesthetics:* Increased sedative effect of hydromorphone
*belladonna alkaloids, difenoxin and atropine, diphenoxylate and atropine, kaolin pectin, loperamide, paregoric:* Increased risk of CNS depression and severe constipation
*buprenorphine, butorphanol, dezocine, nalbuphine, pentazocine:* Possibly potentiated or suppressed symptoms of spontaneous narcotic withdrawal
*CNS depressants, other opioid analgesics:* Additive CNS depression and hypotension
*hydroxyzine:* Increased analgesia, CNS depression, and hypotension
*metoclopramide:* Decreased effect of metoclopramide on GI motility
*naloxone:* Possibly withdrawal symptoms in physically dependent patients
*naltrexone:* Possibly prolonged respiratory depression or cardiac arrest
*neuromuscular blockers:* Additive CNS depression

*alcohol use:* Increased CNS depression

## Adverse Reactions

**CNS:** Anxiety, confusion, dizziness, drowsiness, euphoria, hallucinations, headache, nervousness, restlessness, sedation, somnolence, tremor, weakness
**CV:** Hypertension, orthostatic hypotension, palpitations, tachycardia
**EENT:** Blurred vision, diplopia, dry mouth, laryngeal edema, laryngospasm, nystagmus, tinnitus
**GI:** Abdominal cramps, anorexia, biliary tract spasm, constipation, hepatotoxicity, nausea, vomiting
**GU:** Dysuria, urine retention
**RESP:** Dyspnea, respiratory depression, wheezing
**SKIN:** Diaphoresis, flushing
**Other:** Injection site pain, redness, and swelling; physical and psychological dependence

## Nursing Considerations

• To improve analgesic action, give hydromorphone before pain becomes intense.
• Give I.V. form by direct injection over at least 2 minutes. For infusion, mix drug with $D_5W$, NS, or Ringer's solution.
• Monitor for respiratory depression when using I.V. route. Keep resuscitation equipment and naloxone nearby.
• Rotate I.M. and S.C. injection sites.
• Monitor effectiveness of hydromorphone in relieving pain; consult prescriber as needed.
• Assess patient for constipation.
• Monitor patient for signs of physical dependence or abuse.
• Anticipate that drug may mask or worsen gallbladder pain.
• Be aware that all other around-the-clock opioid analgesics should be stopped when E.R. capsules are prescribed. Expect to give immediate-release nonopioid analgesics for exacerbations of pain and for preventing pain during certain activities.

**PATIENT TEACHING**
• Instruct patient to take hydromorphone exactly as prescribed and before pain is severe.
• Advise patient to take drug with food to avoid GI distress.
• Tell patient not to break open or chew E.R. capsules but to swallow them whole.
• Instruct patient to refrigerate suppositories.
• Caution patient to avoid alcohol and OTC

drugs during therapy, unless prescriber approves.
• Instruct patient to report constipation, difficulty breathing, severe nausea, or vomiting.
• Inform patient that drug may cause drowsiness and sedation. Advise her to avoid potentially hazardous activities until drug's CNS effects are known.
• Tell patient to change position slowly to minimize effects of orthostatic hypotension.
• To avoid withdrawal, instruct physically dependent patient not to stop drug abruptly.

# hydroxychloroquine sulfate

Plaquenil

## Class and Category

*Chemical:* 4-aminoquinoline compound
*Therapeutic:* Antiprotozoal, antirheumatic, lupus erythematosus suppressant
*Pregnancy category:* C

## Indications and Dosages

➤ *To prevent malaria*
**TABLETS**
**Adults.** 400 mg the same day of each week starting 2 wk before entering endemic area and continuing until departure from endemic area. If this isn't possible, initially 800 mg in two divided doses 6 hr apart, followed 1 wk later with 400 mg and then 400 mg on the same day of each week thereafter until departure from endemic area.
**Infants and children.** 5 mg/kg the same day of each week, starting 2 wk before entering endemic area and continuing until departure from endemic area. If this isn't possible, initially 10 mg/kg in two divided doses 6 hr apart, followed 1 wk later with 5 mg/kg and then 5 mg/kg on the same day of each week thereafter until departure from endemic area. *Maximum:* Adult dosage.
➤ *To treat acute attacks of malaria caused by* Plasmodium vivax, P. malariae, P. ovale, *and susceptible strains of* P. falciparum
**TABLETS**
**Adults.** *Initial:* 800 mg, followed by 400 mg in 6 to 8 hr and 400 mg on next 2 consecutive days. Alternatively, 800 mg given as a single dose or an initial dose of 10 mg base/kg (maximum, 620 mg base [800 mg]), followed by 5 mg base/kg (maximum, 310 mg

base [400 mg]) 6 hr after first dose, 5 mg base/kg 18 hr after second dose, and 5 mg base/kg 24 hr after third dose.

**Infants and children.** *Initial:* 10 mg base/kg (maximum, 620 mg base [800 mg]), followed by 5 mg base/kg (maximum, 310 mg base [400 mg]) 6 hr after first dose, 5 mg base/kg 18 hr after second dose, and 5 mg base/kg 24 hr after third dose.

➤ *To treat chronic discoid and systemic lupus erythematosus*

TABLETS

**Adults.** *Initial:* 400 mg q.d. or b.i.d. for several weeks or months. *Maintenance:* 200 to 400 mg q.d.

➤ *To treat acute or chronic rheumatoid arthritis*

TABLETS

**Adults.** *Initial:* 400 to 600 mg q.d. for 4 to 12 wk. *Maintenance:* 200 mg to 400 mg q.d.

**DOSAGE ADJUSTMENT** For patients with rheumatoid arthritis who develop troublesome adverse reactions, initial dosage decreased for 5 to 10 days and then gradually increased to optimum response level.

## Mechanism of Action

May mildly suppress the immune system, inhibiting production of rheumatoid factor and acute phase reactants. Hydroxychloroquine also accumulates in WBCs, stabilizing lysosomal membranes and inhibiting enzymes such as collagenase and the proteases that cause cartilage breakdown. These actions may decrease symptoms of rheumatoid arthritis and lupus erythematosus.

Hydroxychloroquine also binds to and alters the DNA of the malaria parasite to prevent it from reproducing. In addition, it may increase the pH of acid vesicles, which interferes with vesicle function and may inhibit parasitic phospholipid metabolism in erythrocytes, thereby halting plasmodial activity.

## Contraindications

Hypersensitivity to 4-aminoquinoline compounds (including hydroxychloroquine), long-term therapy in children, retinal or visual changes related to 4-aminoquinoline compounds

## Interactions

DRUGS

*aurothioglucose:* Increased risk of blood dyscrasias

*digoxin:* Increased digoxin concentrations

## Adverse Reactions

**CNS:** Abnormal nerve conduction, ataxia, dizziness, emotional lability, headache, irritability, lassitude, nervousness, neuromuscular sensory abnormalities, nightmares, psychosis, seizures, vertigo

**CV:** Cardiomyopathy (with prolonged high doses)

**EENT:** Abnormal pigmentation (bull's eye appearance), blurred vision, central scotoma with decreased visual acuity, corneal deposits, decreased corneal sensitivity, diplopia, irreversible retinal damage (in lupus erythematosus or rheumatoid arthritis), halo vision, lassitude, macular edema or atrophy, nerve-related hearing loss, nystagmus, pericentral or paracentral scotoma, photophobia, retinal fundus changes, tinnitus, visual abnormalities

**ENDO:** Hypoglycemia

**GI:** Abdominal cramps, anorexia, diarrhea, elevated liver function test results, fulminant hepatic failure, nausea, vomiting

**HEME:** Agranulocytosis, aplastic anemia, hemolysis (in patients with glucose-6-phosphate dehydrogenase [G6PD] deficiency), leukopenia, thrombocytopenia

**MS:** Atrophy of proximal skeletal muscle groups, depressed tendon reflexes, muscle weakness

**SKIN:** Acute generalized exanthematous pustulosis, alopecia, altered mucosal and skin pigmentation, bleaching of hair, dermatitis (including exfoliative dermatitis), non–light-sensitive psoriasis, pruritus, psoriasis exacerbation, rash, Stevens-Johnson syndrome, urticaria

**Other:** Porphyria, weight loss

## Nursing Considerations

• Use hydroxychloroquine cautiously in patients with G6PD deficiency, patients with hepatic disease or alcoholism, and patients taking hepatotoxic drugs.

• Monitor children closely for adverse reactions because they are especially sensitive to 4-aminoquinoline compounds.

• Observe patients with psoriasis closely because hydroxychloroquine may lead to severe psoriasis attack. Also monitor patients with

G
H
I

porphyria closely because hydroxychloroquine may worsen the condition. Expect to use hydroxychloroquine in patients with psoriasis or porphyria only after risks and benefits have been considered.

• During prolonged therapy, obtain periodic blood cell counts, as ordered, to detect adverse hematologic effects. Expect to stop hydroxychloroquine if severe adverse effects occur.

• Monitor patient's vision when giving hydroxychloroquine for lupus erythematosus or rheumatoid arthritis because irreversible retinal damage may occur in some patients during long-term or high-dose therapy. Ask regularly about visual abnormalities, such as light flashes or streaks, that may indicate retinopathy. Expect patient to have an initial ophthalmologic examination, followed by examinations every 3 months. Report changes to prescriber immediately, and expect drug to be stopped. Retinal changes may progress even after therapy stops.

• Monitor patient on long-term therapy for muscle weakness and abnormal knee and ankle reflexes. If present, notify prescriber and expect drug to be stopped.

• Expect drug to be stopped if patient with rheumatoid arthritis shows no improvement, such as reduced joint swelling or increased mobility, in 6 months.

• If serious adverse reactions occur, notify prescriber immediately. Expect drug to be stopped. Also expect to give ammonium chloride (8 g daily in divided doses for adults) 3 or 4 days weekly for several months because acidification of urine increases renal excretion of drug.

PATIENT TEACHING

• Instruct patient to take drug with meals or milk to minimize stomach upset.

• Tell patient to take hydroxychloroquine exactly as prescribed because taking too much may cause serious adverse reactions and taking too little or skipping doses decreases effectiveness.

• Caution patient to notify prescriber about troublesome adverse reactions; dosage may need to be adjusted or drug stopped.

• Caution patient who takes hydroxychloroquine for rheumatoid arthritis or lupus erythematosus about possible visual reactions and the need for periodic eye examinations. Tell patient to notify prescriber about abnormal visual changes, including blurred vision, halos around lights, and light flashes or streaks; explain that drug will need to be stopped.

• Tell patient receiving prolonged therapy about the need for periodic blood tests to detect adverse effects.

• Advise patient to notify prescriber if muscle weakness develops.

# hydroxyzine hydrochloride

Apo-Hydroxyzine (CAN), Atarax, Multipax (CAN), Novo-Hydroxyzin (CAN)

## hydroxyzine pamoate

Vistaril

## Class and Category

*Chemical:* Piperazine derivative
*Therapeutic:* Antianxiety, antiemetic, antihistamine, sedative-hypnotic
*Pregnancy category:* C

## Indications and Dosages

➤ *To relieve anxiety and induce sedation and hypnosis*

CAPSULES, ORAL SUSPENSION, SYRUP, TABLETS

**Adults and adolescents.** 50 to 100 mg as a single dose.

**Children.** 600 mcg/kg as a single dose.

I.M. INJECTION

**Adults and adolescents.** 50 to 100 mg q 4 to 6 hr, p.r.n. (antianxiety); 50 mg as a single dose (sedative-hypnotic).

➤ *To treat pruritus*

CAPSULES, ORAL SUSPENSION, SYRUP, TABLETS

**Adults and adolescents.** 25 to 100 mg t.i.d. or q.i.d., p.r.n.

**Children.** 500 mcg/kg q 6 hr, p.r.n.

➤ *To provide antiemetic effects*

CAPSULES, ORAL SUSPENSION, SYRUP, TABLETS

**Adults and adolescents.** 25 to 100 mg t.i.d. or q.i.d., p.r.n.

**Children.** 500 mcg/kg q 6 hr, p.r.n.

I.M. INJECTION

**Adults and adolescents.** 25 to 100 mg, p.r.n.

**Children.** 1.1 mg/kg as a single dose.

➤ *As adjunct to permit reduction in pre-operative and postoperative narcotic dosage*

**I.M. INJECTION**
**Adults and adolescents.** 25 to 100 mg given with prescribed narcotic.
**Children.** 1.1 mg/kg given with prescribed narcotic.
**DOSAGE ADJUSTMENT** For elderly patients, treatment is started at lowest possible dosage.

| Route | Onset | Peak | Duration |
|-------|-------|------|----------|
| P.O. | 15 to 60 min | Unknown | 4 to 6 hr |
| I.M. | 20 to 30 min | Unknown | 4 to 6 hr |

### Mechanism of Action
Competes with histamine for histamine$_1$ receptor sites on the surfaces of effector cells. This suppresses the results of histaminic activity, including edema, flare, and pruritus. Hydroxyzine's antiemetic effect may stem from its central anticholinergic actions. Its sedative actions occur at the subcortical level of the CNS and are dose-related.

### Contraindications
Breast-feeding; early pregnancy; hypersensitivity to cetirizine, hydroxyzine, or their components

### Interactions
**DRUGS**
*CNS depressants:* Increased CNS depression
**ACTIVITIES**
*alcohol use:* Increased CNS depression

### Adverse Reactions
**CNS:** Drowsiness, hallucinations, headache, involuntary motor activity, seizures, tremor
**EENT:** Dry mouth
**SKIN:** Pruritus, rash, urticaria
**Other:** Allergic reaction, injection site pain

### Nursing Considerations
• Don't give hydroxyzine by S.C. or I.V. route because tissue necrosis may occur.
• Inject I.M. form deep into a large muscle, using the Z-track method.
• Observe for oversedation if patient takes another CNS depressant.
**PATIENT TEACHING**
• Urge patient to avoid alcohol.

• Caution patient about drowsiness; tell her to avoid potentially hazardous activities until drug's CNS effects are known.
• Instruct female patient to tell prescriber if she is or could be pregnant because drug is contraindicated in early pregnancy.

# hyoscyamine sulfate

Anaspaz, A-Spas S/L, Cystospaz, Cystospaz-M, Donnamar, ED-SPAZ, Gastrosed, Levbid, Levsin, Levsinex Timecaps, Levsin/SL, Symax SL, Symax SR

### Class and Category
*Chemical:* Belladonna alkaloid, tertiary amine
*Therapeutic:* Antimuscarinic, antispasmodic
*Pregnancy category:* C

### Indications and Dosages
➤ *To treat peptic ulcers and GI tract disorders caused by spasm*
**ELIXIR, ORAL SOLUTION**
**Adults and adolescents.** 0.125 to 0.25 mg q 4 to 6 hr.
**Children.** Dosage individualized by weight.
**E.R. CAPSULES**
**Adults and adolescents.** 0.375 mg q 12 hr.
**E.R. TABLETS**
**Adults and adolescents.** 0.375 to 0.75 mg q 12 hr. *Maximum:* 1.5 mg/day.
**TABLETS**
**Adults and adolescents.** 0.125 to 0.5 mg t.i.d. or q.i.d.
**Children.** Dosage individualized by weight.
**I.V., I.M., OR S.C. INJECTION**
**Adults and adolescents.** 0.25 to 0.5 mg q 4 to 6 hr.
**Children.** Dosage individualized by weight.

➤ *To control salivation and excessive secretions during surgical procedures*
**I.V. INJECTION**
**Adults and adolescents.** 0.5 mg 30 to 60 min before procedure.

### Contraindications
Acute hemorrhage and hemodynamic instability; angle-closure glaucoma; hepatic disease; hypersensitivity to hyoscyamine, other anticholinergics, or their components; ileus; intestinal atony; myasthenia gravis; myocardial ischemia; obstructive GI disease; obstructive uropathy; renal disease; severe ulcerative colitis; tachycardia; toxic megacolon

G
H
I

| Route | Onset | Peak | Duration |
|-------|-------|------|----------|
| P.O.* | 20 to 30 min | 30 to 60 min | 4 hr |
| P.O. (E.R.)† | 20 to 30 min | 40 to 90 min | 12 hr |
| I.V., I.M., S.C. | 2 to 3 min | 15 to 30 min | 4 hr |

## Mechanism of Action

Competitively inhibits acetylcholine at autonomic postganglionic cholinergic receptors. Because the most sensitive receptors are in the salivary, bronchial, and sweat glands, hyoscyamine acts mainly to reduce salivary, bronchial, and sweat gland secretions. It also causes GI smooth muscle to contract and decreases gastric secretion and GI motility. In addition, hyoscyamine causes the bladder detrusor muscle to contract; reduces nasal and oropharyngeal secretions; and decreases airway resistance from relaxation of smooth muscle in the bronchi and bronchioles.

## Interactions

### DRUGS

*anticholinergics:* Possibly increased anti-cholingeric effects
*antidiarrheals (adsorbent):* Possibly decreased therapeutic effects of hyoscyamine
*calcium- and magnesium-containing antacids, carbonic anhydrase inhibitors, citrates, sodium bicarbonate, urinary alkalinizers:* Possibly potentiated therapeutic and adverse effects of hyoscyamine
*haloperidol:* Possibly decreased therapeutic effects of haloperidol
*ketoconazole:* Possibly reduced ketoconazole absorption
*metoclopramide:* Possibly antagonized therapeutic effects of metoclopramide
*opioid analgesics:* Increased risk of severe constipation and ileus

---

* For tablets only; for elixir and oral solution, onset is 5 to 20 min, and peak and duration are unknown.
† For E.R. tablets only; for E.R. capsules, onset and peak are unknown, and duration is 12 hr.

## Adverse Reactions

**CNS:** Drowsiness, insomnia
**EENT:** Blurred vision; dry mouth, nose, and throat; photophobia
**ENDO:** Decreased lactation
**GI:** Constipation
**GU:** Impotence, urine retention
**SKIN:** Decreased sweating
**Other:** Heatstroke, injection site redness and urticaria

## Nursing Considerations

• Use hyoscyamine cautiously in patients with arrhythmias, autonomic neuropathy, coronary artery disease, heart failure, hiatal hernia with reflux esophagitis, hypertension, hyperthyroidism, renal failure, or tachycardia.
• Give drug 30 to 60 minutes before meals and at bedtime. Give bedtime dose at least 2 hours after the day's last meal.
• Anticipate that tablets may not disintegrate and may appear in stool.
• WARNING Expect an increased risk of drug-induced heatstroke in hot or humid weather because hyoscyamine decreases sweating.
• WARNING Be aware that lower doses may paradoxically decrease the heart rate and that higher doses affect nicotinic receptors in autonomic ganglia, causing delirium, disorientation, hallucinations, and restlessness.
• Monitor urine output, and be alert for urine retention.

### PATIENT TEACHING

• Instruct patient to void before taking each dose and to notify prescriber if she has trouble urinating during hyoscyamine therapy.
• Advise patient to take drug 30 to 60 minutes before meals and at bedtime. Bedtime dose should be taken at least 2 hours after the day's last meal.
• Inform patient that drug may cause drowsiness. Advise her to avoid potentially hazardous activities until drug's CNS effects are known.
• If patient reports dry mouth, suggest using sugarless hard candy or gum.
• Inform male patient that drug may cause impotence. If it occurs, suggest that he discuss it with prescriber.
• Advise patient to avoid exposure to high temperatures and to increase fluid intake, unless contraindicated.

# ibuprofen

Actiprofen Caplets (CAN), Advil, Apo-Ibuprofen (CAN), Bayer Select Ibuprofen Pain Relief Formula Caplets, Children's Advil, Children's Motrin, Dolgesic, Excedrin IB, Genpril, Haltran, Ibifon 600 Caplets, Ibuprin, Ibuprohm Caplets, Ibu-Tab, Medipren, Midol IB, Motrin, Motrin-IB, Novo-Profen (CAN), Nu-Ibuprofen (CAN), Nuprin, Pamprin-IB, Q-Profen, Rufen, Trendar

## Class and Category

*Chemical:* Propionic acid derivative
*Therapeutic:* Analgesic, anti-inflammatory, antipyretic
*Pregnancy category:* Not rated

## Indications and Dosages

➤ *To relieve pain in rheumatoid arthritis and osteoarthritis*

**CAPSULES, CHEWABLE TABLETS, ORAL SUSPENSION, TABLETS**
**Adults.** 300 mg q.i.d., or 400, 600, or 800 mg t.i.d. or q.i.d. *Range:* 1.2 to 3.2 g/day.

➤ *To relieve mild to moderate pain*

**CAPSULES, CHEWABLE TABLETS, ORAL SUSPENSION, TABLETS**
**Adults.** 400 mg q 4 to 6 hr, p.r.n.

➤ *To relieve acute migraine pain*

**CAPSULES, CHEWABLE TABLETS, ORAL SUSPENSION, TABLETS**
**Adults.** 200 to 400 mg at onset of migraine pain. *Maximum:* 400 mg/day.

➤ *To relieve pain in primary dysmenorrhea*

**CAPSULES, CHEWABLE TABLETS, ORAL SUSPENSION, TABLETS**
**Adults.** 400 mg q 4 hr, p.r.n.

➤ *To relieve pain in juvenile arthritis*

**CAPSULES, CHEWABLE TABLETS, ORAL SUSPENSION, TABLETS**
**Children.** 30 to 70 mg/kg/day in divided doses t.i.d. or q.i.d.; 20 mg/kg/day for mild disease.

➤ *To relieve minor aches, pains, and dysmenorrhea and to reduce fever*

**CAPSULES, CHEWABLE TABLETS, ORAL SUSPENSION, TABLETS**
**Adults.** 200 to 400 mg q 4 to 6 hr. *Maximum:* 1.2 g/day.

➤ *To reduce fever*

**CAPSULES, CHEWABLE TABLETS, ORAL SUSPENSION, TABLETS**
**Children ages 6 months to 12 years.** 5 to 10 mg/kg q 4 to 6 hr. *Maximum:* 40 mg/kg/day.

## Contraindications

Angioedema, asthma, bronchospasm, nasal polyps, rhinitis, or urticaria caused by hypersensitivity to aspirin, ibuprofen, iodides, or other NSAIDs

| Route | Onset | Peak | Duration |
|---|---|---|---|
| P.O.* | 30 min | Unknown | 4 to 6 hr |
| P.O.† | Up to 7 days | 1 to 2 wk | Unknown |
| P.O.‡ | In 1 hr | 2 to 4 hr | 6 to 8 hr |

## Mechanism of Action

Blocks the activity of cyclooxygenase, the enzyme needed to synthesize prostaglandins, which mediate the inflammatory response and cause local vasodilation, swelling, and pain. By inhibiting prostaglandins, this NSAID reduces inflammatory symptoms and relieves pain. Ibuprofen's antipyretic action probably stems from its effect on the hypothalamus, which increases peripheral blood flow, causing vasodilation and encouraging heat dissipation.

## Interactions

**DRUGS**

*acetaminophen:* Possibly increased renal effects with long-term use of both drugs
*antihypertensives:* Decreased effectiveness of these drugs
*aspirin, other NSAIDs:* Increased risk of bleeding and adverse GI effects
*bone marrow depressants:* Possibly increased leukopenic and thrombocytopenic effects of bone marrow depressants
*cefamandole, cefoperazone, cefotetan:* Increased risk of hypoprothrombinemia and bleeding
*colchicine, platelet aggregation inhibitors:* Increased risk of GI bleeding, hemorrhage, and ulcers
*corticosteroids, potassium supplements:* Increased risk of adverse GI effects
*cyclosporine:* Increased risk of nephrotoxicity from both drugs, increased blood cyclosporine level
*digoxin:* Increased blood digoxin level and risk of digitalis toxicity
*diuretics (loop, potassium-sparing, and thiazide):* Decreased diuretic and antihypertensive effects
*gold compounds, nephrotoxic drugs:* Increased risk of adverse renal effects

* For analgesic effects.
† For anti-inflammatory effects.
‡ For antipyretic effects.

G
H
I

*heparin, oral anticoagulants, thrombolytics:* Increased anticoagulant effects, increased risk of hemorrhage
*insulin, oral antidiabetic drugs:* Possibly increased hypoglycemic effects of these drugs
*lithium:* Increased blood lithium level
*methotrexate:* Decreased methotrexate clearance, increased risk of methotrexate toxicity
*plicamycin, valproic acid:* Increased risk of hypoprothrombinemia and GI bleeding, hemorrhage, and ulcers
*probenecid:* Possibly increased blood level, effectiveness, and risk of toxicity of ibuprofen

**ACTIVITIES**
*alcohol use:* Increased risk of adverse GI effects

## Adverse Reactions

**CNS:** Aseptic meningitis, dizziness, headache, nervousness, seizures, stroke
**CV:** Fluid retention, heart failure, hypertension, MI, peripheral edema, tachycardia
**EENT:** Amblyopia, epistaxis, stomatitis, tinnitus
**GI:** Abdominal cramps, distention, or pain; anorexia; constipation; diarrhea; diverticulitis; dyspepsia; dysphagia; elevated liver function test results; epigastric discomfort; esophagitis; flatulence; gastritis; gastroenteritis; gastroesophageal reflux disease; GI bleeding, hemorrhage, perforation, or ulceration; heartburn; hemorrhoids; hepatic failure; hepatitis; hiatal hernia; indigestion; melena; nausea; stomatitis; vomiting
**GU:** Cystitis, hematuria, renal failure (acute)
**HEME:** Agranulocytosis, anemia, aplastic anemia, eosinophilia, hemolytic anemia, leukopenia, neutropenia, pancytopenia, prolonged bleeding time, thrombocytopenia
**RESP:** Bronchospasm, dyspnea, wheezing
**SKIN:** Blisters, erythema multiforme, photosensitivity, pruritus, rash, Stevens-Johnson syndrome, toxic epidermal necrolysis, urticaria
**Other:** Anaphylaxis, angioedema, flulike symptoms, weight gain

## Nursing Considerations

• Use ibuprofen with extreme caution in patients with a history of ulcer disease or GI bleeding because NSAIDs such as ibuprofen increase the risk of GI bleeding and ulceration. Expect to use ibuprofen for the shortest time possible in these patients.
• Be aware that serious GI tract ulceration, bleeding, and perforation may occur without warning symptoms. Elderly patients are at greater risk. To minimize risk, give drug with food. If GI distress occurs, withhold drug and notify prescriber immediately.
• Use ibuprofen cautiously in patients with hypertension, and monitor blood pressure closely throughout therapy. Drug may cause hypertension or worsen it.
• **WARNING** Monitor patient closely for thrombotic events, including MI and stroke, because NSAIDs increase the risk.
• Monitor patient—especially if he's elderly or receiving long-term ibuprofen therapy—for less common but serious adverse GI reactions, including anorexia, constipation, diverticulitis, dysphagia, esophagitis, gastritis, gastroenteritis, gastroesophageal reflux disease, hemorrhoids, hiatal hernia, melena, stomatitis, and vomiting.
• Monitor liver function test results because, in rare cases, elevations may progress to severe hepatic reactions, including fatal hepatitis, liver necrosis, and hepatic failure.
• Monitor BUN and serum creatinine levels in elderly patients, patients taking diuretics or ACE inhibitors, and patients with heart failure, impaired renal function, or hepatic dysfunction; drug may cause renal failure.
• Monitor CBC for decreased hemoglobin and hematocrit because drug may worsen anemia.
• **WARNING** If patient has bone marrow suppression or is receiving an antineoplastic drug, monitor laboratory results (including WBC count), and watch for evidence of infection because anti-inflammatory and antipyretic actions of ibuprofen may mask signs and symptoms, such as fever and pain.
• Assess patient's skin regularly for signs of rash or other hypersensitivity reaction because ibuprofen is an NSAID and may cause serious skin reactions without warning, even in patients with no history of NSAID sensitivity. At first sign of reaction, stop drug and notify prescriber.
• Although drug's analgesic effect occurs at low doses, expect to give at least 400 mg four times a day for anti-inflammatory effect.
• Expect higher doses for rheumatoid arthritis than for osteoarthritis.
• Be aware that ibuprofen oral suspension may contain sucrose, which may affect blood glucose level in patients with diabetes.

**PATIENT TEACHING**
• Instruct patient to take tablets with a full

glass of water, and caution him not to lie down for 15 to 30 minutes to prevent esophageal irritation.

•Advise patient to take drug with food or after meals to reduce GI distress.

•Urge patient not to take more than prescribed because stomach bleeding may occur.

•Instruct patient to consult prescriber if he needs to take drug for more than 3 days for fever or 10 days for pain; if stomach problems (heartburn, upset, pain) recur; if he has a history of ulcers, bleeding problems, hypertension, or heart or renal disease; if he takes a diuretic; or if he's older than age 65.

•Inform patient with phenylketonuria that Motrin chewable tablets contain aspartame.

•Inform patient that full therapeutic effect for arthritis may take 2 weeks or longer.

•Advise patient to avoid taking two different NSAIDs at the same time, unless directed.

•Urge patient to avoid alcohol, aspirin, and corticosteroids while taking ibuprofen.

•Suggest that patient wear sunscreen and protective clothing when outdoors.

•Advise patient to report flulike symptoms, rash, signs of GI bleeding, swelling, vision changes, and weight gain.

•Urge parents to tell prescriber promptly if child receiving drug develops a severe or persistent sore throat, high fever, headache, persistent diarrhea, nausea, or vomiting or hasn't been drinking fluids.

•Advise parents to consult prescriber before giving OTC ibuprofen to a child if the child has ulcers, bleeding problems, high blood pressure, heart or kidney disease, a need for diuretic therapy, serious adverse effects from previous use of fever reducers or pain relievers, or persistent stomach problems, such as heartburn, upset stomach, or stomach pain.

•Caution pregnant patient not to take NSAIDs such as ibuprofen during the last trimester because they may cause premature closure of the ductus arteriosus.

•Explain that ibuprofen may increase the risk of serious adverse cardiovascular reactions; urge patient to seek immediate medical attention if signs or symptoms arise, such as chest pain, shortness of breath, weakness, and slurring of speech.

•Explain that ibuprofen may increase the risk of serious adverse GI reactions; stress the importance of seeking immediate medical attention for such signs and symptoms as epigastric or abdominal pain, indigestion,

black or tarry stools, or vomiting blood or material that looks like coffee grounds.

•Alert patient to rare but serious skin reactions. Urge him to seek immediate medical attention for rash, blisters, itching, fever, or other indications of hypersensitivity.

# ibutilide fumarate

Corvert

## Class and Category

*Chemical:* Methanesulfonanilide derivative
*Therapeutic:* Class III antiarrhythmic
*Pregnancy category:* C

## Indications and Dosages

➤ *To rapidly convert recent-onset atrial flutter or fibrillation to sinus rhythm*

**I.V. INFUSION**

**Adults who weigh 60 kg (132 lb) or more.** 1 mg over 10 min. Dose repeated 10 min after first dose is finished if arrhythmia persists.

**Adults who weigh less than 60 kg.** 0.01 mg/kg over 10 min. Dose is repeated 10 min after first dose is completed if arrhythmia persists.

DOSAGE ADJUSTMENT Infusion stopped if arrhythmia is terminated or if sustained or nonsustained ventricular tachycardia or prolonged QT or QTc interval develops.

## Mechanism of Action

May promote sodium movement through slow inward sodium channels in myocardial cell membranes. Ibutilide also may inhibit potassium channels in myocardial cell membranes involved in cardiac repolarization. These actions prolong the cardiac action potential by delaying repolarization and increasing atrial and ventricular refractoriness. As a result, the sinus rate slows and AV conduction is delayed.

## Contraindications

Hypersensitivity to ibutilide or components

## Interactions

**DRUGS**

*amiodarone, astemizole, disopyramide, maprotiline, phenothiazines, procainamide, quinidine, sotalol, tricyclic antidepressants:* Possibly prolonged QT interval, leading to increased risk of proarrhythmias

## Adverse Reactions
**CNS:** Headache, syncope
**CV:** AV block, bradycardia, bundle-branch block, heart failure, hypertension, hypotension, idioventricular rhythm, orthostatic hypotension, palpitations, prolonged QT interval, sinus and supraventricular tachycardia, supraventricular arrhythmias, ventricular arrhythmias, ventricular tachycardia (sustained and nonsustained)
**GI:** Nausea
**GU:** Renal failure

## Nursing Considerations
•Before giving ibutilide, check serum electrolyte levels and expect to correct abnormalities, as prescribed. Be especially alert for hypokalemia and hypomagnesemia, which can lead to arrhythmias.
•Give drug undiluted, or dilute it in 50 ml of NS or $D_5W$. Add contents of 10-ml vial (0.1 mg/ml) to 50 ml of solution to obtain 0.017 mg/ml. Use polyvinyl chloride plastic bags or polyolefin bags for admixtures. Give drug within 24 hours (48 hours if refrigerated).
•Infuse drug slowly over 10 minutes.
•As ordered, monitor patient's cardiac rhythm continuously during drug infusion and for at least 4 hours afterward—longer if arrhythmias appear or if patient has abnormal hepatic function. Observe patient for ventricular ectopy.
•Make sure that a defibrillator and drugs to treat sustained ventricular tachycardia are available during therapy and when monitoring patient after therapy.
**PATIENT TEACHING**
•Inform patient that ibutilide will be administered by I.V. infusion and that his heart rhythm will be monitored continuously during the infusion.
•Ask patient to report chest pain, faintness, numbness, tingling, palpitations, and shortness of breath.
•Advise patient to keep follow-up appointments to monitor heart rhythm.

# iloprost

Ventavis

## Class and Category
*Chemical:* Synthetic analogue of prostacyclin PGI2
*Therapeutic:* Pulmonary arterial antihypertensive
*Pregnancy category:* C

## Indications and Dosages
➤ *To improve symptoms and exercise tolerance and prevent further deterioration from pulmonary arterial hypertension in patients with NYHA Class III or IV symptoms*
**INHALATION SOLUTION**
**Adults.** *Initial:* 2.5 mcg as one-time dose. If tolerated well for 2 hr, dosage increased to 5 mcg. *Maintenance:* 5 mcg six to nine times daily during waking hours with at least 2 hr separating each dose. *Maximum:* 45 mcg daily.

---

### Mechanism of Action
Dilates systemic and pulmonary arterial vascular beds, which lowers blood pressure in the pulmonary arterial system.

---

## Contraindications
Hypersensitivity to iloprost or its components

## Interactions
**DRUGS**
*anticoagulants:* Increased risk of bleeding
*antihypertensives, vasodilators:* Increased hypotensive effect

## Adverse Reactions
**CNS:** Apathy, dizziness, headache, insomnia, restlessness, syncope
**CV:** Chest pain, congestive heart failure, hypotension, palpitations, peripheral edema, supraventricular tachycardia, thrombosis, vasodilation
**EENT:** Tongue pain
**ENDO:** Hyperglycemia
**GI:** Abdominal cramps, diarrhea, nausea, vomiting
**GU:** Renal failure
**MS:** Back pain, muscle spasms
**RESP:** Dyspnea, hemoptysis, increased cough, pneumonia
**SKIN:** Flushing
**Other:** Flulike symptoms, increased alkaline phosphatase level

## Nursing Considerations
•Use iloprost cautiously in patients with hepatic or renal impairment.
•Give iloprost only with the Prodose AAD System, a pulmonary drug delivery device. Avoid contact between solution and skin or eyes.

•**WARNING** Don't give iloprost if patient's systolic blood pressure is less than 85 mm Hg.
•Notify prescriber if patient develops exertional syncope because dosage may need to be adjusted.
•**WARNING** Stop iloprost immediately if patient develops signs of pulmonary edema, such as shortness of breath, anxiety, restlessness, and abnormal breath sounds. Notify prescriber and provide supportive care, as prescribed.
•Monitor patient's vital signs while initiating iloprost therapy because drug may cause syncope.

**PATIENT TEACHING**
•Instruct patient to use iloprost inhalation therapy exactly as prescribed. Tell patient that at least 2 hours must elapse between doses but that the benefits of iloprost therapy may not last for 2 hours.
•Teach patient how to administer iloprost via the Prodose AAD System. Tell patient to have a backup system available in case of equipment malfunction.
•Advise patient to stand up slowly because drug may cause dizziness or faintness. If these symptoms persist or worsen, tell patient to notify prescriber because a dosage adjustment may be required.

# imipenem and cilastatin sodium

Primaxin (CAN), Primaxin ADD-Vantage, Primaxin IM, Primaxin IV

## Class and Category

*Chemical:* Thienamycin derivative (imipenem), heptenoic acid derivative (cilastatin sodium)
*Therapeutic:* Antibiotic
*Pregnancy category:* C

## Indications and Dosages

➤ *To treat severe or life-threatening bacterial infections (including endocarditis, pneumonia, and septicemia as well as bone, joint, intra-abdominal, skin, and soft-tissue infections) caused by gram-positive anaerobic organisms, such as most staphylococci and streptococci and some enterococci (including* Enterococcus faecalis); *most strains of* Enterobacteriaceae *(including* Citrobacter *sp.,* Enterobacter *sp.,* Escherichia coli, Klebsiella *sp.,* Morganella morganii, Proteus mirabilis, Providencia stuartii, *and* Serratia marcescens); *and many gram-negative aerobic and anaerobic species (including* Bacteroides *sp.,* Campylobacter *sp.,* Clostridium *sp.,* Haemophilus influenzae, Legionella *sp.,* Neisseria gonorrhoeae, *and* Pseudomonas aeruginosa)

**I.V. INFUSION (DOSAGES BASED ON IMIPENEM CONTENT)**
**Adults and adolescents.** 500 mg q 6 hr to 1,000 mg q 6 to 8 hr. *Maximum:* 50 mg/kg or 4 g/day, whichever is lower.
**Children age 3 months and older.** 15 to 25 mg/kg q 6 hr. *Maximum:* 2,000 to 4,000 mg/day.
**Infants ages 4 weeks to 3 months who weigh 1,500 g (3 lb, 3 oz) or more.** 25 mg/kg q 6 hr. *Maximum:* 2,000 to 4,000 mg/day.
**Neonates ages 1 to 4 weeks who weigh 1,500 g or more.** 25 mg/kg q 8 hr. *Maximum:* 2,000 to 4,000 mg/day.
**Neonates under age 1 week who weigh 1,500 g or more.** 25 mg/kg q 12 hr. *Maximum:* 2,000 to 4,000 mg/day.
➤ *To treat moderate infections caused by the organisms listed above*
**I.V. INFUSION (DOSAGES BASED ON IMIPENEM CONTENT)**
**Adults and adolescents.** 500 mg q 6 to 8 hr up to 1,000 mg q 8 hr. *Maximum:* 50 mg/kg or 4 g/day, whichever is lower.
**Children age 3 months and older.** 15 to 25 mg/kg q 6 hr. *Maximum:* 2,000 to 4,000 mg/day.
**Infants ages 4 weeks to 3 months who weigh 1,500 g or more.** 25 mg/kg q 6 hr. *Maximum:* 2,000 to 4,000 mg/day.
**Neonates ages 1 to 4 weeks who weigh 1,500 g or more.** 25 mg/kg q 8 hr. *Maximum:* 2,000 to 4,000 mg/day.
**Neonates under age 1 week who weigh 1,500 g or more.** 25 mg/kg q 12 hr. *Maximum:* 2,000 to 4,000 mg/day.
**I.M. INJECTION (DOSAGES BASED ON IMIPENEM CONTENT)**
**Adults and adolescents.** 500 to 750 mg q 12 hr. *Maximum:* 1,500 mg/day.
**Children.** 10 to 15 mg/kg q 6 hr.
➤ *To treat mild infections caused by the organisms listed above*
**I.V. INFUSION (DOSAGES BASED ON IMIPENEM CONTENT)**
**Adults and adolescents.** 250 to 500 mg q 6 hr. *Maximum:* 50 mg/kg or 4 g/day, whichever is lower.
**Children age 3 months and older.** 15 to 25 mg/kg q 6 hr. *Maximum:* 2,000 (for fully suscep-

G
H
I

tible organisms) to 4,000 (for moderately susceptible organisms) mg/day.
**Infants ages 4 weeks to 3 months who weigh 1,500 g or more.** 25 mg/kg q 6 hr. *Maximum:* 2,000 to 4,000 mg/day.
**Neonates ages 1 to 4 weeks who weigh 1,500 g or more.** 25 mg/kg q 8 hr. *Maximum:* 2,000 to 4,000 mg/day.
**Neonates under age 1 week who weigh 1,500 g or more.** 25 mg/kg q 12 hr. *Maximum:* 2,000 to 4,000 mg/day.
**I.M. INJECTION (DOSAGES BASED ON IMIPENEM CONTENT)**
**Adults and adolescents.** 500 to 750 mg q 12 hr. *Maximum:* 1,500 mg/day.
**Children.** 10 to 15 mg/kg q 6 hr.

➤ *To treat uncomplicated UTIs caused by the organisms listed above*
**I.V. INFUSION (DOSAGES BASED ON IMIPENEM CONTENT)**
**Adults and adolescents.** 250 mg q 6 hr. *Maximum:* 50 mg/kg or 4 g/day, whichever is lower.
➤ *To treat complicated UTIs caused by the organisms listed above*
**I.V. INFUSION (DOSAGES BASED ON IMIPENEM CONTENT)**
**Adults and adolescents.** 500 mg q 6 hr. *Maximum:* 50 mg/kg or 4 g/day, whichever is lower.
**DOSAGE ADJUSTMENT** Dosage reduced based on creatinine clearance for patients with impaired renal function.

## Mechanism of Action
Produces two related actions. During bacterial cell wall synthesis, imipenem selectively binds to penicillin-binding proteins that are responsible for cell wall formation. This action causes bacterial cells to rapidly lyse and die. Cilastatin sodium inhibits imipenem's breakdown in the kidneys, thus maintaining a high imipenem level in the urinary tract.

## Incompatibilities
Don't administer imipenem and cilastatin through same I.V. line as beta-lactam antibiotics or aminoglycosides.

## Contraindications
Hypersensitivity to imipenem, its components, other beta–lactam antibiotics, or amide-type local anesthetics (I.M.); meningitis (I.V.); severe heart block or shock (I.M.)

## Interactions
**DRUGS**
*cyclosporine:* Increased adverse CNS effects of both drugs
*ganciclovir:* Increased risk of seizures
*probenecid:* Slightly increased blood level and half-life of imipenem

## Adverse Reactions
**CNS:** Confusion, dizziness, fever, seizures, somnolence, tremor, weakness
**CV:** Hypotension
**EENT:** Oral candidiasis
**GI:** Diarrhea, nausea, pseudomembranous colitis, vomiting
**RESP:** Wheezing
**SKIN:** Diaphoresis, pruritus, rash, urticaria
**Other:** Anaphylaxis, injection site thrombophlebitis

## Nursing Considerations
•Obtain body fluid and tissue specimens for culture and sensitivity testing, as ordered, before giving first dose of imipenem and cilastatin. Expect to start therapy before test results are available.
•For I.V. administration, add about 10 ml of diluent to each 250- or 500-mg vial and shake well. Transfer this reconstituted drug to at least 100 ml of prescribed I.V. solution. After the transfer, add another 10 ml of diluent to each vial, shake, and then transfer to infusion container. Shake infusion container until clear. To reconstitute piggyback bottles, add 100 ml of diluent to each 250- or 500-mg infusion bottle, and shake well.
•Administer reconstituted drug within 4 to 10 hours, depending on diluent used (24 to 48 hours if refrigerated). Color may range from clear to yellow; don't administer solution that contains particles.
•Infuse 500-mg or smaller dose over 20 to 30 minutes and 750- to 1,000-mg dose over 40 to 60 minutes.
•Inject I.M. form into a large muscle mass.
•Expect increased risk of imipenem-induced seizures in patients with brain lesions, head trauma, or history of CNS disorders and in those receiving more than 2 g of drug daily.
•Assess patient for signs and symptoms of allergic reaction and bacterial or fungal superinfection.
**PATIENT TEACHING**
•Inform patient that imipenem and cilastatin must be given by infusion or injection.

• Instruct patient to report discomfort at I.V. insertion site.

• Advise patient to report itching, signs of superinfection (such as diarrhea and sore mouth), and hives.

# imipramine hydrochloride

Apo-Imipramine (CAN), Impril (CAN), Norfranil, Novopramine (CAN), Tipramine, Tofranil

## imipramine pamoate

Tofranil-PM

### Class and Category
*Chemical:* Dibenzazepine derivative
*Therapeutic:* Antidepressant
*Pregnancy category:* Not rated

### Indications and Dosages
➤ *To treat depression*

**CAPSULES**

**Adults.** *Initial:* 75 mg/day h.s., gradually increased as needed and tolerated. *Maximum:* 300 mg/day (hospitalized patients), 200 mg/day (outpatients).

**TABLETS**

**Adults.** *Initial:* 25 to 50 mg t.i.d. or q.i.d., gradually increased as needed and tolerated. *Maximum:* 300 mg/day (hospitalized patients), 200 mg/day (outpatients).

DOSAGE ADJUSTMENT Initial dosage reduced to 25 mg h.s. for depressed elderly patients and then adjusted as needed and tolerated up to 100 mg/day in divided doses.

**Adolescents.** *Initial:* 25 to 50 mg/day in divided doses, adjusted as needed and tolerated. *Maximum:* 100 mg/day.

**Children ages 6 to 12.** 10 to 30 mg/day in divided doses b.i.d.

➤ *As adjunct to treat childhood enuresis*

**TABLETS**

**Children age 6 and older.** 25 mg 1 hr before h.s. Increased to 50 mg if no response occurs within 1 wk and child is under age 12; increased to 75 mg if child is age 12 or older. *Maximum:* 2.5 mg/kg/day.

| Route | Onset | Peak | Duration |
|-------|-------|------|----------|
| P.O. | 2 to 3 wk* | Unknown | Unknown |

---

* For antidepressant effect.

### Mechanism of Action
May interfere with reuptake of serotonin (and possibly other neurotransmitters) at presynaptic neurons, thus enhancing serotonin's effects at postsynaptic receptors. Mood elevation may result from restoration of normal levels of neurotransmitters at nerve synapses. This tricyclic antidepressant also blocks acetylcholine receptors, which may explain how it relieves enuresis.

### Contraindications
Acute recovery period after MI; hypersensitivity to imipramine, other tricyclic antidepressants, or their components; use within 2 weeks of MAO inhibitor therapy

### Interactions
**DRUGS**

*amantadine, anticholinergics, antidyskinetics, antihistamines:* Risk of increased anticholinergic effects, including confusion, hallucinations, and nightmares

*anticonvulsants:* Increased risk of CNS depression, increased risk of seizures, decreased effectiveness of imipramine

*antithyroid drugs:* Possibly agranulocytosis

*barbiturates, carbamazepine:* Possibly decreased blood level and effectiveness of imipramine

*cimetidine, fluoxetine:* Possibly increased blood imipramine level

*clonidine, guanadrel, guanethidine:* Possibly decreased antihypertensive effects of these drugs, increased CNS depression (clonidine)

*CNS depressants:* Increased CNS depression, respiratory depression, and hypotension

*disulfiram, ethchlorvynol:* Risk of delirium, increased CNS depression (ethchlorvynol)

*estramustine, estrogen-containing oral contraceptives, estrogens:* Risk of increased bioavailability of imipramine, increased depression

*MAO inhibitors:* Increased risk of hypertensive crisis, severe seizures, and death

*oral anticoagulants:* Possibly increased anticoagulant activity

*pimozide, probucol:* Risk of arrhythmias

*sympathomimetics (including ophthalmic epinephrine and vasoconstrictive local anesthetics):* Increased risk of arrhythmias, hyperpyrexia, hypertension, tachycardia

*thyroid hormones:* Risk of increased therapeutic and adverse effects of both drugs

G
H
I

*alcohol use:* Increased CNS depression, increased alcohol effects
*sun exposure:* Increased risk of photosensitivity

## Adverse Reactions

**CNS:** Anxiety, ataxia, chills, confusion, CVA, delirium, dizziness, drowsiness, excitation, extrapyramidal reactions, fever, hallucinations, headache, insomnia, nervousness, nightmares, parkinsonism, seizures, tremor
**CV:** Arrhythmias, orthostatic hypotension, palpitations
**EENT:** Blurred vision, dry mouth, increased intraocular pressure, pharyngitis, taste perversion, tinnitus, tongue swelling
**ENDO:** Gynecomastia, syndrome of inappropriate ADH secretion
**GI:** Constipation, diarrhea, heartburn, ileus, increased appetite, nausea, vomiting
**GU:** Impotence, libido changes, testicular swelling, urine retention
**HEME:** Agranulocytosis, bone marrow depression
**RESP:** Wheezing
**SKIN:** Alopecia, diaphoresis, jaundice, photosensitivity, pruritus, rash, urticaria
**Other:** Allergic reaction, facial edema, weight gain

## Nursing Considerations

•Use imipramine cautiously in patients with a history of urine retention or angle-closure glaucoma because drug's anticholinergic effects may cause urine retention and increased intraocular pressure.
•**WARNING** Don't give MAO inhibitors within 2 weeks of imipramine. Patient may experience hypertensive crisis, seizures, and death.
•Frequently assess for adverse reactions during first 2 hours of therapy.
•Check supine and standing blood pressure for orthostatic hypotension before and during imipramine therapy and before dosage increases.
•Anticipate an increased risk of arrhythmias in patients with a history of cardiac disease.
•When drug is used for depression, expect mood elevation to take 2 to 3 weeks. Watch patient closely for suicidal tendencies, especially children and adolescents and especially when therapy starts or dosage changes, because depression may worsen temporarily.
•Avoid abrupt withdrawal of drug in patients who receive long-term therapy. Such

withdrawal may cause headache, malaise, nausea, sleep disturbance, and vomiting.
•Taper drug gradually, as ordered, a few days before surgery to avoid the risk of hypertension during surgery.
•Obtain CBC, as ordered, if patient experiences signs and symptoms of infection, such as fever or pharyngitis.
•Limit amount of drug given to potentially suicidal patient.

PATIENT TEACHING
•Advise patient to take imipramine exactly as prescribed. Warn him that stopping drug abruptly may cause headache, malaise, nausea, trouble sleeping, and vomiting.
•Caution parents to monitor child or adolescent closely for suicidal tendencies, especially when therapy starts or dosage changes.
•Urge patient to report chills, trouble urinating, dizziness, excess sedation, fever, palpitations, signs of allergic reaction, and sore throat.
•Caution patient to avoid potentially hazardous activities until drug's CNS effects are known.
•Urge patient to avoid alcohol during imipramine therapy because it increases CNS depression and alcohol effects.
•Suggest that patient eat small, frequent meals to help relieve nausea.
•Instruct patient to avoid prolonged exposure to sunlight because of the risk of photosensitivity.
•Inform male patient about possible impotence and increased or decreased libido.
•If patient reports dry mouth, suggest sugarless candy or gum to relieve it. Tell him to check with prescriber if dry mouth persists after 2 weeks.

# immune globulin intramuscular (human)

## (gamma globulin, IG)

BayGam, WinRho SDF

# immune globulin intravenous (human)

## (IGIV, immune serum globulin, ISG, IVIG)

Gamimune N 5% S/D, Gamimune N 10% S/D, Gammagard Liquid, Gammagard S/D,

Gammagard S/D 0.5 g, Gammar-P IV, Gamunex 10%, Iveegam EN, Octagam 5%, Polygam S/D, Sandoglobulin, Venoglobulin-I, Venoglobulin-S 5%, Venoglobulin-S 10%, WinRho SDF

## Class and Category
*Chemical:* Polyvalent antibody
*Therapeutic:* Antibacterial, anti–Kawasaki disease agent, antipolyneuropathy agent, antiviral, immunizing agent, platelet count stimulator
*Pregnancy category:* C

## Indications and Dosages
➤ *To treat primary immunodeficiency*
**I.M. INJECTION (BAYGAM)**
**Adults.** 0.66 ml/kg (at least 200 mg/kg) q 3 to 4 wk; initial dose may be doubled.
**I.V. INFUSION (GAMIMUNE N 5% S/D OR 10% S/D)**
**Adults.** 100 to 200 mg/kg q mo. If response is inadequate, dose may be increased to as high as 400 mg/kg or dosing frequency may be increased.
**I.V. INFUSION (GAMMAGARD S/D, POLYGAM S/D)**
**Adults.** 200 to 400 mg/kg initially, then at least 100 mg/kg q mo thereafter. If response is inadequate, dose or frequency may be adjusted.
**I.V. INFUSION (GAMMAR-P IV)**
**Adults.** 200 to 400 mg/kg q 3 to 4 wk.
**Adolescents and children.** 200 mg/kg q 3 to 4 wk.
**I.V. INFUSION (GAMUNEX 10%)**
**Adults.** 300 to 600 mg/kg q 3 or 4 wk.
**I.V. INFUSION (IVEEGAM EN)**
**Adults.** 200 mg/kg q mo.
**I.V. INFUSION (OCTAGAM 5%)**
**Adults.** *Initial:* 30 mg/kg/hr for first 30 minutes; increased, if tolerated, to 60 mg/kg/hr for second 30 minutes and, if tolerated, to 120 mg/kg/hr for another 30 minutes; followed by maintenance infusion of up to 200 mg/kg/hr.
**I.V. INFUSION (SANDOGLOBULIN)**
**Adults and children.** 200 mg/kg q mo. If response is inadequate, dose may be increased to 300 mg/kg or dosing frequency may be increased.
**I.V. INFUSION (VENOGLOBULIN-I)**
**Adults and children.** 200 mg/kg q mo. If response is inadequate, dose may be increased to 300 to 400 mg/kg q mo or dosing frequency may be increased.
**I.V. INFUSION (VENOGLOBULIN-S 5% OR 10%)**
**Adults and children.** 200 mg/kg q mo. If response is inadequate, dose may be increased

to as high as 400 mg/kg or dosing frequency may be increased.
➤ *To treat primary immunodeficiency disorders associated with defects in humoral immunity*
**I.V. INFUSION (GAMMAGARD LIQUID)**
**Adults and children.** 300 to 600 mg/kg/day q 3 to 4 wk.
➤ *To treat idiopathic thrombocytopenic purpura (ITP)*
**I.V. INFUSION (GAMIMUNE N 5% S/D)**
**Adults and children.** 400 mg/kg/day for 5 days. Alternatively, 1,000 mg/kg for 1 or 2 days for patients not at risk for increased fluid volume.
**I.V. INFUSION (GAMIMUNE N 10% S/D)**
**Adults and children.** 1,000 mg/kg for 1 or 2 days for patients not at risk for increased fluid volume.
**I.V. INFUSION (GAMUNEX 10%)**
**Adults.** 1 g/kg q.d. for 2 consecutive days (second dose may be withheld if adequate increase in platelet count occurs 24 hours after first dose). Alternatively, 0.4 g/kg q.d. for 5 consecutive days.
**DOSAGE ADJUSTMENT** In acute ITP of childhood, I.V. Sandoglobulin therapy may be discontinued after 2nd day of 5-day course if initial platelet count response is adequate (30,000 to 50,000/mm$^3$). In chronic ITP, an additional I.V. infusion of 400 mg/kg (of either Sandoglobulin or Gamimune) may be prescribed if platelet count falls below 30,000/mm$^3$ or if patient develops significant bleeding. If response remains inadequate, an additional I.V. infusion of 800 to 1,000 mg/kg may be given.
**I.V. INFUSION (GAMMAGARD S/D)**
**Adults.** 1 g/kg. If response is inadequate, up to three separate doses may be administered on alternate days.
**I.V. INFUSION (SANDOGLOBULIN)**
**Adults and adolescents.** 400 mg/kg/day for 2 to 5 consecutive days.
**I.V. INFUSION (VENOGLOBULIN-I)**
**Adults and children.** *Induction:* Cumulative dose up to 2 g/kg over 2 to 7 consecutive days. *Maintenance (adults):* 2 g/kg as a single dose q 2 wk as needed to maintain platelet count above 30,000/mm$^3$ or prevent bleeding episodes. *Maintenance (children):* 1 g/kg as a single dose q 2 wk as needed to maintain platelet count above 30,000/mm$^3$ or prevent bleeding episodes.

G
H
I

**I.V. INFUSION (VENOGLOBULIN-S 5% OR 10%)**

**Adults and children.** Cumulative dose up to 2,000 mg/kg over 5 consecutive days.

DOSAGE ADJUSTMENT An additional I.V. infusion of 1,000 mg/kg may be administered to maintain a platelet count of 30,000/mm³ in children or 20,000/mm³ in adults or to prevent bleeding episodes.

➤ *To treat acute or chronic pediatric immune thrombocytopenia purpura; to treat chronic adult-onset immune thrombocytopenia purpura; to treat prediatric- and adult-onset immune thrombocytopenia purpura secondary to HIV infection*

**I.V. INJECTION (WINRHO SDF)**

**Adults and children.** *Initial:* 250 IU/kg given as a single injection over 3 to 5 min. Or 125 IU/kg given as a single injection over 3 to 5 min and repeated once on a separate day. *Maintenance:* Frequency and dosage highly individualized based on patient's hemoglobin and platelet levels.

DOSAGE ADJUSTMENT For patients with a hemoglobin level less than 10 g/dl, dose reduced to 125 to 200 IU/kg.

➤ *As adjunct to treat Kawasaki disease*

**I.V. INFUSION (GAMMAGARD S/D)**

**Adults and adolescents.** 1 g/kg as a single dose; alternatively, 400 mg/kg/day for 4 consecutive days.

**I.V. INFUSION (IVEEGAM EN, VENOGLOBULIN-S 5% OR 10%)**

**Adults and adolescents.** 2 g/kg as a single dose; alternatively, Iveegam EN may be given at 400 mg/kg q.d. for 4 days.

➤ *To decrease the risk of graft-versus-host disease, interstitial pneumonia, septicemia, and other infections during first 100 days after bone marrow transplantation*

**I.V. INFUSION (GAMIMUNE N 5% S/D OR 10% S/D)**

**Adults over age 20.** 500 mg/kg on 7th and 2nd days before transplant (or at time conditioning therapy for transplantation begins), and then weekly through 90th day after transplant.

➤ *As adjunct to treat bacterial infections secondary to B-cell chronic lymphocytic leukemia*

**I.V. INFUSION (GAMMAGARD S/D, POLYGAM S/D)**

**Adults and adolescents.** 400 mg/kg q 3 to 4 wk.

➤ *To prevent bacterial infection in children with HIV who are immunosuppressed*

**I.V. INFUSION (GAMIMUNE N 5% S/D OR 10% S/D)**

**Children.** 400 mg/kg q.d. every 28 days.

➤ *To prevent hepatitis A*

**I.M. INJECTION (BAYGAM)**

**Adults with household or institutional contacts.** 0.02 ml/kg (0.01 ml/lb).

**Adults traveling to areas where hepatitis A is common.** 0.02 ml/kg if staying less than 3 mo, 0.06 ml/kg (repeated q 4 to 6 mo) if staying 3 mo or longer.

➤ *To prevent or lessen severity of measles (rubeola) in susceptible persons*

**I.M. INJECTION (BAYGAM)**

**Adults.** 0.2 ml/kg (0.11 ml/lb) for persons exposed fewer than 6 days previously.

➤ *To provide passive immunization against varicella in immunosuppressed patients*

**I.M. INJECTION (BAYGAM)**

**Adults.** 0.6 to 1.2 ml/kg if varicella-zoster immune globulin (human) is unavailable.

➤ *To reduce the risk of infection and fetal damage in women who have been exposed to rubella in early pregnancy*

**I.M. INJECTION (BAYGAM)**

**Adults.** 0.55 ml/kg.

➤ *To suppress Rh isoimmunization*

**I.M. INJECTION (WINRHO SDF)**

**Adult pregnant females.** 1,500 IU as a single dose 28 wk gestation followed by 600 IU within 72 hr after delivery of an Rh-positive newborn.

**I.V. INJECTION (WINRHO SDF)**

**Adult pregnant females.** 1,500 IU as a single dose infused over 3 to 5 min at 28 wk gestation followed by 600 IU infused over 3 to 5 min within 72 hr after delivery of an Rh-positive newborn.

DOSAGE ADJUSTMENT For patients who are more than 34 wk gestation and are having an abortion, amniocentesis, or other manipulative procedure, 600 IU given within 72 hr but preferably immediately after procedure. For patients who are 34 wk gestation or less and are having amniocentesis or chorionic villus sampling, 1,500 IU given immediately after procedure and repeated q 12 wk for duration of pregnancy. For patients with a threatened abortion at any stage of pregnancy, 1,500 IU given immediately.

➤ *To treat incompatible blood transfusions or massive fetal hemorrhage*

## I.M. INJECTION (WINRHO SDF)
**Adults exposed to Rh-positive whole blood.** 6,000 IU q 12 hr until total dose (60 IU/ml of blood) is given.
**Adults exposed to Rh-positive RBCs.** 6,000 IU q 12 hr until total dose (120 IU/ml of cells) is given.
### I.V. INJECTION (WINRHO SDF)
**Adults exposed to Rh-positive whole blood.** 3,000 IU infused over 3 to 5 min q 8 hr until total dose (45 IU/ml of blood) is given.
**Adults exposed to Rh-positive RBCs.** 3,000 IU infused over 3 to 5 min q 8 hr until total dose (90 IU/ml of cells) is given.

| Route | Onset | Peak | Duration |
|---|---|---|---|
| I.V. | Unknown | Unknown | 21 to 28 days |

## Mechanism of Action
Releases antibody-specific globulins to produce an antibody-antigen reaction that results in bacterial lysis and facilitates bacterial phagocytosis. In treatment of ITP, immune globulin blocks iron receptors on macrophages to increase immunoglobulin action. Immune globulin also increases cytokine production and improves B-cell immune function by regulating T-cell and macrophage activity. Newly formed antigen-antibody complexes produce split complement components that cause bacterial lysis.

In Kawasaki disease and bacterial infections secondary to B-cell chronic lymphocytic leukemia, immune globulin neutralizes bacterial and viral toxins that harm the immune and inflammatory responses.

## Incompatibilities
Don't mix immune globulin with any other drugs, including other immune globulins, or with any I.V. solutions other than D₅W or manufacturer's supplied diluent because effects of doing so are unknown.

## Contraindications
Hypersensitivity to immune globulin (human) or its components, IgA deficiency in patients with known antibody to IgA

## Interactions
### DRUGS
*vaccines, live-virus:* Possibly decreased response to vaccine

## Adverse Reactions
**CNS:** Headache, malaise
**CV:** Tachycardia
**GI:** Nausea, vomiting
**MS:** Arthralgia, back pain, myalgia
**RESP:** Dyspnea

## Nursing Considerations
•Before administering immune globulin, monitor patient's fluid volume and BUN and serum creatinine levels, as ordered, to determine if he's at risk for acute renal failure. Those at increased risk include patients with renal insufficiency, diabetes mellitus, volume depletion, sepsis, or paraproteinemia; those taking nephrotoxic drugs; and those over age 65. Expect drug to be discontinued if renal function deteriorates.
•When preparing drug for administration, verify that the appropriate form of immune globulin is being used—either immune globulin intramuscular for I.M. injection or immune globulin intravenous for I.V. infusion.
•To reconstitute drug (except Gammagard Liquid, which doesn't need reconstitution), follow manufacturer's guidelines and use only diluent recommended by manufacturer. Don't shake solution; excessive shaking causes foaming. If drug or diluent is cold, drug may take up to 20 minutes to dissolve.
•If drug is reconstituted outside of sterile laminar airflow conditions, administer it immediately and discard unused portions.
•Consult manufacturer's guidelines to determine appropriate flow rate for starting infusion. Expect to increase flow rate after 15 to 30 minutes, according to guidelines.
•When giving drug by I.M. injection, inject it only into the deltoid muscle of the upper arm or the anterolateral aspect of the upper thigh.
•**WARNING** Watch for an acute inflammatory reaction in patients who have never received immune globulin therapy before, in those whose last treatment was more than 8 weeks before, and in those whose initial infusion rate exceeded 1 ml/minute. Within 30 minutes to 1 hour after beginning of infusion, assess for chills, fever, facial flushing, feeling of tightness in chest, dizziness, nausea and vomiting, diaphoresis, and hypotension. Notify prescriber immediately if such symptoms occur, and be prepared to stop infusion until symptoms have subsided.

•**WARNING** After immune globulin administration, monitor patient closely for aseptic meningitis. Notify prescriber if patient develops drowsiness, fever, nausea and vomiting, nuchal rigidity, photophobia, painful eye movements, or severe headache.

•Be aware that immune globulin intravenous is made from human plasma and therefore may contain infectious agents, such as viruses. However, the risk of transmitting a virus by infusion has been reduced by screening blood donors, testing donated blood, and inactivating or removing certain viruses from the product.

•For patient receiving WinRho SDF to treat immune thrombocytopenia purpura, assess clinical response by monitoring patient's platelet count, RBC count, hemoglobin level, and reticulocyte level.

•For patient receiving WinRho SDF for exposure to incompatible blood transfusions or massive fetal hemorrhage, give drug within 72 hours of incident.

**PATIENT TEACHING**
•Instruct patient to immediately report any symptoms he experiences after receiving immune globulin.

•Inform patient that he'll need to postpone live-virus vaccinations for up to 11 months after receiving immune globulin because drug may delay or inhibit his response to vaccine.

# inamrinone

## (amrinone)

Inocor

## Class and Category

*Chemical:* Bipyridine derivative
*Therapeutic:* Cardiac inotrope
*Pregnancy category:* C

## Indications and Dosages

➤ *To treat heart failure in patients who haven't responded sufficiently to digoxin, diuretics, or vasodilators*

**I.V. INFUSION**

**Adults.** *Initial:* 0.75 mg/kg by bolus administered over 2 to 3 min and repeated after 30 min, if needed. *Maintenance:* 5 to 10 mcg/kg/min by infusion. *Maximum:* 10 mg/kg/day.

| Route | Onset | Peak | Duration |
|-------|-------|------|----------|
| I.V. | 2 to 5 min | In 10 min | 30 min to 2 hr |

## Mechanism of Action

Inhibits phosphodiesterase enzymes that normally degrade myocardial cAMP. This action increases intracellular levels of cAMP, which regulates intracellular and extracellular calcium balance. An increased intracellular cAMP level enhances the influx of calcium into the cell, thereby increasing the force of myocardial contractions. Inamrinone also acts directly on peripheral vascular smooth-muscle cells, causing relaxation and dilation. This action reduces preload and afterload.

## Incompatibilities

Don't administer inamrinone through same I.V. line as furosemide to prevent precipitate formation. Don't dilute inamrinone in solution that contains dextrose because a chemical interaction occurs over 24 hours.

## Contraindications

Hypersensitivity to inamrinone, bisulfites, or their components; severe aortic or pulmonary valvular disease

## Interactions

**DRUGS**
*disopyramide:* Possibly severe hypotension

## Adverse Reactions

**CNS:** Fever
**CV:** Chest pain, hypotension, pericarditis, supraventricular tachycardia, ventricular arrhythmias
**GI:** Abdominal pain, anorexia, elevated liver function test results, hepatotoxicity, nausea, vomiting
**HEME:** Elevated erythrocyte sedimentation rate, thrombocytopenia (especially with high-dose or prolonged treatment)
**MS:** Myositis
**RESP:** Hypoxemia, pleuritis
**SKIN:** Jaundice
**Other:** Infusion site burning

## Nursing Considerations

•**WARNING** Be aware that inamrinone may increase the risk of ventricular arrhythmias in patients with atrial flutter or fibrillation. To minimize this risk, expect to pretreat such patients with digoxin.

•Administer inamrinone undiluted or diluted in NS or 0.45NS to a concentration of 1 to 3 mg/ml, as prescribed. Use diluted solution within 24 hours.

•**WARNING** Monitor vital signs regularly. If blood pressure falls significantly, slow or stop inamrinone infusion and notify prescriber.

•Monitor weight, cardiac index, central venous pressure, pulmonary artery wedge pressure, and fluid intake and output as appropriate to assess effectiveness of therapy.

•**WARNING** Assess frequently for signs of thrombocytopenia, such as bruising or bleeding and altered platelet count. If signs appear, expect to decrease inamrinone dose or discontinue drug.

**PATIENT TEACHING**

•Instruct patient to notify you or another nurse if he becomes dizzy, which may indicate hypotension.

# indapamide

Apo-Indapamide (CAN), Gen-Indapamide (CAN), Lozide (CAN), Lozol, Novo-Indapamide (CAN), Nu-Indapamide (CAN)

## Class and Category
*Chemical:* Sulfonamide
*Therapeutic:* Antihypertensive, diuretic
*Pregnancy category:* B

## Indications and Dosages

➤ *To treat edema caused by heart failure*
**TABLETS**
**Adults.** 2.5 mg q.d. in the morning, increased to 5 mg/day after 1 wk, if indicated.

➤ *To manage hypertension*
**TABLETS**
**Adults.** 2.5 mg q.d., increased to 5 mg after 4 wk, if needed.

| Route | Onset | Peak | Duration |
|---|---|---|---|
| P.O.* | 1 to 2 hr | Unknown | 36 hr |
| P.O.† | 1 to 2 wk | 8 to 12 wk | Up to 8 wk |

## Contraindications
Anuria; hypersensitivity to thiazide or related diuretics or to sulfonamide-derived drugs

---

* For edema.
† For hypertension (with multiple doses).

## Mechanism of Action
Acts mainly on the distal convoluted tubules, where it enhances excretion of sodium, chloride, and water by inhibiting sodium ion movement across renal tubules. The resulting decrease in plasma and extracellular fluid volume decreases peripheral vascular resistance and reduces blood pressure. This thiazide diuretic also may cause arterial vasodilation by blocking calcium channels in smooth-muscle cells.

## Interactions
**DRUGS**
*amiodarone:* Increased risk of arrhythmias if hypokalemia develops
*cholestyramine, colestipol:* Decreased indapamide absorption
*diazoxide:* Increased risk of hyperglycemia
*digoxin:* Increased risk of digitalis toxicity if hypokalemia develops
*hypotension-producing drugs:* Increased antihypertensive or diuretic effects
*lithium:* Increased risk of lithium toxicity
*neuromuscular blockers:* Possibly increased neuromuscular blockade, risk of respiratory depression
*oral anticoagulants:* Possibly decreased anticoagulant effects

## Adverse Reactions
**CNS:** Anxiety, dizziness, drowsiness, fatigue, fever, headache, mood changes, nervousness, sleep disturbance, vertigo, weakness
**CV:** Arrhythmias, hypercholesterolemia, orthostatic hypotension, palpitations
**EENT:** Dry mouth
**ENDO:** Hyperglycemia, hypoglycemia
**GI:** Anorexia, constipation, diarrhea, hepatitis, nausea, pancreatitis, thirst, vomiting
**GU:** Impotence, nocturia
**MS:** Gout, muscle spasms
**SKIN:** Jaundice, necrotizing vasculitis, photosensitivity, pruritus, rash, urticaria
**Other:** Dilutional hypochloremia and hyponatremia, hypokalemia, metabolic alkalosis, weight loss

## Nursing Considerations
•Administer indapamide with food or milk to reduce adverse GI reactions.
•Give drug early in the day to avoid nocturia.

G
H
I

•Weigh patient daily, and monitor fluid intake and output, blood pressure, and serum electrolyte levels.
•Monitor BUN and serum creatinine levels regularly, as appropriate.
•If muscle cramps and weakness develop from hypokalemia, expect prescriber to order a potassium supplement or potassium-sparing diuretic.
•When managing hypertension, expect therapeutic response to take several weeks.

**PATIENT TEACHING**
•Advise patient to take indapamide early in the day to avoid nighttime urination and to take it with food or milk to minimize GI distress.
•Encourage patient to eat high-potassium foods, such as oranges and bananas.
•Direct patient to change position slowly to minimize the effects of orthostatic hypotension.
•Instruct patient to weigh himself daily at the same time and wearing similar clothing. Direct him to report a weight gain of more than 2 lb (0.9 kg) per day or 5 lb (2.3 kg) per week.
•Inform patient about possible photosensitivity.
•If patient complains of a dry mouth, suggest sugarless gum or hard candy to relieve it.

# indomethacin

Apo-Indomethacin (CAN), Indocid (CAN), Indocin, Indocin SR, Novo-Methacin (CAN), Nu-Indo (CAN)

# indomethacin sodium trihydrate

Apo-Indomethacin (CAN), Indameth, Indocid (CAN), Indocid PDA (CAN), Indocin, Indocin I.V., Novomethacin (CAN)

## Class and Category
*Chemical:* Indoleacetic acid derivative
*Therapeutic:* Antigout, anti-inflammatory, antirheumatic
*Pregnancy category:* Not rated

## Indications and Dosages
➤ *To relieve symptoms of ankylosing spondylitis, osteoarthritis, and rheumatoid arthritis*

**CAPSULES, ORAL SUSPENSION**
**Adults.** 25 to 50 mg b.i.d. to q.i.d., increased by 25 or 50 mg/day q wk, if needed. *Maximum:* 200 mg/day. After adequate response, dosage reduced as low as possible.
**E.R. CAPSULES (ANTIRHEUMATIC)**
**Adults.** 75 mg q.d., increased to 75 mg b.i.d, if needed.
**SUPPOSITORIES**
**Adults.** 50 mg up to q.i.d.
➤ *To relieve symptoms of juvenile arthritis*
**CAPSULES, ORAL SUSPENSION, SUPPOSITORIES**
**Children.** 1.5 to 2.5 mg/kg/day in divided doses t.i.d. or q.i.d. *Maximum:* 4 mg/kg/day or 150 to 200 mg/day, whichever is less. After adequate response, oral dosage reduced as low as possible.
➤ *To relieve symptoms of acute gouty arthritis*
**CAPSULES, ORAL SUSPENSION**
**Adults.** *Initial:* 100 mg. Increased up to 50 mg t.i.d. *Maximum:* 200 mg/day. After pain relief achieved, dosage tapered until drug is discontinued altogether.
**SUPPOSITORIES**
**Adults.** 50 mg up to q.i.d. *Maximum:* 200 mg/day.
➤ *To treat inflammation and relieve acute shoulder pain from bursitis or tendinitis*
**CAPSULES, ORAL SUSPENSION**
**Adults.** 75 to 150 mg/day in divided doses t.i.d. or q.i.d. for 7 to 14 days.
**SUPPOSITORIES**
**Adults.** 50 mg up to q.i.d. *Maximum:* 200 mg/day.
**DOSAGE ADJUSTMENT** Dosage reduced for elderly patients.
➤ *To treat hemodynamically significant patent ductus arteriosus in premature infants who weigh 500 to 1,750 g (1 to 3.9 lb)*
**I.V. INJECTION**
**Infants over age 7 days.** *Initial:* 200 mcg/kg (0.2 mg/kg) over 5 to 10 sec; 1 or 2 additional doses of 250 mcg/kg (0.25 mg/kg) given at 12- to 24-hr intervals, if needed.
**Neonates ages 2 to 7 days.** *Initial:* 200 mcg/kg (0.2 mg/kg) over 5 to 10 sec; 1 or 2 additional doses of 200 mcg/kg (0.2 mg/kg) given at 12- to 24-hr intervals, if needed.
**Neonates under age 48 hours.** *Initial:* 200 mcg/kg (0.2 mg/kg) over 5 to 10 sec; 1 or 2 additional doses of 100 mcg/kg (0.1 mg/kg) given at 12- to 24-hr intervals, if needed.

| Route | Onset | Peak | Duration |
|---|---|---|---|
| P.O.* | 2 to 4 hr | 2 to 5 days | Unknown |
| P.O.† | 30 min | Unknown | 4 to 6 hr |
| P.O.‡ | In 7 days | 1 to 2 wk | Unknown |

## Mechanism of Action

Blocks the activity of cyclooxygenase, the enzyme needed to synthesize prostaglandins, which mediate the inflammatory response and cause local vasodilation, swelling, and pain. By blocking cyclooxygenase and inhibiting prostaglandins, this NSAID reduces inflammatory symptoms and helps relieve pain.

## Incompatibilities

Don't give indomethacin suspension with alkaline antacids or liquids. Don't mix reconstituted indomethacin sodium with I.V. infusion solutions.

## Contraindications

Allergy or hypersensitivity to aspirin, indomethacin, iodides, other NSAIDs, or their components; history of proctitis or recent rectal bleeding (suppositories)

## Interactions

**DRUGS**

*Note:* All effects listed are for oral forms and suppositories unless indicated.

*acetaminophen:* Increased risk of adverse renal effects (with long-term use of both drugs)

*aluminum- and magnesium-containing antacids:* Possibly decreased blood indomethacin level

*aminoglycosides:* Increased risk of aminoglycoside toxicity

*antihypertensives:* Decreased effectiveness of these drugs

*aspirin, other NSAIDs:* Increased risk of adverse GI effects and non-GI bleeding

*bone marrow depressants:* Possibly increased leukopenic or thrombocytopenic effects of these drugs

*cefamandole, cefoperazone, cefotetan:* In-

creased risk of hypoprothrombinemia and bleeding

*colchicine, platelet aggregation inhibitors:* Increased risk of GI bleeding, hemorrhage, and ulcers

*corticosteroids, potassium supplements:* Increased risk of adverse GI effects

*cyclosporine:* Increased risk of nephrotoxicity from both drugs, increased blood cyclosporine level

*diflunisal:* Increased blood indomethacin level and risk of GI bleeding

*digoxin:* Increased blood digoxin level and risk of digitalis toxicity (all forms)

*diuretics (thiazide, loop, and potassium-sparing):* Decreased diuretic and antihypertensive effects

*gold compounds, nephrotoxic drugs:* Increased risk of adverse renal effects

*heparin, oral anticoagulants, thrombolytics:* Possibly increased anticoagulant effects and risk of hemorrhage

*lithium:* Increased blood lithium level and risk of toxicity

*methotrexate:* Increased risk of methotrexate toxicity

*plicamycin, valproic acid:* Increased risk of hypoprothrombinemia and GI bleeding, hemorrhage, and ulcers

*probenecid:* Increased blood level and effectiveness of indomethacin, increased risk of indomethacin toxicity

*zidovudine:* Increased blood zidovudine level and risk of toxicity, increased risk of indomethacin toxicity

**ACTIVITIES**

*alcohol use:* Increased risk of adverse GI effects

## Adverse Reactions

*Note:* All reactions are for oral forms and suppositories unless indicated.

**CNS:** Confusion, depression, dizziness, drowsiness, fatigue, hallucinations, headache, intraventricular hemorrhage (I.V.), peripheral neuropathy, seizures, stroke, syncope, vertigo

**CV:** Arrhythmias, chest pain, edema, fluid retention (all forms), heart failure, hypertension, MI, pulmonary hypertension (I.V.), tachycardia

**EENT:** Blurred vision, corneal and retinal damage, epistaxis, hearing loss, tinnitus

**ENDO:** Hypoglycemia (I.V.)

---

* For antigout effects.
† For anti-inflammatory effects.
‡ For antirheumatic effects.

**GI:** Abdominal cramps or pain, abdominal distention (I.V.), anorexia, constipation, diarrhea, diverticulitis, dyspepsia, dysphagia, epigastric discomfort, esophagitis, gastritis, gastroenteritis, gastroesophageal reflux disease, GI bleeding and ulceration (all forms), hemorrhoids, hepatic dysfunction (I.V.), hepatic failure, hiatal hernia, ileus (I.V.), indigestion, melena, nausea, necrotizing enterocolitis (I.V.), pancreatitis, peptic ulcer, perforation of stomach or intestine, stomatitis, vomiting (all forms)

**GU:** Acute renal falure, hematuria, interstitial nephritis, nephrotic syndrome, oliguria (I.V.), proteinuria, renal dysfunction (I.V.), vaginal bleeding

**HEME:** Agranulocytosis, anemia, aplastic anemia, bone marrow depression, disseminated intravascular coagulation, hemolytic anemia, iron deficiency anemia, leukopenia, neutropenia, pancytopenia, thrombocytopenia, unusual bleeding or bruising (all forms)

**RESP:** Asthma, respiratory depression

**SKIN:** Ecchymosis, erythema multiforme, erythema nodosum, photosensitivity, pruritus, rash, Stevens-Johnson syndrome, toxic epidermal necrolysis, urticaria

**Other:** Anaphylaxis, angioedema, hyperkalemia (I.V.), hyponatremia (I.V.), injection site irritation

## Nursing Considerations

• Use indomethacin with extreme caution in patients with a history of ulcer disease or GI bleeding because NSAIDs such as indomethacin increase the risk of GI bleeding and ulceration. Expect to use indomethacin for the shortest time possible in these patients.

• Be aware that serious GI tract ulceration, bleeding, and perforation may occur without warning symptoms. Elderly patients are at greater risk. To minimize risk, give oral indomethacin with food, a full glass of water (not suspension), or an antacid to reduce GI distress.

• If GI distress occurs, withhold drug and notify prescriber immediately.

• Use indomethacin cautiously in patients with hypertension, and monitor blood pressure closely throughout therapy. Drug may cause hypertension or worsen it.

• Shake suspension well before administering.

• Give up to 100 mg of daily dose (not E.R. capsules) at bedtime to reduce nighttime pain and morning stiffness in arthritis patients.

• Make sure suppository stays in rectum at least 1 hour to improve absorption.

• To reconstitute I.V. form, add 1 to 2 ml of preservative-free sodium chloride for injection or preservative-free sterile water to vial. Solution made with 1 ml of diluent contains 100 mcg (0.1 mg) of indomethacin/0.1 ml. Solution made with 2 ml of diluent contains 50 mcg (0.05 mg) of indomethacin/0.1 ml. Use solution immediately because it contains no preservatives. Discard unused portion.

• Be aware that scheduled I.V. doses may be withheld if infant or neonate has anuria or a significant decrease in urine output (less than 0.6 ml/kg/hr).

• When using I.V. form, avoid extravasation to protect surrounding tissue.

• Anticipate a second course (another 3 doses) of I.V. indomethacin if patent ductus arteriosus fails to close or reopens. After two courses, surgery may be performed.

• **WARNING** Monitor patient closely for thrombotic events, including MI and stroke, because NSAIDs increase the risk.

• Monitor patient—especially if he's elderly or receiving long-term indomethacin therapy—for less common but serious adverse GI reactions, including anorexia, constipation, diverticulitis, dysphagia, esophagitis, gastritis, gastroenteritis, gastroesophageal reflux disease, hemorrhoids, hiatal hernia, melena, stomatitis, and vomiting.

• Monitor liver function test results because, in rare cases, elevations may progress to severe hepatic reactions, including fatal hepatitis, liver necrosis, and hepatic failure.

• Monitor BUN and serum creatinine levels in elderly patients, patients taking diuretics or ACE inhibitors, and patients with heart failure, impaired renal function, or hepatic dysfunction; drug may cause renal failure.

• Monitor CBC for decreased hemoglobin and hematocrit because drug may worsen anemia.

• **WARNING** If patient has bone marrow suppression or is receiving an antineoplastic drug, monitor laboratory results (including WBC count), and watch for evidence of infection because anti-inflammatory and antipyretic actions of indomethacin may mask signs and symptoms, such as fever and pain.

• Assess patient's skin regularly for signs of rash or other hypersensitivity reaction because indomethacin is an NSAID and may cause serious skin reactions without warning, even in patients with no history of NSAID sensivitity. At first sign of reaction, stop drug and notify prescriber.

•Because indomethacin causes sodium retention, monitor weight and blood pressure, especially if patient has hypertension.

•When drug is used to treat gouty arthritis, expect its action to peak in 24 to 36 hours and significant swelling to gradually disappear over 3 to 5 days.

•Be aware that E.R. form shouldn't be used to treat gouty arthritis.

•Expect to use suppositories for patients who can't swallow oral form.

•To evaluate drug effectiveness, assess for reduced pain and inflammation and improved joint mobility.

•Expect patient to have intermittent checkups during long-term therapy and an ophthalmologic examination if vision changes develop.

**PATIENT TEACHING**
•Advise patient to take indomethacin capsules with a full glass of water and to avoid lying down for 15 to 30 minutes after taking drug. This helps prevent drug from lodging in esophagus and causing irritation. Caution him not to open or crush capsules.

•Instruct patient to take drug with food or an antacid to reduce GI distress.

•Instruct patient to make sure suppository stays in rectum at least 1 hour.

•Urge patient to avoid alcohol during therapy.

•Remind patient that improvement may not occur for 2 to 4 weeks after starting indomethacin and that he should continue taking drug, as prescribed.

•Inform breast-feeding patient that drug appears in breast milk and may cause seizures in infants. Urge her to use another feeding method during indomethacin therapy.

•Caution against prolonged sun exposure during therapy.

•Urge patient to notify prescriber immediately about changes in vision or hearing, fever, itching, rash, sore throat, swelling in arms or legs, and weight gain.

•Stress the importance of undergoing ordered laboratory tests and eye examinations during long-term therapy.

•Caution pregnant patient not to take NSAIDs such as indomethacin during the last trimester because they may cause premature closure of the ductus arteriosus.

•Explain that indomethacin may increase

the risk of serious adverse cardiovascular reactions; urge patient to seek immediate medical attention if signs or symptoms arise, such as chest pain, shortness of breath, weakness, and slurring of speech.

•Explain that indomethacin may increase the risk of serious adverse GI reactions; stress the importance of seeking immediate medical attention for such signs and symptoms as epigastric or abdominal pain, indigestion, black or tarry stools, or vomiting blood or material that looks like coffee grounds.

•Alert patient to rare but serious skin reactions. Urge him to seek immediate medical attention for rash, blisters, itching, fever, or other indications of hypersensitivity.

# infliximab

Remicade

## Class and Category
*Chemical:* Monoclonal antibody
*Therapeutic:* Anti-inflammatory
*Pregnancy category:* C

## Indications and Dosages
➤ *To control moderate to severe Crohn's disease long term, to reduce number of draining enterocutaneous and rectovaginal fistulas, to maintain fistula closure in fistulizing Crohn's disease, to treat moderate to severe ulcerative colitis in patients with an inadequate response to conventional therapy*

**I.V. INFUSION**
**Adults.** *Induction:* 5 mg/kg over 2 hr, repeated 2 and 6 wk after first infusion. *Maintenance:* 5 mg/kg over 2 hr q 8 wk.
**DOSAGE ADJUSTMENT** For patients who respond and then lose response, dosage may be increased up to 10 mg/kg.

➤ *As adjunct to reduce signs and symptoms, inhibit progression of structural damage, and improve physical function in patients with moderate to severe active rheumatoid arthritis*

**I.V. INFUSION**
**Adults.** 3 mg/kg, with methotrexate, repeated 2 and 6 wk after first infusion and then q 8 wk thereafter.
**DOSAGE ADJUSTMENT** For patients with inadequate response to combination treatment, in-

G
H
I

fliximab increased to 10 mg/kg or frequency increased to q 4 wk.

➤ *To treat active ankylosing spondylitis*
**I.V. INFUSION**
**Adults.** 5 mg/kg, repeated 2 and 6 wk after first infusion and then q 6 wk thereafter.

➤ *To treat psoriatic arthritis*
**I.V. INFUSION**
**Adults.** 5 mg/kg, repeated 2 and 6 wk after first infusion and then q 8 wk thereafter.

## Mechanism of Action
Binds with cytokine tumor necrosis factor-alpha (TNF-alpha), preventing it from binding with its receptors. As a result, TNF-alpha can't produce proinflammatory cytokines and endothelial permeability. Infiltration of inflammatory cells into inflamed intestine and joints declines.

## Incompatibilities
Don't infuse infliximab in same I.V. line with other drugs or through plasticized polyvinyl chloride infusion equipment or devices.

## Contraindications
Hypersensitivity to infliximab, murine proteins, or their components; moderate or severe (NYHA Class III or IV) heart failure

## Drug Interactions
*anakinra, etanercept:* Increased risk of neutropenia and serious infections

## Adverse Reactions
**CNS:** Chills, dizziness, fatigue, fever, headache, paresthesia, syncope
**CV:** Chest pain, hypertension, hypotension
**EENT:** Oral candidiasis, pharyngitis, rhinitis, sinusitis, visual changes
**GI:** Abdominal hernia; abdominal pain; acute hepatic failure; cholecystitis; cholestasis; diarrhea; dyspepsia; hepatitis; hepatotoxicity; intestinal obstruction, perforation, or stenosis; nausea; splenic infarction; splenomegaly; vomiting
**GU:** Kidney infection, ureteral obstruction, UTI, vaginal candidiasis, vaginitis
**HEME:** Leukopenia, neutropenia, pancytopenia, thrombocytopenia
**MS:** Arthralgia, back pain, extremity weakness, myalgia

**RESP:** Bronchitis, cough, dyspnea, pneumonia, tuberculosis, upper respiratory tract infection, wheezing
**SKIN:** Facial flushing, jaundice, pruritus, rash, urticaria
**Other:** Lupuslike symptoms, lymphoma

## Nursing Considerations
•**WARNING** Because infliximab increases the risk of developing tuberculosis or reactivating latent tuberculosis, expect prescriber to evaluate patient's risk and start tuberculosis treatment, as needed, before starting infliximab.
•**WARNING** Be aware that infliximab increases the risk of serious or fatal opportunistic infections, including histoplasmosis, listeriosis, and pneumocystosis. Expect prescriber to evaluate patient's risk before starting drug.
•To reconstitute infliximab, use a 21G (or smaller) needle to add 10 ml of sterile water for injection to each vial of drug. Swirl to mix; don't shake. Be aware that solution may foam and be clear or light yellow.
•Withdraw a volume equal to amount of reconstituted drug from a 250-ml glass bottle or polypropylene or polyolefin infusion bag of NS. Then add reconstituted infliximab to bottle to dilute to 250 ml. Use within 3 hours.
•Infuse over at least 2 hours using polyethylene-lined infusion set and in-line, sterile, nonpyrogenic, low-protein-binding filter with pores of 1.2 microns or less. Don't reuse.
•Be prepared to stop infusion if a hypersensitivity or CNS reaction occurs. Keep acetaminophen, antihistamines, corticosteroids, and epinephrine on hand. A reaction may occur 2 hours to 12 days after infusion.
•**WARNING** Watch for infection, especially if patient receives immunosuppressant therapy or has a chronic infection. Upper respiratory tract infections and UTIs are most common, but sepsis and fatal infections have occurred.
•**WARNING** Avoid giving infliximab to patients with NYHA Class III or IV congestive heart failure (CHF) because it may worsen the condition or cause death. If patient does receive infliximab, expect to stop it if CHF worsens.
•Because severe hepatic reactions may occur, monitor liver function. Expect to stop infliximab if jaundice develops or liver enzymes

are 5 times or more the upper limit of normal.

**PATIENT TEACHING**
•Inform patient that infliximab should take effect within 1 to 2 weeks.
•Urge patient to report signs of infection, such as painful urination, cough, and sore throat. Infusion reaction (chest pain, chills, dyspnea, facial flushing, fever, itching, headache, rash) may occur for up to 12 days.
•Explain that infliximab increases the risk of lymphoma; urge prompt medical attention for suspicious signs or symptoms.

# ipecac syrup

Ipecac Syrup

## Class and Category
*Chemical:* Cephaelis acuminata or Cephaelis ipecacuanha derivative
*Therapeutic:* Emetic
*Pregnancy category:* C

## Indications and Dosages
➤ *To induce vomiting after drug overdose and certain types of poisoning*
**SYRUP**
**Adults and children over age 12.** 15 to 30 ml followed by 240 ml of water. Dose repeated if vomiting doesn't begin within 20 to 30 min.
**Children ages 1 to 12.** 15 ml preceded or followed by 120 to 240 ml of water. Dose repeated if vomiting doesn't begin within 20 to 30 min.
**Infants ages 6 months to 1 year.** 5 to 10 ml preceded or followed by 120 to 240 ml of water.

| Route | Onset | Peak | Duration |
|-------|-------|------|----------|
| P.O. | 20 to 30 min | Unknown | 20 to 25 min |

## Mechanism of Action
Induces vomiting by irritating the gastric mucosa and stimulating the medullary chemoreceptor trigger zone in the CNS.

## Contraindications
Loss of gag reflex, poisoning with strychnine or corrosives (such as alkaloid substances, petroleum distillates, and strong acids), seizures, semiconsciousness or unconsciousness, severe inebriation, shock

## Interactions
**DRUGS**
*activated charcoal:* Lack of emetic effect

## Adverse Reactions
**CNS:** Depression, drowsiness
**EENT:** Aspiration of vomitus, coughing
**GI:** Diarrhea, indigestion

## Nursing Considerations
•Give ipecac syrup only to conscious patients, and follow with adequate water. Give young or frightened children water before or after ipecac.
•Expect vomiting to start in 20 to 30 minutes.
•If vomiting doesn't start within 30 minutes of second dose, prepare for gastric lavage.
•Don't give ipecac after ingestion of petroleum distillates, such as gasoline, or caustic substances (to avoid further injury to esophagus).
•If activated charcoal also will be given, expect to do so after patient vomits or 30 minutes after second dose because activated charcoal adsorbs ipecac and inhibits its action.
•Arrhythmias, atrial fibrillation, bradycardia, fatal myocarditis, hypotension, myalgia, or muscle stiffness or weakness may develop if patient takes too much or doesn't vomit.

**PATIENT TEACHING**
•Inform patient of ipecac's effects.
•Tell adult to drink 8 oz (240 ml) of water after taking drug and child to drink 4 to 8 oz (120 to 240 ml) before or after taking drug.
•Inform patient or parents of child that diarrhea may occur after taking drug.
•Urge parents to keep ipecac syrup and phone number of a poison control center.
•**WARNING** Advise parents to replace their ipecac extract or tincture with ipecac syrup. Explain that ipecac fluid extract is 14 times more concentrated than ipecac syrup and can cause serious, possibly toxic, effects if given incorrectly.

# ipratropium bromide

Apo-Ipravent (CAN), Atrovent, Kendral-Ipratropium (CAN)

## Class and Category
*Chemical:* Quaternary *N*-methyl isopropyl derivative of noratropine
*Therapeutic:* Anticholinergic, bronchodilator
*Pregnancy category:* B

G
H
I

## Indications and Dosages

➤ *To treat bronchitis and COPD*

**INHALATION AEROSOL**

**Adults and adolescents.** 2 to 4 inhalations (36 to 72 mcg) t.i.d. or q.i.d. *Maximum:* Up to 12 inhalations (216 mcg)/24 hr.

**INHALATION SOLUTION FOR NEBULIZER**

**Adults and adolescents.** 250 to 500 mcg dissolved in preservative-free sterile NS q 6 to 8 hr. For severe COPD exacerbations, 500 mcg q 4 to 8 hr.

➤ *To treat perennial and allergic rhinitis*

**NASAL SPRAY**

**Adults and children age 6 and older.** 2 sprays of 0.03% (21 mcg/spray) per nostril b.i.d. or t.i.d. *Maximum:* 12 sprays (252 mcg)/24 hr.

➤ *To treat rhinorrhea from common cold*

**NASAL SPRAY**

**Adults and children age 5 and older.** 2 sprays of 0.06% (42 mcg/spray) per nostril t.i.d. or q.i.d. for up to 4 days. *Maximum:* 16 sprays (672 mcg)/24 hr.

| Route | Onset | Peak | Duration |
|---|---|---|---|
| Inhalation | 5 to 15 min | 1 to 2 hr | 3 to 8 hr |
| Nasal | 5 min | 1 to 4 hr | 4 to 8 hr |

## Contraindications

Hypersensitivity to atropine, ipratropium bromide, or their components; hypersensitivity to peanuts, soya lecithin, soybeans, or related products (with aerosol inhaler)

## Interactions

**DRUGS**

*anticholinergics:* Increased anticholinergic effects

*tacrine:* Decreased effects of both drugs

## Adverse Reactions

**CNS:** Dizziness, insomnia

**CV:** Bradycardia (nasal spray), hypertension, palpitations

**EENT:** Dry mouth, laryngospasm, taste perversion (all drug forms); blurred vision, eye irritation and pain, glaucoma or worsening of existing glaucoma (if nasal spray comes in contact with eyes); epistaxis, nasal dryness and irritation, pharyngitis, rhinitis, sinusitis, tinnitus (with nasal spray)

**GI:** Constipation, ileus, nausea

**GU:** Prostatitis, urine retention

**MS:** Arthritis

**RESP:** Bronchitis, bronchospasm, cough, dyspnea, increased sputum production

## Mechanism of Action

After acetylcholine is released from cholinergic fibers, ipratropium prevents it from attaching to muscarinic receptors on membranes of smooth-muscle cells, as shown at right. By blocking acetycholine's effects in the bronchi and bronchioles, ipratropium relaxes smooth muscles and causes bronchodilation.

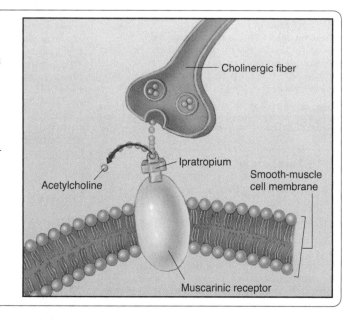

Cholinergic fiber

Ipratropium

Acetylcholine

Smooth-muscle cell membrane

Muscarinic receptor

**SKIN:** Dermatitis, rash, urticaria
**Other:** Anaphylaxis, angioedema, flulike symptoms

## Nursing Considerations
• Use ipratropium cautiously in patients with angle-closure glaucoma, benign prostatic hyperplasia, or bladder neck obstruction.
• As prescribed, mix ipratropium inhalation solution with preservative-free albuterol, and preservative-free ipratropium inhalation solution with cromolyn inhalation solution. Use within 1 hour.
• When using a nebulizer, apply a mouthpiece to prevent drug from leaking out around mask and causing blurred vision or eye pain.

**PATIENT TEACHING**
• Caution patient not to use ipratropium to treat acute bronchospasm.
• Teach patient to use inhaler or nasal spray. Tell him to shake inhaler well with each use.
• Advise patient to keep spray out of his eyes because it may irritate them or blur his vision. If spray comes in contact with his eyes, instruct patient to flush them with cool tap water and to contact prescriber.
• Instruct patient to rinse mouth after each nebulizer or inhaler treatment to help minimize throat dryness and irritation.
• If patient is using 0.06% nasal spray for a common cold, advise him to use it no longer than 4 days.
• Teach patient how to determine whether canister is empty by counting and recording number of doses.
• Advise patient to report decreased response to ipratropium as well as difficulty voiding, eye pain, palpitations, and vision changes.

# ipratropium bromide and albuterol sulfate

Combivent, DuoNeb

## Class and Category
*Chemical:* Quarternary *N*-methyl isopropyl derivative of noratropine (ipratropium); selective beta₂-adrenergic agonist, sympathomimetic (albuterol)
*Therapeutic:* Bronchodilator
*Pregnancy category:* C

## Indications and Dosages
➤ *To treat bronchospasm in patients with COPD who require more than one bronchodilator*

**INHALATION AEROSOL (COMBIVENT)**
**Adults.** 2 inhalations (36 mcg ipratropium, 180 mcg albuterol base) q.i.d. and as needed. *Maximum:* 12 inhalations (216 mcg ipratropium, 1.08 g albuterol base)/24 hr.

**INHALATION SOLUTION FOR NEBULIZER (DUONEB)**
**Adults.** 3 ml (0.5 mg ipratropium, 2.5 mg albuterol base) q.i.d. *Maximum:* 2 additional 3-ml doses/24 hr, p.r.n.

| Route | Onset | Peak | Duration |
|---|---|---|---|
| Inhalation aerosol | In 15 min | 1 hr | 4 to 5 hr |
| Inhalation solution | 5 to 15 min | 1 to 2 hr | Up to 5 hr |

### Mechanism of Action
Prevents acetylcholine (after its release from cholinergic fibers) from attaching to muscarinic receptors on membranes of smooth-muscle cells. By blocking acetylcholine's effects in the bronchi and bronchioles, ipratropium relaxes smooth muscles and causes bronchodilation. Albuterol attaches to beta₂ receptors on bronchial cell membranes, which stimulates the intracellular enzyme adenylate cyclase to convert adenosine triphosphate to cyclic adenosine monophosphate (cAMP). This reaction decreases intracellular calcium level and increases intracellular cAMP. Together, these effects relax bronchial smooth-muscle cells and inhibit histamine release.

## Contraindications
Hypersensitivity to albuterol, ipratropium, or their components; hypersensitivity to atropine or its derivatives; hypersensitivity to peanuts, soya lecithin, soybeans, or related products (with aerosol inhaler)

## Interactions
**DRUGS**
*anticholinergics, such as atropine:* Possibly additive effects of ipratropium

beta blockers: Possibly mutual inhibition of therapeutic effects

MAO inhibitors, tricyclic antidepressants: Possibly potentiation of albuterol's adverse cardiovascular effects

non-potassium-sparing diuretics, such as loop and thiazide diuretics: Increased risk of hypokalemia

sympathomimetic bronchodilators, such as theophylline: Increased risk of adverse cardiovascular effects

## Adverse Reactions

**CNS:** Drowsiness, headache, nervousness, tremor
**CV:** Chest pain, increased heart rate, palpitations
**EENT:** Acute eye pain, altered taste, blurred vision, dry mouth, pharyngitis, sinusitis, sore throat, voice alterations, worsened angle-closure glaucoma
**GI:** Constipation, diarrhea, indigestion, nausea
**GU:** UTI
**MS:** Back pain, leg cramps, muscle aches
**RESP:** Bronchitis, cough, exacerbation of COPD, paradoxical bronchospasm, pneumonia, upper respiratory tract infection, wheezing
**SKIN:** Flushing
**Other:** Hypokalemia

## Nursing Considerations

•Prime the aerosol inhaler with three priming sprays if giving it for the first time or if it hasn't been used for more than 24 hours.
•As prescribed, administer nebulized dose using a mouthpiece or properly fitting face mask attached to a jet nebulizer connected to an air compressor with adequate airflow.
•WARNING Avoid spraying drug directly into patient's eyes because it may cause vision disturbances. In a patient with angle-closure glaucoma, be aware that spraying drug directly into his eyes may precipitate an acute attack or exacerbate the condition.
•Monitor urine output if patient has a history of prostatic hyperplasia or bladder-neck obstruction because drug may aggravate these conditions and cause urine retention.
•Frequently monitor heart rate and rhythm and blood pressure in patients with a history of arrhythmias, coronary artery insufficiency, or hypertension because the drug may cause adverse cardiovascular effects in these pa-

tients. If adverse cardiovascular effects occur, expect to discontinue drug.
•Monitor serum potassium level because drug may cause transient hypokalemia.
•Although immediate hypersensitivity reactions are rare, monitor patient for angioedema, bronchospasm, oropharyngeal edema, pruritus, rash, urticaria, and anaphylaxis.

**PATIENT TEACHING**
•Teach patient how to use inhaler or nebulizer properly. Instruct him to shake aerosol inhaler well before use and to wait 1 minute between inhalations.
•Instruct patient to rinse mouth after each nebulizer or inhaler treatment to help minimize throat dryness and irritation.
•Advise patient to keep drug out of his eyes because it may irritate them or blur his vision. If drug comes in contact with his eyes, instruct patient to flush them with cool tap water and to contact prescriber immediately.
•Caution patient not to use more than the prescribed dose because of the risk of serious adverse reactions and possibly death. Advise patient to contact prescriber immediately if doses become less effective.
•Advise patient to contact prescriber before using other inhaled drugs.

# irbesartan

Avapro

## Class and Category

*Chemical:* Nonpeptide angiotensin II antagonist
*Therapeutic:* Antihypertensive
*Pregnancy category:* C (first trimester), D (later trimesters)

## Indications and Dosages

➤ *To manage hypertension, alone or with other antihypertensives*

**TABLETS**
**Adults and adolescents.** *Initial:* 150 mg q.d. *Maximum:* 300 mg q.d.
**DOSAGE ADJUSTMENT** Initial dosage reduced to 75 mg q.d. for patients with hypovolemia or hyponatremia from such causes as hemodialysis or vigorous diuretic therapy.
**Children ages 6 to 12.** *Initial:* 75 mg q.d. *Maximum:* 150 mg q.d.

➤ *To treat nephropathy in type 2 diabetes mellitus*

**TABLETS**

**Adults.** 300 mg q.d.

| Route | Onset | Peak | Duration |
|-------|-------|------|----------|
| P.O. | Unknown | In 4 to 6 wk | Unknown |

### Mechanism of Action

Selectively blocks binding of the potent vasoconstrictor angiotensin (AT) II to $AT_1$ receptor sites in many tissues, including vascular smooth muscle and adrenal glands. This inhibits the vasoconstrictive and aldosterone-secreting effects of AT II, which reduces blood pressure.

### Contraindications

Hypersensitivity to irbesartan or its components

### Interactions

**DRUGS**

*diuretics:* Possibly additive hypotensive effects

### Adverse Reactions

**CNS:** Anxiety, dizziness, fatigue, headache, nervousness
**CV:** Chest pain, hypotension, peripheral edema, tachycardia
**EENT:** Pharyngitis, rhinitis
**GI:** Abdominal pain, diarrhea, heartburn, indigestion, nausea, vomiting
**GU:** UTI
**MS:** Musculoskeletal pain
**RESP:** Upper respiratory tract infection
**SKIN:** Rash

### Nursing Considerations

•If patient has known or suspected hypovolemia, provide treatment, such as I.V. NS, as prescribed, to correct this condition before beginning irbesartan therapy. Or expect to begin therapy with a lower dosage.
•Frequently monitor blood pressure to evaluate drug's effectiveness.
•If blood pressure isn't controlled with irbesartan alone, expect to also give a diuretic, such as hydrochlorothiazide, as prescribed.
•WARNING If patient receives a diuretic or another antihypertensive during irbesartan therapy, frequently monitor his blood pressure because he's at risk for developing hypotension.

•If patient experiences symptomatic hypotension, expect to discontinue drug temporarily. Immediately place patient in supine position and prepare to administer I.V. NS, as prescribed. Expect to resume drug therapy after blood pressure stabilizes.
•If patient receives a diuretic, provide adequate hydration, as appropriate, to help prevent hypovolemia. Also monitor patient for signs and symptoms of hypovolemia, such as hypotension, dizziness, and fainting.
•WARNING Monitor patient for increased BUN and serum creatinine levels if he has heart failure or impaired renal function because drug may cause acute renal failure. If increases are significant or persistent, notify prescriber immediately.

**PATIENT TEACHING**

•Advise patient to take drug at the same time each day to maintain its therapeutic effect.
•Explain the importance of regular exercise, proper diet, and other lifestyle changes in controlling hypertension.
•Caution patient to avoid hazardous activities until drug's CNS effects are known.
•Instruct patient to consult prescriber before taking any new drug.
•To reduce the risk of dehydration and hypotension, advise patient to drink adequate fluids during hot weather and exercise.
•Instruct patient to contact prescriber if severe nausea, vomiting, or diarrhea occurs and continues because of the risk of dehydration and hypotension.
•Advise female patient to notify prescriber immediately about known or suspected pregnancy. Explain that if she becomes pregnant, prescriber may replace irbesartan with another antihypertensive that's safe to use during pregnancy.
•Urge patient to keep follow-up appointments with prescriber to monitor progress.

## iron dextran

*(contains 50 mg of elemental iron per milliliter)*
DexFerrum, DexIron (CAN), InFeD

### Class and Category

*Chemical:* Iron salt, mineral
*Therapeutic:* Antianemic agent
*Pregnancy category:* C

## Indications and Dosages

➤ *To treat iron deficiency anemia*

**I.V. INFUSION**

**Adults and children who weigh over 15 kg (33 lb).** Dose (ml) = 0.0442 (desired hemoglobin − observed hemoglobin) × lean body weight (in kg) + (0.26 × lean body weight). Alternatively, consult dosage table in package insert. *Maximum:* 2 ml (100 mg)/day.

**Children over age 4 months who weigh 5 to 15 kg (11 to 33 lb).** Dose (ml) = 0.0442 (desired hemoglobin − observed hemoglobin) × weight (kg) + (0.26 × weight). Alternatively, consult dosage table in package insert. *Maximum:* 1 ml (50 mg)/day.

➤ *To replace iron lost in blood loss*

**I.V. INFUSION**

**Adults.** Replacement iron (mg) = ml of blood loss × hematocrit.

### Mechanism of Action

Restores hemoglobin and replenishes iron stores. Iron, an essential component of hemoglobin, myoglobin, and several enzymes (including cytochromes, catalase, and peroxidase), is needed for catecholamine metabolism and normal neutrophil function.

In iron dextran therapy, iron binds to available protein parts after the drug has been split into iron and dextran by cells of the reticuloendothelial system. The bound iron forms hemosiderin or ferritin, physiologic forms of iron, and transferrin, which replenish hemoglobin and depleted iron stores. Dextran is metabolized or excreted.

## Incompatibilities

Don't mix iron dextran with blood for transfusion, other drugs, or parenteral nutrition solutions for I.V. infusion.

## Contraindications

Anemia other than iron deficiency, hypersensitivity to iron dextran or its components

## Interactions

None known.

## Adverse Reactions

**CNS:** Chills, disorientation, dizziness, fever, headache, malaise, paresthesia, seizures, syncope, unconsciousness, weakness

**CV:** Arrhythmias, bradycardia, chest pain, hypertension, hypotension, shock, tachycardia

**EENT:** Altered taste

**GI:** Abdominal pain, diarrhea, nausea, vomiting

**GU:** Hematuria

**HEME:** Leukocytosis

**MS:** Arthralgia, arthritis, backache, myalgia, rhabdomyolysis

**RESP:** Bronchospasm, dyspnea, respiratory arrest, wheezing

**SKIN:** Cyanosis, diaphoresis, rash, pruritus, purpura, urticaria

**Other:** Anaphylaxis, infusion site phlebitis

## Nursing Considerations

• Expect oral iron therapy to stop before iron dextran therapy starts. Iron dextran is given only when oral therapy isn't feasible; it also may be given by I.M. injection.

• Expect to monitor hemoglobin level, hematocrit, serum ferritin level, and transferrin saturation, as ordered, before, during, and after iron dextran therapy.

• **WARNING** Before starting therapy, give a test dose of 0.5 ml of iron dextran gradually over 30 seconds, as prescribed, and monitor patient closely for an anaphylactic reaction.

• Wait 1 to 2 hours before administering the remainder of the dose. Infuse undiluted iron dextran slowly, at a rate not to exceed 1 ml/minute (50 mg/minute).

• **WARNING** Monitor patient closely for signs and symptoms of anaphylaxis (such as severe hypotension, loss of consciousness, collapse, dyspnea, and seizures) during and after infusion. Patients with a history of asthma or allergies are at increased risk for anaphylaxis and, possibly, death. Institute emergency resuscitation measures as needed, including epinephrine administration, as prescribed.

• **WARNING** Assess blood pressure frequently after drug administration because hypotension is a common adverse effect that may be related to infusion rate; avoid rapid infusion.

• Be aware that patient may exhibit adverse reactions, including arthralgia, backache, chills, and vomiting, 1 to 2 days after drug therapy. Symptoms should resolve within 3 to 4 days.

• Assess patients with a history of rheumatoid arthritis for exacerbation of joint pain and swelling.

• If patient has cardiovascular disease, watch for worsening from drug's adverse effects.

• Assess patient for iron overload, characterized by sedation, decreased activity, pale eyes, and bleeding in GI tract and lungs.

• Store iron dextran at 15° to 30° C (59° to 86° F).

**PATIENT TEACHING**

• Instruct patient to immediately report signs of an adverse reaction, such as shortness of breath, wheezing, or rash, during iron dextran therapy.

• Advise patient not to take any oral iron preparations without first consulting prescriber.

• Inform patient that symptoms of iron deficiency may include decreased stamina, learning problems, shortness of breath, and fatigue. Encourage patient to plan periods of activity and rest in order to avoid excessive fatigue.

• Stress the importance of following dosage regimen and of keeping follow-up medical appointments and appointments for laboratory tests.

# iron sucrose

*(contains 100 mg of elemental iron per 5 ml)*
Venofer

## Class and Category

*Chemical:* Iron salt, mineral
*Therapeutic:* Antianemic
*Pregnancy category:* B

## Indications and Dosages

➤ *To treat iron deficiency anemia in hemodialysis patients receiving erythropoietin*

**I.V. INJECTION**

**Adults.** *Initial:* 100 mg of elemental iron injected undiluted over 2 to 5 min during dialysis. *Usual:* 100 mg of elemental iron q wk to three times/wk to a total dose of 1,000 mg. Dosage repeated as needed to maintain target levels of hemoglobin and hematocrit and acceptable blood iron level. *Maximum:* 100 mg/dose.

**I.V. INFUSION**

**Adults.** *Initial:* 100 mg of elemental iron infused diluted over 15 min during dialysis. *Usual:* 100 mg of elemental iron q wk to three times/wk to a total dose of 1,000 mg. Dosage repeated as needed to maintain target levels of hemoglobin and hematocrit and

acceptable blood iron level. *Maximum:* 100 mg/dose.

➤ *To treat iron deficiency anemia in peritoneal dialysis patients receiving erythropoietin*

**I.V. INFUSION**

**Adults.** *Initial:* 300 mg of elemental iron infused diluted over 1.5 hr on days 1 and 14, followed by 400 mg of elemental iron infused over 2.5 hr on day 28. Dosage repeated as needed to maintain target levels of hemoglobin and hematocrit and acceptable blood iron level. *Maximum:* 1,000 mg/ 28 days.

➤ *To treat iron deficiency anemia in non-dialysis patients with chronic renal disease regardless of whether they're receiving erythropoietin*

**I.V. INJECTION**

**Adults.** *Initial:* 200 mg of elemental iron injected undiluted over 2 to 5 min and repeated four more times over a 14-day period for a total dose of 1,000 mg. Dosage repeated as needed to maintain target levels of hemoglobin and hematocrit and acceptable blood iron level. *Maximum:* 1,000 mg/14 days.

**I.V. INFUSION**

**Adults.** 500 mg of elemental iron infused diluted over 3.5 to 5 hr on days 1 and 14. Dosage repeated as needed to maintain target levels of hemoglobin and hematocrit and acceptable blood iron level. *Maximum:* 1,000 mg/14 days.

## Incompatibilities

Don't mix with other drugs or parenteral nutrition solutions for I.V. infusion.

---

## Mechanism of Action

Acts to replenish iron stores lost during dialysis because of increased erythropoiesis and insufficient absorption of iron from the GI tract. Iron is an essential component of hemoglobin, myoglobin, and several enzymes, including cyto-chromes, catalase, and peroxidase, and is needed for catecholamine metabolism and normal neutrophil function. Iron sucrose injection also normalizes RBC production by binding with hemoglobin or being stored as ferritin in reticuloendothelial cells of the liver, spleen, and bone marrow.

G
H
I

## Contraindications
Anemia other than iron deficiency, hypersensitivity to iron salts or their components, iron overload

## Interactions
**DRUGS**
*chloramphenicol:* Possibly decreased effectiveness of iron sucrose
*oral iron preparations:* Possibly reduced absorption of oral iron supplements

## Adverse Reactions
**CNS:** Asthenia, dizziness, fatigue, fever, headache, hypoesthesia, malaise
**CV:** Chest pain, heart failure, hypertension, hypotension, peirpheral edema
**EENT:** Conjunctivitis, ear pain, nasal congestion, nasopharyngitis, rhinitis, sinusitis, taste perversion
**ENDO:** Hyperglycemia, hypoglycemia
**GI:** Abdominal pain, constipation, diarrhea, elevated liver function test results, nausea, occult-positive feces, peritoneal infection, vomiting
**GU:** UTI
**MS:** Arthralgia, arthritis, back pain, leg cramps, muscle pain or weakness, myalgia
**RESP:** Cough, dyspnea, pneumonia, upper respiratory tract infection
**SKIN:** Pruritus, rash
**Other:** Anaphylaxis; fluid overload; gout; hypervolemia; infusion or injection site burning, pain, or redness; sepsis

## Nursing Considerations
•To reconstitute iron sucrose injection for infusion, dilute 100 mg of elemental iron in a maximum of 100 ml of NS for hemodialysis patients or 250 ml of NS for peritoneal dialysis and nondialysis patients immediately before infusion. Discard any unused diluted solution.
•Give drug directly into dialysis line by slow I.V. injection or by infusion.
•WARNING Monitor patient closely for evidence of anaphylaxis, such as severe hypotension, loss of consciousness, collapse, dyspnea, or seizures, during and after therapy. Institute emergency resuscitation measures as needed.
•WARNING Assess blood pressure frequently after drug administration because hypotension is a common adverse reaction that may be related to infusion rate (avoid rapid infusion) or total cumulative dose.

•Monitor hemoglobin, hematocrit, serum ferritin, and transferrin saturation, as ordered, before, during, and after iron sucrose therapy. Serum iron levels must be tested 48 hours after last dose. Notify prescriber and expect to stop therapy if blood iron levels are normal or elevated, to prevent iron toxicity.
•Assess patient for possible iron overload, characterized by sedation, decreased activity, pale eyes, and bleeding in GI tract and lungs.
**PATIENT TEACHING**
•Advise patient not to take any oral iron preparations during iron sucrose therapy without first consulting prescriber.
•Inform patient that symptoms of iron deficiency may include decreased stamina, learning problems, shortness of breath, and fatigue.

# isocarboxazid
Marplan

## Class and Category
*Chemical:* Hydrazine derivative
*Therapeutic:* Antidepressant
*Pregnancy category:* C

## Indications and Dosages
➤ *To treat major depression*
**TABLETS**
**Adults and adolescents over age 16.** *Initial:* 10 mg b.i.d., increased by 10 mg/day every 2 to 4 days, as needed and tolerated. *Maximum:* 60 mg/day.

| Route | Onset | Peak | Duration |
|-------|-------|------|----------|
| P.O. | 7 to 10 days | Unknown | 10 days |

## Contraindications
Cardiovascular disease; cerebrovascular disease; heart failure; hepatic disease; history of headaches; hypersensitivity to isocarboxazid or its components; hypertension; pheochromocytoma; severe renal impairment; use of anesthetics, antihypertensives, bupropion, buspirone, carbamazepine, dextromethorphan, meperidine, selective serotonin reuptake inhibitors, sympathomimetics, or tricyclic antidepressants; use within 14 days of another MAO inhibitor

## Mechanism of Action

Irreversibly binds to MAO, reducing its activity and increasing levels of neurotransmitters, including serotonin and the catecholamine neurotransmitters dopamine, epinephrine, and norepinephrine. This regulation of CNS neurotransmitters helps to ease depression. With long-term use, the drug results in down-regulation (desensitization) of alpha$_2$- or beta-adrenergic and serotonin receptors after 2 to 4 weeks, which also produces an antidepressant effect.

## Interactions

### DRUGS

*anticholinergics, antidyskinetics, antihistamines:* Increased anticholinergic effect, prolonged CNS depression (with antihistamines)
*anticonvulsants:* Increased CNS depression, possibly altered seizure pattern
*antihypertensives, diuretics:* Increased hypotensive effect
*bromocriptine:* Possibly interference with bromocriptine effects
*bupropion:* Increased risk of bupropion toxicity
*buspirone, guanadrel, guanethidine:* Increased risk of hypertension
*caffeine-containing drugs:* Increased risk of dangerous arrhythmias and severe hypertension
*carbamazepine, cyclobenzaprine, maprotiline, other MAO inhibitors:* Increased risk of hyperpyretic crisis, hypertensive crisis, severe seizures, and death; altered pattern of seizures (with carbamazepine)
*CNS depressants:* Increased CNS depression
*dextromethorphan:* Increased risk of excitation, hypertension, and hyperpyrexia
*doxapram:* Increased vasopressor effects of either drug
*fluoxetine, paroxetine, sertraline, trazodone, tricyclic antidepressants:* Increased risk of life-threatening serotonin syndrome
*haloperidol, loxapine, molindone, phenothiazines, pimozide, thioxanthenes:* Prolonged and intensified anticholinergic, hypotensive, and sedative effects of these drugs or isocarboxazid
*insulin, oral antidiabetic drugs:* Increased hypoglycemic effects
*levodopa:* Increased risk of sudden, moderate to severe hypertension
*local anesthetics (with epinephrine or levonordefrin):* Possibly severe hypertension
*meperidine, other opioid analgesics:* Increased risk of coma, hyperpyrexia, hypotension, immediate excitation, rigidity, seizures, severe hypertension, severe respiratory depression, shock, sweating, and death
*methyldopa:* Increased risk of hallucinations, headache, hyperexcitability, and severe hypertension
*methylphenidate:* Increased CNS stimulant effects
*metrizamide:* Decreased seizure threshold and increased risk of seizures
*oral anticoagulants:* Increased anticoagulant activity
*phenylephrine (nasal or ophthalmic):* Potentiated vasopressor effect of phenylephrine
*rauwolfia alkaloids:* Increased risk of moderate to severe hypertension, CNS depression (when isocarboxazid is added to rauwolfia alkaloid therapy), CNS excitation and hypertension (when rauwolfia alkaloid is added to isocarboxazid therapy)
*spinal anesthetics:* Increased risk of hypotension
*sympathomimetics:* Prolonged and intensified cardiac stimulant and vasopressor effects
*tryptophan:* Increased risk of confusion, disorientation, hyperreflexia, hyperthermia, hyperventilation, mania or hypomania, and shivering

### FOODS

*aged cheese; avocados; bananas; fava or broad beans; cured meat or sausage; overripe fruit; pickled or smoked fish, meats or poultry; protein extract; soy sauce; yeast extract; and other foods high in tyramine or other pressor amines:* Increased risk of dangerous arrhythmias and severe hypertensive crisis

### ACTIVITIES

*alcohol-containing products that also may contain tyramine, such as beer (including reduced-alcohol and alcohol-free beer), hard liquor, liqueurs, sherry, and wines (red and white):* Increased risk of developing hypertensive crisis

## Adverse Reactions

**CNS:** Agitation, dizziness, drowsiness, fever, headache, insomnia, intracranial bleeding, overstimulation, restlessness, sedation, tremor, weakness
**CV:** Bradycardia, chest pain, edema, hypertensive crisis, orthostatic hypotension, palpitations, tachycardia
**EENT:** Blurred vision, dry mouth, mydriasis, photophobia, yellowing of sclera

G
H
I

**GI:** Abdominal pain, anorexia, constipation, diarrhea, elevated liver function test results, increased appetite, nausea
**GU:** Darkened urine, oliguria, sexual dysfunction
**HEME:** Leukopenia
**MS:** Muscle spasms, myoclonus, neck stiffness
**SKIN:** Clammy skin, diaphoresis, jaundice, rash
**Other:** Unusual weight gain

## Nursing Considerations

• Monitor patient's blood pressure during isocarboxazid therapy to detect hypertensive crisis and decrease the risk of orthostatic hypotension.

• **WARNING** Notify prescriber immediately if patient has signs and symptoms of hypertensive crisis (drug's most serious adverse effect), such as chest pain, headache, neck stiffness, and palpitations. Expect to stop drug immediately if these occur.

• Keep phentolamine readily available to treat hypertensive crisis. Give 5 mg by slow I.V. infusion, as prescribed, to reduce blood pressure without causing excessive hypotension. Use external cooling measures, as prescribed, to manage fever.

• To avoid hypertensive crisis, expect to wait 10 to 14 days, as prescribed, when switching patient from one MAO inhibitor to another or when switching from a dibenzazepine-related drug, such as amitriptyline or perphenazine.

• Monitor patient with a history of epilepsy for seizures because isocarboxazid may alter seizure threshold. Institute seizure precautions according to facility protocol.

• Monitor liver function test results and assess patient for abdominal pain, darkened urine, and jaundice because isocarboxazid may cause hepatic dysfunction.

• Expect to observe some therapeutic effect in 7 to 10 days, but keep in mind that full effect may not occur for 4 to 8 weeks.

• Be aware that, for maintenance therapy, the smallest dose possible should be used. Once clinical effect has been achieved, expect to decrease the dosage slowly over several weeks.

• Keep dietary restrictions in place for at least 2 weeks after stopping isocarboxazid because of the slow recovery from drug's enzyme-inhibiting effects.

• Ideally, expect to stop drug 10 days before elective surgery, as prescribed, to avoid hypotension.

• Anticipate that coadministration with a selective serotonin reuptake inhibitor may cause confusion, diaphoresis, diarrhea, seizures, and other less severe symptoms.

• Monitor depressed patient for suicidal tendencies, especially when therapy starts or dosage changes, because depression may worsen temporarily. If suicidal tendencies arise, institute suicide precautions, as appropriate and according to facility policy, and notify prescriber immediately.

• Monitor patient for sudden insomnia. If it develops, notify prescriber and be prepared to give drug early in the day.

**PATIENT TEACHING**

• Inform patient and family members that therapeutic effects of isocarboxazid may take several weeks to appear and that he should continue taking drug as prescribed.

• Caution parents to monitor pediatric patients, including adolescents, closely for suicidal tendencies, especially when therapy starts or dosage changes.

• Caution patient to rise slowly from a lying or sitting position to minimize effects of orthostatic hypotension.

• **WARNING** Instruct patient to avoid the following foods, beverages, and drugs during isocarboxazid therapy and for 2 weeks afterward: alcohol-free and reduced-alcohol beer and wine; appetite suppressants; beer; broad beans; cheese (except cottage and cream cheese); chocolate and caffeine in large quantities; dry sausage (including Genoa salami, hard salami, Lebanon bologna, and pepperoni); hay fever drugs; inhaled asthma drugs; liver; meat extract; OTC cold and cough medicines (including those containing dextromethorphan); nasal decongestants (tablets, drops, or spray); pickled herring; products that contain tyramine; protein-rich foods that may have undergone protein changes by aging, fermenting, pickling, or smoking; sauerkraut; sinus drugs; weight-loss preparations; yeast extracts (including brewer's yeast in large quantities); yogurt; and wine.

• Advise patient to notify prescriber immediately about chest pain, dizziness, headache, nausea, neck stiffness, palpitations, rapid heart rate, sweating, and vomiting.

• Advise patient to inform all health care providers (including dentists) that he takes an MAO inhibitor because certain drugs are contraindicated within 2 weeks of therapy.

• Urge patient to avoid potentially hazardous activities until drug's adverse effects are known.

• Urge patient with diabetes mellitus who's taking insulin or an oral antidiabetic drug to monitor blood glucose level frequently during therapy because isocarboxazid may affect glucose control.

• Caution patient not to stop taking drug abruptly to avoid recurrence of original symptoms.

# isoetharine hydrochloride

Arm-a-Med Isoetharine (0.062%, 0.125%, 0.167%, 0.2%, 0.25%), Beta-2 (1%), Bronkosol (1%), Dey-Lute Isoetharine (0.08%, 0.1%, 0.17%, 0.25%)

## isoetharine mesylate

Bronkometer (0.61%)

## Class and Category

*Chemical:* Catecholamine
*Therapeutic:* Bronchodilator
*Pregnancy category:* Not rated

## Indications and Dosages

➤ *To prevent and treat reversible broncho- spasm from chronic bronchitis or em- physema*

**INHALATION AEROSOL**

**Adults and adolescents.** 1 or 2 inhalations (340 or 680 mcg) q 4 hr.

**INHALATION SOLUTION FOR HAND-BULB NEBULIZER**

**Adults.** 3 to 7 inhalations of undiluted 0.5% or 1% solution q 4 hr.

**INHALATION SOLUTION FOR NEBULIZER**

**Adults.** 2.5 to 10 mg over 15 to 20 min. Repeated q 4 hr, p.r.n.

| Route | Onset | Peak | Duration |
|---|---|---|---|
| Inhalation | 5 min | 5 to 15 min | 2 to 3 hr |

## Mechanism of Action

Attaches to beta$_2$ receptors on bronchial cell membranes, which stimulates the intracellular enzyme adenylate cyclase to convert adenosine triphosphate to cyclic adenosine monophosphate (cAMP). Increased intracellular levels of cAMP help relax bronchial smooth-muscle cells, stabilize mast cells, and inhibit histamine release.

## Contraindications

Hypersensitivity to isoetharine, sympathomimetic amines, or their components

## Interactions

**DRUGS**

*beta blockers:* Decreased effects of both drugs
*cyclopropane, halothane:* Increased risk of arrhythmias
*ephedrine:* Increased cardiac stimulation
*epinephrine:* Increased effects of epinephrine
*guanethidine:* Decreased hypotensive effects
*isoproterenol:* Excessive cardiac stimulation
*MAO inhibitors:* Increased risk of hypertensive crisis, increased vascular effects of isoetharine
*methyldopa:* Increased vasopressor response
*nitrates:* Possibly decreased effects of both drugs
*oxytocic drugs:* Increased risk of hypotension
*rauwolfia alkaloids:* Increased risk of hypertension
*tricyclic antidepressants:* Increased risk of arrhythmias

## Adverse Reactions

**CNS:** Anxiety, dizziness, headache, insomnia, tremor, vertigo, weakness
**CV:** Angina, arrhythmias, hypertension, palpitations, tachycardia
**EENT:** Choking sensation, eyelid or lip swelling, laryngospasm, taste perversion
**GI:** Nausea, vomiting
**RESP:** Bronchospasm, cough, paradoxical increased airway resistance (with excessive use), wheezing
**SKIN:** Dermatitis, flushing, pruritus, urticaria
**Other:** Angioedema, facial edema

## Nursing Considerations

• Dilute 1% isoetharine inhalation solution with 1 to 4 ml of sterile NS; 0.062% to 0.25% solutions don't need to be diluted before use.

• Don't use a solution that's pink or darker than light yellow or one that contains precipitate.

• Wait 1 minute after initial inhaler dose to assess whether patient needs a second dose.

• Monitor blood pressure and pulse rate, and observe for arrhythmias during therapy.

**PATIENT TEACHING**

• Teach patient how to use isoetharine inhaler or nebulizer.

• Instruct patient to take drug exactly as directed and not to exceed dosage.

• Instruct patient not to take other drugs, even OTC drugs, unless prescribed.

• Teach patient how to determine when canister needs to be replaced by counting and recording number of doses.

G
H
I

•Instruct patient to report chest pain, difficulty breathing, failure to respond to usual isoetharine dose, irregular heartbeat, productive cough, or tremor.

# isoniazid
## (isonicotinic acid hydrazide, INH)

Isotamine (CAN), Laniazid, Nydrazid, PMS-Isoniazid (CAN)

## Class and Category
*Chemical:* Isonicotinic acid derivative
*Therapeutic:* Antibiotic, antitubercular
*Pregnancy category:* C

## Indications and Dosages
➤ *To prevent tuberculosis*
**SYRUP, TABLETS, I.M. INJECTION**
**Adults and adolescents.** 300 mg q.d.
**Children.** 10 mg/kg q.d. (up to 300 mg).
➤ *As adjunct to treat active tuberculosis*
**SYRUP, TABLETS**
**Adults and adolescents.** 300 mg q.d. or 15 mg/kg (up to 900 mg) 2 or 3 times/wk, based on treatment regimen.
**Children.** 10 to 20 mg/kg (up to 300 mg) q.d. or 20 to 40 mg/kg (up to 900 mg) 2 or 3 times/wk, based on treatment regimen.
**I.M. INJECTION**
**Adults and adolescents.** 5 mg/kg (up to 300 mg) q.d. or 15 mg/kg (up to 900 mg) 2 or 3 times/wk, based on treatment regimen.
**Children.** 10 to 20 mg/kg (up to 300 mg) q.d. or 20 to 40 mg/kg (up to 900 mg) 2 or 3 times/wk, based on treatment regimen.

---

## Mechanism of Action
Interferes with lipid and nucleic acid synthesis in actively growing tubercle bacilli cells. Isoniazid also disrupts bacterial cell wall synthesis and may interfere with mycolic acid synthesis in mycobacterial cells.

---

## Contraindications
History of serious adverse reactions (such as hepatic injury) from isoniazid, hypersensitivity to isoniazid or its components

## Interactions
**DRUGS**
*acetaminophen:* Increased risk of hepatotoxicity and, possibly, nephrotoxicity
*alfentanil:* Decreased alfentanil clearance and increased duration of alfentanil's effects
*aluminum-containing antacids:* Decreased isoniazid absorption
*benzodiazepines:* Decreased benzodiazepine clearance
*carbamazepine:* Increased blood carbamazepine level and toxicity, increased risk of isoniazid toxicity
*corticosteroids:* Decreased isoniazid effects
*cycloserine:* Increased risk of adverse CNS effects and CNS toxicity
*disulfiram:* Changes in behavior and coordination
*enflurane:* Increased risk of high-output renal failure
*halothane:* Increased risk of hepatotoxicity and hepatic encephalopathy
*hepatotoxic drugs, rifampin:* Increased risk of hepatotoxicity
*ketoconazole:* Possibly decreased blood ketoconazole level and resistance to antifungal treatment
*meperidine:* Risk of hypotensive episodes or CNS depression
*nephrotoxic drugs:* Increased risk of nephrotoxicity
*oral anticoagulants:* Increased anticoagulant effects
*phenytoin:* Increased blood phenytoin level, increased risk of phenytoin toxicity
*theophylline:* Increased blood theophylline level
**FOODS**
*tyramine-containing foods, such as cheese and fish:* Increased responses to tyramine contained in foods, possibly resulting in chills; diaphoresis; headache; light-headedness; and red, itchy, clammy skin
**ACTIVITIES**
*alcohol use:* Increased risk of hepatotoxicity and increased isoniazid metabolism

## Adverse Reactions
**CNS:** Clumsiness, confusion, dizziness, encephalopathy, fatigue, fever, hallucinations, neurotoxicity, paresthesia, peripheral neuritis, psychosis, seizures, weakness
**CV:** Vasculitis
**EENT:** Optic neuritis

**ENDO:** Gynecomastia, hyperglycemia
**GI:** Abdominal pain, anorexia, elevated liver function test results, epigastric distress, hepatitis, nausea, vomiting
**GU:** Glycosuria
**HEME:** Agranulocytosis, aplastic anemia, eosinophilia, hemolytic anemia, sideroblastic anemia, thrombocytopenia
**MS:** Arthralgia, joint stiffness
**SKIN:** Jaundice, pruritus, rash
**Other:** Hypocalcemia, hypophosphatemia, injection site irritation, lupus-like symptoms, lymphadenopathy

## Nursing Considerations
• Administer isoniazid cautiously to diabetic, alcoholic, or malnourished patients and those at risk for developing peripheral neuritis.
• Give drug 1 hour before or 2 hours after meals to promote absorption. If GI distress occurs, give drug with a small amount of food or an antacid that doesn't contain aluminum 1 hour before or 2 hours after meal.
• Monitor results of liver enzyme studies, which may be ordered monthly, because isoniazid can cause severe (and possibly fatal) hepatitis.
• Be aware that about 50% of patients metabolize isoniazid more slowly, which may lead to increased toxic effects. Monitor for such adverse reactions as peripheral neuritis; if they occur, expect to decrease dosage.
• Give isoniazid with other antitubercular drugs, as prescribed, to prevent development of resistant organisms.
• Be aware that patients with advanced HIV infection may experience more severe adverse reactions in greater numbers.

**PATIENT TEACHING**
• Instruct patient to take isoniazid exactly as prescribed and not to stop taking it without first consulting prescriber. Explain that treatment may take months or years.
• Direct patient to take drug on an empty stomach 1 hour before or 2 hours after meals. If GI distress occurs, instruct him to take drug with food or an antacid that doesn't contain aluminum.
• Advise patient to watch for and report signs of hepatic dysfunction, including darkened urine, decreased appetite, fatigue, and jaundice.
• Caution patient not to drink alcohol while taking isoniazid because alcohol increases the risk of hepatotoxicity.

• Provide patient with a list of tyramine-containing foods to avoid when taking isoniazid, such as cheese, fish, salami, red wine, and yeast extracts. Inform him that consuming these foods during isoniazid therapy may cause unpleasant adverse reactions, such as chills, pounding heartbeat, and sweating.
• Inform patient that he'll need periodic laboratory tests and physical examinations.
• Instruct patient to report fever, nausea, numbness and tingling in arms and legs, rash, vision changes, vomiting, and yellowing of skin.

# isoproterenol
## (isoprenaline)
Isuprel

## isoproterenol hydrochloride
Isuprel, Isuprel Mistometer

## isoproterenol sulfate
Medihaler-Iso

## Class and Category
*Chemical:* Catecholamine
*Therapeutic:* Antiarrhythmic, bronchodilator
*Pregnancy category:* B (inhalation), C (I.V. infusion)

## Indications and Dosages
➤ *To treat bronchospasm in asthma and to prevent and treat bronchospasm in COPD*

**INHALATION AEROSOL (ISOPROTERENOL HYDROCHLORIDE)**
**Adults and adolescents.** 1 oral inhalation (120 to 131 mcg), repeated in 2 to 5 min. Inhalations repeated q 3 to 4 hr, p.r.n.

**INHALATION AEROSOL (ISOPROTERENOL SULFATE)**
**Adults and adolescents.** 1 oral inhalation (80 mcg), repeated in 2 to 5 min. Inhalations repeated q 4 to 6 hr, p.r.n.

**INHALATION SOLUTION FOR NEBULIZER (ISOPROTERENOL)**
**Adults and adolescents.** 2.5 mg diluted and administered over 10 to 20 min. Repeated q 4 hr, p.r.n.
**Children.** 0.05 to 0.1 mg/kg (up to 1.25 mg) diluted and administered over 10 to 20 min. Repeated q 4 hr, p.r.n.

➤ *To manage bronchospasm during anesthesia*

**I.V. INJECTION (ISOPROTERENOL HYDROCHLORIDE)**
**Adults.** 0.01 to 0.02 mg, repeated p.r.n.

G
H
I

➤ *To treat bradycardia with significant hemodynamic change, such as third-degree heart block or prolonged QT intervals*

**I.V. INFUSION (ISOPROTERENOL HYDROCHLORIDE)**
**Adults.** *Initial:* 2 mcg/min. Titrated according to heart rate, as ordered. *Maximum:* 10 mcg/min.

| Route | Onset | Peak | Duration |
|---|---|---|---|
| I.V.* | Unknown | Unknown | 1 to 2 hr |
| I.V.† | In 5 min | Unknown | 10 min |
| Inhalation | In 5 min | 5 to 15 min | In 3 hr |

## Mechanism of Action
Stimulates beta$_1$ receptors in the myocardium and cardiac conduction system, resulting in positive inotropic and chronotropic effects. Isoproterenol also shortens the AV conduction time and refractory period in patients with AV block. This action increases the ventricular rate and halts bradycardia and associated syncope.

In addition, isoproterenol attaches to beta$_2$ receptors on bronchial cell membranes. This action stimulates the intracellular enzyme adenylate cyclase to convert adenosine triphosphate to cyclic adenosine monophosphate (cAMP). An increased intracellular level of cAMP relaxes bronchial smooth-muscle cells, stabilizes mast cells, and inhibits histamine release.

## Contraindications
Angina pectoris, heart block or tachycardia from digitalis toxicity, ventricular arrhythmias that require inotropic therapy (I.V. form); hypersensitivity to isoproterenol or its components, such as sulfite in some preparations (inhalation form); tachyarrhythmias (I.V. and inhalation forms)

## Interactions
**DRUGS**
*Note:* All interactions listed are for I.V. form unless indicated.
*alpha blockers, other drugs with this action:* Possibly decreased peripheral vasoconstrict-

---

*For treatment of bronchospasm.
†For treatment of bradycardia.

ing and hypertensive effects of isoproterenol
*anesthetics (hydrocarbon inhalation):* Increased risk of atrial and ventricular arrhythmias
*astemizole, cisapride, drugs that prolong QTc interval, terfenadine:* Possibly prolonged QTc interval
*beta blockers (ophthalmic):* Decreased effects of isoproterenol, increased risk of bronchospasm, wheezing, decreased pulmonary function, and respiratory failure
*beta blockers (systemic):* Increased risk of bronchospasm, decreased effects of both drugs (including inhalation form of isoproterenol)
*digoxin:* Increased risk of arrhythmias, hypokalemia, and digitalis toxicity
*diuretics, other antihypertensives:* Possibly decreased antihypertensive effects
*ergot alkaloids:* Increased vasoconstriction and vasopressor effects
*MAO inhibitors:* Intensified and extended cardiac stimulation and vasopressor effects
*quinidine, other drugs that affect myocardial reaction to sympathomimetics:* Increased risk of arrhythmias
*theophylline:* Increased risk of cardiotoxicity, decreased blood theophylline level
*thyroid hormones:* Increased effects of both drugs, increased risk of coronary insufficiency in patients with coronary artery disease
*tricyclic antidepressants:* Increased vasopressor response, increased risk of prolonged QTc interval and arrhythmias

## Adverse Reactions
**CNS:** Dizziness, headache, insomnia, nervousness, syncope, tremor, weakness
**CV:** Angina, arrhythmias, bradycardia, hypertension, hypotension, palpitations, tachycardia, ventricular arrhythmias
**EENT:** Dry mouth, oropharyngeal edema, taste perversion
**ENDO:** Hyperglycemia
**GI:** Heartburn, nausea, vomiting
**MS:** Muscle spasms and twitching
**RESP:** Bronchitis, bronchospasm, cough, dyspnea, increased sputum production, pulmonary edema, wheezing
**SKIN:** Dermatitis, diaphoresis, erythema multiforme, flushing, pallor, pruritus, rash, Stevens-Johnson syndrome, urticaria
**Other:** Angioedema, hypokalemia

## Nursing Considerations
•Expect to give lowest possible dose of iso-

proterenol for shortest possible time to minimize tolerance.
•Don't administer I.V. form if it is pink or brown or contains precipitate.
•Administer infusion through large vein, and monitor for signs of extravasation.
•Monitor blood pressure, cardiac rhythm, central venous pressure, and urine output when giving I.V. drug. Adjust infusion rate to response, as ordered.
•Notify prescriber immediately if heart rate increases significantly or exceeds 110 beats/minute during I.V. infusion.
•Know that drug may increase pulse pressure and cause hypotension. Expect to reduce I.V. infusion slowly to decrease risk of hypotension.
•WARNING Be aware that isoproterenol markedly increases the risk of arrhythmias. If an arrhythmia develops, expect to give a cardio-selective beta blocker, such as atenolol, as prescribed.
•Be aware that isoproterenol isn't used regularly to treat asthma, decreased cardiac output, hypotension, or shock because it increases the risk of arrhythmias, hypotension, and ischemia.
•WARNING If isoproterenol aggravates a ventilation-perfusion problem, expect patient's blood oxygen level to fall even as his breathing seems to improve.

**PATIENT TEACHING**
•Instruct patient not to use isoproterenol inhaler more often than prescribed because excessive use may cause cardiac and respiratory problems.
•Teach patient how to use the inhaler, and observe his technique. Provide a spacer, as needed.
•Instruct patient to wait 2 to 5 minutes before taking second inhalation.
•Advise patient to rinse his mouth after inhalation to remove drug residue and minimize mouth dryness.
•Inform patient that saliva may appear pink after inhalation.
•If patient also uses a corticosteroid inhaler, tell him to take isoproterenol first and then wait at least 2 minutes before taking corticosteroid.
•Instruct patient to report chest pain, dizziness, hyperglycemic symptoms (such as abdominal cramps, lethargy, nausea, and vomiting), insomnia, irregular heartbeat, palpitations, tremor, and weakness.

•Advise patient to also report reduced drug effectiveness, increased use of inhaler, and increased symptoms after taking drug.

# isosorbide dinitrate

Apo-ISDN (CAN), Cedocard-SR (CAN), Coradur (CAN), Coronex (CAN), Dilatrate-SR, Isordil Tembids, Isordil Titradose, Sorbitrate

## isosorbide mononitrate

IMDUR, ISMO, Monoket

## Class and Category
*Chemical:* Organic nitrate
*Therapeutic:* Antianginal, vasodilator
*Pregnancy category:* C

## Indications and Dosages
➤ *To treat or prevent angina*
**CHEWABLE TABLETS**
**Adults.** 5 mg q 2 to 3 hr, p.r.n. (dinitrate).
**E.R. CAPSULES**
**Adults.** 40 to 80 mg q 8 to 12 hr (dinitrate).
**E.R. TABLETS**
**Adults.** 20 to 80 mg q 8 to 12 hr (dinitrate); 30 to 60 mg q.d., increased gradually as tolerated to 120 mg q.d. (mononitrate).
**S.L. TABLETS**
**Adults.** 2.5 to 5 mg q 2 to 3 hr, p.r.n. (dinitrate).
**TABLETS**
**Adults.** 5 to 40 mg q 6 hr, adjusted as needed (dinitrate); 20 mg in 2 doses given 7 hr apart (mononitrate).

| Route | Onset | Peak | Duration |
|---|---|---|---|
| P.O.* | 1 hr† | Unknown | 5 to 6 hr |
| P.O. (chewable)* | In 3 min | Unknown | 30 min to 2 hr |
| P.O. (E.R.)* | 30 min | Unknown | 6 to 8 hr |
| P.O. (S.L.)* | In 3 min | Unknown | 2 hr |

## Contraindications
Angle-closure glaucoma; cerebral hemorrhage; concurrent use of sildenafil; head trauma; hypersensitivity to isosorbide, other

*For dinitrate.
†For mononitrate, onset also is 1 hr; peak and duration are unknown.

nitrates, or their components; orthostatic hypotension; severe anemia

## Interactions

**DRUGS**

*acetylcholine, norepinephrine:* Possibly decreased effectiveness of these drugs
*antihypertensives, calcium channel blockers, opioid analgesics, other vasodilators:* Increased risk of orthostatic hypotension
*aspirin:* Increased blood level and pharmacologic action of isosorbide
*sildenafil:* Increased risk of hypotension and death
*sympathomimetics:* Increased risk of hypotension, possibly decreased therapeutic effects of isosorbide

**ACTIVITIES**

*alcohol use:* Increased risk of orthostatic hypotension

## Adverse Reactions

**CNS:** Agitation, confusion, dizziness, headache, insomnia, restlessness, syncope, vertigo, weakness
**CV:** Arrhythmias, orthostatic hypotension, palpitations, peripheral edema, tachycardia
**EENT:** Blurred vision, diplopia (all drug forms); sublingual burning (S.L. form)
**GI:** Abdominal pain, diarrhea, indigestion, nausea, vomiting
**GU:** Dysuria, impotence, urinary frequency
**HEME:** Hemolytic anemia
**MS:** Arthralgia, muscle twitching
**RESP:** Bronchitis, pneumonia, upper respiratory tract infection
**SKIN:** Diaphoresis, flushing, rash

## Nursing Considerations

•Use isosorbide cautiously in patients with hypovolemia or mild hypotension. Monitor for increased hypotension and reduced cardiac output.
•Give drug 1 hour before or 2 hours after meals. Give with meals if patient experiences severe headaches or adverse GI reactions.
•Know that patient may experience daily headaches from isosorbide's vasodilating effects. Give acetaminophen, as prescribed, to relieve pain.
•**WARNING** Be aware that abrupt drug discontinuation may cause angina and increase the risk of MI.

## Mechanism of Action

Isosorbide may interact with nitrate receptors in vascular smooth-muscle cell membranes. By interacting with nitrate receptors' sulfhydryl groups, the drug is reduced to nitric oxide. Nitric oxide activates the enzyme guanylate cyclase, increasing intracellular formation of cyclic guanosine monophosphate (cGMP). An increased cGMP level may relax vascular smooth muscle by forcing calcium out of muscle cells, causing vasodilation. This improves cardiac output by reducing primarily preload but also afterload.

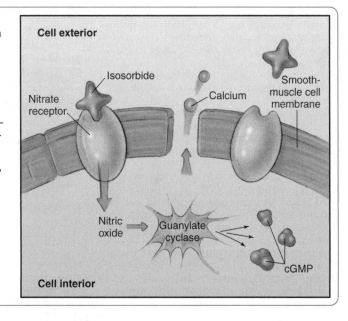

•Monitor blood pressure frequently during isosorbide therapy, especially in the elderly; the drug may cause severe hypotension.
•Keep drug away from heat and light.
**PATIENT TEACHING**
•Teach patient and family to recognize signs and symptoms of angina, including chest pain, fullness, or pressure, which commonly is accompanied by sweating and nausea. Pain may radiate down the left arm or into the neck or jaw. Inform female patients and those with diabetes mellitus or hypertension that they may experience only fatigue and shortness of breath.
•Advise patient not to crush or chew isosorbide E.R. capsules or tablets or S.L. tablets unless specifically ordered to do so.
•Instruct patient to place S.L. tablet under tongue and not to swallow it, but to let it dissolve. Explain that moisture in mouth promotes drug absorption and that tingling or burning in the mouth indicates drug effectiveness.
•Advise patient to chew chewable tablets well and to keep them in his mouth for 1 to 2 minutes before swallowing to enhance drug absorption.
•Instruct patient to take drug before any situation or activity that might precipitate angina.
•Advise patient to carry isosorbide with him at all times.
•Caution patient that abrupt drug discontinuation may cause angina and increase the risk of MI.
•Instruct patient to report blurred vision, fainting, increased angina attacks, rash, and severe or persistent headaches.
•Teach patient to reduce the effects of orthostatic hypotension by changing position slowly. Advise him to lie down if he becomes dizzy.
•Inform patient that drug commonly causes headache, which typically resolves after a few days of continuous therapy. Suggest that patient take acetaminophen as needed and as prescribed.
•Advise patient to avoid potentially hazardous activities until drug's CNS effects are known.
•Urge patient to avoid alcohol consumption.
•Instruct patient to store drug in a tightly closed container away from light and heat.

# isotretinoin

Accutane

## Class and Category

*Chemical:* Retinoid
*Therapeutic:* Acne inhibitor
*Pregnancy category:* X

## Indications and Dosages

➤ *To treat severe recalcitrant nodular acne*
**CAPSULES**
**Adults.** *Initial:* 0.5 mg to 1 mg/kg/day in two divided doses, increased as needed up to 2 mg/kg/day given in two divided doses. *Maximum:* 2 mg/kg/day. Course of therapy given for 15 to 20 wk with second course given, as needed, after a period of 2 mo or more off therapy.

---

### Mechanism of Action

Inhibits sebaceous gland function and keratinization, which results in diminished nodular formation associated with recalcitrant nodular acne.

---

## Contraindications

Hypersensitivity to isotretinoin or any of its components, hypersensitivity to parabens, pregnancy

## Interactions

**DRUGS**
*corticosteroids (systemic):* Possibly increased risk of osteoporosis
*oral contraceptives including microdosed progesterone preparations, medroxyprogesterone injection, levonorgestrel implants:* Possibly decreased effectiveness of contraceptive
*phenytoin:* Possibly increased risk of osteomalacia
*tetracyclines:* Increased risk of benign intracranial hypertension
*vitamin A supplements:* Increased risk of additive toxic effects

## Adverse Reactions

**CNS:** Aggressive or violent behavior, depression, dizziness, drowsiness, emotional instability, fatigue, headache, insomnia, lethargy, malaise, nervousness, paresthesias, pseudotumor cerebri, psychosis, seizures, stroke, suicidal ideation, syncope, weakness
**CV:** Chest pain, decreased high-density

**G**
**H**
**I**

lipoprotein level, edema, elevated creatinine phosphokinase level, hypercholesteremia, hypertriglyceridemia, palpitation, stroke, tachycardia, vascular thrombotic disease, vasculitis

**ENDO:** Abnormal menses, alterations in blood glucose levels

**EENT:** Bleeding and inflammation of gums, cataracts, color vision disorder, conjunctivitis, corneal opacities, decreased night vision, dry mouth or nose, dry eyes, epistaxis, eyelid inflammation, hearing impairment, keratitis, optic neuritis, photophobia, tinnitus, visual disturbances, voice alteration

**GI:** Colitis, hepatitis, ileitis, inflammatory bowel disease, liver enzyme elevation, nausea, pancreatitis

**GU:** Glomerulonephritis, hematuria, proteinuria, WBCs in urine

**HEME:** Anemia, agranulocytosis, neutropenia, platelet count elevation, sedimentation rate elevation, thrombocytopenia

**MS:** Arthralgia, arthritis, back pain (children), bone abnormalities, calcification of tendons and ligaments, premature epiphyseal closure, tendonitis

**RESP:** Bronchospasms, respiratory infection

**SKIN:** Alopecia, bruising, disseminated herpes simplex, dry lips or skin, eczema, eruptive xanthomas, facial erythema, flushing, fulminant acne, hair abnormalities, hirsutism, hyperpigmentation, hypopigmentation, increased sunburn susceptibility, infections, nail dystrophy, paronychia, peeling of palms and soles, photoallergic or photosensitizing reactions, pruritus, pyogenic granuloma, rash, seborrhea, skin fragility, sweating, urticaria

**Other:** Abnormal wound healing, alkaline phosphatase increase, allergic reactions, hyperuricemia, lymphadenopathy, weight loss

## Nursing Considerations

•Ensure that women of childbearing age have had two negative urine or serum pregnancy tests with a sensitivity of at least 50 mIU/ml, joined the Accutane Survey, signed the consent form, and watched the videotape provided by manufacturer prior to beginning isotretinoin therapy.

•WARNING Notify prescriber if elevated serum triglyceride levels can't be controlled or if symptoms of pancreatitis occur (abdominal pain, nausea, vomiting). Drug may need

to be discontinued because fatal hemorrhagic pancreatitis has occurred with drug use.

•Obtain serum lipid level before therapy and periodically thereafter, as ordered, to detect elevated lipid levels that result from isotretinoin therapy.

•Monitor liver enzyme levels periodically, as ordered, because drug can cause hepatitis.

•Assess patient frequently for adverse reactions and report to prescriber any that occur; drug may have serious adverse effects that require discontinuation.

**PATIENT TEACHING**

•Instruct patient to take isotretinoin with food or milk.

•Advise women of child-bearing age that two forms of contraceptives must be used simultaneously (unless absolute abstinence is a chosen method) 1 month before therapy and for 1 month after therapy has stopped because of potential for fetal harm. Inform women who use oral contraceptives that drug may lessen effectiveness of oral contraceptives. Urge patient to notify prescriber immediately if pregnancy occurs.

•Urge patient to report headache, nausea, vomiting and visual disturbances immediately to prescriber because drug will need to be discontinued immediately and the patient referred to a neurologist.

•Caution patient and family that isotretinoin may cause aggressive or violent behavior, depression, psychosis, and suicidal ideation. Instruct patient to notify prescriber immediately if changes in mood occur.

•Tell patient to report hearing changes or tinnitus, visual difficulties, abdominal pain, rectal bleeding, or severe diarrhea to prescriber because drug may need to be discontinued.

•Advise patient to avoid potentially hazardous activities until drug's CNS effects are known. Caution her that changes in night vision may occur suddenly.

•Caution patient not to donate blood during therapy and for one month after therapy has stopped because blood might be given to a pregnant woman.

•Warn patient that transient exacerbation of acne may occur, especially during initial therapy and to notify prescriber if this occurs.

•Instruct patient to avoid wax epilation and skin resurfacing procedures during therapy and for at least 6 months thereafter because of scarring potential.

•Caution patient to avoid exposure to direct sunlight or UV light and to wear sunscreen when outdoors.
•Inform patient that decreased tolerance to contact lenses may occur during and after therapy.
•Alert patient to the potential for mild musculoskeletal adverse reactions that may occur with therapy, which usually clear rapidly after drug is discontinued. Urge patient to notify prescriber if symptoms become bothersome or serious because drug may need to be discontinued.
•Advise patient not to take vitamin A supplements while on drug therapy because of potential additive toxic effects.
•Instruct patient to notify all prescribers of isotretinoin use because of potential interactions.
•Inform patient of need for frequent laboratory tests and importance of complying with scheduled appointments.

# isradipine

DynaCirc

## Class and Category

*Chemical:* Dihydropyridine derivative
*Therapeutic:* Antihypertensive
*Pregnancy category:* C

## Indications and Dosages

➤ *To manage essential hypertension*
**CAPSULES**
**Adults.** *Initial:* 2.5 mg b.i.d., increased by 5 mg q 2 to 4 wk, if needed. *Maximum:* 20 mg/day.

| Route | Onset | Peak | Duration |
|-------|-------|------|----------|
| P.O. | 2 to 3 hr | 2 to 4 wk | Unknown |

## Mechanism of Action

Inhibits calcium movement into coronary vascular smooth-muscle cells by blocking the slow calcium channels in their membranes. By decreasing the intracellular calcium level, isradipine inhibits smooth-muscle cell contractions. The result is relaxation of coronary and vascular smooth muscle, decreased peripheral vascular resistance, and reduced systolic and diastolic blood pressure, all of which decrease myocardial oxygen demand.

## Contraindications

Hypersensitivity to isradipine or its components

## Interactions

**DRUGS**
*anesthetics (hydrocarbon inhalation), antihypertensives, hydrochlorothiazide, prazocin:* Increased risk of hypotension
*beta blockers:* Increased adverse effects of beta blockers
*cimetidine:* Increased blood level and bioavailability of isradipine
*digoxin:* Transiently increased blood digoxin level and risk of digitalis toxicity
*estrogens:* Possibly increased fluid retention and decreased therapeutic effects of isradipine
*lithium:* Increased risk of neurotoxicity
*NSAIDs, sympathomimetics:* Possibly decreased therapeutic effects of isradipine
*procainamide, quinidine:* Increased risk of prolonged QT interval
**FOODS**
*grapefruit juice:* Doubled isradipine bioavailability
*other foods:* Prolonged time to achieve peak blood level

## Adverse Reactions

**CNS:** Asthenia, dizziness, fatigue, headache, paresthesia, somnolence, stroke, syncope, transient ischemic attack, weakness
**CV:** Angina, atrial fibrillation, heart failure, hypotension, MI, orthostatic hypotension, palpitations, peripheral edema, tachycardia, ventricular fibrillation
**EENT:** Gingival hyperplasia, pharyngitis, rhinitis
**GI:** Abdominal cramps, constipation, diarrhea, elevated liver function test results, indigestion, nausea, vomiting
**HEME:** Leukopenia
**MS:** Back pain
**RESP:** Cough
**SKIN:** Flushing, photosensitivity, rash, urticaria
**Other:** Angioedema

## Nursing Considerations

•Monitor blood pressure and heart rate frequently during isradipine therapy.
•Monitor patient with impaired hepatic or renal function for an increased blood isradipine level.

G
H
I

•Avoid giving drug with food, which increases time to peak effect by about 1 hour.
•Observe for mild peripheral edema caused by vasodilation of small blood vessels. Know that this type of edema doesn't result from fluid retention or heart failure.

**PATIENT TEACHING**

•Inform patient that isradipine therapy will be long-term and will require laboratory tests and follow-up visits to monitor drug effects.
•Instruct patient to take drug exactly as prescribed and to swallow capsules whole, not crush or chew them.
•Advise patient to take drug on an empty stomach 1 hour before or 2 hours after meals.
•Instruct patient to take a missed dose as soon as remembered unless it's nearly time for the next dose. If it is, advise him to wait and take the next scheduled dose, but not to double the dose. If more than one dose is missed, tell him to contact prescriber.
•**WARNING** Urge patient not to stop taking drug suddenly. Doing so may lead to life-threatening problems.
•Inform patient that fragments of capsules may be visible in stool.
•Caution patient not to drink grapefruit juice during isradipine therapy.
•Urge patient to avoid potentially hazardous activities until drug's CNS effects are known.
•Caution patient to change position slowly to minimize effects of orthostatic hypotension.
•Urge patient to contact prescriber if he experiences chest pain, fainting, irregular heartbeat, rash, or swollen ankles.
•Instruct patient to maintain good oral hygiene, perform gum massage, and see his dentist every 6 months to prevent gum bleeding and gum disorders.
•To help prevent photosensitivity reactions, caution patient to avoid direct sunlight and to wear protective clothing and apply sunscreen when outdoors.
•Instruct patient to store drug at room temperature in a dry place.

# itraconazole

Sporanox

## Class and Category

*Chemical:* Triazole derivative
*Therapeutic:* Antifungal
*Pregnancy category:* C

## Indications and Dosages

➤ *To treat blastomycosis caused by* Blastomyces dermatitidis *and histoplasmosis caused by* Histoplasma capsulatum

**CAPSULES**

**Adults and adolescents.** *Initial:* 200 mg q.d., increased by 100 mg/day, if needed. *Maximum:* 400 mg/day, with dosage greater than 200 mg given in divided doses b.i.d.

➤ *To treat aspergillosis unresponsive to amphotericin B*

**CAPSULES**

**Adults and adolescents.** 200 to 400 mg/day, with dosage greater than 200 mg/day given in divided doses b.i.d.

➤ *To treat pulmonary and extrapulmonary blastomycosis, histoplasmosis, and refractory aspergillosis*

**I.V. INFUSION**

**Adults and adolescents.** 200 mg infused over 1 hr q 12 hr for 4 doses; then 200 mg q.d. Drug changed to P.O. form within 14 days and therapy continued for at least 3 mo.

**DOSAGE ADJUSTMENT** In life-threatening situations, loading dose adjusted to 200 mg P.O. or I.V. t.i.d. for 3 days. Be aware that I.V. itraconazole shouldn't be used in patients with creatinine clearance less than 30 ml/min/1.73 m$^2$.

➤ *To treat oropharyngeal candidiasis*

**ORAL SOLUTION**

**Adults and adolescents.** 100 mg b.i.d. for 7 to 14 days.

➤ *To treat esophageal candidiasis*

**ORAL SOLUTION**

**Adults and adolescents.** 100 mg q.d. for at least 3 wk and continued for 2 wk after symptoms resolve.

➤ *To treat onychomycosis of toenails only or of toenails and fingernails*

**CAPSULES**

**Adults and adolescents.** 200 mg q.d. for 12 wk.

➤ *To treat onychomycosis of fingernails only*

**CAPSULES**

**Adults and adolescents.** 200 mg b.i.d. for 7 days, then repeated after 3 wk.

## Incompatibilities

Don't administer itraconazole through same I.V. line with other drugs. Don't mix I.V. itraconazole with D$_5$W or solutions that contain LR.

## Mechanism of Action

Inhibits the synthesis of ergosterol, an essential component of fungal cell membranes, by binding with a cytochrome P-450 enzyme needed to convert lanosterol to ergosterol. The lack of ergosterol results in increased cellular permeability and leakage of cell contents. Itraconazole also may lead to fungal cell death by inhibiting fungal respiration under aerobic conditions.

## Contraindications

Concurrent therapy with cisapride, dofetilide, ergot alkaloids, HMG-CoA inhibitors (lovastatin and simvastatin), levomethadyl, oral midazolam, pimozide, quinidine, or triazolam; evidence of ventricular dysfunction, as in congestive heart failure (CHF) or a history of it (onychomycosis treatment); hypersensitivity to itraconazole or its components; planning for pregnancy during onychomycosis treatment

## Interactions

### DRUGS

*alfentanil, buspirone, busulfan, carbamazepine, cyclosporine, digoxin, docetaxel, dofetilide, indinavir, methylprednisolone, phenytoin, pimozide, quinidine, rifabutin, ritonavir, saquinavir, sirolimus, tacrolimus, trimetrexate, vinca alkaloids:* Possibly increased blood levels of these drugs
*alprazolam, diazepam, oral midazolam, triazolam:* Elevated blood levels and possibly prolonged sedative effects of these drugs
*antacids, anticholinergics, H₂-receptor antagonists, omeprazole, sucralfate:* Possibly decreased itraconazole absorption
*atorvastatin, lovastatin, simvastatin:* Increased blood levels of these drugs; possibly rhabdomyolysis
*calcium channel blockers:* Possibly edema and increased blood levels of these drugs
*carbamazepine, isoniazid, nevirapine, phenobarbital, phenytoin, rifabutin, rifampin:* Possibly decreased blood itraconazole level
*cisapride, pimozide, levomethadyl, quinidine:* Possibly life-threatening cardiovascular complications as well as sudden death
*clarithromycin, erythromycin, indinavir, ritonavir:* Possibly increased blood itraconazole level

*didanosine:* Possibly decreased therapeutic effects of itraconazole
*oral antidiabetic drugs:* Possibly increased blood levels of these drugs and risk of hypoglycemia
*warfarin:* Increased anticoagulant effect of warfarin

## Adverse Reactions

**CNS:** Dizziness, drowsiness, fatigue, fever, headache, peripheral neuropathy, vertigo
**CV:** CHF, hypertriglyceridemia, hypertension, peripheral edema
**GI:** Abdominal pain, anorexia, constipation, diarrhea, elevated liver function test results, flatulence, hepatic failure, hepatitis, hepatotoxicity, hyperbilirubinemia, indigestion, nausea, vomiting
**GU:** Menstrual irregularities
**HEME:** Neutropenia
**RESP:** Cough, dyspnea, pulmonary edema
**SKIN:** Alopecia, diaphoresis, photosensitivity, pruritus, rash, Stevens-Johnson syndrome, urticaria
**Other:** Angioedema, anaphylaxis, hypokalemia

## Nursing Considerations

• Because itraconazole has been linked to serious adverse cardiac and hepatic effects, expect to send appropriate nail specimens for laboratory testing to confirm onychomycosis before beginning therapy.
• Be aware that I.V. itraconazole is for infusion only. Don't administer by bolus.
• **WARNING** Keep in mind that itraconazole is a potent inhibitor of the cytochrome P-450 3A4 (CYP3A4) isoenzyme system, which may increase blood levels of drugs metabolized by this system. Patients using such drugs as cisapride with itraconazole or other CYP3A4 inhibitors have experienced life-threatening cardiovascular complications, such as prolonged QT interval, torsades de pointes, and ventricular tachycardia, as well as sudden death.
• Administer itraconazole capsules (but not oral solution) with a meal to ensure maximal absorption.
• Infuse each I.V. dose over 1 hour.
• Keep in mind that a patient with AIDS may have hypochlorhydria, which reduces drug absorption. For such a patient, expect to administer higher doses of itraconazole.
• Monitor liver function test results in patients with impaired hepatic function and

G
H
I

those who have experienced hepatotoxicity with other drugs.

• If patient develops signs and symptoms of peripheral neuropathy or CHF, such as fatigue, dyspnea, and peripheral edema, expect to discontinue drug.

• Assess patient for rash every 8 hours during therapy; notify prescriber if rash occurs.

• If patient also receives warfarin, monitor PT and assess patient for signs and symptoms of bleeding.

• If patient also receives digoxin, monitor blood digoxin level as appropriate to detect toxic level, and assess patient for signs and symptoms of digitalis toxicity, such as nausea and yellow vision.

**PATIENT TEACHING**

• Instruct patient to take itraconazole capsules with a meal, but oral solution without food.

• If patient also takes an oral antidiabetic drug, instruct him to monitor his blood glucose level frequently because of the increased risk of hypoglycemia.

• Advise patient to avoid taking antacids with oral itraconazole.

• Advise patient to notify prescriber immediately of changes in other drugs, such as new drugs and dosage changes.

• Advise patient to notify prescriber immediately about abdominal pain, diarrhea, headache, nausea, peripheral neuropathy, rash, or vomiting.

• Instruct patient to notify prescriber if he experiences signs of liver problems, such as abdominal pain, dark urine, fatigue, loss of appetite, pale stools, weakness, or yellow eyes or skin.

• Caution breast-feeding patient to consult prescriber about continuation of breast-feeding during itraconazole therapy.

# J·K·L

## kanamycin sulfate

Kantrex

### Class and Category
*Chemical:* Aminoglycoside
*Therapeutic:* Antibiotic
*Pregnancy category:* D

### Indications and Dosages
➤ *To treat infections caused by gram-negative organisms (including* Acinetobacter *sp.,* Enterobacter aerogenes, Escherichia coli, Haemophilus influenzae, Klebsiella pneumoniae, Neisseria *sp.,* Proteus *sp.,* Providencia *sp.,* Salmonella *sp.,* Serratia marcescens, Shigella *sp., and* Yersinia *sp.) and gram-positive organisms (including* Staphylococcus aureus *and* Staphylococcus epidermidis)

**I.M. INJECTION**
**Adults and children.** 3.75 mg/kg q 6 hr, 5 mg/kg q 8 hr, or 7.5 mg/kg q 12 hr for 7 to 10 days. *Maximum:* 1.5 g/day.

**I.V. INFUSION**
**Adults and children.** 5 mg/kg q 8 hr or 7.5 mg/kg q 12 hr for 7 to 10 days. *Maximum:* 1.5 g/day.

➤ *As adjunct to suppress intestinal bacterial growth*

**CAPSULES**
**Adults.** 1 g/hr for 4 hr and then 1 g q 6 hr for 36 to 72 hr.

➤ *To treat hepatic coma*

**CAPSULES**
**Adults.** 8 to 12 g/day administered in divided doses.

➤ *To treat respiratory tract infection*

**INHALATION NEBULIZER**
**Adults.** 250 mg b.i.d. to q.i.d. *Maximum:* 1.5 g/day.
**DOSAGE ADJUSTMENT** For elderly patients and those with renal failure, dosage reduced and blood kanamycin level and renal function test results monitored.

### Contraindications
Hypersensitivity to kanamycin, other aminoglycosides, or their components; intestinal obstruction (oral form)

### Mechanism of Action
Binds to negatively charged sites on bacterial outer cell membranes, which disrupts cell membrane integrity. Kanamycin also binds to bacterial ribosomal subunits and inhibits protein synthesis; these actions lead to cell death.

| Route | Onset | Peak | Duration |
|-------|-------|------|----------|
| P.O. | Slow | Unknown | Unknown |
| I.V. | Rapid | Unknown | Unknown |
| I.M. | Unknown | 1 to 2 hr | Unknown |

### Incompatibilities
Don't mix kanamycin in same syringe or administer through same I.V. line as other antibiotics.

### Interactions
**DRUGS**
*cephalosporins, vancomycin:* Increased risk of nephrotoxicity
*digoxin, loop diuretics:* Increased ototoxic and nephrotoxic effects of kanamycin
*general anesthetics, neuromuscular blockers:* Increased risk of neuromuscular blockade
*penicillins:* Inactivation of kanamycin or synergistic effects

### Adverse Reactions
**CNS:** Ataxia, dizziness, headache
**EENT:** Hearing loss
**GI:** Diarrhea
**GU:** Elevated BUN and serum creatinine levels, oliguria, proteinuria
**MS:** Muscle paralysis
**RESP:** Apnea
**SKIN:** Injection site irritation or pain

### Nursing Considerations
• Obtain body fluid or tissue specimen for culture and sensitivity testing before kanamycin therapy begins, as indicated. Therapy may begin before test results are available.
• Administer I.M. injection deep into upper outer quadrant of gluteus maximus. Rotate injection sites.
• Be aware that oral kanamycin is minimally absorbed from intact GI mucosa but may be more extensively absorbed from mechanically irrigated areas of the GI tract.

J
K
L

• For I.V. use, dilute 500-mg vial with 100 to 200 ml of NS or D$_5$W, or 1-g vial with 200 to 400 ml of NS or D$_5$W, and infuse over 30 to 60 min. Be aware that vial contents may darken during storage but potency isn't affected.
• Keep patient well hydrated before and during therapy.
• Monitor blood kanamycin level periodically during therapy, as appropriate.
• Be aware that prolonged treatment increases the risk of ototoxicity and nephrotoxicity. Monitor hearing and renal function if therapy lasts longer than 10 days.

### PATIENT TEACHING
• Explain the need to take kanamycin at prescribed intervals around the clock until patient completes full course of therapy.
• Advise patient to report dizziness, hearing loss, and severe diarrhea or headache to prescriber.


# ketoprofen

Actron, Apo-Keto (CAN), Orudis, Orudis KT, Orudis-SR (CAN), Oruvail, Rhodis

## Class and Category
*Chemical:* Propionic acid derivative
*Therapeutic:* Analgesic, anti-inflammatory
*Pregnancy category:* B

## Indications and Dosages
➤ *To treat symptoms of rheumatoid arthritis*

### CAPSULES, TABLETS
**Adults.** *Initial:* 75 mg t.i.d. or 50 mg q.i.d. *Maximum:* 300 mg/day.

### E.R. CAPSULES
**Adults.** *Maintenance:* 150 to 200 mg q.d. *Maximum:* 300 mg/day.

➤ *To relieve pain associated with dysmenorrhea*

### TABLETS
**Adults.** *Initial:* 25 to 50 mg q 6 to 8 hr p.r.n. *Maximum:* 300 mg/day.
DOSAGE ADJUSTMENT Dosage reduced by 33% to 50% for patients with renal impairment.

## Contraindications
Angioedema; aspirin-, iodide-, or NSAID-induced asthma, bronchospasm, nasal polyps, rhinitis, or urticaria; hypersensitivity to ketoprofen or its components

## Mechanism of Action
Blocks the activity of cyclooxygenase, the enzyme needed for prostaglandin synthesis. Prostaglandins, important mediators of the inflammatory response, cause local vasodilation with swelling and pain. By blocking cyclooxygenase and inhibiting prostaglandins, this NSAID reduces inflammatory symptoms and relieves pain.

## Interactions
### DRUGS
*ACE inhibitors:* Possibly decreased hypotensive effect of ACE inhibitors
*acetaminophen:* Possibly increased adverse renal effects with long-term acetaminophen use
*aspirin, other NSAIDs:* Increased risk of bleeding and adverse GI effects, increased and prolonged blood ketoprofen levels
*cefamandole, cefoperazone, cefotetan:* Increased risk of hypoprothrombinemia and bleeding
*colchicine, platelet aggregation inhibitors:* Increased risk of GI bleeding, hemorrhage, and ulcers
*corticosteroids, potassium supplements:* Increased risk of adverse GI effects
*cyclosporine:* Increased risk of nephrotoxicity from both drugs, increased blood cyclosporine level
*diuretics (loop, potassium-sparing, and thiazide):* Decreased diuretic and antihypertensive effects
*gold compounds, nephrotoxic drugs:* Increased risk of adverse renal effects
*heparin, oral anticoagulants, thrombolytics:* Increased anticoagulant effects, increased risk of hemorrhage
*insulin, oral antidiabetic drugs:* Possibly increased hypoglycemic effects of these drugs
*lithium:* Increased blood lithium level and possibly toxicity
*methotrexate:* Decreased methotrexate clearance, increased risk of methotrexate toxicity
*plicamycin, valproic acid:* Increased risk of hypoprothrombinemia and GI bleeding, hemorrhage, and ulcers
*probenecid:* Possibly increased blood level, effectiveness, and risk of toxicity of ketoprofen

### ACTIVITIES
*alcohol use:* Increased risk of adverse GI effects

## Adverse Reactions

**CNS:** CVA, headache, irritability, nervousness, seizures
**CV:** Edema, fluid retention, hypertension, MI, tachycardia
**EENT:** Tinnitus, vision changes
**GI:** Abdominal pain, anorexia, constipation, diarrhea, diverticulitis, dyspepsia, dysphagia, flatulence, gastritis, gastroenteritis, gastroesophageal reflux disease, GI bleeding and ulceration, hepatic failure, hiatal hernia, indigestion, melena, nausea, perforation of stomach or intestines, stomatitis, vomiting
**GU:** Acute renal failure, decreased urine output
**HEME:** Agranulocytosis, anemia, easy bruising, hemolytic anemia, leukopenia, neutropenia, pancytopenia, thrombocytopenia
**RESP:** Asthma, respiratory depression
**SKIN:** Erythema multiforme, Stevens-Johnson syndrome, toxic epidermal necrolysis, rash
**Other:** Anaphylaxis, angioedema, rapid weight gain

## Nursing Considerations

•Use ketoprofen with extreme caution in patients with a history of ulcer disease or GI bleeding because NSAIDs such as ketoprofen increase the risk of GI bleeding and ulceration. Expect to use ketoprofen for the shortest time possible in these patients.
•Be aware that serious GI tract ulceration, bleeding, and perforation may occur without warning symptoms. Elderly patients are at greater risk. To minimize risk, give drug with food. If GI distress occurs, withhold drug and notify prescriber immediately.
•Use ketoprofen cautiously in patients with hypertension, and monitor blood pressure closely throughout therapy. Drug may cause hypertension or worsen it.
•**WARNING** Monitor patient closely for thrombotic events, including MI and stroke, because NSAIDs increase the risk.
•Monitor patient—especially if he's elderly or receiving long-term ketoprofen therapy—for less common but serious adverse GI reactions, including anorexia, constipation, diverticulitis, dysphagia, esophagitis, gastritis, gastroenteritis, gastroesophageal reflux disease, hemorrhoids, hiatal hernia, melena, stomatitis, and vomiting.
•Monitor liver function test results because,

in rare cases, elevations may progress to severe hepatic reactions, including fatal hepatitis, liver necrosis, and hepatic failure.
•Monitor BUN and serum creatinine levels in elderly patients, patients taking diuretics or ACE inhibitors, and patients with heart failure, impaired renal function, or hepatic dysfunction; drug may cause renal failure.
•Monitor CBC for decreased hemoglobin level and hematocrit because drug may worsen anemia.
•**WARNING** If patient has bone marrow suppression or is receiving an antineoplastic drug, monitor laboratory results (including WBC count), and watch for evidence of infection because anti-inflammatory and antipyretic actions of ketoprofen may mask signs and symptoms, such as fever and pain.
•Assess patient's skin regularly for signs of rash or other hypersensitivity reaction because ketoprofen is an NSAID and may cause serious skin reactions without warning, even in patients with no history of NSAID sensivitity. At first sign of reaction, stop drug and notify prescriber.
•If patient takes acetaminophen, monitor fluid intake and output, BUN level, and serum creatinine level for evidence of adverse renal effects.

**PATIENT TEACHING**
•Instruct patient to take ketoprofen with food or after meals to prevent GI upset. Advise him to take drug with a full glass of water and to avoid lying down for 15 to 30 minutes afterward to prevent drug from lodging in esophagus and causing irritation.
•Advise patient to swallow drug whole and not to crush, break, chew, or open capsules.
•Instruct patient to avoid aspirin, aspirin-containing products, and alcohol while taking ketoprofen to decrease the risk of adverse GI effects.
•Tell patient not to take more drug than prescribed because stomach bleeding may occur.
•If patient takes an anticoagulant, tell him to watch for and immediately report bleeding problems, such as bloody or tarry stools and bloody vomitus.
•If patient takes insulin or an oral antidiabetic, advise him to monitor his blood glucose levels closely. Urge him to carry candy or other simple sugars to treat mild hypoglycemia. If he has frequent or severe episodes, instruct him to consult with his prescriber.

J
K
L

• Inform patient that he may be nervous and irritable while taking ketoprofen.

• Instruct patient to notify prescriber immediately if he develops a rash, decreased urine output, dark yellow or brown urine, or signs of fluid retention, including swelling of extremities and unexplained rapid weight gain.

• Caution pregnant patient not to take NSAIDs such as ketoprofen during the last trimester because they may cause premature closure of the ductus arteriosus.

• Explain that ketoprofen may increase the risk of serious adverse cardiovascular reactions; urge patient to seek immediate medical attention if signs or symptoms arise, such as chest pain, shortness of breath, weakness, and slurring of speech.

• Explain that ketoprofen may increase the risk of serious adverse GI reactions; stress the importance of seeking immediate medical attention for such signs and symptoms as epigastric or abdominal pain, indigestion, black or tarry stools, or vomiting blood or material that looks like coffee grounds.

• Alert patient to rare but serious skin reactions. Urge him to seek immediate medical attention for rash, blisters, itching, fever, or other indications of hypersensitivity.

# ketorolac tromethamine

Toradol

## Class and Category

*Chemical:* Acetic acid derivative
*Therapeutic:* Analgesic, anti-inflammatory
*Pregnancy category:* C

## Indications and Dosages

➤ *To treat moderate to severe pain*

**TABLETS**

**Adults ages 16 to 64.** *Initial:* 20 mg as a single dose, followed by 10 mg q 4 to 6 hr p.r.n., up to 4 times a day. *Maximum:* 40 mg/day for no more than 5 days.

**DOSAGE ADJUSTMENT** For patients who weigh less than 50 kg, elderly patients, and patients with impaired renal function, initial dose reduced to 10 mg.

**I.M. INJECTION**

**Adults ages 16 to 64.** *Initial:* 60 mg as a single dose, followed by oral ketorolac if needed; or 30 mg q 6 hr p.r.n. *Maximum:* 120 mg/day for no more than 5 days.

**DOSAGE ADJUSTMENT** For patients who weigh less than 50 kg, elderly patients, and patients with impaired renal function, initial dose reduced to 30 mg, followed by oral ketorolac if needed; or 15 mg q 6 hr p.r.n., up to maximum of 60 mg/day for no more than 5 days.

**I.V. INJECTION**

**Adults ages 16 to 64.** *Initial:* 30 mg as a single dose, followed by oral ketorolac if needed; or 30 mg q 6 hr p.r.n. *Maximum:* 120 mg/day for no more than 5 days.

**DOSAGE ADJUSTMENT** For patients who weigh less than 50 kg, elderly patients, and patients with impaired renal function, initial dose reduced to 15 mg, followed by oral ketorolac if needed; or 15 mg q 6 hr p.r.n., up to maximum of 60 mg/day for no more than 5 days.

| Route | Onset | Peak | Duration |
|---|---|---|---|
| P.O. | 30 to 60 min | 2 to 3 hr | 5 to 6 hr |
| I.M., I.V. | 30 to 60 min | 1 to 2 hr | 4 to 6 hr |

## Mechanism of Action

Blocks cyclooxygenase, an enzyme needed to synthesize prostaglandins. Prostaglandins mediate the inflammatory response and cause local vasodilation, swelling, and pain. They also promote pain transmission from the periphery to the spinal cord. By blocking cyclooxygenase and inhibiting prostaglandins, this NSAID reduces inflammation and relieves pain.

## Contraindications

Advanced renal impairment or risk of renal impairment due to volume depletion; before or during surgery if hemostasis is critical; breast-feeding; cerebrovascular bleeding; concurrent use of aspirin or other salicylates, other NSAIDs, or probenecid; hemorrhagic diathesis; history of GI bleeding, GI perforation, or peptic ulcer disease; hemophilia or other bleeding problems, including coagulation or platelet function disorders; hypersensitivity to ketorolac tromethamine, aspirin, other NSAIDs, or their components; incomplete hemostasis; labor and delivery

## Interactions

**DRUGS**

*ACE inhibitors:* Increased risk of renal impairment

*acetaminophen, gold compounds:* Increased risk of adverse renal effects
*amphotericin, penicillamine, and other nephrotoxic drugs:* Increased risk or severity of adverse renal reactions
*corticosteroids, potassium supplements:* Increased risk of gastric ulcers or hemorrhage
*antihypertensives, diuretics:* Possibly reduced effects of these drugs
*aspirin and other salicylates, other NSAIDs:* Additive toxicity
*cefamandole, cefoperazone, cefotetan:* Possibly hypoprothrombinemia
*furosemide:* Decreased effects of furosemide
*heparin, oral anticoagulants, platelet aggregation inhibitors, thrombolytics:* Increased risk of GI bleeding and I.M. hematoma formation
*lithium:* Possibly increased blood lithium level and increased risk of lithium toxicity
*methotrexate:* Possibly methotrexate toxicity
*plicamycin, valproic acid:* Possibly hypoprothrombinemia and increased risk of bleeding
*probenecid:* Decreased elimination of ketorolac, increased risk of adverse effects

**ACTIVITIES**
*alcohol use:* Increased risk of adverse GI effects

### Adverse Reactions
**CNS:** Dizziness, drowsiness, headache
**CV:** Edema, fluid retention, hypertension
**EENT:** Stomatitis
**GI:** Abdominal pain; bloating; constipation; diarrhea; flatulence; GI bleeding, perforation, or ulceration; hepatic failure; indigestion; nausea; vomiting
**SKIN:** Diaphoresis, pruritus, rash
**Other:** Anaphylaxis, injection site pain, unusual weight gain

### Nursing Considerations
• Read ketorolac label carefully. Don't use I.M. form for I.V. route. Be aware that ketorolac isn't for intrathecal or epidural use.
• Inject I.M. ketorolac slowly, deep into a large muscle mass. Monitor site for bleeding, bruising, or hematoma.
• Administer I.V. injection over at least 15 seconds.
• Notify prescriber if pain relief is inadequate or if breakthrough pain occurs between doses because supplemental doses of an opioid analgesic may be required.

•**WARNING** Monitor liver function test results. If elevated levels persist or worsen, notify prescriber and expect to stop drug, as ordered, to prevent hepatic impairment.
•**WARNING** Monitor patients with a history of peripheral edema, heart failure, or hypertension for adequate fluid balance because drug can promote fluid retention and worsen these conditions. Assess patient for dyspnea, edema, unexplained rapid weight gain, and decreased activity tolerance. Notify prescriber if such symptoms develop.

**PATIENT TEACHING**
• Instruct patient to take ketorolac tablets with a meal, snack, or antacid to prevent stomach upset. Advise him to take drug with a full glass of water and to remain upright for at least 15 minutes after taking tablet.
• Advise patient not to use aspirin, other salicylates, or other NSAIDs while taking ketorolac without consulting prescriber. Encourage patient to limit use of acetaminophen to only a few days during ketorolac therapy and to notify prescriber of use.
• Caution patient to avoid hazardous activities until drug's CNS effects are known.
• Urge patient to avoid alcohol while taking drug.
• Encourage patient to have dental procedures performed before starting drug therapy because of increased risk of bleeding.
• Teach patient proper oral hygiene measures, and encourage him to use a soft-bristled toothbrush while taking ketorolac.

# labetalol hydrochloride

Normodyne, Trandate

### Class and Category
*Chemical:* Benzamine derivative
*Therapeutic:* Antihypertensive
*Pregnancy category:* C

### Indications and Dosages
➤ *To manage hypertension*
**TABLETS**
**Adults.** *Initial:* 100 mg b.i.d., increased by 100 mg b.i.d. as needed and tolerated q 2 to 3 days. *Maintenance:* 200 to 400 mg b.i.d. For severe hypertension, 1.2 to 2.4 g/day in divided doses b.i.d. or t.i.d.

➤ *To manage severe hypertension and treat hypertensive emergencies*

**I.V. INFUSION**
**Adults.** 200 mg diluted in 160 ml of D$_5$W and infused at 2 mg/min until desired response occurs.
**I.V. INJECTION**
**Adults.** 20 mg given over 2 min; additional doses given in increments of 40 to 80 mg q 10 min as indicated until desired response occurs. *Maximum:* 300 mg.

| Route | Onset | Peak | Duration |
|-------|-------|------|----------|
| P.O. | 20 min to 2 hr | 1 to 4 hr | 8 to 24 hr |
| I.V. | 2 to 5 min | 5 to 15 min | 2 to 4 hr |

## Mechanism of Action
Selectively blocks alpha$_1$ and beta$_2$ receptors in vascular smooth muscle and beta$_1$ receptors in the heart. These actions reduce peripheral vascular resistance and blood pressure. Potent beta blockade prevents reflex tachycardia, which commonly occurs when alpha blockers reduce the resting heart rate, cardiac output, or stroke volume.

## Incompatibilities
Don't dilute labetalol in sodium bicarbonate solution or administer through same I.V. line as alkaline drugs, such as furosemide; doing so may cause white precipitate to form.

## Contraindications
Asthma, cardiogenic shock, heart failure, hypersensitivity to labetalol or its components, second- or third-degree heart block, severe bradycardia

## Interactions
**DRUGS**
*allergen immunotherapy, allergenic extracts for skin testing:* Increased risk of serious systemic reaction or anaphylaxis
*calcium channel blockers, clonidine, diazoxide, guanabenz, reserpine:* Possibly hypotension
*cimetidine:* Possibly increased labetalol effects
*estrogens, NSAIDs:* Possibly reduced antihypertensive effect of labetalol
*general anesthetics:* Increased risk of hypotension and myocardial depression
*insulin, oral antidiabetic drugs:* Increased risk of hyperglycemia

*nitroglycerin:* Possibly hypertension
*phenoxybenzamine, phentolamine:* Possibly additive alpha$_1$-blocking effects
*sympathomimetics with alpha- and beta-adrenergic effects (such as pseudoephedrine):* Possibly hypertension, excessive bradycardia, or heart block
*xanthines (aminophylline and theophylline):* Possibly decreased therapeutic effects of both drugs
**FOODS**
*all food:* Increased blood labetalol level
**ACTIVITIES**
*alcohol use:* Increased labetalol effects

## Adverse Reactions
**CNS:** Anxiety, confusion, depression, dizziness, drowsiness, fatigue, paresthesia, syncope, vertigo, weakness, yawning
**CV:** Bradycardia, chest pain, edema, heart block, heart failure, hypotension, orthostatic hypotension, ventricular arrhythmias
**EENT:** Nasal congestion, taste perversion
**GI:** Elevated liver function test results, hepatic necrosis, hepatitis, indigestion, nausea, vomiting
**GU:** Ejaculation failure, impotence
**RESP:** Dyspnea, wheezing
**SKIN:** Jaundice, pruritus, rash, scalp tingling

## Nursing Considerations
•During I.V. labetalol administration, monitor blood pressure according to facility policy, usually every 5 minutes for 30 minutes, then every 30 minutes for 2 hours, and then every hour for 6 hours.
•Keep patient in supine position for 3 hours after I.V. administration.
•**WARNING** Be aware that labetalol masks common signs of shock.
•Monitor blood glucose level in diabetic patient because labetalol may conceal symptoms of hypoglycemia.
•Be aware that stopping labetalol tablets abruptly after long-term therapy could result in angina, MI, or ventricular arrhythmias. Expect to taper dosage over 2 weeks while monitoring response.
**PATIENT TEACHING**
•Advise patient to report confusion, difficulty breathing, rash, slow pulse, and swelling in arms or legs.

•Caution patient not to discontinue drug abruptly because doing so could cause angina and rebound hypertension.
•Suggest that patient minimize effects of orthostatic hypotension by rising slowly, avoiding sudden position changes, and taking drug at bedtime, if approved by prescriber.
•Instruct diabetic patient to monitor blood glucose level frequently and to be alert for signs of hypoglycemia.
•Inform patient that scalp tingling may occur during the early phase of treatment but is transient.
•Urge patient to avoid alcohol during labetalol therapy.

# lactulose

Acilac (CAN), Cephulac, Cholac, Chronulac, Constilac, Constulose, Duphalac, Enulose, Evalose, Heptalac, Lactulax (CAN), Laxilose (CAN), PMS-Lactulose (CAN), Portalac

## Class and Category
*Chemical:* Synthetic disaccharide sugar
*Therapeutic:* Ammonia reducer, laxative
*Pregnancy category:* B

## Indications and Dosages
➤ *To treat constipation*
**POWDER, SYRUP**
**Adults.** *Initial:* 10 to 20 g/day, increased p.r.n. *Maximum:* 40 g/day.
➤ *To prevent and treat hepatic encephalopathy*
**POWDER, SYRUP**
**Adults.** *Initial:* 20 to 30 g t.i.d. or q.i.d. until two or three soft stools occur daily. *Usual:* 60 to 100 g/day in divided doses. For acute episodes, 20 to 30 g q 2 hr initially to achieve rapid laxative effect and then reduced to usual dosage.
**RETENTION ENEMA**
**Adults.** 200 g (300 ml) diluted in 700 ml of water or NS and given q 4 to 6 hr, as needed.

| Route | Onset | Peak | Duration |
|-------|-------|------|----------|
| P.O. | 24 to 48 hr | Unknown | Unknown |

## Contraindications
Hypersensitivity to lactulose or its components, low-galactose diet

## Mechanism of Action
Arrives unchanged in the colon, where it breaks down into lactic acid and small amounts of formic and acetic acids, acidifying fecal contents. Acidification leads to increased osmotic pressure in the colon, which, in turn, increases stool water content and softens stool.

Also, lactulose makes the intestinal contents more acidic than blood. This prevents ammonia diffusion from the intestines into the blood, as occurs in hepatic encephalopathy. The trapped ammonia is converted into ammonia ions and, by lactulose's cathartic effect, is expelled in the feces (with other nitrogenous wastes).

## Interactions
**DRUGS**
*antacids, antibiotics (especially oral neomycin), other laxatives:* Decreased effectiveness of lactulose

## Adverse Reactions
**GI:** Abdominal cramps and distention, diarrhea, flatulence
**ENDO:** Hyperglycemia
**Other:** Hypernatremia, hypokalemia, hypovolemia

## Nursing Considerations
•When giving lactulose by retention enema, use a rectal tube with a balloon to help patient retain enema for 30 to 60 minutes. If not retained for at least 30 minutes, repeat dose. Be sure to deflate the balloon and remove the rectal tube after administration has been completed.
•Expect to periodically check serum electrolyte levels of elderly or debilitated patient who uses oral drug longer than 6 months.
•Monitor blood ammonia level in patient with hepatic encephalopathy. Also monitor for dehydration, hypernatremia, and hypokalemia when giving higher lactulose doses to treat this condition.
•Monitor diabetic patient for hyperglycemia because lactulose contains galactose and lactose.
•Plan to replace fluids if frequent bowel movements cause hypovolemia.

J
K
L

PATIENT TEACHING
• Advise patient to take lactulose with food or to dilute it with juice to minimize sweet taste.
• Direct patient not to use other laxatives while taking lactulose.
• Instruct patient to report abdominal distention or severe diarrhea.
• Advise diabetic patient to monitor blood glucose level frequently and to report hyperglycemia.
• Instruct patient to increase fluid intake if frequent bowel movements occur.
• Teach patient with chronic constipation the importance of exercising, increasing fiber in her diet, and increasing fluid intake.
• Inform patient that because oral lactulose must reach the colon to work, bowel movement may not occur for 24 to 48 hours after taking drug.

# lamotrigine

Lamictal

## Class and Category
*Chemical:* Phenyltriazine
*Therapeutic:* Anticonvulsant
*Pregnancy category:* C

## Indications and Dosages
➤ *As adjunct to treat partial seizures and Lennox-Gastaut syndrome*
CHEWABLE TABLETS, TABLETS
**Adults and children age 12 and older also taking enzyme-inducing anticonvulsants.** 50 mg q.d. for 2 wk and then 100 mg/day in divided doses b.i.d. for 2 wk. Increased by 100 mg q 1 to 2 wk, if needed. *Maintenance:* 300 to 500 mg/day in divided doses b.i.d. *Maximum:* 700 mg/day in divided doses b.i.d.
**Children ages 2 to 12 also taking enzyme-inducing anticonvulsants.** 0.6 mg/kg/day in divided doses b.i.d. for 2 wk and then 1.2 mg/kg/day in divided doses b.i.d. for 2 wk. Increased by 1.2 mg/kg q 1 to 2 wk, if needed to reach maintenance dosage. *Maintenance:* 5 to 15 mg/kg/day in divided doses b.i.d. *Maximum:* 400 mg/day.
**Adults and children age 12 and older also taking enzyme-inducing anticonvulsants and valproic acid.** 25 mg q.o.d. for 2 wk, followed by 25 mg q.d. for 2 wk. Increased by 25 to 50 mg q 1 to 2 wk, if needed. *Maintenance:* 100 to 400 mg/day as a single dose or in divided doses b.i.d. *Maximum:* 400 mg/day.

**Children ages 2 to 12 also taking enzyme-inducing anticonvulsants and valproic acid.** 0.15 mg/kg/day as a single dose or in divided doses b.i.d. for 2 wk and then 0.3 mg/kg/day as a single dose or in divided doses b.i.d. for next 2 wk. Increased by 0.3 mg/kg q 1 to 2 wk, if needed to reach maintenance dosage. *Maintenance:* 1 to 5 mg/kg/day as a single dose or in divided doses b.i.d. *Maximum:* 200 mg/day.
➤ *To treat partial seizures after conversion from an enzyme-inducing anticonvulsant*
CHEWABLE TABLETS, TABLETS
**Adults.** With enzyme-inducing anticonvulsant, 50 mg q.d. for 2 wk, followed by 100 mg q.d. for next 2 wk. Increased by 100 mg q 1 to 2 wk (while continuing to take enzyme-inducing anticonvulsant), if needed until usual maintenance dosage—500 mg/day in divided doses b.i.d.—is achieved. Then, enzyme-inducing anticonvulsant is tapered over 4 wk and discontinued.
➤ *To delay the time to occurrence of mood episodes (depression, mania, hypomania, mixed episodes) as maintenance therapy for bipolar I disorder*
CHEWABLE TABLETS, TABLETS
**Adults.** 25 mg q.d. for 2 wk, followed by 50 mg q.d. for 2 wk, followed by 100 mg q.d. for 1 wk and then increased to 200 mg q.d. as maintenance dose. *Maximum:* 200 mg/day. Adults also taking valproic acid. 25 mg q.o.d. for 2 wk, followed by 25 mg q.d. for 2 wk, followed by 50 mg q.d. for 1 wk, and then increased to 100 mg q.d. as maintenance dose.
DOSAGE ADJUSTMENT If valproic acid is discontinued, lamotrigine dosage is doubled over a 2-wk period in equal weekly increments.
**Adults taking carbamazepine or other enzyme-inducing drugs, excluding valproic acid.** 50 mg q.d. for 2 wk, followed by 100 mg q.d. in divided doses for 2 wk, followed by 200 mg q.d. in divided doses for 1 wk, followed by 300 mg q.d. in divided doses for 1 wk, and then increased up to 400 mg q.d. in divided doses as maintenance dose.
DOSAGE ADJUSTMENT If carbamazepine or other enzyme-inducing drug is discontinued, lamotrigine dosage is kept constant for 1 wk, then decreased by 50% over a 2-wk period in equal weekly increments.

| Route | Onset | Peak | Duration |
|-------|-------|------|----------|
| P.O. | Days to wks | Unknown | Unknown |

## Mechanism of Action
May stabilize neuron membranes by blocking their sodium channels and inhibiting release of excitatory neurotransmitters, such as glutamate and aspartate, through these channels. By blocking the release of neurotransmitters, lamotrigine inhibits the spread of seizure activity in the brain and reduces seizure frequency.

## Contraindications
Hypersensitivity to lamotrigine or its components

## Interactions
**DRUGS**
*acetaminophen (long-term use):* Possibly decreased blood lamotrigine level
*carbamazepine, phenobarbital, phenytoin, primidone:* Decreased blood lamotrigine level, possibly increased CNS depression
*folate inhibitors, such as co-trimoxazole and methotrexate:* Increased blood lamotrigine level
*valproic acid:* Increased blood lamotrigine level, decreased lamotrigine clearance, decreased blood valproic acid level
**ACTIVITIES**
*alcohol use:* Possibly increased CNS depression

## Adverse Reactions
**CNS:** Amnesia, anxiety, ataxia, confusion, depression, dizziness, drowsiness, emotional lability, fever, headache, increased seizure activity, lack of coordination
**CV:** Chest pain
**EENT:** Blurred vision, diplopia, dry mouth, nystagmus
**GI:** Abdominal pain, anorexia, constipation, diarrhea, vomiting
**HEME:** Anemia, eosinophilia, leukopenia, thrombocytopenia
**SKIN:** Petechiae, photosensitivity, pruritus, rash, Stevens-Johnson syndrome, toxic epidermal necrolysis
**Other:** Angioedema, flulike symptoms, lymphadenopathy

## Nursing Considerations
•**WARNING** Lamotrigine may cause potentially life-threatening rash. Notify prescriber at first sign, and expect to discontinue drug.
•Monitor for seizure activity during therapy.
•Be aware that abrupt discontinuation of lamotrigine may cause increased seizure activity. Expect to taper dosage over at least 2 weeks even for treatment of bipolar disorder.
**PATIENT TEACHING**
•Advise patient to take lamotrigine exactly as prescribed and not to stop drug abruptly because seizure activity may increase.
•Advise patient to notify prescriber immediately if rash occurs.
•Instruct patient to report increased seizure activity, vision changes, and vomiting.
•Caution patient to avoid potentially hazardous activities until drug's CNS effects are known.
•Advise patient to avoid direct sunlight and to wear protective clothing to minimize the risk of photosensitivity.
•Instruct patient to wear medical identification stating that she takes an anticonvulsant.

# lansoprazole
Prevacid, Prevacid I.V., Prevacid SoluTab

## Class and Category
*Chemical:* Substituted benzimidazole
*Therapeutic:* Antisecretory, antiulcer
*Pregnancy category:* B

## Indications and Dosages
➤ *To treat duodenal ulcers and maintain healed duodenal ulcers*
**DELAYED-RELEASE CAPSULES, DELAYED-RELEASE SUSPENSION, DELAYED-RELEASE ORALLY DISINTEGRATING TABLETS**
**Adults.** 15 to 30 mg q.d. a.c. in the morning for 4 wk. *Maximum:* 30 mg/day.
➤ *To treat gastric ulcers*
**DELAYED-RELEASE CAPSULES, DELAYED-RELEASE SUSPENSION, DELAYED-RELEASE ORALLY DISINTEGRATING TABLETS**
**Adults.** 15 to 30 mg q.d. a.c. in the morning for up to 8 wk.
➤ *To treat gastroesophageal reflux disease*
**DELAYED-RELEASE CAPSULES, DELAYED-RELEASE SUSPENSION, DELAYED-RELEASE ORALLY DISINTEGRATING TABLETS**
**Adults.** 15 mg q.d. a.c. in the morning for up to 8 wk.

J K L

▶ *To treat erosive esophagitis*
DELAYED-RELEASE CAPSULES, DELAYED-RELEASE SUSPEN-
SION, DELAYED-RELEASE ORALLY DISINTEGRATING TABLETS
**Adults.** *Initial:* 30 mg q.d. a.c. in the morning
for up to 8 wk. Continued an additional 8
wk if indicated. *Maintenance:* 15 mg q.d.

▶ *To treat erosive esophagitis short-term*
*(up to 7 days) in patients unable to take*
*oral medication*
**I.V.** INFUSION
**Adults.** 30 mg q.d. infused over 30 min for
up to 7 days.

▶ *To treat pathological hypersecretory*
*conditions, such as Zollinger-Ellison*
*syndrome*
DELAYED-RELEASE CAPSULES, DELAYED-RELEASE SUSPEN-
SION, DELAYED-RELEASE ORALLY DISINTEGRATING TABLETS
**Adults.** *Initial:* 60 mg q.d. a.c. in the morning, increased as needed according to patient's condition. Doses exceeding 120 mg/
day administered in divided doses. *Maxi-*
*mum:* 180 mg/day.

▶ *To eradicate* Helicobacter pylori *and*
*reduce risk of duodenal ulcer recur-*
*rence*
DELAYED-RELEASE CAPSULES, DELAYED-RELEASE SUSPEN-
SION, DELAYED-RELEASE ORALLY DISINTEGRATING TABLETS
**Adults.** 30 mg plus 1 g of amoxicillin and
500 mg of clarithromycin q 12 hr a.c. for 10
to 14 days. Alternatively, 30 mg plus 1 g of
amoxicillin t.i.d. a.c. for 14 days.

▶ *To treat symptomatic pediatric gastro-*
*esophageal reflux disease*
DELAYED-RELEASE CAPSULES, DELAYED-RELEASE SUSPEN-
SION, DELAYED-RELEASE ORALLY DISINTEGRATING TABLETS
**Children ages 12 to 17.** 15 mg q.d. for up to
8 wk.
**Children ages 1 to 11 weighing 30 kg (66 lb)**
**or less.** 15 mg q.d. for up to 12 wk.
**Children ages 1 to 11 weighing more than**
**30 kg.** 30 mg q.d. for up to 12 wk.

▶ *To treat symptomatic pediatric erosive*
*esophagitis*
DELAYED-RELEASE CAPSULES, DELAYED-RELEASE SUSPEN-
SION, DELAYED-RELEASE ORALLY DISINTEGRATING TABLETS
**Children ages 12 to 17.** 30 mg q.d. for up to
8 wk.
**Children ages 1 to 11 weighing 30 kg (66 lb)**
**or less.** 15 mg q.d. for up to 12 wk.
**Children ages 1 to 11 weighing more than**
**30 kg.** 30 mg q.d. for up to 12 wk.

| Route | Onset | Peak | Duration |
|-------|-------|------|----------|
| P.O. | 1 to 3 hr | Unknown | Over 24 hr |

## Mechanism of Action
Binds to and inactivates the hydrogen-
potassium adenosine triphosphate enzyme
system (also called the proton pump) in
gastric parietal cells. This action blocks
the final step of gastric acid production.

## Incompatibilities
Don't give any other drugs with parenteral
lansoprazole, and dilute only with solutions
recommended by manufacturer (sterile water
for initial reconstitution and NS, LR, or $D_5W$
for further dilution).

## Contraindications
Hypersensitivity to lansoprazole or its components

## Interactions
DRUGS
*ampicillin, digoxin, iron salts, ketoconazole,*
*other drugs that depend on low gastric pH*
*for bioavailability:* Inhibited absorption of
these drugs
*sucralfate:* Delayed lansoprazole absorption
*theophylline:* Slightly decreased blood theophylline level

## Adverse Reactions
**CNS:** Dizziness, headache
**GI:** Abdominal pain, anorexia, diarrhea, he-
patotoxicity, increased appetite, nausea, pan-
creatitis, pseudomembranous colitis, vomiting
**GU:** Urine retention
**HEME:** Agranulocytosis, aplastic anemia, he-
molytic anemia, leukopenia, neutropenia,
pancytopenia, thrombocytopenia, thrombotic
thrombocytopenic purpura
**MS:** Arthralgia
**SKIN:** Erythema multiforme, pruritus, rash,
Stevens-Johnson syndrome, toxic epidermal
necrolysis
**Other:** Anaphylaxis, injection site reaction

## Nursing Considerations
•Give patient lansoprazole before meals.
Antacids may be given as well, if needed.
•If patient is prescribed capsules and has
trouble swallowing, open capsule and sprin-

kle granules on applesauce, Ensure pudding, cottage cheese, yogurt, or strained pears. Don't crush the granules, and have patient swallow the mixture immediately. Or empty granules into 2 ounces of apple, orange, or tomato juice; mix quickly, and have patient swallow immediately. Then add 2 or more ounces of juice to glass and have patient drink immediately to ensure a full dose.
•For patient prescribed delayed-release orally disintegrating tablets, place tablet on tongue and let it dissolve, with or without water, until patient can swallow particles.
•For patient with NG tube, don't use oral suspension. Instead use capsules or orally disintegrating tablets. For capsule form, open capsule, mix granules in 40 ml of apple juice only, and inject through tube. Then flush tube with apple juice only. For disintegrating tablets, place tablet in syringe and draw up 4 ml (for 15-mg tablet) or 8 ml (for 30-mg tablet) of water. Shake gently, and inject through tube within 15 minutes. Then refill syringe with 5 ml of water, shake gently, and inject through tube.
•For delayed-release oral suspension, empty packet contents into a container with 2 tablespoons of water (no other liquids or foods should be used), stir well, and have patient drink immediately. If any particles remain in container, add more water, stir, and have patient drink again immediately.
•Reconstitute parenteral form by injecting 5 ml of sterile water into 30-mg vial of drug. Mix gently until powder dissolves. Use within 1 hour. After reconstitution, dilute with 50 ml of NS, LR, or $D_5W$. Give within 12 hours if mixed with $D_5W$ or 24 hours if mixed with NS or LR.
•Give parenteral drug with a filter following manufacturer's guidelines. Change filter every 24 hours. Give as an I.V. infusion over 30 minutes. Flush the line with NS, LR, or $D_5W$ before and after giving lansoprazole.
•Expect to use lansoprazole with antibiotics because decreased gastric acid secretion helps antibiotics eradicate *H. pylori*.
•If given with antibiotics, watch for diarrhea from possible pseudomembranous colitis.

**PATIENT TEACHING**
•Urge patient to take lansoprazole as prescribed, usually before a meal (preferably breakfast) to decrease gastric acid output.

•Tell patient who has trouble swallowing capsules to open them and sprinkle granules on applesauce, Ensure pudding, cottage cheese, yogurt, or strained pears. Tell her not to chew granules but to swallow immediately. Or she may empty granules into 2 ounces of apple, orange, or tomato juice; mix quickly; and swallow immediately. Tell her to refill glass with 2 or more ounces of juice and drink immediately to ensure a full dose.
•Tell patient prescribed delayed-release orally disintegrating tablets to place the tablet on her tongue, let it dissolve with or without water, and swallow the particles.
•Tell patient prescribed delayed-release oral suspension to empty contents of packet into a container with 2 tablespoons of water (no other liquids or foods), stir well, and drink immediately. If she notices any particles remaining in container, tell her to add more water, stir, and drink immediately.
•Inform patient that she may take antacids with lansoprazole.
•Advise patient to report diarrhea, severe headache, or worsening of symptoms immediately to prescriber.

# lanthanum carbonate

Fosrenol

## Class and Category
*Chemical:* Rare earth element
*Therapeutic:* Phosphate binder
*Pregnancy category:* C

## Indications and Dosages
➤ *To reduce serum phosphate levels in patients with end-stage renal disease*
**TABLETS**
**Adults.** *Initial:* 250 to 500 mg t.i.d. with meals; increased, as needed, by 750 mg daily q 2 to 3 wk until an acceptable serum phosphate level is reached.

## Contraindications
Bowel obstruction, hypersensitivity to lanthanum carbonate or any of its components, hypophosphatemia

## Interactions
None known.

## Mechanism of Action

During digestion, phosphate is released into the upper GI tract (below left) and absorbed into the bloodstream, increasing serum phosphate levels. In patients with end-stage renal disease, however, inefficient phosphate clearance from the blood leads to abnormally elevated levels.

Lanthanum dissociates in the upper GI tract, releasing ions that attach to unbound phosphate to form an insoluble complex (below right). Unabsorbed into the bloodstream, these altered phosphate molecules can't elevate the patient's serum phosphate level.

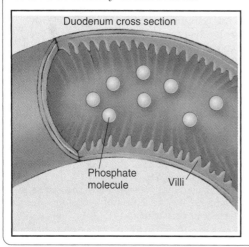

Duodenum cross section

Phosphate molecule    Villi

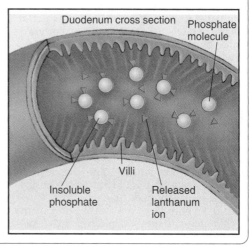

Duodenum cross section    Phosphate molecule

Villi

Insoluble phosphate    Released lanthanum ion

## Adverse Reactions

**CNS:** Headache
**CV:** Hypotension
**EENT:** Rhinitis
**ENDO:** Hypercalcemia
**GI:** Abdominal pain, constipation, diarrhea, nausea, vomiting
**GU:** Dialysis graft occlusion
**RESP:** Bronchitis

## Nursing Considerations

•Use lanthanum carbonate cautiously in patients with acute peptic ulcer, ulcerative colitis, Crohn's disease, or bowel obstruction because drug effects are unknown in these patients.
•Monitor the patient's serum phosphate levels, as ordered, especially during dosage titration, to determine effectiveness of lanthanum carbonate therapy. Serum phosphate levels should fall below 6.0 mg/dl.

### PATIENT TEACHING

•Instruct patient to take lanthanum carbonate with or immediately after meals.

•Advise patient to chew each tablet thoroughly before swallowing.
•Urge patient to take drug exactly as prescribed, and explain that it may take weeks to reach a desired serum phosphate level.

# leflunomide

Arava

## Class and Category

*Chemical:* Malonitrilamide immunomodulator
*Therapeutic:* Antirheumatic
*Pregnancy category:* X

## Indications and Dosages

➤ *To relieve symptoms of active rheumatoid arthritis, improve physical function and slow disease progression*

### TABLETS

**Adults.** *Loading:* 100 mg q.d. for 3 days. *Maintenance:* 20 mg q.d., reduced to 10 mg q.d. if poorly tolerated. *Maximum:* 20 mg/day.

## Mechanism of Action
Inhibits dihydroorotate dehydrogenase, the enzyme in the autoimmune process that leads to rheumatoid arthritis. This action relieves inflammation and prevents alteration of the autoimmune process.

## Contraindications
Hypersensitivity to leflunomide or its components, pregnancy

## Interactions
**DRUGS**
*activated charcoal, cholestyramine:* Decreased blood leflunomide level
*methotrexate:* Risk of hepatotoxicity
*NSAIDs:* Possibly impaired NSAID metabolism
*rifampin, tolbutamide:* Increased blood leflunomide level
*vaccines (live-virus):* Possibly adverse reactions to vaccines caused by leflunomide-induced immunosuppression

## Adverse Reactions
**CNS:** Anxiety, dizziness, drowsiness, fatigue, fever, headache, paresthesia
**CV:** Chest pain, hypertension, palpitations, tachycardia
**EENT:** Blurred vision, conjunctivitis, dry mouth, epistaxis, mouth ulcers, pharyngitis, rhinitis, sinusitis
**GI:** Abdominal pain, cholestasis, constipation, diarrhea, elevated liver function test results, flatulence, gastritis, gastroenteritis, hepatic failure, hepatitis, nausea, vomiting
**GU:** UTI
**HEME:** Agranulocytosis, anemia, pancytopenia, thrombocytopenia
**MS:** Back pain, synovitis, tendinitis
**RESP:** Asthma, bronchitis, dyspnea, interstitial lung disease, respiratory tract infection
**SKIN:** Alopecia (transient), erythematous rash, jaundice, pruritus, urticaria
**Other:** Sepsis, weight loss

## Nursing Considerations
• Assess liver enzyme (ALT and AST) levels at start of therapy, monthly during first 6 months, and if stable, every 6 to 8 weeks thereafter, as ordered. Expect to stop drug if hepatic dysfunction develops.
• Obtain platelet count, WBC count, and hemoglobin or hematocrit at beginning of therapy and every 4 to 8 weeks thereafter, as ordered.

• Notify prescriber if patient develops a serious infection because leflunomide may need to be interrupted and cholestyramine or charcoal may be required to eliminate drug rapidly.
• **WARNING** Monitor patient's respiratory function closely because drug may cause interstitial lung disease that could become life-threatening. If patient develops a cough and dyspnea, notify prescriber; drug may need to be stopped, and patient may need cholestyramine or charcoal to eliminate drug rapidly.

**PATIENT TEACHING**
• Advise patient that leflunomide doesn't cure arthritis but may relieve its symptoms and improve physical function.
• Inform patient that reversible hair loss may occur.
• Caution female patient of childbearing potential not to become pregnant while taking drug because of the high risk of birth defects.
• Instruct patient to report signs of hepatotoxicity, such as mouth ulcers, unusual bleeding or bruising, and yellow skin or eyes.
• Tell patient to report signs of respiratory dysfunction, such as cough and dyspnea.
• Advise patient to avoid live vaccines during leflunomide therapy.
• Instruct patient to notify prescriber if she develops an infection.

# lepirudin
Refludan

## Class and Category
*Chemical:* Yeast-derived recombinant form of hirudin
*Therapeutic:* Anticoagulant
*Pregnancy category:* B

## Indications and Dosages
➤ *To prevent thromboembolic complications in patients with heparin-induced thrombocytopenia and associated thromboembolic disease*

**I.V. INFUSION AND INJECTION**
**Adults.** *Initial:* 0.4 mg/kg, but no more than 44 mg, given by bolus over 15 to 20 sec, followed by continuous infusion of 0.15 mg/kg/hr for 2 to 10 days or longer, as indicated. *Maximum:* 0.21 mg/kg/hr.
**DOSAGE ADJUSTMENT** For patients with renal insufficiency, bolus dose decreased to 0.2 mg/kg and infusion rate adjusted as follows: for

creatinine clearance of 45 to 60 ml/min/ 1.73 m$^2$, 50% of standard infusion rate; for creatinine clearance of 30 to 44 ml/min/ 1.73 m$^2$, 30% of standard infusion rate; for creatinine clearance of 15 to 29 ml/min/ 1.73 m$^2$, 15% of standard infusion rate; for clearance of less than 15 ml/min/1.73 m$^2$, expect drug to be stopped.

| Route | Onset | Peak | Duration |
|-------|-------|------|----------|
| I.V. | Immediate | Unknown | Unknown |

## Mechanism of Action
Forms a tight bond with thrombin, neutralizing this enzyme's actions, even when the enzyme is trapped within clots. One molecule of lepirudin binds with one molecule of thrombin. Thrombin causes fibrinogen to convert to fibrin, which is essential for clot formation.

## Incompatibilities
Don't mix lepirudin in same I.V. line with other drugs.

## Contraindications
Hypersensitivity to lepirudin or other hirudins

## Interactions
*oral anticoagulants, platelet aggregation inhibitors, thrombolytics:* Increased risk of bleeding complications and enhanced effects of lepirudin

## Adverse Reactions
**CNS:** Chills, fever, intracranial hemorrhage
**CV:** Heart failure
**EENT:** Epistaxis
**GI:** GI or rectal bleeding, hepatic dysfunction
**GU:** Hematuria, vaginal bleeding
**HEME:** Anemia, easy bruising, hematoma
**RESP:** Hemoptysis, pneumonia
**SKIN:** Excessive bleeding from wounds, rash, pruritus, urticaria
**Other:** Anaphylaxis, injection site bleeding, sepsis

## Nursing Considerations
• Be aware that patients with heparin-induced thrombocytopenia have low platelet counts, which can lead to severe bleeding and even death. Lepirudin prevents clotting without further reducing platelet count.

• To reconstitute, mix drug with NS or sterile water for injection. Warm solution to room temperature before administering.
• For I.V. bolus, reconstitute 50 mg with 1 ml of sterile water for injection or sodium chloride for injection. Then further dilute by withdrawing reconstituted solution into a 10-ml syringe and adding enough sterile water for injection, sodium chloride for injection, or D$_5$W to produce a total volume of 10 ml, or 5 mg of lepirudin/ml. Administer prescribed dose over 15 to 20 seconds.
• For I.V. infusion, reconstitute 2 vials of drug and transfer to infusion bag that contains 250 or 500 ml of NS or D$_5$W. Concentration will be 0.4 or 0.2 mg/ml.
• Adjust infusion rate as prescribed, according to patient's APTT ratio, which is APTT divided by a control value. Target APTT ratio during treatment is 1.5 to 2.5.
• Expect to obtain first APTT 4 hours after starting infusion and to obtain follow-up APTT daily (more often for patients with hepatic or renal impairment).
• Stop infusion for 2 hours, as ordered, if APTT is above target range. Expect to decrease infusion rate by one-half when restarting. If APTT is below target range, expect to increase rate in 20% increments and recheck APTT in 4 hours.
• Avoid I.M. injections or needle sticks during therapy to minimize risk of hematoma.
• Observe I.M. injection sites, I.V. infusion sites, and wounds for bleeding.
• Monitor for ecchymoses on arms and legs, epistaxis, hematemesis, hematuria, melena, and vaginal bleeding.

**PATIENT TEACHING**
• Tell patient to report unexpected bleeding, such as blood in urine, easy bruising, nosebleeds, tarry stools, and vaginal bleeding.
• Advise patient to avoid bumping arms and legs because of the risk of bruising.
• Encourage patient to use an electric razor and a soft toothbrush to reduce the risk of bleeding.

# leuprolide acetate

Eligard 7.5 mg, Eligard 22.5 mg, Lupron, Lupron Depot, Lupron Depot-3 Month 11.25 mg, Lupron Depot-3 Month 22.5 mg, Lupron Depot-4 Month 30 mg, Lupron Depot-Ped, Lupron-3 Month SR Depot 22.5 mg, Viadur

## Class and Category
*Chemical:* Synthetic peptide gonadotropin-releasing hormone analogue
*Therapeutic:* Antianemic, antiendometrionic agent, antineoplastic, gonadotropin inhibitor
*Pregnancy category:* X

## Indications and Dosages
➤ *To treat prostate cancer*
**I.M. INJECTION (LEUPROLIDE ACETATE FOR INJECTION)**
**Adults.** 7.5 mg/mo, 22.5 mg q 3 mo, or 45 mg q 4 mo.
**S.C. INJECTION (LEUPROLIDE ACETATE FOR INJECTABLE SUSPENSION)**
**Adults.** 7.5 mg/mo.
**S.C. INJECTION (LEUPROLIDE ACETATE INJECTION)**
**Adults.** 1 mg q.d.
➤ *To provide palliative treatment of advanced prostate cancer*
**IMPLANT (VIADUR)**
**Adults.** 1 implant q 12 mo.
**S.C. INJECTION (ELIGARD FOR INJECTABLE SUSPENSION)**
**Adults.** 7.5 mg/mo. 22.5 mg q 3 mo, or 45 mg q 6 mo.
➤ *To treat precocious central puberty*
**I.M. INJECTION (LEUPROLIDE ACETATE FOR INJECTION)**
**Children who weigh more than 37.5 kg (83 lb).** *Initial:* 15 mg q 4 wk. *Maintenance:* Dosage increased as needed in increments of 3.75 mg q 4 wk. *Maximum:* 15 mg q 4 wk.
**Children who weigh 25 to 37.5 kg (55 to 83 lb).** *Initial:* 11.25 mg q 4 wk. *Maintenance:* Dosage increased as needed in increments of 3.75 mg q 4 wk. *Maximum:* 15 mg q 4 wk.
**Children who weigh less than 25 kg.** *Initial:* 7.5 mg q 4 wk. *Maintenance:* Dosage increased as needed in increments of 3.75 mg q 4 wk. *Maximum:* 15 mg q 4 wk.
**S.C. INJECTION (LEUPROLIDE ACETATE INJECTION)**
**Children.** 50 mcg/kg/day. Dosage increased in increments of 10 mcg/kg/day.
➤ *To treat endometriosis*
**I.M. INJECTION (LEUPROLIDE ACETATE FOR INJECTION)**
**Adults.** 3.75 mg q mo or 11.25 mg q 3 mo for up to 6 mo. *Maximum:* 33.75 mg total dose.
➤ *As adjunct to treat anemia due to uterine leiomyomas*
**I.M. INJECTION (LEUPROLIDE ACETATE FOR INJECTION)**
**Adults.** 3.75 mg q mo up to 3 mo or 11.25 mg single dose. *Maximum:* 11.25 mg total dose.

## Contraindications
Women and children (leuprolide acetate injectable suspension); hypersensitivity to benzyl alcohol, gonadorelin, and gonadotropin-releasing hormone analogues, including leu-prolide, and their components; pregnancy; undiagnosed abnormal vaginal bleeding

## Adverse Reactions
**CNS:** Dizziness, fatigue, headache, insomnia, malaise, memory loss, paresthesia, peripheral neuropathy, syncope (all adults); anxiety, depression, mood changes, nervousness (adult females)
**CV:** Arrhythmias, edema, hypotension, palpitations (all adults); angina, MI, thrombophlebitis (adult males), vasodilation
**EENT:** Blurred vision (all adults)
**ENDO:** Breast tenderness or swelling (all adults); amenorrhea, androgenic effects (adult females); decreased size of testicles (adult males)
**GI:** Hepatic dysfunction, nausea, vomiting (all adults); constipation, gastroenteritis (adult males)
**GU:** Decreased libido (all adults); endometriosis flareup, vaginitis (adult females); impotence, prostate cancer flareup, prostate pain (adult males); uterine bleeding, vaginal discharge (female children)
**HEME:** Leukopenia
**MS:** Arthralgia, bone density loss, bone pain, myalgia, tenosynovitis (all adults); body pain (children)
**RESP:** Asthma, dyspnea, pulmonary embolism
**SKIN:** Photosensitivity, rash, urticaria
**Other:** Anaphylaxis, hot flashes, weight gain (all adults); injection site abscess, burning, edema, induration, itching, pain, or redness (adults and children)

| Route | Onset | Peak | Duration |
|---|---|---|---|
| I.M., S.C.* | 1 wk | Unknown | 4 to 12 wk after therapy |
| I.M., S.C.† | 2 to 4 wk | After 1 to 2 mo | 60 to 90 days after therapy |

*Gonadotropin inhibitor.
†Antiendometrionic, antineoplastic.

J
K
L

## Mechanism of Action

After stimulating follicle-stimulating hormone (FSH) and luteinizing hormone (LH), continuous leuprolide therapy suppresses secretion of gonadotropin-releasing hormone, decreasing testosterone and estradiol levels. In children with central precocious puberty, this stops menses and reproductive organ development.

In adult males, continuous suppression decreases testosterone levels and causes pharmacologic castration, which slows the activity of prostatic neoplastic cells. In women with endometriosis or uterine leiomyomas, leuprolide suppresses ovarian function, inactivating endometrial tissues and resulting in amenorrhea.

## Nursing Considerations

• Reconstitute leuprolide acetate depot suspension with diluent provided by manufacturer. Add diluent to powder for suspension and thoroughly shake vials to disperse particles into a uniform milky suspension. Use immediately after mixing, and discard any unused portion. If using a prefilled dual-chamber syringe, follow manufacturer's instructions to release diluent into chamber containing powder. Shake gently after diluted to disperse particles evenly in solution. Be aware that no dilution or reconstitution is needed for leuprolide acetate injection for S.C. administration. Rotate injection sites.

• **WARNING** Be aware that leuprolide acetate for injectable suspension (Eligard) is approved only for use in males for the palliative treatment of prostate cancer. Use the provided syringes and delivery system, and read and follow the instructions carefully to ensure proper mixing of the product; shaking alone is inadequate to mix the product.

• **WARNING** Monitor patient for possible allergic reaction (erythema and induration) at injection site because leuprolide injections contain benzyl alcohol. Be aware that manufacturer recommends that injection be administered by physician.

• For patient prescribed a leuprolide implant (Viadur), follow manufacturer's guidelines in preparing inner aspect of upper arm and loading implanter. Be aware that implant must be removed in 12 months. A new implant may then be inserted if needed.

• During first weeks of leuprolide therapy, monitor patient being treated for prostate cancer for initial worsening of symptoms, such as increased bone pain, difficult urination, and paresthesia or paralysis (in patients with vertebral metastasis).

• During treatment for prostate cancer, monitor patient's serum testosterone and PSA levels periodically, as ordered, to determine response to leuprolide therapy.

• Expect to stop drug before age 11 in females and age 12 in males treated for precocious central puberty.

• Monitor bone density test results, as ordered, of women at risk for osteoporosis who are receiving leuprolide because of potential for drug-induced estrogen loss, which may result in decreased bone density.

• Be aware that therapeutic doses of leuprolide suppress the pituitary-gonadal system and that normal function doesn't return until 4 to 12 weeks after drug is stopped.

**PATIENT TEACHING**

• Instruct patient who is self-administering leuprolide injection to use syringe provided by manufacturer. If manufacturer's syringe is unavailable, advise her to use only a 0.5-ml disposable, low-dose, U-100 insulin syringe to ensure accurate dosage. Substitution of syringes is not recommended for leuprolide acetate for injectable suspension.

• Inform patient prescribed Viadur that implant will be inserted under his skin on inside of his upper arm, where it can remain for up to 12 months. Reassure him that the area will be anesthetized before insertion. After insertion, tell patient to avoid heavy lifting and to keep site clean and dry for 24 hours. Also tell him that the surgical closure strip can be removed as soon as the small incision has healed (in about 3 days). Reinforce the need to make an appointment in 12 months to have the implant removed and a new one inserted.

• Advise women to immediately report monthly menses or breakthrough bleeding to prescriber.

• Instruct female patient of childbearing age to use a nonhormonal form of contraception during leuprolide therapy. Advise her to stop taking drug and notify prescriber at once if she becomes pregnant.

• Inform patient with osteoporosis or at risk for developing it that drug may increase bone density loss.

• Inform parents of child being treated for central precocious puberty that they should ex-

pect normal gonadal-pituitary function to return 4 to 12 weeks after drug is discontinued.
• Advise patient to report symptoms of depression or memory problems.
• Caution patient being treated for prostate cancer that drug may initially worsen such symptoms as bone pain and that it may cause new signs or symptoms to occur during first few weeks of treatment. Reassure patient that this is transient.

# levalbuterol hydrochloride

Xopenex, Xopenex HFA

## Class and Category

*Chemical:* Sympathomimetic amine
*Therapeutic:* Bronchodilator
*Pregnancy category:* C

## Indications and Dosages

➤ *To prevent or treat bronchospasm in reversible obstructive airway disease*
INHALATION AEROSOL
**Adults and children age 4 and older.** 45 or 90 mcg (1 or 2 inhalations) q 4 to 6 hr.
INHALATION SOLUTION
**Adults and children age 12 and older.** 0.63 to 1.25 mg t.i.d. q 6 to 8 hr. *Maximum:* 1.25 mg t.i.d.
**Children ages 6 to 11.** 0.31 to 0.63 mg t.i.d. *Maximum:* 0.63 mg t.i.d.
DOSAGE ADJUSTMENT For elderly patients, dosage limited to 0.63 mg t.i.d. q 6 to 8 hr.

| Route | Onset | Peak | Duration |
|-------|-------|------|----------|
| Inhalation | 10 to 17 min | 1.5 hr | 5 to 6 hr |

## Contraindications

Hypersensitivity to levalbuterol, other sympathomimetic amines, or their components

## Mechanism of Action

Attaches to beta$_2$ receptors on bronchial cell membranes, which stimulates the intracellular enzyme adenyl cyclase to convert adenosine triphosphate to cAMP. An increased intracellular cAMP level relaxes bronchial smooth muscle and inhibits histamine release from mast cells.

## Interactions

DRUGS
*beta blockers:* Blocked effects of both drugs
*digoxin:* Decreased blood digoxin level
*loop or thiazide diuretics:* Increased risk of hypokalemia
*MAO inhibitors, sympathomimetics, tricyclic antidepressants:* Increased risk of adverse cardiovascular effects

## Adverse Reactions

**CNS:** Anxiety, chills, dizziness, hypertonia, insomnia, migraine headache, nervousness, paresthesia, syncope, tremor
**CV:** Chest pain, hypertension, hypotension, tachycardia
**EENT:** Dry mouth and throat, rhinitis, sinusitis
**GI:** Diarrhea, indigestion, nausea, vomiting
**MS:** Leg cramps, myalgia
**RESP:** Asthma exacerbation, cough, dyspnea, paradoxical bronchospasm
**Other:** Flulike symptoms, lymphadenopathy

## Nursing Considerations

• Use levalbuterol cautiously in patients with arrhythmias, diabetes mellitus, hypertension, hyperthyroidism, or a history of seizures.
• Give oral solution form only by nebulizer.
• Monitor the patient's pulse rate and blood pressure before and after nebulizer treatment.
• Because drug may provoke paradoxical bronchospasm, observe for dyspnea, wheezing, and increased coughing.
PATIENT TEACHING
• Teach patient how to use levalbuterol nebulizer and to measure correct dose.
• Tell patient to prime inhaler before using it for the first time or when it hasn't been used for more than 3 days by releasing 4 test sprays into the air, away from her face.
• Show patient how to clean nebulizer or inhaler, and explain the need to do so at least once weekly.
• Instruct patient to notify prescriber if drug fails to work or if she needs more frequent treatments because her asthma is worsening.
• Instruct patient not to increase the dosage or frequency unless advised to do so by prescriber.
• Urge patient to stop drug and contact prescriber if paradoxical bronchospasm occurs.

J
K
L

•Instruct patient to use inhalation solution within 2 weeks of opening the foil pouch and to protect drug from light and heat.
•Urge patient to consult prescriber before using OTC or other drugs.

# levetiracetam

Keppra

## Class and Category
*Chemical:* Pyrrolidine derivative
*Therapeutic:* Anticonvulsant
*Pregnancy category:* C

## Indications and Dosages
➤ *As adjunct to treat partial seizures in patients with epilepsy*
**ORAL SOLUTION, TABLETS**
**Adults and adolescents over age 16.** *Initial:* 500 mg b.i.d., increased by 1,000 mg/day q 2 wk if needed. *Maximum:* 3,000 mg/day.
**DOSAGE ADJUSTMENT** Maximum dosage reduced to 2,000 mg/day if creatinine clearance is 50 to 80 ml/min/1.73 m$^2$; reeduced to 1,500 mg/ day if clearance is 30 to 49 ml/min/1.73 m$^2$; and reduced to 1,000 mg/day if clearance is less than 30 ml/min/1.73 m$^2$. For patients with end-stage renal disease who are receiving dialysis, expect to give another 250 to 500 mg/dose, as prescribed, after each session.
**Children ages 4 to 16.** *Initial:* 10 mg/kg b.i.d., increased by 20 mg/kg/day q 2 wk until recommended daily dose of 60 mg/kg/day is reached.
**DOSAGE ADJUSTMENT** For children who can't tolerate a daily dose of 60 mg/kg/day, dosage reduced to point of tolerance.

## Mechanism of Action
May protect against secondary generalized seizure activity by preventing coordination of epileptiform burst firing. Levetiracetam doesn't seem to involve inhibitory and excitatory neurotransmission.

## Contraindications
Hypersensitivity to levetiracetam or its components

## Adverse Reactions
**CNS:** Aggression, agitation, anger, anxiety, apathy, asthenia, ataxia, confusion, depression, dizziness, emotional lability, fatigue, headache, hostility, increased reflexes, irritability, mental or mood changes, nervousness, neurosis, paresthesia, personality disorder, somnolence, vertigo
**EENT:** Amblyopia, conjunctivitis, diplopia, ear pain, pharyngitis, rhinitis, sinusitis
**GI:** Anorexia, constipation, diarrhea, gastroenteritis, pancreatitis, vomiting
**GU:** Albuminuria
**HEME:** Leukopenia, neutropenia, pancytopenia, thrombocytopenia
**MS:** Neck pain
**RESP:** Asthma, cough
**SKIN:** Alopecia, ecchymosis, pruritus, skin discoloration, vesiculobullous rash
**Other:** Dehydration, facial edema, infection

## Nursing Considerations
•Know that children who weigh 20 kg or less should be given only the oral solution form.
•Assess compliance during first 4 weeks of therapy, when adverse reactions are most common.
•Monitor patient for seizure activity during levetiracetam therapy. As appropriate, implement seizure precautions according to facility policy.
•Stopping drug may increase seizure activity. Expect to taper dosage gradually.
**PATIENT TEACHING**
•Caution patient that levetiracetam may cause dizziness and drowsiness, especially during first 4 weeks of therapy.
•Advise patient to avoid hazardous activities until drug's full CNS effects are known.
•Caution patient not to stop taking levetiracetam abruptly; inform her that drug dosage should be tapered under prescriber's direction to reduce the risk of breakthrough seizures.
•Advise patient to keep taking other anticonvulsants, as ordered, while taking levetiracetam.
•Encourage patient to avoid alcohol during therapy because alcohol can increase incidence of drowsiness and dizziness.
•Instruct patient to see prescriber regularly so that her progress can be monitored.

# levodopa

Dopar, Larodopa

## Class and Category

*Chemical:* Dihydroxyphenylalanine isomer, metabolic precursor of dopamine
*Therapeutic:* Antidyskinetic
*Pregnancy category:* Not rated

## Indications and Dosages

➤ *To manage symptoms of primary Parkinson's disease, postencephalitic parkinsonism, and parkinsonism caused by CNS injury from carbon monoxide or manganese intoxication*

**CAPSULES, TABLETS**

**Adults and children age 12 and older.** *Initial:* 250 mg/day in divided doses b.i.d. to q.i.d. Increased by 100 to 750 mg q 3 to 7 days, as indicated. *Maximum:* 8 g/day.

| Route | Onset | Peak | Duration |
|-------|-------|------|----------|
| P.O. | 14 to 21 days* | Unknown | 5 hr |

## Contraindications

Angle-closure glaucoma, history of melanoma, hypersensitivity to levodopa or its components, suspicious undiagnosed skin lesions, use within 14 days of MAO inhibitor therapy

## Interactions

**DRUGS**

*antacids:* Increased blood levodopa level
*antihypertensives:* Risk of orthostatic hypotension
*benzodiazepines:* Possibly decreased therapeutic effects of levodopa
*bromocriptine:* Possibly additive effects of levodopa
*furazolidone, MAO inhibitors, procarbazine:* Risk of severe hypertension
*haloperidol, loxapine, molindone, papaverine, phenothiazines, phenytoin, rauwolfia alkaloids:* Decreased effects of levodopa
*inhaled anesthetics, sympathomimetics:* Increased risk of arrhythmias
*iron salts:* Possibly decreased blood level and effectiveness of levodopa
*methyldopa:* Possibly toxic CNS effects

*metoclopramide:* Possibly worsening of Parkinson's disease and decreased therapeutic effects of metoclopramide
*pyridoxine (vitamin B$_6$):* Decreased antidyskinetic effect of levodopa

**FOODS**

*high-protein food:* Decreased levodopa absorption

**ACTIVITIES**

*cocaine use:* Increased risk of arrhythmias

## Adverse Reactions

**CNS:** Aggressiveness, anxiety, ataxia, confusion, delusions, dizziness, dream disturbances, dyskinesia, dystonia, euphoria, hallucinations, headache, increased tremor, insomnia, malaise, mood changes, severe depression, suicidal tendencies, syncope, weakness
**CV:** Arrhythmias, hot flashes, orthostatic hypotension, palpitations
**EENT:** Bitter aftertaste, blurred vision, darkened saliva, diplopia, dry mouth, increased salivation, mydriasis, tooth clenching and grinding
**GI:** Abdominal pain, anorexia, constipation, diarrhea, flatulence, GI bleeding, hepatotoxicity, hiccups, indigestion, nausea, vomiting
**GU:** Darkened urine, priapism, urine retention
**SKIN:** Darkened sweat, diaphoresis, rash

## Nursing Considerations

•Expect to discontinue levodopa 6 to 8 hours before surgery to avoid interactions with anesthetics.
•Observe patient for mental or behavioral changes and suicidal tendencies. Notify prescriber immediately if they occur.
•Monitor for muscle twitching and blepharospasm (eyelid spasm), which are early signs of overdose. Report these signs immediately.
•Expect patient to be tested for acromegaly and diabetes during long-term levodopa therapy. Also expect to monitor hematopoietic, hepatic, and renal function.

**PATIENT TEACHING**

•Advise patient to take levodopa with meals if she experiences adverse GI reactions.
•Because protein impairs drug absorption, instruct patient to avoid high-protein meals during levodopa therapy and to distribute protein intake equally throughout the day.

---

* With multiple doses.

## Mechanism of Action

By supplementing a low level of endogenous dopamine, levodopa helps control alterations in voluntary muscle movement (such as tremors and rigidity) associated with Parkinson's disease. Dopamine, a neurotransmitter that's synthesized and released by neurons leading from substantia nigra to basal ganglia, is essential for normal motor function. By stimulating peripheral and central dopaminergic$_2$ (D$_2$) receptors on postsynaptic cells, dopamine inhibits the firing of striatal neurons (such as cholinergic neurons). In Parkinson's disease, progressive degeneration of these neurons substantially reduces the supply of intrasynaptic dopamine. Levodopa, a dopamine precursor, increases the dopamine supply in neurons, making more available to stimulate dopaminergic receptors.

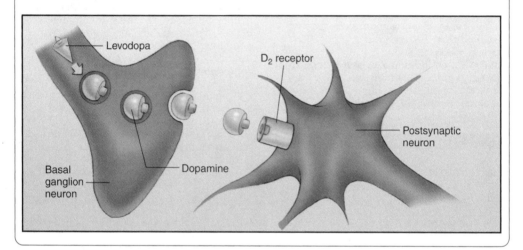

- Caution patient to avoid excessive use of vitamins and fortified cereals that contain vitamin B$_6$ or iron, which can reduce levodopa's effects.
- Instruct patient to report fainting, increased muscle tremor, difficult urination, and severe or persistent nausea and vomiting.
- Urge patient to continue taking drug as prescribed even if results of therapy aren't evident immediately.
- Inform patient that saliva, sweat, and urine may darken but that this isn't harmful.
- Direct patient to protect drug from heat, light, and moisture and to discard darkened pills because they have lost their potency.
- Advise patient to change position slowly to minimize effects of orthostatic hypotension.
- Caution male patient about risk of priapism (persistent, painful erection), and urge him to seek medical treatment immediately if it occurs.

# levofloxacin

Levaquin

## Class and Category

*Chemical:* Fluoroquinolone
*Therapeutic:* Antibiotic
*Pregnancy category:* C

## Indications and Dosages

➤ *To treat acute maxillary sinusitis caused by* Haemophilus influenzae, Moraxella catarrhalis, *or* Streptococcus pneumoniae

**TABLETS, I.V. INFUSION, ORAL SOLUTION**

**Adults.** 500 mg q.d. (over 60 to 90 min for I.V. infusion) for 10 to 14 days. Or 759 mg q.d. for 5 days.

➤ *To treat acute exacerbations of chronic bacterial bronchitis caused by* H. influenzae, Haemophilus parainfluenzae,

M. catarrhalis, S. pneumoniae, *or*
Staphylococcus aureus
**TABLETS, I.V. INFUSION, ORAL SOLUTION**
**Adults.** 500 mg q.d. (over 60 to 90 min for
I.V. infusion) for 7 days.

➤ *To treat community-acquired pneumonia
caused by* Chlamydia pneumoniae, H.
influenzae, H. parainfluenzae, Klebsiella
pneumoniae, Legionella pneumophila,
M. catarrhalis, Mycoplasma pneumoniae, S. aureus, *or* S. pneumoniae
**TABLETS, I.V. INFUSION, ORAL SOLUTION**
**Adults.** 500 mg q.d. (over 60 to 90 min for
I.V. infusion) for 7 to 14 days. Alternatively,
for infection caused by *C. pneumoniae, H.
influenzae, H. parainfluenzae, M. pneumoniae,* or *S. pneumoniae,* 750 mg q.d. (over 60
to 90 min for I.V. infusion) for 5 days.

➤ *To treat uncomplicated UTIs caused by*
Escherichia coli, K. pneumoniae, *or*
Staphylococcus saprophyticus
**TABLETS, I.V. INFUSION, ORAL SOLUTION**
**Adults.** 250 mg q.d. (over 60 to 90 min for
I.V. infusion) for 3 days.

➤ *To treat complicated UTIs and acute
pyelonephritis caused by* E. coli
**TABLETS, I.V. INFUSION, ORAL SOLUTION**
**Adults.** 250 mg q.d. (over 60 to 90 min for
I.V. infusion) for 10 days.

➤ *To treat mild to moderate skin and soft-
tissue infections caused by* S. aureus *or*
Streptococcus pyogenes
**TABLETS, I.V. INFUSION, ORAL SOLUTION**
**Adults.** 500 mg q.d. (over 60 to 90 min for
I.V. infusion) for 7 to 10 days.

➤ *To treat complicated skin and soft-tissue
infections caused by methicillin-sensi-
tive* Enterococcus faecalis, Proteus
mirabilis, S. aureus, *or* S. pyogenes; *to
treat nosocomial pneumonia caused by*
S. aureus, Pseudomonas aeruginosa,
Serratia marcescens, E. coli, K. pneumoniae, H. influenzae, *or* S. pneumoniae
**TABLETS, I.V. INFUSION, ORAL SOLUTION**
**Adults.** 750 mg q.d. (over 60 to 90 min for
I.V. infusion) for 7 to 14 days.

➤ *To treat chronic bacterial prostatitis caused
by* E. coli, E. faecalis, *or* S. epidermidis
**TABLETS, I.V. INFUSION, ORAL SOLUTION**
**Adults.** 500 mg q.d. (over 60 to 90 min for
I.V. infusion) for 28 days.

**DOSAGE ADJUSTMENT** For complicated UTIs
in patients with creatinine clearance of 10 to
19 ml/min/1.73 m$^2$, 250 mg initially and then
maintenance dosage of 250 mg q 48 hr. For
complicated skin and soft-tissue infections
and nosocomial pneumonia when creatinine
clearance is 19 ml/min/1.73 m$^2$ or less,
750 mg initially and then maintenance dosage of 500 mg q 48 hr; when creatinine
clearance is 20 to 49 ml/min/1.73 m$^2$,
750 mg initially and then maintenance dosage of 750 mg q 48 hr. For all other indications, when creatinine clearance is 19 ml/
min/1.73 m$^2$ or less, 500 mg initially and
then maintenance dosage of 250 mg q 48 hr;
when creatinine clearance is 20 to 49 ml/
min/1.73 m$^2$, 500 mg initially and then maintenance dosage of 250 mg q 24 hr.

## Mechanism of Action
Interferes with bacterial cell replication
by inhibiting the bacterial enzyme DNA
gyrase, which is essential for replication
and repair of bacterial DNA.

## Contraindications
Hypersensitivity to levofloxacin, other fluoroquinolones, or their components

## Interactions
**DRUGS**
*aluminum-, calcium-, or magnesium-contain-
ing antacids; didanosine; iron; sucralfate;
zinc:* Reduced GI absorption of levofloxacin
*antineoplastics:* Decreased blood levofloxacin
level
*cimetidine:* Increased blood levofloxacin level
*cyclosporine:* Increased risk of nephrotoxicity
*NSAIDs:* Possibly increased CNS stimulation
and risk of seizures
*oral anticoagulants:* Increased anticoagulant
effect and risk of bleeding
*oral antidiabetic drugs:* Possibly hyperglycemia or hypoglycemia
*theophylline:* Increased blood theophylline
level and risk of toxicity
**ACTIVITIES**
*sun exposure:* Increased risk of photosensitity

## Adverse Reactions
**CNS:** Anxiety, CNS stimulation, dizziness,
headache, increased ICP, light-headedness,
nervousness, peripheral neuropathy, psychosis, seizures, sleep disturbance

J
K
L

**CV:** Arrhythmias, prolonged QT interval
**EENT:** Taste perversion
**ENDO:** Hyperglycemia, hypoglycemia
**GI:** Abdominal pain, anorexia, constipation, diarrhea, flatulence, indigestion, nausea, pseudomembranous colitis, vomiting
**GU:** Crystalluria, vaginal candidiasis
**HEME:** Eosinophilia, hemolytic anemia
**MS:** Back pain, rhabdomyolysis, tendon rupture
**SKIN:** Photosensitivity, pruritus, rash, urticaria
**Other:** Anaphylaxis

## Nursing Considerations
•Use levofloxacin cautiously in patients with renal insufficiency. Monitor renal function as appropriate during levofloxacin treatment.
•Use drug cautiously in patients with CNS disorders that may lower the seizure threshold, such as epilepsy.
•Expect to obtain culture and sensitivity tests before levofloxacin treatment begins.
•Avoid giving drug within 2 hours of antacids.
•Give parenteral form over 60 to 90 minutes, depending on dosage, because bolus or rapid I.V. delivery may cause hypotension.
•**WARNING** Stop levofloxacin at the first sign of hypersensitivity, including rash, because it may lead to anaphylaxis. Reaction may occur after the first dose. Expect to give epinephrine, and provide supportive care.
•Monitor blood glucose level, especially in diabetic patient who takes an oral antidiabetic or insulin, because levfloxacin may alter blood glucose levels. If so, notify prescriber, stop drug immediately for hypoglycemia, and provide prescribed treatment.
•Monitor QT interval if needed. If it lengthens, notify prescriber immediately and stop drug. Patients with hypokalemia, significant bradycardia, or cardiomyopathy and those receiving a class Ia or III antiarrhythmic shouldn't receive levofloxacin.
•Notify prescriber if patient has symptoms of peripheral neuropathy (pain, burning, tingling, numbness, weakness, or altered sensations of light touch, pain, temperature, position sense, or vibration sense), which could be permanent; tendon rupture, which requires immediate rest; or CNS abnormalities (seizures, psychosis, increased ICP or CNS stimulation), which may lead to more serious adverse reactions, such as suicidal thoughts. In each case, expect to stop levofloxacin.

•Monitor patient's bowel elimination. If diarrhea develops, obtain stool culture to check for pseudomembranous colitis. If confirmed, expect to stop drug and give fluid, electrolytes, and antibiotics effective against *Clostridium difficile.*

### PATIENT TEACHING
•If patient will take oral solution, tell him to take it 1 hour before or 2 hours after eating.
•Advise patient to increase fluid intake during levofloxacin therapy to prevent crystalluria.
•Direct patient to take an antacid, didanosine, iron, sucralfate, or zinc at least 2 hours before or after levofloxacin.
•Tell patient to complete the drug as prescribed, even if symptoms subside.
•Advise patient to avoid excessive exposure to sunlight and to wear sunscreen because of increased risk of photosensitivity. Tell patient to notify prescriber at first sign of photosensitivity.
•Caution patient to avoid hazardous activities until drug's CNS effects are known.
•Tell patient to stop drug and notify prescriber if he develops tendon pain or inflammation or abnormal changes in motor or sensory function.
•Urge patient to stop drug and tell prescriber if a rash or other allergic reaction develops.
•Advise diabetic patient to monitor blood glucose level and notify prescriber about changes.

# levorphanol tartrate
Levo-Dromoran

## Class, Category, and Schedule
*Chemical:* Morphinan derivative
*Therapeutic:* Analgesic, anesthesia adjunct
*Pregnancy category:* Not rated
*Controlled substance:* Schedule II

## Indications and Dosages
➤ *To relieve moderate to severe pain*
**TABLETS**
**Adults.** 2 mg q 6 to 8 hr, p.r.n. Increased to 3 mg q 6 to 8 hr, if indicated.
**I.V. INJECTION**
**Adults.** Up to 1 mg q 3 to 6 hr, p.r.n. *Maximum:* 8 mg/day for non-opioid-dependent patients.

**I.M. OR S.C. INJECTION**

**Adults.** 1 to 2 mg q 6 to 8 hr, p.r.n. *Maximum:* 8 mg/day for non-opioid-dependent patients.

➤ *To provide preoperative sedation*

**I.M. OR S.C. INJECTION**

**Adults.** 1 to 2 mg 60 to 90 min before procedure.

| Route | Onset | Peak | Duration |
|-------|-------|------|----------|
| P.O. | 10 to 60 min | 90 to 120 min | 4 to 5 hr |
| I.V. | Unknown | In 20 min | 4 to 5 hr |
| I.M. | Unknown | 60 min | 4 to 5 hr |
| S.C. | Unknown | 60 to 90 min | 4 to 5 hr |

## Mechanism of Action

Decreases intracellular level of cyclic adenosine monophosphate by inhibiting adenylate cyclase, which regulates release of pain neurotransmitters, such as substance P, gamma-aminobutyric acid, dopamine, acetylcholine, and noradrenaline. Levorphanol also stimulates mu and kappa opioid receptors, altering perception of and emotional response to pain.

## Incompatibilities

Don't mix levorphanol tartrate with solutions that contain aminophylline, ammonium chloride, amobarbital sodium, chlorothiazide sodium, heparin sodium, methicillin sodium, nitrofurantoin sodium, novobiacin sodium, pentobarbital sodium, perphenazine, phenobarbital sodium, phenytoin, secobarbital sodium, sodium bicarbonate, sodium iodide, sulfadiazine sodium, sulfisoxazole diethanolamine, or thiopental sodium.

## Contraindications

Acute alcoholism, acute or severe asthma, anoxia, hypersensitivity to levorphanol tartrate or its components, increased intracranial pressure, respiratory depression, upper airway obstruction

## Interactions

**DRUGS**

*alfentanil, CNS depressants, fentanyl, sufentanil:* Possibly increased CNS and respiratory depression and hypotension

*anticholinergics:* Increased risk of severe constipation

*antidiarrheals, such as difenoxin and atropine, kaolin, and loperamide:* Increased risk of severe constipation and increased CNS depression

*antihypertensives:* Increased risk of hypotension

*buprenorphine:* Possibly decreased therapeutic effects of levorphanol and increased risk of respiratory depression

*hydroxyzine:* Increased risk of CNS depression and hypotension

*metoclopramide:* Possibly antagonized effects of metoclopramide

*naloxone, naltrexone:* Decreased therapeutic effects of levorphanol

*neuromuscular blockers:* Increased risk of prolonged CNS and respiratory depression

**ACTIVITIES**

*alcohol use:* Possibly increased CNS and respiratory depression and hypotension

## Adverse Reactions

**CNS:** Amnesia, coma, confusion, delusions, depression, dizziness, drowsiness, dyskinesia, hypokinesia, insomnia, nervousness, personality disorder, seizures

**CV:** Bradycardia, cardiac arrest, hypotension, orthostatic hypotension, palpitations, shock, tachycardia

**EENT:** Abnormal vision, diplopia, dry mouth

**GI:** Abdominal pain, biliary tract spasm, constipation, hepatic failure, indigestion, nausea, vomiting

**GU:** Dysuria, urine retention

**RESP:** Apnea, hyperventilation

**SKIN:** Cyanosis, pruritus, rash, urticaria

**Other:** Injection site pain, redness, and swelling; physical and psychological dependence

## Nursing Considerations

• **WARNING** Be aware that levorphanol may be habit-forming.

• Administer drug with food if GI distress occurs.

• If respiratory depression occurs, expect to administer naloxone to reverse it.

• Monitor supine and standing blood pressure, and notify prescriber of orthostatic hypotension.

• Carefully assess for adverse reactions in elderly patients; they are especially sensitive to drug and are at increased risk for constipation.

**PATIENT TEACHING**

• Advise patient to avoid potentially hazardous activities until drug's CNS effects are known.

• Instruct patient to avoid alcoholic beverages while taking levorphanol.

J
K
L

•Direct patient to change position slowly to minimize effects of orthostatic hypotension.
•Advise patient to notify prescriber if constipation, nausea, or vomiting occurs.
•If patient reports dry mouth, suggest that she use sugarless candy or gum or ice chips.

# levothyroxine sodium

## (L-thyroxine sodium, T₄, thyroxine sodium)

Eltroxin (CAN), Levo-T, Levothroid, Levoxyl, PMS-Levothyroxine Sodium (CAN), Synthroid, Unithroid

### Class and Category
*Chemical:* Synthetic thyroxine (T₄)
*Therapeutic:* Thyroid hormone replacement
*Pregnancy category:* A

### Indications and Dosages
➤ *To treat mild hypothyroidism*
**TABLETS**
**Adults.** *Initial:* 50 mcg q.d., increased by 25 to 50 mcg q 2 to 3 wk until desired response occurs or therapeutic blood level is reached. *Maintenance:* 75 to 125 mcg q.d.
**DOSAGE ADJUSTMENT** For elderly patients and those with cardiovascular disease or chronic hypothyroidism, initial dosage usually reduced to 12.5 to 25 mcg q.d. and then increased by 12.5 to 25 mcg q 3 to 4 wk until desired response occurs. For elderly patients, maintenance dosage is limited to 75 mcg q.d.
**Children over age 10.** 2 to 3 mcg/kg q.d. *Usual:* 150 to 200 mcg/day.
**Children ages 6 to 10.** 4 to 5 mcg/kg q.d. *Usual:* 100 to 150 mcg/day.
**Children ages 1 to 5.** 3 to 5 mcg/kg q.d. *Usual:* 75 to 100 mcg/day.
**Infants ages 6 to 12 months.** 5 to 6 mcg/kg q.d. *Usual:* 50 to 75 mcg q.d.
**Infants under age 6 months.** 5 to 6 mcg/kg q.d. *Usual:* 25 to 50 mcg q.d.
➤ *To treat severe hypothyroidism*
**TABLETS**
**Adults.** *Initial:* 12.5 to 25 mcg q.d. Increased by 25 mcg q 2 to 3 wk until desired response occurs or therapeutic blood level is reached. *Maintenance:* 75 to 125 mcg q.d. *Maximum:* 200 mcg q.d.
**Children over age 10.** 2 to 3 mcg/kg q.d. *Usual:* 150 to 200 mcg/day.

**Children ages 6 to 10.** 4 to 5 mcg/kg q.d. *Usual:* 100 to 150 mcg/day.
**Children ages 1 to 5.** 3 to 5 mcg/kg q.d. *Usual:* 75 to 100 mcg/day.
**Infants ages 6 to 12 months.** 5 to 6 mcg/kg q.d. *Usual:* 50 to 75 mcg q.d.
**Infants under age 6 months.** 5 to 6 mcg/kg q.d. *Usual:* 25 to 50 mcg q.d.
**I.V. OR I.M. INJECTION**
**Adults.** 50 to 100 mcg q.d. until therapeutic blood level is reached.
**Children.** 75% of usual P.O. dose q.d. until therapeutic blood level is reached.
➤ *To treat myxedema coma*
**I.V. INJECTION**
**Adults.** 200 to 500 mcg on day 1. If no significant improvement, 100 to 300 mcg on day 2. Daily dose continued as prescribed until therapeutic blood level is reached and P.O. administration is tolerated.
**Children.** 75% of usual P.O. dose q.d. until therapeutic blood level is reached and P.O. administration is tolerated.

| Route | Onset | Peak | Duration |
|-------|-------|------|----------|
| P.O. | 3 to 5 days | 3 to 4 wk | 1 to 3 wk |
| I.V. | 6 to 8 hr | 24 hr | Unknown |
| I.M. | Unknown | Unknown | 1 to 3 wk |

### Mechanism of Action
Replaces endogenous thyroid hormone, which may exert its physiologic effects by controlling DNA transcription and protein synthesis. Levothyroxine exhibits all of the following actions of endogenous thyroid hormone. The drug:
•increases energy expenditure
•accelerates the rate of cellular oxidation, which stimulates body tissue growth, maturation, and metabolism
•regulates differentiation and proliferation of stem cells
•aids in myelination of nerves and development of synaptic processes in the nervous system
•regulates growth
•decreases blood and hepatic cholesterol concentrations
•enhances carbohydrate and protein metabolism, increasing gluconeogenesis and protein synthesis.

## Contraindications
Acute MI (unless caused or complicated by hyperthyroidism), hypersensitivity to levothyroxine or its components, uncorrected adrenal insufficiency, untreated thyrotoxicosis

## Interactions
**DRUGS**
*adrenocorticoids:* Possibly adrenocorticoid dosage adjustments as thyroid status changes
*aluminum- and magnesium-containing antacids, bile acid sequestrants, calcium carbonate, cation exchange resins, cholestyramine, colestipol, ferrous sulfate, kayexalate, sucralfate:* Possibly reduced effects of levothyroxine
*amiodarone, iodide:* Possibly hyperthyroidism
*beta blockers:* Possibly impaired action of beta blockers and decreased conversion of $T_4$ to triiodothyronine ($T_3$)
*cholestyramine, colestipol:* Delayed or inhibited levothyroxine absorption
*digoxin:* Reduced therapeutic effects of digoxin
*estrogen, phenylbutazone, phenytoin:* Reduced binding of levothyroxine to protein, possibly requiring increased levothyroxine dosage
*insulin, oral antidiabetic drugs:* Possibly uncontrolled diabetes mellitus, requiring increased dosage of insulin or oral antidiabetic drug
*ketamine:* Possibly hypertension and tachycardia
*maprotiline:* Increased risk of arrhythmias
*oral anticoagulants:* Altered anticoagulant activity, possibly need for anticoagulant dosage adjustment
*selective serotonin reuptake inhibitors, tricyclic and tetracyclic antidepressants:* Increased therapeutic and toxic effects of both drugs
*sympathomimetics:* Increased risk of coronary insufficiency in patients with coronary artery disease
*theophylline:* Decreased theophylline clearance
**FOODS**
*dietary fiber, soybean flour (infant formula), walnuts:* Possibly decreased absorption of levothyroxine from GI tract

## Adverse Reactions
**CNS:** Fatigue, headache, insomnia, somnolence
**ENDO:** Hyperthyroidism (with overdose)
**GI:** Dysphagia
**MS:** Muscle weakness, myalgia, slipped capital femoral epiphysis
**SKIN:** Alopecia (transient), rash, urticaria
**Other:** Weight gain

## Nursing Considerations
•Administer levothyroxine tablets as a single daily dose 30 to 60 minutes before breakfast. If patient has difficulty swallowing, crush tablet and suspend in a small amount of water or food.
•To prevent decreased drug absorption, administer oral levothyroxine at least 4 hours before or after aluminum- or magnesium-containing antacids, bile acid sequestrants, calcium carbonate, cation exchange resins, cholestyramine, colestipol, ferrous sulfate, kayexalate, or sucralfate.
•Expect to give drug I.V. or I.M. if patient can't take tablets. Be aware that drug shouldn't be given S.C.
•For I.V. use, reconstitute drug by adding 5 ml of NS.
•Monitor PT of patient who is receiving anticoagulants; she may require a dosage adjustment.
•Monitor blood glucose level of diabetic patient. Prescriber may reduce antidiabetic drug dosage as thyroid hormone level enters therapeutic range.
•Expect patient to undergo regular thyroid function tests during levothyroxine therapy.
**PATIENT TEACHING**
•Inform patient that levothyroxine replaces a hormone that is normally produced by the thyroid gland and that she'll probably need to take drug for life.
•Instruct patient to take drug at least 30 minutes before breakfast because drug absorption is increased on an empty stomach and evening doses may cause insomnia.
•Stress the need to take levothyroxine with a full glass of water to avoid choking, gagging, having tablet stick in throat, and developing heartburn afterward.
•Inform patient that drug may require a few weeks to take effect.
•Advise patient not to stop drug or change dosage unless told to do so by prescriber.
•Instruct patient to report signs of hyperthyroidism, such as diarrhea, excessive sweating, heat intolerance, insomnia, palpitations, weight loss, chest pain, shortness of breath, leg cramps, headache, nervousness, irritability, tremors, changes in appetite, vomiting, fever, and changes in menstrual periods.
•Tell patient to notify prescriber if rash or hives develop during drug use.
•Inform patient that transient hair loss may occur during first few months of therapy.

•Instruct female patient of childbearing age to notify prescriber immediately if she becomes pregnant because levothyroxine dosage may need to be increased.

# levothyroxine sodium and liothyronine sodium

## (liotrix, T₃ [liothyronine], T₄ [levothyroxine])

Thyrolar-¼, Thyrolar-½, Thyrolar-1, Thyrolar-2, Thyrolar-3

## Class and Category

*Chemical:* Thyroid hormones (levothyroxine, liothyronine)
*Therapeutic:* Thyroid hormone replacement
*Pregnancy category:* A

## Indications and Dosages

➤ To *treat hypothyroidism without myxedema*

**TABLETS**

**Adults.** *Initial:* 25 mcg levothyroxine and 6.25 mcg liothyronine (1 tablet of Thyrolar-½) q.d., increased q 2 to 3 wks by 12.5 mcg levothyroxine and 3.1 mcg liothyronine until therapeutic effects occur. *Maintenance:* 50 mcg levothyroxine and 12.5 mcg liothyronine (1 tablet of Thyrolar-1) to 100 mcg levothyroxine and 25 mcg liothyronine (1 tablet of Thyrolar-2) q.d.

➤ To *treat long-standing myxedema or hypothyroidism in patients with cardiovascular disease*

**TABLETS**

**Adults.** *Initial:* 12.5 mcg levothyroxine and 3.1 mcg liothyronine (1 tablet of Thyrolar-¼) q.d., increased q 2 to 3 wk by 12.5 mcg levothyroxine and 3.1 mcg liothyronine until therapeutic effects occur. *Maintenance:* 50 mcg levothyroxine and 12.5 mcg liothyronine (1 tablet of Thyrolar-1) to 100 mcg levothyroxine and 25 mcg liothyronine (1 tablet of Thyrolar-2) q.d.

**DOSAGE ADJUSTMENT** For elderly patients, initial dose usually reduced to 25% to 50% of adult dose; dosage then doubled q 6 to 8 wk until therapeutic effects occur.

➤ To *treat congenital hypothyroidism in children*

**TABLETS**

**Children age 12 and older.** 75 mcg levothy-

roxine and 18.75 mcg liothyronine (1 tablet of Thyrolar 1 and 1 tablet of Thyrolar-½) q.d.

**Children ages 6 to 12.** 50 mcg levothyroxine and 12.5 mcg liothyronine (1 tablet of Thyrolar-1) q.d. to 75 mcg levothyroxine and 18.75 mcg liothyronine (1 tablet of Thyrolar-1 and 1 tablet of Thyrolar-½) q.d.

**Children ages 1 to 6.** 37.5 mcg levothyroxine and 9.35 mcg liothyronine (1 tablet of Thyrolar-½ and 1 tablet of Thyrolar-¼) q.d. to 50 mcg levothyroxine and 12.5 mcg liothyronine (1 tablet of Thyrolar-1) q.d.

**Children ages 6 months to 12 months.** 25 mcg levothyroxine and 6.25 mcg liothyronine (1 tablet of Thyrolar-½) q.d. to 37.5 mcg levo-thyroxine and 9.35 mcg liothyronine (1 tablet of Thyrolar-½ and 1 tablet of Thyrolar-¼) q.d.

**Newborn infants to age 6 months.** 12.5 mcg levothyroxine and 3.1 mcg liothyronine (1 tablet of Thyrolar-¼) q.d. to 25 mcg levothyroxine and 6.25 mcg liothyronine (1 tablet of Thyrolar-½) q.d.

---

## Mechanism of Action

Thyroid hormones, levothyroxine and liothyronine replace endogenous thyroid hormone, which may exert its physiologic effects by controlling DNA transcription and protein synthesis. These hormones exhibit all of the actions of endogenous thyroid hormone. The combination drug:
•increases energy expenditure
•accelerates the rate of cellular oxidation, which stimulates growth, maturation, and metabolism of body tissues
•aids in myelination of nerves and development of synaptic processes in the nervous system
•enhances carbohydrate and protein metabolism, increasing gluconeogenesis and protein synthesis.

---

## Contraindications

Hypersensitivity to levothyroxine, liothyronine, or their components; uncorrected adrenal insufficiency; untreated thyrotoxicosis

## Interactions

**DRUGS**
**levothyroxine and liothyronine**
*adrenocorticoids:* Possibly a need for adrenocorticoid dosage adjustments as thyroid status changes

*cholestyramine, colestipol:* Decreased absorption of levothyroxine and liothyronine
*digoxin:* Possibly a need for digoxin dosage adjustment as thyroid status changes
*estrogen:* Reduced binding of levothyroxine and liothyronine to protein, possibly requiring increased thyroid hormone dosage
*insulin, oral antidiabetic drugs:* Possibly a need for insulin or oral antidiabetic dosage adjustment as thyroid status changes
*ketamine:* Possibly hypertension and tachycardia
*maprotiline:* Increased risk of arrhythmias
*oral anticoagulants:* Altered anticoagulant activity; possibly a need for anticoagulant dosage adjustment
*sympathomimetics:* Increased effects of either drug; risk of coronary insufficiency in patients with coronary artery disease

### Adverse Reactions
**CNS:** Anxiety, asthenia, depression, fatigue, headache, insomnia, sluggish feeling, tremor
**CV:** Arrhythmias, chest pain, hypertension, palpitations, tachycardia
**EENT:** Keratoconjunctivitis sicca
**ENDO:** Hyperthyroidism (with overdose), hypothyroidism, increase or decrease in TSH
**GI:** Nausea
**MS:** Arthralgia, myalgia
**SKIN:** Alopecia (transient), dry skin, hyperhidrosis, pruritus, rash, urticaria
**Other:** Allergic reactions, increased weight

### Nursing Considerations
• Administer levothyroxine and liothyronine as a single daily dose before breakfast.
• Expect patient to undergo periodic thyroid function tests during levothyroxine and liothyronine therapy.
• Monitor PT of patient taking an anticoagulant; she may require a dosage adjustment.
• Frequently monitor blood glucose level of diabetic patient. Prescriber may adjust antidiabetic drug dosage as thyroid hormone replacement is achieved.

**PATIENT TEACHING**
• Inform patient that she'll probably take levothyroxine and liothyronine for life. Caution her not to stop drug or change dosage unless instructed by prescriber.
• Tell patient to take drug before breakfast because evening doses may cause insomnia.
• Advise patient to store tablets in refrigerator in a tightly sealed, light-resistant container.

• Instruct patient to report signs of hyperthyroidism, such as chest pain, excessive sweating, heat intolerance, insomnia, palpitations, and weight loss.
• Advise diabetic patient to monitor blood glucose level frequently because antidiabetic drug dosage may need to be adjusted.
• Inform patient that transient hair loss may occur during first few months of therapy.
• Inform patient of need for periodic thyroid hormone blood tests to monitor drug effectiveness.

# lidocaine hydrochloride
## (lignocaine hydrochloride)
Alphacaine (CAN), Anestacon, DermaFlex, Dilocaine, L-Caine, Xylocaine, Xylocard (CAN)

### Class and Category
*Chemical:* Aminoacetamide
*Therapeutic:* Class IB antiarrhythmic, local anesthetic
*Pregnancy category:* B

### Indications and Dosages
➤ *To treat ventricular tachycardia or ventricular fibrillation*
**I.V. INFUSION AND INJECTION**
**Adults.** *Loading:* 50 to 100 mg (or 1 to 1.5 mg/kg), administered at 25 to 50 mg/min. If desired response isn't achieved after 5 to 10 min, second dose of 25 to 50 mg (or 0.5 to 0.75 mg/kg) is given q 5 to 10 min until maximum loading dose (300 mg in 1 hr) has been given. *Maintenance:* 20 to 50 mcg/kg/min (1 to 4 mg/min) by continuous infusion. Smaller bolus dose repeated 15 to 20 min after start of infusion if needed to maintain therapeutic blood level. *Maximum:* 300 mg (or 3 mg/kg) over 1 hr.
**Children.** *Loading:* 1 mg/kg. *Maintenance:* 30 mcg/kg/min by continuous infusion. *Maximum:* 3 mg/kg.
**DOSAGE ADJUSTMENT** For elderly patients receiving I.V. lidocaine to treat arrhythmias and for patients with acute hepatitis or decompensated cirrhosis, loading dose and continuous infusion rate reduced by 50%.
**I.M. INJECTION**
**Adults.** 300 mg, repeated after 60 to 90 min, if needed.
➤ *To provide topical anesthesia for skin or mucous membranes*

FILM-FORMING GEL, JELLY, OR OINTMENT
**FILM-FORMING GEL, JELLY, OR OINTMENT**
**Adults.** Thin layer applied to skin or mucous membranes as needed before procedure.

| Route | Onset | Peak | Duration |
|---|---|---|---|
| I.V. | 45 to 90 sec | Immediate | 10 to 20 min |
| I.M. | 5 to 15 min | Unknown | 60 to 90 min |
| Topical | 2 to 5 min | Unknown | 0.5 to 1 hr |

## Mechanism of Action
Combines with fast sodium channels in myocardial cell membranes, which inhibits sodium influx into cells and decreases ventricular depolarization, automaticity, and excitability during diastole. Lidocaine also blocks nerve impulses by decreasing the permeability of neuronal membranes to sodium. This action produces local anesthesia.

## Contraindications
Adams-Stokes syndrome; hypersensitivity to lidocaine, amide anesthetics, or their components; severe heart block (without artificial pacemaker); Wolff-Parkinson-White syndrome

## Interactions
**DRUGS**
*beta blockers, cimetidine:* Increased blood lidocaine level and risk of toxicity
*MAO inhibitors, tricyclic antidepressants:* Risk of severe, prolonged hypertension
*mexiletine, tocainide:* Additive cardiac effects
*neuromuscular blockers:* Possibly increased neuromuscular blockade
*phenytoin, procainamide:* Increased cardiac depression

## Adverse Reactions
**CNS:** Anxiety, confusion, difficulty speaking, dizziness, hallucinations, lethargy, paresthesia, seizures
**CV:** Bradycardia, cardiac arrest, hypotension, new or worsening arrhythmias
**EENT:** Blurred vision, diplopia, tinnitus
**GI:** Nausea
**MS:** Muscle weakness, myalgia
**RESP:** Respiratory arrest or depression
**Other:** Injection site burning, irritation, stinging, swelling, and tenderness

## Nursing Considerations
•Observe for respiratory depression after bolus injection and during I.V. infusion of lidocaine.
•Keep life-support equipment and vasopressors nearby during I.V. administration in case respiratory depression or other reactions occur.
•Carefully check prefilled syringes before using. Use only syringes labeled "for cardiac arrhythmias" for I.V. administration.
•As prescribed, titrate I.V. dose to minimum amount needed to prevent arrhythmias.
•During I.V. administration, place patient on cardiac monitor, as ordered, and closely observe her at all times. Monitor for worsening arrhythmias, widening QRS complex, and prolonged PR interval—possible signs of drug toxicity.
•Monitor blood lidocaine level, as ordered. Check for therapeutic level of 2 to 5 mcg/ml.
•If signs of toxicity, such as dizziness, occur, notify prescriber and expect to discontinue or slow infusion.
•Give I.M. injection in deltoid muscle only.
•Apply lidocaine jelly or ointment to gauze or bandage before applying to skin.
•Monitor vital signs as well as BUN and serum creatinine and electrolyte levels during and after therapy.
**PATIENT TEACHING**
•Inform patient who receives lidocaine as an anesthetic that she'll experience numbness.
•Advise patient to report difficulty speaking, dizziness, injection site pain, nausea, numbness or tingling, and vision changes.

# lincomycin hydrochloride
Lincocin

## Class and Category
*Chemical:* Lincosamide
*Therapeutic:* Bacteriostatic or bactericidal antibiotic
*Pregnancy category:* C

## Indications and Dosages
➤ *To treat serious respiratory, skin, and soft-tissue infections caused by susceptible strains of streptococci, pneumococci, and staphylococci*

CAPSULES
**Adults and adolescents.** 500 mg q 6 to 8 hr.
**Children over age 1 month.** 7.5 to 15 mg/kg q
6 hr; alternatively, 10 to 20 mg/kg q 8 hr.
**I.V. INFUSION**
**Adults.** 600 mg to 1 g q 8 to 12 hr. *Maximum:*
8 g/day in divided doses for life-threatening
infection.
**Children over age 1 month.** 10 to 20 mg/kg/
day in divided doses q 8 to 12 hr, depending
on severity of infection.
**I.M. INJECTION**
**Adults and adolescents.** 600 mg q 12 to
24 hr.
**Children over age 1 month.** 10 mg/kg q 12 to
24 hr.
DOSAGE ADJUSTMENT Dosage reduced by 25%
to 30% for patients with severely impaired
renal function.

## Mechanism of Action
Inhibits protein synthesis in susceptible
bacteria by binding to the 50S subunit of
bacterial ribosomes and preventing peptide bond formation, thus causing bacterial cells to die.

## Incompatibilities
Don't administer lincomycin with novobiocin
or kanamycin.

## Contraindications
Hypersensitivity to lincomycin, clindamycin,
or their components

## Interactions
DRUGS
*antimyasthenic drugs:* Possibly antagonized
effects of these drugs
*chloramphenicol, clindamycin, erythromycin:*
Possibly blocked access of lincomycin to its
site of action
*hydrocarbon inhalation anesthetics, neuro-
muscular blockers:* Increased neuromuscular
blockade, possibly severe respiratory depression
*opioid analgesics:* Increased risk of prolonged or increased respiratory depression

## Adverse Reactions
CNS: Fever, vertigo
CV: Cardiac arrest and hypotension (with
rapid administration)

EENT: Glossitis, stomatitis, tinnitus
GI: Abdominal cramps, colitis, diarrhea,
nausea, pseudomembranous colitis, rectal
candidiasis, vomiting
GU: Vaginal candidiasis
HEME: Agranulocytosis, eosinophilia,
leukopenia, neutropenia, thrombocytopenic
purpura
SKIN: Erythema multiforme, rash, Stevens-
Johnson syndrome, urticaria
Other: Anaphylaxis, angioedema, super-
infection

## Nursing Considerations
•Expect to obtain a specimen for culture and
sensitivity testing before administering first
dose of lincomycin.
•WARNING Be aware that some preparations
of lincomycin contain benzyl alcohol, which
can cause a fatal toxic syndrome in neonates
or premature infants, characterized by CNS,
respiratory, circulatory, and renal impairment
and metabolic acidosis. Because lincomycin
has appeared in breast milk, breast-feeding
patient may be required to stop drug or stop
breast-feeding.
•Dilute 600-mg dose in at least 100 ml
of $D_5W$, $D_{10}W$, NS, $D_5NS$, or other compatible diluent recommended by manufacturer.
Dilute higher doses in 100 ml of a compatible diluent for each gram being administered—for example, dilute a 3-g dose in at
least 300 ml of diluent. Use diluted solution
within 24 hours if stored at room temperature.
•WARNING Administer lincomycin over at
least 1 hour for each gram being administered. For example, infuse 1 g over 1 hour
and 3 g over 3 hours. Too-rapid infusion
may result in cardiac arrest or hypotension.
•WARNING Monitor patient for a hypersensitivity reaction, such as rash, pruritus, wheezing, and dysphagia due to laryngeal edema.
If such reactions occur, discontinue infusion
and notify prescriber immediately. If anaphylaxis occurs, administer epinephrine, antihistamines, oxygen, and corticosteroids, as
prescribed. Be aware that patients with a
history of asthma or significant allergies are
at increased risk for a hypersensitivity reaction.
•Observe patient for signs of superinfection,
such as vaginal itching and sore mouth.

J
K
L

• Monitor patient for signs of pseudomembranous colitis, such as watery, loose stools. Patients with a history of GI disease, particularly colitis or regional enteritis, are at increased risk for colitis. Be aware that antibiotic-related diarrhea may be more severe and less well tolerated in elderly patients. Expect to stop lincomycin if patient develops diarrhea.

• Monitor results of liver and renal function tests, CBC, and platelet counts periodically during lincomycin therapy.

• Before diluting drug, store it at a controlled room temperature of 20° to 25° C (68° to 77° F).

**PATIENT TEACHING**

• Advise patient to take lincomycin capsules with a full glass of water on an empty stomach 1 hour before or 2 hours after meals to maximize drug's effectiveness.

• Review with patient possibly serious adverse reactions associated with lincomycin use, such as difficulty breathing, rash, and chest tightness, and tell her to report any that occur.

• Inform patient that yogurt or buttermilk can help maintain intestinal flora and may decrease the risk of diarrhea.

• Stress the importance of following dosage regimen and keeping follow-up medical and laboratory appointments.


# lindane

Bio-Well, GBH, G-well, Hexit (CAN), Kildane, Kwell, Kwellada (CAN), Kwildane, PMS-Lindane (CAN), Scabene, Thionex

## Class and Category

*Chemical:* Benzene derivative
*Therapeutic:* Pediculicide, scabicide
*Pregnancy category:* B

## Indications and Dosages

➤ *To treat scabies and pediculosis*

**CREAM, LOTION**

**Adults and children.** For scabies, thin layer applied once over entire skin surface. For pediculosis, thin layer applied once to affected skin and hair.

**SHAMPOO**

**Adults and children.** 30 ml (for short hair) or 45 ml (for long hair) applied to dry hair and worked into lather for 4 to 5 min.

## Mechanism of Action

Penetrates parasite skeleton and inhibits neuronal membrane function, causing seizures and death. Lindane also kills parasite eggs.

## Contraindications

Hypersensitivity to lindane or its components, prematurity (in neonates), seizure disorders

## Interactions

**ACTIVITIES**

*use of oil-based hair products:* Possibly increased absorption of lindane

## Adverse Reactions

**CNS:** Dizziness, irritability, nervousness, restlessness, seizures, unsteadiness
**SKIN:** Erythema, pruritus, rash, urticaria

## Nursing Considerations

• Use lindane cautiously in patients at risk for CNS toxicity, such as infants and elderly patients, and in patients weighing less than 110 lb (50 kg).

• Wear gloves when applying drug. If another person will apply drug, supply gloves for use.

• For scabies, apply thin layer of preparation to dry skin and rub in thoroughly. Trim patient's nails, and apply under nails with toothbrush. Apply to body from neck down, including soles. Leave drug on for 8 to 12 hours (usually overnight), and then remove with bath or shower.

• Expect to reduce application time for infants and children to 6 to 8 hours, as prescribed, because of the risk of systemic absorption.

• Keep lindane away from mouth and eyes. Don't use on open wounds, cuts, or sores.

• Expect to administer topical steroids or oral antihistamines to reduce pruritus, which may continue for several weeks with scabies.

• For hospitalized patients, use special linen-handling precautions until treatment is completed.

• **WARNING** Be aware that lindane may cause seizures or other adverse CNS reactions; therefore, use it only after other treatments have been tried.

• Monitor immunocompromised patients closely because they're at increased risk for adverse reactions.

## PATIENT TEACHING

•Inform patient that lindane is for one-time use but may be reapplied after 1 week if she finds live lice or nits (eggs).

•Caution patient to avoid eyes, mucous membranes, and open areas of skin when applying drug and not to inhale vapors.

•Instruct patient (or parents of a child) to wear gloves when applying drug.

•For scabies, instruct patient to shake lotion bottle well before using and to apply lotion or cream in a thin layer all over body from the neck down, avoiding face and scalp. Direct her to leave drug on for 8 to 12 hours and then wash it off in the bath or shower. Explain that itching may persist for several weeks after treatment.

•For pubic lice, instruct patient to shake lotion bottle well before using and to apply a thin layer of lotion to pubic hair and skin as well as to groin, thighs, and lower stomach if they're also affected. Direct her to leave lotion on for 12 hours and then thoroughly wash it off in the bath or shower.

•For head lice, instruct patient to shake lotion bottle well before using and to apply lotion to affected areas of head and scalp as well as nearby hairy areas and rub it in well. Tell her to leave lotion on for 12 hours and then thoroughly wash it off.

•For head or pubic lice, instruct patient to wash and dry her hair before applying lindane shampoo, especially if she uses oil-based hair products. Instruct her to shake bottle well before using and then apply shampoo to dry hair, working it in thoroughly and adding a small amount of water if needed to form good lather. Direct her to wait 4 minutes, rinse her hair well, and then dry it with a clean towel. Instruct her to use a fine-toothed comb or tweezers to remove nits or nit shells. Direct patient not to use shampoo again for 7 days and then only if she finds live lice. Caution patient not to use shampoo in the shower to avoid getting it in her eyes and mouth.

•Advise patient to wash lindane off her skin and to contact prescriber if irritation (severe itching, hives, or redness) occurs.

•Explain that if lice come back, the problem is probably reinfestation rather than treatment failure.

•Advise patient to notify family members and sexual contacts about infestation.

# linezolid

Zyvox

## Class and Category

*Chemical:* Oxazolidinone
*Therapeutic:* Antibiotic
*Pregnancy category:* C

## Indications and Dosages

➤ *To treat vancomycin-resistant* Enterococcus faecium *infections, including bacteremia*

ORAL SUSPENSION, TABLETS, I.V. INFUSION

**Adults and adolescents.** 600 mg q 12 hr for 14 to 28 days.

**Infants and children.** 10 mg/kg q 8 hr for 14 to 28 days.

➤ *To treat nosocomial pneumonia caused by* Staphylococcus aureus *(methicillin-susceptible and -resistant strains) or* Streptococcus pneumoniae *(penicillin-susceptible strains only) and community-acquired pneumonia, including accompanying bacteremia, caused by* S. aureus *(methicillin-susceptible strains only) or* S. pneumoniae *(penicillin-susceptible strains only); to treat complicated skin and soft-tissue infections, including diabetic foot infections without concomitant osteomyelitis, caused by* S. aureus *(methicillin-susceptible and -resistant strains),* Streptococcus pyogenes, *or* Streptococcus agalactiae

ORAL SUSPENSION, TABLETS, I.V. INFUSION

**Adults and adolescents.** 600 mg q 12 hr for 10 to 14 days.

**Infants and children.** 10 mg/kg q 8 hr for 10 to 14 days.

➤ *To treat uncomplicated skin and soft-tissue infections caused by* S. aureus *(methicillin-susceptible strains only) or* S. pyogenes

ORAL SUSPENSION, TABLETS

**Adults.** 400 mg q 12 hr for 10 to 14 days.
**Adolescents.** 600 mg q 12 hr for 10 to 14 days.
**Children age 5 to 11 years.** 10 mg/kg q 12 hr for 10 to 14 days.
**Infants and children to age 5 years.** 10 mg/kg q 8 hr.

## Incompatibilities

Don't add other drugs to linezolid solution. Don't infuse linezolid in the same I.V. line as amphotericin B, chlorpromazine hydrochlo-

J
K
L

ride, co-trimoxazole, diazepam, erythromycin lactobionate, pentamidine isethionate, or phenytoin sodium because these drugs are physically incompatible. Don't infuse linezolid with ceftriaxone sodium because these drugs are chemically incompatible.

## Contraindications

Hypersensitivity to linezolid or its components; phenylketonuria (oral suspension)

## Interactions

**DRUGS**

*adrenergics, including pseudoephedrine and phenylpropanolamine:* Enhanced vasopressor response of adrenergics, resulting in increased blood pressure
*serotonergics:* Possibly serotonin syndrome

**FOODS**

*tyramine-containing foods and beverages:* Possibly hypertension

## Adverse Reactions

**CNS:** Dizziness, fever, headache, insomnia, optic and peripheral neuropathy, serotonin syndrome
**CV:** Hypertension
**EENT:** Oral candidiasis, tongue discoloration
**GI:** Abdominal pain, constipation, diarrhea, indigestion, nausea, pseudomembranous colitis, vomiting
**GU:** Vaginal candidiasis
**HEME:** Anemia, leukopenia, pancytopenia, thrombocytopenia
**SKIN:** Pruritus, rash
**Other:** Lactic acidosis

## Mechanism of Action

Linezolid inhibits bacterial protein synthesis by interfering with translation of ribonucleic acid (RNA) to protein. In bacteria, protein synthesis begins with binding of a 30S ribosomal subunit and a 50S ribosomal subunit to a messenger RNA (mRNA) molecule to form a 70S initiation complex. The 50S ribosomal subunit consists of 23S ribosomal RNA (rRNA) and other ribosomal subunits. Then translation begins. Transfer RNA (tRNA) attaches to the 50S subunit and brings specific amino acids into place. As the tRNA and amino acids fall into place, they are joined together by peptide bonds and elongate to form a polypeptide chain, as shown below left. This chain eventually combines with other polypeptide chains to form a complete protein molecule. After translation is complete, the ribosomal subunits fall away and are ready to combine with more mRNA to start the translation process over again.

Linezolid binds to a site on the bacterial 23S rRNA of the 50S subunit. This action prevents formation of a functional 70S initiation complex, an essential component of the bacterial translation. Without proper protein production, as shown below right, susceptible bacteria can't multiply. Linezolid is bacteriostatic against staphylococci and enterococci and bactericidal against most streptococci.

## Nursing Considerations
- Obtain body tissue and fluid specimens for culture and sensitivity tests, as ordered, before giving first dose of linezolid. Expect to begin drug before test results are known.
- Infuse I.V. solution over 30 to 120 minutes with $D_5W$, NS, or LR.
- **WARNING** Monitor CBC weekly, as ordered, to detect or track worsening myelosuppression in patients who need more than 2 weeks of therapy, who have preexisting myelosuppression and are receiving drugs that produce bone marrow suppression, or who have chronic infection and are receiving or have received antibiotic therapy.
- Notify prescriber if patient develops visual impairment that suggests optic neuropathy, such as changes in visual acuity or color vision, blurred vision, lost vision, or visual field defect. If optic or peripheral neuropathy develops, the drug may need to be stopped.
- Monitor bowel pattern daily. Assess patient for secondary infection, including oral candidiasis and profuse, watery diarrhea.

### PATIENT TEACHING
- Caution patient with phenylketonuria that oral suspension contains phenylalanine.
- Advise patient not to take OTC cold remedies without consulting prescriber because medications that contain pseudoephedrine or propanolamine may cause or worsen hypertension.
- Instruct patient to avoid foods and beverages that contain large amounts of tyramine, including aged cheese, fermented or air-dried meats, sauerkraut, soy sauce, tap beers, red wines, and protein-rich foods that have been stored for long periods or poorly refrigerated.
- Instruct patient to notify prescriber immediately about severe diarrhea, vision changes, or changes in limb sensation (such as pins and needles, numbness, or tingling) because drug may need to be stopped.

# liothyronine sodium
## (L-triiodothyronine, sodium L-triiodothyronine, $T_3$, thyronine sodium)

Cytomel, Triostat

## Class and Category
*Chemical:* Synthetic triiodothyronine ($T_3$)
*Therapeutic:* Thyroid hormone replacement
*Pregnancy category:* A

## Indications and Dosages
➤ *To treat mild hypothyroidism*
### TABLETS
**Adults.** *Initial:* 25 mcg q.d. Increased by 12.5 to 25 mcg q 1 to 2 wk until desired response occurs. *Maintenance:* 25 to 50 mcg/day.
**DOSAGE ADJUSTMENT** For elderly patients and those with cardiovascular disease, initial dose reduced to 5 mcg q.d. and then increased by 5 mcg q 2 wk.

➤ *To treat congenital hypothyroidism*
### TABLETS
**Adults and children.** *Initial:* 5 mcg q.d. Increased by 5 mcg q 3 to 4 days until desired response occurs. *Maintenance:* Highly individualized.

➤ *To treat simple nontoxic goiter*
### TABLETS
**Adults.** *Initial:* 5 mcg q.d. Increased by 5 to 10 mcg q 1 to 2 wk up to 25 mcg/day. Then increased by 12.5 to 25 mcg/wk, as indicated. *Maintenance:* 50 to 100 mcg/day.

➤ *To treat myxedema*
### TABLETS
**Adults.** *Initial:* 2.5 to 5 mcg q.d. Increased by 5 to 10 mcg q 1 to 2 wk up to 25 mcg/day. Then increased by 12.5 to 25 mcg q 1 to 2 wk, as indicated. *Maintenance:* 25 to 50 mcg/day.

➤ *To treat myxedema coma or premyxedema coma (severe hypothyroidism)*
### I.V. INJECTION
**Adults.** *Initial:* 25 to 50 mcg. Repeated q 4 to 12 hr as indicated by patient's response. Then P.O. therapy is resumed as soon as possible.
**DOSAGE ADJUSTMENT** When treating myxedema coma in patients with known or suspected cardiovascular disease, initial dose decreased to 10 to 20 mcg.

➤ *To differentiate hyperthyroidism from euthyroidism ($T_3$ suppression test)*
### TABLETS
**Adults.** 75 to 100 mcg/day for 7 days.

| Route | Onset | Peak | Duration |
|---|---|---|---|
| P.O. | 24 to 72 hr | 48 to 72 hr | Up to 72 hr |
| I.V. | 2 to 4 hr | 2 days | Unknown |

## Contraindications
Acute MI (unless caused or complicated by hypothyroidism), hypersensitivity to liothyronine or its components, uncorrected adrenal insufficiency, untreated thyrotoxicosis

J
K
L

## Mechanism of Action

Replaces endogenous thyroid hormone, which may exert its physiologic effects by controlling DNA transcription and protein synthesis. Like endogenous thyroid hormone, liothyronine:

• increases energy expenditure
• accelerates the rate of cellular oxidation, which stimulates body tissue growth, maturation, and metabolism
• regulates differentiation and proliferation of stem cells
• aids in myelination of nerves and development of synaptic processes in the nervous system
• regulates growth
• decreases blood and hepatic cholesterol concentrations
• enhances carbohydrate and protein metabolism, increasing gluconeogenesis and protein synthesis.

## Interactions
### DRUGS

*adrenocorticoids:* Possibly need for adrenocorticoid dosage adjustments as thyroid status changes
*beta blockers:* Possibly impaired action of beta blockers
*cholestyramine, colestipol:* Decreased liothyronine absorption
*digoxin:* Reduced therapeutic effects of digoxin
*estrogen, phenylbutazone, phenytoin:* Reduced binding of liothyronine to protein, possibly requiring increased liothyronine dosage
*insulin, oral antidiabetic drugs:* Possibly uncontrolled diabetes mellitus, requiring increased dosage of insulin or oral antidiabetic drug
*ketamine:* Possibly hypertension and tachycardia
*maprotiline:* Increased risk of arrhythmias
*oral anticoagulants:* Altered anticoagulant activity, possibly need for anticoagulant dosage adjustment
*sympathomimetics:* Increased risk of coronary insufficiency in patients with coronary artery disease
*theophylline:* Decreased theophylline clearance
*tricyclic antidepressants:* Increased therapeutic and toxic effects of both drugs

## Adverse Reactions

**CNS:** Insomnia
**ENDO:** Hyperthyroidism (with overdose)
**SKIN:** Alopecia (transient), rash, urticaria

## Nursing Considerations

• Be aware that liothyronine is used most often when rapid onset or rapidly reversible thyroid hormone replacement is needed.
• Administer tablet as a single daily dose before breakfast.
• Give I.V. injections more than 4 hours but less than 12 hours apart.
• Evaluate response to therapy by monitoring pulse rate and blood pressure.
• Expect patient to undergo regular tests of thyroid function during liothyronine therapy.
• Monitor PT of patient receiving anticoagulants because she may require a dosage adjustment.
• Frequently monitor blood glucose level of diabetic patient. Prescriber may reduce antidiabetic drug dosage as thyroid hormone level enters therapeutic range.
• Be aware that liothyronine is used in $T_3$ suppression test to differentiate hyperthyroidism from euthyroidism (normal thyroid function). For this test, $^{131}I$ uptake test is performed before and after liothyronine administration. Suppression of $^{131}I$ uptake by 50% indicates normal thyroid function.

### PATIENT TEACHING

• Inform patient that liothyronine usually is taken for life. Caution her not to discontinue drug or change dosage unless instructed by prescriber.
• Instruct patient to take drug before breakfast; evening doses may cause insomnia.
• Advise patient to report signs of hyperthyroidism, such as chest pain, excessive sweating, heat intolerance, increased pulse rate, nervousness, and palpitations.
• Inform patient that transient hair loss may occur during first few months of therapy.
• Instruct diabetic patient to monitor blood glucose level frequently because antidiabetic drug dosage may need to be reduced.
• Inform patient of need for periodic blood tests to monitor drug effectiveness.

# lisinopril

Prinivil, Zestril

| Route | Onset | Peak | Duration |
|---|---|---|---|
| P.O. | 1 hr | 6 to 8 hr | 24 hr |

## Class and Category

*Chemical:* Lysine ester of enalaprilat
*Therapeutic:* Antihypertensive, vasodilator
*Pregnancy category:* C (first trimester), D (later trimesters)

## Indications and Dosages

➤ *To manage uncomplicated essential hypertension*

**TABLETS**

**Adults.** *Initial:* 10 mg/day. *Maintenance:* 20 to 40 mg/day. *Maximum:* 80 mg/day.
DOSAGE ADJUSTMENT For patients with renal failure, initial dosage reduced to 5 mg/day if creatinine clearance is 10 to 30 ml/min/ 1.73 m$^2$, and to 2.5 mg/day if creatinine clearance is less than 10 ml/min/1.73 m$^2$. For patients receiving a diuretic, initial dosage reduced to 5 mg/day.

**Children age 6 and older with a GFR of at least 30 ml/min/1.73 m$^2$.** *Initial:* 0.07 mg/kg q.d., adjusted according to blood pressure response up to 5 mg daily. *Maximum:* 0.61 mg/kg or 40 mg/day.

➤ *To treat heart failure, along with digoxin and diuretics*

**TABLETS**

**Adults.** *Initial:* 5 mg/day. *Maintenance:* 5 to 20 mg/day. *Maximum:* 80 mg/day.
DOSAGE ADJUSTMENT For patients with hyponatremia or creatinine clearance of 30 ml/ min/1.73 m$^2$ or less, initial dosage reduced to 2.5 mg/day.

➤ *To improve survival in hemodynamically stable patient after acute MI*

**TABLETS**

**Adults.** 5 mg within 24 hr after onset of symptoms, followed by 5 mg after 24 hr and 10 mg after 48 hr. *Maintenance:* 10 mg/day for 6 wk. *Maximum:* 80 mg/day.
DOSAGE ADJUSTMENT For patients with baseline systolic blood pressure of 120 mm Hg or less, initial dosage decreased to 2.5 mg/day for first 3 days after MI. If systolic blood pressure falls to 100 mm Hg or less during therapy, maintenance dosage decreased to 2.5 to 5 mg as tolerated; if systolic blood pressure is 90 mm Hg or less for more than 1 hr, drug is discontinued.

## Mechanism of Action

May reduce blood pressure by inhibiting the conversion of angiotensin I to angiotensin II. Angiotensin II is a potent vasoconstrictor that also stimulates the adrenal cortex to secrete aldosterone. Lisinopril may also inhibit renal and vascular production of angiotensin II. Decreased release of aldosterone reduces sodium and water reabsorption and increases their excretion, thereby reducing blood pressure.

## Contraindications

Hypersensitivity to lisinopril, other ACE inhibitors, or their components; history of angioedema related to previous treatment with an ACE inhibitor; hereditary or idiopathic angioedema

## Interactions

**DRUGS**

*allopurinol, bone marrow depressants (such as methotrexate), procainamide, systemic corticosteroids:* Increased risk of potentially fatal neutropenia or agranulocytosis
*cyclosporine, potassium-sparing diuretics, potassium supplements:* Increased risk of hyperkalemia
*diuretics, other antihypertensives:* Increased hypotensive effect
*lithium:* Increased blood lithium level and risk of lithium toxicity
*NSAIDs:* Possibly reduced antihypertensive effect, reduced renal function in patients with preexisting renal dysfunction
*sympathomimetics:* Possibly reduced antihypertensive effect

**FOODS**

*high-potassium diet, potassium-containing salt substitutes:* Increased risk of hyperkalemia

**ACTIVITIES**

*alcohol use:* Possibly increased hypotensive effect

## Adverse Reactions

**CNS:** Ataxia, confusion, CVA, dizziness, fatigue, headache, syncope, transient ischemic attack, vertigo

J
K
L

**CV:** Arrhythmias, chest pain, hypotension, MI, orthostatic hypotension, palpitations, peripheral edema, vasculitis
**ENDO:** Hyperglycemia
**GI:** Abdominal pain, anorexia, cholestatic jaundice, diarrhea, elevated liver enzymes, fulminant hepatic necrosis, gastritis, hepatitis, indigestion, nausea, pancreatitis, vomiting
**GU:** Acute renal failure, decreased libido, impotence, pyelonephritis
**HEME:** Agranulocytosis, anemia, hemolytic anemia, neutropenia, thrombocytopenia
**MS:** Muscle spasms, myalgia
**RESP:** Bronchospasm, cough, dyspnea, paroxysmal nocturnal dyspnea, pulmonary embolism and infarction, upper respiratory tract infection
**SKIN:** Pruritus, rash, Stevens-Johnson syndrome, toxic epidermal necrolysis, urticaria
**Other:** Anaphylaxis, angioedema

## Nursing Considerations
• Use lisinopril cautiously in patients with fluid volume deficit, heart failure, impaired renal function, or sodium depletion.
• To prepare pediatric suspension, add 10 ml of purified water to a polyethylene terephthalate (PET) bottle containing ten 20-mg tablets and shake for at least 1 minute. Add 30 ml of Bicitra diluent and 160 ml of Ora-Sweet SF to the concentrate in the PET bottle, and shake gently for several seconds. Store in refrigerator for up to 4 weeks. Shake the suspension before each use.
• Monitor blood pressure often, especially early in treatment. If excessive hypotension develops, expect to withhold drug for several days.
• WARNING If angioedema affects face, glottis, larynx, limbs, lips, mucous membranes, or tongue, notify prescriber immediately and expect to stop lisinopril and start appropriate therapy at once. If airway obstruction threatens, promptly give 0.3 to 0.5 ml of epinephrine 1:1,000 solution S.C., as prescribed.
• Notify prescriber if patient has persistent, nonproductive cough, a common adverse effect of ACE inhibitors such as lisinopril.
• Monitor for dehydration, which can lead to hypotension. Be aware that diarrhea and vomiting can cause dehydration.
• Monitor patient for hepatic dysfunction because lisinopril, an ACE inhibitor, may rarely cause a syndrome that starts with cholestatic jaundice or hepatitis and progresses to fulminant hepatic necrosis. If patient develops jaundice or marked elevation in liver enzymes, withhold drug and notify prescriber.

**PATIENT TEACHING**
• Explain to patient that lisinopril helps to control but doesn't cure hypertension and that she may need lifelong therapy.
• Advise patient to take lisinopril at the same time every day.
• Emphasize the importance of taking drug as ordered, even if patient feels well; caution her not to stop drug without consulting prescriber.
• Instruct patient to report dizziness, especially during the first few days of therapy.
• Inform patient that a persistent, nonproductive cough may develop during lisinopril therapy. Urge her to notify prescriber immediately if cough becomes difficult to tolerate.
• Advise patient to drink adequate fluid and avoid excessive sweating, which can lead to dehydration and hypotension. Make sure she understands that diarrhea and vomiting also can cause hypotension.
• Caution patient not to use salt substitutes that contain potassium.
• Instruct patient to report signs of infection, such as fever and sore throat, which may indicate neutropenia.
• Advise patient to change position slowly to minimize effects of orthostatic hypotension.

# lithium carbonate

Carbolith (CAN), Duralith (CAN), Eskalith, Eskalith CR, Lithane, Lithizine (CAN), Lithobid, Lithonate, Lithotabs

## lithium citrate
Cibalith-S

## Class and Category
*Chemical:* Alkaline metal, monovalent cation
*Therapeutic:* Antidepressant, antimanic
*Pregnancy category:* D

## Indications and Dosages
➤ *To treat recurrent bipolar affective disorder, to prevent bipolar disorder depression*

CAPSULES, TABLETS

**Adults and children age 12 and older.** *Initial:* 300 to 600 mg t.i.d. *Maintenance:* 300 mg t.i.d. or q.i.d. *Maximum:* 2,400 g/day.
**Children up to age 12.** 15 to 20 mg/kg/day in divided doses b.i.d. or t.i.d.

E.R. TABLETS

**Adults and children age 12 and older.** *Initial:* 900 to 1,800 mg/day in divided doses b.i.d. or t.i.d. *Maintenance:* 450 mg b.i.d. or 300 mg t.i.d. *Maximum:* 2,400 g/day.

SLOW-RELEASE CAPSULES

**Adults and children age 12 and older.** 600 to 900 mg on day 1, increased to 1,200 to 1,800 mg/day in divided doses t.i.d. *Maintenance:* 900 to 1,200 mg/day in divided doses t.i.d. *Maximum:* 2,400 g/day.

SYRUP (LITHIUM CITRATE)

**Adults and children age 12 and older.** 8 to 16 mEq (equivalent of 300 to 600 mg of lithium carbonate) t.i.d. *Maintenance:* Equivalent of 300 mg of lithium carbonate t.i.d. or q.i.d. *Maximum:* Equivalent of 2,400 g/day of lithium carbonate.
**Children up to age 12.** 0.4 to 0.5 mEq (equivalent of 15 to 20 mg of lithium carbonate)/kg/day in divided doses b.i.d. or t.i.d.

| Route | Onset | Peak | Duration |
|-------|-------|------|----------|
| P.O. | 1 to 3 wk | Unknown | Unknown |

### Mechanism of Action

May increase presynaptic degradation of the catecholamine neurotransmitters serotonin, dopamine, and norepinephrine; inhibit their release at neuronal synapses; and decrease postsynaptic receptor sensitivity. These actions may correct overactive catecholamine systems in patients with mania.

Antidepressant action may result from enhanced serotonergic activity.

## Contraindications

Blood dyscrasias, bone marrow depression, brain damage, cerebrovascular disease, coma, coronary artery disease, excessive intake of other CNS depressants, hypersensitivity to lithium or its components, impaired hepatic function, myeloproliferative disorders, severe depression, severe hypertension or hypotension

## Interactions

DRUGS

*ACE inhibitors, NSAIDs, piroxicam:* Possibly increased blood lithium level and increased risk of toxicity
*acetazolamide, sodium bicarbonate, urea, xanthines:* Decreased blood lithium level
*calcium channel blockers, molindone:* Increased risk of neurotoxicity from lithium
*calcium iodide, iodinated glycerol, potassium iodide:* Possibly increased hypothyroid effects of both drugs
*carbamazepine:* Possibly increased therapeutic effects of carbamazepine and neurotoxic effect of lithium
*chlorpromazine, other phenothiazines:* Possibly impaired GI absorption and decreased blood levels of these drugs; possibly masking of early signs of lithium toxicity
*desmopressin, lypressin, vasopressin:* Possibly impaired antidiuretic effects of these drugs
*diuretics (loop and osmotic):* Increased lithium reabsorption by kidneys, possibly leading to lithium toxicity
*fluoxetine, methyldopa, metronidazole:* Increased risk of lithium toxicity from reduced renal clearance of lithiun
*haloperidol and other antipyschotics:* Increased risk of irreversible neurotoxicity and brain damage
*neuromuscular blockers:* Risk of prolonged paralysis or weakness
*norepinephrine:* Possibly decreased therapeutic effects of norepinephrine and severe respiratory depression
*selective serotonin reuptake inhibitors:* Increased risk of adverse effects, such as diarrhea, confusion, dizziness, agitation, and tremor
*thyroid hormones:* Possibly hypothyroidism
*tricyclic antidepressants:* Possibly severe mood swings from mania to depression

FOODS

*high-sodium foods:* Increased excretion and possibly decreased therapeutic effects of lithium

## Adverse Reactions

**CNS:** Ataxia, coma, confusion, depression, dizziness, drowsiness, headache, lethargy, mania, seizures, syncope, tremor (in hands), vertigo
**CV:** Arrhythmias (including bradycardia and tachycardia), ECG changes, edema

J
K
L

**EENT:** Dental caries, dry mouth, exophthalmos
**ENDO:** Diabetes insipidus, euthyroid goiter, hypothyroidism, myxedema
**GI:** Abdominal distention and pain, anorexia, diarrhea, nausea, thirst
**GU:** Stress incontinence, urinary frequency
**HEME:** Leukocytosis
**MS:** Muscle twitching and weakness
**RESP:** Dyspnea
**SKIN:** Acne; alopecia; dry, thin hair; pruritus; rash
**Other:** Cold sensitivity, weight gain or loss

## Nursing Considerations

• Administer lithium after meals to slow absorption from GI tract and reduce adverse reactions. Dilute syrup with juice or other flavored drink before giving.
• Note that 5 ml of lithium citrate equals 8 mEq of lithium ion or 300 mg of lithium carbonate.
• Expect to monitor blood lithium level two or three times weekly during first month, and then weekly to monthly during maintenance therapy and when initiating or discontinuing NSAID therapy. In uncomplicated cases, plan to monitor lithium level every 2 to 3 months.
• Be aware that lithium has a narrow therapeutic range. Even a slightly high blood level is dangerous, and some patients exhibit signs of toxicity at normal levels.
• Expect prescriber to decrease dosage after acute manic episode is controlled.
• **WARNING** Be aware that lithium affects the normal shifting of intracellular and extracellular potassium ions, which can cause ECG changes, such as flattened or inverted T waves; lithium also can increase the risk of cardiac arrest.
• Monitor ECGs, renal and thyroid function test results, and serum electrolyte levels, as appropriate, during lithium treatment.
• **WARNING** Be aware that lithium can cause reversible leukocytosis, which usually peaks within 7 to 10 days of initiating therapy; WBC count typically returns to baseline within 10 days after lithium is discontinued.
• Weigh patient daily to detect sudden weight changes.
• Frequently monitor blood glucose level in diabetic patient because lithium alters glucose tolerance.
• Palpate thyroid gland to detect enlargement because drug may cause goiter.

• Ensure that patient's fluid and sodium intake is adequate during treatment.

**PATIENT TEACHING**

• Advise patient to take lithium with or after meals to minimize adverse reactions.
• Instruct patient to swallow E.R. or slow-release form whole.
• Direct patient to mix syrup form with juice or other flavored drink before taking.
• Inform patient that frequent urination, nausea, and thirst may occur during the first few days of treatment.
• Caution patient not to stop taking lithium or adjust dosage without first consulting prescriber.
• Instruct patient to report signs of toxicity, such as diarrhea, drowsiness, muscle weakness, tremor, uncoordinated body movements, and vomiting.
• Urge patient to avoid potentially hazardous activities until drug's CNS effects are known.
• Advise patient to maintain normal fluid and sodium intake.
• Emphasize importance of complying with scheduled checkups and laboratory tests.

# lomefloxacin hydrochloride

Maxaquin

## Class and Category

*Chemical:* Fluoroquinolone
*Therapeutic:* Antibiotic
*Pregnancy category:* C

## Indications and Dosage

➤ *To treat mild to moderate lower respiratory tract infections caused by susceptible organisms, including* Haemophilus influenzae *and* Moraxella catarrhalis

**TABLETS**

**Adults.** 400 mg q.d. for 10 days.

➤ *To treat uncomplicated cystitis caused by* Escherichia coli; *to treat uncomplicated cystitis caused by* Klebsiella pneumoniae, Proteus mirabilis, *or* Staphylococcus saprophyticus

**TABLETS**

**Adults.** 400 mg q.d. for 3 days.

➤ *To treat complicated UTIs caused by* Citrobacter diversus, *Enterobacteriaceae,* E. coli, K. pneumoniae, P. mirabilis, *or* Pseudomonas aeruginosa

TABLETS

**Adults.** 400 mg q.d. for 14 days.

➤ *To provide prophylaxis for transurethral surgery*

TABLETS

**Adults.** 400 mg as a single dose 2 to 6 hr before surgery.

➤ *To provide prophylaxis for transrectal biopsy*

TABLETS

**Adults.** 400 mg as a single dose 1 to 6 hr before surgery.

➤ *To treat gonorrhea (as alternative to ciprofloxacin or ofloxacin)*

TABLETS

**Adults.** 400 mg as a single dose.

DOSAGE ADJUSTMENT For patients with creatinine clearance between 11 and 39 ml/min/1.73 m$^2$, loading dose of 400 mg given on day 1 and followed by 200 mg q.d.

---

## Mechanism of Action

Inhibits the bacterial enzyme DNA gyrase, which normally is responsible for the unwinding and supercoiling of bacterial DNA before it replicates. By inhibiting this enzyme, lomefloxacin interferes with bacterial cell replication and causes cell death.

---

## Contraindications

History of tendinitis or tendon rupture, hypersensitivity to lomefloxacin or any quinolone derivative

## Interactions

DRUGS

*aluminum-, calcium-, or magnesium-containing antacids; iron salts; sucralfate; zinc:* Decreased absorption and blood level of lomefloxacin

*cyclosporine:* Possibly increased blood cyclosporine level, increased nephrotoxicity

*probenecid:* Decreased lomefloxacin excretion, increased risk of toxicity

*warfarin:* Possibly increased anticoagulant effect and risk of bleeding

## Adverse Reactions

**CNS:** Ataxia, cerebral thrombosis, dizziness, drowsiness, hallucinations, headache, insomnia, nervousness, peripheral neuropathy, phobia, vertigo

**CV:** Prolonged QT interval, torsades de pointes, vasculitis

**EENT:** Diplopia, laryngeal edema, oral candidiasis, painful oral mucosa, taste perversion

**GI:** Abdominal pain, diarrhea, hepatitis, indigestion, nausea, pseudomembranous colitis, vomiting

**GU:** Interstitial nephritis, polyuria, renal failure, urine retention, vaginal candidiasis

**HEME:** Hemolytic anemia

**MS:** Tendinitis, tendon rupture

**RESP:** Pulmonary edema

**SKIN:** Exfolitaive dermatitis, hyperpigmentation, photosensitivity, Stevens-Johnson syndrome, toxic epidermal necrolysis

**Other:** Anaphylaxis

## Nursing Considerations

•Know that lomefloxacin shouldn't be given to patients with QT-interval prolongation or hypokalemia or to patients taking class IA antiarrhythmic drugs (such as quinidine or procainamide) or class III antiarrhythmic drugs (such as amiodarone or sotalol) because of the increased risk of torsades de pointes.

•Expect to obtain body fluid or tissue sample for culture and sensitivity testing and to review results, if possible, before lomefloxacin therapy begins.

•If patient's culture test results are positive for gonorrhea, expect to obtain serologic test for syphilis at diagnosis and to repeat test 3 months after lomefloxacin therapy.

•Give drug with meals and a full glass of water.

•Ensure that patient maintains adequate fluid intake during therapy.

•Observe for signs of secondary infections, such as sore mouth or vaginal discharge.

•Notify prescriber if patient experiences severe or prolonged diarrhea, which may indicate pseudomembranous colitis.

•Be aware that prolonged use may lead to growth of drug-resistant organisms.

•Notify prescriber and expect to stop lomefloxacin if patient develops symptoms of peripheral neuropathy (pain, burning, tingling, numbness, weakness, or changes in sensations of light touch, pain, temperature, position, or vibration) to prevent an irreversible condition or tendon rupture that requires immediate rest and avoidance of exercise involving the affected area.

PATIENT TEACHING

•Advise patient to take lomefloxacin at the same time each day with meals and with a full glass of water.

J
K
L

•Caution patient not to take antacids, iron, sucralfate, or zinc 1 hour before or 2 hours after taking lomefloxacin because these preparations impair drug absorption.

•Urge patient to drink plenty of fluids during treatment.

•Instruct patient to complete the full course of therapy, even if symptoms subside.

•Advise patient to notify prescriber if symptoms don't improve within a few days after starting lomefloxacin or if severe GI distress or diarrhea develops.

•Instruct patient to notify prescriber and stop taking drug if she experiences tendon inflammation or pain; advise her to rest until tendinitis and tendon rupture have been ruled out.

•Urge patient to avoid direct sunlight, to wear protective clothing, and to use sunscreen because photosensitivity reactions can occur during therapy and for several days afterward.

•Explain that risk of photosensitivity can be decreased by taking lomefloxacin at least 12 hours before sun exposure. Urge patient to stop drug and notify prescriber at first sign of photosensitivity, such as skin burning, redness, swelling, blisters, rash, itching, or dermatitis.

•Inform patient that an allergic reaction may occur after a single dose. Stress that patient should stop lomefloxacin and notify prescriber if rash or other allergic reaction develops.

•Caution patient to avoid potentially hazardous activities until drug's CNS effects are known.

# loracarbef

Lorabid

## Class and Category

*Chemical:* Carbacephem
*Therapeutic:* Antibiotic
*Pregnancy category:* B

## Indications and Dosages

➤ *To treat acute bronchitis caused by* Haemophilus influenzae, Moraxella catarrhalis, *or* Streptococcus pneumoniae

**CAPSULES, ORAL SUSPENSION**

**Adults and adolescents.** 200 to 400 mg q 12 hr for 7 days.

➤ *To treat chronic bronchitis exacerbations caused by* H. influenzae, M. catarrhalis, *or* S. pneumoniae

**CAPSULES, ORAL SUSPENSION**

**Adults and adolescents.** 400 mg q 12 hr for 7 days.

➤ *To treat pneumonia caused by* H. influenzae *or* S. pneumoniae

**CAPSULES, ORAL SUSPENSION**

**Adults and adolescents.** 400 mg q 12 hr for 14 days.

➤ *To treat pharyngitis, sinusitis, or tonsillitis caused by* Streptococcus pyogenes

**CAPSULES, ORAL SUSPENSION**

**Adults and adolescents.** 200 to 400 mg q 12 hr for 10 days.

**Children.** 7.5 mg/kg q 12 hr for 10 days.

➤ *To treat acute otitis media caused by* H. influenzae, M. catarrhalis, S. pneumoniae, *or* S. pyogenes

**ORAL SUSPENSION**

**Children.** 15 mg/kg q 12 hr for 10 days.

➤ *To treat uncomplicated skin and soft-tissue infections caused by* Staphylococcus aureus *or* S. pyogenes

**CAPSULES, ORAL SUSPENSION**

**Adults and adolescents.** 200 mg q 12 hr for 7 days.

**ORAL SUSPENSION**

**Children.** 7.5 mg/kg q 12 hr for 7 days.

➤ *To treat uncomplicated cystitis caused by* Escherichia coli *or* Staphylococcus saprophyticus

**CAPSULES, ORAL SUSPENSION**

**Adults and adolescents.** 200 mg q.d. for 7 days.

➤ *To treat uncomplicated pyelonephritis caused by* E. coli

**CAPSULES, ORAL SUSPENSION**

**Adults and adolescents.** 400 mg q 12 hr for 14 days.

DOSAGE ADJUSTMENT If creatinine clearance is 10 to 49 ml/min/1.73 m$^2$, 50% of usual dose given at normal interval or usual dose given at twice the normal interval; if clearance is less than 10 ml/min/1.73 m$^2$, usual adult dosage given q 3 to 5 days.

## Contraindications

Hypersensitivity to loracarbef, other cephalosporins, or their components

## Mechanism of Action

Interferes with bacterial cell wall synthesis by inhibiting the final step in the cross-linking of peptidoglycan strands. Peptidoglycan makes the bacterial cell membrane rigid and protective. Without it, bacterial cells rupture and die.

## Interactions
**DRUGS**
*probenecid:* Inhibited renal excretion of loracarbef, resulting in increased blood level
**FOODS**
*all foods:* Inhibited drug absorption

## Adverse Reactions

**CNS:** Dizziness, drowsiness, headache, insomnia, nervousness, seizures
**EENT:** Oral candidiasis
**GI:** Abdominal pain, anorexia, diarrhea, nausea, pseudomembranous colitis, vomiting
**GU:** Vaginal candidiasis
**SKIN:** Pruritus, rash, urticaria

## Nursing Considerations

•Expect to obtain body fluid or tissue sample for culture and sensitivity testing and to review results, if possible, before giving first dose of loracarbef.
•Be aware that oral suspension is absorbed more rapidly and produces a higher peak plasma level than capsules.
•Monitor patient for signs of secondary infections, such as sore mouth and vaginal discharge.
•Monitor for seizures, especially if patient has impaired renal function.
**PATIENT TEACHING**
•Advise patient to take loracarbef at least 1 hour before or 2 hours after meals.
•Instruct patient to complete the full course of therapy as prescribed, even if symptoms decrease.
•Instruct patient to discard unused oral solution after 14 days.
•Advise patient to report diarrhea, hives, or severe rash to prescriber.

# lorazepam

Apo-Lorazepam (CAN), Ativan, Lorazepam Intensol, Novo-Lorazem (CAN), Nu-Loraz (CAN)

## Class, Category, and Schedule
*Chemical:* Benzodiazepine
*Therapeutic:* Amnestic, antianxiety, anticonvulsant, sedative
*Pregnancy category:* D (parenteral), Not rated (oral)
*Controlled substance:* Schedule IV

## Indications and Dosages
➤ *To treat anxiety*
**ORAL CONCENTRATE, TABLETS**
**Adults and adolescents.** 1 to 3 mg b.i.d. or t.i.d. *Maximum:* 10 mg/day.
DOSAGE ADJUSTMENT For elderly or debilitated patients, initial dosage possibly reduced to 0.5 to 2 mg/day in divided doses.

➤ *To treat insomnia caused by anxiety*
**ORAL CONCENTRATE, TABLETS**
**Adults and adolescents.** 2 to 4 mg h.s.
DOSAGE ADJUSTMENT Dosage possibly reduced for elderly or debilitated patients.

➤ *To provide preoperative sedation*
**I.V. INJECTION**
**Adults and adolescents.** 0.044 mg/kg or 2 mg, whichever is less, given 2 hr before procedure. *Maximum:* 0.05 mg/kg or total of 4 mg.
**I.M. INJECTION**
**Adults and adolescents.** 0.05 mg/kg 2 hr before procedure. *Maximum:* 4 mg.

➤ *To treat status epilepticus*
**I.V. INJECTION**
**Adults and adolescents.** *Initial:* 4 mg at a rate of 2 mg/min. Repeated in 10 to 15 min if seizures don't subside. *Maximum:* 8 mg/24 hr.

| Route | Onset | Peak | Duration |
|-------|-------|------|----------|
| I.V. | 5 min | Unknown | 12 to 24 hr |
| I.M. | 15 to 30 min | Unknown | 12 to 24 hr |

## Incompatibilities
Don't mix I.V. lorazepam in same syringe as buprenorphine.

## Contraindications
Acute angle-closure glaucoma, hypersensitivity to lorazepam or its components, intraarterial administration, psychosis

## Interactions
**DRUGS**
*CNS depressants:* Additive CNS depression
*digoxin:* Possibly increased blood digoxin level and risk of digitalis toxicity

*fentanyl:* Possibly decreased therapeutic effects of fentanyl
*probenecid:* Possibly increased therapeutic and adverse effects of lorazepam
**ACTIVITIES**
*alcohol use:* Increased CNS depression

---

**Mechanism of Action**

May potentiate the effects of gamma-aminobutyric acid (GABA) and other inhibitory neurotransmitters by binding to specific benzodiazepine receptors in the limbic and cortical areas of the CNS. GABA inhibits excitatory stimulation, which helps control emotional behavior. The limbic system contains a highly dense area of benzodiazepine receptors, which may explain the drug's antianxiety effects. Also, lorazepam hyperpolarizes neuronal cells, thereby interfering with their ability to generate seizures.

---

**Adverse Reactions**

**CNS:** Amnesia, anxiety, ataxia, confusion, delusions, depression, dizziness, drowsiness, euphoria, headache, hypokinesia, irritability, malaise, nervousness, slurred speech, tremor
**CV:** Chest pain, palpitations, tachycardia
**EENT:** Blurred vision, dry mouth, increased salivation, photophobia
**GI:** Abdominal pain, constipation, diarrhea, nausea, thirst, vomiting
**GU:** Libido changes
**SKIN:** Diaphoresis
**Other:** Injection site pain (I.M.) or phlebitis (I.V.), physical and psychological dependence, withdrawal symptoms

**Nursing Considerations**

• Use extreme caution when giving lorazepam to elderly patients because it can cause hypoventilation.
• Inject I.M. lorazepam deep into a large muscle mass, such as the gluteus maximus.
• Dilute I.V. drug with equal amount of sterile water for injection, sodium chloride for injection, or $D_5W$. Give diluted drug slowly, at a rate not to exceed 2 mg/min.
• During I.V. use, monitor respirations every 5 to 15 minutes and keep emergency resuscitation equipment readily available.

• Because abrupt drug discontinuation increases the risk of withdrawal symptoms, expect to taper dosage gradually, especially in epileptic patients.

**PATIENT TEACHING**

• Instruct patient to take lorazepam exactly as prescribed and not to stop drug without consulting prescriber because of the risk of withdrawal symptoms.
• Advise patient to avoid potentially hazardous activities until drug's CNS effects are known.
• Urge patient to avoid alcohol while taking lorazepam because it increases drug's CNS depressant effects.
• Instruct patient to report excessive drowsiness and nausea.

# losartan potassium

Cozaar

**Class and Category**

*Chemical:* Angiotensin II receptor antagonist
*Therapeutic:* Antihypertensive
*Pregnancy category:* C (first trimester), D (later trimesters)

**Indications and Dosages**

➤ *To manage hypertension*
**TABLETS**
**Adults.** *Initial:* 50 mg q.d. *Maintenance:* 25 to 100 mg as a single dose or in divided doses b.i.d.

➤ *To treat nephropathy in patients with type 2 diabetes mellitus and hypertension*
**TABLETS**
**Adults.** *Initial:* 50 mg q.d., increased to 100 mg q.d., as needed.

➤ *To reduce stroke risk in patients with hypertension and left ventricular hypertrophy*
**TABLETS**
**Adults.** *Initial:* 50 mg q.d., followed by 12.5 mg hydrochlorothiazide q.d. Dosage increased to 100 mg q.d., as needed, followed by 25 mg hydrochlorothiazide q.d., as needed.
**Children age 6 and older.** *Initial:* 0.7 mg/kg to a maximum of 50 mg q.d. *Maximum:* 1.4 mg/kg or 100 mg q.d.
**DOSAGE ADJUSTMENT** Initial dosage reduced to 25 mg q.d. for patients with impaired hepatic function or volume depletion.

| Route | Onset | Peak | Duration |
|---|---|---|---|
| P.O. | Unknown | 6 hr | Over 24 hr |

## Mechanism of Action
Blocks binding of angiotensin II to receptor sites in many tissues, including vascular smooth muscle and adrenal glands. Angiotensin II is a potent vasoconstrictor that also stimulates the adrenal cortex to secrete aldosterone. The inhibiting effects of angiotensin II reduce blood pressure.

## Contraindications
Hypersensitivity to losartan or its components

## Interactions
**DRUGS**
*cyclosporine, potassium-sparing diuretics, potassium supplements:* Increased risk of hyperkalemia
*diuretics, other antihypertensives:* Possibly hypotension
*indomethacin, NSAIDs, sympathomimetics:* Possibly decreased antihypertensive effect of losartan
**FOODS**
*high-potassium diet, potassium-containing salt substitutes:* Increased risk of hyperkalemia

## Adverse Reactions
**CNS:** Dizziness, fatigue, headache, insomnia
**CV:** Hypotension
**EENT:** Nasal congestion
**GI:** Diarrhea, indigestion, nausea, vomiting
**HEME:** Thrombocytopenia
**MS:** Back pain, leg pain, muscle spasms
**RESP:** Cough, upper respiratory tract infection
**Other:** Angioedema, hyperkalemia, hyponatremia

## Nursing Considerations
•Be aware that losartan is more effective in some patients when given in two divided doses daily; it may be used with other antihypertensives.
•Know that patients of African descent with hypertension and left ventricular hypertrophy may not benefit from losartan to reduce stroke risk.
•WARNING Be aware that patients with severe heart failure or renal artery stenosis may ex-

perience acute renal failure because losartan inhibits the angiotensin-aldosterone system, on which renal function depends.
•Monitor patient's blood pressure and renal function studies to evaluate drug effectiveness.
•Periodically monitor patient's serum potassium level, as appropriate, to detect hyperkalemia.
•Monitor patient for muscle pain; rarely, rhabdomyolysis develops in patients taking other angiotensin II receptor blockers.
**PATIENT TEACHING**
•Instruct patient taking losartan to avoid potassium-containing salt substitutes, which can increase the risk of hyperkalemia.
•Advise patient to avoid exercising in hot weather and drinking excessive amounts of alcohol; instruct her to notify prescriber if she experiences prolonged diarrhea, nausea, or vomiting.

# lovastatin
## (mevinolin)
Altoprev, Mevacor

## Class and Category
*Chemical:* Mevinic acid derivative
*Therapeutic:* Antihyperlipidemic
*Pregnancy category:* X

## Indications and Dosages
➤ *To reduce LDL and total cholesterol levels in patients with primary hypercholesterolemia*
**TABLETS**
**Adults.** *Initial:* 20 mg as a single dose with evening meal. *Maintenance:* 20 to 80 mg/day as a single dose or in divided doses with meals. *Maximum:* 80 mg/day.
DOSAGE ADJUSTMENT For patients who also take immunosuppressants, initial dosage decreased to 10 mg q.d. and maximum dosage limited to 20 mg q.d.
**E.R. TABLETS**
**Adults.** *Initial:* 10 mg, 20 mg, 40 mg, or 60 mg as single dose h.s., increased, as needed, q 4 wk, up to maximum dose. *Maintenance:* 10 to 60 mg/day as single dose. *Maximum:* 60 mg/day.

➤ *To reduce LDL, total cholesterol, and apolipoprotein B levels in adolescents with heterozygous familial hypercholesterolemia*

**TABLETS**

**Adolescents 1 yr postmenarche (ages 10 to 17).** *Initial:* 20 mg/day for LDL reduction of 20% or more, 10 mg/day for LDL reduction of less than 20%; dosage adjusted after at least 4 wk. *Maintenance:* 10 to 40 mg/day. *Maximum:* 40 mg/day.

**DOSAGE ADJUSTMENT** For patients who also take amiodarone or verapamil, maximum dosage limited to 40 mg/day. For patients who also take cyclorsporine, gemfibrozil or other fibrates or lipid-lowering drugs such as niacin (1 g or more daily), maximum dosage of lovastatin limited to 20 mg/day. For patients with creatinine clearance less than 30 ml/min/1.73 m², maximum dosage limited to 20 mg/day.

| Route | Onset | Peak | Duration |
|-------|-------|------|----------|
| P.O. | In 2 wk | Unknown | 4 to 6 wk |

## Mechanism of Action

Interferes with the hepatic enzyme hydroxymethylglutaryl-coenzyme A reductase. By doing so, lovastatin reduces the formation of mevalonic acid (a cholesterol precursor), thus interrupting the pathway by which cholesterol is synthesized. When the cholesterol level declines in hepatic cells, LDLs are consumed, which also reduces the amount of circulating total cholesterol and serum triglycerides. The decrease in LDLs may result in a decreased level of apolipoprotein B, which is found within each LDL particle.

## Contraindications

Acute hepatic disease, breast-feeding, hypersensitivity to lovastatin or its components, pregnancy, unexplained elevated liver function test results

## Interactions

**DRUGS**

*amiodarone, clarithromycin, cyclosporine, danazol, erythromycin, fibric acid derivatives, gemfibrozil and other fibrates, HIV protease inhibitors, immunosuppressants, itraconazole, ketoconazole, nefazodone, niacin (1 g/day or more), telithromycin, verapamil:* Increased risk of severe myopathy or rhabdomyolysis

*bile acid sequestrants, cholestyramine, colestipol:* Decreased bioavailability of lovastatin

*isradipine:* Increased hepatic clearance of lovastatin

*itraconazole, ketoconazole:* Increased lovastatin blood level

*oral anticoagulants:* Increased anticoagulant effect and risk of bleeding

**FOODS**

*all foods:* Increased lovastatin absorption

*grapefruit juice (more than 1 qt/day):* Increased risk of myopathy or rhabdomyolysis

**ACTIVITIES**

*alcohol use:* Increased lovastatin blood level

## Adverse Reactions

**CNS:** Dizziness, fatigue, headache, insomnia

**EENT:** Blurred vision, cataracts, pharyngitis, rhinitis, sinusitis

**GI:** Abdominal cramps and pain, constipation, diarrhea, elevated liver function test results, flatulence, indigestion, nausea, vomiting

**MS:** Arthritis, back pain, myalgia, myopathy, myositis, rhabdomyolysis

**RESP:** Cough, upper respiratory tract infection

**SKIN:** Dermatomyositis, erythema multiforme, pruritus, rash, Stevens-Johnson syndrome, toxic epidermal necrolysis

**Other:** Anaphylaxis, angioedema

## Nursing Considerations

•Use lovastatin cautiously in patients with a history of liver disease and patients who consume large amounts of alcohol.

•Monitor liver function test results before and during lovastatin therapy. If serum transaminase levels rise, expect to measure them more often, as ordered. If AST or ALT level reaches or exceeds three times the upper limit of normal and persists at that level, expect to stop drug.

•Administer lovastatin 1 hour before or 4 hours after giving bile acid sequestrant, cholestyramine, or colestipol.

•Expect patient to follow a standard low-cholesterol diet during therapy.

•Be aware that drug exerts effects mainly on total cholesterol and LDL levels and has only slight effects on HDL and triglyceride levels.

**PATIENT TEACHING**

•Instruct patient who takes drug once daily to do so with evening meal to enhance absorption.

•Advise patient to report muscle aches, pains, tenderness, or weakness; severe GI distress; and vision changes.

•Urge patient to avoid consuming alcohol or more than 1 quart of grapefruit juice daily while taking drug.

•Direct patient to follow a low-cholesterol diet as adjunct to therapy. Recommend weight loss and exercise programs as appropriate.

•Stress the importance of periodic eye examinations during therapy.

•Teach female patients appropriate contraceptive methods and the need to report suspected pregnancy immediately.

# loxapine hydrochloride

Loxapac (CAN), Loxitane, Loxitane C, Loxitane IM

## loxapine succinate

Loxapac (CAN), Loxitane

## Class and Category

*Chemical:* Dibenzoxazepine derivative
*Therapeutic:* Antipsychotic
*Pregnancy category:* C

## Indications and Dosages

➤ *To treat psychotic disorders and schizophrenia*

**CAPSULES, ORAL SOLUTION**

**Adults.** *Initial:* 10 mg b.i.d., increased over 7 days. *Maintenance:* 15 to 25 mg b.i.d. to q.i.d. *Maximum:* 250 mg/day.

**DOSAGE ADJUSTMENT** For elderly patients, dosage reduced to 3 to 5 mg b.i.d.

➤ *To treat acute exacerbations of psychotic disorders*

**I.M. INJECTION**

**Adults.** 12.5 to 50 mg q 4 to 6 hr or longer. *Maximum:* 250 mg/day.

| Route | Onset | Peak | Duration |
|-------|-------|------|----------|
| P.O. | 20 to 30 min | 1.5 to 3 hr | 12 hr |

## Mechanism of Action

May treat psychotic disorders by blocking dopamine at postsynaptic receptors in the brain. With prolonged use, loxapine enhances antipsychotic effects by causing depolarization blockade of dopamine tracts, resulting in decreased dopamine neurotransmission.

## Contraindications

Blood dyscrasias, bone marrow depression, cerebrovascular disease, coma, coronary artery disease, hypersensitivity to loxapine or its components, impaired hepatic function, myeloproliferative disorders, severe drug-induced CNS depression, severe hypertension or hypotension

## Interactions

**DRUGS**

*amphetamines, ephedrine:* Decreased effects of these drugs

*antacids, antidiarrheals (adsorbent):* Possibly decreased absorption of oral loxapine

*anticholinergics:* Possibly increased anticholinergic effects

*anticonvulsants:* Lowered seizure threshold, increased risk of seizures

*antidyskinetics:* Possibly antagonized therapeutic effects of these drugs

*bromocriptine:* Possibly decreased therapeutic effects of bromocriptine

*CNS depressants:* Increased CNS depression

*dopamine:* Possibly decreased alpha-adrenergic effects of dopamine

*epinephrine:* Possibly severe hypotension or tachycardia, decreased effects of epinephrine

*guanadrel, guanethidine, levodopa:* Possibly decreased therapeutic effects of these drugs

*MAO inhibitors, tricyclic antidepressants:* Possibly increased blood levels of these drugs and increased CNS depressant and anticholinergic effects of these drugs and loxapine

*metaraminol:* Possibly decreased vasopressor effect of metaraminol

*methoxamine:* Possibly decreased vasopressor effect and duration of action of methoxamine

J
K
L

*alcohol use:* Increased CNS depression

## Adverse Reactions
**CNS:** Confusion, drowsiness, dystonia, involuntary motor activity, neuroleptic malignant syndrome, pseudoparkinsonism, sleep disturbance, tardive dyskinesia
**CV:** Orthostatic hypotension
**EENT:** Blurred vision, dry mouth
**ENDO:** Galactorrhea, gynecomastia
**GI:** Constipation, ileus, nausea, vomiting
**GU:** Menstrual irregularities, sexual dysfunction, urine retention
**SKIN:** Photosensitivity (mild), rash
**Other:** Weight gain

## Nursing Considerations
• Be aware that loxapine's full antipsychotic effect may require weeks.
• Assess for signs of tardive dyskinesia, including involuntary protrusion of tongue and chewing movements. These signs may appear months or years after loxapine therapy begins and may not disappear with dosage reduction.
• Observe for extrapyramidal reactions or parkinsonian symptoms, such as excessive salivation, masklike facies, rigidity, and tremor, especially in first few days of treatment. Prescriber may reduce dosage to control these symptoms.
• **WARNING** Monitor for neuroleptic malignant syndrome, a rare but possibly fatal adverse reaction. Early signs include altered mental status, arrhythmias, fever, and muscle rigidity.
**PATIENT TEACHING**
• Instruct patient to dilute loxapine oral solution with orange or grapefruit juice just before taking. Advise her to use the calibrated dropper that accompanies the solution to ensure correct dosage.
• Direct patient to avoid taking antacids and antidiarrheals 2 hours before or after taking loxapine.
• Caution patient to avoid alcohol while taking loxapine.
• Advise patient to change position slowly to minimize effects of orthostatic hypotension.
• Urge patient to avoid potentially hazardous activities until drug's CNS effects are known.

• Advise patient to avoid prolonged exposure to sun and to use sunscreen to minimize the risk of photosensitivity.
• Encourage patient to have periodic eye examinations during therapy.

# lypressin
Diapid

## Class and Category
*Chemical:* Synthetic vasopressin analogue
*Therapeutic:* Antidiuretic
*Pregnancy category:* C

## Indications and Dosages
➤ *To control and prevent dehydration, polydipsia, and polyuria in patients with neurogenic diabetes insipidus that is unresponsive to other therapy*
**NASAL SOLUTION**
**Adults and adolescents.** 1 or 2 sprays q.i.d. If more drug is needed, interval between doses is decreased rather than increasing number of sprays/dose.

| Route | Onset | Peak | Duration |
|---|---|---|---|
| Intranasal | In 1 hr | 0.5 to 2 hr | 3 to 4 hr |

### Mechanism of Action
Increases cellular permeability of collecting ducts in kidneys, leading to increased urine osmolality and decreased urine output.

## Contraindications
Hypersensitivity to lypressin or its components

## Interactions
**DRUGS**
*carbamazepine, chlorpropamide, clofibrate:* Possibly increased antidiuretic effect
*demeclocycline, lithium, norepinephrine:* Decreased antidiuretic effect of lypressin

## Adverse Reactions
**CNS:** Headache
**EENT:** Conjunctivitis; nasal congestion, irritation, and itching; periorbital edema and itching; rhinorrhea
**GI:** Abdominal cramps, diarrhea, heartburn

(if excessive intranasal use causes dripping into pharynx)
**RESP:** Cough, transient dyspnea (if drug is accidentally inhaled)
**Other:** Water intoxication

## Nursing Considerations
•Assess patient for nasal congestion or upper respiratory tract infection, which can reduce lypressin absorption and require larger doses or adjunct therapy.
•Administer final spray of drug at bedtime to help control nocturia.
•**WARNING** Be aware that inadvertent inhalation, although rare, may cause chest tightness, continuous cough, and dyspnea.
•Observe for nasal irritation during long-term therapy.
•Monitor patient for signs and symptoms of water intoxication, including coma, confusion, drowsiness, persistent headache, seizures, urine retention, and weight gain.

### PATIENT TEACHING
•Teach patient how to administer lypressin correctly by holding head upright and bottle in a vertical position and spraying 1 or 2 sprays in each nostril with each dose.
•Instruct patient to take last dose of day at bedtime to control nocturia.
•Instruct patient to use drug exactly as prescribed. Explain that using extra sprays wastes drug.
•Advise patient to report abdominal cramps, heartburn, persistent headache, severe nasal irritation, and shortness of breath.

# M

## magnesium chloride

*(contains 64 mg of elemental magnesium per tablet, 100 mg of elemental magnesium per enteric-coated tablet, 64 mg of elemental magnesium per E.R. tablet, and 200 mg of elemental magnesium per 1 ml of injection)*

Chloromag, Mag-L-100, Slow-Mag

## magnesium citrate (citrate of magnesia)

*(contains 40.5 to 47 mg of elemental magnesium per 5 ml of oral solution)*

Citroma, Citro-Mag (CAN)

## magnesium gluconate

*(contains 54 mg of elemental magnesium per 5 ml of oral solution and 27 to 29.3 mg of elemental magnesium per tablet)*

Almora, Maglucate (CAN), Magonate, Magtrate

## magnesium hydroxide (milk of magnesia)

*(contains 135 mg of elemental magnesium per tablet, 129 to 130 mg of elemental magnesium per chewable tablet, and 164 to 328 mg of elemental magnesium per 5 ml of liquid, liquid concentrate, or oral solution)*

Phillips' Chewable Tablets, Phillips' Magnesia Tablets (CAN), Phillips' Milk of Magnesia, Phillips' Milk of Magnesia Concentrate

## magnesium lactate

*(contains 84 mg of elemental magnesium per E.R. tablet)*

Mag-Tab SR Caplets

## magnesium oxide

*(contains 84.5 mg of elemental magnesium per capsule and 50 to 302 mg of elemental magnesium per tablet)*

Mag-200, Mag-Ox 400, Maox, Uro-Mag

## magnesium sulfate

*(contains 100 to 500 mg of elemental magnesium per 1 ml of injection, 1 to 5 g of elemental magnesium per 10 ml of injection, and 40 mEq per 5 mg of crystals)*

## Class and Category

*Chemical:* Cation, electrolyte
*Therapeutic:* Antacid, antiarrhythmic, anticonvulsant, electrolyte replacement, laxative
*Pregnancy category:* A (parenteral magnesium sulfate), Not rated (others)

## Indications and Dosages

➤ *To correct magnesium deficiency caused by alcoholism, magnesium-depleting drugs, malnutrition, or restricted diet; to prevent magnesium deficiency based on U.S. and Canadian recommended daily allowances*

CAPSULES, CHEWABLE TABLETS, CRYSTALS, ENTERIC-COATED TABLETS, E.R. TABLETS, LIQUID, LIQUID CONCENTRATE, ORAL SOLUTION, TABLETS (MAGNESIUM CHLORIDE, CITRATE, GLUCONATE, HYDROXIDE, LACTATE [EXCEPT IN CHILDREN], OXIDE, SULFATE)

Dosage individualized based on severity of deficiency and normal recommended daily allowances listed below.

**Male adults and children over age 10.** 270 to 400 mg/day (130 to 250 mg/day Canadian).

**Female adults and children over age 10.** 280 to 300 mg/day (135 to 210 mg/day Canadian).

**Pregnant females.** 320 mg/day (195 to 245 mg/day Canadian).

**Breast-feeding females.** 340 to 355 mg/day (245 to 265 mg/day Canadian).

**Children ages 7 to 10.** 170 mg/day (100 to 135 mg/day Canadian).

**Children ages 4 to 6.** 120 mg/day (65 mg/day Canadian).

**Children from birth to age 3.** 40 to 80 mg/day (20 to 50 mg/day Canadian).

➤ *To treat mild magnesium deficiency*

**I.M. INJECTION (MAGNESIUM SULFATE)**

**Adults and adolescents.** 1 g q 6 hr for 4 doses.

➤ *To treat severe hypomagnesemia*

**I.V. INFUSION (MAGNESIUM CHLORIDE)**

**Adults.** 4 g diluted in 250 ml of $D_5W$ and infused at a rate not to exceed 3 ml/min. *Maximum:* 40 g/day.

**I.V. INFUSION (MAGNESIUM SULFATE)**

**Adults and adolescents.** 5 g diluted in 1 L of I.V. solution and infused over 3 hr.

➤ *To provide supplemental magnesium in total parenteral nutrition*

**I.V. INFUSION (MAGNESIUM SULFATE)**

**Adults.** 1 to 3 g/day.

**Children.** 0.25 mg to 1.25 g/day.

**DOSAGE ADJUSTMENT** Adult dosage may be increased to 6 g/day for certain conditions, such as short-bowel syndrome.

**I.M. INJECTION (MAGNESIUM SULFATE)**

**Adults and adolescents.** Up to 250 mg/kg q 4 hr, p.r.n.

➤ *To prevent and control seizures in preeclampsia or eclampsia as well as seizures caused by epilepsy, glomerulonephritis, or hypothyroidism*

**I.V. INFUSION OR INJECTION (MAGNESIUM SULFATE)**

**Adults.** *Loading:* 4 g diluted in 250 ml of compatible solution and infused over 30 min. *Maintenance:* 1 to 2 g/hr by continuous infusion.

**I.M. INJECTION (MAGNESIUM SULFATE)**

**Adults.** 4 to 5 g q 4 hr, p.r.n.

**Children.** 20 to 40 mg/kg, repeated p.r.n.

➤ *To relieve indigestion associated with hyperacidity*

**CHEWABLE TABLETS, LIQUID, LIQUID CONCENTRATE, ORAL SOLUTION TABLETS (MAGNESIUM HYDROXIDE)**

**Adults and adolescents.** 400 to 1,200 mg (5 to 15 ml liquid or 2.5 to 7.5 ml liquid concentrate) up to 4 times/day with water, or 622 to 1,244 mg (tablets or chewable tablets) up to 4 times/day.

**CAPSULES, TABLETS (MAGNESIUM OXIDE)**

**Adults and adolescents.** 140 mg (capsules) t.i.d. or q.i.d. with water or milk, or 400 to 800 mg/day (tablets).

➤ *To relieve constipation, to evacuate colon for rectal or bowel examination*

**LIQUID, LIQUID CONCENTRATE (MAGNESIUM HYDROXIDE)**

**Adults and children age 12 and older.** 2.4 to 4.8 g (30 to 60 ml)/day as a single dose or in divided doses.

**Children ages 6 to 11.** 1.2 to 2.4 g (15 to 30 ml)/day as a single dose or in divided doses.

**Children ages 2 to 5.** 0.4 to 1.2 g (5 to 15 ml)/day as a single dose or in divided doses.

**ORAL SOLUTION (MAGNESIUM CITRATE)**

**Adults and children age 12 and older.** 11 to 25 g/day as a single dose or in divided doses.

**Children ages 6 to 11.** 5.5 to 12.5 g/day as a single dose or in divided doses.

**Children ages 2 to 5.** 2.7 to 6.25 g/day as a single dose or in divided doses.

**CRYSTALS (MAGNESIUM SULFATE)**

**Adults and children age 12 and older.** 10 to 30 g/day as a single dose or in divided doses.

**DOSAGE ADJUSTMENT** Dosage limited to 20 g of magnesium sulfate q 48 hr for patients with severe renal impairment.

**Children ages 6 to 11.** 5 to 10 g/day as a single dose or in divided doses.

**Children ages 2 to 5.** 2.5 to 5 g/day as a single dose or in divided doses.

**CAPSULES, TABLETS (MAGNESIUM OXIDE)**

**Adults.** 2 to 4 g with a full glass of water or milk, usually h.s.

| Route | Onset | Peak | Duration |
|---|---|---|---|
| P.O.* | 0.5 to 3 hr | Unknown | Unknown |
| P.O.† | 20 min | Unknown | 20 to 180 min |
| I.M.‡ | 1 hr | Unknown | 3 to 4 hr |
| I.V.‡ | Immediate | Unknown | About 30 min |

## Mechanism of Action

Assists all enzymes involved in phosphate transfer reactions that use adenosine triphosphate (ATP). Magnesium is required for normal function of the ATP-dependent sodium-potassium pump in muscle membranes. It may effectively treat digitalis glycoside–induced arrhythmias because correction of hypomagnesemia improves the sodium-potassium pump's ability to distribute potassium into intracellular spaces and because magnesium decreases calcium uptake and potassium outflow through myocardial cell membranes.

As a laxative, magnesium exerts a hyperosmotic effect in the small intestine. It causes water retention that distends the bowel and causes the duodenum to secrete cholecystokinin. This substance stimulates fluid secretion and intestinal motility.

As an antacid, magnesium reacts with water, converting magnesium oxide to magnesium hydroxide. Magnesium hydroxide rapidly reacts with gastric acid to form water and magnesium chloride, which increases gastric pH.

As an anticonvulsant, magnesium depresses the CNS and blocks peripheral neuromuscular impulse transmission by decreasing the amount of available acetylcholine.

## Incompatibilities

Don't combine magnesium sulfate with alkali carbonates and bicarbonates, alkali hydroxides, arsenates, calcium, clindamycin phosphate, dobutamine, fat emulsions, heavy

---

* For laxative effect.
† For antacid effect.
‡ For anticonvulsant effect.

metals, hydrocortisone sodium succinate, phosphates, polymyxin B, procaine hydrochloride, salicylates, sodium bicarbonate, strontium, and tartrates.

## Contraindications
Hypersensitivity to magnesium salts or any component of magnesium-containing preparations
*For magnesium chloride:* Coma, heart disease, renal impairment
*For magnesium sulfate:* Heart block, MI, preeclampsia 2 hours or less before delivery (I.V. form)
*For magnesium used as laxative:* Acute abdominal problem (as indicated by abdominal pain, nausea, or vomiting), diverticulitis, fecal impaction, intestinal obstruction or perforation, presence of colostomy or ileostomy, severe renal impairment, ulcerative colitis

## Interactions
**DRUGS**
*amphotericin B, cisplatin, cyclosporine, gentamicin:* Possibly magnesium wasting and need for magnesium dosage adjustment
*anticholinergics:* Possibly decreased absorption and therapeutic effects of these drugs
*calcium salts (I.V.):* Possibly neutralization of magnesium sulfate's effects
*cellulose sodium phosphate:* Possibly binding with magnesium, possibly decreased therapeutic effectiveness of cellulose
*CNS depressants:* Possibly increased CNS depression
*digoxin (I.V.):* Possibly heart block and conduction changes, especially when calcium salts are also administered
*digoxin, fluoroquinolones, folic acid, H₂-receptor blockers, iron preparations, isoniazid, ketoconazole, penicillamine, phenothiazines, phenytoin, phosphates (oral), tetracyclines:* Possibly decreased absorption and blood levels of these drugs
*diuretics (loop or thiazide):* Possibly hypomagnesemia
*edetate sodium, sodium polystyrene sulfonate:* Possibly binding with magnesium
*enteric-coated drugs:* Possibly quicker dissolution of these drugs and increased risk of adverse GI reactions
*etidronate (oral):* Decreased etidronate absorption
*mecamylamine:* Possibly prolonged effects of mecamylamine
*methenamine, streptomycin, sucralfate, tetracyclines, tobramycin (oral), urinary acidifiers:*

Possibly decreased therapeutic effects of these drugs
*misoprostol:* Increased misoprostol-induced diarrhea
*neuromuscular blockers:* Possibly increased neuromuscular blockade
*nifedipine:* Possibly increased hypotensive effects when taken with magnesium sulfate
*potassium-sparing diuretics:* Increased risk of hypermagnesemia
*salicylates:* Possibly increased excretion and lower blood levels of salicylates
*sodium polystyrene sulfonate resin:* Possibly metabolic alkalosis
**FOODS**
*high-glucose intake:* Increased urinary excretion of magnesium
**ACTIVITIES**
*alcohol use:* Increased urinary excretion of magnesium

## Adverse Reactions
**CNS:** Confusion, decreased reflexes, dizziness, syncope
**CV:** Arrhythmias, Hypotension
**GI:** Flatulence, vomiting
**MS:** Muscle cramps
**RESP:** Dyspnea, respiratory depression or paralysis
**SKIN:** Diaphoresis
**Other:** Allergic reaction, hypermagnesemia, injection site pain or irritation (I.M. form), laxative dependence, magnesium toxicity

## Nursing Considerations
•Be aware that magnesium sulfate is the elemental form of magnesium. Oral preparations aren't all equivalent.
•Be aware that drug isn't metabolized. Drug remaining in the GI tract produces watery stool within 30 minutes to 3 hours.
•Make sure patient chews magnesium chewable tablets thoroughly before swallowing.
•Avoid giving other oral drugs within 2 hours of a magnesium-containing antacid.
•Before administering drug as a laxative, shake oral solution, liquid, or liquid concentrate well and give with a large amount of water.
•WARNING Observe for and report to prescriber early signs of hypermagnesemia: bradycardia, depressed deep tendon reflexes, diplopia, dyspnea, flushing, hypotension, nausea, slurred speech, vomiting, and weakness.
•WARNING Be aware that magnesium may precipitate myasthenic crisis by decreasing patient's sensitivity to acetylcholine.

•Frequently assess cardiac status of patient taking drugs that lower heart rate, such as beta blockers, because magnesium may aggravate symptoms of heart block.

•**WARNING** Be aware that magnesium chloride for injection contains the preservative benzyl alcohol, which may cause fatal toxic syndrome in neonates and premature infants.

•Provide adequate diet, exercise, and fluids for patient being treated for constipation.

•Monitor serum electrolyte levels in patients with renal insufficiency because they're at risk for magnesium toxicity.

•Be aware that magnesium salts aren't intended for long-term use.

**PATIENT TEACHING**

•Advise patient to chew magnesium chewable tablets thoroughly before swallowing and to follow with a full glass of water. Mention that these tablets have a chalky taste.

•Instruct patient to take magnesium-containing antacid between meals and at bedtime. Urge him not to take other drugs within 2 hours of a magnesium-containing antacid.

•Tell patient to notify prescriber and avoid using a magnesium-containing laxative if he experiences abdominal pain, nausea, or vomiting.

•Instruct patient to refrigerate magnesium citrate solution.

•Caution patient about the risk of dependence with long-term laxative use.

•Teach patient to prevent constipation by increasing dietary fiber and fluid intake and exercising regularly.

• Inform patient that magnesium supplements used to replace electrolytes can cause diarrhea.

# mannitol

Osmitrol, Resectisol

## Class and Category

*Chemical:* Hexahydroxy alcohol
*Therapeutic:* Antiglaucoma, diagnostic agent, osmotic diuretic, urinary irrigant
*Pregnancy category:* B

## Indications and Dosages

➤ *To reduce intracranial or intraocular pressure*

**I.V. INFUSION**

**Adults and adolescents.** 0.25 to 2 g/kg as 15% to 25% solution given over 30 to 60 min. If used before eye surgery, 1.5 to 2 g/kg 60 to 90 min before procedure. *Maximum:* 6 g/kg/day.

**DOSAGE ADJUSTMENT** For small or debilitated patients, dosage reduced to 0.5 g/kg.

➤ *To diagnose oliguria or inadequate renal function*

**I.V. INFUSION**

**Adults and adolescents.** 200 mg/kg or 12.5 g as 15% to 20% solution given over 3 to 5 min. Second dose given only if patient fails to excrete 30 to 50 ml of urine in 2 to 3 hr. Drug discontinued if no response after second dose. Alternatively, 100 ml of 20% solution diluted in 180 ml of NS (forming 280 ml of 7.2% solution) and infused at 20 ml/min; followed by measurement of urine output. *Maximum:* 6 g/kg/day.

➤ *To prevent oliguria or acute renal failure*

**I.V. INFUSION**

**Adults and adolescents.** 50 to 100 g as 5% to 25% solution. *Maximum:* 6 g/kg/day.

➤ *To treat oliguria*

**I.V. INFUSION**

**Adults and adolescents.** 50 to 100 g as 15% to 25% solution given over 90 min to several hr. *Maximum:* 6 g/kg/day.

➤ *To promote diuresis in drug toxicity*

**I.V. INFUSION**

**Adults and adolescents.** *Loading:* 25 g. *Maintenance:* Up to 200 g as 5% to 25% solution given continuously to maintain urine output of 100 to 500 ml/hr with positive fluid balance of 1 to 2 L. *Maximum:* 6 g/kg/day.

➤ *To promote diuresis in hemolytic transfusion reaction*

**I.V. INFUSION**

**Adults.** 20 g given over 5 min and repeated if needed. *Maximum:* 6 g/kg/day.

➤ *To provide irrigation during transurethral resection of prostate gland*

**IRRIGATION SOLUTION**

**Adults.** 2.5% or 5% solution, as needed.

| Route | Onset | Peak | Duration |
|---|---|---|---|
| I.V.* | 1 to 3 hr | Unknown | Up to 8 hr |
| I.V.† | 30 to 60 min | Unknown | 4 to 8 hr |
| I.V.‡ | In 15 min | Unknown | 3 to 8 hr |

* To produce diuresis.
† To decrease intraocular pressure.
‡ To decrease intracranial pressure.

## Mechanism of Action

Elevates plasma osmolality, causing water to flow from tissues, such as the brain and eyes, and from CSF, into extracellular fluid, thereby decreasing intracranial and intraocular pressure.

As an osmotic diuretic, mannitol increases the osmolarity of glomerular filtrate, which decreases water reabsorption. This leads to increased excretion of water, sodium, chloride, and toxic substances.

As an irrigant, mannitol minimizes the hemolytic effects of water used as an irrigant and reduces the movement of hemolyzed blood from the urethra to the systemic circulation, which prevents hemoglobinemia and serious renal complications.

## Incompatibilities

Don't administer mannitol through same I.V. line as blood or blood products.

## Contraindications

Active intracranial bleeding (except during craniotomy), anuria, hepatic failure, hypersensitivity to mannitol or its components, pulmonary edema, severe dehydration, severe heart failure, severe pulmonary congestion, severe renal insufficiency

## Interactions
### Drugs

*digoxin:* Increased risk of digitalis toxicity from hypokalemia
*diuretics:* Possibly increased therapeutic effects of mannitol

## Adverse Reactions

**CNS:** Chills, dizziness, fever, headache, seizures
**CV:** Chest pain, heart failure, hypertension, tachycardia, thrombophlebitis
**EENT:** Blurred vision, dry mouth, rhinitis
**GI:** Diarrhea, nausea, thirst, vomiting
**GU:** Polyuria, urine retention
**RESP:** Pulmonary edema
**SKIN:** Extravasation with edema and tissue necrosis, rash, urticaria
**Other:** Dehydration, hyperkalemia, hypernatremia, hypervolemia, hypokalemia, hyponatremia (dilutional), metabolic acidosis, water intoxication

## Nursing Considerations

• If crystals form in mannitol solution exposed to low temperature, place solution in hot-water bath to redissolve crystals.

• Use a 5-micron in-line filter when administering drug solution of 15% or greater.
• During I.V. infusion of mannitol, monitor vital signs, central venous pressure, and fluid intake and output every hour. Measure urine output with indwelling urinary catheter, as appropriate.
• Check weight and monitor BUN and serum creatinine electrolyte levels daily.
• Provide frequent mouth care to relieve thirst and dry mouth.

### Patient Teaching

• Inform patient that he may experience dry mouth and thirst during mannitol therapy.
• Instruct patient to report chest pain, difficulty breathing, or pain at I.V. site.

# maprotiline hydrochloride

Ludiomil

## Class and Category

*Chemical:* Dibenzobicyclooctadiene derivative
*Therapeutic:* Antidepressant, tricyclic antidepressant
*Pregnancy category:* B

## Indications and Dosages

➤ *To treat mild to moderate depression*
### Tablets

**Adults and adolescents.** *Initial:* 75 mg/day in divided doses for 2 wk. Increased in 25-mg increments as needed and tolerated. *Maintenance:* 150 to 225 mg/day in divided doses; for prolonged therapy, possibly 75 to 150 mg/day in divided doses.

➤ *To treat severe depression in hospitalized patients*
### Tablets

**Adults and adolescents.** *Initial:* 100 to 150 mg/day in divided doses, increased as needed and tolerated. *Maintenance:* 150 to 225 mg/day in divided doses; for prolonged therapy, possibly 75 to 150 mg/day in divided doses.
DOSAGE ADJUSTMENT For patients over age 60, initial dosage reduced to 25 mg/day and then increased by 25 mg/wk up to maintenance dosage of 50 to 75 mg/day in divided doses.

| Route | Onset | Peak | Duration |
|---|---|---|---|
| P.O. | 1 to 3 wk | 3 to 6 wk | Unknown |

M

## Mechanism of Action

Blocks norepinephrine's reuptake at adrenergic nerve fibers. Normally, when a nerve impulse reaches an adrenergic nerve fiber, norepinephrine is released from its storage sites and metabolized in the nerve or at the synapse. Some norepinephrine reaches receptor sites on target organs and tissues, but most is taken back into the nerve and stored by way of the reuptake mechanism. By blocking norepinephrine reuptake, maprotiline increases its level at nerve synapses. An elevated norepinephrine level may improve mood and, consequently, decrease depression.

## Contraindications

Hypersensitivity to maprotiline, mirtazapine, or their components; use within 14 days of MAO inhibitor therapy

## Interactions

**DRUGS**

*anticholinergics, antihistamines:* Increased atropine-like adverse effects, such as blurred vision, constipation, dizziness, and dry mouth
*anticonvulsants:* Increased risk of CNS depression, possibly lower seizure threshhold and increased risk of seizures
*bupropion, clozapine, haloperidol, loxapine, molindone, other tricyclic antidepressants, phenothiazines, pimozide, thioxanthenes, trazodone:* Possibly increased anticholinergic effects, possibly lowered seizure threshhold and increased risk of seizures
*cimetidine:* Possibly increased blood maprotiline level
*clonidine, guanadrel, guanethidine:* Possibly decreased antihypertensive effects of these drugs, possibly increased CNS depression (with clonidine)
*CNS depressants:* Increased risk of CNS depression
*estrogens, oral contraceptives containing estrogen:* Possibly decreased therapeutic effects and increased adverse effects of maprotiline
*MAO inhibitors:* Increased risk of hyperpyrexia, hypertensive crisis, severe seizures, or death
*sympathomimetics:* Increased risk of arrhythmias, hyperpyrexia, hypertension, or tachycardia
*thyroid hormones:* Increased risk of arrhythmias

**ACTIVITIES**
*alcohol use:* Increased risk of CNS depression

## Adverse Reactions

**CNS:** Agitation, dizziness, drowsiness, fatigue, headache, insomnia, seizures, tremor, weakness
**EENT:** Blurred vision, dry mouth, increased intraocular pressure
**ENDO:** Gynecomastia
**GI:** Constipation, diarrhea, epigastric distress, increased appetite, nausea, vomiting
**GU:** Impotence, libido changes, testicular swelling, urinary hesitancy, urine retention
**HEME:** Agranulocytosis
**SKIN:** Diaphoresis, photosensitivity, pruritus, rash
**Other:** Weight loss

## Nursing Considerations

•Give largest dose of maprotiline at bedtime if daytime drowsiness occurs.
•Check CBC as ordered, if fever, sore throat, or other signs of agranulocytosis develop.
•Take seizure precautions according to facility policy.
•Expect to taper drug dosage gradually because abrupt drug discontinuation may produce withdrawal symptoms.

**PATIENT TEACHING**

•Advise patient to take maprotiline exactly as prescribed. Caution him not to stop taking drug abruptly because of the risk of withdrawal symptoms, including headache, nausea, nightmares, and vertigo.
•Inform patient that he may not feel drug's effects for several weeks.
•Suggest that patient take drug with food if adverse GI reactions develop.
•Urge patient to report difficulty urinating, excessive drowsiness, fever, or sore throat.
•Advise patient to avoid potentially hazardous activities until drug's CNS effects are known.
•Urge patient to avoid alcohol and other CNS depressants while taking drug.

# mecamylamine hydrochloride

Inversine

## Class and Category

*Chemical:* Ganglionic blocker, secondary amine
*Therapeutic:* Antihypertensive
*Pregnancy category:* C

## Indications and Dosages

➤ *To manage moderately severe to severe hypertension, to treat uncomplicated malignant hypertension*

TABLETS

Adults. *Initial:* 2.5 mg b.i.d. Total dosage increased by 2.5 mg q 2 days until desired response occurs. *Maintenance:* 25 mg/day in divided doses t.i.d.

| Route | Onset | Peak | Duration |
|---|---|---|---|
| P.O. | 0.5 to 2 hr | 3 to 5 hr | 6 to 12 hr |

### Mechanism of Action

Reduces blood pressure by blocking acetylcholine's effects at autonomic ganglia. This action decreases the effects of the sympathetic and parasympathetic nervous systems, reduces sympathetic tone in blood vessels, and causes vasodilation.

## Contraindications

Chronic pyelonephritis; concurrent use of antibiotics or sulfonamides; coronary insufficiency; glaucoma; hypersensitivity to mecamylamine; mild, moderate, or labile hypertension; organic pyloric stenosis; recent MI; uncooperative behavior; uremia

## Interactions

DRUGS

*diuretics, other antihypertensives:* Increased antihypertensive effects
*urinary alkalinizers:* Increased risk of mecamylamine toxicity

ACTIVITIES

*alcohol use:* Possibly increased effects of mecamylamine
*vigorous exercise:* Increased effects of mecamylamine

## Adverse Reactions

CNS: Choreiform movements, confusion, dizziness, fatigue, headache, nervousness, paresthesia, seizures, syncope, tremor, weakness
CV: Hypotension, orthostatic hypotension
EENT: Blurred vision, dry mouth, mydriasis
GI: Anorexia, constipation, diarrhea, ileus, nausea, vomiting
GU: Decreased libido, impotence, urine retention
RESP: Interstitial pulmonary edema and fibrosis

## Nursing Considerations

• Use mecamylamine cautiously in patients with coronary artery disease and those who have had a CVA because drug may reduce blood flow to heart and brain.
• Also use drug cautiously in patients with renal insufficiency because drug may further impair renal function and may accumulate in blood.
• Give drug after meals for more gradual absorption and more constant blood pressure control.
• Give largest doses of drug at noon and in the evening.
• Monitor blood pressure with patient standing at start of treatment to determine drug's effectiveness and need for increased dosage. Check blood pressure 3 to 5 hours after dose, during drug's peak effect.
• Expect to reduce dosage for patients with conditions that may decrease drug requirements, such as fever, infection, and sodium depletion.
• Monitor for orthostatic hypotension, especially in the morning, during hot weather, and after exercise.
• Assess bowel function and be alert for signs of ileus (abdominal cramps and distention, constipation, and diarrhea).
• Expect to discontinue drug gradually to prevent rebound hypertension.

PATIENT TEACHING

• Instruct patient to take mecamylamine after meals and at the same time every day.
• Urge patient not to use alcohol while taking drug.
• Instruct patient to change position slowly to minimize effects of orthostatic hypotension.
• Inform patient that excessive sweating, vigorous exercise, hot weather, and salt depletion can cause dizziness and hypotension.
• Caution patient to avoid potentially hazardous activities until drug's CNS effects are known.
• Instruct patient to report abdominal cramps or distention, blurred vision, persistent constipation or liquid stools, severe dizziness, shortness of breath, or tremor.
• Inform male patient that drug may cause decreased libido and impotence.
• If possible, teach patient how to monitor his blood pressure daily at home and provide guidelines for calling prescriber.

M

# meclizine hydrochloride

## (meclozine hydrochloride)

Antivert, Bonamine (CAN), Bonine, Dizmiss, Dramamine II, Meclicot, Medivert, Meni-D

### Class and Category
*Chemical:* Piperazine derivative
*Therapeutic:* Antiemetic, antivertigo
*Pregnancy category:* B

### Indications and Dosages
➤ *To prevent and treat vertigo*
CAPSULES, CHEWABLE TABLETS, TABLETS
**Adults and adolescents.** 25 to 100 mg/day, p.r.n., in divided doses.

➤ *To treat motion sickness*
CAPSULES, TABLETS
**Adults.** 25 to 50 mg 1 hr before travel and then q 24 hr, p.r.n., for duration of trip.

| Route | Onset | Peak | Duration |
|-------|-------|------|----------|
| P.O. | 1 hr | Unknown | 8 to 24 hr |

### Mechanism of Action
May inhibit nausea and vomiting by reducing the sensitivity of the labyrinthine apparatus and blocking cholinergic synapses in the brain's vomiting center.

### Contraindications
Hypersensitivity to meclizine or its components

### Interactions
**DRUGS**
*anticholinergics:* Possibly potentiated anticholinergic effects
*apomorphine:* Possibly decreased emetic response to apomorphine
*CNS depressants:* Possibly potentiated CNS depression
**ACTIVITIES**
*alcohol use:* Possibly potentiated CNS depression

### Adverse Reactions
**CNS:** Dizziness, drowsiness, euphoria, excitement, fatigue, hallucinations, headache, insomnia, nervousness, restlessness, vertigo
**CV:** Hypotension, palpitations, tachycardia
**EENT:** Blurred vision; diplopia; dry mouth, nose, and throat; tinnitus
**GI:** Abdominal pain, anorexia, constipation, diarrhea, nausea, vomiting

**GU:** Urinary frequency and hesitancy, urine retention
**RESP:** Bronchospasm, thickening of respiratory secretions
**SKIN:** Jaundice, rash, urticaria

### Nursing Considerations
• Use meclizine cautiously in patients with asthma, glaucoma, or prostate enlargement.
• Be aware that drug may mask signs of brain tumor, intestinal obstruction, or ototoxicity.
PATIENT TEACHING
• Inform patient that drug works best for motion sickness when taken before travel.
• Instruct patient to chew meclizine chewable tablets thoroughly before swallowing.
• Instruct patient to report blurred vision or drowsiness.
• Urge patient to avoid alcohol while taking drug.
• Caution patient to avoid potentially hazardous activities until drug's CNS effects are known.
• Advise patient to have regular eye examinations during long-term therapy.

# meclofenamate sodium

Meclomen

### Class and Category
*Chemical:* Fenamate (anthranilic acid) derivative
*Therapeutic:* Analgesic, antidysmenorrheal, anti-inflammatory, antirheumatic
*Pregnancy category:* Not rated

### Indications and Dosages
➤ *To relieve pain and inflammation in rheumatoid arthritis and osteoarthritis*
CAPSULES
**Adults and adolescents over age 14.** 50 to 100 mg q 6 to 8 hr, p.r.n. *Maximum:* 400 mg/day.

➤ *To relieve mild to moderate pain*
CAPSULES
**Adults and adolescents over age 14.** 50 mg q 4 to 6 hr, p.r.n. Increased to 100 mg q 4 to 6 hr, if needed. *Maximum:* 400 mg/day.

➤ *To treat hypermenorrhea and primary dysmenorrhea*

CAPSULES
**Adults and adolescents over age 14.** 100 mg
t.i.d. for up to 6 days.

| Route | Onset | Peak | Duration |
|---|---|---|---|
| P.O.* | 1 hr | 0.5 to 2 hr | 4 to 6 hr |
| P.O.† | Few days | 2 to 3 wk | Unknown |

## Mechanism of Action
Blocks cyclooxygenase, the enzyme needed
to synthesize prostaglandins, which mediate the inflammatory response and cause
local vasodilation, swelling, and pain. By
inhibiting prostaglandins, this NSAID reduces inflammatory symptoms. It also relieves pain because prostaglandins promote pain transmission from the periphery
to the spinal cord.

## Contraindications
Hypersensitivity to aspirin, iodides, meclofenamate, other NSAIDs, or their components

## Interactions
DRUGS
*acetaminophen:* Increased risk of adverse
renal effects with long-term use of both drugs
*anticoagulants, thrombolytics:* Prolonged PT
and increased risk of bleeding
*antihypertensives:* Decreased effectiveness of
antihypertensives
*beta blockers:* Impaired antihypertensive effect of beta blockers
*cefamandole, cefoperazone, cefotetan, plica-
mycin, valproic acid:* Hypoprothrombinemia
and increased risk of bleeding
*cimetidine:* Altered blood meclofenamate
level
*colchicine, glucocorticoids, potassium supple-
ments:* Increased GI irritability and bleeding
*cyclosporine, gold compounds, nephrotoxic
drugs:* Increased risk of nephrotoxicity
*digoxin:* Increased blood digoxin level
*insulin, oral antidiabetic drugs:* Decreased
effectiveness of these drugs
*lithium:* Increased risk of lithium toxicity
*loop diuretics:* Decreased effects of these drugs
*methotrexate:* Increased risk of methotrexate
toxicity

---

* For analgesic effect.
† For antirheumatic effect.

*NSAIDs, salicylates:* Increased GI irritability
and risk of bleeding, decreased meclofenamate effectiveness
*phenytoin:* Increased blood phenytoin level
*probenecid:* Increased risk of meclofenamate
toxicity
ACTIVITIES
*alcohol use:* Increased GI irritability and
bleeding

## Adverse Reactions
**CNS:** Dizziness, drowsiness, fatigue, headache, insomnia, seizures, stroke
**CV:** Hypertension, MI, peripheral edema,
tachycardia
**EENT:** Stomatitis, tinnitus
**GI:** Abdominal pain; anorexia; constipation;
diarrhea; diverticulitis; dyspepsia; dysphagia;
elevated liver function test results; esophagitis; flatulence; gastritis; gastroenteritis; gastroesophageal reflux disease; GI bleeding,
perforation, and ulceration; hepatic failure;
indigestion; jaundice; melena; nausea; perforation of stomach or intestines; stomatitis;
vomiting
**GU:** Acute renal failure, dysuria, elevated
BUN and serum creatinine levels
**HEME:** Agranulocytosis, anemia, easy bruising, hemolytic anemia, leukopenia, neutropenia, pancytopenia, thrombocytopenia
**RESP:** Asthma, respiratory depression
**SKIN:** Erythema multiforme, pruritus, rash,
Stevens-Johnson syndrome, toxic epidermal
necrolysis, urticaria
**Other:** Anaphylaxis, angioedema

## Nursing Considerations
•Use meclofenamate with extreme caution in
patients with a history of ulcer disease or GI
bleeding because NSAIDs such as meclofenamate increase the risk of GI bleeding and
ulceration. Expect to use meclofenamate for
the shortest time possible in these patients.
•Be aware that serious GI tract ulceration,
bleeding, and perforation may occur without
warning symptoms. Elderly patients are at
greater risk. To minimize risk, give drug
with food and a full glass of water. If GI distress occurs, withhold drug and notify prescriber immediately.
•Use meclofenamate cautiously in patients
with hypertension, and monitor blood pressure closely throughout therapy. Drug may
cause hypertension or worsen it.

M

•**WARNING** Monitor patient closely for thrombotic events, including MI and stroke, because NSAIDs increase the risk.

•Monitor patient—especially if he's elderly or receiving long-term meclofenamate therapy—for less common but serious adverse GI reactions, including anorexia, constipation, diverticulitis, dysphagia, esophagitis, gastritis, gastroenteritis, gastroesophageal reflux disease, hemorrhoids, hiatal hernia, melena, stomatitis, and vomiting.

•Monitor liver function test results because, in rare cases, elevations may progress to severe hepatic reactions, including fatal hepatitis, liver necrosis, and hepatic failure.

•Monitor BUN and serum creatinine levels in elderly patients, patients taking diuretics or ACE inhibitors, and patients with heart failure, impaired renal function, or hepatic dysfunction; drug may cause renal failure.

•Monitor CBC for decreased hemoglobin and hematocrit because drug may worsen anemia.

•**WARNING** If patient has bone marrow suppression or is receiving an antineoplastic drug, monitor laboratory results (including WBC count), and watch for evidence of infection because anti-inflammatory and antipyretic actions of meclofenamate may mask signs and symptoms, such as fever and pain.

•Assess patient's skin regularly for signs of rash or other hypersensitivity reaction because meclofenamate is an NSAID and may cause serious skin reactions without warning, even in patients with no history of NSAID sensitivity. At first sign of reaction, stop drug and notify prescriber.

•Expect lower doses of meclofenamate to be used for long-term therapy.

**PATIENT TEACHING**

•Tell patient to take drug with a full glass of water to keep it from lodging in esophagus and causing irritation. Also suggest taking drug with food or milk to avoid GI distress.

•Instruct patient to report itching, rash, severe diarrhea, and swelling in ankles or fingers.

•Caution patient to avoid potentially hazardous activities until drug's CNS effects are known.

•Caution pregnant patient not to take NSAIDs such as meclofenamate during the last trimester because they may cause premature closure of the ductus arteriosus.

•Explain that meclofenamate may increase the risk of serious adverse cardiovascular reactions; urge patient to seek immediate medical attention if signs or symptoms arise, such as chest pain, shortness of breath, weakness, and slurring of speech.

•Explain that meclofenamate may increase the risk of serious adverse GI reactions; stress the importance of seeking immediate medical attention for such signs and symptoms as epigastric or abdominal pain, indigestion, black or tarry stools, or vomiting blood or material that looks like coffee grounds.

•Alert patient to rare but serious skin reactions. Urge him to seek immediate medical attention for rash, blisters, itching, fever, or other indications of hypersensitivity.

# meloxicam

Mobic

## Class and Category

*Chemical:* Oxicam derivative
*Therapeutic:* Anti-inflammatory
*Pregnancy category:* C

## Indications and Dosages

➤ *To relieve signs and symptoms of osteoarthritis and rheumatoid arthritis*

**ORAL SUSPENSION, TABLETS**

**Adults.** 7.5 mg q.d. *Maximum:* 15 mg/day.

➤ *To relieve pauciarticular or polyarticular signs and symptoms of juvenile rheumatoid arthritis*

**ORAL SUSPENSION, TABLETS**

**Children age 2 and older.** 0.125 mg/kg q.d. *Maximum:* 7.5 mg/day.

---

### Mechanism of Action

Blocks cyclooxygenase, the enzyme needed to synthesize prostaglandins, which mediate the inflammatory response and cause local vasodilation, swelling, and pain. By inhibiting prostaglandins, the NSAID meloxicam reduces inflammatory symptoms. It also relieves pain because prostaglandins promote pain transmission from the periphery to the spinal cord.

---

## Contraindications

Angioedema, asthma, bronchospasm, nasal polyps, rhinitis, or urticaria induced by hypersensitivity to aspirin, meloxicam, other NSAIDs, or their components

## Interactions

### DRUGS

*ACE inhibitors:* Decreased antihypertensive effect, increased risk of renal failure
*aspirin:* Increased risk of GI ulceration
*furosemide:* Decreased diuretic effect of furosemide, possibly renal impairment
*lithium:* Elevated blood lithium level, possibly lithium toxicity
*warfarin and other oral anticoagulants:* Increased risk of bleeding

### ACTIVITIES

*alcohol use, smoking:* Increased risk of GI bleeding

## Adverse Reactions

**CNS:** Dizziness, headache, seizures, stroke
**CV:** Hypertension, MI, tachycardia
**EENT:** Laryngitis, pharyngitis, sinusitis
**GI:** Abdominal pain, anorexia, diarrhea, diverticulitis, dyspepsia, dysphagia, elevated liver function test results, esophagitis, flatulence, gastritis, gastroenteritis, gastroesophageal reflux disease, GI bleeding and ulceration, hepatic failure, indigestion, melena, nausea, perforation of stomach or intestines, stomatitis, vomiting
**GU:** Acute renal failure
**HEME:** Agranulocytosis, anemia, easy bruising, hemolytic anemia, leukopenia, neutropenia, pancytopenia, thrombocytopenia
**MS:** Arthralgia; back pain; joint crepitation, effusion, or swelling; muscle spasms; myalgia
**RESP:** Asthma, respiratory depression
**SKIN:** Erythema multiforme, pruritus, rash, Stevens-Johnson syndrome, toxic epidermal necrolysis
**Other:** Anaphylaxis, angioedema, flulike symptoms

## Nursing Considerations

•Use meloxicam with extreme caution in patients with a history of ulcer disease or GI bleeding because NSAIDs such as meloxicam increase the risk of GI bleeding and ulceration. Expect to use meloxicam for the shortest time possible in these patients.
•Be aware that serious GI tract ulceration, bleeding, and perforation may occur without warning symptoms. Elderly patients are at greater risk. To minimize risk, give drug with food and a full glass of water. If GI distress occurs, withhold drug and notify prescriber immediately.
•Use meloxicam cautiously in patients with hypertension, and monitor blood pressure closely throughout therapy. Drug may cause hypertension or worsen it.
•**WARNING** Monitor patient closely for thrombotic events, including MI and stroke, because NSAIDs increase the risk.
•Monitor patient—especially if he's elderly or receiving long-term meloxicam therapy—for less common but serious adverse GI reactions, including anorexia, constipation, diverticulitis, dysphagia, esophagitis, gastritis, gastroenteritis, gastroesophageal reflux disease, hemorrhoids, hiatal hernia, melena, stomatitis, and vomiting.
•Monitor liver function test results because, in rare cases, elevations may progress to severe hepatic reactions, including fatal hepatitis, liver necrosis, and hepatic failure.
•Monitor BUN and serum creatinine levels in elderly patients, patients taking diuretics or ACE inhibitors, and patients with heart failure, impaired renal function, or hepatic dysfunction; drug may cause renal failure.
•Monitor CBC for decreased hemoglobin and hematocrit because drug may worsen anemia.
•**WARNING** If patient has bone marrow suppression or is receiving an antineoplastic drug, monitor laboratory results (including WBC count), and watch for evidence of infection because anti-inflammatory and antipyretic actions of meloxicam may mask signs and symptoms, such as fever and pain.
•Assess patient's skin regularly for signs of rash or other hypersensitivity reaction because meloxicam is an NSAID and may cause serious skin reactions without warning, even in patients with no history of NSAID sensitivity. At first sign of reaction, stop drug and notify prescriber.
•Monitor patient for adequate hydration before beginning meloxicam therapy to decrease risk of renal dysfunction.

### PATIENT TEACHING

•Instruct patient to take meloxicam with food or after meals if stomach upset occurs.
•If oral suspension is prescribed, tell patient to shake container gently before use.
•Caution patient to avoid using other NSAIDs, aspirin, or products containing aspirin while taking meloxicam.

M

•Advise patient to refrain from smoking and alcohol use because these activities may increase the risk of adverse GI reactions.

•Instruct patient to notify prescriber if he develops signs or symptoms of hepatic dysfunction, such as dark yellow or brown urine, fatigue, fever, itching, lethargy, nausea, or yellowing of eyes or skin.

•Advise patient, especially if he's taking an oral anticoagulant such as warfarin, to report immediately signs of bleeding, such as easy bruising, stomach pain, blood in urine, or black tarry stools.

•Caution pregnant patient not to take NSAIDs such as meloxicam during the last trimester because they may cause premature closure of the ductus arteriosus.

•Explain that meloxicam may increase the risk of serious adverse cardiovascular reactions; urge patient to seek immediate medical attention if signs or symptoms arise, such as chest pain, shortness of breath, weakness, and slurring of speech.

•Explain that meloxicam may increase the risk of serious adverse GI reactions; stress the importance of seeking immediate medical attention for such signs and symptoms as epigastric or abdominal pain, indigestion, black or tarry stools, or vomiting blood or material that looks like coffee grounds.

•Alert patient to rare but serious skin reactions. Urge him to seek immediate medical attention for rash, blisters, itching, fever, or other indications of hypersensitivity.

# memantine hydrochloride

Namenda

## Class and Category

*Chemical:* N-methyl-D-aspartate (NMDA) receptor antagonist
*Therapeutic:* Antidementia agent
*Pregnancy category:* B

## Indications and Dosages

➤ *To treat moderate-to-severe dementia of the Alzheimer's type*

**TABLETS**

**Adults.** *Initial:* 5 mg q.d. P.O., increased by 5 mg/wk, as needed, to 10 mg/day in two divided doses; then 15 mg/day with one 5-mg and one 10-mg dose/day; then 20 mg/day in two divided doses. *Maintenance:* 20 mg/day. DOSAGE ADJUSTMENT Dosage reduction probable for patients with renal impairment.

## Contraindications

Hypersensitivity to memantine, amantadine, or their components

## Interactions

**DRUGS**

*amantadine, dextromethorphan, ketamine:* Possibly additive effects
*carbonic anhydrase inhibitors, sodium bicarbonate:* Decreased memantine clearance, leading to increased blood drug levels and risk of adverse effects
*cimetidine, hydrochlorothiazide, metformin, nicotinic acid, quinidine, ranitidine, triamterene:* Possibly increased blood levels of both agents

## Adverse Reactions

**CNS:** Abnormal gait, agitation, akathisia, anxiety, confusion, delirium, delusions, depression, dizziness, drowsiness, fatigue, hallucinations, headache, hyperexcitability, insomnia, psychosis, restlessness, somnolence
**CV:** Hypertension, peripheral edema, tachycardia
**GI:** Anorexia, constipation, diarrhea, nausea, vomiting
**GU:** Urinary incontinence, UTI
**MS:** Arthralgia, back pain
**RESP:** Bronchitis, cough, dyspnea, upper respiratory tract infection
**Other:** Generalized pain, flulike symptoms

## Nursing Considerations

•Use memantine with caution in patients with renal tubular acidosis or severe UTI because these conditions cause urine to become alkaline, thereby reducing memantine excretion and increasing the risk of adverse reactions.

•Monitor patient's response to memantine, and notify prescriber if serious or bothersome adverse reactions occur.

**PATIENT TEACHING**

•Advise patient to avoid a diet excessively high in fruits and vegetables because these foods contribute to alkaline urine, which can alter memantine clearance and increase adverse reactions.

•Caution patient to avoid potentially hazardous activities until drug's CNS effects are known.

## Mechanism of Action

Memantine blocks the action of the excitatory amino acid glutamate on N-methyl-D-aspartate (NMDA) receptor cells in the central nervous system. In Alzheimer's disease, glutamate levels are abnormally high when brain cells are both at rest and active. Normally, when certain brain cells are resting, magnesium ions block NMDA receptors and prevent the influx of sodium and calcium ions and the outflow of potassium ions. When learning and memory cells in the brain are active, glutamate engages with NMDA receptors, magnesium ions are removed from NMDA receptors, and the cells are depolarized. During depolarization, sodium and calcium ions enter brain cells and potassium ions leave. In Alzheimer's disease, excessive circulating glutamate permanently removes magnesium ions and opens ion channels. The excessive influx of calcium may damage brain cells and play a major role in Alzheimer's disease. What's more, dying brain cells release additional glutamate, worsening the cycle of brain cell destruction.

Memantine replaces magnesium on the NMDA receptors of brain cells, closing ion channels and preventing calcium influx and the resulting damage to brain cells. By preventing excessive brain cell death, memantine slows the progression of Alzheimer's disease.

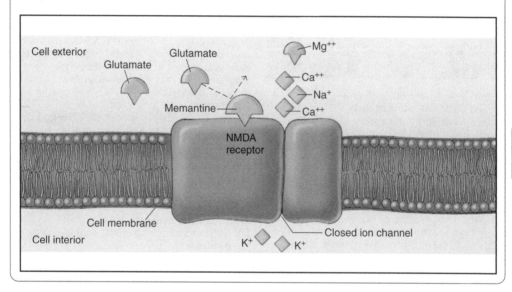

M

# meperidine hydrochloride

## (pethidine hydrochloride)

Demerol

### Class, Category, and Schedule
*Chemical:* Phenylpiperidine derivative opioid
*Therapeutic:* Analgesic
*Pregnancy category:* C
*Controlled substance:* Schedule II

## Indications and Dosages

➤ *To relieve moderate to severe pain*
SYRUP, TABLETS, I.M. OR S.C. INJECTION
**Adults.** 50 to 150 mg q 3 to 4 hr, p.r.n.
**Children.** 1.1 to 1.8 mg/kg q 3 to 4 hr, p.r.n.

➤ *To provide preoperative sedation*
I.V. INJECTION
**Adults.** 15 to 35 mg/hr, p.r.n.
I.M. OR S.C. INJECTION
**Adults.** 50 to 100 mg 30 to 90 min before surgery.

**Children.** 1 to 2 mg/kg 30 to 90 min before surgery. *Maximum:* 100 mg q 3 to 4 hr.

➤ *As adjunct to anesthesia*
**I.V. INFUSION OR INJECTION**
**Adults.** Individualized. Repeated slow injections of 10 mg/ml solution or continuous infusion of dilute solution (1 mg/ml) titrated as needed.

➤ *To provide obstetric analgesia*
**I.M. OR S.C. INJECTION**
**Adults.** 50 to 100 mg given with regular, painful contractions; repeated q 1 to 3 hr.
**DOSAGE ADJUSTMENT** For patients with creatinine clearance of 10 to 50 ml/min/1.73 m$^2$, 75% of usual dose is used; with creatinine clearance of less than 10 ml/min/1.73 m$^2$, 50% of usual dose is used.

| Route | Onset | Peak | Duration |
|---|---|---|---|
| P.O. | 15 min | 1 to 1.5 hr | 2 to 4 hr |
| I.V. | 1 min | 5 to 7 min | 2 to 4 hr |
| I.M., S.C. | 10 to 15 min | 30 to 50 min | 2 to 4 hr |

## Mechanism of Action
Binds with opiate receptors in the spinal cord and higher levels of the CNS. In this way, meperidine stimulates mu and kappa receptors, which alters the perception of and emotional response to pain.

## Incompatibilities
Don't mix meperidine in same syringe with aminophylline, barbiturates, heparin, iodides, methicillin, morphine sulfate, phenytoin, sodium bicarbonate, sulfadiazine, or sulfisoxazole.

## Contraindications
Acute asthma; hypersensitivity to meperidine, narcotics, or their components; increased intracranial pressure; severe respiratory depression; upper respiratory tract obstruction; use within 14 days of MAO inhibitor therapy

## Interactions
**DRUGS**
*acyclovir, ritonavir:* Possibly increased blood meperidine level
*alfentanil, CNS depressants, fentanyl, sufentanil:* Increased risk of CNS and respiratory depression and hypotension
*amphetamines, MAO inhibitors:* Risk of increased CNS excitation or depression with possibly fatal reactions
*anticholinergics:* Increased risk of severe constipation
*antidiarrheals (such as loperamide and difenoxin and atropine):* Increased risk of severe constipation and increased CNS depression
*antihypertensives:* Increased risk of hypotension
*buprenorphine:* Possibly decreased therapeutic effects of meperidine and increased risk of respiratory depression
*cimetidine:* Reduced clearance and volume of distribution of meperidine
*hydroxyzine:* Increased risk of CNS depression and hypotension
*metoclopramide:* Possibly decreased effects of metoclopramide
*naloxone, naltrexone:* Decreased pharmacologic effects of meperidine
*neuromuscular blockers:* Increased risk of prolonged respiratory and CNS depression
*oral anticoagulants:* Possibly increased anticoagulant effect and risk of bleeding
*phenytoin:* Possibly enhanced hepatic metabolism of meperidine
**ACTIVITIES**
*alcohol use:* Possibly increased CNS and respiratory depression and hypotension

## Adverse Reactions
**CNS:** Confusion, depression, dizziness, drowsiness, euphoria, headache, increased intracranial pressure, lack of coordination, malaise, nervousness, nightmares, restlessness, seizures, syncope, tremor
**CV:** Hypotension, orthostatic hypotension, tachycardia
**EENT:** Blurred vision, diplopia, dry mouth
**GI:** Abdominal cramps or pain, anorexia, constipation, ileus, nausea, vomiting
**GU:** Dysuria, urinary frequency, urine retention
**RESP:** Dyspnea, respiratory arrest or depression, wheezing
**SKIN:** Diaphoresis, flushing, pruritus, rash, urticaria
**Other:** Injection site pain, redness, and swelling; physical and psychological dependence

## Nursing Considerations
•Use meperidine with extreme caution in patients with acute abdominal conditions,

hepatic or renal disorders, hypothyroidism, prostatic hyperplasia, seizures, or supraventricular tachycardia.
•To minimize local anesthetic effect, dilute syrup with water before administration.
•Give I.V. dose slowly by direct injection or as a slow continuous infusion. Mix with $D_5W$, NS, or Ringer's or LR solution.
•Keep naloxone available when giving I.V. meperidine.
•Be aware that S.C. injection is painful and isn't recommended.
•Be aware that oral form of meperidine is less than half as effective as parenteral meperidine. Give I.M. form when possible, and expect to increase dosage when switching patient to oral form.
•Monitor patient's respiratory and cardiovascular status during treatment. Notify prescriber immediately and expect to discontinue drug if respiratory rate falls to less than 12 breaths/minute or if respiratory depth decreases.
•Monitor bowel function to detect constipation, and assess the need for stool softeners.
•Assess for signs of physical dependence and abuse.
•Expect withdrawal symptoms to occur if drug is abruptly withdrawn after long-term use.

**PATIENT TEACHING**
•Inform patient that meperidine is a controlled substance and that he'll need identification to purchase it.
•Advise patient to take drug exactly as prescribed.
•Instruct patient to report constipation, severe nausea, and shortness or breath.
•Advise patient to avoid potentially hazardous activities until drug's CNS effects are known.
•Instruct patient to prevent postoperative atelectasis by turning, coughing, and deep-breathing.
•Urge patient to avoid alcohol, sedatives, and tranquilizers during meperidine therapy.

# mephentermine sulfate

Wyamine

## Class and Category
*Chemical:* Sympathomimetic amine
*Therapeutic:* Vasopressor
*Pregnancy category:* C

## Indications and Dosages
➤ *To treat hypotension secondary to spinal anesthesia*

**I.V. INJECTION**
**Adults.** 30 to 45 mg (15 mg for obstetric patients); may be repeated, as needed, to maintain blood pressure.

**I.V. INFUSION**
**Adults.** Dosage individualized based on patient response to therapy. Average dose is 1 to 5 mg/min.

| Route | Onset | Peak | Duration |
|-------|-------|------|----------|
| I.V. | Almost immediate | Unknown | 15 to 30 min |

## Mechanism of Action
Stimulates alpha-adrenergic receptors directly and indirectly, resulting in positive inotropic and chronotropic effects. Indirect stimulation occurs by the release of norepinephrine from its storage sites in the heart and other tissues. By enhancing cardiac contraction, mephentermine improves cardiac output, thereby increasing blood pressure. Increased peripheral resistance from peripheral vasoconstriction may also contribute to increased blood pressure. Mephentermine can affect the heart rate but the change is variable, based on vagal tone. It may also stimulate beta-adrenergic receptors.

## Contraindications
Hypersensitivity to mephentermine, phenothiazine-induced hypotension, use within 14 days of MAO inhibitor therapy

## Interactions
**DRUGS**
*alpha blockers and other drugs with alpha-blocking effects:* Possibly decreased peripheral vasoconstrictive and hypertensive effects of mephentermine
*beta blockers (ophthalmic):* Decreased effects of mephentermine; increased risk of bronchospasm, wheezing, decreased pulmonary function, and respiratory failure
*beta blockers (systemic):* Increased risk of bronchospasm, decreased effects of both drugs
*diuretics and other antihypertensives:* Possibly reduced effectiveness of these drugs

*doxapram:* Possibly increased vasopressor effects of either drug

*ergot alkaloids:* Increased vasopressor effects

*guanadrel, guanethidine, mecamylamine, methyldopa, reserpine:* Possibly decreased effects of these drugs and increased risk of adverse effects

*hydrocarbon inhalation anesthetics:* Increased risk of atrial and ventricular arrhythmias

*MAO inhibitors:* Intensified and extended cardiac stimulation and vasopressor effects, possibly severe headache and hypertensive crisis

*maprotiline, tricyclic antidepressants:* Increased vasopressor response; increased risk of prolonged QTc interval, arrhythmias, hypertension, and hyperpyrexia

*methylphenidate:* Possibly increased vasopressor effect of mephentermine

*nitrates:* Possibly reduced antianginal effects of nitrates and decreased vasopressor effect

*other sympathomimetics (such as dopamine):* Possibly increased cardiac effects and adverse reactions

*oxytocin:* Possibly severe hypertension

*thyroid hormones:* Increased effects of both drugs, increased risk of coronary insufficiency in patients with coronary artery disease

## Adverse Reactions

**CNS:** Anxiety, dizziness, drowsiness, euphoria, headache, incoherence, nervousness, psychosis, restlessness, seizures, weakness
**CV:** Angina, arrhythmias (including bradycardia, tachycardia, and ventricular arrhythmias), hypertension, hypotension, palpitations, peripheral vasoconstriction
**GI:** Nausea, vomiting
**RESP:** Dyspnea
**SKIN:** Peripheral necrosis

## Nursing Considerations

•Before administering mephentermine, expect to intervene, as ordered, to correct hemorrhage, hypovolemia, metabolic acidosis, or hypoxia.
•Discard vial if you observe discoloration or precipitate.
•Using $D_5W$ or NS, prepare a 1-mg/ml concentration solution for infusion.
•Administer drug using an infusion pump to provide a controlled rate.
•Monitor blood pressure, cardiac rate and rhythm, central venous pressure (if appropri-

ate), and urine output during administration. Adjust infusion rate according to patient response, as ordered. Be aware that patients with a history of cardiovascular disease (including hypertension) or hyperthyroidism and chronically ill patients are at increased risk for mephentermine's adverse cardiovascular effects.
•Assess patients with angle-closure glaucoma for signs of an exacerbation, such as eye pain or blurred vision.
•Assess circulation in patients with a history of occlusive vascular disease, such as atherosclerosis and Raynaud's disease, because mephentermine may cause decreased circulation and increase the risk of necrosis or gangrene. Inspect I.V. site periodically for signs of extravasation.
•**WARNING** Be aware that weeping, excitability, seizures, and hallucinations are some of the symptoms of mephentermine overdose. Contact prescriber immediately if patient experiences such symptoms, and expect to provide supportive treatment.
•Be aware that mephentermine can increase contractions in pregnant women, especially during the third trimester. Expect drug to be prescribed only when benefits outweigh potential adverse effects.
•Store drug at 15° to 30° C (59° to 86° F); don't freeze.

**PATIENT TEACHING**
•Instruct patient receiving mephentermine to report adverse reactions, including chest pain, difficulty breathing, dizziness, irregular heartbeat, headache, and weakness.

# mephenytoin

Mesantoin

## Class and Category
*Chemical:* Hydantoin derivative
*Therapeutic:* Anticonvulsant
*Pregnancy category:* Not rated

## Indications and Dosages
➤ *To control generalized tonic-clonic, focal, and jacksonian seizures when other drugs are ineffective*

**TABLETS**
**Adults.** *Initial:* 50 to 100 mg/day during first wk. Increased by 50 to 100 mg at 1-wk intervals until desired response is reached. *Main-*

*tenance:* 200 to 600 mg/day in equally divided doses. *Maximum:* 1.2 g/day.
**Children.** *Initial:* 20 to 50 mg/day. Increased by 25 to 50 mg at 1-wk intervals until desired response occurs. *Maintenance:* 100 to 400 mg/day in equally divided doses. *Maximum:* 400 mg/day.

➤ *To replace other anticonvulsants*
**TABLETS**
**Adults.** 50 to 100 mg q.d. during first wk. Dosage gradually increased while decreasing dosage of other drug over 3 to 6 wk.

| Route | Onset | Peak | Duration |
|-------|-------|------|----------|
| P.O. | 30 min | Unknown | 24 to 48 hr |

## Mechanism of Action
Limits the spread of seizure activity and the start of new seizures by:
• regulating voltage-dependent sodium and calcium channels in neurons
• inhibiting calcium movement across neuronal membranes
• enhancing sodium-potassium adenosine triphosphatase activity in neurons and glial cells.
   These actions may result from mephenytoin's ability to slow the recovery rate of inactivated sodium channels.

## Contraindications
Hypersensitivity to mephenytoin, phenytoin, other hydantoins, or their components

## Interactions
**DRUGS**
*acetaminophen:* Increased risk of hepatotoxicity with long-term acetaminophen use
*amiodarone:* Possibly increased blood mephenytoin level and risk of toxicity
*antacids:* Possibly decreased mephenytoin effectiveness
*antineoplastics:* Increased mephenytoin metabolism
*bupropion, clozapine, loxapine, MAO inhibitors, maprotiline, phenothiazines, pimozide, thioxanthenes:* Possibly lowered seizure threshold and decreased therapeutic effects of mephenytoin, possibly intensified CNS depressant effects of these drugs
*calcium channel blockers, fluconazole, itraconazole, ketoconazole, miconazole, omeprazole:* Possibly increased blood phenytoin level

*carbamazepine:* Decreased blood carbamazepine level, possibly increased blood phenytoin level and risk of toxicity
*chloramphenicol, cimetidine, disulfiram, isoniazid, methylphenidate, metronidazole, phenylbutazone, ranitidine, salicylates, sulfonamides, trimethoprim:* Possibly impaired metabolism of these drugs and increased risk of mephenytoin toxicity
*corticosteroids, cyclosporine, digoxin, disopyramide, doxycycline, furosemide, levodopa, mexiletine, quinidine:* Decreased therapeutic effects of these drugs
*diazoxide:* Possibly decreased therapeutic effects of both drugs
*estrogens, progestins:* Decreased therapeutic effects of these drugs, increased blood phenytoin level
*felbamate:* Possibly impaired metabolism and increased blood level of phenytoin
*fluoxetine:* Possibly increased blood phenytoin level and risk of toxicity
*folic acid:* Increased mephenytoin metabolism, decreased seizure control
*haloperidol:* Possibly lowered seizure threshold and decreased therapeutic effects of mephenytoin; possibly decreased blood haloperidol level
*insulin, oral antidiabetic drugs:* Possibly increased blood glucose level and decreased therapeutic effects of these drugs
*lamotrigine:* Possibly decreased therapeutic effects of lamotrigine
*lithium:* Increased risk of lithium toxicity
*methadone:* Possibly increased methadone metabolism, leading to withdrawal symptoms
*molindone:* Possibly lowered seizure threshold, impaired absorption, and decreased therapeutic effects of mephenytoin
*oral anticoagulants:* Possibly impaired metabolism of these drugs and increased risk of mephenytoin toxicity; possibly increased anticoagulant effect initially, but decreased effect with prolonged therapy
*oral contraceptives containing estrogen and progestin:* Possibly breakthrough bleeding and decreased contraceptive effectiveness
*rifampin:* Possibly decreased therapeutic effects of mephenytoin
*streptozocin:* Possibly decreased therapeutic effects of streptozocin
*sucralfate:* Possibly decreased mephenytoin absorption

*tricyclic antidepressants:* Possibly lowered seizure threshold and decreased therapeutic effects of mephenytoin; possibly decreased blood level of tricyclic antidepressants
*valproic acid:* Decreased blood phenytoin level, increased blood valproic acid level
*vitamin D analogues:* Decreased vitamin D analogue activity, risk of anticonvulsant-induced rickets and osteomalacia
*xanthines:* Possibly inhibited mephenytoin absorption and increased clearance of xanthines
*zaleplon:* Increased clearance and decreased effectiveness of zaleplon

**ACTIVITIES**
*alcohol use:* Possibly decreased mephenytoin effectiveness

## Adverse Reactions
**CNS:** Ataxia, choreoathetoid movements, confusion, dizziness, drowsiness, excitement, fatigue, fever, headache, peripheral neuropathy, sedation, slurred speech, stuttering, tremor
**EENT:** Gingival hyperplasia, nystagmus
**GI:** Constipation, diarrhea, nausea, vomiting
**HEME:** Agranulocytosis, leukopenia, thrombocytopenia
**MS:** Muscle twitching
**SKIN:** Rash, Stevens-Johnson syndrome, toxic epidermal necrolysis
**Other:** Lymphadenopathy, systemic lupus erythematosus

## Nursing Considerations
•Because of mephenytoin's potentially dangerous adverse effects, expect to use it only when other drugs are ineffective.
•Keep in mind that mephenytoin doesn't control absence seizures.
•**WARNING** Be aware that drug shouldn't be abruptly discontinued because doing so may cause status epilepticus. Plan to reduce dosage gradually or substitute another drug, as prescribed, when discontinuing mephenytoin.
•Obtain CBC and differential before treatment, after 2 weeks of treatment, and then monthly during first year of treatment, as ordered.
•Notify prescriber immediately and expect to discontinue mephenytoin and substitute another drug if depressed blood counts, enlarged lymph nodes, or rash develops.
**PATIENT TEACHING**
•Urge patient to take mephenytoin exactly as prescribed and not to stop it abruptly.

•Advise patient to take drug with food to enhance absorption and reduce adverse GI reactions.
•Caution patient on once-a-day therapy to be especially careful not to miss a dose.
•Advise patient to report impaired coordination, persistent headache, rash, severe GI distress, swollen gums or lymph nodes, or unusual bleeding or bruising.
•Encourage patient to maintain good oral hygiene and to have regular dental checkups to reduce the risk of gum disease.
•Instruct patient to keep medical appointments to monitor drug effectiveness and check for adverse reactions. Explain the need for periodic laboratory tests.
•Advise patient to wear medical identification stating that he has epilepsy and takes mephenytoin to prevent seizures.

# mephobarbital

Mebaral

## Class, Category, and Schedule
*Chemical:* Barbiturate derivative
*Therapeutic:* Anticonvulsant, sedative
*Pregnancy category:* D
*Controlled substance:* Schedule IV

## Indications and Dosages
➤ *To treat seizures*
**TABLETS**
**Adults.** 400 to 600 mg/day as a single dose or in divided doses, usually beginning with low dose and increasing over 4 to 5 days until optimum dosage is determined.
**Children over age 5.** 32 to 64 mg t.i.d. or q.i.d.
**Children under age 5.** 16 to 32 mg t.i.d. or q.i.d.
➤ *To provide sedation*
**TABLETS**
**Adults.** 32 to 100 mg t.i.d. or q.i.d.
**Children.** 16 to 32 mg t.i.d. or q.i.d.

| Route | Onset | Peak | Duration |
|---|---|---|---|
| P.O. | 30 to 60 min | Unknown | 10 to 16 hr |

## Contraindications
Hepatic disease or failure; history of addiction to sedatives or hypnotics; hypersensitivity to mephobarbital, other barbiturates, or their components; nephritis; porphyria; severe respiratory disease with obstruction or dyspnea

## Mechanism of Action

May reduce seizure activity by reducing transmission of monosynaptic and polysynaptic nerve impulses, which causes decreased excitability in nerve cells. As a sedative, mephobarbital inhibits upward conduction of nerve impulses to the reticular formation of the brain, which disrupts impulse transmission to the cortex. As a result, mephobarbital depresses the CNS and produces drowsiness, hypnosis, and sedation.

## Interactions

### DRUGS

*acetaminophen:* Possibly decreased effects of acetaminophen (with long-term mephobarbital use)

*anesthetics (halogenated hydrocarbon):* Increased risk of hepatotoxicity (with long-term mephobarbital use)

*carbamazepine, chloramphenicol, corticosteroids, cyclosporine, dacarbazine, digoxin, disopyramide, doxycycline, griseofulvin, metronidazole, oral contraceptives, phenylbutazone, quinidine, theophyllines, vitamin D:* Decreased effectiveness of these drugs

*CNS depressants:* Increased CNS depression

*divalproex sodium, valproic acid:* Increased risk of CNS depression and neurotoxicity

*guanadrel, guanethidine:* Increased risk of orthostatic hypotension

*haloperidol:* Possibly decreased blood haloperidol level and change in seizure pattern

*hydantoins:* Possibly interference with hydantoin metabolism

*leucovorin:* Possibly decreased anticonvulsant effect of mephobarbital

*maprotiline:* Possibly increased CNS depression and decreased therapeutic effects of mephobarbital

*mexiletine:* Possibly decreased blood mexiletine level

*oral anticoagulants:* Possibly decreased therapeutic effects of anticoagulants, possibly increased risk of bleeding when mephobarbital is discontinued

*tricyclic antidepressants:* Possibly decreased therapeutic effects of tricyclic antidepressants

### ACTIVITIES

*alcohol use:* Increased CNS depression

## Adverse Reactions

**CNS:** Agitation, anxiety, ataxia, confusion, delusions, depression, dizziness, drowsiness, fever, hallucinations, headache, insomnia, irritability, nervousness, nightmares, paradoxical stimulation, seizures, syncope, tremor
**CV:** Orthostatic hypotension
**EENT:** Vision changes
**GI:** Anorexia, constipation, hepatic dysfunction, nausea, vomiting
**HEME:** Agranulocytosis
**MS:** Arthralgia, bone pain, muscle twitching or weakness
**RESP:** Respiratory depression
**SKIN:** Exfoliative dermatitis, rash, Stevens-Johnson syndrome
**Other:** Physical and psychological dependence, weight loss

## Nursing Considerations

• Observe for signs of physical and psychological dependence, especially with prolonged use of mephobarbital at high doses.
• Observe for signs of chronic barbiturate intoxication, including confusion, insomnia, poor judgment, slurred speech, and unsteady gait.
• Assess for paradoxical stimulation in patient who receives drug for acute or chronic pain.
• **WARNING** Expect to taper dosage gradually when discontinuing drug. Be aware that withdrawal symptoms can be severe and may cause death. Mild signs and symptoms, including anxiety, muscle twitching, nausea, orthostatic hypotension, and progressive weakness, may appear 8 to 12 hours after last drug dose. More severe signs include delirium and seizures.

### PATIENT TEACHING

• Advise patient to take mephobarbital exactly as prescribed. Caution him not to stop taking drug abruptly because of the risk of withdrawal symptoms and, for epileptic patients, seizures.
• Instruct patient to avoid alcohol, sleeping pills, and other sedatives while taking mephobarbital because of the risk of increased CNS depression.
• Advise patient to avoid potentially hazardous activities until drug's CNS effects are known.
• Advise patient to change position slowly to minimize effects of orthostatic hypotension.
• Urge patient to report confusion, fever, rash, or severe dizziness.

M

# meprobamate

Apo-Meprobamate (CAN), Equanil, MB-Tab, Meprospan, Miltown, Neuramate

## Class, Category, and Schedule
*Chemical:* Carbamate derivative
*Therapeutic:* Antianxiety
*Pregnancy category:* Not rated
*Controlled substance:* Schedule IV

## Indications and Dosages
➤ *To treat anxiety*
**S.R. CAPSULES**
**Adults and adolescents.** 400 to 800 mg q morning and h.s. *Maximum:* 2,400 mg/day.
**Children ages 6 to 12.** 200 mg q morning and h.s.
**TABLETS**
**Adults and adolescents.** 1,200 to 1,600 mg/day in divided doses t.i.d. or q.i.d. *Maximum:* 2,400 mg/day.
**DOSAGE ADJUSTMENT** For patients with creatinine clearance of 10 to 50 ml/min/1.73 m$^2$, drug administered q 12 hr; with creatinine clearance of less than 10 ml/min/1.73 m$^2$, drug administered q 18 hr.
**Children ages 6 to 12.** 200 to 600 mg/day in divided doses b.i.d. or t.i.d.

| Route | Onset | Peak | Duration |
|-------|-------|------|----------|
| P.O. | 1 hr | Unknown | Unknown |

### Mechanism of Action
May act at multiple sites in the CNS, including the thalamus and limbic system. Meprobamate inhibits spinal reflexes, causing CNS relaxation; its sedative effects may account for its anticonvulsant action. It also has muscle relaxant properties.

## Contraindications
Hypersensitivity to meprobromate or related drugs, such as carisoprodol; porphyria

## Interactions
**DRUGS**
*CNS depressants:* Increased CNS depression
**ACTIVITIES**
*alcohol use:* Increased CNS depression

## Adverse Reactions
**CNS:** Ataxia, dizziness, drowsiness, euphoria, headache, paradoxical stimulation, paresthesia, slurred speech, syncope, vertigo, weakness
**CV:** Arrhythmias, including tachycardia; hypotension; palpitations
**EENT:** Impaired visual accommodation
**GI:** Diarrhea, nausea, vomiting
**SKIN:** Erythematous maculopapular rash, pruritus, urticaria
**Other:** Physical dependence

## Nursing Considerations
•Use meprobamate cautiously in patients with impaired hepatic or renal function, seizure disorders, or suicidal tendencies.
•Also use drug cautiously in patients with a history of drug dependence or abuse because meprobamate use can lead to physical dependence and abuse.
•Observe for signs of chronic drug intoxication, such as ataxia, slurred speech, and vertigo.
•**WARNING** Expect to taper dosage gradually over 2 weeks when discontinuing meprobamate because abrupt drug discontinuation can exacerbate previous symptoms, such as anxiety, or cause withdrawal symptoms, such as confusion, hallucinations, muscle twitching, tremor, and vomiting.

**PATIENT TEACHING**
•Instruct patient to take meprobamate exactly as directed and not to stop taking it abruptly.
•Advise patient not to crush or chew S.R. capsules.
•Instruct patient to avoid potentially hazardous activities until drug's CNS effects are known.
•Direct patient to avoid alcohol, sedatives, and other CNS depressants while taking meprobamate.
•Inform patient that meprobamate may become less effective after several months of treatment.
•Instruct patient to report development of a rash.

# meropenem

Merrem I.V.

## Class and Category
*Chemical:* Carbapenem
*Therapeutic:* Antibiotic
*Pregnancy category:* B

# Indications and Dosages

➤ *To treat complicated appendicitis and peritonitis caused by susceptible strains of alpha-hemolytic streptococci,* Bacteroides fragilis, Bacteroides thetaiotaomicron, Escherichia coli, Klebsiella pneumoniae, Peptostreptococcus *sp., or* Pseudomonas aeruginosa

**I.V. INFUSION OR INJECTION**

**Adults and children weighing more than 50 kg (110 lb).** 1 g q 8 hr infused over 15 to 30 min or given as a bolus over 3 to 5 min.

**Children older than age 3 months weighing less than 50 kg.** 20 mg/kg q 8 hr infused over 15 to 30 min or given as a bolus over 3 to 5 min. *Maximum:* 1 g q 8 hr.

**DOSAGE ADJUSTMENT** For patients with creatinine clearance of 26 to 50 ml/min/1.73 m$^2$, dosage reduced to 1 g q 12 hr. For those with creatinine clearance of 10 to 25 ml/min/1.73 m$^2$, dosage reduced to 500 mg q 12 hr. For those with creatinine clearance of less than 10 ml/min/1.73 m$^2$, dosage reduced to 500 mg q 24 hr.

➤ *To treat complicated skin and skin structure infections caused by* Staphylococcus aureus, Streptococcus agalactiae, Streptococcus pyogenes, *viridans group streptococci,* Enterococcus faecalis *(excluding vancomycin-resistant isolates),* Pseudo-monas aeruginosa, Escherichia coli, Proteus mirabilis, Bacteroides fragilis, *and* Peptostreptococcus species

**I.V. INFUSION**

**Adults and children weighing more than 50 kg (110 lb).** 500 mg q 8 hr infused over 15 to 30 min.

**Children older than age 3 months weighing less than 50 kg.** 10 mg/kg q 8 hr infused over 15 to 30 min. *Maximum:* 500 mg q 8 hr.

**DOSAGE ADJUSTMENT** For patients with creatinine clearance of 26 to 50 ml/min/1.73 m$^2$, dosage reduced to 500 mg q 12 hr. For those with creatinine clearance of 10 to 25 ml/min/1.73 m$^2$, dosage reduced to 250 mg q 12 hr. For those with creatinine clearance of less than 10 ml/min/1.73 m$^2$, dosage reduced to 250 mg q 24 hr.

➤ *To treat bacterial meningitis caused by* Haemophilus influenzae, Neisseria meningitidis, *or* Streptococcus pneumoniae *in children*

**I.V. INFUSION OR INJECTION**

**Children weighing more than 50 kg.** 2 g q 8 hr infused over 15 to 30 min or given as a bolus over 3 to 5 min.

**Children older than age 3 months weighing less than 50 kg.** 40 mg/kg q 8 hr infused over 15 to 30 min or given as a bolus over 3 to 5 min. *Maximum:* 2 g q 8 hr.

## Mechanism of Action

Penetrates cell walls of most gram-negative and gram-positive bacteria, inactivating penicillin-binding proteins. This action inhibits bacterial cell wall synthesis and causes cell death.

## Incompatibilities

Don't mix meropenem in same solution with other drugs.

## Contraindications

Hypersensitivity to meropenem, other carbapenem drugs, beta lactams, or their components

## Interactions

**DRUGS**

*probenecid:* Inhibited renal excretion of meropenem

*valproic acid:* Possibly reduced blood level of valproic acid to subtherapeutic level

## Adverse Reactions

**CNS:** Headache, seizures

**CV:** Shock

**EENT:** Epistaxis, glossitis, oral candidiasis

**GI:** Anorexia, constipation, diarrhea, elevated liver function test results, nausea, pseudomembranous colitis, vomiting

**GU:** Elevated BUN and serum creatinine levels, hematuria, renal failure

**HEME:** Agranulocytosis, leukopenia, neutropenia

**RESP:** Apnea, dyspnea

**SKIN:** Diaper rash from candidiasis (children), erythema multiforme, pruritus, rash, Stevens-Johnson syndrome, toxic epidermal necrolysis

**Other:** Anaphylaxis; angioedema; injection site inflammation, pain, phlebitis, or thrombophlebitis; sepsis

## Nursing Considerations

•Obtain body fluid and tissue samples, as ordered, for culture and sensitivity testing.

Expect to review test results, if possible, before giving first dose of meropenem.

•For I.V. bolus, add 10 ml of sterile water for injection to 500 mg/20-ml vial, or 20 ml of diluent to 1 g/30-ml vial of drug. Shake to dissolve.

•**WARNING** Be aware that fatal hypersensitivity reactions have occurred with meropenem. Determine whether patient has had previous reactions to antibiotics or other allergens.

•Be prepared to administer emergency treatment for anaphylaxis.

•Institute seizure precautions, according to facility policy, for patients with bacterial meningitis or CNS or renal disorders because they're at increased risk for seizures with meropenem.

•Monitor patient with creatinine clearance of 10 to 26 ml/min/1.73 m² for signs and symptoms of seizures, heart failure, renal failure, or shock.

PATIENT TEACHING

•Tell patient to report trouble breathing, diarrhea, injection site pain, or mouth soreness.

# mesalamine

Asacol, Canasa, Mesasal (CAN), Pentasa, Rowasa, Salofalk (CAN)

## Class and Category

*Chemical:* 5-Aminosalicylic acid derivative
*Therapeutic:* Anti-inflammatory
*Pregnancy category:* B

## Indications and Dosages

➤ *To treat and maintain remission of ulcerative colitis*

DELAYED-RELEASE TABLETS (ASACOL)

**Adults.** *Initial:* 0.8 g t.i.d. for 6 wk. *Maintenance:* 1.6 g/day in divided doses.

DELAYED-RELEASE TABLETS (MESASAL)

**Adults.** 1.5 to 3 g/day in divided doses for 6 wk.

DELAYED-RELEASE TABLETS (SALOFALK)

**Adults.** 1 g t.i.d. or q.i.d. for 6 wk.

E.R. CAPSULES

**Adults.** 1 g q.i.d. for up to 8 wk.

➤ *To treat mild to moderate distal ulcerative colitis, proctitis, and proctosigmoiditis*

RECTAL SUSPENSION

**Adults.** 4 g (60 ml) q.d. h.s. for 3 to 6 wk.

➤ *To treat active ulcerative proctitis*

SUPPOSITORIES (CANASA)

**Adults.** 0.5 g b.i.d. or t.i.d. for 3 to 6 wk. Or 1 g h.s. for 3 to 6 wk.

## Contraindications

Hypersensitivity to mesalamine, salicylates, or their components

## Interactions

DRUGS

*digoxin:* Possibly decreased absorption and bioavailability of digoxin
*lactulose:* Possibly interference with delayed-release tablets or E.R. capsules
*omeprazole:* Increased mesalamine absorption

## Adverse Reactions

**CNS:** Chills, dizziness, fatigue, fever, headache (severe), weakness
**EENT:** Rhinitis
**GI:** Abdominal cramps or pain (severe), anorexia, bloody diarrhea, colitis, diarrhea, elevated liver function test results, flatulence, indigestion, nausea, pancreatitis, rectal pain, vomiting
**GU:** Nephrotoxicity
**HEME:** Agranulocytosis
**MS:** Back pain, dysarthria
**RESP:** Fibrosing alveolitis
**SKIN:** Acne, alopecia, pruritus, rash

## Nursing Considerations

•Use mesalamine cautiously in patients with sulfite sensitivity. Some drug formulations contain sulfites, which may cause hypersensitivity reactions in these patients.

•Ensure that suppository is firm before inserting it. If it's too soft, chill in refrigerator for 30 minutes or run under cold water before removing wrapper. Moisten it with water-soluble lubricant or tap water before

---

### Mechanism of Action

May reduce inflammation by inhibiting the enzyme cyclooxygenase and decreasing production of arachidonic acid metabolites, which may be increased in patients with inflammatory bowel disease. Cyclooxygenase is needed to form prostaglandins from arachidonic acid. Prostaglandins mediate inflammatory activity and produce signs and symptoms of inflammation. Mesala-mine also may reduce inflammation by interfering with leukotriene synthesis and by inhibiting the enzyme lipoxygenase, both of which take part in inflammatory response.

insertion. Have patient retain suppository for
1 to 3 hours, as directed.
• Administer rectal suspension at bedtime,
and have patient retain it for the prescribed
time—about 8 hours, if possible. Retention
time ranges from 3.5 to 12 hours.
• Be aware that rectal suspension may darken slightly over time but that this change
doesn't affect potency. Discard rectal suspension that turns dark brown.
• Assess patient for evidence of acute intolerance similar to flare-up of inflammatory
bowel disease: acute abdominal cramps and
pain, bloody diarrhea, and, possibly, fever,
headache, and rash.
• For patients with impaired renal function,
expect to monitor renal function test results
periodically during long-term therapy because drug may cause nephrotoxicity.
• Monitor patient's CBC with differential for
eosinophilia, which may indicate an allergic
reaction.

**PATIENT TEACHING**
• Instruct patient taking oral drug to swallow
tablets or capsules whole and not to break
outer coating.
• Teach patient how to administer rectal suspension or suppositories correctly. Emphasize
shaking suspension bottle well before using.
• Advise patient to notify prescriber immediately about abdominal cramps or pain,
bloody diarrhea, fever, headache, or rash.

# mesoridazine besylate

Serentil

## Class and Category

*Chemical:* Alkylpiperidine phenothiazine
derivative
*Therapeutic:* Antipsychotic
*Pregnancy category:* Not rated

## Indications and Dosages

➤ *To treat schizophrenia in patients who
failed to respond to other antipsychotic
drugs, either because those drugs were
ineffective or because intolerable adverse effects prevented attainment of an
effective dose*

**ORAL SOLUTION, TABLETS**
**Adults and adolescents.** 50 mg t.i.d., increased as needed and tolerated. *Maximum:*
400 mg/day.

**I.M. INJECTION**
**Adults and adolescents.** 25 mg, repeated in
30 to 60 min, as needed. *Maximum:* 200 mg/
day.

| Route | Onset | Peak | Duration |
|---|---|---|---|
| P.O., I.M. | Up to several wk | 6 wk to 6 mo | 4 to 8 hr |

## Mechanism of Action

Depresses brain areas that control activity
and aggression—including the cerebral
cortex, hypothalamus, and limbic system—by an unknown mechanism.

## Contraindications

Blood dyscrasias; bone marrow depression;
cerebral arteriosclerosis; coma; concurrent
use of high doses of CNS depressants; concurrent use of other drugs that prolong the
QTc interval, such as disopyramide, procainamide, and quinidine; congenital long-QT
syndrome; coronary artery disease; hepatic
dysfunction; history of arrhythmias; hypersensitivity to mesoridazine, other phenothiazines, or their components; myeloproliferative disorders; severe CNS depression; severe
hypertension or hypotension; subcortical
brain damage

## Interactions

**DRUGS**
*aluminum- or magnesium-containing antacids, antidiarrheals (adsorbent):* Decreased
mesoridazine absorption
*amantadine, anticholinergics:* Increased anticholinergic effects, and possibly decreased
therapeutic effects of mesoridazine
*aminoglycosides, ototoxic drugs:* Masked
symptoms of ototoxicity, such as dizziness,
tinnitus, and vertigo
*anticonvulsants:* Possibly lowered seizure
threshold
*antithyroid drugs:* Increased risk of agranulocytosis
*appetite suppressants:* Possibly antagonized
anorectic effect
*astemizole, cisapride, disopyramide, erythromycin, pimozide, probucol, procainamide,
quinidine:* Increased risk of prolonged QT interval and life-threatening arrhythmias
*beta blockers:* Increased blood levels of both
drugs, possibly resulting in additive hypoten-

sion, retinopathy, arrhythmias, and tardive dyskinesia

*CNS depressants, general anesthetics:* Increased CNS depression

*dextroamphetamine:* Possibly interference with action of either drug

*levodopa:* Possibly inhibited effects of levodopa

*lithium:* Possibly decreased absorption of mesoridazine

*opioid analgesics:* Possibly decreased mesoridazine effects; increased CNS and respiratory depression and orthostatic hypotension; increased risk of severe constipation

*oral anticoagulants:* Possibly decreased therapeutic effects of anticoagulants

*sympathomimetics:* Possibly decreased therapeutic effects of these drugs and increased risk of hypotension

*thiazide diuretics:* Possibly orthostatic hypotension, hyponatremia, and water intoxication

*tricyclic antidepressants:* Increased tricyclic antidepressant levels, inhibited mesoridazine metabolism, increased risk of neuroleptic malignant syndrome

**ACTIVITIES**

*alcohol use:* Increased CNS depression

## Adverse Reactions

**CNS:** Ataxia, dizziness, drowsiness, extrapyramidal reactions (tardive dyskinesia, pseudoparkinsonism), fever, neuroleptic malignant syndrome, restlessness, seizures, slurred speech, syncope, tremor, weakness

**CV:** Hypotension, orthostatic hypotension, prolonged QTc interval, torsades de pointes

**EENT:** Blurred vision, dry mouth, hypertrophic papillae of tongue, increased salivation, photophobia

**ENDO:** Galactorrhea, gynecomastia

**GI:** Constipation, hepatotoxicity, nausea, vomiting

**GU:** Dysuria, ejaculation disorders, impotence, menstrual irregularities, priapism

**HEME:** Agranulocytosis, leukopenia, thrombocytopenia

**SKIN:** Contact dermatitis, decreased sweating, jaundice, photosensitivity, rash

**Other:** Injection site pain, weight gain

## Nursing Considerations

• Before beginning mesoridazine therapy, expect to perform a 12-lead ECG to detect prolonged QTc interval. If patient's QTc interval is greater than 450 msec, expect to withhold drug because of the risk of life-threatening torsades de pointes.

• Wear gloves when working with liquid and parenteral forms of mesoridazine, and avoid contact with clothing or skin; drug may cause contact dermatitis.

• Discard injection solution if it's frankly discolored or contains precipitate; slightly yellow color is acceptable.

• Inject I.M. drug deep into upper outer quadrant of buttocks; massage area afterward to prevent sterile abscess.

• Implement continuous ECG monitoring, as ordered, to detect arrhythmias. Expect to discontinue mesoridazine if the QTc interval exceeds 500 msec.

• Monitor serum potassium level before and during therapy, and administer potassium supplements as prescribed.

• Assess patient for hypotension and orthostatic hypotension, especially during I.M. therapy. Notify prescriber if either develops.

• **WARNING** Monitor patient for evidence of neuroleptic malignant syndrome, a potentially fatal reaction to antipsychotic drugs, and notify prescriber if they develop. Early signs include altered mental status, fever, hypertension or hypotension, muscle rigidity, and tachycardia.

• Assess patient for signs of blood dyscrasias, including cellulitis, fever, and pharyngitis. If they develop, discontinue drug, as directed.

• Monitor patient for signs of tardive dyskinesia, even after treatment stops. Notify prescriber if they develop.

• Expect to taper drug dosage before discontinuation to avoid adverse reactions, such as dizziness, nausea, tremor, and vomiting.

**PATIENT TEACHING**

• Instruct patient to take mesoridazine exactly as prescribed and not to stop it abruptly.

• Inform patient that I.M. injection may be painful.

• Caution patient to avoid potentially hazardous activities until drug's CNS effects are known.

• Advise patient to change position slowly to minimize effects of orthostatic hypotension.

• Instruct patient to report fever, involuntary facial movements, sore throat, unusual bleeding or bruising, and yellowing of eyes or skin.

• Urge patient to avoid alcohol and prolonged sun exposure during therapy.
• If patient requires long-term therapy, explain the risk of tardive dyskinesia. Also advise him to have regular eye examinations.

# metaproterenol sulfate

Alupent, Arm-a-Med Metaproterenol,
Dey-Lute Metaproterenol

## Class and Category

*Chemical:* Sympathomimetic amine
*Therapeutic:* Antiasthmatic, bronchodilator
*Pregnancy category:* C

## Indications and Dosages

➤ *To treat bronchospasm*

SYRUP, TABLETS

**Adults and children age 9 or older who weigh more than 27 kg (59 lb).** 20 mg q 6 to 8 hr.
**Children ages 6 to 9 who weigh 27 kg or less.** 10 mg q 6 to 8 hr.

INHALATION AEROSOL

**Adults and adolescents.** 2 to 3 inhalations (1.3 to 1.95 mg) q 3 to 4 hr. *Maximum:* 12 inhalations/day.
**Children ages 6 to 12.** 1 to 3 inhalations (0.65 to 1.95 mg) q 3 to 4 hr. *Maximum:* 12 inhalations/day.

INHALATION NEBULIZER

**Adults and adolescents.** 0.2 to 0.3 ml of 5% solution diluted in 2.5 ml of NS t.i.d. or q.i.d., p.r.n., but not more frequently than q 4 hr.
**Children ages 6 to 12.** 0.1 to 0.2 ml of 5% solution diluted in NS to a total volume of 3 ml t.i.d. or q.i.d., p.r.n., but not more frequently than q 4 hr.

| Route | Onset | Peak | Duration |
|---|---|---|---|
| P.O. | 15 min | 1 hr | 4 hr or longer |
| Inhalation (aerosol) | 1 min | 1 hr | 4 hr or longer |
| Inhalation (nebulizer) | 5 to 30 min | Unknown | 4 hr or longer |

## Contraindications

Angina, cerebral arteriosclerosis, dilated heart failure, heart block from digitalis toxicity, hypersensitivity to metaproterenol or its components, labor, local anesthesia, organic brain damage, tachyarrhythmias

## Mechanism of Action

Attaches to beta$_2$ receptors on bronchial cell membranes. This stimulates the intracellular enzyme adenyl cyclase to convert adenosine triphosphate to cyclic adenosine monophosphate (cAMP). An increased intracellular level of cAMP relaxes bronchial smooth-muscle cells and inhibits histamine release.

## Interactions

DRUGS

*beta blockers:* Increased risk of bronchospasm
*MAO inhibitors, tricyclic antidepressants:* Possibly potentiated cardiovascular effects of metaproterenol
*other sympathomimetics:* Possibly additive effects of both drugs and risk of toxicity
*theophylline:* Increased risk of arrhythmias

## Adverse Reactions

**CNS:** Dizziness, fatigue, headache, insomnia, malaise, nervousness, tremor
**CV:** ECG changes, hypertension, palpitations, tachycardia
**EENT:** Dry mouth, pharyngitis, taste perversion
**GI:** Diarrhea, nausea, vomiting
**RESP:** Asthma exacerbation, cough

## Nursing Considerations

• Anticipate that a single dose of nebulized metaproterenol may not completely stop an acute asthma attack.
• Monitor for adverse reactions and signs of toxicity, especially if patient uses tablets and aerosol. Notify prescriber if they develop.
• Be aware that tolerance may occur with continued use.

PATIENT TEACHING

• Caution patient not to use metaproterenol inhaler or nebulizer more often than prescribed.
• Teach patient to use inhaler correctly, to hold breath during second half of inhalation, and to wait 2 minutes between inhalations.
• Instruct parents to use spacer with their child's metered-dose inhaler.
• Advise patient to use metaproterenol 5 minutes before using corticosteroid inhaler, if prescribed, to maximize airway opening.
• Instruct patient to notify prescriber immediately if diarrhea, increased shortness of breath, insomnia, or irregular heartbeat occurs.
• Instruct patient to notify prescriber if drug becomes less effective.

M

# metaxalone

Skelaxin

## Class and Category

*Chemical:* Oxazolidinone derivative
*Therapeutic:* Skeletal muscle relaxant
*Pregnancy category:* Not rated

## Indications and Dosages

➤ *To relieve discomfort caused by acute, painful musculoskeletal conditions*

**TABLETS**

**Adults and children over age 12.** 800 mg t.i.d. or q.i.d.

| Route | Onset | Peak | Duration |
|-------|-------|------|----------|
| P.O. | Usually in 1 hr | Unknown | 4 to 6 hr |

### Mechanism of Action

May depress the CNS, resulting in sedation, which in turn may reduce skeletal muscle spasms to provide pain relief. Metaxalone does not directly relax tense skeletal muscles.

## Contraindications

Hypersensitivity to metaxalone or its components, significant renal or hepatic disease, tendency to develop drug-induced, hemolytic, or other anemias

## Interactions

**DRUGS**

*CNS depressants:* Increased CNS depression

**ACTIVITIES**

*alcohol use:* Increased CNS depression

## Adverse Reactions

**CNS:** Dizziness, drowsiness, excitement, headache, insomnia, irritability, nervousness, restlessness
**GI:** Abdominal cramps or pain, GI upset, jaundice, hepatotoxicity, nausea, vomiting
**HEME:** Hemolytic anemia, leukopenia
**SKIN:** Pruritus, rash

## Nursing Considerations

• Be aware that metaxalone may not be prescribed for women who are or may become pregnant unless the potential benefits outweigh the risks because drug's effect on fetus is unknown.
• Monitor patient for excessive drowsiness, which may lead to respiratory depression.
• Caution patient to consult prescriber before taking other drugs, such as sleeping pills, cold or allergy preparations, opioid analgesics, and antidepressants.
• Monitor liver function test results for elevations, especially in patients with preexisting hepatic disease.
• Monitor renal function test results, as prescribed, for signs of impaired renal function because drug is excreted by the kidneys.
• Provide rest and other pain-relief measures.
• Store drug at 15° to 30° C (59° to 86° F).

**PATIENT TEACHING**

• Advise patient to take metaxalone tablets exactly as prescribed and not to increase dosage or frequency.
• Caution patient to avoid potentially hazardous activities, such as driving or operating machinery, until drug's CNS effects are known.
• Instruct patient to avoid alcohol and other CNS depressants during metaxalone therapy.
• Urge patient to notify prescriber if he notices a rash or itching, which may signify a hypersensitivity reaction, or if he develops signs of hepatotoxicity, such as tiredness, nausea, yellow skin, or flulike symptoms.

# metformin hydrochloride

Gen-Metformin (CAN), Glucophage, Glucophage XR, Glumetza, Glycon (CAN), Novo-Metformin (CAN), Riomet

## Class and Category

*Chemical:* Dimethylbiguanide
*Therapeutic:* Antidiabetic
*Pregnancy category:* B

## Indications and Dosages

➤ *To reduce blood glucose level in type 2 diabetes mellitus*

**ORAL SOLUTION, TABLETS**

**Adults and children age 10 and older.** *Initial:* 500 mg b.i.d. or 850 mg q.d. Dosage increased as prescribed by 500 mg/wk or by 850 mg q 2 wk until desired response occurs. *Usual:* 500 to 850 mg b.i.d. or t.i.d. *Maximum:* 2,550 mg/day (adults and adolescents age 17 and older); 2,000 mg/day (children ages 10 to 16).

DOSAGE ADJUSTMENT If patient takes insulin, initial dosage reduced to 500 mg q.d. and then increased as prescribed by 500 mg q wk until blood glucose level is controlled.

**E.R. TABLETS**

**Adults and adolescents age 18 and older.**
*Initial:* 500 mg q.d. (Glucophage XR) or 1,000 mg q.d. (Glumetza) with evening meal. Increased as prescribed by 500 mg/wk. *Maximum:* 2,000 mg q.d.
DOSAGE ADJUSTMENT If control isn't achieved with maximum once-daily E.R. dosage, regimen may be changed to 1,000 mg b.i.d. If control is not achieved after 4 wk of maximum dosage, an oral sulfonylurea may be prescribed.

➤ *As adjunct to insulin therapy in type 2 diabetes mellitus*

**ORAL SOLUTION, TABLETS, E.R. TABLETS**

**Adults.** *Initial:* 500 mg (Glucophage, Glucophage XR) or 1,000 mg (Glumetza) q.d. in addition to current dose of insulin. Increased by 500 mg/wk, as needed. *Maximum:* 2,000 mg for Glucophage XR and Glumetza; 2,500 mg for Glucophage.
DOSAGE ADJUSTMENT If fasting blood glucose level drops below 120 mg/dl, insulin dosage decreased by 10% to 25%. Subsequent insulin dosage decrease may be needed based upon patient's continued response.

## Contraindications
Hypersensitivity to metformin or its components, impaired renal function, metabolic acidosis, use of iodinated contrast media within preceding 48 hours

| Route | Onset | Peak | Duration |
|---|---|---|---|
| P.O. (tablets) | Unknown | Up to 2 wk | 2 wk after drug discontinued |

## Mechanism of Action
May promote the storage of excess glucose as glycogen in the liver, which reduces glucose production. Metformin also may improve glucose use by skeletal muscle and adipose tissue by increasing glucose transport across cell membranes. This drug also may increase the number of insulin receptors on cell membranes and make them more sensitive to insulin. In addition, metformin modestly decreases blood triglyceride and total cholesterol levels.

## Interactions
**DRUGS**
*calcium channel blockers, corticosteroids, estrogens, isoniazid, nicotinic acid, oral contraceptives, phenothiazines, phenytoin, sympathomimetics, thiazide and other diuretics, thyroid drugs:* Possibly hyperglycemia
*cationic drugs (such as amiloride, cimetidine, digoxin, morphine, procainamide, quinidine, quinine, ranitidine, triamterene, trimethoprim, vancomycin), nifedipine:* Increased blood metformin level
*clofibrate, MAO inhibitors, probenecid, propranolol, rifabutin, rifampin, salicylates, sulfonamides, sulfonylureas:* Increased risk of hypoglycemia

**FOODS**
*all foods:* Possibly delayed metformin absorption

**ACTIVITIES**
*alcohol use:* Increased risk of hypoglycemia and lactate formation

## Adverse Reactions
**CNS:** Headache
**EENT:** Metallic taste
**ENDO:** Hypoglycemia
**GI:** Abdominal distention, anorexia, constipation, diarrhea, flatulence, indigestion, nausea, vomiting
**HEME:** Aplastic anemia, megaloblastic anemia, thrombocytopenia
**SKIN:** Photosensitivity, rash
**Other:** Lactic acidosis, weight loss

## Nursing Considerations
• Administer metformin tablets with food, which decreases and slightly delays absorption, thus reducing the risk of adverse GI reactions. Administer E.R. tablets with evening meal; don't break or crush them.
• Expect prescriber to alter dosage if patient has a condition that decreases or delays gastric emptying, such as diarrhea, gastroparesis, GI obstruction, ileus, or vomiting.
• Assess BUN and serum creatinine level, as appropriate, before and during long-term therapy in those at increased risk for lactic acidosis.
• Monitor patient's hepatic function, as ordered, because impaired hepatic function may significantly reduce the liver's ability to clear lactate, predisposing the patient to lactic acidosis.
• Monitor blood glucose level to evaluate drug effectiveness. Assess for hyperglycemia

M

and the need for insulin during times of increased stress, such as infection and surgery.
•Withhold drug, as ordered, if patient becomes dehydrated or develops hypoxemia or sepsis because these conditions increase the risk of lactic acidosis.
•Be aware that iodinated contrast media used in radiographic studies increase the risk of renal failure and lactic acidosis during metformin therapy. Expect to withhold metformin for 48 hours before and after testing.

**PATIENT TEACHING**
•Instruct patient to take metformin tablets with meals: at breakfast if taking drug once a day, or at breakfast and dinner if taking drug twice a day. Instruct him to take E.R. tablets once daily with evening meal and to swallow them whole, not crush or chew them.
•Direct patient to take drug exactly as prescribed and not to change the dosage or frequency unless instructed.
•Stress the importance of following prescribed diet, exercising regularly, controlling weight, and checking blood glucose level.
•Teach patient how to measure his blood glucose level and recognize signs of hyperglycemia and hypoglycemia. Urge him to notify prescriber of abnormal blood glucose level.
•Caution patient to avoid alcohol, which can increase the risk of hypoglycemia.
•Instruct patient to watch for early signs of lactic acidosis, including drowsiness, hyperventilation, malaise, and muscle pain, and notify prescriber if such signs develop.
•Advise patient to expect laboratory monitoring of glycosylated hemoglobin level every 3 months until blood glucose level is controlled.

# methadone hydrochloride

Dolophine, Methadose

## Class, Category, and Schedule
*Chemical:* Phenylheptylamine
*Therapeutic:* Synthetic opiate agonist
*Pregnancy category:* C
*Controlled substance:* Schedule II

## Indications and Dosages
➤ *To manage narcotic detoxification*

**DISPERSIBLE TABLETS, ORAL CONCENTRATE, I.M. OR S.C. INJECTION**
**Adults.** *Initial:* 15 to 40 mg q.d. or as needed. *Usual:* Dosage individualized based on clinical response. *Maximum:* 120 mg/day.
**Children.** Dosage individualized based on age and size. *Maximum:* 120 mg/day.

➤ *To maintain narcotic abstinence*
**DISPERSIBLE TABLETS, ORAL CONCENTRATE**
**Adults.** Dosage individualized based on clinical response. *Maximum:* 120 mg/day.
**Children.** Dosage individualized based on age and size. *Maximum:* 120 mg/day.

➤ *To treat severe or chronic pain*
**ORAL CONCENTRATE, ORAL SOLUTION**
**Adults.** 5 to 20 mg q 4 to 8 hr. Dosage increased or dosing interval decreased, as prescribed and as needed. *Maximum:* 120 mg/day.
**Children.** Dosage individualized based on age and size.

**TABLETS, I.M. OR S.C. INJECTION**
**Adults.** 2.5 to 10 mg q 3 to 4 hr as needed. For chronic pain, dosage and dosing interval may be adjusted, as prescribed and as needed.
**Children.** Dosage individualized based on age and size.

**DOSAGE ADJUSTMENT** Elderly patients, debilitated patients, and patients with severe hepatic or renal dysfunction, hypothyroidism, Addison's disease, prostatic hyperplasia, or urethral stricture need individualized reduced dosages.

| Route | Onset | Peak | Duration |
|-------|-------|------|----------|
| P.O. | 30 to 60 min | 1.5 to 2 hr | 4 to 6 hr |
| I.M. | 10 to 20 min | 1 to 2 hr | 4 to 5 hr |

## Mechanism of Action
Binds with and activates opioid receptors (primarily mu receptors) in the spinal cord and in higher levels of the CNS to produce analgesia and euphoric effects.

## Contraindications
Acute or postoperative pain, acute or severe asthma, chronic respiratory disease, diarrhea associated with pseudomembranous colitis or poisoning, hypersensitivity to methadone or its components, respiratory depression, severe inflammatory bowel disease

# Interactions

**DRUGS**

*ammonium chloride, ascorbic acid, potassium, sodium phosphate:* May precipitate methadone withdrawal symptoms
*amitriptyline, chloripramine, nortriptyline:* Increased CNS and respiratory depression
*anticholinergics:* Possibly severe constipation leading to ileus; urine retention
*antiemetics, general anesthetics, hypnotics, phenothiazines, sedatives, tranquilizers:* Possibly coma, hypotension, respiratory depression, and severe sedation
*antihistamines, choral hydrate, glutethimide, MAO inhibitors, methocarbamol:* Increased CNS and respiratory depressant effects of methadone
*antihypertensives, hypotension-producing drugs:* Increased hypotension, risk of orthostatic hypotension
*azole antifungals, macrolide antibiotics:* Increased or prolonged opioid effect
*buprenorphine:* Decreased therapeutic effect of methadone, increased respiratory depression, possibly withdrawal symptoms
*calcium channel blockers, class Ia and class III antiarrhythmics, diuretics, laxatives, mineralocorticoid hormones, neuroleptics, tricyclic antidepressants:* Increased risk of electrolyte disturbances and prolonged QT interval
*carbamazepine, phenobarbital, St. John's wort:* Possibly precipitation of withdrawal symptoms
*cimetidine:* Increased analgesic and CNS and respiratory depressant effects of methadone
*desipramine:* Increased plasma desipramine level
*didanosine, stavudine:* Decreased plasma levels of these drugs
*diuretics:* Decreased diuresis
*efavirenz, nevirapine, ritonavir, ritonavir and lopinavir:* Decreased blood methadone level
*hydroxyzine:* Increased analgesic, CNS depressant, and hypotensive effects of methadone
*loperamide, paregoric:* Increased CNS depression, possibly severe constipation
*MAO inhibitors:* Possibly increased risk of severe adverse reactions
*metoclopramide:* Possibly antagonized metoclopramide effects on GI motility
*mixed agonist-antagonist analgesics:* Possibly withdrawal symptoms

*naloxone:* Antagonized analgesic and CNS and respiratory depressant effects of methadone, possibly withdrawal symptoms
*naltrexone:* Possibly induction or worsening of withdrawal symptoms if methadone given within 7 days before naltrexone
*neuromuscular blockers:* Increased or prolonged respiratory depression
*opioid analgesics (such as alfentanil and sufentanil):* Increased CNS and respiratory depression, increased hypotension
*phenytoin, rifampin:* May precipitate withdrawal symptoms
*selective serotonin reuptake inhibitors:* Possibly increased blood methadone levels and increased risk of methadone toxicity
*zidovudine:* Increased blood zidovudine level and risk of toxicity

**ACTIVITIES**

*alcohol use:* Increased CNS and respiratory depression, possibly hypotension

# Adverse Reactions

**CNS:** Agitation, amnesia, anxiety, asthenia, coma, confusion, decreased concentration, delirium, delusions, depression, dizziness, drowsiness, euphoria, fever, hallucinations, headache, insomnia, lethargy, light-headedness, malaise, psychosis, restlessness, sedation, seizures, syncope, tremor
**CV:** Bradycardia, cardiac arrest, cardiomyopathy, edema, heart failure, hypotension, orthostatic hypotension, palpitations, phlebitis, prolonged QT interval, shock, tachycardia, torsades de pointes, T-wave inversion on ECG, ventricular fibrillation or tachycardia
**EENT:** Blurred vision, diplopia, dry mouth, glossitis, laryngeal edema or laryngospasm (allergic), miosis, nystagmus, rhinitis
**GI:** Abdominal cramps or pain, anorexia, biliary tract spasm, constipation, diarrhea, dysphagia, elevated liver function test results, gastroesophageal reflux, hiccups, ileus and toxic megacolon (in patients with inflammatory bowel disease), indigestion, nausea, vomiting
**GU:** Amenorrhea, decreased ejaculate potency, decreased libido, difficult ejaculation, impotence, prolonged labor, urinary hesitancy, urine retention
**HEME:** Anemia, leukopenia, thrombocytopenia
**MS:** Arthralgia

**RESP:** Apnea, asthma exacerbation, atelectasis, bronchospasm, depressed cough reflex, hypoventilation, pulmonary edema, respiratory arrest and depression, wheezing
**SKIN:** Diaphoresis, flushing
**Other:** Allergic reaction; facial edema; hypokalemia; hypomagnesemia; injection site edema, pain, rash, or redness; physical and psychological dependence; weight gain; withdrawal symptoms

## Nursing Considerations
•Before giving methadone, make sure opioid antagonist and equipment for administering oxygen and controlling respiration are nearby.
•Before therapy begins, assess patient's current drug use, including all prescription and OTC drugs.
•WARNING Give drug cautiously to patients at risk for a prolonged QT interval, such as those with cardiac hypertrophy, hypokalemia, or hypomagnesemia; those with a history of cardiac conduction abnormalities; and those taking diuretics or medications that affect cardiac conduction.
•Dilute oral concentrate with water or another liquid to a volume of at least 30 ml, but preferably to 90 ml or more, before administration. Dissolve dispersible tablets in water or another liquid before administration.
•Monitor patient for expected excessive drowsiness, unsteadiness, or confusion during first 3 to 5 days of therapy, and notify prescriber if effects continue to worsen or persist beyond this time.
•WARNING Monitor respiratory and circulatory status carefully and at frequent intervals during methadone therapy because respiratory depression, circulatory depression, respiratory arrest, shock, hypotension, and cardiac arrest are potential hazards of therapy. Monitor children frequently for respiratory depression and paradoxical CNS excitation because of their increased sensitivity to drug. Assess for excessive or persistent sedation; dosage may need to be adjusted.
•Monitor for drug tolerance, especially in patients with a history of chronic drug abuse, because methadone can cause physical and psychological dependence.
•Monitor patient for pain because maintenance dosage doesn't provide pain relief; patients who have developed a tolerance to opiate agonists, including those with chronic cancer pain, may require a higher dosage.
•Monitor patients who are pregnant or who have liver or renal impairment for increased adverse effects from methadone because drug may have a prolonged duration and cumulative effect in these patients. Methadone may prolong labor by reducing strength, duration, and frequency of uterine contractions, so expect dosage to be tapered before third trimester of pregnancy. Breast-feeding mothers on maintenance therapy put their infants at risk of withdrawal symptoms if they abruptly stop breast-feeding or discontinue methadone therapy. Methadone also accumulates in CNS tissue, increasing the risk of seizures in infants.
•Check plasma amylase and lipase levels in patients who develop biliary tract spasms because levels may increase up to 15 times normal. Notify prescriber immediately of any significant or sustained increase.
•Monitor patients who have head injuries or other conditions that may increase intracranial pressure (ICP) because methadone may further increase ICP.
•Assess patient for withdrawal symptoms and tolerance to therapy because physiologic dependence can occur with long-term methadone use. Avoid abrupt discontinuation because withdrawal symptoms will occur within 3 to 4 days after last dose.
•Monitor patients, especially the elderly, for cardiac arrhythmias, hypotension, hypovolemia, orthostatic hypotension, and vasovagal syncope because drug may produce cholinergic effects in patients with cardiac disease, resulting in bradycardia and peripheral vasodilation; dosage decrease may be indicated.
•Monitor patients with prostatic hypertrophy, urethral stricture, or renal disease for urine retention and oliguria because drug can increase tension of detrusor muscle.
•Be prepared to treat symptoms of anxiety. Be aware that anxiety may be confused with symptoms of opiate abstinence and that methadone doesn't have antianxiety effects.

**PATIENT TEACHING**
•Instruct patient taking oral concentrate form of methadone to dilute it with water or another liquid to a volume of at least 30 ml and preferably to 90 ml or more before administration.

•Instruct patient to dissolve dispersible tablets in water or other liquid before administration.

•Advise patient to notify prescriber of all other drugs he's currently taking and to avoid alcohol and other depressants, such as sleeping pills and tranquilizers, because they may increase drug's CNS depressant effects.

•Instruct patient to take drug only as prescribed and not to change dosage without prescriber approval. Inform patient that abrupt cessation of methadone therapy can precipitate withdrawal symptoms. Urge him to notify prescriber if he develops any concerns over therapy.

•Urge patient to notify prescriber if he experiences palpitations, dizziness, light-headedness, or syncope, which may be caused by methadone-induced arrhythmias.

•Instruct patient to avoid activities that require mental alertness because methadone therapy may cause drowsiness or sleepiness.

•Teach patient to change positions slowly to minimize effects of orthostatic hypotension.

•Instruct patient to notify prescriber of worsening or breakthrough pain because dosage may need to be adjusted.

•Inform parents that a child on methadone maintenance therapy may become unusually excited or restless; advise them to notify prescriber of changes in child's behavior.

•Instruct female patient to notify prescriber immediately if she becomes pregnant during methadone therapy because drug may cause physical dependence in fetus and withdrawal symptoms in neonate.

•Caution patient who is breast-feeding not to stop doing so abruptly and not to stop taking methadone without prescriber's approval because infant may experience withdrawal symptoms.

# methamphetamine hydrochloride

Desoxyn, Desoxyn Gradumet

## Class, Category, and Schedule
*Chemical:* Amphetamine
*Therapeutic:* CNS stimulant
*Pregnancy category:* C
*Controlled substance:* Schedule II

## Indications and Dosages

➤ *To treat attention-deficit hyperactivity disorder (ADHD)*

**E.R. TABLETS**

**Children age 6 and older.** 20 to 25 mg q.d.

**TABLETS**

**Children age 6 and older.** *Initial:* 5 mg q.d. or b.i.d. Increased by 5 mg q wk. *Maintenance:* 20 to 25 mg/day in divided doses b.i.d.

| Route | Onset | Peak | Duration |
|-------|-------|------|----------|
| P.O. | Unknown | Unknown | 6 to 24 hr |

## Mechanism of Action

May produce CNS stimulation by facilitating norepinephrine's release and blocking its reuptake at adrenergic nerve terminals and by directly stimulating alpha and beta receptors in the peripheral nervous system. Methamphetamine also promotes dopamine release and blocks its reuptake in the brain's limbic regions. The drug appears to act mainly in the cerebral cortex and, possibly, the reticular activating system. These actions decrease motor restlessness, increase alertness, and diminish drowsiness and fatigue. The drug's peripheral actions include increased blood pressure and mild bronchodilation and respiratory stimulation.

## Contraindications

Advanced arteriosclerosis; glaucoma; hypersensitivity to methamphetamine, sympathomimetic amines, or their components; hyperthyroidism; history of drug abuse; moderate to severe hypertension; severe agitation; symptomatic cardiovascular disease; use within 14 days of MAO inhibitor therapy

## Interactions

**DRUGS**

*ascorbic acid:* Decreased methamphetamine absorption and therapeutic effect

*beta blockers:* Increased risk of heart block, hypotension, and severe bradycardia

*CNS stimulants:* Increased CNS stimulation and risk of adverse reactions

*digoxin, levodopa:* Increased risk of arrhythmias

*diuretics, other antihypertensives:* Possibly decreased antihypertensive effect

*ethosuximide, phenobarbital, phenytoin:* Possibly delayed absorption of these drugs
*haloperidol, phenothiazines:* Possibly interference with these drugs' therapeutic effects and with methamphetamine's CNS stimulant effects
*inhalation anesthetics:* Increased risk of ventricular arrhythmias
*insulin:* Altered insulin requirements
*lithium:* Possibly antagonized CNS stimulant effects of methamphetamine
*MAO inhibitors:* Possibly severe hypertension, risk of hypertensive crisis, increased vasopressor effect of methamphetamine
*meperidine:* Increased risk of hypotension and life-threatening interactions, such as severe respiratory depression and coma
*metrizamide (intrathecal):* Increased risk of seizures
*thyroid hormones:* Enhanced effects of both drugs
*tricyclic antidepressants:* Increased risk of arrhythmias and severe hypertension
*urinary acidifiers:* Increased metabolism and shortened pharmacologic effects of methamphetamine
*urinary alkalinizers:* Decreased metabolism and prolonged pharmacologic effects of methamphetamine

**FOODS**
*caffeine:* Increased methamphetamine effects

## Adverse Reactions
**CNS:** Dizziness, euphoria, headache, hyperactivity, insomnia, irritability, nervousness, psychotic episodes, restlessness, talkativeness, tremor
**CV:** Arrhythmias, chest pain, hypertension, hypotension, palpitations, tachycardia
**EENT:** Blurred vision, dry mouth, taste perversion
**GI:** Abdominal cramps, anorexia, constipation, diarrhea, nausea, vomiting
**GU:** Impotence, libido changes
**SKIN:** Diaphoresis, urticaria
**Other:** Physical and psychological dependence

## Nursing Considerations
• Use methamphetamine cautiously in patients with a history of psychiatric problems or suicidal or homicidal tendencies.
• Assess for seizures in patients with a history of seizure disorders because drug may lower seizure threshold.

• Observe for signs of drug tolerance and, possibly, extreme dependence, which may develop after a few weeks. Be aware that methamphetamine abuse may occur.
• Expect treatment for ADHD to include psychological, educational, and social measures in addition to drug therapy.
• Watch for signs of chronic methamphetamine intoxication, including hyperactivity, insomnia, irritability, and personality changes. Notify prescriber if such signs occur.

**PATIENT TEACHING**
• Instruct parent of patient to give methamphetamine at least 6 hours before bedtime to prevent insomnia.
• Explain the high risk of abuse with this drug. Instruct parent of patient not to increase dosage unless advised to do so by prescriber and not to give drug to prevent fatigue.
• Caution parent that patient should not crush or chew E.R. tablets.
• Advise parent that patient should avoid caffeine, which increases drug's effects.
• Instruct parent of patient to report signs of overstimulation, such as diarrhea, hyperactivity, insomnia, and irritability.

# methazolamide
MZM, Neptazane

## Class and Category
*Chemical:* Sulfonamide derivative
*Therapeutic:* Antiglaucoma
*Pregnancy category:* C

## Indications and Dosages
➤ *To treat open-angle glaucoma*
**TABLETS**
**Adults.** 50 to 100 mg b.i.d. or t.i.d.

| Route | Onset | Peak | Duration |
|-------|-------|------|----------|
| P.O. | 2 to 4 hr | 6 to 8 hr | 10 to 18 hr |

### Mechanism of Action
Inhibits the enyzme carbonic anhydrase, which normally appears in renal proximal tubule cells, choroid plexus of the brain, and ciliary processes of the eye. By inhibiting this enzyme in the eyes, methazolamide decreases aqueous humor secretion, which reduces intraocular pressure.

## Contraindications

Cirrhosis; hyperchloremic acidosis; hypersensitivity to methazolamide, other carbonic anhydrase inhibitors, or their components; hypokalemia; hyponatremia; severe adrenocortical, hepatic, or renal impairment

## Interactions

**DRUGS**

*amphetamines, anticholinergics, mecamylamine, procainamide, quinidine:* Decreased renal clearance of these drugs, increased risk of toxicity

*amphotericin B, corticosteroids:* Increased risk of severe hypokalemia

*barbiturates, carbamazepine, phenytoin, primidone:* Increased risk of osteopenia

*digoxin:* Increased risk of hypokalemia and digitalis toxicity

*ephedrine:* Possibly prolonged duration of action of ephedrine

*insulin, oral antidiabetic drugs:* Increased risk of glycosuria and hyperglycemia

*lithium:* Increased lithium excretion

*mannitol:* Increased diuresis and further reduction of intraocular pressure

*methenamine compounds:* Decreased methenamine effectiveness

*mexiletine:* Possibly impaired renal excretion of mexiletine

*neuromuscular blockers:* Possibly prolonged duration of action of blockers from methazolamide-induced hypokalemia, increased risk of prolonged respiratory paralysis and depression

*salicylates:* Possibly CNS depression and metabolic acidosis, increased risk of methazolamide toxicity

## Adverse Reactions

**CNS:** Confusion, depression, drowsiness, fatigue, fever, malaise, paresthesia, seizures, weakness

**EENT:** Hearing loss, myopia (transient), taste perversion, tinnitus

**GI:** Anorexia, diarrhea, nausea, vomiting

**GU:** Crystalluria, nephrotoxicity, renal calculi

**SKIN:** Photosensitivity, pruritus, rash, Stevens-Johnson syndrome, urticaria

**Other:** Metabolic acidosis

## Nursing Considerations

• Use methazolamide cautiously in patients with obstructive pulmonary disease.

• Monitor fluid intake and output, weight, and serum electrolyte levels during methazolamide therapy.

**PATIENT TEACHING**

• Direct patient to take methazolamide exactly as prescribed because increasing dosage may lead to metabolic acidosis.

• Advise patient to take drug with food if GI distress occurs.

• Instruct patient to notify prescriber if rash develops.

• Caution patient to avoid potentially hazardous activities until drug's CNS effects are known.

• Stress the importance of regular eye examinations during methazolamide therapy.

# methenamine hippurate

Hiprex, Urex

# methenamine mandelate

Mandelamine

## Class and Category

*Chemical:* Formaldehyde precursor, hexamethylenetetramine

*Therapeutic:* Antibiotic

*Pregnancy category:* C

## Indications and Dosages

➤ *To prevent or suppress frequently recurring UTIs caused by a wide variety of gram-negative and gram-positive bacteria (including enterococci,* Escherichia coli, Micrococcus pyogenes, *and staphylococci) in intermittently catheterized patients with neurogenic bladder*

**ENTERIC-COATED TABLETS, ORAL SUSPENSION (METHENAMINE MANDELATE)**

**Adults and adolescents.** 1 g q.i.d. a.c. and h.s.

**Children ages 6 to 12.** 500 mg q.i.d., or 50 mg/kg/day in divided doses.

**Children under age 6.** 18.4 mg/kg q.i.d.

**TABLETS (METHENAMINE HIPPURATE)**

**Adults and adolescents.** 1 g b.i.d.

**Children ages 6 to 12.** 0.5 to 1 g q 12 hr.

## Contraindications

Concurrent therapy with sulfonamides, hypersensitivity to methenamine, renal insufficiency, severe dehydration, severe hepatic disease

M

## Mechanism of Action

Hydrolyzes to formaldehyde and ammonia in an acidic environment, such as urine, producing greater amounts of formaldehyde as pH decreases. Formaldehyde exerts a bactericidal action, possibly by denaturing proteins. To facilitate hydrolysis, methenamine is formulated with a weak organic acid, such as hippuric acid or mandelic acid.

## Interactions

**DRUGS**
*bicarbonate-containing antacids, urinary alkalinizers:* Decreased methenamine effectiveness
*sulfonamides, such as sulfamethizole:* Possibly formation of insoluble precipitate in urine
**FOODS**
*milk, milk products, most fruits:* Possibly decreased effectiveness of methenamine

## Adverse Reactions

**CNS:** Headache
**CV:** Edema
**EENT:** Stomatitis
**GI:** Abdominal cramps, anorexia, diarrhea, nausea, vomiting
**GU:** Bladder irritation, crystalluria, dysuria, hematuria, proteinuria, urinary frequency
**RESP:** Pulmonary hypersensitivity (dyspnea, pneumonitis)
**SKIN:** Pruritus, rash, urticaria

## Nursing Considerations

• Be aware that methenamine is used for prophylaxis; it isn't recommended as primary treatment for UTI.
• Be aware that drug shouldn't be given to patients whose creatinine clearance is less than 50 ml/min/1.73 m$^2$.
• Before giving first dose, expect to obtain urine specimen for culture and sensitivity tests, as ordered, and to review test results if available.
• Plan to give methenamine mandelate around the clock to maintain a therapeutic blood level.
• Make sure patient receives adequate fluids.
• Expect to repeat culture and sensitivity tests if patient fails to improve.
**PATIENT TEACHING**
• Instruct patient to take methenamine with food to avoid GI distress.

• Direct patient to drink extra fluids; avoid alkaline foods, such as milk, milk products, and most fruits; and avoid antacids that contain sodium bicarbonate or carbonate during methenamine therapy.
• Instruct patient to report painful urination, rash, or severe GI distress.
• Urge patient to comply with order for urine testing before and during long-term therapy.

# methicillin sodium

Staphcillin

## Class and Category

*Chemical:* Penicillinase-resistant penicillin
*Therapeutic:* Antibiotic
*Pregnancy category:* B

## Indications and Dosages

➤ *To treat general infections, such as sepsis, sinusitis, and skin and soft-tissue infections, caused by susceptible organisms (including penicillinase-producing and non-penicillinase-producing strains of* Staphylococcus epidermidis, Staphylococcus saprophyticus, *and* Streptococcus pneumoniae)
**I.V. INFUSION, I.M. INJECTION**
**Adults and children weighing 40 kg (88 lb) or more.** 1 g q 4 to 6 hr (I.M.) or 1 g q 6 hr (I.V.). *Maximum:* 24 g/day.
**Children weighing less than 40 kg.** 25 mg/kg q 6 hr.
**DOSAGE ADJUSTMENT** For adults and children with cystic fibrosis, dosage adjusted to 50 mg/kg q 6 hr.
➤ *To treat bacterial meningitis*
**I.V. INFUSION, I.M. INJECTION**
**Neonates weighing 2 kg (4.4 lb) or more.** 50 mg/kg q 8 hr for first wk after birth and then 50 mg/kg q 6 hr.
**Neonates weighing less than 2 kg.** 25 to 50 mg/kg q 12 hr for first wk after birth and then 50 mg/kg q 8 hr.

## Incompatibilities

Don't mix methicillin in same syringe or I.V. solution with other drugs. Don't mix methicillin with dextrose solutions because their low acidity may damage drug. Administer methicillin at least 1 hour before or after aminoglycosides and at different sites; otherwise, mutual inactivation can occur.

## Mechanism of Action
Kills bacterial cells by inhibiting bacterial cell wall synthesis. In susceptible bacteria, the rigid, cross-linked cell wall is assembled in several steps. In the final stage of cross-linking, methicillin binds with and inactivates penicillin-binding proteins (enzymes responsible for linking cell wall strands), resulting in bacterial cell lysis and death. *Staphylococcus aureus* has developed resistance to methicillin by altering its penicillin-binding proteins.

## Contraindications
Hypersensitivity to methicillin sodium, other penicillins, or their components

## Interactions
### DRUGS
*aminoglycosides:* Substantial aminoglycoside inactivation
*chloramphenicol, erythromycins, sulfonamides, tetracyclines:* Possibly decreased therapeutic effects of methicillin
*methotrexate:* Increased risk of methotrexate toxicity
*probenecid:* Possibly decreased renal clearance, increased blood level, and increased risk of toxicity of methicillin

## Adverse Reactions
**CNS:** Aggressiveness, agitation, anxiety, confusion, depression, headache, seizures
**EENT:** Oral candidiasis
**GI:** Abdominal pain, diarrhea, hepatotoxicity, nausea, pseudomembranous colitis, vomiting
**GU:** Interstitial nephritis, vaginitis
**HEME:** Leukopenia, neutropenia, thrombocytopenia
**SKIN:** Exfoliative dermatitis, pruritus, rash, urticaria
**Other:** Anaphylaxis; infusion site redness, swelling, and tenderness; injection site pain, redness, and swelling; serum sickness–like reaction

## Nursing Considerations
•**WARNING** Be aware that methicillin is not a first-line treatment for the indications above because of the prevalence of methicillin-resistant *Staphylococcus aureus.*
•Before giving first dose, obtain appropriate body fluid or tissue specimens for culture and sensitivity tests, as ordered, and review test results if available.
•Inject I.M. form deep into gluteal muscle.
•During I.V. use, observe infusion site closely for redness, swelling, and tenderness.
•Monitor fluid intake and output and renal function test results during methicillin therapy.
•Observe for signs of superinfection, such as diarrhea, vaginal itching, and white patches or sores in mouth or on tongue. Notify prescriber if they occur.
•Closely monitor renal function test results, including serum creatinine level; about one-third of patients experience interstitial nephritis after 10 days of methicillin therapy.
•Monitor liver function test results, and observe for signs of hepatotoxicity, such as fever and nausea. Notify prescriber if they develop.
### PATIENT TEACHING
•Inform patient that I.M. injection may be painful.
•Unless contraindicated, instruct patient to drink extra fluids during methicillin therapy.
•Advise patient to report diarrhea, injection site pain, mouth sores, or rash.

# methimazole

Tapazole

## Class and Category
*Chemical:* Thioimidazole derivative
*Therapeutic:* Antithyroid
*Pregnancy category:* D

## Indications and Dosages
➤ *To treat mild hyperthyroidism*
### TABLETS
**Adults and adolescents.** *Initial:* 15 mg/day as a single dose or in divided doses b.i.d. for 6 to 8 wk or until euthyroid level is reached. *Maintenance:* 5 to 30 mg/day as a single dose or in divided doses b.i.d.
**Children.** *Initial:* 0.4 mg/kg/day as a single dose or in divided doses b.i.d. *Maintenance:* 0.2 mg/kg/day as a single dose or in divided doses b.i.d.
➤ *To treat moderate hyperthyroidism*
### TABLETS
**Adults and adolescents.** *Initial:* 30 to 40 mg/day as a single dose or in divided doses b.i.d. for 6 to 8 wk or until euthyroid level is reached. *Maintenance:* 5 to 30 mg/day as a single dose or in divided doses b.i.d.

**Children.** *Initial:* 0.4 mg/kg/day as a single dose or in divided doses b.i.d. *Maintenance:* 0.2 mg/kg/day as a single dose or in divided doses b.i.d.

➤ *To treat severe hyperthyroidism*
**TABLETS**
**Adults and adolescents.** *Initial:* 60 mg/day as a single dose or in divided doses b.i.d. for 6 to 8 wk or until euthyroid level is reached. *Maintenance:* 5 to 30 mg/day as a single dose or in divided doses b.i.d.
**Children.** *Initial:* 0.4 mg/kg/day as a single dose or in divided doses b.i.d. *Maintenance:* 0.2 mg/kg/day as a single dose or in divided doses b.i.d.

➤ *As adjunct to treat thyrotoxicosis*
**SUPPOSITORIES**
**Adults and adolescents.** 15 to 20 mg q 4 hr on first day and then adjusted based on patient response.
**Children.** 0.4 mg/kg/day as a single dose or in divided doses b.i.d.

| Route | Onset | Peak | Duration |
|-------|-------|------|----------|
| P.O. | 5 days | 7 wk | Unknown |

**Mechanism of Action**

Directly interferes with thyroid hormone synthesis in the thyroid gland by inhibiting iodide incorporation into thyroglobulin. Iodination of thyroglobulin is an important step in synthesizing the thyroid hormones thyroxine and triiodothyronine. Eventually, thyroglobulin is depleted and the circulating thyroid hormone level drops.

**Contraindications**

Breast-feeding; hypersensitivity to methimazole, other antithyroid drugs, or their components

**Interactions**
**DRUGS**
*amiodarone, iodine, potassium iodide:* Decreased response to methimazole
*digoxin:* Possibly increased blood digoxin level
*oral anticoagulants:* Possibly a need for altered anticoagulant dosage

**Adverse Reactions**
**CNS:** Drowsiness, headache, paresthesia, vertigo
**CV:** Edema

**EENT:** Loss of taste
**ENDO:** Hypothyroidism
**GI:** Diarrhea, indigestion, nausea, vomiting
**HEME:** Agranulocytosis, aplastic anemia, leukopenia, thrombocytopenia
**MS:** Arthralgia, myalgia
**SKIN:** Alopecia, jaundice, pruritus, rash, skin discoloration, urticaria
**Other:** Lupus-like symptoms, lymphadenopathy

**Nursing Considerations**
•Closely monitor thyroid function test results during methimazole therapy.
•Check CBC results to detect abnormalities caused by inhibition of myelopoiesis.
•Watch for signs of hypothyroidism, such as cold intolerance, depression, and edema.
•Be aware that hyperthyroidism may increase metabolic clearance of beta blockers and theophylline and that dosages of these drugs may need to be reduced as the patient's thyroid condition becomes corrected.
**PATIENT TEACHING**
•Instruct patient to take drug with meals to avoid adverse GI reactions.
•Explain about possible hair loss or thinning during and for months after therapy.
•Instruct patient to notify prescriber immediately about cold intolerance, fever, sore throat, tiredness, and unusual bleeding or bruising.

# methocarbamol

Carbacot, Robaxin, Robaxin 750, Skelex

**Class and Category**
*Chemical:* Carbamate derivative of guaifenesin
*Therapeutic:* Skeletal muscle relaxant
*Pregnancy category:* C

**Indications and Dosages**
➤ *To relieve discomfort caused by acute, painful musculoskeletal conditions*
**TABLETS**
**Adults and adolescents.** *Initial:* 1,500 mg q.i.d. for 2 to 3 days; for severe discomfort, 8,000 mg/day. *Maintenance:* 750 mg q 4 hr, 1,000 mg q.i.d., or 1,500 mg t.i.d.
**I.V. INJECTION (100 MG/ML)**
**Adults and adolescents.** Up to 3,000 mg/day administered at 8-hr intervals for 3 consecutive days. Regimen repeated as prescribed after patient is drug-free for 48 hr.

**I.M. INJECTION (100 MG/ML)**
**Adults and adolescents.** 1,000 to 3,000 mg/
day administered at 8-hr intervals for 3 con-
secutive days. Regimen repeated as pre-
scribed after patient is drug-free for 48 hr.
➤ *To provide supportive therapy for tetanus*
**TABLETS**
**Adults and adolescents.** 24,000 mg/day given
by NG tube.
**I.V. INFUSION OR INJECTION (100 MG/ML)**
**Adults and adolescents.** 1,000 to 3,000 mg by
infusion or 1,000 to 2,000 mg by direct injec-
tion q 6 hr. *Maximum:* 300 mg (3 ml)/min.
**Children.** 15 mg/kg q 6 hr.

| Route | Onset | Peak | Duration |
|-------|-------|------|----------|
| P.O. | 30 min | Unknown | Unknown |
| I.V. | Immediate | Unknown | Unknown |

---

**Mechanism of Action**
May depress the CNS, which leads to sedation and reduced skeletal muscle
spasms. Methocarbamol also alters the
perception of pain.

---

**Contraindications**
Hypersensitivity to methocarbamol or its
components, renal disease (injectable form)

**Interactions**
**DRUGS**
*CNS depressants:* Increased CNS depression
**ACTIVITIES**
*alcohol use:* Increased CNS depression

**Adverse Reactions**
**CNS:** Dizziness, drowsiness, fever, headache,
light-headedness, seizures (I.V.), syncope,
vertigo, weakness
**CV:** Bradycardia, hypotension, and thrombophlebitis (parenteral)
**EENT:** Blurred vision, conjunctivitis, diplopia, metallic taste, nasal congestion, nystagmus
**GI:** Nausea
**GU:** Black, brown, or green urine
**SKIN:** Flushing, pruritus, rash, urticaria
**Other:** Anaphylaxis (parenteral), angioedema,
injection site irritation or pain (I.M.), injection site sloughing (I.V.)

**Nursing Considerations**
•If needed, crush tablets and mix with water
for administration by NG tube.

•Administer I.V. form directly through infusion line at 3 ml/min. To prepare solution,
add 10 ml to no more than 250 ml of D₅W or
NS. Infuse at no more than 300 mg (3 ml)/
min to avoid hypotension and seizures.
•Keep patient recumbent during I.V. administration and for at least 15 minutes afterward. Then have him rise slowly.
•Monitor I.V. site regularly for signs of
phlebitis.
•Inject I.M. form deep into large muscle,
such as gluteus. Give no more than 5 ml/dose
every 8 hours. One dose is usually adequate.
•Don't give drug by S.C. route.
•Keep epinephrine, antihistamines, and corticosteroids available in case patient experiences anaphylactic reaction.
•Be aware that the parenteral dosage form
shouldn't be used in patients with renal dysfunction because the polyethylene glycol 300
vehicle is nephrotoxic.
**PATIENT TEACHING**
•Tell patient to take drug exactly as prescribed.
•Advise patient to take drug with food or
milk to avoid nausea.
•Inform patient that urine may turn green,
black, or brown until drug is discontinued.
•Advise patient to avoid potentially hazardous activities until drug's CNS effects are
known.
•Instruct patient to avoid alcohol and other
CNS depressants during therapy.

# methotrexate (amethopterin)

Rheumatrex

## methotrexate sodium

Folex, Folex PFS, Mexate, Mexate-AQ

## Class and Category
*Chemical:* Folic acid analogue
*Therapeutic:* Antipsoriatic, antirheumatic
*Pregnancy category:* X

## Indications and Dosages
➤ *To treat severe psoriasis unresponsive to other therapy*
**TABLETS (METHOTREXATE)**
**Adults.** 2.5 to 5 mg q 12 hr for 3 doses/wk,
increased as ordered by 2.5 mg/wk. *Maxi-
mum:* 20 mg/wk.

I.V. OR I.M. INJECTION (METHOTREXATE SODIUM)
**Adults.** 10 mg/wk. *Maximum:* 25 mg/wk.

➤ *To treat severe rheumatoid arthritis unresponsive to other therapy*

TABLETS (METHOTREXATE)
**Adults.** 2.5 to 5 mg q 12 hr for 3 doses/wk, increased as ordered by 2.5 mg/wk. *Maximum:* 20 mg/wk.

| Route | Onset | Peak | Duration |
|-------|-------|------|----------|
| P.O., I.V., I.M. | 3 to 6 wk | Unknown | Unknown |

## Mechanism of Action

May exert immunosuppressive effects by inhibiting replication and function of T and possibly B lymphocytes. Methotrexate also slows the growth of rapidly proliferating cells, such as epithelial skin cells associated with psoriasis. This action may result from the drug's ability to inhibit dihydrofolate reductase, the enzyme that reduces folic acid to tetrahydrofolic acid. Inhibition of tetrahydrofolic acid interferes with DNA synthesis and cell reproduction in rapidly proliferating cells.

## Contraindications

Breast-feeding, hypersensitivity to methotrexate or its components, pregnancy

## Interactions

DRUGS
*bone marrow depressants:* Possibly increased bone marrow depression
*co-trimoxazole:* Possibly increased bone marrow suppression
*folic acid:* Possibly decreased effectiveness of methotrexate
*hepatotoxic drugs:* Increased risk of hepatotoxicity
*chloramphenicol, neomycin, tetracycline:* Possibly decreased absorption of methotrexate
*NSAIDs, penicillins, phenylbutazone, phenytoin, probenecid, salicylates, sulfonamides:* Increased risk of methotrexate toxicity
*oral anticoagulants:* Increased risk of bleeding
*sulfonamides:* Increased risk of hepatotoxicity
*theophylline:* Possibly increased risk of theophylline toxicity
*vaccines:* Risk of disseminated infection with live-virus vaccines, risk of suppressed response to killed-virus vaccines

ACTIVITIES
*alcohol use:* Increased risk of hepatotoxicity

## Adverse Reactions

**CNS:** Aphasia, cerebral thrombosis, chills, dizziness, drowsiness, fatigue, fever, headache, hemiparesis, leukoencephalopathy, malaise, paresis, seizures
**CV:** Chest pain, deep vein thrombosis, hypotension, pericardial effusion, pericarditis, thromboembolism
**ENDO:** Gynecomastia
**EENT:** Blurred vision, conjunctivitis, gingivitis, glossitis, pharyngitis, stomatitis, transient blindness, tinnitus
**GI:** Abdominal pain, anorexia, cirrhosis, diarrhea, elevated liver function test results, enteritis, GI bleeding and ulceration, hepatitis, hepatotoxicity, nausea, pancreatitis, vomiting
**GU:** Cystitis, hematuria, infertility, menstrual dysfunction, nephropathy, renal failure, tubular necrosis, vaginal discharge
**HEME:** Anemia, aplastic anemia, leukopenia, neutropenia, pancytopenia, thrombocytopenia
**MS:** Arthralgia, dysarthia, myalgia, stress fracture
**RESP:** Dry nonproductive cough, dyspnea, interstitial pneumonitis, pneumonia, pulmonary fibrosis or failure, pulmonary infiltrates
**SKIN:** Acne, alopecia, altered skin pigmentation, ecchymosis, erythema multiforme, exfoliative dermatitis, furunculosis, necrosis, photosensitivity, pruritus, psoriatic lesions, rash, Stevens-Johnson syndrome, telangiectasia, toxic epidermal necrolysis, ulceration, urticaria
**Other:** Anaphylaxis, increased risk of infection, lymphadenopathy, lymphoproliferative disease

## Nursing Considerations

•Follow facility policy for preparing and handling drug; parenteral form poses a risk of carcinogenicity, mutagenicity, and teratogenicity. Avoid skin contact.
•Monitor results of CBC, chest X-ray, liver and renal function tests, and urinalysis before and during treatment.
•Unless contraindicated, increase patient's fluid intake to 2 to 3 L/day to reduce the risk of adverse GU reactions.
•Assess patient for signs of bleeding and infection.

•**WARNING** Expect renal impairment to severely alter drug elimination.
•Be aware that high doses of methotrexate can impair renal elimination by forming crystals that obstruct urine flow. To prevent drug precipitation, alkalinize patient's urine with sodium bicarbonate tablets, as ordered.
•Follow standard precautions because drug can cause immunosuppression.
•If patient becomes dehydrated from vomiting, notify prescriber and expect to withhold drug until patient recovers.
•If patient receives high doses of drug, keep leucovorin readily available to use as antidote.
•Be aware that methotrexate resistance may develop with prolonged use.
**PATIENT TEACHING**
•Prepare a calendar of treatment days for patient, and stress the importance of following instructions exactly.
•Instruct patient to avoid alcohol during methotrexate therapy.
•Encourage frequent mouth care to reduce the risk of mouth sores.
•Instruct patient to use sunblock when exposed to sunlight.
•Advise patient to notify prescriber about bruising, chills, cough, fever, dark or bloody urine, mouth sores, shortness of breath, sore throat, and yellow skin or eyes.
•Urge women of childbearing age to use contraception during methotrexate therapy.

# methscopolamine bromide

Pamine, Pamine Forte

## Class and Category
*Chemical:* Quaternary ammonium derivative of scopolamine
*Therapeutic:* Anticholingeric
*Pregnancy category:* C

## Indications and Dosages
➤ *As adjunct to treat peptic ulcer*
**TABLETS**
**Adults.** For mild to moderate symptoms, 2.5 mg 30 min before meals and 2.5 to 5 mg h.s.; for severe symptoms, 5 mg 30 min. before meals and h.s.

| Route | Onset | Peak | Duration |
|-------|-------|------|----------|
| P.O. | 1 hr | Unknown | 4 to 6 hr |

## Mechanism of Action
Reduces volume and total acid content of gastric secretions, which may have a beneficial effect in treating peptic ulcer. Drug also reduces GI motility and inhibits salivation, which may produce additional beneficial effects.

## Contraindications
Glaucoma, hypersensitivity to methscopolamine bromide or its components, intestinal atony (elderly or debilitated patients), myasthenia gravis, obstructive disease of GI or GU tract, paralytic ileus, severe ulcerative colitis, toxic megacolon complicating ulcerative colitis, unstable cardiovascular status in acute hemorrhage

## Interactions
**DRUGS**
*antacids:* Possibly decreased methscopolamine absorption
*anticholinergics, antipsychotics, tricyclic antidepressants*: Possibly increased anti-cholinergic effects

## Adverse Reactions
**CNS:** Confusion, dizziness, drowsiness, headache, insomnia, nervousness, weakness
**CV:** Palpitations, tachycardia
**EENT:** Blurred vision, cycloplegia, dry mouth, increased intraocular pressure, loss of taste, pupil dilation
**ENDO**: Suppression of lactation
**GI:** Bloating, constipation, nausea, vomiting
**GU:** Impotence, urinary hesitancy, urine retention
**SKIN:** Decreased sweating, urticaria
**Other:** Anaphylaxis

## Nursing Considerations
•Use with caution in elderly patients and in patients with autonomic neuropathy, congestive heart failure, coronary artery disease, hepatic or renal disease, hypertension, hyperthyroidism, prostatic hypertrophy, tachycardia, or ulcerative colitis.
•Notify prescriber if diarrhea occurs because it may be an early sign of incomplete intestinal obstruction.
**PATIENT TEACHING**
•Advise patient to avoid excessive exposure to heat to reduce the risk of heat prostration and heatstroke because methscopolamine decreases sweating.

M

•Caution patient to avoid antacids because antacids may interfere with the drug's absorption.
•Advise patient to avoid potentially hazardous activities until drug's CNS effects are known.

# methsuximide

Celontin

## Class and Category
*Chemical:* Succinimide derivative
*Therapeutic:* Anticonvulsant
*Pregnancy category:* Not rated

## Indications and Dosages
➤ *To treat absence seizures unresponsive to other drugs*
CAPSULES
**Adults and children.** *Initial:* 300 mg q.d. Increased by 150 to 300 mg/day q 1 to 2 weeks until control is achieved with minimal adverse reactions. *Maximum:* 1.2 g/day in divided doses.

---

### Mechanism of Action
Elevates seizure threshold and reduces frequency of seizures by depressing the motor cortex and elevating the threshold of CNS response to convulsive stimuli. Methsuximide is metabolized to the active metabolite *N*-demethylmethsuximide, which may add to the anticonvulsant effects of the drug.

---

## Contraindications
Hypersensitivity to methsuximide, succinimides, or their components

## Interactions
DRUGS
*carbamazepine, phenobarbital, phenytoin, primidone:* Possibly decreased blood methsuximide level
*CNS depressants:* Possibly increased CNS depression
*haloperidol:* Altered seizure pattern; possibly decreased blood haloperidol level
*loxapine, MAO inhibitors, maprotiline, molindone, phenothiazines, pimozide, thioxanthenes, tricyclic antidepressants:* Possibly lowered seizure threshold and reduced therapeutic effect of methsuximide
ACTIVITIES
*alcohol use:* Possibly increased CNS depression

## Adverse Reactions
**CNS:** Aggressiveness, ataxia, decreased concentration, dizziness, drowsiness, fatigue, fever, headache, insomnia, irritability, mental depression, nightmares, seizures
**EENT:** Periorbital edema, pharyngitis
**GI:** Abdominal and epigastric pain, abdominal cramps, abnormal liver function test results, anorexia, diarrhea, hiccups, nausea, vomiting
**GU:** Microscopic hematuria, proteinuria
**HEME:** Agranulocytosis, aplastic anemia, eosinophilia, leukopenia, pancytopenia
**MS:** Muscle pain
**SKIN:** Erythematous and pruritic rash, Stevens-Johnson syndrome, systemic lupus erythematosus, urticaria
**Other:** Lymphadenopathy

## Nursing Considerations
•Monitor CBC and platelet count and assess patient for signs of infection, such as cough, fever, and pharyngitis, because methsuximide may cause blood dyscrasias.
•Monitor liver function test results and urinalysis results in patients with a history of hepatic or renal disease; methsuximide may cause functional changes in the liver and kidneys.
•When administering drug to patient with a history of mixed-type epilepsy, institute seizure precautions because drug may increase risk of generalized tonic-clonic seizures.
•Expect the dosage to be carefully and slowly adjusted according to patient's response and needs and withdrawn slowly to avoid precipitating seizures.
•Plan to use the 150-mg capsule when making dosage adjustments for small children.
•Notify prescriber if patient develops depression or aggressiveness.
PATIENT TEACHING
•Advise patient to take a missed dose as soon as he remembers unless it's nearly time for the next dose. Warn him not to double the dose.
•Instruct patient to take the drug with milk or food to reduce gastric irritation.
•Advise patient to notify prescriber if he develops cough, fever, or pharyngitis.
•Urge patient to avoid alcohol because of the increased risk of CNS depression.
•Instruct patient to avoid potentially hazardous activities until drug's adverse effects are known.
•Caution patient not to stop taking drug abruptly to avoid the risk of absence seizures.

# methyldopa

Aldomet, Apo-Methyldopa (CAN), Dopamet (CAN), Nu-Medopa (CAN)

## methyldopate hydrochloride

Aldomet

## Class and Category

*Chemical:* 3,4-dihydroxyphenylalanine (DOPA) analogue
*Therapeutic:* Antihypertensive
*Pregnancy category:* B (oral form), C (parenteral form)

## Indications and Dosages

➤ *To manage hypertension, to treat hypertensive crisis*

ORAL SUSPENSION, TABLETS (METHYLDOPA)

**Adults.** *Initial:* 250 mg b.i.d. or t.i.d. for first 48 hr, increased as ordered after 2 days. *Maintenance:* 500 to 2,000 mg/day in divided doses b.i.d. to q.i.d. *Maximum:* 3,000 mg/day.

**Children.** *Initial:* 10 mg/kg/day in divided doses b.i.d. to q.i.d. for first 48 hr, increased as ordered after 2 days. *Maximum:* 65 mg/kg or 3,000 mg/day.

I.V. INFUSION (METHYLDOPATE HYDROCHLORIDE)

**Adults.** 250 to 500 mg diluted in $D_5W$ and infused over 30 to 60 min q 6 hr. *Maximum:* 1,000 mg q 6 hr.

**Children.** 20 to 40 mg/kg infused over 30 to 60 min q 6 hr. *Maximum:* 65 mg/kg or 3,000 mg/day.

| Route | Onset | Peak | Duration |
|---|---|---|---|
| P.O. | Unknown | 4 to 6 hr* | 12 to 24 hr† |
| I.V. | Unknown | 4 to 6 hr | 10 to 16 hr |

## Incompatibilities

Don't administer methyldopa through same I.V. line as barbiturates or sulfonamides.

## Contraindications

Active hepatic disease, hypersensitivity to methyldopa or its components, impaired hepatic function from previous methyldopa therapy, use within 14 days of MAO inhibitor therapy

---

\* For single dose; 2 to 3 days for multiple doses.
† For single dose; 24 to 48 hr for multiple doses.

## Mechanism of Action

Is decarboxylated in the body to produce alpha-methylnorepinephrine, a metabolite that stimulates central inhibitory alpha-adrenergic receptors. This action may reduce blood pressure by decreasing sympathetic stimulation of the heart and peripheral vascular system.

## Interactions

DRUGS

*antihypertensives:* Increased hypotension
*appetite suppressants, NSAIDs, tricyclic antidepressants:* Possibly decreased therapeutic effects of methyldopa
*central anesthetics:* Possibly need for reduced anesthetic dosage
*CNS depressants:* Possibly increased CNS depression
*haloperidol:* Increased risk of adverse CNS effects
*levodopa:* Possibly decreased therapeutic effects of levodopa and increased risk of adverse CNS effects
*lithium:* Increased risk of lithium toxicity
*MAO inhibitors:* Possibly hallucinations, headaches, hyperexcitability, and severe hypertension
*oral anticoagulants:* Possibly increased therapeutic effects of anticoagulants
*sympathomimetics:* Possibly decreased therapeutic effects of methyldopa and increased vasopressor effects of sympathomimetics

ACTIVITIES

*alcohol use:* Possibly increased CNS depression

## Adverse Reactions

**CNS:** Decreased concentration, depression, dizziness, drowsiness, fever, headache, involuntary motor activity, memory loss (transient), nightmares, paresthesia, parkinsonism, sedation, vertigo, weakness
**CV:** Angina, bradycardia, edema, heart failure, myocarditis, orthostatic hypotension
**EENT:** Black or sore tongue, dry mouth, nasal congestion
**ENDO:** Gynecomastia
**GI:** Constipation, diarrhea, flatulence, hepatic necrosis, hepatitis, nausea, pancreatitis, vomiting
**GU:** Decreased libido, impotence
**HEME:** Agranulocytosis, hemolytic anemia, leukopenia, positive Coombs' test, positive

M

tests for ANA and rheumatoid factor, thrombocytopenia
**SKIN:** Eczema, rash, urticaria
**Other:** Weight gain

## Nursing Considerations
•For I.V. infusion, add methyldopate to 100 ml of $D_5W$ and administer over 30 to 60 minutes.
•Expect to monitor CBC and differential results before and periodically during methyldopa therapy.
•Monitor blood pressure regularly during therapy.
•Monitor results of Coombs' test; a positive result after several months of treatment indicates that patient has hemolytic anemia. Expect prescriber to discontinue drug.
•Assess for weight gain and edema. If they develop, administer a diuretic, as prescribed.
•Notify prescriber if patient experiences signs of heart failure (dyspnea, edema, hypertension) or involuntary, rapid, jerky movements.
•Be aware that hypertension may return within 48 hours after stopping drug.

### PATIENT TEACHING
•Instruct patient to take methyldopa exactly as prescribed and not to skip a dose. Explain that hypertension can return within 48 hours after stopping drug.
•Suggest that patient take drug at bedtime to minimize daytime drowsiness.
•Instruct patient to weigh himself daily and to report a gain of more than 5 lb (2.3 kg) in 2 days.
•Advise patient to change position slowly to minimize effects of orthostatic hypotension.
•Direct patient to notify prescriber about bruising, chest pain, fever, involuntary jerky movements, prolonged dizziness, rash, and yellow eyes or skin.
•Caution patient not to discontinue drug abruptly; doing so may precipitate withdrawal symptoms, such as headache, hypertension, increased sweating, nausea, and tremor.

# methylphenidate hydrochloride

Concerta, Metadate, Metadate CD, Metadate ER, Methylin, Methylin ER, PMS-Methylphenidate (CAN), Riphenidate (CAN), Ritalin, Ritalin-LA, Ritalin SR (CAN), Ritalin-SR

## Class, Category, and Schedule
*Chemical:* Piperidine derivative
*Therapeutic:* CNS stimulant
*Pregnancy category:* C
*Controlled substance:* Schedule II

## Indications and Dosages
➤ *To treat attention-deficit hyperactivity disorder (ADHD)*
CAPSULES, E.R. TABLETS, ORAL SOLUTION, S.R. TABLETS, TABLETS
**Adults and adolescents.** 5 to 20 mg b.i.d. or t.i.d. *Maximum:* 90 mg/day.
**Children ages 6 to 12.** 5 mg b.i.d. before breakfast and lunch; increased by 5 to 10 mg/day at 1–wk intervals. *Maximum:* 60 mg/day.

**E.R. ONCE-DAILY TABLETS (CONCERTA)**
**Adults and adolescents.** 18 mg q.d.; increased in 18-mg increments at 1-wk intervals. *Maximum:* 72 mg/day, not to exceed 2 mg/kg/day.
**Children ages 6 to 12.** 18 mg q.d. *Maximum:* 54 mg/day.

**E.R. ONCE-DAILY CAPSULES (METADATE CD)**
**Children age 6 and over.** 20 mg q.d. Dosage titrated to 40 or 60 mg q.d. based on individual response. *Maximum:* 60 mg/day.
**DOSAGE ADJUSTMENT** Dosage reduced or drug stopped if no improvement in symptoms in 1 mo. When maintenance dosage is achieved with tablets, regimen may be switched to E.R. or S.R. tablets.

➤ *To treat narcolepsy*
ORAL SOLUTION, TABLETS
**Adults and adolescents.** 5 to 20 mg b.i.d. or t.i.d. *Maximum:* 90 mg/day.

| Route | Onset | Peak | Duration |
|---|---|---|---|
| P.O. (tablets) | Unknown | Unknown | 3 to 6 hr |
| P.O. (E.R., S.R.) | Unknown | Unknown | About 8 hr |
| P.O. (E.R. once-daily) | Unknown | Unknown | About 12 hr |

## Contraindications
Anxiety, depression, glaucoma, hypersensitivity to methylphenidate or its components, motor tics, severe agitation, tension, Tourette syndrome or family history of it, use within 14 days of MAO inhibitor therapy

## Mechanism of Action

Blocks the reuptake mechanism of dopaminergic neurons in the cerebral cortex and subcortical structures of the brain, including the thalamus, decreasing motor restlessness and improving concentration.

Methylphenidate also may trigger sympathomimetic activity. This action produces increased motor activity, alertness, mild euphoria, and decreased fatigue in patients with narcolepsy.

## Interactions

### DRUGS

*anticholinergics:* Possibly increased anticholinergic effects of both drugs
*anticonvulsants, oral anticoagulants, phenylbutazone, tricyclic antidepressants:* Inhibited metabolism and increased blood levels of these drugs
*diuretics, antihypertensives:* Decreased therapeutic effects of these drugs
*MAO inhibitors:* Possibly increased adverse effects of methylphenidate, possibly severe hypertension

### FOODS

*caffeine:* Increased methylphenidate effects

## Adverse Reactions

**CNS:** Dizziness, fever, headache, hyperactivity, insomnia, nervousness, psychosis, Tourette syndrome
**CV:** Angina, bradycardia, hypertension, hypotension, palpitations, tachycardia
**EENT:** Dry throat, pharyngitis, rhinitis, sinusitis, vision changes
**ENDO:** Dysmenorrhea, growth suppression in children (with long-term use)
**GI:** Abdominal pain, anorexia, diarrhea, hepatotoxicity, nausea, vomiting
**HEME:** Anemia, leukopenia, thrombocytopenia, thrombocytopenic purpura
**MS:** Arthralgia
**RESP:** Increased cough, upper respiratory tract infection
**SKIN:** Erythema multiforme, exfoliative dermatitis, rash, urticaria
**Other:** Physical and psychological dependence, weight loss

## Nursing Considerations

• WARNING Be aware that methylphenidate may induce CNS stimulation and psychosis and may worsen behavior disturbances and thought disorders. Use drug cautiously in children with psychosis.
• WARNING Know that the E.R. tablet form (Concerta) shouldn't be administered to patients with esophageal motility disorders; drug may cause GI obstruction because the tablet doesn't change shape in GI tract.
• Monitor blood pressure and pulse rate to detect hypertension and signs of excessive stimulation. Notify prescriber if you detect such signs. For patient with hypertension, expect to increase antihypertensive dosage or add another antihypertensive to existing regimen.
• WARNING Watch for signs of physical or psychological dependence. Methylphenidate's abuse potential is similar to that of amphetamines; use cautiously in patients with a history of drug abuse.
• Stopping drug abruptly after long-term use may unmask dysphoria, paranoia, severe depression, or suicidal thoughts.
• Expect patient currently taking methylphenidate tablets b.i.d. or t.i.d., or E.R. tablets at doses of 20 to 60 mg/day, to be switched to E.R. once-daily tablets, as prescribed.
• Monitor growth in children. Report failure to grow or gain weight, and expect to stop drug.

### PATIENT TEACHING

• Tell patient not to chew or crush E.R. tablets.
• Advise patient to take tablets at least 6 hours before bedtime to avoid insomnia and to take E.R. once-daily tablets in the morning.
• Advise patient taking E.R. once-daily tablets (Concerta) not to be alarmed if he notices intact tablet in stool. Inform him that drug is slowly released from nonabsorbable tablet shell.
• Inform patient taking capsule form to swallow it whole or sprinkle the capsule contents onto a tablespoon of applesauce and take immediately, followed by a liquid such as water.
• Direct patient to notify prescriber about excessive nervousness, fever, insomnia, palpitations, rash, or vomiting.
• Warn patient with seizure disorder that drug may cause seizures.
• Inform parents of children on long-term therapy that drug may delay growth.

M

# methylprednisolone
Medrol, Meprolone

# methylprednisolone acetate
depMedalone, Depoject, Depo-Medrol, Depopred, Depo-Predate, Methylcotolone

# methylprednisolone sodium succinate
A-methaPred, Solu-Medrol

## Class and Category
*Chemical:* Synthetic glucocorticoid
*Therapeutic:* Anti-inflammatory, immunosuppressant
*Pregnancy category:* Not rated

## Indications and Dosages
➤ *To treat ulcerative colitis*
**I.V. INFUSION (METHYLPREDNISOLONE SODIUM SUCCINATE)**
**Adults.** 40 to 120 mg 3 to 7 times/wk for 2 or more wk. Later doses given I.V. or I.M., based on patient's condition and response.
**Children.** 0.14 to 0.84 mg/kg/day in divided doses q 12 to 24 hr.
➤ *To treat a wide range of immune and inflammatory disorders, including allergic rhinitis, asthma, Crohn's disease, and systemic lupus erythematosus*
**TABLETS (METHYLPREDNISOLONE)**
**Adults.** 4 to 48 mg/day as a single dose or in divided doses.
**Children.** 0.42 to 1.67 mg/kg/day in divided doses t.i.d. or q.i.d.
**I.V. INFUSION, I.M. INJECTION (METHYLPREDNISOLONE SODIUM SUCCINATE)**
**Adults.** *Initial:* 10 to 40 mg infused over several min. Later doses given I.V. or I.M., based on patient's condition and response.
**Children.** 0.14 to 0.84 mg/kg q 12 to 24 hr.
**I.M. INJECTION (METHYLPREDNISOLONE ACETATE)**
**Adults.** 40 to 120 mg q.d. to q 2 wk, according to clinical response.
**Children.** 0.14 to 0.84 mg/kg q 12 to 24 hr.
**INTRA-ARTICULAR, INTRALESIONAL, OR SOFT-TISSUE INJECTION (METHYLPREDNISOLONE ACETATE)**
**Adults.** 4 to 80 mg q 1 to 5 wk, according to clinical response.
➤ *To treat adrenal hyperplasia*
**I.M. INJECTION (METHYLPREDNISOLONE ACETATE)**
**Adults.** 40 mg q 2 wk.
**Children.** 0.14 to 0.84 mg/kg q 12 to 24 hr.

➤ *To treat acute exacerbations of multiple sclerosis*
**TABLETS (METHYLPREDNISOLONE)**
**Adults.** 160 mg q.d. for 7 days followed by 64 mg q.o.d. for 1 mo.
**I.V. OR I.M. INJECTION (METHYLPREDNISOLONE ACETATE, METHYLPREDNISOLONE SODIUM SUCCINATE)**
**Adults.** 160 mg q.d. for 1 wk followed by 64 mg q.o.d. for 1 mo.
➤ *To treat adrenocortical insufficiency*
**TABLETS (METHYLPREDNISOLONE), I.M. INJECTION (METHYLPREDNISOLONE SODIUM SUCCINATE)**
**Children.** 0.18 mg/kg/day in divided doses t.i.d.
**I.M. INJECTION (METHYLPREDNISOLONE ACETATE)**
**Children.** 0.12 mg/kg q 3 days or 0.039 to 0.059 mg/kg q.d.

| Route | Onset | Peak | Duration |
|-------|-------|------|----------|
| P.O. | In 60 min | 1 to 2 hr | 1.25 to 1.5 days |
| I.V. | Rapid | 30 min | Unknown |
| I.M. | 6 to 48 hr | 4 to 8 days | 1 to 4 wk |

## Mechanism of Action
Binds to intracellular glucocorticoid receptors and suppresses inflammatory and immune responses by inhibiting accumulation of neutrophils and monocytes at inflammation sites, stabilizing lysosomal membranes, suppressing the antigen response of macrophages and helper T cells, and inhibiting the synthesis of inflammatory response mediators, such as cytokines, interleukins, and prostaglandins.

## Incompatibilities
Don't mix methylprednisolone with any drug without first consulting pharmacist. Don't dilute methylprednisolone acetate with any other drug.

## Contraindications
Fungal infection, hypersensitivity to methylprednisolone or its components, idiopathic thrombocytopenic purpura (I.M.)

## Interactions
**DRUGS**
*acetaminophen:* Increased risk of hepatotoxicity
*amphotericin B, carbonic anhydrase inhibitors:* Possibly severe hypokalemia
*anabolic steroids, androgens:* Increased risk of edema and worsening of acne

*anticholinergics:* Possibly increased intraocular pressure

*asparaginase:* Increased risk of hyperglycemia and toxicity

*aspirin, NSAIDs:* Increased risk of adverse GI effects and bleeding

*cyclosporine:* Increased risk of seizures

*digoxin:* Possibly hypokalemia-induced arrhythmias and digitalis toxicity

*ephedrine, phenobarbital, phenytoin, rifampin:* Decreased blood methylprednisolone level

*estrogens, oral contraceptives:* Possibly increased therapeutic and toxic effects of methylprednisolone

*insulin, oral antidiabetic drugs:* Possibly increased blood glucose level

*isoniazid:* Possibly decreased therapeutic effects of isoniazid

*mexiletine:* Possibly decreased blood mexiletine level

*neuromuscular blockers:* Possibly increased neuromuscular blockade, causing respiratory depression or apnea

*oral anticoagulants, thrombolytics:* Increased risk of GI ulceration and hemorrhage, possibly decreased therapeutic effects of these drugs

*potassium-depleting drugs, such as thiazide diuretics:* Possibly severe hypokalemia

*potassium supplements:* Possibly decreased effects of these supplements

*somatrem, somatropin:* Possibly decreased therapeutic effects of these drugs

*streptozocin:* Increased risk of hyperglycemia

*troleandomycin:* Increased blood methylprednisolone level

*vaccines:* Decreased antibody response and increased risk of neurologic complications

**ACTIVITIES**

*alcohol use:* Increased risk of adverse GI effects and bleeding

## Adverse Reactions

**CNS:** Ataxia, behavioral changes, depression, dizziness, euphoria, fatigue, headache, increased intracranial pressure with papilledema, insomnia, malaise, mood changes, paresthesia, restlessness, seizures, steroid psychosis, syncope, vertigo

**CV:** Arrhythmias (from hypokalemia), edema, fat embolism, heart failure, hypertension, hypotension, thromboembolism, thrombophlebitis

**EENT:** Exophthalmos, glaucoma, increased intraocular pressure, nystagmus, posterior subcapsular cataracts

**ENDO:** Adrenal insufficiency, cushingoid symptoms (moon face, buffalo hump, central obesity, supraclavicular fat pad enlargement), diabetes mellitus, growth suppression in children, hyperglycemia, negative nitrogen balance from protein catabolism

**GI:** Abdominal distention, hiccups, increased appetite, melena, nausea, pancreatitis, peptic ulcer, ulcerative esophagitis, vomiting

**GU:** Amenorrhea, glycosuria, menstrual irregularities, perineal burning or tingling

**HEME:** Easy bruising, leukocytosis

**MS:** Arthralgia; aseptic necrosis of femoral and humeral heads; compression fractures; muscle atrophy, twitching, or weakness; myalgia; osteoporosis; spontaneous fractures; steroid myopathy; tendon rupture

**SKIN:** Acne; altered skin pigmentation; diaphoresis; erythema; hirsutism; necrotizing vasculitis; petechiae; purpura; rash; scarring; sterile abscess; striae; subcutaneous fat atrophy; thin, fragile skin; urticaria

**Other:** Anaphylaxis, hypocalcemia, hypokalemia, hypokalemic alkalosis, impaired wound healing, masking of signs of infection, metabolic alkalosis, suppressed skin test reaction, weight gain

## Nursing Considerations

• Give methylprednisolone tablets with food to minimize indigestion and GI irritation. For once-daily dosing, administer in the morning to coincide with normal cortisol secretion. Expect prescriber to add an antacid or $H_2$-receptor antagonist to regimen.

• Discard parenteral products that are discolored or contain particles.

• Inject I.M. form deep into gluteal muscle.

• Arrange for low-sodium diet with added potassium, as prescribed.

• Protect patient from falling, especially elderly patient at risk for fractures from osteoporosis.

• Closely monitor for signs of infection because drug may mask them.

• Assess for possible depression or psychotic episodes during therapy.

• Monitor blood glucose level; dosage of insulin or oral antidiabetic drug may need to be adjusted in diabetic patient.

• **WARNING** To avoid possibly fatal acute adrenocortical insufficiency, expect to taper long-term therapy when it must be discontinued.

## PATIENT TEACHING

• Caution patient not to stop taking methylprednisolone abruptly or to change dosage without consulting prescriber.
• Instruct patient to take a missed dose as soon as he remembers unless it's nearly time for the next dose. Caution against double-dosing.
• Urge patient to notify prescriber immediately about dark or tarry stools; signs of impending adrenocortical insufficiency, such as anorexia, dizziness, fainting, fatigue, fever, joint pain, muscle weakness, or nausea; and sudden weight gain or swelling.
• Instruct patient not to obtain vaccinations unless approved by prescriber.
• Urge patient to take vitamin D, calcium supplements, or both if recommended by prescriber.
• Inform patient that insomnia and restlessness usually resolve after 1 to 3 weeks of therapy.
• Caution patient to avoid people with contagious diseases.
• Discuss the need for regular exercise or physical therapy to maintain muscle mass.
• Advise patient to carry medical identification that documents his need for long-term corticosteroid therapy.

# metoclopramide hydrochloride

Apo-Metoclop (CAN), Maxeran (CAN), Metoclopramide Intensol, Octamide, PMS-Metoclopramide (CAN), Reglan

## Class and Category

*Chemical:* Benzamide
*Therapeutic:* Antiemetic, upper GI stimulant
*Pregnancy category:* B

## Indications and Dosages

➤ *To treat diabetic gastroparesis*
**ORAL SOLUTION, ORAL SOLUTION CONCENTRATE, TABLETS**
**Adults and adolescents.** 10 mg 30 min a.c. and h.s. up to q.i.d.
**I.V. OR I.M. INJECTION**
**Adults and adolescents.** 10 mg t.i.d. or q.i.d. for severe symptoms; dosage adjusted as needed.
➤ *To treat gastroesophageal reflux disease*
**ORAL SOLUTION, ORAL SOLUTION CONCENTRATE, TABLETS**
**Adults and adolescents.** 10 to 15 mg 30 min a.c. and h.s.
➤ *To prevent chemotherapy-induced vomiting*
**I.V. INFUSION**
**Adults and adolescents.** 3 mg/kg before chemotherapy and then 0.5 mg/kg/hr for 8 hr.

**I.V. INJECTION**
**Adults and adolescents.** 1 to 2 mg/kg 30 min before chemotherapy and then repeated q 2 to 3 hr, as needed.
**Children.** 1 mg/kg as a single dose, repeated in 1 hr. *Maximum:* 2 mg/kg.
➤ *To prevent postoperative nausea and vomiting*
**I.M. INJECTION**
**Adults and adolescents.** 10 to 20 mg near end of procedure.
**DOSAGE ADJUSTMENT** Reduced by half if creatinine clearance is less than 40 ml/min/1.73 m$^2$.

| Route | Onset | Peak | Duration |
|-------|-------|------|----------|
| P.O. | 30 to 60 min | Unknown | 1 to 2 hr |
| I.V. | 1 to 3 min | Unknown | 1 to 2 hr |
| I.M. | 10 to 15 min | Unknown | 1 to 2 hr |

## Mechanism of Action

Antagonizes the inhibitory effect of dopamine on GI smooth muscle. This causes gastric contraction, which promotes gastric emptying and peristalsis, thus reducing gastroesophageal reflux. Metoclopramide also blocks dopaminergic receptors in the chemoreceptor trigger zone, preventing nausea and vomiting.

## Incompatibilities

Don't administer metoclopramide through same I.V. line as calcium gluconate, cephalothin sodium, chloramphenicol sodium, cisplatin, erythromycin lactobionate, furosemide, methotrexate, penicillin G potassium, or sodium bicarbonate.

## Contraindications

Concurrent use of butyrophenones, phenothiazines, or other drugs that may cause extrapyramidal reactions; GI hemorrhage, mechanical obstruction, or perforation; hypersensitivity to metoclopramide or its components; pheochromocytoma; seizure disorders

## Interactions

**DRUGS**
*anticholinergics, opioid analgesics:* Possibly decreased therapeutic effects of metoclopramide
*apomorphine:* Possibly decreased antiemetic effect of apomorphine, possibly increased CNS depression

*bromocriptine, pergolide:* Possibly decreased therapeutic effects of these drugs
*cimetidine:* Possibly decreased absorption and therapeutic effects of cimetidine
*CNS depressants:* Possibly increased CNS depression
*cyclosporine:* Increased blood cyclosporine level
*digoxin:* Decreased gastric digoxin absorption
*levodopa:* Possibly decreased levodopa effects
*MAO inhibitors:* Increased risk of severe hypertension if patient has essential hypertension
*mexiletine:* Possibly faster mexiletene absorption
*succinylcholine:* Possibly prolonged therapeutic action of succinylcholine

**ACTIVITIES**
*alcohol use:* Increased risk of excessive sedation

## Adverse Reactions

**CNS:** Agitation, anxiety, depression, dizziness, drowsiness, extrapyramidal reactions (motor restlessness, parkinsonism, tardive dyskinesia), fatigue, headache, insomnia, irritability, lassitude, neuroleptic malignant syndrome, panic reaction, restlessness
**CV:** AV block, fluid retention, heart failure, hypertension, hypotension, supraventricular tachycardia
**EENT:** Dry mouth
**ENDO:** Galactorrhea, gynecomastia
**GI:** Constipation, diarrhea, nausea
**GU:** Menstrual irregularities
**HEME:** Agranulocytosis
**SKIN:** Rash
**Other:** Restless leg syndrome

## Nursing Considerations
•Use metoclopramide cautiously in patients with hypertension because it may increase catecholamine levels.
•Use drug cautiously in elderly patients because they have an increased risk of tardive dyskinesia and parkinsonian effects. Expect to stop drug if these symptoms develop.
•Monitor patient with NADH-cytochrome b5 reductase deficiency because metoclopramide increases the risk of methemoglobinemia and sulfhemoglobinemia and patient can't receive methylene blue.
•Assess patient for signs of intestinal obstruction, such as abnormal bowel sounds, diarrhea, nausea, and vomiting, before administering metoclopramide. Notify prescriber if you detect them.

•For I.V. administration, you needn't dilute doses of 10 mg or less. Give drug over 1 to 2 minutes. For doses larger than 10 mg, dilute in 50 ml of NS, 0.45NS, $D_5W$, or LR solution and infuse over at least 15 minutes.
•Avoid rapid I.V. delivery because it may cause anxiety, restlessness, and drowsiness.
•**WARNING** Notify prescriber if patient displays signs of toxicity, such as disorientation, drowsiness, and extrapyramidal reactions.
•Monitor patient, especially one with heart failure or cirrhosis, for possible signs of fluid retention or volume overload due to transient increase in plasma aldosterone level.
•Monitor patient closely for neuroleptic malignant syndrome, a rare but potentially fatal disorder characterized by hyperthermia, muscle rigidity, altered level of consciousness, irregular pulse or blood pressure, tachycardia, diaphoresis, and arrhythmias.
•Store drug in a light-resistant container; discard if discolored or contains particulate.

**PATIENT TEACHING**
•Advise against activities that require alertness for about 2 hours after each dose.
•Urge patient to avoid alcohol and CNS depressants while taking metoclopramide because they may increase CNS depression.
•Tell patient to immediately report involuntary movements of face, eyes, tongue, or hands.
•Explain that stopping metoclopramide may cause withdrawal symptoms that include dizziness, nervousness, and headache.

# metolazone
Diulo, Mykrox, Zaroxolyn

## Class and Category
*Chemical:* Quinazoline derivative
*Therapeutic:* Antihypertensive, diuretic
*Pregnancy category:* B

## Indications and Dosages
➤ *To manage mild to moderate hypertension*
**EXTENDED TABLETS**
**Adults.** 2.5 to 5 mg q.d.
**PROMPT TABLETS (MYKROX)**
**Adults.** 0.5 mg q.d. *Maintenance:* 0.5 to 1 mg q.d. *Maximum:* 1 mg/day.
➤ *To manage edema from heart failure or renal disease*
**EXTENDED TABLETS**
**Adults.** 5 to 20 mg q.d.

| Route | Onset | Peak | Duration |
|-------|-------|------|----------|
| P.O. | 1 hr | 2 hr | 12 to 24 hr |

## Mechanism of Action
Promotes renal excretion of water and sodium by inhibiting their reabsorption in distal convoluted tubules. The resulting reduction in plasma and extracellular fluid volume reduces blood pressure. Metolazone also helps reduce blood pressure by decreasing peripheral vascular resistance.

## Contraindications
Anuria; hepatic coma; hypersensitivity to metolazone, other sulfonamide derivatives, quinethazones, thiazides, or their components; renal failure

## Interactions
**DRUGS**
*allopurinol:* Increased risk of hypersensitivity to allopurinol
*amiodarone:* Increased risk of arrhythmias from hypokalemia
*amphotericin B:* Increased risk of electrolyte imbalances
*anesthetics:* Increased effects of anesthetics
*antigout drugs:* Increased blood uric acid level and risk of gout attack
*antihypertensives:* Increased hypotension
*antineoplastics:* Prolonged antineoplastic-induced leukopenia
*calcium salts:* Increased risk of hypercalcemia
*cholestyramine, colestipol:* Decreased metolazone absorption
*diazoxide:* Increased risk of hyperglycemia
*digoxin:* Increased risk of electrolyte imbalances and digoxin-induced arrhythmias
*diuretics:* Additive effects of both drugs, possibly leading to severe hypovolemia and electrolyte imbalances
*dopamine:* Increased diuretic effect
*insulin, oral antidiabetic drugs:* Decreased effectiveness of these drugs, increased risk of hyperglycemia
*lithium:* Increased risk of lithium toxicity
*methenamine:* Decreased metolazone effectiveness from urinary alkalinization
*methyldopa:* Possibly hemolytic anemia
*neuromuscular blockers:* Increased risk of hypokalemia and neuromuscular blockade, increased risk of respiratory depression

*NSAIDs, sympathomimetics:* Possibly decreased metolazone effectiveness
*oral anticoagulants:* Decreased anticoagulation
*vitamin D:* Increased vitamin D action, increased risk of hypercalcemia

## Adverse Reactions
**CNS:** Anxiety, chills, depression, dizziness, drowsiness, headache, insomnia, neuropathy, paresthesia, restlessness, syncope, weakness
**CV:** Chest pain, cold extremities, orthostatic hypotension, palpitations, peripheral edema, vasculitis, venous thrombosis
**EENT:** Bitter taste, blurred vision, dry mouth, epistaxis, pharyngitis, sinus congestion, tinnitus
**ENDO:** Hyperglycemia
**GI:** Abdominal pain, anorexia, cholecystitis, constipation, diarrhea, hepatic dysfunction, hepatitis, indigestion, nausea, pancreatitis, vomiting
**GU:** Decreased libido, glycosuria, impotence
**HEME:** Agranulocytosis, aplastic anemia, leukopenia, thrombocytopenia
**MS:** Arthralgia, gout, myalgia
**RESP:** Cough
**SKIN:** Dry skin, necrosis, petechiae, photosensitivity, pruritus, rash, urticaria
**Other:** Hypochloremia, hypokalemia, hyponatremia, hypovolemia, metabolic alkalosis

## Nursing Considerations
•**WARNING** Be aware that Mykrox prompt tablets shouldn't be substituted for Diulo or Zaroxolyn extended tablets because they aren't equivalent.
•Anticipate giving metolazone with a loop diuretic if patient responds poorly to loop diuretic alone.
•To monitor drug's diuretic effect, measure fluid intake and output and daily weight.
•If response to 1 mg of Mykrox is inadequate, expect to add another drug rather than increase dosage.
•Monitor blood chemistry test results and assess for signs and symptoms of hypochloremia, hypokalemia, and, possibly, mild metabolic alkalosis.
•Monitor serum calcium and uric acid levels, especially if patient has a history of gout or renal calculi. Metolazone may slightly increase calcium reabsorption and decrease uric acid excretion.

- Inform patient that metolazone controls but doesn't cure hypertension. Discuss possible need for lifelong therapy and consequences of uncontrolled hypertension.
- Instruct patient to take drug at the same time each day.
- Direct patient to take drug with food or milk to minimize adverse GI reactions.
- Advise patient to change position slowly to minimize effects of orthostatic hypotension.
- Urge patient to notify prescriber about persistent, severe diarrhea, nausea, or vomiting, which can cause dehydration and increase the risk of orthostatic hypotension.
- Stress the importance of weight and diet control, especially limiting sodium intake.
- Inform diabetic patient that drug may increase blood glucose level and that he should check his blood glucose level frequently.

# metoprolol succinate

Toprol-XL

# metoprolol tartrate

Apo-Metoprolol (CAN), Betaloc (CAN), Betaloc Durules (CAN), Lopresor (CAN), Lopresor SR (CAN), Lopressor, Novometoprol (CAN)

## Class and Category

*Chemical:* Beta$_1$-adrenergic antagonist
*Therapeutic:* Antianginal, antihypertensive, MI prophylaxis and treatment
*Pregnancy category:* C

## Indications and Dosages

➤ *To manage hypertension, alone or with other antihypertensives*

**E.R. TABLETS (METOPROLOL SUCCINATE)**
**Adults.** *Initial:* 25 to 100 mg q.d., adjusted weekly as prescribed. *Maximum:* 400 mg q.d.

**E.R. TABLETS (METOPROLOL TARTRATE)**
**Adults.** *Maintenance:* 100 to 400 mg q.d. to maintain blood pressure control after therapeutic level has been achieved with immediate-release tablets.

**TABLETS (METOPROLOL TARTRATE)**
**Adults.** *Initial:* 100 mg q.d., adjusted weekly as prescribed. *Maximum:* 450 mg/day as a single dose or in divided doses.

➤ *To treat acute MI or evolving acute MI*

**TABLETS (METOPROLOL TARTRATE), I.V. INJECTION (METOPROLOL TARTRATE)**
**Adults.** *Initial:* 5 mg by I.V. bolus q 2 min for 3 doses followed by 50 mg P.O. for patients who tolerate total I.V. dose (or 25 to 50 mg P.O. for patients who can't tolerate total I.V. dose) q 6 hr for 48 hr, starting 15 min after final I.V. dose; after 48 hr, 100 mg b.i.d. followed by maintenance dosage. *Maintenance:* 100 mg P.O. b.i.d. for at least 3 mo.

➤ *To treat angina pectoris and chronic stable angina*

**E.R. TABLETS (METOPROLOL SUCCINATE)**
**Adults.** 100 mg q.d., increased weekly as prescribed. *Maximum:* 400 mg/day as a single dose or in divided doses.

**E.R. TABLETS (METOPROLOL TARTRATE)**
**Adults.** *Initial:* 100 mg q.d., adjusted weekly as prescribed. *Maximum:* 450 mg/day.

**TABLETS (METOPROLOL TARTRATE)**
**Adults.** *Initial:* 50 mg b.i.d., adjusted weekly as prescribed. *Maximum:* 450 mg/day.

➤ *To treat stable, symptomatic (New York Heart Association [NYHA] Class II or III), ischemic, hypertensive, or cardiomyopathic heart failure*

**E.R. TABLETS (METOPROLOL SUCCINATE)**
**Adults.** *Initial:* 25 mg q.d. (NYHA Class II) or 12.5 mg q.d. (NYHA Class III or more severe heart failure) for 2 wk. Then dosage doubled every 2 wk as tolerated. *Maximum:* 200 mg/day.

| Route | Onset | Peak | Duration |
|---|---|---|---|
| P.O. | 60 min | 1 to 2 hr | Unknown |
| P.O. (E.R.) | Unknown | 6 to 12 hr | Unknown |
| I.V. | Unknown | 20 min | Unknown |

## Mechanism of Action

Inhibits stimulation of beta$_1$-receptor sites, located mainly in the heart, resulting in decreased cardiac excitability, cardiac output, and myocardial oxygen demand. These effects help relieve angina. Metoprolol also helps reduce blood pressure by decreasing renal release of renin.

## Contraindications

Acute heart failure, bradycardia of less than 45 beats/minute, cardiogenic shock, hypersensitivity to metoprolol or its components, second- or third-degree AV block

M

## Interactions

**DRUGS**

*aluminum salts, barbiturates, calcium salts, cholestyramine, colestipol, NSAIDs, rifampin, salicylates, sulfinpyrazone:* Decreased therapeutic effects of metoprolol
*amiodarone, digoxin, diltiazem, verapamil:* Increased risk of complete AV block
*calcium channel blockers:* Increased risk of heart failure, increased effects of both drugs
*cimetidine:* Increased blood metoprolol level
*clonidine, diazoxide, guanabenz:* Increased risk of hypotension
*estrogens:* Possibly decreased antihypertensive effect of metoprolol
*general anesthetics:* Increased risk of hypotension and heart failure
*insulin, oral antidiabetic drugs:* Decreased blood glucose control, possibly masking of signs and symptoms of hypoglycemia (by metoprolol)
*lidocaine:* Increased risk of lidocaine toxicity
*MAO inhibitors:* Increased risk of hypertension
*neuromuscular blockers:* Possibly enhanced and prolonged neuromuscular blockade
*other antihypertensives:* Additive hypotensive effect
*phenothiazines:* Possibly increased blood levels of both drugs
*propafenone:* Increased blood level and half-life of metoprolol
*sympathomimetics, xanthines:* Possibly decreased therapeutic effects of these drugs or metoprolol

**FOODS**

*all foods:* Increased bioavailability of metoprolol

## Adverse Reactions

**CNS:** Anxiety, confusion, depression, dizziness, drowsiness, fatigue, hallucinations, headache, insomnia, weakness
**CV:** Angina, arrhythmias (including AV block and bradycardia), chest pain, heart failure, hypertension, orthostatic hypotension
**EENT:** Nasal congestion, taste disturbance
**GI:** Constipation, diarrhea, hepatitis, nausea, vomiting
**GU:** Impotence
**HEME:** Leukopenia, thrombocytopenia
**MS:** Arthralgia, back pain, myalgia
**RESP:** Bronchospasm, dyspnea
**SKIN:** Diaphoresis, photosensitivity, rash, urticaria

## Nursing Considerations

•For patient with acute MI who can't tolerate initial dosage or who delays treatment, start with maintenance dosage, as prescribed and tolerated.
•Before starting therapy for heart failure, expect to give a diuretic, an ACE inhibitor, and digoxin to stabilize patient.
•Be aware that the metoprolol dosage for heart failure is highly individualized. Monitor patient for signs and symptoms of worsening heart failure during dosage increases. If heart failure worsens, expect to increase the diuretic dosage and possibly decrease the metoprolol dosage or temporarily discontinue drug, as prescribed. Be aware that the metoprolol dosage shouldn't be increased until signs and symptoms of worsening heart failure have been stabilized.
•If patient with heart failure develops symptomatic bradycardia, expect to decrease the metoprolol dosage.
•**WARNING** If dosage exceeds 400 mg/day, monitor patient for bronchospasm and dyspnea because metoprolol competitively blocks beta$_2$-adrenergic receptors in bronchial and vascular smooth muscles.
•**WARNING** When substituting metoprolol for clonidine, expect to gradually reduce clonidine dosage and increase metoprolol dosage over several days. Giving these drugs together causes additive hypotensive effects.
•Be aware that patients who take metoprolol may be at risk for AV block. If AV block results from depressed AV node conduction, prepare to administer appropriate drug, as prescribed, or assist with insertion of temporary pacemaker.
•Check for signs of poor glucose control in patient with diabetes mellitus. Metoprolol may interfere with therapeutic effects of insulin and oral antidiabetic drugs. It also may mask evidence of hypoglycemia, such as palpitations, tachycardia, and tremor.
•Monitor patient with peripheral vascular disease for signs and symptoms of arterial insufficiency (pain, pallor, and coldness in affected extremity) because metoprolol can precipitate or aggravate peripheral vascular disease.
•Be aware that abrupt withdrawal of drug can precipitate thyroid storm in patient with hyperthyroidism or thyrotoxicosis.
•**WARNING** Expect to taper metoprolol dosage when drug is discontinued; abrupt discontinuation can cause myocardial ischemia, MI, ven-

tricular arrhythmias, or severe hypertension, especially in patients with cardiac disease.

**PATIENT TEACHING**
• Instruct patient to take metoprolol with food at the same time each day—once daily for E.R. tablets. Inform him that he may halve tablets but not chew or crush them.
• Advise patient to notify prescriber if pulse rate falls below 60 beats/minute or is significantly lower than usual.
• Urge diabetic patient to check blood glucose level frequently during metoprolol therapy.
• Caution patient not to stop taking drug abruptly.

# metronidazole

Apo-Metronidazole (CAN), Flagyl, Flagyl I.V. RTU, Metric 21, MetroGel, MetroGel-Vaginal, Nidagel (CAN), Novonidazol (CAN), Protostat, Trikacide (CAN)

## metronidazole hydrochloride

Flagyl I.V.

### Class and Category
*Chemical:* Nitroimidazole derivative
*Therapeutic:* Antibiotic, antiprotozoal
*Pregnancy category:* B

### Indications and Dosages
➤ *To treat systemic anaerobic infections caused by* Bacteroides fragilis, Clostridium difficile, Clostridium perfringens, Eubacterium, Fusobacterium, Peptococcus, Peptostreptococcus, *and* Veillonella *sp.*

**CAPSULES, TABLETS**
**Adults and adolescents.** 7.5 mg/kg up to 1,000 mg q 6 hr for 7 days or longer. *Maximum:* 4,000 mg/day.
**Children.** 7.5 mg/kg q 6 hr or 10 mg/kg q 8 hr.

**I.V. INFUSION**
**Adults and adolescents.** *Initial:* 15 mg/kg and then 7.5 mg/kg up to 1,000 mg q 6 hr for 7 days or longer. *Maximum:* 4,000 mg/day.
**Children.** 7.5 mg/kg q 6 hr or 10 mg/kg q 8 hr.
➤ *To treat amebiasis (*Entamoeba histolytica*)*

**CAPSULES, TABLETS**
**Adults.** 500 to 750 mg t.i.d. for 5 to 10 days.
**Children.** 11.6 to 16.7 mg/kg t.i.d. for 10 days.

➤ *To treat trichomoniasis (*Trichomonas vaginalis)*

**CAPSULES, TABLETS**
**Adults.** 2,000 mg as a single dose, 1,000 mg b.i.d. for 24 hr, or 250 mg t.i.d. for 7 days.
**Children.** 5 mg/kg t.i.d. for 7 days.
➤ *To prevent perioperative bowel infection*

**I.V. INFUSION**
**Adults and adolescents.** 15 mg/kg 1 hr before surgery and then 7.5 mg/kg 6 and 12 hr after initial dose.
➤ *To treat acne in patients with rosacea*

**TOPICAL GEL**
**Adults.** Thin film applied to affected area b.i.d. for 9 wk.
➤ *To treat bacterial vaginosis*

**VAGINAL CREAM**
**Adults.** 500 mg (1 applicatorful) q.d. or b.i.d. for 10 to 20 days.

**VAGINAL GEL**
**Adults.** 37.5 mg (1 applicatorful) q.d. or b.i.d. for 5 days.

**VAGINAL TABLETS**
**Adults.** 500 mg h.s. for 10 to 20 days.

### Mechanism of Action
Undergoes intracellular chemical reduction during anaerobic metabolism. After metronidazole is reduced, it damages DNA's helical structure and breaks its strands, which inhibits bacterial nucleic acid synthesis and causes cell death.

### Incompatibilities
Don't administer I.V. metronidazole with aluminum needles or hubs or through same I.V. line as other drugs.

### Contraindications
Breast-feeding, hypersensitivity to metronidazole or its components, trichomoniasis during first trimester of pregnancy

### Interactions
**DRUGS**
*cimetidine:* Possibly delayed elimination and increased blood level of metronidazole
*disulfiram:* Possibly combined toxicity, resulting in confusion and psychotic reactions
*neurotoxic drugs:* Increased risk of neurotoxicity
*oral anticoagulants:* Possibly increased anticoagulant effect

*phenobarbital:* Increased metabolism and decreased blood level and half-life of metronidazole

*phenytoin:* Decreased phenytoin clearance

**ACTIVITIES**

*alcohol use:* Possibly disulfiram-like effects

## Adverse Reactions

**CNS:** Ataxia, dizziness, encephalopathy, fever, headache, light-headedness, peripheral neuropathy, seizures (high doses)

**EENT:** Dry mouth, lacrimation (topical form), metallic taste, pharyngitis

**GI:** Abdominal cramps or pain, anorexia, diarrhea, nausea, pancreatitis, vomiting

**GU:** Darkened urine, vaginal candidiasis (oral, parenteral, and topical forms); burning or irritation of sexual partner's penis, candidal cervicitis or vaginitis, dysuria, urinary frequency, vulvitis (vaginal form)

**HEME:** Leukopenia

**MS:** Back pain

**SKIN:** Burning sensation, stinging sensation, dry skin (topical form); erythema, pruritus, rash, urticaria (oral and parenteral forms)

**Other:** Injection site edema, pain, or tenderness

## Nursing Considerations

• Give I.V. drug by slow infusion over 1 hour; don't give by direct I.V. injection.

• Discontinue primary I.V. infusion during metronidazole infusion.

• **WARNING** If patient has adverse CNS reactions, such as seizures or peripheral neuropathy, tell prescriber and stop drug immediately.

• Monitor patient with severe liver disease because slowed metronidazole metabolism may cause drug to accumulate in body and increase the risk of adverse effects.

• If skin irritation occurs, apply topical gel less frequently or discontinue it, as ordered.

• Monitor CBC and culture and sensitivity tests if therapy lasts longer than 10 days or if second course of treatment is needed.

**PATIENT TEACHING**

• Instruct female patient to notify prescriber if she is pregnant, intends to get pregnant, or is breast-feeding.

• Direct patient to take metronidazole at evenly spaced intervals throughout the day and with food to minimize adverse GI reactions.

• Urge patient to complete the entire course of therapy.

• Caution patient to avoid alcohol during therapy and for at least 3 days afterward.

• Advise patient to avoid hazardous activities until drug's CNS effects are known.

• If patient reports dry mouth, suggest ice chips or sugarless hard candy or gum; suggest a dental visit if dryness lasts longer than 2 weeks.

• Instruct patient to notify prescriber if no improvement occurs within a few days of taking tablets or capsules.

• Direct patient using topical gel to wash hands and affected area with a mild, nonirritating cleaner; to rinse well and pat dry; and then to apply a thin film of drug and wash hands again.

• Advise patient with rosacea to keep topical gel away from eyes. If drug gets into eyes, urge him to wash his eyes immediately with large amounts of cool tap water and to call prescriber if eyes continue to hurt or burn.

• Instruct patient with rosacea to notify prescriber if no improvement occurs after 3 weeks of topical use; full therapeutic effect may take 9 weeks.

• Teach patient how to fill, insert, and clean vaginal cream or gel applicator after use. Instruct her to wash her hands before and after administration.

• To help vaginal tablets dissolve, instruct patient to run tap water over unwrapped tablet for a few seconds before insertion.

• Inform patient with trichomoniasis that male sexual partners should wear condoms during her treatment and may need treatment themselves to prevent reinfection.

• Caution patient that vaginal cream and tablets (not gel) may contain oils that damage latex condoms.

• Urge patient to follow up with prescriber to make sure infection is gone.

# metyrosine

Demser

## Class and Category

*Chemical:* Alpha-methyl tyrosine

*Therapeutic:* Antipheochromocytoma agent

*Pregnancy category:* C

## Indications and Dosages

➤ *To control hypertension and related symptoms until pheochromocytomectomy is performed, to treat chronic malignant pheochromocytoma*

**CAPSULES**
**Adults and adolescents.** *Initial:* 250 mg q.i.d., increased as ordered by 250 to 500 mg/day. *Maintenance:* 2,000 to 3,000 mg/day in divided doses q.i.d. Preoperative dosage given for at least 7 days. *Maximum:* 4,000 mg/day in divided doses.

---

**Mechanism of Action**
Blocks the activity of tyrosine hydroxylase, the enzyme that controls the rate of catecholamine synthesis. This action decreases production of the catecholamines epinephrine and norepinephrine, which, in patients with pheochromocytoma, are produced in excessive amounts.

---

**Contraindications**
Hypersensitivity to metyrosine or its components

**Interactions**
**DRUGS**
*CNS depressants:* Increased sedation
*haloperidol, phenothiazines:* Increased extrapyramidal effects
**ACTIVITIES**
*alcohol use:* Increased sedation

**Adverse Reactions**
**CNS:** Anxiety, confusion, depression, disorientation, extrapyramidal reactions (difficulty speaking, drooling, parkinsonism, tremor, trismus), hallucinations, headache, sedation
**CV:** Peripheral edema
**EENT:** Dry mouth, nasal congestion, pharyngeal edema
**ENDO:** Galactorrhea, gynecomastia
**GI:** Abdominal pain, diarrhea, elevated serum AST level, nausea, vomiting
**GU:** Crystalluria, dysuria (transient), ejaculation failure, hematuria, impotence, urolithiasis
**HEME:** Anemia, eosinophilia, thrombocytopenia, thrombocytosis
**SKIN:** Urticaria

**Nursing Considerations**
•Expect patient taking metyrosine to experience moderate to severe sedation at low and high dosages. Sedation begins during first 24 hours, peaks after 2 to 3 days, and tends to wane during next few days. It usually subsides after 1 week unless dosage is increased or exceeds 2 g/day.
•Obtain urine specimens as ordered to check for crystalluria and urolithiasis. If crystalluria develops, increase fluid intake to achieve daily urine output of 2,000 ml or more with doses above 2 g/day. If crystalluria persists, reduce dosage or stop drug, as ordered.
•Expect to adjust dosage, as prescribed, based on clinical response and urine catecholamine level.
•If signs and symptoms aren't adequately controlled by metyrosine, expect to add an alpha-adrenergic blocker, such as phenoxybenzamine, as prescribed.
**PATIENT TEACHING**
•Inform patient about metyrosine's sedative effects. Advise him to avoid alcohol and CNS depressants, which may increase sedation.
•Instruct patient to increase fluid intake, as appropriate.
•Urge patient to notify prescriber about drooling, severe diarrhea, trembling and shaking of hands and fingers, or trouble speaking.
•Inform patient that he may experience changes in sleep pattern for 2 to 3 days after stopping drug.
•Advise patient to keep regular visits with prescriber to monitor progress.

# mexiletine hydrochloride
Mexitil

**Class and Category**
*Chemical:* Lidocaine analogue
*Therapeutic:* Class IB antiarrhythmic
*Pregnancy category:* C

**Indications and Dosages**
➤ *To treat life-threatening ventricular arrhythmias*
**CAPSULES**
**Adults.** *Initial:* 200 mg q 8 hr, adjusted, as ordered, by 50 to 100 mg/dose q 2 to 3 days, as tolerated. If patient tolerates 300 mg or less q 8 hr, total dosage may be divided and given q 12 hr. If patient continues to experience arrhythmias, dosage frequency may be changed to q.i.d. *Maximum:* 1,200 mg/day when given q 8 hr (400 mg/dose); 900 mg/day when given q 12 hr (450 mg/dose).

➤ *To rapidly control life-threatening ventricular arrhythmias*
**CAPSULES**
**Adults.** *Initial:* 400 mg followed by 200 mg after 8 hr. *Maintenance:* 200 mg q 8 hr, adjusted, as ordered, by 50 to 100 mg/dose q 2 to 3 days, as tolerated. If patient tolerates 300 mg or less q 8 hr, total dosage may be divided and given q 12 hr. If patient continues to experience arrhythmias, dosage frequency may be changed to q.i.d.
**DOSAGE ADJUSTMENT** For patients with severe hepatic disease or heart failure, dosage reduced and adjusted q 2 or 3 days.

| Route | Onset | Peak | Duration |
|-------|-------|------|----------|
| P.O. | 0.5 to 2 hr | 2 to 3 hr | 8 to 12 hr |

## Mechanism of Action

Produces antiarrhythmic effect by inhibiting fast sodium channels in myocardial cell membranes, especially in the His-Purkinje system. This action decreases the duration of the action potential and effective refractory period of the His-Purkinje system. The myocardium, which becomes refractory again after the resting membrane potential is restored, is less likely to generate and respond to ectopic ventricular impulses.

## Contraindications

Cardiogenic shock, second- or third-degree AV block without a pacemaker

## Interactions
**DRUGS**
*aluminum- or magnesium-containing antacids:* Delayed mexiletine absorption
*antiarrhythmics:* Increased cardiac effects
*cimetidine:* Possibly increased or decreased blood mexiletine level
*hepatic enzyme inducers:* Accelerated metabolism and decreased blood level of mexiletine
*metoclopramide:* Accelerated mexiletine absorption
*rifampin:* Decreased blood mexiletine level
*theophylline:* Increased blood theophylline level
*urine acidifiers:* Accelerated renal excretion of mexiletine
*urine alkalinizers:* Delayed mexiletine excretion

**FOODS**
*caffeine:* Possibly decreased clearance and increased effects of caffeine
*foods that may acidify urine (such as cheese, cranberries, eggs, fish, grains, meats, plums, poultry, and prunes):* Accelerated renal excretion of mexiletine
*foods that may alkalinize urine (such as milk and all vegetables and fruits except cranberries, plums, and prunes):* Delayed renal excretion of mexiletine
**ACTIVITIES**
*smoking:* Reduced mexiletine half-life

## Adverse Reactions

**CNS:** Confusion, dizziness, fatigue, headache, lack of coordination, light-headedness, nervousness, paresthesia, seizures, sleep disturbance, syncope, tremor, weakness
**CV:** Atrial arrhythmias, AV conduction disorders, bradycardia, cardiogenic shock, chest pain, heart failure, hypotension, palpitations, PVCs, ventricular arrhythmias (increased)
**EENT:** Blurred vision, dry mouth, tinnitus
**GI:** Constipation, diarrhea, heartburn, nausea, vomiting
**HEME:** Agranulocytosis, leukopenia, thrombocytopenia
**RESP:** Dyspnea
**SKIN:** Rash

## Nursing Considerations

• If mexiletine is replacing another antiarrhythmic, expect to give the first dose 6 to 12 hours after the last dose of quinidine sulfate or disopyramide, 3 to 6 hours after the last dose of procainamide, or 8 to 12 hours after the last dose of tocainide, as prescribed.
• If mexiletine is replacing parenteral lidocaine, expect to reduce or withdraw lidocaine 1 to 2 hours after starting mexiletine, as prescribed.
• Monitor continuous ECG and serum mexiletine level.
• Assess for signs of thrombocytopenia, which may occur within a few days after mexiletine therapy starts. Expect platelet count to return to normal within 1 month after mexiletine therapy stops.
**PATIENT TEACHING**
• Instruct patient to take mexiletine at evenly spaced intervals, to avoid missing doses, and to take drug as prescribed, even if he's feeling well.

•Advise patient to take drug with food to reduce adverse GI reactions.

•Inform patient that nausea and vomiting may occur within 2 hours after dose but tend to lessen as treatment continues.

•Advise patient to avoid potentially hazardous activities until drug's CNS effects are known.

•Teach patient how to measure pulse rate, and advise him to contact prescriber if rate falls below 50 beats/minute or if rhythm becomes irregular.

•Urge patient to notify prescriber immediately about chest pain, chills, fast or irregular heartbeat, fever, shortness of breath, and unusual bleeding or bruising.

•Advise patient to avoid dramatically increasing intake of foods that may acidify urine (cheese, cranberries, eggs, fish, grains, meats, plums, poultry, prunes) or alkalinize urine (milk, all vegetables, all fruits except cranberries, plums, and prunes).

•Encourage patient to keep regular visits with prescriber to monitor progress.

## mezlocillin sodium

Mezlin

### Class and Category

*Chemical:* Acyclaminopenicillin
*Therapeutic:* Antibiotic
*Pregnancy category:* B

### Indications and Dosages

➤ *To treat moderate to severe infections, including bacteremia, bone and joint infections, gynecologic infections (such as endometritis, pelvic cellulitis, and pelvic inflammatory disease), intra-abdominal infections (such as cholangitis, cholecystitis, hepatic abscess, intra-abdominal abscess, and peritonitis), lower respiratory tract infections (such as pneumonia and lung abscess), meningitis, septicemia caused by susceptible bacteria, or skin and soft-tissue infections (such as cellulitis and diabetic foot ulcer); to manage febrile neutropenia*

**I.V. INFUSION, I.M. INJECTION**

**Adults and adolescents.** 3 g q 4 hr or 4 g q 6 hr.

➤ *To treat life-threatening infections of the types listed above*

**I.V. INFUSION, I.M. INJECTION**

**Adults and adolescents.** Up to 350 mg/kg/day. *Maximum:* 24,000 mg/day.

**Children and infants.** 50 mg/kg q 4 hr (or infused over 30 min q 4 hr).

**Neonates over age 7 days weighing 2,000 g (4.4 lb) or less.** 75 mg/kg I.V. q 8 hr.

**Neonates age 7 days or less weighing 2,000 g or less.** 75 mg/kg I.V. q 12 hr.

**Neonates age 7 days or less weighing more than 2,000 g.** 75 mg/kg I.V. q 6 hr.

➤ *To treat uncomplicated UTI*

**I.V. INFUSION, I.M. INJECTION**

**Adults.** 1.5 to 2 g q 6 hr.

➤ *To treat complicated UTI*

**I.V. INFUSION**

**Adults.** 3 g q 6 hr.

**DOSAGE ADJUSTMENT** Dosing interval extended to q 6 to 8 hr if needed for patients with creatinine clearance of 10 to 30 ml/min/1.73 m$^2$. Dosing interval extended and dosage reduced to 1.5 to 2 g for patients with creatinine clearance below 10 ml/min/1.73 m$^2$.

➤ *To treat uncomplicated gonorrhea caused by susceptible strains of* Neisseria gonorrhoeae

**I.V. INFUSION, I.M. INJECTION**

**Adults.** 1 to 2 g as a single dose given with 1 g of probenecid P.O. (or probenecid given up to 30 min before mezlocillin).

➤ *To prevent infection from potentially contaminated surgical procedures*

**I.V. INFUSION**

**Adults.** 4 g 30 min before surgery and then 4 g q 6 hr for 2 more doses.

➤ *To prevent infection in cesarean section*

**I.V. INFUSION**

**Adults.** 4 g as soon as umbilical cord is clamped; then 4 g q 4 hr for 2 more doses, starting 4 hr after initial dose.

### Mechanism of Action

Inhibits bacterial cell wall synthesis. In susceptible bacteria, the rigid, cross-linked cell wall is assembled in several steps. Mezlocillin exerts its effects in the final stage of the cross-linking process by binding with and inactivating penicillin-binding proteins (enzymes responsible for linking cell wall strands). This action causes bacterial cell lysis and death.

M

## Incompatibilities

Administer mezlocillin at separate sites and at least 1 hour before or after aminoglycosides. Don't mix mezlocillin in same I.V. bag, bottle, or tubing as other drugs.

## Contraindications

Hypersensitivity to mezlocillin, other penicillins, or their components

## Interactions

**DRUGS**

*aminoglycosides:* Substantial aminoglycoside inactivation
*chloramphenicol, erythromycins, sulfonamides, tetracyclines:* Possibly decreased therapeutic effects of mezlocillin
*methotrexate:* Increased risk of methotrexate toxicity
*probenecid:* Increased blood level and prolonged half-life of mezlocillin

## Adverse Reactions

**CNS:** Depression, headache, seizures
**EENT:** Oral candidiasis
**GI:** Abdominal pain, diarrhea, pseudomembranous colitis, nausea, vomiting
**GU:** Vaginitis
**HEME:** Leukopenia, neutropenia
**SKIN:** Exfoliative dermatitis, pruritus, rash, urticaria
**Other:** Anaphylaxis; hypokalemia; injection site pain, redness, and swelling; serum sickness-like reaction

## Nursing Considerations

•**WARNING** Before starting mezlocillin therapy, make sure patient has had no previous hypersensitivity reactions to penicillins.
•Anticipate that mezlocillin therapy will last for at least 2 days after signs and symptoms have resolved—typically 7 to 10 days, depending on severity of infection. Complicated infections may need longer treatment. Group A beta-hemolytic streptococcal infections usually are treated for at least 10 days to reduce the risk of rheumatic fever or glomerulonephritis.
•For I.M. injection, reconstitute each gram of mezlocillin with 3 to 4 ml of sterile water for injection and shake vigorously. Inject no more than 2 g into a large muscle, such as the gluteus maximus, over 12 to 15 seconds to minimize discomfort.
•Although drug may be given I.M., expect to use intermittent I.V. infusion, as directed, for serious infections.

•For I.V. use, reconstitute each gram of mezlocillin with 9 to 10 ml of sterile water for injection, $D_5W$, or sodium chloride for injection and shake vigorously. Inject directly into I.V. tubing over 3 to 5 minutes.
•For intermittent infusion, further dilute to desired volume (50 to 100 ml) with an appropriate I.V. solution and administer over 30 minutes. Discontinue other infusions during mezlocillin administration.
•Be aware that mezlocillin powder and reconstituted solution may darken slightly but that potency isn't affected.
•Periodically monitor serum potassium level in patient receiving long-term therapy, as appropriate.
•During long-term therapy, monitor for signs and symptoms of superinfection, such as oral candidiasis and vaginitis.

**PATIENT TEACHING**

•Instruct patient taking mezlocillin to notify prescriber immediately if increased bruising or other bleeding tendencies develop.
•Advise patient to notify prescriber if diarrhea occurs and to check with prescriber before taking an antidiarrheal because of the risk of masking pseudomembranous colitis.

# micafungin sodium

Mycamine

## Class and Category

*Chemical:* Semisynthetic lipopeptide echinocandin
*Therapeutic:* Antifungal
*Pregnancy category:* C

## Indications and Dosages

➤ *To treat esophageal candidiasis*

**I.V. INFUSION**

**Adults.** 150 mg infused over 1 hr daily.

➤ *To prevent* Candida *infection in patients undergoing hematopoietic stem cell transplantation*

**I.V. INFUSION**

**Adults.** 50 mg infused over 1 hr daily.

| Route | Onset | Peak | Duration |
|-------|-------|------|----------|
| I.V. | Unknown | Unknown | Unknown |

## Contraindications

Hypersensitivity to micafungin or its components

## Mechanism of Action
Inhibits synthesis of 1,3-beta-D-glucan, which is an essential component of the *Candida* fungal cell wall. Without 1,3-beta-D-glucan, the fungal cell dies.

## Incompatibilities
Mixing or infusing with other drugs may cause micafungin to precipitate.

## Interactions
### DRUGS
*immunosuppressants:* Possibly additive adverse hematologic effects
*nifedipine, sirolimus:* Increased plasma nifedipine and sirolimus levels

## Adverse Reactions
**CNS:** Delirium, dizziness, dysgeusia, fatigue, fever, headache, rigors, somnolence
**CV:** Hypertension, hypotension, shock, vasodilation
**EENT:** Mucosal inflammation
**GI:** Abdominal pain, anorexia, constipation, diarrhea, dyspepsia, elevated liver enzyme levels, hepatic dysfunction, hiccups, hyperbilirubinemia, nausea, vomiting
**GU:** Acute renal failure, elevated serum creatinine and blood urea levels
**HEME:** Anemia, eosinophilia, hemolytic anemia, leukopenia, lymphopenia, neutropenia, thrombocytopenia
**SKIN:** Flushing, pruritus, rash, urticaria
**Other:** Anaphylaxis, angioedema, hypocalcemia, hypokalemia, hypomagnesemia, hypophosphatemia, injection site reactions including phlebitis and thrombophlebitis

## Nursing Considerations
• Use cautiously in patients with hepatic or renal insufficiency.
• Reconstitute micafungin by adding 5 ml of NS to each 50-mg vial being used to yield a concentration of 10 mg micafungin/ml. Swirl vial gently to minimize excessive foaming. Add reconstituted solution to 100 ml of NS and administer over 1 hour. Protect diluted solution from light, although you need not cover the infusion drip chamber or tubing.
• Always flush an existing intravenous line with NS before administering micafungin through that line.
• Monitor infusion rate carefully because infusions that took less than 1 hour to infuse

have been associated with more frequent hypersensitivity reactions.
• **WARNING** Monitor patient closely for hypersensitivity reactions including anaphylaxis and angioedema. Discontinue micafungin infusion immediately if present, notify prescriber, and provide supportive care, as prescribed.
• Monitor patient's liver and renal function closely throughout therapy because liver and renal abnormalities may occur in patients receiving micafungin.
• Monitor patient's hematologic status closely because a variety of hematologic abnormalities may occur. If abnormalities are detected, monitor patient closely. If condition worsens, expect micafungin to be discontinued.

### PATIENT TEACHING
• Instruct patient to report any infusion site discomfort immediately.
• Tell patient to report any unusual or persistent signs and symptoms to prescriber.

# midazolam hydrochloride
Versed

## Class, Category, and Schedule
*Chemical:* Benzodiazepine
*Therapeutic:* Sedative-hypnotic
*Pregnancy category:* D
*Controlled substance:* Schedule IV

## Indications and Dosages
➤ *To induce preoperative sedation or amnesia, to control preoperative anxiety*
### ORAL SOLUTION
**Children ages 6 months to 16 years.** 0.25 to 0.5 mg/kg as a single dose 30 to 45 min before surgery. *Usual:* 0.5 mg/kg. *Maximum:* 20 mg.
### I.V. INJECTION
**Adults age 60 and older.** 1.5 mg over 2 min immediately before procedure. After 2-min waiting period, dosage adjusted to desired level in 25% increments, as ordered. *Maximum:* 1 mg in 2 min.
**Adults under age 60 and adolescents.** Up to 2.5 mg over 2 min immediately before procedure. After 2-min waiting period, dosage adjusted to desired level in 25% increments, as ordered. *Maximum:* 5 mg.

M

**Children ages 6 to 12.** *Initial:* 0.025 to 0.05 mg/kg, up to 0.4 mg/kg, if needed. *Maximum:* 10 mg.
**Children ages 6 months to 5 years.** *Initial:* 0.05 to 0.1 mg/kg, up to 0.6 mg/kg, if needed. *Maximum:* 6 mg.

**I.M. INJECTION**
**Adults age 60 and older.** 0.02 to 0.05 mg/kg as a single dose 30 to 60 min before surgery.
**Adults under age 60 and adolescents.** 0.07 to 0.08 mg/kg as a single dose 30 to 60 min before surgery.
**Children ages 6 months to 12 years.** 0.1 to 0.15 mg/kg, up to 0.5 mg/kg for more anxious patients. *Maximum:* 10 mg.

➤ *To relieve agitation and anxiety in mechanically ventilated patients*

**I.V. INFUSION**
**Adults.** *Initial:* 0.01 to 0.05 mg/kg infused over several min, repeated at 10- to 15-min intervals until adequate sedation occurs. *Maintenance:* 0.02 to 0.1 mg/kg/hr initially, adjusted to desired level in 25% to 50% increments, as ordered. After achieving desired level of sedation, infusion rate decreased by 10% to 25% every few hr, as ordered, until minimum effective infusion rate is determined.
**Children.** *Initial:* 50 to 200 mcg/kg over 2 to 3 min followed by 1 to 2 mcg/kg/min by continuous infusion. *Maintenance:* 0.4 to 6 mcg/kg/min.
**Infants over age 32 weeks.** 1 mcg/kg/min by continuous infusion.
**Infants under age 32 weeks.** 0.5 mcg/kg/min by continuous infusion.

| Route | Onset | Peak | Duration |
|-------|-------|------|----------|
| I.V.* | 1.5 to 5 min | Rapid | 2 to 6 hr |
| I.M.* | 5 to 15 min | 15 to 60 min | 2 to 6 hr |
| I.M.† | 30 to 60 min | Unknown | Unknown |

## Contraindications

Acute angle-closure glaucoma; alcohol intoxication; coma; hypersensitivity to midazolam, other benzodiazepines, or their components; shock

---

* For sedation.
† For amnesia.

## Mechanism of Action

May exert its sedating effect by increasing the activity of gamma-aminobutyric acid, a major inhibitory neurotransmitter in the brain. As a result, midazolam produces a calming effect, relaxes skeletal muscles, and—at high doses—induces sleep.

## Interactions

**DRUGS**
*antihypertensives:* Increased risk of hypotension
*cimetidine, diltiazem, erythromycin, fluconazole, indinavir, itraconazole, ketoconazole, ranitidine, ritonavir, saquinavir, verapamil:* Intense and prolonged sedation caused by reduced midazolam metabolism
*CNS depressants:* Possibly increased CNS and respiratory depression and hypotension
*rifampin:* Decreased blood midazolam level
**FOODS**
*grapefruit, grapefruit juice:* Possibly increased blood midazolam level and risk of toxicity
**ACTIVITIES**
*alcohol use:* Possibly intense, prolonged sedative effect and increased respiratory depression and hypotension

## Adverse Reactions

**CNS:** Agitation, delirium, or dreaming during emergence from anesthesia; anxiety; ataxia; chills; combativeness; confusion; dizziness; drowsiness; euphoria; excessive sedation; headache; insomnia; lethargy; nervousness; nightmares; paresthesia; prolonged emergence from anesthesia; restlessness; retrograde amnesia; sleep disturbance; slurred speech; weakness; yawning
**CV:** Cardiac arrest, hypotension, nodal rhythm, PVCs, tachycardia, vasovagal episodes
**EENT:** Blurred vision, diplopia, or other vision changes; increased salivation; laryngospasm; miosis; nystagmus; toothache
**GI:** Hiccups, nausea, retching, vomiting
**RESP:** Airway obstruction, bradypnea, bronchospasm, coughing, decreased tidal volume, dyspnea, hyperventilation, respiratory arrest, shallow breathing, tachypnea, wheezing
**SKIN:** Pruritus, rash, urticaria
**Other:** Injection site burning, edema, induration, pain, redness, and tenderness

## Nursing Considerations

•Before administering midazolam, determine whether patient consumes alcohol or takes antihypertensives, antibiotics, or protease inhibitors because these substances can produce an intense and prolonged sedative effect when taken during midazolam therapy.

•WARNING Be aware that I.V. midazolam is given only in hospital or ambulatory care settings that allow continuous monitoring of respiratory and cardiac function. Keep resuscitative drugs and equipment readily available.

•As needed, combine midazolam injection with $D_5W$, NS, or LR solution. With $D_5W$ and NS, solution is stable for 24 hours. With LR, solution is stable for 4 hours.

•As needed, mix injection in same syringe with atropine sulfate, meperidine hydrochloride, morphine sulfate, or scopolamine hydrobromide. The resulting solution is stable for 30 minutes.

•Assess level of consciousness frequently because the range between sedation and unconsciousness or disorientation is narrow with midazolam.

•Be aware that recovery time is usually 2 hours but may be up to 6 hours.

PATIENT TEACHING

•Inform patient that he may not remember procedure because midazolam produces amnesia.

•Advise patient to avoid potentially hazardous activities until drug's adverse CNS effects, such as dizziness and drowsiness, have worn off.

•Instruct patient to avoid alcohol and other CNS depressants for 24 hours after receiving drug, unless directed otherwise by prescriber.

# midodrine hydrochloride

ProAmatine

## Class and Category

*Chemical:* Desglymidodrine prodrug
*Therapeutic:* Antihypotensive, vasopressor
*Pregnancy category:* C

## Indications and Dosages

➤ *To treat symptomatic orthostatic hypotension*

TABLETS

**Adults.** 10 mg t.i.d. in 3- to 4-hr intervals.

DOSAGE ADJUSTMENT Initial dose possibly reduced to 2.5 mg for patients with renal impairment.

| Route | Onset | Peak | Duration |
|-------|-------|------|----------|
| P.O. | Unknown | 30 min | 2 to 3 hr |

### Mechanism of Action

Is broken down into the active metabolite desglymidodrine. Desglymidodrine directly stimulates alpha-adrenergic receptors in arteries and veins. This action increases total peripheral vascular resistance, which in turn increases systolic and diastolic blood pressure.

## Contraindications

Acute renal disease, hypersensitivity to midodrine or its components, initial supine systolic pressure above 180 mm Hg, persistent and excessive supine hypertension, pheochromocytoma, severe heart disease, thyrotoxicosis, urine retention

## Interactions

DRUGS

*beta blockers, digoxin:* Enhanced or precipitated bradycardia, AV block, arrhythmias
*cimetidine, flecainide, metformin, procainamide, quinidine, ranitidine, triamterene:* Possibly decreased renal clearance of these drugs
*dihydroergotamine, ephedrine, phenylephrine, phenylpropanolamine, pseudoephedrine:* Increased vasopressor effects
*doxazosin, prazosin, terazosin:* Antagonized midodrine effects
*fludrocortisone acetate:* Increased risk of supine hypertension

## Adverse Reactions

**CNS:** Anxiety, asthenia, chills, confusion, delusions, dizziness, feeling of pressure or fullness in head, headache, hyperesthesia, insomnia, nervousness, paresthesia, somnolence
**CV:** Hypertension (sitting and supine), vasodilation
**EENT:** Canker sore, dry mouth, vision changes
**GI:** Flatulence, indigestion, nausea
**GU:** Dysuria, urinary frequency and urgency, urine retention
**MS:** Back pain, leg cramps

M

**SKIN:** Dry skin, erythema multiforme, facial flushing, piloerection, rash, scalp pruritus

## Nursing Considerations
•Monitor hepatic and renal function, as ordered, before and during midodrine therapy.
•Administer drug at 3- to 4-hour intervals, if needed and ordered, to control symptoms. Don't give after evening meal, less than 4 hours before bed, or more often than every 3 hours.
•**WARNING** Monitor for severe, persistent systolic supine hypertension, which may develop with single doses up to 20 mg.
•Avoid placing patient flat in bed for any length of time. Elevate head of bed when he's supine.
•Monitor supine and sitting blood pressure frequently during midodrine therapy.

**PATIENT TEACHING**
•Instruct patient to take midodrine every 3 to 4 hours during daytime but not to take final dose after evening meal or within 4 hours of going to bed.
•Advise patient to elevate head of bed when he lies supine. Caution him not to remain flat for any length of time.
•Direct patient to notify prescriber immediately about headache, increased dizziness, urine retention, or vision changes.
•Encourage patient to keep follow-up appointments to monitor blood pressure and hepatic and renal function.

# miglitol

Glyset

## Class and Category
*Chemical:* Desoxynojirimycin derivative
*Therapeutic:* Alpha-glucosidase inhibitor, antidiabetic drug
*Pregnancy category:* B

## Indications and Dosages
➤ *To manage type 2 diabetes mellitus*
**TABLETS**
**Adults.** *Initial:* 25 mg t.i.d. with first bite of each meal. Alternatively, 25 mg q.d., gradually increased to 25 mg t.i.d. *Maximum:* 100 mg t.i.d.
**DOSAGE ADJUSTMENT** After 4 to 8 wk, dosage increased, if ordered, to 50 mg t.i.d. for about 3 mo; then dosage adjusted based on glycosylated hemoglobin (HbA$_{1C}$) level.

| Route | Onset | Peak | Duration |
|-------|-------|------|----------|
| P.O. | Rapid | 2 to 3 hr | Unknown |

## Mechanism of Action
Inhibits intestinal glucoside hydrolase enzymes, which normally hydrolyze oligosaccharides and disaccharides to glucose and other monosaccharides. This action delays carbohydrate digestion and absorption and reduces the postprandial blood glucose level.

## Contraindications
Acute or chronic bowel disorder, diabetic ketoacidosis, hypersensitivity to miglitol or its components

## Interactions
**DRUGS**
*digestive enzyme preparations, intestinal adsorbents (activated charcoal):* Decreased miglitol effects
*digoxin:* Decreased blood digoxin level
*propranolol, ranitidine:* Decreased bioavailability of these drugs

## Adverse Reactions
**GI:** Abdominal pain, diarrhea, flatulence, hepatotoxicity
**HEME:** Low serum iron level
**SKIN:** Rash (transient)

## Nursing Considerations
•Use miglitol cautiously in patient with serum creatinine level above 2 mg/dl.
•Be aware that some patients with type 2 diabetes also may receive a sulfonylurea as an adjunct to miglitol therapy.
•Give miglitol with first bite of each meal. Drug must be at site of enzymatic action when carbohydrates reach small intestine.
•Review patient's HbA$_{1C}$ level, as appropriate, to monitor long-term glucose control.
•Monitor for signs of overdose, such as transient increases in abdominal discomfort, diarrhea, and flatulence (but not hypoglycemia).

**PATIENT TEACHING**
•Explain that miglitol is an adjunct to diet, which is the primary treatment for type 2 diabetes mellitus.
•Instruct patient to take drug with first bite of each meal.

• Describe signs and symptoms of hypoglycemia and pathophysiology of diabetes to patient and family members.

• If miglitol is the only drug patient takes to control blood glucose level, explain that it won't cause hypoglycemia.

• If patient takes a sulfonylurea or insulin with miglitol, suggest that he keep a source of glucose readily available to reverse hypoglycemia.

• Explain the importance of monitoring blood and urine glucose levels.

• Inform patient that adverse GI reactions usually decrease in frequency and intensity over time.

• Teach obese patient about weight loss, calorie restriction, diet, and regular exercise, as indicated.

# milrinone lactate

Primacor

## Class and Category

*Chemical:* Bipyridine derivative

*Therapeutic:* Inotropic, vasodilator
*Pregnancy category:* C

## Indications and Dosages

➤ *To provide short-term treatment of acute heart failure*

**I.V. INFUSION**

**Adults.** *Loading:* 50 mcg/kg over 10 min (at least 0.375 mcg/kg/min). *Usual:* 0.375 to 0.75 mcg/kg/min. *Maximum:* 1.13 mg/kg/day.

**DOSAGE ADJUSTMENT** Dosage adjusted according to cardiac output, pulmonary artery wedge pressure (PAWP), and clinical response. For patients with creatinine clearance of 30 to 39 ml/min/1.73 m², infusion rate reduced to 0.33 mcg/kg/min; of 20 to 29 ml/min/1.73 m², to 0.28 mcg/kg/min; of 10 to 19 ml/min/1.73 m², to 0.23 mcg/kg/min; and of less than 9 ml/min/1.73 m², to 0.20 mcg/kg/min.

| Route | Onset | Peak | Duration |
|---|---|---|---|
| I.V. | 5 to 15 min | Unknown | 3 to 6 hr |

## Mechanism of Action

An inotropic drug, milrinone increases the force of myocardial contraction—and cardiac output—by blocking the enzyme phosphodiesterase. Normally, this enzyme is activated by hormones binding to cell membrane receptors. As shown below left, phosphodiesterase normally degrades intracellular cAMP, which restricts calcium movement into myocardial cells. By inhibiting phosphodiesterase, as shown below right, milrinone slows the rate of cAMP degradation, increasing the intracellular cAMP level and the amount of calcium that enters myocardial cells. In blood vessels, increased cAMP causes smooth-muscle relaxation, which improves cardiac output by reducing preload and afterload.

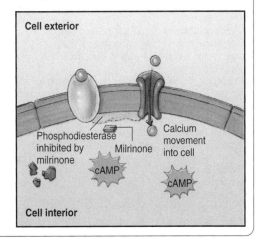

## Incompatibilities
Don't administer milrinone through same I.V. line as furosemide because precipitate will form. Don't add other drugs to premixed milrinone flexible containers.

## Contraindications
Hypersensitivity to milrinone or its components

## Interactions
**DRUGS**
*antihypertensives:* Possibly hypotension

## Adverse Reactions
**CNS:** Headache, tremor
**CV:** Angina, hypotension, supraventricular arrhythmias, ventricular ectopic activity, ventricular fibrillation, ventricular tachycardia, torsades de pointes
**GI:** Liver function test abnormalities
**HEME:** Thrombocytopenia
**RESP:** Bronchospasm
**SKIN:** Rash
**Other:** Anaphylactic shock, hypokalemia

## Nursing Considerations
•Make sure ECG equipment is available for continuous monitoring during milrinone therapy.
•Discard drug if it's discolored or contains particles.
•For loading dose, directly infuse undiluted drug into I.V. line with a compatible infusing solution. For continuous infusion, dilute drug with 0.45NS, NS, or D$_5$W. Dilution isn't needed when using premixed milrinone flexible containers.
•Check platelet count before and periodically during infusion, as ordered. Expect to discontinue drug if platelet count falls below 150,000/mm$^3$.
•Administer loading dose using a controlled-rate infusion device. For continuous infusion, use a calibrated electronic infusion device.
•Monitor cardiac output, pulmonary artery wedge pressure, blood pressure, heart rate, weight, and fluid status during therapy to determine drug effectiveness.
•Monitor renal and liver function test results and serum electrolyte levels. Notify prescriber of abnormalities.
•If severe hypotension develops, notify prescriber immediately and expect to stop drug.

•Expect patient to receive digoxin before starting milrinone, which can increase ventricular response rate.
**PATIENT TEACHING**
•Reassure patient that you'll be present and he'll be monitored constantly during therapy.

# minocycline
Minocin

# minocycline hydrochloride
Alti-Minocycline (CAN), Apo-Minocycline (CAN), Dynacin, Gen-Minocycline (CAN), Minocin, Novo-Minocycline (CAN), Vectrin

## Class and Category
*Chemical:* Tetracycline
*Therapeutic:* Antibiotic, antiprotozoal
*Pregnancy category:* D

## Indications and Dosages
➤ *To treat bartonellosis, brucellosis, chancroid, granuloma inguinale, inclusion conjunctivitis, lymphogranuloma venereum, nongonococcal urethritis, plague, psittacosis, Q fever, relapsing fever, respiratory tract infections (including pneumonia), rickettsial pox, Rocky Mountain spotted fever, tularemia, typhus, and UTIs caused by gram-negative organisms (including* Bartonella bacilliformis, Brucella *sp.,* Haemophilus ducreyi, Haemophilus influenzae, Vibrio cholerae, *and* Yersinia pestis)*, susceptible gram-positive organisms (including certain strains of* Streptococcus pneumoniae)*, and other organisms (including* Actinomyces *sp.,* Bacillus anthracis, Borrelia recurrentis, Chlamydia *sp.,* Mycoplasma pneumoniae, *and* Rickettsiae)*; as adjunct to treat intestinal amebiasis and as alternative to treat listeriosis caused by* Listeria monocytogenes, *syphilis caused by* Treponema pallidum, *and yaws caused by* Treponema pertenue *for nonpregnant patients allergic to penicillin*
**CAPSULES, ORAL SUSPENSION**
**Adults and adolescents.** *Initial:* 200 mg. *Maintenance:* 100 mg q 12 hr. Or 100 to 200 mg initially followed by 50 mg q 6 hr.

**Children over age 8.** *Initial:* 4 mg/kg. *Maintenance:* 2 mg/kg q 12 hr.
**I.V. INJECTION**
**Adults and adolescents.** *Initial:* 200 mg.
*Maintenance:* 100 mg q 12 hr. *Maximum:*
400 mg q.d.
**Children over age 8.** *Initial:* 4 mg/kg. *Maintenance:* 2 mg/kg q 12 hr.
**DOSAGE ADJUSTMENT** If patient has renal impairment, don't exceed 200 mg daily.
➤ *As adjunct to treat inflammatory acne vulgaris that's unresponsive to oral tetracycline or erythromycin*
**CAPSULES, ORAL SUSPENSION**
**Adults and adolescents.** 50 mg q.d. to t.i.d.
➤ *To treat uncomplicated gonorrhea caused by* Neisseria gonorrhoeae *in nonpregnant patients allergic to penicillin*
**CAPSULES, ORAL SUSPENSION**
**Adults and adolescents.** *Initial:* 200 mg.
*Maintenance:* 100 mg q 12 hr for at least 4 days.
➤ *To treat uncomplicated gonococcal urethritis in men*
**CAPSULES, ORAL SUSPENSION**
**Adults and adolescents.** 100 mg b.i.d. for 5 days.
➤ *To treat asymptomatic meningococcal carriers with* Neisseria meningitidis *in nasopharynx*
**CAPSULES, ORAL SUSPENSION**
**Adults and adolescents.** 100 mg q 12 hr for 5 days.
**Children over age 8.** *Initial:* 4 mg/kg. *Maintenance:* 2 mg/kg q 12 hr for 5 days.
➤ *To treat infections caused by* Mycobacterium marinum
**CAPSULES, ORAL SUSPENSION**
**Adults.** 100 mg q 12 hr for 6 to 8 wk.

| Route | Onset | Peak | Duration |
|-------|-------|------|----------|
| P.O. | Unknown | 2 to 4 hr | 6 to 12 hr |
| I.V. | Unknown | Unknown | 6 to 12 hr |

## Incompatibilities
Don't mix minocycline in same syringe with solution that contains calcium because precipitate will form.

## Contraindications
Hypersensitivity to minocycline, other tetracyclines, or their components

## Mechanism of Action
Inhibits bacterial protein synthesis by competitively binding to the 30S ribosomal subunit of the mRNA-ribosome complex of certain organisms.

## Interactions
**DRUGS**
*aluminum-, calcium-, or magnesium-containing antacids; calcium supplements; choline and magnesium salicylates; iron-containing preparations; magnesium-containing laxatives; sodium bicarbonate:* Possibly formation of nonabsorbable complex, impaired minocycline absorption
*cholestyramine, colestipol:* Possibly impaired cholestyramine or colestipol absorption
*cimetidine:* Possibly decreased GI absorption and effectiveness of minocycline
*digoxin:* Possibly increased blood digoxin level and risk of digitalis toxicity
*insulin:* Possibly decreased need for insulin
*iron salts:* Possibly decreased GI absorption and antimicrobial effect of minocycline
*lithium:* Possibly altered blood lithium level
*methoxyflurane:* Increased risk of nephrotoxicity
*oral anticoagulants:* Possibly potentiated anticoagulant effects
*oral contraceptives containing estrogen:* Decreased contraceptive effectiveness, increased risk of breakthrough bleeding
*penicillin:* Interference with bactericidal action of penicillin
*vitamin A:* Possibly benign intracranial hypertension

## Adverse Reactions
**CNS:** Dizziness, fever, headache, light-headedness, unsteadiness, vertigo
**CV:** Pericarditis
**EENT:** Blurred vision, darkened or discolored tongue, glossitis, papilledema, tooth discoloration, vision changes
**GI:** Abdominal cramps or pain, anorexia, diarrhea, dysphagia, enterocolitis, esophageal irritation and ulceration, hepatitis, hepatotoxicity, indigestion, nausea, pancreatitis, vomiting
**GU:** Genital candidiasis, nephrotoxicity
**HEME:** Eosinophilia, hemolytic anemia, neutropenia, thrombocytopenia, thrombocytopenic purpura
**MS:** Arthralgia, myopathy (transient)

M

**RESP:** Pulmonary infiltrates (with eosinophilia)
**SKIN:** Erythema multiforme, exfoliative dermatitis, brown pigmentation of skin and mucous membranes, erythematous and maculopapular rash, jaundice, onycholysis, photosensitivity, pruritus, purpura (anaphylactoid), Stevens-Johnson syndrome, urticaria
**Other:** Anaphylaxis, angioedema, serum sickness-like reaction, systemic lupus erythematosus exacerbation

## Nursing Considerations
• Use minocycline cautiously in patients with renal or hepatic dysfunction and in those taking other hepatotoxic drugs because drug may cause nephrotoxicity or hepatotoxicity.
• **WARNING** Notify prescriber if patient is breast-feeding because minocycline appears in breast milk and may have toxic effects.
• Monitor blood, renal, and hepatic tests before and during long-term therapy.
• Shake oral suspension well before use.
• To prepare drug for I.V. use, reconstitute each 100-mg vial with 5 to 10 ml of sterile water for injection. Further dilute in 500 to 1,000 ml of NS, $D_5W$, $D_5NS$, or Ringer's or LR solution. Administer final dilution immediately, but avoid rapid administration.
• Store reconstituted drug at room temperature and use within 24 hours.
• Assess patient for signs of superinfection; if they appear, notify prescriber, discontinue minocycline, and start appropriate therapy, as ordered.
• Monitor PT in patient who also takes an anticoagulant during minocycline therapy.

**PATIENT TEACHING**
• Instruct patient to shake oral suspension well and to use calibrated measuring device.
• Advise patient to take minocycline with a full glass of water, with food or milk, and in an upright position to minimize esophageal and GI irritation.
• Direct patient to take a missed dose as soon as he remembers unless it's nearly time for the next dose. Caution against double-dosing.
• Instruct patient not to take minocycline within 2 hours of an antacid or 3 hours of an iron preparation.
• Urge patient to complete full course of treatment even if he feels better beforehand.
• Instruct patient to notify prescriber if no improvement occurs in a few days.

• Advise patient to avoid prolonged exposure to sun or sunlamps during therapy.
• Counsel female patient to avoid becoming pregnant because minocycline should be avoided, if possible, during tooth development (last half of gestation up to age 8). Drug may permanently turn teeth yellow, gray, or brown and cause enamel hypoplasia. It also may slow skeletal growth and cause congenital anomalies, including limb reduction.
• Encourage patient who uses an oral contraceptive to use additional contraceptive method during minocycline therapy.
• Instruct patient to notify prescriber immediately about blurred vision, dizziness, headache, known or suspected pregnancy, and unsteadiness.

# minoxidil (oral)
Loniten

## minoxidil (topical)
Apo-Gain (CAN), Gen-Minoxidil (CAN), Minox (CAN), Minoxigaine (CAN), Rogaine (CAN), Rogaine ES for Men, Rogaine for Men, Rogaine for Women

## Class and Category
*Chemical:* Piperidinopyrimidine derivative
*Therapeutic:* Antihypertensive (oral), hair-growth stimulant (topical)
*Pregnancy category:* C

## Indications and Dosages
➤ *To manage severe symptomatic hypertension or hypertension with target organ damage that's unresponsive to other treatment*

**TABLETS**
**Adults and adolescents.** *Initial:* 5 mg as single dose or divided doses b.i.d. Increased, as directed, after at least 3 days. *Maintenance:* 10 to 40 mg/day. *Maximum:* 100 mg/day.
**Children.** *Initial:* 0.2 mg/kg q.d. Increased, as directed, after at least 3 days. *Maintenance:* 0.25 to 1 mg/kg/day as a single dose or in divided doses b.i.d. *Maximum:* 50-mg starting dose, 50 mg/day.
**DOSAGE ADJUSTMENT** Dosage possibly reduced for elderly patients and patients who have renal failure or are undergoing dialysis.

➤ *To treat alopecia*

TOPICAL 2%
**Adults up to age 65.** 1 ml applied b.i.d. to area of desired hair growth.
TOPICAL 5%
**Adult men up to age 65.** 1 ml applied b.i.d. to area of desired hair growth.

| Route | Onset | Peak | Duration |
|---|---|---|---|
| P.O. | 30 min | 2 to 3 hr | 24 to 48 hr |
| Topical 2% | 4 mo | 1 yr | Unknown |
| Topical 5% | 2 mo | 1 yr | Unknown |

## Mechanism of Action

Reduces blood pressure by inhibiting intracellular phosphodiesterase, an enzyme that facilitates hydrolysis of cAMP and cGMP. This action decreases intracellular cAMP level, relaxes arterial smooth muscles, and lowers blood pressure. Oral minoxidil produces greater dilation in arteries than in veins. It also reduces peripheral resistance and increases the heart rate, cardiac output, and stroke volume.

Topical minoxidil may cause hair regrowth by increasing cutaneous blood flow and stimulating resting hair follicles.

## Contraindications

Acute MI; dissecting aortic aneurysm; hypersensitivity to minoxidil or its components, including propylene glycol; pheochromocytoma; skin irritation or abrasions (topical)

## Interactions
### DRUGS

*guanethidine:* Possibly severe hypotension, increased risk of orthostatic hypotension (oral)
*nitrates, other hypotension-producing drugs, potent parenteral antihypertensives:* Possibly severe hypotension
*NSAIDs, sympathomimetics:* Decreased antihypertensive effects
*topical petrolatum, topical steroids:* Increased absorption of topical minoxidil if used on same area
*topical retinoids:* Increased absorption of topical minoxidil and, possibly, formation of granulation tissue

## Adverse Reactions

**CNS:** Fatigue, paresthesia (oral); light-headedness, neuritis (topical); headache (both)

**CV:** ECG changes, heart failure, pericardial tamponade, pericarditis, rebound hypertension (oral); cardiac tamponade, hypotension, palpitations, reflex hypertension (topical); angina, edema, fast or irregular heartbeat, pericardial effusion (both)
**EENT:** Vision changes (topical)
**ENDO:** Breast tenderness (oral)
**GI:** Abdominal distention, ascites, nausea, vomiting (oral)
**GU:** Elevated BUN and serum creatinine levels (oral); sexual dysfunction (topical)
**HEME:** Leukopenia; thrombocytopenia; transient decrease in hematocrit, hemoglobin, and erythrocyte counts (oral)
**RESP:** Dyspnea, pulmonary hypertension (oral)
**SKIN:** Flushing, hyperpigmentation, Stevens-Johnson syndrome (oral); allergic contact dermatitis, alopecia, dry or flaky skin, eczema, erythema, folliculitis, scalp burning (topical); hypertrichosis, rash (both)
**Other:** Facial edema (topical); sodium and water retention, weight gain (both)

## Nursing Considerations

•**WARNING** Be aware that patient who receives guanethidine should be hospitalized before starting oral minoxidil therapy so that his blood pressure can be monitored.
•Be aware that drug isn't usually prescribed for mild hypertension.
•For rapid management of hypertension, expect to adjust dosage up to every 6 hours and to monitor patient as prescribed. Also expect to give a beta blocker and diuretic.
•Monitor progress by measuring blood pressure frequently and weight daily. Evaluate for signs of fluid and sodium retention and for other systemic adverse reactions.
•Watch for signs of pericardial effusion. Be prepared to stop oral minoxidil, if ordered.
•Expect to discontinue oral minoxidil gradually because abrupt discontinuation may lead to rebound hypertension.
•Apply topical drug only on healthy scalp. Avoid using on sunburned or abraded scalp.
•Use gloves when applying solution.
•When using spray applicator, avoid inhaling mist.
•Expect minoxidil to be least effective in men with mainly frontal hair loss.
•Expect topical form to have little effect on blood pressure in patients who don't have hypertension.

M

•Inform patient that oral minoxidil controls but doesn't cure hypertension.
•Advise him to take tablets at the same time every day.
•Teach patient how to take his radial pulse, and advise him to measure it daily. Instruct him to notify prescriber if it exceeds normal rate by 20 beats/minute or more.
•Stress the importance of daily blood pressure and weight measurements.
•Instruct patient to notify prescriber immediately about bloating, breathing problems, a fast or irregular heartbeat, flushed or red skin, swelling of feet or lower legs, or weight gain of more than 5 lb (2.3 kg) in 1 day.
•Advise patient to have regular checkups with prescriber to monitor progress.
•Urge patient to consult prescriber before taking other prescription or OTC drugs.
•Reassure patient that body hair thickening and darkening reverses after oral minoxidil is discontinued.
•For patient using topical minoxidil, teach proper application technique and provide manufacturer's written instructions. Advise him to wear gloves when applying drug and to make sure hair and scalp are dry first.
•Instruct patient to start applying drug at center of balding area, to let drug dry for 2 to 4 hours, and not to use hairdryer to help it dry faster.
•Warn patient to avoid applying drug to abraded, irritated, or sunburned areas of scalp; to avoid inhaling mist when using a spray applicator; and to avoid getting drug in his eyes, nose, or mouth. If accidental contact does occur, advise him to flush the area with large amounts of cool tap water.
•Instruct patient not to shampoo his hair for at least 4 hours after application and to avoid using other skin products on treated skin. Direct him to avoid using minoxidil 24 hours before and after applying chemical hair products, such as dyes and relaxers.
•Caution patient not to use more drug or apply it more often than prescribed and not to apply it to other body areas. Explain the risk of adverse systemic reactions with excessive topical use.
•Caution patient to keep topical minoxidil away from heat or flame; it's flammable.
•Inform patient that minoxidil may stain clothing, hats, or bed linens before it's dry.

•Instruct patient to notify prescriber if burning, itching, or redness develops after application. For severe reactions, advise patient to wash drug off and consult prescriber before applying it again.
•Urge patient to consult prescriber if hair loss continues after 2 weeks or if growth fails to increase in 4 months.
•Inform patient that new hair growth may be lost 3 to 4 months after stopping topical minoxidil and that progressive hair loss will resume.

# mirtazapine

Remeron, Remeron SolTab

## Class and Category
*Chemical:* Piperazinoazepine
*Therapeutic:* Antidepressant
*Pregnancy category:* C

## Indications and Dosages
➤ *To treat major depression*
DISINTEGRATING TABLETS, TABLETS
**Adults.** *Initial:* 15 mg q.d., preferably h.s. Increased as needed and tolerated at 1- to 2-wk intervals. *Maximum:* 45 mg/day.

| Route | Onset | Peak | Duration |
|-------|-------|------|----------|
| P.O. | 1 to 2 wk | 6 wk or longer | Unknown |

### Mechanism of Action
May inhibit neuronal reuptake of norepinephrine and serotonin. By doing so, this tetracyclic antidepressant increases the action of these neurotransmitters in nerve cells. Increased neuronal serotonin and norepinephrine levels may elevate mood.

## Contraindications
Hypersensitivity to mirtazapine or its components, use within 14 days of an MAO inhibitor

## Interactions
DRUGS
*antihypertensives:* Increased hypotensive effects of these drugs or enhanced mirtazapine effects
*anxiolytics, hypnotics, other CNS depressants (including sedatives):* Increased CNS depression
*MAO inhibitors:* Possibly hyperpyrexia, hypertension, seizures

**ACTIVITIES**
*alcohol use:* Increased CNS depression

## Adverse Reactions
**CNS:** Agitation, amnesia, anxiety, apathy, asthenia, ataxia, cerebral ischemia, chills, confusion, delirium, delusions, depersonalization, depression, dizziness, dream disturbances, drowsiness, dyskinesia, dystonia, emotional lability, euphoria, extrapyramidal reactions, fever, hallucinations, hostility, hyperkinesia, hyperreflexia, hypoesthesia, hypokinesia, lack of coordination, malaise, mania, migraine headache, neurosis, paranoia, paresthesia, seizures, somnolence, syncope, tremor, vertigo
**CV:** Angina, bradycardia, edema, hypercholesterolemia, hypertension, hypertriglyceridemia, hypotension, MI, orthostatic hypotension, peripheral edema, PVCs, vasodilation
**EENT:** Accommodation disturbances, conjunctivitis, dry mouth, earache, epistaxis, eye pain, glaucoma, gingival bleeding, glossitis, hearing loss, hyperacusis, keratoconjunctivitis, lacrimation, pharyngitis, sinusitis, stomatitis
**ENDO:** Breast pain
**GI:** Abdominal distention and pain, anorexia, cholecystitis, colitis, constipation, elevated ALT level, eructation, increased appetite, nausea, thirst, vomiting
**GU:** Amenorrhea, cystitis, dysmenorrhea, dysuria, hematuria, impotence, increased libido, leukorrhea, renal calculi, urinary frequency and incontinence, urine retention, UTI, vaginitis
**HEME:** Agranulocytosis, neutropenia
**MS:** Arthralgia, back pain, dysarthria, muscle twitching, myalgia, myasthenia, neck pain and rigidity
**RESP:** Asthma, bronchitis, cough, dyspnea, pneumonia
**SKIN:** Acne, alopecia, dry skin, exfoliative dermatitis, photosensitivity, pruritus, rash
**Other:** Dehydration, facial edema, flulike symptoms, herpes simplex, weight gain or loss

## Nursing Considerations
• Administer mirtazapine before bedtime.
• Expect disintegrating tablet to dissolve on patient's tongue within 30 seconds.
• **WARNING** Don't give drug within 14 days of an MAO inhibitor to avoid serious, possibly fatal, reaction.
• If patient takes drug for depression, watch closely for suicidal tendencies, especially when therapy starts or dosage changes, because depression may temporarily worsen.
• Monitor patient closely for infection (fever, pharyngitis, stomatitis), which may be linked to a low WBC count. If these signs occur, notify prescriber and expect to stop drug.
• Expect mirtazapine therapy to last 6 months or longer for acute depression.

**PATIENT TEACHING**
• Instruct patient not to swallow disintegrating tablet. Tell him to hold tablet on tongue and allow it to dissolve. Inform him that tablet will dissolve within 30 seconds.
• Inform phenylketonuric patient that mirtazapine disintegrating tablets contain phenylalanine 2.6 mg per 15-mg tablet, 5.2 mg per 30-mg tablet, and 7.8 mg per 45-mg tablet.
• Instruct patient to avoid alcohol and other CNS depressants during mirtazapine therapy and for up to 7 days after drug is discontinued.
• Advise patient to avoid potentially hazardous activities until drug's CNS effects are known.
• Direct patient to change position slowly to minimize effects of orthostatic hypotension.
• Instruct patient to notify prescriber immediately about chills, fever, mouth irritation, sore throat, and other signs of infection.
• Encourage patient to visit prescriber regularly during therapy to monitor progress.

# misoprostol
Cytotec

## Class and Category
*Chemical:* Prostaglandin $E_1$ analogue
*Therapeutic:* Antiulcer, gastric antisecretory
*Pregnancy category:* X

## Indications and Dosages
➤ *To prevent NSAID-induced gastric ulcers*
**TABLETS**
**Adults.** 200 mcg q.i.d. or 400 mcg b.i.d. with food, with last dose h.s. every day.
**DOSAGE ADJUSTMENT** Dosage reduced to 100 mcg q.i.d. if patient can't tolerate 200-mcg dose.

| Route | Onset | Peak | Duration |
|---|---|---|---|
| P.O. | 30 min | 60 to 90 min | 3 to 6 hr |

## Mechanism of Action

May protect the stomach from NSAID-induced mucosal damage by increasing gastric mucus production and mucosal bicarbonate secretion. Misoprostol also inhibits gastric acid secretion caused by such stimuli as food, coffee, and histamine.

## Contraindications

Breast-feeding, hypersensitivity to prostaglandins or their analogues, in pregnant women (to prevent NSAID-induced gastric ulcers)

## Interactions
**DRUGS**
*magnesium-containing antacids:* Increased misoprostol-induced diarrhea

## Adverse Reactions

**CNS:** Headache, syncope
**CV:** Arrhythmias, chest pain, edema, hypertension, hypotension, increased cardiac enzyme levels, MI, phlebitis, thromboembolism
**GI:** Abdominal pain, constipation, diarrhea, flatulence, indigestion, nausea, vomiting
**GU:** Dysmenorrhea, hypermenorrhea, menstrual irregularities, vaginal bleeding
**Skin:** Diaphoresis

## Nursing Considerations

•**WARNING** Ask female patient if she is or may be pregnant. If so, notify prescriber because misoprostol may cause uterine bleeding, contractions, and spontaneous abortion as well as teratogenic effects in the fetus.
•Use drug cautiously in patients with cerebrovascular disease, coronary artery disease, or uncontrolled epilepsy because of the risk of severe complications.
•Also use misoprostol cautiously in patients with inflammatory bowel disease because drug may worsen intestinal inflammation and cause diarrhea. If diarrhea causes severe dehydration, drug may be discontinued.
**PATIENT TEACHING**
•Caution female patient about the risk of taking misoprostol during pregnancy, and urge her to use reliable contraception during therapy. Urge her to notify prescriber immediately if she is or might be pregnant.
•Instruct patient to take misoprostol with meals and at bedtime.
•Advise patient that he may take NSAIDs, if prescribed, during misoprostol therapy.

•Explain that diarrhea is dose related and usually resolves after 8 days. Tell patient to avoid magnesium-containing antacids because they may worsen diarrhea and to call prescriber if diarrhea lasts more than 8 days.
•Urge female patient to notify prescriber immediately about postmenopausal bleeding; she may need diagnostic tests.

# mitoxantrone hydrochloride

Novantrone

## Class and Category

*Chemical:* Anthracenedione
*Therapeutic:* Antineoplastic
*Pregnancy category:* D

## Indications and Dosages

➤ *To reduce neurologic disability and frequency of relapses in patients with secondary (chronic) progressive, progressive relapsing, or worsening relapsing-remitting multiple sclerosis (patients whose neurologic status is significantly abnormal between relapses)*
**I.V. INFUSION**
**Adults.** 12 mg/m$^2$ over 5 to 15 min q 3 mo. *Maximum:* Cumulative dose of 140 mg/m$^2$.

➤ *As adjunct to treat pain related to advanced hormone-refractory prostate cancer*
**I.V. INFUSION**
**Adults.** 12 to 14 mg/m$^2$ over 5 to 15 min q 21 days.

➤ *As adjunct to treat acute nonlymphocytic leukemia (ANLL)*
**I.V. INFUSION**
**Adults.** *Initial:* 12 mg/m$^2$ over at least 3 min on days 1 to 3 with 100 mg/m$^2$ of cytarabine as a continuous 24-hr infusion on days 1 to 7. If patient's antileukemic response is inadequate or incomplete, a second induction course is given at the same dosage. *Maintenance:* 6 wk after induction, 12 mg/m$^2$ over at least 3 min on days 1 and 2 with 100 mg/m$^2$ of cytarabine as a continuous 24-hr infusion on days 1 to 5. A second maintenance course is given 4 wk after the first if needed and tolerated.

## Mechanism of Action

Binds to DNA, causing cross-linkage and strand breakage, interfering with RNA synthesis, and inhibiting topoisomerase II, an enzyme that uncoils and repairs damaged DNA. Mitoxantrone produces a cytocidal effect on proliferating and nonproliferating cells and doesn't appear to be cell-cycle specific. It's known to inhibit B-cell, T-cell, and macrophage proliferation and impair antigen function.

## Incompatibilities

Don't mix mitoxantrone in the same infusion as heparin (because a precipitate may form); don't mix with any other drugs.

## Contraindications

Hypersensitivity to mitoxantrone or its components

## Interactions

**DRUGS**

*allopurinol, colchicine, probenecid, sulfinpyrazone:* Possibly interference with antihyperuricemic action of these drugs
*blood-dyscrasia–causing drugs (such as cephalosporins and sulfasalazine):* Increased risk of leukopenia and thrombocytopenia
*bone marrow depressants, such as carboplatin and lomustine:* Possibly additive bone marrow depression
*daunorubicin, doxorubicin:* Increased risk of cardiotoxicity
*methotrexate and other antineoplastics:* Risk of developing leukemia
*vaccines, killed virus:* Decreased antibody response to vaccine
*vaccines, live virus:* Increased risk of replication of and adverse effects of vaccine virus, decreased antibody response to vaccine

## Adverse Reactions

**CNS:** Headache, seizures
**CV:** Arrhythmias, chest pain, congestive heart failure, decreased left ventricular ejection fraction, ECG changes
**EENT:** Blue-colored cornea, conjunctivitis, mucositis, stomatitis
**GI:** Abdominal pain, diarrhea, GI bleeding, nausea, vomiting
**GU:** Blue-green urine, renal failure
**HEME:** Acute myelogenous leukemia, leukopenia, other leukemias, thrombocytopenia

**MS:** Myelodysplasia
**RESP:** Cough, dyspnea
**SKIN:** Alopecia, extravasation, jaundice
**Other:** Allergic reaction, anaphylaxis, hyperuricemia, infection, infusion site pain or redness

## Nursing Considerations

•Before and during therapy, expect patient to have an echocardiogram, ECG, and radionuclide angiography to evaluate cardiac status. Expect to obtain hematocrit, hemoglobin level, and CBC with platelet count.
•Be aware that drug shouldn't be given to patient with multiple sclerosis whose neutrophil count is less than $1,500/mm^3$.
•Obtain liver function test results, as ordered, before each course of therapy. Expect that drug won't be given to patient with multiple sclerosis and abnormal liver function.
•Anticipate obtaining pregnancy test before each course of therapy for women of childbearing age who have multiple sclerosis.
•Follow facility policy for handling antineoplastics. Be aware that manufacturer recommends goggles, gloves, and a gown during drug preparation and administration.
•Before infusing drug, dilute it in at least 50 ml of NS or $D_5W$.
•**WARNING** Be aware that drug shouldn't be given intrathecally because paralysis may occur.
•If mitoxantrone solution contacts your skin or mucosa, wash thoroughly with warm water. If it contacts your eyes, irrigate them thoroughly with water or NS.
•Discard unused diluted solution because it contains no preservatives. After penetration of the stopper, store undiluted drug for up to 7 days at room temperature or 14 days under refrigeration. Avoid freezing drug.
•If extravasation occurs, stop the infusion immediately and notify prescriber. Reinsert the I.V. line in another vein and resume the infusion. Although mitoxantrone is a nonvesicant, observe the extravasation site for signs of necrosis or phlebitis.
•Monitor patients with chickenpox or recent exposure to it and patients with herpes zoster for severe, generalized disease.
•Watch for evidence of cardiotoxicity, such as arrhythmias and chest pain, in patient with heart disease. Risk increases when cumulative dose reaches $140 mg/m^2$ in cancer patient, $100 mg/m^2$ in multiple sclerosis patient.

M

•Monitor blood uric acid level for hyperuricemia in patients with a history of gout or renal calculi. Expect to give allopurinol, as prescribed, to patients with leukemia or lymphoma who have elevated blood uric acid level to prevent uric acid nephropathy.

•**WARNING** If severe or life-threatening nonhematologic or hematologic toxicity occurs during the first induction course, expect to withhold the second course until it resolves.

•If patient develops thrombocytopenia, take precautions according to facility policy.

•Assess patient for evidence of infection, such as fever, if leukopenia occurs. Expect to obtain appropriate specimens for culture and sensitivity testing.

•Be aware that patients receiving mitoxantrone in combination with other antineoplastics or radiation therapy are at risk for developing secondary leukemia, including acute myelogenous leukemia.

**PATIENT TEACHING**

•Advise patient to complete dental work, if possible, before treatment begins or defer it until blood counts return to normal; drug may delay healing and cause gingival bleeding. Teach patient proper oral hygiene, and advise use of a toothbrush with soft bristles.

•Urge patient to drink plenty of fluid to increase urine output and uric acid excretion.

•Advise patient to contact prescriber immediately if GI upset occurs, but to continue taking drug unless otherwise directed.

•Stress the importance of complying with the dosage regimen and keeping follow-up medical and laboratory appointments.

•Explain that urine may appear blue-green for 24 hours after treatment and that the whites of the eyes may appear blue. Stress that these effects are temporary and harmless. Explain that hair loss is possible, but that hair should return after therapy ends.

•Caution patient not to receive immunizations unless approved by prescriber. Also, advise persons who live in same household as patient to avoid receiving immunization with oral polio vaccine. Tell patient to avoid persons who recently received the oral polio vaccine or to wear a mask over his nose and mouth.

•Instruct patient to avoid persons with infections if bone marrow depression occurs. Advise patient to contact prescriber if fever, chills, cough, hoarseness, lower back or side pain, or painful or difficult urination occurs; these changes may signal an infection.

•Tell patient to contact prescriber immediately if he notices unusual bleeding or bruising, black or tarry stools, blood in urine or stool, or pinpoint red spots on his skin.

•Urge patient not to touch his eyes or inside his nose unless he has just washed his hands.

•Stress the need to avoid accidental cuts, as from a razor or fingernail clippers, because they may cause excessive bleeding or infection.

•Caution patient to avoid contact sports or activities that may cause bruising or injury.

# modafinil

Provigil

## Class, Category, and Schedule

*Chemical:* Benzhydryl sulfinylacetamide derivative
*Therapeutic:* CNS stimulant
*Pregnancy category:* C
*Controlled substance:* Schedule IV

## Indications and Dosages

➤ *To improve daytime wakefulness in patients with narcolepsy, obstructive sleep apnea hypopnea syndrome, and shift work sleep disorder*

**TABLETS**

**Adults and adolescents age 16 and older.** 200 mg q.d. in the morning or 1 hr before starting work shift *Maximum:* 400 mg/day.

**DOSAGE ADJUSTMENT** For patients with severe hepatic impairment, dosage should be reduced by 50%.

## Contraindications

Hypersensitivity to modafinil or its components

## Mechanism of Action

May inhibit the release of gamma-aminobutyric acid (GABA), the most common inhibitory neurotransmitter, or CNS depressant, in the brain. Modafinil also increases the release of glutamate, an excitatory neurotransmitter, or CNS stimulant, in the thalamus and hippocampus. These two actions may improve wakefulness.

# Interactions

## DRUGS

*amitriptyline, citalopram, clomipramine, diazepam, imipramine, propranolol, tolbutamide, topiramate:* Possibly prolonged elimination time and increased blood levels of these drugs
*carbamazepine:* Possibly decreased modafinil effectiveness and decreased blood carbamazepine level
*cimetidine, clarithromycin, erythromycin, fluconazole, fluoxetine, fluvoxamine, itraconazole, ketoconazole, nefazodone, sertraline:* Possibly inhibited metabolism, decreased clearance, and increased blood level of modafinil
*contraceptive-containing implants or devices, oral contraceptives:* Possibly contraceptive failure
*cyclosporine:* Possibly decreased blood cyclosporine level and increased risk of organ transplant rejection
*dexamethasone, phenobarbital and other barbiturates, primidone, rifabutin, rifampin:* Possibly decreased blood level and effectiveness of modafinil
*dextroamphetamine, methylphenidate:* Possibly 1-hour delay in modafinil absorption when these drugs are administered together
*fosphenytoin, mephenytoin, phenytoin:* Possibly decreased effectiveness of modafinil, increased blood phenytoin level, and increased risk of phenytoin toxicity
*theophylline:* Possibly decreased blood level and effectiveness of theophylline
*triazolam:* Possibly decreased effectiveness of triazolam
*warfarin:* Possibly decreased warfarin metabolism and increased risk of bleeding

## FOODS

*all foods:* 1-hour delay in modafinil absorption and possibly delayed onset of action
*caffeine:* Increased CNS stimulation
*grapefruit juice:* Possibly decreased modafinil metabolism

# Adverse Reactions

**CNS:** Anxiety, depression, headache, insomnia, mania, nervousness, psychosis
**GI:** Nausea
**HEME:** Agranulocytosis
**Other:** Infection

# Nursing Considerations

•Be aware that modafinil shouldn't be given to patients with mitral valve prolapse syndrome or a history of left ventricular hypertrophy because drug may cause ischemic changes.
•**WARNING** Monitor patient with a history of alcoholism, stimulant abuse, or other substance abuse for compliance with modafinil therapy. Observe for signs of misuse or abuse, including frequent prescription refill requests, increased frequency of dosing, or drug-seeking behavior. Also watch for evidence of excessive modafinil dosage, including aggressiveness, anxiety, confusion, decreased prothrombin time, diarrhea, irritability, nausea, nervousness, palpitations, sleep disturbances, and tremor.
•Be aware that modafinil, like other CNS stimulants, may alter mood, perception, thinking, judgment, feelings, motor skills, and signs that patient needs sleep.
•If giving drug to patient with a history of psychosis, emotional instability, or psychological illness with psychotic features, be prepared to perform baseline behavioral assessments or frequent clinical observation.

## PATIENT TEACHING

•Inform patient that modafinil can help, but not cure, narcolepsy and that drug's full effects may not be seen right away.
•Advise patient to avoid taking modafinil within 1 hour of eating because food may delay drug's absorption and onset of action. If he drinks grapefruit juice, encourage him to drink a consistent amount daily.
•Inform patient that drug can affect his concentration and function and can hide signs of fatigue. Urge him not to drive or perform activities that require mental alertness until drug's full CNS effects are known.
•Because alcohol may decrease alertness, advise patient to avoid it while taking modafinil.
•Encourage a regular sleeping pattern.
•Caution patient to avoid excessive intake of foods, beverages, and over-the-counter drugs that contain caffeine because caffeine may lead to increased CNS stimulation.
•Inform female patient that modafinil can decrease the effectiveness of certain contraceptives, including birth control pills and implantable hormonal contraceptives. If she uses such contraceptives, urge her to use an alternate birth control method during mo-

M

dafinil therapy and for up to 1 month after she stops taking the drug.
•Advise patient to keep follow-up appointments with prescriber so that her progress can be monitored.

# moexipril hydrochloride
Univasc

## Class and Category
*Chemical:* Prodrug of moexiprilat
*Therapeutic:* Antihypertensive
*Pregnancy category:* C (first trimester), D (later trimesters)

## Indications and Dosages
➤ *To manage hypertension without diuretic therapy*
**TABLETS**
**Adults.** *Initial:* 7.5 mg q.d. 1 hr a.c. *Maintenance:* 7.5 to 30 mg as a single dose or in divided doses b.i.d. 1 hr a.c. *Maximum:* 30 mg/day.
**DOSAGE ADJUSTMENT** For patients with creatinine clearance of less than 40 ml/min/1.73 m$^2$, initial dosage reduced to 3.75 mg q.d. and increased, as ordered, to maximum of 15 mg/day.
➤ *To manage hypertension with diuretic therapy*
**TABLETS**
**Adults.** *Initial:* 3.75 mg q.d. 1 hr a.c. Increased gradually, as ordered, until blood pressure is controlled.

| Route | Onset | Peak | Duration |
|-------|-------|------|----------|
| P.O. | 1 hr | 3 to 6 hr | 24 hr |

## Mechanism of Action
Is converted to the active metabolite moexiprilat, which reduces blood pressure by inhibiting ACE activity. ACE normally catalyzes the conversion of angiotensin I to angiotensin II—a vasoconstrictor that stimulates aldosterone secretion by the adrenal cortex and directly suppresses renin release. Inhibited ACE activity results in decreased peripheral arterial resistance, increased plasma renin activity, and decreased aldosterone secretion. Decreased aldosterone secretion causes water and sodium excretion.

## Contraindications
History of angioedema with previous ACE inhibitor use, hypersensitivity to moexipril or its components

## Interactions
**DRUGS**
*allopurinol, bone marrow depressants, corticosteroids (systemic), cytostatic drugs, procainamide:* Increased risk of possibly fatal neutropenia or agranulocytosis
*antacids:* Possibly decreased moexipril bioavailability
*cyclosporine, heparin, potassium-containing drugs, potassium-sparing diuretics, potassium supplements:* Increased risk of hyperkalemia
*digoxin:* Possibly increased blood digoxin level
*diuretics, other hypotension-producing drugs:* Hypotension, risk of renal failure (from sodium or volume depletion caused by diuretics), possibly decreased secondary aldosteronism and hypokalemia caused by diuretics
*lithium:* Increased blood lithium level and risk of lithium toxicity
*NSAIDs (especially indomethacin), sympathomimetics:* Decreased antihypertensive effect of moexipril
*phenothiazines:* Increased pharmacologic effects of moexipril
**FOODS**
*all foods:* Decreased moexipril absorption
*low-salt milk, salt substitutes:* Possibly hyperkalemia
**ACTIVITIES**
*alcohol use:* Possibly hypotension

## Adverse Reactions
**CNS:** Anxiety, chills, confusion, CVA, dizziness, drowsiness, fatigue, fever, headache, malaise, mood changes, nervousness, sleep disturbance, syncope
**CV:** Angina, arrhythmias, chest pain, hypotension, MI, orthostatic hypotension, palpitations, peripheral edema
**EENT:** Dry mouth, hoarseness, laryngeal edema, mouth or tongue swelling, pharyngitis, rhinitis, sinusitis, taste perversion, tinnitus
**GI:** Abdominal distention or pain, anorexia, constipation, diarrhea, dysphagia, elevated liver function test results, hepatitis, increased appetite, nausea, pancreatitis, vomiting

**GU:** Azotemia, elevated BUN and serum creatinine and uric acid levels, interstitial nephritis, oliguria, proteinuria, renal insufficiency, urinary frequency
**HEME:** Agranulocytosis, bone marrow depression, elevated erythrocyte sedimentation rate, hemolytic anemia, leukocytosis, leukopenia, neutropenia, thrombocytopenia
**MS:** Arthralgia, leg heaviness or weakness, myalgia, myositis
**RESP:** Bronchospasm, cough, dyspnea, upper respiratory tract infection
**SKIN:** Alopecia, diaphoresis, flushing, onycholysis, pallor, pemphigus, photosensitivity, pruritus, rash, Stevens-Johnson syndrome, urticaria
**Other:** Anaphylaxis, angioedema (of arms, face, larynx, legs, lips, mucous membranes, tongue), flulike symptoms, hyperkalemia, hyponatremia, positive ANA titer

## Nursing Considerations

•WARNING Contact prescriber if patient is or may be pregnant. Moexipril may cause fetal or neonatal harm or death if used during second or third trimester.
•Be aware that patient who already takes a diuretic should be medically supervised for several hours after first dose of moexipril.
•Administer drug 1 hour before meals.
•Monitor blood pressure, leukocyte count, and liver and renal function test results during moexipril therapy.
•Be aware that black patients may be less responsive to drug's antihypertensive effect if moexipril is used alone to control blood pressure.

**PATIENT TEACHING**
•Urge female patient to notify prescriber immediately if she is or may be pregnant.
•Instruct patient to take moexipril at the same time each day, 1 hour before meals.
•Direct patient to take a missed dose as soon as he remembers unless it's nearly time for the next dose. Caution against doubling the dose.
•WARNING Instruct patient to stop drug and seek immediate medical attention for hoarseness; swelling of tongue, glottis, larynx, face, hands, or feet; or sudden difficulty swallowing or breathing.
•Caution patient not to stop drug without consulting prescriber even if he feels better.

•Inform patient about possible dizziness, especially after first dose and if he takes a diuretic.
•Advise patient to change position slowly to minimize effects of orthostatic hypotension.
•Caution patient to avoid potentially hazardous activities until drug's CNS effects are known.
•Instruct patient to notify prescriber if he faints or experiences persistent dizziness.
•Instruct patient to report evidence of infection (such as chills, fever, and sore throat) as well as diarrhea, nausea, or vomiting, which may lead to dehydration-induced hypotension.
•Advise patient to avoid alcohol during moexipril therapy because it may cause hypotension.
•Instruct patient to check with prescriber before taking OTC drugs.
•Urge patient to avoid potassium supplements and potassium-containing salt substitutes unless prescriber allows them.
•Advise patient to visit prescriber regularly to monitor progress.
•Discuss the importance of weight control and low-salt diet in managing hypertension.

# molindone hydrochloride

Moban, Moban Concentrate

## Class and Category
*Chemical:* Dihydroindolone derivative
*Therapeutic:* Antipsychotic drug
*Pregnancy category:* Not rated

## Indications and Dosages
➤ *To manage symptoms of psychotic disorders*
**ORAL SOLUTION, TABLETS**
**Adults and children age 12 and older.** *Initial:* 50 to 75 mg q.d. in divided doses t.i.d. or q.i.d. Dosage increased to 100 mg/day in 3 to 4 days as needed. *Maintenance:* For mild psychosis, 5 to 15 mg t.i.d. or q.i.d.; for moderate psychosis, 10 to 25 mg t.i.d. or q.i.d.; for severe psychosis, 225 mg/day in divided doses. *Maximum:* 225 mg/day.
DOSAGE ADJUSTMENT Initial dosage reduced for elderly or debilitated patients.

| Route | Onset | Peak | Duration |
|-------|-------|------|----------|
| P.O. | Unknown | Unknown | 24 to 36 hr |

## Mechanism of Action

Occupies dopamine receptor sites in the reticular activating and limbic systems in the CNS. By blocking dopamine activity in these areas, molindone reduces the symptoms of psychosis, helping the patient to think and behave more coherently.

## Contraindications

Hypersensitivity to molindone, its components, or other antipsychotic drugs, including haloperidol, loxapine, phenothiazines, and thioxanthenes

## Interactions

### DRUGS

*amphetamines:* Decreased amphetamine effectiveness, decreased antipsychotic effectiveness of molindone

*anesthetics, barbiturates, benzodiazepines, CNS depressants, opioid analgesics:* Possibly prolonged and intensified CNS depressant effects

*antacids, antidiarrheals:* Decreased molindone absorption

*anticholinergics, antidyskinetics, antihistamines:* Possibly increased anticholinergic effects

*beta blockers:* Possibly increased effect of beta blocker

*bromocriptine:* Possibly decreased therapeutic effects of bromocriptine and increased serum prolactin level

*extrapyramidal reaction–causing drugs, such as amoxapine, haloperidol, loxapine, metoclopramide, olanzapine, phenothiazines, pimozide, rauwolfia alkaloids, risperidone, tacrine, and thioxanthenes:* Increased severity of extrapyramidal effects

*insulin, oral antidiabetic drugs:* Possibly increased serum glucose level

*levodopa:* Inhibited antidyskinetic effects of levodopa, possibly decreased antipsychotic effects of molindone

*lithium:* Increased risk of neurotoxicity, increased extrapyramidal effects

*MAO inhibitors, maprotiline, trazodone, tricyclic antidepressants:* Possibly prolonged and intensified sedative or anticholinergic effects of all drugs

*phenytoin, tetracycline:* Interference with absorption of phenytoin and tetracycline

### ACTIVITIES

*alcohol use:* Prolonged and intensified CNS depression

## Adverse Reactions

**CNS:** Depression, drowsiness, euphoria, extrapyramidal reactions (such as dystonia, motor restlessness, pseudoparkinsonism, and tardive dyskinesia), headache, lack of coordination, neuroleptic malignant syndrome, tiredness
**CV:** Orthostatic hypotension, tachycardia, unstable blood pressure
**EENT:** Blinking or eyelid spasm, blurred vision, dry mouth, inability to move eyes, nasal congestion
**ENDO:** Breast engorgement, lactation
**GI:** Constipation, nausea
**GU:** Decreased libido, menstrual irregularities, urine retention
**MS:** Muscle spasms of back, face, and neck; muscle twitching; twisting movements of the body; weakness or stiffness of limbs
**RESP:** Dyspnea
**SKIN:** Diaphoresis, pallor, rash
**Other:** Heatstroke

## Nursing Considerations

•**WARNING** Assess patient for signs and symptoms of neuroleptic malignant syndrome, such as diaphoresis, dyspnea, fatigue, fever, incontinence, pallor, severe muscle stiffness, tachycardia, and unstable blood pressure; notify prescriber immediately if they occur. Expect to discontinue drug and begin intensive medical treatment. Monitor patient carefully for recurrence if antipsychotic therapy resumes.
•Be aware that molindone shouldn't be administered to patients who have severe CNS depression or who are comatose because of drug's CNS depressant effects.
•Monitor elderly patients for orthostatic hypotension and symptoms of tardive dyskinesia, including blinking or eyelid spasms, involuntary movements of the limbs, and unusual facial expressions, because these patients may be sensitive to drug's anticholinergic and extrapyramidal effects. Expect to reduce dosage or discontinue drug.
•Administer oral solution undiluted or mixed with water, carbonated beverage, fruit juice, or milk.

### PATIENT TEACHING

•Instruct patient to follow treatment regimen and to notify prescriber before discon-

tinuing drug because gradual dosage reduction may be needed.
•Instruct patient not to take drug within 2 hours of taking an antacid. Advise him to take drug with food or a full glass of milk or water to reduce gastric irritation.
•Instruct patient to take oral solution undiluted or mixed with water, carbonated beverage, fruit juice, or milk.
•Urge patient to avoid alcohol because of possible additive effects and hypotension.
•Advise patient, especially if elderly, to rise slowly from a supine or seated position to avoid dizziness, light-headedness, and fainting.
•Explain that drug may reduce the body's response to heat. Tell patient to avoid temperature extremes, such as a hot shower, hot tub, or sauna. Urge him to use caution during exercise.
•Caution patient not to take OTC drugs for colds or allergies because they can increase the risk of heatstroke and increase anticholinergic effects, such as blurred vision, constipation, dry mouth, and urine retention.
•Inform patient and family members that maximum clinical improvement in symptoms.may take several weeks or months.

# mometasone furoate monohydrate

Nasonex

## Class and Category
*Chemical:* Glucocorticoid
*Therapeutic:* Anti-inflammatory
*Pregnancy category:* C

## Indications and Dosages
➤ *To manage symptoms of seasonal or perennial allergic rhinitis*
**NASAL SPRAY**
**Adults and children 12 years and over.** 100 mcg (2 sprays) in each nostril q.d.
**Children ages 2 to 12.** 50 mcg (1 spray) in each nostril q.d.

---

### Mechanism of Action
Inhibits the activity of cells and mediators active in the inflammatory response, possibly by decreasing influx of inflammatory cells into nasal passages and thereby decreasing nasal inflammation.

---

## Contraindications
Hypersensitivity to mometasone or its components; recent septal ulcers, nasal surgery, or nasal trauma

## Adverse Reactions
**CNS:** Headache
**CV:** Chest pain
**EENT:** Bad taste, conjunctivitis, dry mouth, earache, epistaxis, nasal irritation, oral candidiasis, otitis media, pharyngitis, rhinitis, sinusitis
**ENDO:** Dysmenorrhea, growth suppression
**GI:** Diarrhea, dyspepsia, nausea, vomiting
**MS:** Arthralgia, myalgia, musculoskeletal pain
**RESP:** Asthma, bronchitis, increased cough, upper respiratory tract infection, wheezing
**Other:** Angioedema, flu-like symptoms, viral infection

## Nursing Considerations
•Use mometasone cautiously if patient has tubercular infection; untreated fungal, bacterial, or systemic viral infection; or ocular herpes simplex.
•Closely monitor a child's growth pattern; drug may stunt growth.
•**WARNING** Assess patient who switches from a systemic corticosteroid to an intranasal preparation, such as mometasone, for signs of adrenal insufficiency (fatigue, lassitude, weakness, nausea, vomiting, and hypotension), which may be life-threatening. Hypothalamic-pituitary-adrenal axis function may take several months to recover after systemic corticosteroids are discontinued. Abrupt withdrawal of mometasone also may precipitate adrenal insufficiency.

**PATIENT TEACHING**
•Instruct patient to shake container before each use. Instruct her to blow her nose, tilt her head slightly forward, and insert tube into a nostril, pointing toward inner corner of eye, away from nasal septum. Tell her to hold the other nostril closed and spray while inhaling gently. Then have her repeat the procedure in the other nostril.
•Instruct patient to contact prescriber if symptoms persist or have worsened after 3 weeks.
•Caution patient to avoid exposure to chickenpox and measles and, if exposed, to contact prescriber immediately.

M

# montelukast sodium

Singulair

## Class and Category

*Chemical:* Leukotriene receptor antagonist
*Therapeutic:* Antiasthmatic
*Pregnancy category:* B

## Indications and Dosages

➤ *To prevent or treat asthma*

ORAL GRANULES

**Children ages 12 to 23 mo.** 4 mg q.d. in the evening. *Maximum:* 4 mg/day.

CHEWABLE TABLETS

**Children ages 6 to 14.** 5 mg q.d. in the evening. *Maximum:* 5 mg/day.
**Children ages 2 to 5.** 4 mg q.d. in the evening. *Maximum:* 4 mg/day.

TABLETS

**Adults and adolescents age 15 and older.** 10 mg q.d. in the evening. *Maximum:* 10 mg/day.

➤ *To treat seasonal allergic rhinitis*

ORAL GRANULES

**Children ages 2 to 5.** 4 mg q.d.

CHEWABLE TABLETS

**Children ages 6 to 14.** 5 mg q.d.
**Children ages 2 to 5.** 4 mg q.d.

TABLETS

**Adults and adolescents age 15 and older.** 10 mg q.d.

➤ *To treat perennial allergic rhinitis*

ORAL GRANULES

**Children ages 6 months to 5 years.** 4 mg q.d.

CHEWABLE TABLETS

**Children ages 6 to 14.** 5 mg q.d.
**Children ages 2 to 5.** 4 mg q.d.

TABLETS

**Adults and adolescents age 15 and older.** 10 mg q.d.

| Route | Onset | Peak | Duration |
|-------|-------|------|----------|
| P.O. | Unknown | Unknown | 24 hr |

## Contraindications

Hypersensitivity to montelukast or its components

## Interactions

DRUGS

*phenobarbital:* Decreased amount of circulating montelukast

## Mechanism of Action

Antagonizes receptors for cysteinyl leukotrienes, which are produced by arachidonic acid metabolism and released from mast cells, eosinophils, and other cells. When cysteinyl leukotrienes bind to their receptor sites in bronchial airways, they increase endothelial membrane permeability, which leads to airway edema, smooth-muscle contraction, and altered activity of the cells involved in asthma's inflammatory process. Montelukast blocks these effects.

## Adverse Reactions

**CNS:** Asthenia, dizziness, fatigue, fever, headache, hypoesthesia, paresthesia (in all patients)
**EENT:** Dental pain, epistaxis, nasal congestion (in all patients); laryngitis, otitis media, pharyngitis, sinusitis
**GI:** Abdominal pain, cholestatic hepatitis, dyspepsia, elevated liver function test results, hepatotoxicity, indigestion, infectious gastroenteritis (in all patients); diarrhea, nausea (in children)
**GU:** Pyuria
**RESP:** Cough, upper respiratory tract infection
**SKIN:** Pruritus, rash, urticaria
**Other:** Anaphylaxis, angioedema (in all patients); flulike syndrome, viral infection (in children)

## Nursing Considerations

•WARNING Be aware that drug shouldn't be given for acute asthma attack or status asthmaticus.
•Be aware that montelukast shouldn't be abruptly substituted for inhaled or oral corticosteroids; expect to taper corticosteroid dosage gradually, as directed.
•Monitor for adverse reactions, such as cardiac and pulmonary symptoms, eosinophilia, and vasculitis, in patient undergoing corticosteroid withdrawal. Notify prescriber if such reactions occur.

PATIENT TEACHING

•Advise patient to take montelukast daily as prescribed, even when he feels well. Urge him not to decrease dosage or stop taking other prescribed asthma drugs unless instructed by prescriber.
•Caution patient not to use drug for acute asthma attack or status asthmaticus; make

sure he has appropriate short-acting rescue drug available.

• Tell parents administering oral granules to pour contents directly into the child's mouth or mix with ice cream or cold or room temperature applesauce, carrots, or rice—but not liquids or other foods—just prior to administration. Liquids may be given after drug has been administered. Once packet is opened, the full dose must be administered within 15 minutes. Drug must not be stored for future use if mixed with food.

• Instruct patient to notify prescriber if he needs to use short-acting inhaled bronchodilator more often than usual, or more often than prescribed, to control symptoms.

• Teach patient to use peak flowmeter to determine personal best expiratory volume.

• Caution patient with aspirin sensitivity to avoid aspirin and NSAIDs during montelukast therapy. Montelukast may not effectively reduce bronchospasm in such a patient.

• Inform patient (or parents of child) with phenylketonuria that chewable tablet contains phenylalanine.

# moricizine hydrochloride

Ethmozine

## Class and Category

*Chemical:* Phenothiazine derivative
*Therapeutic:* Class I antiarrhythmic
*Pregnancy category:* B

## Indications and Dosages

➤ *To treat life-threatening ventricular arrhythmias*

**TABLETS**

**Adults.** 200 to 300 mg q 8 hr. *Maximum:* 900 mg/day.

**DOSAGE ADJUSTMENT** For patients with hepatic or renal impairment, initial dosage possibly reduced to 600 mg/day or less.

| Route | Onset | Peak | Duration |
|-------|-------|------|----------|
| P.O. | 2 hr | 6 to 14 hr | 10 to 24 hr |

## Contraindications

Cardiogenic shock, hypersensitivity to moricizine or its components, right bundle-branch block with left hemiblock (bifascicular block) unless pacemaker is present, second- or third-degree AV block unless pacemaker is present

## Mechanism of Action

Exerts potent local anesthetic activity and stabilizes myocardial cell membranes, thus reducing ventricular arrhythmias. Moricizine prolongs the PR interval, AV nodal conduction time, infranodal conduction time, and intraventricular conduction time by inhibiting sodium influx across myocardial cell membranes. These effects decrease myocardial excitability, conduction velocity, and automaticity. Prolonged conduction decreases the refractory period and increases the ratio of refractory period to action potential duration, thus preventing arrhythmias.

## Interactions

**DRUGS**

*cimetidine:* Decreased moricizine clearance, increased blood moricizine level
*digoxin:* Prolonged PR interval
*other antiarrhythmics:* Increased risk of adverse cardiac effects
*propranolol:* Slightly prolonged PR interval
*theophylline:* Increased theophylline clearance, decreased blood theophylline level

## Adverse Reactions

**CNS:** Abnormal gait, agitation, akathisia, anxiety, asthenia, ataxia, coma, confusion, depression, dizziness, dyskinesia, euphoria, fatigue, hallucinations, headache, hypoesthesia, hypothermia, lack of coordination, memory loss, nervousness, paresthesia, seizures, sleep disturbance, somnolence, tremor, vertigo

**CV:** Angina, AV block, bradycardia, cardiac arrest, heart failure, hypertension, hypotension, junctional rhythm, MI, palpitations, proarrhythmias (new rhythm disturbances or worsened existing arrhythmias), pulmonary embolism, sinus pause or arrest, supraventricular arrhythmias (including atrial fibrillation and flutter), thrombophlebitis, vasodilation, ventricular tachycardia (sustained)

**EENT:** Bitter taste, blurred vision, diplopia, dry mouth, eye pain, lip or tongue swelling, nystagmus, periorbital edema, pharyngitis, sinusitis, tinnitus

**GI:** Abdominal pain, anorexia, diarrhea, dysphagia, elevated liver function test results, flatulence, hepatotoxicity, ileus, indigestion, nausea, vomiting

M

**GU:** Decreased libido, dysuria, flank pain, impotence, urinary frequency and incontinence, urine retention
**MS:** Myalgia
**RESP:** Apnea, asthma, cough, dyspnea, hyperventilation
**SKIN:** Diaphoresis, dry skin, pruritus, rash, urticaria
**Other:** Drug-induced fever

## Nursing Considerations
• Expect moricizine therapy to start in hospital because of the risk of proarrhythmias.
• Expect prescriber to discontinue previous antiarrhythmic one to two plasma half-lives before starting moricizine therapy.
• If needed to increase compliance, consult prescriber about changing to 12-hour dosing interval.
• Monitor liver and renal function test results for changes; expect prescriber to lower dose for patient with hepatic or renal impairment.
• Expect proarrhythmic effects to occur during first week of therapy, regardless of dosage.
• Anticipate higher risk of ventricular tachyarrhythmias in patients with cardiomegaly, coronary artery disease, heart failure, history of MI, or sustained ventricular tachycardia.
• Monitor ECG during therapy because drug may cause decreased JT interval and increased PR and QRS intervals. Notify prescriber if you detect such changes.
• **WARNING** Expect to discontinue drug if second- or third-degree AV block develops and patient doesn't have a ventricular pacemaker.
• Monitor serum electrolyte levels during therapy and correct imbalances, as prescribed.
• Expect an increased risk of dizziness and nausea with higher doses.

**PATIENT TEACHING**
• Instruct patient to take moricizine at evenly spaced intervals, as prescribed, even if he feels well.
• Advise patient to take a missed dose as soon as he remembers if it's 4 hours or more before the next scheduled dose. Caution against double-dosing.
• Teach patient how to check his pulse rate, and direct him to do so daily. Urge him to notify prescriber about significant changes.
• Advise patient to avoid hazardous activities until drug's CNS effects are known.
• Instruct patient to notify prescriber about chest pain, fast or irregular heartbeat, shortness of breath, and swelling of feet or lower legs.
• Urge patient to visit prescriber regularly to monitor progress.

# morphine sulfate
Astramorph PF, Avinza, Duramorph, Epimorph (CAN), Kadian, M-Eslon (CAN), Morphine Extra-Forte (CAN), Morphine Forte (CAN), Morphine H.P. (CAN), Morphitec (CAN), MS Contin, MSIR, MS/L, MS/L Concentrate, MS/S, OMS Concentrate, Oramorph SR, Rescudose, RMS Uniserts, Roxanol, Roxanol 100, Roxanol UD, Statex (CAN)

## Class, Category, and Schedule
*Chemical:* Phenanthrene derivative
*Therapeutic:* Analgesic
*Pregnancy category:* C
*Controlled substance:* Schedule II

## Indications and Dosages
➤ *To relieve acute or chronic moderate to severe pain; as adjunct to treat pulmonary edema caused by left-sided heart failure; to supplement general, local, or regional anesthesia*
**CAPSULES, ORAL SOLUTION, SYRUP, TABLETS**
**Adults.** *Initial:* 10 to 30 mg q 4 hr, p.r.n.
**Children.** Individualized dosage based on patient's age, size, and need.
**I.V. INFUSION**
**Adults.** *Initial:* 15 mg (or more) followed by 0.8 to 10 mg/hr, increased as needed for effectiveness. *Maintenance:* 0.8 to 80 mg/hr.
**Children.** 0.01 to 0.04 mg/kg/hr postoperatively, 0.025 to 2.6 mg/kg/hr for severe chronic cancer pain, or 0.03 to 0.15 mg/kg/hr for sickle cell crisis.
**Neonates.** *Initial:* 0.010 mg/kg/hr (10 mcg/kg/hr) postoperatively. *Maintenance:* 0.015 to 0.02 mg/kg/hr (15 to 20 mcg/kg/hr).
**I.V. INJECTION**
**Adults.** 2.5 to 15 mg injected slowly.
**Children.** 0.5 to 0.1 mg/kg administered slowly.
**I.M. OR S.C. INJECTION**
**Adults.** *Initial:* 10 mg (based on 70-kg [154-lb] adult) q 4 hr. *Maintenance:* 5 to 20 mg.
**Children.** *Initial:* 0.1 to 0.2 mg/kg q 4 hr. *Maximum:* 15 mg/dose.
**EPIDURAL INFUSION (PRESERVATIVE-FREE)**
**Adults.** *Initial:* 2 to 4 mg/24 hr, increased by 1 to 2 mg/24 hr, as directed.

EPIDURAL INJECTION (PRESERVATIVE-FREE)

**Adults.** *Initial:* 5 mg into lumbar region. If pain isn't relieved after 1 hr, 1- to 2-mg doses given at appropriate intervals to relieve pain. *Maximum:* 10 mg/24 hr.

INTRATHECAL INJECTION (PRESERVATIVE-FREE)

**Adults.** 0.2 to 1 mg as a single dose.

SUPPOSITORIES

**Adults.** 10 to 30 mg q 4 hr, p.r.n.

**Children.** Individualized dosage based on patient's age, size, and need.

➤ *To relieve chronic moderate to severe pain that requires opioids for more than a few days*

E.R. CAPSULES

**Adults.** Individualized dosage given q 12 to 24 hr.

E.R. TABLETS

**Adults.** 30 mg q 12 hr. Dosage increased based on patient's response.

➤ *To relieve MI pain*

I.V. INJECTION

**Adults.** 1 to 4 mg by slow I.V. injection. Repeated up to q 5 min, if needed. *Maximum:* 2 to 15 mg.

➤ *To provide preoperative analgesia*

I.M. OR S.C. INJECTION

**Adults.** 5 to 20 mg given 45 to 60 min before surgery.

**Children.** 0.05 to 0.1 mg/kg given 45 to 60 min before surgery. *Maximum:* 10 mg.

➤ *To provide analgesia during labor*

I.M. OR S.C. INJECTION

**Adults.** 10 mg, with subsequent doses based on patient's response.

| Route | Onset | Peak | Duration |
|---|---|---|---|
| P.O. | Unknown | 1 to 2 hr | 4 to 5 hr |
| P.O. (E.R.) | Unknown | Unknown | 8 to 12 hr |
| I.V. | Unknown | 20 min | 4 to 5 hr |
| I.M. | 10 to 30 min | 30 to 60 min | 4 to 5 hr |
| S.C. | 10 to 30 min | 50 to 90 min | 4 to 5 hr |
| Epidural | 15 to 60 min | Unknown | Up to 24 hr |
| Intrathecal | 15 to 60 min | Unknown | Up to 24 hr |
| P.R. | 20 to 60 min | Unknown | Unknown |

## Mechanism of Action

Binds with and activates opioid receptors (mainly mu receptors) in brain and spinal cord to produce analgesia and euphoria.

## Contraindications

*For all drug forms:* Asthma, hypersensitivity to morphine or its components, labor (premature delivery), prematurity (in infants), respiratory depression, upper airway obstruction

*For oral solution:* Acute abdominal disorders, acute alcoholism, alcohol withdrawal syndrome, arrhythmias, brain tumor, head injuries, heart failure caused by chronic lung disease, increased intracranial or cerebrospinal pressure, recent biliary tract surgery, respiratory insufficiency, seizure disorders, severe CNS depression, surgical anastomosis, use within 14 days of an MAO inhibitor

*For I.V., I.M., or S.C. injection:* Acute alcoholism, alcohol withdrawal syndrome, arrhythmias, brain tumor, heart failure caused by chronic lung disease, seizure disorders

*For epidural or intrathecal injection:* Anticoagulant therapy, bleeding tendency, injection site infection, parenteral corticosteroid treatment (or other treatment or condition that prohibits drug administration by intrathecal or epidural route) within 2 weeks

## Interactions

DRUGS

*amitriptyline, clomipramine, nortriptyline:* Increased CNS and respiratory depression

*anticholinergics:* Possibly severe constipation leading to ileus, urine retention

*antidiarrheals (such as loperamide and paregoric):* CNS depression, possibly severe constipation

*antihistamines, chloral hydrate, glutethimide, MAO inhibitors, methocarbamol:* Increased CNS and respiratory depressant effects of morphine

*antihypertensives, hypotension-producing drugs:* Increased hypotension, risk of orthostatic hypotension

*buprenorphine:* Decreased therapeutic effects of morphine, increased respiratory depression, possibly withdrawal symptoms

*cimetidine:* Increased analgesic and CNS and respiratory depressant effects of morphine

*CNS depressants (antiemetics, general anesthetics, hypnotics, phenothiazines, sedatives,*

**M**

*tranquilizers):* Possibly coma, hypotension, respiratory depression, severe sedation
*diuretics:* Decreased diuretic efficacy
*hydroxyzine:* Increased analgesic, CNS depressant, and hypotensive effects of morphine
*metoclopramide:* Possibly antagonized metoclopramide effect on GI motility
*mixed agonist-antagonist analgesics:* Possibly withdrawal symptoms
*naloxone:* Antagonized analgesic and CNS and respiratory depressant effects of morphine, possibly withdrawal symptoms
*naltrexone:* Possibly induction or worsening of withdrawal symptoms if morphine given within 7 to 10 days before naltrexone
*neuromuscular blockers:* Increased or prolonged respiratory depression
*opioid analgesics (such as alfentanil and sufentanil):* Increased CNS and respiratory depression, increased hypotension
*zidovudine:* Decreased zidovudine clearance

**ACTIVITIES**
*alcohol use:* Increased CNS and respiratory depression, increased hypotension

## Adverse Reactions

**CNS:** Amnesia, anxiety, coma, confusion, decreased concentration, delirium, delusions, depression, dizziness, drowsiness, euphoria, fever, hallucinations, headache, insomnia, lethargy, light-headedness, malaise, psychosis, restlessness, sedation, seizures, syncope, tremor
**CV:** Bradycardia, cardiac arrest, hypotension, orthostatic hypotension, palpitations, shock, tachycardia
**EENT:** Blurred vision, diplopia, dry mouth, laryngeal edema or laryngospasm (allergic), miosis, nystagmus, rhinitis
**GI:** Abdominal cramps or pain, anorexia, biliary tract spasm, constipation, diarrhea, dysphagia, elevated liver function test results, gastroesophageal reflux, hiccups, ileus and toxic megacolon (in patients with inflammatory bowel disease), intestinal obstruction, indigestion, nausea, vomiting
**GU:** Decreased ejaculate potency, decreased libido, difficult ejaculation, impotence, menstrual irregularities, oliguria, prolonged labor, urinary hesitancy, urine retention
**HEME:** Anemia, leukopenia, thrombocytopenia
**MS:** Arthralgia
**RESP:** Apnea, asthma exacerbation, atelectasis, bronchospasm, depressed cough reflex, hypoventilation, pulmonary edema, respiratory arrest and depression, wheezing
**SKIN:** Diaphoresis, flushing, pallor, pruritus, urticaria
**Other:** Allergic reaction; anaphylaxis; facial edema; injection site edema, pain, rash, or redness; physical and psychological dependence; withdrawal symptoms

## Nursing Considerations

• Store morphine sulfate at room temperature.
• Before giving morphine, make sure opioid antagonist and equipment for giving oxygen and controlling respiration are available.
• Before therapy, assess patient's drug use, including all prescription and OTC drugs.
• Expect prescriber to start patient who has never received opioids on immediate-release form and then switch to E.R. form if therapy must last longer than a few days.
• Give oral form with food or milk to minimize adverse GI reactions, if needed. If desired, mix oral solution with fruit juice to improve taste.
• If needed, open E.R. capsules and sprinkle contents on applesauce (at room temperature or cooler) just before giving to patient. Make sure patient doesn't chew or crush capsules or dissolve capsule's pellets in his mouth.
• Be aware that E.R. forms of morphine aren't interchangeable.
• Discard injection solution that is discolored or darker than pale yellow or that contains precipitates that don't dissolve with shaking.
• **WARNING** Don't use highly concentrated morphine solutions (such as 10 to 25 mg/ml) for single-dose I.V., I.M., or S.C. administration. These solutions are intended for use in continuous, controlled microinfusion devices.
• For direct I.V. injection, dilute appropriate dose with 4 to 5 ml of sterile water for injection. Inject 2.5 to 15 mg directly into tubing of free-flowing I.V. solution over 4 to 5 minutes. Rapid I.V. injection may increase adverse reactions.
• For continuous I.V. infusion, dilute drug in $D_5W$ and administer with infusion-control device. Adjust dose and rate based on patient response, as prescribed.
• Avoid I.M. route for long-term therapy because of injection site irritation.
• During S.C. injection, take care to avoid injecting drug intradermally.

•For intrathecal injection, expect prescriber to give no more than 2 ml of 0.5-mg/ml solution or 1 ml of 1-mg/ml solution. Expect intrathecal dosage to be about one-tenth of epidural dosage.

•If rectal suppository is too soft to insert, chill it in refrigerator for 30 minutes or run wrapped suppository under cold tap water.

•**WARNING** Monitor respiratory and cardiovascular status carefully and frequently during morphine therapy. Be alert for respiratory depression and hypotension.

•Monitor patient for excessive or persistent sedation; dosage may need to be adjusted.

•If patient is receiving a continuous morphine infusion, watch for and notify prescriber about new neurologic signs or symptoms. Inflammatory masses (such as granulomas) have caused serious neurologic reactions, including paralysis.

•Expect morphine to cause physical and psychological dependence; watch for drug tolerance and withdrawal symptoms, such as body aches, diaphoresis, diarrhea, fever, piloerection, rhinorrhea, sneezing, and yawning.

•If tolerance to morphine develops, expect prescriber to increase dosage.

•Morphine may have a prolonged duration and cumulative effect in patients with impaired hepatic or renal function. It also may prolong labor by reducing strength, duration, and frequency of uterine contractions.

•When discontinuing morphine in patients receiving more than 30 mg/day, expect prescriber to reduce daily dose by about one-half for 2 days and then by 25% every 2 days thereafter until total dose reaches initial amount recommended for patients who haven't received opioids (15 to 30 mg/day). This regimen minimizes the risk of withdrawal symptoms.

**PATIENT TEACHING**

•Instruct patient to take morphine exactly as prescribed and not to change dosage without consulting prescriber.

•Inform patient that he may take tablets or capsules with food or milk to relieve GI distress and may mix oral solution with juice to improve taste.

•Urge patient not to break, chew, or crush E.R. capsules and tablets to avoid rapid release and, possibly, toxicity.

•For patient who has difficulty swallowing, suggest that he open E.R. capsules and sprinkle contents on food or liquids. Urge him to take drug immediately and not let capsule contents dissolve in his mouth.

•Instruct patient to moisten rectal suppository before inserting it.

•Urge patient to avoid alcohol and other CNS depressants during morphine therapy.

•Advise patient to avoid potentially hazardous activities during morphine therapy.

•Tell patient to change positions slowly to minimize the effects of orthostatic hypotension.

•Instruct patient to notify prescriber about worsening or breakthrough pain.

•Inform patient that morphine may be habit-forming. Urge him to notify prescriber if he experiences anxiety, decreased appetite, excessive tearing, irritability, muscle aches or twitching, rapid heart rate, or yawning.

•Advise female patient to notify prescriber if she becomes pregnant. Regular morphine use during pregnancy may cause physical dependence in fetus and withdrawal in neonate.

# moxifloxacin hydrochloride

Avelox, Avelox IV

## Class and Category

*Chemical:* Fluoroquinolone
*Therapeutic:* Antibiotic
*Pregnancy category:* C

## Indications and Dosages

➤ *To treat acute sinusitis caused by* Haemophilus influenzae, Moraxella catarrhalis, *or* Streptococcus pneumoniae; *to treat mild to moderate community-acquired pneumonia caused by* Chlamydia pneumoniae, H. influenzae, M. catarrhalis, Mycoplasma pneumoniae, *or* S. pneumoniae *(including penicillin- or multi-drug-resistant strains)*

**TABLETS, I.V. INFUSION**

**Adults.** 400 mg q 24 hr for 10 days.

➤ *To treat acute exacerbation of chronic bronchitis caused by* H. influenzae, H. parainfluenzae, Klebsiella pneumoniae, M. catarrhalis, S. pneumoniae, *or* Staphylococcus aureus

TABLETS, I.V. INFUSION
**Adults.** 400 mg q 24 hr for 5 days.

➤ *To treat uncomplicated skin and soft-tissue infections caused by* S. aureus *or* Streptococcus pyogenes
TABLETS, I.V. INFUSION
**Adults.** 400 mg q 24 hr for 7 days.

➤ *To treat complicated skin and skin structure infections caused by* S. aureus, E. coli, K. pneumoniae, *or* Enterobacter cloacae
TABLETS, I.V. INFUSION
**Adults.** 400 mg q 24 hr for 7 to 21 days.

➤ *To treat complicated intra-abdominal infections, including polymicrobial infections such as abscesses caused by* E.coli, Bacteroides fragilis, Streptococcus anginosus, Streptococcus constellatus, Enterococcus faecalis, Proteus mirabilis, Clostridium perfringens, Bacteroides thetaiotaomicron, *or* Peptostreptococcus *species*
TABLETS, I.V. INFUSION
**Adults.** 400 mg q 24 hr for 5 to 14 days with initial dosage given as I.V. infusion.

## Incompatibilities
Do not infuse I.V. form of moxifloxacin simultaneously through the same I.V. line with other I.V. substances, additives, or drugs.

---

### Mechanism of Action
Inhibits synthesis of the bacterial enzyme DNA gyrase by counteracting the excessive supercoiling of DNA during replication or transcription. Inhibition of DNA gyrase causes rapid- and slow-growing bacterial cells to die.

---

## Contraindications
Hypersensitivity to moxifloxacin, other fluoroquinolones, or their components

## Interactions
**DRUGS**
*aluminum- or magnesium-containing antacids; drug formulations with divalent or trivalent cations, such as didanosine chewable buffered tablets or powder for oral solution; metal cations, such as iron; multivitamins containing iron or zinc; sucralfate:* Possibly substantial interference with moxi-floxacin absorption, causing low blood moxifloxacin level
*class Ia antiarrhythmics, such as quinidine; class III antiarrhythmics, such as sotalol; other drugs known to prolong QTc interval, such as disopyramide and pentamidine:* Possibly prolonged QTc interval
*corticosteroids:* Increased risk of Achilles and other tendon ruptures
*NSAIDs:* Increased risk of CNS stimulation and seizures
*warfarin:* Possibly increased anticoagulation

## Adverse Reactions
**CNS:** Dizziness, headache, psychosis, psychotic reaction, seizures, syncope
**CV:** Hypertension, hypotension, palpitations, peripheral edema, tachycardia, vasodilation, ventricular tachyarrhythmias
**EENT:** Altered taste
**GI:** Abdominal pain, abnormal liver function test results, cholestatic hepatitis, diarrhea, dyspepsia, hepatitis, nausea, pseudomembranous colitis, vomiting
**HEME:** Anemia, eosinophilia, leukopenia, prolonged PT, thrombocytopenia
**MS:** Tendon inflammation, pain, or rupture
**Skin:** Stevens-Johnson syndrome
**Other:** Anaphylaxis, anaphylactic shock, angioedema

## Nursing Considerations
• Obtain a fluid or tissue specimen for culture and sensitivity, as ordered. Expect to begin therapy before results are available.
• **WARNING** Before starting therapy, determine if patient receives a class Ia antiarrhythmic, such as quinidine; a class III antiarrhythmic, such as sotalol; or other drugs that prolong the QTc interval. Be aware that these drugs should be avoided in patients taking moxifloxacin because they may prolong the QTc interval and lead to life-threatening ventricular tachycardia or torsades de pointes.
• Infuse over 60 minutes with ready-to-use flexible bags with 400 mg of moxifloxacin in 250 ml of 0.8% saline. Don't dilute further.
• If giving through Y-type tubing or piggyback method, stop other solutions during moxifloxacin infusion, and flush the line before and after infusion with a compatible solution, such as 0.9% NaCl, 1M NaCl, 5% dextrose, sterile water for injection, 10% dextrose, or lactated Ringer's. Also flush line

before and after giving other drugs in the same I.V. line.

• Don't refrigerate I.V. moxifloxacin ready-to-use bags because precipitation will occur. Discard any unused portion; premixed bags are for single-use only.

• Expect to obtain a 12-lead ECG to assess patient for a prolonged QTc interval. Ask patient if he or a blood relative has a history of prolonged QTc interval.

• If patient has hypokalemia, expect to correct it before beginning moxifloxacin therapy to prevent arrhythmias.

• Determine if patient has a history of a CNS disorder, such as cerebral arteriosclerosis or epilepsy, because drug may lower the seizure threshold. Notify prescriber before therapy starts, and take seizure precautions.

• If profuse, watery diarrhea develops, contact prescriber and expect to obtain a stool specimen to rule out pseudomembranous colitis.

• Monitor serum potassium level, as ordered, during therapy to assess for hypokalemia.

• Keep emergency resuscitation equipment readily available, and observe for evidence of hypersensitivity, such as angioedema, dyspnea, and urticaria. If you suspect anaphylaxis, prepare to give epinephrine, corticosteroids, and diphenhydramine, as prescribed.

**PATIENT TEACHING**

• Advise patient to notify prescriber immediately about palpitations or fainting because they may indicate a serious arrhythmia.

• Teach patient to take drug at least 4 hours before and 8 hours after aluminum- or magnesium-containing antacids, didanosine chewable buffered tablets or oral solution prepared from powder, multivitamins containing iron or zinc, or sucralfate.

• Urge patient to drink plenty of fluids while taking moxifloxacin.

• Caution patient to stop taking drug and notify prescriber if he experiences difficulty breathing, a rash, or other signs of an allergic reaction.

• Urge patient to stop any exercise and contact prescriber immediately if he develops tendon inflammation, pain, or rupture.

• Caution patient to avoid activities of mental alertness until adverse CNS effects are known.

• Urge patient to tell prescriber about diarrhea.

• Caution patient to complete the prescribed course of therapy even if he feels better.

# mycophenolate mofetil

CellCept, CellCept Oral Suspension

## mycophenolate mofetil hydrochloride

CellCept Intravenous

## mycophenolic acid

Myfortic

## Class and Category

*Chemical:* 2-morpholinoethyl ester of mycophenolic acid
*Therapeutic:* Immunosuppressant
*Pregnancy category:* C

## Indications and Dosages

➤ *To prevent organ rejection in patients receiving allogenic kidney transplants*

**CAPSULES, ORAL SUSPENSION, TABLETS, I.V. INFUSION**

**Adults.** 1 g (over 2 hr for I.V. infusion) b.i.d.

**E.R. TABLETS**

**Adults.** 720 mg b.i.d.

**SUSPENSION**

**Children with body surface area less than 1.25 m².** 600 mg/m² b.i.d. *Maximum:* 2 g (10 ml) daily.

**CAPSULES**

**Children with body surface area of 1.25 m² to 1.5 m².** 750 mg b.i.d.

**CAPSULES, TABLETS**

**Children with body surface area greater than 1.5 m².** 1 g b.i.d.

➤ *To prevent organ rejection in patients receiving allogenic heart transplants*

**CAPSULES, ORAL SUSPENSION, TABLETS, I.V. INFUSION**

**Adults.** 1.5 g (over 2 hr for I.V. infusion) b.i.d.

➤ *To prevent organ rejection in patients receiving allogenic liver transplants*

**I.V. INFUSION**

**Adults.** 1 g infused over 2 hr b.i.d.

**CAPSULES, ORAL SUSPENSION, TABLETS**

**Adults.** 1.5 g b.i.d.

## Incompatibilities

Don't mix or administer mycophenolate mofetil hydrochloride in the same infusion catheter with other I.V. drugs or admixtures.

## Contraindications

Hypersensitivity to mycophenolate mofetil, mycophenolic acid, or any of its components; hypersensitivity to polysorbate 80 (I.V. form)

M

## Mechanism of Action

Hydrolyzes to form mycophenolic acid (MPA), which inhibits guanosine nucleotide synthesis and proliferation of T and B lymphocytes. MPA also suppresses antibody formation by B lymphocytes and prevents glycosylation of lymphocyte and monocyte glycoproteins involved in adhesion to endothelial cells. MPA also may inhibit leukocytes from sites of inflammation and graft rejection, which may explain how mycophenolate mofetil prolongs allogeneic transplant survival.

## Interactions
### DRUGS

*acyclovir, ganciclovir, probenecid:* Increased plasma levels of both drugs
*antacids with magnesium and aluminum hydroxides:* Decreased absorption of oral mycophenolate mofetil
*azathioprine:* Increased bone marrow suppression
*cholestyramine:* Decreased plasma level of mycophenolate mofetil
*live vaccines:* Decreased effectiveness of live vaccines
*oral contraceptives:* Possibly decreased effectiveness of oral contraceptives

## Adverse Reactions

**CNS:** Agitation, anxiety, chills, confusion, delirium, depression, dizziness, emotional lability, fever, hallucinations, headache, hypertonia, hypesthesia, insomnia, malaise, nervousness, neuropathy, paresthesia, psychosis, seizure, somnolence, syncope, thinking abnormality, tremor, vertigo
**CV:** Angina pectoris, arrhythmias, arterial thrombosis, atrial fibrillation or flutter, bradycardia, cardiac arrest, cardiovascular disorder, congestive heart failure, extrasystole, generalized edema, hemorrhage, hypercholesteremia, hyperlipemia, hypertension, hypotension, increased lactic dehydrogenase, increased SGOT and SGPT, increased venous pressure, palpitation, pericardial effusion, peripheral edema, peripheral vascular disorder, postural hypotension, pulmonary edema or hypertension, supraventricular tachycardia, thrombosis, vasodilation, vasospasm, ventricular extrasystole, ventricular tachycardia

**EENT:** Amblyopia, cataract, conjunctivitis, deafness, dry mouth, ear disorder or pain, epistaxis, eye hemorrhage, gingivitis, gum hyperplasia, lacrimation disorder, mouth ulceration, oral moniliasis, pharyngitis, rhinitis, sinusitis, stomatitis, tinnitus, vision abnormality, voice alteration
**ENDO:** Cushing's syndrome, diabetes mellitus, hypercalcemia, hypocalcemia, hypoglycemia, hypothyroidism, parathyroid disorder
**GI:** Abdomen enlargement or pain, anorexia, ascites, cholangitis, cholestatic jaundice, constipation, diarrhea, dyspepsia, dysphagia, esophagitis, flatulence, gastritis, gastroenteritis, gastrointestinal hemorrhage, gastrointestinal infection, gastrointestinal moniliasis, hepatitis, hernia, ileus, jaundice, liver damage, liver function test abnormalities, melena, nausea, peritonitis, rectal disorder, stomach ulcer, vomiting
**GU:** Albuminuria; bilirubinemia; dysuria; hematuria; hydronephrosis; impotence; increased BUN or creatinine levels; kidney tubular necrosis; nocturia; oliguria; pain; prostatic disorder; pyelonephritis; renal failure; scrotal edema, urinary tract disorder or infection; urine abnormality, frequency, incontinence, or retention
**HEME:** anemia, coagulation disorder, hypochromic anemia, increased prothrombin time or thromboplastin time, leukocytosis, leukopenia, polyhemia, thrombocytopenia
**MS:** Arthralgia; back, neck or pelvic pain; joint disorder; leg cramps; myalgia; myasthenia; osteoporosis
**RESP:** Apnea; asthma; atelectasis; bronchitis; cough; dyspnea; hemoptysis; hyperventilation; hypoxia; lung edema; pleural effusion; pneumonia; pneumothorax; respiratory acidosis, moniliasis, neoplasm, or pain; sputum increase
**SKIN:** Abscess; acne; cellulite; ecchymosis; fungal dermatitis; pallor; petechia; pruritus; rash; benign neoplasm, carcinoma, hypertrophy, or ulcer; sweating; vesiculobullous rash
**Other:** Abnormal healing, accidental injury, acidosis, alkalosis, alopecia, cyst, dehydration, facial edema, flulike syndrome, gout, hiccup, hirsutism, hyperkalemia, hyperuricemia, hypervolemia, hypochloremia, hypokalemia, hypomagnesemia, hyponatremia, hypoproteinemia, hypophosphatemia, increased alkaline phosphatase, increased

gamma glutamyl transpeptidase, infection, sepsis, thirst, weight gain or loss

## Nursing Considerations
• Expect to give I.V. form within 24 hours of transplantation and for no longer than 14 days. Expect to switch patient to oral form as soon as possible, as ordered.
• Expect to administer oral form of drug as soon as possible following transplantation.
• When preparing oral suspension or I.V. form, avoid inhalation or direct contact with skin or mucous membranes. If contact occurs, wash area thoroughly with soap and water and rinse eyes with water.
• To prepare oral suspension, tap closed bottle several times to loosen powder and then measure 94 ml of water in a graduated cylinder. Add half of the water to the bottle and shake for about 1 minute. Then add reminder of water and shake again for 1 minute. Remove child-resistant cap and push bottle adapter into neck of bottle. Close bottle tightly with child-resistant cap. Be aware that the suspension bottle may become cold immediately after reconstitution.
• Know that oral suspension can be administered by 8F or larger nasogastric tube.
• When giving oral suspension, don't mix with any other drugs. Ask patient about history of phenylketonuria before initial administration because oral suspension contains aspartame.
• Don't open or crush capsules. If necessary, use the oral suspension.
• Handle I.V. form similarly to a chemotherapeutic drug because mycophenolate mofetil is genotoxic and embryotoxic and may have mutagenic properties.
• Know that I.V. form must be reconstituted and diluted to 6 mg/ml using 5% dextrose injection USP. Inject 14 ml of 5% dextrose injection USP into each vial (two vials will be needed for each 1-g dose; three vials for each 1.5-g dose), then shake gently. Further dilute a 1-g dose by adding two reconstituted vials to 140 ml of 5% dextrose injection USP; dilute a 1.5-g dose by adding three reconstituted vials to 210 ml of 5% dextrose injection USP.
• Be aware that I.V. should be administered within 4 hours of constitution as an infusion over no less than 2 hours. Never administer by rapid or bolus I.V. injection.

• Know that cyclosporine and corticosteroids should be used with mycophenolate mofetil therapy.
• Obtain CBC weekly during first month of therapy, twice monthly for the second and third months of therapy, and then monthly through the first year, as ordered.
• Monitor patient closely for adverse reactions because drug has many adverse effects, some of which can be serious or severe.
• Expect to stop drug or reduce the dose and provide supportive care, as ordered, if neutropenia develops.

**PATIENT TEACHING**
• Advise women of childbearing age that two forms of contraceptives should be used simultaneously before beginning mycophenolate mofetil therapy and for 6 weeks following discontinuation of therapy because of potential for fetal harm. Inform women who use oral contraceptives that drug may decrease effectiveness of oral contraceptives. Urge patient to notify prescriber immediately if pregnancy occurs.
• Tell patient to take oral form of drug on an empty stomach.
• Instruct patient not to crush tablets or capsules or open capsules.
• Inform patient not to receive live vaccines during therapy. Urge him to avoid people who have received such vaccines or to wear a protective mask when he's around them.
• Caution patient to avoid contact with people who have infections because drug causes immunosuppression.
• Tell patient to report any signs of infection, unexpected bruising or bleeding, or any other sign of bone marrow depression immediately.
• Advise patient to avoid exposure to direct sunlight and UV light and to wear sunscreen when outdoors because of increased risk for skin cancer.
• Advise patient not to take antacids at the same time as oral mycophenolate mofetil because some antacids can decrease drug's absorption.
• Stress importance of follow-up care to monitor the drug's effectiveness and possible adverse effects because of the increased risk for cancer and infections as a result of immunosuppression. Inform patient of the need for periodic laboratory tests.

# N·O

# nabumetone

Relafen

## Class and Category

*Chemical:* Naphthylalkanone derivative
*Therapeutic:* Anti-inflammatory, antirheumatic
*Pregnancy category:* C (first trimester), Not rated (later trimesters)

## Indications and Dosages

➤ *To relieve symptoms of acute and chronic osteoarthritis and rheumatoid arthritis*

**TABLETS**

**Adults.** *Initial:* 1 g/day as a single dose or in divided doses b.i.d., increased to 1.5 to 2 g/day in divided doses b.i.d. *Maintenance:* Adjusted according to clinical response. *Maximum:* 2 g/day.

---

### Mechanism of Action

Blocks activity of cyclooxygenase, the enzyme needed to synthesize prostaglandins, which mediate the inflammatory response and cause local vasodilation, swelling, and pain. Prostaglandins also promote pain transmission from the periphery to the spinal cord. By blocking cyclooxygenase and inhibiting prostaglandins, the NSAID nabumetone reduces inflammatory symptoms and relieves pain.

---

## Contraindications

Angioedema, asthma, bronchospasm, nasal polyps, rhinitis, or urticaria induced by aspirin, iodides, or other NSAIDs

## Interactions

**DRUGS**

*acetaminophen (long-term use):* Increased risk of adverse renal effects
*anticoagulants, thrombolytics:* Increased risk of GI bleeding
*antihypertensives:* Decreased antihypertensive effectiveness
*beta blockers:* Decreased antihypertensive effects of beta blockers

*bone marrow depressants, such as aldesleukin and cisplatin:* Increased risk of leukopenia and thrombocytopenia
*cefamandole, cefoperazone, cefotetan, plicamycin, valproic acid:* Increased risk of hypoprothrombinemia and bleeding
*colchicine, other NSAIDs, salicylates:* Increased GI irritability and bleeding
*cyclosporine, gold compounds, nephrotoxic drugs:* Increased risk of nephrotoxicity
*digoxin:* Increased blood digoxin level and risk of digitalis toxicity
*diuretics:* Decreased diuretic effectiveness
*glucocorticoids, potassium supplements:* Increased GI irritability and bleeding
*insulin, oral antidiabetic drugs:* Increased effectiveness of these drugs; risk of hypoglycemia
*lithium:* Increased risk of lithium toxicity
*methotrexate:* Increased risk of methotrexate toxicity
*probenecid:* Increased risk of nabumetone toxicity

**ACTIVITIES**

*alcohol use:* Increased GI irritability and bleeding

## Adverse Reactions

**CNS:** Drowsiness, fatigue, fever, headache, nervousness, seizures, stroke, vertigo
**CV:** Edema, hypertension, MI, tachycardia
**EENT:** Dry mouth, pharyngitis, stomatitis, tinnitus
**GI:** Abdominal pain, anorexia, constipation, diarrhea, diverticulitis, dyspepsia, dysphagia, esophagitis, flatulence, gastritis, gastroenteritis, gastroesophageal reflux disease, GI bleeding and ulceration, hepatic dysfunction, indigestion, jaundice, melena, nausea, perforation of stomach or intestines, stomatitis, vomiting
**GU:** Albuminuria, azotemia, interstitial nephritis, nephrotic syndrome
**HEME:** Agranulocytosis, anemia, eosinophilia, granulocytopenia, hemolytic anemia, leukopenia, neutropenia, pancytopenia, thrombocytopenia
**MS:** Muscle spasms, myalgia
**RESP:** Asthma, pneumonitis, respiratory depression
**SKIN:** Alopecia, erythema multiforme, photosensitivity, pruritus, rash, Stevens-Johnson syndrome, toxic epidermal necrolysis
**Other:** Anaphylaxis, angioedema

**N**
**O**

## Nursing Considerations

• Use nabumetone with extreme caution in patients with a history of ulcer disease or GI bleeding because NSAIDs such as nabumetone increase the risk of GI bleeding and ulceration. Expect to use nabumetone for the shortest time possible in these patients.

• Be aware that serious GI tract ulceration, bleeding, and perforation may occur without warning symptoms. Elderly patients are at greater risk. To minimize risk, give drug with food. If GI distress occurs, withhold drug and notify prescriber immediately.

• Use nabumetone cautiously in patients with hypertension, and monitor blood pressure closely throughout therapy. Drug may cause hypertension or worsen it.

•**WARNING** Monitor patient closely for thrombotic events, including MI and stroke, because NSAIDs increase the risk.

• Monitor patient—especially if he's elderly or receiving long-term nabumetone therapy—for less common but serious adverse GI reactions, including anorexia, constipation, diverticulitis, dysphagia, esophagitis, gastritis, gastroenteritis, gastroesophageal reflux disease, hemorrhoids, hiatal hernia, melena, stomatitis, and vomiting.

• Monitor liver function test results because, in rare cases, elevations may progress to severe hepatic reactions, including fatal hepatitis, liver necrosis, and hepatic failure.

• Monitor BUN and serum creatinine levels in elderly patients, patients taking diuretics or ACE inhibitors, and patients with heart failure, impaired renal function, or hepatic dysfunction; nabumetone may cause renal failure.

• Monitor CBC for decreased hemoglobin and hematocrit because drug may worsen anemia.

•**WARNING** If patient has bone marrow suppression or is receiving treatment with an antineoplastic, monitor laboratory results (including WBC count), and watch for evidence of infection because anti-inflammatory and antipyretic actions of nabumetone may mask signs and symptoms, such as fever and pain.

• Assess patient's skin regularly for signs of rash or other hypersensitivity reaction because nabumetone is an NSAID and may cause serious skin reactions without warning, even in patients with no history of NSAID sensitivity. At first sign of reaction, stop drug and notify prescriber.

• Assess patient for severe hepatic reactions, including jaundice. Stop drug, as prescribed, if symptoms persist.

**PATIENT TEACHING**

• Instruct patient to take nabumetone with food to reduce GI distress.

• Advise patient to take drug with a full glass of water and to remain upright for 15 to 30 minutes afterward to prevent drug from lodging in the esophagus and causing irritation.

• Caution patient not to increase dosage or frequency of use without consulting prescriber.

• Urge patient to avoid alcohol to reduce risk of GI bleeding.

• Inform patient that regular laboratory tests are needed to check for drug toxicity during long-term therapy.

• Caution pregnant patient not to take NSAIDs such as nabumetone during the last trimester because they may cause premature closure of the ductus arteriosus.

• Explain that nabumetone may increase the risk of serious adverse cardiovascular reactions; urge patient to seek immediate medical attention if signs or symptoms arise, such as chest pain, shortness of breath, weakness, and slurring of speech.

• Explain that nabumetone may increase the risk of serious adverse GI reactions; stress the importance of seeking immediate medical attention for such signs and symptoms as epigastric or abdominal pain, indigestion, black or tarry stools, or vomiting blood or material that looks like coffee grounds.

• Alert patient to rare but serious skin reactions. Urge her to seek immediate medical attention for rash, blisters, itching, fever, or other indications of hypersensitivity.

# nadolol

Corgard, Syn-Nadolol (CAN)

## Class and Category

*Chemical:* Nonselective beta blocker
*Therapeutic:* Antianginal, antihypertensive
*Pregnancy category:* C

## Indications and Dosages

➤ *To manage hypertension, alone or with other antihypertensives*

**TABLETS**
**Adults.** *Initial:* 40 mg q.d., increased by 40 to 80 mg/day q 7 days, as prescribed. *Maintenance:* 40 to 80 mg/day. *Maximum:* 320 mg/day.

➤ *To manage angina pectoris as long-term therapy*
**TABLETS**
**Adults.** *Initial:* 40 mg q.d., increased by 40 to 80 mg/day q 3 to 7 days, as prescribed. *Maintenance:* 40 to 80 mg/day. *Maximum:* 240 mg/day.
DOSAGE ADJUSTMENT Interval possibly increased to q 24 to 36 hr if creatinine clearance is 31 to 50 ml/min/1.73 m$^2$; to q 24 to 48 hr if it's 10 to 30 ml/min/1.73 m$^2$; or to q 40 to 60 hr if it's less than 10 ml/min/1.73 m$^2$.

| Route | Onset | Peak | Duration |
|-------|-------|------|----------|
| P.O. | Up to 5 days | 4 hr | 24 hr |

**Mechanism of Action**
Selectively blocks alpha$_1$ and beta$_2$ receptors in vascular smooth muscle and beta$_1$ receptors in the heart, thereby reducing peripheral vascular resistance and blood pressure. Potent beta blockade decreases cardiac excitability, cardiac output, and myocardial oxygen demand, thus reducing angina. It also prevents reflex tachycardia, which typically occurs with most alpha blockers.

**Contraindications**
Asthma; bronchospasm; cardiogenic shock; heart failure; hypersensitivity to nadolol, other beta blockers, or their components; second- or third-degree AV block; severe COPD; sinus bradycardia

**Interactions**
**DRUGS**
*allergen immunotherapy, allergenic extracts for skin testing:* Increased risk of serious systemic reactions or anaphylaxis
*amiodarone:* Increased risk of conduction abnormalities and negative inotropic effects
*calcium channel blockers:* Increased risk of bradycardia
*cimetidine:* Possibly increased effects of nadolol

*clonidine, guanabenz:* Impaired blood pressure control
*diazoxide, nitroglycerin:* Increased risk of hypotension
*estrogens, NSAIDs:* Possibly reduced antihypertensive effect of nadolol
*general anesthetics:* Increased risk of hypotension and myocardial depression
*insulin, oral antidiabetic drugs:* Possibly increased risk of hyperglycemia and impaired recovery from hypoglycemia, masking of signs of hypoglycemia
*lidocaine:* Increased risk of lidocaine toxicity
*neuromuscular blockers:* Possibly prolonged action of these drugs
*phenothiazines:* Possibly increased blood levels of both drugs
*reserpine:* Increased risk of bradycardia and hypotension
*sympathomimetics with alpha- and beta-adrenergic effects, such as pseudoephedrine:* Possibly hypertension, excessive bradycardia, and heart block
*xanthines, such as theophyllines:* Possibly decreased therapeutic effects of both drugs

**Adverse Reactions**
**CNS:** Anxiety, depression, dizziness, drowsiness, fatigue, headache, paresthesia, syncope, vertigo, weakness, yawning
**CV:** Bradycardia, chest pain, edema, heart block, heart failure, hypotension, orthostatic hypotension, ventricular arrhythmias
**EENT:** Nasal congestion, taste perversion
**GI:** Dyspepsia, elevated liver function test results, hepatic necrosis, hepatitis, nausea, vomiting
**GU:** Ejaculation failure, impotence
**RESP:** Cough, dyspnea, wheezing
**SKIN:** Jaundice, pruritus, scalp tingling

**Nursing Complications**
•Use nadolol cautiously in patients with diabetes mellitus because it may prolong or worsen hypoglycemia by interfering with glycogenolysis.
•Anticipate that drug may worsen psoriasis and, in patients with myasthenia gravis, muscle weakness and diplopia.
•WARNING Withdraw drug gradually over 2 weeks, or as ordered, to avoid MI caused by unopposed beta stimulation or thyroid storm caused by underlying hyperthyroidism. Expect drug to mask tachycardia caused by hyperthyroidism.

•Teach patient how to take her radial pulse, and direct her to do so before each dose of nadolol.
•Instruct patient to notify prescriber if pulse rate falls below 60 beats/minute.
•Caution patient not to stop taking drug abruptly or change dosage. Direct her to take a missed dose as soon as possible unless it's within 8 hours of the next scheduled dose.
•Advise patient with diabetes to monitor blood glucose level frequently because nadolol may mask signs of hypoglycemia, such as tachycardia.
•Review signs of impending heart failure, and urge patient to notify prescriber immediately if they occur.

# nafarelin acetate

Synarel

## Class and Category

*Chemical:* Decapeptide, gonadotropin-releasing hormone analogue
*Therapeutic:* Antiendometriotic, gonadal hormone inhibitor
*Pregnancy category:* X

## Indications and Dosages

➤ *To treat endometriosis*
NASAL INHALATION
**Adults.** 1 spray (200 mcg) into one nostril q morning and 1 spray into other nostril q evening for up to 6 mo. If amenorrhea doesn't occur in 2 mo, dosage increased, as prescribed, to 800 mcg/day in divided doses.

➤ *To treat gonadotropin-dependent precocious puberty*
NASAL INHALATION
**Children at puberty.** 2 sprays (400 mcg) into each nostril q morning and evening. *Maximum:* 1,800 mcg/day in divided doses t.i.d.

| Route | Onset | Peak | Duration |
|-------|-------|------|----------|
| Nasal | 60 to 120 days* | 20 days† | 3 to 6 mo† |

## Contraindications

Breast-feeding; hypersensitivity to gonadotropin-releasing hormones, gonadotropin-releasing hormone analogues, nafarelin, or their components; pregnancy; undiagnosed vaginal bleeding

## Mechanism of Action

Stimulates the release of the gonadotropins luteinizing hormone (LH) and follicle-stimulating hormone (FSH), which temporarily increase ovarian steroidogenesis. Within 1 month, however, repeated administration of nafarelin halts pituitary gland stimulation and decreases LH and FSH secretion. This action decreases the estrogen level, which improves symptoms of endometriosis. In children, repeated nafarelin administration returns LH and FSH to prepubescent levels, stopping development of secondary sex characteristics and slowing bone growth.

## Interactions
DRUGS
*nasal decongestants:* Possibly impaired nafarelin absorption

## Adverse Reactions

**CNS:** Asthenia, depression, fever, headache, mood changes, paresthesia
**CV:** Chest pain, edema, hot flashes, palpitations
**EENT:** Eye pain, rhinitis
**ENDO:** Galactorrhea, gynecomastia, transient increase in pubic hair growth
**GU:** Hypermenorrhea, hypertrophy of female genitalia, impotence, libido changes, menstrual irregularities, ovarian cysts, uterine bleeding, vaginal dryness, vaginal spotting between menses
**MS:** Arthralgia, decreased bone density, myalgia
**RESP:** Dyspnea
**SKIN:** Acne, hirsutism, rash, seborrhea, skin discoloration (brown)
**Other:** Body odor

## Nursing Considerations

•Be aware that nafarelin isn't recommended for use in breast-feeding women.
•Expect to start treatment for endometriosis between days 2 and 4 of menstrual cycle. Menses should cease after 6 weeks of treat-

---

* For gonadal hormone inhibitor effects, 4 wk
† For antiendometriotic effects.

ment. Continued menses may indicate lack of compliance.
•Know that bone loss may increase if endometriosis treatment lasts longer than 6 months. Safety of retreatment after 6 months is unknown.
•Avoid giving nasal decongestant within 2 hours after nafarelin administration because it may impair nafarelin absorption.
•Be aware that prescriber will regularly monitor serum hormone levels in patient with gonadotropin-dependent precocious puberty, especially during first 6 to 8 weeks of therapy, to ensure rapid suppression of pituitary function.

**PATIENT TEACHING**
•Instruct patient to comply with prescriber's instructions for administering nafarelin to obtain desired drug effects.
•Instruct patient to tilt her head back while administering nafarelin to enhance absorption; urge her to try not to sneeze afterward.
•Caution patient not to change dosage without consulting prescriber.
•Counsel patient to notify prescriber if she is or could be pregnant.
•Direct patient not to use nasal decongestant within 2 hours after using nafarelin. If rhinitis occurs, urge her to contact prescriber for instructions.
•Teach patient how to cope with adverse reactions to help maximize compliance.
•Inform patient with endometriosis that drug should cause menses to stop. Urge her to notify prescriber if periods fail to stop even though she's taking drug exactly as prescribed.
•Advise patient with endometriosis to avoid alcohol and tobacco during therapy because they increase bone loss.
•Inform patient with gonadotropin-dependent precocious puberty that signs of puberty will persist during first month of treatment. If they don't resolve within 2 months, advise patient or parents to notify prescriber.
•Inform patient with gonadotropin-dependent precocious puberty that prescriber will assess bone growth velocity and bone age during first 3 to 6 months of therapy.
•Reassure parents of child with precocious puberty that child will resume growing when treatment stops.

# nafcillin sodium

Nafcil, Nallpen, Unipen

## Class and Category
*Chemical:* Penicillin
*Therapeutic:* Antibiotic
*Pregnancy category:* B

## Indications and Dosages
➤ *To treat infections caused by penicillinase-producing* Staphylococcus aureus
**CAPSULES, TABLETS**
**Adults and adolescents.** 250 to 1,000 mg q 4 to 6 hr. *Maximum:* 6,000 mg/day.
**Children over age 1 month.** 6.25 to 12.5 mg/kg q 6 hr.
**Neonates.** 10 mg/kg q 6 to 8 hr.
**I.V. INFUSION**
**Adults and adolescents.** 500 to 1,500 mg q 4 hr. *Maximum:* 20,000 mg/day.
**Children from birth to age 12.** 10 to 20 mg/kg q 4 hr, or 20 to 40 mg/kg q 8 hr.
**I.M. INJECTION**
**Adults and adolescents.** 500 mg q 4 to 6 hr. *Maximum:* 12,000 mg/day.
**Children over age 1 month.** 25 mg/kg q 12 hr.
**Neonates.** 10 mg/kg q 12 hr.
➤ *To treat streptococcal pharyngitis*
**CAPSULES, TABLETS**
**Children.** 250 mg q 8 hr.
➤ *To treat bone and joint infections, endocarditis, meningitis, and pericarditis caused by susceptible organisms*
**I.V. INFUSION**
**Adults and adolescents.** 1,500 to 2,000 mg q 4 to 6 hr. *Maximum:* 20,000 mg/day.
**I.V. INFUSION, I.M. INJECTION**
**Children from birth to age 12.** 10 to 20 mg/kg q 4 hr or 20 to 40 mg/kg q 8 hr. For meningitis in neonates weighing up to 2 kg (4.4 lb), 25 to 50 mg/kg q 12 hr for first week after birth and then 50 mg/kg q 8 hr. For neonates weighing 2 kg or more, 50 mg/kg q 8 hr during first week after birth and then 50 mg/kg q 6 hr.

## Incompatibilities
Don't mix nafcillin in same I.V. bag as aminoglycosides; they're chemically incompatible.

## Contraindications
Hypersensitivity to nafcillin, other penicillins, or their components

N
O

## Mechanism of Action

Binds to certain penicillin-binding proteins in bacterial cell walls, thereby inhibiting the final stage of bacterial cell wall synthesis. The result is cell lysis. Nafcillin's action is bolstered by its chemical composition; its unique side chain resists destruction by beta-lactamases.

## Interactions

**DRUGS**
*aminoglycosides:* Substantial mutual inactivation
*chloramphenicol, erythromycins, sulfonamides, tetracyclines:* Possibly decreased therapeutic effects of nafcillin
*hepatotoxic drugs:* Increased risk of hepatotoxicity
*methotrexate:* Increased risk of methotrexate toxicity
*probenecid:* Increased blood nafcillin level
**FOODS**
*all foods:* Decreased nafcillin absorption

## Adverse Reactions

**CNS:** Depression, headache, seizures
**EENT:** Oral candidiasis
**GI:** Abdominal pain, diarrhea, nausea, pseudomembranous colitis, vomiting
**GU:** Vaginitis
**HEME:** Leukopenia, neutropenia
**SKIN:** Exfoliative dermatitis, pruritus, rash, urticaria
**Other:** Anaphylaxis; hypokalemia; injection site pain, redness, and swelling; serum sickness–like reaction

## Nursing Considerations

• Obtain body fluid or tissue samples for culture and sensitivity testing, as prescribed, and obtain test results, if possible, before giving nafcillin, as ordered.
• Give capsules or tablets at least 1 hour before meals or 2 hours afterward.
• For I.M. injection, use only reconstituted solutions from vials. Inject deep into large muscle, preferably upper outer quadrant of gluteus maximus or lateral part of thigh.
• For intermittent I.V. infusion, infuse over 30 to 60 minutes.

• Give nafcillin at least 1 hour before or after aminoglycosides, especially if patient has renal disease.
• When giving nafcillin to patient at risk for hypertension or fluid overload, be aware that each gram contains 2.5 mEq of sodium.
• **WARNING** Avoid giving nafcillin to premature neonate if drug was reconstituted with bacteriostatic water that contains benzyl alcohol. Doing so can cause potentially fatal metabolic acidosis and circulatory, CNS, renal, and respiratory dysfunction.
• Monitor serum nafcillin levels closely in children, as ordered, because the liver and biliary tract, principal routes of nafcillin elimination, function immaturely in children.
• Monitor for signs of superinfection, such as oral candidiasis and pseudomembranous colitis, especially in elderly, immunocompromised, or debilitated patients who receive large doses of nafcillin.

**PATIENT TEACHING**
• Instruct patient to take nafcillin capsules or tablets on an empty stomach.
• Urge patient to complete entire prescription, even if she feels better.
• Advise patient to notify prescriber if she experiences chills, fever, GI distress, or rash.

# nalbuphine hydrochloride

Nubain

## Class and Category

*Chemical:* Phenanthrene derivative
*Therapeutic:* Analgesic, anesthesia adjunct
*Pregnancy category:* B

## Indications and Dosages

➤ *To relieve moderate to severe pain*
**I.V., I.M., OR S.C. INJECTION**
**Adults who weigh 70 kg (154 lb).** 10 mg q 3 to 6 hr, p.r.n. Dosage adjusted for patients who weigh more or less.
➤ *As adjunct to anesthesia*
**I.V. INJECTION**
**Adults.** 0.3 to 3 mg/kg over 10 to 15 min followed by 0.25 to 0.5 mg/kg, as needed.
**DOSAGE ADJUSTMENT** For patients who have repeatedly received an opioid agonist, initial dose possibly reduced to 25% of usual dos-

age. For patients in whom tolerance to drug's effects hasn't developed, maximum usually is 20 mg/dose or 160 mg/day.

| Route | Onset | Peak | Duration |
|-------|-------|------|----------|
| I.V. | 2 to 3 min | 30 min | 3 to 4 hr |
| I.M. | In 15 min | 1 hr | 3 to 6 hr |
| S.C. | In 15 min | Unknown | 3 to 6 hr |

### Mechanism of Action
Binds with and stimulates mu and kappa opiate receptors in the spinal cord and higher levels in the CNS. In this way, nalbuphine alters the perception of and emotional response to pain.

## Incompatibilities
Don't administer nalbuphine with diazepam or pentobarbital. Use separate I.V. line or flush line well before and after administration.

## Contraindications
Hypersensitivity to nalbuphine or its components

## Interactions
**DRUGS**
*alfentanil, CNS depressants, fentanyl, sufentanil:* Increased risk of hypotension and CNS and respiratory depression
*anticholinergics:* Increased risk of severe constipation and urine retention
*antidiarrheals, such as difenoxin and atropine, loperamide, and paregoric:* Increased risk of severe constipation and increased CNS depression
*antihypertensives:* Increased risk of hypotension
*buprenorphine:* Possibly decreased therapeutic effects of nalbuphine and increased risk of respiratory depression
*hydroxyzine:* Increased risk of CNS depression and hypotension
*MAO inhibitors:* Risk of possibly fatal increased CNS excitation or depression
*metoclopramide:* Possibly antagonized effects of metoclopramide
*naloxone, naltrexone:* Decreased pharmacologic effects of nalbuphine
*neuromuscular blockers:* Increased risk of prolonged CNS and respiratory depression

**ACTIVITIES**
*alcohol use:* Increased risk of coma, hypotension, profound sedation, and respiratory depression

## Adverse Reactions
**CNS:** Confusion, depression, dizziness, euphoria, fatigue, hallucinations, headache, nervousness, restlessness, seizures, syncope, tiredness, weakness
**CV:** Hypertension, hypotension, tachycardia
**EENT:** Blurred vision, diplopia, dry mouth
**GI:** Abdominal cramps, anorexia, constipation, nausea, vomiting
**GU:** Decreased urine output, ureteral spasm
**RESP:** Dyspnea, pulmonary edema, respiratory depression, wheezing
**SKIN:** Diaphoresis, flushing, pruritus, rash, sensation of warmth, urticaria
**Other:** Injection site burning, pain, redness, swelling, and warmth

## Nursing Considerations
• Use nalbuphine cautiously in patients taking other drugs that can cause respiratory depression.
• Keep resuscitation equipment and naloxone readily available to reverse nalbuphine's effects, if needed.
• For direct I.V. injection through an I.V. line with a compatible infusing solution, give drug slowly—no more than 10 mg over 3 to 5 minutes. Inject into free-flowing NS, D$_5$W, or LR solution.
• During prolonged use, expect to give a stool softener to minimize constipation.
• If patient is opioid-dependent, expect drug to cause withdrawal symptoms, such as abdominal cramps, anorexia, anxiety, backache, bone or joint pain, confusion, depression, diaphoresis, dysphoria, erythema, fear, fever, irritability, labile blood pressure and pulse, lacrimation, muscle spasms, myalgia, mydriasis, nasal congestion, nausea, opioid craving, piloerection, restlessness, rhinorrhea, sensation of crawling skin, sleep disturbances, tremor, uneasiness, vomiting, and yawning.
• **WARNING** Be aware that drug may obscure neurologic assessment findings if patient has a cerebral aneurysm, head injury, or increased intracranial pressure.

## PATIENT TEACHING

• Advise patient to avoid potentially hazardous activities until nalbuphine's CNS effects are known.
• Counsel patient against making important decisions while receiving drug because it may cloud her judgment.

# nalidixic acid

NegGram

## Class and Category

*Chemical:* Naphthyridine derivative quinolone
*Therapeutic:* Antibiotic
*Pregnancy category:* Not rated (first trimester), B (later trimesters)

## Indications and Dosages

➤ *To treat UTIs caused by gram-negative bacteria, such as most* Enterobacter *sp.,* Escherichia coli, Klebsiella *sp.,* Morganella morganii, Proteus mirabilis, Proteus vulgaris, *and* Providencia rettgeri

ORAL SUSPENSION, TABLETS

**Adults and children age 12 and older.** *Initial:* 1,000 mg q 6 hr for 1 to 2 wk. *Maintenance:* 500 mg q 6 hr. *Maximum:* 4,000 mg/day.
**Children ages 3 months to 12 years.** *Initial:* 55 mg/kg/day in divided doses q.i.d. for 1 to 2 wk. *Maintenance:* 33 mg/kg/day in divided doses q.i.d.

---

### Mechanism of Action

Inhibits the enzyme DNA gyrase, which is responsible for the unwinding and supercoiling of bacterial DNA before it replicates. By inhibiting this enzyme, nalidixic acid causes bacterial cells to die.

---

## Contraindications

Hypersensitivity to nalidixic acid or its components, porphyria, seizure disorder, use with melphalan or other related chemotherapeutic alkylating drugs

## Interactions

DRUGS

*aluminum-, calcium-, and magnesium-containing antacids; didanosine; multivitamins containing iron or zinc; sucralfate:* Possibly interference with nalidixic acid absorption
*chloramphenicol, nitrofurantoin, tetracycline:* Decreased effects of nalidixic acid
*cyclosporine:* Possibly increased blood cyclosporine level
*melphalan:* Possibly increased risk of serious GI toxicity
*oral anticoagulants:* Increased anticoagulant effects
*probenecid:* Decreased effects of nalidixic acid and increased risk of adverse reactions
*theophylline:* Possibly increased blood theophylline level

FOODS

*caffeine:* Decreased clearance and prolonged half-life of caffeine

## Adverse Reactions

**CNS:** Confusion, drowsiness, hallucinations, headache, increased intracranial pressure with bulging fontanels (in infants and children), light-headedness, malaise, paresthesia, peripheral neuropathy, psychosis, restlessness, seizures, tremor, weakness
**EENT:** Altered color perception, blurred vision, diplopia, halo vision, photophobia
**GI:** Abdominal pain, diarrhea, nausea, pseudomembranous colitis, vomiting
**HEME:** Eosinophilia, hemolytic anemia, leukopenia, thrombocytopenia
**MS:** Tendon rupture
**SKIN:** Jaundice, photosensitivity, pruritus, rash, Stevens-Johnson syndrome, urticaria
**Other:** Anaphylaxis, metabolic acidosis

## Nursing Considerations

• Be aware that nalidixic acid shouldn't be given to patient with creatinine clearance below 10 ml/min/1.73 $m^2$ because of the increased risk of drug toxicity and should be used cautiously in patients with liver disease, epilepsy, glucose-6-phosphate dehydrogenase deficiency, or severe cerebral arteriosclerosis or renal failure.
• Avoid giving drug within 2 hours of giving didanosine; multivitamin that contains iron or zinc; sucralfate; or antacid that contains aluminum, calcium, or magnesium.
• If nalidixic acid therapy exceeds 2 weeks, monitor patient's blood counts and renal and liver function test results periodically, as ordered.
• **WARNING** Stop nalidixic acid at first sign of hypersensitivity, including rash, because it may indicate anaphylaxis. Reaction may occur with first dose. Expect to give epinephrine and supportive care.

•If patient also takes cyclosporine or theophylline, monitor blood level of these drugs and adjust dosage, as prescribed.

•If patient has a history of seizures or cerebral arteriosclerosis, monitor for seizures during nalidixic acid therapy.

•Notify prescriber if patient has symptoms of peripheral neuropathy (pain, burning, tingling, numbness, weakness, or altered sensations of light touch, pain, temperature, position sense, or vibration sense), which could be permanent; or tendon rupture, which requires immediate rest. In each case, expect to stop nalidixic acid.

**PATIENT TEACHING**

•Encourage patient to drink plenty of fluids during therapy unless directed otherwise by prescriber.

•Urge patient to finish entire prescription, even if she feels better before it's finished.

•Advise patient to protect skin from sunlight.

•Urge patient to notify prescriber immediately about vision changes or such adverse CNS reactions as confusion, drowsiness, hallucinations, psychosis, and seizures.

•Urge patient to stop drug and notify prescriber if rash or other evidence of hypersensitivity develops.

•Tell patient to take drug at least 2 hours before or after aluminum-, calcium-, or magnesium-containing antacids; didanosine chewable buffered tablets or oral solution prepared from powder; multivitamins that contain iron or zinc; or sucralfate.

•Caution patient to avoid hazardous tasks until CNS effects of drug are known.

•Instruct patient to limit caffeine intake while taking nalidixic acid.

•Tell patient to stop drug and notify prescriber if she develops tendon pain or inflammation or abnormal changes in motor or sensory function.

# nalmefene hydrochloride

Revex

## Class and Category

*Chemical:* 6-Methylene analogue of naltrexone
*Therapeutic:* Opioid antagonist
*Pregnancy category:* B

## Indications and Dosages

➤ *To treat known or suspected opioid overdose*

**I.V. , I.M., OR S.C. INJECTION**

**Adults.** 500 mcg/70 kg (154 lb) followed by second dose of 1,000 mcg/70 kg in 2 to 5 min, as indicated. *Maximum:* 1,500 mcg/70 kg.

➤ *To treat postoperative opioid-induced respiratory depression*

**I.V. INJECTION**

**Adults.** *Initial:* 0.25 mcg/kg q 2 to 5 min until desired degree of reversal is achieved. *Maximum:* 1 mcg/kg.

**DOSAGE ADJUSTMENT** Initial and subsequent doses possibly reduced to 0.1 mcg/kg for patients at increased risk for cardiovascular complications.

| Route | Onset | Peak | Duration |
|---|---|---|---|
| I.V. | 2 to 5 min | Unknown | 30 to 60 min* |
| I.M., S.C. | 5 to 15 min | Unknown | Several hr |

## Mechanism of Action

Antagonizes mu, kappa, and sigma receptors in the CNS, thus reversing the analgesia, hypotension, respiratory depression, and sedation caused by most opioids. Mu receptors are responsible for analgesia, euphoria, miosis, and respiratory depression; kappa receptors for analgesia and sedation; and sigma receptors for controlling dysphoria and other delusional states.

## Contraindications

Hypersensitivity to nalmefene or its components

## Interactions

**DRUGS**

*opioid analgesics (including alfentanil, fentanyl, and sufentanil):* Reversal of these drugs' analgesic and adverse effects, possibly withdrawal symptoms in opioid-dependent patients

## Adverse Reactions

**CNS:** Agitation, chills, confusion, depression, dizziness, fever, hallucinations, headache, nervousness, somnolence, tremor

---

* For partial reversal of opioid effects; up to several hr for full reversal.

**CV:** Arrhythmias, hypertension, hypotension, tachycardia, vasodilation
**EENT:** Dry mouth, pharyngitis
**GI:** Diarrhea, nausea, vomiting
**GU:** Urine retention
**SKIN:** Pruritus
**Other:** Withdrawal symptoms

## Nursing Considerations

•Use nalmefene cautiously in patients with hepatic or renal dysfunction because drug is metabolized by liver and excreted by kidneys.
•Also use drug cautiously in patients who have received a cardiotoxic drug and in those at increased risk for cardiovascular complications.
•**WARNING** Monitor for withdrawal symptoms, especially when giving nalmefene to opioid-dependent patient. Symptoms may include abdominal cramps, anorexia, anxiety, backache, bone or joint pain, confusion, depression, diaphoresis, dysphoria, erythema, fear, fever, irritability, labile blood pressure and pulse, lacrimation, muscle spasms, myalgia, mydriasis, nasal congestion, nausea, opioid craving, piloerection, restlessness, rhinorrhea, sensation of crawling skin, sleep disturbances, tremor, uneasiness, vomiting, and yawning.
•Be prepared to provide mechanical or assisted ventilation if reversal of opioid-induced respiratory depression is incomplete.

**PATIENT TEACHING**
•Urge opioid-dependent patient to seek drug rehabilitation.

# naloxone hydrochloride

Narcan

## Class and Category

*Chemical:* Thebaine derivative
*Therapeutic:* Opioid antagonist
*Pregnancy category:* B

## Indications and Dosages

➤ *To treat known or suspected opioid overdose*
**I.V. INJECTION**
**Adults and children age 5 and older who weigh more than 20 kg (44 lb).** 0.4 to 2 mg repeated q 2 to 3 min, p.r.n. If no response after 10 mg, patient may not have narcotic-induced respiratory depression.
**Infants and children under age 5.** 0.01 mg/kg as a single dose; if no improvement, another

0.1 mg/kg, as prescribed. Alternatively, 0.1 mg/kg repeated q 2 to 3 min, as needed
**I.V., I.M., OR S.C. INJECTION**
**Neonates.** 0.01 mg/kg repeated I.V. q 2 to 3 min, as prescribed, until desired response occurs. Alternatively, initial I.V. dose of 0.1 mg/kg.

➤ *To treat postoperative opioid-induced respiratory depression*
**I.V. INJECTION**
**Adults and adolescents.** *Initial:* 0.1 to 0.2 mg q 2 to 3 min until desired response occurs. Additional doses given q 1 to 2 hr, if needed, based on patient response.
**Children.** *Initial:* 0.005 to 0.01 mg q 2 to 3 min until desired response occurs. Additional doses given q 1 to 2 hr, if needed, based on patient response.

➤ *To reverse opioid-induced asphyxia*
**I.V., I.M., OR S.C. INJECTION**
**Neonates.** *Initial:* 0.01 mg/kg q 2 to 3 min until desired response occurs. Additional doses given q 1 to 2 hr, if needed, based on patient response.

➤ *As adjunct to treat hypotension caused by septic shock*
**I.V. INFUSION OR INJECTION**
**Adults.** 0.03 to 0.2 mg/kg over 5 min followed by continuous infusion of 0.03 to 0.3 mg/kg/ hr for 1 to 24 hr, as needed, based on patient response.

| Route | Onset | Peak | Duration |
|---|---|---|---|
| I.V. | 1 to 2 min | 5 to 15 min | 45 min or longer |
| I.M., S.C. | 2 to 5 min | 5 to 15 min | 45 min or longer |

## Mechanism of Action

Briefly and competitively antagonizes mu, kappa, and sigma receptors in the CNS, thus reversing the analgesia, hypotension, respiratory depression, and sedation caused by most opioids. Mu receptors are responsible for analgesia, euphoria, miosis, and respiratory depression. Kappa receptors are responsible for analgesia and sedation. Sigma receptors control dysphoria and other delusional states.

## Incompatibilities

Don't mix naloxone with any other solution unless you verify that drugs are compatible;

drug is incompatible with alkaline, bisulfite, and metabisulfite solutions.

## Contraindications
Hypersensitivity to naloxone or its components

## Interactions
**DRUGS**
*butorphanol, nalbuphine, pentazocine:* Reversal of these drugs' analgesic and adverse effects
*opioid analgesics:* Reversal of these drugs' analgesic and adverse effects, possibly withdrawal symptoms in opioid-dependent patients

## Adverse Reactions
**CNS:** Excitement, irritability, nervousness, restlessness, seizures, tremor, violent behavior
**CV:** Hypertension (severe), hypotension, ventricular fibrillation, ventricular tachycardia
**GI:** Nausea, vomiting
**RESP:** Pulmonary edema
**SKIN:** Diaphoresis
**Other:** Withdrawal symptoms

## Nursing Considerations
•Keep resuscitation equipment readily available during naloxone administration.
•Administer drug by I.V. route whenever possible.
•Give repeat doses as prescribed, depending on patient's response.
•Anticipate that rapid reversal of opioid effects can cause diaphoresis, nausea, and vomiting.
•**WARNING** Monitor for withdrawal symptoms, especially when giving naloxone to opioid-dependent patient. Symptoms may include abdominal cramps, anorexia, anxiety, backache, bone or joint pain, confusion, depression, diaphoresis, dysphoria, erythema, fear, fever, irritability, labile blood pressure and pulse, lacrimation, muscle spasms, myalgia, mydriasis, nasal congestion, nausea, opioid craving, piloerection, restlessness, rhinorrhea, sensation of crawling skin, sleep disturbances, tremor, uneasiness, vomiting, and yawning.
•Expect patient with hepatic or renal dysfunction to have increased circulating blood naloxone level.
**PATIENT TEACHING**
•Inform patient or family that naloxone will reverse opioid-induced adverse reactions.
•Urge opioid-dependent patient to seek drug rehabilitation.

# naltrexone hydrochloride
ReVia

## Class and Category
*Chemical:* Thebaine derivative
*Therapeutic:* Opioid antagonist
*Pregnancy category:* C

## Indications and Dosages
➤ *To treat opioid dependence*
**TABLETS**
**Adults.** *Initial:* 25 mg, repeated within 1 hr, if needed and if no withdrawal symptoms occur. *Maintenance:* 50 to 150 mg q.d. or 350 mg/wk by intermittent dosing regimen.
➤ *As adjunct to treat alcoholism*
**TABLETS**
**Adults.** 50 mg q.d. (up to 100 mg/day for some patients) for 12 wk.

| Route | Onset | Peak | Duration |
|-------|-------|------|----------|
| P.O. | 15 to 30 min | In 12 hr | 24 hr* |

## Mechanism of Action
Displaces opioid agonists from—or blocks them from binding with—mu, kappa, and delta receptors. Opioid receptor blockade reverses the euphoric effect of opioids. Naltrexone also inhibits the effects of endogenous opioids, thus reducing alcohol craving.

## Contraindications
Acute hepatitis, acute opioid withdrawal, concurrent use of opioid analgesics (including opiate agonists, such as methadone or levo-alpha-acetyl-methadol [LAAM]), hepatic failure, hypersensitivity to naltrexone or its components, opioid dependence

## Interactions
**DRUGS**
*opioid analgesics:* Reversal of the analgesic and adverse effects of these drugs, possibly withdrawal symptoms in opioid-dependent patients
*thioridazine:* Increased somnolence and lethargy

---

* For 50 mg; 48 hr for 100 mg; 72 hr for 150 mg.

## Adverse Reactions

**CNS:** Anxiety, chills, confusion, depression, dizziness, fatigue, fever, hallucinations, headache, insomnia, irritability, nervousness, restlessness
**CV:** Chest pain, edema, hypertension, tachycardia
**EENT:** Blurred vision, burning eyes, eyelid swelling, hoarseness, pharyngitis, rhinitis, sneezing, tinnitus
**GI:** Abdominal cramps, anorexia, constipation, diarrhea, GI ulceration, nausea, thirst, vomiting
**GU:** Difficult ejaculation, urinary frequency
**MS:** Arthralgia, myalgia
**RESP:** Cough, dyspnea
**SKIN:** Pruritus, rash

## Nursing Considerations

• To avoid withdrawal symptoms, wait 7 to 10 days after last opioid dose, as prescribed, before starting patient on naltrexone.
• Give drug with food or antacids to decrease adverse GI reactions.
• Anticipate that some patients may require treatment for up to 1 year.

**PATIENT TEACHING**

• WARNING Caution patient against taking opioids during naltrexone therapy or in the future because she'll be more sensitive to them. In fact, strongly warn patient that taking large doses of heroin or any other opioid (including methadone or LAAM) while taking naltrexone could lead to coma, serious injury, or death.
• Urge patient to undergo comprehensive rehabilitation in addition to receiving naltrexone.
• Inform patient about nonopioid treatments for cough, diarrhea, and pain.
• Instruct patient to carry medical identification that lists naltrexone therapy.

# nandrolone decanoate

Deca-Durabolin, Hybolin Decanoate, Kabolin

## Class, Category, and Schedule

*Chemical:* Testosterone derivative
*Therapeutic:* Antianemic
*Pregnancy category:* X
*Controlled substance:* Schedule III

## Indications and Dosages

➤ *To manage anemia caused by chronic renal failure*

**I.M. INJECTION**
**Adults and adolescents age 14 and older.**
50 to 100 mg q 1 to 4 wk for females; 50 to 200 mg q 1 to 4 wk for males.
**Children ages 2 to 13.** 25 to 50 mg q 3 to 4 wk.

### Mechanism of Action

Increases production of erythropoietin, a precursor of RBCs. Nandrolone also increases hemoglobin level and RBC volume.

## Contraindications

Breast cancer in females with hypercalcemia; breast or prostate cancer in males; hypersensitivity to nandrolone, anabolic steroids, or their components; known or suspected pregnancy; nephrosis; nephrotic phase of nephritis; severe hepatic dysfunction

## Interactions

**DRUGS**
*corticosteroids:* Increased risk of edema and severe acne
*drugs with sodium:* Increased risk of edema
*hepatotoxic drugs:* Increased risk of hepatotoxicity
*insulin, oral antidiabetic drugs:* Possibly hypoglycemia
*NSAIDs, oral anticoagulants, salicylates:* Increased anticoagulant effects
*somatrem, somatropin:* Possibly accelerated epiphyseal maturation

**FOODS**
*food with sodium:* Increased risk of edema

## Adverse Reactions

**CNS:** Excitement, depression, insomnia
**CV:** Edema, hyperlipidemia
**ENDO:** Feminization in postpubertal males (epididymitis, gynecomastia, impotence, oligospermia, priapism, testicular atrophy); glucose intolerance; virilism in females (acne, clitoral enlargement, decreased breast size, deepened voice, diaphoresis, emotional lability, flushing, hirsutism, hoarseness, libido changes, male-pattern baldness, menstrual irregularities, nervousness, oily hair or skin, vaginitis, weight gain); virilism in prepubertal males (acne, decreased ejaculatory volume, epididymitis, penis enlargement, prepubertal closure of epiphyseal plates, priapism, unnatural growth of body and facial hair)

**GI:** Diarrhea, elevated liver function test results, hepatocellular carcinoma, nausea, vomiting
**GU:** Urinary frequency
**HEME:** Unusual bleeding
**SKIN:** Jaundice
**Other:** Injection site induration and pain, physical and psychological dependence

## Nursing Considerations

•Provide adequate calories and protein, as ordered, to maintain a positive nitrogen balance. Also provide adequate iron intake to ensure optimal response to nandrolone.
•Weigh patient daily to detect fluid retention, which can lead to edema. If patient retains fluid, expect to place her on sodium-restricted diet or diuretic therapy, as ordered.
•Assess boys younger than age 7 for secondary sexual characteristics, and notify prescriber.
•Assess patient for signs of virilism, and notify prescriber if they develop.
•Monitor diabetic patient for decreased glucose control; notify prescriber of hyperglycemia.
•Be aware that some people use nandrolone as a sports aid; long-term use may lead to abuse, addiction, and such adverse reactions as antisocial behavior, cardiovascular complications, hepatotoxicity, and libido changes.
•If no improvement occurs after 6 months, expect prescriber to discontinue nandrolone.

**PATIENT TEACHING**
•Review signs of virilism with patient, and urge her to notify prescriber if they develop. Explain that some changes may be permanent.
•To prevent vaginitis, advise women to wash after intercourse and to wear cotton underwear.
•Instruct patient to notify prescriber immediately about menstrual changes.
•Advise patient to notify prescriber about sudden weight gain—a sign of edema, which may cause significant problems in patients with cardiac or renal disorders.
•Inform adolescent males that they may need to undergo semen evaluation every 3 to 4 months.
•Instruct diabetic patient to monitor blood glucose level often, to watch for signs of hyperglycemia, and to report significant changes.

## naproxen

Apo-Naproxen (CAN), EC-Naprosyn, Naprosyn, Naprosyn-E (CAN), Naxen (CAN), Novo-Naprox (CAN), Nu-Naprox (CAN)

## naproxen sodium

Aleve, Anaprox, Anaprox DS, Apo-Napro-Na (CAN), Naprelan, Naprosyn-SR (CAN), Novo-Naprox Sodium (CAN)

## Class and Category

*Chemical:* Propionic acid derivative
*Therapeutic:* Analgesic, anti-inflammatory, antipyretic
*Pregnancy category:* C

## Indications and Dosages

➤ *To relieve mild to moderate musculo-skeletal inflammation, including ankylosing spondylitis, osteoarthritis, and rheumatoid arthritis*

**DELAYED-RELEASE TABLETS, ORAL SUSPENSION, TABLETS (NAPROXEN)**
**Adults.** 250 to 500 mg b.i.d. *Maximum:* 1,500 mg/day for limited periods, as prescribed.

**E.R. TABLETS (NAPROXEN SODIUM)**
**Adults.** 750 to 1,000 mg q.d. *Maximum:* 1,500 mg/day.

**TABLETS (NAPROXEN SODIUM)**
**Adults.** 275 to 550 mg b.i.d. *Maximum:* 1,650 mg/day for limited periods, as prescribed.

**SUPPOSITORIES (NAPROXEN SODIUM)**
**Adults.** 500 mg h.s. in addition to daytime P.O. administration. *Maximum:* 1,500 mg/day (P.O. and suppository combined).

➤ *To relieve symptoms of juvenile rheumatoid arthritis and other inflammatory conditions in children*

**ORAL SUSPENSION, TABLETS (NAPROXEN)**
**Children.** 10 mg/kg/day in divided doses b.i.d.

➤ *To relieve symptoms of acute gouty arthritis*

**DELAYED-RELEASE TABLETS, ORAL SUSPENSION, TABLETS (NAPROXEN)**
**Adults.** *Initial:* 750 mg, then 250 mg q 8 hr until symptoms subside.

**E.R. TABLETS (NAPROXEN SODIUM)**
**Adults.** *Initial:* 1,000 to 1,500 mg on day 1, then 1,000 mg q.d. until symptoms subside. *Maximum:* 1,500 mg/day.

**TABLETS (NAPROXEN SODIUM)**
**Adults.** *Initial:* 825 mg, then 275 mg q 8 hr until symptoms subside.

➤ *To relieve mild to moderate pain, including acute tendinitis and bursitis, arthralgia, dysmenorrhea, and myalgia*

N
O

**Adults.** *Initial:* 1,000 mg q.d. *Maximum:* 1,500 mg/day.
**E.R. TABLETS (NAPROXEN SODIUM)**
**Adults.** *Initial:* 1,100 mg q.d., increased as prescribed. *Maximum:* 1,500 mg/day.
**ORAL SUSPENSION, TABLETS (NAPROXEN)**
**Adults.** *Initial:* 500 mg, then 250 mg q 6 to 8 hr, p.r.n. *Maximum:* 1,250 mg/day.
**TABLETS (NAPROXEN SODIUM)**
**Adults.** *Initial:* 550 mg, then 275 mg q 6 to 8 hr, p.r.n. *Maximum:* 1,375 mg/day.

➤ *To relieve fever and mild to moderate musculoskeletal inflammation or pain*
**TABLETS (OTC NAPROXEN SODIUM)**
**Adults.** 220 mg q 8 to 12 hr; or 440 mg and 220 mg 12 hr later. *Maximum:* 660 mg/day for 10 days unless directed otherwise.
**DOSAGE ADJUSTMENT** For patients older than age 65, 220 mg q 12 hr. *Maximum:* 440 mg for 10 days unless directed otherwise.

| Route | Onset | Peak | Duration |
|---|---|---|---|
| P.O. (naproxen)* | 1 hr† | 2 to 4 hr†‡ | 7 to 12 hr† |
| P.O. (naproxen sodium)* | 30 min† | 1 hr†‡ | 7 to 12 hr† |

## Mechanism of Action
Blocks cyclooxygenase, the enzyme needed to synthesize prostaglandins, which mediate the inflammatory response and cause local vasodilation, swelling, and pain. Thus, naproxen, an NSAID, reduces symptoms of inflammation and relieves pain. Antipyretic action probably stems from its effect on the hypothalamus, which increases peripheral blood flow, causing vasodilation and heat dissipation.

## Contraindications
Angioedema, asthma, bronchospasm, nasal polyps, rhinitis, or urticaria induced by aspirin, iodides, or other NSAIDs; hypersensitivity to naproxen or its components

---

* For antirheumatism, onset is in 14 days, peak is unknown, and duration is 2 to 4 wk.
† For analgesia.
‡ For gout, 1 to 2 days.

## Interactions
**DRUGS**
*ACE inhibitors:* Decreased antihypertensive effects; increased risk of renal dysfunction
*acetaminophen:* Increased risk of adverse renal effects with combined long-term use
*anticoagulants, thrombolytics:* Prolonged PT, increased risk of bleeding
*antihypertensives:* Decreased effectiveness of antihypertensive
*aspirin:* Decreased aspirin effectiveness from lowered plasma and peak aspirin levels
*beta blockers:* Decreased antihypertensive effects of these drugs
*bone marrow depressants, such as aldesleukin and cisplatin:* Increased risk of leukopenia and thrombocytopenia
*cefamandole, cefoperazone, cefotetan, plicamycin, valproic acid:* Increased risk of hypoprothrombinemia and bleeding
*cimetidine:* Altered blood naproxen level
*colchicine, glucocorticoids, other NSAIDs, potassium supplements, salicylates:* Increased GI irritability and bleeding
*cyclosporine, gold compounds, nephrotoxic drugs:* Increased risk of nephrotoxicity
*digoxin:* Increased blood digoxin level and risk of digitalis toxicity
*diuretics:* Decreased diuretic effectiveness
*furosemide:* Decreased natriuretic effect
*insulin, oral antidiabetic drugs:* Increased effectiveness of these drugs; risk of hypoglycemia
*lithium:* Increased risk of lithium toxicity
*methotrexate:* Increased risk of methotrexate toxicity
*naproxen-containing products:* Increased risk of toxicity
*phenytoin:* Increased blood phenytoin level
*probenecid:* Increased risk of naproxen toxicity
**ACTIVITIES**
*alcohol use, smoking:* Increased risk of naproxen-induced GI ulceration

## Adverse Reactions
**CNS:** Aseptic meningitis, chills, cognitive impairment, decreased concentration, depression, dizziness, dream disturbances, drowsiness, fever, headache, insomnia, lightheadedness, malaise, seizures, stroke, vertigo
**CV:** Edema, heart failure, hypertension, MI, palpitations, tachycardia, vasculitis
**EENT:** Stomatitis, tinnitus, vision or hearing changes
**ENDO:** Hyperglycemia, hypoglycemia

**GI:** Abdominal pain, anorexia, colitis, constipation, diarrhea, diverticulitis, dyspepsia, dysphagia, elevated liver function test results, esophagitis, flatulence, gastritis, gastroenteritis, gastroesophageal reflux disease, GI bleeding and ulceration, heartburn, hematemesis, indigestion, melena, nausea, pancreatitis, perforation of stomach or intestines, stomatitis, vomiting

**GU:** Glomerulonephritis, hematuria, interstitial nephritis, menstrual irregularities, nephrotic syndrome, renal failure, renal papillary necrosis

**HEME:** Agranulocytosis, anemia, aplastic anemia, eosinophilia, granulocytopenia, hemolytic anemia, leukopenia, neutropenia, pancytopenia, thrombocytopenia

**MS:** Muscle weakness, myalgia

**RESP:** Asthma, dyspnea, eosinophilic pneumonitis, respiratory depression

**SKIN:** Alopecia, diaphoresis, ecchymosis, erythema multiforme, photosensitivity, pruritus, pseudoporphyria, purpura, rash, Stevens-Johnson syndrome, toxic epidermal necrolysis, urticaria

**Other:** Anaphylaxis, angioedema, hyperkalemia

## Nursing Considerations

• Use naproxen with extreme caution in patients with a history of ulcer disease or GI bleeding because NSAIDs such as naproxen increase the risk of GI bleeding and ulceration. Expect to use naproxen for the shortest time possible in these patients.

• Be aware that serious GI tract ulceration, bleeding, and perforation may occur without warning symptoms. Elderly patients are at greater risk. To minimize risk, give drug with food. If GI distress occurs, withhold drug and notify prescriber immediately.

• Use naproxen cautiously in patients with hypertension, and monitor blood pressure closely. Drug may cause hypertension or worsen it. Because of naproxen's sodium content, watch for fluid retention.

• Rehydrate a dehydrated patient before giving drug. If patient has renal disease, monitor renal function closely during therapy.

• Naproxen isn't recommended for patients with advanced renal disease.

•**WARNING** Monitor patient closely for thrombotic events, including MI and stroke, because NSAIDs increase the risk.

• Monitor patient—especially if she's elderly or receiving long-term naproxen therapy—for less common but serious adverse GI reactions, including anorexia, constipation, diverticulitis, dysphagia, esophagitis, gastritis, gastroenteritis, gastroesophageal reflux disease, hemorrhoids, hiatal hernia, melena, stomatitis, and vomiting.

• Monitor liver function test results because, in rare cases, elevations may progress to severe hepatic reactions, including fatal hepatitis, liver necrosis, and hepatic failure.

• Monitor BUN and serum creatinine levels in elderly patients, patients taking diuretics or ACE inhibitors, and patients with heart failure, impaired renal function, or hepatic dysfunction; naproxen may cause renal failure.

• Monitor CBC for decreased hemoglobin and hematocrit because drug may worsen anemia.

•**WARNING** If patient has bone marrow suppression or is receiving treatment with an antineoplastic drug, monitor laboratory results (including WBC count), and watch for evidence of infection because anti-inflammatory and antipyretic actions of naproxen may mask signs and symptoms, such as fever and pain.

• Assess patient's skin regularly for signs of rash or other hypersensitivity reaction because naproxen is an NSAID and may cause serious skin reactions without warning, even in patients with no history of NSAID sensivitity. At first sign of reaction, stop drug and notify prescriber.

• Assess drug effectiveness in ankylosing spondylitis: decreased night pain, morning stiffness, and pain at rest; in osteoarthritis: decreased joint pain or tenderness and increased mobility, range of motion, and ability to perform daily activities; in rheumatoid arthritis: increased mobility and decreased joint swelling and morning stiffness; in acute gouty arthritis: decreased heat, pain, swelling, and tenderness in affected joints.

• Tell prescriber if patient complains of vision changes; patient may need ophthalmic exam.

### PATIENT TEACHING

• Caution patient not to exceed recommended dose; serious adverse reactions may occur.

• Tell patient to swallow delayed-release tablets whole and not to break, crush, or chew.

•Advise patient to take drug with food to reduce GI distress.

•Tell patient to take drug with a full glass of water and to remain upright for 15 to 30 minutes afterward to prevent drug from lodging in esophagus and causing irritation.

•Caution patient to avoid hazardous activities until drug's CNS effects are known.

•Urge patient to keep scheduled appointments with prescriber to monitor progress.

•Tell pregnant patient to avoid naproxen-containing products late in pregnancy.

•Advise against taking naproxen for more than 10 days without consulting prescriber.

•Explain that naproxen may increase the risk of serious adverse cardiovascular reactions; urge patient to seek immediate medical attention if signs or symptoms arise, such as chest pain, shortness of breath, weakness, and slurring of speech.

•Explain that naproxen may increase the risk of serious adverse GI reactions; stress the importance of seeking immediate medical attention for such signs and symptoms as epigastric or abdominal pain, indigestion, black or tarry stools, or vomiting blood or material that looks like coffee grounds.

•Alert patient to rare but serious skin reactions. Urge her to seek immediate medical attention for rash, blisters, itching, fever, or other indications of hypersensitivity.

# naratriptan hydrochloride

Amerge

## Class and Category

*Chemical:* Selective serotonin 5-HT receptor agonist
*Therapeutic:* Antimigraine
*Pregnancy category:* C

## Indications and Dosages

➤ *To relieve acute migraine with or without aura*

**TABLETS**

**Adults.** 1 to 2.5 mg as a single dose, repeated in 4 hr p.r.n. if only partial relief obtained. *Maximum:* 5 mg/day.

**DOSAGE ADJUSTMENT** For patients with mild to moderate renal or hepatic impairment, maximum dosage reduced to 2.5 mg/day.

## Mechanism of Action

Binds to receptors on intracranial blood vessels and sensory nerves in the trigeminal-vascular system to stimulate negative feedback, which halts serotonin release. Thus, naratriptan selectively constricts inflamed and dilated cranial vessels in the carotid circulation and inhibits production of proinflammatory neuropeptides.

## Contraindications

Basilar or hemiplegic migraine; cerebrovascular, peripheral vascular, or coronary artery disease (ischemic or vasospastic); hypersensitivity to naratriptan or its components; hypertension (uncontrolled); severe hepatic or renal dysfunction; use within 24 hours of another 5-HT agonist or an ergotamine-containing or ergot-type drug, such as dihydroergotamine or methysergide

## Interactions
**DRUGS**

*ergot-containing drugs:* Possibly prolonged or additive vasospastic reactions
*fluoxetine, fluvoxamine, paroxetine, sertraline:* Possibly weakness, hyperreflexia, and incoordination
*oral contraceptives:* Possibly reduced clearance and increased blood level of naratriptan
*other selective serotonin 5-HT receptor agonists (including rizatriptan, sumatriptan, and zolmitriptan):* Possibly additive effects

## Adverse Reactions

**CNS:** Dizziness, drowsiness, fatigue, malaise, paresthesia
**CV:** Chest pain, pressure, or heaviness
**EENT:** Decreased salivation, otitis media, pharyngitis, photophobia, rhinitis, throat tightness
**GI:** Nausea, vomiting

## Nursing Considerations

•**WARNING** Because naratriptan therapy can cause coronary artery vasospasm, monitor patient with coronary artery disease for signs or symptoms of angina while taking drug. Because naratriptan may also cause peripheral vasospastic reactions, such as ischemic bowel disease, monitor patient for abdominal pain and bloody diarrhea.

•Monitor patient for hypertension during naratriptan therapy. Drug may increase sys-

tolic blood pressure by as much as 32 mm Hg.
•Be prepared to perform a complete neu-
rovascular assessment in any patient who reports an unusual headache or who fails to
respond to first dose of naratriptan.

**PATIENT TEACHING**
•Inform patient that naratriptan is used to
treat acute migraine attacks and that it
won't prevent or reduce the number of migraines.
•Advise patient not to take more than maximum prescribed dosage during any 24-hour
period.
•If patient experiences no relief from initial
dose of naratriptan, instruct her to notify
prescriber rather than taking another dose in
4 hours because she may need a different
drug.
•Advise patient to seek reevaluation by prescriber if she experiences more than four
headaches during any 30-day period while
taking naratriptan.

# nateglinide

Starlix

## Class and Category
*Chemical:* Amino acid derivative
*Therapeutic:* Antidiabetic
*Pregnancy category:* C

## Indications and Dosages
➤ *To control blood glucose level in type 2*
  *diabetes mellitus as monotherapy or in*
  *combination with metformin or a thia-*
  *zolidinedione*

**TABLETS**
**Adults.** 120 mg t.i.d. 1 to 30 min a.c.
**DOSAGE ADJUSTMENT** Dosage reduced to 60
mg t.i.d. in patients with near-goal glycosylated hemoglobin ($HbA_{1c}$) level.

| Route | Onset | Peak | Duration |
|-------|-------|------|----------|
| P.O. | 20 min | 1 hr | 4 hr |

## Mechanism of Action
Nateglinide stimulates the release of insulin
from functioning beta cells of the pancreas.
In patients with type 2 diabetes mellitus, a
lack of functioning beta cells diminishes
blood levels of insulin and causes glucose
intolerance. By interacting with the adenosine triphosphatase (ATP)–potassium channel on the beta cell membrane, nateglinide
prevents potassium ($K^+$) from leaving the
cell. This causes the beta cell to depolarize
and the cell membrane's calcium channel to
open. Consequently, calcium ($Ca^{++}$) moves
into the cell and insulin moves out of it.
The extent of insulin release is glucose dependent; the lower the glucose level, the
less insulin is secreted from the cell.

By promoting insulin secretion in patients with type 2 diabetes mellitus,
nateglinide improves glucose tolerance.

Outside beta cell
Ca++   Ca++
ATP-potassium channel
Nateglinide
Calcium channel
ATP
Insulin secretion
Ca++
K+
K+
Inside beta cell
Insulin

## Contraindications
Diabetic ketoacidosis, hypersensitivity to nateglinide or its components, type 1 diabetes mellitus

## Interactions
**DRUGS**
*corticosteroids, sympathomimetics, thiazide diuretics, thyroid products:* Possibly reduced hypoglycemic effects of nateglinide
*MAO inhibitors, nonselective beta-adrenergic blockers, NSAIDs, salicylates:* Possibly additive hypoglycemic effects of nateglinide

## Adverse Reactions
**CNS:** Dizziness
**ENDO:** Hypoglycemia
**GI:** Diarrhea
**MS:** Accidental trauma, arthropathy, back pain
**RESP:** Bronchitis, cough, upper respiratory tract infection
**SKIN:** Pruritus, rash, urticaria
**Other:** Flulike symptoms

## Nursing Considerations
• Administer nateglinide 1 to 30 minutes before meals to reduce the risk of hypoglycemia.
• Monitor fasting glucose and HbA$_{1c}$ levels periodically, as ordered, to evaluate treatment effectiveness.
• Monitor patient frequently in event of fever, infection, trauma, or surgery because transient loss of glucose control may occur, requiring an alteration in therapy.
**PATIENT TEACHING**
• Instruct patient to take nateglinide 1 to 30 minutes before meals. Advise her to skip scheduled dose if she skips a meal to reduce the risk of hypoglycemia.
• Teach patient how to measure blood glucose level and recognize signs of hyperglycemia and hypoglycemia. Advise her to notify prescriber if blood glucose level is abnormal.
• Inform patient that strenuous exercise, insufficient caloric intake, and consumption of alcohol increase the risk of hypoglycemia.
• Advise patient to monitor blood glucose levels as prescribed and to maintain follow-up appointments to monitor HbA$_{1c}$ level because drug may become less effective over time.

# nedocromil sodium
Tilade

## Class and Category
*Chemical:* Pyranoquinoline dicarboxylic acid derivative
*Therapeutic:* Antiasthmatic, anti-inflammatory
*Pregnancy category:* B

## Indications and Dosages
➤ *To control mild to moderate chronic asthma*
**ORAL INHALATION**
**Adults and children age 6 and older.** 2 inhalations (3.5 mg) q.i.d. Dosage frequency possibly reduced to b.i.d. or t.i.d. once desired response occurs.

| Route | Onset | Peak | Duration |
|---|---|---|---|
| Inhalation | 2 to 4 wk | Unknown | 6 to 12 hr |

### Mechanism of Action
Inhibits the activation and release of inflammatory mediators—such as histamine, leukotrienes, and prostaglandins—in the lumen and mucosa of the bronchi and bronchioles. As a result, nedocromil inhibits allergen-induced early and late asthmatic reactions when administered directly to the bronchial mucosa. The drug also may inhibit axon reflexes and release sensory neuropeptides in the lungs. This action:
• suppresses bradykinin-induced bronchoconstriction
• decreases localized tissue edema and mucus secretion
• mobilizes anti-inflammatory cells.

## Contraindications
Hypersensitivity to nedocromil or its components

## Adverse Reactions
**CNS:** Dizziness, fatigue, headache (possibly severe), tremor
**CV:** Chest pain
**EENT:** Dry mouth, hoarseness, pharyngitis, rhinitis, taste perversion
**GI:** Abdominal pain, diarrhea, elevated liver function test results, indigestion, nausea, vomiting

**HEME:** Leukopenia, neutropenia
**MS:** Arthritis
**RESP:** Bronchospasm, cough, upper respiratory tract infection
**SKIN:** Rash, sensation of warmth

## Nursing Considerations
•Be aware that nedocromil may be used alone or with other drugs, such as bronchodilators and corticosteroids.
•Avoid using nedocromil to reverse acute bronchospasm because drug doesn't have bronchodilator effects.
•Continue nedocromil therapy during acute exacerbations unless patient becomes intolerant of inhaled form. Intolerance is characterized by bronchospasm, cough, and wheezing.
•**WARNING** Monitor for life-threatening bronchospasm immediately after administration. If it occurs, notify prescriber and expect to discontinue nedocromil therapy and start a different drug.

### PATIENT TEACHING
•Advise patient to store nedocromil at room temperature and to shake it before use.
•Instruct patient to prime drug canister with three sprays before first use and after more than 7 days of disuse.
•If patient has trouble coordinating inhalation with each spray, suggest using a spacer.
•Urge patient to take drug regularly, even when she has no symptoms.
•Inform patient that drug's full effect may not occur for 1 or more weeks after therapy starts.
•If patient uses other inhalers, instruct her to use bronchodilator first and wait 5 minutes before using nedocromil.
•Caution patient not to spray nedocromil into eyes.
•Instruct patient to wash mouthpiece after each use and not to use nedocromil mouthpiece with other aerosol drugs.
•Advise patient to gargle or rinse mouth after inhalation to relieve dry mouth, hoarseness, throat irritation, and unpleasant taste.
•Instruct patient to discard canister after 104 metered sprays.
•Urge patient to notify prescriber if symptoms worsen or fail to improve; caution against increasing the number of inhalations without consulting prescriber.

# nefazodone hydrochloride
Serzone

## Class and Category
*Chemical:* Phenylpiperazine derivative
*Therapeutic:* Antidepressant
*Pregnancy category:* C

## Indications and Dosages
➤*To treat major depression*
### TABLETS
**Adults.** *Initial:* 100 mg b.i.d., increased by 100 to 200 mg/day q wk, as prescribed. *Maintenance:* 150 to 300 mg b.i.d. *Maximum:* 600 mg/day.
**DOSAGE ADJUSTMENT** Initial dosage possibly reduced to 50 mg b.i.d. for elderly or debilitated patients; then dosage adjusted as ordered, based on patient response.

| Route | Onset | Peak | Duration |
|-------|-------|------|----------|
| P.O. | Several wk | Unknown | Unknown |

### Mechanism of Action
Believed to inhibit serotonin reuptake at presynaptic neurons, which may increase the neuronal level of serotonin, an inhibitory neurotransmitter that is thought to regulate mood. Nefazodone also may act as a postsynaptic serotonin receptor antagonist, further increasing the amount of synaptic serotonin that's available.

## Contraindications
Concurrent use of astemizole, cisapride, or terfenadine; hypersensitivity to nefazodone, other phenylpiperazine antidepressants, or their components; restarting nefazodone therapy that was discontinued because of liver injury; use within 14 days of MAO inhibitor therapy

## Interactions
### DRUGS
*alprazolam, buspirone, carbamazepine, cyclosporine, modafinil, triazolam:* Increased blood levels of these drugs
*antihypertensives:* Increased risk of hypotension
*astemizole, cisapride, terfenadine:* Increased blood levels of these drugs, prolonged QT interval, and, possibly, serious cardiovascular

effects, including death from ventricular tachycardia

*cilostazol:* Decreased cilostazol clearance, increased adverse effects of cilostazol, such as headache

*dextromethorphan, sibutramine, tramadol, trazodone:* Increased risk of serotonin syndrome

*digoxin:* Increased blood digoxin level, increased risk of digitalis toxicity

*haloperidol:* Decreased haloperidol clearance

*indinavir:* Inhibited indinavir metabolism

*levobupivacaine:* Increased blood levobupivacaine level, possibly toxicity

*lovastatin, simvastatin:* Increased risk of rhabdomyolysis and myositis

*MAO inhibitors:* Possibly fatal reactions, including autonomic instability (with rapidly fluctuating vital signs), hyperthermia, mental status changes (such as severe agitation progressing to delirium and coma), muscle rigidity, and myoclonus

*methadone:* Increased blood level and adverse effects of methadone, additive CNS effects

*nevirapine:* Increased nefazodone metabolism, inhibited nevirapine metabolism

*ritonavir:* Inhibited nefazodone and ritonavir metabolism

*sildenafil:* Decreased sildenafil clearance

*tacrolimus:* Decreased tacrolimus clearance and increased adverse effects, including delirium and renal failure

**ACTIVITIES**

*alcohol use:* Increased risk of CNS depression

## Adverse Reactions

**CNS:** Abnormal gait, apathy, asthenia, ataxia, chills, confusion, decreased concentration, delusions, depersonalization, dizziness, dream disturbances, euphoria, fever, hallucinations, headache, hostility, hypotonia, insomnia, light-headedness, malaise, memory loss, myoclonic jerks, neuralgia, paranoia, paresthesia, somnolence, suicidal ideation, syncope, tremor, vertigo

**CV:** Angina, hypertension, hypotension, peripheral edema, orthostatic hypotension, tachycardia, vasodilation, ventricular arrhythmias

**EENT:** Abnormal vision, blurred vision, conjunctivitis, diplopia, dry eyes and mouth, earache, epistaxis, eye pain, gingivitis, halitosis, hyperacusis, laryngitis, mydriasis, neck

rigidity, periodontal abscess, pharyngitis, photophobia, stomatitis, taste perversion, tinnitus, visual field defects

**ENDO:** Breast pain, gynecomastia, lymphadenopathy

**GI:** Abdominal distention, colitis, constipation, diarrhea, elevated liver function test results, eructation, esophagitis, gastritis, gastroenteritis, hernia, hepatotoxicity, hiccups, increased appetite, indigestion, life-threatening hepatic failure, nausea, peptic ulcer, rectal bleeding, thirst, vomiting

**GU:** Abnormal ejaculation; amenorrhea; cystitis; hematuria; hypermenorrhea; impotence; libido changes; nocturia; pelvic pain; polyuria; renal calculi; urinary frequency, incontinence, or urgency; urine retention; UTI; vaginal bleeding; vaginitis

**HEME:** Anemia, leukopenia

**MS:** Arthralgia, arthritis, bursitis, dysarthria, gout, muscle stiffness, tenosynovitis

**RESP:** Asthma, bronchitis, cough, dyspnea, pneumonia

**SKIN:** Acne, alopecia, dry skin, ecchymosis, eczema, maculopapular rash, photosensitivity, pruritus, rash, urticaria

**Other:** Allergic reaction, dehydration, infection, serotonin syndrome, weight loss

## Nursing Considerations

•**WARNING** Be aware that nefazodone should not be given with astemizole, cisapride, MAO inhibitors, or terfenadine; serious, even fatal, reactions may occur.

•**WARNING** Be aware that life-threatening hepatic failure has occurred during nefazodone therapy, resulting in need for transplant or even death. Monitor patient for signs of hepatic failure, such as jaundice, malaise, and elevated liver function test results.

•Assess for signs of serotonin syndrome, such as abdominal cramps, aggressive behavior, agitation, chills, diarrhea, headache, insomnia, lack of coordination, nausea, palpitations, paresthesia, poor concentration, and worsening of obsessive thoughts.

•Monitor patient closely for suicidal tendencies, especially when therapy starts or dosage changes, because depression may worsen temporarily. Follow facility policy.

**PATIENT TEACHING**

•Instruct patient to take nefazodone exactly as prescribed and not to alter dosage.

•Urge patient to immediately report signs of hepatic failure, such as jaundice, dark urine, lack of appetite, nausea, or abdominal pain.
•Inform patient that antidepressant effects may not occur for several weeks and that treatment may last 6 months or longer.
•Caution patient to avoid alcohol during nefazodone therapy.
•Advise patient to avoid potentially hazardous activities until drug's CNS effects are known.
•Suggest that patient try sugarless gum or hard candy for dry mouth. Urge her to notify prescriber if dry mouth persists.

# neomycin sulfate

Mycifradin, Neo-Fradin

## Class and Category

*Chemical:* Aminoglycoside
*Therapeutic:* Antibiotic
*Pregnancy category:* D

## Indications and Dosages

➤ *To suppress intestinal bacterial growth in preoperative bowel preparation*

**TABLETS (24-HR REGIMEN)**

**Adults.** 1 g q hr for 4 doses and then 1 g q 4 hr for remainder of 24 hr before surgery. Alternatively, for 8 a.m. surgery, 1 g of neomycin with erythromycin at 1 p.m., 2 p.m., and 11 p.m. the day before surgery.

**Children.** 25 mg/kg at 1 p.m., 2 p.m., and 11 p.m. the day before surgery.

**TABLETS (2- TO 3-DAY REGIMEN)**

**Adults and children.** 88 mg/kg q 4 hr in 6 equally divided doses for 2 to 3 days before surgery.

➤ *As adjunct in hepatic encephalopathy*

**TABLETS**

**Adults.** 4 to 12 g/day in divided doses q 6 hr for 5 to 6 days.

**Children.** 50 to 100 mg/kg/day in divided doses q 6 hr for 5 to 6 days.

➤ *To treat infectious diarrhea caused by enteropathic* Escherichia coli

**TABLETS**

**Adults and children.** 50 mg/kg/day in divided doses q.i.d. for 2 to 3 days.

## Mechanism of Action

Is transported into bacterial cells, where it competes with messenger RNA to bind with a specific receptor protein on the 30S ribosomal subunit of DNA. This action causes abnormal, nonfunctioning proteins to form. A lack of functional proteins causes bacterial cell death.

## Contraindications

Hypersensitivity or serious reaction to neomycin, other aminoglycosides, or their components; inflammatory or ulcerative GI disease; intestinal obstruction

## Interactions

**DRUGS**

*digoxin, spironolactone:* Possibly reduced absorption rate of these drugs
*dimenhydrinate:* Possibly masked symptoms of neomycin-induced ototoxicity
*methotrexate:* Possibly decreased absorption and bioavailability of methotrexate
*neuromuscular blockers:* Potentiated neuromuscular blockade, increased risk of prolonged respiratory depression
*oral anticoagulants:* Possibly potentiated anticoagulant effects

## Adverse Reactions

**EENT:** Ototoxicity
**GI:** Diarrhea, malabsorption syndrome (decreased serum carotene level and xylose absorption, increased fecal fat and flatulence), nausea, pseudomembranous colitis, vomiting
**GU:** Nephrotoxicity

## Nursing Considerations

•Monitor BUN and serum creatinine levels to assess renal function before and during neomycin therapy. Expect to decrease dosage or stop drug if nephrotoxicity develops.
•Monitor blood neomycin level, as directed, to assess for therapeutic range of 5 to 10 mcg/ml.
•**WARNING** Neomycin is highly ototoxic and may cause hearing loss and tinnitus.
•Monitor for signs of pseudomembranous colitis, such as severe abdominal cramps and severe, watery diarrhea.
•Anticipate that neomycin's curare-like effect may worsen muscle weakness in patients with neuromuscular disorders, such as myasthenia gravis and parkinsonism.

N
O

• Urge patient to complete the full course of neomycin therapy.
• Unless contraindicated, urge patient to drink plenty of fluids to prevent nephrotoxicity.
• Urge patient undergoing bowel preparation to comply with recommended regimen, including low-residue diet, bisacodyl enema administration, and neomycin use.
• Advise patient to notify prescriber about hearing loss or ringing in ears.

# neostigmine bromide

Prostigmin

## neostigmine methylsulfate

Prostigmin

## Class and Category

*Chemical:* Quaternary ammonium compound
*Therapeutic:* Anticholinesterase, curare antidote
*Pregnancy category:* C

## Indications and Dosages

➤ *To treat symptoms of myasthenia gravis*
**TABLETS (NEOSTIGMINE BROMIDE)**
**Adults.** *Initial:* 15 mg q 3 to 4 hr. Dosage adjusted based on clinical response. *Maintenance:* 150 mg/day in divided doses based on clinical response.
**Children.** 2 mg/kg/day in 6 to 8 divided doses.
**I.M. OR S.C. INJECTION (NEOSTIGMINE METHYLSULFATE)**
**Adults.** *Initial:* 0.5 mg. Dosage adjusted based on clinical response.
**Children.** 0.01 to 0.04 mg/kg q 2 to 3 hr.

➤ *To reverse nondepolarizing neuromuscular blockade*
**I.V. INJECTION (NEOSTIGMINE METHYLSULFATE)**
**Adults.** 0.5 to 2 mg by slow push, repeated as needed up to 5 mg; 0.6 to 1.2 mg of atropine or 0.2 to 0.6 mg of glycopyrrolate is given with or a few minutes before neostigmine, as ordered.
**Children.** 0.04 mg/kg by slow push; 0.02 mg of atropine/kg is given I.M. or S.C. with each dose or alternate doses.

➤ *To prevent postoperative, nonobstructive urine retention and abdominal distention (adynamic ileus)*

**I.M. OR S.C. INJECTION (NEOSTIGMINE METHYLSULFATE)**
**Adults.** 0.25 mg immediately after surgery and repeated q 4 to 6 hr for 2 to 3 days.

➤ *To treat postoperative, nonobstructive urine retention and abdominal distention (adynamic ileus)*
**I.M. OR S.C. INJECTION (NEOSTIGMINE METHYLSULFATE)**
**Adults.** 0.5 mg; injections repeated q 3 hr for at least 5 doses if patient has voided or bladder has emptied within 1 hr.

| Route | Onset | Peak | Duration |
|-------|-------|------|----------|
| P.O. | 45 to 75 min* | Unknown | 3 to 6 hr |
| I.V. | 4 to 8 min† | 30 min | 2 to 4 hr |
| I.M. | 20 to 30 min† | 30 min | 2 to 4 hr |

## Mechanism of Action
Inhibits the action of cholinesterase, an enzyme that destroys acetylcholine at myoneuronal junctions, thereby increasing acetylcholine accumulation at myoneuronal junctions and facilitating nerve impulse transmission across the junctions. This action:
• helps prevent or relieve urine retention by increasing detrusor muscle tone in the bladder and causing bladder contractions strong enough to induce urination
• prevents or treats postoperative abdominal distention by increasing gastric motility and tone
• improves muscle strength and increases muscle response to repetitive nerve stimulation in myasthenia gravis.

## Contraindications
Hypersensitivity to neostigmine, other anticholinesterases, bromides, or their components; mechanical obstruction of intestinal or urinary tract; peritonitis

## Interactions
**DRUGS**
*aminoglycosides, anesthetics, capreomycin, colistimethate, colistin, lidocaine, lincomycins, polymyxin B, quinine:* Increased risk of neuromuscular blockade
*anticholinergics:* Possibly masked signs of cholinergic crisis

---

\* For adynamic ileus, 2 to 4 hr.
† For adynamic ileus, 10 to 30 min.

*guanadrel, guanethidine, mecamylamine, tri-methaphan:* Possibly antagonized effects of neostigmine, possibly decreased antihypertensive effects

*neuromuscular blockers:* Possibly prolonged action of depolarizing—and antagonized action of nondepolarizing—neuromuscular blockers

*procainamide, quinidine:* Possibly antagonized effects of neostigmine

*quinine:* Decreased neostigmine effectiveness

## Adverse Reactions
**CNS:** Dizziness, drowsiness, headache, seizures, syncope, weakness
**CV:** Arrhythmias (AV block, bradycardia, nodal rhythm, tachycardia), cardiac arrest, ECG changes, hypotension
**EENT:** Increased salivation, lacrimation, miosis, vision changes
**GI:** Abdominal cramps, diarrhea, flatulence, increased peristalsis, nausea, vomiting
**GU:** Urinary frequency
**MS:** Arthralgia, dysarthria, muscle spasms
**RESP:** Bronchospasm, dyspnea, increased bronchial secretions, respiratory arrest or depression
**SKIN:** Flushing, diaphoresis, rash, urticaria

## Nursing Considerations
• Be aware that 15 mg of oral neostigmine bromide is equivalent to 0.5 mg of parenteral neostigmine methylsulfate.
• If also giving atropine, be sure to administer it before neostigmine, as prescribed.
• When giving neostigmine I.V., make sure patient is well ventilated and airway remains patent until normal respiration is assured.
• If patient has myasthenia gravis, give drug night and day, as ordered, with larger portions of daily dose during periods of increased fatigue. If patient's condition becomes refractory to neostigmine, expect to reduce dosage or discontinue drug, as prescribed, for a few days.
• **WARNING** Monitor for signs of neostigmine overdose, which can cause possibly fatal cholinergic crisis (increased muscle weakness, including respiratory muscles). Expect to stop neostigmine and atropine, as ordered.

### PATIENT TEACHING
• Instruct patient to take neostigmine exactly as prescribed.
• Advise patient to take drug with food or milk to reduce adverse GI reactions.

• Suggest that patient with myasthenia gravis keep a daily record of doses and adverse reactions during therapy.
• Instruct patient to schedule activities to minimize fatigue.

# nesiritide
Natrecor

## Class and Category
*Chemical:* Human B-type natriuretic peptide
*Therapeutic:* Arterial and venous smooth muscle cell relaxant
*Pregnancy category:* C

## Indications and Dosages
➤ *To reduce dyspnea at rest or with minimal activity in patients with acute decompensated congestive heart failure*
**I.V. INFUSION, I.V. INJECTION**
**Adults.** 2-mcg/kg bolus followed by continuous infusion of 0.01 mcg/kg/min for up to 48 hr.

| Route | Onset | Peak | Duration |
|-------|-------|------|----------|
| I.V. | In 15 min | 1 hr | 3 hr |

### Mechanism of Action
Binds to the guanylate cyclase receptor of vascular smooth muscle and endothelial cells. This action increases intracellular levels of cyclic guanosine monophosphate, which leads to arterial and venous smooth muscle cell relaxation. Ultimately, nesiritide reduces pulmonary capillary wedge pressure and systemic arterial pressure in patients with congestive heart failure, which decreases the heart's workload and subsequently relieves dyspnea.

## Incompatibilities
Don't infuse nesiritide through same I.V. line as bumetanide, enalaprilat, ethacrynate sodium, furosemide, heparin, hydralazine, or insulin because these drugs are chemically and physically incompatible with nesiritide. Don't infuse drugs that contain the preservative sodium metabisulfite through same I.V. line as nesiritide.

## Contraindications
Hypersensitivity to nesiritide or its components; primary therapy for cardiogenic

shock; systolic blood pressure less of than 90 mm Hg

## Interactions
**DRUGS**
*ACE inhibitors:* Increased risk of symptomatic hypotension

## Adverse Reactions
**CNS:** Anxiety, dizziness, headache, insomnia
**CV:** Angina, bradycardia, hypotension, PVCs, ventricular tachycardia
**GI:** Abdominal pain, nausea, vomiting
**GU:** Elevated serum creatinine level
**MS:** Back pain

## Nursing Considerations
•**WARNING** Be aware that nesiritide isn't recommended for patients suspected to have low cardiac filling pressures or patients for whom vasodilating drugs aren't appropriate, such as those with constrictive pericarditis, pericardial tamponade, restrictive or obstructive cardiomyopathy, significant valvular stenosis, or other conditions in which cardiac output depends on venous return.
•Reconstitute 1.5-mg vial by adding 5 ml of diluent removed from a 250-ml plastic I.V. bag containing preservative-free $D_5W$, NS, $D_5.45NS$, or $D_5.2NS$.
•Don't shake vial. Rock it gently so that all surfaces, including the stopper, are in contact with the diluent to ensure complete reconstitution. Inspect drug for particulate matter and discoloration; if present, discard drug.
•Withdraw entire contents of the reconstituted solution and add it to the same 250-ml plastic I.V. bag used to withdraw the diluent to yield a solution of about 6 mcg/ml. Invert the I.V. bag several times to ensure complete mixing.
•After preparing the infusion bag, withdraw the bolus volume from the infusion bag and administer it over about 60 seconds. Immediately after the bolus, infuse drug at 0.1 ml/kg/hr, which will deliver 0.01 mcg/ kg/min.
•Prime I.V. tubing with 25 ml of solution before connecting to the I.V. line and before administering the bolus dose or starting the infusion.
•Flush the I.V. line between doses of nesiritide and incompatible drugs.

•Because nesiritide binds to heparin and therefore could bind to the heparin lining of a heparin-coated catheter, don't give it through a central heparin-coated catheter.
•Store reconstituted vials at room temperature (20° to 25° C [68° to 77° F]) or refrigerate (2° to 8° C [36° to 46° F]) for up to 24 hours.
•Because nesiritide contains no antimicrobial preservatives, discard the reconstituted solution after 24 hours.
•Monitor blood pressure and heart rate and rhythm frequently during therapy.
•If hypotension occurs, notify prescriber and expect to reduce dosage or discontinued the drug. Implement measures to support blood pressure as prescribed.
•Assess patient's breath sounds and respiratory rate, rhythm, depth, and quality frequently during drug therapy.
•Monitor serum creatinine level during drug therapy and notify prescriber of abnormal results.
•Store unopened drug at controlled room temperature or refrigerate. Keep in carton until time of use.
**PATIENT TEACHING**
•Instruct patient to notify you or another nurse if she becomes dizzy because this may indicate hypotension.
•Reassure patient that her blood pressure, heart rate, and breathing will be monitored frequently.

# netilmicin sulfate

Netromycin

## Class and Category
*Chemical:* Aminoglycoside
*Therapeutic:* Antibiotic
*Pregnancy category:* D

## Indications and Dosages
➤ *To treat serious systemic infections, such as intra-abdominal infections, lower respiratory tract infections, septicemia, and skin and soft-tissue infections, caused by* Enterobacter aerogenes, Escherichia coli, Klebsiella pneumoniae, Proteus mirabilis, Pseudomonas aeruginosa, Serratia *sp., and* Staphylococcus aureus

**I.V. INFUSION, I.M. INJECTION**

**Adults and children age 12 and older.** 1.3 to 2.2 mg/kg q 8 hr or 2 to 3.25 mg/kg q 12 hr for 7 to 14 days. *Maximum:* 7.5 mg/kg/day.
**Children ages 6 weeks to 12 years.** 1.8 to 2.7 mg/kg q 8 hr or 2.7 to 4 mg/kg q 12 hr for 7 to 14 days.
**Infants up to age 6 weeks.** 2 to 3.25 mg/kg q 12 hr for 7 to 14 days.

➤ *To treat complicated UTIs caused by* Citrobacter *sp.,* Enterobacter *sp.,* E. coli, K. pneumoniae, P. mirabilis, P. aeruginosa, Serratia *sp., and* Staphylococcus *sp.*

**I.V. INFUSION, I.M. INJECTION**

**Adults and adolescents.** 1.5 to 2 mg/kg q 12 hr for 7 to 14 days. *Maximum:* 7.5 mg/kg/day.

## Incompatibilities

Don't mix netilmicin with beta-lactam antibiotics (penicillins and cephalosporins) because substantial mutual inactivation may result. If prescribed concurrently, administer these drugs at separate sites.

## Mechanism of Action

Is transported into bacterial cells, where it competes with messenger RNA to bind with a specific receptor protein on the 30S ribosomal subunit of DNA. This action causes abnormal, nonfunctioning proteins to form. A lack of functional proteins causes bacterial cell death.

## Contraindications

Hypersensitivity to netilmicin, other aminoglycosides, or their components

## Interactions

**DRUGS**

*capreomycin, other aminoglycosides:* Increased risk of nephrotoxicity, neuromuscular blockade, and ototoxicity
*cephalosporins, nephrotoxic drugs:* Increased risk of nephrotoxicity
*loop diuretics, ototoxic drugs:* Increased risk of ototoxicity
*methoxyflurane, polymyxins (parenteral):* Increased risk of nephrotoxicity and neuromuscular blockade
*neuromuscular blockers:* Increased neuromuscular blockade

## Adverse Reactions

**CNS:** Disorientation, dizziness, encephalopathy, headache, myasthenia gravis–like syndrome, neuromuscular blockade (acute muscle paralysis and apnea), paresthesia, peripheral neuropathy, seizures, vertigo, weakness
**CV:** Hypotension, palpitations
**EENT:** Blurred vision, hearing loss, nystagmus, tinnitus
**GI:** Diarrhea, elevated liver function tests results, nausea, vomiting
**GU:** Elevated BUN and serum creatinine levels, nephrotoxicity, oliguria, proteinuria
**HEME:** Anemia, eosinophilia, leukopenia, prolonged PT, thrombocytopenia, thrombocytosis
**MS:** Muscle twitching
**RESP:** Apnea
**SKIN:** Allergic dermatitis, erythema, pruritus, rash
**Other:** Angioedema; hyperkalemia; injection site hematoma, induration, and pain

## Nursing Considerations

•To prepare netilmicin for I.V. use, dilute each dose in 50 to 200 ml of suitable diluent, such as NS, $D_5W$, or LR solution, and administer slowly over 30 to 60 minutes.
•Ensure adequate hydration during therapy to maintain adequate renal function.
•Monitor blood netilmicin level; optimum peak level is 6 to 10 mcg/ml and trough level is 0.5 to 2 mcg/ml.
•Check BUN and serum creatinine levels, urine specific gravity, and creatinine clearance during netilmicin therapy, as ordered.
•Anticipate higher risk of nephrotoxicity in elderly patients, those with impaired renal function, and those who receive high doses or prolonged netilmicin therapy.
•Reduce dosage or discontinue drug, as ordered, if signs of drug-induced auditory or vestibular toxicity develop; the damage may be permanent.

**PATIENT TEACHING**

•Encourage patient to drink plenty of fluids during netilmicin therapy.
•Instruct patient to notify prescriber immediately about dizziness, hearing loss, muscle twitching, nausea, numbness and tingling, ringing or buzzing in ears, seizures, significant changes in amount of urine or frequency of urination, and vomiting.
•Urge patient to keep follow-up appointments to monitor progress.

N
O

# nicardipine hydrochloride
Cardene, Cardene SR

## Class and Category
*Chemical:* Dihydropyridine derivative
*Therapeutic:* Antianginal, antihypertensive
*Pregnancy category:* C

## Indications and Dosages
➤ *To manage angina pectoris and Prinz-metal's angina, to manage hypertension*
CAPSULES
**Adults and adolescents.** 20 to 40 mg t.i.d., increased q 3 days, as prescribed.
E.R. CAPSULES
**Adults.** 30 mg b.i.d.
I.V. INFUSION
**Adults.** 0.5 to 2.2 mg/hr by continuous infusion.
➤ *To control acute hypertension*
I.V. INFUSION
**Adults.** *Initial:* 5 mg/hr by continuous infusion; increased by 2.5 mg/hr q 5 to 15 min, as prescribed. *Maximum:* 15 mg/hr.

| Route | Onset | Peak | Duration |
|---|---|---|---|
| P.O. | 20 min | 1 to 2 hr | Unknown |
| P.O. (E.R.) | 20 min | 1 to 2 hr | 12 hr |
| I.V. | Immediate | Unknown | Unknown |

## Mechanism of Action
May slow extracellular calcium movement into myocardial and vascular smooth-muscle cells by deforming calcium channels in cell membranes, inhibiting ion-controlled gating mechanisms, and interfering with calcium release from the sarcoplasmic reticulum. By decreasing the intracellular calcium level, nicardipine inhibits smooth-muscle cell contraction and dilates coronary and systemic arteries. As with other calcium channel blockers, these actions lead to decreased myocardial oxygen requirements and reduced peripheral resistance, blood pressure, and afterload.

## Incompatibilities
Don't mix nicardipine with sodium bicarbonate or LR solution, and don't administer through same I.V. line.

## Contraindications
Advanced aortic stenosis, hypersensitivity to any calcium channel blocker, second- or third-degree AV block in patient without artificial pacemaker

## Interactions
DRUGS
*anesthetics (hydrocarbon inhalation):* Possibly hypotension
*beta blockers, other antihypertensives, prazocin:* Increased risk of hypotension
*calcium supplements:* Possibly impaired action of nicardipine
*cimetidine:* Increased nicardipine bioavailability
*digoxin:* Transiently increased blood digoxin level, increased risk of digitalis toxicity
*disopyramide, flecainide:* Increased risk of bradycardia, conduction defects, and heart failure
*estrogens:* Possibly increased fluid retention and decreased therapeutic effects of nicardipine
*lithium:* Increased risk of neurotoxicity
*NSAIDs, sympathomimetics:* Possibly decreased therapeutic effects of nicardipine
*procainamide, quinidine:* Possibly prolonged QT interval
FOODS
*grapefruit, grapefruit juice:* Possibly increased bioavailability of nicardipine
*high-fat meals:* Decreased blood nicardipine level
ACTIVITIES
*alcohol use:* Increased hypotensive effect

## Adverse Reactions
**CNS:** Anxiety, asthenia, ataxia, confusion, dizziness, drowsiness, headache, nervousness, paresthesia, psychiatric disturbance, syncope, tremor, weakness
**CV:** Arrhythmias (bradycardia, tachycardia), chest pain, heart failure, hypotension, orthostatic hypotension, palpitations, peripheral edema
**EENT:** Altered taste, blurred vision, dry mouth, epistaxis, gingival hyperplasia, pharyngitis, rhinitis, tinnitus
**ENDO:** Gynecomastia, hyperglycemia
**GI:** Anorexia, constipation, diarrhea, elevated liver function test results, indigestion, nausea, thirst, vomiting

**GU:** Dysuria, nocturia, polyuria, sexual dysfunction, urinary frequency
**HEME:** Anemia, leukopenia, thrombocytopenia
**MS:** Joint stiffness, muscle spasms
**RESP:** Bronchitis, cough, upper respiratory tract infection
**SKIN:** Dermatitis, diaphoresis, erythema multiforme, flushing, photosensitivity, pruritus, rash, Stevens-Johnson syndrome, urticaria
**Other:** Hypokalemia, weight gain

## Nursing Considerations
• Check blood pressure and pulse rate before nicardipine therapy begins, during dosage changes, and periodically throughout therapy. During prolonged therapy, periodically assess ECG tracings for arrhythmias and other changes.
• Dilute each 25-mg ampule of nicardipine with 240 ml of solution to yield 0.1 mg/ml. Mixture is stable at room temperature for 24 hours.
• Administer continuous infusion by I.V. pump or controller, and adjust according to patient's blood pressure, as prescribed.
• Change peripheral I.V. site every 12 hours, if feasible.
• Give first dose of oral nicardipine 1 hour before stopping I.V. infusion, as prescribed.
• Monitor fluid intake and output and daily weight for signs of fluid retention, which may precipitate heart failure. Also assess for signs of heart failure, such as crackles, dyspnea, jugular vein distention, peripheral edema, and weight gain.
• During prolonged therapy, periodically monitor liver and renal function test results. Expect elevated liver function test results to return to normal after drug is discontinued.
• Monitor serum potassium level during prolonged therapy. Hypokalemia increases the risk of arrhythmias.
• Because of drug's negative inotropic effect on some patients, closely monitor patients who take a beta blocker or have heart failure or significant left ventricular dysfunction.
• WARNING Expect to taper dosage gradually before discontinuing drug. Otherwise, angina or dangerously high blood pressure could result.
**PATIENT TEACHING**
• Urge patient to take nicardipine as prescribed, even if she feels well.
• Instruct patient to swallow E.R. capsules whole, not to chew, crush, cut, or open them.

• Advise patient not to take drug within 1 hour of eating a high-fat meal or grapefruit product. Urge her not to alter the amount of grapefruit products in her diet without consulting prescriber.
• WARNING Caution patient against stopping nicardipine abruptly because angina or dangerously high blood pressure could result.
• Teach patient how to take her pulse, and urge her to notify prescriber immediately if it falls below 50 beats/minute.
• Teach patient how to measure her blood pressure, and advise her to do so weekly if nicardipine was prescribed for hypertension. Suggest that she keep a log of blood pressure readings to take to follow-up visits.
• Advise patient to change position slowly to minimize effects of orthostatic hypotension.
• Urge patient to avoid potentially hazardous activities until drug's CNS effects are known.
• Advise patient to notify prescriber immediately about chest pain that's not relieved by rest or nitroglycerin, constipation, irregular heartbeats, nausea, pronounced dizziness, severe or persistent headache, and swelling of hands or feet.
• Encourage patient to comply with suggested lifestyle changes, such as alcohol moderation, low-sodium or low-fat diet, regular exercise, smoking cessation, stress management, and weight reduction.
• Inform patient that saunas, hot tubs, and prolonged hot showers may cause dizziness or fainting.
• Instruct patient to avoid prolonged sun exposure and to use sunscreen when going outdoors.

# niclosamide
Niclocide

## Class and Category
*Chemical:* Salicylanilide derivative
*Therapeutic:* Anthelmintic
*Pregnancy category:* B

## Indications and Dosages
➤ *To treat beef* (Taenia saginata), *fish* (Diphyllobothrium latum), *or pork* (Taenia solium) *tapeworm infestations*

**CHEWABLE TABLETS**
**Adults.** 2 g as a single dose; repeated in 7 days, if needed. *Maximum:* 2 g/day.
**Children who weigh more than 34 kg (75 lb).** 1.5 g as a single dose; repeated in 7 days, if needed. *Maximum:* 2 g/day.
**Children who weigh 11 (24 lb) to 34 kg.** 1 g as a single dose; repeated in 7 days, if needed. *Maximum:* 2 g/day.

➤ *To treat dwarf tapeworm* (Hymenolepsis nana) *infestations*
**CHEWABLE TABLETS**
**Adults.** 2 g/day for 7 days; repeated in 7 to 14 days, if needed.
**Children who weigh more than 34 kg.** 1.5 g on day 1 and then 1 g/day for the next 6 days; repeated in 7 to 14 days, if needed. *Maximum:* 2 g/day.
**Children who weigh 11 to 34 kg.** 1 g on day 1 and then 500 mg/day for the next 6 days; repeated in 7 to 14 days, if needed. *Maximum:* 2 g/day.

---

**Mechanism of Action**
May alter anaerobic energy production in tapeworms by inhibiting oxidative phosphorylation in their mitochondria, which decreases the synthesis of ATP. Niclosamide causes the scolex (headlike segment) and proximal segment of the tapeworm to detach from the intestinal wall, which leads to parasite evacuation from the intestines through normal peristalsis.

---

**Contraindications**
Age under 2 years; hypersensitivity to niclosamide, other anthelmintics, or their components

**Interactions**
**ACTIVITIES**
*alcohol use:* Decreased niclosamide effects

**Adverse Reactions**
**CNS:** Dizziness, drowsiness, headache, lightheadedness
**EENT:** Taste perversion
**GI:** Abdominal distress, anorexia, constipation, diarrhea, nausea, vomiting
**SKIN:** Anal pruritus, rash

**Nursing Considerations**
•To determine type of infestation, collect several stool specimens before starting niclosamide therapy, as ordered, because eggs and parasite segments are released irregularly.
•If patient can't chew tablets thoroughly, crush them and give with small amount of water.
•For young child, crush tablets to fine powder and mix with small amount of water to make paste.
•Be aware that treatment isn't considered successful until stools have shown no eggs or parasites for at least 3 months.

**PATIENT TEACHING**
•Instruct patient to take niclosamide after a light meal.
•For young child, instruct parent to crush tablets to fine powder and mix with small amount of water to make paste.
•Urge patient to complete entire course of niclosamide therapy.
•Advise patient to avoid potentially hazardous activities until drug's CNS effects are known.
•Advise patient to store niclosamide in a cool, dry, dark place. Caution against storing in bathroom, near kitchen sink, or in other damp places because heat and moisture break down drug.
•Inform patient that stool may need to be examined on day 7 of treatment and again 1 and 3 months after treatment.
•Instruct patient to wash her hands thoroughly, to wash all bedding, and to use meticulous personal and environmental hygiene to decrease the risk of autoinfection.
•Caution patient against eating undercooked fish, pork, or beef.

# nicotine for inhalation
Nicotrol Inhaler

## nicotine nasal solution
Nicotrol NS

## nicotine polacrilex
Nicorette, Nicorette Plus (CAN)

## nicotine transdermal system
Habitrol, Nicoderm, NicoDerm CQ, Nicotrol, ProStep

## Class and Category
*Chemical:* Pyridine alkaloid
*Therapeutic:* Smoking cessation adjunct

*Pregnancy category:* C (nicotine polacrilex), D (other forms of nicotine)

## Indications and Dosages

➤ *To relieve nicotine withdrawal symptoms, including craving*

CHEWING GUM

**Adults.** *Initial:* 2 or 4 mg p.r.n. or q 1 to 2 hr, adjusted to complete withdrawal by 4 to 6 mo. *Maximum:* 30 pieces of 2-mg gum/day or 20 pieces of 4-mg gum/day.

NASAL SOLUTION

**Adults.** 1 to 2 sprays (1 to 2 mg) in each nostril/hr. *Maximum:* 5 mg/hr or 40 mg/day for up to 3 mo.

ORAL INHALATION

**Adults and adolescents.** 6 to 16 cartridges (24 to 64 mg)/day for up to 12 wk; then dosage gradually reduced over 12 wk or less. *Maximum:* 16 cartridges (64 mg)/day for 6 mo.

TRANSDERMAL SYSTEM

**Adults.** *Initial:* 14 to 22 mg q.d., adjusted to lower-dose systems over 2 to 5 mo.

DOSAGE ADJUSTMENT For adolescents and for adults who weigh less than 45 kg (100 lb) and who smoke less than 10 cigarettes daily or have heart disease, initial dosage reduced to 11 to 14 mg q.d. and adjusted to lower-dose systems over 2 to 5 mo.

---

### Mechanism of Action

Binds selectively to nicotinic-cholinergic receptors at autonomic ganglia, in the adrenal medulla, at neuromuscular junctions, and in the brain. By providing a lower dose of nicotine than cigarettes, this drug reduces nicotine craving and withdrawal symptoms.

---

## Contraindications

Hypersensitivity to nicotine, its components, or components of transdermal system; life-threatening arrhythmias; nonsmokers; recovery from acute MI; severe angina pectoris; skin disorders (transdermal); temporomandibular joint disease (chewing gum)

## Interactions

DRUGS

*acetaminophen, beta blockers, imipramine, insulin, oxazepam, pentazocine, theophylline:* Possibly increased therapeutic effects of these drugs (chewing gum, nasal spray, transdermal system)

*alpha blockers, bronchodilators:* Possibly increased therapeutic effects of these drugs (chewing gum, transdermal system)

*bupropion:* Potentiated therapeutic effects of nicotine, possibly increased risk of hypertension

*sympathomimetics:* Possibly decreased therapeutic effects of these drugs (chewing gum, transdermal system)

*theophylline, tricyclic antidepressants:* Possibly altered pharmacologic actions of these drugs (oral inhalation)

FOODS

*acidic beverages (citrus juices, coffee, soft drinks, tea, wine):* Decreased nicotine absorption from gum if beverages consumed within 15 minutes before or while chewing gum

*caffeine:* Increased effects of caffeine (chewing gum, nasal spray, transdermal system)

## Adverse Reactions

**CNS:** Dizziness, dream disturbances, drowsiness, headache, irritability, light-headedness, nervousness (chewing gum, transdermal system); amnesia, confusion, difficulty speaking, headache, migraine headache, paresthesia (nasal spray); chills, fever, headache, paresthesia (oral inhalation)

**CV:** Arrhythmias (all forms); hypertension (chewing gum, transdermal system); peripheral edema (nasal spray)

**EENT:** Increased salivation, injury to teeth or dental work, mouth injury, pharyngitis, stomatitis (chewing gum); altered taste, dry mouth (chewing gum, transdermal system); altered smell and taste, burning eyes, dry mouth, earache, epistaxis, gum disorders, hoarseness, lacrimation, mouth and tongue swelling, nasal blisters, nasal irritation or ulceration, pharyngitis, rhinitis, sinus problems, sneezing, vision changes (nasal spray); altered taste, lacrimation, pharyngitis, rhinitis, sinusitis, stomatitis (oral inhalation)

**GI:** Eructation (chewing gum); abdominal pain, constipation, diarrhea, flatulence, increased appetite, indigestion, nausea, vomiting (chewing gum, transdermal system); abdominal pain, constipation, diarrhea, flatulence, hiccups, indigestion, nausea (nasal spray); diarrhea, flatulence, hiccups, indigestion, nausea, vomiting (oral inhalation)

N
O

**GU:** Dysmenorrhea (chewing gum, transdermal system); menstrual irregularities (nasal spray)
**MS:** Jaw and neck pain (chewing gum); arthralgia, myalgia (chewing gum, transdermal system); arthralgia, back pain, myalgia (nasal spray); back pain (oral inhalation)
**RESP:** Cough (chewing gum, transdermal system); bronchitis, bronchospasm, chest tightness, cough, dyspnea, increased sputum production (nasal spray); chest tightness, cough, dyspnea, wheezing (oral inhalation)
**SKIN:** Diaphoresis, erythema, pruritus, rash, urticaria (chewing gum, transdermal system); acne, flushing of face, pruritus, purpura, rash (nasal spray); pruritus, rash, urticaria (oral inhalation)
**Other:** Allergic reaction (chewing gum, transdermal system); physical dependence (nasal spray); flulike symptoms, generalized pain, withdrawal symptoms (oral inhalation)

## Nursing Considerations
• When administering nicotine by oral inhalation, expect optimal effect to result from continuous puffing for 20 minutes.
**PATIENT TEACHING**
• Instruct patient to read and follow package instructions to obtain best results with nicotine product.
• Advise patient to notify prescriber about other drugs she takes.
• Stress that patient must stop smoking as soon as treatment starts to avoid toxicity.
• For chewing gum therapy, instruct patient to wait at least 15 minutes after drinking coffee, juice, soft drink, tea, or wine. Advise her to chew gum until she detects a tingling sensation or peppery taste and then to place the gum between her cheek and gum until tingling or peppery taste subsides. Then direct her to move the gum to a different site until tingling or taste subsides, repeating until she no longer feels the sensation—usually about 30 minutes. Caution against swallowing the gum.
• For nasal spray, tell patient to tilt her head back and spray into a nostril. Caution against sniffing, swallowing, or inhaling spray because nicotine is absorbed through nasal mucosa.
• Warn patient that prolonged use of nasal form may cause dependence.
• For oral inhalation, tell patient to use 6 to 16 cartridges daily to prevent or relieve

withdrawal symptoms and craving. Starting with 1 or 2 cartridges daily yields poor success. Direct patient to inhale through device like a cigarette, puffing often for 20 minutes.
• For transdermal system, tell patient not to open package until just before use because nicotine is lost in the air. Advise her to apply system to clean, hairless, dry site on upper outer arm or upper body. Instruct her to change systems and rotate sites every 24 hours and not to use the same site for 7 days.
• **WARNING** Urge patient to keep all unused nicotine forms safely away from children and pets and to discard used forms carefully. (Enough nicotine may remain in used systems to poison children and pets.) Instruct her to contact a poison control center immediately if she suspects that a child has ingested nicotine.
• Explain to patient with asthma or COPD that nicotine may cause bronchospasm.
• Inform patient that it may take several attempts to successfully stop smoking. Urge her to join a smoking cessation program.

# nifedipine

Adalat, Adalat CC, Adalat PA (CAN), Adalat XL (CAN), Apo-Nifed (CAN), Novo-Nifedin (CAN), Nu-Nifed (CAN), Procardia, Procardia XL

## Class and Category
*Chemical:* Dihydropyridine derivative
*Therapeutic:* Antianginal, antihypertensive
*Pregnancy category:* C

## Indications and Dosages
➤ *To manage angina*
**CAPSULES (ADALAT, APO-NIFED, NOVO-NIFEDIN, NU-NIFED, PROCARDIA)**
**Adults.** *Initial:* 10 mg t.i.d., increased over 1 to 2 wk as needed. *Maintenance:* 10 to 20 mg t.i.d. *Maximum:* 180 mg/day, 30 mg/dose.
**E.R. TABLETS (ADALAT XL, PROCARDIA XL)**
**Adults.** *Initial:* 30 to 60 mg q.d., increased or decreased over 7 to 14 days based on patient response. *Maximum:* 90 mg/day.
➤ *To manage hypertension*
**E.R. TABLETS (ADALAT CC)**
**Adults.** *Initial:* 30 mg q.d. *Maintenance:* 30 to 60 mg q.d., increased or decreased over 7 to 14 days based on patient response. *Maximum:* 90 mg/day.

### E.R. TABLETS (ADALAT PA)
**Adults.** *Initial:* 10 to 20 mg b.i.d., increased q 3 wk based on patient response. *Maintenance:* 20 mg b.i.d. *Maximum:* 80 mg/day.

### E.R. TABLETS (ADALAT XL)
**Adults.** *Initial:* 30 to 60 mg q.d., increased or decreased over 7 to 14 days based on patient response. *Maintenance:* 60 to 90 mg q.d. *Maximum:* 120 mg/day.

### E.R. TABLETS (PROCARDIA XL)
**Adults.** 30 to 60 mg q.d., increased or decreased over 7 to 14 days based on patient response. *Maximum:* 120 mg/day.

DOSAGE ADJUSTMENT Dosage possibly reduced for elderly patients and those with heart failure or impaired hepatic or renal function.

| Route | Onset | Peak | Duration |
|-------|-------|------|----------|
| P.O. (cap) | 20 min | Unknown | Unknown |

## Mechanism of Action
May slow movement of calcium into myocardial and vascular smooth-muscle cells by deforming calcium channels in cell membranes, inhibiting ion-controlled gating mechanisms, and disrupting calcium release from sarcoplasmic reticulum. Decreasing intracellular calcium level inhibits smooth-muscle cell contraction and dilates arteries, which decreases myocardial oxygen demand, peripheral resistance, blood pressure, and afterload.

## Contraindications
Hypersensitivity to a calcium channel blocker, second- or third-degree AV block without artificial pacemaker, sick sinus syndrome

## Interactions
### DRUGS
*anesthetics (hydrocarbon inhalation):* Possibly hypotension
*antiviral drugs, cimetidine, dalfopristin, diltiazem, erythromycin, fluconazole, itraconazole, ketoconazole, nefazodone, other antihypertensives, prazocin, quinupristin, timolol, valproic acid, verapamil:* Increased risk of hypotension
*benazepril:* Possibly increased heart rate and hypotensive effect
*beta blockers:* Increased risk of profound hypotension, heart failure, worsening of angina

*calcium supplements:* Possibly interference with action of nifedipine
*carbamazepine, NSAIDs, phenobarbitone, phenytoin, rifampin, rifapentine, St. John's wort, sympathomimetics:* Possibly decreased therapeutic effects of nifedipine
*digoxin:* Transiently increased blood digoxin level, increased risk of digitalis toxicity
*disopyramide, flecainide:* Increased risk of bradycardia, conduction defects, and heart failure
*doxazocin:* Decreased doxazocin effectiveness; increased nifedipine effectiveness
*estrogens:* Possibly increased fluid retention and decreased therapeutic effects of nifedipine
*lithium:* Increased risk of neurotoxicity
*metformin:* Increased metformin absorption and plasma level
*tacrolimus:* Decreased tacrolimus metabolism

### FOODS
*grapefruit, grapefruit juice:* Possibly increased bioavailability of nifedipine
*high-fat meals:* Possibly delayed nifedipine absorption

### ACTIVITIES
*alcohol use:* Additive hypotensive effect

## Adverse Reactions
**CNS:** Anxiety, ataxia, confusion, dizziness, drowsiness, headache, nervousness (possibly extreme), nightmares, paresthesia, psychiatric disturbance, syncope, tremor, weakness
**CV:** Arrhythmias (bradycardia, tachycardia), chest pain, heart failure, hypotension, palpitations, peripheral edema
**EENT:** Altered taste, blurred vision, dry mouth, epistaxis, gingival hyperplasia, nasal congestion, pharyngitis, sinusitis, tinnitus
**ENDO:** Gynecomastia, hyperglycemia
**GI:** Anorexia, constipation, diarrhea, dyspepsia, elevated liver function test results, hepatitis, nausea, vomiting
**GU:** Dysuria, nocturia, polyuria, sexual dysfunction, urinary frequency
**HEME:** Anemia, leukopenia, positive Coombs' test, thrombocytopenia
**MS:** Joint stiffness, muscle cramps
**RESP:** Chest congestion, cough, dyspnea, respiratory tract infection, wheezing
**SKIN:** Dermatitis, diaphoresis, erythema multiforme, flushing, photosensitivity, pruritus, rash, urticaria

N
O

## Nursing Considerations

- When starting and stopping nifedipine therapy, taper it, as prescribed, over 7 to 14 days.
- For closely monitored hospitalized patient with angina, dosage may be increased 10 mg every 4 to 6 hours to control chest pain.
- Because of drug's negative inotropic effect on some patients, frequently monitor heart rate and rhythm and blood pressure in patients who take a beta blocker or have heart failure or significant left ventricular dysfunction.
- Monitor fluid intake and output and daily weight; fluid retention may lead to heart failure. Also assess for signs of heart failure, such as crackles, dyspnea, jugular vein distention, peripheral edema, and weight gain.

**PATIENT TEACHING**

- Instruct patient to swallow E.R. tablets whole, not to crush, chew, or break them. Inform her that their empty shells may appear in stool.
- Urge patient to take nifedipine exactly as prescribed, even when she's feeling well. Advise her to notify prescriber if she misses two or more doses.
- Urge patient not to take drug within 1 hour of a high-fat meal or grapefruit. Urge her not to alter the amount of grapefruit in her diet without consulting prescriber.
- **WARNING** Caution patient against stopping nifedipine abruptly because angina or dangerously high blood pressure could result.
- Teach patient how to measure her pulse rate and blood pressure, and advise her to call prescriber if they drop below accepted levels. Suggest that she keep a log of weekly measurements and take it to follow-up visits.
- Instruct patient to notify prescriber immediately about chest pain, difficulty breathing, ringing in ears, and swollen gums.
- Advise patient to avoid potentially hazardous activities until drug's CNS effects are known.
- Urge patient to avoid alcoholic beverages because they may worsen dizziness, drowsiness, and hypotension.
- Teach patient to minimize constipation by increasing her intake of fluids, if allowed, and dietary fiber.
- Emphasize the need to comply with prescribed lifestyle changes, such as alcohol moderation, low-fat or low-sodium diet, regular exercise, smoking cessation, stress reduction, and weight reduction.

- Stress the need for good oral hygiene and regular dental visits.
- Caution patient that hot tubs, saunas, and prolonged hot showers may cause dizziness and fainting.
- Advise patient to avoid prolonged sun exposure and to wear sunscreen when outdoors.

# nimodipine

Nimotop

## Class and Category

*Chemical:* Dihydropyridine derivative
*Therapeutic:* Cerebral vasodilator
*Pregnancy category:* C

## Indications and Dosages

➤ *To treat neurologic deficits associated with subarachnoid hemorrhage*

**CAPSULES**

**Adults.** 60 mg q 4 hr within 96 hr of hemorrhage and continued for 21 days.

**DOSAGE ADJUSTMENT** Dosage reduced to 30 mg q 4 hr for patients with hepatic impairment.

---

### Mechanism of Action

Inhibits calcium ion transfer into smooth muscle cells, thereby inhibiting contraction of vascular smooth muscle. By relieving or preventing reactive vasodilation, nimodipine may prevent cerebral arterial spasms after hemorrhage.

---

## Contraindications

Cardiogenic shock, hepatic function impairment, hypersensitivity to nimodipine or its components

## Interactions

**DRUGS**

*anesthetics (hydrocarbon inhalation):* Possibly hypotension
*antihypertensives, prazocin:* Increased risk of hypotension
*beta blockers:* Increased adverse effects of beta blockers
*cimetidine:* Increased nimodipine bioavailability
*digoxin:* Transiently increased blood digoxin level and risk of digitalis toxicity

*estrogens:* Possibly increased fluid retention and decreased therapeutic effect of nimodipine
*lithium:* Increased risk of neurotoxicity
*NSAIDs, sympathomimetics:* Possibly decreased therapeutic effect of nimodipine
*procainamide, quinidine:* Increased risk of prolonged QT interval

## Adverse Reactions
**CNS:** Dizziness, headache
**CV:** Hypotension, edema
**GI:** Diarrhea, nausea
**SKIN:** Rash

## Nursing Considerations
•For patients who can't take oral nimodipine, be prepared to extract drug from capsule using an 18G needle and syringe, to administer drug through a nasogastric or percutaneous esophagogastrostomy tube, and then to flush tube with 30 ml of NS.
•WARNING Assess patients with cardiac history for progressive hemodynamic instability and cardiac arrhythmias because of nimodipine's potential effects on heart rate and conduction.
•Monitor blood pressure throughout drug therapy for possible hypotension.
•Monitor fluid intake and output and assess for signs of edema, which may indicate fluid retention, because drug promotes peripheral vasodilation. Notify prescriber if edema persists or if patient develops a negative fluid balance.
**PATIENT TEACHING**
•Instruct patient to swallow nimodipine capsules whole and not to crush or chew them.
•Teach patient how to monitor pulse and blood pressure. Suggest that she keep a log of weekly measurements and take it to follow-up office appointment.
•Advise patient to notify prescriber immediately if she experiences pronounced dizziness or headache or swelling of hands or feet.

# nisoldipine

Sular

## Class and Category
*Chemical:* Dihydropyridine derivative
*Therapeutic:* Antihypertensive
*Pregnancy category:* C

## Indications and Dosages
➤ *To manage hypertension*

**E.R. TABLETS**
**Adults.** 20 mg q.d., increased by 10 mg q 7 days, as prescribed. *Maintenance:* 20 to 40 mg/day. *Maximum:* 60 mg/day.
DOSAGE ADJUSTMENT For patients over age 65 and patients with hepatic impairment, initial dosage reduced to 10 mg q.d.

## Mechanism of Action
May slow extracellular calcium movement into myocardial and vascular smooth-muscle cells by deforming calcium channels in cell membranes, inhibiting ion-controlled gating mechanisms, and interfering with calcium release from the sarcoplasmic reticulum. By decreasing the intracellular calcium level, nisoldipine inhibits smooth-muscle cell contraction and dilates coronary and systemic arteries. As with other calcium channel blockers, these actions lead to decreased myocardial oxygen requirements and reduced peripheral resistance, blood pressure, and afterload.

## Contraindications
Hypersensitivity to any calcium channel blocker, second- or third-degree AV block without artificial pacemaker, sick sinus syndrome

## Interactions
**DRUGS**
*beta blockers:* Possibly increased risk of hypotension
*cimetidine, ranitidine:* Increased blood nisoldipine level
*NSAIDs:* Decreased antihypertensive effect of nisoldipine
*quinidine:* Possibly decreased blood nisoldipine level
**FOODS**
*grapefruit, grapefruit juice:* Possibly increased bioavailability of nisoldipine
*high-fat meals:* Possibly delayed nisoldipine absorption
**ACTIVITIES**
*alcohol use:* Additive hypotensive effect

## Adverse Reactions
**CNS:** Dizziness, headache
**CV:** Angina, hypotension, palpitations, peripheral edema

**EENT:** Pharyngitis, sinusitis
**GI:** Constipation, nausea
**RESP:** Dyspnea
**SKIN:** Rash

## Nursing Considerations
•Monitor pulse rate and rhythm and blood pressure before starting nisoldipine therapy, during dosage adjustments, and periodically throughout therapy.
•Don't break or crush E.R. tablets.
•For optimal absorption, give drug 30 minutes before or 2 hours after meals.
•Monitor fluid intake and output and daily weight to assess for signs of fluid retention, which may lead to heart failure. Also assess for signs of heart failure, such as crackles, dyspnea, jugular vein distention, peripheral edema, and weight gain.
**PATIENT TEACHING**
•Instruct patient to swallow E.R. nisoldipine tablets whole, not to break, crush, or chew them.
•Advise patient not to take drug within 1 hour of eating a high-fat meal or grapefruit product. Urge her not to alter the amount of grapefruit products in her diet without consulting prescriber.
•Urge patient to continue taking drug as prescribed, even if she feels well.
•**WARNING** Caution patient against stopping drug abruptly because blood pressure could rise dangerously high.
•Instruct patient to notify prescriber about constipation, difficulty breathing, dizziness, irregular heartbeat, nausea, severe headache, and swelling of hands or feet.
•Teach patient and family how to measure blood pressure, and instruct them to notify prescriber if systolic blood pressure falls below 90 mm Hg. Suggest that patient keep a log of weekly measurements and take it to follow-up visits.
•Advise patient to change positions slowly to minimize the effects of orthostatic hypotension. Inform her that hot tubs, saunas, and prolonged hot showers may worsen this adverse reaction.
•Caution patient to avoid potentially hazardous activities until drug's CNS effects are known.
•Urge patient to avoid alcohol and OTC alcohol-containing drugs without consulting prescriber. Many OTC preparations can raise blood pressure.

•Emphasize the need to adhere to prescribed lifestyle changes, such as alcohol moderation, low-fat and low-sodium diet, regular exercise, smoking cessation, stress reduction, and weight reduction.

# nitazoxanide

Alinia

## Class and Category
*Chemical:* Benzamide
*Therapeutic:* Antiprotozoal
*Pregnancy category:* B

## Indications and Dosages
➤ *To treat diarrhea caused by* Cryptosporidium parvum
**ORAL SUSPENSION, TABLETS**
**Adults and children age 12 and older.** 500 mg q 12 hr with meals for 3 days.
**ORAL SUSPENSION**
**Children ages 4 to 11.** 200 mg (10 ml) q 12 hr with meals for 3 days.
**Children ages 12 months to 47 months.** 100 mg (5 ml) q 12 hr with meals for 3 days.
➤ *To treat diarrhea caused by* Giardia lamblia
**ORAL SUSPENSION, TABLETS**
**Children age 12 and older.** 500 mg q 12 hr with meals for 3 days
**ORAL SUSPENSION**
**Children ages 4 to 11.** 200 mg (10 ml) q 12 hr with meals for 3 days.
**Children ages 12 months to 47 months.** 100 mg (5 ml) q 12 hr with meals for 3 days.

| Route | Onset | Peak | Duration |
|-------|-------|------|----------|
| P.O. | 1 to 4 hr | Unknown | Unknown |

### Mechanism of Action
May destroy *Cryptosporidium parvum* and *Giardia lamblia* by interfering with the enzyme-dependent electron transfer reaction required for their anaerobic energy metabolism. Other unidentified mechanisms may also be involved. With loss of protozoal activity in the intestines, diarrhea ceases.

## Contraindications
Hypersensitivity to nitazoxanide or its components

## Interactions
### DRUGS
*other highly plasma protein–bound drugs with narrow therapeutic indices (such as warfarin and phenytoins):* Possibly increased risk of toxicity of these drugs

## Adverse Reactions
**CNS:** Headache
**GI:** Abdominal pain, anorexia, diarrhea, nausea, vomiting

## Nursing Considerations
• Use nitazoxanide cautiously in children with impaired hepatic function, biliary disease, or renal insufficiency.
• Prepare nitazoxanide suspension by first tapping bottle until powder flows freely. Add 24 ml of tap water to the powder and shake vigorously to suspend powder. Add another 24 ml of water and shake vigorously again. Keep bottle of reconstituted suspension tightly capped.
• Use oral suspension for children age 11 and younger because tablets contain more nitazoxanide than is recommended for children younger than age 12.
### PATIENT TEACHING
• Tell parents of patient to give nitazoxanide with meals.
• Advise parents to keep reconstituted nitazoxanide bottle tightly closed and to shake the bottle well before each use.
• Instruct parents to discard any unused drug after 7 days from first opening bottle.
• Inform parents of diabetic patient that oral nitazoxanide suspension contains 1.48 grams of sucrose/5 ml. Tell them that they should make sure to monitor the patient's blood glucose level closely.
• Tell parents that discoloration of eye or urine, although uncommon, may occur and is harmless.

# nitrofurantoin

Apo-Nitrofurantoin (CAN), Furadantin, Macrobid, Macrodantin, Novo-Furantoin (CAN)

## Class and Category
*Chemical:* Nitrofuran derivative
*Therapeutic:* Antibiotic
*Pregnancy category:* B (except near term)

## Indications and Dosages
➤ *To treat acute cystitis*

### CAPSULES, ORAL SUSPENSION, TABLETS
**Adults.** 50 to 100 mg q 6 hr. *Maximum:* 600 mg/day or 10 mg/kg/day.
**Children over age 1 month.** 0.75 to 1.75 mg/kg q 6 hr.
### E.R. CAPSULES
**Adults and children age 12 and older.** 100 mg q 12 hr for 7 days.

➤ *To suppress chronic cystitis*
### CAPSULES, ORAL SUSPENSION, TABLETS
**Adults.** 50 to 100 mg h.s. *Maximum:* 600 mg/day or 10 mg/kg/day.
**Children over age 1 month.** 1 mg/kg/day h.s.

---

### Mechanism of Action
Inactivates or alters bacterial ribosomal proteins and other macromolecules. This inhibits bacterial protein synthesis, aerobic energy metabolism, DNA synthesis, RNA synthesis, and cell wall synthesis. Nitrofurantoin is bacteriostatic at low doses and bactericidal at higher doses.

---

## Contraindications
Age under 1 month, anuria, creatinine clearance of less than 60 ml/min/1.73 m$^2$, hypersensitivity to nitrofurantoin or parabens, oliguria, pregnancy near term

## Interactions
### DRUGS
*hepatotoxic drugs:* Increased risk of hepatotoxicity
*magnesium trisilicate:* Decreased nitrofurantoin absorption
*methyldopa, procainamide, hemolytics:* Increased risk of toxic effects from nitrofurantoin
*nalidixic acid:* Possibly impaired therapeutic effects of this drug
*neurotoxic drugs:* Increased risk of neurotoxicity
*probenecid, sulfinpyrazone:* Increased blood nitrofurantoin level and increased risk of toxicity

## Adverse Reactions
**CNS:** Chills, confusion, depression, headache, neurotoxicity, peripheral neuropathy
**EENT:** Optic neuritis, parotitis, tooth discoloration
**GI:** Abdominal pain, anorexia, diarrhea, hepatitis, nausea, pancreatitis, pseudomembranous colitis, vomiting
**GU:** Rust-colored to brown urine

N
O

**HEME:** Aplastic anemia, granulocytopenia, hemolytic anemia, leukopenia, megaloblastic anemia, methemoglobinemia, thrombocytopenia
**MS:** Arthralgia, myalgia
**RESP:** Asthma (in asthmatic patients), cyanosis, pneumonitis (acute)
**SKIN:** Alopecia, erythema multiforme, exfoliative dermatitis, jaundice, pruritus, rash, urticaria
**Other:** Anaphylaxis, angioedema, drug-induced fever

## Nursing Considerations

• Obtain a specimen of the patient's urine for culture and sensitivity tests, as ordered; review test results if possible before giving nitrofurantoin.
• Give drug with food or milk to avoid staining teeth.
• Don't crush or break capsules.
• Shake oral suspension before pouring dose, and mix with food or milk, as needed.
• Monitor patient for signs of superinfection, such as abdominal pain, diarrhea, and fever.
• Monitor elderly patients for pulmonary and hepatic abnormalities because rare but severe reactions have occurred with nitrofurantoin use in the elderly.

**PATIENT TEACHING**
• Instruct patient to shake nitrofurantoin oral suspension before measuring dose and to take drug with food or milk.
• Caution patient against taking any preparations that contain magnesium trisilicate during therapy.
• Inform patient that urine may become brown, orange, or rust-colored during therapy.
• Instruct patient to complete the prescribed course of therapy even if symptoms subside.

# nitroglycerin

## (glyceryl trinitrate)

Deponit, Minitran, Nitro-Bid, Nitrocot, Nitro-Dur, Nitrogard, Nitroglyn E-R, Nitroject, Nitrol, Nitrolingual, Nitrong SR, Nitro-par, Nitrostat, Nitro-time, Transderm-Nitro, Tridil

## Class and Category

*Chemical:* Nitrate
*Therapeutic:* Antianginal, antihypertensive, vasodilator
*Pregnancy category:* C

## Indications and Dosages

➤ *To prevent or treat angina*

**E.R. BUCCAL TABLETS**
**Adults.** 1 mg q 5 hr while awake.

**E.R. CAPSULES**
**Adults.** 2.5, 6.5, or 9 mg q 12 hr. Frequency increased to q 8 hr based on patient's response.

**E.R. TABLETS**
**Adults.** 2.6 or 6.5 mg q 12 hr. Frequency increased to q 8 hr based on patient's response.

**S.L. TABLETS**
**Adults.** 0.3 to 0.6 mg, repeated q 5 min. *Maximum:* 3 tabs in 15 min or 10 mg/day.

**TRANSDERMAL OINTMENT**
**Adults.** 1" to 2" (15 to 30 mg) q 8 hr. Frequency increased to q 6 hr if angina occurs between doses. *Maximum:* 5" (75 mg)/application.

**TRANSDERMAL PATCH**
**Adults.** 0.1 to 0.8 mg/hr, worn 12 to 14 hr.

**TRANSLINGUAL SPRAY**
**Adults.** 1 or 2 metered doses (0.4 or 0.8 mg) onto or under tongue, repeated q 5 min as needed. *Maximum:* 3 metered doses in 15 min or 1.2 mg/day.

➤ *To prevent or treat angina, to manage hypertension or heart failure*

**I.V. INFUSION**
**Adults.** 5 mcg/min, increased by 5 mcg/min q 3 to 5 min to 20 mcg/min, as prescribed, and then by 10 to 20 mcg/min q 3 to 5 min until desired effect occurs.

| Route | Onset | Peak | Duration |
|---|---|---|---|
| P.O. (buccal) | 3 min | Unknown | 5 hr |
| P.O. (E.R.) | 20 to 45 min | Unknown | 8 to 12 hr |
| I.V. | 1 to 2 min | Unknown | 3 to 5 min |
| S.L. | 1 to 3 min | Unknown | 30 to 60 min |
| Trans-dermal (ointment) | In 30 min | Unknown | 4 to 8 hr |
| Trans-dermal (patch) | In 30 min | Unknown | 8 to 24 hr |
| Trans-lingual | 2 to 4 min | Unknown | 30 to 60 min |

## Incompatibilities

Don't administer I.V. nitroglycerin through I.V. bags or tubing made of polyvinyl chloride. Don't mix drug with other solutions.

## Mechanism of Action

May interact with nitrate receptors in vascular smooth-muscle cell membranes. This interaction reduces nitroglycerin to nitric oxide, which activates the enzyme guanylate cyclase, increasing intracellular formation of cGMP. The increased cGMP level may relax vascular smooth muscle by forcing calcium out of muscle cells, causing vasodilation. Venous dilation decreases venous return to the heart, reducing left ventricular end-diastolic pressure and pulmonary artery wedge pressure. Arterial dilation decreases systemic vascular resistance, systolic arte-rial pressure, and mean arterial pressure. Thus, nitroglycerin reduces preload and afterload, decreasing myocardial workload and oxygen demand. It also dilates coronary arteries, increasing blood flow to ischemic myocardial tissue.

## Contraindications

Acute MI (S.L.), angle-closure glaucoma, cerebral hemorrhage, concurrent use of phosphodiesterase inhibitors, constrictive pericarditis (I.V.), head trauma, hypersensitivity to adhesive in transdermal form, hypersensitivity to nitrates, hypotension (I.V.), hypovolemia (I.V.), inadequate cerebral circulation (I.V.), increased intracranial pressure, orthostatic hypotension, pericardial tamponade, severe anemia

## Interactions
### DRUGS

*acetylcholine, norepinephrine:* Possibly decreased therapeutic effects of these drugs
*heparin:* Possibly decreased anticoagulant effect of heparin (I.V. nitroglycerin)
*opioid analgesics, other antihypertensives, vasodilators:* Possibly increased orthostatic hypotension
*phosphodiesterase inhibitors, such as sildenafil:* Possibly severe hypotensive effect of nitroglycerin
*sympathomimetics:* Possibly decreased antianginal effect of nitroglycerin and increased risk of hypotension

### ACTIVITIES

*alcohol use:* Possibly increased orthostatic hypotension

## Adverse Reactions

**CNS:** Agitation, anxiety, dizziness, headache, insomnia, restlessness, syncope, weakness

**CV:** Arrhythmias (including tachycardia), edema, hypotension, orthostatic hypotension, palpitations
**EENT:** Blurred vision, burning or tingling in mouth (buccal, S.L. forms), dry mouth
**GI:** Abdominal pain, diarrhea, indigestion, nausea, vomiting
**GU:** Dysuria, impotence, urinary frequency
**HEME:** Methemoglobinemia
**MS:** Arthralgia
**RESP:** Bronchitis, pneumonia
**SKIN:** Contact dermatitis (transdermal forms), flushing of face and neck, rash

## Nursing Considerations

•Use nitroglycerin cautiously in elderly patients, especially those who are volume depleted or taking several medications, because of the increased risk of hypotension and falls. Hypotension may be accompanied by angina and paradoxical slowing of the heart rate. Notify prescriber if these occur, and provide appropriate treatment, as ordered.
•Plan a nitroglycerin-free period of about 10 hours each day, as prescribed, to maintain therapeutic effects and avoid tolerance.
•Place E.R. buccal tablets in buccal pouch with patient in sitting or lying position.
•Don't break or crush E.R. tablets or capsules. Have patient swallow them whole with a full glass of water.
•Place S.L. tablet under patient's tongue and make sure it dissolves completely.
•Be sure to remove cotton from S.L. tablet container to allow quick access to the drug.
•When applying transdermal ointment, apply correct amount on dose-measuring paper. Then place paper on hairless area of body and spread in a thin even layer over an area at least 2 inches by 3 inches. Don't place on cuts or irritated areas. Wash your hands after application. Rotate sites. Store at room temperature.
•Open transdermal patch package immediately before use. Apply patch to hairless area, and press edges to seal. Rotate sites. Store at room temperature. If patient needs cardioversion or defibrillation, remove transdermal patch.
•Don't shake translingual spray container before administering. Have patient inhale and hold her breath, and then spray drug under or on her tongue.
•Be aware that I.V. nitroglycerin should be diluted only in $D_5W$ or NS and shouldn't be

**N O**

mixed with other infusions. The pharmacist should add drug to a glass bottle, not a container made of polyvinyl chloride. Don't use a filter because plastic absorbs drug. Administer with infusion pump.

• Check vital signs before every dosage adjustment and frequently during therapy.

• Frequently monitor heart and breath sounds, level of consciousness, fluid intake and output, and pulmonary artery wedge pressure, if possible.

• Store premixed containers in the dark; don't freeze them.

•**WARNING** Assess for signs of overdose, such as confusion, diaphoresis, dyspnea, flushing, headache, hypotension, nausea, palpitations, tachycardia, vertigo, vision changes, and vomiting. Treat as prescribed by removing nitroglycerin source, if possible; elevating the legs above heart level; and administering an alpha-adrenergic agonist, such as phenylephrine, as prescribed, to treat severe hypotension.

**PATIENT TEACHING**

• Teach patient to recognize signs and symptoms of angina pectoris, including chest fullness, pain, and pressure, which may be accompanied by sweating and nausea. Pain may radiate down left arm or into neck or jaw. Inform female patients and those with diabetes mellitus or hypertension that they may experience only fatigue and shortness of breath.

• Instruct patient to read and follow package instructions to obtain full benefits of drug.

• To prevent drug tolerance, inform patient that prescriber may order a 10- to 12-hour drug-free period at night (or at another time if she has chest pain at night or in the morning).

• Instruct patient to swallow E.R. tablets or capsules whole—not to break, crush, or chew them—with a full glass of water.

• For sublingual or buccal use, advise patient to place a tablet under her tongue or in her buccal pouch when angina starts and then to sit or lie down. Instruct her not to swallow drug, but to let it dissolve. Explain that moisture in her mouth helps drug absorption. If angina doesn't subside, instruct patient to place another tablet under her tongue or in her buccal pouch after 5 minutes and to repeat, if needed, for three doses total. If pain doesn't subside after 20 minutes, urge patient to call 911 or another emergency service.

• Advise patient to carry S.L. tablets in their original brown bottle in a purse or jacket pocket, but not one that will be affected by body heat. Instruct her to store drug in a dry place at room temperature and to discard cotton from container. Advise her to discard and replace S.L. tablets after 6 months.

• Advise patient using transdermal ointment or patch to rotate sites to avoid skin sensitization.

• Inform patient that swimming or bathing doesn't affect transdermal forms but that hot tubs, saunas, prolonged hot showers, electric blankets, and magnetic therapy over site may increase drug absorption and cause dizziness and hypotension.

• Caution against inhaling translingual spray.

• Inform patient that drug commonly causes headache, which typically resolves after a few days of continuous therapy. Suggest that patient take acetaminophen, as needed.

• Advise patient to notify prescriber immediately about blurred vision, dizziness, and severe headache.

• Suggest that patient change positions slowly to minimize effects of orthostatic hypotension.

• Advise patient to avoid potentially hazardous activities until drug's CNS effects are known.

• Urge patient to avoid alcohol and erectile dysfunction drugs during therapy.

# nitroprusside sodium

Nipride, Nitropress

## Class and Category

*Chemical:* Cyanonitrosylferrate
*Therapeutic:* Antihypertensive, vasodilator
*Pregnancy category:* C

## Indications and Dosages

➤ *To treat hypertensive crisis and manage severe heart failure*

**I.V. INFUSION**

**Adults and children.** *Initial:* 0.25 to 0.3 mcg/kg/min, increased gradually q few minutes until blood pressure reaches desired level. *Maintenance:* 3 mcg/kg/min (range, 0.25 to 10 mcg/kg/min). *Maximum:* 10 mcg/kg/min for 10 min.

| Route | Onset | Peak | Duration |
|-------|-------|------|----------|
| I.V. | 1 to 2 min | Immediate | 1 to 10 min |

## Mechanism of Action

May interact with nitrate receptors in vascular smooth-muscle cell membranes. This action reduces nitroprusside to nitric oxide and then activates intracellular guanylate cyclase, which increases the cGMP level. The increased cGMP level may relax vascular smooth muscle by forcing calcium out of muscle cells. Smooth-muscle relaxation causes arteries and veins to dilate, which reduces peripheral vascular resistance and blood pressure.

## Incompatibilities

Don't mix nitroprusside with any other drug.

## Contraindications

Acute heart failure with decreased peripheral vascular resistance, congenital optic atrophy, decreased cerebral perfusion, hypersensitivity to nitroprusside or its components, hypertension from aortic coarctation or AV shunting, tobacco-induced amblyopia

## Interactions

**DRUGS**
*dobutamine:* Increased cardiac output, decreased pulmonary artery wedge pressure
*ganglionic blockers, general anesthetics, hypotension-producing drugs:* Increased hypotensive effect
*sympathomimetics:* Decreased antihypertensive effect of nitroprusside

## Adverse Reactions

**CNS:** Anxiety, dizziness, headache, increased intracranial pressure, nervousness, restlessness
**CV:** Hypotension, tachycardia
**ENDO:** Hypothyroidism
**GI:** Abdominal pain, ileus, nausea, vomiting
**HEME:** Methemoglobinemia
**MS:** Muscle twitching
**SKIN:** Diaphoresis, flushing, rash
**Other:** Infusion site phlebitis

## Nursing Considerations

•Obtain baseline vital signs before administering nitroprusside.
•**WARNING** Don't give drug undiluted. Reconstitute with 2 ml of $D_5W$, and add solution to 250 to 500 ml of $D_5W$ to produce 200 mcg/ml or 100 mcg/ml, respectively.
•Be aware that solution is stable at room temperature for 24 hours when protected from light. Don't use reconstituted solution if it contains particles or is blue, green, red, or darker than faint brown.
•Use an infusion pump. Place opaque covering over infusion container because drug is metabolized by light. I.V. tubing doesn't need to be covered.
•Keep patient supine when starting drug or titrating dose up or down.
•Monitor blood pressure continuously with intra-arterial pressure monitor. Record blood pressure every 5 minutes at start of infusion and every 15 minutes thereafter.
•If patient has severe heart failure, expect to administer an inotropic drug, such as dopamine or dobutamine, as prescribed.
•**WARNING** For patient who receives prolonged nitroprusside therapy or short-term high-dose therapy, monitor for signs of thiocyanate toxicity (ataxia, blurred vision, delirium, dizziness, dyspnea, headache, hyperreflexia, loss of consciousness, nausea, tinnitus, vomiting). Toxicity can cause arrhythmias, metabolic acidosis, severe hypotension, and death.
•Monitor serum thiocyanate level at least every 72 hours; levels above 100 mcg/ml are associated with toxicity.
•**WARNING** Assess for signs of cyanide toxicity (absence of reflexes, coma, distant heart sounds, hypotension, metabolic acidosis, mydriasis, pink skin, shallow respirations, and weak pulse). If you detect such signs, discontinue nitroprusside, as ordered, and give 4 to 6 mg/kg of sodium nitrite over 2 to 4 minutes to convert hemoglobin to methemoglobin. Follow with 150 to 200 mg/kg of sodium thiosulfate. Repeat this regimen at one-half the original doses after 2 hours, as ordered.
**PATIENT TEACHING**
•Advise patient to change position slowly to minimize dizziness from sudden, severe hypotension.

# nizatidine

Apo-Nizatidine (CAN), Axid, Axid AR

## Class and Category

*Chemical:* Ethenediamine derivative
*Therapeutic:* Antiulcer
*Pregnancy category:* B

## Indications and Dosages

➤ *To manage active duodenal ulcer*

**CAPSULES**
**Adults and adolescents.** 300 mg h.s. or 150 mg b.i.d. for 8 wk.
**DOSAGE ADJUSTMENT** Dosage reduced to 150 mg/day for patients with creatinine clearance of 20 to 50 ml/min/1.73 m$^2$; to 150 mg q.o.d. for those with creatinine clearance of less than 20 ml/min/1.73 m$^2$.
➤ *To prevent recurrence of duodenal ulcer*
**CAPSULES**
**Adults and adolescents.** 150 mg h.s.
**DOSAGE ADJUSTMENT** Dosage reduced to 150 mg q.o.d. for patients with creatinine clearance of 20 to 50 ml/min/1.73 m$^2$; to 150 mg q 3 days for those with creatinine clearance of less than 20 ml/min/1.73 m$^2$.
➤ *To manage acute benign gastric ulcer*
**CAPSULES**
**Adults and adolescents.** 300 mg h.s. or 150 mg b.i.d.
➤ *To manage gastroesophageal reflux disease*
**CAPSULES**
**Adults and adolescents.** 150 mg b.i.d.
➤ *To prevent or relieve acid indigestion or heartburn*
**TABLETS**
**Adults and adolescents.** 75 mg 30 min to 1 hr before meals.

| Route | Onset | Peak | Duration |
|-------|-------|------|----------|
| P.O. | Unknown | Unknown | 10 to 12 hr* |

### Mechanism of Action
Inhibits basal and nocturnal secretion of gastric acid by reversibly and competitively blocking H$_2$ receptors, especially those in gastric parietal cells. Nizatidine also inhibits gastric acid secretion in response to stimuli, including food and caffeine.

### Contraindications
Hypersensitivity to nizatidine or other H$_2$-receptor antagonists

### Interactions
**DRUGS**
*antacids:* Decreased nizatidine bioavailability
*itraconazole, ketoconazole:* Decreased absorption of these drugs

---

* For nocturnal acid secretion; up to 4 hr for food-stimulated acid secretion.

*salicylates:* Increased blood level of these drugs
*sucralfate:* Possibly decreased nizatidine absorption

### Adverse Reactions
**CNS:** Agitation, anxiety, confusion, depression, dizziness, fatigue, fever, hallucinations, headache, insomnia, somnolence
**CV:** Arrhythmias, chest pain, vasculitis
**EENT:** Amblyopia, dry mouth, laryngeal edema, pharyngitis, rhinitis, sinusitis
**ENDO:** Gynecomastia
**GI:** Abdominal pain, constipation, diarrhea, hepatitis, nausea, vomiting
**GU:** Decreased libido, hyperuricemia not associated with gout or nephrolithiasis, impotence
**HEME:** Anemia, aplastic anemia, eosinophilia, hemolytic anemia, leukopenia, neutropenia, pancytopenia, thrombocytopenia
**MS:** Back pain, myalgia
**RESP:** Bronchospasm, cough
**SKIN:** Alopecia, diaphoresis, erythema multiforme, exfoliative dermatitis, jaundice, pruritus, rash, Stevens-Johnson syndrome, toxic epidermal necrolysis, urticaria
**Other:** Anaphylaxis, angioedema, serum sickness–like reaction

### Nursing Considerations
•Monitor CBC, BUN and serum creatinine levels, and liver function test results before and periodically during nizatidine therapy.
•Don't give within 1 hour of an antacid.
**PATIENT TEACHING**
•Instruct patient not to take nizatidine within 1 hour of an antacid.
•Urge patient to take drug exactly as prescribed, even if she feels better. Inform her that ulcer may take up to 8 weeks to heal.
•If patient smokes, urge her to stop because smoking increases gastric acid production.
•Teach patient to minimize constipation by drinking plenty of fluids (if allowed), eating high-fiber foods, and exercising regularly.
•Instruct patient to notify prescriber immediately about abdominal pain, easy bruising, extreme fatigue, yellow skin or sclera, trouble swallowing food, bloody vomitus, or bloody or tarry stools.
•Urge patient not to take nizatidine with other acid reducers.

# norepinephrine bitartrate

## (levarterenol bitartrate)

Levophed

## Class and Category

*Chemical:* Catecholamine
*Therapeutic:* Cardiac stimulant, vasopressor
*Pregnancy category:* C

## Indications and Dosages

➤ *To treat acute hypotension, cardiogenic shock, and septic shock*

**I.V. INFUSION**

**Adults.** *Initial:* 0.5 to 1 mcg/min. Increased, as ordered, until systolic blood pressure reaches desired level. *Maintenance:* 2 to 12 mcg/min.

**Children.** 0.1 mcg/kg/min. *Maximum:* 1 mcg/kg/min.

➤ *To treat refractory shock*

**I.V. INFUSION**

**Adults.** Up to 30 mcg/min.

| Route | Onset | Peak | Duration |
|-------|-------|------|----------|
| I.V. | Rapid | Unknown | 1 to 2 min |

## Mechanism of Action

At more than 4 mcg/min, directly stimulates alpha-adrenergic receptors and inhibits adenyl cyclase, which inhibits cAMP production. Inhibition of cAMP contricts arteries and veins and increases peripheral vascular resistance and systolic blood pressure. At less than 2 mcg/min, norepinephrine directly stimulates beta-adrenergic receptors in the myocardium and increases adenyl cyclase activity, producing positive inotropic and chronotropic effects.

## Contraindications

Concurrent use of hydrocarbon inhalation anesthetics, hypersensitivity to norepinephrine or its components, hypovolemia, mesenteric or peripheral vascular thrombosis

## Interactions

**DRUGS**

*alpha blockers:* Decreased vasopressor effects of norepinephrine
*beta blockers:* Decreased cardiac-stimulating effect of norepinephrine, possibly decreased therapeutic effects of both drugs

*digoxin:* Increased risk of arrhythmias, possibly potentiated inotropic effect
*doxapram:* Possibly increased vasopressor effects of both drugs
*ergonovine, ergotamine, methylergonovine, methysergide, oxytocin:* Possibly increased vasoconstriction
*general anesthetics:* Risk of arrhythmias
*guanadrel, guanethidine:* Increased vasopressor response to norepinephrine, possibly severe hypertension
*MAO inhibitors:* Possibly life-threatening arrhythmias, hyperpyrexia, severe headache, severe hypertension, and vomiting
*maprotiline, tricyclic antidepressants:* Possibly potentiated cardiovascular and pressor effects of norepinephrine, including arrhythmias, severe hypertension, and hyperpyrexia
*methylphenidate:* Possibly potentiated vasopressor effect of norepinephrine
*nitrates:* Possibly decreased therapeutic effects of both drugs
*phenoxybenzamine:* Possibly arrhythmias or hypotension
*sympathomimetics:* Increased risk of adverse cardiovascular effects
*thyroid hormones:* Increased risk of coronary insufficiency

## Adverse Reactions

**CNS:** Anxiety, dizziness, headache, insomnia, nervousness, tremor, weakness
**CV:** Angina, bradycardia, ECG changes, edema, hypertension, hypotension, palpitations, peripheral vascular insufficiency (including gangrene), PVCs, sinus tachycardia
**GI:** Nausea, vomiting
**GU:** Decreased renal perfusion
**RESP:** Apnea, dyspnea
**SKIN:** Pallor
**Other:** Infusion site sloughing and tissue necrosis, metabolic acidosis

## Nursing Considerations

• Dilute norepinephrine concentrate for infusion in $D_5W$, $D_5NS$, or NS. Dilutions typically range from 16 to 32 mcg/ml.
• Make sure solution contains no particles and isn't discolored before administering.
• Give drug with a flow-control device.
• Check blood pressure every 2 to 3 minutes, preferably by direct intra-arterial monitoring, until stabilized and then every 5 minutes.

N
O

•**WARNING** Because extravasation can cause severe tissue damage and necrosis, expect prescriber to give multiple S.C. injections of phentolamine (5 to 10 mg diluted in 10 to 15 ml of NS) around extravasated infusion site.
•If blanching occurs along vein, change infusion site and notify prescriber at once.
•Monitor continuous ECG during therapy.
**PATIENT TEACHING**
•Urge patient to notify you at once about burning, leaking, or tingling around I.V. site.

# norfloxacin

Noroxin

## Class and Category
*Chemical:* Fluoroquinolone
*Therapeutic:* Antibiotic
*Pregnancy category:* C

## Indications and Dosages
➤ *To treat uncomplicated UTIs caused by* Escherichia coli, Klebsiella pneumoniae, *or* Proteus mirabilis
**TABLETS**
**Adults.** 400 mg q 12 hr for 3 days.
➤ *To treat uncomplicated UTIs caused by* Citrobacter freundii, Enterobacter aerogenes, Enterobacter cloacae, Enterococcus faecalis, Proteus *sp.*, Pseudomonas aeruginosa, Staphylococcus aureus, Staphylococcus epidermidis, Staphylococcus saprophyticus, *or* Streptococcus agalactiae
**TABLETS**
**Adults.** 400 mg q 12 hr for 7 to 10 days.
➤ *To treat complicated UTIs caused by* E. coli, E. faecalis, K. pneumoniae, P. aeruginosa, P. mirabilis, *or* Serratia marcescens
**TABLETS**
**Adults.** 400 mg q 12 hr for 10 to 21 days. *Maximum:* 800 mg/day.
➤ *To treat uncomplicated gonorrhea*
**TABLETS**
**Adults.** 800 mg as a single dose.
➤ *To treat prostatitis caused by* E. coli
**TABLETS**
**Adults.** 400 mg q 12 hr for 28 days.

**DOSAGE ADJUSTMENT** Dosage reduced to 400 mg q.d. for patients with creatinine clearance of 30 ml/min/1.73 m$^2$ or less.

## Mechanism of Action
Inhibits the enzyme DNA gyrase, which unwinds and supercoils bacterial DNA before it replicates. By inhibiting this enzyme, norfloxacin interferes with bacterial cell replication and causes cell death.

## Contraindications
Hypersensitivity to norfloxacin, other fluoroquinolones, or their components

## Interactions
**DRUGS**
*aluminum-, calcium-, or magnesium-containing antacids; ferrous sulfate; magnesium-containing laxatives; sucralfate; zinc:* Possibly decreased absorption and blood level of norfloxacin
*cyclosporine:* Possibly increased serum creatinine and blood cyclosporine levels
*didanosine:* Possibly decreased norfloxacin absorption
*glyburide:* Risk of severe hypoglycemia
*nitrofurantoin:* Possibly decreased norfloxacin effectiveness
*probenecid:* Decreased norfloxacin excretion and risk of toxicity
*warfarin:* Possibly increased anticoagulant effect and risk of bleeding

## Adverse Reactions
**CNS:** Dizziness, drowsiness, headache, insomnia, peripheral neuropathy, psychosis, seizures, tremors
**CV:** Prolonged QT interval, torsades de pointes
**EENT:** Decreased taste sensation. diplopia, hearing loss, taste perversion, tinnitus
**GI:** Abdominal cramps or pain, diarrhea, elevated liver function test results, hepatitis, nausea, pseudomembranous colitis, vomiting
**GU:** Interstitial nephritis, renal failure, vaginal candidiasis
**HEME:** Agranulocytosis, hemolytic anemia, leukopenia, neutropenia, thrombocytopenia
**MS:** Myasthenia gravis exacerbation; tendinitis; tendon inflammation, pain, or rupture

**SKIN:** Blisters, diaphoresis, erythema, erythema multiforme, exfoliative dermatitis, photosensitivity, pruritus, rash, Stevens-Johnson syndrome, toxic epidermal necrolysis, urticaria
**Other:** Angioedema, anaphylaxis

## Nursing Considerations
•Obtain urine specimen for culture and sensitivity tests before starting drug, if possible.
•Determine if patient has a history of a CNS disorder because drug may lower the seizure threshold. Notify prescriber before starting drug, and institute seizure precautions.
•Give drug on an empty stomach 2 hours before or after antacids, didanosine, sucralfate, or vitamins that contain iron or zinc.
•Keep emergency resuscitation equipment readily available, and watch for signs of hypersensitivity, such as angioedema, dyspnea, and urticaria. If you suspect anaphylaxis, prepare to give epinephrine, corticosteroids, and diphenhydramine, as prescribed.
•If patient has myasthenia gravis, assess her frequently for a change in respiratory status because norfloxacin may lead to life-threatening weakness of respiratory muscles.
•Notify prescriber if patient has symptoms of peripheral neuropathy (pain, burning, tingling, numbness, weakness, or altered sensations of light touch, pain, temperature, position sense, or vibration sense), which could be permanent; or tendon rupture, which requires immediate rest. In each case, expect to stop norfloxacin.

**PATIENT TEACHING**
•Instruct patient to take norfloxacin on an empty stomach with a large glass of water to prevent crystalluria. Urge her to drink several glasses of water every day during therapy.
•Instruct patient to take drug at least 2 hours before or after eating, drinking milk, or taking antacids, didanosine, sucralfate, or vitamins that contain iron or zinc.
•Advise patient to avoid hazardous activities until drug's CNS effects are known.
•Tell patient to stop drug and report tendon pain or inflammation or abnormal changes in motor or sensory function.
•Advise patient to protect skin from sunlight and to report first sign of photosensitivity.
•Tell patient to take drug exactly as prescribed, even if symptoms subside.

# nortriptyline hydrochloride
Aventyl, Pamelor

## Class and Category
*Chemical:* Dibenzocycloheptene derivative
*Therapeutic:* Antidepressant
*Pregnancy category:* D

## Indications and Dosages
➤ *To treat depression*
**CAPSULES, ORAL SOLUTION**
**Adults.** *Initial:* 25 mg t.i.d. or q.i.d. *Maximum:* 150 mg/day.
**Adolescents.** 25 to 50 mg/day or 1 to 3 mg/kg/day in divided doses.
**Children ages 6 to 12.** 10 to 20 mg/day or 1 to 3 mg/kg/day in divided doses.
DOSAGE ADJUSTMENT Dosage possibly reduced to 30 to 50 mg/day (in divided doses or h.s.) for elderly patients.

| Route | Onset | Peak | Duration |
|-------|-------|------|----------|
| P.O. | 2 to 3 wk | Unknown | Unknown |

### Mechanism of Action
May interfere with reuptake of serotonin (and possibly other neurotransmitters) at presynaptic neurons, thus enhancing serotonin's effects at postsynaptic receptors. By restoring normal neurotransmitter levels at nerve synapses, this tricyclic antidepressant may elevate mood.

## Contraindications
Acute recovery phase of CVA or MI; hypersensitivity to nortriptyline, other tricyclic antidepressants, or their components; use within 14 days of MAO inhibitor therapy

## Interactions
**DRUGS**
*amantadine, anticholinergics, antidyskinetics, antihistamines:* Possibly increased anticholinergic effects, confusion, hallucinations, nightmares; increased CNS depression
*anticonvulsants:* Possibly increased CNS depression and risk of seizures, possibly decreased anticonvulsant effectiveness
*antithyroid drugs:* Possibly agranulocytosis
*barbiturates, carbamazepine:* Possibly decreased level and effects of nortriptyline
*bupropion, clozapine, cyclobenzaprine, halo-*

*peridol, loxapine, maprotiline, molindone, phenothiazines, thioxanthenes:* Possibly increased sedative and anticholinergic effects and possibly increased risk of seizures
*cimetidine, fluoxetine:* Possibly increased blood nortriptyline level and risk of toxicity
*clonidine:* Possibly decreased antihypertensive effect and increased CNS depression
*disulfiram:* Possibly delirium
*ethchlorvynol:* Possibly delirium, increased CNS depression
*guanadrel, guanethidine:* Possibly decreased antihypertensive effect of these drugs
*MAO inhibitors:* Increased risk of hypertensive crisis, severe seizures, and death
*oral anticoagulants:* Possibly increased anticoagulant activity
*pimozide, probucol:* Possibly arrhythmias
*sympathomimetics, including ophthalmic epinephrine and vasoconstrictive local anesthetics:* Increased risk of arrhythmias, hyperpyrexia, hypertension, and tachycardia
*thyroid hormones:* Possibly increased therapeutic and toxic effects of both drugs

**ACTIVITIES**
*alcohol use:* Increased CNS and respiratory depression, hypertension, alcohol effects

## Adverse Reactions

**CNS:** Ataxia, confusion, CVA, delirium, dizziness, drowsiness, excitation, hallucinations, headache, insomnia, nervousness, nightmares, parkinsonism, suicidal ideation (children and adolescents), tremor
**CV:** Arrhythmias, orthostatic hypotension
**EENT:** Blurred vision, dry mouth, increased intraocular pressure, taste perversion
**GI:** Constipation, diarrhea, heartburn, ileus, increased appetite, nausea, vomiting
**GU:** Sexual dysfunction, urine retention
**HEME:** Bone marrow depression
**RESP:** Wheezing
**SKIN:** Diaphoresis, urticaria
**Other:** Weight gain

## Nursing Considerations

•Expect to stop MAO inhibitor therapy 10 to 14 days before starting nortriptyline therapy.
•**WARNING** Monitor children and adolescents closely for suicidal thinking and behavior; drug increases the risk in these groups.
•Oral solution (10 mg/5 ml) is 4% alcohol.
•Give drug with food to reduce GI reactions.
•Monitor blood nortriptyline level; therapeu-

tic range is 50 to 150 ng/ml.
•Monitor ECG tracing to detect arrhythmias.
**PATIENT TEACHING**
•Explain that oral solution contains alcohol.
•Discourage alcohol use during therapy.
•Explain that improvement may take weeks.
•Advise patient to avoid hazardous activities until drug's CNS effects are known.
•**WARNING** Urge parents to watch their child or adolescent closely for abnormal thinking or behavior or increased aggression or hostility. Stress importance of notifying prescriber.
•Instruct patient to change position slowly to minimize effects of orthostatic hypotension.
•Suggest that patient minimize constipation by drinking plenty of fluids (if allowed), eating high-fiber foods, and exercising regularly.

# nystatin

Mycostatin, Nadostine (CAN), Nilstat, Nystex, Nystop, Pedi-Dri

## Class and Category

*Chemical:* Amphoteric polyene macrolide
*Therapeutic:* Antifungal
*Pregnancy category:* Not rated (lozenges, oral suspension, tablets, topical), A (vaginal)

## Indications and Dosages

➤ *To treat oropharyngeal candidiasis (thrush)*
**LOZENGES (PASTILLES)**
**Adults and children over age 5.** 200,000 to 400,000 U dissolved in mouth 4 or 5 times/day for up to 14 days.
**ORAL SUSPENSION**
**Adults and children.** 400,000 to 600,000 U swished and swallowed q.i.d. until at least 48 hr after symptoms subside.
**Infants.** 200,000 U to each side of mouth q.i.d. until at least 48 hr after symptoms subside.
**Neonates.** 100,000 U applied to each side of mouth q.i.d. until at least 48 hr after symptoms subside.
**TABLETS**
**Adults and adolescents.** 500,000 to 1,000,000 U t.i.d. until at least 48 hr after symptoms subside.
**Children age 5 and older.** 500,000 U q.i.d. until at least 48 hr after symptoms subside.

➤ *To treat cutaneous and mucocutaneous candidiasis*

CREAM, OINTMENT, POWDER

**Adults and children.** 100,000 U (1 g) on affected area b.i.d. or t.i.d. for at least 2 wk.

➤ *To treat vulvovaginal candidiasis*
VAGINAL TABLETS
**Adults and adolescents.** 100,000 U (1 tab) q.d. or b.i.d. for 14 days.

---

## Mechanism of Action
Binds to sterols in fungal cell membranes, impairing membrane integrity. Cells lose intracellular potassium and other cellular contents and, eventually, die.

---

## Contraindications
Hypersensitivity to nystatin or its components

## Adverse Reactions
**ENDO:** Hyperglycemia (lozenge, oral suspension)
**GI:** Abdominal pain, diarrhea, nausea, vomiting (oral forms)
**GU:** Vaginal burning or itching (vaginal form)
**SKIN:** Irritation (topical forms)

## Nursing Considerations
•Prepare nystatin powder for oral suspension for each dose; it has no preservatives.
•Gently rub nystatin cream or ointment into skin at affected area. Keep area dry and avoid occlusive dressings.
•Don't get topical form in patient's eyes.
•When treating candidal infection of feet, dust patient's shoes, socks, and feet.
•For vaginal form, use applicator supplied by manufacturer.
PATIENT TEACHING
•Instruct patient to let nystatin lozenges dissolve slowly in her mouth, not to chew or swallow them.
•Instruct patient to swish oral suspension in her mouth for as long as possible before swallowing.
•Advise patient to gently rub ointment or cream into skin at affected area, to keep area dry, and to avoid occlusive dressings.
•Caution patient to keep topical form away from her eyes.
•Advise patient with candidal infection of feet to dust her shoes, socks, and feet with nystatin.
•Instruct patient who uses vaginal form to insert it with applicator supplied by manufacturer.

# octreotide acetate
Sandostatin, Sandostatin LAR Depot

## Class and Category
*Chemical:* Cyclic octapeptide, somatostatin analogue
*Therapeutic:* Antidiarrheal, hormone suppressant
*Pregnancy category:* B

## Indications and Dosages
➤ *To control symptoms associated with vasoactive intestinal peptide tumors (watery diarrhea) and metastatic carcinoid tumors (diarrhea and flushing)*
I.M. INJECTION
**Adults currently receiving S.C. injections.** 20 mg q 4 wk for 2 mo, with S.C. doses continued for 2 to 4 wk after I.M. injections start. If patient has positive response to initial 2-mo regimen, dosage reduced to 10 mg q 4 wk. If symptoms persist or increase after initial 2-mo regimen, dosage increased to 30 mg q 4 wk, as prescribed.
S.C. INJECTION
**Adults.** *Initial:* 200 to 300 mcg/day in divided doses b.i.d. to q.i.d. for first 2 wk. *Maintenance:* Individualized. *Maximum:* 450 mcg/day.

➤ *To treat symptoms of acromegaly, to suppress the release of growth hormone from pituitary tumors*
I.V. OR S.C. INJECTION
**Adults.** *Initial:* 50 mcg t.i.d. *Usual:* 100 mcg t.i.d. *Maximum:* 1,500 mcg/day.
I.M. INJECTION
**Adults currently receiving S.C. injections.** 20 mg q 4 wk for 3 mo, then adjusted as prescribed in response to serum growth hormone level. *Maximum:* 40 mg q 4 wk.

| Route | Onset | Peak | Duration |
|-------|-------|------|----------|
| S.C. | Unknown | Unknown | Up to 12 hr |

## Incompatibilities
Don't mix octreotide in same syringe with fat emulsions or total parenteral nutrition solutions.

## Contraindications
Hypersensitivity to octreotide or its components

## Mechanism of Action

Controls many types of secretory diarrhea by inhibiting secretion of serotonin and pituitary and GI hormones (including insulin, glucagon, growth hormone, thyrotropin, and, possibly, thyroid-stimulating hormone) as well as vasoactive intestinal peptides and pancreatic polypeptides (including gastrin, secretin, and motilin). Inhibition of serotonin and peptides increases intestinal absorption of water and electrolytes, decreases pancreatic and gastric acid secretions, and increases intestinal transit time by slowing gastric motility.

By inhibiting hormones involved in vasodilation, octreotide increases splanchnic arterial resistance and decreases GI blood flow, hepatic vein wedge pressure, hepatic blood flow, portal vein pressure, and intravariceal pressure, thus raising seated and standing blood pressures. By inhibiting serotonin secretion, the drug decreases symptoms of acromegaly, including diarrhea, flushing, wheezing, and urinary excretion of 5-hydroxyindoleacetic acid.

## Interactions
### DRUGS

*beta blockers, calcium channel blockers:* Additive cardiovascular effects of these drugs
*bromocriptine:* Increased blood bromocriptine level
*cisapride:* Decreased effectiveness of both drugs
*cyclosporine:* Decreased blood cyclosporine level
*diuretics:* Increased risk of fluid and electrolyte imbalances
*insulin, oral antidiabetic drugs:* Increased risk of hypoglycemia
*quinidine, terfenadine:* Decreased metabolic clearance and increased blood levels of these drugs
*vitamin $B_{12}$:* Decreased blood levels of vitamin $B_{12}$

## Adverse Reactions
**CNS:** Dizziness, drowsiness, fatigue, headache
**CV:** Arrhythmias (including conduction abnormalities), edema, hypotension, orthostatic hypotension
**EENT:** Vision changes
**ENDO:** Hyperglycemia, hypoglycemia
**GI:** Abdominal pain, acute cholecystitis, ascending cholangitis, biliary obstruction, cholelithiasis, cholestatic hepatitis, constipation, flatulence, nausea, pancreatitis, vomiting
**GU:** Increased urine output
**Other:** Dehydration, electrolyte imbalances, injection site irritation

## Nursing Considerations
- Give octreotide by I.V. injection only in an emergency, as prescribed.
- To prepare depot injection (long-acting suspension form), let powder and diluent warm to room temperature and then reconstitute according to manufacturer's instructions. Gently inject 2 ml of supplied diluent down side of vial without disturbing depot powder. Let diluent saturate powder. After 2 to 5 minutes, check sides and bottom of vial without inverting it. Once powder is completely saturated, swirl—don't shake—vial for 30 to 60 seconds to form suspension. Use immediately after reconstituting.
- Don't give depot injection by S.C. route; give only by I.M. route and only to patients who respond to and tolerate S.C. drug, as prescribed.
- To minimize pain, use smallest injection volume to deliver desired dose and rotate injection sites.
- Avoid using deltoid site for I.M. injection because injection site reactions and pain may result. Intragluteal injection is recommended.
- **WARNING** To avoid worsening of symptoms, expect to continue S.C. injections when switching to I.M. injections, as prescribed.
- Be aware that octreotide increases risk of acute cholecystitis, ascending cholangitis, biliary obstruction, cholestatic hepatitis, and pancreatitis.
- Monitor vital signs, bowels sounds, and stool consistency. Assess for abdominal pain and signs of gallbladder disease.
- Monitor serum liver enzyme levels, as appropriate.
- Monitor patient for signs of electrolyte imbalances and dehydration.
- Carefully monitor diabetic patient for altered glucose control.

•If patient has periodic flare-ups of symptoms, expect to give additional S.C. octreotide temporarily, as prescribed.

**PATIENT TEACHING**
•Advise patient to change position slowly to minimize effects of orthostatic hypotension.
•Instruct patient to notify prescriber about adverse reactions, especially abdominal pain, which may indicate pancreatitis.
•Urge diabetic patient to monitor blood glucose level frequently.

# ofloxacin

Floxin

## Class and Category

*Chemical:* Fluoroquinolone
*Therapeutic:* Antibiotic
*Pregnancy category:* C

## Indications and Dosages

➤ *To treat acute, uncomplicated cystitis caused by* Escherichia coli *or* Klebsiella pneumoniae
**TABLETS, I.V. INFUSION**
**Adults.** 200 mg q 12 hr for 3 days.

➤ *To treat uncomplicated cystitis caused by* Citrobacter diversus, Enterobacter aerogenes, Proteus mirabilis, *or* Pseudomonas aeruginosa
**TABLETS, I.V. INFUSION**
**Adults.** 200 mg q 12 hr for 7 days.

➤ *To treat complicated UTIs caused by* C. diversus, E. coli, K. pneumoniae, P. mirabilis, *or* P. aeruginosa
**Adults.** 200 mg q 12 hr for 10 days.

➤ *To treat uncomplicated gonorrhea*
**TABLETS, I.V. INFUSION**
**Adults and adolescents.** 400 mg as single dose.

➤ *To treat urethritis or cervicitis caused by* Chlamydia trachomatis *or* Neisseria gonorrhoeae
**TABLETS, I.V. INFUSION**
**Adults and adolescents.** 300 mg b.i.d. for 7 days as an alternative to doxycycline or azithromycin.

➤ *To treat pelvic inflammatory disease caused by susceptible organisms*
**TABLETS**
**Adults and adolescents.** 400 mg b.i.d. with metronidazole P.O. for 10 to 14 days.

**I.V. INFUSION**
**Adults and adolescents.** 400 mg q 12 hr with metronidazole I.V. and then switched to oral therapy, as prescribed, after 24 hr. Complete course of therapy lasts 14 days.

➤ *To treat prostatitis caused by* E. coli
**TABLETS, I.V. INFUSION**
**Adults.** 300 mg q 12 hr for 6 wk.

➤ *To treat lower respiratory tract infections caused by* Haemophilus influenzae *or* Streptococcus pneumoniae *and skin and soft-tissue infections caused by* Staphylococcus aureus *or* Streptococcus pyogenes
**TABLETS, I.V. INFUSION**
**Adults.** 400 mg q 12 hr for 10 days.
**DOSAGE ADJUSTMENT** If creatinine clearance is 20 to 50 ml/min/1.73 m$^2$, dosing interval possibly reduced to q 24 hr; if clearance is less than 10 ml/min/1.73 m$^2$, dosage possibly reduced by 50% and given q 24 hr.

---

### Mechanism of Action

Inhibits synthesis of the bacterial enzyme DNA gyrase by counteracting the excessive supercoiling of DNA during replication or transcription. Inhibition of DNA gyrase causes rapid- and slow-growing bacterial cells to die.

---

## Incompatibilities

Don't mix ofloxacin with other I.V. drugs or additives.

## Contraindications

Hypersensitivity to ofloxacin, other fluoroquinolones, or their components

## Interactions

**DRUGS**
*aluminum-, calcium-, or magnesium-containing antacids; didanosine; ferrous sulfate; magnesium-containing laxatives; multivitamins; sevelamer; sucralfate; zinc:* Decreased absorption of oral ofloxacin
*probenecid:* Decreased ofloxacin excretion, increased risk of toxicity
*procainamide:* Decreased renal clearance of procainamide
*warfarin:* Possibly increased anticoagulant activity and risk of bleeding

## Adverse Reactions

**CNS:** Dizziness, drowsiness, headache, insomnia, peripheral neuropathy

N
O

**CV:** Arrhythmias, prolonged QT interval
**GI:** Abdominal cramps or pain, diarrhea, nausea, pseudomembranous colitis, vomiting
**GU:** Vaginal candidiasis
**MS:** Tendinitis; tendon inflammation, pain, or rupture
**SKIN:** Blisters, diaphoresis, erythema, erythema multiforme, exfoliative dermatitis, photosensitivity, pruritus, rash, Stevens-Johnson syndrome, toxic epidermal necrolysis, urticaria
**Other:** Infusion site phlebitis

## Nursing Considerations

•For I.V. infusion, dilute drug in NS or $D_5W$ to at least 4 mg/ml, and infuse over 60 minutes to minimize the risk of hypotension. Discard unused portion.
•Notify prescriber if patient has symptoms of peripheral neuropathy (pain, burning, tingling, numbness, weakness, or altered sensations of light touch, pain, temperature, position sense, or vibration sense), which could be permanent; tendon rupture (pain and inflammation), which requires immediate rest; or a severe photosensitivity reaction. In each case, expect to stop ofloxacin.
•Maintain adequate hydration to prevent development of highly concentrated urine and crystalluria.
•Expect an increased risk of toxicity in severe hepatic disease, including cirrhosis.
•Be aware that ofloxacin may stimulate the CNS and aggravate seizure disorders.
•If diarrhea develops, consider the possibility of pseudomembranous colitis.
•Be alert for secondary fungal infection.

**PATIENT TEACHING**
•Encourage patient to take each oral dose with a full glass of water.
•Tell patient to complete full course of ofloxacin therapy exactly as prescribed, even if he feels better before it's complete.
•Urge patient not to take antacids, iron or zinc preparations, or other drugs (such as sucralfate and didanosine), within 2 hours of ofloxacin to prevent decreased or delayed drug absorption.
•Advise patient to avoid hazardous activities until CNS effects of drug are known.
•Tell patient to limit exposure to sun and ultraviolet light to prevent phototoxicity.
•Advise patient to notify prescriber immediately about burning skin, hives, itching, rash,

rapid heart rate, abnormal motor or sensory function, and tendon pain.
•Urge patient to seek medical attention immediately for trouble breathing or swallowing, which may signal an allergic reaction.
•Instruct a diabetic patient who takes insulin or an antidiabetic to notify prescriber immediately if he develops a hypoglycemic reaction; ofloxacin will have to be stopped.

# olanzapine

Zydis, Zyprexa

## Class and Category

*Chemical:* Thienobenzodiazepine derivative
*Therapeutic:* Antipsychotic
*Pregnancy category:* C

## Indications and Dosages

➤ *To treat psychosis*
**ORALLY DISINTEGRATING TABLETS, TABLETS**
**Adults.** *Initial:* 5 to 10 mg q.d. *Usual:* 10 mg/day. *Maximum:* 20 mg/day

➤ *To treat manic phase of acute bipolar disorder*
**ORALLY DISINTEGRATING TABLETS, TABLETS**
**Adults.** *Initial:* 10 to 15 mg q.d.; may be increased or decreased by 5 mg q 24 hr as needed and prescribed. *Usual:* 5 to 20 mg q.d. for 3 to 4 wk. *Maximum:* 20 mg/day.

➤ *As adjunct to treat acute bipolar disorder*
**ORALLY DISINTEGRATING TABLETS, TABLETS**
**Adults.** *Initial:* 10 mg q.d. in conjunction with lithium or valproate sodium; may be increased or decreased by 5 mg q 24 hr, as needed and prescribed. *Usual:* 5 to 20 mg/day for 6 wk. *Maximum:* 20 mg/day.
**DOSAGE ADJUSTMENT** Initial dosage possibly reduced to 5 mg for debilitated patients, those prone to hypotension, and female nonsmokers over age 65.

➤ *To treat agitation associated with schizophrenia and bipolar I mania*
**I.M. INJECTION**
**Adults.** 5 to 10 mg p.r.n. Repeat as needed q 2 to 4 hr.
**DOSAGE ADJUSTMENT** Dosage decreased to 5 mg for elderly patients and 2.5 mg for debilitated patients, those prone to hypotension, and female nonsmokers older than 65.

| Route | Onset | Peak | Duration |
|-------|-------|------|----------|
| P.O. | 1 wk | Unknown | Unknown |
| I.M. | Unknown | Unknown | Unknown |

## Mechanism of Action

May achieve its antipsychotic effects by antagonizing dopamine and serotonin receptors. Anticholinergic effects may result from competitive binding to and antagonism of the muscarinic receptors $M_1$ through $M_5$.

## Contraindications

Blood dyscrasias, bone marrow depression, cerebral arteriosclerosis, coma, coronary artery disease, hepatic dysfunction, high-dose CNS depressants, hypersensitivity to olanzapine or its components, hypertension, hypotension, myeloproliferative disorders, severe CNS depression, subcortical brain damage

## Interactions

**DRUGS**

*anticholinergics:* Increased anticholinergic effects, altered thermoregulation
*antihypertensives:* Increased effects of both drugs, increased risk of hypotension
*carbamazepine, omeprazole, rifampin:* Increased olanzapine clearance
*CNS depressants:* Additive CNS depression, potentiated orthostatic hypotension
*diazepam:* Increased CNS depressant effects
*fluvoxamine:* Decreased olanzapine clearance
*levodopa:* Decreased levodopa efficacy
*lorazepam (parenteral):* Possibly increased somnolence with I.M. injection of olanzapine
**ACTIVITIES**
*alcohol use:* Additive CNS depression, potentiated orthostatic hypotension
*smoking:* Decreased blood olanzapine level

## Adverse Reactions

**CNS:** Abnormal gait, agitation, akathisia, altered thermoregulation, amnesia, anxiety, asthenia, dizziness, euphoria, fever, headache, hypertonia, insomnia, nervousness, neuroleptic malignant syndrome, restlessness, somnolence, stuttering, tardive dyskinesia, tremor
**CV:** Chest pain, hypertension, hypotension, orthostatic hypotension, peripheral edema, tachycardia

**EENT:** Amblyopia, dry mouth, increased salivation, pharyngitis, rhinitis
**ENDO:** Hyperglycemia
**GI:** Abdominal pain, constipation, dysphagia, increased appetite, nausea, thirst, vomiting
**GU:** Urinary incontinence, UTI
**MS:** Arthralgia; back, joint, or limb pain; muscle spasms and twitching
**RESP:** Cough
**SKIN:** Ecchymosis, photosensitivity, pruritus, urticaria
**Other:** Anaphylaxis, angioedema, flulike symptoms, weight gain

## Nursing Considerations

• Reconstitute parenteral olanzapine by dissolving contents of vial in 2.1 ml of sterile water to yield 5 mg/ml. Solution should be clear yellow. Use within 1 hour.
• Inject I.M. olanzapine slowly and deep into muscle mass.
• Keep patient recumbent after I.M. injection of olanzapine if drowsiness or dizziness occurs. Don't let patient sit or stand up until blood pressure and heart rate have returned to baseline.
• Monitor patient's blood pressure routinely during therapy because olanzapine may cause orthostatic hypotension.
• Be aware that olanzapine may worsen such conditions as angle-closure glaucoma, benign prostatic hyperplasia, and seizures.
• Assess daily weight to detect fluid retention.
• Notify prescriber if patient develops tardive dyskinesia or urinary incontinence.
• Be alert for and immediately report to prescriber signs of neuroleptic malignant syndrome.
• Monitor patient for suicidal tendencies. Notify prescriber and implement suicide precautions according to facility policy.
• Monitor patient's blood glucose level routinely because olanzapine use may increase risk of hyperglycemia.

**PATIENT TEACHING**

• Advise patient to avoid alcohol and smoking during olanzapine therapy.
• Teach patient to open the orally disintegrating tablet sachet by peeling back the foil on the blister and not to push tablet through the foil. Immediately after opening the blister, tell him to use dry hands to remove tablet and place it in his mouth. Explain

that tablet will disintegrate rapidly in his saliva so that he can easily swallow it without liquid.
• Caution patient with phenylketonuria that disintegrating tablets contain phenylalanine.
• Urge patient to avoid potentially hazardous activities until drug's CNS effects are known.
• Instruct patient to change position slowly to minimize effects of orthostatic hypotension.

# olanzapine and fluoxetine hydrochloride

Symbyax

## Class and Category
*Chemical:* thienobenzodiazepine derivative (olanzapine) and selective serotonin reuptake inhibitor (fluoxetine)
*Therapeutic:* Antipsychotic
*Pregnancy category:* C

## Indications and Dosages
➤ *To treat depression associated with bipolar disorder*
**CAPSULES**
**Adults.** *Initial:* 6 mg olanzapine/25 mg fluoxetine q.d. in the evening and then dosage increased as needed. *Maximum:* 12 mg olanzapine/50 mg fluoxetine.

## Contraindications
Hypersensitivity to olanzapine, fluoxetine, or other selective serotonin reuptake inhibitors or their components; use within 14 days of MAO inhibitor therapy or within 5 weeks of thioridazine therapy

| Route | Onset | Peak | Duration |
|---|---|---|---|
| P.O. (olan-zapine) | Unknown | 6 hr | Unknown |
| P.O. (fluox-etine) | Unknown | 6 to 8 hr | Unknown |

### Mechanism of Action
May activate the monoaminergic neural system's serotonin, norepinephrine, and dopamine release in the prefrontal cortex to produce an enhanced antidepressant effect.

## Interactions
**DRUGS**
*almotriptan:* Increased risk of weakness, hyperreflexia, and incoordination
*alprazolam, diazepam:* Possibly prolonged half-life of these drugs
*anticholinergics:* Increased anticholinergic effects, altered thermoregulation
*antihypertensives:* Increased effects of both drugs
*aspirin, NSAIDS, warfarin:* Increased risk of bleeding
*astemizole:* Increased risk of serious arrhythmias
*buspirone:* Decreased buspirone effects
*carbamazepine, omeprazole, rifampin:* Increased olanzapine clearance
*clozapine, fluphenazine, haloperidol, maprotiline, trazodone:* Increased risk of adverse effects
*CNS depressants:* Additive CNS depression, potentiated orthostatic hypotension
*diazepam:* Increased CNS depressant effects
*fluvoxamine:* Decreased olanzapine clearance
*levodopa:* Decreased levodopa efficacy
*lithium:* Increased or decreased blood lithium level
*MAO inhibitors:* Possibly life-threatening adverse effects
*phenytoin:* Increased blood phenytoin level and risk of toxicity
*pimozide:* Possibly bradycardia
*serotonergics (such as amphetamines and other psychostimulants, antidepressants, and dopamine agonists):* Serotonin syndrome
*thioridazine:* Increased risk of serious ventricular arrhythmias
*tricyclic antidepressants:* Increased risk of adverse effects, including seizures
*tryptophan:* Increased risk of central and peripheral toxicity
**ACTIVITIES**
alcohol use: Additive CNS depression, potentiated orthostatic hypotension
smoking: Decreased blood olanzapine level

## Adverse Reactions
**CNS:** Amnesia, asthenia, chills, fever, hyperkinesia, migraine, neuroleptic malignant syndrome, personality changes, seizures, serotonin syndrome, sleep disturbance, somnolence, speech alteration, tardive dyskinesia, tremor

**CV:** Bradycardia, chest pain, edema, hypertension, orthostatic hypotension, tachycardia, vasodilation
**EENT:** Abnormal vision, amblyopia, dry mouth, ear pain, increased salivation, otitis media, pharyngitis, taste perversion, tinnitus
**ENDO:** Breast pain, hyperglycemia, increased prolactin level, menorrhagia
**GI:** Diarrhea, elevated liver function test results, increased appetite, thirst
**GU:** Abnormal ejaculation, anorgasmia, decreased libido, impotence, urinary frequency or incontinence, UTI
**MS:** Arthralgia, muscle twitching, neck pain or rigidity,
**RESP:** Bronchitis, dyspnea
**SKIN:** Ecchymosis, photosensitivity, rash, urticaria
**Other:** Anaphylaxis, angioedema, hyponatremia, infection, weight gain or loss

## Nursing Considerations
•Use with caution in patients with cardiovascular or cerebrovascular disease or conditions that would predispose patients to hy potension because of olanzapine and fluoxetine's potential to cause orthostatic hypotension.
•Be aware that the olanzapine component in this combination drug should not be used in patients with dementia-related psychosis because of increased risk of cerebrovascular adverse effects.
•Monitor patient's blood glucose level routinely because drug may increase risk of developing hyperglycemia.
•Monitor patient closely for neuroleptic malignant syndrome (hyperthermia, muscle rigidity, altered level of consciousness, irregular pulse or blood pressure, tachycardia, diaphoresis, and arrhythmias), a rare but potentially fatal adverse effect.
•Monitor hepatic function, as ordered, in patients with hepatic disease because olanzapine and fluoxetine combination can elevate hepatic enzyme levels.
PATIENT TEACHING
•Advise patient to avoid exercise in hot weather to reduce the risk of dehydration and hypotension. Also instruct him to notify prescriber if he experiences prolonged diarrhea, nausea, or vomiting.

•Caution patient to avoid potentially hazardous activities until drug's CNS effects are known.
•Instruct patient to change position slowly to minimize effects of orthostatic hypotension.
•Caution patient to avoid using aspirin or NSAIDs while taking olanzapine and fluoxetine because concomitant use can increase the risk of bleeding.
•Advise patient to avoid alcohol and smoking during therapy because of increased risk of adverse effects.
•Instruct patient to notify prescriber if he develops a rash or hives.

# olmesartan medoxomil
Benicar
## Class and Category
*Chemical:* Angiotensin II receptor antagonist
*Therapeutic:* Antihypertensive
*Pregnancy category:* C (first trimester), D (later trimesters)

## Indications and Dosages
➤ *To manage or as adjunct to manage hypertension*
TABLETS
**Adults.** *Initial:* 20 mg q.d., increased in 2 wk to 40 mg q.d., if needed.
DOSAGE ADJUSTMENT Lower starting dosage is recommended for patients with possible depletion of intravascular volume, such as those treated with diuretics, especially if impaired renal function is present.

## Contraindications
Hypersensitivity to olmesartan medoxomil or its components

## Interactions
None known

## Adverse Reactions
**CNS:** Ashenia, dizziness, fatigue, headache, vertigo
**CV:** Chest pain, hypercholesterolemia, hyperlipidemia, hypertriglyceridemia, insomnia, peripheral edema, tachycardia

## Mechanism of Action

Olmesartan medoxomil blocks angiotensin II from binding to receptor sites in many tissues, including vascular smooth muscle and adrenal glands. Angiotensin II, a potent vasoconstrictor, is then free to stimulate the adrenal cortex to secrete aldosterone, and the inhibiting effects of angiotensin II reduce blood pressure.

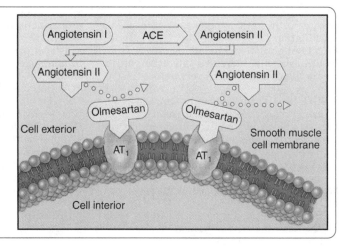

**EENT:** Pharyngitis, rhinitis, sinusitis
**ENDO:** Hyperglycemia, hyperuricemia
**GI:** Abdominal pain, diarrhea, gastroenteritis, indigestion, nausea, vomiting
**GU:** Acute renal failure, elevated BUN and serum creatinine levels, hematuria, UTI
**MS:** Arthralgia, arthritis, back pain, myalgia, rhabdomyolysis, skeletal pain
**RESP:** Bronchitis, cough, upper respiratory tract infection
**SKIN:** Alopecia, pruritus, rash, urticaria
**Other:** Angioedema, increased CK level, flu-like symptoms, pain

## Nursing Considerations

•Expect to provide treatment such as NS solution I.V., as prescribed, to correct known or suspected hypovolemia before beginning olmesartan therapy.
•Monitor patient for increased BUN and serum creatinine levels, especially in a patient with impaired renal function, because drug may cause acute renal failure. If increased levels are significant or persist, notify prescriber immediately.
•Monitor blood pressure frequently to assess effectiveness of therapy. If blood pressure isn't controlled with olmesartan alone, expect to administer a diuretic, such as hydrochlorothiazide, as prescribed.
•**WARNING** Monitor patient's blood pressure frequently if he receives a diuretic or other antihypertensive during olmesartan ther-

apy because of an increased risk of hypotension.
•Expect to discontinue drug temporarily if patient experiences hypotension. If hypotension occurs, place patient in supine position immediately and prepare to administer NS solution I.V., as prescribed. Expect to resume drug therapy after blood pressure stabilizes.
•If patient also receives a diuretic, provide adequate hydration, as appropriate, to help prevent hypovolemia. Monitor him for signs and symptoms of hypovolemia, such as hypotension with dizziness and fainting.

### PATIENT TEACHING

•Advise patient to avoid exercise in hot weather and excessive alcohol use to reduce the risk of dehydration and hypotension. Also instruct him to notify prescriber if he has prolonged diarrhea, nausea, or vomiting.
•Caution patient to avoid potentially hazardous activities until drug's CNS effects are known.
•Explain the importance of regular exercise, proper diet, and other lifestyle changes in controlling hypertension.
•Advise female patient to notify prescriber immediately about known or suspected pregnancy. Explain that if she becomes pregnant, prescriber may replace olmesartan with another antihypertensive that is safe to use during pregnancy.

# olsalazine sodium

Dipentum

## Class and Category

*Chemical:* Salicylate derivative
*Therapeutic:* Bowel disease suppressant
*Pregnancy category:* C

## Indications and Dosages

➤ *To maintain remission of ulcerative colitis*

**CAPSULES, TABLETS**
**Adults and adolescents.** 500 mg b.i.d.

---

### Mechanism of Action

Exerts an anti-inflammatory action in the GI tract after being converted by colonic bacteria to mesalamine (5-aminosalicylic acid), which inhibits cyclooxygenase. Inhibition of cyclooxygenase reduces prostaglandin production in the intestinal mucosa. This in turn reduces production of arachidonic acid metabolites, which may be increased in patients with inflammatory bowel disease. Olsalazine also exerts an anti-inflammatory effect by indirectly inhibiting leukotriene synthesis, which normally catalyzes the production of arachidonic acid.

---

## Contraindications

Hypersensitivity to olsalazine, salicylates, or their components

## Interactions

**DRUGS**
*oral anticoagulants:* Possibly prolonged PT

## Adverse Reactions

**CNS:** Anxiety, depression, dizziness, headache, insomnia
**CV:** Hot flashes, pericarditis, second-degree AV block
**EENT:** Dry eyes and mouth, lacrimation, tinnitus
**GI:** Abdominal pain, anorexia, diarrhea, nausea, vomiting
**GU:** Dysuria, hematuria, nephrotic syndrome, urinary frequency
**HEME:** Hemolytic anemia, lymphopenia, neutropenia
**MS:** Muscle spasms, myalgia
**SKIN:** Acne, alopecia, erythema nodosum, photosensitivity
**Other:** Dehydration

## Nursing Considerations

• Assess for aspirin allergy before giving olsalazine.
• Assess quantity and consistency of stools and frequency of bowel movements before, during, and after therapy.
• Give drug with food to decrease adverse GI reactions.
• Monitor skin turgor for signs of adequate hydration.
• Assess for abdominal pain and hyperactive bowel sounds.
• Monitor renal function studies, as appropriate.

**PATIENT TEACHING**
• Instruct patient to take olsalazine with food.
• Urge patient to continue taking drug as prescribed, even if symptoms improve.
• Advise patient to watch for signs of dehydration.

# omalizumab

Xolair

## Class and Category

*Chemical:* Recombinant IgG1K anti-IgE monoclonal antibody
*Therapeutic:* Antiallergenic
*Pregnancy category:* B

## Indications and Dosages

➤ *To treat moderate to severe persistent asthma in patients with positive skin test or in vitro reactivity to a perennial aeroallergen whose symptoms have been inadequately controlled with inhaled corticosteroids*

**S.C. INJECTION**
**Adults and adolescents age 12 and older.** 150 to 375 mg q 2 or 4 wk. Dose and dosing frequency determined by body weight and blood IgE levels.
**DOSAGE ADJUSTMENT** Dosage adjusted for significant changes in body weight.

## Contraindications

Hypersensitivity to omalizumab or its components

N
O

## Mechanism of Action
In asthma, inflammation results when antigen reexposure causes mast cells to degranulate and release histamine and **other** chemical mediators. Omalizumab helps reduce inflammation by binding to circulating IgE and preventing it from binding to mast cells. This action inhibits degranulation and blocks the release of histamine and other chemical mediators.

## Interactions
**DRUGS**
None reported.

## Adverse Reactions
**CNS:** Dizziness, fatigue, headache, vertigo
**EENT:** Earache, pharyngitis, sinusitis
**MS:** Arm or leg pain, arthralgia, fractures
**RESP:** Upper respiratory tract infection
**SKIN:** Dermatitis, pruritus, urticaria
**Other:** Anaphylaxis; generalized pain; injection site bruising, burning, hive or mass formation, induration, inflammation, itching, pain, redness, stinging, and warmth; malignancies; viral infection

## Nursing Considerations
•Record patient's weight and obtain blood IgE levels, as ordered, before initiating omalizumab therapy because decisions regarding dosage and dosing frequency are based upon these factors.
•Reconstitute using sterile water for injection and allow 15 to 20 minutes on average for the lyophilized product to dissolve. To reconstitute, draw 1.4 ml of sterile water for injection into a 3-ml syringe with a 1" 18-gauge needle. Place omalizumab vial upright and inject sterile water into vial using aseptic technique. Gently swirl the upright vial for about 1 minute to evenly wet the powder. Do not shake. Every 5 minutes, gently swirl the vial for 5 to 10 seconds until you see no gel-like particles in the solution. Discard if powder takes longer than 40 minutes to dissolve, and start again with a new vial. Once reconstituted, solution should appear clear or slightly opalescent and may have a few small bubbles or foam around the edge of the vial. Use reconstituted solution within 8 hours if refrigerated or 4 hours if stored at room temperature.

•To remove reconstituted omalizumab from vial, invert vial for 15 seconds to allow solution to drain toward stopper. Using a new 3-ml syringe equipped with a 1" 18-gauge needle, insert needle into inverted vial and position needle tip at the very bottom of the solution in the vial stopper. Then pull plunger all the way back to end of syringe barrel in order to remove all the solution from the inverted vial. To obtain a full 150-mg dose (1 vial containing 1.2 ml of reconstituted omalizumab), you must withdraw all the product from the vial before expelling any air or excess solution from the syringe.
•Do not administer more than 150 mg per injection site.
•Be prepared to inject omalizumab over 5 to 10 seconds because solution is slightly viscous.
•**WARNING** Monitor patient closely for hypersensitivity reactions after injection because anaphylaxis, although rare, has occurred within 2 hours of omalizumab administration. Have emergency medication and equipment to treat anaphylaxis readily available.
•**WARNING** Monitor patient closely for signs of cancer. Report any abnormal findings to prescriber.

**PATIENT TEACHING**
•Instruct patient to notify prescriber if any signs of hypersensitivity occur, such as a rash.
•Caution patient that any improvement in his asthma may take time.
•Encourage patient to comply with regularly scheduled prescriber visits.
•Inform patient of risk of malignancy and suggest routine cancer screening.
•Instruct patient that omalizumab is not used to treat acute bronchospasm or status asthmaticus.
•Tell patient not to abruptly discontinue any prescribed systemic or inhaled corticosteroid when starting omalizumab therapy because steroid dosage must be tapered gradually under prescriber's supervision.

# omega-3-acid ethyl esters

Omacor

## Class and Category
*Chemical:* Ethyl esters of omega-3 fatty acids
*Therapeutic:* Lipid regulator
*Pregnancy category:* C

## Indications and Dosages
➤ *As adjunct to diet to reduce triglyceride level that exceeds 500 mg/dl*
**CAPSULES**
**Adults.** 4 g q.d. or 2 g b.i.d.

---

### Mechanism of Action
Omega-3-acid ethyl esters are essential fatty acids thought to inhibit very-low-density lipoprotein and triglyceride synthesis in the liver. With less triglyceride synthesis, plasma triglyceride levels decrease.

---

## Contraindications
Hypersensitivity to omega-3-acid ethyl esters or their components

## Interactions
**DRUGS**
*anticogulants:* Possibly increased bleeding time

## Adverse Reactions
**CV:** Angina pectoris
**EENT:** Halitosis, nosebleeds, taste perversion
**GI:** Diarrhea, dyspepsia, eructation, nausea, vomiting
**HEME:** Prolonged bleeding time
**MS:** Back pain
**SKIN:** Bruising, rash
**Other:** Flulike symptoms

## Nursing Considerations
• Be aware that drugs known to increase triglyceride levels—such as beta blockers, thiazide diuretics and estrogens—should be discontinued or changed, if possible, before omega-3 ethyl ester therapy starts.
• Expect to check patient's triglyceride level before starting and periodically throughout omega-3-acid ethyl ester therapy to determine effectiveness.
• Administer drug with meals.
• Expect to stop omega-3-acid ethyl ester therapy after 2 months if patient's trigylceride level doesn't decrease as expected.
**PATIENT TEACHING**
• Stress importance of dietary measures, an exercise program, and controlling other factors—such as blood glucose level—that may contribute to elevated triclyceride levels.
• Advise patient to take drug with meals.
• Explain that patient will need periodic laboratory tests to evaluate the drug's effectiveness.
• Instruct patient to seek immediate medical attention if chest pain occurs.

# omeprazole
Losec (CAN), Prilosec, Zegerid

## Class and Category
*Chemical:* Substituted benzimidazole
*Therapeutic:* Antiulcer
*Pregnancy category:* C

## Indications and Dosages
➤ *To treat gastroesophageal reflux disease (GERD) without esophageal lesions, to prevent erosive esophagitis*
**DELAYED-RELEASE CAPSULES, DELAYED-RELEASE TABLETS, ORAL SUSPENSION**
**Adults.** 20 mg q.d. for 4 wk.
➤ *To treat GERD with erosive esophagitis*
**DELAYED-RELEASE CAPSULES, DELAYED-RELEASE TABLETS, ORAL SUSPENSION**
**Adults.** 20 mg q.d. for 4 to 8 wk.
➤ *To treat pediatric GERD and other acid-related disorders*
**DELAYED-RELEASE CAPSULES**
**Children age 2 and older weighing 20 kg (44 lb) or less.** 10 mg q.d.
**Children age 2 and older weighing more than 20 kg.** 20 mg q.d.
➤ *To provide short-term treatment of active benign gastric ulcer*
**DELAYED-RELEASE CAPSULES**
**Adults.** 40 mg q.d. for 4 to 8 wk.
**DELAYED-RELEASE TABLETS**
**Adults.** 20 mg q.d. for 4 to 8 wk, increased to 40 mg q.d., p.r.n.
➤ *To treat duodenal or gastric ulcer associated with* Helicobacter pylori
**DELAYED-RELEASE CAPSULES, ORAL SUSPENSION**
**Adults.** 40 mg q.d. given with clarithromycin for 14 days, followed by 20 mg q.d. alone for another 14 days. Or, 20 mg b.i.d. given with amoxicillin for 14 days. Or, 20 mg b.i.d. given with amoxicillin and clarithromycin for 10 days.

N
O

## Mechanism of Action

Omeprazole interferes with gastric acid secretion by inhibiting the hydrogen-potassium-adenosine triphosphatase ($H^+K^+$-ATPase) enzyme system, or proton pump, in gastric parietal cells. Normally, the proton pump uses energy from the hydrolysis of adenosine triphosphate to drive hydrogen ($H^+$) and chloride ($Cl^-$) out of parietal cells and into the stomach lumen in exchange for potassium ($K^+$), which leaves the stomach lumen and enters the parietal cells. After this exchange, $H^+$ and $Cl^-$ combine in the stomach to form hydrochloric acid (HCl), as shown below left. Omeprazole irreversibly blocks the exchange of intracellular $H^+$ and extracellular $K^+$, as shown below right. By preventing $H^+$ from entering the stomach lumen, omeprazole prevents additional HCl from forming.

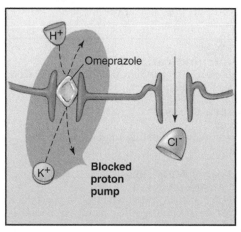

**DELAYED-RELEASE TABLETS**

**Adults.** 20 mg b.i.d. with clarithromycin and amoxicillin or metronidazole for 7 days, followed by 20 mg q.d. for up to 3 wk (for duodenal ulcer) or 20 to 40 mg q.d. for up to 12 wk (for gastric ulcer).

➤ *To provide long-term treatment of gastric hypersecretory conditions, such as multiple endocrine adenoma syndrome, systemic mastocytosis, and Zollinger-Ellison syndrome*

**DELAYED-RELEASE CAPSULES, DELAYED-RELEASE TABLETS**

**Adults.** 60 mg q.d. or in divided doses, as prescribed. *Maximum:* 120 mg t.i.d.

| Route | Onset | Peak | Duration |
|-------|-------|------|----------|
| P.O. | 1 hr | In 2 hr | 72 to 96 hr |

## Contraindications

Hypersensitivity to omeprazole, other proton pump inhibitors, or their components

## Interactions

**DRUGS**

*alprazolam, astemizole, carbamazepine, cisapride, cyclosporine, diazepam, diltiazem, erythromycin, felodipine, lidocaine, lovastatin, midazolam, quinidine, simvastatin, terfenadine, triazolam, verapamil:* Decreased clearance and increased blood levels of these drugs

*ampicillin, iron salts, itraconazole, ketoconazole, vitamin $B_{12}$:* Impaired absorption of these drugs

*cilostazol:* Increased blood cilostazol level

*digoxin:* Increased digoxin bioavailability, possibly digitalis toxicity

*levobupivacaine:* Increased risk of levobupivacaine toxicity

*methotrexate:* Possibly delayed methotrexate elimination

*nifedipine:* Decreased nifedipine clearance, increased risk of hypotension

*phenytoin:* Decreased phenytoin clearance, increased risk of phenytoin toxicity

*sucralfate:* Decreased omeprazole absorption
*warfarin:* Possibly increased risk of abnormal bleeding

## Adverse Reactions

**CNS:** Agitation, asthenia, dizziness, drowsiness, fatigue, headache, psychic disturbances, somnolence
**CV:** Chest pain, hypertension, peripheral eddema
**EENT:** Anterior ischemic optic neuropathy, optic atrophy or neuritis, stomatitis
**ENDO:** Hypoglycemia
**GI:** Abdominal pain, constipation, diarrhea, dyspepsia, elevated liver function test results, flatulence, hepatic dysfunction or failure, indigestion, nausea, pancreatitis, vomiting
**GU:** Interstitial nephritis
**HEME:** Agranulocytosis, anemia, hemolytic anemia, leukopenia, leukocytosis, neutropenia, pancytopenia, thrombocytopenia
**MS:** Back pain
**RESP:** Cough
**SKIN:** Erythema multiforme, photosensitivity, pruritus, rash, Stevens-Johnson syndrome, toxic epidermal necrolysis, urticaria
**Other:** Anaphylaxis, angioedema, hyponatremia

## Nursing Considerations

• Give omeprazole before meals, preferably in the morning for once-daily dosing. If necessary, also give an antacid, as prescribed.
• If needed, open capsule and sprinkle enteric-coated granules on applesauce or yogurt or mix with water or acidic fruit juice, such as apple or cranberry juice. Give immediately.
• To give drug via NG tube, mix granules in acidic juice because enteric coating dissolves in alkaline pH.
• Because drug can interfere with absorption of vitamin $B_{12}$, monitor for macrocytic anemia.
• Be aware that long-term use of omeprazole may increase the risk of gastric carcinoma.

**PATIENT TEACHING**
• Tell patient to take drug before eating—usually before breakfast—and to swallow delayed-release capsules or tablets whole. If needed, patient may sprinkle contents of capsule onto 1 tablespoon of applesauce and swallow immediately without chewing pellets. Tell him to follow with a glass of cool water and not to keep any leftover mixture.
• If patient takes the oral suspension, tell him to empty the package into a small cup containing 2 tablespoons of water (no other beverage should be used), stir the mixture well, drink it immediately, refill the cup with water, and drink again.
• Encourage patient to avoid alcohol, aspirin products, ibuprofen, and foods that may increase gastric secretions during therapy.
• Advise patient to notify prescriber immediately about abdominal pain or diarrhea.
• Urge female patient of childbearing age to use effective contraceptive method during therapy and to inform prescriber immediately if she becomes or suspects she may be pregnant.

# ondansetron hydrochloride

Zofran, Zofran ODT

## Class and Category

*Chemical:* Carbazole
*Therapeutic:* Antiemetic
*Pregnancy category:* B

## Indications and Dosages

➤ *To prevent chemotherapy-induced nausea and vomiting*

**DISINTEGRATING TABLETS, ORAL SOLUTION, TABLETS**
**Adults and children age 12 and older.** *Initial:* 8 mg given 30 min before chemotherapy. *Postchemotherapy:* 8 mg given 8 hr after initial dose, then 8 mg q 12 hr for 1 to 2 days.
**Children ages 4 to 12.** *Initial:* 4 mg given 30 min before chemotherapy. *Postchemotherapy:* 4 mg given 4 and 8 hr after initial dose, then 4 mg q 8 hr for 1 to 2 days.

**I.V. INFUSION**
**Adults.** 32 mg infused over 15 min starting 30 min before chemotherapy; or three 0.15-mg/kg doses, each infused over 15 min, starting with the first dose given 30 min before chemotherapy and second and third doses given 4 and 8 hours after first dose.
**Children ages 6 months to 18 years.** Three 0.15-mg/kg doses, each infused over 15 min, starting with first dose given 30 min before chemotherapy and second and third doses given 4 and 8 hours after first dose.

N
O

➤ *To prevent postoperative nausea and vomiting*

**DISINTEGRATING TABLETS, ORAL SOLUTION, TABLETS**

**Adults.** 16 mg as a single dose 1 hr before anesthesia induction.

**I.V. INJECTION**

**Adults and children age 12 and older.** 4 mg as a single dose over 2 to 5 min just before anesthesia induction or if nausea or vomiting develops shortly after surgery.

**Children ages 2 to 12 who weigh more than 40 kg (88 lb).** 4 mg as a single dose over 2 to 5 min just before anesthesia induction or if nausea or vomiting develops shortly after surgery.

**Children ages 1 month to 12 years who weigh less than 40 kg.** 0.1 mg/kg as a single dose over 2 to 5 min just before or immediately after anesthesia induction or if nausea or vomiting develops shortly after surgery.

**I.M. INJECTION**

**Adults and children age 12 and older.** 4 mg as a single dose just before anesthesia induction or if nausea or vomiting develops shortly after surgery.

➤ *To prevent nausea and vomiting after radiation therapy*

**DISINTEGRATING TABLETS, ORAL SOLUTION, TABLETS**

**Adults and children age 12 and older.** *Initial:* 8 mg as a single dose given 1 to 2 hr before radiation therapy. *Posttherapy:* 8 mg q 8 hr, as needed and tolerated.

DOSAGE ADJUSTMENT For patients with hepatic impairment, maximum dosage limited to 8 mg/day I.V. or P.O.

## Incompatibilities

Don't give ondansetron in same I.V. line as acyclovir, allopurinol, aminophylline, amphotericin B, ampicillin, ampicillin and sulbactam, amsacrine, cefepime, cefoperazone, furosemide, ganciclovir, lorazepam, methylprednisolone, mezlocillin, piperacillin, or sargramostim. Alkaline solutions and highly concentrated fluorouracil solutions are physically incompatible.

## Contraindications

Hypersensitivity to ondansetron or its components

## Interactions

**DRUGS**

*cisplatin, cyclophosphamide:* Possibly altered blood levels of these drugs

**ACTIVITIES**

*alcohol use:* Increased stimulant and sedative effects, including mood and physical sensations

## Mechanism of Action

Blocks serotonin receptors centrally in the chemoreceptor trigger zone and peripherally at vagal nerve terminals in the intestine. This action reduces nausea and vomiting by preventing serotonin release in the small intestine (the probable cause of chemotherapy- and radiation-induced nausea and vomiting) and by blocking signals to the CNS. Ondansetron may also bind to other serotonin receptors and to mu-opioid receptors.

## Adverse Reactions

**CNS:** Agitation, akathisia, anxiety, ataxia, dizziness, drowsiness, fever, headache, hypotension, restlessness, seizures, syncope, somnolence, weakness

**CV:** Arrythmias, chest pain, hypotension, pulmonary embolism, shock, tachycardia

**EENT:** Accommodation disturbances, altered taste, blurred vision, dry mouth, laryngeal edema, laryngospasm

**GI:** Abdominal pain, anorexia, constipation, diarrhea, elevated liver function test results, flatulence, indigestion, intestinal obstruction, thirst

**RESP:** Bronchospasm, shortness of breath

**SKIN:** Flushing, hyperpigmentation, maculopapular rash, pruritus

**Other:** Anaphylaxis, angioedema, injection site burning, pain, and redness

## Nursing Considerations

•WARNING Be aware that oral disintegrating tablets may contain aspartame, which is metabolized to phenylalanine and must be used cautiously in patients with phenylketonuria.

•Place disintegrating tablet on patient's tongue immediately after opening package. It dissolves in seconds.

•Use calibrated container or oral syringe to measure dose of oral solution.

•Give up to 4 mg I.V. diluted in 50 ml of $D_5W$ or NS.

•WARNING Be aware that ondansetron may mask symptoms of adynamic ileus or gastric distention after abdominal surgery.

## PATIENT TEACHING
• Advise patient to use calibrated container or oral syringe to measure oral ondansetron solution.
• Instruct patient to place ondansetron disintegrating tablet on his tongue immediately after opening package and to let it dissolve on his tongue before swallowing.
• Advise patient to notify prescriber immediately about signs of hypersensitivity reaction, such as rash.

# orlistat
Xenical

## Class and Category
*Chemical:* Lipase inhibitor
*Therapeutic:* Antiobesity
*Pregnancy category:* B

## Indications and Dosages
➤ *To promote weight loss in patients with a body mass index above 30 kg (66 lb)/m² 27 kg (59.4 lb)/m² in patients with dia-betes mellitus, hyperlipidemia, or hypertension—and to reduce the risk of weight regain*

### GELCAPS
**Adults.** 120 mg t.i.d. with fat-containing meals.

## Contraindications
Cholestasis, chronic malabsorption syndrome, hypersensitivity to orlistat or its components

## Interactions
### DRUGS
*cyclosporine:* Altered cyclosporine absorption
*fat-soluble vitamins:* Decreased vitamin absorption, especially vitamin E and beta-carotene
*pravastatin:* Potentiated lipid-lowering effect

## Adverse Reactions
**CNS:** Anxiety, depression, dizziness, fatigue, headache, sleep disturbance
**CV:** Pedal edema
**EENT:** Gingival or tooth disorder, otitis
**GI:** Abdominal discomfort or pain, diarrhea (infectious), fatty or oily stool, fecal inconti-

## Mechanism of Action
In the GI tract, orlistat binds with and inactivates gastric and pancreatic enzymes known as lipases, as shown. Normally, lipase enzymes convert ingested triglycerides into absorbable free fatty acids and monoglycerides. By inactivating lipase, orlistat allows undigested triglycerides to pass through the GI tract and exit the body in feces. Blocking the absorption of some of these fats lowers the number of calories the person receives from food, which promotes weight loss.

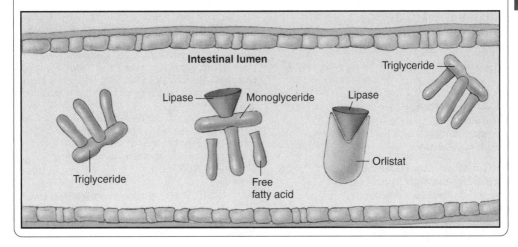

N
O

nence or urgency, flatulence with discharge, increased frequency of bowel movements, nausea, rectal pain, vomiting
**GU:** Menstrual irregularities, UTI, vaginitis
**MS:** Arthralgia, arthritis, back pain, leg pain, myalgia, tendinitis
**RESP:** Respiratory tract infection
**SKIN:** Dry skin, pruritus, rash, urticaria
**Other:** Anaphylaxis, angioedema, flulike symptoms

## Nursing Considerations
•Give orlistat with or up to 1 hour after meals that contain fat.
•Consult prescriber if you think that patient has an eating disorder, such as anorexia nervosa or bulimia.

**PATIENT TEACHING**
•Instruct patient to take orlistat with or shortly after meals that contain fat.
•Advise patient to take a multivitamin that contains fat-soluble vitamins and beta-carotene at least 2 hours before or after taking drug, if indicated.
•Inform patient about drug's adverse GI effects, but explain that reducing dietary fat may decrease them. Instruct him to notify prescriber if they become too unpleasant.
•Help patient plan a reduced-fat diet (less than 30% of daily calories) and an exercise program to promote weight loss.
•Advise patient to weigh himself daily, at the same time and wearing similar clothes, to check his progress in losing weight.

# orphenadrine citrate
Aniflex, Banflex, Flexoject, Miolin, Mio-Rel, Myotrol, Norflex, Orfro, Orphenate

## orphenadrine hydrochloride
Disipal (CAN)

## Class and Category
*Chemical:* Tertiary amine
*Therapeutic:* Skeletal muscle relaxant
*Pregnancy category:* C

## Indications and Dosages
➤ *To relieve muscle spasms in painful musculoskeletal conditions*

**E.R. TABLETS (ORPHENADRINE CITRATE)**
**Adults and adolescents.** 100 mg b.i.d. in the morning and evening.

**TABLETS (ORPHENADRINE HYDROCHLORIDE)**
**Adults and adolescents.** 50 mg t.i.d. *Maximum:* 250 mg/day.

**I.V. OR I.M. INJECTION (ORPHENADRINE CITRATE)**
**Adults and adolescents.** 60 mg q 12 hr, p.r.n.
**DOSAGE ADJUSTMENT** Dosage reduced to 25 to 50 mg t.i.d. or q.i.d. if patient also receives aspirin and caffeine.

| Route | Onset | Peak | Duration |
|---|---|---|---|
| P.O. | In 1 hr | Unknown | 4 to 6 hr* |
| I.V. | Immediate | Unknown | 4 to 6 hr |
| I.M. | 30 min | Unknown | 4 to 6 hr |

## Mechanism of Action
May reduce muscle spasms by acting on the cerebral motor centers or the medulla. Postganglionic anticholinergic effects and some antihistaminic and local anesthetic action contribute to skeletal muscle relaxation.

## Contraindications
Angle-closure glaucoma; hypersensitivity to orphenadrine or its components; myasthenia gravis; obstruction of bladder neck, duodenum, or pylorus; prostatic hypertrophy; stenosing peptic ulcers

## Interactions
**DRUGS**
*amantadine, amitriptyline, amoxapine, antimuscarinics, atropine, bupropion, carbinoxamine, chlorpromazine, clemastine, clomipramine, clozapine, cyclobenzaprine, diphenhydramine, disopyramide, doxepin, imipramine, maprotiline, mesoridazine, methdilazine, nortriptyline, phenothiazines, procainamide, promazine, promethazine, protriptyline, thioridazine, triflupromazine, trimeprazine, trimipramine:* Possibly additive anticholinergic effects
*CNS depressants:* Increased CNS depression
*haloperidol:* Increased schizophrenic symptoms, possibly tardive dyskinesia
*propoxyphene:* Increased risk of anxiety, confusion, and tremor

**ACTIVITIES**
*alcohol use:* Increased CNS depression

---

* 12 hr for extended-release.

## Adverse Reactions
**CNS:** Agitation, confusion, dizziness, drowsiness, light-headedness, syncope, tremor
**CV:** Palpitations, tachycardia
**EENT:** Blurred vision, dry eyes and mouth, increased contact lens awareness
**GI:** Abdominal distention, constipation, nausea, vomiting
**GU:** Urine retention

## Nursing Considerations
•Be aware that orphenadrine shouldn't be given to patients with tachycardia or cardiac insufficiency.
•Administer I.V. form over 5 minutes with patient in supine position. Have patient remain in this position for 5 to 10 minutes to minimize adverse reactions. Then assist him to sitting position.
•Be aware that drug can aggravate myasthenia gravis and cause tachycardia.
•Anticipate that drug's anticholinergic effects may cause blurred vision, dry eyes, and increased contact lens awareness.

**PATIENT TEACHING**
•Advise patient to avoid potentially hazardous activities until orphenadrine's CNS effects are known.
•Inform patient that dry mouth may occur but can be relieved with such measures as increased intake of fluid, ice chips, and sugarless candy or gum.
•Suggest that patient (especially one who wears contact lenses) use artificial tears to avoid discomfort from dry eyes.

# oxacillin sodium

Bactocill, Prostaphlin

## Class and Category
*Chemical:* Penicillin
*Therapeutic class:* Antibiotic
*Pregnancy category:* B

## Indications and Dosages
➤ *To treat bacteremia, bone and joint infections (such as osteomyelitis and infectious arthritis), CNS infections (such as ventriculitis and meningitis), endocarditis, septicemia, skin and soft-tissue infections, upper and lower respiratory tract infections, and UTIs caused by penicillinase-producing strains of* Staphylococcus *or other susceptible organisms*

**CAPSULES, ORAL SOLUTION**
**Adults and children who weigh 40 kg (88 lb) or more.** 500 to 1,000 mg q 4 to 6 hr. *Maximum:* 6 g/day.
**Children who weigh less than 40 kg.** 50 to 100 mg/kg/day in divided doses q 4 to 6 hr.
➤ *To treat mild to moderate infections caused by penicillinase-producing strains of* Staphylococcus *or other susceptible organisms*

**I.V. INFUSION, I.M. INJECTION**
**Adults and children who weigh 40 kg or more.** 250 to 500 mg q 4 to 6 hr.
**Infants and children who weigh less than 40 kg.** 50 mg/kg/day in divided doses q 4 to 6 hr.
**Neonates over age 7 days who weigh more than 2,000 g.** 25 to 50 mg/kg q 6 hr.
**Neonates over age 7 days who weigh less than 2,000 g.** 25 to 50 mg/kg q 8 hr.
**Neonates age 7 days and younger who weigh more than 2,000 g.** 25 to 50 mg/kg q 8 hr.
**Neonates age 7 days and younger who weigh 2,000 g or less.** 25 to 50 mg/kg q 12 hr.
➤ *To treat severe infections caused by penicillinase-producing strains of* Staphylococcus *or other susceptible organisms*

**I.V. INFUSION, I.M. INJECTION**
**Adults and children who weigh 40 kg or more.** 1,000 mg q 4 to 6 hr.
**Infants and children who weigh less than 40 kg.** 100 to 200 mg/kg/day in divided doses q 4 to 6 hr.
**Neonates over age 7 days who weigh more than 2,000 g.** 25 to 50 mg/kg q 6 hr.
**Neonates over age 7 days who weigh less than 2,000 g.** 25 to 50 mg/kg q 8 hr.
**Neonates age 7 days and younger who weigh more than 2,000 g.** 25 to 50 mg/kg q 8 hr.
**Neonates age 7 days and younger who weigh 2,000 g or less.** 25 to 50 mg/kg q 12 hr.
➤ *To treat endocarditis caused by methicillin-susceptible* Staphylococcus aureus *in patients without a prosthetic valve*

**I.V. INFUSION**
**Adults.** 2 g q 4 hr for 4 to 6 wk.
➤ *To treat endocarditis caused by methicillin-susceptible* S. aureus *in patients with a prosthetic valve*

**I.V. INFUSION**
**Adults.** 2 g q 4 hr for at least 6 wk.

## Incompatibilities
Don't give oxacillin at same time or in same admixture as aminoglycosides because they are chemically and physically incompatible and will inactivate each other.

### Mechanism of Action
Inhibits bacterial cell wall synthesis. In susceptible bacteria, the rigid, cross-linked cell wall is assembled in several steps. Oxacillin exerts its effects in the final stage of the cross-linking process by binding with and inactivating penicillin-binding proteins (enzymes responsible for linking the cell wall strands). This action causes bacterial cell lysis and death.

## Contraindications
Hypersensitivity to oxacillin, penicillins, or their components

## Interactions
**DRUGS**
*aminoglycosides:* Inactivation of both drugs
*chloramphenicol, erythromycins, sulfonamides, tetracyclines:* Decreased therapeutic effects of oxacillin
*oral contraceptives:* Decreased contraceptive efficacy
*probenecid:* Increased blood oxacillin level
**FOODS**
*all foods:* Altered absorption of oxacillin

## Adverse Reactions
**CNS:** Anxiety, depression, fatigue, hallucinations, headache, seizures
**EENT:** Oral candidiasis
**GI:** Diarrhea, nausea, pseudomembranous colitis, vomiting
**GU:** Interstitial nephritis, vaginal candidiasis
**HEME:** Agranulocytosis, anemia, granulocytopenia, neutropenia
**SKIN:** Exfoliative dermatitis, pruritus, rash, urticaria
**Other:** Anaphylaxis

## Nursing Considerations
• Administer oxacillin at least 1 hour before other antibiotics.
• Give oral forms on an empty stomach, preferably 1 hour before or 2 hours after a meal, to prevent impaired absorption.

• Before reconstitution, tap bottle several times to loosen powder. For I.M. injection, reconstitute with sterile water for injection, 0.45NS, or NS. Shake until solution is clear.
• For I.V. infusion, reconstitute only with NS or $D_5W$.
• When giving drug to patient at risk for hypertension or fluid overload, be aware that each gram of oxacillin contains 4.02 mEq of sodium.
**PATIENT TEACHING**
• Advise patient to take oxacillin on an empty stomach.
• Instruct patient to notify prescriber immediately should a rash develop.
• Advise female patient who uses an oral contraceptive to use an additional contraceptive method during oxacillin therapy.

# oxandrolone
Oxandrin

## Class, Category, and Schedule
*Chemical:* Testosterone derivative
*Therapeutic:* Appetite stimulant
*Pregnancy category:* X
*Controlled susbstance:* Schedule III

## Indications and Dosages
➤ *To promote weight gain after chronic infection, extensive surgery, failure to maintain weight despite no evidence of pathology, or severe trauma; to offset protein catabolism from prolonged use of corticosteroids*

**TABLETS**
**Adults.** 2.5 to 20 mg in divided doses given b.i.d. to q.i.d. for 2 to 4 wk; intermittent therapy repeated as prescribed. *Maximum:* 20 mg/day.
**Children.** 0.1 mg/kg q.d.; intermittent therapy repeated as prescribed.
**DOSAGE ADJUSTMENT** Dosage shouldn't exceed 5 mg b.i.d. for elderly patients.

### Mechanism of Action
Promotes tissue-building processes and reverses catabolic or tissue-depleting processes by promoting protein anabolism.

## Contraindications

Breast cancer (males); breast cancer with hypercalcemia (females); hypersensitivity to oxandrolone, anabolic steroids, or their components; nephrosis; pregnancy; prostate cancer

## Interactions

**DRUGS**

*corticosteroids:* Increased risk of edema and severe acne
*hepatotoxic drugs:* Increased risk of hepatotoxicity
*insulin, oral antidiabetic drugs:* Possibly hypoglycemia
*NSAIDs, oral anticoagulants, salicylates:* Increased anticoagulant effects
*sodium-containing drugs:* Increased risk of edema
*somatrem, somatropin:* Possibly accelerated epiphyseal closure
*warfarin:* Increased warfarin half-life and risk of bleeding

**FOODS**

*high-sodium foods:* Increased risk of edema

## Adverse Reactions

**CNS:** Depression, excitement, insomnia
**CV:** Decreased serum HDL level, edema, hyperlipidemia, hypertension
**ENDO:** Feminization in postpubertal males (epididymitis, gynecomastia, impotence, oligospermia, priapism, testicular atrophy); glucose intolerance; virilism in females (acne, clitoral enlargement, decreased breast size, deepened voice, diaphoresis, emotional lability, flushing, hirsutism, hoarseness, libido changes, male-pattern baldness, menstrual irregularities, nervousness, oily skin or hair, vaginal bleeding, vaginitis, weight gain), virilism in prepubertal males (acne, decreased ejaculatory volume, penis enlargement, prepubertal closure of epiphyseal plates, unnatural growth of body and facial hair)
**GI:** Diarrhea, elevated liver function test results, hepatocellular carcinoma, nausea, vomiting
**GU:** Benign prostatic hyperplasia, prostate cancer, urinary frequency, urine retention (elderly males)
**HEME:** Iron deficiency anemia, leukemia, prolonged bleeding time
**SKIN:** Jaundice
**Other:** Fluid retention, hypercalcemia (females), physical and psychological dependence, sodium retention

## Nursing Considerations

• Use oxandrolone cautiously in patients with heart disease because drug has hypercholesterolemic effects.
• Provide adequate calories and protein, as ordered, to maintain a positive nitrogen balance during oxandrolone therapy.
• Anticipate an increased risk of fluid and sodium retention in patients with cardiac, hepatic, or renal dysfunction.
• Weigh patient daily to detect fluid retention. If patient has fluid retention, expect a sodium-restricted diet or diuretics.
• **WARNING** Be aware that oxandrolone may suppress spermatogenesis in males and cause permanent virilization in females.
• Monitor blood glucose level frequently in patient with diabetes mellitus.
• If patient takes an oral anticoagulant, check INR or PT as ordered.

**PATIENT TEACHING**

• Advise patient to consume a diet high in protein and calories to achieve maximum therapeutic effect of oxandrolone.
• Urge patient to weigh himself daily during therapy and to notify prescriber immediately about swelling or unexplained weight gain.
• Explain that drug may alter libido.
• Inform female patient that drug may cause permanent physical changes (clitoral enlargement, deepened voice, hair growth).
• Advise female patient of childbearing age to use contraception during therapy and to notify prescriber immediately about suspected or known pregnancy.
• Instruct diabetic patient to monitor blood glucose level frequently.
• If patient takes warfarin, advise bleeding precautions (such as an electric shaver and soft toothbrush). Tell patient to notify prescriber immediately about bleeding.

# oxaprozin

Daypro

## Class and Category

*Chemical:* Proprionic acid derivative
*Therapeutic:* Anti-inflammatory, antirheumatic
*Pregnancy category:* C (first trimester), Not rated (later trimesters)

## Indications and Dosages
➤ *To treat rheumatoid arthritis*
**TABLETS**
**Adults.** 1,200 mg q.d. Dosage adjusted based on patient response. *Maximum:* 1,800 mg/day or 26 mg/kg/day (whichever is less) in divided doses b.i.d. or t.i.d.
➤ *To treat osteoarthritis*
**TABLETS**
**Adults.** 600 to 1,200 mg q.d. *Maximum:* 1,800 mg/day or 26 mg/kg (whichever is less) in divided doses b.i.d. or t.i.d.
**DOSAGE ADJUSTMENT** Initial loading dose of 1,200 to 1,800 mg possibly given to speed onset of action. Initial dose limited to 600 mg q.d. for patients with renal impairment.

| Route | Onset | Peak | Duration |
|-------|-------|------|----------|
| P.O. | In 7 days | Unknown | Unknown |

## Mechanism of Action
Blocks cyclooxygenase, the enzyme needed to synthesize prostaglandins, which mediate the inflammatory response and cause local vasodilation, swelling, and pain. By blocking cyclooxygenase and prostaglandins, the NSAID oxaprozin relieves pain.

## Contraindications
Angioedema, asthma, bronchospasm, nasal polyps, rhinitis, or urticaria induced by aspirin, iodides, or other NSAIDs

## Interactions
**DRUGS**
*ACE inhibitors, antihypertensives:* Decreased antihypertensive response, possibly impaired renal function
*acetaminophen:* Increased risk of adverse renal effects with long-term use of both drugs
*anticoagulants, thrombolytics:* Prolonged PT, increased risk of bleeding
*beta blockers:* Decreased antihypertensive effect
*bone marrow depressants:* Increased risk of leukopenia and thrombocytopenia
*cefamandole, cefoperazone, cefotetan, plicamycin, valproic acid:* Increased risk of hypoprothrombinemia and bleeding
*cimetidine:* Decreased oxaprozin clearance
*corticosteroids, potassium supplements:* Increased risk of adverse GI effects
*digoxin:* Increased blood digoxin level and risk of digitalis toxicity

*diuretics:* Possibly decreased diuretic effect
*insulin, oral antidiabetic drugs:* Increased effectiveness of these drugs; risk of hypoglycemia
*lithium:* Increased blood lithium level
*methotrexate:* Increased blood methotrexate level and risk of methotrexate toxicity
*other NSAIDs, salicylates:* Increased GI irritability and bleeding
*probenecid:* Increased risk of oxaprozin toxicity
**ACTIVITIES**
*alcohol use, smoking:* Increased risk of adverse GI effects

## Adverse Reactions
**CNS**: Aseptic meningitis, cerebral hemorrhage, confusion, dizziness, drowsiness, fatigue, headache, insomnia, ischemic CVA, nervousness, sedation, transient ischemic attacks, vertigo, weakness
**CV**: Deep vein thrombosis, hypertension, hypotension, MI, peripheral edema
**EENT**: Tinnitus
**ENDO**: Hypoglycemia
**GI**: Abdominal pain, constipation, diarrhea, dyspepsia, elevated liver function test results, GI bleeding or ulceration, hepatitis, jaundice, liver failure, nausea, perforation of stomach or intestine, vomiting
**GU**: Acute renal failure, dysuria, interstitial nephritis, urinary frequency
**HEME**: Agranulocytosis, anemia, aplastic anemia, leukopenia, pancytopenia, thrombocytopenia
**SKIN**: Alopecia, erythema multiforme, exfoliative dermatitis, maculopapular rash, photosensitivity, Stevens-Johnson syndrome, toxic epidermal necrolysis
**Other:** Anaphylaxis, angioedema

## Nursing Considerations
• Use oxaprozin with extreme caution in patients with a history of ulcer disease or GI bleeding because NSAIDs such as oxaprozin increase the risk of GI bleeding and ulceration. Expect to use oxaprozin for the shortest time possible in these patients.
• Be aware that serious GI tract ulceration, bleeding, and perforation may occur without warning symptoms. Elderly patients are at greater risk. To minimize risk, give drug with food. If GI distress occurs, withhold drug and notify prescriber immediately.
• Use oxaprozin cautiously in patients with hypertension, and monitor blood pressure

closely throughout therapy. Drug may cause hypertension or worsen it.

•**WARNING** Monitor patient closely for thrombotic events, including MI and stroke, because NSAIDs increase the risk.

•**WARNING** If patient has bone marrow suppression or is receiving antineoplastic drug therapy, monitor laboratory results (including WBC count), and watch for evidence of infection because anti-inflammatory and antipyretic actions of oxaprozin may mask signs and symptoms, such as fever and pain.

•Especially if patient is elderly or taking oxaprozin long-term, watch for less common but serious adverse GI reactions, including anorexia, constipation, diverticulitis, dysphagia, esophagitis, gastritis, gastroenteritis, gastroesophageal reflux disease, hemorrhoids, hiatal hernia, melena, stomatitis, and vomiting.

•Monitor liver function test results because, in rare cases, elevated levels may progress to severe hepatic reactions, including fatal hepatitis, liver necrosis, and hepatic failure.

•Monitor BUN and serum creatinine levels in patients with heart failure, impaired renal function, or hepatic dysfunction; those taking diuretics or ACE inhibitors; and elderly patients because drug may cause renal failure.

•Monitor CBC for decreased hemoglobin level and hematocrit because drug may worsen anemia.

•Assess patient's skin routinely for rash or other signs of hypersensitivity reaction because oxaprozin and other NSAIDs may cause serious skin reactions without warning, even in patients with no history of NSAID hypersensitivity. Stop drug at first sign of reaction, and notify prescriber.

**PATIENT TEACHING**

•Instruct patient to take oxaprozin exactly as prescribed.

•Advise patient to take drug with a full glass of water and to remain upright for 15 to 30 minutes afterward to prevent drug from lodging in esophagus and causing irritation.

•Urge patient to avoid alcohol as well as aspirin and other NSAIDs during oxaprozin therapy to avoid bleeding complications.

•Advise patient to avoid excessive sun exposure to reduce the risk of photosensitivity.

•Caution patient to avoid hazardous activities until drug's CNS effects are known.

•Inform patient that risk of bleeding may continue for up to 2 weeks after stopping drug.

•Explain that oxaprozin may increase the risk of serious adverse cardiovascular reactions; urge patient to seek immediate medical attention if signs or symptoms arise, such as chest pain, shortness of breath, weakness, and slurring of speech.

•Inform patient that oxaprozin also may increase the risk of serious adverse GI reactions; stress the importance of seeking immediate medical attention for such signs and symptoms as epigastric or abdominal pain, indigestion, black or tarry stools, or vomiting blood or material that looks like coffee grounds.

•Alert patient to the possibility of rare but serious skin reactions. Urge him to seek immediate medical attention for rash, blisters, itching, fever, or other indications of hypersensitivity.

# oxazepam

Apo-Oxazepam (CAN), Novoxapam (CAN), Serax

## Class, Category, and Schedule

*Chemical:* Benzodiazepine
*Therapeutic:* Antianxiety, sedative hypnotic
*Pregnancy category:* Not rated
*Controlled substance:* Schedule IV

## Indications and Dosages

➤ *To treat anxiety*

**CAPSULES, TABLETS**

**Adults.** 10 to 15 mg t.i.d. or q.i.d. for mild to moderate anxiety; up to 30 mg t.i.d. or q.i.d. for severe anxiety.

➤ *To help manage acute alcohol withdrawal symptoms*

**CAPSULES, TABLETS**

**Adults.** 15 to 30 mg t.i.d. or q.i.d.

**DOSAGE ADJUSTMENT** For elderly or debilitated patients, initial dose of 10 mg t.i.d. increased cautiously to 15 mg t.i.d. or q.i.d.

## Contraindications

Acute angle-closure glaucoma; concurrent use of itraconazole or ketoconazole; hypersensitivity to oxazepam, benzodiazepines, or their components; psychoses

## Mechanism of Action

May potentiate the effects of gamma-aminobutyric acid (GABA) and other inhibitory neurotransmitters by binding to specific benzodiazepine receptors in the limbic and cortical areas of the CNS. GABA inhibits excitatory stimulation, which helps control emotional behavior. The limbic system contains highly dense areas of benzodiazepine receptors, which may explain oxazepam's antianxiety effects.

## Interactions

**DRUGS**

*cimetidine, oral contraceptives:* Impaired metabolism and elimination of oxazepam
*clozapine:* Increased risk of respiratory depression and arrest
*CNS depressants:* Increased risk of apnea and CNS depression
*levodopa:* Decreased therapeutic effects of levodopa
*probenecid:* Increased therapeutic effects of oxazepam and risk of oversedation

**ACTIVITIES**

*alcohol use:* Increased risk of apnea and CNS depression

## Adverse Reactions

**CNS:** Anxiety (in daytime), ataxia, confusion, depression, dizziness, drowsiness, fatigue, headache, insomnia, nightmares, sleep disturbance, slurred speech, syncope, talkativeness, tremor, vertigo
**GI:** Nausea
**Other:** Drug tolerance, physical and psychological dependence, withdrawal symptoms

## Nursing Considerations

•WARNING Be aware that oxazepam may cause physical and psychological dependence.
•Be aware that drug shouldn't be stopped abruptly after prolonged use; doing so may cause seizures or withdrawal symptoms, such as insomnia, irritability, and nervousness.
•Be aware that withdrawal symptoms can occur when therapy lasts only 1 or 2 weeks.
•WARNING Monitor respiratory status in patients with pulmonary disease (such as severe COPD), respiratory depression, or sleep apnea; drug may worsen ventilatory failure.

•Expect an increased risk of falls among elderly patients from impaired cognition and motor function. Take safety precautions.
•Be aware that drug may worsen acute intermittent porphyria, myasthenia gravis, and severe renal impairment.
•Expect patient with late-stage Parkinson's disease to experience decreased cognition or coordination and, possibly, increased psychosis.

**PATIENT TEACHING**

•Instruct patient to take oxazepam exactly as prescribed and not to stop taking it without consulting prescriber.
•Caution patient about possible drowsiness and reduced coordination.
•Urge patient to avoid alcohol, which increases oxazepam's sedative effects.

# oxcarbazepine

Trileptal

## Class and Category

*Chemical:* Tricyclic iminostilbene derivative
*Therapeutic:* Anticonvulsant
*Pregnancy category:* C

## Indications and Dosages

➤ *As adjunct to treat partial seizures*
**ORAL SUSPENSION, TABLETS**
**Adults and adolescents over age 16.** *Initial:* 300 mg b.i.d. Dosage increased by 600 mg/day q wk. *Usual:* 1,200 mg/day. *Maximum:* 2,400 mg/day.
**Children ages 4 to 16.** *Initial:* 4 to 5 mg/kg b.i.d. to maximum initial dose of 600 mg/day. *Usual:* For children who weigh 20 to 29 kg (44 to 64 lb), 900 mg/day; for 29.1 to 39 kg (65 to 86 lb), 1,200 mg/day; for more than 39 kg, 1,800 mg/day. *Maximum:* 1,800 mg/day.
DOSAGE ADJUSTMENT For patients with creatinine clearance of less than 30 ml/min/1.73 m$^2$, usual initial dosage reduced by 50%.

➤ *As monotherapy to treat partial seizures*
**ORAL SUSPENSION, TABLETS**
**Adults and adolescents over age 16.** *Initial:* 300 mg b.i.d. Dosage increased by 300 mg/day q 3 days as needed. *Usual:* 1,200 mg/day. *Maximum:* 2,400 mg/day.
**Children ages 4 to 16.** *Initial:* 4 to 5 mg/kg b.i.d., increased by 5 mg/kg/day every 3rd day to maximum maintenance dosage, as needed. *Maximum:* For children who weigh 20 to 24.9 kg (44 to 55 lb), 900 mg/day; for 25 to

34.9 kg (55 to 77 lb), 1,200 mg/day; for 35 to 49.9 kg (77 to 110 lb), 1,500 mg/day; for 50 to 59.9 kg (110 to 132 lb), 1,800 mg/day; for 60 to 70 kg (132 to 154 lb), 2,100 mg/day.

➤ *To convert to monotherapy in the treatment of partial seizures*

ORAL SUSPENSION, TABLETS

**Adults and adolescents over age 16.** *Initial:* 300 mg b.i.d. Dosage increased by 600 mg/day q wk over 2 to 4 wk, as needed, while dosage of other anticonvulsant is reduced. *Usual:* 1,200 mg/day. *Maximum:* 2,400 mg/day.

**Children ages 4 to 16.** *Initial:* 4 to 5 mg/kg b.i.d., increased by 10 mg/kg/day weekly as needed to maximum maintenance dosage while dosage of other anticonvulsant is reduced over 3 to 6 wk. *Maximum:* For children who weigh 20 to 24.9 kg (44 to 55 lb), 900 mg/day; for 25 to 34.9 kg (55 to 77 lb), 1,200 mg/day; for 35 to 49.9 kg (77 to 110 lb), 1,500 mg/day; for 50 to 59.9 kg (110 to 132 lb), 1,800 mg/day; for 60 to 70 kg (132 to 154 lb), 2,100 mg/day.

---

### Mechanism of Action

May prevent or halt seizures by closing or blocking sodium channels in the neuronal cell membrane. By preventing sodium from entering the cell, oxcarbazepine may slow nerve impulse transmission, thus decreasing the rate at which neurons fire.

---

## Contraindications

Hypersensitivity to carbamazepine, oxcarbazepine, or their components

## Interactions

DRUGS

*carbamazepine, phenobarbital, phenytoin, valproic acid:* Decreased blood oxcarbazepine level, possibly increased blood levels of phenobarbital and phenytoin
*felodipine, verapamil:* Decreased blood levels of these drugs
*oral contraceptives:* Decreased effectiveness

ACTIVITIES

*alcohol use:* Possibly additive CNS depressant effects

## Adverse Reactions

**CNS:** Abnormal gait, ataxia, dizziness, fatigue, fever, headache, somnolence, tremor

**EENT:** Abnormal vision, diplopia, nystagmus, rhinitis
**GI:** Abdominal pain, indigestion, nausea, vomiting
**SKIN:** Rash, Stevens-Johnson syndrome, toxic epidermal necrolysis
**Other:** Hyponatremia

## Nursing Considerations

• Patient with an allergic reaction to carbamazepine may have hypersensitivity to oxcarbazepine.
• Monitor serum sodium level for signs of hyponatremia, especially during first 3 months.
• Monitor therapeutic oxcarbazepine levels during initiation and titration, and expect to adjust dosage accordingly.
• Implement seizure precautions as needed.
• Monitor patient's skin closely. If a reaction develops, notify prescriber immediately because skin reactions caused by oxcarbazepine may be serious or life-threatening.
• WARNING Monitor patient closely for evidence of multi-organ hypersensitivity, which may include fever, rash, organ dysfunction, lymphadenopathy, hepatitis, liver function abnormalities, hematologic abnormalities, pruritus, nephritis, oliguria, hepato-renal syndrome, arthralgia, and asthenia. If suspected, notify prescriber and expect to stop giving drug. Provide supportive care, as prescribed.

PATIENT TEACHING

• Teach patient to shake suspension well and prepare the dose immediately afterwards. Tell him to then withdraw the prescribed amount using the supplied oral dosing syringe. Instruct him to mix the dose in a small glass of water just before taking it, or tell him that he can swallow drug directly from the syringe. Instruct him to close the bottle and rinse the syringe with warm water and allow it to dry thoroughly.
• Inform patient that he may experience dizziness, double vision, and unsteady gait.
• Instruct patient not to drink alcohol during oxcarbazepine therapy.
• Alert patient to the possibility of hypersensitivity or serious skin reactions and the need to report them to prescriber.
• Warn patient to notify prescriber immediately if he develops a fever, rash, and additional symptoms because drug may need to be stopped and emergency medical care given.

•Alert female patients of childbearing age that oxcarbazepine may render hormonal contraceptives ineffective. Urge patient to use an additional or a different contraceptive during oxcarbazepine therapy.

# oxtriphylline

Apo-Oxtriphylline (CAN), Choledyl, Choledyl SA

## oxtriphylline and guaifenesin

Brondelate, Choledyl Expectorant (CAN)

## Class and Category

*Chemical:* Xanthine derivative
*Therapeutic:* Bronchodilator
*Pregnancy category:* C

## Indications and Dosages

➤ *To treat acute asthma, bronchospasm due to chronic bronchitis or COPD*

**DELAYED-RELEASE TABLETS (OXTRIPHYLLINE), ELIXIR (OXTRIPHYLLINE AND GUAIFENESIN)**

**Adults and children age 6 and older.** 300 mg q.d. for 3 days and then increased to 400 mg q.d. for 3 days. *Maintenance:* 600 mg/day in divided doses q 6 to 8 hr.

**E.R. TABLETS (OXTRIPHYLLINE)**

**Adults and children age 6 and older.** 300 mg q.d. for 3 days and then increased to 400 mg q.d. for 3 days. *Maintenance:* 600 mg/day in divided doses q 12 hr.

---

## Mechanism of Action

Inhibits phosphodiesterase enzymes, causing bronchodilation. Normally, these enzymes inactivate cAMP and cGMP, which are responsible for bronchial smooth-muscle relaxation. Other mechanisms of action may include calcium translocation, prostaglandin antagonism, catecholamine stimulation, inhibition of cGMP metabolism, and adenosine receptor antagonism. Guaifenesin eases expectoration by thinning and loosening sputum and bronchial secretions.

---

## Contraindications

Hypersensitivity to oxtriphylline, guaifenesin, xanthines, or their components; peptic ulcer; seizure disorder unless controlled by an anticonvulsant

## Interactions

**DRUGS**

*activated charcoal, aminoglutethimide, barbiturates, ketoconazole, rifampin, sulfinpyrazone, sympathomimetics:* Decreased blood theophylline level
*allopurinol, beta blockers (nonselective), calcium channel blockers, cimetidine, corticosteroids, disulfiram, ephedrine, influenza virus vaccine, interferon, macrolides, mexiletine, oral contraceptives, quinolones, thiabendazole:* Increased blood theophylline level
*benzodiazepines, propofol:* Possibly antagonized sedative effects of these drugs
*carbamazepine, isoniazid, loop diuretics:* Possibly altered blood theophylline level
*halothane anesthetics:* Increased risk of cardiotoxicity
*hydantoins:* Possibly decreased blood hydantoin level
*ketamine:* Increased risk of seizures
*lithium:* Decreased blood lithium level
*neuromuscular blockers:* Possibly reversal of neuromuscular blockade
*tetracyclines:* Possibly increased adverse effects of theophylline

**FOODS**

*all foods:* Altered bioavailability and absorption of E.R. oxtriphylline
*charcoal broiled beef; low-carbohydrate, high-protein diet:* Increased theophylline elimination
*high-carbohydrate, low-protein diet:* Decreased elimination and prolonged half-life of theophylline

**ACTIVITIES**

*alcohol use:* Increased CNS effects, especially with elixir
*smoking (1 or more packs/day):* Decreased effects of oxtriphylline

## Adverse Reactions

**CNS:** Anxiety, dizziness, headache, insomnia, restlessness, seizures
**CV:** Hypotension, palpitations, sinus tachycardia
**EENT:** Unpleasant taste
**GI:** Anorexia, diarrhea, nausea, vomiting
**RESP:** Tachypnea
**SKIN:** Alopecia, flushing, rash

## Nursing Considerations

•Be aware that oxtriphylline contains 64% anhydrous theophylline, so dosage is based on equivalent of 5 to 6 mg of anhydrous theophylline/kg.

•**WARNING** Be aware that elixir form contains 20% alcohol and shouldn't be used in children or in patients with a history of alcohol abuse.

•Be aware that food delays absorption of delayed-release and E.R. forms and that large volumes of fluid may increase absorption.

•Know that elixir is absorbed more rapidly and that delayed-release and E.R. preparations vary in their absorption rate.

•Monitor blood theophylline level because toxicity may develop at a level only slightly above therapeutic.

**PATIENT TEACHING**

•Tell patient to take elixir on an empty stomach with a full glass of water to enhance absorption.

•If patient complains of GI discomfort, suggest that he take drug with or just after meals.

•Urge patient to stop smoking and to notify prescriber about changes in smoking habits. Also instruct him to avoid alcohol during oxtriphylline therapy.

•Encourage patient to keep follow-up appointments for laboratory studies.

# oxybutynin chloride

Ditropan, Ditropan XL

## Class and Category

*Chemical:* Tertiary amine
*Therapeutic:* Antispasmodic
*Pregnancy category:* B

## Indications and Dosages

➤ *To treat overactive bladder, including neurogenic bladder, with urinary frequency, urgency, or incontinence from involuntary contraction of detrusor muscle*

**E.R. TABLETS**

**Adults.** *Initial:* 5 mg q.d., adjusted by 5 mg/wk, as prescribed. *Maximum:* 30 mg/day.

**SYRUP, TABLETS**

**Adults.** 5 mg b.i.d. or t.i.d. *Maximum:* 5 mg q.i.d. or 20 mg/day.

**Children age 5 and older.** 5 mg b.i.d. *Maximum:* 15 mg t.i.d.

**TRANSDERMAL SYSTEM**

**Adults.** 3.9-mg/day system applied twice/wk.

**DOSAGE ADJUSTMENT** For elderly patients, possibly 2.5 mg b.i.d. initially, increased to maximum of 5 mg t.i.d., as prescribed.

| Route | Onset | Peak | Duration |
|---|---|---|---|
| P.O. | 30 to 60 min | 3 to 6 hr | 6 to 10 hr |
| Transdermal | Unknown | 24 to 48 hr | 96 hr |

## Mechanism of Action

Exerts antimuscarinic (atropine-like) and potent direct antispasmodic (papaverine-like) actions on smooth muscle in the bladder and decreases detrusor muscle contractions. The result is increased bladder capacity and a decreased urge to void.

## Contraindications

Acute hemorrhage, angle-closure glaucoma, GI obstruction, hypersensitivity to oxybutynin or its components, ileus, intestinal atony in elderly or debilitated patients, myasthenia gravis, obstructive uropathy, toxic megacolon with ulcerative colitis

## Interactions

**DRUGS**

*amantadine, amitriptyline, amoxapine, antimuscarinics, brompheniramine, bupropion, carbinoxamine, chlorpheniramine, chlorpromazine, clemastine, clomipramine, clozapine, cyclobenzaprine, dimenhydrinate, diphenhydramine, disopyramide, doxepin, doxylamine, imipramine, maprotiline, mesoridazine, methdilazine, nortriptyline, procainamide, promazine, promethazine, protriptyline, thioridazine, triflupromazine, trimeprazine, trimipramine:* Increased anticholinergic effects

*CNS depressants:* Increased sedation

*ketoconazole:* Possibly altered total absorption rate and blood level of ketoconazole

*opioid agonists:* Increased depressive effects on GI motility and bladder function

*parasympathomimetics:* Decreased antimuscarinic action of oxybutynin

**ACTIVITIES**

*alcohol use:* Increased sedation

## Adverse Reactions

**CNS:** Asthenia, confusion, dizziness, drowsiness, hallucinations, headache, insomnia, nervousness, restlessness, seizures, somnolence

**CV:** Arrhythmias, hypertension, palpitations, peripheral edema, tachycardia, vasodilation

**EENT:** Blurred vision; dry eyes, mouth, nose, and throat; pharyngitis; rhinitis; sinusitis

N
O

**GI:** Abdominal pain, constipation, diarrhea, esophagitis, flatulence, gastroesophageal reflux, indigestion, nausea
**GU:** Cystitis, impotence, urinary hesitancy, urine retention, UTI
**MS:** Arthritis, back pain
**RESP:** Bronchitis, cough, upper respiratory tract infection
**SKIN:** Decreased sweating, dry skin, flushing, rash, urticaria
**Other:** Flulike symptoms, heatstroke

## Nursing Considerations

• Use oxybutynin cautiously in patients with diarrhea because it may signal incomplete GI obstruction, especially in patients with colostomy or ileostomy.
• Assess urinary symptoms before and after treatment.
• Make sure patient swallows E.R. tablets whole and doesn't crush, chew, or divide them. Expect to see portions of drug in stool.
• Apply transdermal system to dry, intact skin of abdomen, hip, or buttock; rotate sites to avoid the same site for at least 7 days.
• **WARNING** Monitor for adverse cardiovascular reactions in patients with arrhythmias, coronary artery disease, heart failure, or hypertension because drug's antimuscarinic effects may increase their risk.
• Decreased GI motility can cause adynamic ileus; assess for abdominal pain and ileus.
• Be aware that drug may aggravate benign prostatic hyperplasia, gastroesophageal reflux disease, and hyperthyroidism.

PATIENT TEACHING
• Instruct patient to take oxybutynin on an empty stomach. If adverse GI reactions develop, suggest that he take drug with food or milk.
• Advise patient to swallow tablets whole and not to chew, crush, or break them.
• Warn of possible decreased alertness, and advise against performing hazardous activities until drug's CNS effects are known.
• Caution patient to avoid strenuous exercise and excessive sun exposure because of increased risk of heatstroke.
• Urge patient to avoid alcohol during therapy

# oxycodone and acetaminophen

Endocet, Oxycocet (CAN), Percocet, Percocet-Demi (CAN), Roxicet, Roxilox, Tylox

## Class, Category, and Schedule
*Chemical:* Phenanthrene derivative (oxycodone), aminophenyl derivative (acetaminophen)
*Therapeutic:* Analgesic
*Pregnancy category:* Not rated
*Controlled substance:* Schedule II

## Indications and Dosages
➤ *To control moderate to moderately severe pain*
CAPSULES, TABLETS
**Adults.** 5 mg of oxycodone and 325 to 500 mg of acetaminophen (1 tab or capsule) q 4 to 6 hr, p.r.n. *Maximum:* 4,000 mg/day of acetaminophen.
ORAL SOLUTION
**Adults.** 5 mg (5 ml) of oxycodone and 325 mg of acetaminophen q 4 to 6 hr, p.r.n. *Maximum:* 4,000 mg/day of acetaminophen.

| Route | Onset | Peak | Duration |
|-------|-------|------|----------|
| P.O. | 30 min | 90 min | 3 to 4 hr |

### Mechanism of Action
Produces a synergistic analgesic effect through two mechanisms of action. Oxycodone, a mu receptor agonist, alters the perception of and emotional response to pain at the spinal cord and higher levels of the CNS by blocking the release of inhibitory neurotransmitters, such as gamma-aminobutyric acid and acetylcholine.

Acetaminophen blocks the activity of cyclooxygenase, an enzyme necessary for prostaglandin synthesis. Prostaglandins, important mediators in the inflammatory response, cause local vasodilation with swelling and pain.

## Contraindications
Hypercapnia; hypersensitivity to oxycodone, acetaminophen, or their components; ileus; use within 14 days of MAO inhibitor therapy

## Interactions

### DRUGS

*antacids:* Decreased and delayed acetaminophen absorption

*antianxiety drugs, benzodiazepines, brompheniramine, carbinoxamine, chlorpheniramine, clemastine, dimenhydrinate, diphenhydramine, doxylamine, general anesthetics, hypnotics, methdilazine, opioid antagonists, phenothiazines, promethazine, sedatives, skeletal muscle relaxants, tramadol, tricyclic antidepressants, trimeprazine:* Potentiated respiratory depression from these drugs and oxycodone

*anticholinergics:* Possibly severe constipation and paralytic ileus

*antidiarrheals:* Possibly severe constipation and additive CNS depression

*antihypertensives:* Possibly exaggerated antihypertensive effects and risk of orthostatic hypotension

*antineoplastics, immunosuppressants:* Risk of masking signs of infection, such as fever and pain

*barbiturates:* Additive CNS depression

*butorphanol, pentazocine:* Possibly acute withdrawal symptoms in opioid-dependent patients, decreased analgesic effect

*carbamazepine, phenobarbital, phenytoin, primidone, rifampin:* Possibly need for increased oxycodone dosage to achieve analgesia and prevent withdrawal symptoms in opioid-dependent patients, possibly increased risk of acetaminophen-induced hepatotoxicity

*cimetidine, ritonavir:* Possibly apnea, confusion, disorientation, and seizures from respiratory depression and impaired CNS function, increased risk of acetaminophen-induced hepatotoxicity (ritonavir)

*MAO inhibitors:* Possibly fatal reactions, including cardiac arrest, coma, respiratory depression, seizures, and severe hypertension

*nalbuphine, nalmefene, naloxone, naltrexone:* Blocked oxycodone effects, withdrawal symptoms in opioid-dependent patients

*verapamil:* Increased constipation

*warfarin:* Increased INR and risk of bleeding

### FOODS

*all foods:* Decreased and delayed acetaminophen absorption

### ACTIVITIES

*alcohol use:* Additive CNS depression, increased risk of acetaminophen-induced hepatotoxicity

## Adverse Reactions

**CNS:** Confusion, dizziness, drowsiness, euphoria, excitation, hallucinations, headache, restlessness, sedation, somnolence

**CV:** Bradycardia, hypotension, orthostatic hypotension, palpitations

**EENT:** Blurred vision, dry eyes, lens opacities, miosis

**GI:** Abdominal pain, constipation, elevated liver function test results, hepatotoxicity, nausea, vomiting

**GU:** Amenorrhea, decreased libido, erectile dysfunction, oliguria, renal tubular necrosis, urinary hesitancy, urine retention

**RESP:** Respiratory depression

**SKIN:** Erythema, flushing, pruritus, urticaria

**Other:** Drug tolerance, hypoprothrombinemia, physical and psychological dependence, withdrawal symptoms

## Nursing Considerations

• **WARNING** Be aware that oxycodone has a high potential for abuse.

• Use drug cautiously in patients with head injury because drug may alter neurologic findings.

• Assess pain level regularly, and give drug as prescribed before pain becomes severe.

• Administer drug with a full glass of water or, to minimize GI distress, with food or milk.

• Adjust dosage to relieve pain as prescribed, keeping in mind the maximum daily dose of acetaminophen. Be prepared to adjust dosage for patient who hasn't previously received opioids until he can tolerate drug's effects.

• Avoid giving drug within 1 to 2 hours of antacids or food because of risk of decreased drug effectiveness.

• Assess for possible respiratory depression or paradoxical excitation during dosage titration.

• Assess for abdominal pain because oxycodone may mask signs and symptoms of underlying GI disorders.

• Increase patient's dietary fiber intake if needed to prevent constipation.

• Anticipate an increased risk of falling during therapy. Institute safety precautions according to facility policy.

### PATIENT TEACHING

• Instruct patient not to take oxycodone and acetaminophen more often than prescribed and not to stop taking drug abruptly after long-term use.

N
O

• Encourage patient to take drug with a full glass of water and with food, if possible.
• Suggest that patient change position slowly to minimize effects of orthostatic hypotension.
• Instruct patient to avoid alcohol and potentially hazardous activities during therapy.
• Advise patient to notify prescriber about possible signs of toxicity or hypersensitivity, such as excessive light-headedness, extreme dizziness, itching, swelling, and trouble breathing.

# oxycodone hydrochloride

OxyContin, Roxicodone, Supeudol (CAN)

## Class, Category, and Schedule
*Chemical:* Phenanthrene derivative
*Therapeutic:* Analgesic
*Pregnancy category:* Not rated
*Controlled substance:* Schedule II

## Indications and Dosages
➤ *To relieve moderate to severe pain*
ORAL SOLUTION
**Adults.** 5 mg q 3 to 6 hr, p.r.n., and increased as needed.
TABLETS
**Adults.** 5 mg q 3 to 6 hr or 10 mg q 6 to 8 hr, p.r.n.
➤ *To manage pain for more than a few days*
CONTROLLED-RELEASE TABLETS, E.R. TABLETS
**Adults who haven't received opioids before.**
*Initial:* 10 to 20 mg q 12 hr, adjusted q 1 to 2 days, as prescribed, based on total amount of oxycodone needed daily to control pain.
**Adults who currently receive an opioid agonist or fixed-ratio combination drugs (opioid agonist plus acetaminophen, aspirin, or NSAID).**
Half the 24-hr oxycodone dose q 12 hr, as prescribed. Be prepared to manage breakthrough pain with immediate-release tablets, p.r.n., and adjust q 1 to 2 days, as prescribed.
**Adults who use fentanyl transdermal patch.**
10 mg oxycodone for each 25 mcg/hr of fentanyl patch dosage q 12 hr, beginning 12 to 18 hr after removing patch.
DOSAGE ADJUSTMENT To provide supplemental analgesia for adults receiving controlled-release oxycodone, one-fourth to one-third the 12-hr controlled-release dose given as tablet q 3 to 6 hr, p.r.n.

## Mechanism of Action
Alters the perception of and emotional response to pain at the spinal cord and higher levels of the CNS by blocking the release of inhibitory neurotransmitters, such as gamma-aminobutyric acid and acetylcholine.

| Route | Onset | Peak | Duration |
|---|---|---|---|
| P.O. | 10 to 15 min | 1 hr | 3 to 4 hr |

## Contraindications
Hypercapnia, hypersensitivity to oxycodone or its components, ileus, use within 14 days of MAO inhibitor therapy

## Interactions
DRUGS
*anticholinergics:* Possibly severe constipation and ileus
*antidiarrheals:* Possibly severe constipation and additive CNS depression
*antihypertensives:* Possibly exaggerated antihypertensive effects and risk of orthostatic hypotension.
*butorphanol, pentazocine:* Possibly acute withdrawal symptoms in opioid-dependent patients, decreased analgesic effects
*carbamazepine, phenytoin, primidone, rifampin:* Possibly need for increased oxycodone dosage to achieve analgesia and prevent withdrawal symptoms in opioid-dependent patients
*cimetidine:* Possibly apnea, confusion, disorientation, and seizures from respiratory depression and impaired CNS function
*CNS depressants:* Possibly increased CNS and respiratory depression and orthostatic hypotension
*MAO inhibitors:* Possibly fatal reactions, including cardiac arrest, coma, respiratory depression, seizures, and severe hypertension
*nalbuphine, nalmefene, naloxone, naltrexone:* Blocked oxycodone effects, withdrawal symptoms in opioid-dependent patients
ACTIVITIES
*alcohol use:* Additive CNS effects

## Adverse Reactions
**CNS:** Dizziness, drowsiness, euphoria, excitation, headache, sedation, somnolence
**CV:** Bradycardia, chest pain, hypotension, or-

thostatic hypotension, palpitations
**EENT:** Blurred vision, dry eyes, lens opacities, miosis
**GI:** Constipation, elevated liver function test results, nausea, vomiting
**GU:** Amenorrhea, decreased libido, erectile dysfunction, oliguria, urinary hesitancy, urine retention
**RESP:** Respiratory depression
**SKIN:** Pruritus
**Other:** Anaphylaxis, drug tolerance, physical and psychological dependence, withdrawal symptoms

## Nursing Considerations

•**WARNING** Be aware that oxycodone has a high potential for abuse.
•**WARNING** Be aware that abuse of crushed controlled-release tablets poses a hazard of overdose and death. If you suspect abuse and determine that patient also is abusing alcohol or illicit substances, notify prescriber immediately because the risk of overdose and death is increased. If you suspect parenteral abuse, be aware that tablet excipients, especially talc, may result in local tissue necrosis, infection, pulmonary granulomas, endocarditis, and valvular heart injury.
•Assess baseline neurologic status before each dose in patient with head injury because drug may obscure progression of his condition.
•Assess pain level regularly, and give drug as prescribed before pain becomes severe.
•Be prepared to adjust dosage for patient who hasn't previously received opioids until he can tolerate drug's effects.
•Expect to give controlled-release tablets only to opioid-tolerant patients who need at least 160 mg/day.
•Assess patient for possible respiratory depression or paradoxical excitation during dosage titration.
•Assess patient for abdominal pain because oxycodone may mask signs and symptoms of underlying GI disorders.

### PATIENT TEACHING

•**WARNING** Strongly warn patient to swallow tablets whole and not to break, chew, or crush them because taking broken, chewed, or crushed tablets leads to rapid release and absorption of a potentially fatal dose.
•Instruct patient not to take oxycodone more often than prescribed and not to stop taking drug abruptly after long-term use.

•Instruct patient to avoid alcohol and hazardous activities during oxycodone therapy.
•Tell patient to notify prescriber about signs of possible toxicity or hypersensitivity, such as excessive light-headedness, extreme dizziness, itching, swelling, and trouble breathing.

# oxycodone hydrochloride and ibuprofen

Combunox

## Class and Category

*Chemical:* Phenanthrene derivative (oxycodone), propionic acid derivative (ibuprofen)
*Therapeutic:* Analgesic
*Pregnancy category:* C
*Controlled substance:* Schedule II

## Indications and Dosages

➤ *For short-term management of acute, moderate to severe pain*

### TABLETS

**Adults.** 5 mg (oxycodone) and 400 mg (ibuprofen) q 6 hr, not to exceed 7 days.

| Route | Onset | Peak | Duration |
|-------|-------|------|----------|
| P.O. | 10 to 15 min | 1 hr | 3 to 6 hr |

### Mechanism of Action

Oxycodone alters the perception of and emotional response to pain at the spinal cord and higher levels of the CNS by blocking release of inhibitory neurotransmitters, such as gamma-aminobutyric acid and acetylcholine.

Ibuprofen blocks cyclooxygenase (mainly cyclooxygenase-1), the enzyme needed to synthesize prostaglandins, which mediate the inflammatory response and cause local vasodilation, swelling, and pain. By inhibiting prostaglandins, this NSAID reduces inflammatory symptoms and relieves pain.

## Contraindications

Angioedema; asthma; bronchospasm; hypercapnia; hypersensitivity to oxycodone, ibuprofen, other opioids, or their components; paralytic ileus; previous allergic reactions to aspirin or other NSAIDs; respiratory

N
O

depression; use within 14 days of MAO inhibitor therapy

## Interactions

### DRUGS

**Oxycodone and ibuprofen**

*antihypertensives:* Possibly exaggerated antihypertensive effects and risk of orthostatic hypotension

*hypnotics, sedatives, opioids:* Possibly additive effects, leading to greater duration of somnolence and, in severe cases, respiratory depression

### ACTIVITIES

*alcohol use:* Additive CNS effects and increased risk of adverse GI effects

**Oxycodone component only**

*anticholinergics:* Possibly severe constipation and ileus

*antidiarrheals:* Possibly severe constipation and additive CNS depression

*butorphanol, pentazocine:* Possibly acute withdrawal symptoms in opioid-dependent patients, decreased analgesic effects

*carbamazepine, phenytoin, primidone, rifampin:* Possibly need for increased oxycodone dosage to achieve analgesia and prevent withdrawal symptoms in opioid-dependent patients

*cimetidine:* Possibly apnea, confusion, disorientation, and seizures from respiratory depression and impaired CNS function

*CNS depressants:* Possibly increased CNS and respiratory depression and orthostatic hypotension

*MAO inhibitors:* Possibly fatal reactions, including cardiac arrest, coma, respiratory depression, seizures, and severe hypertension

*nalbuphine, nalmefene, naloxone, naltrexone:* Blocked oxycodone effects, withdrawal symptoms in opioid-dependent patients

*opioids:* Increased anticholinergic effects and leading to dry eyes, dry mouth, urine retention, and constipation

**Ibuprofen component only**

*ACE inhibitors:* Possibly decreased antihypertensive effect of ACE inhibitors

*acetaminophen:* Possibly increased renal effects with long-term use of both drugs

*aspirin, other NSAIDs:* Increased risk of bleeding and adverse GI effects

*bone marrow depressants:* Possibly increased leukopenic and thrombocytopenic effects of these drugs

*cefamandole, cefoperazone, cefotetan:* Increased risk of hypoprothrombinemia and bleeding

*colchicines, platelet aggregation inhibitors:* Increased risk of GI bleeding, hemorrhage, and ulcers

*corticosteroids, potassium supplements:* Increased risk of adverse GI effects

*cyclosporine:* Increased risk of nephrotoxicity from both drugs, increased blood cyclosporine level

*digoxin:* Increased blood digoxin level and risk of digitalis toxicity

*diuretics (loop, potassium-sparing, and thiazide):* Decreased diuretic and antihypertensive effects

*gold compounds, nephrotoxic drugs:* Increased risk of adverse renal effects

*heparin, oral anticoagulants, thrombolytics:* Increased anticoagulant effects, increased risk of hemorrhage

*insulin, oral antidiabetic drugs:* Possibly increased hypoglycemic effects of these drugs

*lithium:* Increased blood lithium level

*methotrexate:* Decreased methotrexate clearance, increased risk of methotrexate toxicity

*plicamycin, valproic acid:* Increased risk of hypoprothrombinemia and GI bleeding, hemorrhage, and ulcers

*probenecid:* Possibly increased blood level, effectiveness, and risk of toxicity of ibuprofen

*warfarin:* Increased risk of serious GI bleeding because of synergistic effects

## Adverse Reactions

**CNS:** Abnormal thinking, anxiety, aseptic meningitis, asthenia, chills, dizziness, drowsiness, euphoria, excitation, fever, headache, hyperkinesia, hypertonia, nervousness, sedation, somnolence

**CV:** Bradycardia, chest pain, fluid retention, heart failure, hypotension, palpitations, peripheral edema, thrombophlebitis, vasodilation

**EENT:** Amblyopia, blurred vision, dry eyes, epistaxis, lens opacities, miosis, stomatitis, taste perversion, tinnitus

**GI:** Abdominal cramps or pain, abdominal distention, anorexia, constipation, diarrhea, elevated liver function test results, epigastric discomfort, flatulence, gastritis, GI bleeding or ulceration, heartburn, hepatitis, indigestion, nausea, vomiting

**GU:** Acute renal failure, amenorrhea, cystitis, decreased libido, erectile dysfunction, hematuria, oliguria, urinary frequency or hesitancy, urine retention
**HEME:** Agranulocytosis, anemia, aplastic anemia, eosinophilia, hemolytic anemia, neutropenia, prolonged bleeding time, thrombocytopenia
**RESP:** Bronchospasm, dyspnea, respiratory depression, wheezing
**MS:** Arthritis, back pain
**SKIN:** Blisters, diaphoresis, ecchymosis, erythema multiforme, photosensitivity, pruritus, rash, Stevens-Johnson syndrome, urticaria
**Other:** Anaphylaxis, angioedema, drug tolerance, flulike symptoms, hypokalemia, infection, physical and psychological dependence, weight gain, withdrawal symptoms

## Nursing Considerations
•Use oxycodone and ibuprofen with extreme caution in patients with significant COPD or cor pulmonale and in patients who have substantially decreased respiratory reserve, hypoxia, or hypercapnia because oxycodone component can depress respiratory drive.
•Use drug cautiously in elderly or debilitated patients and in those with severe impairment of hepatic or renal function, hypothyroidism, Addison's disease, acute alcoholism, seizure disorders, CNS depression or coma, alcohol withdrawal syndrome, kyphoscoliosis associated with respiratory depression, toxic psychosis, benign prostatic hyperplasia, or urethral stricture because drug can cause hypotension, alter mental state, or depress respirations.
•Monitor patient's blood pressure because opioid analgesics like oxycodone and ibuprofen can cause severe hypotension.
•Monitor patients with biliary tract disease, including pancreatitis, for pain because the drug may cause spasm of the sphincter of Oddi.
•**WARNING** Be aware that oxycodone and ibuprofen has a high potential for abuse.
•Assess patient's pain level regularly, and give drug as prescribed, before pain becomes severe.
•Be prepared to adjust dosage for patient who hasn't previously received opioids until he can tolerate drug's effects.
•Assess patient for possible respiratory depression or paradoxical excitation during dosage adjustment.

•Assess patient for abdominal pain because oxycodone may mask signs and symptoms of underlying GI disorders.
•Be aware that ibuprofen's antipyretic and anti-inflammatory actions may mask signs and symptoms of infection.
**PATIENT TEACHING**
•Tell patient to take oxycodone and ibuprofen with food or after meals to reduce GI distress that may be caused by ibuprofen.
•Urge patient to take drug with a full glass of water and not to lie down for 15 to 30 minutes afterward to prevent esophageal irritation.
•Instruct patient not to take oxycodone and ibuprofen more often than prescribed or for more than 7 days.
•Advise patient to avoid taking another NSAID at the same time, unless directed by prescriber, because of increased risk of adverse reactions.
•Tell patient to avoid alcohol, aspirin, and hazardous activities while taking oxycodone and ibuprofen.
•Advise patient to notify prescriber about signs of possible toxicity or hypersensitivity, such as severe light-headedness or dizziness, itching, swelling, and trouble breathing.
•Suggest that patient wear sunscreen and protective clothing when outdoors to minimize photosensitivity.

# oxymetholone
Anadrol-50, Anapolon-50 (CAN)

## Class, Category, and Schedule
*Chemical:* Testosterone derivative
*Therapeutic:* Antianemic, antiangioedema (hereditary)
*Pregnancy category:* X
*Controlled substance:* Schedule III

## Indications and Dosages
➤ *To treat acquired and congenital aplastic anemias, anemias caused by deficient RBC production, bone marrow failure anemias, hypoplastic anemias caused by myelotoxic drugs, and myelofibrosis; to prevent or treat hereditary angioedema*
**TABLETS**
**Adults and children.** 1 to 2 mg/kg/day for 3 to 6 mo. *Maximum:* 5 mg/kg/day.

## Mechanism of Action
Combats anemia by increasing production of erythropoietin, a precursor of RBCs. Oxymetholone also increases the hemoglobin level and RBC volume.

## Contraindications
Breast or prostate cancer in males patients, hypercalcemia in female patients with breast cancer, hypersensitivity to oxymetholone or anabolic steroids, nephrosis, nephrotic phase of nephritis, pregnancy, severe hepatic dysfunction

## Interactions
**DRUGS**
*corticosteroids*: Increased risk of edema and severe acne
*hepatotoxic drugs:* Increased risk of hepatotoxicity
*insulin, oral antidiabetic drugs:* Possibly hypoglycemia
*NSAIDs, oral anticoagulants, salicylates:* Increased anticoagulant effects
*sodium-containing drugs:* Increased risk of edema
*somatrem, somatropin:* Possibly accelerated epiphyseal maturation
**FOODS**
*high-sodium foods:* Increased risk of edema

## Adverse Reactions
**CNS:** Depression, excitement, insomnia
**CV:** Decreased serum HDL level, edema, hyperlipidemia, hypertension
**ENDO:** Feminization in postpubertal males (epididymitis, gynecomastia, impotence, oligospermia, priapism, testicular atrophy), glucose intolerance, virilism in females (acne, clitoral enlargement, decreased breast size, deepened voice, diaphoresis, emotional lability, flushing, hirsutism, hoarseness, libido changes, male-pattern baldness, menstrual irregularities, nervousness, oily hair or skin, vaginal bleeding, vaginitis, weight gain), virilism in prepubertal males (acne, decreased ejaculatory volume, penis enlargement, prepubertal closure of epiphyseal plates, unnatural growth of body and facial hair)
**GI:** Diarrhea, elevated liver function test results, hepatocellular carcinoma, nausea, vomiting
**GU:** Benign prostatic hyperplasia, prostate cancer, urinary frequency, urine retention (elderly males)

**HEME:** Iron deficiency anemia, leukemia, prolonged bleeding time
**SKIN:** Jaundice
**Other:** Fluid retention, hypercalcemia (females), physical and psychological dependence, sodium retention

## Nursing Considerations
•Be aware that oxymetholone shouldn't be used in patients with a history of hypercalcemia because drug may exacerbate this condition or in patients with prostate problems because drug may promote benign or cancerous tumor growth.
•Anticipate increased risk of fluid and sodium retention in patients with cardiac, hepatic, or renal dysfunction. Monitor for signs and symptoms of fluid retention.
•Monitor daily weight. Expect to place patient with fluid retention on sodium-restricted diet or diuretics, as prescribed.
•**WARNING** Be aware that oxymetholone may suppress spermatogenesis in males and cause permanent virilization in females.
**PATIENT TEACHING**
•Advise patient to consume a diet high in protein and calories to achieve maximum therapeutic effect of oxymetholone.
•Instruct patient to check his weight daily during oxymetholone therapy and to notify prescriber immediately about swelling or unexplained weight gain.
•Inform patient that drug may cause libido changes.
•Advise diabetic patient to monitor blood glucose levels frequently because drug may increase hypoglycemic effect of antidiabetic drugs.
•Inform female patient that drug may cause permanent physical changes, such as clitoral enlargement, deepened voice, and unnatural hair growth.
•Advise female patient of childbearing age to use contraception during therapy and to notify prescriber immediately about suspected or known pregnancy.

# oxymorphone hydrochloride

Numorphan

## Class, Category, and Schedule
*Chemical:* Phenanthrene derivative
*Therapeutic*: Analgesic

*Pregnancy category:* Not rated
*Controlled substance:* Schedule II

## Indications and Dosages

➤ *To relieve moderate to severe pain, to relieve anxiety in patients with dyspnea from pulmonary edema caused by acute left ventricular dysfunction*

**I.V. INJECTION**
**Adults.** *Initial:* 0.5 mg, repeated q 3 to 6 hr, p.r.n.
**I.M. OR S.C. INJECTION**
**Adults.** *Initial:* 1 to 1.5 mg, repeated q 3 to 6 hr, p.r.n.
**SUPPOSITORIES**
**Adults.** 5 mg q 4 to 6 hr, p.r.n.

➤ *To relieve obstetric pain during labor*

**I.M. INJECTION**
**Adults.** 0.5 to 1 mg as a single dose.

| Route | Onset | Peak | Duration |
|-------|-------|------|----------|
| I.V. | 5 to 10 min | 15 to 30 min | 3 to 4 hr |
| I.M. | 10 to 15 min | 30 to 90 min | 3 to 6 hr |
| S.C. | 10 to 20 min | 30 to 90 min | 3 to 6 hr |
| P.R. | 15 to 30 min | 2 hr | 3 to 6 hr |

### Mechanism of Action

Alters the perception of and emotional response to pain at the spinal cord and higher levels of the CNS by blocking the release of inhibitory neurotransmitters, such as gamma-aminobutyric acid and acetylcholine.

## Contraindications

Acute or severe asthma; hypersensitivity to oxymorphone, other morphine analogues, or their components; ileus; pulmonary edema from a chemical respiratory irritant; severe respiratory depression; upper airway obstruction

## Interactions

**DRUGS**
*anticholingerics:* Increased risk of urine retention, severe constipation
*antidiarrheals, antiperistaltics:* Increased risk of severe constipation, CNS depression
*antihypertensives, diuretics, hypotension-producing drugs:* Increased hypotensive effects

*buprenorphine:* Reduced oxymorphone effectiveness if buprenorphine is given first, possibly withdrawal symptoms in oxymorphone-dependent patients
*CNS depressants:* Additive CNS depressant effects, increased risk of habituation
*hydroxyzine, other opioid analgesics:* Increased analgesia, CNS depression, and hypotensive effects
*MAO inhibitors:* Increased risk of unpredictable, severe, sometimes fatal adverse reactions
*metoclopramide:* Antagonized effects of metoclopramide on GI motility
*naloxone:* Antagonized analgesic, CNS, and respiratory depressant effects of oxymorphone
*naltrexone:* Withdrawal symptoms in oxymorphone-dependent patients
*neuromuscular blockers:* Additive respiratory depression

**ACTIVITIES**
*alcohol use:* Additive CNS depressant effects, increased risk of habituation

## Adverse Reactions

**CNS:** Confusion, delusions, depersonalization, dizziness, drowsiness, euphoria, headache, light-headedness, nervousness, nightmares, restlessness, seizures, tiredness, tremor, weakness
**CV:** Bradycardia, hypertension, hypotension, palpitations, tachycardia
**EENT:** Blurred vision, diplopia, dry mouth, laryngeal edema, laryngospasm, tinnitus
**GI:** Abdominal cramps or pain, constipation, hepatotoxicity, nausea, vomiting
**GU:** Decreased urine output, dysuria, urinary frequency
**MS:** Muscle rigidity (with large doses), uncontrolled muscle movements
**RESP:** Atelectasis, bradypnea, bronchospasm, dyspnea, irregular breathing, respiratory depression, wheezing
**SKIN:** Diaphoresis, erythema, flushing of face
**Other:** Injection site burning, pain, redness, and swelling

## Nursing Considerations

•Monitor vital signs during oxymorphone therapy to detect respiratory depression and hypotension.
•Monitor urinary and bowel status; constipation may become so severe that it causes ileus.
•Offer fluids to relieve dry mouth.

• Instruct patient to take oxymorphone exactly as prescribed and not to stop taking drug abruptly; warn him that drug can cause physical dependence.
• Stress the importance of taking drug before pain becomes severe.
• Instruct patient to store suppositories in refrigerator.
• Encourage patient to increase fluid and fiber intake to prevent constipation.
• Urge patient not to drink alcohol or use CNS depressants during therapy without first consulting prescriber.
• Caution patient to avoid potentially hazardous activities until drug's CNS effects are known.
• Advise female patient to stop drug and notify prescriber about known or suspected pregnancy.

# oxytetracycline

Terramycin I.M.

## oxytetracycline hydrochloride

Terramycin

## Class and Category

*Chemical:* Tetracycline derived from *Streptomyces rimosus*
*Therapeutic:* Antibiotic, antiprotozoal
*Pregnancy category:* D

## Indications and Dosages

➤ *To treat systemic bacterial and protozoal infections, such as bronchitis, chlamydial infection, Lyme disease, nongonococcal urethritis, rickettsial infection, traveler's diarrhea, and UTIs*
CAPSULES (OXYTETRACYCLINE HYDROCHLORIDE)
**Adults and adolescents.** 250 to 500 mg q 6 hr. *Maximum:* 4,000 mg/day.
**Children ages 8 to 12.** 6.25 to 12.5 mg/kg q 6 hr.
I.M. INJECTION (OXYTETRACYCLINE)
**Adults and adolescents.** 100 mg q 8 hr, 150 mg q 12 hr, or 250 mg q.d. *Maximum:* 500 mg/day.
**Children ages 8 to 12.** 5 to 8.3 mg/kg q 8 hr or 7.5 to 12.5 mg/kg q 12 hr. *Maximum:* 250 mg/day.
DOSAGE ADJUSTMENT Dosage possibly reduced for patients with renal impairment.

➤ *To treat brucellosis*
CAPSULES (OXYTETRACYCLINE HYDROCHLORIDE)
**Adults and adolescents.** 500 mg q 6 hr for 3 wk with 1,000 mg of streptomycin I.M. q 12 hr in wk 1 and q.d. in wk 2. *Maximum:* 4,000 mg/day.
➤ *To treat uncomplicated gonorrhea*
CAPSULES (OXYTETRACYCLINE HYDROCHLORIDE)
**Adults and adolescents.** *Initial:* 1,500 mg, then 500 mg q 6 hr to total of 9,000 mg for full course of treatment.
➤ *To treat syphilis*
CAPSULES (OXYTETRACYCLINE HYDROCHLORIDE)
**Adults and adolescents.** 500 to 1,000 mg q 6 hr for 10 to 15 days to total of 30 to 40 g for full course of treatment.

## Mechanism of Action
Binds with ribosomal subunits of susceptible bacteria and alters the cytoplasmic membrane, inhibiting bacterial protein synthesis and rendering the organism ineffective.

## Contraindications
Hypersensitivity to tetracyclines or their components

## Interactions
**DRUGS**
*antacids, calcium supplements, cholestyramine, choline salicylates, colestipol, iron supplements, magnesium salicylates:* Possibly decreased absorption of oxytetracycline
*digoxin:* Increased blood digoxin level
*lithium:* Altered blood lithium level
*methoxyflurane:* Increased risk of nephrotoxicity
*oral anticoagulants:* Increased anticoagulant effects
*oral contraceptives:* Decreased contraceptive effectiveness, increased risk of breakthrough bleeding and pregnancy
*penicillins:* Decreased bactericidal effects of penicillins
*sodium bicarbonate:* Possibly decreased absorption of oral oxytetracycline
*vitamin A:* Increased risk of benign intracranial hypertension
**FOODS**
*all foods, especially dairy products:* Possibly interference with oxytetracycline absorption

## Adverse Reactions

**CNS:** Dizziness, light-headedness, tiredness, unsteadiness, weakness
**EENT:** Darkened, discolored, or sore tongue; stomatitis, tooth discoloration (in infants and children under age 8)
**GI:** Abdominal cramps, diarrhea, indigestion, nausea, thirst, vomiting
**GU:** Urinary frequency
**SKIN:** Photosensitivity
**Other:** Superinfection

## Nursing Considerations

•WARNING Be aware that oxytetracycline shouldn't be given to premature infants because it may impair skeletal growth or to children under age 8 because it may permanently discolor teeth and cause enamel hypoplasia.
•Administer I.M. injection in an adult in the upper outer quadrant of the buttocks or mid-lateral thigh; the deltoid muscle may be used but only if well developed. In children, inject only in the mid-lateral thigh.
•Be aware that patient should be switched from parenteral to oral form as soon as possible.

### PATIENT TEACHING

•Instruct patient to take oxytetracycline capsules 1 hour before meals and 3 hours before or after other drugs and dairy products.
•Advise patient to take drug with a full glass of water and in an upright position to minimize adverse GI reactions.
•Urge patient to complete entire course of oxytetracycline therapy, even if he feels better beforehand.
•Caution patient to avoid potentially hazardous activities until drug's CNS effects are known.
•Advise patient to avoid excessive sun exposure and to protect skin when outdoors.
•Urge female patient who uses oral contraceptives to use an additional form of birth control during oxytetracycline therapy.
•Advise patient to discard outdated capsules because drug may become toxic.

N
O

# P

## palonosetron hydrochloride

Aloxi

### Class and Category
*Chemical:* Selective serotonin subtype 3 (5-HT₃) receptor antagonist
*Therapeutic:* Antiemetic
*Pregnancy category:* B

### Indications and Dosages
➤ *To prevent acute and delayed nausea and vomiting from chemotherapy*

**I.V. INJECTION**
**Adults.** 0.25 mg over 30 sec approximately 30 min before start of chemotherapy.

### Incompatibilities
Palonosetron should not be mixed with any other drug.

### Contraindications
Hypersensitivity to palonosetron or its components

### Interactions
**DRUGS**
None reported.

### Adverse Reactions
**CNS:** Anxiety, dizziness, drowsiness, fatigue, headache, insomnia, weakness
**CV:** Bradycardia, hypotension, prolonged QT interval, tachycardia
**GI:** Abdominal pain, constipation, diarrhea
**SKIN:** Dermatitis, pruritus, rash
**Other:** Hyperkalemia

### Nursing Considerations
• Use palonosetron cautiously in patients who have or may develop prolonged cardiac conduction intervals—especially QT interval—such as those with congenital QT syndrome, hypokalemia, or hypomagnesemia; those taking a diuretic known to induce electrolyte abnormalities, an antiarrhythmic, or another drug that may prolong QT interval; and those who have received cumulative high-dose anthracycline therapy. With these patients, obtain a baseline ECG before giving palonosetron; repeat the ECG 15 minutes or 24 hours after giving drug, as ordered. Notify prescriber of any delayed conduction.
• Flush I.V. line before and after palonosetron administration with normal saline solution.
• Closely monitor any patient hypersensitive to other selective serotonin receptor antagonists for a similar reaction. If a reaction occurs, notify prescriber immediately.

**PATIENT TEACHING**
• Advise patient to avoid hazardous activities until drug's CNS effects are known.

### Mechanism of Action
Chemotherapy-induced nausea and vomiting may occur when a chemotherapeutic drug irritates the small intestine's mucosa, causing enterochromaffin cells within the mucosa to release serotonin (5-HT₃). Then, 5-HT₃ stimulates sympathetic receptors on afferent vagal nerve endings and the vagus nerve initiates the vomiting reflex.

Palonosetron selectively blocks 5-HT₃ receptors in afferent vagal nerve endings, preventing the vagus nerve from inducing the vomiting reflex and thereby averting or reducing the nausea and vomiting associated with chemotherapy. Palonosetron may also block 5-HT₃ receptors centrally, in the chemoreceptor trigger zone of the brain's area postrema.

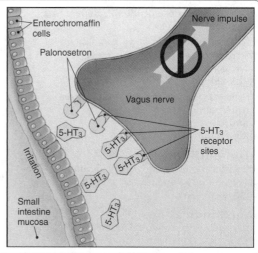

•Instruct patient to notify prescriber of any hypersensitivity reaction, such as rash or allergic dermatitis.

# pamidronate disodium

Aredia

## Class and Category

*Chemical:* Bisphosphonate
*Therapeutic:* Antihypercalcemic, bone resorption inhibitor
*Pregnancy category:* D

## Indications and Dosages

➤ *To treat cancer-induced hypercalcemia that's inadequately managed by oral hydration alone*

**I.V. INFUSION**

**Adults.** 60 to 90 mg over 2 to 24 hr as a single dose when corrected serum calcium level is 12 to 13.5 mg/dl; 90 mg over 2 to 24 hr when corrected serum calcium level is greater than 13.5 mg/dl. May be repeated as prescribed after 7 days if hypercalcemia recurs.

**DOSAGE ADJUSTMENT** For patients with renal failure, dosage is limited to 30 mg over 4 to 24 hr, as prescribed. For patients with cardiac or renal failure, drug is given in a smaller volume of fluid or at a slower rate, as prescribed.

➤ *To treat moderate to severe Paget's disease of bone*

**I.V. INFUSION**

**Adults.** 30 mg/day over 4 hr on 3 consecutive days for a total dose of 90 mg. Repeated as needed and tolerated.

➤ *To treat osteolytic bone metastases of breast cancer*

**I.V. INFUSION**

**Adults.** 90 mg over 2 hr q 3 to 4 wk.

➤ *To treat osteolytic bone metastases of multiple myeloma*

**I.V. INFUSION**

**Adults.** 90 mg over 4 hr q mo.

## Incompatibilities

Don't mix pamidronate with calcium-containing infusion solutions, such as Ringer's solution.

## Contraindications

Hypersensitivity to pamidronate, other bisphosphonates, or their components

## Mechanism of Action

Inhibits bone resorption, possibly by impairing attachment of osteoclast precursors to mineralized bone matrix, thus reducing the rate of bone turnover in Paget's disease and osteolytic metastases. Pamidronate also reduces the flow of calcium from resorbing bone into the bloodstream.

## Interactions

**DRUGS**

*calcium-containing preparations; vitamin D preparations, such as calcifediol and calcitriol:* Antagonized pamidronate effects when used to treat hypercalcemia

## Adverse Reactions

**CNS:** Confusion, fever, psychosis
**CV:** Hypotension
**GI:** Abdominal cramps, anorexia, GI bleeding, indigestion, nausea, vomiting
**GU:** Azotemia
**HEME:** Leukopenia, lymphopenia
**MS:** Bone pain, muscle spasms or stiffness, osteonecrosis (mainly of jaw)
**RESP:** Dyspnea
**Other:** Anaphylaxis, angioedema, hypocalcemia, hypokalemia, hypomagnesemia, hypophosphatemia, injection site pain and swelling

## Nursing Considerations

•Make sure patient has had a dental checkup before invasive dental procedures during pamidronate therapy, especially if patient has cancer; is receiving chemotherapy, head or neck radiation, or a corticosteroid; or has poor oral hygiene because the risk of osteonecrosis is increased in these patients.

•Stay alert for fever during the first 3 days of pamidronate therapy, especially in patients receiving high doses. If fever develops, obtain the patient's CBC with differential, as ordered.

•Obtain serum creatinine level before each treatment. Notify prescriber of abnormal results because drug may need to be withheld or dosage adjusted until creatinine level returns to normal.

•Assess patient with anemia, leukopenia, or thrombocytopenia for worsening of the condition during first 2 weeks of therapy.

PATIENT TEACHING
•Stress the importance of complying with prescribed administration schedule for pamidronate.
•Advise patient to avoid calcium and vitamin D supplements during pamidronate therapy.
•Instruct patient on proper oral hygiene and on need to notify prescriber about invasive dental procedures.

# pancreatin

Donnazyme (contains 500 mg of pancreatin, 1,000 U of lipase, 12,500 U of protease, 12,500 U of amylase), Hi-Vegi-Lip (contains 2,400 mg of pancreatin, 4,800 U of lipase, 60,000 U of protease, 60,000 U of amylase), Pancrezyme 4X (contains 2,400 mg of pancreatin, 12,000 U of lipase, 60,000 U of protease, 60,000 U of amylase), 4X Pancreatin (contains 2,400 mg of pancreatin, 12,000 U of lipase, 60,000 U of protease, 60,000 U of amylase), 8X Pancreatin (contains 7,200 mg of pancreatin, 22,500 U of lipase, 180,000 U of protease, 180,000 U of amylase)

## Class and Category
*Chemical:* Pancreatic enzyme
*Therapeutic:* Digestant, pancreatic enzyme replacement
*Pregnancy category:* C

## Indications and Dosages
➤ *To treat pancreatic insufficiency, including steatorrhea*
CAPSULES, TABLETS
**Adults.** 8,000 to 24,000 U of lipase with meals or snacks, adjusted as prescribed, according to need for steatorrhea control. For severe insufficiency, up to 36,000 U of lipase with meals or snacks.

### Mechanism of Action
Releases the enzymes pancreatin, lipase, amylase, and protease, mainly in the duodenum and upper jejunum. These enzymes facilitate the hydrolysis of fats into glycerol and fatty acids, starches into dextrins and sugars, and proteins into peptides. Pancreatin acts locally in the GI tract but is quickly inactivated by gastric acid.

## Contraindications
Acute exacerbation of chronic pancreatic disease; acute pancreatitis; hypersensitivity to pancreatin, pancrelipase, or pork

## Interactions
DRUGS
*acarbose, miglitol:* Decreased effectiveness of these drugs
*aluminum hydroxide, H₂-receptor antagonists, omeprazole, sodium bicarbonate:* Increased gastric pH, prolonged enzymatic action of pancreatin
*calcium carbonate– and magnesium hydroxide–containing antacids:* Decreased pancreatin effectiveness
*iron supplements:* Decreased iron absorption

## Adverse Reactions
**EENT:** Stomatitis
**GI:** Abdominal cramps or pain, diarrhea, intestinal obstruction, nausea
**SKIN:** Rash, urticaria
**Other:** Hyperuricemia

## Nursing Considerations
•WARNING Don't administer pancreatin to patient who is allergic to pork.
•Assess patient for GI disturbances and hyperuricemia when giving high doses of pancreatin.
•If patient opens capsules and sprinkles contents on food, assess for signs of sensitization (chest tightness, dyspnea, nasal congestion, wheezing), which may result from repeated inadvertent inhalation of powder.
•Be aware that brands of pancreatin aren't interchangeable because the same doses don't contain equivalent amounts of drug.
PATIENT TEACHING
•Instruct patient to take pancreatin before or with meals or snacks to maximize effectiveness.
•To prevent capsule or tablet from lodging in esophagus, advise patient to take drug with a beverage while sitting upright, to swallow it quickly, and to follow with 1 or 2 mouthfuls of solid food.
•Caution patient not to chew tablets; doing so may irritate mouth, lips, and tongue.
•If patient has trouble swallowing capsules, advise her to open the capsule and sprinkle its contents on food without inhaling them.
•Caution patient not to take antacids that contain calcium carbonate or magnesium hydroxide during therapy.

# pancrelipase

Cotazym (contains 8,000 U of lipase, 30,000 U of protease, 30,000 U of amylase), Cotazym-S (contains 5,000 U of lipase, 20,000 U of protease, 20,000 U of amylase), Ilozyme (contains 11,000 U of lipase, 30,000 U of protease, 30,000 U of amylase), Ku-Zyme HP (contains 8,000 U of lipase, 30,000 U of protease, 30,000 U of amylase), Pancrease (contains 4,500 U of lipase, 25,000 U of protease, 20,000 U of amylase), Pancrease MT 4 (contains 4,000 U of lipase, 12,000 U of protease, 12,000 U of amylase), Pancrease MT 10 (contains 10,000 U of lipase, 30,000 U of protease, 30,000 U of amylase), Pancrease MT 16 (contains 16,000 U of lipase, 48,000 U of protease, 48,000 U of amylase), Pancrease MT 20 (contains 20,000 U of lipase, 44,000 U of protease, 56,000 U of amylase), Protilase (contains 4,000 U of lipase, 25,000 U of protease, 20,000 U of amylase), Ultrase MT 12 (contains 12,000 U of lipase, 39,000 U of protease, 39,000 U of amylase), Ultrase MT 20 (contains 20,000 U of lipase, 65,000 U of protease, 65,000 U of amylase), Viokase Tablets (contains 8,000 U of lipase, 30,000 U of protease, 30,000 U of amylase), Viokase Powder (contains 16,800 U of lipase, 70,000 U of protease, 70,000 U of amylase), Zymase (contains 12,000 U of lipase, 24,000 U of protease, 24,000 U of amylase)

## Class and Category

*Chemical:* Porcine pancreatic enzyme
*Therapeutic:* Pancreatic enzyme replacement
*Pregnancy category:* C

## Indications and Dosages

➤ *To treat pancreatic insufficiency, including steatorrhea*

**CAPSULES, DELAYED-RELEASE CAPSULES, POWDER, TABLETS**
**Adults and adolescents.** 33,000 to 44,000 U of lipase before or with meals or snacks; adjusted as prescribed. For patients with severe deficiency, possibly up to 88,000 U of lipase with meals or snacks or dosing frequency increased to q hr.
**Children ages 7 to 12.** 4,000 to 12,000 U of lipase with meals and snacks; adjusted as needed and tolerated.
**Children ages 1 to 6.** 4,000 to 8,000 U of lipase with meals and 4,000 U of lipase with each snack; adjusted as needed and tolerated.

**Infants ages 6 to 11 months.** 2,000 U of lipase with meals; adjusted as needed and tolerated.

## Mechanism of Action

Releases high levels of the enzymes lipase, amylase, and protease, mainly in the duodenum and upper jejunum. These enzymes facilitate the hydrolysis of fats into glycerol and fatty acids, starches into dextrins and sugars, and proteins into peptides.

## Contraindications

Acute exacerbation of chronic pancreatic disease; acute pancreatitis; hypersensitivity to pancreatin, pancrelipase, or pork

## Interactions

**DRUGS**
*acarbose, miglitol:* Decreased effectiveness of these drugs
*aluminum hydroxide, H₂-receptor antagonists, omeprazole, sodium bicarbonate:* Increased gastric pH, prolonged enzymatic action of pancrelipase
*calcium carbonate– and magnesium hydroxide–containing antacids:* Decreased pancrelipase effectiveness
*iron supplements:* Decreased iron absorption

## Adverse Reactions

**EENT:** Stomatitis
**GI:** Abdominal cramps or pain, diarrhea, intestinal obstruction, nausea
**HEME:** Anemia
**SKIN:** Rash, urticaria
**Other:** Hyperuricemia

## Nursing Considerations

• **WARNING** Don't administer pancrelipase to patient who is allergic to pork.
• Be aware that brands of pancrelipase aren't interchangeable because the same doses don't contain equivalent amounts of drug.
• Mix powder with fluid or soft, nondairy food.
• If necessary, open delayed-release capsules and mix contents (enteric-coated spheres, microspheres, or microtablets) with liquids or soft food that requires no chewing. Administer immediately because enteric coating will dissolve after prolonged contact with foods that have a pH greater than 6.

•If patient opens capsules and sprinkles contents on food, assess for signs of sensitization (chest tightness, dyspnea, nasal congestion, wheezing), which may result from repeated inadvertent inhalation of powder.
•Give drug before or with meals and snacks, and follow with a glass of water or juice.
•Expect drug to cause stomatitis if held in mouth.
•Monitor stool for fecal fat content, as ordered.
•Monitor patient for iron deficiency anemia because serum iron level may decline during pancrelipase therapy.

PATIENT TEACHING
•Instruct patient to take pancrelipase before or with meals and snacks and to follow with a glass of water or juice.
•Instruct patient not to chew capsules (or capsule contents) or crush tablets and to swallow immediately because drug may cause irritation if held in mouth.
•Urge patient not to inhale powder from delayed-release capsules because doing so may cause chest tightness, shortness of breath, stuffy nose, trouble breathing, and wheezing.
•Inform patient that sneezing and tearing also may result from contact with powder.
•Caution patient not to use antacids because they may decrease drug effectiveness.
•Inform patient that her stool may smell foul.

# pantoprazole sodium

Pantoloc (CAN), Protonix

## Class and Category
*Chemical:* Substituted benzimidazole
*Therapeutic:* Antiulcer, gastric acid proton pump inhibitor
*Pregnancy category:* B

## Indications and Dosages
➤ *To treat gastroesophageal reflux disease (GERD)*
DELAYED-RELEASE TABLETS
Adults. 40 mg q.d. for up to 8 wk. Repeated for another 4 to 8 wk if healing doesn't occur.
I.V. INFUSION
Adults. 40 mg q.d. infused over 2 min or 15 min for 7 to 10 days, followed by oral doses.

➤ *To maintain healing of erosive esophagitis and reduce relapse of daytime and nighttime symptoms in patients with GERD*
DELAYED-RELEASE TABLETS
Adults. 40 mg q.d. for up to 12 mo.

➤ *To treat pathological hypersecretion associated with Zollinger-Ellison syndrome or other neoplastic conditions*
I.V. INFUSION
Adults. 80 mg q 12 hr infused over 2 min or 15 min; adjusted based on patient's acid output measurements up to 80 mg q 8 hr.

| Route | Onset | Peak | Duration |
|-------|-------|------|----------|
| P.O. | 1 day | 1 wk | 1 wk |
| I.V. | 1 day | Unknown | 1 wk |

## Mechanism of Action
Interferes with gastric acid secretion by inhibiting the hydrogen-potassium-adenosine triphosphatase ($H^+$-$K^+$-ATPase) enzyme system, or proton pump, in gastric parietal cells. Normally, the proton pump uses energy from the hydrolysis of ATPase to drive $H^+$ and chloride ($Cl^-$) out of parietal cells and into the stomach lumen in exchange for potassium ($K^+$), which leaves the stomach lumen and enters parietal cells. After this exchange, $H^+$ and $Cl^-$ combine in the stomach to form hydrochloric acid (HCl). Pantoprazole irreversibly inhibits the final step in gastric acid production by blocking the exchange of intracellular $H^+$ and extracellular $K^+$, thus preventing $H^+$ from entering the stomach and additional HCl from forming.

## Incompatibilities
Midazolam and products containing zinc may cause precipitation or discoloration.

## Contraindications
Hypersensitivity to pantoprazole, substituted benzimidazoles (omeprazole, lansoprazole, rabeprazole sodium), or their components

## Interactions
DRUGS
*ampicillin, cyanocobalamin, digoxin, iron salts, ketoconazole:* Possibly impaired absorption of these drugs
*warfarin:* Increased INR, PT, and bleeding risk

## Adverse Reactions

**CNS:** Anxiety, asthenia, confusion, dizziness, headache, hypertonia, hypokinesia, insomnia, malaise, migraine, speech disorder vertigo
**CV:** Chest pain, hypercholesterolemia, hyperlipidemia
**EENT:** Anterior ischemic optic neuropathy, blurred vision, increased salivation, pharyngitis, rhinitis, sinusitis, tinnitus
**ENDO:** Hyperglycemia
**GI:** Abdominal pain, constipation, diarrhea, elevated liver function tests results, flatulence, gastroenteritis, hepatotoxicity, indigestion, nausea, pancreatitis, vomiting
**GU:** Elevated serum creatinine level, interstitial nephritis
**HEME:** Pancytopenia
**MS:** Arthralgia, back or neck pain, rhabdomyolysis
**RESP:** Bronchitis, dyspnea, increased cough, upper respiratory tract infection
**SKIN:** Erythema multiforme, rash, Stevens-Johnson syndrome, toxic epidermal necrolysis
**Other:** Anaphylaxis, angioedema, elevated creatine kinase and phosphokinase levels, flulike symptoms, generalized pain, hyperuricemia, infection, injection site reaction

## Nursing Considerations

• Ensure the continuity of gastric acid suppression during transition from oral to I.V. pantoprazole (or vice versa) because even a brief interruption of effective suppression can lead to serious complications.
• Don't give pantoprazole within 4 weeks of testing for *Helicobacter pylori* because antibiotics, proton pump inhibitors, and bismuth preparations suppress *H. pylori* and may lead to false-negative results. Be aware that drug may cause false-positive results in urine screening tests for tetrahydrocannabinol. Obtain guidelines regarding pantoprazole use from prescriber before testing.
• Flush I.V. line with $D_5W$, NS, or LR injection before and after giving drug.
• When giving I.V. over 2 minutes, reconstitute with 10 ml of NS injection. Solution may be stored up to 2 hours at room temperature.
• When giving I.V. over 15 minutes, reconstitute with 10 ml NS injection. Then, further reconstitute with 100 ml (for GERD) or 80 ml (for pathological hypersecretion in

Zollinger-Ellison syndrome) of $D_5W$, NS injection, or LR injection. Solution may be stored up to 2 hours before further dilution and up to 22 hours before use.
• Monitor PT or INR during therapy, as ordered, if patient takes an oral anticoagulant.
• Be aware that, if drug is given for more than 3 years, patient may not be able to absorb vitamin $B_{12}$ because of hypochlorhydria or achlorhydria. Treatment for cyanocobalamin deficiency may be needed.

**PATIENT TEACHING**
• Instruct patient to swallow pantoprazole tablets whole and not to chew or crush them.
• Advise patient to expect relief of symptoms within 2 weeks of starting therapy.
• Advise patient who takes warfarin to follow bleeding precautions and to notify prescriber immediately if bleeding occurs.

# paricalcitol

Zemplar

## Class and Category

*Chemical:* Sterol derivative, vitamin D analogue
*Therapeutic:* Antihyperparathyroid
*Pregnancy category:* Not rated

## Indications and Dosages

➤ *To prevent and treat secondary hyperparathyroidism in patients with chronic renal failure stage 3 or 4*

**I.V. INJECTION**
**Adults.** *Initial:* 0.04 to 0.1 mcg/kg (2.8 to 7 mcg) no more than q.o.d. at any time during dialysis. *Maintenance:* If initial dosage doesn't produce a satisfactory response, 2 to 4 mcg given q 2 to 4 wk. *Maximum:* 0.24 mcg/kg/dose or up to 16.8 mcg/dose.
**Children age 5 and older.** *Initial:* 0.04 mcg/kg three times weekly if baseline intact parathyroid hormone (iPTH) level is less than 500 pg/ml, or 0.08 mcg/kg three times weekly if baseline iPTH level equals or exceeds 500 pg/ml. *Maintenance:* If initial dosage isn't adequate, adjust in 0.04-mcg/kg increments as needed.
**DOSAGE ADJUSTMENT** If serum PTH level remains the same or increases, dosage is increased. If serum PTH level decreases by less than 30%, dosage is increased. If serum PTH level decreases by 30% to 60%, dosage is

maintained. If serum PTH level decreases by more than 60%, dosage is decreased. If serum PTH level is 1.5 to 3 times the upper limit of normal, dosage is maintained. **DOSAGE ADJUSTMENT** Dosage is immediately reduced or stopped if serum calcium level is elevated or serum calcium-phosphorus product exceeds 75. Dosage restarted at a lower dose when these levels return to normal.

**CAPSULES**

**Adults.** *Initial:* If baseline iPTH level is less than 500 pg/ml, 1 mcg daily or 2 mcg three times weekly, doses separated by at least 1 day. If iPTH level exceeds 500 pg/ml, 2 mcg daily or 4 mcg three times weekly, doses separated by at least 1 day. *Maintenance:* Dosage adjusted in 1-mcg increments based on iPTH level relative to baseline.

| Route | Onset | Peak | Duration |
|-------|-------|------|----------|
| I.V. | Unknown | Unknown | 15 hr |

### Mechanism of Action

Reduces serum PTH level by an unknown mechanism. In chronic renal failure, decreased renal synthesis of vitamin D leads to chronic hypocalcemia. In response, parathyroid glands secrete PTH to stimulate vitamin D synthesis, but serum calcium levels can't normalize because of renal failure.

## Contraindications

Evidence of vitamin D toxicity, hypercalcemia, hypersensitivity to paricalcitol or components

## Interactions

**DRUGS**

*atazanavir, clarithromycin, indinavir, itraconazole, ketoconazole, nefazodone, nelfinavir, ritonavir, saquinavir, telithromycin, voriconazole:* Increased effects of oral paricalcitol
*drugs, such as cholestyramine, that impair absorption of fat-soluble vitamins:* Possibly impaired absorption of oral paricalcitol

## Adverse Reactions

**CNS:** Arthritis, asthenia, chills, depression, dizziness, fever, headache, insomnia, lightheadedness, malaise, neuropathy, syncope, vertigo
**CV:** Cardiomyopathy, chest pain, congestive heart failure, edema, hypertension, hypotension, MI, orthostatic hypotension, palpitations
**EENT:** Amblopia, bronchitis, dry mouth, epistaxis, pharyngitis, retinal abnormality, rhinitis, sinusitis, taste perversion
**ENDO:** Hypoglycemia
**GI:** Abdominal pain, constipation, diarrhea, dyspepsia, gastritis, gastroenteritis, GI bleeding, nausea, vomiting
**GU:** Abnormal kidney function, uremia, UTI
**MS:** Back pain, leg cramps, myalgia
**RESP:** Increased cough, pneumonia
**SKIN:** Ecchymosis, hypertrophy, pruritus, rash (including vesiculobullous), ulceration, urticaria
**Other:** Acidosis, allergic reaction, dehydration, generalized edema, gout, hyperkalemia, hyperphosphatemia, hypervolemia, hypokalemia, infections, influenza, sepsis

## Nursing Considerations

• Before giving drug, look for particles and discoloration; if present, discard drug.
• Give as I.V. bolus; discard unused portion.
• Monitor serum calcium and phosphorus levels, as ordered, twice weekly to guide dosage adjustments and then monthly.
• **WARNING** Paricalcitol may lead to vitamin D toxicity and hypercalcemia. Look for early evidence, including arthralgia, constipation, dry mouth, headache, metallic taste, myalgia, nausea, somnolence, vomiting, and weakness. Also look for late evidence, including albuminuria, anorexia, arrhythmias, azotemia, conjunctivitis (calcific), decreased libido, elevated BUN and serum ALT and AST levels, vascular calcification, hypercholesterolemia, hypertension, hyperthermia, irritability, mild acidosis, nephrocalcinosis, nocturia, pancreatitis, photophobia, polydipsia, polyuria, pruritus, rhinorrhea, and weight loss.
• If toxicity occurs, notify prescriber immediately and expect to decrease or stop drug. Place patient on bed rest and give fluids, low-calcium diet, and a laxative, as prescribed. If patient has a hypercalcemic crisis and dehydration, expect to infuse NS and a loop diuretic to prompt renal calcium excretion.
• Expect to check patient's serum PTH level every 3 months.
• If patient also takes digoxin, monitor her for evidence of digitalis glycoside toxicity, which is potentiated by hypercalcemia.
• Store drug at 25° C (77° F).

P

**PATIENT TEACHING**
• Advise patient to follow a diet high in calcium and low in phosphorus.
• Explain that patient may need phosphate binders to control serum phosphorus level.
• Review the early evidence of hypercalcemia and vitamin D toxicity. Tell patient to contact prescriber immediately if it develops.
• Urge patient to avoid hazardous activities until drug's adverse CNS effects are known.
• If patient takes digoxin, explain evidence of toxicity and the need to contact prescriber immediately if it develops.

# paroxetine hydrochloride

Paxil, Paxil CR

## paroxetine mesylate

## Class and Category
*Chemical:* Phenylpiperidine derivative
*Therapeutic:* Antidepressant, antiobsessional, antipanic
*Pregnancy category:* C

## Indications and Dosages
➤ *To treat major depression*
**C.R. TABLETS**
**Adults.** *Initial:* 25 mg q.d., increased as prescribed and tolerated by 12.5 mg/day q wk. *Maximum:* 62.5 mg/day.
**ORAL SUSPENSION, TABLETS**
**Adults.** *Initial:* 20 mg q.d., increased as prescribed and tolerated by 10 mg/day q wk. *Maximum:* 50 mg/day.
➤ *To treat obsessive-compulsive disorder*
**ORAL SUSPENSION, TABLETS**
**Adults.** *Initial:* 20 mg q.d., increased as prescribed and tolerated by 10 mg/day q wk. *Usual:* 20 to 60 mg q.d. *Maximum:* 60 mg/day.
➤ *To treat panic disorder*
**C.R. TABLETS**
**Adults.** *Initial:* 12.5 mg q.d., increased by 12.5 mg/day q wk as needed. *Maximum:* 75 mg/day.
**ORAL SUSPENSION, TABLETS**
**Adults.** *Initial:* 10 mg q.d., increased as prescribed and tolerated by 10 mg/day q wk. *Usual:* 10 to 60 mg q.d. *Maximum:* 60 mg/day.

➤ *To treat social anxiety disorder*
**C.R. TABLETS**
**Adults.** *Initial:* 12.5 mg q.d., increased by 12.5 mg/day q wk as needed. *Maximum:* 37.5 mg/day.
**ORAL SUSPENSION, TABLETS (HYDROCHLORIDE)**
**Adults.** *Initial:* 20 mg q.d., increased as prescribed and tolerated by 10 mg/day q wk. *Usual:* 20 to 60 mg q.d. *Maximum:* 60 mg/day.
➤ *To treat generalized anxiety disorder*
**ORAL SUSPENSION, TABLETS (HYDROCHLORIDE)**
**Adults.** *Initial:* 20 mg q.d., increased as prescribed and tolerated by 10 mg/day q wk. *Usual:* 20 to 50 mg q.d. *Maximum:* 60 mg/day.
➤ *To treat posttraumatic stress disorder*
**ORAL SUSPENSION, TABLETS (HYDROCHLORIDE)**
**Adults.** *Initial:* 20 mg q.d., increased as prescribed and tolerated by 10 mg/day q wk. *Usual:* 20 to 50 mg q.d. *Maximum:* 50 mg/day.
➤ *To treat premenstrual dysphoric disorder*
**C.R. TABLETS**
**Adults.** *Initial:* 12.5 mg q.d. in the morning, increased as needed after 1 wk to 25 mg q.d. Or 12.5 mg q.d. in the morning only during luteal phase of menstrual cycle (2-wk period before onset of monthly cycle), increased as needed after 1 wk to 25 mg q.d. in the morning during luteal phase of menstrual cycle.
**DOSAGE ADJUSTMENT** For patients who are elderly, debilitated, or have creatinine clearance less than 30 ml/min/1.73 m$^2$, initially 10 mg/ day; maximum, 40 mg/day. Avoid C.R. form. For patients taking C.R. tablets with creatinine clearance less than 30 ml/min/1.73 m$^2$, initially 12.5 mg/day; maximum, 50 mg/day.

| Route | Onset | Peak | Duration |
|-------|-------|------|----------|
| P.O. | 1 to 4 wk | Unknown | Unknown |

## Mechanism of Action
Exerts antidepressant, antiobsessional, and antipanic effects by potentiating serotonin activity in the CNS and inhibiting serotonin reuptake at presynaptic neuronal membrane. Blocked serotonin reuptake increases levels and prolongs activity of serotonin at synaptic receptor sites.

## Contraindications

Hypersensitivity to paroxetine or its components, use within 14 days of an MAO inhibitor, thioridazine therapy

## Interactions

### DRUGS

*antacids:* Hastened release of C.R. paroxetine
*aspirin, NSAIDs, warfarin:* Increased anticoagulant activity and risk of bleeding
*astemizole:* Increased risk of arrhythmias
*atomoxetine, risperidone, other drugs metabolized by CYP2D6:* Increased plasma levels of these drugs
*barbiturates, primidone:* Decreased blood paroxetine level
*cimetidine:* Possibly increased blood paroxetine level
*cisapride, isoniazid, MAO inhibitors, procarbazine:* Possibly serotonin syndrome
*codeine, haloperidol, metoprolol, perphenazine, propranolol, risperidone, thioridazine:* Decreased metabolism and increased effects of these drugs
*cyproheptadine:* Decreased paroxetine effects
*dextromethorphan:* Decreased dextromethorphan metabolism and increased risk of toxicity
*digoxin:* Possibly decreased digoxin effects
*encainide, flecainide, propafenone, quinidine:* Potentiated toxicity of these drugs
*lithium:* Possibly increased blood paroxetine level, increased risk of serotonin syndrome
*methadone:* Decreased methadone metabolism, increased risk of adverse effects
*phenytoin:* Possibly phenytoin toxicity
*procyclidine:* Increased blood procyclidine level and anticholinergic effects
*theophylline:* Possibly increased blood theophylline level and risk of toxicity
*tramadol:* Increased risk of serotonin syndrome and seizures
*tricyclic antidepressants:* Increased metabolism and blood antidepressant levels; increased risk of toxicity, including seizures
*tryptophan:* Increased risk of serotonin syndrome

## Adverse Reactions

**CNS:** Agitation, asthenia, confusion, decreased concentration, dizziness, drowsiness, emotional lability, headache, insomnia, mania, restlessness, somnolence, tremor
**CV:** Palpitations, tachycardia

**EENT:** Blurred vision, dry mouth, rhinitis, taste perversion
**GI:** Abdominal cramps or pain, anorexia, constipation, diarrhea, flatulence, nausea, vomiting
**GU:** Decreased libido, difficult ejaculation, impotence, sexual dysfunction, urine retention
**MS:** Back pain, myalgia, myasthenia, myopathy
**SKIN:** Diaphoresis, rash
**Other:** Weight gain or loss

## Nursing Considerations

- Shake oral suspension well. Measure with an oral syringe or calibrated device.
- Don't give enteric-coated form with antacids.
- If patient is depressed, watch closely for suicidal tendencies, especially when therapy starts or dosage changes.
- Watch for mania, which may result from any antidepressant in a susceptible patient.
- Monitor patient closely for evidence of GI bleeding, especially if patient also takes a drug known to cause GI bleeding, such as aspirin, an NSAID, or warfarin.
- Paroxetine may cause serotonin syndrome.
- To minimize adverse reactions, expect to taper drug rather than stopping abruptly.

### PATIENT TEACHING

- Advise patient to take paroxetine in the morning to minimize insomnia and to take it with food if adverse GI reactions develop.
- Instruct patient to avoid taking C.R. paroxetine within 2 hours of an antacid.
- Tell patient to swallow C.R. tablets whole and not to cut, crush, or chew them.
- Suggest that patient avoid hazardous activities until drug's CNS effects are known.
- Tell family or caregiver to observe patient closely for suicidal tendencies, especially when therapy starts or dosage changes and especially if patient is a child or teenager.
- Explain that full effect may take 4 weeks.
- Urge patient to avoid alcohol during paroxetine therapy; its effects on drug are unknown.
- Tell patient not to take aspirin or NSAIDs during therapy because they increase the risk of bleeding. If patient takes warfarin, tell her to adopt bleeding precautions and to notify prescriber at once if bleeding occurs.
- Inform patient that episodes of acute depression may persist for months or longer and that they require continued follow-up.
- Instruct patient not to stop drug abruptly but to taper dosage as instructed.

P

•Alert female patients of childbearing age that paroxetine may cause birth defects if taken during the first trimester of pregnancy. Stress the need for effective contraception.

# pegfilgrastim

Neulasta

## Class and Category

*Chemical:* Recombinant granulocyte colony-stimulating factor conjugate
*Therapeutic:* Antineutropenic, hematopoietic stimulator
*Pregnancy category:* C

## Indications and Dosages

➤ *To reduce the risk of infection, as manifested by febrile neutropenia, after myelosuppressive chemotherapy*

**S.C. INJECTION**

**Adults.** 6 mg with each chemotherapy cycle.

### Mechanism of Action

Induces formation of neutrophil progenitor cells by binding to receptors on granulocytes, which then divide. Pegfilgrastim also potentiates the effects of mature neutrophils, thus reducing fever and the risk of infection from severe neutropenia. It is pharmacologically identical to human granulocyte colony-stimulating factor.

## Contraindications

Hypersensitivity to filgrastim, pegfilgrastim, or their components or to proteins derived from *Escherichia coli*

## Interactions

**DRUGS**

*lithium:* Increased neutrophil production

## Adverse Reactions

**CNS:** Fever
**GI:** Elevated liver function test results, splenic rupture, splenomegaly
**GU:** Elevated uric acid level
**HEME:** Leukocytosis, sickle cell crisis
**MS:** Bone pain
**RESP:** Dyspnea, hypoxia, pulmonary infiltrates
**SKIN:** Rash, urticaria
**Other:** Anaphylaxis

## Nursing Considerations

•Avoid giving pegfilgrastim for 14 days before and 24 hours after cytotoxic chemotherapy.
•Check CBC, hematocrit, and platelet count before and periodically during therapy.
•Let drug warm to room temperature before injection. Use prefilled syringe and needles.
•Don't shake the solution.
•Discard drug that contains particles, is discolored, or was stored more than 48 hours at room temperature.
•**WARNING** If signs of allergy occur, stop infusion and notify prescriber at once. If anaphylaxis occurs, give antihistamine, epinephrine, corticosteroid, and bronchodilator, as ordered.
•**WARNING** Be aware that patients receiving filgrastim (parent drug) have had splenic rupture and acute respiratory distress syndrome. Watch for fever, respiratory distress, and upper abdominal or shoulder tip pain.
•Assess patients with sickle cell disease for signs of sickle cell crisis; urge hydration.
•Give nonopioid and opioid analgesics, as ordered, if patient experiences bone pain.
•Store drug at 2° to 8° C (36° to 46° F), and protect from freezing and light.

**PATIENT TEACHING**

•Urge patient to immediately report possibly serious reactions, such as trouble breathing, rash, chest tightness, and left upper abdominal or shoulder tip pain. Also tell her to report signs of infection, such as fever or chills.
•If patient will be giving herself the drug, teach her how to prepare, give, and store it.
•Tell patient to rotate injection sites among thigh, stomach (except for 2″ around navel), buttocks, and outer, upper arms. Caution her to avoid tender, hard, red, or bruised areas.
•Urge patient to discard used needles and syringes in a puncture-resistant container and not to reuse them.
•Stress the importance of follow-up tests.
•Advise patient to store drug in refrigerator and not to freeze it. Tell her to discard drug if left unrefrigerated for more than 48 hours.

# pegvisomant

Somavert

## Class and Category

*Chemical:* Human growth hormone (GH) receptor antagonist
*Therapeutic:* Growth suppressant
*Pregnancy category:* B

## Mechanism of Action

In acromegaly, elevated blood levels of GH overstimulate the liver to produce excessive amounts of insulin-like growth factors, such as IGF-1. Excessive IGFs before puberty stimulate the linear growth of bones, causing the patient's unusual height and extremely long arms and legs. After puberty, the excessive hormone secretion causes periosteal bone proliferation, resulting in widening of the hands and feet, and coarsening of the facial features, as well as other complications.

Pegvisomant selectively blocks GH cell surface receptors. As a result, the liver delivers less IGF-1 and other proteins to the blood, preventing the overgrowth of bone and other tissues.

## Indications and Dosages

➤ *To treat acromegaly in patients with an inadequate response to surgery, radiation, or other medical treatment or for whom such treatment is inappropriate*

**S. C. INJECTION**

**Adults.** *Initial:* 40 mg as loading dose on day 1; then 10 mg q.d. *Maintenance:* Adjusted q 4 to 6 wk in 5-mg increments if insulin-like growth factor-I (IGF-I) levels are above or below normal. *Maximum:* 30 mg daily.

## Contraindications

Hypersensitivity to pegvisomant, its components, or latex

## Interactions

**DRUGS**

*Insulin, oral antidiabetics:* Enhanced action of insulin and oral antidiabetics, possibly resulting in hypoglycemia

*Opioids:* Decreased serum pegvisomant levels

## Adverse Reactions

**CNS:** Dizziness, paresthesia

**CV:** Chest pain, hypertension, peripheral edema

**EENT:** Ear infection, sinusitis

**GI:** Diarrhea, elevated liver function test results, nausea

**MS:** Back pain

**RESP:** Upper respiratory tract infection

**SKIN:** Blisters

**Other:** Cold, flulike symptoms, injection site lipohypertrophy and pain, weight gain

## Nursing Considerations

• Obtain liver enzyme levels before starting pegvisomant, as ordered. If they're elevated but 3 times or less normal, expect to monitor them monthly for 6 months, quarterly for 6 months, and then twice yearly for the next year. If they're more than 3 times normal, expect to withhold drug until the cause of elevation has been determined.

• Reconstitute drug by injecting 1 ml of diluent provided (sterile water for injection) into vial, aiming the stream against vial wall. Hold vial between the palms of both hands and roll gently to dissolve the powder.

Don't shake it. Give dose within 6 hours of reconstitution and discard any remaining amount.
• Watch for evidence of liver dysfunction during therapy. If liver enzyme levels rise to 3 to 5 times normal but patient has no evidence of liver dysfunction (jaundice, bilirubinuria, fatigue, nausea, vomiting, right-upper-quadrant pain, ascites, unexplained edema, easy bruising) or increases in serum total bilirubin level, expect therapy to continue but liver enzymes to be monitored weekly and a complete hepatic workup to be done. If enzyme levels are at least 5 times above normal or transaminase level is at least 3 times above normal with increased total bilirubin (with or without evidence of hepatic dysfunction), notify prescriber immediately and expect to stop drug. If patient develops evidence of hepatic dysfunction, regardless of liver enzyme levels, notify prescriber immediately, and expect a complete liver workup to be performed. If liver damage is confirmed, expect drug to be stopped.
• Monitor patient's IGF-1 levels every 4 to 6 weeks, as ordered, until they've normalized and then every 6 months. Notify prescriber if levels are decreased or elevated. Be aware that GH levels should not be used to make dosage adjustments because pegvisomant interferes with laboratory measurement of GH.

**PATIENT TEACHING**
• Teach patient how to reconstitute and administer pegvisomant.
• Tell patient about the need for frequent laboratory studies and their importance to properly adjust drug dosage and detect abnormalities that might relate to drug therapy.
• Advise patient to stop drug immediately and notify prescriber if her skin or whites of her eyes become yellow or she has other evidence of liver dysfunction, such as dark urine, light-colored stools, little or no appetite for several days, nausea, tiredness, or abdominal pain.
• Instruct female patient of childbearing age to notify prescriber about known or suspected pregnancy.
• Caution patient to tell prescriber about all other drugs she's taking.

# penbutolol sulfate

Levatol

## Class and Category

*Chemical:* Nonselective beta-adrenergic blocker
*Therapeutic:* Antihypertensive
*Pregnancy category:* Not rated

## Indications and Dosages

➤ *To manage hypertension*
**TABLETS**
**Adults.** 20 mg q.d.
**DOSAGE ADJUSTMENT** For elderly patients, dosage individualized according to sensitivity to drug.

| Route | Onset | Peak | Duration |
|-------|-------|------|----------|
| P.O. | Unknown | 1.5 to 3 hr | Unknown |

### Mechanism of Action

May reduce blood pressure by competing with beta-adrenergic receptor agonists, which helps reduce cardiac output, decrease sympathetic outflow to peripheral blood vessels, and inhibit renin release by the kidneys.

## Contraindications

Asthma, bradycardia (fewer than 45 beats/min), cardiogenic shock, heart failure, hypersensitivity to penbutolol or its components, second- or third-degree AV block

## Interactions

**DRUGS**
*allergen immunotherapy, allergenic extracts for skin testing:* Increased risk of serious systemic reaction or anaphylaxis
*amiodarone:* Additive depressant effect on cardiac conduction, negative inotropic effects
*anesthetics (hydrocarbon inhalation):* Increased risk of myocardial depression and hypotension
*calcium channel blockers, clonidine, diazoxide, guanabenz, other hypotension-producing drugs, reserpine:* Additive hypotension and possibly other beta blocker effects
*cimetidine:* Possibly increased blood penbutolol level
*estrogens:* Decreased antihypertensive effect of penbutolol
*fentanyl and its derivatives:* Possibly increased risk of initial bradycardia after in-

duction doses of fentanyl derivative (with long-term penbutolol use)

*insulin, oral antidiabetic drugs:* Possibly impaired glucose control and masking of hypoglycemia symptoms such as tachycardia
*lidocaine:* Decreased lidocaine clearance, increased risk of lidocaine toxicity
*MAO inhibitors:* Increased risk of significant hypertension
*neuromuscular blockers:* Possibly potentiated and prolonged action of these drugs
*NSAIDs:* Possibly decreased hypotensive effect of penbutolol
*other beta blockers:* Additive beta blocker effects
*phenothiazines:* Increased blood levels of both drugs
*phenytoin (parenteral):* Additive cardiac depressant effects
*sympathomimetics, xanthines:* Possibly inhibited effects of penbutolol and these drugs

### Adverse Reactions
**CNS:** Anxiety, depression, dizziness, drowsiness, fatigue, insomnia, light-headedness, nervousness, syncope, weakness
**CV:** Bradycardia, chest pain, edema, peripheral vascular insufficiency
**EENT:** Nasal congestion
**GI:** Constipation, diarrhea, epigastric pain, nausea, vomiting
**GU:** Impotence
**RESP:** Bronchospasm, dyspnea

### Nursing Considerations
• Expect varied drug effectiveness in elderly patients, who may be more sensitive to penbutolol's antihypertensive effects because of reduced drug clearance by kidneys.
• WARNING Avoid discontinuing penbutolol therapy abruptly because doing so may precipitate myocardial infarction, myocardial ischemia, severe hypertension, or ventricular arrhythmias, particularly in patients with known cardiovascular disease. Monitor for tachycardia because drug may also mask certain signs of hyperthyroidism. Be aware that abrupt withdrawal of drug in patients with hyperthyroidism or thyrotoxicosis can precipitate thyroid storm.
• Monitor blood pressure and cardiac output, as appropriate, in patients who have a history of systolic heart failure or left ventricu-

lar dysfunction because drug's negative inotropic effect can depress cardiac output.
• Monitor patients with diabetes mellitus who take antidiabetic drugs because penbutolol can prolong hypoglycemia or promote hyperglycemia. Be aware that penbutolol can also mask signs of hypoglycemia, especially tachycardia, palpitations, and tremor.
• Monitor for impaired circulation in elderly patients with age-related peripheral vascular disease or patients with Raynaud's phenomenon. Keep in mind that elderly patients are also at increased risk for beta blocker–induced hypothermia.
• Monitor drug refill frequency to help determine patient compliance.
**PATIENT TEACHING**
• Instruct patient to take penbutolol at the same time every day and not to change dosage without consulting prescriber.
• Advise patient not to stop taking drug abruptly, but to taper dosage gradually under prescriber's supervision.
• Instruct patient with diabetes mellitus to regularly monitor blood glucose level and test urine for ketones.
• Advise patient to consult prescriber before taking over-the-counter drugs, especially cold remedies.
• Urge patient to avoid potentially hazardous activities until drug's CNS effects are known.
• Instruct patient to inform prescriber of chest pain, fainting, light-headedness, or shortness of breath, any of which may indicate the need for a dosage change.
• Inform patient that penbutolol doesn't cure hypertension. Encourage her to follow recommended diet and lifestyle changes.

# penicillamine
Cuprimine, Depen

### Class and Category
*Chemical:* Degradation product of penicillin
*Therapeutic:* Antirheumatic, antiurolithic, chelating agent
*Pregnancy category:* D

### Indications and Dosages
➤ *To treat cystinuria*
**CAPSULES, TABLETS**
**Adults and adolescents.** 500 mg q.i.d.
**Children.** 7.5 mg/kg q.i.d.

➤ *To treat rheumatoid arthritis*
**CAPSULES, TABLETS**
**Adults and adolescents.** *Initial:* 125 or
250 mg q.d. Dosage increased by 125 or
250 mg/day q 2 to 3 mo. *Maximum:*
1,500 mg/day.

➤ *To treat Wilson's disease*
**CAPSULES, TABLETS**
**Adults and adolescents.** Dosage individualized up to 2 g/day in divided doses q.i.d. by
measuring urinary copper excretion.
**DOSAGE ADJUSTMENT** For elderly patients,
125 mg q.d. initially, then increased by
125 mg/day q 2 to 3 mo, up to maximum of
750 mg/day; for pregnant women, maximum
dose of 1 g/day; for women undergoing
planned cesarean section, dosage limited to
250 mg/day during last 6 wk of pregnancy
and until wound healing completed.

| Route | Onset | Peak | Duration |
|-------|-------|------|----------|
| P.O. | 2 to 3 mo* | Unknown | Unknown |

## Mechanism of Action
Combines with copper to form a ring-
shaped complex that is excreted in urine,
thereby reducing copper levels in the
body. Penicillamine also lowers urine cystine levels by binding with cystine to
form penicillamine-cysteine disulfide,
which is more soluble than cystine and
more easily excreted in urine. The decrease in urine cystine levels also helps
prevent the formation of cystine calculi
and may help existing cystine calculi dissolve over time. In addition, penicillamine
improves lymphocyte function by reducing IgM rheumatoid factor and immune
complexes in serum and synovial fluid,
which may play a role in the treatment of
rheumatoid arthritis.

## Contraindications
Hypersensitivity to penicillin, penicillamine,
or their components; penicillamine-related
aplastic anemia or agranulocytosis; renal insufficiency (for patients with rheumatoid
arthritis)

---

* For rheumatoid arthritis; 1 to 3 mo for
  Wilson's disease.

## Interactions
**DRUGS**
*4-aminoquinolines, bone marrow depressants,
gold compounds, immunosuppressants (excluding glucocorticoids), phenylbutazone:*
Possibly increased risk of serious hematologic or renal adverse reactions
*iron supplements:* Possibly decreased effectiveness of penicillamine
*pyridoxine:* Decreased effectiveness of pyridoxine, possibly increased risk of anemia or
peripheral neuritis reaction

## Adverse Reactions
**CNS:** Agitation, anxiety, fever, mental
changes, myasthenic syndrome, neuropathy
**EENT:** Altered or loss of taste, optic neuritis,
stomatitis, tinnitus
**GI:** Anorexia, diarrhea, hepatic dysfunction,
intrahepatic cholestasis, mild epigastric pain,
pancreatitis, nausea, toxic hepatitis, vomiting
**GU:** Glomerulonephropathy, hematuria, proteinuria, renal failure
**HEME:** Agranulocytosis, aplastic anemia,
hemolytic anemia, leukopenia, thrombocytopenia
**MS:** Arthralgia, dystonia, muscle weakness
**SKIN:** Pemphigus, pruritus, rash, urticaria
**Other:** Lupuslike symptoms, lymphadenopathy

## Nursing Considerations
•Use penicillamine cautiously in elderly patients because they're at greater risk for
rash, altered taste, and renal impairment.
•Administer penicillamine 1 hour before or
2 hours after meals and at least 1 hour before or after any other drug, food, or milk.
Give last dose of day at least 3 hours after
evening meal to ensure maximum absorption.
•For patient who has difficulty swallowing
capsules or tablets, open capsule and mix
contents in 15 to 30 ml of pureed fruit or
fruit juice to mask drug's sulfur odor. Alternatively, request pharmacist to prepare an
elixir for oral administration.
•Expect to administer 25 mg of pyridoxine,
as prescribed, to patients being treated with
penicillamine because penicillamine increases intake requirements for this vitamin.
•Monitor for febrile reactions in patients
who developed a fever during previous penicillamine administration. Expect drug to be

discontinued if patient develops drug-induced fever.

• Assess skin and mucous membranes for possible sensitivity reactions, such as skin lesions and mouth ulcers. Be prepared to discontinue drug as prescribed.

• Expect to monitor urine laboratory test results, as ordered, twice weekly during the first month of therapy, then every 2 weeks for the next 5 months, and monthly thereafter. Watch for proteinuria or hematuria, which may precipitate nephrotic syndrome, especially in patients with renal disease or history of renal insufficiency. Also, weigh patient daily, observe for signs of edema, and monitor intake and output because penicillamine may worsen underlying renal disease.

• **WARNING** Monitor patient's WBC and differential cell count, hemoglobin, and platelet count, as ordered, and assess patient's skin, lymph nodes, and body temperature for abnormalities twice weekly during first month of therapy, then every 2 weeks for the next 5 months, and monthly thereafter because drug may cause potentially serious hematologic reactions.

• Because of the potential for cross-sensitivity between penicillamine and penicillin, monitor for symptoms of an allergic reaction in patients with a history of penicillin allergy.

• Notify prescriber if patient complains of decreased sense of taste, especially for salty and sweet foods. Expect normal taste sensation to be restored (except in patients with Wilson's disease) with administration of 5 to 10 mg of copper a day, as prescribed.

• Monitor patients with diabetes mellitus for reduced insulin requirements to prevent the risk of nighttime hypoglycemia because penicillamine may promote the formation of anti-insulin antibodies.

• Monitor results of patient's liver function studies, as ordered, every 6 months (every 3 months for first year if patient has Wilson's disease) throughout penacillamine therapy because drug may cause serious hepatic dysfunction.

**PATIENT TEACHING**

• Advise patient to take penicillamine on an empty stomach.

• Instruct adult male and nonpregnant female patients with cystinuria to increase their fluid intake and follow the prescribed low-methionine diet to minimize cystine production and

enhance drug's effectiveness. Encourage patient to drink about 1 pint of fluid at bedtime and again during the night because this is when urine is more concentrated.

• Tell patient to notify prescriber immediately if he develops a fever, sore throat, chills, bruising, or bleeding because drug may need to be stopped.

• Instruct patient being treated for Wilson's disease to follow a diet low in copper, avoiding such foods as broccoli, chocolate, copper-enriched cereals, liver, molasses, mushrooms, nuts, and shellfish. Inform her that improvement in her condition may require 1 to 3 months of therapy.

• Advise patient to consult prescriber before having dental work done during penicillamine therapy because drug can promote mouth ulcers.

• Instruct patient to avoid consuming iron during penicillamine therapy because iron can decrease drug's effectiveness.

• Inform patient that her sense of taste may decrease during penicillamine therapy. Advise her to notify prescriber if decreased taste becomes intolerable.

• Inform patient with rheumatoid arthritis that improvement in condition may require 2 to 3 months of therapy.

• Caution female patient to notify prescriber immediately if she becomes or may be pregnant because dosage may need to be reduced to prevent serious birth defects.

# penicillin G benzathine

Bicillin C-R, Bicillin C-R 900/300, Bicillin L-A, Megacillin (CAN), Permapen

## penicillin G potassium

Megacillin (CAN), Pentids, Pfizerpen

## penicillin G procaine

Ayercillin (CAN), Crysticillin 300 AS, Pfizerpen-AS, Wycillin

## penicillin G sodium

## penicillin V potassium

Apo-Pen-VK (CAN), Beepen-VK, Betapen-VK, Ledercillin VK, Nadopen-V 200 (CAN), Nadopen-V 400 (CAN), Novo-Pen-VK (CAN), Nu-Pen VK (CAN), Pen Vee (CAN), Pen Vee K, V-Cillin K (CAN), Veetids

**P**

## Class and Category
*Chemical:* Penicillin
*Therapeutic:* Antibiotic
*Pregnancy category:* B

## Indications and Dosages
➤ *To treat systemic infections caused by gram-positive organisms (including* Bacillus anthracis, Corynebacterium diphtheriae, *enterococci,* Listeria monocytogenes, Staphylococcus aureus, *and* S. epidermidis), *gram-negative organisms (including* Neisseria gonorrhoeae, N. meningitidis, Pasteurella multocida, *and* Streptobacillus moniliformis *[rat-bite fever]), and gram-positive anaerobes (including* Actinomyces israelii *[actinomycosis],* Clostridium perfringens, C. tetani, Peptococcus *sp.,* Peptostreptococcus *sp., and spirochetes, especially* Treponema carateum *[pinta],* T. pallidum, *and* T. pertenue *[yaws]*)

ORAL SOLUTION, TABLETS (PENICILLIN G POTASSIUM)
**Adults and adolescents.** 200,000 to 500,000 U (125 to 312 mg) q 4 to 6 hr. *Maximum:* 2 million U/day.
**Children.** 4,167 to 15,000 U/kg q 4 hr, 6,250 to 22,500 U/kg q 6 hr, or 8,333 to 30,000 U/kg q 8 hr.

TABLETS (PENICILLIN V POTASSIUM)
**Adults and adolescents.** 200,000 to 800,000 U (125 to 500 mg) q 6 to 8 hr. *Maximum:* 11,520,000 U (7,200 mg)/day
**Children.** 4,167 to 13,280 U (2.5 to 8.3 mg)/kg q 4 hr, 6,250 to 20,000 U (3.75 to 12.5 mg)/kg q 6 hr, or 8,333 to 26,720 U (5 to 16.7 mg)/kg q 8 hr.

I.V. INFUSION, I.M. INJECTION (PENICILLIN G POTASSIUM, PENICILLIN G SODIUM)
**Adults and adolescents.** 1 to 5 million U q 4 to 6 hr. *Maximum:* 80 million U/day.
**Children.** 8,333 to 16,667 U/kg q 4 hr or 12,500 to 25,000 U/kg q 6 hr.
**Premature and full-term neonates.** 30,000 U/kg q 12 hr.

I.M. INJECTION (PENICILLIN G PROCAINE)
**Adults and adolescents.** 600,000 to 1,200,000 U/day in divided doses q 12 to 24 hr.
➤ *To treat moderately severe to severe streptococcal infections*
I.M. INJECTION (PENICILLIN G BENZATHINE)
**Adults and children weighing more than 45 kg (100 lb).** 1.2 million U as a single injection.

**Children weighing 27 to 45 kg (59 to 100 lb).** 900,000 U as a single injection.
**Children weighing less than 27 kg.** 300,000 to 600,000 U as a single injection.
➤ *To treat congenital syphilis*
I.M. INJECTION (PENICILLIN G BENZATHINE: BICILLIN L-A ONLY)
**Children under age 2.** 50,000 U/kg as a single injection.
➤ *To treat syphilis of less than 1 year's duration*
I.M. INJECTION (PENICILLIN G BENZATHINE: BICILLIN L-A ONLY)
**Adults and adolescents.** 2.4 million U as a single injection.
**Children.** 50,000 U/kg up to adult dosage as a single injection. *Maximum:* 2.4 million U/dose.
➤ *To treat syphilis of more than 1 year's duration*
I.M. INJECTION (PENICILLIN G BENZATHINE: BICILLIN L-A ONLY)
**Adults and adolescents.** 2.4 million U q wk for 3 wk.
**Children.** 50,000 U/kg q wk for 3 wk.
➤ *To treat bacterial meningitis*
I.V. INFUSION, I.M. INJECTION (PENICILLIN G POTASSIUM)
**Adults.** 50,000 U/kg q 4 hr or 24 million U/day in divided doses q 2 to 4 hr.

---

### Mechanism of Action
Inhibits the final stage of bacterial cell wall synthesis by competitively binding to penicillin-binding proteins inside the cell wall. Penicillin-binding proteins are responsible for various steps in bacterial cell wall synthesis. By binding to these proteins, penicillin leads to cell wall lysis.

---

## Contraindications
Hypersensitivity to penicillin or its components

## Incompatibilities
Don't mix any penicillin in the same syringe or container with aminoglycosides because aminoglycosides will be inactivated. Don't mix penicillin G with drugs that may result in a pH below 5.5 or above 8.

## Interactions
DRUGS
*ACE inhibitors, potassium-containing drugs, potassium-sparing diuretics:* In-

creased risk of hyperkalemia (penicillin G potassium)

*chloramphenicol, erythromycin, sulfonamides, tetracycline, thrombolytics:* Possibly interference with penicillin's bactericidal effect

*cholestyramine, colestipol:* Possibly impaired absorption of oral penicillin G

*methotrexate:* Decreased methotrexate clearance, increased risk of toxicity

*oral contraceptives:* Decreased contraceptive effectiveness (with penicillin V)

*probenecid:* Increased blood penicillin level

**FOODS**

*acidic beverages, such as fruit juices:* Possibly altered effects of oral penicillin G

## Adverse Reactions

**CNS:** Confusion, dizziness, dysphasia, hallucinations, headache, lethargy, sciatic nerve irritation, seizures

**CV:** Labile blood pressure, palpitations

**EENT:** Black "hairy" tongue, oral candidiasis, stomatitis, taste perversion

**GI:** Abdominal pain, diarrhea, elevated liver function test results (transient), indigestion, nausea, pseudomembranous colitis

**GU:** Interstitial nephritis (acute), vaginal candidiasis

**MS:** Muscle twitching

**SKIN:** Rash

**Other:** Electrolyte imbalances; injection site necrosis, pain, or redness

## Nursing Considerations

•Obtain body tissue and fluid samples for culture and sensitivity tests as ordered before giving first dose. Expect to begin drug therapy before test results are known.

•Reconstitute vials of penicillin for injection with sterile water for injection, $D_5W$, or sodium chloride for injection.

•Administer penicillin at least 1 hour before other antibiotics.

•Inject I.M. form deep into large muscle mass. Apply ice to relieve pain.

•**WARNING** Give penicillin G benzathine and penicillin G procaine only by deep I.M. injection; I.V. injection may be fatal, and intraarterial injection may cause extensive tissue and organ necrosis.

•Be aware that I.M. drug is absorbed slowly, which may make allergic reactions difficult to treat.

•Assess patient for signs of secondary infection, such as profuse, watery diarrhea.

•Monitor serum sodium level and assess for early signs of heart failure in patients receiving high doses of penicillin G sodium.

•When giving penicillin G potassium to patient at risk for hypertension or fluid overload, be aware that each gram of pencillin G potassium also contains 1.02 mEq of sodium.

**PATIENT TEACHING**

•Instruct patient to report previous allergies to penicillins and to notify prescriber immediately about adverse reactions, including fever.

•Advise patient who uses oral contraceptives to use an additional form of contraception during penicillin V therapy.

# pentamidine isethionate

NebuPent, Pentacarinat (CAN), Pentam 300, Pneumopent (CAN)

## Class and Category

*Chemical:* Diamidine derivative

*Therapeutic:* Antiprotozoal

*Pregnancy category:* C

## Indications and Dosages

➤ *To prevent* Pneumocystis carinii *pneumonia*

**ORAL INHALATION (NEBUPENT, PENTACARINAT)**

**Adults and adolescents.** 300 mg q 4 wk or 150 mg q 2 wk, using nebulizer and continuing until nebulizer chamber is empty (30 to 45 min).

**ORAL INHALATION (PNEUMOPENT)**

**Adults and adolescents.** *Initial:* 60 mg q 24 to 72 hr for 5 doses over 2 wk, using ultrasonic nebulizer and continuing until nebulizer chamber is empty (about 15 min). *Maintenance:* 60 mg q 2 wk, using ultrasonic nebulizer and continuing until nebulizer chamber is empty.

➤ *To treat* P. carinii *pneumonia*

**I.V. INFUSION, I.M. INJECTION**

**Adults and children.** 4 mg/kg q.d. for 14 to 21 days, given deep I.M. or by I.V. infusion over 1 to 2 hr.

**DOSAGE ADJUSTMENT** Dosage possibly reduced or I.V. infusion time or dosing interval extended for patients with renal failure.

## Incompatibilities

Don't mix pentamidine with other drugs or with saline solutions because precipitation may occur.

## Contraindications

History of anaphylactic reaction to pentamidine or its components (inhalation form)

**P**

## Mechanism of Action
May bind to DNA and inhibit DNA replication in *Pneumocystis carinii*. Pentamidine also may inhibit dihydrofolate reductase, an enzyme needed to convert dihydrofolic acid to tetrahydrofolic acid in this organism. This action inhibits the formation of coenzymes that are essential to the growth and replication of *P. carinii*.

## Interactions
**DRUGS**
*bone marrow depressants, drugs that cause blood dyscrasias:* Increased risk of adverse hematologic effects
*didanosine:* Increased risk of pancreatitis
*erythromycin (I.V.):* Increased risk of torsades de pointes
*foscarnet:* Increased risk of severe but reversible hypocalcemia, hypomagnesemia, and nephrotoxicity
*nephrotoxic drugs:* Increased risk of nephrotoxicity

## Adverse Reactions
**CNS:** Chills, confusion, dizziness, fatigue, fever, hallucinations, headache (I.V., I.M. forms)
**CV:** Arrhythmias, edema, hypotension, prolonged QT interval, torsades de pointes, ventricular tachycardia (I.V., I.M. forms)
**EENT:** Bitter or metallic taste (all forms), pharyngitis (inhalation form)
**ENDO:** Diabetes mellitus, hyperglycemia (I.V., I.M. forms); hypoglycemia (all forms)
**GI:** Abdominal pain, anorexia, diarrhea, elevated liver function test results, nausea, vomiting (I.V., I.M. forms); pancreatitis (all forms)
**GU:** Elevated serum creatinine level (I.V., I.M. forms); renal insufficiency (inhalation form)
**HEME:** Anemia, leukopenia, thrombocytopenia, unusual bleeding or bruising (I.V., I.M. forms)
**MS:** Myalgia (I.V., I.M. forms)
**RESP:** Bronchospasm, chest pain or congestion, cough, dyspnea, extrapulmonary pneumocystosis, pneumothorax (inhalation form)
**SKIN:** Night sweats (I.V., I.M. forms); rash (all forms)
**Other:** Hyperchloremic acidosis; hyperkalemia; hypocalcemia; hypomagnesemia; infusion site sterile abscess (I.V. form); injection site induration, pain, and phlebitis (I.M. form)

## Nursing Considerations
• Store pentamidine at room temperature, protected from light. Use within 24 hours after reconstitution.
• For I.V. use, dissolve contents of 300-mg vial with 3 to 5 ml of sterile water for injection or $D_5W$. Further dilute in 50 to 250 ml of $D_5W$ and infuse over 1 to 2 hours.
• For I.M. use, dissolve contents of vial in 3 ml of sterile water for injection and inject deep into large muscle mass. Be aware that I.M. administration increases the risk of sterile abscess formation at injection site.
• When giving drug I.V. or I.M., keep patient supine and monitor blood pressure frequently during and after administration. Keep emergency resuscitation equipment readily available.
• Assess for hypoglycemia and arrhythmias in patient receiving I.V. or I.M. pentamidine. Although uncommon, these adverse reactions can be severe.
• For inhalation, reconstitute contents of vial with 6 ml of sterile water for injection (if using NebuPent or Pentacarinat) or 3 to 5 ml of sterile water for injection or inhalation (if using Pneumopent). Reconstitute immediately before use. Don't use NS because it causes precipitation. Place reconstituted drug into Respirgard II nebulizer, and set flow rate at 5 to 7 L/min for use with NebuPent or Pentacarinat. Don't mix with any other drugs. For Pneumopent administration, place reconstituted drug in Fisoneb ultrasonic nebulizer and set flow rate at the mid-flow mark.
• Administer aerosolized pentamidine with patient in supine or recumbent position for best distribution of drug.
• If patient who uses inhalation form has a history of asthma or smoking, notify prescriber if bronchospasm or a cough develops. She may need an aerosolized bronchodilator before each dose of pentamidine.
• Monitor CBC; platelet count; liver function test results; BUN, serum creatinine and calcium, and blood glucose levels; and ECG tracing throughout therapy, as ordered.
• Monitor blood glucose level because pentamidine use can induce insulin release from pancreas, causing severe hypoglycemia that can last from 1 day to several weeks.

• Be aware that hyperglycemia and diabetes mellitus can occur up to several months after discontinuation of parenteral therapy.

**PATIENT TEACHING**
• Stress importance of complying with the prescribed administration schedule when pentamidine is used to prevent *P. carinii* pneumonia.
• Advise patient to avoid potentially hazardous activities until drug's CNS effects are known.
• Instruct patient to notify prescriber about unusual bleeding or bruising and to take precautions to avoid bleeding, such as using a soft-bristled toothbrush and an electric shaver.
• Caution patient about possible hypoglycemic effects of pentamidine therapy.
• Advise patient to have follow-up laboratory studies to test for diabetes mellitus, which can occur up to several months after stopping pentamidine therapy.

# pentazocine lactate

Talwin

## pentazocine hydrochloride and naloxone hydrochloride

Talwin-Nx

## Class, Category, and Schedule

*Chemical:* Synthetic opioid
*Therapeutic:* Analgesic
*Pregnancy category:* C
*Controlled substance:* Schedule IV

## Indications and Dosages

➤ *To relieve moderate to severe pain*
**I.V., I.M., OR S.C. INJECTION**
**Adults.** *Initial:* 30 mg q 3 to 4 hr, p.r.n. *Maximum:* 30 mg/single dose I.V., 60 mg/single dose I.M. or S.C., or 360 mg/24 hr for all parenteral forms.
➤ *To relieve obstetric pain*
**I.V. INJECTION**
**Adults.** 20 mg when contractions become regular; repeated 2 or 3 times q 2 to 3 hr, as prescribed.
**I.M. INJECTION**
**Adults.** 30 mg as a single dose.

| Route | Onset | Peak | Duration |
|---|---|---|---|
| I.V. | 2 to 3 min | 15 to 30 min | 2 to 3 hr |
| I.M., S.C. | 15 to 20 min | 30 to 60 min | 2 to 3 hr |

## Mechanism of Action

Binds with opioid receptors, primarily kappa and sigma receptors, at many CNS sites to alter the perception of and emotional response to pain.

## Incompatibilities

Don't mix pentazocine in same syringe with a soluble barbiturate because precipitation will occur.

## Contraindications

Hypersensitivity to pentazocine or its components

## Interactions

**DRUGS**
*anticholinergics:* Increased risk of urine retention and severe constipation
*antidiarrheals, antiperistaltics:* Increased risk of severe constipation and CNS depression
*antihypertensives, diuretics, other hypotension-producing drugs:* Additive hypotensive effects
*buprenorphine:* Decreased pentazocine effectiveness, increased respiratory depression
*CNS depressants:* Increased CNS depression, increased risk of habituation
*hydroxyzine, other opioid analgesics:* Increased analgesia, CNS depression, and hypotensive effects
*MAO inhibitors:* Increased risk of unpredictable, severe, and sometimes fatal adverse reactions
*metoclopramide:* Antagonized metoclopramide effects on GI motility
*naloxone:* Antagonized analgesic, CNS, and respiratory depressant effects of pentazocine
*naltrexone:* Withdrawal symptoms in patients physically dependent on pentazocine
*neuromuscular blockers:* Increased respiratory depression
**ACTIVITIES**
*alcohol use:* Additive CNS depression and increased risk of habituation

## Adverse Reactions

**CNS:** Chills, dizziness, drowsiness, euphoria, fatigue, headache, insomnia, light-headedness, nervousness, nightmares, paresthesia, restlessness, weakness
**CV:** Hypotension, tachycardia
**EENT:** Blurred vision, diplopia, dry mouth, laryngeal edema, laryngospasm

P

**GI:** Constipation, hepatotoxicity, nausea, vomiting
**GU:** Decreased urine output, dysuria, urinary frequency, urine retention
**MS:** Muscle rigidity (with large doses)
**RESP:** Atelectasis, bronchospasm, dyspnea, hypoventilation, wheezing
**SKIN:** Diaphoresis, erythema multiforme, facial flushing, pruritus, rash, Stevens-Johnson syndrome, toxic epidermal necrolysis, urticaria
**Other:** Facial edema; injection site burning, pain, redness, or swelling; physical and psychological dependence

## Nursing Considerations
• Use pentazocine with extreme caution in patients who have head injury, intracranial lesion, or increased intracranial pressure because drug may mask neurologic signs and symptoms.
• Use drug cautiously in patients who are physically dependent on opioid agonists because drug may prompt withdrawal symptoms; in patients with acute MI because drug's cardiovascular effects can increase cardiac workload; in patients with renal or hepatic dysfunction because drug is metabolized in the liver and excreted in urine; and in patients with respiratory conditions because drug depresses the respiratory system.
• When giving repeated parenteral doses, use I.M. or I.V. route when possible and as prescribed because S.C. route may cause severe tissue damage at injection site. Rotate I.M. sites to avoid tissue damage.
• After giving parenteral form, expect to taper dosage gradually, as prescribed, to reduce the risk of withdrawal symptoms.
**PATIENT TEACHING**
• Caution patient that prolonged use of pentazocine may result in drug dependence.
• Advise patient to avoid potentially hazardous activities until drug's CNS effects are known.
• Caution patient not to use alcohol or OTC drugs without consulting prescriber.
• Advise patient to notify prescriber if she notices signs of an allergic reaction, such as a rash or itching.

# pentobarbital sodium
Nembutal, Nova Rectal (CAN), Novopentobarb (CAN)

## Class, Category, and Schedule
*Chemical:* Barbiturate
*Therapeutic:* Anticonvulsant, sedative-hypnotic
*Pregnancy category:* D
*Controlled substance:* Schedule II (oral, parenteral), III (rectal)

## Indications and Dosages
➤ *To provide daytime sedation*
**ELIXIR**
**Adults.** 20 mg t.i.d. or q.i.d.
**Children.** 2 to 6 mg/kg q.d.
**SUPPOSITORIES**
**Adults.** 30 mg b.i.d. to q.i.d.
**Children.** 2 mg/kg t.i.d.
➤ *To provide short-term treatment of insomnia*
**CAPSULES, ELIXIR**
**Adults.** 100 mg h.s.
**I.V. INJECTION**
**Adults.** *Initial:* 100 mg, with additional small doses at 1-min intervals, as prescribed. *Maximum:* 500 mg.
**I.M. INJECTION**
**Adults.** 150 to 200 mg h.s.
**SUPPOSITORIES**
**Adults and adolescents over age 14.** 120 to 200 mg h.s.
**Children ages 12 to 14.** 60 to 120 mg h.s.
**Children ages 5 to 12.** 60 mg h.s.
**Children ages 1 to 4.** 30 to 60 mg h.s.
**Infants ages 2 months to 1 year.** 30 mg h.s.
➤ *To provide preoperative sedation*
**CAPSULES, ELIXIR**
**Adults.** 100 mg before surgery.
**Children.** 2 to 6 mg/kg before surgery. *Maximum:* 100 mg/dose.
**I.M. INJECTION**
**Adults.** 150 to 200 mg before surgery.
**Children.** 2 to 6 mg/kg before surgery. *Maximum:* 100 mg/dose.
**SUPPOSITORIES**
**Children ages 12 to 14.** 60 to 120 mg before surgery.
**Children ages 5 to 12.** 60 mg before surgery.
**Children ages 1 to 4.** 30 to 60 mg before surgery.
**Infants ages 2 months to 1 year.** 30 mg before surgery.
➤ *To provide emergency treatment of seizures associated with eclampsia, meningitis, status epilepticus, tetanus, or toxic*

*reactions to local anesthetics or strych-nine*

**I.V. INJECTION**
**Adults.** 100 mg, with additional small doses at 1-min intervals, as prescribed. *Maximum:* 500 mg.
**Children.** 50 mg, with additional small doses at 1-min intervals, as prescribed, until desired effect occurs.

**I.M. INJECTION**
**Children.** 50 mg, with additional small doses at 1-min intervals, as prescribed, until desired effect occurs.

DOSAGE ADJUSTMENT Dosage possibly reduced for elderly or debilitated patients and those with hepatic dysfunction.

| Route | Onset | Peak | Duration |
|---|---|---|---|
| P.O., P.R. | 15 to 60 min | 1 to 4 hr | 3 to 4 hr |
| I.V. | In 1 min | Unknown | 15 min |
| I.M. | 10 to 25 min | Unknown | 3 to 4 hr |

## Mechanism of Action
Inhibits ascending conduction in the reticular formation, which controls CNS arousal to produce drowsiness, hypnosis, and sedation. Pentobarbital also decreases the spread of seizure activity in the cortex, thalamus, and limbic system. It promotes an increased threshold for electrical stimulation in the motor cortex, which may contribute to its anticonvulsant properties.

## Contraindications
Hepatic disease; history of addiction to hypnotics or sedatives; hypersensitivity to pentobarbital, barbiturates, or their components; nephritis; porphyria; severe respiratory disease with airway obstruction or dyspnea

## Interactions
**DRUGS**
*acetaminophen:* Possibly decreased effects of acetaminophen (with long-term pentobarbital use)
*carbamazepine, chloramphenicol, corticosteroids, cyclosporine, dacarbazine, digoxin, disopyramide, doxycycline, griseofulvin, metronidazole, oral contraceptives, phenyl-butazone, quinidine, theophyllines, vitamin D:* Decreased effectiveness of these drugs
*CNS depressants:* Increased CNS depression and risk of habituation
*divalproex sodium, valproic acid:* Increased risk of CNS toxicity and neurotoxicity
*guanadrel, guanethidine:* Possibly increased risk of orthostatic hypotension
*halogenated hydrocarbon anesthetic:* Increased risk of hepatotoxicity (with long-term pentobarbital use)
*haloperidol:* Possibly decreased blood haloperidol level, possibly altered seizure pattern or frequency
*hydantoins:* Possibly interference with hydantoin metabolism
*leucovorin:* Possibly decreased anticonvulsant effect of pentobarbital
*maprotiline:* Possibly enhanced CNS depression and decreased therapeutic effects of pentobarbital
*mexiletine:* Possibly decreased blood mexiletine level
*oral anticoagulants:* Possibly decreased therapeutic effects of these drugs, possibly increased risk of bleeding when pentobarbital is discontinued
*tricyclic antidepressants:* Possibly decreased therapeutic effects of these drugs
**ACTIVITIES**
*alcohol use:* Increased CNS depression

## Adverse Reactions
**CNS:** Agitation, anxiety, ataxia, confusion, delusions, depression, dizziness, drowsiness, fever, hallucinations, headache, insomnia, irritability, nervousness, nightmares, paradoxical stimulation, seizures, syncope, tremor
**CV:** Orthostatic hypotension
**EENT:** Vision changes
**GI:** Anorexia, constipation, hepatic dysfunction, nausea, vomiting
**HEME:** Agranulocytosis
**MS:** Arthralgia, bone pain, muscle twitching or weakness
**RESP:** Respiratory depression
**SKIN:** Exfoliative dermatitis, rash, Stevens-Johnson syndrome
**Other:** Physical and psychological dependence, weight loss

## Nursing Considerations
•Use pentobarbital with extreme caution in patients with depression, a history of drug abuse, or suicidal tendencies.

P

•Use drug cautiously in elderly or debilitated patients and those with acute or chronic pain because it may induce paradoxical stimulation.
•When using I.V. route, inject drug at 50 mg/min or less to avoid adverse respiratory and circulatory reactions.
•If patient shows premonitory signs of hepatic coma, withhold drug and notify prescriber immediately.
•Monitor I.V. site closely and be careful to avoid extravasation. Drug is highly alkaline and may cause local tissue damage and necrosis.

**PATIENT TEACHING**
•Inform patient that pentobarbital is habit-forming, and stress the importance of taking it exactly as prescribed.
•Instruct patient who takes elixir form to use a calibrated measuring device and to close container tightly after use.
•Instruct patient who uses suppositories to refrigerate them.
•Advise patient to avoid potentially hazardous activities until drug's CNS effects are known.
•Urge patient to avoid alcohol and other CNS depressants because they may increase drug's adverse CNS effects.

# pentosan polysulfate sodium

Elmiron

## Class and Category
*Chemical:* Low-molecular-weight heparin-like compound
*Therapeutic:* Local anti-inflammatory (bladder-specific)
*Pregnancy category:* B

## Indications and Dosages
➤ *To relieve bladder discomfort or pain caused by interstitial cystitis*
**CAPSULES**
**Adults.** 100 mg t.i.d. for up to 3 mo, possibly followed by another 3 mo if no improvement and no adverse reactions occur.

### Mechanism of Action
Adheres to the mucosal membrane of the bladder wall and may block irritating solutes from reaching the cells, thereby decreasing local pain and discomfort.

## Contraindications
Hypersensitivity to pentosan, other structurally related compounds, or their components

## Interactions
**DRUGS**
*alteplase (recombinant), aspirin (high doses), heparin, oral anticoagulants, streptokinase:* Increased risk of hemorrhage

## Adverse Reactions
**CNS:** Depression, dizziness, emotional lability, headache
**GI:** Abdominal pain, diarrhea, hepatic dysfunction, indigestion, nausea, rectal hemorrhage
**HEME:** Unusual bleeding or bruising
**SKIN:** Alopecia, rash

## Nursing Considerations
•Use pentosan with extreme caution in patients with conditions that increase the risk of bleeding, such as aneurysm, diverticula, GI ulceration, hemophilia, polyps, and thrombocytopenia (especially heparin-induced).
•Use drug cautiously in patients with hepatic dysfunction because drug is desulfated in the liver and spleen.
•Monitor for abnormal bleeding, such as unexplained bruises and epistaxis, because drug is a weak anticoagulant.

**PATIENT TEACHING**
•Instruct patient to take pentosan with a full glass of water at least 1 hour before or 2 hours after meals.
•Explain the pattern of exacerbations and remissions associated with interstitial cystitis. Reassure patient that symptoms should improve within 3 months after starting therapy.
•Advise patient to take bleeding precautions during therapy, such as using an electric shaver and a soft-bristled toothbrush.
•If alopecia develops, explain that it's usually confined to a single area.

# pentoxifylline

Trental

## Class and Category
*Chemical:* Xanthine derivative
*Therapeutic:* Blood viscosity reducer
*Pregnancy category:* C

## Indications and Dosages

➤ *To treat peripheral vascular disease*

**E.R. TABLETS**

**Adults.** 400 mg t.i.d. with meals.
DOSAGE ADJUSTMENT Dosage possibly reduced to 400 mg b.i.d. for patients who experience adverse GI or CNS reactions.

| Route | Onset | Peak | Duration |
|---|---|---|---|
| P.O. | 2 to 4 wk | Unknown | Unknown |

### Mechanism of Action

Relieves symptoms of peripheral vascular disease through several actions. Pentoxifylline:
• reduces blood viscosity by decreasing the plasma fibrinogen level and inhibiting RBC and platelet aggregation
• improves erythrocyte flexibility by inhibiting phosphodiesterase and increasing the amount of cAMP in RBCs
• decreases peripheral vascular resistance and improves microcirculatory blood flow and tissue oxygenation.

## Contraindications

Hypersensitivity to pentoxifylline, methylxanthines (such as caffeine, theophylline, and theobromine), or their components; recent cerebral or retinal hemorrhage

## Interactions

**DRUGS**

*antihypertensives:* Potentiated antihypertensive effects
*cefamandole, cefoperazone, cefotetan, heparin, oral anticoagulants, other platelet aggregation inhibitors, plicamycin, thrombolytics, valproic acid:* Increased risk of bleeding
*cimetidine:* Increased blood pentoxifylline level, increased risk of adverse effects
*sympathomimetics, xanthines:* Enhanced CNS stimulation

**ACTIVITIES**

*smoking:* Possibly decreased therapeutic effects of pentoxifylline

## Adverse Reactions

**CNS:** Asceptic meningitis, dizziness, headache
**GI:** Indigestion, nausea, vomiting

## Nursing Considerations

• Use pentoxifylline cautiously in elderly patients and those with hepatic or renal dysfunction.

• Administer drug with meals and, if needed, an antacid to reduce adverse GI reactions.

**PATIENT TEACHING**

• Instruct patient to swallow pentoxifylline E.R. tablets whole and not to crush, break, or chew them.
• Advise patient to take drug with meals to reduce GI irritation. If adverse GI reactions occur anyway, advise her to also take an antacid with meals.
• Although symptoms may not improve for several weeks, urge patient to continue taking drug as prescribed to achieve maximum therapeutic effect.
• Instruct patient not to smoke during therapy because smoking constricts blood vessels and may reduce drug effectiveness.
• Urge patient to notify prescriber about adverse reactions; dosage may need reduction.

# pergolide mesylate

Permax

## Class and Category

*Chemical:* Semisynthetic ergot alkaloid derivative
*Therapeutic:* Antidyskinetic
*Pregnancy category:* B

## Indications and Dosages

➤ *As adjunct to relieve symptoms of Parkinson's disease*

**TABLETS**

**Adults.** *Initial:* 0.05 mg q.d on days 1 and 2, increased by 0.1 or 0.15 mg q 3 days over next 12 days; then increased by 0.25 mg q 3 days until effective. *Maximum:* 5 mg/day.

## Contraindications

Hypersensitivity to pergolide mesylate, other ergot alkaloid derivatives, or their components

### Mechanism of Action

Directly stimulates postsynaptic dopamine receptors to inhibit the firing of striatal neurons (such as cholinergic neurons), which helps control changes in voluntary muscle movement—such as tremors and rigidity—caused by Parkinson's disease.

**P**

## Interactions
**DRUGS**
*antihypertensives, other hypotension-producing drugs:* Possibly additive hypotensive effects *droperidol, haloperidol, loxapine, methyldopa, metoclopramide, molindone, papaverine, phenothiazines, reserpine, thioxanthenes:* Possibly decreased effectiveness of pergolide

## Adverse Reactions
**CNS:** Anxiety, confusion, dizziness, drowsiness, dyskinesia, falling asleep suddenly during activities, fatigue, hallucinations, insomnia, weakness
**CV:** Cardiac valvulopathy, hypertension, hypotension, orthostatic hypotension, peripheral edema
**EENT:** Dry mouth, facial swelling, rhinitis, vision changes
**GI:** Anorexia, constipation, diarrhea, indigestion, nausea, vomiting
**GU:** UTI
**HEME:** Anemia
**RESP:** Pleural effusion, pleuritis, pulmonary fibrosis
**MS:** Low back pain, muscle weakness
**Other:** Flulike symptoms

## Nursing Considerations
•Monitor heart rate and rhythm of patients at risk for cardiac arrhythmias because pergolide increases risk of premature atrial contractions and sinus tachycardia.
•Monitor blood pressure for symptomatic orthostatic hypotension or sustained hypertension, especially during early stages of treatment. Be aware that tolerance usually develops with gradual titration.
•**WARNING** Be aware that stopping drug or changing dosage abruptly may cause neuroleptic malignant syndrome (NMS). When drug is being stopped or dosage changed, assess patient for evidence of NMS, such as difficulty breathing, rapid heartbeat, high fever, labile blood pressure, diaphoresis, loss of bladder control, muscle stiffness, and seizures. Notify prescriber immediately, and prepare to give supportive care.
•Assess patient for mouth discomfort and oral candidiasis, especially if she complains of dry mouth. Notify prescriber immediately if symptoms persist or infection develops.

•If patient has a psychiatric disorder, watch for confusion and hallucinations, which pergolide may worsen.
**PATIENT TEACHING**
•Stress the importance of taking pergolide regularly and in exact dosage prescribed. Caution patient that altering dose or dosing interval may increase the risk of adverse reactions and decrease drug's effectiveness.
•Instruct patient or caregiver to avoid abrupt drug discontinuation because this may precipitate neuroleptic malignant syndrome.
•Inform patient that several weeks or months may pass before drug's therapeutic effects are achieved.
•Inform patient or caregiver that patient may experience orthostatic hypotension early during pergolide treatment but that she'll probably develop a tolerance to it over time.
•Advise patient to rise slowly from a seated or lying position during initial therapy to reduce the risk of dizziness or fainting.
•Alert patient that pergolide may cause her to fall asleep without warning during daily activities. Advise against driving and activities that demand mental alertness until drug's full CNS effects are known, which may take up to 1 year after start of therapy.
•Urge patient to avoid alcohol, especially if she has adverse CNS reactions to drug.
•Advise patient with a history of psychiatric disorders (or caregiver) to notify prescriber immediately if confusion or hallucinations worsen during pergolide therapy.
•Suggest that patient chew sugarless gum or suck on hard candy to prevent dry mouth.
•Suggest regular dental checkups to decrease the risk of gingival disorders from a dry mouth.

# perindopril erbumine
Aceon

## Class and Category
*Chemical:* Perindoprilat prodrug
*Therapeutic:* Antihypertensive
*Pregnancy category:* C (first trimester), D (later trimesters)

## Indications and Dosages
➤ *To manage hypertension*
**TABLETS**
**Adults.** *Initial:* 4 mg/day as a single dose or

in divided doses b.i.d., increased as prescribed until blood pressure is controlled or maximum dosage is reached. *Maintenance:* 4 to 8 mg/day. *Maximum:* 8 mg/day.

DOSAGE ADJUSTMENT If patient takes a diuretic, initial dosage possibly reduced to 2 to 4 mg/day; if patient has renal failure, initial dosage possibly reduced to 2 mg/day.

➤ *To reduce risk of cardiovascular death or nonfatal MI in patients with stable coronary artery disease*

TABLETS

**Adults.** *Initial:* 4 mg q.d. for 2 wk; then increased to 8 mg q.d. *Maintenance:* 8 mg q.d.

DOSAGE ADJUSTMENT If patient is elderly, 2 mg q.d. for 1 wk, increased to 4 mg q.d. for 1 wk and then to 8 mg q.d. if tolerated.

## Mechanism of Action

Is converted to the active metabolite perindoprilat, which competes with angiotensin I binding sites, blocking conversion of angiotensin I to angiotensin II, a potent vasoconstrictor. As a result, this ACE inhibitor reduces vasoconstriction and blood pressure. Decreased angiotensin II also reduces aldosterone secretion, increasing renal excretion of water and sodium.

## Contraindications

History of angioedema with ACE inhibitor treatment; hypersensitivity to perindopril, other ACE inhibitors, or their components

## Interactions

DRUGS

*diuretics:* Increased risk of hypotension
*lithium:* Increased blood lithium level and risk of toxicity
*potassium-sparing diuretics, potassium supplements:* Increased risk of hyperkalemia

## Adverse Reactions

**CNS:** Amnesia, anxiety, dizziness, fatigue, fever, headache, hypertonia, migraine, syncope, vertigo
**CV:** Chest pain, ECG changes, heart murmur, hypotension, orthostatic hypotension, palpitations, PVCs
**EENT:** Conjunctivitis, earache, epistaxis, hoarseness, pharyngitis, rhinitis, sinusitis, sneezing, tinnitus

**GI:** Abdominal pain, diarrhea, elevated liver function test results, flatulence, increased appetite, indigestion
**GU:** Flank pain, renal calculi, urinary frequency and urgency, vaginitis
**HEME:** Hematoma, leukopenia, neutropenia
**MS:** Arthritis, back pain, gout, limb pain, myalgia, neck pain
**RESP:** Cough
**SKIN:** Canker sores, diaphoresis, dry skin, ecchymosis, erythema, pruritus, rash
**Other:** Angioedema, facial edema

## Nursing Considerations

• Use cautiously in patients with heart failure, renal artery stenosis, or renal dysfunction.
• Monitor patients with hepatic dysfunction for enhanced therapeutic drug effects because drug's bioavailability is increased.
• Monitor serum potassium level to detect hyperkalemia, especially in patients with renal insufficiency or diabetes mellitus and those who use a potassium-containing salt substitute or take a potassium-sparing diuretic or potassium supplement.

PATIENT TEACHING

• Instruct patient to take perindopril exactly as prescribed, even if she feels well.
• WARNING Urge patient to stop taking drug and notify prescriber immediately if she experiences signs of angioedema.
• Advise patient to notify prescriber at once about fever, sore throat, or other signs that may indicate neutropenia.
• Urge patient to avoid taking potassium supplements and using potassium-containing salt substitutes unless prescriber approves.
• Instruct patient to avoid hazardous activities until drug's CNS effects are known.
• Advise female patients to notify prescriber promptly about suspected, known, or intended pregnancy.

# perphenazine

Apo-Perphenazine (CAN), PMS Perphenazine (CAN), Trilafon, Trilafon Concentrate

## Class and Category

*Chemical:* Piperazine phenothiazine
*Therapeutic:* Antiemetic, antipyschotic
*Pregnancy category:* Not rated

## Indications and Dosages

➤ *To treat psychotic disorders*

**ORAL SOLUTION**

**Hospitalized adults and adolescents.** 8 to 16 mg b.i.d. to q.i.d., adjusted as prescribed and tolerated. *Maximum:* 64 mg/day.

**TABLETS**

**Adults and adolescents.** 4 to 16 mg b.i.d. to q.i.d., adjusted as prescribed and tolerated. *Maximum:* 64 mg/day.

**I.M. INJECTION**

**Adults and adolescents.** 5 to 10 mg q 6 hr, adjusted as prescribed and tolerated. *Maximum:* 15 mg/day for outpatients, 30 mg/day for hospitalized patients.

➤ *To treat severe nausea and vomiting*

**TABLETS**

**Adults and adolescents.** 8 to 16 mg/day in divided doses, decreased as appropriate. *Maximum:* 24 mg/day.

**I.V. INFUSION OR INJECTION**

**Adults and adolescents.** 1 mg q 1 to 2 min, up to 5 mg total.

**I.M. INJECTION**

**Adults and adolescents.** 5 mg, increased to 10 mg as ordered for rapid control of severe vomiting. *Maximum:* 15 mg/day for outpatients, 30 mg/day for hospitalized patients.

**DOSAGE ADJUSTMENT** Initial dose possibly reduced and gradually increased for elderly, emaciated, or debilitated patients. Adolescents may need lower end of adult dosage range.

| Route | Onset | Peak | Duration |
|-------|-------|------|----------|
| P.O. | Several wk | 4 to 7 days | Unknown |
| I.M. | Unknown | 1 to 2 hr | 6 hr |

### Mechanism of Action

Depresses areas of the brain that control activity and aggression, including the cerebral cortex, hypothalamus, and limbic system, by an unknown mechanism. Perphenazine also prevents nausea and vomiting by inhibiting or blocking dopamine receptors in the medullary chemoreceptor trigger zone and peripherally by blocking the vagus nerve in the GI tract.

## Incompatibilities

Don't mix perphenazine oral solution with beverages that contain caffeine or tannins (such as coffee, colas, and teas) or pectinates (such as apple juice) because they're physically incompatible.

## Contraindications

Blood dyscrasias; bone marrow depression; cerebral arteriosclerosis; coma; concurrent use of CNS depressants (large doses); coronary artery disease; hepatic impairment; hypersensitivity to perphenazine, other phenothiazines, or their components; myeloproliferative disorders; severe CNS depression; severe hypertension or hypotension; subcortical brain damage

## Interactions

**DRUGS**

*aluminum- and magnesium-containing antacids, antidiarrheals (adsorbent):* Decreased absorption of oral perphenazine
*amantadine, anticholinergics, antidyskinetics, antihistamines:* Increased adverse anticholinergic effects
*amphetamines:* Decreased therapeutic effects of both drugs
*anticonvulsants:* Decreased seizure threshold, inhibited metabolism and toxicity of anticonvulsant
*antithyroid drugs:* Increased risk of agranulocytosis
*apomorphine:* Additive CNS depression, decreased emetic response to apomorphine if perphenazine is given first
*appetite suppressants (except phenmetrazine):* Antagonized anorectic effect of appetite suppressants
*beta blockers:* Increased blood levels of both drugs and risk of arrhythmias, hypotension, irreversible retinopathy, and tardive dyskinesia
*bromocriptine:* Possibly interference with bromocriptine's effects
*CNS depressants:* Increased CNS and respiratory depression and hypotensive effects
*dopamine:* Antagonized peripheral vasoconstriction with high doses of dopamine
*ephedrine:* Decreased vasopressor response to ephedrine
*epinephrine:* Blocked alpha-adrenergic effects of epinephrine, possibly causing severe hypotension and tachycardia
*hepatotoxic drugs:* Increased risk of hepatotoxicity
*hypotension-causing drugs:* Increased risk of severe orthostatic hypotension

*levodopa:* Inhibited antidyskinetic effects of levodopa

*lithium:* Possibly neurotoxicity (disorientation, extrapyramidal symptoms, unconsciousness)

*maprotiline, selective serotonin reuptake inhibitors, tricyclic antidepressants:* Prolonged and intensified sedative and anticholinergic effects of these drugs or perphenazine

*metrizamide:* Decreased seizure threshold

*opioid analgesics:* Increased CNS and respiratory depression, increased risk of orthostatic hypotension and severe constipation

*ototoxic drugs, especially antibiotics:* Possibly masking of some symptoms of ototoxicity, such as dizziness, tinnitus, and vertigo

*probucol, other drugs that prolong QT interval:* Prolonged QT interval, which may increase risk of ventricular tachycardia

*thiazide diuretics:* Possibly hyponatremia and water intoxication

**ACTIVITIES**

*alcohol use:* Increased CNS and respiratory depression, hypotensive effects, and risk of heatstroke

## Adverse Reactions

**CNS:** Behavioral changes, cerebral edema, dizziness, drowsiness, extrapyramidal reactions (such as akathisia, dystonia, pseudoparkinsonism), fever, headache, neuroleptic malignant syndrome, seizures, syncope, tardive dyskinesia (persistent)

**CV:** Bradycardia, cardiac arrest, hypertension, hypotension, orthostatic hypotension, tachycardia

**EENT:** Blurred vision, dry mouth, glaucoma, laryngeal edema, miosis, mydriasis, nasal congestion, ocular changes (corneal opacification, retinopathy)

**ENDO:** Decreased libido, galactorrhea, gynecomastia, syndrome of inappropriate ADH secretion

**GI:** Anorexia, constipation, diarrhea, fecal impaction, nausea, vomiting

**GU:** Bladder paralysis, ejaculation failure, menstrual irregularities, polyuria, urinary frequency, urinary incontinence, urine retention

**HEME:** Agranulocytosis, eosinophilia, hemolytic anemia, leukopenia, pancytopenia, thrombocytopenic purpura

**RESP:** Asthma

**SKIN:** Diaphoresis, eczema, erythema, exfoliative dermatitis, hyperpigmentation, jaundice, pallor, photosensitivity, pruritus, urticaria

**Other:** Anaphylaxis, angioedema

## Nursing Considerations

- Use perphenazine cautiously in patients with depression or hepatic, pulmonary, or renal dysfunction and in elderly patients, who are at increased risk for increased plasma concentrations and tardive dyskinesia.
- When using I.V. route, dilute drug to 0.5 mg/ml with sodium chloride for injection. Protect solution from light. Slight yellowing is acceptable, but discard solution if it's markedly discolored or contains precipitate.
- Obtain blood samples for CBC and liver and renal function tests, as ordered, to detect adverse reactions.
- Monitor temperature frequently, and notify prescriber if it rises; a significant increase suggests drug intolerance.
- Monitor blood pressure of patient who takes large doses of perphenazine, especially if surgery is indicated, because of the increased risk of hypotension.

**PATIENT TEACHING**

- Instruct patient to take perphenazine exactly as prescribed to ensure optimal effectiveness and minimize adverse reactions.
- Remind patient who takes oral solution to use a calibrated measuring device.
- Instruct patient taking oral solution to dilute every 5 ml (teaspoon) of drug in 2 fluid oz of water, milk, tomato juice, fruit juice (except apple), soup, or carbonated beverage. Caution her not to mix drug in beverages that contain caffeine or tannins, such as cola, coffee, and tea.
- Caution patient not to spill oral solution on skin or clothing because it can cause contact dermatitis and damage clothing.
- Urge patient to avoid alcohol and other CNS depressants during perphenazine therapy and to avoid potentially hazardous activities until drug's CNS effects are known.
- Advise patient to avoid excessive sun exposure and to protect skin when outdoors.
- Instruct patient to notify prescriber about persistent or severe adverse reactions.
- Urge patient to comply with long-term follow-up to detect adverse reactions and determine possible need for dosage adjustments.

P

# phenazopyridine hydrochloride

Azo-Standard, Baridium, Eridium, Geridium, Phenazo (CAN), Phenazodine, Pyridiate, Pyridium, Urodine, Urogesic, Viridium

## Class and Category

*Chemical:* Azo dye
*Therapeutic:* Urinary analgesic
*Pregnancy category:* B

## Indications and Dosages

➤ *To relieve burning and pain on urination, and urinary frequency and urgency*

TABLETS

**Adults and adolescents.** 200 mg t.i.d. with or without food for no longer than 2 days.
**Children.** 4 mg/kg t.i.d. with food for no longer than 2 days.

### Mechanism of Action

Exerts a topical or local anesthetic effect on the mucosa of the urinary tract as drug is excreted in urine. Phenazopyridine's exact mechanism is unknown.

## Contraindications

Hypersensitivity to phenazopyridine or its components, renal insufficiency

## Adverse Reactions

**CNS:** Headache
**GI:** Indigestion, nausea, vomiting
**GU:** Reddish orange urine
**SKIN:** Pruritus, rash
**Other:** Discoloration of body fluids

## Nursing Considerations

•Notify prescriber if yellowish skin or sclerae develop in patient taking phenazopyridine because this may indicate drug accumulation from impaired renal excretion. Expect prescriber to discontinue drug.
•Be aware that phenazopyridine treatment should be limited to 2 days in patients with UTIs.

PATIENT TEACHING

•Instruct patient not to take phenazopyridine for longer than 2 days and to notify prescriber if symptoms persist beyond that time.
•If GI distress develops, advise patient to take drug with meals.
•Inform patient that drug turns urine orange to red and may discolor other body fluids, such as tears.
•Advise patient not to wear contact lenses during therapy because they may become stained.

# phenelzine sulfate

Nardil

## Class and Category

*Chemical:* Hydrazine derivative
*Therapeutic:* Antidepressant
*Pregnancy category:* C

## Indications and Dosages

➤ *To treat depression*

TABLETS

**Adults.** *Initial:* 1 mg/kg/day, increased gradually as prescribed and tolerated. *Maintenance:* 45 mg/day. *Maximum:* 90 mg/day.
DOSAGE ADJUSTMENT For elderly patients, initial dosage possibly reduced to 0.8 to 1 mg/kg/day in divided doses and increased as prescribed and tolerated to maximum of 60 mg/day.

| Route | Onset | Peak | Duration |
|-------|-------|------|----------|
| P.O. | 7 to 10 days | 4 to 8 wk | 10 days |

## Contraindications

Cardiovascular disease; cerebrovascular disease; heart failure; hepatic disease; history of headaches; hypersensitivity to phenelzine or its components; hypertension; pheochromocytoma; severe renal impairment; use of anesthetics, antihypertensives, bupropion, buspirone, carbamazepine, CNS depressants, cyclobenzaprine, dextromethorphan, meperidine, selective serotonin-reuptake inhibitors, sympathomimetics, or tricyclic antidepressants; use within 14 days of other MAO inhibitor

## Interactions

DRUGS

*anticholinergics, antidyskinetics, antihistamines:* Increased anticholinergic effect, prolonged CNS depression (antihistamines)
*anticonvulsants:* Increased CNS depression, possibly altered pattern of seizures
*beta blockers:* Increased risk of bradycardia
*bromocriptine:* Possibly interference with bromocriptine effects

## Mechanism of Action

Phenelzine relieves symptoms of unipolar depressive disorders by inhibiting the enzyme monoamine oxidase (MAO). Normally, MAO breaks down monoamine neurotransmitters, such as serotonin, as shown below left. By inhibiting this enzyme, phenelzine increases the concentration of serotonin in the vesicles of monoamine nerve endings, allowing more serotonin to be released and engage with receptors on postsynaptic cells, as shown below right. A serotonin deficiency may be responsible in part for endogenous depression.

*bupropion:* Increased risk of bupropion toxicity

*buspirone:* Increased risk of hypertension

*caffeine-containing drugs:* Increased risk of dangerous arrhythmias and severe hypertension

*carbamazepine, cyclobenzaprine, maprotiline, other MAO inhibitors:* Increased risk of hyperpyretic crisis, hypertensive crisis, severe seizures, and death; altered pattern of seizures (with carbamazepine)

*CNS depressants:* Increased CNS depression

*dextromethorphan:* Increased risk of excitation, hypertension, and hyperpyrexia

*diuretics:* Increased hypotensive effect

*doxapram:* Increased vasopressor effects of either drug

*fluoxetine:* Increased risk of agitation, confusion, GI symptoms, hyperpyretic episodes, hypertensive crisis, potentially fatal serotonin syndrome, restlessness, and severe seizures.

*guanadrel, guanethidine:* Increased risk of hypertension

*haloperidol, loxapine, molindone, phenothiazines, pimozide, thioxanthenes:* Prolonged and intensified anticholinergic, hypotensive, and sedative effects of these drugs or phenelzine

*insulin, oral antidiabetic drugs:* Increased hypoglycemic effects

*levodopa:* Increased risk of sudden, moderate to severe hypertension

*local anesthetics (with epinephrine or levonordefrin):* Possibly severe hypertension

*meperidine, other opioid analgesics:* Increased risk of coma, hyperpyrexia, hypotension, immediate excitation, rigidity, seizures, severe hypertension, severe respiratory depression, sweating, vascular collapse, and death

*methyldopa:* Increased risk of hallucinations, headache, hyperexcitability, and severe hypertension

*methylphenidate:* Increased CNS stimulant effect of methylphenidate

*metrizamide:* Decreased seizure threshold, increased risk of seizures *oral anticoagulants:* Increased anticoagulant activity

*paroxetine, sertraline, trazodone, tricyclic antidepressants:* Increased risk of potentially fatal serotonin syndrome

*phenylephrine (nasal or ophthalmic):* Potentiated vasopressor effect of phenylephrine

*rauwolfia alkaloids:* Increased risk of moderate to severe hypertension, CNS depression (when phenelzine is added to rauwolfia alkaloid therapy), CNS excitation and hypertension (when rauwolfia alkaloid is added to phenelzine therapy)

*spinal anesthetics:* Increased risk of hypotension

*succinylcholine:* Possibly increased neuromuscular blockade of succinylcholine

*sympathomimetics:* Prolonged and intensified cardiac stimulant and vasopressor effects

*tryptophan:* Increased risk of confusion, disorientation, hyperreflexia, hyperthermia, hyperventilation, mania or hypomania, and shivering

**FOODS**

*foods and beverages high in tyramine or other pressor amines, such as aged cheese; beer; fava beans or other broad beans; cured meat or sausage; liqueurs; overripe fruit; red and white wine; reduced-alcohol and alcohol-free beer and wine; sauerkraut; sherry; smoked or pickled fish, meats, and poultry; yeast or protein extracts:* Increased risk of sudden, severe hypertension

**ACTIVITIES**

*alcohol use:* Increased CNS depressant effects and hypertensive crisis

## Adverse Reactions

**CNS:** Agitation, dizziness, drowsiness, headache, overstimulation, restlessness, sedation, sleep disturbance, weakness

**CV:** Bradycardia, edema, hypertensive crisis, orthostatic hypotension, palpitations, tachycardia

**EENT:** Blurred vision, dry mouth, photophobia

**GI:** Abdominal pain, constipation, diarrhea, elevated liver function test results, increased appetite, nausea

**GU:** Impotence, priapism, sexual dysfunction, urinary frequency, urine retention

**MS:** Muscle twitching

**SKIN:** Diaphoresis, rash

**Other:** Hypernatremia, weight gain

## Nursing Considerations

•Use phenelzine cautiously in patients with epilepsy because drug may alter seizure threshold.

•Expect to observe some therapeutic effect within 7 to 10 days, but keep in mind that full effect may not occur for 4 to 8 weeks.

•Monitor cardiovascular status closely for changes in heart rate (especially if patient receives more than 30 mg/day) and signs of life-threatening hypertensive crisis. Question patient frequently about headaches and palpitations. If either occurs, notify prescriber and expect to discontinue drug.

•Keep phentolamine readily available to treat hypertensive crisis. Give 5 mg by slow I.V., as prescribed, to reduce blood pressure without causing excessive hypotension. Use external cooling measures, as prescribed, to manage fever.

•To avoid hypertensive crisis, expect to wait 10 to 14 days, as prescribed, when switching patient from one MAO inhibitor to another or when switching from a dibenzazepine-related drug, such as amitriptyline or perphenazine.

**PATIENT TEACHING**

•Inform patient and family members that therapeutic effects of phenelzine may take several weeks to appear and that she should continue taking drug as prescribed.

•Caution patient to rise slowly from a lying or sitting position to minimize effects of orthostatic hypotension.

• **WARNING** Instruct patient to avoid the following foods, beverages, and drugs during phenelzine therapy and for 2 weeks afterward: alcohol-free and reduced-alcohol beer and wine; appetite suppressants; beer; broad beans; cheese (except cottage and cream cheese); chocolate and caffeine in large quantities; dry sausage (including Genoa salami, hard salami, pepperoni, and Lebanon bologna); hay fever drugs; inhaled asthma drugs; liver; meat extract; OTC cold and cough preparations (including those containing dextromethorphan), nasal decongestants (tablets, drops, or spray); pickled herring; products that contain tryptophan; protein-rich foods that may have undergone protein changes by aging, pickling, fermenting, or smoking; sauerkraut; sinus drugs; weight-loss preparations; yeast extracts (including

brewer's yeast in large quantities); yogurt; and wine.
• Advise patient to inform all health care providers (including dentists) that she takes an MAO inhibitor because certain drugs are contraindicated within 2 weeks of therapy.
• Urge patient to avoid potentially hazardous activities until drug's CNS effects are known.
• Stress the importance of reporting headaches and other unusual, persistent, or severe symptoms.
• Urge patient with diabetes mellitus who's taking insulin or oral antidiabetic drug to monitor blood glucose level frequently during therapy because phenelzine may affect glucose control.

# phenobarbital

Ancalixir (CAN), Barbita, Solfoton

## phenobarbital sodium

Luminal

### Class, Category, and Schedule
*Chemical:* Barbiturate
*Therapeutic:* Anticonvulsant, sedative-hypnotic
*Pregnancy category:* D
*Controlled substance:* Schedule IV

### Indications and Dosages
➤ *To treat seizures*
CAPSULES, ELIXIR, TABLETS
**Adults.** 60 to 250 mg/day as a single dose or in divided doses.
**Children.** 1 to 6 mg/kg/day as a single dose or in divided doses.
I.V. INJECTION
**Adults.** 100 to 320 mg, repeated as needed and as prescribed. *Maximum:* 600 mg/day.
**Children.** *Initial:* 10 to 20 mg/kg as a single dose. *Maintenance:* 1 to 6 mg/kg/day.
➤ *To treat status epilepticus*
I.V. INFUSION OR INJECTION
**Adults.** 10 to 20 mg/kg given slowly and repeated as needed and as prescribed.
**Children.** 15 to 20 mg/kg over 10 to 15 min.
➤ *To provide short-term treatment of insomnia*
CAPSULES, ELIXIR, TABLETS
**Adults.** 100 to 320 mg h.s.
I.V., I.M., OR S.C. INJECTION
**Adults.** 100 to 325 mg h.s.

➤ *To provide daytime sedation*
CAPSULES, ELIXIR, TABLETS
**Adults.** 30 to 120 mg/day in divided doses b.i.d. or t.i.d.
**Children.** 2 mg/kg t.i.d.
I.V., I.M., OR S.C. INJECTION
**Adults.** 30 to 120 mg/day in divided doses b.i.d. or t.i.d.
➤ *To provide preoperative sedation*
CAPSULES, ELIXIR, TABLETS
**Children.** 1 to 3 mg/kg before surgery.
I.M. INJECTION
**Adults.** 130 to 200 mg 60 to 90 min before surgery.
I.V. OR I.M. INJECTION
**Children.** 1 to 3 mg/kg 60 to 90 min before surgery.
DOSAGE ADJUSTMENT Dosage possibly reduced for elderly or debilitated patients to minimize confusion, depression, and excitement.

| Route | Onset | Peak | Duration |
|---|---|---|---|
| P.O. | 20 to 60 min | Unknown | Unknown |
| I.V. | 5 min | 30 min | 4 to 6 hr |
| I.M., S.C. | 5 to 20 min | Unknown | 4 to 6 hr |

### Mechanism of Action
Inhibits ascending conduction of impulses in the reticular formation, which controls CNS arousal to produce drowsiness, hypnosis, and sedation. Phenobarbital also decreases the spread of seizure activity in the cortex, thalamus, and limbic system. It promotes an increased threshold for electrical stimulation in the motor cortex, which may contribute to its anticonvulsant properties.

### Contraindications
Hepatic disease; history of addiction to hypnotics or sedatives; hypersensitivity to phenobarbital, other barbiturates, or their components; nephritis; porphyria; severe respiratory disease with airway obstruction or dyspnea

### Interactions
DRUGS
*acetaminophen:* Decreased acetaminophen effectiveness with long-term phenobarbital therapy
*amphetamines:* Delayed intestinal absorption of phenobarbital

*anesthetics (halogenated hydrocarbon):* Possibly hepatotoxicity

*anticonvulsants (hydantoin):* Unpredictable effects on metabolism of anticonvulsant

*anticonvulsants (succinimide), including carbamazepine:* Decreased blood levels and elimination half-lives of these drugs

*calcium channel blockers:* Possibly excessive hypotension

*carbonic anhydrase inhibitors:* Enhanced osteopenia induced by phenobarbital

*chloramphenicol, corticosteroids, cyclosporine, dacarbazine, digoxin, metronidazole, quinidine:* Decreased effectiveness of these drugs from enhanced metabolism

*CNS depressants:* Additive CNS depression

*cyclophosphamide:* Possibly reduced half-life and increased leukopenic activity of cyclophosphamide

*disopyramide:* Possibly ineffectiveness of disopyramide

*doxycycline, fenoprofen:* Shortened half-life of these drugs

*griseofulvin:* Possibly decreased absorption and effectiveness of griseofulvin

*guanadrel, guanethidine:* Possibly increased orthostatic hypotension

*haloperidol:* Decreased seizure threshold, decreased blood haloperidol level

*ketamine (high doses):* Increased risk of hypotension and respiratory depression

*leucovorin:* Interference with phenobarbital's anticonvulsant effect

*levothyroxine, oral contraceptives, phenylbutazone, tricyclic antidepressants:* Decreased effectiveness of these drugs

*loxapine, phenothiazines, thioxanthenes:* Decreased seizure threshold

*MAO inhibitors:* Prolonged phenobarbital effects, possibly altered pattern of seizure activity

*maprotiline:* Increased CNS depression, decreased seizure threshold at high doses, decreased phenobarbital effectiveness

*methoxyflurane:* Possibly hepatotoxicity and nephrotoxicity

*methylphenidate:* Increased risk of phenobarbital toxicity

*mexiletine:* Decreased blood mexiletine level

*oral anticoagulants:* Decreased anticoagulant activity, increased risk of bleeding when phenobarbital is discontinued

*pituitary hormones (posterior):* Increased risk of arrhythmias and coronary insufficiency

*primidone:* Altered pattern of seizures, increased CNS effects of both drugs

*valproate, valproic acid:* Decreased phenobarbital metabolism, increased risk of barbiturate toxicity

*vitamin D:* Decreased phenobarbital effectiveness

*xanthines:* Increased xanthine metabolism, antagonized hypnotic effect of phenobarbital

**ACTIVITIES**

*alcohol use:* Additive CNS depression

## Adverse Reactions

**CNS:** Anxiety, depression, dizziness, drowsiness, headache, irritability, lethargy, mood changes, paradoxical stimulation, sedation, vertigo

**CV:** Hypotension, sinus bradycardia

**EENT:** Miosis, ptosis

**GI:** Constipation, diarrhea, nausea, vomiting

**GU:** Decreased libido, impotence, sexual dysfunction

**MS:** Arthralgia, bone tenderness

**RESP:** Bronchospasm, respiratory depression

**SKIN:** Dermatitis, photosensitivity, rash, urticaria

**Other:** Injection site phlebitis (I.V.), physical and psychological dependence

## Nursing Considerations

•Be aware that phenobarbital shouldn't be given during third trimester of pregnancy because repeated use can cause dependence in neonate. It also shouldn't be given to breast-feeding women because it may cause CNS depression in infants.

•Use I.V. route cautiously in patients with cardiovascular disease, hypotension, pulmonary disease, or shock because drug may cause adverse hemodynamic or respiratory effects.

•Because drug can cause respiratory depression, assess respiratory rate and depth before use, especially in patient with bronchopneumonia, pulmonary disease, respiratory tract infection, or status asthmaticus.

•Give elixir undiluted or mix with water, milk, or fruit juice. Use a calibrated device to measure doses.

•If necessary, crush tablets and mix with food or fluids.

•Reconstitute sterile powder with at least 10 ml of sterile water for injection. Don't use reconstituted solution if it fails to clear within 5 minutes. Further dilute prescribed dose with NS or $D_5W$ and infuse over 30 to 60 minutes.

•Don't administer more rapidly than 60 mg/min by I.V. injection.

•During I.V. administration, monitor blood pressure, respiratory rate, and heart rate and rhythm. Anticipate increased risk of hypotension, even when giving drug at recommended rate. Keep resuscitation equipment readily available.

•During I.M. use, don't inject more than 5 ml into any one I.M. site to prevent sterile abscess formation.

•Be aware that drug may cause physical and psychological dependence.

•Anticipate that phenobarbital's CNS effects may exacerbate major depression, suicidal tendencies, or other mental disorders.

•Take safety precautions for elderly patients, as appropriate, because they're more likely to experience confusion, depression, and excitement as adverse CNS reactions.

•Anticipate that phenobarbital may cause paradoxical stimulation in children.

•Be aware that drug may trigger signs and symptoms in patients with acute intermittent porphyria.

**PATIENT TEACHING**

•Instruct patient to take phenobarbital elixir undiluted or to mix it with water, milk, or fruit juice. Advise her to use a calibrated device to measure doses.

•If patient has trouble swallowing tablets, suggest that she crush them and mix with food or fluid.

•Caution patient about possible drowsiness and reduced alertness. Advise her to avoid potentially hazardous activities until drug's CNS effects are known.

•Urge patient to avoid alcohol during therapy.

•Inform parents that a child may react with paradoxical excitement. Tell them to notify prescriber if this occurs.

•Instruct female patient to notify prescriber about suspected, known, or intended pregnancy. Advise against breast-feeding during therapy.

# phentolamine mesylate

Regitine

## Class and Category

*Chemical:* Imidazoline
*Therapeutic:* Antihypertensive, diagnostic aid, vasodilator
*Pregnancy category:* Not rated

## Indications and Dosages

➤ *To diagnose pheochromocytoma*

**I.V. INJECTION**

**Adults.** 2.5 mg as a single dose. After negative result, repeat test with 5-mg dose, as prescribed.

**Children.** 1 mg as a single dose. After negative result, repeat test with 0.1-mg/kg dose, as prescribed.

➤ *To manage hypertension before or during pheochromocytomectomy*

**I.V. OR I.M. INJECTION**

**Adults.** 5 mg 1 to 2 hr before surgery, repeated as needed and as prescribed. During surgery, 5 mg I.V., as ordered.

**Children.** 1 mg 1 to 2 hr before surgery, repeated as needed and as prescribed. During surgery, 1 mg I.V., as ordered.

➤ *To prevent dermal necrosis or sloughing after extravasation of I.V. norepinephrine*

**I.V. INJECTION**

**Adults, children, and infants.** 10 mg/L of I.V. fluid that contains norepinephrine at rate determined by patient response.

➤ *To treat dermal necrosis or sloughing after extravasation of I.V. norepinephrine*

**INTRADERMAL INJECTION**

**Adults.** 5 to 10 mg in 10 ml of NS infiltrated in affected area within 12 hr of extravasation.

**Children.** 0.1 to 0.2 mg/kg. *Maximum:* 10 mg.

---

### Mechanism of Action

Blocks the actions of circulating epinephrine and norepinephrine by antagonizing alpha$_1$ and alpha$_2$ receptors. Phentolamine causes peripheral vasodilation through direct relaxation of vascular smooth muscle and alpha blockade. Positive inotropic and chronotropic effects increase cardiac output. A positive inotropic effect primarily raises blood pressure, but in larger doses, phentolamine causes peripheral vasodilation and can reduce blood pressure.

In patients with pheochromocytoma, phentolamine causes systolic and diastolic blood pressures to fall dramatically. In those without pheochromocytoma, it causes blood pressure to fall or rise slightly or remain the same.

P

## Contraindications

Angina, hypersensitivity to phentolamine or its components, MI

## Interactions

**DRUGS**

*antihypertensives:* Additive hypotensive effect
*dopamine:* Antagonized vasopressor activity of dopamine
*epinephrine, methoxamine, norepinephrine, phenylephrine:* Inhibited alpha adrenergic effects of these drugs
*metaraminol:* Possibly decreased vasopressor effect of metaraminol

**ACTIVITIES**

*alcohol use:* Additive vasodilation, increased risk of hypotension and tachycardia

## Adverse Reactions

**CNS:** Dizziness
**CV:** Angina; arrhythmias, including tachycardia; hypotension
**EENT:** Nasal congestion
**GI:** Diarrhea, nausea, vomiting
**GU:** Ejaculation disorders, priapism
**MS:** Muscle weakness
**SKIN:** Flushing

## Nursing Considerations

• Reconstitute each 5-mg vial of phentolamine with 1 ml of sterile water for injection.
• Use reconstituted solution immediately; don't store unused portion.
• Dilute 5 to 10 mg of reconstituted solution in 500 ml of $D_5W$.
• Inspect drug for particles and discoloration before administering.
• When using drug to diagnose pheochromocytoma, withhold all nonessential drugs, as ordered, for at least 24 hours (preferably 48 to 72 hours) before test.
• Before giving I.V. test dose for pheochromocytoma, place patient in supine position and determine baseline blood pressure by taking readings every 10 minutes for at least 30 minutes.
• Expect patient with pheochromocytoma to have excessive hypotension after receiving drug.
• Take safety precautions according to facility policy if patient experiences dizziness.

**PATIENT TEACHING**

• Instruct patient to move slowly after phentolamine administration to minimize dizziness and avoid falls.

# phenylephrine hydrochloride

Alconefrin Nasal Drops 12, Alconefrin Nasal Drops 25, Alconefrin Nasal Drops 50, Alconefrin Nasal Spray 25, Doktors, Duration, Neo-Synephrine, Neo-Synephrine Nasal Drops, Neo-Synephrine Nasal Jelly, Neo-Synephrine Nasal Spray, Neo-Synephrine Pediatric Nasal Drops, Nostril Spray Pump, Nostril Spray Pump Mild, Rhinall, Rhinall-10 Children's Flavored Nose Drops, Vicks Sinex

## Class and Category

*Chemical:* Sympathomimetic amine
*Therapeutic:* Antiarrhythmic, decongestant, vasoconstrictor, vasopressor
*Pregnancy category:* C (parenteral), Not rated (nasal)

## Indications and Dosages

➤ *To manage mild to moderate hypotension*
**I.V. INJECTION**
**Adults.** *Initial:* 0.1 to 0.5 mg. *Usual:* 0.2 mg, repeated no more than q 10 to 15 min, as prescribed.
**I.M. OR S.C. INJECTION**
**Adults.** *Initial:* 1 to 5 mg. *Usual:* 2 to 5 mg (range, 1 to 10 mg), repeated no more than q 10 to 15 min, as prescribed.
➤ *To treat severe hypotension or shock*
**I.V. INFUSION**
**Adults.** *Initial:* 100 to 180 mcg/min (0.1 to 0.18 mg/min) until blood pressure is stable. *Maintenance:* 40 to 60 mcg/min (0.04 to 0.06 mg/min). Infusion concentration and flow rate adjusted as prescribed, based on patient response.
➤ *To prevent hypotension during spinal anesthesia*
**I.M. OR S.C. INJECTION**
**Adults.** 2 to 3 mg 3 or 4 min before injection of spinal anesthetic.
**Children.** 0.5 to 1 mg for each 11.3 kg (25 lb).
➤ *To treat hypotension during spinal anesthesia*
**I.V. INJECTION**
**Adults.** *Initial:* 0.2 mg, increased by no more than 0.2 mg, as prescribed. *Maximum:* 0.5 mg/dose.
**Children.** 0.5 to 1 mg for each 11.3 kg (25 lb).
➤ *To treat paroxysmal supraventricular tachycardia*

**I.V. INJECTION**

**Adults.** *Initial:* Up to 0.5 mg by rapid injection; later doses increased 0.1 to 0.2 mg higher than preceding dose, as prescribed. *Maximum:* 1 mg/dose.

➤ *To treat sinus, nasal, and eustachian tube congestion*

**NASAL JELLY OR SOLUTION**

**Adults and children age 12 and older.** 2 or 3 drops or sprays of 0.25% or 0.5% solution q 4 hr, p.r.n., or small quantity of 0.5% nasal jelly in each nostril q 3 to 4 hr, p.r.n. A 1% solution may be used for severe congestion.
**Children ages 6 to 12.** 2 or 3 drops or sprays of 0.25% solution in each nostril q 4 hr, p.r.n.
**Children ages 2 to 6.** 2 or 3 drops or sprays of 0.125% or 0.16% solution in each nostril q 4 hr, p.r.n.

| Route | Onset | Peak | Duration |
|-------|-------|------|----------|
| I.V. | Immediately | Unknown | 15 to 20 min |
| I.M. | 10 to 15 min | Unknown | 30 min to 2 hr |
| S.C. | 10 to 15 min | Unknown | 50 min to 1 hr |
| Nasal | Unknown | Unknown | 30 min to 4 hr |

**Mechanism of Action**

Directly stimulates alpha-adrenergic receptors and inhibits activity of the intracellular enzyme adenyl cyclase, which then inhibits production of cAMP. The inhibition of cAMP causes arterial and venous constriction and increases peripheral vascular resistance and systolic blood pressure. With greater-than-therapeutic doses, phenylephrine directly stimulates beta-adrenergic receptors in the myocardium, which increases the activity of adenyl cyclase and produces a positive inotropic and chronotropic effect. Intranasal administration directly stimulates alpha-adrenergic receptors on the nasal mucosa, constricting local vessels and decreasing blood flow and mucosal edema.

**Incompatibilities**

Don't combine nasal form with alkalies, butacaine, ferrous salts, metals, or oxidizing agents.

**Contraindications**

Hypersensitivity to bisulfites, phenylephrine, or their components; severe coronary artery disease or hypertension; use within 14 days of MAO inhibitor therapy; ventricular tachycardia

**Interactions**

**DRUGS**

*alpha blockers, haloperidol, loxapine, phenothiazines, thioxanthenes:* Possibly decreased vasoconstrictor effect of phenylephrine; decreased decongestant effect of nasal phenylephrine (with phenothiazines)
*antihypertensives, diuretics:* Possibly decreased antihypertensive effects
*atropine:* Possibly enhanced vasopressor effect of phenylephrine
*beta blockers:* Decreased therapeutic effects of both drugs
*bretylium:* Possibly potentiated vasopressor effect and arrhythmias
*doxapram:* Increased vasopressor effect of both drugs
*ergot alkaloids:* Possibly cerebral blood vessel rupture, increased vasopressor effect, peripheral vascular ischemia, and gangrene (with ergotamine)
*guanadrel, guanethidine:* Increased vasopressor effect of phenylephrine, increased risk of severe hypertension and arrhythmias
*hydrocarbon inhalation anesthetics:* Increased risk of serious arrhythmias
*MAO inhibitors:* Increased and prolonged cardiac stimulation, increased vasopressor effect, increased risk of severe cardiovascular and cerebrovascular effects, hyperpyrexia, vomiting
*maprotiline, tricyclic antidepressants:* Increased risk of severe cardiovascular effects (including arrhythmias, hyperpyrexia, severe hypertension); possibly increased or decreased sensitivity to I.V. phenylephrine
*mecamylamine, methyldopa:* Decreased hypotensive effects of these drugs, increased vasopressor effect of phenylephrine
*nitrates:* Possibly decreased vasopressor effect of phenylephrine and decreased antianginal effect of nitrates
*oxytocin:* Possibly severe, persistent hypertension
*phenoxybenzamine:* Decreased vasoconstrictor effect of phenylephrine, possibly hypotension and tachycardia

P

*theophylline:* Possibly enhanced toxicity (including cardiotoxicity); decreased blood theophylline level (with nasal phenylephrine)
*thyroid hormones:* Increased cardiovascular effects of both drugs
*urinary acidifiers:* Possibly increased elimination and decreased therapeutic effects (with nasal phenylephrine)
*urinary alkalizers:* Possibly decreased elimination and toxic effects (with nasal phenylephrine)

## Adverse Reactions

**CNS:** Dizziness, headache, insomnia, nervousness, paresthesia, restlessness, sleep disturbance (nasal), tremor, weakness
**CV:** Angina, bradycardia, hypertension, hypotension, palpitations, peripheral vasoconstriction that may lead to necrosis or gangrene, tachycardia, ventricular arrhythmias
**EENT:** Burning, dry, or stinging nasal mucosa; rebound congestion; and rhinitis (nasal forms)
**GI:** Nausea, vomiting
**RESP:** Dyspnea
**SKIN:** Extravasation with tissue necrosis and sloughing, pallor
**Other:** Allergic reaction

## Nursing Considerations

• Don't dilute phenylephrine for I.M. or S.C. use.
• To reduce the risk of tissue extravasation, don't inject S.C. drug intradermally.
• For I.V. use, dilute with $D_5W$ or sodium chloride for injection and prepare as prescribed—usually 10 mg/500 ml.
• After nasal application, rinse spray bottle tip or nasal dropper with hot water and dry with clean tissue. Wipe tip of nasal jelly tube with clean tissue.
• To prevent transmission of infection, don't use nasal form on more than one patient.
• Assess for signs and symptoms of angina, arrhythmias, and hypertension because phenylephrine may increase myocardial oxygen demand and the risk of proarrhythmias and blood pressure changes.
• WARNING Monitor patient with thyroid disease for increased sensitivity to catecholamines and, possibly, thyrotoxicity or cardiotoxicity.
• WARNING Be aware that extravasation may cause tissue necrosis, gangrene, and other re-

actions around injection site. Expect to use phentolamine if extravasation occurs.
**PATIENT TEACHING**
• Inform patient who uses nasal form of phenylephrine that excessive use may cause rebound congestion. Urge her not to exceed recommended dosage and to use for only 3 to 5 days.
• Teach patient who uses nasal form how to care for spray bottle, dropper, or tube.
• Advise patient to avoid potentially hazardous activities until drug's CNS effects are known.

# phenytoin

Dilantin-30 (CAN), Dilantin-125, Dilantin Infatabs

# phenytoin sodium

Dilantin, Dilantin Kapseals, Phenytex

## Class and Category

*Chemical:* Hydantoin derivative
*Therapeutic:* Anticonvulsant
*Pregnancy category:* C

## Indications and Dosages

➤ *To treat tonic-clonic, simple, or complex partial seizures in patients who have had no prior treatment*
**CHEWABLE TABLETS, ORAL SUSPENSION (PHENYTOIN)**
**Adults and adolescents.** *Initial:* 125 mg suspension or 100 to 125 mg tablet t.i.d., adjusted q 7 to 10 days as needed and tolerated.
**Children.** *Initial:* 5 mg/kg/day in divided doses b.i.d. or t.i.d., adjusted as needed and tolerated. *Maintenance:* 4 to 8 mg/kg/day in divided doses b.i.d. or t.i.d. *Maximum:* 300 mg/day.
**EXTENDED CAPSULES (PHENYTOIN SODIUM)**
**Adults and adolescents.** *Initial:* 100 mg t.i.d., adjusted q 7 to 10 days as needed and tolerated. *Maintenance:* Once seizures are controlled, adjusted dosage given q.d. if needed and tolerated.
DOSAGE ADJUSTMENT For hospitalized patients without hepatic or renal disease, oral loading dose of 400 mg followed in 2 hr by 300 mg and then in 2 more hr by another 300 mg for a total of 1 g.
**Children.** *Initial:* 5 mg/kg/day in divided doses b.i.d. or t.i.d., adjusted as needed and

tolerated. *Maintenance*: 4 to 8 mg/kg/day in divided doses b.i.d. or t.i.d. *Maximum:* 300 mg/day.

**PROMPT CAPSULES (PHENYTOIN SODIUM)**
**Adults and adolescents.** 100 mg t.i.d., adjusted q 7 to 10 days as needed and tolerated.
**Children.** *Initial:* 5 mg/kg/day in divided doses b.i.d. or t.i.d., adjusted as needed and tolerated. *Maintenance*: 4 to 8 mg/kg/day in divided doses b.i.d. or t.i.d. *Maximum:* 300 mg/day.

➤ *To treat status epilepticus*
**I.V. INJECTION (PHENYTOIN SODIUM)**
**Adults and adolescents.** *Initial:* 15 to 20 mg/kg by slow push in 50 ml of sodium chloride for injection at no more than 50 mg/min. *Maintenance*: Beginning within 12 to 24 hr of initial dose, 5 mg/kg/day P.O. in divided doses b.i.d. to q.i.d., or 100 mg I.V. q 6 to 8 hr.
**Children.** 15 to 20 mg/kg at no more than 1 mg/kg/min. *Maximum:* 50 mg/min.
**DOSAGE ADJUSTMENT** For elderly or very ill patients and those with CV or hepatic disease, dosage reduced to 25 mg/min, as prescribed, or possibly as low as 5 to 10 mg/min to reduce the risk of adverse reactions.

➤ *To prevent or treat seizures during neurosurgery*
**I.V. INJECTION (PHENYTOIN SODIUM)**
**Adults.** 100 to 200 mg q 4 hr at no more than 50 mg/min during or immediately after neurosurgery.

## Mechanism of Action
Limits the spread of seizure activity and the start of new seizures by regulating voltage-dependent sodium and calcium channels in neurons, inhibiting calcium movement across neuronal membranes, and enhancing sodium-potassium ATP activity in neurons and glial cells. These actions all help stabilize the neurons.

## Incompatibilities
Don't mix phenytoin in same syringe with any other drugs or with any I.V. solutions other than sodium chloride for injection because precipitate will form.

## Contraindications
Adams-Stokes syndrome, hypersensitivity to phenytoin or its components, SA block, sec-

ond- or third-degree heart block, sinus bradycardia

## Interactions
**DRUGS**
*acetaminophen:* Possibly hepatotoxicity, decreased acetaminophen effects
*activated charcoal, antacids, calcium salts, enteral feedings, sucralfate:* Decreased absorption of oral phenytoin
*allopurinol, benzodiazepines, chloramphenicol, cimetidine, disulfiram, fluconazole, isoniazid, itraconazole, methylphenidate, metronidazole, miconazole, omeprazole, phenacemide, ranitidine, sulfonamides, trazodone, trimethoprim:* Decreased metabolism and increased effects of phenytoin
*amiodarone, ticlopidine:* Possibly increased blood phenytoin level
*antifungals (azole):* Increased blood phenytoin level, decreased blood antifungal level
*antineoplastics, nitrofurantoin, pyridoxine:* Decreased phenytoin effects
*barbiturates:* Variable effects on blood phenytoin level
*bupropion, clozapine, loxapine, MAO inhibitors, maprotiline, molindone, phenothiazines, pimozide, thioxanthenes, tricyclic antidepressants:* Decreased seizure threshold, decreased anticonvulsant effect of phenytoin
*calcium channel blockers:* Increased metabolism and decreased effects of these drugs, possibly increased blood phenytoin level
*carbamazepine:* Decreased blood level and effects of carbamazepine, possibly phenytoin toxicity
*carbonic anhydrase inhibitors:* Increased risk of osteopenia from phenytoin
*chlordiazepoxide, diazepam:* Possibly increased blood phenytoin level, decreased effects of these drugs
*clonazepam:* Possibly decreased blood level and effects of clonazepam, possibly phenytoin toxicity
*corticosteroids, cyclosporine, dicumarol, digoxin, disopyramide, doxycycline, estrogens, furosemide, lamotrigine, levodopa, methadone, metyrapone, mexiletine, oral contraceptives, quinidine, sirolimus, tacrolimus, theophylline:* Increased metabolism and decreased effects of these drugs
*dopamine:* Increased risk of severe hypotension and bradycardia (with I.V. phenytoin)
*fluoxetine:* Increased blood phenytoin level and risk of phenytoin toxicity

P

*folic acid, leucovorin:* Decreased blood phenytoin level, increased risk of seizures
*haloperidol:* Decreased effects of haloperidol, decreased anticonvulsant effect of phenytoin
*halothane anesthetics:* Increased risk of hepatotoxicity and phenytoin toxicity
*ifosfamide:* Decreased phenytoin effects, possibly increased toxicity
*influenza virus vaccine:* Possibly decreased phenytoin effects
*insulin, oral antidiabetic drugs:* Possibly hyperglycemia, increased blood phenytoin level (with tolbutamide)
*levonorgestrel, mebendazole, streptozocin, sulfonylureas:* Decreased effects of these drugs
*lidocaine, propranolol (possibly other beta blockers):* Increased cardiac depressant effects (with I.V. phenytoin), possibly decreased blood level and increased adverse effects of phenytoin
*lithium:* Increased risk of lithium toxicity, increased risk of neurologic symptoms with normal blood lithium level
*meperidine:* Increased metabolism and decreased effects of meperidine, possibly meperidine toxicity
*methadone:* Possibly increased metabolism of methadone and withdrawal symptoms
*neuromuscular blockers:* Shorter duration of action and decreased effects of neuromuscular blockers
*oral anticoagulants:* Decreased metabolism and increased effects of phenytoin; early increase in anticoagulant effect followed by decrease
*paroxetine:* Decreased bioavailability of both drugs
*phenylbutazone, salicylates:* Increased phenytoin effects, possibly phenytoin toxicity
*primidone:* Increased primidone effects, possibly primidone toxicity
*rifampin:* Increased hepatic metabolism of phenytoin
*valproic acid:* Possibly decreased phenytoin metabolism, resulting in increased phenytoin effects; possibly decreased blood valproic acid level
*vitamin D:* Possibly decreased vitamin D effects, resulting in rickets or osteomalacia (with long-term use of phenytoin)

**ACTIVITIES**
*alcohol use:* Additive CNS depression, increased phenytoin clearance

## Adverse Reactions

**CNS:** Ataxia, confusion, depression, dizziness, drowsiness, excitement, fever, headache, involuntary motor activity, lethargy, nervousness, peripheral neuropathy, restlessness, slurred speech, tremor, weakness
**CV:** Cardiac arrest, hypotension, vasculitis
**EENT:** Amblyopia, conjunctivitis, diplopia, earache, epistaxis, eye pain, gingival hyperplasia, hearing loss, loss of taste, nystagmus, pharyngitis, photophobia, rhinitis, sinusitis, taste perversion, tinnitus
**ENDO:** Gynecomastia, hyperglycemia
**GI:** Abdominal pain, anorexia, constipation, diarrhea, epigastric pain, hepatic dysfunction, hepatic necrosis, hepatitis, nausea, vomiting
**GU:** Glycosuria, priapism, renal failure
**HEME:** Acute intermittent porphyria (exacerbation), agranulocytosis, anemia, eosinophilia, leukopenia, pancytopenia, thrombocytopenia
**MS:** Arthralgia, arthropathy, bone fractures, muscle twitching, osteomalacia, polymyositis
**RESP:** Apnea, asthma, bronchitis, cough, dyspnea, hypoxia, increased sputum production, pneumonia, pneumothorax, pulmonary fibrosis
**SKIN:** Exfoliative dermatitis, jaundice, maculopapular or morbilliform rash, purpuric dermatitis, Stevens-Johnson syndrome, toxic epidermal necrolysis, unusual hair growth, urticaria
**Other:** Facial feature enlargement, injection site pain, lupus-like symptoms, lymphadenopathy, polyarteritis, weight gain or loss

## Nursing Considerations

•Be aware that preferred administration routes for phenytoin are oral and I.V. injection. With I.M. administration, phenytoin has a variable absorption rate.
•If patient has difficulty swallowing, open prompt (rapid-release) capsules and mix contents with food or fluid.
•Shake oral suspension before measuring dose, and use a calibrated measuring device.
•To minimize GI distress, give phenytoin with or just after meals.
•Inspect I.V. form for particles and discoloration before administering.
•**WARNING** Avoid rapid I.V. injection because it may cause cardiac arrest, CNS depression, or severe hypotension.
•To decrease vein irritation, follow I.V. injec-

tion with flush of sodium chloride for injection through same I.V. catheter.
• Continuously monitor ECG tracings and blood pressure when administering I.V. phenytoin.
• Frequently assess I.V. site for signs of extravasation because drug can cause tissue necrosis.
• If patient has an NG tube in place, minimize drug absorption by polyvinyl chloride tubing by diluting suspension threefold with sodium chloride for injection, $D_5W$, or sterile water. After administration, flush tube with at least 20 ml of diluent.
• Separate oral phenytoin administration by at least 2 hours from antacids and calcium salts.
• Expect continuous enteral feedings to disrupt phenytoin absorption and, possibly, reduce blood phenytoin level. Discontinue tube feedings 1 to 2 hours before and after phenytoin administration, as prescribed. Anticipate giving increased phenytoin doses to compensate for reduced bioavailability during continuous tube feedings.
• Monitor blood phenytoin level. Therapeutic level ranges from 10 to 20 mcg/L.
• **WARNING** Monitor hematologic status during therapy because phenytoin can cause blood dyscrasias. A patient with a history of agranulocytosis, leukopenia, or pancytopenia may have an increased risk of infection because phenytoin can cause myelosuppression.
• Anticipate that drug may worsen intermittent porphyria.
• Frequently monitor blood glucose level of patient with diabetes mellitus because drug can stimulate glucagon secretion and impair insulin secretion, either of which can raise blood glucose level.
• Monitor blood thyroid hormone levels as appropriate in patient receiving thyroid replacement therapy because phenytoin may decrease circulating thyroid hormone levels and increase thyroid-stimulating hormone level.
• Be aware that long-term phenytoin therapy may increase patient's requirements for folic acid or vitamin D supplements. However, keep in mind that a diet high in folic acid may decrease seizure control.

**PATIENT TEACHING**
• Instruct patient to crush or thoroughly chew phenytoin chewable tablets before swallowing or to shake oral solution well before using.
• Advise patient to take drug exactly as pre-

scribed and not to change brands or dosage or stop taking drug unless instructed by prescriber.
• Instruct patient to avoid taking antacids or calcium products within 2 hours of phenytoin.
• Urge patient to avoid alcohol during therapy.
• Caution patient to avoid potentially hazardous activities until drug's CNS effects are known.
• Inform patient with diabetes mellitus about the increased risk of hyperglycemia and the possible need for increased antidiabetic drug dosage during therapy. Advise her to monitor her blood glucose level frequently.
• Stress the importance of good oral hygiene, and encourage patient to inform her dentist that she's taking phenytoin.
• Encourage patient to obtain medical identification that indicates her diagnosis and drug therapy.

# physostigmine salicylate

Antilirium

## Class and Category
*Chemical:* Salicylic acid derivative
*Therapeutic:* Anticholinergic antidote, cholinesterase inhibitor
*Pregnancy category:* Not rated

## Indications and Dosages
➤ *To counteract toxic anticholinergic effects (anticholinergic syndrome)*
**I.V. OR I.M. INJECTION**
**Adults and adolescents.** 0.5 to 2 mg at no more than 1 mg/min; then 1 to 4 mg, repeated q 20 to 30 min as needed and as prescribed.
**Children.** 0.02 mg/kg I.V. at a rate not to exceed 0.5 mg/min, repeated q 5 to 10 min as needed and as prescribed. *Maximum:* 2 mg/ dose.

| Route | Onset | Peak | Duration |
|-------|-------|------|----------|
| I.V. | 3 to 8 min | 5 min | 30 to 60 min |
| I.M. | 3 to 8 min | 20 to 30 min | 30 to 60 min |

## Contraindications
Asthma; cardiovascular disease; diabetes mellitus; gangrene; GI or GU obstruction; hypersensitivity to physostigmine, sulfites, or their components

## Mechanism of Action

Inhibits the destruction of acetylcholine by acetylcholinesterase. This action increases the concentration of acetylcholine at cholinergic transmission sites and prolongs and exaggerates the effects of acetylcholine that are blocked by toxic doses of anticholinergics.

## Interactions

**DRUGS**

*choline esters:* Enhanced effects of carbachol and bethanechol with concurrent use of physostigmine, enhanced effects of acetylcholine and methacholine with prior use of physostigmine
*succinylcholine:* Prolonged neuromuscular paralysis

## Adverse Reactions

**CNS:** CNS stimulation, fatigue, hallucinations, restlessness, seizures (with too-rapid I.V. administration), weakness
**CV:** Bradycardia (with too-rapid I.V. administration), irregular heartbeat, palpitations
**EENT:** Increased salivation, lacrimation, miosis
**GI:** Abdominal pain, diarrhea, nausea, vomiting
**GU:** Urinary urgency
**MS:** Muscle twitching
**RESP:** Bronchospasm, chest tightness, dyspnea (with too-rapid I.V. administration), increased bronchial secretions, wheezing
**SKIN:** Diaphoresis

## Nursing Considerations

• Use physostigmine cautiously in patients with bradycardia, epilepsy, or Parkinson's disease.
• Avoid rapid I.V. administration because it may lead to bradycardia, respiratory distress, or seizures.
• Frequently monitor pulse and respiratory rates, blood pressure, and neurologic status during therapy.
• Monitor ECG tracing during I.V. administration.
• Closely monitor patient with asthma for asthma attack because drug may precipitate attack by causing bronchoconstriction.
• Monitor for seizures in patient with a history of seizures because drug can induce seizures by causing CNS stimulation.
• **WARNING** Be alert for signs of a life-threatening cholinergic crisis, which may indicate a physostigmine overdose: confusion, diaphoresis, hypotension, miosis, muscle weakness, nausea, paralysis (including respiratory paralysis), salivation, seizures, sinus bradycardia, and vomiting. If you detect such signs, prepare to give atropine (the antidote) and use resuscitation equipment. Keep in mind that atropine counteracts only muscarinic cholinergic effects; paralytic effects may continue.

**PATIENT TEACHING**

• Reassure patient that her vital signs will be monitored frequently to help prevent or detect adverse reactions.
• Instruct patient to notify prescriber immediately about signs of cholinergic crisis.

# pindolol

NovoPindol (CAN), SynPindol (CAN), Visken

## Class and Category

*Chemical:* Nonselective beta blocker
*Therapeutic:* Antihypertensive
*Pregnancy category:* B

## Indications and Dosages

➤ *To manage hypertension*

**TABLETS**

**Adults.** *Initial:* 5 mg b.i.d., increased by 10 mg/day q 3 to 4 wk, as prescribed. *Maintenance:* 10 to 30 mg/day. *Maximum:* 60 mg/day (U.S.), 45 mg/day (Canadian).

| Route | Onset | Peak | Duration |
|-------|-------|------|----------|
| P.O. | Unknown | 1 to 2 hr | Up to 24 hr |

## Mechanism of Action

Blocks sympathetic stimulation of beta$_1$ receptors in the heart and beta$_2$ receptors in vascular and bronchial smooth muscle by competing with adrenergic neurotransmitters, such as catecholamines. Pindolol's negative chronotropic effects slow the resting heart rate and reduce exercise-induced tachycardia. Its negative inotropic effects reduce cardiac output, myocardial contractility, systolic and diastolic blood pressure, and myocardial oxygen consumption during stress or exercise. Among beta blockers, pindolol has the most intrinsic sympathomimetic activity and nonselective antagonism.

## Contraindications

Advanced AV block; asthma; bronchospasm; cardiogenic shock; heart failure; hepatic disease; hypersensitivity to pindolol, other beta blockers, or their components; hypotension (with systolic pressure less than 100 mm Hg); sinus bradycardia

## Interactions

### DRUGS

*allergy extracts or immunotherapy, iodinated contrast media:* Increased risk of systemic reaction or anaphylaxis

*aluminum salts, barbiturates, calcium salts, certain penicillins, cholestyramine, colestipol, NSAIDs, rifampin, salicylates, sulfinpyrazone:* Decreased blood level and effects of pindolol

*antihypertensives:* Additive hypotensive effect

*calcium channel blockers, quinidine:* Possibly increased effects of both drugs, symptomatic bradycardia (with diltiazem or verapamil), excessive hypertension or heart failure (with nifedipine)

*cimetidine:* Increased blood pindolol level

*epinephrine:* Possibly hypertension followed by bradycardia

*ergotamine:* Possibly severe peripheral vasoconstriction with pain and cyanosis

*estrogens:* Decreased antihypertensive effect

*fentanyl, fentanyl derivatives:* Risk of bradycardia after anesthesia induction

*insulin, oral antidiabetic drugs:* Masked symptoms of hypoglycemia, increased risk of hyperglycemia

*lidocaine:* Increased risk of lidocaine toxicity

*MAO inhibitors:* Possibly hypertension

*neuromuscular blockers:* Possibly increased or prolonged neuromuscular blockade

*phenothiazines:* Increased blood levels of both drugs

*phenytoin:* Possibly increased cardiac depressant effects

*prazosin, reserpine:* Increased risk of orthostatic hypotension, bradycardia (with reserpine)

*quinolones:* Possibly increased bioavailability of pindolol

*xanthines:* Possibly decreased effects of both drugs, decreased xanthine clearance

## Adverse Reactions

**CNS:** Anxiety, confusion, CVA, depression, dizziness, fatigue, fever, hallucinations, hypothermia, insomnia, memory loss, paresthesia, peripheral neuropathy, syncope, weakness

**CV:** Arrhythmias (including AV block and bradycardia), chest pain, decreased peripheral circulation, heart failure, hyperlipidemia, hypotension, MI, orthostatic hypotension, peripheral edema and ischemia, thrombosis of renal or mesenteric artery

**EENT:** Pharyngitis

**ENDO:** Hyperglycemia, hypoglycemia

**GI:** Colitis (ischemic), constipation, diarrhea, elevated liver function test results, gastritis, nausea, pancreatitis, vomiting

**GU:** Cystitis, decreased libido, renal colic, renal failure, urinary frequency, urine retention, UTI

**HEME:** Agranulocytosis, bleeding, eosinophilia, leukopenia, nonthrombocytopenic purpura, thrombocytopenia, thrombocytopenic purpura, unusual bleeding or bruising

**MS:** Arthralgia, back pain

**RESP:** Bronchospasm, pulmonary edema, pulmonary emboli

**SKIN:** Acne; alopecia; crusted, red, or scaly skin; diaphoresis; eczema; exfoliative dermatitis; hyperpigmentation; pruritus; purpura; rash

**Other:** Angioedema, positive ANA titer

## Nursing Considerations

• Monitor blood pressure and pulse rate frequently, especially at start of pindolol therapy. Also monitor fluid intake and output and daily weight, and assess for signs of heart failure, such as dyspnea, edema, fatigue, and jugular vein distention.

• Be aware that drug shouldn't be stopped abruptly because MI, myocardial ischemia, severe hypertension, or ventricular arrhythmias may result.

• Expect to discontinue drug up to 2 days before surgery, as prescribed, to reduce the risk of heart failure.

• Assess distal circulation and peripheral pulses in patient with Raynaud's phenomenon or other peripheral vascular disorder because drug can worsen these conditions.

• Be aware that pindolol can mask tachycardia from hyperthyroidism and that abrupt withdrawal can cause thyroid storm. Drug also may potentiate diplopia and muscle weakness in patient with myasthenia gravis; decrease blood glucose level, prolong or mask symptoms of hypoglycemia, and pro-

P

mote hyperglycemia in patient with diabetes mellitus; and worsen psoriasis.

**PATIENT TEACHING**

•Instruct patient to weigh herself daily during pindolol therapy and to notify prescriber if she gains more than 2 lb (0.9 kg) in 1 day or 5 lb (2.3 kg) in 1 week.

•Caution patient not to stop taking drug abruptly.

•Advise patient to rise slowly from a seated or lying position to minimize effects of orthostatic hypotension.

•Advise patient to avoid potentially hazardous activities until drug's CNS effects are known.

•Instruct patient to contact prescriber about bleeding or bruising, cough at night, depression, dizziness, edema, rash, shortness of breath, slow pulse rate, or sore throat.

•Advise diabetic patient to monitor her blood glucose level more often during pindolol therapy because drug may mask symptoms of hypoglycemia.

•Inform patient with psoriasis that drug may aggravate this condition.

# pioglitazone hydrochloride

Actos

## Class and Category

*Chemical:* Thiazolidinedione
*Therapeutic:* Antidiabetic
*Pregnancy category:* C

## Indications and Dosages

➤ *To achieve glucose control in type 2 diabetes mellitus as monotherapy or in combination with insulin, metformin, or a sulfonylurea*

**TABLETS**

**Adults.** *Initial:* 15 or 30 mg q.d. *Maximum:* 45 mg/day.

**DOSAGE ADJUSTMENT** For patients taking insulin, insulin dosage decreased by 10% to 25%, as prescribed, once glucose level reaches 100 mg/dl or less. If hypoglycemia occurs, dosage of any concurrent antidiabetic is reduced, as prescribed.

## Contraindications

Diabetic ketoacidosis, hypersensitivity to pioglitazone or its components, severe hepatic dysfunction, type 1 diabetes mellitus

## Mechanism of Action

Decreases insulin resistance by enhancing the sensitivity of insulin-dependent tissues, such as adipose tissue, skeletal muscle, and the liver, and reduces glucose output from the liver. Drug activates peroxisome proliferator-activated receptor-gamma (PPARγ) receptors, which modulate transcription of insulin-responsive genes involved in glucose control and lipid metabolism. In this way, pioglitazone reduces hyperglycemia, hyperinsulinemia, and hypertriglyceridemia in patients with type 2 diabetes mellitus and insulin resistance. However, to work effectively, pioglitazone needs endogenous insulin. Unlike sulfonylureas, it doesn't increase pancreatic insulin secretion.

## Interactions

**DRUGS**

*ketoconazole:* Possibly decreased metabolism of pioglitazone
*oral contraceptives:* Possibly decreased effectiveness of oral contraceptives

## Adverse Reactions

**CNS:** Headache
**CV:** Congestive heart failure, edema
**EENT:** Pharyngitis, sinusitis, tooth disorders
**HEME:** Decreased hemoglobin level and hematocrit
**MS:** Myalgia
**RESP:** Upper respiratory tract infection
**Other:** Weight gain

## Nursing Considerations

•Be aware that pioglitazone isn't recommended for patients classified by the New York Heart Association with a cardiac status of Class III or IV.

•Be prepared to monitor liver function test results before therapy begins, every 2 months during first year, and annually thereafter, as ordered, because drug is extensively metabolized in the liver. Expect to stop drug if jaundice develops or ALT values exceed 2½ times normal.

• **WARNING** Monitor patient for signs and symptoms of congestive heart failure—such as shortness of breath, rapid weight gain, or edema—because pioglitazone can cause fluid retention that may lead to or worsen heart failure. Notify prescriber immediately of any deterioration in the patient's cardiac status, and expect to discontinue the drug, as ordered.

• Assess for signs and symptoms of hypoglycemia, especially if patient is also taking another antidiabetic drug.

• Monitor fasting glucose level, as ordered, to evaluate effectiveness of therapy.

• Monitor glycosylated hemoglobin level to assess long-term effectiveness of drug therapy.

**PATIENT TEACHING**

• Stress the need for patient to continue exercise program, diet control, and weight management during pioglitazone therapy.

• Advise patient to notify prescriber immediately if she experiences shortness of breath, fluid retention, or sudden weight gain because drug may need to be discontinued.

• Instruct patient to keep appointments for liver function tests, as ordered, typically every 2 months during first year of therapy and annually thereafter.

• Inform female patient who uses oral contraceptives that drug decreases their effectiveness; suggest that she use another method of contraception while taking pioglitazone.

# pioglitazone hydrochloride and metformin hydrochloride

Actoplus Met

## Class and Category

*Chemical:* Thiazolidinedione (pioglitazone), biguanide (metformin)
*Therapeutic:* Antidiabetic (pioglitazone, metformin)
*Pregnancy category:* C

## Indications and Dosages

➤ *To reduce blood glucose level in patients with type 2 diabetes mellitus who have responded well to pioglitazone initially but need additional glycemic control*

**TABLETS**

**Adults.** *Initial:* 15 mg pioglitazone and 500 mg metformin (1 tablet) b.i.d. or 15 mg pioglitazone and 850 mg metformin (1 tablet) q.d., adjusted gradually as needed.

➤ *To reduce blood glucose level in patients who haven't achieved adequate glycemic control with metformin monotherapy*

**TABLETS**

**Adults.** *Initial:* 15 mg pioglitazone and 500 mg metformin (1 tablet) or 15 mg pioglitazone and 850 mg metformin (1 tablet) q.d. or b.i.d., adjusted gradually as needed.

➤ *To reduce blood glucose level in patients who are already taking pioglitazone and metformin separately*

**TABLETS**

**Adults.** *Initial:* 15 mg pioglitazone and 500 mg metformin (1 tablet) or 15 mg pioglitazone and 850 mg metformin (1 tablet) q.d. or b.i.d. based on dose of pioglitazone and metformin already being taken.

---

### Mechanism of Action

Pioglitazone decreases insulin resistance by enhancing the sensitivity of insulin-dependent tissues, such as adipose tissue, skeletal muscle, and the liver, and it reduces glucose output from the liver. It activates peroxisome proliferator-activated receptor-gamma (PPARγ) receptors, which modulate transcription of insulin-responsive genes involved in glucose control and lipid metabolism. In this way, pioglitazone reduces hyperglycemia, hyperinsulinemia, and hypertriglyceridemia in patients with type 2 diabetes mellitus and insulin resistance. Efficacy depends on the presence of endogenous insulin.

Metformin may promote the storage of excess glucose as glycogen in the liver, which reduces glucose production. It also may improve glucose use by skeletal muscle and adipose tissue by increasing glucose transport across cell membranes. It may increase the number of insulin receptors on cell membranes and make them more sensitive to insulin. And it modestly decreases blood triglyceride and total cholesterol levels.

---

## Contraindications

Hypersensitivity to pioglitazone, metformin, or their components; impaired renal function; metabolic acidosis, including diabetic ketoacidosis; severe hepatic dysfunction; type 1 diabetes mellitus; use of iodinated contrast media within preceding 48 hours

## Interactions

**DRUGS**

**pioglitazone component only**

*hormonal contraceptives:* Possibly decreased contraceptive effectiveness

*insulin, other oral antidiabetics:* Increased risk of hypoglycemia

*ketoconazole:* Possibly decreased pioglitazone metabolism

**metformin component only**

*cationic drugs (such as amiloride, cimetidine, digoxin, morphine, procainamide, quinidine, quinine, ranitidine, triamterene, trimethoprim, vancomycin), nifedipine:* Increased metformin level

*calcium channel blockers, corticosteroids, estrogens, hormonal contraceptives, isoniazid, nicotinic acid, phenothiazines, phenytoin, sympathomimetics, thiazide and other diuretics, thyroid drugs:* Possibly hyperglycemia

*clofibrate, MAO inhibitors, probenecid, propranolol, rifabutin, rifampin, salicylates, sulfonamides, sulfonylureas:* Increased risk of hypoglycemia

*furosemide:* Possibly increased blood metformin level, decreased blood furosemide level

**FOODS**

*all foods:* Possibly delayed metformin absorption

**ACTIVITIES**

*alcohol use:* Increased risk of hypoglycemia and lactate formation

## Adverse Reactions

**CNS:** Dizziness, headache

**CV:** Congestive heart failure, edema

**EENT:** Metallic taste, pharyngitis, sinusitis, tooth disorders

**ENDO:** Hyperglycemia, hypoglycemia

**GI:** Abdominal distention, anorexia, constipation, diarrhea, elevated liver transaminase levels, flatulence, indigestion, nausea, vomiting

**GU:** Urinary tract infection

**HEME:** Aplastic anemia, decreased hemoglobin and hematocrit levels, megaloblastic anemia, thrombocytopenia

**MS:** Myalgia

**RESP:** Upper respiratory tract infection

**SKIN:** Photosensitivity, rash

**Other:** Decreased vitamin $B_{12}$ levels, lactic acidosis, weight gain or loss

## Nursing Considerations

•Be aware that the pioglitazone and metformin combination isn't recommended for patients with New York Heart Association cardiac status Class III or IV.

•Use drug cautiously in patients with edema because pioglitazone may cause or worsen edema.

•Give drug with meals to reduce the risk of adverse GI reactions.

•Expect prescriber to alter dosage if patient has a condition that decreases or delays gastric emptying, such as diarrhea, gastroparesis, GI obstruction, ileus, or vomiting.

•Withhold drug, as ordered, if patient becomes dehydrated because dehydration increases the risk of lactic acidosis.

•Be aware that iodinated contrast media increase the risk of renal failure and lactic acidosis during pioglitazone and metformin therapy. Expect to withhold drug for 48 hours before and after radiographic studies.

•Expect to monitor liver function test results before therapy begins, every 2 months during first year of therapy, and annually thereafter, as ordered, because drug is extensively metabolized in the liver. If patient develops jaundice or if ALT values exceed 2½ times normal, expect to stop drug.

•Assess BUN and serum creatinine levels, as appropriate, before and during long-term therapy in patients at increased risk for lactic acidosis because of the metformin component of drug.

•**WARNING** Monitor patient for evidence of heart failure—such as shortness of breath, rapid weight gain, or edema—because pioglitazone can cause fluid retention that may lead to or worsen heart failure. Notify prescriber immediately if patient's cardiac status deteriorates, and expect to stop drug.

•Assess patient for signs and symptoms of hypoglycemia, especially if patient is also taking another antidiabetic drug.

•Monitor fasting glucose level, as ordered, to evaluate effectiveness of therapy. Assess patient for hyperglycemia and the need for insulin during times of increased stress, such as during infection or surgery.

•Monitor glycosylated hemoglobin level to assess long-term effectiveness of therapy.

•Be aware that patients with inadequate vitamin $B_{12}$ or calcium intake or absorption may develop abnormal vitamin $B_{12}$ levels. Routine vitamin $B_{12}$ measurements should be obtained every 2 to 3 years, as ordered, to check for this abnormality.

•Expect to stop drug temporarily, as ordered,

before any surgical procedure that warrants restricted intake of food and fluids and to not resume drug until patient's oral intake has resumed and renal function is normal.

**PATIENT TEACHING**

• Stress the need for patient to continue exercise program, diet control, and weight management during pioglitazone and metformin therapy.

• Instruct patient to take drug at breakfast if taking drug once a day, or at breakfast and dinner if taking drug twice a day.

• Direct patient to take drug exactly as prescribed and not to change the dosage or frequency unless instructed.

• Advise patient to notify prescriber immediately about shortness of breath, fluid retention, or sudden weight gain because drug may need to be stopped.

• Teach patient how to check her blood glucose level and recognize hyperglycemia and hypoglycemia. Urge her to notify prescriber about abnormal blood glucose level.

• Caution patient to avoid alcohol, which can increase the risk of hypoglycemia.

• Instruct patient to watch for early symptoms of lactic acidosis, including drowsiness, hyperventilation, malaise, and muscle pain, and to notify prescriber if they develop.

• Instruct patient to keep appointments for liver function tests, as ordered, typically every 2 months during first year of therapy and annually thereafter.

• Inform female patient who uses hormonal contraceptives that drug decreases their effectiveness; suggest another contraceptive while taking pioglitazone and metformin.

• Warn female patients with irregular periods that pioglitazone and metformin may induce ovulation. Instruct these women to use adequate contraception while taking drug.

# piperacillin sodium

Pipracil

## Class and Category

*Chemical:* Piperazine derivative of ampicillin, acylureidopenicillin
*Therapeutic:* Antibiotic
*Pregnancy category:* B

## Indications and Dosages

➤ *To treat moderate to severe bacterial infections, including bone and joint infec-*tions, gynecologic infections, intra-abdominal infections, lower respiratory tract infections, septicemia, and skin and soft-tissue infections, caused by susceptible strains of Acinetobacter sp., anaerobic cocci, Bacteroides sp., Enterobacter sp., Escherichia coli, Haemophilus influenzae, Klebsiella sp., Proteus sp., Pseudomonas aeruginosa, and Serratia sp.*

**I.V. INFUSION**

**Adults and adolescents.** 12 to 18 g/day or 200 to 300 mg/kg/day in divided doses q 4 to 6 hr. *Maximum:* 24 g/day.

➤ *To treat bacterial meningitis*

**I.V. INFUSION**

**Adults and adolescents.** 4 g q 4 hr or 75 mg/kg q 6 hr. *Maximum:* 24 g/day.

➤ *To treat uncomplicated UTIs and community-acquired pneumonia caused by susceptible organisms, including* E. coli, Klebsiella *sp., and* Serratia *sp.*

**I.V. INFUSION, I.M. INJECTION**

**Adults.** 6 to 8 g/day or 100 to 125 mg/kg/day in divided doses q 6 to 12 hr.

➤ *To treat complicated UTIs caused by susceptible organisms, including* Acinetobacter *sp.,* Klebsiella *sp., and* Serratia *sp.*

**I.V. INFUSION**

**Adults.** 8 to 16 g/day or 125 to 200 mg/kg/day in divided doses q 6 to 8 hr.

➤ *To treat uncomplicated gonorrhea caused by susceptible strains of* Neisseria gonorrhoeae

**I.M. INJECTION**

**Adults.** 2 g as a single dose 30 min after 1-g dose of probenecid P.O.

➤ *To provide surgical prophylaxis in intra-abdominal procedures, including GI and biliary surgery*

**I.V. INFUSION**

**Adults.** 2 g 20 to 30 min before anesthesia, 2 g during surgery, and 2 g q 6 hr for 24 hr after surgery.

➤ *To provide surgical prophylaxis in abdominal hysterectomy*

**I.V. INFUSION**

**Adults.** 2 g 20 to 30 min before anesthesia, 2 g just after surgery, and 2 g 6 hr later.

➤ *To provide surgical prophylaxis in vaginal hysterectomy*

**I.V. INFUSION**

**Adults.** 2 g 20 to 30 min before anesthesia, then 2 g 6 and 12 hr after initial dose.

P

▶ *To provide surgical prophylaxis in cesarean section*

**I.V. INFUSION**

**Adults.** 2 g after cord is clamped, then 2 g 4 and 8 hr after initial dose.

## Mechanism of Action

Binds to specific penicillin-binding proteins and inhibits the third and final stage of bacterial cell wall synthesis by interfering with an autolysin inhibitor. Uninhibited autolytic enzymes destroy the cell wall and result in cell lysis.

## Incompatibilities

Don't mix piperacillin sodium in same container with aminoglycosides because of chemical incompatibility (depending on concentrations, diluents, pH, and temperature). Don't mix with solutions that contain only sodium bicarbonate because of chemical instability.

## Contraindications

Hypersensitivity to cephalosporins, penicillins, or their components

## Interactions

**DRUGS**

*aminoglycosides:* Additive or synergistic effects against some bacteria, possibly mutual inactivation

*anti-inflammatory drugs (including aspirin and NSAIDs), heparin, oral anticoagulants, platelet aggregation inhibitors, sulfinpyrazone, thrombolytics:* Increased risk of bleeding

*hepatotoxic drugs (including labetalol and rifampin):* Increased risk of hepatotoxicity

*methotrexate:* Increased blood methotrexate level and risk of toxicity

*probenecid:* Increased blood piperacillin level and risk of toxicity

*vecuronium:* Possibly prolonged perioperative neuromuscular blockade of vecuronium

## Adverse Reactions

**CNS:** CVA, dizziness, fever, hallucinations, headache, lethargy, seizures

**CV:** Cardiac arrest, hypotension, palpitations, tachycardia, vasodilation, vasovagal reactions

**EENT:** Oral candidiasis, pharyngitis

**GI:** Diarrhea, epigastric distress, intestinal necrosis, nausea, pseudomembranous colitis, vomiting

**GU:** Hematuria, impotence, nephritis, neurogenic bladder, priapism, proteinuria, renal failure, vaginal candidiasis

**HEME:** Agranulocytosis, eosinophilia, hemolytic anemia, leukopenia, neutropenia, pancytopenia, prolonged bleeding time, thrombocytopenia

**MS:** Arthralgia

**RESP:** Dyspnea, pulmonary embolism, pulmonary hypertension

**SKIN:** Exfoliative dermatitis, mottling, rash, toxic epidermal necrolysis, urticaria

**Other:** Anaphylaxis; facial edema; hypokalemia; hyponatremia; injection site pain, phlebitis, and skin ulcer; superinfection

## Nursing Considerations

• Obtain blood, sputum, or other samples for culture and sensitivity testing, as ordered, before giving piperacillin. Expect to begin piperacillin therapy before results are available.

• Be aware that sunlight may darken powder for dilution but won't alter drug potency.

• For initial dilution for I.V. infusion, reconstitute each gram of drug with at least 5 ml of sterile water for injection, sodium chloride for injection, $D_5W$, $D_5NS$, or bacteriostatic water that contains parabens or benzyl alcohol. Shake solution vigorously after adding diluent to help drug dissolve, and inspect for particles and discoloration before giving.

• For further dilution, use sodium chloride for injection, $D_5W$, $D_5NS$, LR solution, or dextran 6% in NS. Solutions diluted with LR solution should be given within 2 hours.

• For intermittent infusion, infuse appropriate dose over 20 to 30 minutes.

• Give aminoglycosides 1 hour before or after piperacillin; use a separate site, I.V. bag, and tubing.

• For I.M. injection, reconstitute each gram of piperacillin with at least 2 ml of an appropriate diluent listed above.

• Don't give more than 2 g I.M. at any one site. Use deltoid area cautiously and only if well developed to avoid injuring the radial nerve.

• Watch for bleeding or excessive bruising because drug can decrease platelet aggregation, especially in patients with renal failure. If bleeding occurs, notify prescriber and expect to stop piperacillin.

• Monitor CBC regularly, as ordered, to detect hematologic abnormalities, such as leukopenia and neutropenia.

•Monitor serum potassium level to detect hypokalemia from urinary potassium loss.
•Check for diarrhea (possible pseudomembranous colitis) during and after therapy.
•Watch closely for hypersensitivity reactions, especially if patient has cystic fibrosis. Notify prescriber, and expect to stop drug.

**PATIENT TEACHING**
•Advise patient to consult prescriber before using OTC drugs during piperacillin therapy because of the risk of interactions.
•Inform patient that increased bruising may occur if she takes anti-inflammatory drugs during piperacillin therapy.
•Advise patient to notify prescriber about signs of superinfection, such as severe diarrhea or white patches on tongue or in mouth.
•Instruct patient to complete full course of therapy, even if symptoms subside.

# piperacillin sodium and tazobactam sodium

Tazocin (CAN), Zosyn

## Class and Category
*Chemical:* Piperazine derivative of ampicillin, acylureidopenicillin (piperacillin); penicillinate sulfone (tazobactam)
*Therapeutic:* Antibiotic
*Pregnancy category:* B

## Indications and Dosages
➤ *To treat moderate to severe gramnegative or anaerobic infections, such as appendicitis, community-acquired pneumonia, diabetic foot ulcers, intraabdominal infections, pelvic inflammatory disease, peritonitis, postpartum endometritis, and uncomplicated or complicated skin or soft-tissue infections caused by susceptible organisms, such as* Bacteroides *sp. (including many strains of* Bacteroides fragilis*),* Clostridium *sp.,* Enterobacter *sp.,* Enterococcus faecalis, Escherichia coli, Haemophilus influenzae, Klebsiella pneumoniae, Morganella morganii, Neisseria gonorrhoeae, Proteus mirabilis, Proteus vulgaris, Pseudomonas aeruginosa, and* Serratia *sp.*

**I.V. INFUSION**
**Adults and adolescents.** 3.375 g q 6 hr. *Maximum:* 4.5 g q 6 to 8 hr.

➤ *To treat nosocomial pneumonia caused by susceptible organisms*
**I.V. INFUSION**
**Adults and adolescents.** 4.5 g q 6 hr in addition to aminoglycoside therapy for 7 to 14 days.
**DOSAGE ADJUSTMENT** Dosage possibly decreased to 2.25 g q 6 hr for patients with creatinine clearance of 20 to 40 ml/min/1.73 m$^2$; to 2.25 g q 8 hr for those with creatinine clearance of less than 20 ml/min/1.73 m$^2$.

## Mechanism of Action
Binds to specific penicillin-binding proteins and inhibits the third and final stage of bacterial cell wall synthesis. Piperacillin does this by interfering with an autolysin inhibitor. Uninhibited autolytic enzymes destroy the cell wall and result in cell lysis.
Tazobactam doesn't change piperacillin's action, but it protects piperacillin against Richmond and Sykes types II, III, IV, and V beta-lactamases; staphylococcal beta-lactamases; and extended-spectrum beta-lactamases.

## Incompatibilities
Don't mix piperacillin and tazobactam in same container with aminoglycosides because of chemical incompatibility (depending on concentrations, diluents, pH, and temperature).

## Contraindications
Hypersensitivity to beta-lactamase inhibitors, cephalosporins, penicillins, piperacillin, tazobactam, or their components

## Interactions
**DRUGS**
*aminoglycosides:* Additive or synergistic effects against some bacteria, possibly mutual inactivation
*anti-inflammatory drugs (including aspirin and NSAIDs), heparin, oral anticoagulants, platelet aggregation inhibitors, sulfinpyrazone, thrombolytics:* Increased risk of bleeding
*hepatotoxic drugs (including labetalol and rifampin):* Increased risk of hepatotoxicity
*methotrexate:* Increased blood methotrexate level and risk of toxicity
*probenecid:* Increased blood piperacillin level and risk of toxicity

P

*vecuronium:* Possibly prolonged neuromuscular blockade in perioperative period

## Adverse Reactions

**CNS:** Chills, CVA, dizziness, fever, hallucinations, headache, lethargy, seizures
**CV:** Cardiac arrest, hypotension, palpitations, tachycardia, vasodilation, vasovagal reactions
**EENT:** Epistaxis, oral candidiasis, pharyngitis
**GI:** Diarrhea, elevated liver function test results, epigastric distress, intestinal necrosis, nausea, pseudomembranous colitis, vomiting
**GU:** Hematuria, impotence, nephritis, neurogenic bladder, priapism, proteinuria, renal failure, vaginal candidiasis
**HEME:** Eosinophilia, leukopenia, neutropenia, thrombocytopenia
**MS:** Arthralgia, prolonged muscle relaxation
**RESP:** Dyspnea, pulmonary embolism, pulmonary hypertension
**SKIN:** Erythema multiforme, exfoliative dermatitis, mottling, rash, Stevens-Johnson syndrome
**Other:** Anaphylaxis, facial edema, hypokalemia, hyponatremia

## Nursing Considerations

•Expect to obtain blood, sputum, or other samples for culture and sensitivity testing before giving piperacillin and tazobactam. Therapy may start before tests are complete.
•Be aware that sunlight may darken powder for dilution but won't alter drug potency.
•Reconstitute with sterile water for injection, sodium chloride for injection, D₅W, or bacteriostatic water or NS that contains parabens or benzyl alcohol.
•For additional dilution (50 to 150 ml except as noted), use appropriate solution, such as sodium chloride for injection, sterile water for injection (no more than 50 ml), D₅W, or dextran 6% in NS.
•Shake solution vigorously after adding diluent to help drug dissolve, and inspect for particles and discoloration before giving.
•Administer over at least 30 minutes.
•Assess for bleeding or excessive bruising because drug can decrease platelet aggregation.
•Monitor serum potassium level; hypokalemia may result from urinary potassium loss.

•Monitor for diarrhea during or shortly after drug therapy; diarrhea may signal pseudomembranous colitis.
•Give aminoglycosides 1 hour before or after piperacillin and tazobactam; use a separate site, I.V. bag, and tubing.

PATIENT TEACHING
•Instruct patient to take drug for as long as prescribed, even after feeling better.
•Inform diabetic patients who test urine glucose level that drug may alter results of copper reduction tests, such as Clinitest. Advise using a test based on enzymatic glucose oxidase reaction, such as Diastix or TesTape.
•Advise patient to consult prescriber before using OTC drugs during treatment with piperacillin and tazobactam because of the risk of interactions.
•Inform patient that increased bruising may occur if she takes anti-inflammatory drugs, such as aspirin and NSAIDs, during piperacillin and tazobactam therapy.
•Advise patient to notify prescriber about signs of superinfection, such as severe diarrhea or white patches on tongue or in mouth.

# pirbuterol acetate

Maxair, Maxair Autohaler

## Class and Category

*Chemical:* Sympathomimetic amine
*Therapeutic:* Bronchodilator
*Pregnancy category:* C

## Indications and Dosages

➤ *To prevent or treat bronchospasm caused by COPD, to treat bronchospasm caused by asthma*

ORAL INHALATION
**Adults and adolescents.** 1 or 2 inhalations (200 to 400 mcg) q 4 to 6 hr. *Maximum:* 12 inhalations (2.4 mg)/day.

| Route | Onset | Peak | Duration |
|-------|-------|------|----------|
| Oral inhalation | In 5 min | In 30 to 90 min | 3 to 6 hr |

## Contraindications

Hypersensitivity to pirbuterol or its components, tachycardia

## Mechanism of Action
Attaches to beta$_2$ receptors on bronchial cell membranes, which stimulates the intracellular enzyme adenyl cyclase to convert adenosine triphosphate (ATP) to cAMP. The increased intracellular level of cAMP relaxes bronchial smooth-muscle cells and inhibits histamine release. Pirbuterol also stabilizes mast cells and inhibits the release of histamine.

## Interactions
**DRUGS**
*beta-adrenergic bronchodilators:* Additive effects
*beta blockers (ophthalmic):* Possibly decreased pirbuterol effects, increased risk of bronchospasm
*beta blockers (systemic):* Decreased effects of both drugs, increased risk of bronchospasm
*MAO inhibitors, tricyclic antidepressants:* Potentiated cardiovascular effects

## Adverse Reactions
**CNS:** Anxiety, confusion, depression, dizziness, headache, nervousness, tiredness, tremor
**CV:** Arrhythmias (including PVCs and tachycardia), chest pain, ECG changes (including flattening of T waves, prolonged QT interval, and ST-segment depression), hypotension, palpitations
**EENT:** Dry mouth
**GI:** Abdominal cramps, diarrhea, nausea, vomiting
**RESP:** Bronchospasm, cough
**SKIN:** Alopecia, rash, urticaria
**Other:** Facial edema, hypokalemia

## Nursing Considerations
•For patient with a cardiovascular disorder, such as arrhythmias, hypertension, or ischemic cardiac disease, monitor blood pressure and heart rate and rhythm to detect significant changes after pirbuterol use.
•Be aware that elderly patients have a greater risk of adverse reactions than younger adults.
•**WARNING** Discontinue drug and notify prescriber immediately if patient experiences paradoxical bronchospasm, a life-threatening adverse reaction.

**PATIENT TEACHING**
•Teach patient how to use an inhaler and spacer correctly, and urge her to keep the inhaler readily available at all times.
•Recommend the use of an autohaler if patient has trouble coordinating inhalations with a regular inhaler.
•Advise patient to clean the inhaler's mouthpiece at least once daily.
•Caution patient against overusing drug because doing so may increase adverse reactions.
•Teach patient how to use a peak flow meter and how to determine her personal best reading.
•**WARNING** Advise patient to notify prescriber if symptoms worsen, if bronchospasm occurs more frequently, if she needs to use the inhaler more often, or if the inhaler becomes less effective.

# piroxicam

Apo-Piroxicam (CAN), Feldene, Novo-Pirocam (CAN), Nu-Pirox (CAN), PMS-Piroxicam (CAN)

## Class and Category
*Chemical:* Oxicam derivative
*Therapeutic:* Anti-inflammatory, antirheumatic
*Pregnancy category:* Not rated

## Indications and Dosages
➤ *To treat acute and chronic osteoarthritis and rheumatoid arthritis*
**CAPSULES**
**Adults.** *Initial:* 20 mg q.d. or 10 mg b.i.d.

| Route | Onset | Peak | Duration | |
|-------|-------|------|----------|---|
| P.O. | Unknown | Several days to 1 wk* | Unknown | P |

## Mechanism of Action
Blocks the activity of cyclooxygenase, the enzyme needed for prostaglandin synthesis. Prostaglandins, important mediators of the inflammatory response, cause local vasodilation with swelling and pain. By blocking cyclooxygenase activity and inhibiting prostaglandins, this NSAID reduces inflammatory symptoms and pain.

---

*With severe inflammation, 2 wk or more.

## Contraindications

Angioedema, asthma, bronchospasm, nasal polyps, rhinitis, or urticaria induced by aspirin, iodides, or other NSAIDs; hypersensitivity to piroxicam or its components

## Interactions

**DRUGS**

*acetaminophen:* Possibly increased adverse renal effects with long-term use of both drugs
*antihypertensives:* Possibly decreased or reversed effects of antihypertensives
*aspirin, other NSAIDs:* Increased risk of bleeding and adverse GI effects, possibly increased blood piroxicam level
*cefamandole, cefoperazone, cefotetan:* Increased risk of hypoprothrombinemia and bleeding
*colchicine:* Increased risk of GI bleeding, hemorrhage, and ulcers
*corticosteroids, potassium supplements:* Increased risk of adverse GI effects
*cyclosporine:* Increased risk of nephrotoxicity from both drugs, increased blood cyclosporine level
*diuretics:* Decreased antihypertensive, diuretic, and natriuretic effects of diuretics
*gold compounds, nephrotoxic drugs:* Increased risk of adverse renal effects
*heparin, oral anticoagulants, thrombolytics:* Increased anticoagulant effects, increased risk of hemorrhage
*insulin, oral antidiabetic drugs:* Possibly increased hypoglycemic effect of these drugs
*lithium:* Possibly increased blood lithium level and toxicity
*methotrexate:* Decreased methotrexate clearance, increased risk of methotrexate toxicity
*platelet aggregation inhibitors:* Increased risk of bleeding and GI ulceration or hemorrhage
*plicamycin, valproic acid:* Increased risk of hypoprothrombinemia and GI bleeding, hemorrhage, and ulceration
*probenecid:* Possibly increased blood level, effectiveness, and risk of toxicity of piroxicam

**ACTIVITIES**

*alcohol use:* Increased risk of adverse GI effects

## Adverse Reactions

**CNS:** Anxiety, aseptic meningitis, asthenia, cerebral hemorrhage, confusion, depression, dizziness, dream disturbances, drowsiness, fever, headache, insomnia, ischemic CVA, malaise, nervousness, paresthesia, somnolence, syncope, transient ischemic attack, tremor, vertigo
**CV:** Deep vein thrombosis, edema, heart failure, hypertension, MI, peripheral edema, tachycardia
**EENT:** Blurred vision, dry mouth, epistaxis, glossitis, stomatitis, tinnitus
**ENDO:** Hypoglycemia
**GI:** Abdominal pain; anorexia; constipation; diarrhea; elevated liver function test results; esophagitis; flatulence; gastritis; GI bleeding, perforation, or ulceration; heartburn; hematemesis; hepatitis; indigestion; jaundice; liver failure; melena; nausea; vomiting
**GU:** Acute renal failure, cystitis, dysuria, elevated serum creatinine level, hematuria, interstitial nephritis, nephrotic syndrome, oliguria, polyuria, proteinuria, renal failure or insufficiency
**HEME:** Agranulocytosis, anemia, aplastic anemia, coagulation abnormalities, eosinophilia, leukopenia, pancytopenia, thrombocytopenia
**RESP:** Asthma, dyspnea
**SKIN:** Alopecia, diaphoresis, ecchymosis, erythema, erythema multiforme, exfoliative dermatitis, photosensitivity, pruritus, purpura, rash, Stevens-Johnson syndrome, toxic epidermal necrolysis, urticaria
**Other:** Anaphylaxis, angioedema, flulike symptoms, hyperkalemia, infection, sepsis, weight loss or gain

## Nursing Considerations

• Administer piroxicam with food to decrease GI upset.
• Use piroxicam with extreme caution in patients with a history of ulcer disease or GI bleeding because NSAIDs such as piroxicam increase the risk of GI bleeding and ulceration. Expect to use piroxicam for the shortest time possible in these patients.
• Be aware that serious GI tract ulceration, bleeding, and perforation may occur without warning symptoms. Elderly patients are at greater risk. To minimize risk, give drug with food. If GI distress occurs, withhold drug and notify prescriber immediately.
• Use piroxicam cautiously in patients with hypertension, and monitor blood pressure closely throughout therapy. Drug may cause hypertension or worsen it.

•**WARNING** Monitor patient closely for thrombotic events, including MI and stroke, because NSAIDs increase the risk.

•**WARNING** If patient has bone marrow suppression or is receiving antineoplastic drug therapy, monitor laboratory results (including WBC count), and watch for evidence of infection because anti-inflammatory and antipyretic actions of piroxicam may mask signs and symptoms, such as fever and pain.

•Especially if patient is elderly or taking piroxicam long-term, watch for less common but serious adverse GI reactions, including anorexia, constipation, diverticulitis, dysphagia, esophagitis, gastritis, gastroenteritis, gastroesophageal reflux disease, hemorrhoids, hiatal hernia, melena, stomatitis, and vomiting.

•Monitor liver function test results because, in rare cases, elevated levels may progress to severe hepatic reactions, including fatal hepatitis, liver necrosis, and hepatic failure.

•Monitor BUN and serum creatinine levels in patients with heart failure, impaired renal function, or hepatic dysfunction; those taking diuretics or ACE inhibitors; and elderly patients because drug may cause renal failure.

•Monitor CBC for decreased hemoglobin and hematocrit because drug may worsen anemia.

•Assess patient's skin routinely for rash or other signs of hypersensitivity reaction because piroxicam and other NSAIDs may cause serious skin reactions without warning, even in patients with no history of NSAID hypersensitivity. Stop drug at first sign of reaction, and notify prescriber.

•**WARNING** Be aware that drug may cause premature closure of ductus arteriosus in growing fetus during third trimester of pregnancy. Be prepared to suggest referral for high-risk pregnancy.

**PATIENT TEACHING**

•Advise patient to take piroxicam with meals to minimize GI distress. Also direct her to take drug with a full glass of water and to remain upright for 30 minutes afterward to decrease the risk of drug lodging in esophagus and causing irritation.

•Instruct patient to swallow capsules whole and not to crush, break, chew, or open them.

•Advise patient to avoid alcohol, aspirin, and other NSAIDs, unless prescribed, while taking piroxicam.

•Caution patient to avoid hazardous activities until drug's CNS effects are known.

•If patient also takes an anticoagulant, advise her to watch for and immediately report bleeding problems, such as bloody or tarry stools and bloody vomitus.

•If patient also takes insulin or an oral antidiabetic, advise her to closely monitor her blood glucose level to prevent hypoglycemia. Encourage her to carry candy or other simple sugars to treat mild hypoglycemia. Advise her to notify prescriber if hypoglycemic episodes are frequent or severe.

•Explain that piroxicam may increase the risk of serious adverse cardiovascular reactions; urge patient to seek immediate medical attention if signs or symptoms arise, such as chest pain, shortness of breath, weakness, and slurring of speech.

•Tell patient that piroxicam may increase the risk of serious adverse GI reactions; stress the need to seek immediate medical attention for such signs and symptoms as epigastric or abdominal pain, indigestion, black or tarry stools, or vomiting blood or material that looks like coffee grounds.

•Alert patient to the possibility of rare but serious skin reactions. Urge her to seek immediate medical attention for rash, blisters, itching, fever, or other indications of hypersensitivity.

•Instruct female patient to consult prescriber if she becomes pregnant because drug may cause premature closure of ductus arteriosus in growing fetus.

# polymyxin B sulfate

Aerosporin

## Class and Category

*Chemical: Bacillus polymyxa* derivative
*Therapeutic:* Antibiotic
*Pregnancy category:* Not rated

## Indications and Dosages

➤ *To treat infections that are resistant to less toxic drugs, such as bacteremia, septicemia, and UTIs caused by susceptible organisms, including* Enterobacter aerogenes, Escherichia coli, Haemophilus influenzae, *and* Klebsiella pneumoniae

## I.V. INFUSION
**Adults and children age 2 and older.**
15,000 to 25,000 U/kg/day in divided doses q 12 hr or as a continuous infusion. *Maximum:* 2 million U/day.
**Infants and children under age 2.** Up to 40,000 U/kg/day in divided doses q 12 hr or as a continuous infusion.

## I.M. INJECTION
**Adults and children age 2 and older.**
25,000 to 30,000 U/kg/day in divided doses q 4 to 6 hr. *Maximum:* 2 million U/day.
**Infants and children under age 2.** Up to 40,000 U/kg/day in divided doses q 4 to 6 hr.

**DOSAGE ADJUSTMENT** Dosage reduced by 50% for patients with creatinine clearance of 5 to 20 ml/min/1.73 m$^2$; by 85% for patients with creatinine clearance of less than 5 ml/min/ 1.73 m$^2$.

➤ *To prevent bacteriuria and bacteremia in patients with an indwelling catheter*

## BLADDER IRRIGATION
**Adults and children age 2 and older.** Combination of 200,000 U (20 mg) of polymyxin B sulfate and 57 mg of neomycin sulfate added to 1,000 ml of NS daily as a continuous bladder irrigation for up to 10 days; rate adjusted as prescribed, based on patient's urine output.

➤ *To treat meningitis caused by susceptible strains of* Pseudomonas aeruginosa *or* H. influenzae

## INTRATHECAL INJECTION
**Adults and children age 2 and older.** 50,000 U q.d. for 3 to 4 days, then 50,000 U q.o.d. for at least 2 wk after CSF cultures are negative and glucose content is normal.
**Infants and children under age 2.** 20,000 U q.d. for 3 to 4 days, then 25,000 U q.o.d. for at least 2 wk after CSF cultures are negative and glucose content is normal.

---

## Mechanism of Action
Binds to cell membrane phospholipids in gram-negative bacteria, increasing the permeability of the cell membrane. Polymyxin B also acts as a cationic detergent, altering the osmotic barrier of the membrane and causing essential intracellular metabolites to leak out. Both actions lead to cell death.

---

## Incompatibilities
Don't mix polymyxin B sulfate with amphotericin B, calcium salts, chloramphenicol, chlorothiazide, heparin sodium, magnesium salts, nitrofurantoin, penicillins, prednisolone, and tetracyclines. They're incompatible.

## Contraindications
Hypersensitivity to polymyxin B or its components

## Interactions
**DRUGS**
*general anesthetics, neuromuscular blockers, skeletal muscle relaxants:* Increased or prolonged skeletal muscle relaxation, possibly respiratory paralysis
*nephrotoxic and neurotoxic drugs (such as aminoglycosides, amphotericin B, colistin, sodium citrate, streptomycin, tobramycin, and vancomycin):* Increased risk of nephrotoxicity and neurotoxicity

## Adverse Reactions
**CNS:** Ataxia, confusion, dizziness, drowsiness, fever, giddiness, headache, increased leukocyte and protein levels in CSF, neurotoxicity, paresthesia (circumoral or peripheral), slurred speech
**CV:** Thrombophlebitis
**EENT:** Blurred vision, nystagmus
**GU:** Albuminuria, azotemia, cylindruria, decreased urine output, hematuria, nephrotoxicity
**HEME:** Eosinophilia
**RESP:** Respiratory muscle paralysis
**SKIN:** Rash, urticaria
**Other**: Anaphylaxis, drug-induced fever, facial flushing, injection site pain, stiff neck (with intrathecal injection), superinfection

## Nursing Considerations
•Be aware that patients receiving polymyxin B sulfate are hospitalized to allow appropriate supervision.
•Obtain blood, urine, or other samples for culture and sensitivity tests, as ordered, before giving drug. Expect to begin polymyxin B therapy before results are known. Keep in mind that baseline renal function tests should have been performed before administration. Check these test results, if available, and notify prescriber of abnormalities.
•For I.M. injection, reconstitute sterile powder with 2 ml of sterile water for injection or sodium chloride for injection.

•Be aware that I.M. route isn't usually recommended (especially for infants and children) because it can cause severe pain at injection site.

•For I.V. infusion, dissolve polymyxin B in 300 to 500 ml of $D_5W$ and infuse over 60 to 90 minutes.

•For intrathecal route, add 10 ml of sodium chloride for injection to vial of polymyxin B.

•Inspect for particles and discoloration before giving drug.

•During therapy, monitor renal function, including BUN and serum creatinine levels, especially in patients with a history of renal insufficiency.

•WARNING Be aware that declining urine output and rising BUN level suggest nephrotoxicity, which also is characterized by albuminuria, azotemia, cylindruria, excessive excretion of electrolytes, hematuria, leukocyturia, and rising blood drug level. Notify prescriber immediately if you detect any of these signs.

•WARNING Notify prescriber immediately if patient experiences blurred vision, circumoral or peripheral paresthesia, confusion, dizziness, drowsiness, facial flushing, giddiness, myasthenia, nystagmus, or slurred speech. These may be signs of neurotoxicity, a serious adverse reaction that may lead to respiratory arrest or paralysis if untreated.

•Assess for signs of superinfection, such as mouth sores, severe diarrhea, and white patches on tongue or in mouth, especially in debilitated or elderly patients.

•Monitor fluid intake and output and provide adequate fluids to reduce the risk of nephrotoxicity.

PATIENT TEACHING
•Encourage patient to maintain adequate fluid intake during polymyxin B therapy.

•Instruct patient to notify prescriber immediately about diarrhea, mouth sores, or vaginitis, which may be early signs of superinfection.

# potassium acetate

*(contains 2 or 4 mEq of elemental potassium per 1 ml of injection)*

## potassium bicarbonate

*(contains 6.5 mEq of elemental potassium per tablet, 20 or 25 mEq of elemental potassium per effervescent tablet for oral solution)*

K+Care ET, K-Electrolyte, K-Ide, Klor-Con/EF, K-Lyte, K-Vescent

## potassium bicarbonate and potassium chloride

*(contains 20 mEq of elemental potassium per 2.8-g granule packet; 20, 25, or 50 mEq of elemental potassium per effervescent tablet for oral solution)*

Klorvess Effervescent Granules, K-Lyte/Cl, K-Lyte/Cl 50, Neo-K (CAN), Potassium Sandoz (CAN)

## potassium bicarbonate and potassium citrate

*(contains 25 or 50 mEq of elemental potassium per effervescent tablet for oral solution)*

Effer-K, K-Lyte DS

## potassium chloride

*(contains 8 or 10 mEq of elemental potassium per E.R. capsule; 6.7, 8, 10, 12, or 20 mEq of elemental potassium per E.R. tablet; 10, 20, 30, or 40 mEq of elemental potassium per 15 ml of oral solution; 10, 15, 20, or 25 mEq of elemental potassium per packet for oral solution; 20 mEq of elemental potassium per packet for oral suspension; 0.1, 0.2, 0.3, 0.4, 1.5, 2, 3, or 10 mEq of elemental potassium per 1 ml of injection)*

Apo-K (CAN), Cena-K, Gen-K, K-8, K-10 (CAN), K+ 10, Kalium Durules (CAN), Kaochlor 10%, Kaochlor S-F 10%, Kaon-Cl, Kato, Kay Ciel, K+ Care, KCL 5% (CAN), K-Dur, K-Ide, K-Lease, K-Long (CAN), K-Lor, Klor-Con 10, Klor-Con Powder, Klor-Con/25 Powder, Klorvess 10% Liquid, Klotrix, K-Lyte/Cl Powder, K-Med 900 (CAN), K-Norm, K-Sol, K-Tab, Micro-K, Micro-K 10, Potasalan, Roychlor 10% (CAN), Rum-K, Slow-K, Ten-K

## potassium gluconate

*(contains 20 mEq of elemental potassium per 15 ml of elixir; 2, 2.3, or 2.5 mEq of elemental potassium per tablet)*

Glu-K, Kaon, Kaylixir, K-G Elixir, Potassium-Rougier (CAN)

## potassium gluconate and potassium chloride

*(contains 20 mEq of elemental potassium per 15 ml of oral solution; 20 mEq of elemental potassium per 5-g packet for oral solution)*

Kolyum

## potassium gluconate and potassium citrate

*(contains 20 mEq of elemental potassium per 15 ml of oral solution)*
Twin-K

## trikates

*(contains 15 mEq of elemental potassium per 5 ml of oral solution)*
Tri-K

## Class and Category

*Chemical:* Electrolyte cation
*Therapeutic:* Electrolyte replacement
*Pregnancy category:* C

## Indications and Dosages

➤ *To prevent or treat hypokalemia in patients who can't ingest sufficient dietary potassium or who are losing potassium because of certain conditions (such as hepatic cirrhosis and prolonged vomiting) or drugs (such as potassium-wasting diuretics and certain antibiotics)*

EFFERVESCENT TABLETS (POTASSIUM BICARBONATE)
**Adults and adolescents.** 25 to 50 mEq/g q.d. or b.i.d., as needed and tolerated. *Maximum:* 100 mEq/day.

EFFERVESCENT TABLETS (POTASSIUM BICARBONATE AND POTASSIUM CHLORIDE)
**Adults and adolescents.** 20, 25, or 50 mEq q.d. or b.i.d., as needed and tolerated. *Maximum:* 100 mEq/day.

EFFERVESCENT TABLETS (POTASSIUM BICARBONATE AND POTASSIUM CITRATE)
**Adults and adolescents.** 25 or 50 mEq q.d. or b.i.d., as needed and tolerated. *Maximum:* 100 mEq/day.

ELIXIR (POTASSIUM GLUCONATE)
**Adults and adolescents.** 20 mEq b.i.d. to q.i.d., as needed and tolerated. *Maximum:* 100 mEq/day.
**Children.** 2 to 3 mEq/kg/day in divided doses.

E.R. CAPSULES (POTASSIUM CHLORIDE)
**Adults and adolescents.** 40 to 100 mEq/day in divided doses b.i.d. or t.i.d. for treatment; 16 to 24 mEq/day in divided doses b.i.d. or. t.i.d. for prevention. *Maximum:* 100 mEq/day.

E.R. TABLETS (POTASSIUM CHLORIDE)
**Adults and adolescents.** 6.7 to 20 mEq t.i.d. *Maximum:* 100 mEq/day.

GRANULE PACKETS (POTASSIUM BICARBONATE AND POTASSIUM CHLORIDE)
**Adults and adolescents.** 20 mEq q.d. or b.i.d., as needed and tolerated. *Maximum:* 100 mEq/day.

GRANULES FOR ORAL SUSPENSION (POTASSIUM CHLORIDE)
**Adults and adolescents.** 20 mEq 1 to 5 times/day, as needed. *Maximum:* 100 mEq/day.

ORAL SOLUTION (POTASSIUM CHLORIDE)
**Adults and adolescents.** 20 mEq q.d. to q.i.d., as needed and tolerated. *Maximum:* 100 mEq/day.
**Children.** 1 to 3 mEq/kg/day in divided doses.

ORAL SOLUTION (POTASSIUM GLUCONATE AND POTASSIUM CHLORIDE, POTASSIUM GLUCONATE AND POTASSIUM CITRATE)
**Adults and adolescents.** 20 mEq b.i.d. to q.i.d., as needed and tolerated. *Maximum:* 100 mEq/day.
**Children.** 2 to 3 mEq/kg/day in divided doses.

POWDER PACKET FOR ORAL SOLUTION (POTASSIUM CHLORIDE)
**Adults.** 15 to 25 mEq b.i.d. to q.i.d., as needed and tolerated. *Maximum:* 100 mEq/day.
**Children.** 1 to 3 mEq/kg/day in divided doses, as needed and tolerated.

POWDER PACKET FOR ORAL SOLUTION (POTASSIUM GLUCONATE AND POTASSIUM CHLORIDE)
**Adults and adolescents.** 20 mEq b.i.d. to q.i.d., as needed and tolerated. *Maximum:* 100 mEq/day.
**Children.** 2 to 3 mEq/kg/day in divided doses.

ORAL TRIKATES SOLUTION (POTASSIUM ACETATE, POTASSIUM BICARBONATE, AND POTASSIUM CITRATE)
**Adults and adolescents.** 15 mEq t.i.d. to q.i.d., as needed and tolerated. *Maximum:* 100 mEq/day.
**Children.** 2 to 3 mEq/kg/day in divided doses.

TABLETS (POTASSIUM GLUCONATE)
**Adults and adolescents.** 5 to 10 mEq b.i.d. to q.i.d., as needed and tolerated. *Maximum:* 100 mEq/day.

I.V. INFUSION (POTASSIUM ACETATE AND POTASSIUM CHLORIDE)
**Adults and adolescents with serum potassium level above 2.5 mEq/L.** Up to 10 mEq/hr. Maximum: 200 mEq/day.
**Adults and adolescents with serum potassium level below 2 mEq/L, ECG changes, or paralysis.** Up to 20 mEq/hr. Maximum: 400 mEq/day.
**Children.** 3 mEq/kg/day.
DOSAGE ADJUSTMENT Dosage adjusted as prescribed based on patient's ECG patterns and serum potassium level.

## Mechanism of Action

Acts as the major cation in intracellular fluid, activating many enzymatic reactions that are essential for physiologic processes, including nerve impulse transmission and cardiac and skeletal muscle contraction. Potassium also helps maintain electroneutrality in cells by controlling the exchange of intracellular and extracellular ions. It also helps maintain normal renal function and acid-base balance.

## Incompatibilities

Don't mix potassium chloride for injection in same syringe with amino acid solutions, lipid solutions, or mannitol because these drugs may precipitate from solution. Administration with blood or blood products can cause lysis of infused RBCs.

## Contraindications

Acute dehydration, Addison's disease (untreated), concurrent use of potassium-sparing diuretics, crush syndrome, heat cramps, hyperkalemia, hypersensitivity to potassium salts or their components, renal impairment with azotemia or oliguria, severe hemolytic anemia

## Interactions

### DRUGS

*ACE inhibitors, beta blockers, blood products, cyclosporine, heparin, NSAIDs, potassium-containing drugs, potassium-sparing diuretics:* Increased risk of hyperkalemia
*amphotericin B, corticosteroids (glucocorticoids or mineralocorticoids), gentamicin, penicillins, polymyxin B:* Possibly hypokalemia
*anticholinergics, drugs with anticholinergic activity:* Increased risk of GI ulceration, stricture, and perforation
*calcium salts (parenteral):* Possibly arrhythmias
*digoxin:* Increased risk of digitalis toxicity
*insulin, laxatives, sodium bicarbonate:* Decreased serum potassium level
*sodium polystyrene sulfonate:* Possibly decreased serum potassium level and fluid retention
*thiazide diuretics:* Possibly hyperkalemia when diuretic is discontinued

### FOODS

*low-salt milk, salt substitutes:* Increased risk of hyperkalemia

## Adverse Reactions

**CNS:** Confusion, paralysis, paresthesia, weakness
**CV:** Arrhythmias, ECG changes
**EENT:** Throat pain when swallowing
**GI:** Abdominal pain; bloody stools; diarrhea; flatulence; GI bleeding, perforation, or ulceration; intestinal obstruction; nausea; vomiting
**RESP:** Dyspnea
**SKIN:** Rash
**Other:** Hyperkalemia

## Nursing Considerations

• Administer oral potassium with or immediately after meals.
• Mix potassium chloride for oral solution or potassium gluconate elixir in cold water, orange juice, tomato juice (if patient isn't sodium restricted), or apple juice, and stir for 1 full minute before administering.
• Mix potassium bicarbonate, potassium bicarbonate and potassium chloride, and potassium bicarbonate and potassium citrate effervescent tablets with cold water and allow to dissolve completely.
• Be aware that liquid form of oral potassium is prescribed for patients with delayed gastric emptying, esophageal compression, or intestinal obstruction or stricture to decrease the risk of tissue damage.
• **WARNING** Be aware that direct injection of a potassium concentrate may be immediately fatal. Dilute potassium concentrate for injection with an adequate volume of solution before I.V. use. Maximum concentration suggested is 40 mEq/L, although stronger concentrations (up to 80 mEq/L) may be used for severe hypokalemia. Inappropriate solutions or improper technique may cause extravasation, fever, hyperkalemia, hypervolemia, I.V. site infection, phlebitis, venospasm, and venous thrombosis.
• Infuse potassium slowly to avoid phlebitis and decrease the risk of adverse cardiac reactions. Keep in mind that different forms of potassium salts contain different amounts of elemental potassium per gram and that not all forms are dosage equivalent.
• Monitor serum potassium level before and during administration of I.V. potassium.
• **WARNING** Be aware that some forms of potassium contain tartrazine, which may cause an allergic reaction, such as asthma.

P

Some forms may also contain aluminum, which may become toxic in a patient with impaired renal function.

•Regularly assess patient for signs of hypokalemia, such as arrhythmias, fatigue, and weakness, and for signs of hyperkalemia, such as arrhythmias, confusion, dyspnea, and paresthesia.

•Because adequate renal function is needed for potassium supplementation, monitor serum creatinine level and urine output during administration. Notify prescriber about signs of decreased renal function.

**PATIENT TEACHING**

•Inform patient that potassium is a normal part of a regular diet and that most meats, seafoods, fruits, and vegetables contain sufficient potassium to meet the recommended daily intake. Also advise her not to exceed the recommended daily amount of potassium.

•Teach patient the correct way to take the prescribed potassium. This can vary from swallowing a tablet with a full glass of water to mixing certain preparations with one-half to a full glass of cold water or juice.

•Caution patient not to crush or chew E.R. forms unless instructed otherwise.

•Instruct patient to take drug with or right after food.

•Teach patient how to take her radial pulse, and advise her to notify prescriber about significant changes in heart rate or rhythm.

•Advise patient to watch stools for changes in color and consistency and to notify prescriber if they become black or tarry or bright red from blood.

•Inform patient that although she may see waxy form of E.R. tablet in stools, she has received all of the potassium.

•Urge patient to keep follow-up laboratory appointments as directed by prescriber to determine serum potassium level.


# potassium iodide

## (KI, SSKI)

Pima, Thyro-Block

## Class and Category

*Chemical:* Iodine
*Therapeutic:* Antithyroid, radiation protectant
*Pregnancy category:* D

## Indications and Dosages

➤ *To prepare for thyroidectomy*
**ORAL SOLUTION**
**Adults and children.** 50 to 250 mg t.i.d. for 10 to 14 days before surgery.
➤ *To manage thyrotoxic crisis*
**ORAL SOLUTION**
**Adults.** 50 to 250 mg t.i.d. or 500 mg q 4 hr.
➤ *To protect thyroid gland during radiation exposure*
**ORAL SOLUTION, SYRUP, TABLETS**
**Adults and adolescents.** 100 to 150 mg 24 hr before administration of or exposure to radioactive isotopes of iodine and q.d. for 3 to 10 days afterward. *Maximum:* 12 g/day.
**Children age 1 and older.** 130 mg q.d. for 10 days after administration of or exposure to radioactive isotopes of iodine.
**Children under age 1.** 65 mg q.d. for 10 days after administration of or exposure to radioactive isotopes of iodine.

| Route | Onset | Peak | Duration |
|---|---|---|---|
| P.O.* | 24 hr | 10 to 15 days | Up to 6 wk |

## Mechanism of Action

Inhibits the release of thyroid hormone into the circulation, thus alleviating symptoms caused by excessive thyroid hormone stimulation. Potassium iodide also blocks thyroidal uptake of radioactive iodine isotopes that are released as a result of radiation exposure.

## Contraindications

Acute bronchitis, Addison's disease, dehydration, heat cramps, hyperkalemia, hypersensitivity to iodides or their components, hyperthyroidism, iodism, renal impairment, tuberculosis

## Interactions

**DRUGS**
*antithyroid drugs, lithium:* Increased risk of hypothyroidism and goiter
*captopril, enalapril, lisinopril, potassium-sparing diuretics:* Increased risk of hyperkalemia

---

*For antithyroid effects.

## Adverse Reactions

**CNS:** Confusion, fatigue, headache, heaviness or weakness in legs, paresthesia
**CV:** Irregular heartbeat
**EENT:** Burning in mouth or throat, increased salivation, metallic taste, sore teeth or gums
**GI:** Diarrhea, epigastric pain, indigestion, nausea, vomiting
**HEME:** Eosinophilia
**MS:** Arthralgia
**SKIN:** Acneiform lesions, urticaria
**Other:** Angioedema, lymphadenopathy

## Nursing Considerations

• Be aware that potassium iodide shouldn't be given to patients with tuberculosis because drug may cause pulmonary irritation and increased secretions.
• **WARNING** Monitor serum potassium level regularly in patients with renal impairment because of the risk of hyperkalemia.
• Monitor thyroid function test results periodically to assess drug's effectiveness.

**PATIENT TEACHING**
• Advise patient taking potassium iodide oral solution or syrup to use a calibrated liquid-measuring device to ensure accurate doses.
• Urge patient to mix solution or syrup in a full glass (8 oz) of water, fruit juice, milk, or broth to improve taste and lessen GI reactions. Advise patient taking tablet form to dissolve each tablet in half a glass (4 oz) of water or milk before ingestion.
• If crystals form in solution, advise patient to place the closed container in warm water and gently shake to dissolve.
• Instruct patient to discard bottle and obtain a new one if solution turns brownish yellow.

# potassium phosphates

K-Phos Original, Neutra-Phos-K

# potassium and sodium phosphates

K-Phos M.F., K-Phos-Neutral, K-Phos No. 2, Neutra-Phos

# sodium phosphates

## Class and Category

*Chemical:* Anion, soluble salts
*Therapeutic:* Antiurolithic, electrolyte replenisher, urinary acidifier
*Pregnancy category:* C

## Indications and Dosages

➤ *As adjunct to treat UTIs, to prevent renal calculus formation*

**MONOBASIC TABLETS (POTASSIUM PHOSPHATES)**
**Adults and adolescents.** 1 g in 180 to 240 ml of water q.i.d., after meals and h.s.

**MONOBASIC TABLETS (POTASSIUM AND SODIUM PHOSPHATES)**
**Adults and adolescents.** 250 mg in 240 ml of water q.i.d., after meals and h.s. Dosage interval may be increased to q 2 hr if urine is difficult to acidify. *Maximum:* 2 g/24 hr.

➤ *To prevent or treat hypophosphatemia*

**CAPSULES (POTASSIUM PHOSPHATES)**
**Adults and children age 4 and older.** 1.45 g in 75 ml of water or juice q.i.d., after meals and h.s.
**Children up to age 4.** 200 mg in 60 ml of water or juice q.i.d., after meals and h.s.

**CAPSULES (POTASSIUM AND SODIUM PHOSPHATES)**
**Adults and children age 4 and older.** 1.25 g in 75 ml of water or juice q.i.d., after meals and h.s.
**Children up to age 4.** 200 mg in 60 ml of water or fruit juice q.i.d., after meals and h.s.

**MONOBASIC TABLETS (POTASSIUM PHOSPHATES)**
**Adults and children age 4 and older.** 1 g in 180 to 240 ml of water q.i.d., after meals and h.s.
**Children up to age 4.** 200 mg in 60 ml of water q.i.d., after meals and h.s.

**MONOBASIC TABLETS (POTASSIUM AND SODIUM PHOSPHATES)**
**Adults and children age 4 and older.** 250 mg in 240 ml of water q.i.d., after meals and h.s.
**Children up to age 4.** 200 mg in 60 ml of water q.i.d., after meals and h.s.

**ORAL SOLUTION (POTASSIUM PHOSPHATES, POTASSIUM AND SODIUM PHOSPHATES)**
**Adults and children age 4 and older.** 250 mg q.i.d., after meals and h.s.
**Children up to age 4.** 200 mg q.i.d., after meals and h.s.

**TABLETS (POTASSIUM AND SODIUM PHOSPHATES)**
**Adults and children age 4 and older.** 250 mg in a full glass of water q.i.d., after meals and h.s.
**Children up to age 4.** 200 mg in 60 ml of water q.i.d., after meals and h.s.

**I.V. INFUSION (SODIUM PHOSPHATES)**
**Adults and adolescents.** 10 to 15 mmol (310 to 465 mg)/day.
**Children.** 1.5 to 2 mmol (46.5 to 62 mg)/kg/day.

## Mechanism of Action

Reverses symptoms of hypophosphatemia by replenishing the body's supply of phosphate; acidifies urine by causing hydrogen to be exchanged for sodium in the renal distal tubule; and inhibits formation of calcium renal calculi by preventing solidification of calcium oxalate.

## Incompatibilities

Don't add phosphates to calcium- or magnesium-containing solutions because precipitate may form.

## Contraindications

Hyperkalemia (potassium formulations only), hypernatremia (sodium formulations only), hyperphosphatemia, magnesium ammonium phosphate urolithiasis accompanied by infection, severe renal insufficiency, UTIs caused by urea-splitting organisms

## Interactions

**DRUGS**

*ACE inhibitors, cyclosporine, heparin (long-term use), NSAIDs, potassium-containing drugs, potassium-sparing diuretics:* Increased risk of hyperkalemia (potassium formulations only)

*aluminum- or magnesium-containing antacids:* Possibly impaired phosphate absorption

*anabolic steroids, androgens, corticosteroids, estrogens:* Increased risk of edema (sodium formulations only)

*calcium-containing drugs:* Increased risk of calcium deposition in soft tissues

*iron supplements:* Decreased absorption of oral iron

*phosphate-containing drugs, vitamin D:* Increased risk of hyperphosphatemia

*salicylates:* Increased blood salicylate level

*zinc supplements:* Reduced zinc absorption

**FOODS**

*low-salt milk, salt substitutes:* Increased risk of hyperkalemia

*oxalates (in spinach and rhubarb), phyates (in bran and whole grains):* Decreased absorption of phosphate

## Adverse Reactions

**CNS:** Anxiety, confusion, dizziness, fatigue, headache, paresthesia, seizures, tremor, weakness

**CV:** Arrhythmias, edema of legs, tachycardia

**GI:** Diarrhea, epigastric pain, nausea, thirst, vomiting

**GU:** Decreased urine output

**MS:** Muscle cramps or weakness

**RESP:** Dyspnea

**Other:** Hyperkalemia, hypernatremia, hyperphosphatemia, hypocalcemia, weight gain

## Nursing Considerations

• Monitor serum phosphorus level, as appropriate, in patient who receives phosphates and has a condition that may be associated with an elevated phosphorus level, such as chronic renal disease, hypoparathyroidism, and rhabdomyolysis; phosphates may further increase serum phosphorus level.

• Monitor serum calcium level, as appropriate, in patient who receives phosphates and has a condition that may be associated with a low calcium level, such as acute pancreatitis, chronic renal disease, hypoparathyroidism, osteomalacia, rhabdomyolysis, and rickets; phosphates may further decrease serum calcium level.

• Monitor serum potassium level, as appropriate, in patient who receives potassium phosphate and has a condition that may be associated with an elevated potassium level, such as acute dehydration, adrenal insufficiency, extensive tissue breakdown (as in severe burns), myotonia congenita, pancreatitis, rhabdomyolysis, and severe renal insufficiency; she may have an increased risk of hyperkalemia.

• Monitor serum sodium level in patient who receives sodium phosphates and has a condition that may be exacerbated by sodium excess, such as heart failure, hypernatremia, hypertension, peripheral or pulmonary edema, preeclampsia, renal impairment, and severe hepatic disease.

• Monitor urine pH, as ordered, to assess drug effectiveness when it's used to acidify urine.

• When administering sodium phosphates, monitor ECG tracing frequently during I.V. infusion to detect arrhythmias.

**PATIENT TEACHING**

• Instruct patient to take phosphates after meals to avoid GI upset and decrease laxative effect.

• Stress the importance of not swallowing capsules or tablets whole; instead, advise patient to soak tablets in water or fruit juice for 2 to 3 minutes to dissolve them.

•Suggest chilling the diluted drug to improve the flavor, but caution against freezing.
•Encourage increased intake of fluids (8 oz/ hour, if not contraindicated) to prevent kidney stones.
•Urge patient to notify prescriber immediately about muscle weakness or cramps, unexplained weight gain, or shortness of breath.
•Instruct patient who needs an iron supplement to take it 1 to 2 hours after taking phosphates.

# pralidoxime chloride

## (2-PAM chloride, 2-pyridine aldoxime methochloride)

Protopam Chloride

### Class and Category
*Chemical:* Quaternary ammonium oxime
*Therapeutic:* Anticholinesterase antidote
*Pregnancy category:* C

### Indications and Dosages
➤ *As adjunct to reverse organophosphate pesticide toxicity*
**I.V. INFUSION, I.M. OR S.C. INJECTION**
**Adults.** *Initial:* 1 to 2 g in 100 ml of NS infused over 15 to 30 min, given concurrently with atropine 2 to 6 mg q 5 to 60 min until muscarinic signs and symptoms disappear; may be repeated in 1 hr and then q 3 to 8 hr if muscle weakness persists. If I.V. route isn't feasible, administer I.M. or S.C.
**Children.** *Initial:* 20 mg/kg in 100 ml of NS infused over 15 to 30 min, given concurrently with atropine (dosage individualized); may be repeated in 1 hr and then q 3 to 8 hr if muscle weakness persists. If I.V. route isn't feasible, administer I.M. or S.C.

➤ *To treat anticholinesterase overdose secondary to myasthenic drugs (including ambenonium, neostigmine, and pyridostigmine)*
**I.V. INJECTION**
**Adults.** *Initial:* 1 to 2 g, followed by 250 mg q 5 min.

➤ *To treat exposure to nerve agents*
**I.V. INJECTION**
**Adults.** *Initial:* 1 atropine-containing autoinjector followed by 1 pralidoxime-containing autoinjector as soon as atropine's effects are evident; both injections repeated q 15 min

for 2 additional doses if nerve agent symptoms persist.
**DOSAGE ADJUSTMENT** Dosage reduced for patients with renal insufficiency.

---

### Mechanism of Action
Reverses muscle paralysis by removing the phosphoryl group from inhibited cholinesterase molecules at the neuromuscular junction of skeletal and respiratory muscles. Reactivation of cholinesterase restores the body's ability to metabolize acetylcholine, which is inhibited by the effects of organophosphate pesticides, anticholinesterase overdose, or nerve agent poisoning.

---

### Contraindications
Hypersensitivity to pralidoxime chloride or its components

### Interactions
**DRUGS**
*aminophylline, morphine, phenothiazines, reserpine, succinylcholine, theophylline:* Increased symptoms of organophosphate poisoning
*barbiturates:* Potentiated barbiturate effects

### Adverse Reactions
**CNS:** Dizziness, drowsiness, headache
**CV:** Increased systolic and diastolic blood pressure, tachycardia
**EENT:** Accommodation disturbances, blurred vision, diplopia
**GI:** Nausea, vomiting
**MS:** Muscle weakness
**RESP:** Hyperventilation
**Other:** Injection site pain

### Nursing Considerations
•Be aware that pralidoxime must be administered within 36 hours of toxicity to be effective.
•Use drug with extreme caution in patients with myasthenia gravis who are being treated for organophosphate poisoning because pralidoxime may precipitate myasthenic crisis.
•Reconstitute drug according to manufacturer's guidelines and administration route.
•For intermittent infusion, further dilute with NS to a volume of 100 ml and infuse over 15 to 30 minutes.

P

•Avoid too-rapid administration, which may cause hypertension, laryngospasm, muscle spasms, neuromuscular blockade, and tachycardia. Also be sure to avoid intradermal injection.

•Closely monitor neuromuscular status during therapy.

•Monitor BUN and serum creatinine levels, as appropriate, in patients with renal insufficiency because drug is excreted in urine.

•When pralidoxime is administered with atropine, expect signs of atropination, such as dry mouth and nose, flushing, mydriasis, and tachycardia, to occur earlier than might be expected when atropine is given alone.

**PATIENT TEACHING**

•Inform patient receiving I.M. pralidoxime that she'll experience pain at the injection site for 40 to 60 minutes afterward.

•Reassure patient that she'll be closely monitored throughout therapy.

# pramipexole dihydrochloride

Mirapex

## Class and Category

*Chemical:* Benzothiazolamine derivative
*Therapeutic:* Antidyskinetic
*Pregnancy category:* C

## Indications and Dosages

➤ *To treat Parkinson's disease, with or without concurrent levodopa therapy*

**TABLETS**

**Adults.** *Initial:* 0.125 mg t.i.d. for 1 wk, increased weekly thereafter as follows: for week 2, 0.25 mg t.i.d.; for week 3, 0.5 mg t.i.d.; for week 4, 0.75 mg t.i.d.; for week 5, 1 mg t.i.d.; for week 6, 1.25 mg t.i.d.; and for week 7, 1.5 mg t.i.d. *Maintenance:* 1.5 to 4.5 mg/day in divided doses t.i.d. *Maximum:* 4.5 mg/day. DOSAGE ADJUSTMENT For patients with renal impairment, dosage reduced as follows: for creatinine clearance of 35 to 59 ml/min/1.73 m$^2$, initial dose of 0.125 mg b.i.d., maximum of 3 mg/day; for creatinine clearance of 15 to 34 ml/min/1.73 m$^2$, initial dose of 0.125 mg q.d., maximum of 1.5 mg/day. Drug should not be given to patients with creatinine clearance of less than 15 ml/min/1.73 m$^2$.

## Mechanism of Action

May stimulate dopamine receptors in the brain, thereby easing symptoms of Parkinson's disease, which is thought to be caused by a dopamine deficiency.

## Contraindications

Hypersensitivity to pramipexole or its components

## Interactions

**DRUGS**

*carbidopa, levodopa:* Possibly increased peak blood levodopa level and potentiation of levodopa's dopaminergic adverse effects
*diltiazem, quinidine, quinine, ranitidine, triamterene, verapamil:* Decreased pramipexole clearance
*haloperidol, metoclopramide, phenothiazines, thioxanthenes:* Decreased pramipexole effectiveness

## Adverse Reactions

**CNS:** Amnesia, anxiety, asthenia, confusion, dream disturbances, drowsiness, dyskinesia, dystonia, fever, hallucinations, insomnia, malaise, paranoia, restlessness
**CV:** Edema, orthostatic hypotension
**EENT:** Diplopia, dry mouth, rhinitis, vision changes
**GI:** Anorexia, constipation, dysphagia, nausea
**GU:** Decreased libido, impotence, urinary frequency, urinary incontinence
**MS:** Arthralgia, myalgia, myasthenia
**RESP:** Pneumonia
**SKIN:** Diaphoresis, rash
**Other:** Weight loss

## Nursing Considerations

•Use pramipexole cautiously in patients with hallucinations, hypotension, or retinal problems (such as macular degeneration) because drug may worsen these conditions.

•Also use cautiously in patients with renal impairment because pramipexole elimination may be decreased.

•Take safety precautions according to facility policy until drug's CNS effects are known.

•Don't discontinue pramipexole therapy abruptly. Sudden withdrawal may cause a symptom complex resembling neuroleptic malignant syndrome, consisting of hyperpyrexia, muscle rigidity, altered level of consciousness, and autonomic instability.

**PATIENT TEACHING**
• Advise patient to take pramipexole with meals if nausea occurs.
• Caution patient about possible dizziness, drowsiness, or light-headedness, which may result from orthostatic hypotension. Advise her not to rise quickly from a lying or sitting position to minimize these effects.
• Instruct patient to notify prescriber immediately about vision problems or urinary frequency or incontinence.
• Inform patient that improvement in motor performance and activities of daily living may take 2 to 3 weeks.

# pramlintide acetate

Symlin

## Class and Category

*Chemical:* Synthetic analogue of human amylin, a pancreatic beta cell hormone
*Therapeutic:* Antidiabetic
*Pregnancy category:* C

## Indications and Dosages

➤ *To achieve euglycemia in patients with type 1 diabetes who use mealtime insulin therapy but have not achieved desired glucose control*

**S.C. INJECTION**

**Adults.** *Initial:* 15 mcg immediately before major meals combined with dosage reduction of preprandial rapid-acting or short-acting insulin, including fixed-mix insulins such as 70/30, by 50%. When nausea has been absent for at least 3 days, dosage increased in increments of 15 mcg. *Maintenance:* 30 to 60 mcg before major meals.
**DOSAGE ADJUSTMENT** Dosage decreased to 30 mcg if nausea occurs and persists at higher dosages.

➤ *To achieve euglycemia in patients with type 2 diabetes who use mealtime insulin, with or without a sulfonylurea and/or metformin, and have not achieved desire glucose control*

**S.C. INJECTION**

**Adults.** *Initial:* 60 mcg immediately before major meals combined with dosage reduction of preprandial rapid-acting or short-acting insulin, including fixed-mix insulins such as 70/30, by 50%. When nausea has been absent

for 3 to 7 days, dosage increased to 120 mcg before major meals.
**DOSAGE ADJUSTMENT** Dosage decreased to 60 mcg before major meals if nausea occurs and persists with 120-mcg dosage.

| Route | Onset | Peak | Duration |
|-------|-------|------|----------|
| S.C. | Unknown | 19 to 21 min | 3 hr |

## Mechanism of Action

Slows the rate at which food is released from the stomach to the small intestine, thus reducing the initial postprandial rise in serum glucose level. Pramlintide also suppresses glucagon secretion and promotes satiety, thus furthering weight loss, which also lowers serum glucose level.
Pramlintide is a synthetic analogue of amylin, a naturally occurring neuroendocrine hormone secreted with insulin by pancreatic beta cells. In diabetes, secretion of insulin and amylin is reduced or absent.

## Contraindications

Gastroparesis, hypersensitivity to pramlintide, cresol or its components; hypoglycemia unawareness

## Incompatibilities

Do not mix in same syringe as insulin because pharmacokinetic parameters of pramlintide become altered.

## Interactions

**DRUGS**

*drugs that alter GI motility (such as anticholinergics) or slow intestinal absorption of nutrients (such as alpha-glucosidase inhibitors):* Altered effects of these drugs
*oral drugs:* Delayed absorption

## Adverse Reactions

**CNS:** Dizziness, fatigue, headache
**EENT:** Blurred vision, pharyngitis
**ENDO:** Insulin-induced hypoglycemia
**GI:** Abdominal pain, anorexia, nausea, vomiting
**MS:** Arthralgia
**RESP:** Coughing
**SKIN:** Diaphoresis
**Other:** Hypersensitivity reactions; local injection site reaction, such as redness, swelling, or pruritus

## Nursing Considerations
•Because of the risks involved with pramlintide therapy, insulin-using patients with type 1 or 2 diabetes must have failed to achieve adequate glycemic control despite individualized insulin management and must be receiving ongoing care under the guidance of the insulin prescriber and a diabetes educator before pramlintide is prescribed.
•Expect that certain patients won't be prescribed pramlintide because its risks may outweigh its benefits. These include patients with poor compliance to the current insulin regimen, poor compliance with monitoring blood glucose level, a glycosylated hemoglobin greater than 9%, recurrent severe hypoglycemia that required assistance during the past 6 months, hypoglycemia unawareness, gastroparesis, concurrent therapy with drugs that stimulate GI motility, and pediatric patients.
•Before pramlintide therapy starts, make sure patient's pre-meal insulin dosage has been reduced by 50%.
•Give pramlintide immediately before major meals.
•Monitor patient's pre- and post-meal blood glucose levels regularly to determine effectiveness of pramlintide and insulin therapy and to detect hypoglycemia.
•For 3 hours after each dose of pramlintide, monitor patient closely for hypoglycemia, which may be severe, especially in patients with type 1 diabetes. Effects may include hunger, headache, sweating, tremor, irritability, and trouble concentrating. They may occur with a rapid decrease in blood glucose level regardless of glucose values.
•Although pramlintide doesn't cause hypoglycemia, it's use with insulin increases the risk of insulin-induced severe hypoglycemia, which can result in loss of consciousness, coma, or seizures. If hypoglycemia occurs, provide supportive care, including glucagon if prescribed, and notify prescriber. Expect insulin dosage accompanying pramlintide to be reduced.
•Keep in mind that early warning symptoms of hypoglycemia may be different or less severe if patient has had diabetes for a long time; has diabetic nerve disease; takes a beta blocker, clonidine, guanethidine, or reserpine; or is under intensified diabetes control.
•Closely monitor patients who are taking oral antidiabetics, ACE inhibitors, disopyramide, fibrates, fluoxetine, MAO inhibitors, pentoxifylline, propoxyphene, salicylates, or sulfonamide antibiotics because of an increased risk of hypoglycemia.
•Expect pramlintide to be stopped if patient develops recurrent hypoglycemia that requires medical assistance, develops persistent nausea, or becomes noncompliant with therapy or follow-up visits.

**PATIENT TEACHING**
•Alert patient that insulin-induced hypoglycemia may occur within 3 hours of injecting pramlintide. Review signs and symptoms and appropriate treatment. Tell patient to notify prescriber if hypoglycemia occurs because insulin dosage will need to be reduced.
•Stress importance of monitoring blood glucose level often, especially before and after eating.
•Tell patient to inject drug subcutaneously immediately before major meals using an insulin syringe to draw up dose and using the same technique as with insulin administration, including rotating sites. Advise patient to inject drug into her abdomen or thigh and not to use her arm as an injection site because absorption may be too variable.
•Warn patient not to mix pramlintide and insulin together in the same syringe.
•Warn patient that nausea is common with pramlintide; urge her to notify prescriber because dosage may need to be decreased.
•Caution patient that if she misses a dose of pramlintide, she should skip the missed dose and continue with the next scheduled dose.
•Instruct patient to keep unopened pramlintide vials in the refrigerator; vials that have been opened may be kept in the refrigerator or at room temperature. Vials should be discarded 28 days after opening.
•Caution patient to avoid hazardous activities that require mental alertness until effects of pramlintide are known.
•Reassure patient that pramlintide won't alter her awareness of or her body's response to insulin-induced hypoglycemia.
•Alert patient that she'll need close follow-up care, at least weekly until a target dose of pramlintide has been reached, she's tolerating the drug well, and her blood glucose level is stable.

•Instruct female patients of childbearing age to notify prescriber about planned, suspected, or known pregnancy because drug therapy will need to be adjusted.
•Tell patient that local injection site reactions, such as redness, swelling or itching, may occur but that they usually resolve within a few weeks.

# pravastatin sodium

Pravachol

## Class and Category

*Chemical*: Mevinic acid derivative
*Therapeutic*: Antihyperlipidemic
*Pregnancy category*: X

## Indications and Dosages

➤ *To prevent coronary and cardiovascular events in patients at risk, to treat hyperlipidemia*

**TABLETS**

**Adults.** *Initial*: 10 to 40 mg q.d. h.s., increased q 4 wk, as needed. *Maintenance*: 10 to 80 mg h.s.
**DOSAGE ADJUSTMENT** For patients with significant renal or hepatic impairment, those taking immunosuppressants, and elderly patients, initial dosage reduced to 10 mg q.d. h.s. For elderly patients and those taking immunosuppressants, maintenance dosage usually limited to 20 mg/day.

➤ *To treat pediatric heterozygous familial hypercholesterolemia*

**TABLETS**

**Adolescents ages 14 to 18.** 40 mg q.d. h.s.
**Children ages 8 to 14.** 20 mg q.d. h.s.

---

### Mechanism of Action

Inhibits cholesterol synthesis in the liver by blocking the enzyme needed to convert hydroxymethylglutaryl-CoA (HMG-CoA) to mevalonate, an early precursor of cholesterol. When cholesterol synthesis is blocked, the liver also increases the breakdown of LDL cholesterol.

---

## Contraindications

Active hepatic disease or unexplained, persistent elevated liver function test results; breast-feeding; hypersensitivity to pravastatin or its components; pregnancy

## Interactions

**DRUGS**

*cholestyramine, colestipol:* Decreased pravastatin bioavailability
*cyclosporine, erythromycin, gemfibrozil, immunosuppressants, niacin:* Increased risk of rhabdomyolysis and acute renal failure
*oral anticoagulants:* Increased bleeding or prolonged PT

## Adverse Reactions

**CNS:** Anxiety, depression, dizziness, fatigue, headache, nervousness, sleep disturbance
**CV:** Angina pectoris, chest pain
**EENT:** Blurred vision, diplopia, rhinitis
**ENDO:** Abnormal thyroid function
**GI:** Abdominal pain, constipation, diarrhea, elevated liver function test results, flatulence, heartburn, indigestion, nausea, pancreatitis, vomiting
**GU:** Dysuria, nocturia, urinary frequency
**MS:** Arthralgia, musculoskeletal cramps or pain, myalgia, myopathy, rhabdomyolysis
**RESP:** Cough, dyspnea, upper respiratory tract infection
**SKIN:** Rash
**Other:** Angioedema

## Nursing Considerations

•Use pravastatin cautiously in patients with renal or hepatic impairment and in elderly patients.
•Monitor liver function test results before pravastatin therapy starts, before dosage increases, and periodically throughout therapy, as prescribed.
•Give drug 1 hour before or 4 hours after giving cholestyramine or colestipol.
•Report unexplained muscle aches or weakness and significant increases in CK level to prescriber because drug rarely causes rhabdomyolysis with acute renal failure caused by myoglobinuria. Expect to stop drug and provide supportive care.
•Monitor BUN and serum creatinine levels periodically for abnormal elevations.
•Monitor blood lipoprotein level, as indicated, to evaluate response to therapy.

**PATIENT TEACHING**

•Instruct patient to take drug at bedtime, without regard to meals.
•Advise patient to notify prescriber immediately about muscle pain, tenderness, weak-

P

ness, and other signs and symptoms of myopathy.
• Urge female patient of childbearing age to use a reliable method of contraception during therapy and to notify prescriber at once if she becomes or might be pregnant.
• Instruct patient not to discontinue drug without consulting prescriber, even when cholesterol level returns to normal.

# prazosin hydrochloride

Minipress

## Class and Category
*Chemical:* Quinazoline derivative
*Therapeutic:* Antihypertensive
*Pregnancy category:* C

## Indications and Dosages
➤ *To manage hypertension*
**CAPSULES**
**Adults.** *Initial:* 1 mg b.i.d. or t.i.d. *Maintenance:* 6 to 15 mg/day in divided doses b.i.d. or t.i.d. *Maximum:* 40 mg/day.
**Children.** *Initial:* 50 to 400 mcg/kg/day in divided doses b.i.d. or t.i.d. *Maximum:* 7 mg/dose, 15 mg/day.
**TABLETS**
**Adults.** *Initial:* 0.5 mg b.i.d. or t.i.d. for at least 3 days, then increased to 1 mg b.i.d. or t.i.d., if tolerated, for an additional 3 days. Subsequent dosages adjusted gradually, as needed and tolerated. *Maintenance:* 6 to 15 mg/day in divided doses b.i.d. or t.i.d. *Maximum:* 40 mg/day.
**Children.** *Initial:* 50 to 400 mcg/kg/day in divided doses b.i.d. or t.i.d. *Maximum:* 7 mg/dose, 15 mg/day.
**DOSAGE ADJUSTMENT** For elderly patients and those with renal impairment, initial dosage possibly reduced to 1 mg q.d. to b.i.d.

| Route | Onset | Peak | Duration |
|-------|-------|------|----------|
| P.O. | 0.5 to 1.5 hr | 2 to 4 hr* | 7 to 10 hr |

## Contraindications
Hypersensitivity to prazosin, other quinazolines, or their components

---

* For a single dose; 3 to 4 wk for multiple doses.

## Mechanism of Action
Selectively and competitively inhibits alpha$_1$-adrenergic receptors. This action promotes peripheral arterial and venous dilation and reduces peripheral vascular resistance, thereby lowering blood pressure.

## Interactions
**DRUGS**
*beta blockers, diuretics, other antihypertensives:* Increased risk of hypotension and syncope
*dopamine:* Antagonized peripheral vasoconstrictive effect of dopamine (with high doses)
*ephedrine:* Decreased vasopressor response to ephedrine
*epinephrine:* Possibly severe hypotension and tachycardia
*metaraminol:* Decreased vasopressor effect of metaraminol
*methoxamine, phenylephrine:* Possibly decreased vasopressor effect and shortened duration of action of these drugs
*NSAIDs, sympathomimetics:* Decreased effectiveness of prazosin

## Adverse Reactions
**CNS:** Dizziness, drowsiness, fatigue, headache, malaise, nervousness, syncope
**CV:** Edema, orthostatic hypotension, palpitations
**EENT:** Dry mouth
**GI:** Nausea
**GU:** Urinary frequency, urinary incontinence

## Nursing Considerations
• Use prazosin cautiously in patients with renal impairment because of increased sensitivity to prazosin's effects; in those with angina pectoris because drug may induce or aggravate angina; in those with narcolepsy because prazosin may exacerbate cataplexy; and in elderly patients because they're at increased risk for drug-induced hypotension.
• Monitor blood pressure regularly to evaluate effectiveness of therapy.
**PATIENT TEACHING**
• Instruct patient who is beginning prazosin therapy to take drug at bedtime to minimize effects of first-dose hypotension.
• Stress the importance of taking drug even when feeling well.

•Advise patient to avoid drinking alcohol, standing for long periods, and exercising in hot weather because these activities increase the risk of orthostatic hypotension.

•Suggest rising slowly from a lying or sitting position to minimize the effects of orthostatic hypotension.

•Urge patient to avoid potentially hazardous activities until drug's CNS effects are known.

•Advise patient to notify prescriber immediately about adverse reactions, especially dizziness and fainting.

•Instruct patient not to take any drugs, including OTC preparations, without first consulting prescriber to avoid serious interactions.

# prednisolone

Cotolone, Delta-Cortef, Prelone

## prednisolone acetate

Articulose-50, Key-Pred, Predacort 50, Predalone 50, Predate 50, Predcor-25, Predcor-50, Pred-Ject 50

## prednisolone sodium phosphate

Pediapred

## prednisolone tebutate

Nor-Pred T.B.A., Predalone T.B.A., Predate TBA, Predcor-TBA

### Class and Category
*Chemical:* Glucocorticoid
*Therapeutic:* Anti-inflammatory, immunosuppressant
*Pregnancy category:* C

### Indications and Dosages
➤ *To treat adrenal insufficiency and acute and chronic inflammatory and immunosuppressive disorders*
SYRUP, TABLETS (PREDNISOLONE); ORAL SOLUTION (PREDNISOLONE SODIUM PHOSPHATE)
**Adults and adolescents.** 5 to 60 mg q.d. or in divided doses. *Maximum:* 250 mg/day.
I.M. INJECTION (PREDNISOLONE ACETATE)
**Adults and adolescents.** 4 to 60 mg/day.
INTRA-ARTICULAR, INTRALESIONAL, OR SOFT-TISSUE INJECTION (PREDNISOLONE ACETATE, PREDNISOLONE TEBUTATE)
**Adults and adolescents.** 4 to 100 mg of prednisolone acetate, repeated as needed, or 4 to 40 mg of prednisolone tebutate, repeated q 1 to 3 wk, as needed.

➤ *To treat adrenocortical insufficiency in children*
SYRUP, TABLETS (PREDNISOLONE); ORAL SOLUTION (PREDNISOLONE SODIUM PHOSPHATE)
**Children.** 0.14 mg/kg/day in divided doses t.i.d.
I.M. INJECTION (PREDNISOLONE ACETATE)
**Children.** 0.14 mg/kg over a 24-hr period in divided doses t.i.d. q third day.

➤ *To treat acute exacerbations of multiple sclerosis*
SYRUP, TABLETS (PREDNISOLONE); ORAL SOLUTION (PREDNISOLONE SODIUM PHOSPHATE)
**Adults.** 200 mg/day for 1 wk, followed by 80 mg q.o.d. for 1 mo.

### Contraindications
Hypersensitivity to prednisolone or its components, idiopathic thrombocytopenic purpura (I.M. form), systemic fungal infection

### Interactions
**DRUGS**
*acetaminophen:* Possibly hepatotoxicity (with long-term use or high doses of acetaminophen)
*acetazolamide:* Possibly hypernatremia or edema
*amphotericin B (parenteral):* Possibly severe hypokalemia
*anabolic steroids, androgens:* Possibly edema and severe acne
*anticholinergics:* Increased intraocular pressure
*asparaginase:* Increased hyperglycemic effect of asparaginase, possibly neuropathy and disturbances in erythropoiesis
*carbonic anhydrase inhibitors:* Possibly hypocalcemia, hypokalemia, and osteoporosis
*digoxin:* Possibly arrhythmias and digitalis toxicity from hypokalemia
*diuretics:* Possibly decreased natriuretic and diuretic effects of diuretics, severe hypokalemia (with potassium-depleting diuretics)
*ephedrine:* Increased metabolic clearance of prednisolone
*estrogens, oral contraceptives:* Decreased clearance, increased elimination half-life, and increased therapeutic and toxic effects of prednisolone
*folic acid:* Increased folic acid requirements (with long-term prednisolone use)
*heparin, oral anticoagulants, streptokinase, urokinase:* Possibly decreased anticoagulant

P

effect and increased risk of GI ulceration and bleeding

*immunosuppressants:* Increased risk of infection, lymphomas, and other lymphoproliferative disorders

*isoniazid:* Decreased blood isoniazid level

*mexiletine:* Possibly accelerated metabolism and decreased blood level of mexiletine

*neuromuscular blockers:* Increased neuromuscular blockade

*NSAIDs:* Increased risk of GI ulceration and bleeding, possibly added therapeutic effect when NSAIDs are used to treat arthritis

*potassium supplements:* Decreased effectiveness of both drugs

*rifampin, other hepatic enzyme inducers:* Decreased prednisolone effect

*ritodrine:* Increased risk of pulmonary edema in pregnant women

*salicylates:* Possibly decreased blood salicylate level, increased risk of GI ulceration and bleeding

*sodium-containing drugs:* Possibly edema and hypertension

*somatrem, somatropin:* Inhibited growth response to somatrem or somatropin

*streptozocin:* Increased risk of hyperglycemia

*toxoids, vaccines:* Possibly loss of antibody response, increased risk of neurologic complications

*tricyclic antidepressants:* Possibly exacerbated adverse psychiatric effects of prednisolone

*troleandomycin:* Increased therapeutic and toxic effects of prednisolone

**FOODS**

*sodium-containing foods:* Increased risk of edema and hypertension

**ACTIVITIES**

*alcohol use:* Increased risk of GI ulceration and bleeding

| Route | Onset | Peak | Duration |
|---|---|---|---|
| P.O. (prednisolone) | Unknown | 1 to 2 hr | 1.25 to 1.5 days |
| I.M. (prednisolone acetate) | Slow | Unknown | Unknown |
| Intra-articular, intralesional, soft-tissue injection (prednisolone tebutate) | 1 to 2 days | Unknown | 1 to 3 wk |

## Mechanism of Action

Binds to intracellular glucocorticoid receptors and suppresses inflammatory and immune responses by:
- inhibiting neutrophil and monocyte accumulation at inflammation site and suppressing their phagocytic and bactericidal activity
- stabilizing lysosomal membranes
- suppressing antigen response of macrophages and helper T cells
- inhibiting synthesis of inflammatory response mediators, such as cytokines, interleukins, and prostaglandins.

## Adverse Reactions

**CNS:** Euphoria, headache, insomnia, nervousness, psychosis, restlessness, seizures, vertigo

**CV:** Edema, heart failure, hypertension

**EENT:** Cataracts, exophthalmos, glaucoma, increased ocular pressure

**ENDO:** Adrenal insufficiency, Cushing's syndrome, growth suppression in children, hyperglycemia

**GI:** Anorexia, GI bleeding and ulceration, increased appetite, indigestion, intestinal perforation, nausea, pancreatitis, vomiting

**GU:** Menstrual irregularities

**MS:** Avascular necrosis of joints, bone fractures, muscle atrophy or weakness, myalgia, osteoporosis, tendon rupture (local injection only)

**SKIN:** Acne; cutaneous or subcutaneous atrophy (with frequent repository injections); diaphoresis; ecchymosis; flushing; petechiae; striae; thin, fragile skin

**Other:** Delayed wound healing, hypernatremia, hypokalemia, injection site scarring, negative nitrogen balance

## Nursing Considerations

- **WARNING** Avoid using prednisolone in patients with a history of active tuberculosis because drug can reactivate the disease.
- Administer once-daily doses in the morning to match the body's normal cortisol secretion schedule.
- Inspect injectable form for particulates and discoloration before administering.
- For I.M. injection, shake suspension well before withdrawing. Notify prescriber if patient has idiopathic thrombocytopenic purpura because I.M. injections are contraindicated.

•For intra-articular injection, attach a 20G to 24G needle to an empty syringe, using aseptic technique, so prescriber can remove a few drops of synovial fluid to confirm that needle is in the joint. The aspirating syringe is then exchanged with a prenisolone-filled syringe to inject drug into joint.

•Because prednisolone can produce many adverse reactions, assess patient regularly for signs and symptoms of such reactions, including heart failure and hypertension. Also monitor patient's intake, output, and daily weight.

•Monitor growth pattern in children because prednisolone may retard bone growth.

•Be aware that prolonged use may cause hypothalamic-pituitary-adrenal suppression.

•**WARNING** Withdraw drug gradually, as ordered, if therapy lasts longer than 2 weeks. Abrupt discontinuation may cause acute adrenal insufficiency or, possibly, death.

•Be aware that patient may be at risk for emotional instability or psychic disturbance while taking prednisolone, especially if she is predisposed to these conditions or is taking high doses.

**PATIENT TEACHING**

•Instruct patient to take oral prednisolone with food to decrease stomach upset and to take once-daily dose in the morning.

•Stress the importance of taking drug exactly as prescribed; taking too much increases the risk of serious adverse reactions.

•Caution patient not to discontinue drug abruptly.

•Urge patient to avoid alcohol during therapy because of increased risk of GI ulcers and bleeding.

•Encourage patient to avoid potentially hazardous activities until drug's CNS effects are known.

•Advise patient to avoid people with contagious infections because drug has an immunosuppressant effect. Urge her to notify prescriber immediately about exposure to measles or chickenpox.

•Caution against receiving vaccinations or other immunizations and coming in contact with people who have recently received the oral poliovirus vaccine.

•Teach patient about potential side effects of prednisolone therapy, including restlessness, mood swings, nervousness, and delayed wound healing.

•Instruct patient to notify prescriber imme-

diately about joint pain, swelling, tarry stools, and visual disturbances. Also instruct her to report signs of infection or injury for up to 12 months after therapy.

•Advise patient to restrict joint use after intra-articular injection and to obtain activity guidelines from prescriber.

•Instruct diabetic patient to monitor her blood glucose level frequently because prednisolone may cause hyperglycemia.

•Advise patient to comply with follow-up visits to assess drug's effectiveness and detect adverse reactions.

•Encourage patient to carry or wear medical identification notifying others of prednisolone therapy.

# prednisone

Apo-Prednisone (CAN), Deltasone Liquid Pred, Meticorten, Orasone 1, Orasone 5, Orasone 10, Prednicen-M, Prednicot, Prednisone Intensol, Sterapred, Sterapred DS, Winpred (CAN)

## Class and Category

*Chemical:* Glucocorticoid
*Therapeutic:* Anti-inflammatory, immunosuppressant
*Pregnancy category:* Not rated

## Indications and Dosages

➤ *To treat adrenal insufficiency and acute and chronic inflammatory and immunosuppressive disorders*

**ORAL SOLUTION, SYRUP, TABLETS**

**Adults and adolescents.** 5 to 60 mg/day as a single dose or in divided doses. *Maximum:* 250 mg/day.

➤ *To treat adrenogenital syndrome*

**ORAL SOLUTION, SYRUP, TABLETS**

**Adults and adolescents.** 5 to 10 mg q.d.
**Children.** 5 mg/m$^2$/day in divided doses b.i.d.

➤ *To treat acute exacerbations of multiple sclerosis*

**ORAL SOLUTION, SYRUP, TABLETS**

**Adults.** 200 mg q.d. for 1 wk, then 80 mg q.o.d. for 1 mo. *Maximum:* 250 mg/day.

➤ *To treat nephrosis in children*

**ORAL SOLUTION, SYRUP, TABLETS**

**Children age 10 and older.** 20 mg q.i.d.
**Children ages 4 to 10.** 15 mg q.i.d.

P

**Children ages 18 months to 4 years.** 7.5 to 10 mg q.i.d.

➤ *To treat rheumatic carditis, leukemia, and tumors in children*

**ORAL SOLUTION, SYRUP, TABLETS**

**Children.** 0.5 mg/kg q.i.d. for 2 to 3 wk, then 0.375 mg/kg q.i.d. for 4 to 6 wk.

➤ *As adjunct to treat tuberculosis in children (with concurrent antitubercular therapy)*

**ORAL SOLUTION, SYRUP, TABLETS**

**Children.** 0.5 mg/kg q.i.d. for 2 mo.

| Route | Onset | Peak | Duration |
|-------|-------|------|----------|
| P.O. | Rapid | 1 to 2 hr | 1.25 to 1.5 days |

## Mechanism of Action

Binds to intracellular glucocorticoid receptors and suppresses inflammatory and immune responses by:
• inhibiting neutrophil and monocyte accumulation at inflammation site and suppressing their phagocytic and bactericidal activity
• stabilizing lysosomal membranes
• suppressing antigen response of macrophages and helper T cells
• inhibiting synthesis of inflammatory response mediators, such as cytokines, interleukins, and prostaglandins.

## Contraindications

Hypersensitivity to prednisone or its components, systemic fungal infection

## Interactions

### DRUGS

*acetaminophen:* Possibly hepatotoxicity (with long-term use or high doses of acetaminophen)
*acetazolamide sodium:* Possibly hypernatremia or edema
*amphotericin B (parenteral):* Possibly severe hypokalemia
*anabolic steroids, androgens:* Possibly edema and severe acne
*antacids:* Decreased absorption of prednisone (with long-term use)
*anticholinergics:* Increased intraocular pressure
*asparaginase:* Increased hyperglycemic effect of asparaginase, possibly neuropathy and disturbances in erythropoiesis

*carbonic anhydrase inhibitors:* Possibly hypocalcemia, hypokalemia, and osteoporosis
*digoxin:* Possibly arrhythmias and digitalis toxicity from hypokalemia
*diuretics:* Possibly decreased natriuretic and diuretic effects of diuretics, severe hypokalemia (with potassium-depleting diuretics)
*ephedrine:* Increased metabolic clearance of prednisone
*estrogens, oral contraceptives:* Decreased clearance, increased elimination half-life, and increased therapeutic and toxic effects of prednisone
*folic acid:* Increased folic acid requirements (with long-term prednisone use)
*heparin, oral anticoagulants, streptokinase, urokinase:* Possibly decreased anticoagulant effect and increased risk of GI ulceration and bleeding
*immunosuppressants:* Increased risk of infection, lymphomas, and other lymphoproliferative disorders
*isoniazid:* Decreased blood isoniazid level
*mexiletine:* Possibly accelerated metabolism and decreased blood level of mexiletine
*neuromuscular blockers:* Increased neuromuscular blockade
*NSAIDs:* Increased risk of GI ulceration and bleeding, possibly added therapeutic effect when NSAIDs are used to treat arthritis
*potassium supplements:* Decreased effectiveness of both drugs
*ritodrine:* Increased risk of pulmonary edema in pregnant women
*salicylates:* Possibly decreased blood salicylate level, increased risk of GI ulceration and bleeding
*sodium-containing drugs:* Possibly edema and hypertension
*somatrem, somatropin:* Inhibited growth response to somatrem or somatropin
*streptozocin:* Increased risk of hyperglycemia
*toxoids, vaccines:* Possibly loss of antibody response, increased risk of neurologic complications
*tricyclic antidepressants:* Possibly exacerbated adverse psychiatric effects of prednisone
*troleandomycin:* Increased therapeutic and toxic effects of prednisone

### FOODS

*sodium-containing foods:* Increased risk of edema and hypertension

**ACTIVITIES**
*alcohol use:* Increased risk of GI ulceration and bleeding

## Adverse Reactions
**CNS:** Euphoria, headache, insomnia, nervousness, psychosis, restlessness, seizures, vertigo
**CV:** Edema, heart failure, hypertension
**EENT:** Cataracts, exophthalmos, glaucoma, increased ocular pressure
**ENDO:** Adrenal insufficiency, Cushing's syndrome, growth suppression in children, hyperglycemia
**GI:** Anorexia, GI bleeding and ulceration, increased appetite, indigestion, intestinal perforation, nausea, pancreatitis, vomiting
**GU:** Menstrual irregularities
**MS:** Avascular necrosis of joints, bone fractures, muscle atrophy or weakness, myalgia, osteoporosis
**SKIN:** Acne; diaphoresis; ecchymosis; flushing; petechiae; striae; thin, fragile skin
**Other:** Delayed wound healing, hypernatremia, hypokalemia, negative nitrogen balance

## Nursing Considerations
•Administer once-daily doses of prednisone in the morning to match the body's normal cortisol secretion schedule.
•Because prednisone can produce many adverse reactions, assess regularly for signs and symptoms of such reactions as heart failure and hypertension. Also monitor fluid intake and output and daily weight.
•Monitor growth pattern in children because prednisone may retard bone growth.
•Be aware that prolonged use of prednisone may cause hypothalamic-pituitary-adrenal suppression.
•**WARNING** Withdraw prednisone gradually, as ordered, if therapy lasts longer than 2 weeks. Abrupt discontinuation may cause acute adrenal insufficiency and, possibly, death.

**PATIENT TEACHING**
•Instruct patient to take prednisone with food to decrease GI distress and to take once-daily dose in the morning.
•Stress the importance of taking drug exactly as prescribed; taking more than prescribed dosage increases the risk of serious adverse reactions.
•Caution patient not to discontinue drug abruptly.

•Urge patient to avoid alcohol during therapy because of the increased risk of GI ulcers and bleeding.
•Encourage patient to avoid potentially hazardous activities until drug's CNS effects are known.
•Advise patient to avoid people with contagious infections because drug has an immunosuppressant effect. Urge her to notify prescriber immediately about possible exposure to measles or chickenpox.
•Caution against receiving vaccinations or other immunizations and coming in contact with people who have recently received the oral poliovirus vaccine.
•Instruct patient to notify prescriber immediately about joint pain, swelling, tarry stools, and visual disturbances. Also instruct her to report signs of infection or injury for up to 12 months after therapy.
•Instruct diabetic patient to monitor her blood glucose level frequently because prednisone may cause hyperglycemia.
•Advise patient to comply with follow-up visits to assess drug effectiveness and detect adverse reactions.
•Encourage patient to carry or wear medical identification to notify others of prednisone therapy.

# pregabalin
Lyrica

## Class and Category
*Chemical:* Structural derivative of gamma-aminobutyric acid (GABA)
*Therapeutic:* Analgesic, anticonvulsant
*Pregnancy category:* C

## Indications and Dosages
➤ *To relieve neuropathic pain associated with diabetic peripheral neuropathy*
**CAPSULES**
**Adults.** *Initial:* 50 mg t.i.d., increased to 100 mg t.i.d. within 1 wk as needed.
➤ *To relieve postherpetic neuralgia; as adjunct therapy to manage partial onset seizures*
**CAPSULES**
**Adults.** *Initial:* 75 mg b.i.d. or 50 mg t.i.d., increased to 150 mg b.i.d. or 100 mg t.i.d. within 1 week as needed. Then increased to

300 mg b.i.d. or 200 mg t.i.d. in 2 to 4 weeks as needed.

DOSAGE ADJUSTMENT If patient's creatinine clearance is 30 to 60 ml/min/1.73 m², daily dosage reduced by 50%. If creatinine clearance is 15 to 30 ml/min/1.73 m², daily dosage reduced by 75% and frequency reduced to q.d. or b.i.d. If creatinine clearance is less than 15 ml/min/1.73 m², daily dosage decreased to as low as 25 mg q.d. If patient has hemodialysis, daily dosage is reduced and supplemental dose given immediately after every 4-hour hemodialysis session as follows: If reduced daily dosage is 25 mg q.d., give supplemental dose of 25 to 50 mg. If reduced daily dosage is 25 to 50 mg q.d., give supplemental dose of 50 to 75 mg. If reduced daily dosage is 75 mg, give supplemental dose of 100 to 150 mg.

| Route | Onset | Peak | Duration |
|-------|-------|------|----------|
| P.O. | Unknown | 1.5 hr | Unknown |

## Mechanism of Action

Binds to the alpha₂-delta site, an auxiliary subunit of voltage calcium channels, in CNS tissue where it may reduce calcium-dependent release of several neurotransmitters, possibly by modulating calcium channel function. With fewer neurotransmitters present, pain sensation and seizure activity are reduced.

## Contraindications

Hypersenstivity to pregabalin or its components

## Interactions

**DRUGS**

*CNS depressants:* Additive CNS effects such as somnolence
*lorazepam, oxycodone:* Additive effects on cognitive and gross motor function
*thiazolidinedione antidiabetics:* Possibly increased risk of peripheral edema and weight gain

**ACTIVITIES**

*alcohol use:* Additive effects on cognitive and gross motor function

## Adverse Reactions

**CNS:** Abnormal gait, amnesia, anxiety, asthenia, ataxia, confusion, difficulty concentrating, dizziness, euphoria, extrapyramidal syndrome, fever, headache, hypertonia, hypesthesia, incoordination, intracranial hypertension, myoclonus, nervousness, neuropathy, paresthesia, psychotic depression, schizophrenic reaction, somnolence, stupor, tremor, twitching, vertigo
**CV:** Chest pain, heart failure, peripheral edema, ventricular fibrillation
**EENT:** Amblyopia, blurred vision, conjunctivitis, decreased visual acuity, diplopia, dry mouth, nystagmus, otitis media, tinnitus, visual field defect
**ENDO:** Hypoglycemia
**GI:** Abdominal pain, constipation, diarrhea, flatulence, gastroenteritis, gastrointestinal hemorrhage, increased appetite, nausea, vomiting
**GU:** Acute renal failure, anorgasmia; decreased libido; glomerulitis, impotence; nephritis; urinary frequency, incontinence, or retention
**HEME:** Decreased platelet count, leukopenia, thrombocytopenia
**MS:** Arthralgia, back pain, elevated creatine kinase levels, leg cramps, myalgia, myasthenia
**RESP:** Apnea, dyspnea
**SKIN:** Ecchymosis, exfoliative dermatitis, pruritus
**Other:** Anaphylaxis, angioedema, facial edema, hypersensitivity reaction, Stevens-Johnson syndrome, weight gain

## Nursing Considerations

•Be aware that pregabalin therapy should not be stopped abruptly but gradually over a minimum of 1 week to decrease the risk of seizure activity and avoid unpleasant symptoms such as diarrhea, headache, insomnia, and nausea.
•Monitor patient closely for adverse reactions. Notify prescriber if significant adverse reactions persist.

**PATIENT TEACHING**

•Warn patient not to stop taking pregabalin abruptly.
•Urge patient to avoid potentially hazardous activities until she knows how drug affects her.
•Instruct patient to notify prescriber if she experiences changes in vision or unexplained muscle pain, tenderness, or weakness, especially if these muscle symptoms are accompanied by malaise or fever.

•Alert patient that drug may cause edema and weight gain.
•If patient also takes a thiazolidinedione antidiabetic drug, tell her these effects may be intensified. If significant, tell patient to notify prescriber.
•Inform male patient who plans to father a child that pregabalin could impair his fertility.
•Instruct diabetic patients to inspect their skin while taking pregabalin.

# primidone

Apo-Primidone (CAN), Myidone, Mysoline, PMS Primidone (CAN), Sertan (CAN)

## Class and Category

*Chemical:* Prodrug of phenobarbital
*Therapeutic:* Anticonvulsant
*Pregnancy category:* Not rated

## Indications and Dosages

➤ *To manage generalized tonic-clonic seizures, nocturnal myoclonic seizures, complex partial seizures, and simple partial seizures caused by epilepsy*

CHEWABLE TABLETS, ORAL SUSPENSION, TABLETS
**Adults and children age 8 and older.** *Initial:* 100 or 125 mg h.s. for first 3 days, then increased to 100 or 125 mg b.i.d. for next 3 days, followed by 100 or 125 mg t.i.d. for next 3 days. On 10th day, begin maintenance dosage as prescribed. *Maintenance:* 250 mg t.i.d. or q.i.d., adjusted as needed. *Maximum:* 2 g/day.
**Children up to age 8.** *Initial:* 50 mg h.s. for first 3 days, then increased to 50 mg b.i.d. for next 3 days, followed by increase to 100 mg b.i.d. for next 3 days. On 10th day, begin maintenance dosage. *Maintenance:* 125 to 250 mg t.i.d., adjusted as needed.

## Contraindications

Hypersensitivity to primidone, phenobarbital, or their components; porphyria

---

## Mechanism of Action

Prevents seizures by decreasing the excitability of neurons and increasing the motor cortex's threshold of electrical stimulation.

---

## Interactions
### DRUGS

*acetaminophen:* Decreased acetaminophen effectiveness, increased risk of hepatotoxicity
*adrenocorticoids, chloramphenicol, cyclosporine, dacarbazine, disopyramide, doxycycline, levothyroxine, metronidazole, mexiletine, oral anticoagulants, oral contraceptives (estrogen-containing), quinidine, tricyclic antidepressants:* Decreased effectiveness of these drugs
*amphetamines:* Possibly delayed absorption of primidone
*anticonvulsants:* Possibly altered pattern of seizures
*carbamazepine:* Decreased effectiveness of primidone
*carbonic anhydrase inhibitors:* Increased risk of osteopenia
*CNS depressants:* Possibly enhanced CNS and respiratory depressant effects of both drugs
*cyclophosphamide:* Reduced half-life and increased leukopenic activity of cyclophosphamide
*enflurane, halothane, methoxyflurane:* Increased risk of hepatotoxicity; increased risk of nephrotoxicity (with methoxyflurane)
*fenoprofen:* Decreased elimination half-life of fenoprofen
*folic acid:* Increased folic acid requirements
*griseofulvin:* Decreased antifungal effects of griseofulvin
*guanadrel, guanethidine:* Possibly aggravated orthostatic hypotension
*haloperidol, loxapine, maprotiline, molindone, phenothiazines, thioxanthenes:* Possibly lowered seizure threshold and increased CNS depression
*leucovorin:* Possibly decreased anticonvulsant effects of primidone (with large doses)
*MAO inhibitors:* Possibly prolonged effects of primidone and altered pattern of seizures
*methylphenidate:* Possibly increased blood primidone level, resulting in toxicity
*phenobarbital:* Increased sedative effects of either drug, possibly altered pattern of seizures
*phenylbutazone:* Decreased primidone effectiveness, increased metabolism and decreased half-life of phenylbutazone
*rifampin:* Decreased blood primidone level
*valproic acid:* Increased blood primidone level, leading to increased CNS depression

P

and neurotoxicity; decreased half-life of valproic acid and enhanced risk of hepatotoxicity
*vitamin D:* Decreased effects of vitamin D
*xanthines:* Increased metabolism and clearance of xanthines (except dyphylline)

**ACTIVITIES**
*alcohol use:* Possibly increased CNS and respiratory depressant effects of primidone

## Adverse Reactions

**CNS:** Ataxia, confusion, dizziness, drowsiness, excitement, mental changes, mood changes, restlessness
**EENT:** Diplopia, nystagmus
**GI:** Anorexia, nausea, vomiting
**GU:** Impotence
**RESP:** Dyspnea
**Other:** Folic acid deficiency

## Nursing Considerations

• Monitor blood levels of primidone and phenobarbital (its active metabolite), as ordered, to determine therapeutic level or detect toxic levels.
• Anticipate that drug may cause confusion, excitement, or mood changes in elderly patients and children.
• Assess for signs of folic acid deficiency: mental dysfunction, neuropathy, tiredness, and weakness.

**PATIENT TEACHING**
• Instruct patient to crush primidone tablets and mix with foods or fluids, as needed.
• Advise patient taking oral suspension to shake the bottle well and measure doses with a calibrated device.
• Suggest that patient take drug with meals to minimize adverse GI reactions.
• Urge patient not to stop taking primidone abruptly because doing so can precipitate seizures.
• Caution patient about possible decreased alertness.
• Advise her to avoid potentially hazardous activities until drug's CNS effects are known.
• Urge patient to avoid alcohol and other CNS depressants during primidone therapy.

# probenecid

Benemid, Benuryl (CAN), Probalan

## Class and Category

*Chemical:* Sulfonamide derivative
*Therapeutic:* Antibiotic adjunct, antigout, uricosuric
*Pregnancy category:* Not rated

## Indications and Dosages

➤ *To treat chronic gouty arthritis and hyperuricemia due to chronic gout*
**TABLETS**
**Adults and adolescents.** *Initial:* 250 mg b.i.d. for 1 wk, then increased to maintenance dosage. *Maintenance:* 500 mg b.i.d.; if not effective or 24-hr uric acid excretion isn't greater than 700 mg, dosage increased by 500 mg/day q 4 wk, as needed and prescribed, up to a maximum of 3 g/day. If no acute attacks of gout occur over next 6 mo and serum uric acid level is within normal limits, dosage decreased, as prescribed, by 500 mg q 6 mo until lowest effective maintenance dose is reached. *Maximum:* 3 g/day.
**DOSAGE ADJUSTMENT** Dosage possibly increased for patients with mild renal dysfunction, except for elderly patients, who require a dosage reduction.

➤ *As adjunct to antibiotic therapy with penicillins and some cephalosporins*
**TABLETS**
**Adults, adolescents age 14 and older, and children weighing more than 50 kg (110 lb).** 500 mg q.i.d.; if given with I.V. or I.M. antibiotic, administer at least 30 min before antibiotic.
**Children ages 2 to 14 weighing up to 50 kg.** 25 mg/kg as a single dose, followed by 10 mg/kg q.i.d.; if given with I.V. or I.M. antibiotic, administer at least 30 min before antibiotic.

➤ *As adjunct to treat sexually transmitted diseases*
**TABLETS**
**Adults and adolescents.** 1 g as a single dose administered together with appropriate antibiotic.

➤ *As adjunct to treat pediatric gonorrhea*
**TABLETS**
**Postpubertal children and children weighing more than 45 kg (99 lb).** 1 g as a single dose administered together with appropriate antibiotic.

➤ *As adjunct to treat neurosyphilis*
**TABLETS**
**Adults and adolescents.** 500 mg q.i.d. concurrently with 1 daily dose (2.4 million U) of penicillin G procaine for 10 to 14 days.

| Route | Onset | Peak | Duration |
|-------|-------|------|----------|
| P.O. | Unknown | 30 min* | 8 hr† |

### Mechanism of Action
Increases urinary excretion of uric acid and lowers serum uric acid level, which may prevent or resolve urate deposits, tophus formation, and joint changes. Eventually, the incidence of acute gout attacks decreases. Probenecid also inhibits renal excretion of penicillins and some cephalosporin antibiotics, thereby increasing their serum concentration and prolonging their duration of action.

### Contraindications
Age less than 2 years, blood dyscrasias, hypersensitivity to probenecid or its components, renal calculi (urate)

### Interactions
**DRUGS**
*acyclovir:* Decreased renal tubular secretion of acyclovir
*allopurinol:* Additive antihyperuricemic effects
*aminosalicylate sodium, cephalosporins, ciprofloxacin, clofibrate, dapsone, ganciclovir, imipenem, methotrexate, nitrofurantoin, norfloxacin, penicillins:* Increased and possibly prolonged blood levels of these drugs, increased risk of toxicity
*antineoplastics (rapidly cytolytic):* Possibly uric acid nephropathy
*diazoxide, mecamylamine, pyrazinamide:* Increased risk of hyperuricemia, decreased probenecid effectiveness
*dyphylline:* Increased half-life of dyphylline
*furosemide:* Increased blood furosemide level
*heparin:* Increased and prolonged anticoagulant effect
*indomethacin, ketoprofen, other NSAIDs:* Possibly increased adverse effects
*lorazepam, oxazepam, temazepam:* Increased effects of these drugs and, possibly, excessive sedation

---

\* For renal clearance of uric acid; 2 hr for effect on blood antibiotic level.
† For effect on blood antibiotic level; unknown for renal clearance of uric acid.

*riboflavin:* Decreased GI absorption of riboflavin
*rifampin, sulfonamides:* Increased blood levels of these drugs and, possibly, toxicity
*salicylates:* Decreased uricosuric effects of probenecid
*sodium benzoate and sodium phenylacetate:* Decreased renal elimination of these drugs
*sulfonylureas:* Increased sulfonylurea half-life
*thiopental:* Prolonged thiopental effect
*zidovudine:* Increased risk of zidovudine toxicity
**ACTIVITIES**
*alcohol use:* Increased risk of hyperuricemia, decreased probenecid effectiveness

### Adverse Reactions
**CNS:** Dizziness, headache
**EENT:** Sore gums
**GI:** Anorexia, nausea, vomiting
**GU:** Hematuria, renal calculi (urate), renal colic, urinary frequency
**MS:** Costovertebral pain; joint pain, redness, and swelling
**SKIN:** Facial flushing, pruritus, rash, urticaria

### Nursing Considerations
•Be aware that probenecid therapy shouldn't be started until acute gout attack has subsided. If acute gout attack begins during therapy, continue drug therapy as prescribed.
•Use drug cautiously in patients with peptic ulcer disease.
•Expect to give sodium bicarbonate (3 to 7.5 g/day) or potassium citrate (7.5 g/day), as prescribed, to keep urine alkaline and prevent renal calculus formation.
•Monitor CBC, serum uric acid level, and liver and renal function test results during therapy.
•Closely monitor patients receiving intermittent therapy because they're more likely to develop allergic reactions.
•Monitor blood glucose level frequently in diabetic patient who takes a sulfonylurea because of the risk of drug interactions.
**PATIENT TEACHING**
•Advise patient to take probenecid with meals to minimize GI distress.
•Encourage patient to increase fluid intake (up to 3 L/day, if not contraindicated) to help prevent renal calculus formation.
•Instruct patient to notify prescriber immediately if she experiences signs of an acute gout attack (joint pain, swelling, and red-

P

ness) or of kidney stones (flank pain and blood in urine).

•Caution patient against taking salicylates while taking probenecid. Instead, advise her to use acetaminophen to treat mild pain or fever.

# probenecid and colchicine

ColBenemid, Col-Probenecid, Proben-C

## Class and Category
*Chemical:* Sulfonamide derivative (probenecid), colchicium alkaloid derivative (colchicine)
*Therapeutic:* Antigout
*Pregnancy category:* Not rated

## Indications and Dosages
➤ *To treat chronic gouty arthritis in patients who experience frequent attacks*

**TABLETS**

**Adults.** *Initial:* 1 tablet (500 mg of probenecid/0.5 mg of colchicine) q.d. for 1 wk, then increased to maintenance dosage. *Maintenance:* 1 tablet b.i.d.; if not effective or 24-hr uric acid excretion isn't greater than 700 mg, dosage increased by 1 tablet/day q 4 wk, as needed and prescribed, up to a maximum of 4 tablets/day. If no acute attacks of gout occur over next 6 mo and serum uric acid level is within normal limits, dosage decreased, as prescribed, by 1 tablet q 6 mo until lowest effective maintenance dose is reached.

**DOSAGE ADJUSTMENT** Dosage possibly increased for patients with mild renal dysfunction.

## Contraindications
Age less than 2 years; blood dyscrasias; hypersensitivity to colchicine, probenecid, or their components; renal calculi (urate)

## Interactions
**DRUGS**

*acyclovir:* Decreased renal tubular secretion of acyclovir
*allopurinol:* Additive antihyperuricemic effects
*aminosalicylate sodium, cephalosporins, ciprofloxacin, clofibrate, dapsone, ganciclovir, imipenem, methotrexate, nitrofurantoin, norfloxacin, penicillins:* Increased and possibly prolonged blood levels of these drugs, increased risk of toxicity
*antineoplastics (rapidly cytolytic):* Possibly uric acid nephropathy

*cyclosporine:* Possibly impaired renal function and risk of nephrotoxicity
*diazoxide, mecamylamine, pyrazinamide:* Increased risk of hyperuricemia, decreased probenecid effectiveness
*dyphylline:* Increased half-life of dyphylline
*erythromycin:* Impaired metabolism of colchicine
*furosemide:* Increased blood furosemide level
*heparin:* Increased and prolonged anticoagulant effect
*indomethacin, ketoprofen, other NSAIDs:* Possibly increased adverse effects
*lorazepam, oxazepam, temazepam:* Increased effects of these drugs and, possibly, excessive sedation
*riboflavin:* Decreased GI absorption of riboflavin
*rifampin, sulfonamides:* Increased blood levels of these drugs and, possibly, toxicity
*salicylates:* Decreased uricosuric effects of probenecid and colchicine
*sodium benzoate and sodium phenylacetate:* Decreased renal elimination of these drugs
*sulfonylureas:* Increased sulfonylurea half-life
*thiopental:* Prolonged thiopental effect
*vitamin $B_{12}$ (cyanocobalamin):* Reversible decrease in blood vitamin $B_{12}$ level
*zidovudine:* Increased risk of zidovudine toxicity

**ACTIVITIES**

*alcohol use:* Increased risk of hyperuricemia, decreased antigout effects

---

## Mechanism of Action
Reduces the frequency of gout attacks through several mechanisms. Probenecid increases urinary excretion of uric acid and reduces the serum level of uric acid, which may prevent or resolve urate deposits, tophus formation, and joint changes. Eventually, the incidence of acute gout attacks may decrease.

Colchicine helps to stop inflammation, probably by disrupting microtubules in leukocytes. Microtubules contribute to cell structure and movement. When colchicine binds to tubulin (the protein from which microtubules are made), it causes microtubules to fall apart. This, in turn, disrupts cell function and prevents leukocytes from continuing to invade joints and produce inflammation.

## Adverse Reactions

**CNS:** Dizziness, fever, headache, peripheral neuritis
**EENT:** Sore gums
**GI:** Abdominal pain, anorexia, diarrhea, hepatic necrosis, nausea, vomiting
**GU:** Hematuria, nephropathy (urate), nephrotic syndrome, renal calculi (urate), renal colic, urinary frequency
**HEME:** Agranulocytosis, anemia, aplastic anemia, hemolytic anemia, leukopenia
**MS:** Back or rib pain, gout attacks, muscle weakness
**SKIN:** Alopecia, dermatitis, flushing, purpura
**Other:** Anaphylaxis

## Nursing Considerations

•Be aware that probenecid and colchicine therapy shouldn't be started until acute gout attack has subsided. If acute gout attack begins during therapy, expect to continue drug therapy.
•Use drug cautiously in patients with peptic ulcer disease.
•Expect to give sodium bicarbonate (3 to 7.5 g/day) or potassium citrate (7.5 g/day), as prescribed, to keep urine alkaline and prevent renal calculus formation.
•Monitor CBC, serum uric acid level, and liver and renal function test results during therapy.
•Closely monitor patients receiving intermittent therapy because they are more prone to allergic reactions.
•Frequently monitor blood glucose level of diabetic patient who takes a sulfonylurea because of the risk of drug interactions.

### PATIENT TEACHING

•Advise patient to take probenecid and colchicine with meals to minimize stomach upset.
•Encourage increased fluid intake (up to 3 L/day, if not contraindicated) to help prevent renal calculus formation.
•Instruct patient to notify prescriber immediately if she experiences a gouty arthritis flare-up (joint pain, swelling, and redness) or signs of kidney stones, such as flank pain and blood in urine.
•Caution patient against taking salicylates while taking drug. Instead, advise her to use acetaminophen to treat mild pain or fever.

# procainamide hydrochloride

Procanbid, Procan SR, Promine, Pronestyl, Pronestyl-SR

## Class and Category

*Chemical:* Ethyl benzamide monohydrochloride
*Therapeutic:* Antiarrhythmic
*Pregnancy category:* C

## Indications and Dosages

➤ *To treat life-threatening ventricular arrhythmias*

### CAPSULES, TABLETS

**Adults.** 50 mg/kg/day in 8 divided doses (q 3 hr), adjusted as needed and tolerated. *Maximum:* 6 g/day (maintenance).
**Children.** 12.5 mg/kg q.i.d.

### E.R. TABLETS

**Adults.** *Maintenance:* 50 mg/kg/day in divided doses q.i.d. (q 6 hr), adjusted as needed and tolerated. *Maximum:* 6 g/day (maintenance).

### I.V. INFUSION OR INJECTION

**Adults.** *Initial:* 100 mg diluted in $D_5W$ and administered at a rate not to exceed 50 mg/min. Dosage repeated q 5 min until arrhythmia is controlled or maximum total dose of 1 g is reached. Alternatively, 10 to 15 mg/kg I.V. bolus administered at a rate of 25 to 50 mg/min. *Maintenance:* 1 to 4 mg/min by continuous infusion.

### I.M. INJECTION

**Adults.** 50 mg/kg/day in divided doses q 3 to 6 hr.

➤ *To treat ventricular extrasystoles and arrhythmias associated with anesthesia and surgery*

### I.V. INFUSION OR INJECTION

**Adults.** *Initial:* 100 mg diluted in $D_5W$ and administered at a rate not to exceed 50 mg/min. Dosage repeated q 5 min until arrhythmia is controlled or maximum total dose of 1 g is reached. Alternatively, 10 to 15 mg/kg I.V. bolus administered at a rate of 25 to 50 mg/min. *Maintenance:* 1 to 4 mg/min by continuous infusion.

### I.M. INJECTION

**Adults.** 100 to 500 mg q 3 to 6 hr.
**DOSAGE ADJUSTMENT** For elderly patients or those with cardiac or hepatic insufficiency, dosage possibly reduced or dosing intervals increased. For patients with creatinine clearance less than 50 ml/min/1.73 $m^2$, initial dosage reduced to 1 to 2 mg/min.

| Route | Onset | Peak | Duration |
|-------|-------|------|----------|
| P.O. | Unknown | Unknown | 60 to 90 min |
| P.O. (E.R.) | Unknown | 60 to 90 min | Unknown |
| I.V. | Unknown | Immediate | Unknown |
| I.M. | 10 to 30 min | 15 to 60 min | Unknown |

## Mechanism of Action

Prolongs the recovery period after myocardial repolarization by inhibiting sodium influx through myocardial cell membranes. This action prolongs the refractory period, causing myocardial automaticity, excitability, and conduction velocity to decline.

## Contraindications

Complete heart block, hypersensitivity to procainamide or its components, systemic lupus erythematosus, torsades de pointes

## Interactions

**DRUGS**

*antiarrhythmics:* Additive cardiac effects
*anticholinergics, antidyskinetics, antihistamines:* Possibly intensified atropine-like adverse effects, increased risk of ileus
*antihypertensives:* Additive hypotensive effects
*antimyasthenics:* Possibly antagonized effect of antimyasthenic on skeletal muscle
*bethanechol:* Possibly antagonized cholinergic effect of bethanechol
*bone marrow depressants:* Possibly increased leukopenic or thrombocytopenic effects
*bretylium:* Possibly decreased inotropic effect of bretylium and enhanced hypotension
*neuromuscular blockers:* Possibly increased or prolonged neuromuscular blockade
*pimozide:* Possibly prolonged QT interval, leading to life-threatening arrhythmias

## Adverse Reactions

**CNS:** Chills, disorientation, dizziness, lightheadedness
**CV:** Heart block (second-degree), hypotension, pericarditis, prolonged QT interval, tachycardia
**EENT:** Bitter taste
**GI:** Abdominal distress, anorexia, diarrhea, nausea, vomiting
**HEME:** Agranulocytosis, neutropenia, thrombocytopenia
**MS:** Arthralgia, myalgia
**RESP:** Pleural effusion
**SKIN:** Pruritus, rash
**Other:** Drug-induced fever

## Nursing Considerations

• Place patient in a supine position before administering procainamide I.M. or I.V. to minimize hypotensive effects. Monitor blood pressure frequently and ECG tracings continuously during administration and for 30 minutes afterward.
• Inspect parenteral solution for particles and discoloration before giving drug; discard if particles are present or solution is darker than light amber.
• When possible, give drug by I.V. infusion or injection, as prescribed, rather than by I.M. injection.
• If drug is to be administered I.M. and patient's platelet count is below 50,000/mm$^3$, notify prescriber immediately because patient may develop bleeding, bruising, or hematomas from procainamide-induced bone marrow suppression and thrombocytopenia. Expect to administer procainamide I.V.
• For I.V. injection, dilute procainamide with $D_5W$ according to manufacturer's instructions before administration.
• For I.V. infusion, dilute 200 to 1,000 mg of procainamide to a concentration of 2 or 4 mg/ml using 50 to 500 ml of $D_5W$.
• Administer I.V. infusion with an infusion pump or other controlled-delivery device.
• Don't exceed 500 mg in 30 minutes by I.V. infusion or 50 mg/min by I.V. injection because heart block or cardiac arrest may occur.
• Anticipate that patient has reached maximum clinical response when ventricular tachycardia resolves, hypotension develops, or QRS complex is 50% wider than original width.
• Expect to administer first oral dose 3 to 4 hours after last I.V. dose.

**PATIENT TEACHING**

• Instruct patient to swallow E.R. procainamide tablets whole, without breaking, crushing, or chewing them.
• If patient has trouble swallowing, advise her to crush regular-release tablets or open capsules and mix contents with food or fluid.
• Instruct patient to take drug 1 hour before or 2 hours after meals with a full glass of water. Inform her that she may take procainamide with food if GI irritation develops.

•Urge patient to obtain needed dental work before therapy starts or after blood count returns to normal because drug can cause myelosuppression and increased risk of bleeding and infection. Stress the need for good oral hygiene during therapy, and urge patient to consult prescriber before scheduling dental procedures.
•Advise patient to notify prescriber immediately about bruising, chills, diarrhea, fever, or rash.

# prochlorperazine

Compazine, Stemetil (CAN)

## prochlorperazine edisylate

Compazine

## prochlorperazine maleate

Compazine Spansule, Nu-Prochlor (CAN), Stemetil (CAN)

## Class and Category

*Chemical:* Phenothiazine, piperazine
*Therapeutic:* Antianxiety, antiemetic, antipsychotic
*Pregnancy category:* Not rated

## Indications and Dosages

➤ *To control nausea and vomiting related to surgery*

**I.V. INFUSION OR INJECTION (PROCHLORPERAZINE EDISYLATE)**
**Adults and adolescents.** 5 to 10 mg at a rate not to exceed 5 mg/ml 15 to 30 min before anesthesia or during or after surgery, as needed. Dosage repeated once, if necessary. *Maximum:* 10 mg/dose, 40 mg/day.

**I.M. INJECTION (PROCHLORPERAZINE EDISYLATE)**
**Adults and adolescents.** 5 to 10 mg 1 to 2 hr before anesthesia or during or after surgery, as needed. Dosage repeated once in 30 min, if necessary. *Maximum:* 10 mg/dose, 40 mg/day.

➤ *To control severe nausea and vomiting*

**E.R. CAPSULES (PROCHLORPERAZINE MALEATE)**
**Adults and adolescents.** 15 to 30 mg q.d. in the morning, or 10 mg q 12 hr. *Maximum:* 40 mg/day.

**ORAL SOLUTION (PROCHLORPERAZINE EDISYLATE)**
**Adults and adolescents.** 5 to 10 mg t.i.d. or q.i.d. *Maximum:* 40 mg/day.
**Children weighing 18 to 39 kg (40 to 86 lb).** 2.5 mg t.i.d. or 5 mg b.i.d. *Maximum:* 15 mg/day.
**Children weighing 14 to 18 kg (31 to 40 lb).** 2.5 mg b.i.d. or t.i.d. *Maximum:* 10 mg/day.

**Children weighing 9 to 14 kg (20 to 31 lb).** 2.5 mg q.d. or b.i.d. *Maximum:* 7.5 mg/day.

**TABLETS (PROCHLORPERAZINE MALEATE)**
**Adults and adolescents.** 5 to 10 mg t.i.d. or q.i.d. *Maximum:* 40 mg/day.

**I.V. INFUSION OR INJECTION (PROCHLORPERAZINE EDISYLATE)**
**Adults and adolescents.** 2.5 to 10 mg at a rate not to exceed 5 mg/min. *Maximum:* 40 mg/day.

**I.M. INJECTION (PROCHLORPERAZINE EDISYLATE)**
**Adults and adolescents.** 5 to 10 mg q 3 to 4 hr, p.r.n. *Maximum:* 40 mg/day.
**Children ages 2 to 12.** 132 mcg/kg/dose to maximum of 10 mg on day 1, then increased as needed. *Maximum:* On day 1, 10 mg for all children; thereafter, 25 mg/day for children ages 6 to 12, 20 mg/day for children ages 2 to 6.

**SUPPOSITORIES (PROCHLORPERAZINE)**
**Adults and adolescents.** 25 mg b.i.d.
**Children weighing 18 to 39 kg.** 2.5 mg t.i.d. or 5 mg b.i.d. *Maximum:* 15 mg/day.
**Children weighing 14 to 18 kg.** 2.5 mg b.i.d. or t.i.d. *Maximum:* 10 mg/day.
**Children weighing 9 to 14 kg.** 2.5 mg q.d. or b.i.d. *Maximum:* 7.5 mg/day.

➤ *To manage psychotic disorders, such as schizophrenia*

**ORAL SOLUTION (PROCHLORPERAZINE EDISYLATE)**
**Adults and adolescents.** 5 to 10 mg t.i.d. or q.i.d., increased gradually q 2 to 3 days, as needed and tolerated. *Maximum:* 150 mg/day.
**Children ages 2 to 12.** 2.5 mg b.i.d. or t.i.d. *Maximum:* On day 1, 10 mg for all children; thereafter, 25 mg/day for children ages 6 to 12, 20 mg/day for children ages 2 to 6.

**TABLETS (PROCHLORPERAZINE MALEATE)**
**Adults and adolescents.** 5 to 10 mg t.i.d. or q.i.d., increased gradually q 2 to 3 days, as needed and tolerated. *Maximum:* 150 mg/day.

**I.M. INJECTION (PROCHLORPERAZINE EDISYLATE)**
**Adults and adolescents.** *Initial:* 10 to 20 mg, repeated q 2 to 4 hr, as prescribed, to bring symptoms under control (usually 3 to 4 doses). *Maintenance:* 10 to 20 mg q 4 to 6 hr. *Maximum:* 200 mg/day.
**Children ages 2 to 12.** 132 mcg/kg/dose on day 1, then increased as needed. *Maximum:* On day 1, 10 mg for all children; thereafter, 25 mg/day for children ages 6 to 12, 20 mg/day for children ages 2 to 6.

P

➤ *To provide short-term treatment of anx-iety*

**E.R. CAPSULES (PROCHLORPERAZINE MALEATE)**

**Adults and adolescents.** 15 mg q.d. in the morning, or 10 mg q 12 hr. *Maximum:* 20 mg/day for no longer than 12 wk.

**ORAL SOLUTION, TABLETS (PROCHLORPERAZINE EDISYLATE)**

**Adults and adolescents.** 5 mg t.i.d. or q.i.d. *Maximum:* 20 mg/day for no longer than 12 wk.

**I.V. INFUSION OR INJECTION (PROCHLORPERAZINE EDISYLATE)**

**Adults and adolescents.** 2.5 to 10 mg at a rate not to exceed 5 mg/min. *Maximum:* 40 mg/day.

**I.M. INJECTION (PROCHLORPERAZINE EDISYLATE)**

**Adults and adolescents.** 5 to 10 mg q 3 to 4 hr, p.r.n.

DOSAGE ADJUSTMENT Initial dose usually reduced and subsequent dosage increased more gradually for elderly, emaciated, and debilitated patients.

| Route | Onset | Peak | Duration |
|---|---|---|---|
| P.O., I.V., I.M., P.R. | Up to several wk* | Up to 6 mo | Unknown |

## Incompatibilities

Don't mix prochlorperazine in same syringe with other drugs. A precipitate may form when prochlorperazine edisylate is mixed in same syringe with morphine sulfate.

## Mechanism of Action

Alleviates psychotic symptoms by blocking dopamine receptors, depressing the release of selected hormones, and producing an alpha-adrenergic blocking effect in the brain.

Prochlorperazine also alleviates nausea and vomiting by centrally blocking dopamine receptors in the medullary chemoreceptor trigger zone and by peripherally blocking the vagus nerve in the GI tract.

Anticholinergic effects and alpha-adrenergic blockade reduce anxiety by decreasing arousal and filtering internal stimuli to the brain stem reticular activating system.

---

* For antipsychotic effects; unknown for other indications.

## Contraindications

Age less than 2 years, blood dyscrasias, bone marrow depression, cerebral arteriosclerosis, coma, coronary artery disease, hepatic dysfunction, hypersensitivity to phenothiazines, myeloproliferative disorders, pediatric surgery, severe CNS depression, severe hypertension or hypotension, subcortical brain damage, use of large quantities of CNS depressants, weight less than 9 kg (20 lb)

## Interactions

**DRUGS**

*aluminum- or magnesium-containing antacids, antidiarrheals (adsorbent):* Possibly inhibited absorption of oral prochlorperazine

*amantadine, anticholinergics, antidyskinetics, antihistamines:* Possibly intensified anticholinergic adverse effects, increased risk of prochlorperazine-induced hyperpyretic effect

*amphetamines:* Decreased stimulant effect of amphetamines, decreased antipsychotic effect of prochlorperazine

*anticonvulsants:* Lowered seizure threshold

*antithyroid drugs:* Increased risk of agranulocytosis

*apomorphine:* Possibly decreased emetic response to apomorphine, additive CNS depression

*appetite suppressants:* Possibly antagonized anorectic effect of appetite suppressants (except for phenmetrazine)

*astemizole, cisapride, disopyramide, erythromycin, pimozide, probucol, procainamide:* Additive QT interval prolongation, increased risk of ventricular tachycardia

*beta blockers:* Increased risk of additive hypotensive effects, irreversible retinopathy, arrhythmias, and tardive dyskinesia

*bromocriptine:* Decreased effectiveness of bromocriptine

*CNS depressants:* Additive CNS depression

*dopamine:* Possibly antagonized peripheral vasoconstriction (with high doses of dopamine)

*ephedrine, epinephrine:* Decreased vasopressor effects of these drugs

*hepatotoxic drugs:* Increased incidence of hepatotoxicity

*hypotension-producing drugs:* Possibly severe hypotension with syncope

*levodopa:* Inhibited antidyskinetic effect of levodopa

*lithium:* Reduced absorption of oral prochlorperazine, increased excretion of lithium, increased extrapyramidal effects, possibly masking of early symptoms of lithium toxicity

*MAO inhibitors, maprotiline, tricyclic antidepressants:* Possibly prolonged and intensified anticholinergic and sedative effects, increased blood antidepressant levels, inhibited prochlorperazine metabolism, and increased risk of neuroleptic malignant syndrome

*mephentermine:* Possibly antagonized antipsychotic effect of prochlorperazine and vasopressor effect of mephentermine

*metrizamide:* Increased risk of seizures

*opioid analgesics:* Increased risk of CNS and respiratory depression, orthostatic hypotension, severe constipation, and urine retention

*ototoxic drugs:* Possibly masking of some symptoms of ototoxicity, such as dizziness, tinnitus, and vertigo

*phenytoin:* Possibly inhibited phenytoin metabolism and increased risk of phenytoin toxicity

*thiazide diuretics:* Possibly potentiated hyponatremia and water intoxication

**ACTIVITIES**
*alcohol use:* Additive CNS depression

## Adverse Reactions

**CNS:** Akathisia, altered temperature regulation, dizziness, drowsiness, extrapyramidal reactions (such as dystonia, pseudoparkinsonism, tardive dyskinesia)
**CV:** Hypotension, orthostatic hypotension, tachycardia
**EENT:** Blurred vision, dry mouth, nasal congestion, ocular changes, pigmentary retinopathy
**ENDO:** Galactorrhea, gynecomastia
**GI:** Constipation, epigastric pain, nausea, vomiting
**GU:** Dysuria, ejaculation disorders, menstrual irregularities, urine retention
**SKIN:** Decreased sweating, photosensitivity, pruritus, rash
**Other:** Weight gain

## Nursing Considerations

• Avoid contact between skin and solution forms of prochlorperazine because contact dermatitis could result.
• Inject I.M. form slowly and deeply into upper outer quadrant of buttocks. Keep patient supine for 30 minutes after injection to minimize hypotensive effects.

• Rotate I.M. injection sites to prevent irritation and sterile abscesses.
• Be aware that I.V. form may be administered undiluted as injection or diluted in isotonic solution as infusion (mesylate form requires dilution in at least 1 L). Both forms should be administered at a rate not to exceed 5 mg/min.
• Protect prochlorperazine from light.
• Be aware that parenteral solution may develop a slight yellowing that won't affect potency. Don't use if discoloration is pronounced or precipitate is present.
• Expect antipsychotic effects to occur in 2 to 3 weeks, although the range is days to months.
• **WARNING** Monitor closely for numerous adverse reactions that may be serious.
• Be aware that adverse reactions may occur for up to 12 weeks after discontinuation of E.R. capsules.

**PATIENT TEACHING**
• Instruct patient to take prochlorperazine with food or a full glass of milk or water to minimize GI distress.
• Advise patient to swallow E.R. capsules whole, not to crush or chew them.
• Instruct patient using a suppository to refrigerate it for 30 minutes or hold it under running cold water before removing the wrapper if it softens during storage.
• Teach patient the correct administration technique for suppository.
• Caution patient receiving long-term therapy not to stop taking prochlorperazine abruptly because doing so may lead to such adverse reactions as nausea, vomiting, and trembling.
• Urge patient to avoid alcohol and OTC drugs that may contain CNS depressants.
• Advise patient to rise slowly from lying and sitting positions to minimize effects of orthostatic hypotension.
• Urge patient to avoid potentially hazardous activities because of the risk of drowsiness and impaired judgment and coordination.
• Instruct patient to avoid excessive sun exposure and to wear sunscreen when outdoors.
• Urge patient to notify prescriber about involuntary movements and restlessness.
• Inform patient that adverse reactions may occur for up to 12 weeks after discontinuing E.R. capsules.

**P**

# procyclidine hydrochloride

Kemadrin, PMS-Procyclidine (CAN), Procyclid (CAN)

## Class and Category

*Chemical:* Synthetic tertiary amine
*Therapeutic:* Antidyskinetic
*Pregnancy category:* C

## Indications and Dosages

➤ *To treat parkinsonism*

**ELIXIR, TABLETS**

**Adults and adolescents.** *Initial:* 2.5 mg t.i.d. after meals; may be increased gradually to 5 mg t.i.d., as needed. If necessary, a 4$^{th}$ dose of 5 mg may be given h.s.

➤ *To treat drug-induced extrapyramidal symptoms*

**ELIXIR, TABLETS**

**Adults and adolescents.** *Initial:* 2.5 mg t.i.d.; dosage increased in daily increments of 2.5 mg, as needed and tolerated.

| Route | Onset | Peak | Duration |
|-------|-------|------|----------|
| P.O. | Unknown | Unknown | 4 hr |

### Mechanism of Action

Competes with acetylcholine to block muscarinic cholinergic receptors in the CNS, which may decrease salivation and relax smooth muscle. Procyclidine also may block dopamine reuptake and storage in CNS cells, thus prolonging dopamine's effects.

## Contraindications

Achalasia, angle-closure glaucoma, bladder neck obstructions, hypersensitivity to procyclidine or its components, megacolon, myasthenia gravis, prostatic hypertrophy, pyloric or duodenal obstruction, stenosing peptic ulcers

## Interactions

**DRUGS**

*amantadine, other anticholinergics, MAO inhibitors:* Additive anticholinergic effects
*antidiarrheals (adsorbent):* Decreased therapeutic effect of procyclidine
*carbidopa-levodopa, levodopa:* Potentiated dopaminergic effects of levodopa

*chlorpromazine:* Decreased blood chlorpromazine level
*CNS depressants:* Increased sedative effects
*digoxin:* Increased risk of digitalis toxicity
*haloperidol:* Possibly worsening of schizophrenic symptoms, decreased blood haloperidol level, tardive dyskinesia

**ACTIVITIES**

*alcohol use:* Increased sedative effects

## Adverse Reactions

**CNS:** Drowsiness, euphoria, headache, memory loss, nervousness, paresthesia, unusual excitement
**CV:** Orthostatic hypotension, tachycardia
**EENT:** Blurred vision; dry mouth, nose, or throat
**GI:** Constipation, indigestion, nausea, vomiting
**GU:** Dysuria
**MS:** Muscle cramps
**SKIN:** Decreased sweating, photosensitivity

## Nursing Considerations

•Use procyclidine cautiously in patients with cardiac disorders because of drug's anticholinergic effects. Frequently monitor blood pressure and heart rate and rhythm.
•Monitor for drug abuse because procyclidine provides a false sense of well-being that may tempt patient to abuse it.

**PATIENT TEACHING**

•Instruct patient to take procyclidine after meals to minimize GI distress.
•Advise patient to avoid alcohol and OTC drugs that may contain CNS depressants because of potential for drug interactions.
•Urge patient to avoid potentially hazardous activities because of risk of drowsiness and reduced alertness.
•Caution patient not to stop taking procyclidine abruptly because doing so may cause sudden adverse reactions.
•If patient reports dry mouth, suggest sugarless hard candy or gum and increased fluid intake.
•Inform patient that exercise and increased fluid intake can help prevent constipation.
•Encourage patient to avoid extreme temperatures because procyclidine may cause decreased sweating, thereby increasing the risk of heatstroke. Also advise patient to wear sunscreen when outdoors.
•Explain to contact lens wearer that drug

may increase lens awareness or blur vision. Suggest using artificial tears for relief.
•Instruct patient to notify prescriber about adverse reactions.

# progestins

### hydroxyprogesterone caproate

Gesterol LA 250, Hy/Gestrone, Hylutin, Prodrox, Pro-Span

### levonorgestrel

Norplant System

### medrogestone

Colprone (CAN)

### medroxyprogesterone acetate

Alti-MPA (CAN), Amen, Curretab, Cycrin, Depo-Provera, Gen-Medroxy (CAN), Novo-Medrone (CAN), Provera

### megestrol acetate

Apo-Megestrol (CAN), Megace, Megace OS (CAN)

### norethindrone

Aygestin, Norlutate (CAN)

### norgestrel

Ovrette

### progesterone

Crinone, Gesterol 50, PMS-Progesterone (CAN), Prometrium

## Class and Category

*Chemical:* Progesterone derivative, steroid hormone
*Therapeutic:* Antianorectic, anticachectic, antineoplastic, ovarian hormone replacement
*Pregnancy category:* D (hydroxyprogesterone, megestrol [tablets], progesterone); X (levonorgestrel, medroxyprogesterone [parenteral], megestrol [parenteral and suspension], norethindrone, norgestrel); NR (medrogestone, medroxyprogesterone [tablets])

## Indications and Dosages

➤ *To treat renal cancer*
**I.M. INJECTION (MEDROXYPROGESTERONE)**
**Adults and adolescents.** *Initial:* 400 mg to 1 g q wk until improvement and stabilization occur. *Maintenance:* 400 mg or more q mo.

➤ *To treat breast cancer*
**TABLETS (MEGESTROL)**
**Adults and adolescents.** 160 mg q.d. as single dose or in divided doses.
➤ *To treat endometrial cancer*
**TABLETS (MEGESTROL)**
**Adult and adolescent women.** 40 to 320 mg q.d. in divided doses.
**I.M. INJECTION (MEDROXYPROGESTERONE)**
**Adults and adolescents.** *Initial:* 400 mg to 1 g q wk until improvement and stabilization occur. *Maintenance:* 400 mg or more q mo.
➤ *To treat anorexia, cachexia, or significant weight loss in patients who have AIDS*
**SUSPENSION (MEGESTROL)**
**Adults and adolescents.** 800 mg q.d. for the first mo, and then 400 or 800 mg q.d. for the next 3 mo.
➤ *To treat endometriosis*
**TABLETS (NORETHINDRONE ACETATE)**
**Adult and adolescent women.** *Initial:* 5 mg q.d. for 2 wk, increased by 2.5 mg/day at 2 wk intervals to total dose of 15 mg/day. *Maintenance:* 15 mg q.d. for 6 to 9 mo unless temporarily discontinued because of breakthrough menstrual bleeding.
➤ *As adjunct to treat endometrial shedding in menopausal women*
**TABLETS (MEDROGESTONE)**
**Adult and adolescent women.** 5 to 10 mg q.d. on days 15 through 25 of menstrual cycle.
➤ *To treat secondary amenorrhea*
**TABLETS (MEDROGESTONE)**
**Adult and adolescent women.** 5 to 10 mg q.d. on days 15 through 25 of menstrual cycle.
**TABLETS (MEDROXYPROGESTERONE)**
**Adult and adolescent women.** 5 to 10 mg q.d. for 5 to 10 days, starting anytime during menstrual cycle.
**TABLETS (NORETHINDRONE ACETATE)**
**Adult and adolescent women.** 2.5 to 10 mg q.d. on days 5 through 25 of menstrual cycle. Alternatively, 2.5 to 10 mg q.d. for 5 to 10 days during last half of menstrual cycle.
**CAPSULES (PROGESTERONE)**
**Adult and adolescent women.** 400 mg q.d. in evening for 10 days.
**I.M. INJECTION (HYDROXYPROGESTERONE)**
**Adult and adolescent women.** 375 mg as one-time dose.
**I.M. INJECTION (PROGESTERONE)**
**Adult and adolescent women.** 5 to 10 mg q.d. for 6 to 10 days. Alternatively, 100 to 150 mg injected as single dose.

P

VAGINAL GEL (PROGESTERONE)
**Adult and adolescent women.** 45 mg (1 applicatorful of 4% vaginal gel) q.o.d. for up to 6 doses. Dosage increased, as needed, to 90 mg (1 applicatorful of 8% vaginal gel) q.o.d. for up to 6 doses.

➤ *To treat dysfunctional uterine bleeding*
TABLETS (MEDROGESTONE)
**Adult and adolescent women.** 5 to 10 mg q.d. on days 15 through 25 of menstrual cycle.
TABLETS (MEDROXYPROGESTERONE)
**Adult and adolescent women.** 5 to 10 mg q.d. for 5 to 10 days, starting on day 16 or 21 of menstrual cycle.
TABLETS (NORETHINDRONE ACETATE)
**Adult and adolescent women.** 2.5 to 10 mg q.d. on days 5 through 25 of menstrual cycle. Alternatively, 2.5 to 10 mg q.d. for 5 to 10 days during last half of menstrual cycle.
I.M. INJECTION (HYDROXYPROGESTERONE)
**Adult and adolescent women.** 375 mg as one-time dose.
I.M. INJECTION (PROGESTERONE)
**Adult and adolescent women.** 5 to 10 mg q.d. for 6 consecutive days.

➤ *To induce menses*
TABLETS (MEDROGESTONE)
**Adult and adolescent women.** 5 to 10 mg q.d. on days 15 through 25 of the menstrual cycle.
TABLETS (MEDROXYPROGESTERONE)
**Adult and adolescent women.** 10 mg q.d. for 10 days, starting on day 16 of menstrual cycle. Repeated for two or more cycles if bleeding is satisfactorily controlled.
I.M. INJECTION (HYDROXYPROGESTERONE)
**Adult and adolescent women.** 125 to 250 mg on day 10 of menstrual cycle, repeated q 7 days until suppression is no longer desired.

➤ *To prevent pregnancy (postcoital)*
TABLETS (LEVONORGESTREL)
**Adult and adolescent women.** 0.75 mg as soon as possible within 72 hr of intercourse. Second dose given 12 hr later.

➤ *To prevent pregnancy*
TABLETS (NORETHINDRONE)
**Adult and adolescent women.** 0.35 mg q.d., starting on day 1 of menstrual cycle and continuing uninterrupted through the year, whether or not menstrual bleeding occurs.
TABLETS (NORGESTREL)
**Adult and adolescent women.** 0.075 mg q.d. starting on day 1 of menstrual cycle and continuing uninterrupted throughout the year, whether or not menstrual bleeding occurs.

I.M. INJECTION (MEDROXYPROGESTERONE)
**Adult and adolescent women.** 150 mg q 3 mo.
SUBDERMAL IMPLANT (LEVONORGESTREL)
**Adult and adolescent women.** One set of implants surgically inserted q 2 yr.

## Contraindications
Active thromboembolic disorder; thrombophlebitis; significant hepatic disease; hypersensitivity to peanuts (progesterone); progestins, or their components; known or suspected breast cancer; pregnancy; undiagnosed genital, uterine, or urinary tract bleeding

## Interactions
DRUGS
*aminoglutethimide:* Possibly decreased blood level of medroxyprogesterone
*carbamazepine, phenobarbital, phenytoin, rifabutin, rifampin:* Possibly decreased effectiveness of progestin

## Adverse Reactions
**CNS:** Change in or loss of coordination or speech, depression, dizziness, drowsiness, fatigue, headache, irritability, migraine, mood changes, nervousness, postmenopausal dementia, syncope, unusual tiredness or weakness
**CV:** Ankle or foot edema; hypotension; numbness or pain in chest, arm, or leg; thromboembolism
**ENDO:** Adrenal insufficiency or suppression, breast pain or tenderness, Cushing's syndrome, delayed return of fertility in women, galactorrhea, hyperglycemia, vaginal spotting
**EENT:** Gingival bleeding, swelling, or tenderness; vision changes or loss
**GI:** Abdominal cramps or pain, diarrhea, nausea, vomiting
**GU:** Amenorrhea, breakthrough bleeding or metromenorrhagia, decreased libido, hypermenorrhea, ovarian enlargement or cysts
**MS:** Back pain, decreased bone density, osteoporosis, osteoporotic fractures
**RESP:** Dyspnea
**SKIN:** Acne, alopecia, melasma, rash
**Other:** Anaphylaxis; facial fullness; hot flashes; injection or implantation site irritation, pain, or redness; weight gain

## Mechanism of Action

Selected progestins may diminish the response to endogenous hormones in tumor cells by decreasing the number of steroid hormone receptors, causing a direct cytotoxic effect or antiproliferative effect on cell cycle growth and increased terminal cell differentiation. At higher doses, some progestins decrease adrenal production of estradiol and androstenedione, which may decrease estrogen- or testosterone-sensitive tumors. Megestrol stimulates appetite and metabolic effects, which promotes weight gain. Progestins also bind to cytostolic receptors that are loosely bound in the cell nucleus, resulting in increased protein synthesis that improves cachexia.

Progestins affect other hormones, especially estrogen, by reducing the availability or stability of the hormone receptor complex, shutting off estrogen-responsive genes, or causing a negative feedback mechanism that decreases the number of functioning estrogen receptors. These actions allow the menstrual cycle to function normally, alleviating amenorrhea and dysfunctional uterine bleeding and inducing menses. Progestins also act to transform a proliferative uterine endometrium into a more differentiated, secretory one, which is the basis for using medroxypro-gesterone to treat some types of amenorrhea. In a normal ovulatory cycle not resulting in pregnancy, the decline in pro-gesterone secretion caused by degeneration of the corpus luteum in the late luteal phase results in endometrial sloughing. A similar sloughing occurs after 5 to 10 days of medroxyprogesterone, provided that adequate estrogen-stimulated proliferation has occurred during the follicular phase.

Selected progestins also inhibit the secretion of gonadotropins from the pituitary gland, which prevents ovulation, follicular maturation, thickening of cervical mucus to prevent sperm penetration, and creation of an atrophic endometrium, resulting in a contraceptive effect.

## Nursing Considerations

• Use progestins cautiously in patients with a history of thrombosis or CNS disorders, such as depression or seizures.

• Be aware that drug causes significant loss of bone mineral density in adolescence and early adulthood and isn't recommended for long-term contraception. If other contraceptive methods are inadequate, evaluate bone mineral density routinely, as ordered.

• Confirm that patient isn't pregnant before giving progestin as a contraceptive.

• Shake container vigorously before giving medroxyprogesterone acetate injection suspension or megestrol acetate oral suspension.

• Inject parenteral medroxyprogesterone into the deltoid muscle rather than the gluteal muscle to lessen absorption problems that may occur when patient inadvertently sits on the injection site.

• Be aware that cyclical use of progestins is based on a menstrual cycle of 28 days.

• **WARNING** Notify prescriber immediately if patient develops sudden vision loss, abnormal protrusion of eyeball, diplopia, papilledema, migraine, or other signs of thrombotic events. Expect to discontinue progestin if such signs occur.

• Monitor patient for adrenal suppression, especially with megestrol therapy. If suspected, notify prescriber.

### PATIENT TEACHING

• Instruct female patient to notify prescriber if uterine bleeding continues for longer than 3 months or if menstruation is delayed by 45 days.

• Warn patient taking progestin for noncontraceptive purposes to use a contraceptive method to prevent pregnancy because drug may harm fetus.

• Advise female patient to contact prescriber immediately if she suspects pregnancy or misses a menstrual period.

• Stress the importance of using a second method of birth control when taking other drugs that could reduce the contraceptive effectiveness of progestins.

• Advise female patient who vomits shortly after taking the progestin-only oral contraceptive pill not to take another dose immediately thereafter but to wait until next scheduled dose before resuming therapy and to use an additional contraceptive method for 48 hours afterward.

• Caution female patient who vomits within 1 hour of taking progestin for emergency contraception to contact prescriber about whether to repeat dose.

P

•Teach female patient how to administer vaginal gel, if prescribed. Tell her to avoid using other vaginal products for 6 hours before and after administration to ensure the gel's complete absorption.

•Direct patient to alert all prescribers about progestin therapy because certain blood tests may be affected.

•Emphasize importance of good dental hygiene and regular dental checkups because elevated progestin blood level increases the growth of normal oral flora, which may lead to gum tenderness, bleeding, or swelling.

•Caution postmenopausal women about increased risk of dementia associated with progestin therapy.

# promethazine hydrochloride

Anergan 25, Anergan 50, Antinaus 50, Histantil (CAN), Pentazine, Phenazine 25, Phenazine 50, Phencen-50, Phenergan, Phenergan Fortis, Phenergan Plain, Phenerzine, Phenoject-50, Pro-50, Promacot, Pro-Med 50, Promet, Prorex-25, Prorex-50, Prothazine, Shogan, V-Gan-25, V-Gan-50

## Class and Category

*Chemical:* Phenothiazine derivative
*Therapeutic:* Antiemetic, antihistamine, antivertigo, sedative-hypnotic
*Pregnancy category:* C

## Indications and Dosages

➤ *To prevent or treat motion sickness*
SYRUP, TABLETS
**Adults and adolescents.** 25 mg 30 to 60 min before travel and repeated 8 to 12 hr later, if needed. *Maximum:* 150 mg/day.

➤ *To treat vertigo*
SYRUP, TABLETS
**Adults and adolescents.** 25 mg b.i.d., p.r.n. *Maximum:* 150 mg/day.
**Children age 2 and older.** 0.5 mg/kg or 10 to 25 mg q 12 hr, p.r.n.
SUPPOSITORIES
**Adults and adolescents.** 25 mg b.i.d., p.r.n. *Maximum:* 150 mg/day.
**Children age 2 and older.** 0.5 mg/kg or 12.5 to 25 mg q 12 hr.

➤ *To prevent or treat nausea and vomiting associated with certain types of anesthesia and surgery*

SYRUP, TABLETS
**Adults and adolescents.** *Initial:* 25 mg, then 10 to 25 mg q 4 to 6 hr, p.r.n. *Maximum:* 150 mg/day.
**Children age 2 and older.** 0.25 to 0.5 mg/kg or 10 to 25 mg q 4 to 6 hr, p.r.n.
I.V. OR I.M. INJECTION
**Adults and adolescents.** 12.5 to 25 mg q 4 hr, p.r.n. *Maximum:* 150 mg/day.
I.M. INJECTION
**Children age 2 and older.** 0.25 to 0.5 mg/kg or 12.5 to 25 mg q 4 to 6 hr, p.r.n.
SUPPOSITORIES
**Adults and adolescents.** *Initial:* 25 mg, then 12.5 to 25 mg q 4 to 6 hr, p.r.n. *Maximum:* 150 mg/day.
**Children age 2 and older.** 0.25 to 0.5 mg/kg or 12.5 to 25 mg q 4 to 6 hr.

➤ *To treat signs and symptoms of allergic response*
SYRUP, TABLETS
**Adults and adolescents.** 10 to 12.5 mg q.i.d. before meals and h.s., p.r.n. Alternatively, 25 mg h.s., p.r.n. *Maximum:* 150 mg/day.
**Children age 2 and older.** 0.125 mg/kg q 4 to 6 hr or 5 to 12.5 mg t.i.d., p.r.n. Alternatively, 0.5 mg/kg or 25 mg h.s., p.r.n.
I.V. INJECTION
**Adults and adolescents.** 25 mg, repeated within 2 hr, if needed.
I.M. INJECTION, SUPPOSITORIES
**Adults and adolescents.** 25 mg, repeated in 2 hr, p.r.n. *Maximum:* 150 mg/day.
**Children age 2 and older.** 0.125 mg/kg q 4 to 6 hr or 6.25 to 12.5 mg t.i.d., p.r.n. Alternatively, 0.5 mg/kg or 25 mg h.s., p.r.n.

➤ *To provide nighttime, preoperative, or postoperative sedation*
SYRUP, TABLETS
**Adults and adolescents.** 25 to 50 mg as a single dose. *Maximum:* 150 mg/day.
**Children age 2 and older.** 0.5 to 1 mg/kg or 10 to 25 mg as a single dose. Alternatively, for preoperative sedation, 1.1 mg/kg along with 1.1 mg/kg of meperidine and appropriate dose of an atropine-like drug.
I.V. INJECTION
**Adults and adolescents.** 25 to 50 mg as a single dose. Alternatively, for preoperative and postoperative sedation, 25 to 50 mg combined with appropriately reduced dosages of analgesics and anticholinergics.
I.M. INJECTION, SUPPOSITORIES
**Adults and adolescents.** 25 to 50 mg as a single dose. Alternatively, for preoperative and

postoperative sedation, 25 to 50 mg combined with appropriately reduced dosages of analgesics and anticholinergics.
**Children age 2 and older.** 0.5 to 1 mg/kg or 12.5 to 25 mg as a single dose. Alternatively, for preoperative sedation, 1.1 mg/kg along with 1.1 mg/kg of meperidine and an appropriate dose of an atropine-like drug.

➤ *To relieve apprehension and promote sleep the night before surgery*
**SYRUP, TABLETS, SUPPOSITORIES**
**Adults and adolescents.** 50 mg along with 50 mg of meperidine and an appropriate dose of an atropine-like drug h.s. on the night before surgery.
**DOSAGE ADJUSTMENT** Dosage usually decreased for elderly patients.

➤ *To provide obstetric sedation*
**I.V. OR I.M. INJECTION**
**Adults and adolescents.** 50 mg for early stages of labor, followed by 1 or 2 doses of 25 to 75 mg after labor is definitely established, repeated q 4 hr during normal labor.

| Route | Onset | Peak | Duration |
|---|---|---|---|
| P.O. | 15 to 60 min | Unknown | 4 to 6 hr |
| I.V. | 3 to 5 min | Unknown | 4 to 6 hr |
| I.M., P.R. | 20 min | Unknown | 4 to 6 hr |

**Mechanism of Action**
Competes with histamine for $H_1$-receptor sites, thereby antagonizing many histamine effects and reducing allergy signs and symptoms. Promethazine also prevents motion sickness, nausea, and vertigo by acting centrally on the medullary chemoreceptive trigger zone and by decreasing vestibular stimulation and labyrinthine function in the inner ear. In addition, it promotes sedation and relieves anxiety by blocking receptor sites within the CNS, directly reducing stimuli to the brain.

**Contraindications**
Angle-closure glaucoma; benign prostatic hyperplasia; bladder neck obstruction; bone marrow depression; breast-feeding; children younger than age 2; coma; hypersensitivity or history of idiosyncratic reaction to promethazine, other phenothiazines, or their components; hypertensive crisis; lower respiratory tract disorders (including asthma) when used as an antihistamine; pyloroduode-

nal obstruction; stenosing peptic ulcer; use of large quantities of CNS depressants

**Interactions**
**DRUGS**
*amphetamines:* Decreased stimulant effect of amphetamines
*anticholinergics:* Possibly intensified anticholinergic adverse effects
*anticonvulsants:* Lowered seizure threshold
*appetite suppressants:* Possibly antagonized anorectic effect of appetite suppressants
*beta blockers:* Increased risk of additive hypotensive effects, irreversible retinopathy, arrhythmias, and tardive dyskinesia
*bromocriptine:* Decreased effectiveness of bromocriptine
*CNS depressants:* Additive CNS depression
*dopamine:* Possibly antagonized peripheral vasoconstriction (with high doses of dopamine)
*ephedrine, metaraminol, methoxamine:* Decreased vasopressor response to these drugs
*epinephrine:* Blocked alpha-adrenergic effects of epinephrine, increased risk of hypotension
*guanadrel, guanethidine:* Decreased antihypertensive effects of these drugs
*hepatotoxic drugs:* Increased risk of hepatotoxicity
*hypotension-producing drugs:* Possibly severe hypotension with syncope
*levodopa:* Inhibited antidyskinetic effects of levodopa
*MAO inhibitors:* Possibly prolonged and intensified anticholinergic and CNS depressant effects of promethazine
*metrizamide:* Increased risk of seizures
*ototoxic drugs:* Possibly masking of some symptoms of ototoxicity, such as dizziness, tinnitus, and vertigo
*quinidine:* Additive cardiac effects
*riboflavin:* Increased riboflavin requirements
**ACTIVITIES**
*alcohol use:* Additive CNS depression

**Adverse Reactions**
**CNS:** Akathisia, CNS stimulation, confusion, dizziness, drowsiness, dystonia, euphoria, excitation, fatigue, hallucinations, hysteria, incoordination, insomnia, irritability, nervousness, neuroleptic malignant syndrome, paradoxical stimulation, pseudoparkinsonism, restlessness, sedation, seizures, syncope, tardive dyskinesia, tremor
**CV:** Bradycardia, hypertension, hypotension, tachycardia

**830** propafenone hydrochloride

**EENT:** Blurred vision; diplopia; dry mouth, nose, and throat; nasal congestion; tinnitus; vision changes
**ENDO:** Hyperglycemia
**GI:** Anorexia, cholestatic jaundice, ileus, nausea, rectal burning or stinging (suppository form), vomiting
**GU:** Dysuria
**HEME:** Agranulocytosis, leukopenia, thrombocytopenia, thrombocytopenic purpura
**RESP:** Apnea, respiratory depression, tenacious bronchial secretions
**SKIN:** Dermatitis, diaphoresis, jaundice, photosensitivity, rash, urticaria
**Other:** Angioedema, paradoxical reactions

## Nursing Considerations
•Use promethazine cautiously in children and elderly patients because they may be more sensitive to drug effects and in patients with cardiovascular disease or hepatic dysfunction because of potential adverse effects.
•Also use drug cautiously in patients with asthma because of its anticholinergic effects and in patients with seizure disorders or those who use medication that may affect seizure threshold because drug may lower patient's seizure threshold.
•Inject I.M. form deep into large muscle mass and rotate sites.
•**WARNING** Avoid inadvertent intra-arterial injection of promethazine because it can cause arteriospasm; gangrene may develop from impaired circulation.
•Give I.V. injection at a rate not to exceed 25 mg/min; rapid I.V. administration may produce a transient fall in blood pressure.
•**WARNING** Monitor respiratory function because drug may suppress cough reflex and cause thickening of bronchial secretions, aggravating such conditions as asthma and COPD, and, in rare cases, may depress respirations and induce apnea.
•Monitor patient's hematologic status as ordered because promethazine may cause bone marrow depression, especially when used with other known marrow-toxic agents. Assess patient for signs and symptoms of infection or bleeding.
•**WARNING** Monitor patient for signs and symptoms of neuroleptic malignant syndrome, such as fever, hypertension or hypotension, involuntary motor activity, mental changes, muscle rigidity, tachycardia, and tachypnea. Be prepared to provide support-

ive treatment and additional drug therapy, as prescribed.
•Be aware that patient shouldn't have intradermal allergen tests within 72 hours of receiving promethazine because drug may significantly alter flare response.

**PATIENT TEACHING**
•Tell patient to use a calibrated device to ensure accurate doses of promethazine syrup.
•Teach patient correct administration technique for suppository, if needed.
•Advise patient to avoid OTC drugs unless approved by prescriber.
•Instruct patient to notify prescriber immediately if she experiences involuntary movements and restlessness.
•Urge patient to avoid alcohol and other CNS depressants while taking promethazine.
•Instruct patient to avoid hazardous activities until drug's CNS effects are known.
•Suggest frequent rinsing and use of sugarless gum or hard candy to relieve dry mouth.
•Advise patient to avoid excessive sun exposure and to use sunscreen when outdoors.

# propafenone hydrochloride

Rythmol

## Class and Category
*Chemical:* 3-Phenylpropriophenone
*Therapeutic:* Class IC antiarrhythmic
*Pregnancy category:* C

## Indications and Dosages
➤ *To treat life-threatening ventricular arrhythmias*
**TABLETS**
**Adults.** *Initial:* 150 mg q 8 hr; after 3 or 4 days, increased to 225 mg q 8 hr (in the U.S.) or 300 mg q 12 hr (in Canada), if needed; after an additional 3 or 4 days, further increased to 300 mg q 8 hr, if needed. *Maximum:* 900 mg/day.

## Contraindications
Bronchospastic disorders, such as asthma; cardiogenic shock; electrolyte imbalances; heart failure (uncontrolled); hypersensitivity to propafenone or its components; severe hypotension; sinus bradycardia or AV conduction disturbances (in patient without artificial pacemaker)

## Mechanism of Action
Prolongs the recovery period after myocardial repolarization by inhibiting sodium influx through myocardial cell membranes. This action prolongs the refractory period, causing myocardial automaticity, excitability, and conduction velocity to decline.

## Interactions
**DRUGS**
*amiodarone:* Possibly altered cardiac conduction and repolarization; possibly increased blood propafenone level
*anesthetics (local):* Increased risk of adverse CNS effects
*antiarrhythmics, fluoxetine:* Increased propafenone levels and risk of adverse CV effects
*cimetidine, erythromycin, ketoconazole, paroxetine, ritonavir, saquinavir, sertraline:* Possibly increased blood propafenone level
*desipramine:* Possibly increased blood level of desipramine or propafenone
*digoxin:* Increased risk of digitalis toxicity
*haloperidol, imipramine, venlafaxine:* Possibly increased blood levels of these drugs
*metoprolol, propranolol:* Increased blood level and half-life of these drugs
*orlistat:* Possibly decreased absorption of propafenone
*quinidine:* Inhibited propafenone metabolism
*rifampin:* Possibly decreased propafenone level
*warfarin:* Increased blood warfarin level and risk of bleeding
**FOODS**
*grapefruit juice:* Possibly increased blood propafenone level

## Adverse Reactions
**CNS:** Dizziness, fatigue, headache
**CV:** Angina, AV block, bradycardia, heart failure, irregular heartbeat, tachycardia, ventricular arrhythmias
**EENT:** Altered taste, blurred vision, dry mouth
**GI:** Constipation, diarrhea, nausea, vomiting
**SKIN:** Rash

## Nursing Considerations
•Assess for electrolyte imbalances, such as hyperkalemia, before beginning therapy with propafenone or any antiarrhythmic to reduce the risk of adverse cardiac reactions.

•Use propafenone cautiously in patients with heart failure or myocardial dysfunction because drug's beta-blocking activity may further depress myocardial contractility.
•Monitor ECG tracings, blood pressure, and pulse rate, particularly at the start of therapy and with dosage increases.
**PATIENT TEACHING**
•Instruct patient to take a missed dose of propafenone if she remembers within 4 hours; otherwise, tell her to skip the missed dose and to resume the regular dosing schedule.
•Advise patient not to discontinue propafenone or change dosage without consulting prescriber.
•Urge patient to carry or wear medical identification indicating that she takes propafenone.
•Advise patient to avoid potentially hazardous activities until drug's CNS effects are known.
•Encourage patient to increase fluid intake and add fiber to diet if she becomes constipated.
•Inform patient that drug may cause an unusual taste in her mouth. Advise her to notify prescriber if taste interferes with compliance.

# propantheline bromide
Pro-Banthine, Propanthel (CAN)

## Class and Category
*Chemical:* Quaternary amine
*Therapeutic:* Anticholinergic
*Pregnancy category:* C

## Indications and Dosages
➤ *As adjunct to treat peptic ulcer disease*
**TABLETS**
**Adults.** 15 mg t.i.d. before meals and 30 mg h.s., adjusted as needed and tolerated. *Maximum:* 120 mg/day.
**Children.** 0.375 mg/kg q.i.d., adjusted as needed and tolerated.
**DOSAGE ADJUSTMENT** For elderly patients with mild symptoms or patients of below-average weight, dosage possibly reduced to 7.5 mg t.i.d. or q.i.d.

| Route | Onset | Peak | Duration |
|-------|-------|------|----------|
| P.O. | Unknown | Unknown | 6 hr |

## Mechanism of Action

Prevents the neurotransmitter acetylcholine from combining with receptors on the postganglionic parasympathetic nerve terminal, thereby reducing smooth-muscle spasms in the GI system, slowing GI motility, and inhibiting gastric acid secretion. All these effects help to heal peptic ulcers.

## Contraindications

Adhesions between iris and lens, angle-closure glaucoma, hemorrhage accompanied by hemodynamic instability, hepatic dysfunction, hypersensitivity to propantheline or its components, ileus, myasthenia gravis, myocardial ischemia, obstructive GI or urinary disease, renal dysfunction, severe ulcerative colitis, tachycardia

## Interactions

**DRUGS**

*amantadine, other anticholinergics, tricyclic antidepressants:* Additive anticholinergic effects
*antacids, antidiarrheals (adsorbent):* Possibly reduced absorption of propantheline
*antimyasthenics:* Possibly further reduction in intestinal motility
*atenolol:* Increased effects of atenolol
*cyclopropane:* Possibly ventricular arrhythmias
*digoxin:* Possibly digitalis toxicity
*haloperidol:* Decreased antipsychotic effect of haloperidol in schizophrenic patients
*ketoconazole:* Decreased ketoconazole absorption
*metoclopramide:* Possibly decreased metoclopramide effect on GI motility
*opioid analgesics:* Increased risk of severe constipation and urine retention
*phenothiazines:* Possibly decreased antipsychotic effects
*potassium chloride:* Possibly increased severity of potassium chloride–induced GI ulceration, stricture, or perforation
*urinary alkalizers:* Delayed urinary excretion of propantheline

## Adverse Reactions

**CNS:** Dizziness, excitement, insomnia, nervousness, paradoxical CNS stimulation
**CV:** Palpitations, tachycardia
**EENT:** Blurred vision; dry mouth, nose, and throat
**GI:** Constipation, dysphagia, heartburn, ileus, nausea, vomiting
**GU:** Impotence, urinary hesitancy, urine retention
**SKIN:** Decreased sweating, dry skin, flushing

## Nursing Considerations

•Don't administer propantheline within 1 hour of antacids or antidiarrheals.
•Monitor elderly patients closely because they may respond to usual drug dose with agitation, confusion, drowsiness, or excitement.
•**WARNING** Be aware that drug can interfere with sweating reflex, thereby increasing the risk of heatstroke.

**PATIENT TEACHING**

•Instruct patient to take propantheline 30 to 60 minutes before meals and at bedtime, as prescribed.
•Inform patient that drug may cause dizziness. Advise her not to perform potentially hazardous activities until drug's CNS effects are known.
•Encourage patient to increase her fluid and fiber intake to decrease constipation. Instruct her to report persistent constipation and urine retention.
•Advise patient to avoid excessive exposure to heat to reduce the risk of heat prostration and heatstroke, because propantheline decreases sweating.
•Suggest that patient relieve dry mouth with frequent rinsing and sugar-free hard candy or gum.

# propofol

## (disoprofol)

Diprivan

## Class and Category

*Chemical:* 2,6-diisopropylphenol derivative
*Therapeutic:* Sedative-hypnotic
*Pregnancy category:* B

➤ *To provide sedation for critically ill patients in intensive care*

**I.V. INFUSION**

**Adults.** 2.8 to 130 mcg/kg/min. *Usual:* 27 mcg/kg/min.

| Route | Onset | Peak | Duration |
|-------|-------|------|----------|
| I.V. | Within 40 sec | Unknown | 3 to 5 min |

## Mechanism of Action
Decreases cerebral blood flow, cerebral metabolic oxygen consumption, and intracranial pressure and increases cerebrovascular resistance, which may play a role in propofol's hypnotic effects.

## Incompatibilities
Don't mix propofol with other drugs before administration. Don't administer propofol through same I.V. line as blood or plasma products because globular component of emulsion will aggregate.

## Contraindications
Hypersensitivity to propofol or its components

## Interactions
**DRUGS**
*CNS depressants:* Additive CNS depressant, respiratory depressant, and hypotensive effects; possibly decreased emetic effects of opioids
*droperidol:* Possibly decreased control of nausea and vomiting
**ACTIVITIES**
*alcohol use:* Additive CNS depressant, respiratory depressant, and hypotensive effects

## Adverse Reactions
**CV:** Bradycardia, hypotension
**GI:** Nausea, vomiting
**MS:** Involuntary muscle movements (transient)
**RESP:** Apnea
**Other:** Injection site burning, pain, or stinging

## Nursing Considerations
•Use propofol cautiously in patients with cardiac disease, peripheral vascular disease, impaired cerebral circulation, or increased intracranial pressure because drug may aggravate these disorders.
•If ordered to dilute drug before administration, use only $D_5W$ to yield a final concentration of 2 mg/ml or more.
•Consult prescriber about pretreating injection site with 1 ml of 1% lidocaine to minimize pain, burning, or stinging that may

occur with propofol administration. Administering drug through a larger vein in the forearm or antecubital fossa may also minimize injection site discomfort.
•Shake container well before using and administer drug promptly after opening.
•Use a drop counter, syringe pump, or volumetric pump to safely control infusion rate. Don't infuse drug through filter with a pore size of less than 5 microns because doing so could cause emulsion to break down.
•Discard all unused portions of propofol solution as well as reservoirs, I.V. tubing, and solutions immediately after or within 12 hours of administration (6 hours if propofol was transferred from original container) to prevent bacterial growth in stagnant solution. Also, protect solution from light.
•Expect patient to recover from sedation within 8 minutes.
**PATIENT TEACHING**
•Encourage patient and family to voice concerns and ask questions before propofol administration.
•Reassure patient that she'll be closely monitored throughout drug administration and that her vital functions, including breathing, will be supported as needed.

# propoxyphene hydrochloride
Cotanol-65, Darvon, PP-Cap

## propoxyphene hydrochloride and acetaminophen
E-Lor, Wygesic

## propoxyphene hydrochloride, aspirin, and caffeine
Darvon Compound-65, PC-Cap, Propoxyphene Compound-65

## propoxyphene napsylate
Darvon-N

## propoxyphene napsylate and acetaminophen
Darvocet-N 50, Darvocet-N 100, Propacet 100

## propoxyphene napsylate and aspirin
Darvon-N with A.S.A. (CAN)

## propoxyphene napsylate, aspirin, and caffeine

Darvon-N Compound (CAN)

### Class, Category, and Schedule
*Chemical:* Synthetic opioid
*Therapeutic:* Analgesic
*Pregnancy category:* Not rated
*Controlled substance:* Schedule IV

### Indications and Dosages
➤ *To relieve mild to moderate pain*
**CAPSULES (PROPOXYPHENE HYDROCHLORIDE, ASPIRIN, AND CAFFEINE)**
**Adults.** 1 capsule (65 mg of propoxyphene/ 389 mg of aspirin/32.4 mg of caffeine) q 4 hr, p.r.n. *Maximum:* 390 mg of propoxyphene hydrochloride/day.
**CAPSULES (PROPOXYPHENE NAPSYLATE AND ASPIRIN)**
**Adults.** 1 capsule (100 mg of propoxyphene/ 325 mg of aspirin) q 4 hr, p.r.n. *Maximum:* 600 mg of propoxyphene napsylate/day.
**CAPSULES (PROPOXYPHENE NAPSYLATE, ASPIRIN, AND CAFFEINE)**
**Adults.** 1 capsule (100 mg of propoxyphene/ 375 mg of aspirin/30 mg of caffeine) q 4 hr, p.r.n. *Maximum:* 600 mg of propoxyphene napsylate/day.
**CAPSULES, ORAL SUSPENSION, TABLETS (PROPOXYPHENE NAPSYLATE)**
**Adults.** 100 mg q 4 hr, p.r.n. *Maximum:* 600 mg/day.
**CAPSULES, TABLETS (PROPOXYPHENE HYDROCHLORIDE)**
**Adults.** 65 mg q 4 hr, p.r.n. *Maximum:* 390 mg/day.

**TABLETS (PROPOXYPHENE HYDROCHLORIDE AND ACETAMINOPHEN)**
**Adults.** 1 tablet (65 mg of propoxyphene/ 650 mg of acetaminophen) q 4 hr, p.r.n.
**TABLETS (PROPOXYPHENE HYDROCHLORIDE, ASPIRIN, AND CAFFEINE)**
**Adults.** 1 tablet (65 mg of propoxyphene/ 375 mg of aspirin/30 mg of caffeine) q 4 hr, p.r.n. *Maximum:* 390 mg of propoxyphene hydrochloride/day.
**TABLETS (PROPOXYPHENE NAPSYLATE AND ACETAMINOPHEN)**
**Adults.** 1 tablet (100 mg of propoxyphene/ 650 mg of acetaminophen) or 2 tablets (each containing 50 mg of propoxyphene/325 mg of acetaminophen) q 4 hr, p.r.n.

| Route | Onset | Peak | Duration |
|-------|-------|------|----------|
| P.O. | 15 to 60 min | 2 hr | 4 to 6 hr |

### Contraindications
Hypersensitivity to propoxyphene or its components (including acetaminophen and aspirin), respiratory depression, severe asthma, upper airway obstruction, use within 14 days of MAO inhibitor therapy

### Interactions
**DRUGS**
*amphetamines:* Possibly fatal seizures (with propoxyphene overdose)
*anticholinergics:* Increased risk of severe constipation and urine retention
*antidiarrheals:* Severe constipation, possibly increased CNS depression
*antihypertensives:* Possibly exaggerated antihypertensive response

### Mechanism of Action
Produces analgesia through a synergistic analgesic effect.

Propoxyphene strongly agonizes mu receptors, blocking the release of such inhibitory neurotransmitters as gamma-aminobutyric acid (GABA) and acetylcholine. It also mediates analgesia by changing pain perception at the spinal cord and higher CNS levels and by altering the emotional response to pain.

Acetaminophen acts centrally to increase the pain threshold by inhibiting cyclooxygenase, an enzyme involved in prostaglandin synthesis.

Aspirin possesses analgesic, anti-inflammatory, antiplatelet, and antipyretic properties. It interferes with arachidonate metabolism as it acetylates proteins and inhibits prostaglandin synthesis by irreversibly inhibiting cyclooxygenase-2, one of two major enzymes that act on arachidonic acid. Aspirin also decreases the perception of pain.

Caffeine exhibits a direct stimulant effect at all levels of the CNS and cardiovascular system. It stimulates the medullary respiratory center, relaxes bronchial smooth muscle, stimulates gastric acid secretion, increases renal blood flow, and acts as a mild diuretic.

*buprenorphine:* Possibly decreased propoxyphene effectiveness, increased respiratory depression
*carbamazepine:* Possibly carbamazepine toxicity
*CNS depressants:* Increased CNS and respiratory depression, hypotensive effects, and risk of habituation
*hydroxyzine:* Increased analgesic, CNS depressant, and hypotensive effects of propoxyphene
*MAO inhibitors:* Severe, possibly fatal reactions, including hypertensive crisis
*metoclopramide:* Possibly antagonized effects of metoclopramide on GI motility
*naloxone:* Antagonized analgesic and CNS and respiratory depressant effects of propoxyphene
*naltrexone:* Risk of withdrawal symptoms in patients who are dependent on propoxyphene, possibly decreased analgesic effect of propoxyphene
*neuromuscular blockers:* Additive respiratory depressant effects
*opioid analgesics:* Additive CNS and respiratory depressant and hypotensive effects
*warfarin:* Increased anticoagulation effects

**ACTIVITIES**
*alcohol use:* Increased CNS and respiratory depression, hypotensive effects, and risk of habituation
*nicotine chewing gum, other smoking deterrents, smoking cessation:* Decreased effectiveness of propoxyphene

### Adverse Reactions
**CNS:** Dizziness, drowsiness, fatigue, insomnia, light-headedness, malaise, nervousness, sedation, tremor
**CV:** Orthostatic hypotension, tachycardia
**EENT:** Blurred vision, diplopia, dry mouth, tinnitus
**GI:** Abdominal cramps, anorexia, constipation, nausea, vomiting
**GU:** Decreased urine output
**MS:** Muscle weakness
**RESP:** Dyspnea, respiratory depression, wheezing
**SKIN:** Flushing of face, pruritus, rash, urticaria
**Other:** Psychological dependence

### Nursing Considerations
•Use propoxyphene cautiously in patients with hepatic or renal dysfunction because delayed elimination may occur. Monitor hepatic and renal function test results.

•**WARNING** Be aware that long-term, high-dose propoxyphene therapy may lead to psychological dependence in some patients. Assess for opioid and alcohol use, which increase the risk of drug abuse or dependence.
•Be aware that abruptly discontinuing drug can result in withdrawal symptoms.
**PATIENT TEACHING**
•Inform patient that she may take propoxyphene with food if she experiences GI distress.
•Instruct patient not to take more than the prescribed amount because drug may be addictive.
•Inform patient that drug may cause blurred vision, drowsiness, dizziness, and impaired judgment and coordination. Urge her to avoid potentially hazardous activities until drug's CNS effects are known.
•Instruct patient to avoid alcohol and other sedatives while taking drug.
•Advise smokers to inform prescriber if they attempt to stop smoking during propoxyphene therapy because increased drug dosage may be required for effective analgesia.
•Urge patient to notify prescriber immediately if pain isn't relieved or worsens.

# propranolol hydrochloride

Apo-Propranolol (CAN), Detensol (CAN), Inderal, Inderal LA, Novopranol (CAN), pms Propranolol (CAN)

### Class and Category
*Chemical:* Beta-adrenergic blocker
*Therapeutic:* Antianginal, antiarrhythmic, antihypertensive, anti-MI, antimigraine, antitremor, hypertrophic cardiomyopathy and pheochromocytoma therapy adjunct
*Pregnancy category:* C

### Indications and Dosages
➤ *To manage hypertension*
**E.R. TABLETS**
**Adults.** *Initial:* 80 mg q.d., increased gradually up to 160 mg q.d. *Maximum:* 640 mg/day.
**ORAL SOLUTION, TABLETS**
**Adults.** *Initial:* 40 mg b.i.d., increased gradually to 120 to 240 mg/day, as needed. *Maximum:* 640 mg/day.
**Children.** *Initial:* 0.5 to 1 mg/kg/day in divided doses b.i.d. to q.i.d., adjusted as needed. *Maintenance:* 2 to 4 mg/kg/day in divided doses b.i.d.

➤ *To treat chronic angina*

**E.R. TABLETS**

**Adults.** *Initial:* 80 mg q.d., increased q 3 to 7 days, as prescribed. *Maximum:* 320 mg/day.

**ORAL SOLUTION, TABLETS**

**Adults.** 80 to 320 mg/day in divided doses b.i.d., t.i.d., or q.i.d.

➤ *To treat supraventricular arrhythmias and ventricular tachycardia*

**ORAL SOLUTION, TABLETS**

**Adults.** 10 to 30 mg t.i.d. or q.i.d., adjusted as needed.

**I.V. INJECTION**

**Adults.** 1 to 3 mg at a rate not to exceed 1 mg/min; repeated after 2 min and again after 4 hr, if needed.

**Children.** 0.01 to 0.1 mg/kg at a rate not to exceed 1 mg/min; repeated q 6 to 8 hr, as needed. *Maximum:* 1 mg/dose.

➤ *To control tremor*

**ORAL SOLUTION, TABLETS**

**Adults.** *Initial:* 40 mg b.i.d., adjusted as needed and prescribed. *Maximum:* 320 mg/day.

➤ *To prevent vascular migraine headaches*

**E.R. TABLETS**

**Adults.** *Initial:* 80 mg q.d., increased gradually, as needed. *Maximum:* 240 mg/day.

**ORAL SOLUTION, TABLETS**

**Adults.** *Initial:* 20 mg q.i.d., increased gradually, as needed. *Maximum:* 240 mg/day.

➤ *As adjunct to treat hypertrophic cardiomyopathy*

**ORAL SOLUTION, TABLETS**

**Adults.** 20 to 40 mg t.i.d. or q.i.d., adjusted as needed.

➤ *As adjunct to manage pheochromocytoma*

**ORAL SOLUTION, TABLETS**

**Adults.** For operable tumors, 20 mg t.i.d. to 40 mg t.i.d. or q.i.d. for 3 days before surgery, concomitantly with an alpha blocker. For inoperable tumors, 30 to 160 mg/day in divided doses.

➤ *To prevent MI*

**ORAL SOLUTION, TABLETS**

**Adults.** 180 to 240 mg/day in divided doses.

**DOSAGE ADJUSTMENT** Dosage increased or decreased for elderly patients, depending on sensitivity to propranolol.

| Route | Onset | Peak | Duration |
|---|---|---|---|
| P.O. | Unknown | 1 to 1.5 hr* | Unknown |

## Mechanism of Action

Exerts the following effects through its beta-blocking actions:

• prevents arterial dilation and inhibits renin secretion, resulting in decreased blood pressure (in hypertension and pheochromocytoma) and relief of migraine headaches

• decreases the heart rate, which helps resolve tachyarrhythmias

• improves myocardial contractility, which helps ease the symptoms of hypertrophic cardiomyopathy

• decreases myocardial oxygen demand, which helps prevent angina pain and death of myocardial tissue

In addition, peripheral beta-adrenergic blockade may play a role in propranolol's ability to alleviate tremor.

## Contraindications

Asthma, cardiogenic shock, greater than first-degree AV block, heart failure (unless secondary to tachyarrhythmia that's responsive to propranolol), hypersensitivity to propranolol or its components, sinus bradycardia

## Interactions

**DRUGS**

*allergen immunotherapy, allergenic extracts for skin testing:* Increased risk of serious systemic adverse reactions or anaphylaxis

*amiodarone:* Additive depressant effects on conduction, negative inotropic effects

*anesthetics (hydrocarbon inhalation):* Increased risk of myocardial depression and hypotension

*beta blockers:* Additive beta blockade effects

*calcium channel blockers, clonidine, diazoxide, guanabenz, resperpine, other hypotension-producing drugs:* Additive hypotensive effect and, possibly, other beta blockade effects

*cimetidine:* Possibly interference with propranolol clearance

---

* For regular-release form; unknown for E.R. form.

*estrogens:* Decreased antihypertensive effect of propranolol

*fentanyl, fentanyl derivatives:* Possibly increased risk of initial bradycardia after induction doses of fentanyl or a derivative (with long-term propranolol use)

*glucagon:* Possibly blunted hyperglycemic response

*insulin, oral antidiabetic drugs:* Possibly impaired glucose control, masking of tachycardia in response to hypoglycemia

*lidocaine:* Decreased lidocaine clearance, increased risk of lidocaine toxicity

*MAO inhibitors:* Increased risk of significant hypertension

*neuromuscular blockers:* Possibly potentiated and prolonged action of these drugs

*NSAIDs:* Possibly decreased hypotensive effects

*phenothiazines:* Increased blood levels of both drugs

*phenytoin:* Additive cardiac depressant effects (with parenteral phenytoin)

*propafenone:* Increased blood level and half-life of propranolol

*sympathomimetics, xanthines:* Possibly mutual inhibition of therapeutic effects

**ACTIVITIES**
*nicotine chewing gum, smoking cessation, smoking deterrents:* Increased therapeutic effects of propranolol

## Adverse Reactions

**CNS:** Anxiety, depression, dizziness, drowsiness, fatigue, fever, insomnia, lethargy, nervousness, weakness

**CV:** AV conduction disorders, cold extremities, heart failure, hypotension, sinus bradycardia

**EENT:** Laryngospasm, nasal congestion, pharyngitis

**GI:** Abdominal pain, constipation, diarrhea, nausea, vomiting

**GU:** Sexual dysfunction

**HEME:** Agranulocytosis

**MS:** Muscle weakness

**RESP:** Bronchospasm, dyspnea, respiratory distress, wheezing

**SKIN:** Erythema multiforme, erythematous rash, exfoliative dermatitis, Stevens-Johnson syndrome, toxic epidermal necrolysis, urticaria

**Other:** Anaphylaxis, flulike symptoms

## Nursing Considerations

• Monitor blood pressure, apical and radial pulses, fluid intake and output, daily weight, respiration, and circulation in extremities before and during propranolol therapy.

• Give I.V. injection at no more than 1 mg/minute.

• **WARNING** Monitor ECG continuously, as ordered, when giving I.V. injection. Have emergency drugs and equipment available in case of hypotension or cardiac arrest.

• Protect injection solution from light.

• Because drug's negative inotropic effect can depress cardiac output, monitor cardiac output in patients with heart failure, particularly those with severely compromised left ventricular dysfunction.

• Be aware that propranolol can mask tachycardia that occurs in hyperthyroidism and that abrupt withdrawal of drug in patients with hyperthyroidism or thyrotoxicosis can precipitate thyroid storm.

• Monitor diabetic patient who is receiving antidiabetic drugs because propranolol can prolong hypoglycemia or promote hyperglycemia. Propranolol also can mask signs of hypoglycemia, especially tachycardia, palpitations, and tremor, but it doesn't suppress diaphoresis or hypertensive response to hypoglycemia.

• **WARNING** Be aware that abruptly stopping drug may cause myocardial ischemia, MI, ventricular arrhythmias, or severe hypertension, especially in patients with cardiac disease.

**PATIENT TEACHING**
• Instruct patient to take propranolol at the same time every day.

• Caution patient not to change dosage without consulting prescriber and not to stop taking drug abruptly.

• Advise patient to notify prescriber immediately if she experiences shortness of breath.

• Instruct diabetic patient to regularly monitor blood glucose level and urine for ketones.

• Advise patient to consult prescriber before taking OTC drugs, especially cold remedies.

• Urge patient to avoid potentially hazardous activities until drug's CNS effects are known.

• Advise smoker to notify prescriber immediately if she stops smoking because smoking cessation may decrease drug metabolism, calling for dosage adjustments.

**P**

# propylthiouracil

## (PTU)

Propyl-Thyracil (CAN)

## Class and Category

*Chemical:* Thiourea derivative
*Therapeutic:* Antithyroid
*Pregnancy category:* D

## Indications and Dosages

➤ *To treat hyperthyroidism*

**TABLETS**

**Adults and adolescents.** *Initial:* For mild to moderate hyperthyroidism, 300 to 900 mg/day in 1 to 4 divided doses until patient becomes euthyroid; for severe hyperthyroidism, 300 to 1,200 mg/day in 1 to 4 divided doses until patient becomes euthyroid. *Maintenance:* 50 to 600 mg/day in 1 to 4 divided doses.

**Children age 10 and older.** *Initial:* 50 to 300 mg/ day in 1 to 4 divided doses. *Maintenance:* Adjusted based on response to initial dosage.

**Children ages 6 to 10.** *Initial:* 50 to 150 mg/ day in 1 to 4 divided doses. *Maintenance:* Adjusted based on response to initial dosage.

**Neonates.** 10 mg/kg/day in divided doses.

➤ *As adjunct to treat thyrotoxic crisis*

**TABLETS**

**Adults and adolescents.** 200 to 400 mg q 4 hr on day 1 along with other measures. Dosage gradually decreased as crisis subsides.

**DOSAGE ADJUSTMENT** For patients with creatinine clearance of 10 to 50 ml/min/1.73 m$^2$, recommended dosage reduced by 25%; for creatinine clearance of less than 10 ml/min/ 1.73 m$^2$, recommended dosage reduced by 50%.

| Route | Onset | Peak | Duration |
|---|---|---|---|
| P.O. | Unknown | 17 wk | Unknown |

## Mechanism of Action

Inhibits conversion of peripheral thyroxine to triiodothyronine by interfering with incorporation of iodide into thyroglobulin; drug remains iodinated and degraded in the thyroid gland. Diversion of oxidized iodine away from thyroglobulin diminishes thyroid hormone synthesis and levels of circulating thyroid hormone.

## Contraindications

Breast-feeding, hypersensitivity to propylthiouracil or its components

## Interactions

**DRUGS**

*amiodarone, iodinated glycerol, iodine, potassium iodide:* Decreased efficacy of propylthiouracil

*digoxin:* Risk of digitalis toxicity

*oral anticoagulants:* Possibly enhanced anticoagulant effect

*sodium iodide 131 (radioactive iodine, $^{131}I$):* Decreased thyroid uptake of $^{131}I$

## Adverse Reactions

**CNS:** Dizziness, paresthesia, peripheral neuropathy
**CV:** Vasculitis
**ENDO:** Hypothyroidism
**GI:** Abdominal pain, nausea, vomiting
**HEME:** Agranulocytosis, leukopenia
**MS:** Arthralgia, joint redness or swelling
**SKIN:** Pruritus, rash, urticaria
**Other:** Lupuslike symptoms

## Nursing Considerations

•Monitor CBC, PT, and liver and thyroid function test results in patients taking propylthiouracil. Elevated serum triiodothyronine (T$_3$) level may be the sole indicator of inadequate treatment.

•Expect to stop drug 3 to 4 days before $^{131}I$ treatment to prevent decreased thyroid uptake of $^{131}I$; therapy may be resumed 3 to 5 days after radiation, if needed.

•Be aware that serum T$_3$ and thyroxine levels should decrease after about 3 weeks of therapy.

•Expect prescriber to decrease beta blocker or theophylline dosage once patient is euthyroid.

**PATIENT TEACHING**

•Instruct patient to take propylthiouracil with meals to decrease adverse GI reactions.

•Advise patient to avoid dietary sources of iodine, such as iodized salt and shellfish.

•Instruct patient to monitor pulse rate and weight daily and to report increased heart rate and excessive weight loss to prescriber.

•Urge patient to report signs of infection, such as fever and sore throat, or possible signs of hepatic dysfunction, such as anorexia and right-upper-quadrant pain.

•Instruct patient to notify prescriber immediately if she becomes pregnant.
•Advise patient to report signs and symptoms of hypothyroidism, such as cold intolerance, depression, and increased fatigue.
•Tell patient to ask prescriber before using OTC cold remedies (some contain iodides).

# protamine sulfate

## Class and Category
*Chemical:* Simple low-molecular-weight protein
*Therapeutic:* Heparin antagonist
*Pregnancy category:* C

## Indications and Dosages
➤ *To treat heparin toxicity or hemorrhage associated with heparin therapy*
**I.V. INJECTION**
**Adults and children.** 1 mg for each 100 U of heparin to be neutralized, or as indicated by coagulation test results. *Maximum:* 100 mg (within 2-hr period).

| Route | Onset | Peak | Duration |
|-------|-------|------|----------|
| I.V. | 5 min | Unknown | 2 hr |

### Mechanism of Action
Neutralizes anticoagulant activity. A strong basic polypeptide, protamine combines with strongly acidic heparin complex to form an inactive stable salt, thereby neutralizing the anticoagulant activity of both drugs.

## Incompatibilities
Don't mix protamine sulfate in same syringe with other drugs unless they're known to be compatible. Several cephalosporins, penicillins, and other antibiotics are incompatible.

## Contraindications
Allergy to fish, hypersensitivity to protamine or its components

## Interactions
**DRUGS**
*heparin:* Neutralized anticoagulant effect of both drugs

## Adverse Reactions
**CNS:** Weakness
**CV:** Bradycardia, hypertension, hypotension, shock

**GI:** Nausea, vomiting
**HEME:** Unusual bleeding or bruising
**RESP:** Dyspnea, pulmonary edema (noncardiogenic), pulmonary hypertension
**SKIN:** Flushing, sensation of warmth
**Other:** Anaphylaxis

## Nursing Considerations
•Expect to administer I.V. protamine undiluted. However, dilute drug if needed (for patients other than neonates) with 5 ml of bacteriostatic water for injection containing 0.9% benzyl alcohol. For neonates, reconstitute with preservative-free sterile water for injection.
•Inject drug slowly at a rate of 5 mg/minute; administer no more than 50 mg in 10 minutes or 100 mg in 2 hours.
•**WARNING** Be aware that rapid administration may cause severe hypotension and anaphylaxis.
•Be prepared to obtain coagulation studies (APTT, activated clotting time) 5 to 15 minutes after administering drug and to repeat studies in 2 to 8 hours to assess for heparin-rebound hypotension, shock, and bleeding.
•Monitor vital signs, hemodynamic parameters, and fluid intake and output, and assess for flushing sensation.
•Have fluids—epinephrine 1:1,000, dobutamine, or dopamine—available for allergic or hypotensive reactions.
•Be aware that vasectomized males have an increased risk of hypersensitivity reaction because of possible accumulation of antiprotamine antibodies.
**PATIENT TEACHING**
•Instruct patient to report adverse reactions immediately.

# protriptyline hydrochloride

Triptil (CAN), Vivactil

## Class and Category
*Chemical:* Dibenzocycloheptene derivative
*Therapeutic:* Antidepressant
*Pregnancy category:* Not rated

## Indications and Dosages
➤ *To treat depression*
**TABLETS**
**Adults.** *Initial:* 5 to 10 mg t.i.d. or q.i.d., increased q wk by 10 mg/day, as needed. *Maximum:* 60 mg/day.

**Children age 12 and older.** *Initial:* 5 mg t.i.d., increased as needed.

DOSAGE ADJUSTMENT For elderly patients, initial dosage limited to 5 mg t.i.d., then adjusted as needed.

| Route | Onset | Peak | Duration |
|-------|-------|------|----------|
| P.O. | 2 to 3 wk | Unknown | Unknown |

## Mechanism of Action
May block the reuptake of norepinephrine and serotonin (and possibly other neurotransmitters) at neuronal membranes, thus enhancing their effects at postsynaptic receptors. These neurotransmitters may play a role in relieving symptoms of depression.

## Contraindications
Acute recovery phase after MI, hypersensitivity to protriptyline or its components, use within 14 days of MAO inhibitor therapy

## Interactions
**DRUGS**
*amantadine, anticholinergics, antidyskinetics, antihistamines:* Additive anticholinergic effects, potentiated effects of antihistamines or protriptyline, possibly impaired detoxification of atropine and related drugs
*anticonvulsants:* Possibly lowered seizure threshold and decreased anticonvulsant effectiveness; enhanced CNS depression
*antithyroid drugs:* Possibly agranulocytosis
*barbiturates, carbamazepine:* Decreased therapeutic effects of protriptyline
*bupropion, clozapine, cyclobenzaprine, haloperidol, loxapine, maprotiline, molindone, phenothiazines, thioxanthenes:* Prolonged and intensified anticholinergic and sedative effects, lowered seizure threshold, increased risk of neuroleptic malignant syndrome; increased blood protriptyline level and inhibited phenothiazine metabolism (with phenothiazine use)
*cimetidine:* Increased risk of protriptyline toxicity
*clonidine, guanadrel, guanethidine:* Decreased hypotensive effects of these drugs; increased CNS depression (with clonidine use)
*CNS depressants:* Possibly serious potentiation of CNS and respiratory depression and hypotensive effect

*disulfiram, ethchlorvynol:* Possibly transient delirium; increased CNS depression (with ethchlorvynol use)
*fluoxetine:* Increased blood protriptyline level
*MAO inhibitors:* Increased risk of hyperpyretic crisis, severe seizures, and death
*methylphenidate:* Possibly antagonized effects of methylphenidate and increased blood protriptyline level
*metrizamide:* Increased risk of seizures
*naphazoline, oxymetazoline, phenylephrine, xylometazoline:* Possibly increased vasopressor effects of these drugs
*oral anticoagulants:* Possibly increased anticoagulant activity
*pimozide, probucol:* Possibly prolonged QT interval and ventricular tachycardia
*sympathomimetics:* Possibly potentiated cardiovascular effects, decreased vasopressor effects of ephedrine and mephentermine
*thyroid hormones:* Increased therapeutic and toxic effects of both drugs
**ACTIVITIES**
*alcohol use:* Possibly increased response to alcohol

## Adverse Reactions
**CNS:** Agitation, ataxia, confusion, dizziness, drowsiness, exacerbation of psychosis, extrapyramidal reactions, fatigue, lack of coordination, paresthesia, peripheral neuropathy, tremor, weakness
**CV:** Arrhythmias, including heart block and tachycardia; CVA; hypertension; hypotension; MI; orthostatic hypotension; palpitations
**EENT:** Black tongue, blurred vision, dry mouth, increased intraocular pressure, lacrimation, stomatitis, tongue swelling
**ENDO:** Hyperglycemia, hypoglycemia
**GI:** Abdominal cramps, anorexia, constipation, diarrhea, epigastric discomfort, hepatic dysfunction, nausea, vomiting
**GU:** Impotence, libido changes, nocturia, urinary frequency and hesitancy, urine retention
**SKIN:** Diaphoresis, petechiae, photosensitivity, rash, urticaria
**Other:** Facial edema, weight gain or loss

## Nursing Considerations
•Use protriptyline cautiously in patients with a history of seizures because drug can lower seizure threshold.

• Use drug cautiously in patients with a history of urine retention or increased intraocular pressure because of drug's autonomic activity.
• **WARNING** Avoid administering protriptyline with an MAO inhibitor. If patient is being switched from an MAO inhibitor to protriptyline, ensure that MAO inhibitor has been discontinued for 14 days before starting protriptyline.

**PATIENT TEACHING**
• Inform patient that protriptyline therapy may take several weeks to reach full effect.
• Instruct patient to avoid potentially hazardous activities until drug's CNS effects are known.
• Advise patient to change position slowly to minimize effects of orthostatic hypotension.
• Urge patient to avoid alcohol while taking drug.
• Suggest that patient drink water and use sugarless gum or hard candy to relieve dry mouth.
• Advise patient to avoid sunlight and tanning booths and to wear protective clothing, a hat, and sunscreen when outdoors.
• Instruct diabetic patient to check blood glucose level frequently during first few weeks of protriptyline therapy.


# pyrazinamide

pms-Pyrazinamide (CAN), Tebrazid (CAN)

## Class and Category
*Chemical:* Pyrazine analogue of nicotinamide
*Therapeutic:* Antitubercular
*Pregnancy category:* C

## Indications and Dosages
➤ *As adjunct to treat tuberculosis, along with other antitubercular drugs*

**TABLETS**
**Adults and children.** 15 to 30 mg/kg q.d.; alternatively, 50 to 70 mg/kg 2 or 3 times/wk.
*Maximum:* 2 g/day for daily regimen, 4 g/day for 2 times/wk regimen, and 3 g/day for 3 times/wk regimen.
**DOSAGE ADJUSTMENT** For patients with HIV infection, 20 to 30 mg/kg/day for first 2 mo of therapy.

## Mechanism of Action
Inhibits the growth of *Mycobacterium tuberculosis* organisms by decreasing the pH level; exhibits bactericidal or bacteriostatic action, depending on blood pyrazinamide level.

## Contraindications
Acute gout, hypersensitivity to pyrazinamide or its components, severe hepatic damage

## Interactions
**DRUGS**
*allopurinol, colchicine, probenecid, sulfinpyrazone:* Possibly increased blood uric acid level and decreased efficacy of antigout therapy
*cyclosporine:* Possibly decreased blood level and therapeutic effects of cyclosporine

## Adverse Reactions
**CNS:** Fever
**GI:** Anorexia, hepatotoxicity, nausea, vomiting
**GU:** Dysuria
**HEME:** Porphyria
**MS:** Arthralgia, gout, myalgia
**SKIN:** Acne, photosensitivity, pruritus, rash, urticaria

## Nursing Considerations
• Review liver function test results before and every 2 to 4 weeks during pyrazinamide therapy.
• Be aware that drug can affect the accuracy of certain urine ketone strip test results.
• Because drug is metabolized by liver, monitor for signs of hepatotoxicity, such as darkened urine, fever, jaundice, malaise, nausea, severe pain in feet or toes, and vomiting.

**PATIENT TEACHING**
• Explain the importance of complying with long-term pyrazinamide therapy.
• Advise diabetic patient to use alternative methods of ketone determination while taking drug.
• Instruct patient to report darkened urine, fever, malaise, nausea, severe pain in feet or toes, vomiting, and yellowing of skin or eyes.
• Inform patient of need for regular blood tests and follow-up visits with prescriber.
• Urge patient to minimize exposure to sun and to wear protective clothing, hat, sunglasses, and sunscreen when outdoors.

# pyridostigmine bromide
Mestinon, Mestinon-SR (CAN), Mestinon
Timespans, Regonol (CAN)

## Class and Category
*Chemical:* Bromide dimethylcarbamate
*Therapeutic:* Antimyasthenic
*Pregnancy category:* Not rated

## Indications and Dosages
➤ *To treat symptoms of myasthenia gravis*
**E.R. TABLETS**
**Adults and adolescents.** 180 to 540 mg q.d.
or b.i.d. (with at least 6 hr between doses).
**SYRUP, TABLETS**
**Adults and adolescents.** *Initial:* 30 to 60 mg
q 3 to 4 hr, adjusted as needed. *Maintenance:*
60 mg to 1.5 g/day.
**Children.** 7 mg/kg/day in 5 or 6 divided
doses.
**I.V. OR I.M. INJECTION**
**Adults and adolescents.** 2 mg q 2 to 3 hr.
**I.M. INJECTION**
**Neonates of myasthenic mothers.** 0.05 to 0.15
mg/kg q 4 to 6 hr.
➤ *To reverse the effects of neuromuscular*
*blockers*
**I.V. INJECTION**
**Adults and adolescents.** 10 to 20 mg after
0.6 to 1.2 mg of I.V. atropine has been
given.
**DOSAGE ADJUSTMENT** Dosage possibly re-
duced for patients with renal impairment.

| Route | Onset | Peak | Duration |
|---|---|---|---|
| P.O. | 30 to 45 min | 1 to 2 hr | 3 to 6 hr |
| P.O. (E.R.) | 30 to 60 min | 1 to 2 hr | 6 to 12 hr |
| I.V. | 2 to 5 min | Unknown | 2 to 4 hr |
| I.M. | 15 min | Unknown | 2 to 4 hr |

## Mechanism of Action
Improves muscle strength compromised by
myasthenia gravis or neuromuscular blockade by competing with acetylcholine for its
binding site on acetylcholinesterase. This
action potentiates the effects of acetylcholine on skeletal muscle and the GI tract.
Inhibited destruction of acetylcholine allows freer transmission of nerve impulses
across the neuromuscular junction.

## Contraindications
Hypersensitivity to pyridostigmine or its
components, mechanical obstruction of GI or
urinary tract

## Interactions
**DRUGS**
*aminoglycosides (systemic), anesthetics (hy-
drocarbon inhalation), capreomycin, lidocaine
(I.V.), lincomycins, polymyxins, quinine:* Possibly antagonized effect of pyridostigmine on
skeletal muscle; possibly decreased neuromuscular blocking activity of these drugs
(with large doses of pyridostigmine)
*anesthetics (local):* Inhibited neuronal transmission, increased anesthesia effects
*anticholinergics:* Possibly masking of signs of
pyridostigmine overdose and reduced intestinal motility
*cholinesterase inhibitors:* Increased risk of
additive toxicity
*edrophonium:* Possibly worsening of patient's
condition
*guanadrel, guanethidine, mecamylamine,
neuromuscular blockers, procainamide:* Possibly prolonged phase I blocking effect or reversal of nondepolarization blockade
*quinidine, trimethaphan:* Possibly antagonized effects of pyridostigmine

## Adverse Reactions
**EENT:** Increased salivation, lacrimation, miosis
**GI:** Abdominal cramps, diarrhea, increased
peristalsis, nausea, vomiting
**GU:** Urinary frequency, incontinence, or
urgency
**MS:** Fasciculations, muscle spasms or weak-
ness
**RESP:** Increased tracheobronchial secretions
**SKIN:** Diaphoresis

## Nursing Considerations
• Use pyridostigmine cautiously in patients
with renal disease because drug is mainly
excreted unchanged by kidneys. Monitor
BUN and serum creatinine levels as appropriate.
• **WARNING** Maintain a rigid dosing schedule
because a missed or late dose can precipitate
myasthenic crisis.
• Observe for cholinergic reactions when administering drug I.V. or I.M.
• **WARNING** Be aware that pyridostigmine
overdose may obscure the diagnosis of myas-

thenic crisis because the primary symptom in both is muscle weakness. Respiratory muscle involvement can lead to death. Be prepared to treat cholinergic crisis by immediately stopping anticholinesterase therapy, administering atropine as prescribed, and assisting with endotracheal intubation and mechanical ventilation, if needed.

•Be aware that reversal of neuromuscular blockade usually occurs in 15 to 30 minutes. Be prepared to maintain patent airway and ventilation until normal voluntary respiration returns completely. Assess respiratory measurements and muscle tone with peripheral nerve stimulator device, as indicated.

**PATIENT TEACHING**

•Instruct patient to take pyridostigmine as directed and on schedule. Explain that a late or missed dose can precipitate a crisis. Suggest the use of a battery-operated alarm clock as a reminder.

•Advise patient to take the oral form with a full glass of water or with food or milk if GI distress occurs.

•Instruct patient not to crush or chew E.R. tablets.

•Ask patient to record pyridostigmine dosage, times taken, and effects to help determine optimal dosage and schedule for her needs.

•Urge patient to carry medical identification describing her condition and drug regimen.

# Q·R·S

## quazepam

Doral

### Class, Category, and Schedule

*Chemical:* Benzodiazepine
*Therapeutic:* Sedative-hypnotic
*Pregnancy category:* X
*Controlled substance:* Schedule IV

### Indications and Dosages

➤ *To treat insomnia*

**TABLETS**

**Adults.** 15 mg h.s.

**DOSAGE ADJUSTMENT** In elderly and debilitated patients, dosage possibly reduced to 7.5 mg h.s. after 1 or 2 nights of therapy.

---

### Mechanism of Action

May antagonize mu receptors at limbic, thalamic, and hypothalamic regions of the brain, blocking release of such inhibitory neurotransmitters as gamma-aminobutyric acid (GABA) and acetylcholine. Central receptors interact with GABA receptors, allowing for greater influx of chloride into the neuron, thereby suppressing neuronal excitability. GABA effects may inhibit spinal afferent pathways and block the cortical and limbic arousal that normally occurs when reticular pathways are stimulated. These effects result in various levels of CNS depression, including sleep.

---

### Contraindications

Hypersensitivity to quazepam or its components, pregnancy, sleep apnea (known or suspected)

### Interactions

**DRUGS**

*addictive drugs:* Possibly habituation
*carbamazepine:* Decreased blood quazepam level, possibly increased blood carbamazepine level
*cimetidine, diltiazem, disulfiram, erythromycin, fluoxetine, fluvoxamine, isoniazid, itraconazole, ketoconazole, nefazodone, oral con-*
*traceptives, propoxyphene, ranitidine, verapamil:* Possibly potentiated effects of quazepam
*clozapine:* Possibly syncope, with respiratory depression or arrest
*CNS depressants, tricyclic antidepressants:* Increased CNS depression
*digoxin:* Possibly increased blood digoxin level and risk of digitalis toxicity
*levodopa:* Possibly decreased therapeutic effects of levodopa
*phenytoin:* Increased risk of phenytoin toxicity
*theophyllines:* Possibly antagonized effects of quazepam
*zidovudine:* Increased risk of zidovudine toxicity

**FOODS**

*grapefruit juice:* Increased blood quazepam level

**ACTIVITIES**

*alcohol use:* Additive CNS depression
*smoking:* Possibly decreased effectiveness of quazepam

### Adverse Reactions

**CNS:** Amnesia (anterograde), anxiety, ataxia, confusion, depression, dizziness, drowsiness, euphoria, fatigue, headache, light-headedness, paresthesia, slurred speech, tremor, weakness
**CV:** Chest pain, palpitations, tachycardia
**EENT:** Blurred vision, dry mouth, hyperacusis, photophobia, worsening of glaucoma
**GI:** Abdominal cramps, constipation, diarrhea, heartburn, nausea, thirst, vomiting
**GU:** Renal dysfunction, urinary incontinence, urine retention
**MS:** Muscle spasms
**RESP:** Increased tracheobronchial secretions

### Nursing Considerations

• Use quazepam cautiously in patients with angle-closure glaucoma because of drug's anticholinergic effects; in patients with hepatic dysfunction because this condition may prolong quazepam's half-life; in patients with myasthenia gravis because drug may worsen condition; in patients with severe COPD because adverse effects of quazepam may compromise respiratory function; in patients with renal dysfunction because accumulation of metabolites may result in toxicity; and in elderly patients because of age-related decreases in hepatic, renal, and cardiac function.
• **WARNING** Notify prescriber if eye pain develops in patient with angle-closure glaucoma.

•**WARNING** Be aware that quazepam may intensify signs and symptoms of depression. Monitor closely for suicidal ideation and institute suicide precautions, as needed

**PATIENT TEACHING**
•Urge patient to avoid alcohol during quazepam therapy because sedation may increase.
•Instruct patient not to discontinue drug abruptly after prolonged use (6 weeks or more).
•Instruct female patient of childbearing age to use effective contraception during therapy and to notify prescriber immediately of known or suspected pregnancy.

# quetiapine fumarate

Seroquel

## Class and Category

*Chemical:* Dibenzothiazepine derivative
*Therapeutic:* Antipsychotic
*Pregnancy category:* C

## Indications and Dosages

➤ *To manage psychotic disorders, including schizophrenia*

**TABLETS**

**Adults.** *Initial:* 25 mg b.i.d. on day 1. Dosage increased by 25 to 50 mg b.i.d. or t.i.d. on days 2 and 3. *Usual:* 300 to 400 mg/day by day 4, in divided doses b.i.d. or t.i.d. Dosage increased q 2 days in increments of 25 to 50 mg b.i.d., as needed. *Maximum:* 800 mg/day.

---

### Mechanism of Action

May produce antipsychotic effects by interfering with dopamine binding to dopamine type 2 ($D_2$)-receptor sites in the brain and by antagonizing serotonin 5-$HT_2$, dopamine type 1 ($D_1$), histamine $H_1$, and adrenergic alpha$_1$ and alpha$_2$ receptors.

---

## Contraindications

Hypersensitivity to quetiapine or its components

## Interactions

**DRUGS**

*antihypertensives:* Possibly enhanced antihypertensive effects of these drugs
*cimetidine, erythromycin, fluconazole, itraconazole, ketoconazole:* Decreased clearance and possibly increased effects of quetiapine
*CNS depressants:* Possibly increased CNS depression

*lorazepam:* Possibly increased effects of lorazepam
*phenytoin, thioridazine:* Increased clearance and possibly decreased effectiveness of quetiapine

**ACTIVITIES**

*alcohol use:* Possibly enhanced CNS depression

## Adverse Reactions

**CNS:** Dizziness, drowsiness, extrapyramidal reactions, hypertonia, tardive dyskinesia
**CV:** Hypercholesterolemia, orthostatic hypotension, palpitations
**EENT:** Dry mouth, pharyngitis, rhinitis
**ENDO:** Hyperglycemia
**GI:** Anorexia, constipation, indigestion
**HEME:** Leukopenia
**MS:** Dysarthria, muscle weakness
**RESP:** Cough, dyspnea
**SKIN:** Diaphoresis
**Other:** Flulike symptoms, weight gain

## Nursing Considerations

•**WARNING** Monitor patient taking quetiapine for predisposing factors for neuroleptic malignant syndrome, such as heat stress, physical exhaustion, dehydration, and organic brain disease. The syndrome includes hyperpyrexia, muscle rigidity, altered mental status, and autonomic instability (which may include irregular pulse or blood pressure, tachycardia, diaphoresis, and arrhythmias).
•Monitor patient for signs of tardive dyskinesia, a potentially irreversible complication characterized by involuntary, dyskinetic movements of tongue, mouth, jaw, eyelids, or face. Notify prescriber if such signs develop because quetiapine may need to be stopped.
•Monitor for orthostatic hypotension, especially during initial dosage titration period. Be prepared to correct underlying conditions, such as hypovolemia and dehydration, before starting therapy, as prescribed.
•Assess patient for hypothyroidism because drug can cause dose-dependent decreases in total and free thyroxine ($T_4$) levels.
•Monitor laboratory results during first 3 weeks of therapy for transient elevations in hepatic enzyme levels. Notify prescriber if they persist or worsen.
•Monitor patient's blood glucose and lipid levels routinely, as ordered, because drug increases the risk of hyperglycemia and hypercholesterolemia.

• Instruct patient to take quetiapine with food to reduce stomach upset.
• Advise patient not to stop taking quetiapine suddenly because doing so may exacerbate his symptoms.
• Inform patient that drug may cause dizziness or drowsiness. Advise him not to drive or perform other activities that require alertness until drug's full CNS effects are known.
• Instruct patient to rise slowly from a seated or lying position to reduce the risk of dizziness or fainting.
• Urge patient to avoid consuming alcoholic beverages because they can increase dizziness and drowsiness.
• Encourage patient on long-term therapy to have regular eye examinations so that cataracts can be detected.

# quinapril hydrochloride

Accupril

## Class and Catgeory

*Chemical:* Ethylester of quinaprilat
*Therapeutic:* Antihypertensive
*Pregnancy category:* C (first trimester), D (later trimesters)

## Indications and Dosages

➤ *To treat hypertension*
TABLETS
**Adults.** *Initial:* 10 or 20 mg q.d., adjusted q 2 wk based on clinical response. *Maintenance:* 20 to 80 mg q.d. or in divided doses b.i.d.
DOSAGE ADJUSTMENT Initial dosage reduced to 5 mg q.d. for patients who are dehydrated from previous diuretic therapy, those who are still receiving diuretic therapy, and those with creatinine clearance of 30 to 60 ml/min/ 1.73 m². Dosage reduced to 2.5 mg q.d. for patients with creatinine clearance of 10 to 30 ml/min/1.73 m².

| Route | Onset | Peak | Duration |
|-------|-------|------|----------|
| P.O. | In 1 hr | 2 to 4 hr | Up to 24 hr |

## Contraindications

History of angioedema related to previous treatment with ACE inhibitor, hypersensitivity to quinapril or its components

## Mechanism of Action

Blocks conversion of angiotensin I to angiotensin II, leading to vasodilation, and reduces aldosterone secretion, which prevents water retention. Quinapril also reduces peripheral arterial resistance. These combined actions lead to a reduction in blood pressure.

## Interactions
DRUGS
*allopurinol, bone marrow depressants, corticosteroids (systemic), procainamide:* Increased risk of fatal neutropenia or agranulocytosis
*CNS depressants, other hypotension-producing drugs:* Additive hypotensive effects
*cyclosporine, potassium preparations, potassium-sparing diuretics:* Possibly hyperkalemia
*lithium:* Possibly increased blood lithium level and risk of toxicity
*NSAIDs, sympathomimetics:* Decreased antihypertensive effect of quinapril
*tetracyclines:* Reduced tetracycline absorption
FOODS
*low-salt milk, salt substitutes:* Increased risk of hyperkalemia
ACTIVITIES
*alcohol use:* Additive hypotensive effects

## Adverse Reactions
**CNS:** Depression, dizziness, drowsiness, fatigue, fever, headache, insomnia, light-headedness, malaise, paresthesia, sleep disturbance, syncope, vertigo
**CV:** Chest pain, hypotension, orthostatic hypotension, palpitations, tachycardia
**EENT:** Amblyopia, dry mouth, loss of taste, pharyngitis
**GI:** Abdominal pain, constipation, diarrhea, indigestion, nausea, vomiting
**GU:** Impotence
**MS:** Arthralgia, back pain, myalgia
**RESP:** Cough, dyspnea
**SKIN:** Alopecia, diaphoresis, flushing, photosensitivity, pruritus, rash, urticaria
**Other:** Anaphylaxis, angioedema

## Nursing Considerations
• Use quinapril cautiously in patients with renal impairment.
• WARNING Be aware that patients with heart failure, hyponatremia, or severe volume or salt depletion; those who've recently received

Q
R
S

intensive diuresis or an increase in diuretic dosage; and those undergoing dialysis may be at risk for excessive hypotension. Monitor blood pressure frequently for first 2 weeks of therapy and whenever quinapril or diuretic dosage increases. If excessive hypotension occurs, notify prescriber immediately, place patient in a supine position, and, if prescribed, infuse NS.

•WARNING Because of the risk of angioedema, be prepared to discontinue drug and administer emergency measures, including S.C. epinephrine 1:1,000 (0.3 to 0.5 ml), if swelling of tongue, glottis, or larynx causes airway obstruction.

•Monitor blood pressure frequently to assess drug's effectiveness.

**PATIENT TEACHING**

•Instruct patient to notify prescriber immediately and stop taking quinapril if he experiences swelling of the face, eyes, lips, or tongue or difficulty breathing.

•Explain that drug may cause dizziness and light-headedness, especially during first few days of therapy. Advise patient to avoid potentially hazardous activities until drug's CNS effects are known and to notify prescriber immediately if he faints.

•Inform female patient of childbearing age of risks of taking quinapril during pregnancy, especially during the second and third trimesters. Caution her to use effective contraception and to notify prescriber immediately of known or suspected pregnancy.

•Advise patient planning to undergo surgery or anesthesia to inform specialist that he's taking quinapril.

•Instruct patient to consult prescriber before using potassium supplements or salt substitutes that contain potassium.

# quinidine gluconate

Quinaglute Dura-tabs, Quinate (CAN), Quin-Release

# quinidine polygalacturonate

Cardioquin

# quinidine sulfate

Apo-Quinidine (CAN), Novoquinidin (CAN), Quinidex Extentabs

## Class and Category

*Chemical:* Dextrorotatory isomer of quinine
*Therapeutic:* Class IA antiarrhythmic
*Pregnancy category:* C

## Indications and Dosages

➤ *To prevent or treat cardiac arrhythmias, including established atrial fibrillation, atrial flutter, paroxysmal atrial fibrillation, paroxysmal atrial tachycardia, paroxysmal atrioventricular junctional rhythm, paroxysmal ventricular tachycardia not associated with complete heart block, and premature atrial and ventricular contractions*

**E.R. TABLETS (QUINIDINE GLUCONATE)**

**Adults.** 324 to 660 mg q 8 to 12 hr. *Maximum:* 1,944 mg/day.

**E.R. TABLETS (QUINIDINE SULFATE)**

**Adults.** 300 to 600 mg q 8 to 12 hr.

**TABLETS (QUINIDINE GLUCONATE)**

**Adults.** *Initial:* 325 mg q 2 to 3 hr for 5 to 8 doses, gradually increasing dosage as needed and prescribed. *Maintenance:* 325 to 488 mg t.i.d. or q.i.d.

**TABLETS (QUINIDINE POLYGALACTURONATE)**

**Adults.** *Initial:* 275 to 825 mg q 3 to 4 hr for 3 or 4 doses, then increased by 137.5 to 275 mg q 3rd or 4th dose until rhythm is restored or toxic effects occur. *Maintenance:* 275 mg b.i.d. or t.i.d.

**TABLETS (QUINIDINE SULFATE)**

**Adults.** *Initial:* For premature atrial and ventricular contractions, 200 to 300 mg t.i.d. or q.i.d.; for paroxysmal supraventricular tachycardia, 400 to 600 mg q 2 to 3 hr until terminated; for atrial flutter, individual titration after digitalization; for conversion of atrial fibrillation, 200 mg q 2 to 3 hr for 5 to 8 doses, followed by subsequent daily increases, as needed. *Maintenance:* 200 to 400 mg t.i.d. or q.i.d.

**Children.** 6 mg/kg 5 times/day.

**I.V. INFUSION (QUINIDINE GLUCONATE)**

**Adults.** 800 mg in 40 ml of $D_5W$ at a rate of up to 0.25 mg/kg/min.

**I.M. INJECTION (QUINIDINE SULFATE)**

**Adults.** 190 to 380 mg q 2 to 4 hr. *Maximum:* 3 g/day.

| Route | Onset | Peak | Duration |
|---|---|---|---|
| P.O. | Unknown | Unknown | 6 to 8 hr |
| P.O. (E.R.) | Unknown | Unknown | 12 hr |

## Mechanism of Action

Depresses excitability, conduction velocity, and contractility of the myocardium and increases the effective refractory period to suppress arrhythmic activity in the atria, ventricles, and His-Purkinje system.

## Contraindications

Digitalis toxicity; history of quinidine-induced thrombocytopenic purpura or torsades de pointes; hypersensitivity to quinidine, other cinchona derivatives, or their components; long-QT syndrome; myasthenia gravis; pacemaker-dependent conduction disturbances

## Interactions

### DRUGS

*antiarrhythmics, phenothiazines, rauwolfia alkaloids:* Additive cardiac effects
*anticholinergics:* Possibly intensified atropine-like adverse effects
*antimyasthenics:* Antagonized antimyasthenic effects on skeletal muscle
*barbiturates, rifampin:* Possibly accelerated elimination and decreased effectiveness of quinidine
*cimetidine:* Increased elimination half-life, possibly leading to quinidine toxicity
*digoxin:* Possibly digitalis toxicity
*hepatic enzyme inducers:* Possibly decreased blood quinidine level
*neuromuscular blockers:* Possibly potentiated neuromuscular blockade
*oral anticoagulants:* Additive hypoprothrombinemia, increased risk of bleeding
*pimozide:* Risk of arrhythmias
*quinine:* Increased risk of quinidine toxicity
*urinary alkalizers (such as antacids, carbonic anhydrase inhibitors, citrates, sodium bicarbonate, thiazide diuretics):* Increased renal tubular reabsorption of quinidine, possibly leading to quinidine toxicity
*verapamil:* Possibly AV block, bradycardia, pulmonary edema, significant hypotension, and ventricular tachycardia

## Adverse Reactions

**CNS:** Anxiety, asthenia, ataxia, confusion, delirium, difficulty speaking, dizziness, drowsiness, extrapyramidal reactions, fever, headache, hypertonia, syncope, vertigo
**CV:** Complete heart block, orthostatic hypotension, palpitations, peripheral edema, prolonged QT interval, torsades de pointes, vasculitis, ventricular arrhythmias, widening QRS complex
**EENT:** Blurred vision, change in color perception, diplopia, dry mouth, hearing loss (high-frequency), pharyngitis, photophobia, rhinitis, tinnitus
**GI:** Abdominal pain, anorexia, constipation, diarrhea, indigestion, nausea, vomiting
**HEME:** Agranulocytosis, hemolytic anemia, leukopenia, neutropenia, thrombocytopenia, thrombocytopenic purpura
**MS:** Arthralgia, myalgia
**RESP:** Dyspnea
**SKIN:** Diaphoresis, eczema, exfoliative dermatitis, flushing, hyperpigmentation, photosensitivity, pruritus, psoriasis, purpura, rash, urticaria
**Other:** Angioedema, flulike symptoms, weight gain

## Nursing Considerations

• Administer I.M. form of quinidine undiluted.
• For intermittent I.V. infusion, dilute drug in 40 ml of $D_5W$ and administer using an infusion pump at a rate of 0.25 mg/kg/min or less. Rapid administration may cause hypotension. Monitor ECG tracings and blood pressure throughout administration.
• Monitor therapeutic blood level of quinidine, as ordered, in all patients receiving drug.
• Monitor heart rate and rhythm closely because quinidine may cause serious adverse reactions and can be cardiotoxic, especially at dosages exceeding 2.4 g/day. Implement continuous cardiac monitoring, as ordered.
• Assess for early signs and symptoms of cinchonism, including blurred vision, change in color perception, confusion, diplopia, headache, and tinnitus, which may indicate quinidine toxicity.

### PATIENT TEACHING

• Advise patient to take quinidine at the same times every day and at evenly spaced intervals.
• Instruct patient to swallow E.R. tablets whole, with a full glass of water, preferably while sitting upright.
• Advise patient to take drug with food if GI upset occurs.
• Urge patient to inform prescriber immediately of blurred or double vision, change in color perception, confusion, diarrhea, fever, headache, loss of hearing, or tinnitus.

Q
R
S

# quinine sulfate

## Class and Category
*Chemical:* Cinchona alkaloid
*Therapeutic:* Antimalarial
*Pregnancy category:* X

## Indications and Dosages
➤ *As adjunct to treat chloroquine-resistant malaria caused by* Plasmodium falciparum
**CAPSULES, TABLETS**
**Adults.** 600 to 650 mg q 8 hr for at least 3 days with one of the following: 250 mg of tetracycline q 6 hr for 7 days; 1.5 g of sulfadoxine and 75 mg of pyrimethamine combined as a single dose; 900 mg of clindamycin q 8 hr for 3 days; or 100 mg of doxycycline q 12 hr for 7 days.
**Children over age 8.** 8.3 mg/kg q 8 hr for at least 3 days with one of the following: 5 mg/kg of tetracycline q 6 hr for 7 days; 6.7 to 13.3 mg/kg of clindamycin q 8 hr for 3 days; or 1.25 mg/kg of pyrimethamine and 25 mg/kg of sulfadoxine combined as a single dose.

### Mechanism of Action
May disrupt function in malarial parasite by elevating intracellular pH in parasitic acid vesicles.

## Contraindications
G6PD deficiency, history of quinine-induced blackwater fever or thrombocytopenic purpura, hypersensitivity to quinine or its components, optic neuritis, pregnancy, tinnitus

## Interactions
**DRUGS**
*acetazolamide, sodium bicarbonate:* Increased risk of quinine toxicity
*aluminum-containing antacids:* Possibly delayed or decreased quinine absorption
*antimyasthenics:* Possibly antagonized antimyasthenic effect on skeletal muscle
*cimetidine:* Possibly reduced clearance of quinine
*digoxin:* Increased blood digoxin level
*hemolytics, neurotoxic drugs, ototoxic drugs:* Increased risk of toxicity of these drugs
*hepatic enzyme inducers:* Possibly decreased blood quinine level
*mefloquine:* Increased risk of seizures

*neuromuscular blockers:* Potentiated neuromuscular blockade
*oral anticoagulants:* Possibly increased anticoagulant effects and risk of bleeding
*quinidine:* Increased risk of prolonged QT interval

## Adverse Reactions
**CNS:** Headache
**EENT:** Blurred vision, hearing loss, tinnitus, vision changes
**ENDO:** Hypoglycemia
**GI:** Abdominal or epigastric pain, diarrhea, nausea, vomiting
**HEME:** Thrombocytopenia

## Nursing Considerations
• Be aware that quinine shouldn't be used in patients with blackwater fever, which can follow chronic malaria, because they're at increased risk for anemia and hemolysis with renal failure.
• Be aware that quinine shouldn't be given I.M. Doing so may cause bleeding, bruising, or hematomas because of quinine's effect on platelets.
• Monitor patient with type 2 diabetes mellitus for alterations in blood glucose level because quinine stimulates release of insulin and may promote hypoglycemia.
• Be aware that quinine can exacerbate optic neuritis or tinnitus. It may also exacerbate muscle weakness and cause dysphagia and respiratory distress in myasthenic patients.
• Assess for early signs and symptoms of cinchonism, including blurred vision, confusion, diplopia, fever, headache, loss of hearing, and tinnitus, which may indicate quinine toxicity.

**PATIENT TEACHING**
• Instruct patient not to crush or chew quinine tablets; they taste bitter and can irritate the mouth and throat.
• Advise patient to take drug with food or after meals to minimize GI irritation.
• Urge patient to notify prescriber immediately if he experiences blurred or double vision, confusion, fever, headache, loss of hearing, or tinnitus, which are indicators of quinine toxicity.
• Advise patient to avoid potentially hazardous activities until he knows how quinine will affect his vision.

# quinupristin and dalfopristin

Synercid

## Class and Category

*Chemical:* Pristinamycin I and IIa derivative, streptogramin
*Therapeutic:* Antibiotic
*Pregnancy category:* B

## Indications and Dosages

➤ *To treat serious or life-threatening infections, such as bacteremia caused by vancomycin-resistant* Enterococcus faecium

**I.V. INFUSION**
**Adults and adolescents age 16 and older.**
7.5 mg/kg q 8 hr.

➤ *To treat complicated skin and soft-tissue infections caused by methicillin-susceptible strains of* Staphylococcus aureus *or* Streptococcus pyogenes

**I.V. INFUSION**
**Adults and adolescents age 16 and older.**
7.5 mg/kg q 12 hr for at least 7 days.

---

### Mechanism of Action

Inhibits bacterial protein synthesis by irreversibly blocking ribosome functioning.

Quinupristin inhibits the late phase of protein synthesis by binding to the 50S ribosomal subunit. Dalfopristin inhibits the early phase of protein synthesis by binding to the 70S or 50S ribosomal subunit. Additionally, this combined activity inhibits transfer RNA (tRNA) synthetase activity, which decreases the amount of free tRNA within the cell. Without tRNA, the bacterial cell cannot incorporate amino acids into peptide chains, resulting in bacterial cell death.

---

## Incompatibilities

Don't mix quinupristin and dalfopristin in saline solutions, including NS, .45NS, 3% sodium chloride, and 5% sodium chloride, because drug is physically incompatible with these solutions.

## Contraindications

Hypersensitivity to quinupristin or dalfopristin, other streptogramin antibiotics, or their components

## Interactions

**DRUGS**
*alfentanil, alprazolam, carbamazepine, delavirdine, diazepam, diltiazem, disopyramide, dofetilide, donepezil, erythromycin, ethinyl estradiol, felodipine, fexofenadine, indinavir, lidocaine, lovastatin, methylprednisolone, nevirapine, norethindrone, quinidine, ritonavir, saquinavir, simvastatin, tacrolimus, triazolam, trimetrexate, verapamil, vinblastine:* Decreased elimination of these drugs, possibly resulting in toxicity
*astemizole, cisapride, terfenadine:* Decreased elimination of these drugs, possibly prolonged QT interval
*cyclosporine, midazolam, nifedipine, terfenadine:* Possibly increased blood levels of these drugs

## Adverse Reactions

**CNS:** Anxiety, confusion, dizziness, fever, headache, hypertonia, insomnia, paresthesia
**CV:** Chest pain, palpitations, peripheral edema, thrombophlebitis, vasodilation
**EENT:** Oral candidiasis, stomatitis
**GI:** Abdominal pain, constipation, diarrhea, elevated liver function test results, indigestion, nausea, pancreatitis, pseudomembranous colitis, vomiting
**GU:** Hematuria, vaginitis
**MS:** Arthralgia, gout, muscle spasms, myalgia, myasthenia
**RESP:** Dyspnea, pleural effusion
**SKIN:** Diaphoresis, pruritus, rash, urticaria
**Other:** Injection site edema, inflammation, pain, or thrombophlebitis

## Nursing Considerations

•Store unopened vials of quinupristin and dalfopristin in refrigerator.
•**WARNING** Reconstitute and further dilute drug with dextrose in water or sterile water for injection only. Don't use saline solutions because drug is physically incompatible with them.
•Dilute prescribed dose in 250 ml dextrose 5% in water ($D_5W$), and infuse over 1 hour through a peripheral I.V. line. If administered by central venous catheter, dilute prescribed dose in 100 ml of $D_5W$. Central venous administration may decrease incidence of infusion site reaction. Use an infusion pump or device to control rate of infusion.
•Further dilute reconstituted solution within

Q
R
S

30 minutes. Vials are for single use only. Discard any unused portion.
- Don't flush I.V. catheter with saline or heparin flush solution because of possible incompatibility. Flush I.V. catheter only with $D_5W$ before and after drug administration.
- Monitor patient for diarrhea, a possible indication of overgrowth of normal intestinal flora, such as *Clostridium difficile*. Be aware that pseudomembranous colitis may result from a toxin produced by *C. difficile*.
- If you suspect that patient has pseudomembranous colitis, notify prescriber and expect to stop drug immediately.
- If patient develops pseudomembranous colitis, be aware that drugs that inhibit peristalsis are contraindicated because of the risk of toxic megacolon.

**PATIENT TEACHING**
- Instruct patient to complete the full course of quinupristin and dalfopristin therapy, as prescribed.
- Advise patient to notify prescriber at once if he develops diarrhea or abdominal pains.
- Inform patient that if he requires long-term therapy, drug will be given in hospital or clinic or by a home health care nurse.

# rabeprazole sodium

AcipHex

## Class and Category
*Chemical:* Substituted benzimidazole
*Therapeutic:* Antiulcer
*Pregnancy category:* B

## Indications and Dosages
➤ *To provide short-term treatment of erosive esophagitis or ulcerative gastroesophageal reflux disease (GERD)*
**DELAYED-RELEASE TABLETS**
**Adults.** For mild to moderate disease, 20 mg q.d. for 4 to 8 wk; course may be repeated if healing has not occurred at the end of 8 wk. For severe reflux with ulceration or stricture formation, 40 mg q.d. for 4 to 8 wk.
➤ *To treat symptomatic GERD*
**DELAYED-RELEASE TABLETS**
**Adults.** 20 mg q.d. for 4 wk. Course may be repeated if symptoms aren't completely resolved.
➤ *To provide maintenance treatment of erosive esophagitis or GERD*

**DELAYED-RELEASE TABLETS**
**Adults.** 20 mg q.d.
➤ *To promote healing of duodenal ulcer, as adjunct to treat* Helicobacter pylori–*positive duodenal ulcer*
**DELAYED-RELEASE TABLETS**
**Adults.** 20 mg q.d. after breakfast for up to 4 wk for ulcer healing and 2 wk when used with antibiotic therapy for *H. pylori.*
➤ *As adjunct to reduce the risk of duodenal ulcer recurrence by eradicating* H. pylori
**DELAYED-RELEASE TABLETS**
**Adults.** 20 mg b.i.d with morning and evening meals in conjunction with amoxicillin 1000 mg b.i.d for 7 days and clarithromycin 500 mg b.i.d. for 7 days.
➤ *To treat hypersecretory conditions, such as Zollinger-Ellison syndrome*
**DELAYED-RELEASE TABLETS**
**Adults.** *Initial:* 60 mg q.d.; may be increased, if needed, to 100 mg q.d. or 60 mg b.i.d.
**DOSAGE ADJUSTMENT** Dosage reduction may be needed if patient has severe hepatic dysfunction.

## Mechanism of Action
Decreases gastric acid secretion by suppressing its release at the secretory surface of gastric parietal cells. Rabeprazole also increases gastric pH and decreases basal acid output, which helps to heal ulcerated areas. In gastric parietal cells, it's transformed to an active sulfonamide, which increases the clearance rate of *Helicobacter pylori.*

## Contraindications
Hypersensitivity to rabeprazole, other substituted benzimidazoles (omeprazole, lansoprazole), or their components

## Interactions
**DRUGS**
*cyclosporine:* Possibly inhibited cyclosporine metabolism
*digoxin:* Increased risk of digitalis toxicity

## Adverse Reactions
**CNS:** Dizziness, headache, malaise
**GI:** Diarrhea, nausea, vomiting
**SKIN:** Erythema multiforme, rash, Stevens-Johnson syndrome, toxic epidermal necrolysis

## Nursing Considerations
•Use rabeprazole cautiously in patients with hepatic dysfunction.
•Monitor serum gastrin level during long-term therapy, as ordered, to detect elevation.
•Closely monitor Japanese men receiving rabeprazole for adverse reactions because they're more likely than other patients to have increased blood drug levels.

PATIENT TEACHING
•Instruct patient to swallow delayed-release rabeprazole tablets whole.
•Inform patients with hypersecretory conditions, such as Zollinger-Ellison syndrome, that treatment can last as long as 1 year.

# raloxifene hydrochloride

## (keoxifene hydrochloride)

Evista

## Class and Category
*Chemical:* Benzothiophene derivative
*Therapeutic:* Osteoporosis prophylactic
*Pregnancy category:* X

## Indications and Dosages
➤ *To prevent osteoporosis in postmenopausal women*
TABLETS
**Adults.** 60 mg q.d.

### Mechanism of Action
Prevents osteoporosis by binding to estrogen receptors, which decreases bone resorption and increases bone mineral density in postmenopausal women.

## Contraindications
History of thromboembolic disease, hypersensitivity to raloxifene or its components, pregnancy

## Interactions
DRUGS
*ampicillin, cholestyramine:* Decreased raloxifene absorption
*warfarin:* Possibly decreased PT

## Adverse Reactions
**CNS:** Depression, fever, insomnia, migraine
**CV:** Chest pain, hot flashes, peripheral edema, thromboembolism

**EENT:** Laryngitis, pharyngitis, sinusitis
**GI:** Abdominal pain, flatulence, indigestion, nausea, vomiting
**GU:** Cystitis, infertility, leukorrhea, UTI, vaginitis
**MS:** Arthralgia, arthritis, leg cramps, myalgia
**RESP:** Cough, pneumonia
**SKIN:** Diaphoresis, rash
**Other:** Flulike symptoms, weight gain

## Nursing Considerations
•WARNING Monitor limbs for impaired circulation and pain (possible thromboembolism).
•Expect prescriber to stop drug at least 72 hours before and during periods of prolonged immobilization. Resume drug as prescribed after patient is fully ambulatory.

PATIENT TEACHING
•Advise patient to avoid lengthy immobility during travel while taking raloxifene because of the increased risk of thromboembolism.
•Instruct patient to report adverse reactions she experiences to prescriber.
•Stress the importance of compliance with long-term raloxifene therapy.

# ramelteon

Rozerem

## Class and Category
*Chemical:* Melatonin receptor agonist
*Therapeutic:* Hypnotic
*Pregnancy category:* C

## Indications and Dosages
➤ *To treat insomnia in patients having difficulty falling asleep*
TABLETS
**Adults.** 8 mg 30 min before h.s.

| Route | Onset | Peak | Duration |
|-------|-------|------|----------|
| P.O. | Unknown | 0.5 to 1.5 hr | Unknown |

### Mechanism of Action
Binds to melatonin receptors MT1 and MT2 in the suprachiasmatic nucleus (SCN) of the hypothalamus. The SCN regulates the sleep-wake cycle, and endogenous melatonin probably is involved in maintaining the circadian rhythm underlying that cycle.

Q
R
S

## Contraindications

Hypersensitivity to ramelteon or its components, severe hepatic dysfunction

## Interactions

**DRUGS**

*benzodiazepines, melatonin, other sedative-hypnotics:* Possible additive sedative effects
*fluconazole, fluvoxamine, ketoconazole:* Increased plasma ramelteon levels
*rifampin:* Decreased ramelteon effectiveness

**ACTIVITIES**

*alcohol use:* Possibly additive CNS effect

## Adverse Reactions

**CNS:** Depression, dizziness, fatigue, headache, insomnia exacerbation, somnolence
**ENDO:** Decreased testosterone levels, increased prolactin levels
**GI:** Diarrhea, dysgeusia, nausea
**MS:** Arthralgia, myalgia
**RESP:** Upper respiratory tract infection

## Nursing Considerations

•Be aware that ramelteon therapy is not recommended for patients with severe sleep apnea or COPD because its effects have not been studied in these patient populations.
•Use cautiously in patients with mild to moderate hepatic dysfunction. Drug is contraindicated in severe hepatic dysfunction.
•Ramelteon is the first approved hypnotic not classified as a controlled substance.
•Monitor depressed patient closely for evidence of worsening of depression. Athough depression has not been identified as an adverse reaction of ramelteon, the drug is a hypnotic and hypnotics worsen depression, including causing suicidal ideation.

**PATIENT TEACHING**

•Instruct patient not to take ramelteon with or immediately after a high fat meal.
•Caution patient to avoid hazardous activities after taking ramelteon; drug's intended effect is to decrease alertness.
•Advise limiting alcohol intake during therapy.
•Tell patient to notify prescriber if insomnia worsens or new signs or symptoms occur.
•Inform patient that drug may affect reproductive hormones; urge patient to report cessation of menses or galactorrhea (females) or decreased libido or problems with infertility.

# ramipril

Altace

## Class and Category

*Chemical:* Ethylester of ramiprilat
*Therapeutic:* Antihypertensive
*Pregnancy category:* C (first trimester), D (later trimesters)

## Indications and Dosages

➤ *To treat heart failure after MI*
**CAPSULES**

**Adults.** *Initial:* 1.25 to 2.5 mg b.i.d. *Maintenance:* 5 mg b.i.d.

➤ *To treat hypertension*
**CAPSULES**

**Adults.** *Initial:* 2.5 mg q.d. *Maintenance:* 2.5 to 20 mg q.d. or in divided doses b.i.d.
**DOSAGE ADJUSTMENT** Initial dosage reduced to 1.25 mg q.d. for patients dehydrated from diuretics, those receiving diuretics, and those with creatinine clearance less than 40 ml/min/1.73 m² ; dosage then slowly increased until blood pressure is under control or maximum daily dose of 5 mg is reached.

| Route | Onset | Peak | Duration |
|-------|-------|------|----------|
| P.O. | 1 to 2 hr | 4 to 6.5 hr | 24 hr |

## Mechanism of Action

Blocks conversion of angiotensin I to angiotensin II, causing vasodilation, and reduces aldosterone secretion, which prevents water retention. Ramipril also reduces peripheral arterial resistance. Combined, these actions reduce blood pressure.

## Contraindications

Hypersensitivity to ramipril, its components, or any other ACE inhibitors

## Interactions

**DRUGS**

*allopurinol, bone marrow depressants, corticosteroids (systemic), procainamide:* Increased risk of fatal neutropenia or agranulocytosis
*CNS depressants, other hypotension-producing drugs:* Additive hypotensive effect
*cyclosporine, potassium preparations, potassium-sparing diuretics:* Possibly hyperkalemia
*insulin, oral antidiabetics:* Increased risk of hypoglycemia

*lithium:* Increased risk of lithium toxicity
*NSAIDs, sympathomimetics:* Decreased antihypertensive effect of ramipril
*tetracyclines:* Reduced tetracycline absorption
**FOODS**
*low-salt milk, salt substitutes:* Increased risk of hyperkalemia
**ACTIVITIES**
*alcohol use:* Additive hypotensive effects

### Adverse Reactions
**CNS:** Depression, dizziness, drowsiness, fatigue, fever, headache, insomnia, light-headedness, malaise, paresthesia, sleep disturbance, syncope, vertigo
**CV:** Chest pain, hypotension, orthostatic hypotension, palpitations, tachycardia
**EENT:** Amblyopia, dry mouth, loss of taste, pharyngitis
**GI:** Abdominal pain, constipation, diarrhea, elevated liver function test results, hepatic failure, hepatitis, nausea, vomiting
**GU:** Acute renal failure, elevated BUN and serum creatinine levels, impotence, oliguria, progressive azotemia
**HEME:** Agranulocytosis, anemia, bone marrow depression, pancytopenia
**MS:** Arthralgia, back pain, myalgia
**RESP:** Cough, dyspnea
**SKIN:** Alopecia, diaphoresis, flushing, jaundice, onycholysis, pemphigoid, photosensitivity, pruritus, rash, Stevens-Johnson syndrome, toxic epidermal necrolysis, urticaria
**Other:** Angioedema

### Nursing Considerations
•Use ramipril cautiously in patients with renal or hepatic impairment.
•**WARNING** Be aware that patients with dehydration, heart failure, or hyponatremia; those who've recently received intensive diuresis or an increase in diuretic dosage; and those undergoing dialysis may be at risk for excessive hypotension. Monitor such patients closely the first 2 weeks of therapy and whenever ramipril or diuretic dosage increases. If excessive hypotension occurs, notify prescriber immediately, place patient in a supine position, and, if prescribed, infuse NS.
•**WARNING** Because of the risk of angioedema, be prepared to stop drug and provide emergency measures, including S.C. epinephrine 1:1,000 (0.3 to 0.5 ml), if swelling of tongue, glottis, or larynx causes airway obstruction.

•Monitor blood pressure frequently during therapy to assess drug's effectiveness.
•Monitor patient's renal and hepatic function closely during therapy.
**PATIENT TEACHING**
•Advise patient to stop taking ramipril and inform prescriber immediately if she experiences swelling of the face, eyes, lips, or tongue or has difficulty breathing.
•Explain that drug may cause dizziness and light-headedness, especially during first few days of therapy. Instruct patient to notify prescriber immediately if she faints.
•Inform female patient of childbearing age of the risks of taking ramipril during pregnancy, especially during the second and third trimesters. Caution patient to use effective contraception and to report known or suspected pregnancy immediately.
•Urge patient to tell providers that she takes ramipril before having surgery or anesthesia.
•Tell patient to ask prescriber before using supplements or salt substitutes that contain potassium.

# ranitidine hydrochloride

Apo-Ranitidine (CAN), Gen-Ranitidine (CAN), Novo-Ranitidine (CAN), Nu-Ranit (CAN), Zantac, Zantac EFFERdose Tablets, Zantac 150 GELdose, Zantac 300 GELdose

### Class and Category
*Chemical:* Aminoalkyl-substituted furan derivative
*Therapeutic:* Antiulcer agent, gastric acid secretion inhibitor
*Pregnancy category:* B

### Indications and Dosages
➤ *To prevent duodenal and gastric ulcers*
**CAPSULES, EFFERVESCENT GRANULES, EFFERVESCENT TABLETS, SYRUP, TABLETS**
**Adults and adolescents.** 150 mg h.s.
➤ *To provide short-term treatment of active duodenal and benign gastric ulcers*
**CAPSULES, EFFERVESCENT GRANULES, EFFERVESCENT TABLETS, SYRUP, TABLETS**
**Adults and adolescents.** 150 mg b.i.d. for gastric ulcers; 150 mg b.i.d. or 300 mg h.s. for duodenal ulcers.
**Children age 1 month to 16 years.** 2 to 4 mg/kg b.i.d. up to 300 mg/day. *Maintenance:* 2 to 4 mg/kg q.d. up to 150 mg/day.

**Q**
**R**
**S**

CONTINUOUS I.V. INFUSION

**Adults and adolescents.** 6.25 mg/hr. *Maximum:* 400 mg/day.

INTERMITTENT I.V. INFUSION

**Adults and adolescents.** 50 mg diluted to total volume of 100 ml and infused over 15 to 20 min q 6 to 8 hr. *Maximum:* 400 mg/day.

**Children.** 2 to 4 mg/kg/day diluted to a suitable volume and infused over 15 to 20 min.

I.V. INJECTION

**Adults and adolescents.** 50 mg diluted to total volume of 20 ml and injected slowly over no less than 5 min q 6 to 8 hr. *Maximum:* 400 mg/day.

I.M. INJECTION

**Adults and adolescents.** 50 mg q 6 to 8 hr. *Maximum:* 400 mg/day.

➤ *To treat acute gastroesophageal reflux disease*

CAPSULES, EFFERVESCENT GRANULES, EFFERVESCENT TABLETS, SYRUP, TABLETS

**Adults and adolescents.** 150 mg b.i.d.

EFFERVESCENT TABLETS

**Children age 1 month to 16 years.** 2.5 to 5 mg/kg b.i.d.

INTERMITTENT I.V. INFUSION

**Children.** 2 to 8 mg/kg diluted to suitable volume and infused over 15 to 20 min t.i.d.

➤ *To treat erosive esophagitis*

CAPSULES, EFFERVESCENT GRANULES, EFFERVESCENT TABLETS, SYRUP, TABLETS

**Adults and adolescents.** 150 mg q.i.d.

EFFERVESCENT TABLETS

**Children age 1 month to 16 years.** 2.5 to 5 mg/kg b.i.d.

➤ *To treat hypersecretory GI conditions, such as Zollinger-Ellison syndrome, systemic mastocytosis, and multiple endocrine adenoma syndrome*

CAPSULES, EFFERVESCENT GRANULES, EFFERVESCENT TABLETS, SYRUP, TABLETS

**Adults and adolescents.** *Initial:* 150 mg b.i.d., adjusted as needed. *Maximum:* 6 g/day in divided doses.

CONTINUOUS I.V. INFUSION

**Adults and adolescents.** *Initial:* 1 mg/kg/hr, increased by 0.5 mg/kg/hr up to 2.5 mg/kg/hr. *Maximum:* 400 mg/day.

INTERMITTENT I.V. INFUSION

**Adults.** 50 mg diluted to total volume of 100 ml and infused over 15 to 20 min q 6 to 8 hr. *Maximum:* 400 mg/day.

I.V. INJECTION

**Adults and adolescents.** 50 mg diluted to total of 20 ml and injected slowly over at least 5 min q 6 to 8 hr. *Maximum:* 400 mg/day.

I.M. INJECTION

**Adults.** 50 mg q 6 to 8 hr.

➤ *To prevent acid indigestion, heartburn, and sour stomach caused by eating certain foods or drinking certain beverages*

TABLETS

**Adults and adolescents.** 75 mg 30 to 60 min before food or beverages expected to cause symptoms. *Maximum:* 150 mg/day over no more than 2 continuous wk.

➤ *To treat acid indigestion, heartburn, and sour stomach*

TABLETS

**Adults and adolescents.** 75 mg when symptoms start; repeated once within 24 hr, if needed.

DOSAGE ADJUSTMENT For patients whose creatinine clearance is less than 50 ml/min/1.73 m$^2$, 150 mg P.O. q 24 hr with dosage interval increased thereafter to q 12 hr, as needed. Or 50 mg I.V. q 18 to 24 hr with dosage interval increased to q 12 hr, as needed. Dosage reduction may also be necessary for patients with hepatic dysfunction.

| Route | Onset | Peak | Duration |
|---|---|---|---|
| P.O., I.V., I.M. | Unknown | 1 to 3 hr | 13 hr |

## Mechanism of Action

Inhibits basal and nocturnal secretion of gastric acid and pepsin by competitively inhibiting the action of histamine at H$_2$ receptors on gastric parietal cells. This action reduces total volume of gastric juices and, thus, irritation of GI mucosa.

## Contraindications

Acute porphyria, hypersensitivity to ranitidine or its components

## Interactions

DRUGS

*antacids:* Decreased ranitidine absorption
*bone marrow depressants:* Increased risk of neutropenia or other blood dyscrasias
*diazepam, itraconazole, ketoconazole, sucralfate:* Decreased absorption of these drugs

*glipizide, glyburide, metoprolol, midazolam, nifedipine, phenytoin, theophylline, warfarin:* Increased effects of these drugs, possibly leading to toxic reactions

**ACTIVITIES**

*alcohol use:* Increased blood alcohol level (with oral ranitidine)

## Adverse Reactions

**CNS:** Dizziness, drowsiness, headache, insomnia
**CV:** Vasculitis
**GI:** Abdominal distress, constipation, diarrhea, nausea, vomiting
**GU:** Impotence
**MS:** Arthralgia, myalgia
**SKIN:** Alopecia, erythema multiforme, rash

## Nursing Considerations

•Be aware that ranitidine must be diluted for I.V. use if not using premixed solution. For I.V. injection, dilute to total of 20 ml with NS, $D_5W$, $D_{10}W$, LR, or 5% sodium bicarbonate. For I.V. infusion, dilute to total volume of 100 ml of same solutions.
•Give I.V. injection at no more than 4 ml/min, intermittent I.V. infusion at 5 to 7 ml/min, and continuous I.V. infusion at 6.25 mg/hr (except in patients with hypersecretory conditions, for whom initial infusion rate is 1 mg/kg/hr, gradually increased after 4 hours, as needed, in increments of 0.5 mg/kg/hr).
•Don't add additives to premixed solution.
•Stop primary I.V. solution infusion during piggyback administration.

**PATIENT TEACHING**

•Tell patient to dissolve 150-mg effervescent tablets or granules in 6 to 8 oz water or 25-mg effervescent tablets in at least 5 ml water.
•Advise patient (or parent) to wait until effervescent tablet is completely dissolved before taking (or giving to child or infant).
•Stress the importance of not chewing effervescent tablets, swallowing them whole, or letting them dissolve on the tongue before swallowing.
•Alert phenylketonurics that effervescent tablets and granules contain phenylalanine.
•Tell patient she may take drug with food.
•Tell patient to stop drug and contact prescriber if she has trouble swallowing, vomits blood, or passes black or bloody stools.
•If needed, advise patient to take antacids, 2 hours before or after ranitidine; advise against taking other acid reducers with drug.

•If patient takes drug to prevent heartburn, tell her to contact prescriber about frequent chest pain or wheezing with heartburn; stomach pain; unexplained weight loss; nausea; vomiting; heartburn for more than 3 months; heartburn with light-headedness, dizziness, or sweating; chest or shoulder pain with shortness of breath, sweating, light-headedness, or pain spreading to arms, neck, or shoulders. These problems could be serious.
•Inform patient that healing of an ulcer may require 4 to 8 weeks of therapy.

# rasburicase

Elitek

## Class and Category

*Chemical:* Tetrameric protein
*Therapeutic:* Uric acid reducer
*Pregnancy category:* C

## Indications and Dosages

➤ *To manage plasma uric acid levels initially in pediatric patients with leukemia, lymphoma, or solid tumor malignancies who receive anticancer therapy that elevates plasma uric acid*

**I.V. INFUSION**

**Children.** 0.15 or 0.20 mg/kg infused over 30 min q.d. for 5 days.

---

### Mechanism of Action

Converts uric acid into an inactive and soluble metabolite at the end of the purine catabolic pathway. This prevents plasma uric acid levels from rising due to tumor lysis from anticancer therapy.

---

## Contraindications

Glucose-6-phosphatase dehydrogenase (G6PD) deficiency; history of anaphylaxis or hypersensitivity reactions, hemolytic reactions, or methemoglobinemia reactions; hypersensitivity to rasburicase or its components

## Interactions

None known

## Adverse Reactions

**CNS:** Anxiety, fever, headache, paresthesia, rigors, seizures

**CV:** Arrhythmia, cardiac failure or arrest, cerebrovascular disorder, chest pain, hemorrhage, hypotension, myocardial infarction, pulmonary edema, thrombophlebitis, thrombosis
**EENT:** Mucositis, retinal hemorrhage
**ENDO:** Hot flashes
**GI:** Abdominal pain, constipation, diarrhea, ileus, intestinal obstruction, nausea, vomiting
**GU:** Acute renal failure
**HEME:** Anemia, hemolysis, methemoglobinemia, neutropenia, pancytopenia
**RESP:** Cyanosis, dyspnea, pneumonia, pulmonary hypertension, respiratory distress
**SKIN:** Cellulitis, rash
**Other:** Anaphylaxis, dehydration, infection, sepsis

## Nursing Considerations

• Be aware that children at high risk for G6PD, such as patients of African or Mediterranean ancestry, should be screened before administering rasburicase because severe hemolysis can occur.
• Expect to administer only one course of therapy because of the high risk for severe allergic reactions.
• Reconstitute rasburicase using only the diluent provided. Add 1 ml of the diluent to each vial needed, and mix by swirling very gently. Don't shake vial or mix by turning it from top to bottom.
• Inject reconstituted solution into an infusion bag containing the appropriate volume of 0.9% NaCl to obtain a final volume of 50 ml. Infuse over 30 minutes using a different line than for the infusion of other drugs. If a separate line isn't possible, flush the line with at least 15 ml of NS solution before and after rasburicase infusion. Don't use filters for the infusion.
• Store reconstituted solution at 2° to 8° C (36° to 46° F) for no longer than 24 hours. Protect drug from light.
• **WARNING** Monitor patient closely for severe hypersensitivity reactions, including anaphylaxis (chest pain, dyspnea, hypotension, urticaria), hemolysis (severe anxiety, pain, dyspnea), and methemoglobinemia (anxiety, hypoxemia, shortness of breath). If such a reaction occurs, discontinue rasburicase immediately, notify prescriber, and institute emergency treatment. Rasburicase shouldn't be reinstituted at any time after such a reaction occurs.
• Ensure that blood samples to measure uric acid levels are collected in pre-chilled tubes containing heparin anticoagulant and are immediately immersed and maintained in ice water until analysis is done (within 4 hours); blood samples left at room temperature will result in low uric acid levels because of enzyme degradation of uric acid at room temperature.

**PATIENT TEACHING**
• Inform child and parents that chemotherapy will start 4 to 24 hours after rasburicase.
• Stress the importance of reporting any adverse reaction immediately.

# remifentanil hydrochloride

Ultiva

## Class, Category, and Schedule

*Chemical:* Fentanyl analogue
*Therapeutic:* Anesthesia adjunct
*Pregnancy category:* C
*Controlled substance:* Schedule II

## Indications and Dosages

➤ *As adjunct to induce general anesthesia*
**INTERMITTENT I.V. INFUSION**
**Adults and children age 2 and older.** 0.5 to 1 mcg/kg in addition to inhalation or I.V. anesthetic.

➤ *To maintain general anesthesia*
**INTERMITTENT I.V. INFUSION**
**Adults and children age 2 and older.** 0.05 to 0.2 mcg/kg, followed by 0.5 to 1 mcg/kg q 2 to 5 min, as needed.

➤ *To continue analgesic effect in immediate postoperative period*
**CONTINUOUS I.V. INFUSION**
**Adults and children age 2 and older.** *Initial:* 0.1 mcg/kg/min, adjusted by 0.025 mcg/kg/min q 5 min, as prescribed, to balance level of analgesia and respiratory rate. *Maximum:* 0.2 mcg/kg/min.

➤ *To supplement local or regional anesthesia in a monitored anesthetic setting*
**I.V. INFUSION**
**Adults and children age 2 and older.** *With a benzodiazepine:* 0.05 mcg/kg/min, beginning

5 min before placement of local or regional block; after placement of block, decreased to 0.025 mcg/kg/min and then further adjusted q 5 min in increments of 0.025 mcg/kg/min, as needed. *Without a benzodiazepine:* 0.1 mcg/kg/min, beginning 5 min before placement of local or regional block; after placement of block, decreased to 0.05 mcg/kg/min and then further adjusted q 5 min in increments of 0.025 mcg/kg/min, as needed.

**I.V. INJECTION**

**Adults and children age 2 and older.** *With a benzodiazepine:* 0.5 mcg/kg administered over 30 to 60 sec as a single dose 60 to 90 sec before local anesthetic is administered. *Without a benzodiazepine:* 1 mcg/kg administered over 30 to 60 sec as a single dose 60 to 90 sec before local anesthetic is administered.

DOSAGE ADJUSTMENT For elderly patients, starting dose possibly reduced by half. If patient is more than 30% over ideal body weight, starting dose based on ideal body weight.

| Route | Onset | Peak | Duration |
|-------|-------|------|----------|
| I.V. | 1 min | 1 to 2 min | 5 to 10 min |

## Incompatibilities

Don't administer remifentanil through same I.V. line as blood because nonspecific esterases in blood products may inactivate drug.

## Contraindications

Epidural or intrathecal administration, hypersensitivity to fentanyl analogues

## Interactions

**DRUGS**

*anesthetics (barbiturate, inhalation), benzodiazepines, propofol:* Possibly synergistic effects, increasing risk of hypotension and respiratory depression

*atropine, glycopyrrolate:* Possibly reversal of remifentanil-induced bradycardia

*ephedrine, epinephrine, norepinephrine:* Possibly reversal of remifentanil-induced hypotension

*neuromuscular blockers:* Prolonged remifentanil-induced skeletal muscle rigidity

*opioid antagonists:* Possibly reversal of remifentanil's effects

## Adverse Reactions

**CNS:** Headache, shivering
**CV:** Asystole, bradycardia, hypotension

## Mechanism of Action

Remifentanil decreases the transmission and perception of pain by stimulating mu-opioid receptors in neurons. This action decreases the activity of adenyl cyclase in neurons, which in turn decreases cAMP production. With less cAMP available, potassium (K⁺) is forced out of neurons, and calcium (Ca⁺⁺) is prevented from entering neurons. As a result, neuron excitability declines, and fewer neurotransmitters (such as substance P) leave the neurons, thereby decreasing pain transmission.

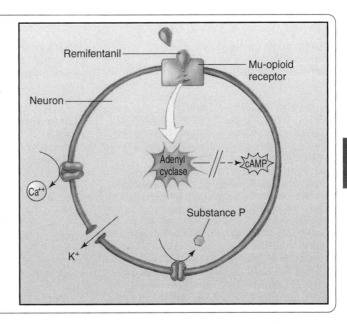

**GI:** Nausea, vomiting
**MS:** Skeletal muscle rigidity
**RESP:** Apnea, cough, dyspnea, respiratory depression, stridor, wheezing
**Other:** Anaphylaxis

## Nursing Considerations

•Inject remifentanil into I.V. tubing at or as close as possible to venous cannula.
•Use infusion device for continuous infusion.
•Monitor vital signs and oxygenation continuously during administration.
•Expect analgesic effects to dissipate rapidly when drug is discontinued. Expect to start adequate postoperative analgesia, as prescribed, before stopping drug.
•**WARNING** After stopping drug, clear I.V. tubing to prevent inadvertent later administration.
•Monitor respiratory status continuously because of risk of respiratory depression from residual effects of other anesthetics for up to 30 minutes after infusion stops.

**PATIENT TEACHING**
•Explain expected drug effects to patient, and reassure her that she'll be monitored continuously during drug administration.

# repaglinide

Prandin

## Class and Category

*Chemical:* Meglitinide
*Therapeutic:* Antidiabetic drug
*Pregnancy category:* C

## Indications and Dosages

➤ *To achieve glucose control in type 2 diabetes mellitus as monotherapy in patients whose glycosylated hemoglobin (HbA₁c) level is less than 8%*

**TABLETS**
**Adults.** *Initial:* 0.5 mg 15 to 30 min before meals b.i.d. Dosage doubled, as needed, q wk until adequate glucose response obtained. *Maintenance:* 0.5 to 4 mg/dose up to q.i.d. *Maximum:* 16 mg/day in divided doses of not more than 4 mg/dose.
➤ *To achieve glucose control in type 2 diabetes mellitus as monotherapy in patients whose HbA₁c is 8% or greater and in combination with metformin or thia-*
*zolidinedione (pioglitazone hydrochloride, rosiglitazone maleate) therapy*

**TABLETS**
**Adults.** *Initial:* 1 or 2 mg 15 to 30 min before meals b.i.d. Dosage doubled, as needed, q wk until adequate glucose response obtained. *Maintenance:* 1 to 4 mg/dose up to q.i.d. *Maximum:* 16 mg/day in divided doses of not more than 4 mg/dose.

**DOSAGE ADJUSTMENT** For patients with moderate to severe hepatic or renal impairment, increased time between dosage adjustments.

## Mechanism of Action

Stimulates release of insulin from functioning pancreatic beta cells. In patients with type 2 diabetes mellitus, a shortage of these cells decreases blood insulin levels and causes glucose intolerance. By interacting with the adenosine triphosphatase (ATP)–potassium channel on the beta cell membrane, repaglinide prevents potassium from leaving the cell. This causes the beta cell to depolarize and the cell membrane's calcium channel to open. As a result, calcium moves into the cell and insulin moves out. The extent of insulin release is glucose dependent; the lower the glucose level, the less insulin is secreted from the cell.

## Contraindications

Diabetic ketoacidosis, hypersensitivity to repaglinide or its components, severe hepatic or renal impairment, type 1 diabetes mellitus

## Interactions

**DRUGS**
*barbiturates, carbamazepine, rifampin, troglitazone:* Possibly increased repaglinide metabolism
*beta blockers, chloramphenicol, clarithromycin, MAO inhibitors, NSAIDs, oral anticoagulants, probenecid, salicylates, sulfonamides:* Enhanced hypoglycemic effects
*calcium channel blockers, corticosteroids, diuretics, estrogens, isoniazid, niacin, oral contraceptives, phenothiazines, phenytoin, sympathomimetics, thyroid hormones:* Possibly loss of glucose control
*erythromycin, ketoconazole, miconazole:* Pos-

sibly inhibited repaglinide metabolism
*gemfibrozil:* Increased blood repaglinide
level, resulting in enhanced and prolonged
blood glucose–lowering effects
*NPH insulin:* Possibly increased risk of
angina

## Adverse Reactions
**CNS:** Headache
**CV:** Angina
**EENT:** Rhinitis, sinusitis
**ENDO:** Hypoglycemia
**GI:** Diarrhea, elevated liver enzymes, nausea
**HEME:** Leukopenia, thrombocytopenia
**MS:** Arthralgia, back pain
**RESP:** Bronchitis, upper respiratory tract infection
**Other:** Anaphylaxis

## Nursing Considerations
•Be aware that repaglinide shouldn't be used
with NPH insulin because the combination
may increase the risk of angina.
•Expect to check HbA$_{1c}$ level every 3 months,
as ordered, to assess patient's long-term control of blood glucose level.
•During increased stress, such as infection,
surgery, and trauma, monitor blood glucose
level often assess need for additional insulin.

**PATIENT TEACHING**
•Instruct patient to take repaglinide 15 to
30 minutes before meals and to skip dose
whenever she skips a meal.
•Explain that repaglinide is an adjunct to
diet in managing type 2 diabetes mellitus.
•Teach patient how to monitor her blood
glucose level and when to notify prescriber.
•Review signs and symptoms of hyperglycemia and hypoglycemia with patient and
family. Instruct patient to notify prescriber
immediately if she experiences anxiety, confusion, dizziness, excessive sweating, headache, increased thirst, increased urination, or
nausea.
•Advise patient to carry identification indicating that she has diabetes. Encourage her
to carry candy or other simple carbohydrates
with her to treat mild episodes of hypoglycemia.
•Inform patient that her HbA$_{1c}$ level will be
tested every 3 to 6 months until her blood
glucose level is controlled.

# reserpine
Novoreserpine (CAN), Reserfia (CAN), Serpalan,
Serpasil (CAN)

## Class and Category
*Chemical:* Rauwolfia alkaloid
*Therapeutic:* Antihypertensive
*Pregnancy category:* C

## Indications and Dosages
➤ *To treat hypertension*
**TABLETS**
**Adults.** 0.1 to 0.25 mg q.d.
**Children.** 0.005 to 0.02 mg/kg/day q.d. or in
divided doses b.i.d.
**DOSAGE ADJUSTMENT** Lower dosage possibly
required for elderly or severely debilitated
patients.

| Route | Onset | Peak | Duration |
|-------|-------|------|----------|
| P.O. | Days to 3 wk | 3 to 6 wk | 1 to 6 wk |

## Contraindications
Active peptic ulcer, electroconvulsive therapy, hypersensitivity to reserpine or its components, mental depression (current or history of), ulcerative colitis

## Interactions
**DRUGS**
*anticholinergics:* Decreased effectiveness of
anticholinergics
*barbiturates:* Increased CNS depression
*beta blockers:* Additive and, possibly, excessive beta-adrenergic blockade
*bromocriptine:* Possibly interference with
bromocriptine's effects
*digoxin, procainamide, quinidine:* Increased
risk of arrhythmias
*hypotension-producing drugs:* Increased antihypertensive effect; increased risk of orthostatic hypotension or bradycardia (with guanadrel or guanethidine)
*levodopa:* Decreased levodopa effectiveness
*MAO inhibitors:* Increased risk of severe hypertension and hyperpyrexia, additive CNS
depression
*NSAIDs:* Decreased antihypertensive effect
*sympathomimetics:* Increased vasopressor effects, decreased antihypertensive effect

**ACTIVITIES**
*alcohol use:* Increased CNS depression

Q
R
S

## Mechanism of Action

Reserpine reduces blood pressure by decreasing norepinephrine stores in presynaptic sympathetic neurons.

Normally, when a nerve impulse activates a sympathetic neuron, the nerve ending releases norepinephrine, which stimulates alpha or beta receptors on target cell membranes, as shown below left. Stimulation of alpha receptors may produce vasoconstriction; stimulation of beta receptors may increase the heart rate and force of myocardial contraction, which raises cardiac output. Through a reuptake mechanism, some norepinephrine returns to the neuron and is stored in vesicles for reuse.

Reserpine displaces norepinephrine from vesicles in the nerve fiber, and MAO degrades the displaced norepinephrine, as shown below right. These actions reduce the amount of norepinephrine available to stimulate postsynaptic alpha and beta receptors, leading to a reduction in vasoconstriction, cardiac output, and blood pressure.

## Adverse Reactions

**CNS:** Anxiety, depression, dizziness, drowsiness, headache, nervousness, nightmares, sleep disturbance, syncope, weakness
**CV:** Arrhythmias, such as bradycardia; chest pain; peripheral edema
**EENT:** Conjunctival injection, dry mouth, epistaxis, glaucoma, hearing loss, nasal congestion, optic atrophy, uveitis
**ENDO:** Breast engorgement
**GI:** Abdominal cramps or pain, anorexia, diarrhea, increased gastric secretions, melena, nausea, vomiting
**GU:** Decreased libido, galactorrhea, gynecomastia, impotence
**MS:** Myalgia
**RESP:** Dyspnea
**SKIN:** Purpura
**Other:** Weight gain

## Nursing Considerations

• Use reserpine cautiously in patients with a history of depression because drug may cause depression that is masked as somatic complaints.
• Monitor blood pressure frequently during drug therapy.
• Alert anesthesiologist if patient is scheduled for surgery. Drug may cause circulatory instability even if withheld before procedure.
**PATIENT TEACHING**
• Instruct patient to take reserpine with food or milk to minimize stomach upset.
• Caution patient about possible drowsiness, and advise her to avoid potentially hazardous activities until drug's CNS effects are known.
• Explain the need for frequent appointments to monitor blood pressure and adjust dosage at start of therapy.

# reteplase

Retavase

## Class and Category

*Chemical:* Recombinant plasminogen activator (r-PA)
*Therapeutic:* Thrombolytic
*Pregnancy category:* C

## Indications and Dosages

➤ *To improve ventricular function, prevent heart failure, and reduce mortality after acute MI*

**I.V. INJECTION**
**Adults.** 10 U over 2 min; repeated after 30 min.

## Incompatibilities

Don't add other drugs to reteplase injection solution or administer them through same I.V. line as reteplase.

### Mechanism of Action

Converts plasminogen to plasmin, which works to break up fibrin clots that have formed in the coronary arteries. Elimination of the clots improves cardiac blood and oxygen flow to the area, thus improving ventricular function.

## Contraindications

Active internal bleeding, aneurysm, arteriovenous malformation, bleeding diathesis, brain tumor, history of CVA or other cerebrovascular disease, hypersensitivity to reteplase or its components, intracranial or intraspinal surgery or trauma during previous 2 months, severe uncontrolled hypertension (systolic 200 mm Hg or higher, diastolic 110 mm Hg or higher)

## Interactions

**DRUGS**

*antifibrinolytics (including aminocaproic acid, aprotinin, and tranexamic acid):* Decreased effectiveness of reteplase
*antineoplastics, antithymocyte globulin, certain cephalosporins (such as cefamandole, cefoperazone, and cefotetan), heparin, oral anticoagulants, platelet aggregation inhibitors (such as abciximab, aspirin, and dipyridamole), strontium-89 chloride, sulfinpyrazone, valproic acid:* Increased risk of bleeding

## Adverse Reactions

**CNS:** Intracranial hemorrhage
**GI:** GI bleeding, nausea, vomiting
**HEME:** Thrombocytopenia
**RESP:** Hemoptysis
**SKIN:** Bleeding from wounds, ecchymosis, hematoma, purpura
**Other:** Allergic reaction, injection site bleeding

## Nursing Considerations

• Expect to begin reteplase therapy, as prescribed, as soon as possible after MI symptoms begin.
• Closely monitor patient with atrial fibrillation, severe hypertension, or other cardiac disease for signs and symptoms of cerebral embolism.
• To reconstitute, use diluent, syringe, needle, and dispensing pin provided. Withdraw 10 ml of preservative-free sterile water for injection. Remove and discard needle from syringe, and connect dispensing pin to syringe. Remove protective cap from spike end of dispensing pin, and insert spike into reteplase vial. Inject 10 ml of sterile water into the vial. With the spike still in the vial, swirl gently to dissolve the powder. Don't shake. Expect to see slight foaming. Let the vial stand for several minutes. When the bubbles dissipate, withdraw 10 ml of reconstituted solution into the syringe (about 0.7 ml may remain in the vial). Now detach the syringe from the dispensing pin and attach the 20G needle.
• Use the solution within 4 hours. Discard if it's discolored or contains particulates.
• Don't administer heparin and reteplase in the same solution. Instead, flush the heparin line with NS or $D_5W$ before and after reteplase injection.
• Because fibrin is lysed during therapy, closely monitor all possible bleeding sites (catheter insertions, arterial and venous punctures, cutdowns, and needle punctures).
• Avoid I.M. injections, venipunctures, and nonessential handling of patient during therapy.
• If arterial puncture is necessary, use an arm vessel that can be compressed, if possible. After sample is obtained, apply pressure for at least 30 minutes, and then apply a pressure dressing. Check site frequently for bleeding.

Q
R
S

•If bleeding occurs and can't be controlled by local pressure, notify prescriber immediately. Be prepared to stop concurrent anticoagulant therapy immediately and to discontinue second reteplase bolus, as prescribed.
•Anticipate that reperfusion arrhythmias—premature ventricular contractions, ventricular tachycardia—may follow coronary thrombolysis.

**PATIENT TEACHING**
•Advise patient to report adverse reactions immediately.

# rifabutin

Mycobutin

## Class and Category

*Chemical:* Spiropiperidyl derivative
*Therapeutic:* Antimycobacterial antibiotic
*Pregnancy category:* B

## Indications and Dosages

➤ *To prevent disseminated* Mycobacterium avium *complex in patients with advanced HIV infection*

**CAPSULES**
**Adults.** 300 mg q.d. or 150 mg b.i.d.

---

### Mechanism of Action

Suppresses RNA synthesis by inhibiting DNA-dependent RNA polymerase in a wide variety of bacteria, including *Mycobacterium avium.* Exhibits dose-dependent bactericidal or bacteriostatic action.

---

## Contraindications

Hypersensitivity to rifabutin or rifamycins

## Interactions

**DRUGS**
*aminophylline, barbiturates, beta blockers, chloramphenicol, clofibrate, corticosteroids, cyclosporine, dapsone, diazepam, digoxin, disopyramide, estramustine, estrogens, ketoconazole, mexiletine, oral anticoagulants, oral antidiabetic drugs, oral contraceptives (containing estrogen), oxtriphylline, phenytoin, quinidine, theophylline, tocainide, verapamil (oral):* Reduced therapeutic effects of these drugs
*fluconazole:* Increased blood rifabutin level
*methadone:* Possibly withdrawal symptoms
*zidovudine:* Decreased blood zidovudine level

## Adverse Reactions

**CNS:** Asthenia, fever, headache, insomnia
**CV:** Chest pain
**EENT:** Discolored saliva, tears, and sputum
**GI:** Abdominal pain, anorexia, diarrhea, discolored feces, elevated liver function test results, eructation, flatulence, indigestion, nausea, vomiting
**GU:** Discolored urine
**HEME:** Neutropenia, thrombocytopenia
**MS:** Myalgia
**SKIN:** Discolored skin and sweat, rash

## Nursing Considerations

•Monitor laboratory values during rifabutin therapy to detect neutropenia and thrombocytopenia.
•Expect drug to cause reddish orange to reddish brown discoloration of skin and body fluids.
•Be aware that drug may cause myelosuppression and increased risk of infection. Notify prescriber immediately if signs of infection, such as fever, develop.

**PATIENT TEACHING**
•Advise patient to take rifabutin with food if GI distress develops.
•Encourage patient to have any necessary dental work done before rifabutin therapy starts to reduce the risk of bleeding or infection.
•Explain that drug may turn urine, feces, saliva, sputum, sweat, tears, and skin reddish orange to reddish brown.
•Caution patient against wearing soft contact lenses during therapy because drug may permanently stain them.
•Advise patient to notify prescriber about signs of *Mycobacterium avium* complex (chills, fever, night sweats, weight loss), tuberculosis, myositis, or uveitis.
•Advise woman of childbearing age who is using an oral contraceptive to change to a nonhormonal method of birth control because rifabutin may decrease contraceptive's effectiveness.

# rifampin

## (rifampicin)

Rifadin, Rifadin IV, Rimactane, Rofact (CAN)

## Class and Category

*Chemical:* Semisynthetic antibiotic derivative of rifamycin
*Therapeutic:* Antimycobacterial antitubercular
*Pregnancy category:* C

## Indications and Dosages

➤ *As adjunct to treat tuberculosis caused by all strains of* Mycobacterium tuberculosis

CAPSULES, ORAL SUSPENSION, I.V. INFUSION

**Adults.** 10 mg/kg q.d. in combination with other antitubercular drugs for 2 mo. *Maximum:* 600 mg/day.

**Infants and children.** 10 to 20 mg/kg q.d. in combination with other antitubercular drugs for 2 mo. *Maximum:* 600 mg/day.

➤ *To eliminate meningococci from nasopharynx of asymptomatic carriers of* Neisseria meningitidis

CAPSULES, ORAL SUSPENSION, I.V. INFUSION

**Adults.** 600 mg q 12 hr for 2 days (total of 4 doses).

**Infants age 1 month and older and children.** 10 mg/kg q 12 hr for 2 days (total of 4 doses). *Maximum:* 600 mg/day.

**Infants under age 1 month.** 5 mg/kg q 12 hr for 2 days (total of 4 doses). *Maximum:* 600 mg/day.

DOSAGE ADJUSTMENT For patients with hepatic impairment, maximum dosage of 8 mg/kg/day. For patients with creatinine clearance of 10 ml/min/1.73 m$^2$ or less, recommended dosage usually decreased by 50%.

---

### Mechanism of Action

Inhibits bacterial and mycobacterial RNA synthesis by binding to DNA-dependent RNA polymerase, thereby blocking RNA transcription. Exhibits dose-dependent bactericidal or bacteriostatic action. Rifampin is highly effective against rapidly dividing bacilli in extracellular cavitary lesions, such as those found in the nasopharynx.

---

## Incompatibilities

Don't administer rifampin in the same I.V. line as diltiazem.

## Contraindications

Concurrent use of nonnucleoside reverse transcriptase inhibitors or protease inhibitors by patients with HIV, hypersensitivity to rifamycins

## Interactions

DRUGS

*aminophylline, oxtriphylline, theophylline:* Increased metabolism and clearance of these theophylline preparations

*anesthetics (hydrocarbon inhalation, except isoflurane), hepatotoxic drugs, isoniazid:* Increased risk of hepatotoxicity

*beta blockers, chloramphenicol, clofibrate, corticosteroids, cyclosporine, dapsone, digitalis glycosides, disopyramide, hexobarbital, itraconazole, ketoconazole, mexiletine, oral anticoagulants, oral antidiabetic drugs, phenytoin, propafenone, quinidine, tocainide, verapamil (oral):* Increased metabolism, resulting in lower blood levels of these drugs

*bone marrow depressants:* Increased leukopenic or thrombocytopenic effects

*clofazimine:* Reduced absorption of rifampin, delaying its peak concentration and increasing its half-life

*diazepam:* Enhanced elimination of diazepam, resulting in decreased drug effectiveness

*estramustine, estrogens, oral contraceptives:* Decreased estrogenic effects

*methadone:* Possibly impaired absorption of methadone, leading to withdrawal symptoms

*probenecid:* Increased blood level or prolonged duration of rifampin, increasing risk of toxicity

*nonnucleoside reverse transcriptase inhibitors, protease inhibitors (indinavir, nelfinavir, ritonavir, saquinavir):* Accelerated metabolism of these drugs (by patients with HIV), resulting in subtherapeutic levels; delayed metabolism of rifampin, increasing risk of toxicity

*trimethoprim:* Increased elimination and shortened elimination half-life of trimethoprim

*vitamin D:* Increased metabolism and decreased efficacy of vitamin D, leading to decreased serum calcium and phosphate levels and increased parathyroid hormone levels

ACTIVITIES

*alcohol use:* Increased risk of hepatotoxicity

## Adverse Reactions

**CNS:** Chills, dizziness, drowsiness, fatigue, headache, paresthesia

**EENT:** Discolored saliva, tears, and sputum; mouth or tongue soreness; periorbital edema

**GI:** Abdominal cramps, anorexia, diarrhea, discolored feces, elevated liver function test results, epigastric discomfort, flatulence, heartburn, hepatitis, nausea, pseudomembranous colitis, vomiting

**GU:** Discolored urine

**MS:** Arthralgia, myalgia

**SKIN:** Discolored skin and sweat

**Other:** Facial edema, flulike symptoms

Q
R
S

## Nursing Considerations
•Obtain blood samples or other specimens for culture and sensitivity testing, as ordered, before giving rifampin and throughout therapy to monitor response to drug.
•Expect to monitor liver function test results before and every 2 to 4 weeks during therapy. Immediately report abnormalities.
•For I.V. infusion, reconstitute by adding 10 ml of sterile water for injection to 600-mg vial of rifampin. Swirl gently to dissolve. Withdraw appropriate dose and add to 500 ml of D₅W (preferred solution) or NS and infuse over 3 hours. Alternatively, withdraw appropriate dose and add to 100 ml of D₅W (preferred solution) or NS and infuse over 30 minutes. Use reconstituted drug promptly because rifampin may precipitate out of D₅W solution after 4 hours. NS solution is stable for up to 24 hours at room temperature.
•Be aware that patient receiving intermittent therapy (once or twice weekly) is at increased risk for adverse reactions.
•Expect drug to discolor skin and body fluids reddish orange to reddish brown.
•Be aware that rifampin can cause myelosuppression and increase risk of infection. Notify prescriber immediately if signs of infection, such as fever, develop.

### PATIENT TEACHING
•Instruct patient to take rifampin 1 hour before or 2 hours after a meal with a full glass of water.
•Stress the need to take drug exactly as prescribed. Explain that interruptions can lead to increased adverse reactions.
•Explain that drug may turn urine, feces, saliva, sputum, sweat, tears, and skin reddish orange to reddish brown.
•Caution patient against wearing soft contact lenses during therapy because drug may permanently stain them.
•Advise patient who takes an oral contraceptive to use an additional form of birth control during rifampin therapy.
•Urge patient to notify prescriber about flu-like symptoms, anorexia, darkened urine, fever, joint pain or swelling, malaise, nausea, vomiting, and yellowish skin or eyes, which may indicate hepatitis.
•Advise patient to avoid alcohol during rifampin therapy.
•Instruct patient to notify prescriber if no improvement occurs within 2 to 3 weeks.

# riluzole
Rilutek

## Class and Category
*Chemical:* Benzothiazole
*Therapeutic:* Amyotrophic lateral sclerosis treatment agent
*Pregnancy category:* C

## Indications and Dosages
➤ *To treat amyotrophic lateral sclerosis*
**TABLETS**
**Adults.** 50 mg q 12 hr.

---

### Mechanism of Action
Inhibits release of glutamic acid, an excitatory amino acid neurotransmitter, in the CNS, thus reducing its effects on target cells. Glutamic acid affects degeneration of neurons; reducing its level may help slow amyotrophic lateral sclerosis.

---

## Contraindications
Hypersensitivity to riluzole or its components

## Interactions
### DRUGS
*allopurinol, hepatotoxic drugs, methyldopa, sulfasalazine:* Increased risk of hepatotoxicity
*amitriptyline, phenacetin, quinolones, tacrine, theophylline:* Delayed elimination of riluzole
*omeprazole, rifampin:* Increased riluzole clearance
### FOODS
*charbroiled foods:* Increased riluzole elimination
### ACTIVITIES
*alcohol use:* Increased risk of hepatotoxicity
*smoking:* Increased riluzole elimination

## Adverse Reactions
**CNS:** Asthenia, dizziness, headache, insomnia, paresthesia (circumoral), somnolence, spasticity, vertigo
**CV:** Peripheral edema
**EENT:** Dry mouth, rhinitis, stomatitis
**GI:** Abdominal pain, anorexia, constipation, diarrhea, elevated liver function test results, flatulence, indigestion, nausea, vomiting
**HEME:** Neutropenia
**MS:** Back or muscle pain or stiffness
**RESP:** Dyspnea, increased cough, pneumonia
**SKIN:** Alopecia, eczema, pruritus

## Nursing Considerations
- Use riluzole cautiously in patients with impaired hepatic or renal function.
- Also use cautiously in elderly patients, women, and Japanese patients because of increased risk of toxicity from decreased drug clearance.
- Monitor liver function test results before and during riluzole therapy.

**PATIENT TEACHING**
- Instruct patient to take riluzole regularly, every 12 hours, 1 hour before or 2 hours after a meal, and at the same time each day.
- Instruct patient to store riluzole at room temperature, protected from bright light.
- Urge patient to minimize alcohol, smoking, and charred foods; they speed drug excretion.
- Tell patient to report fever.

# risedronate sodium

Actonel

## Class and Category
*Chemical:* Pyridinyl bisphosphonate
*Therapeutic:* Bone resorption inhibitor
*Pregnancy category:* C

## Indications and Dosages
➤ *To treat Paget's disease of bone when serum alkaline phosphatase level is at least twice normal and patient is symptomatic or at risk for complications*

**TABLETS**
**Adults.** 30 mg q.d. for 2 mo. Repeated after 2 mo if relapse occurs or if serum alkaline phosphatase level fails to normalize.

➤ *To prevent or treat postmenopausal or glucocorticoid-induced osteoporosis*

**TABLETS**
**Adults.** 5 mg q.d. Alternatively, for postmenopausal osteoporosis, 35 mg once/wk.

| Route | Onset | Peak | Duration |
|-------|-------|------|----------|
| P.O. | Unknown | 3 mo | 16 mo |

### Mechanism of Action
Hinders excessive bone remodeling characteristic of Paget's disease by binding to bone and reducing the rate at which osteoclasts are resorbed by bone.

## Contraindications
Hypersensitivity to risedronate or its components, hypocalcemia

## Interactions
**DRUGS**
*aspirin, NSAIDs:* Increased risk of GI irritation
*calcium-containing preparations, including antacids:* Impaired absorption of risedronate
**FOODS**
*all foods:* Decreased risedronate bioavailability

## Adverse Reactions
**CNS:** Dizziness, headache, weakness
**CV:** Chest pain, peripheral edema
**EENT:** Amblyopia, dry eyes, sinusitis, tinnitus
**GI:** Abdominal pain, colitis, constipation, diarrhea, eructation, nausea
**MS:** Arthralgia, leg cramps, myasthenia
**RESP:** Bronchitis
**SKIN:** Bullous reaction, rash
**Other:** Angioedema, flulike symptoms

## Nursing Considerations
- Give supplemental calcium and vitamin D, as prescribed, during risedronate therapy if patient's dietary intake is inadequate.
- Give calcium supplements and antacids at different time of day than risedronate administration to avoid impaired drug absorption and altered effectiveness.
- Watch for rare but possibly severe rash, bullous skin reactions, and angioedema.

**PATIENT TEACHING**
- Instruct patient to take risedronate at least 1 hour before first food or drink of day (except water) while in an upright position and with 6 to 8 oz of water. Caution against lying down for at least 30 minutes after taking drug to prevent it from lodging in esophagus and causing irritation.
- Tell patient to take calcium supplements or antacids at different times than risedronate.
- Urge women of childbearing age to tell prescriber about planned, suspected, or known pregnancy because of risk to fetal skeleton.
- Tell patient to stop drug and contact prescriber about swelling or skin abnormalities.

# risperidone

Risperdal, Risperdal Consta

## Class and Category
*Chemical:* Benzisoxazole derivative
*Therapeutic:* Antipsychotic
*Pregnancy category:* C

## Indications and Dosages
➤ *To manage psychotic disorders*

ORAL SOLUTION, ORALLY DISINTEGRATING TABLETS, TABLETS

**Adults.** 1 mg b.i.d. on day 1; 2 mg b.i.d. on day 2; 3 mg b.i.d. on day 3. Or, 2 mg q.d on day 1; 4 mg q.d. on day 2; 6 mg q.d. on day 3. Then increased by 1 to 2 mg/day at 1- to 2-wk intervals, as needed. *Maximum:* 16 mg/day.

I.M. INJECTION

**Adults.** *Initial:* 25 mg q 2 wk, increased as needed q 4 wk to 37.5 or 50 mg. *Maximum:* 50 mg q 2 wk.

➤ *To treat bipolar mania*

ORAL SOLUTION, ORALLY DISINTEGRATING TABLETS, TABLETS

**Adults.** *Initial:* 2 or 3 mg q.d., increased as needed by 1 mg daily up to 6 mg. Maximum: 6 mg daily for no more than 3 wk.

DOSAGE ADJUSTMENT Initial dose 0.5 mg b.i.d. for elderly or debilitated patients, those with renal or hepatic impairment, and those at risk for hypotension. Increased by 0.5 mg b.i.d. q wk, as needed. Given q.d. after target dosage maintained for 2 or 3 days. Maximum for patients with severe hepatic dysfunction, 4 mg/day; for elderly patients, 3 mg/day.

---

## Mechanism of Action

Selectively blocks serotonin and dopamine receptors in the mesocortical tract of the CNS to suppress psychotic symptoms.

---

## Incompatibilities

Don't mix oral solution with cola or tea.

## Contraindications

Hypersensitivity to risperidone or its components

## Interactions

DRUGS

*antihypertensives:* Increased antihypertensive effects

*bromocriptine, levodopa, pergolide:* Possibly antagonized effects of these drugs

*carbamazepine:* Increased risperidone clearance with long-term concurrent use

*clozapine:* Decreased risperidone clearance with long-term concurrent use

*CNS depressants:* Additive CNS depression

ACTIVITIES

*alcohol use:* Additive CNS depression

## Adverse Reactions

**CNS:** Aggressiveness, agitation, anxiety, asthenia, decreased concentration, dizziness, dream disturbances, drowsiness, dystonia, fatigue, headache, lassitude, memory loss, nervousness, neuroleptic malignant syndrome, parkinsonism, restlessness, somnolence

**CV:** Chest pain, hypercholesterolemia, orthostatic hypotension, palpitations, tachycardia

**EENT:** Decreased or increased salivation, dry mouth, pharyngitis, rhinitis, sinusitis, vision changes

**ENDO:** Galactorrhea, hyperglycemia

**GI:** Abdominal pain, constipation, diarrhea, indigestion, nausea, vomiting

**GU:** Amenorrhea, decreased libido, dysmenorrhea, dysuria, hypermenorrhea, polyuria, sexual dysfunction

**MS:** Arthralgia, back pain

**RESP:** Cough, dyspnea

**SKIN:** Diaphoresis, dry skin, hyperpigmentation, photosensitivity, pruritus, rash, seborrhea

**Other:** Injection site induration, pain, redness, or swelling; weight gain or loss

## Nursing Considerations

• Use risperidone cautiously in patients with hepatic or renal dysfunction or hypotension and in debilitated or elderly patients because of their increased sensitivity to drug.

• Be aware that oral risperidone or another antipsychotic should be continued for 3 weeks after long-acting I.M. form of risperidone is first administered to provide an adequate therapeutic plasma level until risperidone release from injection site has begun. If the patient has never received oral risperidone, an oral trial should be prescribed before use of I.M. form to determine patient's tolerance of the drug.

• Remove I.M. form of risperidone from refrigerator and allow it to come to room temperature before reconstitution. Follow manufacturer's guidelines for reconstitution, using only the diluent supplied in the dose pack.

• Give I.M. form using only the needle supplied in the dose pack. Inject entire contents of syringe into the upper outer quadrant of gluteal area within 2 minutes of reconstitution. If drug can't be given right after reconstitution, shake the upright vial vigorously back and forth until particles are resuspended. Discard reconstituted drug if not

used within 6 hours. Never administer I.M. form intravenously.
•Monitor for orthostatic hypotension, especially in patients with cardiac or cerebrovascular disease.
•WARNING Immediately notify prescriber and expect to stop drug if patient shows signs of neuroleptic malignant syndrome (altered mental status, autonomic instability, hyperpyrexia, muscle rigidity), which can be fatal.
•Monitor blood glucose and lipid levels as ordered because drug increases the risk of hyperglycemia and hypercholesterolemia.

**PATIENT TEACHING**
•Instruct patient to dilute risperidone oral solution with water, coffee, orange juice, or low-fat milk but not with cola or tea.
•Tell patient prescribed orally disintegrating tablets to break open the blister unit with dry hands by peeling back foil to expose the tablet. Stress the importance of not pushing tablet through the foil because this could damage the tablet. Once patient has removed tablet, she should place immediately on her tongue, where it will dissolve within seconds. Tell patient not to chew orally disintegrating tablet or attempt to spit it out of her mouth.
•Urge patient to avoid alcohol because of its additive CNS effects.
•Caution diabetic patient to monitor blood glucose level closely because risperidone may increase it.

# rivastigmine tartrate
Exelon

## Class and Category
*Chemical:* Carbamate derivative
*Therapeutic:* Antidementia
*Pregnancy category:* B

## Indications and Dosages
➤ *To treat mild to moderate Alzheimer's-type dementia*

**CAPSULES**
**Adults.** *Initial:* 1.5 mg b.i.d. Dosage increased by 3 mg/day q 2 wk, as needed. *Maximum:* 12 mg/day.
DOSAGE ADJUSTMENT If patient develops nausea or vomiting during therapy, treatment should be discontinued for several doses, as prescribed, and restarted at lowest dose and increased by 3 mg/day q 2 wk, as needed.

## Mechanism of Action
May slow the decline of cognitive function in patients with Alzheimer's disease by increasing the concentration of acetylcholine at cholinergic transmission sites. This action prolongs and exaggerates the effects of acetylcholine that are otherwise blocked by toxic levels of anticholinergics. The cognitive decline in these patients is partially related to cholinergic deficits along neuronal pathways projecting from the basal forebrain to the cerebral cortex and hippocampus that are involved in memory, attention, learning, and cognition.

## Contraindications
Hypersensitivity to carbamate derivatives, rivastigmine, or their components

## Interactions
**DRUGS**
*anticholinergics:* Possibly decreased effectiveness of anticholinergics
*bethanechol, succinylcholine:* Possibly synergistic effects

## Adverse Reactions
**CNS:** Aggression, anxiety, asthenia, confusion, depression, dizziness, fatigue, fever, hallucinations, headache, insomnia, malaise, seizures, somnolence, tremor
**CV:** Hypertension
**EENT:** Rhinitis
**GI:** Abdominal pain, anorexia, constipation, diarrhea, flatulence, indigestion, nausea, vomiting
**GU:** UTI
**SKIN:** Increased sweating
**Other:** Flulike symptoms, weight loss

## Nursing Considerations
•WARNING Be aware that rivastigmine should be started at lowest recommended dosage and adjusted to an effective maintenance dosage because initial therapy at high dosage can cause serious adverse GI reactions, including anorexia, nausea, and weight loss. Also, higher than recommended starting dosage may cause severe vomiting and possibly esophageal rupture. If treatment is interrupted for longer than several days, expect to restart drug at lowest recommended dosage.
•Be aware that drug shouldn't be discontin-

Q
R
S

ued abruptly because doing so may increase behavioral disturbances and precipitate a further decline in cognitive function.

•Monitor respiratory status of patients with pulmonary disease, including asthma, chronic bronchitis, and emphysema, because rivastigmine has a weak affinity for peripheral cholinesterase, which may increase bronchoconstriction and bronchial secretions.

•Monitor patient for adequate urine output because cholinomimetics, such as rivastigmine, may induce or exacerbate urinary tract or bladder obstruction.

•Monitor patients with Parkinson's disease for exaggerated parkinsonian symptoms, which may result from drug's increased cholinergic effects on CNS.

**PATIENT TEACHING**

•Explain to patient and family that rivastigmine can't cure Alzheimer's disease but may slow the progressive deterioration of memory and improve patient's ability to perform activities of daily living.

•Advise patient and family that drug should be taken with food to reduce adverse GI effects.

•Instruct a family member to supervise patient's use of rivastigmine.

•Urge caregiver to contact prescriber and to withhold drug if patient stops taking it for more than several days.


# rizatriptan benzoate

Maxalt, Maxalt-MLT

## Class and Category

*Chemical:* Selective 5-hydroxytryptamine
*Therapeutic:* Antimigraine
*Pregnancy category:* C

## Indications and Dosages

➤ *To relieve acute migraine headache*

**DISINTEGRATING TABLETS, TABLETS**

**Adults.** 5 to 10 mg when migraine starts; repeated q 2 hr, p.r.n. *Maximum:* 30 mg/day.
**DOSAGE ADJUSTMENT** For patients taking propranolol, initial dosage reduced to 5 mg, then repeated q 2 hr, p.r.n., up to maximum of 15 mg/day.

## Contraindications

Basilar or hemiplegic migraine, hypersensitivity to rizatriptan or its components, isch-
emic coronary artery disease, uncontrolled hypertension, use within 14 days of MAO inhibitor therapy, use within 24 hours of other serotonin-receptor agonists or ergotamine-containing or ergot-type drugs

## Mechanism of Action

Binds to selective 5-hydroxytryptamine receptor sites on cerebral blood vessels, causing vessels to constrict. This may decrease the characteristic pulsing sensation and thus relieve the pain of migraine headaches. Rizatriptan also may relieve pain by inhibiting the release of proinflammatory neuropeptides and reducing transmission of trigeminal nerve impulses from sensory nerve endings during a migraine attack.

## Interactions

**DRUGS**

*ergot-containing drugs:* Prolonged vasospastic reactions
*MAO inhibitors, propranolol:* Increased blood rizatriptan level
*selective serotonin-reuptake inhibitors:* Increased risk of weakness, hyperreflexia, and lack of coordination
*serotonin-receptor agonists:* Additive vasospastic effects

## Adverse Reactions

**CNS:** Altered temperature sensation, anxiety, asthenia, ataxia, chills, confusion, depression, disorientation, dizziness, dream disturbances, drowsiness, euphoria, fatigue, hangover, headache, hypoesthesia, insomnia, mental impairment, nervousness, paresthesia, somnolence, tremor, vertigo
**CV:** Arrhythmias, such as bradycardia and tachycardia; chest pain; hot flashes; hypertension; palpitations
**EENT:** Blurred vision; burning eyes; dry eyes, mouth, and throat; earache; eye pain or irritation; lacrimation; nasal congestion and irritation; pharyngeal edema; pharyngitis; tinnitus; tongue swelling
**GI:** Abdominal distention, constipation, diarrhea, dysphagia, flatulence, heartburn, indigestion, nausea, thirst, vomiting
**GU:** Menstrual irregularities, polyuria, urinary frequency
**MS:** Arthralgia; dysarthria; muscle spasms, stiffness, or weakness; myalgia
**RESP:** Dyspnea, upper respiratory tract infection, wheezing

**SKIN:** Diaphoresis, flushing, pruritus, rash, urticaria
**Other:** Angioedema, dehydration, facial edema

## Nursing Considerations

•Use rizatriptan cautiously in patients with renal or hepatic dysfunction because of impaired drug metabolism or excretion. Monitor patient's BUN and serum creatinine levels and liver function test results, as appropriate.
•Also use cautiously in patients with peripheral vascular disease because drug may cause vasospastic reactions, leading to vascular and colonic ischemia with abdominal pain and bloody diarrhea. Assess peripheral circulation and bowel sounds frequently during therapy.
•Assess cardiovascular status and institute continuous ECG monitoring, as ordered, immediately after rizatriptan administration in patients with cardiovascular risk factors because of possible asymptomatic cardiac ischemia.
•Monitor blood pressure regularly in patients with hypertension because rizatriptan may increase blood pressure.

**PATIENT TEACHING**
•Instruct patient taking rizatriptan disintegrating tablets to remove tablet from blister pack with dry hands just before taking, to place tablet on tongue, and to allow it to dissolve and be swallowed with saliva.
•Advise phenylketonuric patient not to use disintegrating tablet form because it contains phenylalanine.
•Instruct patient to seek emergency care immediately if cardiac symptoms, such as chest pain, occur after administration.
•Caution patient about possible adverse CNS reactions, and advise her to avoid potentially hazardous activities until drug's CNS effects are known.

# ropinirole hydrochloride

Requip

## Class and Category

*Chemical:* Non-ergot alkaloid dopamine agonist
*Therapeutic:* Antidyskinetic
*Pregnancy category:* C

## Indications and Dosages

➤ *To treat signs and symptoms of Parkinson's disease*

**TABLETS**
**Adults.** *Initial:* 0.25 mg t.i.d. Dosage titrated upward q wk according to the following schedule: 0.25 mg t.i.d. in wk 1; 0.5 mg t.i.d. in wk 2; 0.75 mg t.i.d. in wk 3; 1 mg t.i.d. in wk 4. After wk 4, dosage increased by 1.5 mg/day q wk up to 9 mg/day, then by 3 mg/day up to 24 mg/day. *Maximum:* 24 mg/day.

➤ *To treat moderate to severe primary restless legs syndrome*
**TABLETS**
**Adults.** *Initial:* 0.25 mg 1 to 3 hr before h.s. Dosage increased after 2 days to 0.5 mg and then to 1 mg at the end of the first wk. If nedded, dosage further increased in 0.5-mg increments q wk. *Maximum:* 4 mg daily.

---

### Mechanism of Action

Directly stimulates postsynaptic dopamine type 2 ($D_2$) receptors within the brain and acts as an agonist at peripheral $D_2$ receptors. These actions inhibit the firing of striatal cholinergic neurons, thus helping to control alterations in voluntary muscle movement (such as tremors and rigidity) associated with Parkinson's disease.

---

## Contraindications

Hypersensitivity to ropinirole or its components

## Interactions
**DRUGS**
*carbamazepine, cimetidine, ciprofloxacin, clarithromycin, diltiazem, enoxacin, erythromycin, fluvoxamine, mexiletine, norfloxacin, omeprazole, phenobarbital, phenytoin, rifampin, ritonavir, troleandomycin:* Altered drug clearance and increased blood level of ropinirole
*chlorprothixene, domperidone, droperidol, haloperidol, metoclopramide, phenothiazines, thiothixene:* Possibly decreased effectiveness of ropinirole
*CNS depressants:* Additive effects
*ethinyl estradiol:* Possibly reduced clearance of ropinirole
**ACTIVITIES**
*alcohol use:* Additive effects

## Adverse Reactions
**CNS:** Asthenia, confusion, dizziness, falling asleep during activities of daily living, fatigue, hallucinations, headache, hypoesthesia,

Q
R
S

malaise, neuralgia, paresthesia, rigors, somnolence, syncope, transient ischemic attack, vertigo
**CV:** Acute coronary syndrome, angina, bradycardia, cardiac failure, chest pain, hypertension, MI, orthostatic hypotension, palpitations, peripheral edema, sick sinus syndrome, tachycardia
**EENT:** Abnormal vision, dry mouth, nasal congestion, nasopharyngitis, rhinitis, toothache
**GI:** Abdominal pain, constipation, diarrhea, dyspepsia, gastric hemorrhage, gastroenteritis, indigestion, intestinal obstruction, ischemic hepatitis, nausea, pancreatitis, vomiting
**GU:** Elevated BUN level, erectile dysfunction, UTI
**HEME:** Anemia
**MS:** Arthralgia; arthritis; exacerbation of restless leg syndrome in the early-morning hours; limb pain; muscle cramps, spasms, or stiffness; myalgia; neck pain; osteoarthritis; tendinitis
**RESP:** Asthma, bronchitis, cough, upper respiratory tract infection
**SKIN:** Diaphoresis, flushing, hot flashes, night sweats, rash
**Other:** Influenza, viral infection, weight loss

## Nursing Considerations
•WARNING Expect to reassess patient periodically during ropinirole treatment for excessive sedation. Patient may develop excessive and acute drowsiness as late as 1 year after beginning therapy.
•When ropinirole is given as adjunct to levodopa, expect concurrent dosage of levodopa to be gradually decreased as tolerated.
•Expect to stop ropinirole gradually over 7 days, as follows: over first 4 days, frequency should be reduced from t.i.d to b.i.d.; during last 3 days, frequency should be reduced to q.d., followed by complete withdrawal of drug.
•WARNING Monitor patient for altered mental status during drug withdrawal. Rapid reduction of dosage may lead to a symptom complex resembling neuroleptic malignant syndrome that includes fever, muscle rigidity, altered level of consciousness, and autonomic instability.
•Watch for orthostatic hypotension, especially in patient with early Parkinson's disease. Orthostatic hypotension can occur more than 4 weeks after start of therapy or after a dosage reduction because ropinirole may impair systemic regulation of blood pressure.
•Monitor patient for hallucinations, especially if patient has Parkinson's disease, is elderly, or takes levodopa because incidence of this adverse effect is higher among these patients.
•Monitor patient for worsening of preexisting dyskinesia; ropinirole may potentiate dopaminergic adverse effects of levodopa.
•Avoid giving CNS depressants, sleep aids, and other CNS-interacting drugs during ropinirole therapy because they increase the risk of somnolence.

**PATIENT TEACHING**
•Inform patient with Parkinson's disease that ropinirole helps to improve muscle control and movement but doesn't cure Parkinson's disease.
•Encourage patient to take ropinirole with food to decrease risk of adverse GI effects.
•Caution patient to avoid hazardous activities until CNS effects of drug—including sedation—are known.
•If patient falls asleep during normal activities, advise her to notify prescriber.
•Encourage patient to avoid using alcohol and other sedating drugs (such as sleep aids) during ropinirole therapy because they may enhance drug's CNS depressant effects.
•If patient has restless legs syndrome, explain that symptoms might appear in early morning during ropinirole therapy and could be worse or spread to other limbs. Urge patient to notify prescriber if this occurs.
•Instruct patient to change positions slowly to minimize effect of ropinirole on blood pressure.


# rosiglitazone maleate
Avandia

## Class and Category
*Chemical:* Thiazolidinedione
*Therapeutic:* Antidiabetic drug
*Pregnancy category:* C

## Indications and Dosages
➤ *To achieve glucose control in type 2 diabetes mellitus as monotherapy or in combination with metformin*

TABLETS
**Adults.** *Initial:* 4 mg q.d. or 2 mg b.i.d., increased to 8 mg q.d. or 4 mg b.i.d. if glucose control is inadequate after 12 wk. *Maximum:* 8 mg q.d.
➤ *To achieve glucose control in type 2 diabetes mellitus in combination with insulin therapy*
TABLETS
**Adults.** 4 mg q.d. with no change in insulin dosage. Insulin dosage decreased by 10% to 25% if hypoglycemia occurs or fasting plasma concentrations decrease to less than 100 mg/dl with combination therapy.

---

**Mechanism of Action**
Increases tissue sensitivity to insulin. This peroxisome proliferator-activated receptor agonist regulates the transcription of insulin-responsive genes found in key target tissues, such as adipose tissue, skeletal muscle, and the liver. Enhanced tissue sensitivity to insulin lowers the blood glucose level.

---

**Contraindications**
Hypersensitivity to rosiglitazone or its components

**Interactions**
DRUGS
*CYP2C8 inducers, such as rifampin:* Possibly decreased effects of rosiglitazone
*CYP2C8 inhibitors, such as gemfibrozil:* Possibly increased effects of rosiglitazone

**Adverse Reactions**
**CNS:** Fatigue, headache
**CV:** Congestive heart failure, edema
**EENT:** Sinusitis
**ENDO:** Hyperglycemia, hypoglycemia
**GI:** Diarrhea, hepatotoxicity
**HEME:** Anemia
**MS:** Back pain
**RESP:** Upper respiratory tract infection
**SKIN:** Urticaria
**Other:** Angioedema, weight gain

**Nursing Considerations**
• Use rosiglitazone cautiously in patients with edema, heart failure, or hepatic impairment because of potential adverse reactions.
• Be aware that drug isn't recommended for patients with New York Heart Association Class III or IV cardiac status.

• Evaluate patient's liver function before starting drug and periodically throughout therapy, as ordered. Notify prescriber about abnormalities, such as nausea, vomiting, abdominal pain, fatigue, anorexia, and dark urine. Drug may need to be stopped.
•**WARNING** Monitor patient for evidence of congestive heart failure—such as shortness of breath, rapid weight gain, or edema—because rosiglitazone can cause fluid retention that may lead to or worsen heart failure. Notify prescriber immediately if the patient's cardiac status deteriorates, and expect to stop the drug, as ordered.
• Monitor fasting glucose and glycosylated hemoglobin $A_{1c}$ levels periodically, as ordered, to evaluate the effectiveness of rosiglitazone treatment.
• Be aware that drug is effective only in the presence of endogenous insulin.
PATIENT TEACHING
• Stress the need to follow an exercise program and a diet control program during rosiglitazone therapy.
• Advise patient to notify prescriber immediately if she experiences shortness of breath, fluid retention, or sudden weight gain because drug may need to be discontinued.
• Instruct patient to have liver function tests, as prescribed, about every 2 months for first year and then annually.
• Inform premenopausal, anovulatory patient that drug may induce ovulation, increasing risk of pregnancy.

# rosiglitazone maleate and metformin hydrochloride

Avandamet

**Class and Category**
*Chemical:* Thiazolidinedione (rosiglitazone), dimethylbiguanide (metformin)
*Therapeutic:* Antidiabetic
*Pregnancy category:* C

**Indications and Dosages**
➤ *To reduce blood glucose level as initial therapy in patients with type 2 diabetes mellitus who aren't adequately controlled with rosiglitazone alone*

Q
R
S

TABLETS
**Adults.** *Initial:* 2 mg/500 mg b.i.d if patient was taking 4 mg q.d. of rosiglitazone monotherapy; 4 mg/500 mg b.i.d. if 8 mg q.d. of rosiglitazone monotherapy. Increased as needed after 1 to 2 wk if metformin dosage isn't sufficient or 8 to 12 wk if rosiglitazone dosage isn't sufficient. *Maximum:* 8 mg/2,000 mg/day.

➤ *To reduce blood glucose level as initial therapy in patients with type 2 diabetes mellitus who aren't adequately controlled with metformin alone*

TABLETS
**Adults.** *Initial:* 2 mg/500 mg b.i.d if patient was taking 1,000 mg/day of metformin monotherapy; individualized if patient was taking 1,000 to 2,000 mg/day of metformin monotherapy; or 2 mg/1,000 mg (two tablets of 1-mg/500-mg strength) b.i.d. if patient was taking 2,000 mg/day of metformin monotherapy. Dosage increased, as needed, after 1 to 2 wk if metformin dosage isn't sufficient or after 8 to 12 wk if rosiglitazone dosage isn't sufficient. *Maximum:* 8 mg/2,000 mg/day.

DOSAGE ADJUSTMENT If patient has been taking rosiglitazone and metformin as separate tablets, usual starting dose of combination drug is that of rosiglitazone and metformin already being taken individually.

| Route | Onset | Peak | Duration |
|---|---|---|---|
| P.O. (metformin) | Days to 1 wk | 2 wk | 2 wk after drug is stopped |

## Contraindications

Diabetic coma; heart failure requiring drug treatment; hypersensitivity to metformin, rosiglitazone, or their components; ketoacidosis; metabolic acidosis (acute or chronic); renal disease or dysfunction (serum creatinine level of 1.5 mg/dl or more in men or 1.4 mg/dl or more in women); type 1 diabetes mellitus

## Interactions

DRUGS
**rosiglitazone maleate and metformin hydrochloride**
None known.
**rosiglitazone component only**
*CYP2C8 inducers, such as rifampin:* Possibly decreased effects of rosiglitazone
*CYP2C8 inhibitors, such as gemfibrozil:* Pos-

sibly increased effects of rosiglitazone
**metformin component only**
*cimetidine:* Increased blood metformin level, possibly increased risk of hypoglycemia
*furosemide:* Increased blood metformin level, decreased blood furosemide level
*nifedipine:* Enhanced absorption of metformin
FOODS
*all foods:* Delayed and reduced absorption of metformin
ACTIVITIES
*alcohol use:* Altered blood glucose control (usually hyperglycemia), possibly potentiated effect of metformin on lactate metabolism

## Mechanism of Action

Rosiglitazone and metformin each improve glucose control. Rosiglitazone increases tissue sensitivity to insulin. A peroxisome proliferator-activated receptor agonist, it regulates transcription of insulin-responsive genes in key target tissues, such as adipose tissue, skeletal muscle, and liver. Enhanced insulin sensitivity lowers blood glucose level.

Metformin may promote storage of excess glucose as glycogen in the liver, thus reducing glucose production. It also may improve glucose use by skeletal muscle and adipose tissue by facilitating glucose transport across cell membranes. Metformin also may increase the number of insulin receptors on cell membranes and make them more sensitive to insulin.

## Adverse Reactions

**CNS:** Fatigue, headache
**CV:** Edema, heart failure
**EENT:** Sinusitis
**ENDO:** Hyperglycemia, hypoglycemia
**GI:** Diarrhea, elevated liver function test results, hepatotoxicity
**HEME:** Anemia
**MS:** Arthralgia, back pain
**RESP:** Upper respiratory tract infection
**SKIN:** Urticaria
**Other:** Angioedema, lactic acidosis, viral infection, weight gain

## Nursing Considerations

•WARNING Monitor renal function, as ordered, before beginning rosiglitazone and metformin therapy and at least annually thereafter because significant renal impairment can result in tissue hypoperfusion and hypoxemia, leading to lactic acidosis.

•Evaluate patient's liver function before starting drug and periodically throughout therapy, as ordered. Notify prescriber about abnormalities, such as nausea, vomiting, abdominal pain, fatigue, anorexia, and dark urine. Drug may need to be stopped.

•**WARNING** Expect to stop rosiglitazone and metformin for 48 hours before and after radiographic tests involving I.V. iodinated contrast media because of an increased risk of renal failure and lactic acidosis.

•**WARNING** Monitor malnourished or debilitated patients and those with renal, hepatic, pituitary, or adrenal insufficiency because they have an increased risk of hypoglycemia.

•Expect to monitor vitamin $B_{12}$ blood levels at least every 2 to 3 years in patients with inadequate vitamin $B_{12}$ or calcium intake or absorption because prolonged drug use may impair vitamin $B_{12}$ absorption.

•Monitor fasting blood glucose level to determine patient's response to drug. Expect to monitor glycosylated hemoglobin ($HbA_{1c}$) level every 3 to 6 months, as ordered, to evaluate long-term blood glucose control.

•Monitor blood glucose level often to detect hyperglycemia and assess the need for supplemental insulin during periods of increased stress, such as infection, surgery, and trauma.

•Arrange for instruction about diabetes and consultation with a dietitian or certified diabetes educator, if possible.

•Monitor patient for evidence of heart failure, such as difficulty breathing, fatigue, abnormal heart sounds, and edema. Notify prescriber if such evidence occurs, and expect to stop drug.

### PATIENT TEACHING

•Instruct patient to take rosiglitazone and metformin with morning and evening meals. Caution her not to skip the meal after taking the drug.

•Inform patient that drug is used with diet and exercise therapy and is not a substitute for these additional measures.

•Advise patient not to skip doses, stop drug, or take OTC drugs without first consulting prescriber because of risk of hyperglycemia.

•Inform patient that the most common adverse effects are minor and typically occur during first few weeks of therapy.

•Teach patient how to monitor blood glucose level and when to report changes.

•Advise patient to expect laboratory monitoring of $HbA_{1c}$ level every 3 months until blood glucose level is controlled.

•Instruct patient to report signs of hypoglycemia, such as anxiety, confusion, dizziness, excessive sweating, headache, and nausea.

•Advise patient to carry identification indicating that she has diabetes.

•Advise patient to avoid alcohol because it increases the risk of hypoglycemia.

•Instruct female patient of childbearing age to report suspected or confirmed pregnancy to prescriber because she may need to discontinue rosiglitazone and metformin and switch to insulin therapy, as prescribed, during pregnancy.

# rosuvastatin calcium

Crestor

## Class and Category

*Chemical:* HMG-CoA reductase inhibitor
*Therapeutic:* Antihyperlipidemic
*Pregnancy category:* X

## Indications and Dosages

➤ *To treat heterozygous familial and nonfamilial hypercholesterolemia and mixed dyslipidemia (Fredrickson Type IIa and IIb)*

**TABLETS**

**Adults.** *Initial:* 5 to 20 mg q.d., increased q 2 to 4 wk, as needed. *Maximum:* 40 mg q.d.

➤ *To treat homozygous familial hypercholesterolemia*

**TABLETS**

**Adults.** *Initial:* 20 mg q.d., increased q 2 to 4 wk, as needed. *Maximum:* 40 mg q.d.

**DOSAGE ADJUSTMENT** For patients taking cyclosporine, dosage should not exceed 5 mg q.d.; for Asian patients, initial dosage should be limited to 5 mg q.d.; for patients taking gemfibrozil, 10 mg q.d.; for patients with severe renal impairment (creatinine clearance greater than 30 ml/min/1.73 $m^2$) who are not undergoing hemodialysis, dosage should start at 5 mg q.d. but not exceed 10 mg q.d.

| Route | Onset | Peak | Duration |
|-------|-------|------|----------|
| P.O. | Unknown | 3 to 5 hr | Unknown |

Q
R
S

## Mechanism of Action

Cholesterol and triglycerides circulate in the blood as part of lipoprotein complexes. Rosuvastatin inhibits the enzyme 3-hydroxy-3-methylglutaryl-coenzyme A (HMG-CoA) reductase. This inhibition reduces lipid levels by increasing the number of hepatic low-density-lipoprotein (LDL) receptors on the cell surface to increase uptake and catabolism of LDL. It also inhibits hepatic synthesis of very-low-density lipoprotein (VLDL), which decreases the total number of VLDL and LDL particles.

## Contraindications

Active liver disease, breast-feeding, hypersensitivity to rosuvastatin or its components, pregnancy, unexplained persistent elevations of serum transaminase levels

## Interactions

**DRUGS**

*antacids:* Decreased blood rosuvastatin level if given within 2 hours of rosuvastatin
*cyclosporine, gemfibrozil:* Increased blood rosuvastatin level
*oral contraceptives:* Increased blood ethinyl estradiol and norgestrel levels
*warfarin:* Increased INR

## Adverse Reactions

**CNS:** Asthenia, depression, dizziness, headache, hypertonia, insomnia, paresthesia
**CV:** Chest pain, hypertension, peripheral edema
**EENT:** Pharyngitis, rhinitis, sinusitis
**GI:** Abdominal pain, constipation, diarrhea, elevated liver function test results, gastroenteritis, jaundice, nausea
**GU:** Proteinuria, UTI
**MS:** Arthralgia, arthritis, back pain, myalgia, myopathy, rhabdomyolysis
**RESP:** Bronchitis, increased cough
**SKIN:** Rash
**Other:** Flulike symptoms, generalized pain, infection

## Nursing Considerations

• Use rosuvastatin cautiously in patients who consume large quantities of alcohol or have a history of liver disease because drug is contraindicated in patients with active liver disease or unexplained persistent elevations of transaminase levels.

• Also use cautiously in patients with risk factors for myopathy, such as renal impairment, advanced age, and hypothyroidism.
• Obtain baseline liver function test results and expect to monitor them every 3 months for abnormal elevations. Notify prescriber if elevations occur. If ALT or AST levels increase to more than three times the normal range, expect dosage to be reduced or drug discontinued.
• Monitor serum lipoprotein levels, as ordered, to evaluate patient's response to therapy.
• Expect rosuvastatin to be temporarily withheld if patient develops any condition that may be related to myopathy or that predisposes her to renal failure, such as sepsis, hypotension, major surgery, trauma, uncontrolled seizures, or severe metabolic, endocrine, or electrolyte disorders.
• Notify prescriber if proteinuria or hematuria appears on routine urinalysis because rosuvastatin dosage may need to be reduced.

**PATIENT TEACHING**

• Encourage patient to follow a low-fat, low-cholesterol diet.
• Tell patient to wait at least 2 hours after taking rosuvastatin before taking antacids.
• Instruct patient to notify prescriber immediately about muscle pain, tenderness, or weakness, especially if accompanied by malaise or fever.
• Inform female patient of childbearing age of need to use reliable contraceptive method while taking drug. Instruct her to notify prescriber at once if she suspects she may be pregnant.

# salmeterol xinafoate

Serevent Diskus

## Class and Category

*Chemical:* Sympathomimetic amine
*Therapeutic:* Bronchodilator
*Pregnancy category:* C

## Indications and Dosages

➤ *To prevent asthma-induced bronchospasm*

**ORAL INHALATION POWDER**

**Adults and children age 4 and older.** 1 inhalation (50 mcg) q 12 hr.

➤ *To prevent COPD-induced bronchospasm*

**ORAL INHALATION POWDER**

**Adults.** 1 inhalation (50 mcg) q 12 hr.

➤ *To prevent exercise-induced broncho-spasm*

ORAL INHALATION POWDER

**Adults and children age 4 and older.** 1 inhalation (50 mcg) at least 30 min before exercise.

| Route | Onset | Peak | Duration |
|---|---|---|---|
| Inhalation | 10 to 20 min | 3 to 4 hr | 12 hr |

## Mechanism of Action

Attaches to beta$_2$ receptors on bronchial cell membranes, stimulating the intracellular enzyme adenylate cyclase to convert adenosine triphosphate to cAMP. The resulting increase in the intracellular cAMP level relaxes bronchial smooth-muscle cells, stabilizes mast cells, and inhibits histamine release.

## Contraindications

Hypersensitivity to salmeterol or its components

## Interactions

DRUGS

*beta blockers:* Mutual inhibition of therapeutic effects

*loop or thiazide diuretics:* Increased risk of hypokalemia and potentially life-threatening arrhythmias

*MAO inhibitors, tricyclic antidepressants:* Potentiated adverse vascular effects, such as hypertensive crisis

## Adverse Reactions

**CNS:** Dizziness, fever, headache, nervousness, paresthesia, tremor

**CV:** Tachycardia

**EENT:** Dry mouth, nose, and throat; sinus problems

**GI:** Nausea

**MS:** Arthralgia

**RESP:** Cough, paradoxical bronchospasm

**SKIN:** Contact dermatitis, eczema, rash, urticaria

**Other:** Angioedema, generalized aches and pains

## Nursing Considerations

•Be aware that salmeterol shouldn't be used to relieve bronchospasm quickly because of its prolonged onset of action and that patients already taking drug twice daily shouldn't take additional doses for exercise-induced bronchospasm.

•WARNING Be aware that a recent study suggests asthma-related deaths may increase in African-American patients receiving salmeterol. Monitor this patient population closely throughout salmeterol therapy, and notify prescriber immediately of any changes in patient's respiratory status.

•Watch for arrhythmias and changes in blood pressure after use in patients with cardiovascular disorders, including ischemic cardiac disease, hypertension, and arrhythmias, because of drug's beta-adrenergic effects.

•Be aware that Serevent Diskus delivers full dose of salmeterol in only one inhalation.

•WARNING Stop salmeterol immediately and notify prescriber if patient develops paradoxical bronchospasm. Risk is greatest with first use of a new canister or vial used as an inhalant.

PATIENT TEACHING

•Advise patient who is using salmeterol to prevent asthma-induced bronchospasm to take doses 12 hours apart for optimum effect. Caution against using drug more than every 12 hours.

•Teach patient how to use the diskus by instructing him to slide the lever only once when preparing dose to avoid wasting doses. Advise him to exhale immediately before using the diskus and then to place the mouthpiece to his lips and inhale through his mouth, not his nose. Then he should remove the mouthpiece from his mouth, hold his breath for at least 10 seconds, and exhale slowly.

•Advise patient to rinse his mouth with water after each dose to minimize dry mouth.

•Advise patient to discard diskus 6 weeks after removing it from overwrap or when dose indicator reads zero.

•Instruct patient to notify prescriber if he needs four or more oral inhalations of rapid-acting inhaled bronchodilator a day for 2 or more consecutive days, or if he uses more than one canister of rapid-acting bronchodilator in an 8-week period.

# salsalate

## (salicylsalicylic acid)

Amigesic, Anaflex 750, Argesic-SA, Disalcid, Marthritic, Mono-Gesic, Salflex, Salsitab

## Class and Category

*Chemical:* Salicylic acid ester
*Therapeutic:* Analgesic, anti-inflammatory
*Pregnancy category:* C

## Indications and Dosages

➤ *To relieve symptoms of rheumatoid arthritis and related rheumatic disorders*

CAPSULES

**Adults and adolescents.** *Initial:* 1 g t.i.d.; dosage then titrated, as needed.

TABLETS

**Adults and adolescents.** *Initial:* 0.5 to 1 g b.i.d. or t.i.d.; dosage then titrated, as needed.

| Route | Onset | Peak | Duration |
|-------|-------|------|----------|
| P.O. | Unknown | 2 to 3 wk | Unknown |

### Mechanism of Action

Exerts peripherally induced analgesic and anti-inflammatory effects by blocking pain impulses and inhibiting prostaglandin synthesis.

## Contraindications

Bleeding disorders; hypersensitivity to NSAIDs, salicylates, or their components

## Interactions

DRUGS

*acetaminophen:* Increased risk of renal dysfunction with prolonged use of both drugs
*anticoagulants, thrombolytics:* Increased risk and severity of GI bleeding
*antiemetics:* Masked symptoms of salicylate-induced ototoxicity
*bismuth subsalicylate:* Increased risk of salicylate toxicity with large doses of salsalate
*cefamandole, cefoperazone, cefotetan, platelet aggregation inhibitors, plicamycin, valproic acid:* Possibly hypoprothrombinemia
*corticosteroids:* Possibly decreased blood salsalate level; additive therapeutic effects when both drugs are used to treat arthritis
*furosemide:* Increased risk of ototoxicity and salicylate toxicity
*hydantoins:* Possibly decreased hydantoin metabolism, leading to toxicity
*insulin, oral antidiabetic drugs:* Potentiated hypoglycemic effect
*laxatives (cellulose-containing):* Possibly reduced salsalate effectiveness due to impaired absorption
*methotrexate:* Increased risk of methotrexate toxicity
*NSAIDs:* Increased risk of adverse GI effects
*ototoxic drugs, vancomycin:* Increased risk of ototoxicity
*probenecid, sulfinpyrazone:* Decreased uricosuric effects

*topical salicylic acid, other salicylates:* Increased risk of salicylate toxicity if significant quantities are absorbed
*urinary acidifiers (ammonium chloride, ascorbic acid, potassium or sodium phosphates):* Decreased salicylate excretion, possibly leading to salicylate toxicity
*urinary alkalizers (antacids [long-term high-dose use], carbonic anhydrase inhibitors, citrates, sodium bicarbonate):* Increased salicylate excretion, leading to reduced effectiveness and shortened half-life; increased risk of salicylate toxicity with carbonic anhydrase inhibitor–induced metabolic acidosis
*vitamin K:* Increased vitamin K requirements

ACTIVITIES

*alcohol use:* Increased risk of GI bleeding

## Adverse Reactions

**CNS:** CNS depression, confusion, dizziness, drowsiness, fever, headache, lassitude
**EENT:** Hearing loss, tinnitus, vision changes
**GI:** Anorexia, diarrhea, epigastric discomfort, GI bleeding, heartburn, hepatotoxicity, indigestion, nausea, thirst, vomiting
**HEME:** Hemolytic anemia, leukopenia, prolonged bleeding time, thrombocytopenia
**SKIN:** Diaphoresis, purpura, rash, urticaria
**Other:** Angioedema, Reye's syndrome

## Nursing Considerations

• Avoid using salsalate in patients with hypoprothrombinemia or vitamin K deficiency because drug's hypoprothrombinemic effect may precipitate bleeding.
• Monitor hepatic and renal function, as appropriate, during long-term salsalate therapy.
• Assess for signs and symptoms of GI bleeding, such as abdominal pain or black, tarry stools, especially in patient with peptic ulcer disease.
• Assess for symptoms of ototoxicity, such as ringing or roaring in ears.

PATIENT TEACHING

• Instruct patient to take salsalate with food or a full glass of water and to remain upright for 1 hour after administration to prevent drug from lodging in esophagus and causing irritation.
• Inform patient that therapeutic response may not occur for 2 to 3 weeks.
• Urge patient to notify prescriber immediately of abdominal pain or black, tarry stools; these symptoms may indicate GI bleeding or drug toxicity.

# scopolamine hydrobromide

## scopolamine transdermal system

Transderm-Scōp, Transderm-V (CAN)

### Class and Category

*Chemical:* Belladonna alkaloid, tertiary amine
*Therapeutic:* Anesthesia adjunct, anticholinergic, antiemetic, antispasmodic, antivertigo
*Pregnancy category:* C

### Indications and Dosages

➤ *To treat biliary tract disorders, enuresis, nausea and vomiting, and nocturia*

I.V., I.M., OR S.C. INJECTION (HYDROBROMIDE)
**Adults and adolescents.** 300 to 600 mcg (0.3 to 0.6 mg) as a single dose.
**Children.** 6 mcg (0.006 mg)/kg as a single dose.

➤ *To prevent excessive salivation and respiratory tract secretions during anesthesia*

I.M. INJECTION (HYDROBROMIDE)
**Adults and adolescents.** 0.2 to 0.6 mg 30 to 60 min before induction of anesthesia.
**Children ages 8 to 12.** 0.3 mg 45 to 60 min before induction of anesthesia.
**Children ages 3 to 8.** 0.2 mg 45 to 60 min before induction of anesthesia.
**Children ages 7 months to 3 years.** 0.15 mg 45 to 60 min before induction of anesthesia.
**Infants ages 4 to 7 months.** 0.1 mg 45 to 60 min before induction of anesthesia.

➤ *As adjunct to anesthesia to induce sleep and calmness*

I.V., I.M., OR S.C. INJECTION (HYDROBROMIDE)
**Adults and adolescents.** 0.6 mg t.i.d. or q.i.d.

➤ *As adjunct to anesthesia to induce amnesia*

I.V., I.M., OR S.C. INJECTION (HYDROBROMIDE)
**Adults and adolescents.** 0.32 to 0.65 mg.

➤ *To prevent nausea, vomiting, and vertigo associated with motion sickness*

TRANSDERMAL SYSTEM
**Adults and adolescents.** 1 U.S. transdermal system (0.5 mg) applied behind ear for 3-day period, beginning at least 4 hr before antiemetic effect is required. Alternatively, 1 Canadian transdermal system (1 mg) applied behind ear for 3-day period, beginning at least 12 hr before antiemetic effect is required.

**DOSAGE ADJUSTMENT** Dosage reduction possible for elderly patients because of their increased sensitivity to scopolamine.

### Contraindications

Angle-closure glaucoma; hemorrhage with hemodynamic instability; hepatic dysfunction; hypersensitivity to barbiturates, scopolamine, other belladonna alkaloids, or their components; ileus; intestinal atony; myasthenia gravis; myocardial ischemia; obstructive GI disease, such as pyloric stenosis; obstructive uropathy, as in prostatic hyperplasia; renal impairment; tachycardia; toxic megacolon; ulcerative colitis

| Route | Onset | Peak | Duration |
|---|---|---|---|
| I.V., I.M., S.C.* | 30 min | 1 to 2 hr | 4 to 6 hr |
| I.V.† | 10 min | 50 to 80 min | 2 hr |
| I.M.‡ | 15 to 30 min | Unknown | 4 hr |
| Transdermal | 4 hr | Unknown | 72 hr |

### Mechanism of Action

Competitively inhibits acetylcholine at autonomic postganglionic cholinergic receptors. Because the most sensitive receptors are in the salivary, bronchial, and sweat glands, this action reduces secretions from these glands. Scopolamine reduces GI smooth-muscle tone; decreases gastric secretions and GI motility; reduces bladder detrusor muscle tone; reduces nasal, oropharyngeal, and bronchial secretions; and decreases airway resistance by relaxing smooth muscles in the bronchi and bronchioles.

Scopolamine also blocks neural pathways in the inner ear to relieve motion sickness and depresses the cerebral cortex to produce sedation and hypnotic effects.

Q
R
S

---

* For inhibition of saliva.
† For amnesia.
‡ For antiemesis.

## Interactions

**DRUGS**
*adsorbent antidiarrheals, antacids:* Decreased absorption and therapeutic effects of scopolamine
*anticholinergics (other):* Possibly intensified anticholinergic effects
*antimyasthenics:* Possibly reduced intestinal motility
*CNS depressants:* Possibly potentiated effects of either drug, resulting in additive sedation
*cyclopropane:* Increased risk of ventricular arrhythmias (with I.V. scopolamine)
*haloperidol:* Decreased antipsychotic effect of haloperidol
*ketoconazole:* Decreased ketoconazole absorption
*lorazepam (parenteral):* Possibly hallucinations, irrational behavior, and sedation
*metoclopramide:* Possibly antagonized effect of metoclopramide on GI motility
*opioid analgesics:* Increased risk of severe constipation and ileus
*potassium chloride:* Possibly increased severity of potassium chloride–induced GI lesions
*urinary alkalizers (antacids, carbonic anhydrase inhibitors, citrates, sodium bicarbonate):* Delayed excretion of scopolamine, possibly leading to increased therapeutic and adverse effects

**ACTIVITIES**
*alcohol use:* Additive CNS effects

## Adverse Reactions

**CNS:** Dizziness, drowsiness, euphoria, insomnia, memory loss, paradoxical stimulation
**CV:** Palpitations, tachycardia
**EENT:** Blurred vision; dry eyes, mouth, nose, and throat; mydriasis
**GI:** Constipation, dysphagia
**GU:** Urinary hesitancy, urine retention
**SKIN:** Decreased sweating, dry skin, flushing
**Other:** Injection site irritation or redness

## Nursing Considerations

• For I.V. injection, dilute scopolamine with sterile water for injection.
• Assess for bladder distention and monitor urine output because drug's antimuscarinic effects can cause urine retention.
• Monitor for pain. In presence of pain, drug may act as a stimulant and produce delirium if used without morphine or meperidine.
• Monitor heart rate for transient tachycardia, which may occur with high doses of drug. Rate should return to normal within 30 minutes.

**PATIENT TEACHING**
• Instruct patient to apply scopolamine transdermal patch on hairless area behind ear and to wash hands thoroughly with soap and water before and after applying.
• Advise patient to avoid potentially hazardous activities until drug's CNS effects are known.
• Instruct patient to avoid alcohol while taking oral forms of scopolamine.
• If patient complains of dry eyes, suggest lubricating drops.

# secobarbital sodium

Novosecobarb (CAN), Seconal

## Class, Category, and Schedule
*Chemical:* Barbiturate
*Therapeutic:* Sedative-hypnotic
*Pregnancy category:* D
*Controlled substance:* Schedule II

## Indications and Dosages

➤ *To induce sedation before surgery*
**CAPSULES**
**Adults.** 200 to 300 mg 1 to 2 hr before surgery.
**Children.** 2 to 6 mg/kg 1 to 2 hr before surgery. *Maximum:* 100 mg.

➤ *To provide short-term treatment of insomnia*
**CAPSULES**
**Adults.** 100 mg h.s.

➤ *To relieve apprehension, daytime anxiety, and tension*
**CAPSULES**
**Adults.** 30 to 50 mg t.i.d. or q.i.d.
**Children.** 2 mg/kg t.i.d.
DOSAGE ADJUSTMENT Reduced dosage required for elderly or debilitated patients and those with renal or hepatic dysfunction.

| Route | Onset | Peak | Duration |
|-------|-------|------|----------|
| P.O. | 10 to 15 min | 15 to 30 min | 1 to 4 hr |

## Contraindications
History of barbiturate addiction; hypersensitivity to secobarbital, other barbiturates, or their components; nephritis; porphyria; severe hepatic or respiratory impairment

## Mechanism of Action

Inhibits upward conduction of nerve impulses to the reticular formation of the brain, thereby disrupting impulse transmission to the cortex. This action depresses the CNS, producing drowsiness, hypnosis, and sedation.

## Interactions

**DRUGS**

*acetaminophen, adrenocorticoids, beta blockers, chloramphenicol, cyclosporine, dacarbazine, digoxin, disopyramide, estrogens, metronidazole, oral anticoagulants, oral contraceptives, quinidine, thyroid hormones, tricyclic antidepressants:* Decreased effectiveness of these drugs
*addictive drugs:* Increased risk of addiction
*calcium channel blockers:* Possibly excessive hypotension
*carbamazepine, succinimide anticonvulsants:* Decreased blood levels and increased elimination of these drugs
*carbonic anhydrase inhibitors:* Increased risk of osteopenia
*CNS depressants:* Increased CNS depressant effects
*cyclophosphamide:* Increased risk of leukopenic activity and reduced half-life of cyclophosphamide
*divalproex sodium, valproic acid:* Increased CNS depression and neurologic toxicity
*doxycycline, fenoprofen:* Increased elimination of these drugs
*general anesthetics (enflurane, halothane, methoxyflurane):* Increased risk of hepatotoxicity; increased risk of nephrotoxicity (with methoxyflurane)
*griseofulvin:* Decreased griseofulvin absorption
*guanadrel, guanethidine:* Possibly increased orthostatic hypotension
*haloperidol:* Possibly altered pattern or frequency of seizures, decreased blood haloperidol level
*ketamine:* Increased risk of hypotension or respiratory depression (when secobarbital is used as preanesthetic)
*leucovorin (large doses):* Decreased anticonvulsant effect of secobarbital
*loxapine, phenothiazines, thioxanthenes:* Possibly lowered seizure threshold

*MAO inhibitors:* Possibly prolonged CNS depressant effects of secobarbital
*maprotiline:* Increased CNS depressant effect; possibly lowered seizure threshold and decreased anticonvulsant effect with high doses of maprotiline
*methylphenidate:* Increased risk of barbiturate toxicity
*mexiletine:* Decreased blood mexiletine level
*phenylbutazone:* Decreased effectiveness of secobarbital
*posterior pituitary hormones:* Increased risk of arrhythmias and coronary insufficiency
*primidone:* Increased sedative effect of either drug, change in seizure pattern
*vitamin D:* Decreased vitamin D effects
*xanthines (aminophylline, oxtriphylline, theophylline):* Increased metabolism of xanthines (except dyphylline), decreased hypnotic effect of secobarbital

**FOODS**

*caffeine:* Increased caffeine metabolism, decreased hypnotic effect of secobarbital

**ACTIVITIES**

*alcohol use:* Increased CNS depression

## Adverse Reactions

**CNS:** Anxiety, clumsiness, confusion, depression, dizziness, drowsiness, hangover, headache, insomnia, irritability, lethargy, nervousness, nightmares, paradoxical stimulation, syncope
**CV:** Hypotension
**EENT:** Laryngospasm
**GI:** Anorexia, constipation, nausea, vomiting
**MS:** Arthralgia, muscle weakness
**RESP:** Apnea, bronchospasm, respiratory depression
**SKIN:** Jaundice
**Other:** Drug dependence, weight loss

## Nursing Considerations

•Be aware that prolonged use of secobarbital may lead to tolerance and physical and psychological dependence.
•**WARNING** To avoid withdrawal symptoms, expect to taper drug after long-term therapy. Withdrawal symptoms usually appear 8 to 12 hours after stopping drug and may include anxiety, insomnia, muscle twitching, nausea, orthostatic hypotension, vomiting, weakness, and weight loss. Severe symptoms may include delirium, hallucinations, and seizures. Generalized tonic-clonic seizures may occur within 16 hours or up to 5 days after last dose.

Q
R
S

•Assess patient for signs and symptoms of barbiturate toxicity, including dyspnea, severe confusion, and severe drowsiness. Notify prescriber immediately if they appear because barbiturate toxicity may be life-threatening.
•Expect prescriber to provide patient with the least possible quantity of secobarbital to minimize the risk of acute or chronic overdosage. For patients who are depressed, suicidal, or drug-dependent or who have a history of drug abuse, institute precautions to prevent drug hoarding and overdosage.

**PATIENT TEACHING**
•Instruct patient to take secobarbital exactly as prescribed because of the risk of addiction.
•Inform patient that taking drug with food may reduce adverse GI effects.
•Advise patient to avoid alcohol and caffeine and potentially hazardous activities during therapy.
•Inform patient about possible hangover effect.
•If patient takes an oral contraceptive, recommend using an additional form of birth control during therapy.
•Caution patient not to stop taking drug abruptly.
•Instruct patient to notify prescriber of bone pain, muscle weakness, or unexplained weight loss during therapy.

# secobarbital sodium and amobarbital sodium

Tuinal

## Class, Category, and Schedule
*Chemical:* Barbiturate
*Therapeutic:* Sedative-hypnotic
*Pregnancy category:* D
*Controlled substance:* Schedule II

## Indications and Dosages
➤ *To provide short-term treatment of insomnia*
**CAPSULES**
**Adults.** 100 to 200 mg (50 to 100 mg each of secobarbital sodium and amobarbital sodium) h.s.
➤ *To induce sedation before surgery*
**CAPSULES**
**Adults.** 100 to 200 mg (50 to 100 mg each of secobarbital sodium and amobarbital sodium) 1 hr before surgery.

**DOSAGE ADJUSTMENT** Dosage possibly reduced for elderly or debilitated patients and for those with renal or hepatic dysfunction.

| Route | Onset | Peak | Duration |
|---|---|---|---|
| P.O.* | 10 to 15 min | 15 to 30 min | 1 to 4 hr |
| P.O.† | 45 to 60 min | Unknown | 6 to 8 hr |

## Mechanism of Action
Nonselectively acts on the CNS to alter cerebral function, decrease motor activity, depress the sensory cortex, and produce drowsiness, hypnosis, and sedation. Drug appears to reduce wakefulness and alertness by acting in the thalamus, where it depresses the reticular activating system and interferes with impulse transmission from the periphery to the cortex. It produces CNS depressant effects, ranging from mild sedation and reduction of anxiety to anesthesia and coma, depending on the dosage, route, and individual patient's response. Secobarbital and amobarbital have different rates of action and dissipation. When used together, they provide a balanced sedative-hypnotic effect.

## Contraindications
History of barbiturate addiction; hypersensitivity to secobarbital, amobarbital, or their components; nephritis; porphyria; severe hepatic or respiratory dysfunction

## Interactions
**DRUGS**
*antihistamines, CNS depressants:* Additive CNS depressant effects
*corticosteroids, oral anticoagulants:* Increased metabolism of these drugs, causing decreased anticoagulant response
*doxycycline:* Shortened half-life and increased elimination of doxycycline
*estradiol, estrone, progesterone, other steroidal hormones:* Increased metabolism of these hormones, leading to decreased effectiveness
*griseofulvin:* Decreased absorption of griseofulvin

---

* Secobarbital.
† Amobarbital.

*MAO inhibitors:* Inhibited metabolism of secobarbital and amobarbital, causing prolonged CNS depressant effects
*phenytoin:* Possibly accelerated metabolism of phenytoin
*sodium valproate, valproic acid:* Decreased metabolism of secobarbital and amobarbital
*vitamin D:* Decreased effects of vitamin D
**FOODS**
*caffeine:* Increased metabolism of caffeine; decreased hypnotic effect of secobarbital and amobarbital
**ACTIVITIES**
*alcohol use:* Increased CNS depressant effects

## Adverse Reactions
**CNS:** Anxiety, clumsiness, CNS depression, confusion, dizziness, drowsiness, hallucinations, hangover, headache, insomnia, irritability, light-headedness, nervousness, nightmares, paradoxical stimulation, syncope, unsteadiness
**CV:** Bradycardia, hypotension
**GI:** Constipation, hepatic dysfunction, nausea, vomiting
**HEME:** Agranulocytosis, megaloblastic anemia, thrombocytopenia
**MS:** Osteopenia, rickets
**RESP:** Apnea, hypoventilation
**SKIN:** Exfoliative dermatitis, rash, Stevens-Johnson syndrome
**Other:** Angioedema, physical and psychological dependence, potentially fatal withdrawal syndrome, tolerance

## Nursing Considerations
•Be aware that this combination drug is used for short-term treatment of insomnia because drug loses its effectiveness after 2 weeks.
•Monitor patient for paradoxical drug effects, such as confusion, excitement, or mental depression, especially in elderly patients.
•Be aware that drug has the potential to exaggerate depression, suicidal tendencies, and other mental disorders.
•Be aware that drug shouldn't be discontinued abruptly because withdrawal symptoms can occur.
•Assess patient for signs and symptoms of possible exfoliative dermatitis, such as fever and red, scaly, or thickened skin. If this occurs, notify prescriber and expect to discontinue drug immediately because this condition may indicate a potentially fatal hypersensitivity reaction.

•Be aware that drug may cause physical and psychological dependence.
**PATIENT TEACHING**
•Instruct patient to take secobarbital and amobarbital exactly as prescribed because of the risk of addiction.
•Instruct patient to report severe dizziness, persistent drowsiness, rash, or skin lesions.
•Advise patient to use caution when driving or performing tasks that require alertness.
•Instruct patient not to consume alcohol or other CNS depressants (unless prescribed) because they increase drug's effects.
•If female patient takes an oral contraceptive, recommend that she use an added form of birth control during therapy. Advise patient to notify prescriber immediately of known or suspected pregnancy. Also, caution against breast-feeding while taking drug.
•Encourage patient to use other nondrug therapies to treat insomnia. Offer suggestions for improved sleep, such as getting moderate exercise during the day, setting regular sleep habits, and using relaxation techniques.

# selegiline hydrochloride
Apo-Selegiline (CAN), Carbex, Eldepryl, Gen-Selegiline (CAN), Novo-Selegiline (CAN), Nu-Selegiline (CAN), SD Deprenyl (CAN), Selegiline-5 (CAN)

## Class and Category
*Chemical:* Phenethylamine derivative
*Therapeutic:* Antidyskinetic
*Pregnancy category:* C

## Indications and Dosages
➤ *As adjunct to carbidopa-levodopa therapy to treat Parkinson's disease*
**CAPSULES, TABLETS**
**Adults.** 10 mg q.d., or 5 mg b.i.d. with breakfast and lunch.
**DOSAGE ADJUSTMENT** For patient with levodopa-induced adverse effects, 2.5 mg q.i.d.

## Contraindications
Hypersensitivity to selegiline or its components, use within 14 days of meperidine

## Interactions
**DRUGS**
*fluoxetine, fluvoxamine, nefazodone, paroxetine, sertraline, venlafaxine:* Increased risk of

adverse reactions similar to those of serotonin syndrome (confusion, hypomania, restlessness, myoclonus), autonomic instability, delirium, muscle rigidity, and severe agitation

*levodopa:* Increased risk of confusion, dyskinesia, hallucinations, nausea, and orthostatic hypotension

*meperidine, possibly other opioid agonists:* Increased risk of diaphoresis, excitation, muscle rigidity, and severe hypertension

*tricyclic antidepressants:* Possibly serious CNS reactions, including decreased level of consciousness, hyperpyrexia, hypertension, muscle rigidity, seizures, and syncope

**FOODS**

*caffeine:* Increased risk of hypertension

*foods that contain tyramine or other high-pressor amines:* Increased risk of sudden and severe hypertension

**ACTIVITIES**

*alcohol use:* Increased risk of hypertension

---

**Mechanism of Action**

Reduces dopamine metabolism by noncompetitively inhibiting the brain enzyme monoamine oxidase type B. This increases the amount of dopamine available to relieve symptoms associated with parkinsonism. Selegiline's metabolites may also enhance dopamine transmission by inhibiting its reuptake at synapses.

---

**Adverse Reactions**

**CNS:** Anxiety, chills, confusion, dizziness, drowsiness, dyskinesia, euphoria, extrapyramidal reactions, fatigue, hallucinations, headache, insomnia, irritability, lethargy, memory loss, mood changes, nervousness, paresthesia, restlessness, syncope, tremor, weakness

**CV:** Arrhythmias, chest pain, hypertension, orthostatic hypotension, palpitations, peripheral edema

**EENT:** Altered taste, blepharospasm, blurred vision, burning lips or mouth, diplopia, dry mouth, tinnitus

**GI:** Abdominal pain, anorexia, constipation, diarrhea, GI bleeding, heartburn, nausea, vomiting

**GU:** Dysuria, urinary hesitancy, urinary urgency, urine retention

**MS:** Arthralgia, back and leg pain, muscle fatigue and spasms

**RESP:** Asthma

**SKIN:** Diaphoresis, photosensitivity, rash

**Nursing Considerations**

•Assess patient for mental status and mood changes because selegiline can worsen such conditions as dementia, severe psychosis, tardive dyskinesia, and tremor.

•Monitor patient who is also taking levodopa for levodopa-induced adverse reactions, including confusion, dyskinesia, hallucinations, nausea, and orthostatic hypotension.

•Monitor for decreased symptoms of Parkinson's disease to evaluate drug's effectiveness.

•Be aware that drug can reactivate gastric ulcers because it prevents breakdown of gastric histamine. Assess for related signs and symptoms, such as abdominal pain.

**PATIENT TEACHING**

•Advise patient to avoid taking selegiline in the late afternoon or evening because it may interfere with sleep.

•Caution patient to take only prescribed amount because increased dosage may cause severe adverse reactions.

•Urge patient to avoid potentially hazardous activities until drug's CNS effects are known.

•Advise patient to change positions slowly to minimize the effects of orthostatic hypotension.

•Suggest that patient elevate his legs when sitting to reduce ankle swelling.

•Urge patient to avoid excessive sun exposure.

•Instruct patient to notify prescriber if symptoms develop that could indicate overdose, including muscle twitching and eye spasms.

•Urge patient to notify prescriber if dry mouth lasts longer than 2 weeks. Advise him to have routine dental checkups.

# sertraline hydrochloride

Zoloft

**Class and Category**

*Chemical:* Naphthylamine derivative
*Therapeutic:* Antidepressant, antiobsessant, antipanic
*Pregnancy category:* C

**Indications and Dosages**

➤ *To treat major depression*

**ORAL CONCENTRATE, TABLETS**
**Adults.** *Initial:* 50 mg/day, increased after several wk in increments of 50 mg/day q wk, as needed. *Maximum:* 200 mg/day.

➤ *To treat obsessive-compulsive disorder*
**ORAL CONCENTRATE, TABLETS**
**Adults and adolescents.** *Initial:* 50 mg/day, increased after several wk in increments of 50 mg/day q wk, as needed. *Maximum:* 200 mg/day.
**Children ages 6 to 12.** *Initial:* 25 mg/day, increased q wk, as needed. *Maximum:* 200 mg/day.

➤ *To treat panic disorder, with or without agoraphobia; to treat posttraumatic stress disorder*
**ORAL CONCENTRATE, TABLETS**
**Adults.** *Initial:* 25 mg q.d., increased to 50 mg q.d. after 1 wk; then increased by 50 mg/day q wk, as needed. *Maximum:* 200 mg/day.
**DOSAGE ADJUSTMENT** Initial dosage reduction recommended for elderly patients and those with hepatic impairment.

➤ *To treat premenstrual dysphoric disease (PMDD)*
**ORAL CONCENTRATE, TABLETS**
**Adult women.** *Initial:* 50 mg q.d., in morning or evening, throughout menstrual cycle; or 50 mg q.d., in morning or evening, during luteal phase of menstrual cycle only. Dosage increased each menstrual cycle in 50 mg increments up to 150 mg/day, or each luteal phase up to 100 mg/day, as needed. Once 100 mg/day dosage established for luteal phase, each successive cycle requires a 50 mg titration step for 3 days at the beginning of each luteal phase. *Maximum:* 150 mg/day for dosing throughout menstrual cycle, or 100 mg/day for dosing during luteal phase only.

| Route | Onset | Peak | Duration |
|-------|-------|------|----------|
| P.O. | 2 to 4 wk* | Unknown | Unknown |

**Contraindications**
Concurrent use of disulfiram (oral concentrate) or pimozide; hypersensitivity to sertraline or its components; use within 14 days of an MAO inhibitor

---

* For antidepressant and antipanic effects; for antiobsessant effect, longer than 4 wk.

**Mechanism of Action**
Inhibits reuptake of the neurotransmitter serotonin by CNS neurons, thereby increasing the amount of serotonin available in nerve synapses. An elevated serotonin level may result in elevated mood and reduced depression. This action may also relieve symptoms of other psychiatric conditions attributed to serotonin deficiency.

**Interactions**
**DRUGS**
*aspirin, NSAIDs, warfarin:* Increased anticoagulant activity and risk of bleeding
*astemizole, terfenadine:* Possibly increased blood levels of these drugs, leading to increased risk of arrhythmias
*cimetidine:* Increased sertraline half-life
*MAO inhibitors:* Possibly hyperpyretic episodes, hypertensive crisis, serotonin syndrome, and severe seizures
*moclobemide, serotonergics:* Increased risk of potentially fatal serotonin syndrome
*tolbutamide:* Possibly hypoglycemia
*tricyclic antidepressants:* Possibly impaired metabolism of tricyclic antidepressants, resulting in increased risk of toxicity

**Adverse Reactions**
**CNS:** Aggressiveness, agitation, anxiety, dizziness, drowsiness, fatigue, fever, headache, hyperkinesia, insomnia, nervousness, paresthesia, tremor, weakness, yawning
**CV:** Palpitations
**EENT:** Dry mouth, epistaxis, sinusitis, vision changes
**ENDO:** Syndrome of inappropriate ADH secretion
**GI:** Abdominal cramps, anorexia, constipation, diarrhea, flatulence, increased appetite, indigestion, nausea, vomiting
**GU:** Anorgasmia, decreased libido, ejaculation disorders, impotence, urinary incontinence
**SKIN:** Diaphoresis, flushing, purpura, rash
**Other:** Weight loss

**Nursing Considerations**
• Monitor liver function test results and BUN and serum creatinine levels, as appropriate, in patients with hepatic or renal dysfunction.
• Monitor patient for hypo-osmolarity of serum and urine and for hyponatremia, which may indicate sertraline-induced syndrome of inappropriate ADH secretion.

Q
R
S

•Be aware that effective antidepressant therapy can promote mania in predisposed people. If mania develops, notify prescriber immediately and expect to withhold sertraline.
•Watch closely for suicidal tendencies, especially when therapy starts and dosage changes and especially in children and adolescents.
•Monitor patient closely for evidence of GI bleeding, especially if patient takes a drug known to cause it, such as aspirin, an NSAID, or warfarin.
•When theray stops, expect to taper dosage to minimize adverse effects rather than stopping drug abruptly.

**PATIENT TEACHING**
•Teach patient to dilute oral concentrate before taking it. Tell him to use supplied dropper to remove prescribed amount and mix it with 4 oz (½ cup) of water, ginger ale, lemon or lime soda, lemonade, or orange juice. Warn him not to mix oral concentrate with anything else. Explain that it's normal for mixture to be slightly hazy.
•Tell patient to take dose immediately after mixing it.
•If patient has latex sensitivity, advise him to use an alternate dispenser because the supplied dropper dispenser contains dry natural rubber.
•Advise patient to avoid potentially hazardous activities until drug's CNS effects are known.
•Warn family or caregiver to watch patient closely for suicidal tendencies, especially when therapy starts or dosage changes, and especially if patient is a child or adolescent.
•Caution patient not to stop taking drug abruptly. Explain that gradual tapering helps to avoid withdrawal symptoms.

# sevelamer hydrochloride

Renagel

## Class and Category

*Chemical:* Polyallylamine-epichlorhydrin polymer
*Therapeutic:* Antihyperphosphatemic
*Pregnancy category:* C

## Indications and Dosages

➤ *To lower serum phosphate level during end-stage renal disease*

**CAPSULES**
**Adults.** 2 capsules (806 mg) t.i.d. if serum phosphorus level is 6 to 7.5 mg/dl; 3 capsules (1,209 mg) t.i.d. if serum phosphorus level is 7.6 to 8.9 mg/dl; or 4 capsules (1,612 mg) t.i.d. if serum phosphorus level is 9 mg/dl or more. Dosage increased or decreased gradually by 1 capsule (403 mg)/meal, as needed. *Maximum:* 30 capsules (12.1 g)/day.

---

### Mechanism of Action
Inhibits phosphate absorption in the intestine by binding dietary phosphate, thereby lowering serum phosphorus level.

---

## Contraindications

Fecal impaction, GI obstruction, hypersensitivity to sevelamer or its components, hypophosphatemia, ileus

## Interactions
**DRUGS**
*antiarrhythmics, anticonvulsants, digoxin, levothyroxine, liothyronine, quinolones, tetracyclines, theophylline, warfarin:* Possibly altered absorption of these drugs
*phosphate salts, phosphorus salts:* Neutralized therapeutic effects of sevelamer
*ciprofloxacin:* Decreased ciprofloxacin effectiveness

## Adverse Reactions

**CNS:** Headache, fever
**CV:** Hypertension, hypotension, thrombosis
**EENT:** Nasopharyngitis
**GI:** Constipation, diarrhea, flatulence, indigestion, nausea, vomiting
**RESP:** Bronchitis, dyspnea, increased cough, upper respiratory tract infection
**MS:** Arthralgia, back or limb pain
**SKIN:** Pruritus
**Other:** Infection

## Nursing Considerations

•Give other drugs at least 1 hour before or 3 hours after sevelamer to prevent interaction.
•Be aware that severe hypophosphatemia may occur in patient with dysphagia, major GI tract surgery, or severe GI motility disorder because drug prevents phosphate absorption.
•Monitor blood pressure frequently.
•Monitor serum phosphorus level to deter-

mine drug's effectiveness; monitor other serum electrolyte levels to detect imbalances.

**PATIENT TEACHING**
•Tell patient to take sevelamer with meals and to swallow capsules whole with water, not to open or chew them.
•Caution patient to take other drugs 1 hour before or 3 hours after sevelamer.
•Review symptoms of thrombosis, and advise patient to report them immediately.

# sibutramine hydrochloride monohydrate

Meridia

## Class, Category, and Schedule
*Chemical:* Cyclobutanemethanamine
*Therapeutic:* Antiobesity
*Pregnancy category:* C
*Controlled substance:* Schedule IV

## Indications and Dosages
➤ *As adjunct to dieting to manage obesity*
**CAPSULES**
**Adults.** *Initial:* 10 mg q.d., increased to 15 mg/day after 4 wk if weight loss is inadequate. *Maximum:* 15 mg q.d.
**DOSAGE ADJUSTMENT** Reduction to 5 mg/day may be needed if patient can't tolerate 10-mg dose.

---

### Mechanism of Action
Inhibits central reuptake of dopamine, norepinephrine, and serotonin, thereby suppressing appetite and lowering food intake, leading to weight loss.

---

## Contraindications
Anorexia nervosa, concomitant use of other centrally acting appetite suppressants, hypersensitivity to sibutramine or its components, use within 14 days of MAO inhibitor therapy

## Interactions
**DRUGS**
*certain decongestants and cough, cold, and allergy drugs; ephedrine; phenylpropanolamine; pseudoephedrine:* Increased risk of elevated blood pressure or heart rate
*certain opioid analgesics (dextromethorphan, fentanyl, meperidine, pentazocine), dihydroergotamine, lithium, MAO inhibitors, sero-* *nergics, sumatriptan, tryptophan, zolmitriptan:* Increased risk of serotonin syndrome
*erythromycin, ketoconazole:* Possibly decreased sibutramine clearance

## Adverse Reactions
**CNS:** Anxiety, depression, dizziness, drowsiness, headache, insomnia, nervousness, paresthesia, somnolence
**CV:** Chest pain, edema, hypertension, palpitations, tachycardia
**EENT:** Dry mouth, earache, rhinitis, sinusitis, taste perversion
**GI:** Abdominal pain, anorexia, constipation, diarrhea, gastritis, increased appetite, indigestion, nausea, thirst, vomiting
**GU:** Dysmenorrhea, urine retention, UTI, vaginal candidiasis
**HEME:** Bleeding
**MS:** Arthralgia, back or neck pain, myalgia, tenosynovitis
**SKIN:** Acne, diaphoresis, ecchymosis, flushing, urticaria
**Other:** Anaphylaxis, angioedema, flulike symptoms

## Nursing Considerations
•Use sibutramine cautiously in patients with mild to moderate renal impairment, and expect to not use it in patients with severe renal impairment, including those with end-stage renal disease receiving hemodialysis.
•**WARNING** Use drug cautiously in patients with a history of substance abuse, and watch for signs of misuse.
•Measure blood pressure and pulse rate before and during sibutramine therapy.
•Because serotonin release from nerve terminals has been linked to cardiac valve dysfunction, assess for development of third heart sound.
•**WARNING** If patient takes drugs for migraine, notify prescriber immediately if evidence of serotonin syndrome develops: agitation, anxiety, ataxia, chills, confusion, diaphoresis, disorientation, dysarthria, emesis, excitement, hemiballismus, hyperreflexia, hyperthermia, hypomania, lack of coordination, loss of consciousness, mydriasis, myoclonus, restlessness, tachycardia, tremor, and weakness.
•Because drug decreases salivary flow, monitor patient for adverse dental effects.

**PATIENT TEACHING**
•Caution patient not to take sibutramine more often than prescribed.

Q
R
S

•Teach patient how to measure his blood pressure and pulse rate during therapy.
•Explain that sibutramine is an adjunct to reduced-calorie diet, not a replacement for it.
•Advise patient to report unusual bleeding or bruising.
•Caution against taking OTC products that contain ephedrine because of the increased risk of hypertension.
•Urge patient to avoid potentially hazardous activities until drug's CNS effects are known.
•If patient reports dry mouth, suggest sugar-free hard candy or gum or a saliva substitute.

# sildenafil citrate

Revatio, Viagra

## Class and Category

*Chemical:* Pyrazolopyrimidinone derivative
*Therapeutic:* Antihypertensive (pulmonary arterial), anti-impotence
*Pregnancy category:* B

## Indications and Dosages

➤ *To treat erectile dysfunction*

TABLETS

**Adults.** 50 mg q.d., taken 1 hr before sexual activity; increased as prescribed, based on clinical response. *Maximum:* 100 mg/day.
DOSAGE ADJUSTMENT Initially 25 mg for elderly patients, those with hepatic cirrhosis or creatinine clearance less than 30 ml/min/1.73 m², and those taking potent cytochrome P-450 3A4 inhibitors or ritonavir. Dosage reduced to 25 mg if taken within 4 hr of an alpha-blocker. *Maximum:* 25 mg/48 hr.

➤ *To treat pulmonary arterial hypertension in order to improve exercise ability in patients classified as group 1 by the World Health Organization*

TABLETS

**Adults.** 20 mg t.i.d.

| Route | Onset | Peak | Duration |
|-------|-------|------|----------|
| P.O. | In 30 min | Unknown | 4 hr |

## Mechanism of Action

Enhances the effect of nitric oxide released in the penis by stimulation. Nitric oxide increases the cGMP level, relaxes smooth muscle, and increases blood flow to the corpus cavernosum, thus producing an erection.

## Contraindications

Continuous or intermittent nitrate therapy, hypersensitivity to sildenafil or components

## Interactions

DRUGS

*barbiturates, bosentan, carabamazepine, efavirenza, nevirapine, phenytoin, rifabutin, rifampin:* Altered plasma level of either drug
*cimetidine, erythromycin, itraconazole, keto-conazole, mibefradil:* Prolonged sildenafil effect
*doxazosin and other alpha-blockers:* Increased risk of symptomatic hypotension
*nitrates:* Profound hypotension
*protease inhibitors:* Increased sildenafil effect
*rifampin:* Decreased sildenafil effect

FOODS

*high-fat meals:* Drug absorption delayed by up to 60 minutes

## Adverse Reactions

**CNS:** Cerebrovascular, intracerebral, or subarachnoid hemorrhage; dizziness; headache; migraine; syncope; transient ischemic attack
**CV:** Heart failure, hypertension, hypotension, myocardial infarction or ischemia, orthostatic hypotension, palpitations, sudden cardiac death, tachycardia, ventricular arrhythmias
**EENT:** Blurred vision; change in color perception; diplopia; epistaxis; increased intraocular pressure; nasal congestion; nonarteritic anterior ischemic optic neuropathy; ocular burning, pressure, redness or swelling; paramacular edema; photophobia; retinal vascular bleeding or disease; visual decrease or temporary vision loss; vitreous detachment
**ENDO:** Uncontrolled diabetes mellitus
**GI:** Diarrhea, indigestion
**GU:** Cystitis, dysuria, painful erection, priapism, UTI
**MS:** Arthralgia, back pain
**RESP:** Pulmonary hemorrhage, upper respiratory tract infection
**SKIN:** Flushing, photosensitivity

## Nursing Considerations

•Use sildenafil cautiously in patients with renal or hepatic dysfunction, in elderly patients, and in men with penile abnormalities that may predispose them to priapism.
•Also use cautiously in patients with left ventricular outflow obstruction, such as aortic stenosis and idiopathic hypertrophic

subaortic stenosis, and those with severely impaired autonomic control of blood pressure because these conditions increase patient's sensitivity to vasodilators such as sildenafil.

•Monitor patient's blood pressure and heart rate and rhythm before and frequently during therapy.

•Monitor vision, especially in patients who are older than age 50; who have diabetes, hypertension, coronary artery disease, or hyperlipidemia; or who smoke because sildenafil has rarely been associated with nonarteritic anterior ischemic optic neuropathy that may lead to decreased vision or permanent vision loss.

### PATIENT TEACHING

•Explain that sildenafil used to treat erectile dysfunction may be taken up to 4 hours before sexual activity but that taking it 1 hour beforehand provides most effective results.

•**WARNING** Instruct patient not to take sildenafil if he also takes any form of organic nitrate, either continuously or intermittently, because profound hypotension and death could result. Also caution patient taking sildenafil for erectile dysfunction not to take more than 25 mg within 4 hours of taking an alpha blocker, such as doxazosin, because symptomatic orthostatic hypotension can occur.

•Tell patient to stop taking sildenafil and contact prescriber if vision decreases suddenly in one or both eyes.

•Advise patient taking sildenafil for erectile dysfunction to seek sexual counseling to enhance the drug's effects.

•To avoid possible penile damage and permanent loss of erectile function, urge patient to notify prescriber immediately if erection is painful or lasts longer than 4 hours.

•Instruct diabetic patient to monitor his blood glucose level frequently because drug may affect glucose control.

# simvastatin

Zocor

## Class and Category

*Chemical:* Synthetically derived fermentation product of *Aspergillus terreus*
*Therapeutic:* Antihyperlipidemic
*Pregnancy category:* X

## Indications and Dosages

➤ *To treat hyperlipidemia*

**TABLETS**

**Adults.** *Initial:* 20 to 40 mg/day in the evening. Dosage adjusted at 4-wk intervals, as needed, to achieve target LDL-cholesterol level. *Maintenance:* 5 to 80 mg/day. *Maximum:* 80 mg/day.

➤ *To treat homozygous familial hypercholesterolemia*

**TABLETS**

**Adults.** 40 mg/day in the evening, or 80 mg/day in 3 divided doses—20 mg, 20 mg, and 40 mg (in the evening). Dosage adjusted q 4 wk, as needed, to achieve target LDL-cholesterol level. *Maintenance:* 5 to 40 mg/day. *Maximum:* 80 mg/day.

**DOSAGE ADJUSTMENT** Patients taking cyclosporine or who have severe renal insufficiency should initially receive 5 mg/day and be increased as needed to no more than 10 mg/day. Maximum dosage of 10 mg/day should also not be exceeded in patients who are concomitantly taking fibrates or niacin.

➤ *To treat adolescent heterozygous familial hypercholesterolemia*

**TABLETS**

**Children ages 10 to 17 at least 1 year postmenarche.** *Initial:* 10 mg/day in the evening. Dosage adjusted q 4 wk, as needed, to achieve target LDL-cholesterol level. *Maintenance:* 10 to 40 mg/day. *Maximum:* 40 mg/day.

**DOSAGE ADJUSTMENT** For patients who take cyclosporine, initial dosage reduced to 5 mg/day and maximum dosage reduced to 10 mg/day. For elderly patients and those with renal impairment, initial dosage reduced to 5 mg/day. For patients who take danazol, fibric-acid derivative lipid-lowering drugs, such as gemfibrozil, or lipid-lowering doses of niacin (1 g/day or more), maximum dosage reduced to 10 mg/day. For patients who take amiodarone or verapamil, maximum dosage shouldn't exceed 20 mg/day.

| Route | Onset | Peak | Duration |
|---|---|---|---|
| P.O. | 2 wk | 4 to 6 wk | Unknown |

## Contraindications

Active hepatic disease; pregnancy; breastfeeding; concurrent use with clarithromycin, erythromycin, more than 1 quart of grapefruit juice daily, HIV protease inhibitors, itraconazole, ketoconazole, nefazodone, or telithromycin; hypersensitivity to simvastatin or its components

---

## Mechanism of Action

Interferes with the hepatic enzyme hydroxymethylglutaryl-coenzyme A reductase. This action reduces the formation of mevalonic acid, a cholesterol precursor, thus interrupting the pathway necessary for cholesterol synthesis. When the cholesterol level declines in hepatic cells, LDLs are consumed, which in turn reduces the levels of circulating total cholesterol and serum triglycerides.

---

## Interactions
### DRUGS

*amiodarone, antiretroviral protease inhibitors (amprenavir, indinavir, nelfinavir, ritonavir, saquinavir), clarithromycin, cyclosporine, danazol, gemfibrozil and other fibrates, itraconazole, ketoconazole, erythromycin, nefazodone, niacin (1 g/day or more), telithromycin, verapamil:* Increased risk of myopathy or rhabdomyolysis
*azole antifungals, cyclosporine, gemfibrozil, immunosuppressants, macrolide antibiotics (including erythromycin), niacin, verapamil:* Increased risk of acute renal failure
*bile acid sequestrants, cholestyramine, colestipol:* Decreased simvastatin bioavailability
*digoxin:* Possibly slight elevation in blood digoxin level
*diltiazem, verapamil:* Possibly increased blood simvastatin level, increased risk of myopathy
*oral anticoagulants:* Increased bleeding or prolonged PT
### FOODS
*grapefruit juice (1 or more quarts/day):* Possibly increased blood simvastatin level

## Adverse Reactions
**CNS:** Asthenia, dizziness, fatigue, headache
**CV:** Chest pain
**EENT:** Cataracts, rhinitis
**GI:** Abdominal pain, constipation, diarrhea, elevated liver function test results, flatulence, heartburn, indigestion, nausea, pancreatitis, vomiting
**MS:** Myalgia, myopathy, rhabdomyolysis
**RESP:** Upper respiratory tract infection
**SKIN:** Eczema, pruritus, rash

## Nursing Considerations
•Use simvastatin cautiously in elderly patients and those with renal or hepatic impairment.
•Give drug 1 hour before or 4 hours after giving bile acid sequestrant, cholestyramine, or colestipol.
•Expect to monitor liver function test results every 3 to 6 months for abnormal elevations.
•Monitor serum lipoprotein level, as ordered, to evaluate response to therapy.
### PATIENT TEACHING
•Urge patient to take drug in the evening.
•Encourage patient to follow a low-fat, cholesterol-lowering diet.
•Urge patient to notify prescriber immediately about muscle pain, tenderness, and weakness and other symptoms of myopathy.
•Inform female patient of childbearing age of need to use reliable contraceptive method while taking drug. Instruct her to notify prescriber at once if she suspects pregnancy.
•Advise patient to avoid grapefruit juice to decrease risk of drug toxicity.

# sirolimus
## (rapamycin)

Rapamune

## Class and Category
*Chemical:* Macrocyclic lactone
*Therapeutic:* Immunosuppressant
*Pregnancy category:* C

## Indications and Dosages
➤ *To prevent rejection of kidney transplantation*
### ORAL SOLUTION
**Adults and adolescents over age 13 weighing 40 kg or more.** *Initial:* 6-mg loading dose. *Maintenance:* 2 mg q.d.
**Adolescents over age 13 weighing less than 40 kg.** *Initial:* 3-mg/m$^2$ loading dose. *Maintenance:* 1 mg/m$^2$ q.d.
DOSAGE ADJUSTMENT Maintenance dosage reduced by one-third for patients with impaired hepatic function. Maintenance dosage increased by as much as 400% for patients discontinuing concomitant cyclosporine therapy in order to maintain blood sirolimus trough concentration of 12 to 24 ng/ml

| Route | Onset | Peak | Duration |
|-------|-------|------|----------|
| P.O. | Unknown | Unknown | Up to 6 mo after discontinuation |

## Mechanism of Action

Inhibits activation and proliferation of T lymphocytes and antibody production. Sirolimus also inhibits cell cycle progression from the G1 to the S phase, possibly by inhibiting a key regulatory kinase believed to suppress cytokine-driven T-cell proliferation.

## Contraindications

Hypersensitivity to sirolimus or its components, malignancy

## Interactions

### DRUGS

*aminoglycosides, amphotericin B, cyclosporine:* Possibly impaired renal function
*bromocriptine, cimetidine, cisapride, clarithromycin, clotrimazole, cyclosporine, danazol, diltiazem, erythromycin, fluconazole, indinavir, itraconazole, ketoconazole, metoclopramide, nicardipine, ritonavir, troleandomycin, verapamil:* Possibly increased blood sirolimus level and toxicity
*calcineurin inhibitors, corticosteroids:* Increased risk of deteriorating renal function, serum lipid abnormalities, and UTI
*carbamazepine, phenobarbital, phenytoin, rifabutin, rifapentine, St. John's wort:* Possibly decreased blood sirolimus level
*HMG-CoA reductase inhibitors:* Increased risk of rhabdomyolysis when administered concurrently with sirolimus and cyclosporine
*rifampin:* Significantly increased sirolimus clearance
*vaccines (killed virus):* Possibly decreased immune response to vaccines
*vaccines (live virus):* Increased risk of contracting disease from live virus

### FOODS

*grapefruit juice:* Possibly decreased metabolism of sirolimus
*high-fat diet:* Reduced rate of sirolimus absorption

## Adverse Reactions

**CNS:** Asthenia, fever, headache, insomnia, tremor
**CV:** Atrial fibrillation, chest pain, hyperlipidemia, hypertension, peripheral edema
**GI:** Abdominal pain, constipation, diarrhea, hepatotoxicity, nausea, vomiting
**GU:** Elevated serum creatinine level, UTI
**HEME:** Anemia, lymphoma, neutropenia, pancytopenia, thrombocytopenia
**MS:** Arthralgia, low back or flank pain
**RESP:** Dyspnea on exertion, interstitial lung disease
**SKIN:** Acne, rash
**Other:** Anaphylaxis, delayed wound healing, hypercholesterolemia, hypokalemia, hypophosphatemia, weight gain or loss

## Nursing Considerations

• Use sirolimus cautiously in patients who are receiving other drugs known to adversely affect renal function, such as aminoglycosides and amphotericin B; together, they may further decrease renal function.
• Monitor patients with existing or recent (including recent exposure to) chickenpox and patients with herpes zoster for worsening symptoms because they have an increased risk of developing severe generalized disease while taking sirolimus.
• Mix oral sirolimus with at least 2 oz (60 ml) of water or orange juice in a glass or plastic container. Don't dilute drug in grapefruit juice or any other liquid.
• Stir well and have patient drink solution immediately. Then rinse glass with at least 4 oz (120 ml) of additional liquid, stir well, and have patient drink that liquid to make sure that all of drug is taken.
• Give initial dose as soon after transplantation as possible and daily dose 4 hours after cyclosporine, as prescribed.
• Monitor whole blood sirolimus concentrations, as ordered, in patients receiving concentrated form of drug, patients who weigh less than 40 kg (88 lb), patients with hepatic impairment, and those receiving potent CYP3A4 inducers or inhibitors concurrently.
• Monitor serum creatinine level, as ordered, in patients receiving sirolimus and cyclosporine because this combination may impair renal function. Notify prescriber of any increases in serum creatinine level because sirolimus or cyclosporine dosage may need to be adjusted or discontinued.
• Monitor patient for signs and symptoms of infection and check CBC results, as ordered,

Q
R
S

to detect sirolimus-induced blood dyscrasias or changes in neutrophil count, which may indicate infection.

• For patients with hyperlipidemia, be prepared to institute dietary changes, an exercise program, or a lipid-lowering drug regimen if blood cholesterol or triglyceride levels increase because drug may aggravate hyperlipidemia.

**PATIENT TEACHING**

• Advise patient to take sirolimus consistently either with or without food (but not food high in fat) to prevent changes in absorption rate.

• Instruct patient to take daily dose with at least 2 oz (60 ml) of water or orange juice. Caution him not to dilute drug in grapefruit juice or any other liquid. Advise him to stir mixture well and drink immediately, then to add at least another 4 oz (120 ml) of liquid to empty container, stir mixture again, and drink that liquid to ensure that he has swallowed all of drug.

• Urge patient to avoid people with colds, flu, or other infections because his immunosuppressed state makes him more vulnerable to infection.

• Instruct patient not to take live vaccines, such as measles, mumps, rubella, oral polio, bacille Calmette-Guçrin, yellow fever, varicella, and TY21a typhoid, during sirolimus therapy.

• Advise patient to keep follow-up appointments for blood tests, as ordered.

# sodium bicarbonate

Arm and Hammer Pure Baking Soda, Bell/ans, Citrocarbonate, Soda Mint

## Class and Category

*Chemical:* Electrolyte
*Therapeutic:* Antacid, electrolyte replenisher, systemic and urinary alkalizer
*Pregnancy category:* C

## Indications and Dosages

➤ *To treat hyperacidity*

**EFFERVESCENT POWDER**

**Adults and adolescents.** 3.9 to 10 g in a glass of water after meals. *Maximum:* 19.5 g/day.

**Children ages 6 to 12.** 1 to 1.9 g in a glass of water after meals.

**ORAL POWDER**

**Adults and adolescents.** ½ tsp in a glass of water q 2 hr, p.r.n. *Maximum:* 4 tsp/day in patients up to age 60.

**TABLETS**

**Adults and adolescents.** 325 mg to 2 g q.d. to q.i.d., p.r.n. *Maximum:* 16 g/day.

**Children ages 6 to 12.** 520 mg, repeated once after 30 min, p.r.n.

➤ *To provide urinary alkalization*

**ORAL POWDER**

**Adults and adolescents.** 1 tsp in a glass of water q 4 hr. *Maximum:* 4 tsp/day in patients up to age 60.

**TABLETS**

**Adults and adolescents.** *Initial:* 4 g, then 1 to 2 g q 4 hr. *Maximum:* 16 g/day.

**Children.** 23 to 230 mg/kg/day, adjusted p.r.n.

**I.V. INFUSION**

**Adults and children.** 2 to 5 mEq/kg over 4 to 8 hr.

➤ *To treat metabolic acidosis during cardiac arrest*

**I.V. INJECTION**

**Adults and children.** *Initial:* 1 mEq/kg, followed by 0.5 mEq/kg q 10 min while arrest continues.

➤ *To treat less urgent forms of metabolic acidosis*

**I.V. INFUSION**

**Adults and children.** 2 to 5 mEq/kg over 4 to 8 hr.

**DOSAGE ADJUSTMENT** Dosage reduction possible for elderly patients because of age-related renal impairment.

## Incompatibilities

Don't admix I.V. form of sodium bicarbonate in same solution or administer through same I.V. line as other drugs because precipitate may form.

> ## Mechanism of Action
>
> Increases plasma bicarbonate level, buffers excess hydrogen ions, and raises blood pH, thereby reversing metabolic acidosis. Sodium bicarbonate also increases the excretion of free bicarbonate ions in urine, raising urine pH; increased alkalinity of urine may help to dissolve uric acid calculi. In addition, it relieves symptoms of hyperacidity by neutralizing or buffering existing stomach acid, thereby increasing the pH of stomach contents.

## Contraindications

Hypocalcemia in which alkalosis may lead to tetany; hypochloremic alkalosis secondary to vomiting, diuretics, or nasogastric suction; preexisting metabolic or respiratory alkalosis

## Interactions

**DRUGS**

*amphetamines, quinidine:* Decreased urinary excretion of these drugs, possibly resulting in toxicity

*anticholinergics:* Decreased anticholinergic absorption and effectiveness

*calcium-containing products:* Increased risk of milk-alkali syndrome

*chlorpropamide, lithium, salicylates, tetracyclines:* Increased renal excretion and decreased absorption of these drugs

*ciprofloxacin, norfloxacin, ofloxacin:* Decreased solubility of these drugs, leading to crystalluria and nephrotoxicity

*citrates:* Increased risk of systemic alkalosis; increased risk of calcium calculus formation and hypernatremia in patients with history of uric acid calculi

*digoxin:* Possibly elevated blood digoxin level

*enteric-coated drugs:* Increased risk of gastric or duodenal irritation from rapid removal of enteric coating

*ephedrine:* Increased ephedrine half-life and duration of action

*H₂-receptor antagonists, iron supplements or preparations, ketoconazole:* Decreased absorption of these drugs

*mecamylamine:* Decreased excretion and prolonged effect of mecamylamine

*methenamine:* Decreased methenamine effectiveness

*mexiletine:* Possibly mexiletine toxicity

*potassium supplements:* Decreased serum potassium level

*sucralfate:* Interference with binding of sucralfate to gastric mucosa

*urinary acidifiers (ammonium chloride, ascorbic acid, potassium and sodium phosphates):* Counteracted effects of urinary acidifiers

**FOODS**

*dairy products:* Increased risk of milk-alkali syndrome with prolonged use of sodium bicarbonate

## Adverse Reactions

**CNS:** Mental or mood changes

**CV:** Irregular heartbeat, peripheral edema (with large doses), weak pulse
**EENT:** Dry mouth
**GI:** Abdominal cramps, thirst
**MS:** Muscle spasms, myalgia
**SKIN:** Extravasation with necrosis, tissue sloughing, or ulceration

## Nursing Considerations

•Monitor sodium intake of patient taking sodium bicarbonate because effervescent powder contains 700.6 mg of sodium/3.9 g; oral powder contains 952 mg of sodium/tsp; and tablets contain 325 mg/3.9-mEq tablet, 520 mg/6.2-mEq tablet, and 650 mg/7.7-mEq tablet.

•For I.V. infusion, dilute drug with NS, D₅W, or other standard electrolyte solution before administration.

•Avoid rapid I.V. infusion, which can cause severe alkalosis. Be aware that during cardiac arrest, risk of death from acidosis may outweigh risks of rapid infusion.

•Monitor urine pH, as ordered, to determine drug's effectiveness as urinary alkalizer.

•If patient receiving long-term sodium bicarbonate therapy is on a diet that includes calcium or milk, monitor for milk-alkali syndrome, characterized by anorexia, confusion, headache, hypercalcemia, metabolic acidosis, nausea, renal insufficiency, and vomiting.

•Be aware that parenteral formulations are hypertonic and that increased sodium intake can produce edema and weight gain.

•Assess I.V. site frequently for signs and symptoms of extravasation. If this occurs, notify prescriber immediately and remove I.V. catheter. Elevate the extremity, apply warm compresses, and expect prescriber to administer a local injection of hyaluronidase or lidocaine.

**PATIENT TEACHING**

•Advise patient not to take sodium bicarbonate with large amounts of dairy products or for longer than 2 weeks, unless directed by prescriber.

•Caution patient not to take more than the prescribed amount of drug to avoid adverse reactions.

•Direct patient not to take drug within 2 hours of other oral drugs.

•Advise patient to avoid taking OTC drugs without prescriber's approval because many drugs interact with sodium bicarbonate.

# sodium ferric gluconate

*(contains 62.5 mg of elemental iron per 5 ml)*

Ferrlecit

## Class and Category

*Chemical:* Iron salt, mineral
*Therapeutic:* Antianemic
*Pregnancy category:* B

## Indications and Dosages

➤ *To treat iron deficiency anemia in patients receiving long-term hemodialysis and erythropoietin*

**I.V. INFUSION OR INJECTION**

**Adults.** 125 mg of elemental iron. *Usual:* Minimum cumulative dose of 1 g of elemental iron given over eight sequential dialysis treatment. Dosage repeated at lowest dosage necessary to maintain target levels of hemoglobin and hematocrit and acceptable limits of blood iron levels.

## Incompatibilities

Don't mix sodium ferric gluconate with other drugs or parenteral nutrition solutions for I.V. infusion.

## Mechanism of Action

Acts to replenish iron stores lost during hemodialysis because of increased blood loss or increased iron utilization from epoetin therapy. Iron is an essential component of hemoglobin, myoglobin, and several enzymes, including cytochromes, catalase, and peroxidase, and is needed for catecholamine metabolism and normal neutrophil function. Sodium ferric gluconate also normalizes RBC production by binding with hemoglobin or being stored as ferritin in reticuloendothelial cells of the liver, spleen, and bone marrow.

## Contraindications

Anemia other than iron deficiency, hypersensitivity to iron salts or their components, iron overload

## Interactions

**DRUGS**

*oral iron preparations:* Possibly reduced absorption of oral iron supplements

## Adverse Reactions

**CNS:** Asthenia, dizziness, fatigue, fever, headache, hypertonia, nervousness, paresthesia, syncope
**CV:** Chest pain, generalized edema, hypertension, hypotension, tachycardia
**EENT:** Dry mouth
**GI:** Abdominal pain, diarrhea, nausea, vomiting
**HEME:** Hemorrhage
**MS:** Back pain, leg cramps
**RESP:** Cough, dyspnea, upper respiratory tract infection
**SKIN:** Pruritus
**Other:** Generalized pain, hyperkalemia, hypersensitivity, infusion or injection site reaction

## Nursing Considerations

• To reconstitute sodium ferric gluconate for I.V. infusion, dilute prescribed dosage in 100 ml of NS immediately before infusion. Infuse over 1 hour. Discard any unused diluted solution.

• Inspect drug for particles and discoloration before administration and discard if present.

• Administer undiluted drug by slow I.V. injection at a rate up to 12.5 mg/min, not to exceed 125 mg per injection.

• Be aware that most patients need a minimum cumulative dose of 1 gram of elemental iron administered over eight sequential dialysis treatments.

• **WARNING** Assess patient for signs and symptoms of an allergic reaction, including chills, facial flushing, pruritus, and rash, and of a hypersensitivity reaction, including diaphoresis, dyspnea, nausea, severe lower back pain, vomiting, and wheezing. Discontinue drug and notify prescriber immediately if patient develops an allergic or hypersensitivity reaction, and be prepared to provide emergency interventions.

• **WARNING** Assess blood pressure frequently after drug administration because hypotension may occur and may be related to infusion rate or total cumulative dose. Avoid rapid infusion and be prepared to provide I.V. fluids for volume expansion.

• Expect to monitor blood hemoglobin level, hematocrit, serum ferritin level, and transferrin saturation, as ordered, before, during, and after sodium ferric gluconate therapy. Make

sure that serum iron level is tested 48 hours after last dose. To prevent iron toxicity, notify prescriber and expect to discontinue therapy if blood iron level is normal or elevated.
•Assess patient for possible iron overload, characterized by bleeding in GI tract and lungs, decreased activity, pale conjunctivae, and sedation.

**PATIENT TEACHING**
•Warn patient not to take any oral iron preparations during sodium ferric gluconate therapy without first consulting prescriber.
•Inform patient that symptoms of iron deficiency may include decreased stamina, learning problems, shortness of breath, and fatigue.

# sodium phenylbutyrate

Buphenyl

## Class and Category
*Chemical:* Phenylacetate prodrug
*Therapeutic:* Antihyperammonemic
*Pregnancy category:* C

## Indications and Dosages
➤ *As adjunct to treat urea cycle disorders in combination with low-protein diet*
**POWDER, TABLETS**
**Adults and children who weigh more than 20 kg (44 lb).** 9.9 to 13 g/m$^2$/day in 4 to 6 divided doses with meals.
**Children who weigh up to 20 kg.** 450 to 600 mg/kg/day in 4 to 6 divided doses with meals.

---

### Mechanism of Action
Provides alternate pathway for eliminating waste nitrogen by forming phenylacetate, an active metabolite that conjugates with glutamine to produce phenylacetylglutamine, which is excreted by the kidneys.

---

## Contraindications
Acute hyperammonemia, hypersensitivity to sodium phenylbutyrate or its components

## Interactions
**DRUGS**
*corticosteroids:* Increased serum ammonia level
*haloperidol, valproate:* Increased risk of hyperammonemia
*probenecid:* Decreased excretion of conjugated product of sodium phenylbutyrate

## Adverse Reactions
**CNS:** Depression, disorientation, fatigue, headache, light-headedness, memory loss, syncope
**CV:** Arrhythmias
**EENT:** Hypoacusis, taste perversion
**GI:** Abdominal pain, anorexia, constipation, elevated liver function test results, gastritis, nausea, peptic ulcer, rectal bleeding, vomiting
**GU:** Amenorrhea, menstrual irregularities
**HEME:** Anemia, aplastic anemia, leukocytosis, leukopenia, thrombocytopenia
**SKIN:** Rash
**Other:** Body odor, hyperchloremia, hypoalbuminemia, hypophosphatemia, metabolic acidosis, metabolic alkalosis, weight gain

## Nursing Considerations
•Mix powder form of sodium phenylbutyrate with food or liquid, but not with acidic beverages such as coffee and tea.
•Be aware that drug shouldn't be used to treat acute hyperammonemia, which is a medical emergency.
•Monitor patient with history of heart failure or severe renal failure for fluid retention because of drug's sodium content.

**PATIENT TEACHING**
•Instruct patient to take sodium phenylbutyrate with meals but not to mix it with acidic beverages such as coffee and tea.
•Advise patient to comply with follow-up laboratory tests, as prescribed.
•Urge patient to notify prescriber immediately about changes in body odor because they may be early signs of metabolic imbalance.

# sodium phosphate monobasic monohydrate and sodium phosphate dibasic anhydrous

*(contains 1.5 g of sodium phosphate per tablet)*
Visicol

## Class and Category
*Chemical:* Acid salt
*Therapeutic:* Hyperosmotic laxative
*Pregnancy category:* C

## Indications and Dosages

➤ *To cleanse colon in preparation for colonoscopy*

**TABLETS**

**Adults.** A total of 40 tablets (60 g of sodium phosphate) taken as follows: the evening before scheduled colonoscopy, 3 tablets q 15 min with 2 tablets as last dose; the day of the procedure (starting 3 to 5 hr beforehand), 3 tablets q 15 min with 2 tablets as last dose.

| Route | Onset | Peak | Duration |
|-------|-------|------|----------|
| P.O. | Unknown | Unknown | 1 to 3 hr |

## Mechanism of Action

Increases the concentration gradient and osmotic pressure within the bowel by drawing large amounts of water into the small intestine. Bowel distention and increased fluid accumulation loosen stool and stimulate peristalsis, promoting bowel evacuation. Sodium phosphate also causes the release of cholecystokinin from the intestinal mucosa, which enhances the drug's laxative effect.

## Contraindications

Acute colitis; ascites; bowel perforation; disorders associated with hypomotility, such as hypothyroidism and scleroderma; gastric retention; heart failure; hypersensitivity to sodium phosphate salts or their components; ileus, acute obstruction, or pseudo-obstruction; severe chronic constipation; toxic megacolon; unstable angina pectoris

## Interactions

**DRUGS**

*all oral drugs:* Possibly malabsorption of these drugs

*potassium-sparing diuretics, potassium supplements:* Possibly decreased blood potassium level with long-term use of sodium phosphate; possibly decreased effects of potassium-sparing diuretics

## Adverse Reactions

**CNS:** Dizziness, headache, loss of consciousness, seizures

**GI:** Abdominal cramps, distention, or pain; diarrhea; nausea; rectal irritation; thirst; vomiting

**Other:** Hypernatremia, hyperphosphatemia, hypocalcemia, hypokalemia

## Nursing Considerations

• Expect to correct electrolyte abnormalities, such as hypocalcemia, hypokalemia, hypernatremia, or hyperphosphatemia, as ordered, before beginning sodium phosphate therapy.

• Ensure that patient maintains a clear liquid diet for 12 hours before first dose, as ordered.

• Administer each dose with 8 oz of clear liquid to prevent excessive fluid loss and hypovolemia.

• Be aware that drug should not be given within 7 days of prior use.

• **WARNING** Monitor patient for hypocalcemia, hypokalemia, hypernatremia, and hyperphosphatemia during therapy. Notify prescriber at once if patient develops an electrolyte imbalance, and prepare to administer corrective therapy as prescribed. Expect electrolyte imbalances to return to baseline within 48 to 72 hours.

• During drug administration and for up to 72 hours afterward, monitor serum electrolyte levels, as ordered, of patients with impaired renal function, those with preexisting electrolyte disturbances, and those taking drugs that may affect electrolyte levels.

• Monitor patients at risk for severe electrolyte imbalance, including hypokalemia and hypocalcemia, for prolonged QT interval because serious arrhythmias may occur.

• Monitor fluid intake and output during bowel preparation to prevent or detect excessive fluid loss and hypovolemia.

• Monitor patient for seizure activity and mental status because drug may cause seizures and loss of consciousness in patients with no history of them. Take safety precautions as needed.

• Monitor patients with a history of inflammatory bowel disease for persistent acute abdominal pain, which may indicate ulceration of colonic mucosa. Notify prescriber immediately if pain persists or intensifies.

• Be aware that undigested or partially digested tablets may be visible in watery stools or during colonoscopy.

**PATIENT TEACHING**

• Instruct patient to maintain a clear liquid diet for 12 hours before first dose of sodium phosphate, as ordered.

• Teach patient prescribed dosage and dosing interval. Inform him that bowel preparation will begin the evening before the scheduled procedure and will continue 3 to 5 hours be-

forehand. Encourage him to drink at least 8 oz of clear liquids every time he takes drug to prevent dehydration.
•Instruct patient not to use additional bowel-cleansing agents, especially those containing sodium phosphate, while he's taking this drug.
•Inform patient that stools may be watery during and immediately after drug therapy.
•Explain that he may see undigested or partially digested tablets (either of sodium phosphate or of other drugs) in stools; reassure him that this is a normal occurrence.
•Caution patient to avoid hazardous activities until drug's effects on him are known.

# sodium polystyrene sulfonate

Kayexalate, K-Exit (CAN), Kionex, PMS-Sodium Polystyrene Sulfonate (CAN), SPS Suspension

## Class and Category
*Chemical:* Sulfonated cation-exchange resin
*Therapeutic:* Antihyperkalemic
*Pregnancy category:* C

## Indications and Dosages
➤ *To treat hyperkalemia*
ORAL POWDER, SUSPENSION
**Adults.** 15 g (4 level tsp) q.d. to q.i.d. *Maximum:* 40 g q.i.d.
**Children.** 1 g/kg/dose, as needed.
RECTAL POWDER, SUSPENSION
**Adults.** 25 to 100 g as retention enema, as needed.
**Children.** 1 g/kg/dose as retention enema, as needed.

| Route | Onset | Peak | Duration |
|-------|-------|------|----------|
| P.O. | 2 to 12 hr | Unknown | Unknown |

## Contraindications
Hypersensitivity to sodium polystyrene sulfonate or its components, hypokalemia, obstructive bowel disease, reduced gut motility in neonates, oral administration in neonates

## Interactions
DRUGS
*antacids, laxatives:* Increased risk of metabolic alkalosis
*potassium-sparing diuretics, potassium supplements:* Increased risk of fluid retention

## Mechanism of Action
Releases sodium ions in exchange for other cations in intestines. Resin enters large intestine and releases sodium ions in exchange for hydrogen ions. As the resin moves through the intestines, hydrogen ions are then exchanged for potassium ions, which are in greater concentration. Bound resin leaves the body in feces, carrying potassium and other ions with it, thereby reducing serum potassium level.

## Adverse Reactions
**CV:** Peripheral edema
**GI:** Abdominal cramps, anorexia, constipation, epigastric pain, fecal impaction, indigestion, nausea, vomiting
**GU:** Decreased urine output
**Other:** Hypernatremia, hypocalcemia, hypokalemia, weight gain

## Nursing Considerations
•Use sodium polystyrene sulfonate cautiously in patients with heart failure, hypertension, or marked edema.
•Be aware that drug is available as powdered resin or as solution that contains sorbitol to facilitate movement of resin through intestines. As a result, patient may experience abdominal cramps, diarrhea, nausea, and vomiting.
•Because the drug doesn't take effect for several hours, be aware that it's inappropriate for acute, life-threatening hyperkalemia.
•If patient has hypokalemia or hypocalcemia, notify prescriber immediately and expect to withhold drug because it reduces potassium and calcium levels. Evidence of hypokalemia includes abdominal cramps, acidic urine, anorexia, drowsiness, ECG changes, hypotension, hypoventilation, muscle weakness, and tachycardia. Evidence of hypocalcemia includes abdominal pain, agitation, anxiety, ECG changes, hypotension, muscle twitching, psychosis, seizures, and tetany.
•To administer powdered resin as oral suspension, mix in water, syrup (such as sorbitol), or food and give promptly. If necessary, administer through gastric feeding tube.
•Precede rectal administration with a cleansing enema, as ordered.
•When giving rectally, suspend powdered resin in 100 ml of aqueous solution warmed to body temperature, in bag connected to soft, large

Q
R
S

(French 28) catheter. Have patient lie on his left side with his lower leg straight and upper leg flexed or with his knees to his chest. Gently insert the tube into the rectum and well into the sigmoid colon. The solution should flow into the colon by way of gravity and be retained for 30 to 60 minutes or longer, if possible. After patient is unable to retain the solution any longer, administer a non-sodium-containing cleansing enema, as prescribed.

• After administration, assess for constipation and fecal impaction.

**PATIENT TEACHING**

• Instruct patient not to mix oral form of sodium polystyrene sulfonate with foods and liquids high in potassium content, such as bananas and orange juice.

• Teach patient who will self-administer the rectal solution the correct technique and body position. Remind him to let the solution flow into the colon by gravity and to retain it 30 to 60 minutes, longer if possible.

• Advise patient to notify prescriber immediately about abdominal cramps, nausea, and vomiting.

# sodium thiosalicylate

Rexolate, Tusal

## Class and Category

*Chemical:* Salicylic acid derivative
*Therapeutic:* Analgesic, anti-inflammatory
*Pregnancy category:* Not rated

## Indications and Dosages

➤ *To relieve symptoms of acute gout*
**I.V. OR I.M. INJECTION**
**Adults.** *Initial:* 100 mg q 3 to 4 hr for 2 days, then 100 mg/day.

➤ *To relieve pain from musculoskeletal conditions*
**I.V. OR I.M. INJECTION**
**Adults.** 50 to 100 mg q.d. or q.o.d.

➤ *To relieve symptoms of osteoarthritis*
**I.V. OR I.M. INJECTION**
**Adults.** 100 mg 3 times/wk for several wk, then once/wk, usually up to a total dosage of 2.5 g. After 1 to 2 wk, another course of treatment may be given.

➤ *To treat rheumatic fever*
**I.V. OR I.M. INJECTION**
**Adults.** *Initial:* 100 to 150 mg q 4 to 8 hr for 3 days, then 100 mg b.i.d.

## Mechanism of Action

Exerts peripherally induced analgesic and anti-inflammatory effects by blocking pain impulses and inhibiting prostaglandin synthesis.

## Contraindications

GI bleeding; hemophilia; hemorrhage; hypersensitivity to sodium thiosalicylate, NSAIDs, or their components; Reye's syndrome

## Interactions

**DRUGS**

*ACE inhibitors, beta blockers:* Decreased antihypertensive effect of these drugs
*activated charcoal:* Decreased sodium thiosalicylate absorption
*antacids, urinary alkalizers:* Increased excretion of sodium thiosalicylate, leading to reduced drug effectiveness and shortened half-life
*carbonic anhydrase inhibitors (such as acetazolamide):* Increased risk of salicylate toxicity; possibly displacement of acetazolamide from protein-binding sites, resulting in toxicity
*corticosteroids:* Possibly increased sodium thiosalicylate excretion
*insulin, oral antidiabetic drugs:* Altered glucose control (with large sodium thiosalicylate doses)
*loop diuretics:* Possibly decreased effectiveness of loop diuretics in patients with renal or hepatic impairment
*methotrexate:* Increased risk of methotrexate toxicity
*nizatidine:* Increased blood sodium thiosalicylate level
*probenecid, sulfinpyrazone:* Decreased uricosuric effects
*spironolactone:* Possibly inhibited diuretic effect of spironolactone
*urinary acidifiers (including ammonium chloride, ascorbic acid, methionine):* Decreased sodium thiosalicylate excretion, possibly leading to salicylate toxicity

**ACTIVITIES**

*alcohol use:* Increased risk of gastrointestinal ulceration

## Adverse Reactions

**GI:** Anorexia, diarrhea, GI bleeding, heartburn, hepatotoxicity, indigestion, nausea, thirst, vomiting

**HEME:** Leukopenia, platelet dysfunction, prolonged bleeding time, thrombocytopenia
**RESP:** Bronchospasm
**SKIN:** Rash, urticaria
**Other:** Angioedema

## Nursing Considerations

• Use drug cautiously in patients with asthma, chronic urticaria, or nasal polyps because these patients are more prone to hypersensitivity.
• Expect to monitor patient's hepatic and renal function during long-term drug therapy.
• After repeated administration or large doses, assess patient for signs of salicylate toxicity: CNS depression, confusion, diaphoresis, diarrhea, difficulty hearing, dizziness, headache, hyperventilation, lassitude, tinnitus, and vomiting.
• Be aware that tinnitus usually means that the blood sodium thiosalicylate level has reached or exceeded the upper limit for therapeutic effects.

**PATIENT TEACHING**
• Instruct patient to notify prescriber immediately about bleeding or symptoms of salicylate toxicity.

# solifenacin succinate

VESIcare

## Class and Category

*Chemical:* Muscarinic receptor antagonist
*Therapeutic:* Bladder antispasmodic
*Pregnancy category:* C

## Indications and Dosages

➤ *To treat overactive urinary bladder with symptoms of urge incontinence, urgency, and frequency*

**TABLETS**
**Adults.** 5 mg q.d.; if tolerated well, increased to 10 mg q.d.
**DOSAGE ADJUSTMENT** For patients with severe renal impairment or moderate hepatic impairment or patients taking ketoconazole or other potent CYP3A4 inhibitors, dosage limited to 5 mg q.d.

| Route | Onset | Peak | Duration |
|-------|-------|------|----------|
| P.O. | Unknown | 3 to 8 hr | Unknown |

## Contraindications

Gastric retention, hypersensitivity to solifenacin or its components, uncontrolled angle-closure glaucoma, urine retention

---

### Mechanism of Action

Antagonizes the effect of acetylcholine on muscarinic receptors in detrusor muscle, decreasing the muscle spasms that cause inappropriate bladder emptying. This action increases bladder capacity and volume, which relieves the sensation of urgency and frequency and enhances bladder control.

---

## Interactions

**DRUGS**
*ketoconazole, other potent CYP3A4 inhibitors:* Possibly decreased metabolism of solifenacin and increased risk of adverse effects

## Adverse Reactions

**CNS:** Depression, dizziness, fatigue, headache
**CV:** Hypertension, prolonged QT interval, peripheral edema
**EENT:** Blurred vision, dry eyes or mouth, pharyngitis
**GI:** Abdominal pain, constipation, indigestion, nausea, vomiting
**GU:** UTI, uriney retention
**RESP:** Cough
**Other:** Angioedema, influenza

## Nursing Considerations

• Use cautiously in patients with ulcerative colitis, intestinal atony, or myasthenia gravis because solifenacin may decrease GI motility; in patients with significant bladder outflow obstruction because solifenacin may cause urine retention; in patients with hepatic impairment because solifenacin is metabolized in the liver; and in patients with renal impairment because solifenacin excretion may be impaired.
• Monitor elderly patients, especially those age 75 and older, for adverse reactions because they're at increased risk for solifenacin-induced adverse reactions.

**PATIENT TEACHING**
• Instruct patient to take solifenacin with a full glass of water and to swallow the tablet whole.

Q
R
S

•Caution patient to avoid exertion in a warm or hot environment because sweating may be delayed, which could increase body temperature and increase risk of heatstroke.
•Advise patient to avoid hazardous activities until drug's CNS effects are known.
•Inform patient that alcohol may cause drowsiness; urge patient to limit or avoid alcoholic beverages while taking solifenacin.

# somatropin

Genotropin, Humatrope, Norditropin, Nutropin, Nutropin AQ, Saizen, Serostim, Tev-Tropin

## Class and Category

*Chemical:* Recombinant DNA product
*Therapeutic:* Growth hormone
*Pregnancy category:* B (Serostim) or C (Genotropin, Humatrope, Norditropin, Nutropin, Nutropin AQ, Saizen)

## Indications and Dosages

➤ *To treat growth failure caused by growth hormone deficiency*

**S.C. INJECTION (NUTROPIN, NUTROPIN AQ)**
**Adults.** 0.3 mg (0.9 IU)/kg/wk.
**S.C. INJECTION (SAIZEN)**
**Adults.** *Initial:* 0.005 mg/kg/day, increased after 4 wk by no more than 0.01 mg/kg/day, as needed.
**I.M. OR S.C. INJECTION (HUMATROPE, NUTROPIN, SAIZEN)**
**Children.** 0.18 to 0.3 mg (0.54 to 0.9 IU)/kg/wk, divided into equal doses given q.d. or q.o.d. over 6 to 7 days.
**S.C. INJECTION (NORDITROPIN)**
**Adults.** *Initial:* 0.004 mg/kg/day, increased after 6 wk by no more than 0.016 mg/kg/day, as needed.
**S.C. INJECTION (GENOTROPIN, NORDITROPIN)**
**Children.** 0.16 to 0.24 mg (0.48 to 0.72 IU)/kg/wk, divided into equal doses given q.d. over 6 to 7 days.
**S.C. INJECTION (TEV-TROPIN)**
**Children.** Up to 0.1 mg/kg three times/wk.

➤ *To treat growth failure caused by chronic renal insufficiency*

**S.C. INJECTION (NUTROPIN, NUTROPIN AQ)**
**Children.** Up to 0.35 mg (1.05 IU)/kg/wk, divided into equal doses given q.d.

➤ *To treat growth failure caused by Turner's syndrome*

**S.C. INJECTION (NUTROPIN, NUTROPIN AQ)**
**Adults and children.** Up to 0.375 mg (1.125 IU)/kg/wk, divided into equal doses given q.d. or q.o.d. over 7 days.

➤ *To provide long-term treatment of growth failure in children born small for gestational age and no catch-up growth by age 2*

**S.C. INJECTION (GENOTROPIN)**
**Children.** 0.48 mg/kg/wk, divided into equal doses and administered q.d. over 6 to 7 days.
**S.C. INJECTION (HUMATROPE)**
**Children.** Up to 0.37 mg/kg/wk, divided into equal doses and administered q.d. over 6 to 7 days.

➤ *To treat growth factor failure due to Prader-Willi syndrome*

**S.C. INJECTION (GENOTROPIN)**
**Children.** 0.24 mg/kg/wk.

➤ *To treat AIDS-associated cachexia or weight loss*

**S.C. INJECTION (SEROSTIM)**
**Adults who weigh more than 55 kg (121 lb).** 6 mg h.s.
**Adults who weigh 45 to 55 kg (99 to 121 lb).** 5 mg h.s.
**Adults who weigh 35 to 45 kg (77 to 99 lb).** 4 mg h.s.
**Adults who weigh less than 35 kg.** 0.1 mg/kg h.s.
**DOSAGE ADJUSTMENT** For patients at increased risk for adverse effects related to Serostim therapy, 0.1 mg/kg q.o.d.

| Route | Onset | Peak | Duration |
|---|---|---|---|
| I.M., S.C. | Unknown | Unknown | 12 to 48 hr |

## Mechanism of Action

Increases production of somatomedins (or insulin-like growth factor) in the liver and other tissues, which mediates somatropin's anabolic and growth-promoting effects. The drug binds to specific receptors throughout the body, stimulating amino acid transport; DNA, RNA, and protein synthesis; cell proliferation; and growth of bone and soft tissue.

It also decreases insulin cell receptor sensitivity, thereby increasing blood glucose level; stimulates triglyceride hydrolysis in adipose tissue and hepatic glucose output; and aids bone growth by promoting a positive calcium balance and retention of sodium and potassium.

## Contraindications

Active neoplasia; acute critical illness due to complications following open-heart or abdominal surgery; acute respiratory failure; cancer; closed epiphyses; hypersensitivity to somatropin, its components, or benzyl alcohol; multiple accidental trauma; Prader-Willi syndrome coupled with severe obesity or severe respiratory impairment; proliferative or preproliferative diabetic retinopathy

## Interactions

**DRUGS**

*anabolic steroids, androgens, estrogens, thyroid hormones:* Possibly accelerated epiphyseal closure

*corticosteroids, corticotropin:* Inhibited growth response to somatropin

## Adverse Reactions

**CNS:** Depression, dizziness, headache, hypoesthesia, insomnia, paresthesia, weakness
**CV:** Chest pain, edema
**EENT:** Papilledema, rhinitis, vision changes
**ENDO:** Gynecomastia, hyperglycemia, hypothyroidism
**GI:** Nausea, vomiting
**MS:** Arthralgia, back or bone pain, carpal tunnel syndrome, myalgia
**RESP:** Upper respiratory tract infection
**SKIN:** Increased growth of nevi, rash
**Other:** Flulike symptoms, injection site inflammation

## Nursing Considerations

• Be aware that somatropin shouldn't be used in patients with malignancy and, if currently prescribed, should be stopped if patient is diagnosed with malignancy. Cancer treatment must be completed with evidence of remission before somatropin can be started or restarted.
• Make sure patient with Prader-Willi syndrome has been evaluated for upper airway obstruction and sleep apnea before somatropin therapy starts because of increased risk of respiratory arrest. Notify prescriber immediately and expect to stop somatropin if patient starts snoring, if snoring increases, or if other evidence of upper airway obstruction develops.
• Reconstitute somatropin according to package directions. (Nutropin AQ and forms available in cartridges, such as Norditropin NordiFlex, don't require reconstitution.) In general, swirl vial gently to dissolve contents rather than shaking it.
• Don't reconstitute with diluent that contains benzyl alcohol if drug will be given to neonate; don't use supplied diluent for Humatrope for patients sensitive to Metacresol or glycerin. Instead, use sterile water for injection.
• Store Nutropin AQ vials and cartridges refrigerated in a dark place.
• **WARNING** Anticipate possible headache, nausea, papilledema, vision changes, and vomiting, especially during first 8 weeks of therapy.
• Because somatropin is a protein, monitor patient for a local or systemic allergic reaction.

**PATIENT TEACHING**

• Instruct diabetic patient who takes insulin to monitor blood glucose level frequently; somatropin may induce insulin resistance.
• Inform parents of a child with Turner's syndrome about the increased risk of ear infections.
• Advise family or cargiver to observe patient for limping, which may indicate a slipped epiphysis.

# sotalol hydrochloride

Betapace, Betapace AF, Sotacor (CAN)

## Class and Category

*Chemical:* Methanesulfonanilide
*Therapeutic:* Class III antiarrhythmic
*Pregnancy category:* B

## Indications and Dosages

➤ *To treat life-threatening ventricular arrhythmias*

**TABLETS**

**Adults.** *Initial:* 80 mg b.i.d. *Maintenance:* 160 to 320 mg/day in divided doses b.i.d. or t.i.d. *Maximum:* 640 mg/day.
**DOSAGE ADJUSTMENT** If creatinine clearance is 30 to 60 ml/min/1.73 m², dosage interval extended to q 24 hr; if creatinine clearance is less than 30 ml/min/ 1.73 m², dosage interval extended to q 36 to 48 hr, according to response; if creatinine clearance less than 10 ml/min/ 1.73 m², dosage adjusted as prescribed.

➤ *To maintain normal sinus rhythm in patients with highly symptomatic atrial fibrillation who are currently in sinus rhythm*

**TABLETS**

**Adults.** *Initial:* 80 mg q.d. if creatinine clearance is 40 to 60 ml/min/1.73 m², or 80 mg b.i.d.

Q
R
S

if creatinine clearance exceeds 60 ml/min/1.73 m². *Maintenance:* After at least 3 days (five or six doses given q.d.), if 80-mg dose is tolerated and QT interval less than 500 msec, dosage maintained and patient discharged. Or hospitalized patient monitored closely to determine maintenance dosage while increasing to 120 mg b.i.d. for 3 days (five or six doses if q.d. dosing). *Maximum:* 160 mg b.i.d. if creatinine clearance exceeds 60 ml/min/1.73 m².

DOSAGE ADJUSTMENT If 80-mg q.d. or b.i.d dosage doesn't reduce frequency of atrial fibrillation relapses and is tolerated without excessive QT interval prolongation (greater than 520 msec), dosage increased to 120 mg q.d. or b.i.d., depending on creatinine clearance. If 120-mg dose doesn't reduce frequency of early relapse and is tolerated using same criteria, dosage increased to 160 mg q.d. or b.i.d., depending on creatinine clearance.

DOSAGE ADJUSTMENT Dosage reduced if QT interval is 520 msec or more until it returns to less than 520 msec. Drug stopped if QT interval exceeds 520 msec with lowest maintenance dosage of 80 mg. Daily dose reduced by half and given q.d. if renal function deteriorates.

| Route | Onset | Peak | Duration |
|-------|-------|------|----------|
| P.O. | Unknown | 2 to 3 hr | Unknown |

## Mechanism of Action

Combines class II and class III antiarrhythmic activity to increase sinus cycle length. This beta blocker decreases AV nodal conduction and increases AV nodal refractoriness. Suppression of SA node automaticity and AV node conductivity decreases atrial and ventricular ectopy.

## Contraindications

Asthma, atrial arrhythmias (if baseline QT interval exceeds 450 msec or creatinine clearance is less than 40 ml/min/1.73 m²), cardiogenic shock, congenital or acquired QT syndromes, COPD, heart failure (unless it results from tachyarrhythmia that's treatable by sotalol), hypersensitivity to sotalol or its components, second- or third-degree AV block without functioning pacemaker, sinus bradycardia

## Interactions

**DRUGS**

*allergen immunotherapy, allergenic extracts for skin testing:* Increased risk of serious systemic adverse reaction or anaphylaxis
*amiodarone:* Additive depressant effect on conduction, negative inotropic effect
*anesthetics (hydrocarbon inhalation):* Increased risk of myocardial depression and hypotension
*antacids:* Altered sotalol effectiveness
*astemizole, class I antiarrhythmics, phenothiazines, terfenadine, tricyclic antidepressants:* Prolonged QT interval, life-threatening torsades de pointes
*beta blockers (other):* Additive beta blockade
*beta₂-receptor stimulants:* Decreased effectiveness of these drugs
*calcium channel blockers, clonidine, diazoxide, guanabenz, reserpine and other antihypertensives:* Additive antihypertensive effect and, possibly, other beta-blocking effects
*cimetidine:* Possibly impaired sotalol clearance
*glucagon:* Possibly blunted hyperglycemic response
*insulin, oral antidiabetic drugs:* Impaired glucose control, increased risk of hyperglycemia
*lidocaine:* Decreased lidocaine clearance, increased risk of lidocaine toxicity
*MAO inhibitors:* Increased risk of significant hypertension
*neuromuscular blockers:* Possibly potentiated and prolonged neuromuscular blockade
*phenothiazines:* Increased blood levels of both drugs
*propafenone:* Increased blood level and half-life of sotalol
*sympathomimetics, xanthines:* Possibly mutual inhibition of therapeutic effects

## Adverse Reactions

**CNS:** Anxiety, depression, dizziness, drowsiness, fatigue, insomnia, lethargy, nervousness, weakness
**CV:** AV conduction disorders, bradycardia, heart failure, hypotension, peripheral vascular insufficiency
**EENT:** Nasal congestion
**ENDO:** Hyperglycemia, hypoglycemia
**GI:** Abdominal pain, constipation, diarrhea, nausea, vomiting
**GU:** Sexual dysfunction
**MS:** Muscle weakness
**RESP:** Bronchospasm, dyspnea, wheezing

## Nursing Considerations
• Obtain baseline creatinine clearance and QT interval before starting sotalol, as ordered.
• Monitor blood pressure, apical and radial pulse rates, fluid intake and output, daily weight, and respiratory rate, and assess circulation in extremities before and during sotalol therapy.
• If prescriber is stopping amiodarone, be aware that sotalol shouldn't be started until QT interval has returned to baseline because of possible adverse cardiac effects.
• Be aware that stopping sotalol abruptly may cause life-threatening reactions.
• Monitor serum electrolyte levels because drug can increase risk of torsades de pointes in patients with electrolyte imbalances, especially hypokalemia or hypomagnesemia.
• Assess carefully if patient has diabetes mellitus or thyrotoxicosis because they may mask hypoglycemia and hyperthyroidism.

### PATIENT TEACHING
• Advise patient to notify prescriber immediately if he has difficulty breathing.
• Encourage patient to consult with prescriber before taking OTC drugs, especially cold remedies, which may decrease sotalol's effectiveness.
• Urge patient to avoid potentially hazardous activities until drug's CNS effects are known.

# sparfloxacin

Zagam

## Class and Category
*Chemical:* Fluoroquinolone
*Therapeutic:* Antibiotic
*Pregnancy category:* C

## Indications and Dosages
➤ *To treat community-acquired pneumonia caused by* Chlamydia pneumoniae, Haemophilus influenzae, H. parainfluenzae, Moraxella catarrhalis, Mycoplasma pneumoniae, *or* Streptococcus pneumoniae *and acute bacterial exacerbations of chronic bronchitis caused by* C. pneumoniae, Enterobacter cloacae, H. influenzae, H. parainfluenzae, Klebsiella pneumoniae, M. catarrhalis, Staphylococcus aureus, *or* S. pneumoniae

### TABLETS
**Adults.** 400 mg on day 1, followed by 200 mg/day for 10 days.
**DOSAGE ADJUSTMENT** For patients with creatinine clearance less than 50 ml/min/1.73 m$^2$, 400 mg on day 1 and then dosing interval extended to 200 mg q 48 hr for 9 days.

### Mechanism of Action
Causes bacterial cells to die by inhibiting the enzyme DNA gyrase, which is responsible for unwinding and supercoiling bacterial DNA before it replicates.

## Contraindications
History of photosensitivity, hypersensitivity to quinolone derivatives, job or lifestyle that precludes compliance with measures to prevent phototoxicity, prolonged QTc interval or use of drugs that can prolong QTc interval

## Interactions
### DRUGS
*aluminum-, calcium-, or magnesium-containing antacids; ferrous sulfate; magnesium-containing laxatives; sucralfate; zinc:* Decreased bioavailability of sparfloxacin
*amiodarone, astemizole, bepridil, cisapride, class IA antiarrhythmics (disopyramide, quinidine, procainamide), class III antiarrhythmics (ibutilide, sotalol), erythromycin, pentamidine, phenothiazines, terfenadine, tricyclic antidepressants, other drugs that can prolong QTc interval:* Possibly prolonged QTc interval and torsades de pointes

## Adverse Reactions
**CNS:** Asthenia, cerebral thrombosis, dizziness, drowsiness, headache, insomnia, lightheadedness, nervousness, seizures, somnolence
**CV:** Cardiopulmonary arrest, embolism, prolonged QTc interval, torsades de pointes, vasodilation
**EENT:** Laryngeal edema, taste perversion
**GI:** Abdominal pain, diarrhea, hepatic necrosis or failure, hepatitis, intestinal perforation, nausea, pseudomembranous colitis, vomiting
**GU:** Acute renal failure, vaginal candidiasis
**HEME:** Agranulocytosis, hemolytic anemia, pancytopenia, thrombocytopenia
**MS:** Rhabdomyolysis, tendinitis, tendon rupture
**RESP:** Interstitial pneumonia, pulmonary edema
**SKIN:** Photosensitivity, pruritus, rash,

Q
R
S

Stevens-Johnson syndrome, toxic epidermal necrolysis

**Other:** Acidosis, anaphylaxis, angioedema, squamous cell carcinoma

### Nursing Considerations
• Use sparfloxacin cautiously in patients with known or suspected CNS disorders because of risk of seizures. Institute seizure precautions according to facility policy.
• Monitor renal and liver function test results, as appropriate, during prolonged therapy.
• Measure QTc interval regularly because sparfloxacin has been found to increase QTc interval and risk of torsades de pointes.
• Severe diarrhea may indicate pseudomembranous colitis; give fluid, electrolyte, and protein replacement, as ordered.

**PATIENT TEACHING**
• Urge patient to avoid hazardous activities until sparfloxacin's CNS effects are known.
• Advise patient to notify prescriber immediately about aching or throbbing tendon pain.
• Instruct patient to wait 4 hours after taking sparfloxacin before taking antacids that contain aluminum, calcium, or magnesium; laxatives that contain magnesium; or vitamins that contain iron or zinc.
• Caution patient to avoid exposure to sunlight, bright natural light, and other sources of ultraviolet light during therapy and for 5 days afterward. Urge him to wear sunscreen and protective clothing when outdoors.
• Urge patient to notify prescriber at first sign of photosensitivity reaction (blistering, burning or swelling sensation, itching, rash, redness).

# spectinomycin hydrochloride

Trobicin

### Class and Category
*Chemical:* Aminocyclitol, aminoglycoside derivative
*Therapeutic:* Antibiotic
*Pregnancy category:* Not rated

### Indications and Dosages
➤ *To treat acute endocervical, rectal, and urethral gonorrhea caused by susceptible strains of* Neisseria gonorrhoeae

**I.M. INJECTION**
**Adults and children who weigh 45 kg (99 lb) or more.** 2 g as a single dose, repeated as prescribed for adult if reinfection occurs or

is strongly suspected. *Maximum:* 4 g for adults, 2 g for children.
**Children who weigh less than 45 kg (except infants).** 40 mg/kg as a single dose.

---

### Mechanism of Action
Binds to negatively charged sites on bacterial outer cell membrane, disrupting cell integrity, and binds to bacterial ribosomal subunits, inhibiting protein synthesis. Both actions lead to bacterial cell death.

---

### Contraindications
Hypersensitivity to spectinomycin or its components

### Interactions
None known

### Adverse Reactions
**CNS:** Dizziness, insomnia
**GI:** Abdominal cramps, nausea, vomiting
**Other:** Injection site pain

### Nursing Considerations
• To reconstitute spectinomycin, add 3.2 ml of bacteriostatic water for injection (with benzyl alcohol) to each 2-g vial or 6.2 ml of diluent to each 4-g vial. Shake vial vigorously before withdrawing dose.
• Administer I.M. injection deep into large muscle mass, preferably upper outer quadrant of gluteal muscle.

**PATIENT TEACHING**
• Tell patient he'll be tested for syphilis at the start of treatment and 3 months later because spectinomycin treatment may mask or delay syphilis symptoms.
• Explain risk factors for sexually transmitted diseases, and teach correct use of condoms.
• Advise patient to encourage sexual partner to be tested for gonorrhea.
• Instruct patient to notify prescriber if symptoms fail to improve within a few days.

# spironolactone

Aldactone, Novospiroton (CAN)

### Class and Category
*Chemical:* Aldosterone antagonist
*Therapeutic:* Aldosterone antagonist, antihypertensive, diagnostic aid for primary hyperaldosteronism, diuretic
*Pregnancy category:* Not rated

## Mechanism of Action

Normally, aldosterone attaches to receptors on the walls of distal convoluted tubule cells, causing sodium (Na⁺) and water (H₂0) reabsorption in the blood, as shown at left.
Spironolactone competes with aldoste-rone for these receptors, thereby preventing sodium and water reabsorption and causing their excretion through the distal convoluted tubules, as shown below right. Increased urinary excretion of sodium and water reduces blood volume and blood pressure.

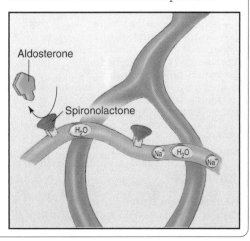

## Indications and Dosages

➤ *To treat edema due to heart failure, hepatic cirrhosis, or nephrotic syndrome*
**TABLETS**
**Adults.** *Initial:* 25 to 200 mg/day in divided doses b.i.d. to q.i.d. for at least 5 days. *Maintenance:* 75 to 400 mg/day in divided doses b.i.d. to q.i.d. *Maximum:* 400 mg/day.
**Children.** *Initial:* 1 to 3 mg/kg/day as a single dose or in divided doses b.i.d. to q.i.d. for at least 2 wk; adjusted, as needed, after 5 days. *Maximum:* 3 times initial dose.
➤ *To treat hypertension*
**TABLETS**
**Adults.** *Initial:* 50 to 100 mg/day as a single dose or in divided doses b.i.d. to q.i.d. for at least 2 wk; gradually adjusted q 2 wk, as needed, to control blood pressure, up to 200 mg/day. *Maximum:* 400 mg/day.
**Children.** *Initial:* 1 to 3 mg/kg/day as a single dose or in divided doses b.i.d. to q.i.d. for at least 2 wk; adjusted, as needed, after 5 days. *Maximum:* 3 times initial dose.
➤ *To aid in the diagnosis of primary hyperaldosteronism*
**TABLETS**
**Adults.** For long test, 400 mg/day in divided doses b.i.d. to q.i.d. for 3 to 4 wk; for short test, 400 mg/day in divided doses b.i.d. to q.i.d. for 4 days.
➤ *To treat primary hyperaldosteronism*
**TABLETS**
**Adults.** 100 to 400 mg/day in divided doses b.i.d. to q.i.d. before surgery. *Maximum:* 400 mg/day.
**DOSAGE ADJUSTMENT** Long-term maintenance dosage decreased for patients at risk for complications during surgery.

➤ *To substitute as therapy for diuretic-induced hypokalemia*
**TABLETS**
**Adults.** 25 to 100 mg/day as a single dose or in divided doses b.i.d. to q.i.d. *Maximum:* 400 mg/day.

| Route | Onset | Peak | Duration |
|-------|-------|------|----------|
| P.O.* | Unknown | 2 to 3 days | 2 to 3 days |

## Contraindications

Acute renal insufficiency, anuria, hyperkalemia, hypersensitivity to spironolactone or its components

---

* For diuretic effect; others unknown.

## Interactions
**DRUGS**

*ACE inhibitors, cyclosporine, other potassium-sparing diuretics, potassium-containing drugs, potassium supplements:* Increased risk of hyperkalemia
*digoxin:* Possibly increased half-life of digoxin
*exchange resins (sodium cycle), such as sodium polystyrene sulfonate:* Increased risk of hypokalemia and fluid retention
*heparin, oral anticoagulants:* Decreased anticoagulant effect of these drugs
*hypotension-producing drugs:* Possibly potentiated antihypertensive or diuretic effect of spironolactone
*lithium:* Possibly lithium toxicity
*NSAIDs, sympathomimetics:* Decreased antihypertensive effect of spironolactone
**FOODS**
*low-salt milk, salt substitutes:* Increased risk of hyperkalemia

## Adverse Reactions
**CNS:** Dizziness, encephalopathy, fatigue, headache
**EENT:** Increased intraocular pressure, nasal congestion, tinnitus, vision changes
**ENDO:** Gynecomastia
**GI:** Abdominal pain, anorexia, constipation, diarrhea, flatulence, nausea, vomiting
**GU:** Impotence
**HEME:** Aplastic anemia, neutropenia
**RESP:** Cough, dyspnea
**MS:** Arthralgia, back and leg pain, muscle weakness, myalgia
**Other:** Hyperkalemia

## Nursing Considerations
• Be aware that for children or patients who have difficulty swallowing, pharmacist may crush spironolactone tablets, mix with a flavored syrup, and dispense as a suspension that is stable for 1 month when refrigerated.
• During diagnosis for primary aldosteronism, the test is considered positive if patient's serum potassium level rises when drug is given and falls when it's discontinued.
• Monitor serum potassium level, as appropriate. Withhold drug and notify prescriber if hyperkalemia develops.
• Evaluate spironolactone's effectiveness by monitoring blood pressure and assessing for edema.

• Stop drug for several days, as prescribed, before patient undergoes adrenal vein catheterization to measure serum aldosterone level and plasma renin activity.
**PATIENT TEACHING**
• Instruct patient to take spironolactone with meals or milk.
• If patient has trouble swallowing tablets, mention that pharmacist can crush them, mix them with a flavored syrup, and dispense as a suspension.
• Teach patient who takes drug for hypertension how to measure his blood pressure. Urge him to monitor it regularly and report measurements greater than 140 mm Hg systolic or 90 mm Hg diastolic to prescriber.
• Caution patient that he may experience dizziness during spironolactone therapy if fluid balance is altered.

# streptokinase

Kabikinase, Streptase

## Class and Category
*Chemical:* Purified beta-hemolytic *Streptococcus* filtrate
*Therapeutic:* Thrombolytic
*Pregnancy category:* C

## Indications and Dosages
➤ *To lyse coronary artery thrombi*
**I.V. INFUSION**
**Adults.** 1,500,000 IU within 60 min of event.
**INTRACORONARY INFUSION**
**Adults.** 20,000-IU bolus, followed by 2,000 IU/min for 60 min for total dose of 140,000 IU.

➤ *To lyse acute arterial thromboembolism or thrombosis, acute pulmonary embolism, or deep vein thrombosis*
**I.V. INFUSION**
**Adults.** 250,000-IU bolus over 30 min, followed by 100,000 IU/hr for 24 to 72 hr.

➤ *To clear occluded arteriovenous cannula*
**I.V. INJECTION**
**Adults.** 100,000 to 250,000 IU instilled slowly into each occluded lumen.

| Route | Onset | Peak | Duration |
|-------|-------|------|----------|
| I.V. | Immediate | 20 to 120 min | 4 hr |

## Mechanism of Action
Binds to fibrin in thrombus and converts trapped plasminogen to plasmin. Plasmin breaks down fibrin, fibrinogen, and other clotting factors, thereby dissolving the thrombus.

## Incompatibilities
Don't mix streptokinase in same syringe or administer through same I.V. line as other drugs.

## Contraindications
Active internal bleeding, AV malformation or aneurysm, bleeding diathesis, history of CVA or intracranial or intraspinal surgery within the past 2 months, hypersensitivity to streptokinase or its components, intracranial cancer, severe uncontrolled hypertension

## Interactions
**DRUGS**
*anticoagulants, enoxaparin, heparin, NSAIDs, platelet aggregation inhibitors:* Increased risk of bleeding
*antifibrinolytics:* Antagonized effects of both drugs
*antihypertensives:* Increased risk of severe hypotension, especially when streptokinase is administered rapidly to treat coronary artery occlusion
*cefamandole, cefoperazone, cefotetan, plicamycin, valproic acid:* Possibly hypoprothrombinemia and increased risk of severe hemorrhage
*corticosteroids, ethacrynic acid, salicylates:* Possibly GI ulceration or bleeding

## Adverse Reactions
**CNS:** Chills, fever
**CV:** Arrhythmias, hypotension
**HEME:** Unusual bleeding or bruising

## Nursing Considerations
• Obtain hematocrit, platelet count, APTT, PT, and INR, as ordered, before giving streptokinase.
• To prevent foaming, don't shake drug during reconstitution.
• Frequently assess for bleeding at I.V. site and for blood in urine and stool. Perform neurologic assessment to detect intracranial bleeding.

• If serious spontaneous bleeding (not controlled by local pressure) occurs, stop streptokinase infusion immediately and notify prescriber.
• Monitor heart rate and rhythm by continuous ECG, as ordered.
• Treat fever with acetaminophen, as prescribed, rather than aspirin to reduce the risk of bleeding.
**PATIENT TEACHING**
• Explain to patient that he'll be on bed rest during streptokinase therapy.
• Inform patient that minor bleeding may occur at arterial puncture or surgical sites. Reassure him that appropriate care measures will be taken if bleeding occurs.
• Advise patient to obtain medical alert identification stating that he takes streptokinase.
• Inform patient that if he experiences chest pain within 12 months of therapy, he should notify health care providers that he has received streptokinase because repeated administration within 12 months may be ineffective.

# streptomycin sulfate

## Class and Category
*Chemical:* Aminoglycoside
*Therapeutic:* Antibiotic
*Pregnancy category:* D

## Indications and Dosages
➤ *To treat gram-negative bacillary bacteremia, meningeal infections, pneumonia, systemic infections, and UTIs caused by susceptible strains of* Aerobacter aerogenes, Brucella, Calymmatobacterium granulomatis, Enterococcus faecalis, Escherichia coli, Haemophilus ducreyi, H. influenzae, Klebsiella pneumoniae, *and* Proteus
**I.M. INJECTION**
**Adults.** 1 to 2 g/day in divided doses q 6 to 12 hr. *Maximum:* 2 g/day.
**Children.** 20 to 40 mg/kg/day in divided doses q 6 to 12 hr.
➤ *As adjunct to treat endocarditis caused by* Streptococcus viridans *or* E. faecalis
**I.M. INJECTION**
**Adults.** 1 g b.i.d. for 1 wk *(S. viridans)* or 2 wk *(E. faecalis)* in conjunction with a peni-

Q
R
S

cillin. Then, 500 mg b.i.d. for 1 wk *(S. viridans)* or 4 wk *(E. faecalis)*.

➤ *As adjunct to treat tuberculosis caused by* Mycobacterium tuberculosis

**I.M. INJECTION**

**Adults.** 1 g/day in combination with other antibiotics; dosage reduced to 1 g 2 or 3 times/wk, as appropriate and prescribed. *Maximum:* 2 g/day.

**Children.** 20 mg/kg/day in combination with other antibiotics. *Maximum:* 1 g/day.

**DOSAGE ADJUSTMENT** For elderly patients, dosage decreased to 500 to 750 mg/day in combination with other antibiotics.

➤ *To treat plague caused by* Yersinia pestis

**I.M. INJECTION**

**Adults.** 2 g/day in 2 equally divided doses for at least 10 days.

**Children.** 30 mg/kg/day in divided doses b.i.d. or t.i.d. for 10 days.

➤ *To treat tularemia caused by* Francisella tularensis

**I.M. INJECTION**

**Adults.** 1 to 2 g/day in divided doses for 7 to 14 days.

**DOSAGE ADJUSTMENT** For patients with creatinine clearance of 50 to 80 ml/min/1.73 m$^2$, dosage reduced to 7.5 mg/kg I.M. q 24 hr; for creatinine clearance of 10 to 49 ml/min/1.73 m$^2$, 7.5 mg/kg I.M. q 24 to 72 hr; for creatinine clearance less than 10 ml/min/1.73 m$^2$, 7.5 mg/kg I.M. q 72 to 96 hr.

---

**Mechanism of Action**

Binds to negatively charged sites on the bacteria's outer cell membrane, disrupting cell integrity. Streptomycin also binds to bacterial ribosomal subunits and inhibits protein synthesis. Both actions lead to bacterial cell death.

---

## Incompatibilities

Don't mix streptomycin in same solution or administer through same I.V. line as other antibiotics.

## Contraindications

Hypersensitivity to streptomycin or other aminoglycosides

## Interactions

**DRUGS**

*antimyasthenics:* Possibly decreased effect of antimyasthenics on skeletal muscle

*beta-lactam antibiotics:* Inactivation of streptomycin

*capreomycin, other aminoglycosides:* Increased potential for ototoxicity, nephrotoxicity, and neuromuscular blockade

*indomethacin (I.V.):* Decreased renal clearance of streptomycin when given to premature neonates, possibly leading to aminoglycoside toxicity

*methoxyflurane, polymyxins (parenteral):* Increased risk of nephrotoxicity and neuromuscular blockade

*nephrotoxic and ototoxic drugs:* Increased risk of nephrotoxicity and ototoxicity

*neuromuscular blockers:* Increased neuromuscular blockade

## Adverse Reactions

**CNS:** Clumsiness, dizziness, neurotoxicity, paresthesia, peripheral neuropathy, seizures, unsteadiness, vertigo

**EENT:** Hearing loss, sensation of fullness in ears, tinnitus, vision loss

**GI:** Anorexia, nausea, thirst, vomiting

**GU:** Decreased or increased urine output, nephrotoxicity

**MS:** Muscle twitching

**SKIN:** Erythema, pruritus, rash, urticaria

## Nursing Considerations

• Use streptomycin cautiously in patients with renal impairment. In severely uremic patients, single dose can produce high blood level of drug for several days; cumulative effects may produce ototoxicity.

• Expect prescriber to order baseline renal function studies and to assess cranial nerve VIII function (responsible for hearing) at start of streptomycin therapy to allow for later comparisons.

• Monitor serum peak and trough levels, as ordered, to ensure adequate but not toxic drug level.

• Be aware that streptomycin should be given only by I.M. injection.

• To reconstitute streptomycin, add 4.2 to 4.5 ml of sodium chloride for injection or sterile water for injection to each 1-g vial to provide a concentration of 200 mg/ml, or add 3.2 to 3.5 ml of diluent to each 5-g vial to provide a concentration of 250 mg/ml. Alternatively, add 6.5 ml of diluent to each 5-g vial to provide a concentration of 500 mg/ml.

• Don't give a concentration greater than 500 mg/ml.

- Rotate injection sites to prevent sterile abscess formation.

**PATIENT TEACHING**
- Advise patient to refrigerate streptomycin solution at 36° to 46° F (2° to 8° C).
- Inform patient that treatment for tuberculosis lasts at least 1 year.
- Urge patient to notify prescriber if he experiences fullness or ringing in ears, hearing loss, or vertigo.

# sucralfate

Apo-sucralfate (CAN), Carafate, Sulcrate (CAN), Sulcrate Suspension Plus (CAN)

## Class and Category
*Chemical:* Disulfated disaccharide, aluminum salt
*Therapeutic:* Antiulcer
*Pregnancy category:* B

## Indications and Dosages
➤ *To prevent duodenal ulcer*
**TABLETS**
**Adults and adolescents.** 1 g b.i.d.
➤ *To treat active duodenal ulcer*
**ORAL SUSPENSION**
**Adults and adolescents.** 1 g q.i.d. 1 hr before meals and h.s. for 4 to 8 wk or, possibly, less. Alternatively, 2 g b.i.d. on empty stomach on waking and h.s. for 4 to 8 wk or, possibly, less.
**TABLETS**
**Adults and adolescents.** 1 g q.i.d. 1 hr before meals and h.s. for 4 to 8 wk or, possibly, less.

---

### Mechanism of Action
May react with hydrochloric acid in the stomach to form a complex that buffers acid. The complex adheres electrostatically to proteins on the ulcer's surface and creates a protective barrier at the ulcer site. Sucralfate also inhibits back-diffusion of hydrogen ions and adsorbs pepsin and bile acids, actions that promote healing of an existing duodenal ulcer and prevent ulcer formation.

---

## Interactions
**DRUGS**
*aluminum-containing drugs (such as antacids, antidiarrheals, buffered aspirin with alumi-*
*num, and vaginal douches):* Possibly aluminum toxicity in patients with renal failure
*antacids:* Possibly interference with binding of sucralfate to GI mucosa
*cimetidine, ciprofloxacin, digoxin, norfloxacin, ofloxacin, phenytoin, ranitidine, tetracycline, theophylline:* Decreased bioavailability of these drugs

## Adverse Reactions
**CNS:** Dizziness, drowsiness, light-headedness
**EENT:** Dry mouth
**GI:** Constipation, diarrhea, indigestion, nausea, vomiting
**MS:** Back pain
**SKIN:** Pruritus, rash, urticaria

## Nursing Considerations
- Use sucralfate cautiously in patients with chronic renal failure because of increased risk of aluminum toxicity.
- Administer drug to patient when he has an empty stomach.

**PATIENT TEACHING**
- Instruct patient to take sucralfate on an empty stomach at least 1 hour before meals and at bedtime.
- Advise patient not to take antacids within 30 minutes of sucralfate.
- Caution patient to check with prescriber before taking another drug within 2 hours of sucralfate.

# sulfadiazine

## Class and Category
*Chemical:* Sulfonamide
*Therapeutic:* Antibiotic, antiprotozoal
*Pregnancy category:* C

## Indications and Dosages
➤ *To treat asymptomatic carriers of meningitis*
**TABLETS**
**Adults and adolescents.** 1 g q 12 hr for 2 days.
**Children ages 1 to 12.** 500 mg q 12 hr for 2 days.
**Children ages 2 to 12 months.** 500 mg q.d. for 2 days.
➤ *To prevent recurrent rheumatic fever*
**TABLETS**
**Adults and adolescents.** 500 mg q.d. (for patients weighing less than 30 kg [66 lb]) to 1 g q.d. (for patients weighing 30 kg or more).
➤ *To treat inclusive nocardiosis*

Q
R
S

**TABLETS**
**Adults and adolescents.** 4 to 8 g/day for at least 6 wk.

➤ *As adjunct to treat toxoplasmosis in patients with AIDS*
**TABLETS**
**Adults and adolescents.** 1 to 2 g q 6 hr, together with 50 to 100 mg/day of pyrimethamine and 10 to 25 mg/day of leucovorin.
**Children age 2 months and older.** 50 mg/kg b.i.d. for 12 mo, together with 2 mg/kg/day of pyrimethamine for 2 days, then 1 mg/kg/day of pyrimethamine for 2 to 6 mo, then 1 mg/kg/day of pyrimethamine 3 times/wk for remainder of 12 mo; in addition, 5 mg of leucovorin given 3 times/wk for 12 mo. *Maximum:* 6 g/day.

➤ *To treat toxoplasmosis in pregnant women after week 16 of gestation*
**TABLETS**
**Adults.** 1 g q 6 hr, together with 25 mg/day of pyrimethamine and 5 to 15 mg/day of leucovorin.

### Mechanism of Action
Inhibits para-aminobenzoic acid, a bacterial enzyme responsible for synthesizing folic acid, which susceptible bacteria require for growth. By inactivating bacteria, sulfadiazine prevents or alleviates infection.

## Contraindications
Breast-feeding; hypersensitivity to sulfadiazine, its components, or other chemically related drugs, such as sulfonamides; pregnancy at term

## Interactions
**DRUGS**
*bone marrow depressants:* Increased risk of leukopenic or thrombocytopenic effects
*cyclosporine:* Decreased blood cyclosporine level, increased risk of nephrotoxicity
*estrogen-containing oral contraceptives:* Increased risk of breakthrough bleeding and pregnancy
*hemolytics:* Increased risk of adverse effects
*hepatotoxic drugs:* Increased risk of hepatotoxicity
*hydantoins, oral anticoagulants, oral antidiabetic drugs:* Increased or prolonged effects of these drugs, possibly toxicity

*indomethacin, probenecid, salicylates:* Increased blood level of free sulfadiazine caused by displacement from plasma protein-binding sites
*methotrexate:* Increased risk of leukopenic or thrombocytopenic effects of methotrexate
*phenylbutazone, sulfinpyrazone:* Increased blood sulfadiazine level
*uricosuric drugs:* Potentiated uricosuric action

## Adverse Reactions
**CNS:** Dizziness, fatigue, fever, headache, lethargy, weakness
**EENT:** Pharyngitis
**GI:** Anorexia, diarrhea, dysphagia, nausea, vomiting
**GU:** Crystalluria
**HEME:** Agranulocytosis, aplastic anemia, hemolytic anemia, leukopenia, thrombocytopenia, unusual bleeding or bruising
**MS:** Arthralgia, myalgia
**SKIN:** Blisters, erythema, jaundice, pallor, photosensitivity, pruritus, rash
**Other:** Drug-induced fever

## Nursing Considerations
• Use sulfadiazine cautiously in patients with blood dyscrasias or megaloblastic anemia from folate deficiency because drug may cause blood dyscrasias; in those with G6PD deficiency because hemolysis may occur; in those with hepatic or renal impairment because of increased risk of toxicity; and in those with porphyria because drug may precipitate an acute attack.
• Obtain blood sample for CBC and body tissue or fluid specimen for culture and sensitivity tests, as ordered, before giving drug. Expect first dose to be given before results are available.
• ▪WARNING Monitor patient for drug-induced fever, which may develop 7 to 10 days after he starts taking sulfadiazine. Signs and symptoms include abdominal pain, anorexia, ataxia, depression, diarrhea, headache, insomnia, nausea, peripheral neuropathy, tinnitus, and vomiting.
• Monitor fluid intake and output during therapy. Altered fluid balance may increase risk of crystalluria.
• Frequently monitor blood glucose level and assess for signs and symptoms of hypoglycemia in patients who take an oral antidiabetic drug. Be prepared to respond if hypoglycemia develops.

## PATIENT TEACHING
• Instruct patient to take sulfadiazine exactly as prescribed and to complete the full course even if he feels better.
• Advise patient to take drug with a full glass of water and to drink plenty of fluids during therapy.
• Urge patient to notify prescriber if urine turns reddish brown; this may indicate crystalluria.
• Inform patient about possible dizziness, and urge him to avoid potentially hazardous activities until drug's CNS effects are known.
• Advise patient to avoid prolonged exposure to sunlight and to wear sunscreen and protective clothing when outdoors.
• Urge patient who takes oral contraceptives to use an additional method of birth control during therapy.
• Advise patient who takes an oral antidiabetic drug to check his blood glucose level frequently because of the increased risk of hypoglycemia during therapy.

# sulfamethizole

Thiosulfil Forte

## Class and Category
*Chemical:* Sulfonamide
*Therapeutic:* Antibiotic
*Pregnancy category:* C

## Indications and Dosages
➤ *To treat cystitis and other UTIs caused by* Enterobacter *sp.,* Escherichia coli, Klebsiella *sp.,* Proteus mirabilis, P. vulgaris, *or* Staphylococcus aureus

### TABLETS
**Adults.** 0.5 to 1 g q 6 to 8 hr.
**Children age 2 months and older.** 7.5 to 11.25 mg/kg q 6 hr.
**DOSAGE ADJUSTMENT** Dosage usually reduced for patients with impaired renal function.

---

### Mechanism of Action
Inhibits para-aminobenzoic acid, a bacterial enzyme responsible for synthesizing folic acid, which susceptible bacteria require for growth. By inactivating bacteria, sulfamethizole prevents or alleviates infection.

---

## Contraindications
Breast-feeding; hypersensitivity to sulfamethizole, its components, or other chemically related drugs, such as sulfonamides; pregnancy at term

## Interactions
### DRUGS
*bone marrow depressants:* Increased risk of leukopenic or thrombocytopenic effects
*cyclosporine:* Decreased blood cyclosporine level, increased risk of nephrotoxicity
*estrogen-containing oral contraceptives:* Increased risk of breakthrough bleeding and pregnancy
*hemolytics:* Increased risk of adverse effects
*hepatotoxic drugs:* Increased risk of hepatotoxicity
*hydantoins, oral anticoagulants, oral antidiabetic drugs:* Increased or prolonged effects of these drugs, possibly toxicity
*indomethacin, probenecid, salicylates:* Increased blood level of free sulfamethizole caused by displacement from plasma protein-binding sites
*methotrexate:* Increased risk of leukopenic or thrombocytopenic effects of methotrexate
*phenylbutazone, sulfinpyrazone:* Increased blood sulfamethizole level
*uricosuric drugs:* Potentiated uricosuric action

## Adverse Reactions
**CNS:** Dizziness, fatigue, fever, headache, lethargy, weakness
**EENT:** Pharyngitis
**GI:** Anorexia, diarrhea, dysphagia, nausea, vomiting
**GU:** Crystalluria
**HEME:** Agranulocytosis, aplastic anemia, hemolytic anemia, leukopenia, thrombocytopenia, unusual bleeding or bruising
**MS:** Arthralgia, myalgia
**SKIN:** Blisters, erythema, jaundice, pallor, photosensitivity, pruritus, rash
**Other:** Drug-induced fever

## Nursing Considerations
• Use sulfamethizole cautiously in patients with blood dyscrasias or megaloblastic anemia from folate deficiency because drug may cause blood dyscrasias; in those with G6PD deficiency because hemolysis may occur; in those with hepatic or renal impairment because of increased risk of toxicity; and in those with porphyria because drug may precipitate an acute attack.

•Obtain blood sample for CBC and body tissue or fluid specimen for culture and sensitivity tests, as ordered, before giving drug. Expect first dose to be given before results are available.

•**WARNING** Monitor patient for drug-induced fever, which may develop 7 to 10 days after he starts taking sulfamethizole. Signs and symptoms include abdominal pain, anorexia, ataxia, depression, diarrhea, headache, insomnia, nausea, peripheral neuropathy, tinnitus, and vomiting.

•Monitor fluid intake and output during therapy. Altered fluid balance may increase risk of crystalluria.

•Frequently monitor blood glucose level and assess for signs and symptoms of hypoglycemia in patients who take an oral antidiabetic drug. Be prepared to respond if hypoglycemia develops.

**PATIENT TEACHING**

•Instruct patient to take sulfamethizole exactly as prescribed and to complete the full course even if he feels better.

•Advise patient to take drug with a full glass of water and to drink plenty of fluids during therapy.

•Urge patient to notify prescriber if urine turns reddish brown; this may indicate crystalluria.

•Inform patient about possible dizziness, and urge him to avoid potentially hazardous activities until drug's CNS effects are known.

•Advise patient to avoid prolonged exposure to sunlight and to wear sunscreen and protective clothing when outdoors.

•Urge patient who takes oral contraceptives to use an additional method of birth control during therapy.

•Advise patient who takes an oral antidiabetic drug to check his blood glucose level frequently because of the increased risk of hypoglycemia during therapy.

# sulfamethoxazole

Apo-Sulfamethoxazole (CAN), Gantanol, Urobak

## Class and Category

*Chemical:* Sulfonamide
*Therapeutic:* Antibiotic, antiprotozoal
*Pregnancy category:* C

## Indications and Dosages

➤ *To treat chlamydial conjunctivitis; malaria (as adjunct to quinine sulfate and pyrimethamine); toxoplasmosis (as adjunct to pyrimethamine); and UTIs, including pyelonephritis and cystitis, caused by susceptible organisms*

**TABLETS**

**Adults.** *Initial:* 2 g, then 1 g q 8 to 12 hr.
**Children age 2 months and older.** *Initial:* 50 to 60 mg/kg, then 25 to 30 mg/kg q 12 hr. *Maximum:* 2 g for initial dose, 75 mg/kg/day for subsequent doses.

**DOSAGE ADJUSTMENT** Dosage reduction usually needed for patients with impaired renal function.

➤ *To treat uncomplicated urethritis, cervicitis, and proctitis caused by* Chlamydia trachomatis

**TABLETS**

**Adults.** 1 g q 12 hr for 10 days.

**DOSAGE ADJUSTMENT** For patients with creatinine clearance of 10 to 30 ml/min/1.73 m$^2$, recommended dose reduced by 50% or dosing interval extended; for creatinine clearance of less than 10 ml/min/1.73 m$^2$, recommended dose reduced by 75% or dosing interval extended, as prescribed.

### Mechanism of Action

Inhibits para-aminobenzoic acid, a bacterial enzyme responsible for synthesizing folic acid, which susceptible bacteria require for growth. By inactivating bacteria, sulfamethoxazole prevents or alleviates infection.

## Contraindications

Breast-feeding; hypersensitivity to sulfamethoxazole, its components, or other chemically related drugs, such as sulfonamides; pregnancy at term

## Interactions

**DRUGS**

*bone marrow depressants:* Increased risk of leukopenic or thrombocytopenic effects
*cyclosporine:* Decreased blood cyclosporine level, increased risk of nephrotoxicity
*estrogen-containing oral contraceptives:* Increased risk of breakthrough bleeding and pregnancy
*hemolytics:* Increased risk of adverse effects
*hepatotoxic drugs:* Increased risk of hepatotoxicity

*hydantoins, oral anticoagulants, oral antidiabetic drugs:* Increased or prolonged effects of these drugs, possibly toxicity

*indomethacin, probenecid, salicylates:* Increased blood level of free sulfamethoxazole caused by displacement from plasma protein-binding sites

*methotrexate:* Increased risk of leukopenic or thrombocytopenic effects of methotrexate

*phenylbutazone, sulfinpyrazone:* Increased blood sulfamethoxazole level

*uricosuric drugs:* Potentiated uricosuric action

## Adverse Reactions

**CNS:** Dizziness, fatigue, fever, headache, lethargy, weakness
**EENT:** Pharyngitis
**GI:** Anorexia, diarrhea, dysphagia, nausea, vomiting
**GU:** Crystalluria
**HEME:** Agranulocytosis, aplastic anemia, hemolytic anemia, leukopenia, thrombocytopenia, unusual bleeding or bruising
**MS:** Arthralgia, myalgia
**SKIN:** Blisters, erythema, jaundice, pallor, photosensitivity, pruritus, rash
**Other:** Drug-induced fever

## Nursing Considerations

•Use sulfamethoxazole cautiously in patients with blood dyscrasias or megaloblastic anemia from folate deficiency because drug may cause blood dyscrasias; in those with G6PD deficiency because hemolysis may occur; in those with hepatic or renal impairment because of increased risk of toxicity; and in those with porphyria because drug may precipitate an acute attack.

•Obtain blood sample for CBC and body tissue or fluid specimen for culture and sensitivity tests, as ordered, before giving drug. Expect first dose to be given before results are available.

•**WARNING** Monitor patient for drug-induced fever, which may develop 7 to 10 days after he starts taking sulfamethoxazole. Signs and symptoms include abdominal pain, anorexia, ataxia, depression, diarrhea, headache, insomnia, nausea, peripheral neuropathy, tinnitus, and vomiting.

•Monitor fluid intake and output during therapy. Altered fluid balance may increase risk of crystalluria.

•Frequently monitor blood glucose level and assess for signs and symptoms of hypoglycemia in patients who take an oral antidiabetic drug. Be prepared to respond if hypoglycemia develops.

**PATIENT TEACHING**

•Instruct patient to take sulfamethoxazole exactly as prescribed and to complete the full course even if he feels better.

•Advise patient to take drug with a full glass of water and to drink plenty of fluids during therapy.

•Urge patient to notify prescriber if urine turns reddish brown; this may indicate crystalluria.

•Inform patient about possible dizziness, and urge him to avoid potentially hazardous activities until drug's CNS effects are known.

•Advise patient to avoid prolonged exposure to sunlight and to wear sunscreen and protective clothing when outdoors.

•Urge patient who takes oral contraceptives to use an additional method of birth control during therapy.

•Advise patient who takes an oral antidiabetic drug to check his blood glucose level frequently because of increased risk of hypoglycemia during therapy.

# sulfasalazine

Alti-Sulfasalazine (CAN), Azulfidine, Azulfidine EN-Tabs, PMS-Sulfasalazine (CAN), PMS-Sulfasalazine E.C. (CAN), Salazopyrin EN-Tabs (CAN), S.A.S.-500 (CAN), S.A.S. Enteric-500 (CAN)

## Class and Category

*Chemical:* Salicylate, sulfonamide
*Therapeutic:* Anti-inflammatory, antirheumatic, immunomodulator
*Pregnancy category:* B

## Indications and Dosages

➤ *To treat inflammatory bowel diseases, such as ulcerative colitis, and to maintain or prolong remission*
**DELAYED-RELEASE TABLETS, TABLETS**
**Adults and adolescents.** *Initial:* 500 to 1,000 mg q 6 to 8 hr. Or 500 mg q 6 to 12 hr to decrease adverse GI reactions. *Maintenance:* 500 mg q 6 hr.
**Children over age 6.** *Initial:* 6.7 to 10 mg/kg q 4 hr, 10 to 15 mg/kg q 6 hr, or 13.3 to 20 mg/kg q 8 hr. *Maintenance:* 7.5 mg/kg q 6 hr.
➤ *To treat rheumatoid arthritis*
**DELAYED-RELEASE TABLETS, TABLETS**
**Adults.** *Initial:* 500 to 1,000 mg q.d. during wk 1, increased by 500 mg/day q wk, as

needed, up to 2,000 mg/day in divided doses. If no response after 12 wk, increased to 3,000 mg/day. *Maintenance:* 1,000 mg q 12 hr. *Maximum:* 3,000 mg/day.

➤ *To treat juvenile rheumatoid arthritis in patients who have not responded to salicylates or other NSAIDs*

**DELAYED-RELEASE TABLETS**

**Children ages 6 to 16.** 30 to 50 mg/kg/day in divided doses b.i.d. *Maximum:* 2 g/day.

## Mechanism of Action

Sulfasalazine is a prodrug of sulfapyridine and 5-aminosalicylic acid (mesalamine) that delivers more sulfapyridine and mesalamine to the colon than either metabolite could provide alone. Sulfapyridine provides antibacterial action along the intestinal wall; mesalamine inhibits cyclooxygenase, thereby decreasing the production of arachidonic acid metabolites and reducing colonic inflammation.

## Contraindications

Hypersensitivity to salicylates, sulfasalazine, sulfonamides, chemically related drugs, or their components; intestinal or urinary obstruction; porphyria

## Interactions

**DRUGS**

*bone marrow depressants:* Increased leukopenic and thrombocytopenic effects of both drugs

*digoxin:* Possibly inhibited absorption and decreased blood level of digoxin

*folic acid (vitamin B₉):* Decreased folic acid absorption

*hepatotoxic drugs:* Increased risk of hepatotoxicity

*hydantoins, oral anticoagulants, oral antidiabetic drugs:* Increased, prolonged, or toxic effects of these drugs

*methotrexate, phenylbutazone, sulfinpyrazone:* Possibly potentiated effects of these drugs

## Adverse Reactions

**CNS:** Ataxia, chills, depression, fatigue, fever, Guillain-Barré syndrome, headache, insomnia, meningitis, peripheral neuropathy, seizures, vertigo, weakness

**EENT:** Hearing loss, orange-yellow tears, pharyngitis, tinnitus

**GI:** Abdominal pain, anorexia, diarrhea, hepatitis, indigestion, nausea, pancreatitis, ulcerative colitis exacerbation, vomiting

**GU:** Crystalluria, decreased ejaculatory volume, male infertility, nephritis, nephrotic syndrome, orange-yellow urine, toxic nephrosis

**HEME:** Agranulocytosis, aplastic anemia, Heinz body or hemolytic anemia, leukopenia, neutropenia, thrombocytopenia, unusual bleeding or bruising

**MS:** Arthralgia

**RESP:** Idiopathic pulmonary fibrosis, lymphocytic interstitial pneumonitis

**SKIN:** Cyanosis, jaundice, photosensitivity, pruritus, purpura, rash, Stevens-Johnson syndrome, toxic epidermal necrolysis, urticaria

## Nursing Considerations

•Monitor CBC, liver function test results, and BUN and serum creatinine levels before and periodically during prolonged sulfasalazine therapy.

•Be aware that sulfasalazine doses over 4 g or a blood level over 50 mcg/ml increases the risk of adverse and toxic reactions.

•Monitor fluid intake and output and urine color, pH, and consistency. Acidic urine may require alkalization to prevent crystalluria.

**PATIENT TEACHING**

•Instruct patient to take sulfasalazine with meals, milk, or an antacid to decrease GI distress, and to swallow tablets whole.

•Advise patient to prevent crystalluria by taking drug with a full glass of water and drinking at least 64 oz of fluid per day.

•Instruct patient and family to administer drug around the clock.

•Inform patient that symptom relief may take 2 to 5 days for ulcerative colitis and 4 to 12 weeks for rheumatoid arthritis.

•Alert patient that drug may turn urine and skin orange-yellow.

•Advise contact lens wearer to consider wearing glasses during therapy because drug can permanently stain contact lenses yellow.

•Instruct patient to avoid prolonged sun exposure and to wear protective clothing and sunscreen when outdoors.

•Advise patient to brush with a soft-bristled toothbrush and to use dental floss and toothpicks gently because leukopenic and thrombocytopenic drug effects increase the risk of infections and gingival bleeding.

•Urge patient to return periodically for laboratory tests and follow-up visits to monitor drug's effect.

# sulfinpyrazone

Anturane, Apo-Sulfinpyrazone (CAN),
Novopyrazone (CAN)

## Class and Category

*Chemical:* Pyrazalone derivative
*Therapeutic:* Antigout, uricosuric
*Pregnancy category:* Not rated

## Indications and Dosages

➤ *To treat chronic or intermittent gouty arthritis*

**CAPSULES, TABLETS**

**Adults.** *Initial:* 100 to 200 mg b.i.d., increased by 200 mg/day q 2 to 4 days, if needed. *Maintenance:* 100 to 200 mg b.i.d. *Maximum:* 400 mg b.i.d. during wk 1; then 200 to 400 mg b.i.d. until serum urate level is controlled.

| Route | Onset | Peak | Duration |
|-------|-------|------|----------|
| P.O. | Unknown | Unknown | 4 to 10 hr |

## Mechanism of Action

Inhibits renal tubular reabsorption of uric acid, thereby increasing uric acid excretion and decreasing serum urate level. Decreased serum urate level prevents urate deposition, tophus formation, and chronic joint changes. It also helps resolve existing urate deposits and eventually reduces the number of gouty arthritis attacks.

## Contraindications

Active peptic ulcer disease, blood dyscrasias, hypersensitivity to sulfinpyrazone or its components, symptoms of GI inflammation or ulceration

## Interactions

**DRUGS**

*acetaminophen:* Increased risk of hepatotoxicity, decreased acetaminophen effects
*aminosalicylate sodium:* Increased blood level and prolonged duration of this drug, possibly leading to toxicity
*antineoplastics:* Increased risk of uric acid nephropathy
*bismuth subsalicylate and other salicylates:* Decreased sulfinpyrazone effects
*cefamandole, cefoperazone, cefotetan, moxalactam, plicamycin, valproic acid:* Possibly hypoprothrombinemia, increased risk of severe hemorrhage

*diazoxide, mecamylamine, pyrazinamide:* Possibly increased serum uric acid level
*hydantoins:* Increased blood hydantoin level, possibly leading to hydantoin toxicity
*niacin:* Possibly decreased uricosuric effect of sulfinpyrazone
*nitrofurantoin:* Decreased nitrofurantoin effectiveness, possibly nitrofurantoin toxicity
*NSAIDs, oral anticoagulants, platelet aggregation inhibitors, thrombolytics:* Increased risk of bleeding
*oral antidiabetic drugs:* Increased risk of hypoglycemia
*probenecid:* Increased sulfinpyrazone effects
*theophylline:* Possibly decreased blood theophylline level
*verapamil:* Increased clearance and decreased bioavailability of verapamil

**ACTIVITIES**

*alcohol use:* Possibly increased serum uric acid level

## Adverse Reactions

**CNS:** Dizziness
**EENT:** Tinnitus
**GI:** Abdominal pain, epigastric discomfort, GI bleeding, indigestion, nausea, vomiting
**GU:** Dysuria, flank pain, hematuria, renal calculi, renal colic, renal failure
**HEME:** Agranulocytosis, anemia, aplastic anemia, leukopenia, thrombocytopenia
**MS:** Arthralgia, gouty arthritis (acute attack)
**RESP:** Bronchospasm, dyspnea, wheezing
**SKIN:** Erythema, rash

## Nursing Considerations

•Expect to administer full maintenance dose immediately, as prescribed, for patient who is switched to sulfinpyrazone from another uricosuric.
•Monitor serum uric acid level periodically, as ordered, to evaluate drug effectiveness.
•Assess for signs of acute gouty arthritis, especially during first few months of therapy.

**PATIENT TEACHING**

•Instruct patient to take sulfinpyrazone with food, milk, or an antacid to prevent GI distress.
•Stress the importance of taking drug every day, even when feeling better, to prevent acute gouty arthritis attacks.
•Inform patient that acute gouty arthritis may worsen during initial therapy but should improve as treatment continues. Explain that he may not experience drug's full therapeutic effect for 6 months.

Q
R
S

• If an acute gouty arthritis attack occurs, advise patient to seek additional treatment but to continue taking sulfinpyrazone, as prescribed, to help prevent exacerbation.
• Advise patient to drink at least 80 oz of fluids per day to decrease the risk of renal calculus formation.
• Instruct patient to consult prescriber before taking OTC products that contain aspirin or acetaminophen.
• Advise patient to avoid alcohol while taking sulfinpyrazone.
• Encourage patient to return for ordered follow-up laboratory tests to check for blood dyscrasias.

# sulfisoxazole

Apo-Sulfisoxazole (CAN), Gantrisin, Novo-Soxazole (CAN), Sulfizole (CAN)

## sulfisoxazole acetyl

Gantrisin

## Class and Category

*Chemical:* Sulfonamide
*Therapeutic:* Antibiotic, antiprotozoal
*Pregnancy category:* C

## Indications and Dosages

➤ *To treat nocardiosis; plague; malaria (as adjunct to quinine sulfate and pyrimethamine); and UTIs, including pyelonephritis and cystitis, caused by susceptible organisms*

ORAL SUSPENSION, ORAL SYRUP, TABLETS

**Adults and adolescents.** *Initial:* 2 to 4 g/day in divided doses. *Maintenance:* 4 to 8 g/day in divided doses q 4 to 6 hr. *Maximum:* 8 g/day.
**Children over age 2 months.** *Initial:* 75 mg/kg, followed by 120 to 150 mg/kg/day in divided doses q 4 to 6 hr. *Maximum:* 6 g/day.

➤ *To treat uncomplicated cystitis in women*

ORAL SUSPENSION, ORAL SYRUP, TABLETS

**Adults.** 2 g as a single dose.

➤ *To treat acute or recurrent otitis media in combination with erythromycin in penicillin-allergic patients*

ORAL SUSPENSION, ORAL SYRUP, TABLETS

**Children.** 150 mg of sulfisoxazole/kg/day and 50 mg of erythromycin/kg/day in divided doses q.i.d.

➤ *To treat lymphogranuloma venereum*

ORAL SUSPENSION, ORAL SYRUP, TABLETS

**Adults.** 500 mg q 6 hr for 21 days.

➤ *To treat uncomplicated urethritis, cervicitis, or proctitis caused by* Chlamydia trachomatis

ORAL SUSPENSION, ORAL SYRUP, TABLETS

**Adults.** 500 mg q 6 hr.

DOSAGE ADJUSTMENT For patients with renal impairment, dosing interval changed to q 8 to 24 hr, as prescribed.

### Mechanism of Action

Inhibits para-aminobenzoic acid, a bacterial enzyme responsible for synthesizing folic acid, which susceptible bacteria require for growth. By inactivating bacteria, sulfisoxazole prevents or alleviates infection.

## Contraindications

Breast-feeding; hypersensitivity to sulfisoxazole, other chemically related drugs, such as sulfonamides, or their components; pregnancy at term

## Interactions

DRUGS

*bone marrow depressants, methotrexate:* Increased risk of leukopenia or thrombocytopenia
*cyclosporine:* Increased risk of nephrotoxicity
*diuretics:* Increased incidence of thrombocytopenic purpura
*hemolytics (such as doxapram and methyldopa):* Increased risk of toxic reaction
*hepatotoxic drugs (such as amiodarone):* Increased risk of hepatotoxicity
*hydantoins, oral anticoagulants, oral antidiabetic drugs:* Increased or prolonged effects of these drugs, possibly toxicity
*indomethacin, probenecid, salicylates:* Increased blood sulfisoxazole level
*oral contraceptives:* Increased risk of breakthrough bleeding with long-term sulfisoxazole use
*phenylbutazone, sulfinpyrazone:* Risk of increased blood sulfisoxazole level
*thiopental:* Increased anesthetic effect of thiopental
*tolbutamide:* Prolonged half-life of tolbutamide
*uricosurics:* Potentiated uricosuric action

## Adverse Reactions

**CNS:** Dizziness, fatigue, fever, headache, lethargy, weakness

**EENT:** Pharyngitis
**GI:** Anorexia, diarrhea, dysphagia, nausea, vomiting
**GU:** Crystalluria
**HEME:** Agranulocytosis, aplastic anemia, hemolytic anemia, leukopenia, thrombocytopenia, unusual bleeding or bruising
**MS:** Arthralgia, myalgia
**SKIN:** Blisters, erythema, jaundice, pallor, photosensitivity, pruritus, rash
**Other:** Drug-induced fever

## Nursing Considerations
• Use sulfisoxazole cautiously in patients with blood dyscrasias or megaloblastic anemia from folate deficiency because drug may cause blood dyscrasias; in those with G6PD deficiency because hemolysis may occur; in those with hepatic or renal impairment because of increased risk of toxicity; and in those with porphyria because drug may precipitate an acute attack.
• Obtain blood sample for CBC and tissue or fluid specimen for culture and sensitivity testing, as ordered, before beginning sulfisoxazole therapy. Expect to give first dose before results are available.
• **WARNING** Expect prescriber to discontinue sulfisoxazole if patient exhibits signs of blood dyscrasias, including fever, jaundice, maculopapular or other rash, pallor, pharyngitis, or purpura.
• Monitor CBC frequently, as appropriate, during treatment for signs of adverse reactions.
• Closely monitor patients with AIDS, who are at increased risk for adverse reactions.
• **WARNING** Monitor patient for drug-induced fever, which may develop 7 to 10 days after he starts taking sulfisoxazole. Signs and symptoms include abdominal pain, anorexia, ataxia, depression, diarrhea, headache, insomnia, nausea, peripheral neuropathy, tinnitus, and vomiting.
• Monitor fluid intake and output. Unless contraindicated, provide sufficient fluids to maintain a daily urine output of at least 1,200 ml.
• For otitis media caused by *Haemophilus influenzae*, expect to give drug with erythromycin, as prescribed.
• Frequently monitor blood glucose level and assess for signs of hypoglycemia in patients who take oral antidiabetic drugs.

**PATIENT TEACHING**
• Instruct patient to take sulfisoxazole exactly as prescribed and to complete the full course of therapy even if he feels better.
• Advise patient to take drug with a full glass of water.
• Inform patient that tablet may be chewed or crushed and mixed with liquid to ease swallowing.
• Advise patient to shake oral suspension well before use and to measure oral suspension or syrup dose with calibrated device to ensure accuracy.
• Inform patient that oral suspension or syrup may be stored at room temperature.
• Advise patient to drink 2 to 3 L of fluid daily to maintain hydration, unless contraindicated.
• Advise patient to avoid potentially hazardous activities until drug's CNS effects are known.
• Instruct patient who takes an oral antidiabetic drug to monitor blood glucose level frequently because of the risk of hypoglycemia.
• Advise patient to avoid prolonged exposure to sunlight and to use sunscreen and wear protective clothing when outdoors.

# sulindac

Apo-Sulin (CAN), Clinoril, Novo-Sundac (CAN)

## Class and Category
*Chemical:* Pyrroleacetic acid derivative
*Therapeutic:* Antigout, anti-inflammatory, antirheumatic
*Pregnancy category:* Not rated

## Indications and Dosages
➤ *To decrease pain and inflammation in ankylosing spondylitis, acute attacks of gout or pseudogout, bursitis, moderately painful arthralgia, osteoarthritis, rheumatoid arthritis, and tendinitis*
**TABLETS**
**Adults and adolescents over age 14.** *Initial:* 150 to 200 mg b.i.d., adjusted based on patient's response. *Maximum:* 200 mg b.i.d.
➤ *To relieve symptoms of acute gouty arthritis, acute subacromial bursitis, and supraspinatus tendinitis*
**TABLETS**
**Adults and adolescents over age 14.** 200 mg b.i.d. for 7 to 14 days; decreased to lowest effective dosage after satisfactory response occurs.
**DOSAGE ADJUSTMENT** For elderly patients, dosage reduced to 50% of usual adult dosage, if needed.

**Q**
**R**
**S**

| Route | Onset | Peak | Duration |
|-------|-------|------|----------|
| P.O. | In 1 wk* | 2 to 3 wk* | Unknown |

## Mechanism of Action

May block the activity of cyclooxygenase, an enzyme needed to synthesize prostaglandins, which mediate the inflammatory response and cause local vasodilation, swelling, and pain. By blocking cyclooxygenase and inhibiting prostaglandins, this NSAID reduces inflammatory symptoms and pain.

## Contraindications

Angioedema, asthma, bronchospasm, nasal polyps, rhinitis, or urticaria induced by aspirin, iodides, or other NSAIDs

## Interactions

**DRUGS**

*acetaminophen, cyclosporine, gold compounds, nephrotoxic drugs:* Increased risk of adverse renal effects
*antacids:* Decreased blood level and effects of sulindac
*antihypertensives:* Risk of decreased antihypertensive effect
*aspirin, salicylates:* Decreased sulindac effects, increased risk of GI hemorrhage
*bone marrow depressants:* Increased risk of leukopenia and thrombocytopenia
*cefamandole, cefoperazone, cefotetan, colchicine, oral anticoagulants, plicamycin, thrombolytics, valproic acid:* Increased risk of bleeding
*cimetidine, ranitidine:* Increased bioavailability of both drugs
*digoxin:* Increased blood digoxin level and risk of digitalis toxicity
*dimethyl sulfoxide (DMSO):* Decreased sulindac effectiveness, possibly peripheral neuropathy with topical application of DMSO
*diuretics:* Possibly decreased loop diuretic effects and increased thiazide diuretic effects
*glucocorticoids, other NSAIDs, potassium supplements:* Increased risk of adverse GI effects
*hydantoins:* Increased blood hydantoin level and risk of phenytoin toxicity

---

* For antirheumatic effects; unknown for antigout or anti-inflammatory effects.

*insulin, oral antidiabetic drugs:* Increased risk of hypoglycemia
*lithium:* Possibly increased blood level and toxic effects of lithium
*methotrexate:* Decreased methotrexate excretion, possibly leading to toxicity
*platelet aggregation inhibitors:* Increased risk of bleeding, additive effects of these drugs
*probenecid:* Increased blood level and adverse and toxic effects of sulindac

**ACTIVITIES**

*alcohol use:* Increased risk of adverse GI effects, including GI bleeding

## Adverse Reactions

**CNS:** Aseptic meningitis, cerebral hemorrhage, chills, drowsiness, fever, headache, ischemic CVA, malaise, nervousness, transient ischemic attack
**CV:** Deep vein thrombosis, edema, heart failure, hypertension, MI, palpitations, peripheral edema
**EENT:** Tinnitus
**ENDO:** Hypoglycemia
**GI:** Abdominal cramps or pain, anorexia, constipation, diarrhea, esophageal irritation, flatulence, gastritis, gastrointestinal bleeding or ulceration, hepatic failure, hepatitis, hepatotoxicity, indigestion, jaundice, liver failure, nausea, perforation of stomach or intestines, vomiting
**GU:** Acute renal failure, decreased urine output, interstitial nephritis, nephrotic syndrome, polyuria, proteinuria
**HEME:** Agranulocytosis, aplastic anemia, leukopenia, pancytopenia
**RESP:** Pulmonary edema, wheezing
**SKIN:** Diaphoresis, erythema multiforme, exfoliative dermatitis, maculopapular rash, pruritus, purpura, Stevens-Johnson syndrome, toxic epidermal necrolysis
**Other:** Anaphylaxis, angioedema, facial edema

## Nursing Considerations

• Use sulindac with extreme caution in patients with a history of ulcer disease or GI bleeding because NSAIDs such as sulindac increase the risk of GI bleeding and ulceration. Expect to use sulindac for the shortest time possible in these patients.
• Be aware that serious GI tract ulceration, bleeding, and perforation may occur without warning symptoms. Elderly patients are at greater risk. To minimize risk, give drug

with food. If GI distress occurs, withhold drug and notify prescriber immediately.

•Use sulindac cautiously in patients with hypertension, and monitor blood pressure closely throughout therapy. Drug may cause hypertension or worsen it.

•WARNING Monitor patient closely for thrombotic events, including MI and stroke, because NSAIDs increase the risk.

•WARNING If patient has bone marrow suppression or is receiving antineoplastic drug therapy, monitor laboratory results (including WBC count), and watch for evidence of infection because anti-inflammatory and antipyretic actions of sulindac may mask signs and symptoms, such as fever and pain.

•Especially if patient is elderly or taking sulindac long-term, watch for less common but serious adverse GI reactions, including anorexia, constipation, diverticulitis, dysphagia, esophagitis, gastritis, gastroenteritis, gastroesophageal reflux disease, hemorrhoids, hiatal hernia, melena, stomatitis, and vomiting.

•Monitor liver function test results because, in rare cases, elevated levels may progress to severe hepatic reactions, including fatal hepatitis, liver necrosis, and hepatic failure.

•Monitor BUN and serum creatinine levels in patients with heart failure, impaired renal function, or hepatic dysfunction; those taking diuretics or ACE inhibitors; and elderly patients because drug may cause renal failure.

•Monitor CBC for decreased hemoglobin and hematocrit because drug may worsen anemia.

•Assess patient's skin routinely for rash or other signs of hypersensitivity reaction because sulindac and other NSAIDs may cause serious skin reactions without warning, even in patients with no history of NSAID hypersensitivity. Stop drug at first sign of reaction, and notify prescriber.

•WARNING Monitor patient for adventitious breath sounds and dyspnea; sulindac may cause fluid retention, which may precipitate heart failure in susceptible patients.

•Expect patient to undergo audiometric examinations before and periodically during prolonged therapy, as ordered.

### PATIENT TEACHING

•Instruct patient to take sulindac exactly as prescribed. Explain that higher doses don't increase effectiveness and may increase risk of adverse reactions.

•Advise patient to crush tablet and mix with food, if needed, to aid in swallowing.

•Instruct patient to take drug with or immediately after meals to decrease GI distress, to take with a full glass of water, and to remain upright for 20 to 30 minutes after administration to prevent drug from lodging in esophagus and causing esophageal irritation.

•Urge patient to notify prescriber immediately of chills, fever, rash, or sweating, which may indicate hypersensitivity.

•Advise patient to consult prescriber before using acetaminophen, alcohol, aspirin, other NSAIDs, or any OTC drugs during sulindac therapy.

•Caution patient to avoid potentially hazardous activities until drug's CNS effects are known.

•Inform patient of need for periodic physical examinations and laboratory tests during prolonged therapy to monitor drug effectiveness.

•Explain that sulindac may increase the risk of serious adverse cardiovascular reactions; urge patient to seek immediate medical attention if signs or symptoms arise, such as chest pain, shortness of breath, weakness, and slurring of speech.

•Tell patient that sulindac also may increase the risk of serious adverse GI reactions; stress the importance of seeking immediate medical attention for such signs and symptoms as epigastric or abdominal pain, indigestion, black or tarry stools, or vomiting blood or material that looks like coffee grounds.

•Alert patient to the possibility of rare but serious skin reactions. Urge him to seek immediate medical attention for rash, blisters, itching, fever, or other indications of hypersensitivity.

Q
R
S

# sumatriptan succinate

Imitrex

## Class and Category

*Chemical:* Serotonin 5-HT$_1$-receptor agonist
*Therapeutic:* Antimigraine
*Pregnancy category:* C

## Indications and Dosages

➤ *To relieve acute migraine attacks, with or without aura, or cluster headaches*

TABLETS

**Adults.** 25 to 100 mg as a single dose as soon as possible after onset of symptoms, repeated q 2 hr, as needed and prescribed. *Maximum:* 300 mg/day.

DOSAGE ADJUSTMENT For patients with hepatic dysfunction, 50 mg is maximum single dose.

S.C. INJECTION

**Adults.** *Initial:* 6 mg, repeated after 1 or 2 hr, if needed. *Maximum:* 2 (6-mg) injections/ 24 hr. If migraine symptoms return after initial S.C. injection, 50 mg P.O. q 2 hr up to 200 mg/day.

NASAL SPRAY

**Adults.** 1 or 2 sprays (5 or 10 mg) into one nostril as a single dose or 1 spray (20 mg) into one nostril as a single dose. One additional dose may be taken if another attack occurs after at least 2 hr. *Maximum:* 40 mg q.d.

| Route | Onset | Peak | Duration |
|---|---|---|---|
| P.O. | In 30 min | 2 to 4 hr | Up to 24 hr |
| S.C. | In 10 min | 1 to 2 hr | Up to 24 hr |
| Nasal | In 15 min | Unknown | Up to 24 hr |

### Mechanism of Action

May stimulate $5-HT_1$ receptors, causing selective vasoconstriction of inflamed and dilated cranial blood vessels in carotid circulation, thus decreasing carotid arterial blood flow and relieving acute migraines.

## Contraindications

Basilar or hemiplegic migraine, cardiovascular disease, concurrent use of ergotamine-containing drugs, hypersensitivity to sumatriptan or its components, ischemic heart disease, Prinzmetal's angina, use within 14 days of MAO inhibitor therapy, use within 24 hours of another serotonin $5-HT_1$-receptor agonist

## Interactions

DRUGS

*antidepressants, lithium:* Increased risk of serious adverse effects

*ergotamine-containing drugs:* Possibly additive or prolonged vasoconstrictive effects

*fluoxetine, fluvoxamine, paroxetine, sertraline:* Possibly incoordination, hyperreflexia, and weakness

*MAO inhibitors:* Risk of decreased sumatriptan clearance, increased risk of serious adverse effects

## Adverse Reactions

**CNS:** Dizziness, drowsiness, fatigue, fever, headache, malaise, sedation, seizures, vertigo, weakness
**CV:** Arrhythmias; chest heaviness, pain, pressure, or tightness; coronary artery vasospasm; ECG changes; hypertension; hypotension; palpitations
**EENT:** Abnormal vision; nasal burning (P.O., S.C.); jaw or mouth discomfort; nasal irritation (nasal); nose or throat discomfort; photophobia (P.O., S.C.); taste perversion (nasal); tongue numbness or soreness
**SKIN:** Dermatitis, diaphoresis, erythema, flushing, pallor, photosensitivity (P.O., S.C.), pruritus, rash, urticaria
**Other:** Injection site burning, pain, and redness

## Nursing Considerations

• Be aware that sumatriptan shouldn't be given to elderly patients because they're more likely to have decreased hepatic function, coronary artery disease (CAD), and more pronounced blood pressure increases.
• Assess patient for chest pain, and monitor blood pressure in patients with CAD before and for at least 1 hour after sumatriptan administration.
• Don't give sumatriptan within 24 hours of another $5-HT_1$-receptor agonist, such as naratriptan, rizatriptan, or zolmitriptan.
• After nasal administration, rinse tip of bottle with hot water (don't suction water into bottle) and dry with a clean tissue. Replace cap after cleaning.
• Inspect injection solution for particles and discoloration before administering. Discard solution if you detect these changes.
• Be aware that drug shouldn't be administered I.V. because this may precipitate coronary artery vasospasm.
• Assess patients with risk factors for CAD for arrhythmias, chest pain, and other signs of heart disease.

•For patients with seizure disorder, institute seizure precautions according to facility policy because sumatriptan may lower seizure threshold.

**PATIENT TEACHING**

•Advise patient to use sumatriptan as soon as possible after the onset of migraine symptoms.

•Urge patient to contact prescriber and avoid taking sumatriptan if headache symptoms aren't typical.

•Remind patient not to exceed prescribed daily dosage.

•Advise patient to swallow tablets whole and drink fluids to disguise unpleasant taste.

•Show patient suitable sites for S.C. injection, and teach him how to load, administer, and discard autoinjector.

•Instruct patient to administer no more than two S.C. doses in 24 hours and not to take a second dose if first dose doesn't provide significant relief.

•Inform patient that he may experience burning, pain, and redness for 10 to 30 minutes after S.C. injection. Suggest that he apply ice to relieve pain and redness.

•Teach patient how to use nasal form correctly.

•To avoid cross-contamination, advise patient not to use the same nasal container for more than one person.

•Encourage patient to lie down in a dark, quiet room after taking drug to help relieve migraine.

•Instruct patient to seek emergency care for chest, jaw, or neck tightness after drug use because drug may cause coronary artery vasospasm; subsequent doses may require ECG monitoring.

•Urge patient to report palpitations or rash to prescriber.

•Advise patient to avoid potentially hazardous activities until drug's CNS effects are known.

•Alert patient with seizure disorder that drug may lower seizure threshold.

•Encourage yearly ophthalmologic examinations for patients who require prolonged drug therapy.

# T

# tacrine hydrochloride

## (tetrahydroaminoacridine, THA)

Cognex

## Class and Category

*Chemical:* Monoamine acridine
*Therapeutic:* Dementia treatment
*Pregnancy category:* C

## Indications and Dosages
➤ *To treat mild to moderate Alzheimer's type dementia*

**CAPSULES**
**Adults.** *Initial:* 10 mg q.i.d. for 4 wk, increased to 20 mg q.i.d. and adjusted q 4 wk

as prescribed. *Maximum:* 160 mg/day in 4 divided doses.

## Contraindications
Hypersensitivity to tacrine, other acridine derivatives, or their components; jaundice from previous tacrine use; serum bilirubin level that exceeds 3 mg/dl

## Interactions
**DRUGS**
*anticholinergics:* Decreased effects of both drugs
*cholinergics, other cholinesterase inhibitors:* Increased effects of these drugs and tacrine, possibly leading to toxicity
*cimetidine:* Increased blood tacrine level, possibly leading to toxicity
*neuromuscular blockers:* Prolonged or exaggerated muscle relaxation
*NSAIDs:* Increased gastric acid secretion, possibly GI irritation and bleeding
*theophylline:* Increased blood theophylline level, possibly leading to toxicity

## Mechanism of Action

Tacrine may relieve dementia in Alzheimer's disease, by increasing the acetylcholine level in the CNS. In Alzheimer's disease, some cholinergic neurons lose their ability to function, which decreases the acetylcholine level. The remaining functioning cholinergic neurons release acetylcholine, but it's enzymatically broken down by cholinesterases into acetic acid and choline, as shown below left. Without acetyl-

choline to activate muscarinic (M) and nicotinic (N) receptors on postsynaptic cell membranes, nerve transmission and excitability decrease.

Tacrine binds with and inhibits cholinesterases, making more intact acetylcholine available in cholinergic synapses, as shown below right. This prolongs and enhances acetylcholine's effects, which increases nerve transmission and reduces symptoms of dementia.

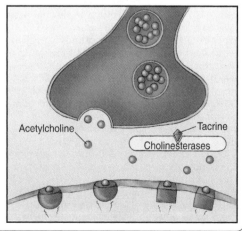

T

**FOODS**

*all foods:* Reduced tacrine bioavailability

**ACTIVITIES**

*smoking:* Possibly decreased tacrine effectiveness

## Adverse Reactions

**CNS:** Agitation, anxiety, asthenia, ataxia, confusion, depression, dizziness, fatigue, hallucinations, headache, hostility, insomnia, seizures, somnolence, syncope, tremor
**CV:** Arrhythmias, chest pain, conduction disturbances, hypertension, hypotension, palpitations, peripheral edema, sick sinus syndrome
**EENT:** Rhinitis
**GI:** Abdominal pain, anorexia, constipation, diarrhea, elevated liver function test results, flatulence, indigestion, nausea, vomiting
**GU:** Bladder obstruction, urinary frequency and incontinence, UTI
**MS:** Back pain, muscle stiffness, myalgia
**RESP:** Asthma, cough, upper respiratory tract infection, wheezing
**SKIN:** Flushing, jaundice, purpura, rash
**Other:** Weight loss

## Nursing Considerations

•Monitor patients with asthma for wheezing and increased mucus production because drug may increase bronchoconstriction and bronchial secretions.
•Expect to monitor hepatic enzyme levels (specifically ALT), as ordered, every other week from at least week 4 to week 16 of tacrine therapy.
•If patient has elevated serum ALT level, monitor for signs and symptoms of hepatitis, such as jaundice and right-upper-quadrant pain. ALT level should return to normal 4 to 6 weeks after therapy stops.
•Once ALT level returns to normal, expect to begin tacrine again (starting at 10 mg q.i.d.) as prescribed, and check hepatic enzyme levels weekly for 16 weeks, monthly for 2 months, and every 3 months thereafter, as ordered.
•Monitor patient for bradyarrhythmias, conduction disturbances, and sick sinus syndrome because tacrine may have a vagotonic effect on the heart rate.
•**WARNING** Be aware that tacrine's cholinergic effects may exacerbate seizures or parkinsonian symptoms.
•Monitor patient's urine output and assess for abdominal distention and abnormal bowel sounds because drug's cholinergic effects may exacerbate conditions involving urinary tract or GI obstruction or ileus.
•Be aware that patients with peptic ulcer disease and those receiving NSAIDs are at increased risk for developing diarrhea, nausea, and vomiting because tacrine increases gastric acid secretion.
•Asess patient for increased symptoms because drug becomes less effective as Alzheimer's disease progresses and the number of intact cholinergic neurons declines.

**PATIENT TEACHING**

•Instruct patient to take tacrine on an empty stomach, and advise caregiver to make sure that drug is swallowed.
•If patient experiences GI distress, suggest taking drug with meals. Mention that drug's effects may be delayed.
•Urge patient to seek assistance when walking and changing position until drug's effects are known. Instruct her to avoid potentially hazardous activities during this period.
•Advise patient not to smoke because it decreases drug's effectiveness.
•Caution patient not to stop taking drug abruptly. Doing so may impair cognitive ability.
•Inform caregiver that drug becomes less effective as Alzheimer's disease progresses.
•Urge caregiver to make sure patient returns regularly for follow-up visits and laboratory tests to monitor drug effectiveness.

# tadalafil

Cialis

## Class and Category

*Chemical:* Phosphodiesterase inhibitor
*Therapeutic:* Anti-impotence
*Pregnancy category:* B

## Indications and Dosages

➤ *To treat erectile dysfunction*

**TABLETS**

**Adults.** *Initial:* 10 mg q.d. taken 1 hr before sexual activity; dosage decreased to 5 mg or increased to 20 mg, as prescribed, based on clinical response. *Maximum:* 20 mg/day.
**DOSAGE ADJUSTMENT** For patients taking potent CYP3A4 inhibitors such as ketoconazole, itraconazole, and ritonavir, dosage should not exceed 10 mg q 72 hr; for patients with moderate to severe renal insufficiency, dosage should not exceed 5 mg q.d.;

for patients with mild to moderate hepatic impairment, dosage should not exceed 10 mg q.d.

| Route | Onset | Peak | Duration |
|-------|-------|------|----------|
| P.O. | Unknown | 30 min to 6 hr | Unknown |

## Mechanism of Action
Enhances the effect of nitric oxide released in the penis during sexual stimulation. Nitric oxide activates the enzyme guanylate cyclase, which causes increased levels of cGMP in the corpus cavernosum. This leads to increased blood flow to the penis, thus producing an erection.

## Contraindications
Continuous or intermittent nitrate therapy, hypersensitivity to tadalafil or its components, retinitis pigmentosa

## Interactions
**DRUGS**
*carbamazepine, phenytoin, phenobarbitol:* Possibly decreased tadalafil effects
*doxazosin, tamsulosin and other alpha blockers:* Increased risk of symptomatic hypotension
*erythromycin, itraconazole, ketoconazole, ritonavir:* Prolonged tadalafil effects
*nitrates:* Profound hypotension
*protease inhibitors (other than ritonavir):* Possibly prolonged tadalafil effects
*rifampin:* Decreased tadalafil effects
**FOODS**
*grapefruit juice:* Possibly prolonged tadalafil effects
**ACTIVITIES**
*alcohol use:* Potentiated blood pressure lowering effects

## Adverse Reactions
**CNS:** Asthenia, dizziness, fatigue, headache, hypesthesia, insomnia, paresthesia, somnolence, stroke, syncope, vertigo
**CV:** Angina pectoris, chest pain, hypotension, hypertension, MI, postural hypotension, palpitations, sudden cardiac death, tachycardia
**EENT:** Blurred vision, changes in color vision, conjunctivitis, dry mouth, epistaxis, eyelid swelling, eye pain, increased lacrimation, nasal congestion, nonarteritic anterior ishcemic optic neuropathy, pharyngitis, retinal artery or vein occlusion, visual field defects
**GI:** Abnormal liver function studies, diarrhea, dysphagia, dyspepsia, esophagitis, gastroesophageal reflux, gastritis, increased gamma-glutamyl transpeptidase levels, nausea, upper abdominal pain, vomiting
**GU:** Priapism, spontaneous penile erection
**MS:** Arthralgia, back or neck pain, extremity pain, myalgia
**RESP:** Dyspnea
**SKIN:** Diaphoresis, exfoliative dermatitis, flushing, pruritus, rash, Stevens-Johnson syndrome
**Other:** Facial edema, hypersensitivity reactions

## Nursing Considerations
•Know that patients with hereditary degenerative retinal disorders, including retinitis pigmentosa, should not receive tadalafil because of the risk of serious ophthalmic adverse reactions.
•Patients with severe hepatic impairment should not receive tadalafil because its effects in these patients are unknown.
•Use tadalafil cautiously in patients with left ventricular outflow obstruction, such as aortic stenosis and idiopathic hypertrophic subaortic stenosis, and those with severely impaired autonomic control of blood pressure because these conditions increase sensitivity to vasodilators such as tadalafil.
•Use tadalafil cautiously in patients with conditions that may predispose them to priapism, such as sickle cell anemia, multiple myeloma, leukemia, or penile deformities (such as angulation, cavernosal fibrosis, or Peyronie's disease).
•Monitor blood pressure and heart rate and rhythm before and during therapy.
**PATIENT TEACHING**
•Explain that tadalafil should be taken 1 hour before sexual activity to provide the most effective results.
•**WARNING** Tell patient not to take tadalafil if he takes any form of organic nitrate, either continuously or intermittently, because profound hypotension and death could result. Tell him to seek immediate medical attention if he has a sudden loss of vision.
•Advise patient to seek sexual counseling to enhance drug's effects.

T

•To avoid possible penile damage and permanent loss of erectile function, urge patient to notify prescriber immediately if erection is painful or lasts longer than 4 hours.
•Advise patient to limit alcohol consumption while taking tadalafil.

# tamoxifen citrate

Apo-Tamox (CAN), Gen-Tamoxifen (CAN), Nolvadex, Novo-Tamoxifen (CAN), Tamofen (CAN), Tamone (CAN)

## Class and Category

*Chemical:* Triphenylethylene derivative
*Therapeutic:* Nonsteroidal antiestrogen agent, partial estrogen agonist
*Pregnancy category:* D

## Indications and Dosages

➤ *To treat metastatic breast cancer in men and women; to treat node-negative breast cancer in women, or node-positive breast cancer in postmenopausal women, after total or segmental mastectomy, axillary dissection, and breast irradiation*

**TABLETS**

**Adults.** 20 to 40 mg q.d. Dosages greater than 20 mg administered b.i.d.

➤ *To reduce the risk of invasive breast cancer in women with ductal carcinoma in situ (DCIS) after surgery and radiation, to reduce the risk of breast cancer in women at high risk*

**TABLETS**

**Adults.** 20 mg q.d. for 5 yr.

---

### Mechanism of Action

Believed to block the effects of estrogen on breast tissue by competing with estrogen for estrogen-receptor binding sites. Estrogen is thought to stimulate the growth of cancer cells.

---

## Contraindications

Hypersensitivity to tamoxifen or its components; women at high risk for breast cancer and women with DCIS who have a history of deep vein thrombosis or pulmonary embolus or who require concomitant coumarin-type anticoagulant therapy

## Interactions

**DRUGS**

*bromocriptine:* Possibly increased blood tamoxifen level
*estrogens:* Possibly altered therapeutic effect of tamoxifen
*warfarin and other coumarin-type anticoagulants:* Increased anticoagulant effect of these drugs

## Adverse Reactions

**CNS:** Confusion, CVA, depression, dizziness, fatigue, headache, light-headedness, somnolence, weakness
**CV:** Edema, hyperlipidemia, thrombosis
**EENT:** Keratopathy, ocular toxicity (including cataracts), optic neuritis, retinopathy
**GI:** Elevated liver function test results, hepatotoxicity, nausea, vomiting
**GU:** Endometrial cancer, endometrial hyperplasia, endometrial polyps, genital itching, menstrual irregularities, ovarian cysts, uterine malignancies, vaginal discharge (females); impotence, decreased libido (males)
**HEME:** Anemia, leukopenia, thrombocytopenia
**MS:** Transient bone or tumor pain
**RESP:** Pulmonary embolism
**SKIN:** Bullous pemphigoid, dry skin, erythema multiforme, rash, Stevens-Johnson syndrome, thinning hair
**Other:** Angioedema, hot flashes, hypercalcemia, weight gain

## Nursing Considerations

•**WARNING** Ensure that patient has been informed of serious or potentially life-threatening adverse effects associated with tamoxifen before therapy begins. Be aware that women with ductal carcinoma in situ or those at high risk for breast cancer are more likely to develop uterine cancer, stroke, or pulmonary emboli than others receiving tamoxifen.
•If patient is premenopausal, begin drug therapy in the middle of menstruation; if patient's menstrual cycles are irregular, verify that she has had a negative pregnancy test before therapy starts.
•Expect patient to undergo an ophthalmic examination before and periodically during tamoxifen therapy. Also expect to monitor patient for adverse ocular reactions, such as cataracts.

•Assess patient for signs and symptoms of thromboembolic events, such as shortness of breath, leg pain, and change in mental status.
•Periodically monitor platelet and WBC count, cholesterol and triglyceride levels, and liver function test results, as ordered.
•Monitor blood calcium level and assess patient for signs and symptoms of hypercalcemia, such as nausea, vomiting, and thirst; tamoxifen may cause hypercalcemia in breast cancer patients with bone metastasis within a few weeks of starting treatment.
•Store tamoxifen in a closed, light-resistant container at room temperature.

**PATIENT TEACHING**
•Advise patient to swallow tamoxifen tablet whole with water.
•Instruct premenopausal patient to use a nonhormonal form of contraception, such as a condom or diaphragm, during tamoxifen therapy. Emphasize that she shouldn't become pregnant while taking drug and for 2 months afterward. Advise her to notify prescriber at once if she becomes pregnant during therapy.
•Inform patient of the most common side effects—hot flashes, vaginal discharge, and irregular menses.
•Urge patient to immediately notify prescriber if she notices a rash, itching, difficulty breathing, or facial swelling, which may signify a hypersensitivity reaction.
•Advise patient to notify prescriber if she experiences leg pain or calf swelling, which may indicate a blood clot.
•Instruct patient to report signs of hepatotoxicity, such as tiredness, nausea, yellow skin, and flulike symptoms.
•Advise patient to have regular gynecologic checkups and to report abnormal symptoms, including abdominal or pelvic pain, new breast lumps, and unusual vaginal discharge or bleeding.
•Urge patients taking tamoxifen for prophylaxis to obtain regular mammograms because drug doesn't prevent all cancers.
•Stress the importance of taking tamoxifen regularly. Urge patient to consult prescriber if adverse reactions, such as nausea and vomiting, are interfering with dosage schedule. These symptoms may be a sign of hypercalcemia.
•Inform women who wish to breast-feed that tamoxifen my appear in breast milk and cause serious adverse effects in the infant.

# tamsulosin hydrochloride

Flomax

## Class and Category
*Chemical:* Sulfamoylphenethylamine derivative
*Therapeutic:* Benign prostatic hyperplasia (BPH) treatment
*Pregnancy category:* B

## Indications and Dosages
➤ *To treat BPH*
**CAPSULES**
**Adults.** *Initial:* 0.4 mg q.d. 30 min p.c. for 2 to 4 wk, increased to 0.8 mg q.d. if no response to initial dosage. *Maximum:* 0.8 mg q.d.

---

### Mechanism of Action
Blocks alpha$_1$-adrenergic receptors in the prostate. This action inhibits smooth-muscle contraction in the prostate, prostatic capsule, prostatic urethra, and bladder neck, which improves the rate of urine flow and reduces the symptoms of BPH.

---

## Contraindications
Hypersensitivity to tamsulosin, quinazolines, or their components

## Interactions
**DRUGS**
*alpha blockers:* Additive effects of both drugs
*cimetidine:* Risk of decreased tamsulosin clearance

## Adverse Reactions
**CNS:** Asthenia, dizziness, drowsiness, headache, insomnia, syncope, vertigo
**CV:** Chest pain, orthostatic hypotension
**EENT:** Amblyopia, diplopia, pharyngitis, rhinitis
**GI:** Diarrhea, nausea
**GU:** Decreased libido, ejaculation disorders
**MS:** Back pain
**SKIN:** Pruritus, rash, urticaria

## Nursing Considerations
•Be aware that prostate cancer should be ruled out before tamsulosin therapy begins.
•Give drug about 30 minutes after the same meal each day.
•If patient takes drug on an empty stomach, monitor his blood pressure because of the increased risk of orthostatic hypotension.

T

•If patient doesn't take drug for several days, resume therapy at 0.4 mg/dose, as prescribed.

**PATIENT TEACHING**
•Instruct patient not to open, crush, or chew tamsulosin capsules and to take drug about 30 minutes after the same meal each day.
•Instruct patient to notify prescriber if he misses several days of therapy; caution him against restarting drug at previous dosage.
•Advise patient to avoid potentially hazardous activities until drug's CNS effects are known. Mention the need for caution if dosage is increased.
•Advise patient to change position slowly, especially after initial dose and each dosage increase, to minimize effects of orthostatic hypotension.

# tegaserod maleate

Zelnorm

## Class and Category

*Chemical:* 3-(5-methoxy-1H-indol-3-ylmethylene)-N-pentylcarbazimidamide hydrogen maleate
*Therapeutic:* Gastrointestinal 5-HT$_4$ receptor partial agonist
*Pregnancy category:* B

## Indications and Dosages

➤ *To treat constipation in women with irritable bowel syndrome short term when it is the primary symptom*

**TABLETS**

**Adult females.** 6 mg b.i.d. before meals for 4 to 6 wk; may continue for another 4 to 6 wk, as needed, if initial response is positive.

➤ *To treat chronic idiopathic constipation in patients younger than age 65*

**TABLETS**

**Adults.** 6 mg b.i.d. before meals.

---

### Mechanism of Action

Activates 5-HT$_4$ receptors in the GI tract to stimulate peristaltic reflex and intestinal secretion and to inhibit visceral sensitivity. These actions enhance basal motor activity and normalize impaired motility throughout the GI tract.

---

## Contraindications

History of abdominal adhesions, bowel obstruction, symptomatic gallbladder disease, or suspected sphincter of Oddi dysfunction; hypersensitivity to tegaserod maleate or its components; moderate or severe hepatic impairment; severe renal impairment

## Interactions

None known

## Adverse Reactions

**CNS:** Dizziness, headache, migraine, syncope
**CV:** Hypotension
**GI:** Abdominal pain, cholecystitis, diarrhea, flatulence, gangrenous bowel, ischemic colitis, nausea, rectal bleeding
**MS:** Arthropathy, back or leg pain
**SKIN:** Pruritus, rash, urticaria
**Other:** Accidental trauma, electrolyte imbalances, hypovolemia, type I allergic reaction

## Nursing Considerations

•Monitor elderly patients closely for diarrhea because they're at increased risk of developing chronic idiopathic constipation, for which diarrhea is the main symptom.
•Be aware that tegaserod shouldn't be given to patients who have diarrhea currently or frequently.
•Give drug at least 1 hour before or 2 to 3 hours after a meal because food reduces the drug's bioavailablity.
•**WARNING** Stop tegaserod immediately if patient develops new or sudden worsening of abdominal pain, rectal bleeding, bloody or severe diarrhea, hypotension, or syncope. Provide appropriate treatment, as ordered.

**PATIENT TEACHING**
•Tell patient to take tegaserod at least 1 hour before meals.
•Advise patient not to take 2 tablets to make up for a missed dose but to skip the missed dose and then resume the regular dosage schedule.
•Instruct patient to notify prescriber if severe diarrhea occurs during therapy or if diarrhea is accompanied by severe cramping, abdominal pain, or dizziness.
•Advise patient to notify prescriber about new or worsening abdominal pain with or without rectal bleeding.
•Inform patient about possible dizziness. Advise against potentially hazardous activities until CNS effects of drug are known.

# telithromycin

Ketek

## Class and Category

*Chemical:* Semisynthetic ketolide
*Therapeutic:* Antibiotic
*Pregnancy category:* C

## Indications and Dosages

➤ *To treat acute bacterial exacerbation of chronic bronchitis caused by* Streptococcus pneumoniae, Haemophilus influenzae, *or* Moraxella catarrhalis; *acute bacterial sinusitis caused by* S. pneumoniae, H. influenzae, M. catarrhalis, *or* Staphylococcus aureus; *or mild-to-moderate community-acquired pneumonia caused by* S. pneumoniae, H. influenzae, M. catarrhalis, Chlamydophila pneumoniae, *or* Mycoplasma pneumoniae

**TABLETS**

**Adults.** 800 mg q.d. P.O. for 5 days (7 to 10 days for community-acquired pneumonia).

| Route | Onset | Peak | Duration |
|-------|-------|------|----------|
| P.O. | Unknown | 1 hr | Unknown |

### Mechanism of Action

Binds to domains II and V of the 50S ribosomal subunit in many aerobic, anaerobic, gram-positive, and gram-negative bacteria of the respiratory tract. Telithromycin may also inhibit the assembly of nascent ribosomal units. These actions inhibit RNA-dependent protein synthesis in bacterial cells, causing them to die.

## Contraindications

Cisapride or pimozide therapy; hypersensitivity to telithromycin, macrolide antibiotics, or their components

## Interactions

**DRUGS**

*atorvastatin, lovastatin, midazolam, pimozide, simvastatin:* Possibly increased blood levels of these drugs
*cisapride, dofetilide, procainamide, quinidine:* Increased risk of prolonged QT interval
*itraconazole, ketoconazole:* Increased blood level of telithromycin
*oral anticoagulants:* Possibly potentiated effects of oral anticoagulants

*rifampin:* Decreased blood level of telithromycin
*sotalol:* Decreased sotalol absorption
*theophylline:* Increased risk of adverse GI reactions

## Adverse Reactions

**CNS:** Dizziness, fatigue, headache, insomnia, somnolence, vertigo
**CV:** Atrial arrhythmias, prolonged QT interval, torsades de pointes
**EENT:** Blurred vision, difficulty focusing eyes, diplopia, dry mouth, glossitis, oral candidiasis, stomatitis
**GI:** Abdominal distention or pain, anorexia, constipation, diarrhea, elevated liver function test results, flatulence, gastroenteritis, gastritis, hepatitis, nausea, pseudomembranous colitis, taste perversion, vomiting
**GU:** Vaginal candidiasis, vaginitis, vaginosis (fungal)
**HEME:** Increased platelet count
**MS:** Exacerbated myasthenia gravis, muscle cramps
**SKIN:** Diaphoresis, rash
**Other:** Angioedema, anaphylaxis

## Nursing Considerations

• Be aware that telithromycin therapy should not be used in patients who have congenital prolonged QT interval or ongoing proarrhythmic conditions (such as uncorrected hypokalemia or hypomagnesemia, or serious bradycardia) or in those receiving concurrent therapy with class IA or class III antiarrhythmics because telithromycin increases the risk of QT prolongation, which may lead to ventricular arrhythmias, including torsades de pointes.
• Use drug cautiously in patients with a history of hepatitis or jaundice from the use of telithromycin.
• Before administering the first telithromycin dose, expect to obtain respiratory specimens for culture and sensitivity testing.
• When no alternative to telithromycin is available for patients with myasthenia gravis, closely monitor patient for worsening, such as respiratory distress, especially during first few hours after first telithromycin dose. If present, notify prescriber immediately and expect to stop telithromycin therapy.
• Monitor patient closely for diarrhea, which may indicate pseudomembranous colitis. If it occurs, notify prescriber and expect to with-

T

hold drug and give fluids, electrolytes, protein, and an antibiotic effective against *Clostridium difficile.*

**PATIENT TEACHING**
•Stress need to take drug for prescribed duration even if patient feels better before prescription is finished.
•Caution patient to avoid hazardous activities until drug's CNS and visual effects are known. Explain that telithromycin can cause trouble focusing eyes, especially for first 30 minutes after a dose.
•Instruct patient to notify prescriber if visual disturbances occur and to avoid quick changes in viewing near and distant objects.
•Tell patient to alert prescriber if she faints because drug may alter heart rhythm.

# telmisartan

Micardis

## Class and Category
*Chemical:* Nonpeptide angiotensin II antagonist
*Therapeutic:* Antihypertensive
*Pregnancy category:* C (first trimester), D (later trimesters)

## Indications and Dosages
➤ *To manage hypertension, alone or with other antihypertensives*

**TABLETS**
**Adults.** *Initial:* 40 mg q.d. *Maintenance:* 20 to 80 mg q.d. *Maximum:* 80 mg/day.

| Route | Onset | Peak | Duration |
|-------|-------|------|----------|
| P.O. | Unknown | In 4 wk | Unknown |

### Mechanism of Action
Blocks angiotensin II from binding to receptor sites in many tissues, including vascular smooth muscle and adrenal glands. This action inhibits the vasoconstrictive and aldosterone-secreting effects of angiotensin II, which reduces blood pressure.

## Contraindications
Hypersensitivity to telmisartan or its components

## Interactions
**DRUGS**
*digoxin:* Increased peak blood digoxin level and risk of digitalis toxicity
*diuretics, other antihypertensives:* Enhanced hypotensive effect

## Adverse Reactions
**CNS:** Asthenia, dizziness, fatigue, headache, syncope, weakness
**CV:** Atrial fibrillation, chest pain, congestive heart failure, hypertension, hypotension, MI, orthostatic hypotension, peripheral edema
**EENT:** Pharyngitis, sinusitis
**GI:** Abdominal pain, diarrhea, indigestion, nausea, vomiting
**GU:** Erectile dysfunction, renal dysfunction, UTI
**MS:** Back pain, leg or muscle cramps, myalgia
**RESP:** ACE cough, upper respiratory tract infection
**SKIN:** Diaphoresis, erythema, urticaria
**Other:** Angioedema, flulike symptoms, hyperkalemia, hypovolemia

## Nursing Considerations
•Administer telmisartan cautiously to patients with dehydration or hyponatremia.
•Expect prescriber to add a diuretic to regimen if patient's blood pressure isn't well controlled by telmisartan.
•Be prepared to treat symptomatic hypotension by placing patient in a supine position and administering NS, as prescribed.
•Monitor BUN and serum creatinine levels and urine output in patients with impaired renal function because they're at increased risk for oliguria, progressive azotemia, and possibly acute renal failure.
•Monitor liver function test results, as appropriate, and assess for signs of drug toxicity in patients with severe hepatic disease because they're at increased risk for toxicity from increased drug accumulation.
•Avoid using telmisartan in pregnant women during second and third trimesters because drug can increase the risk of fetal harm.

**PATIENT TEACHING**
•Advise patient to avoid hazardous activities until telmisartan's CNS effects are known.
•Instruct patient to change position slowly to minimize effects of orthostatic hypotension.
•Urge patient to immediately report diarrhea, dizziness, severe nausea, or vomiting.

•Instruct patient to consult prescriber before taking any new drug.
•Advise patient to drink adequate fluids during hot weather and when exercising.
•Advise female patients of childbearing age to notify presciber immediately about known or suspected pregnancy.

# temazepam

Apo-Temazepam (CAN), Novo-Temazepam (CAN), Restoril

## Class, Category, and Schedule
*Chemical:* Benzodiazepine
*Therapeutic:* Sedative-hypnotic
*Pregnancy category:* X
*Controlled substance:* Schedule IV

## Indications and Dosages
➤ *To provide short-term management of insomnia*
**CAPSULES**
**Adults.** 7.5 to 30 mg 30 min before h.s. *Maximum:* 30 mg/day.
**DOSAGE ADJUSTMENT** For elderly or debilitated patients, 7.5 mg 30 min before bedtime. *Maximum:* 15 mg/day.

> ### Mechanism of Action
> May potentiate the effects of gamma-aminobutyric acid (GABA) and other inhibitory neurotransmitters by binding to specific benzodiazepine receptor sites in the limbic and cortical areas of the CNS. By binding to these receptor sites, temazepam increases GABA's inhibitory effects and blocks cortical and limbic arousal.

## Contraindications
Hypersensitivity to temazepam, other benzodiazepines, or their components; pregnancy

## Interactions
**DRUGS**
*antihistamines (such as brompheniramine, carbinoxamine, chlorpheniramine, clemastine, cyproheptadine, diphenhydramine, trimeprazine), anxiolytics, barbiturates, general anesthetics, opioid analgesics, phenothiazines, promethazine, sedative-hypnotics, tramadol, tricyclic antidepressants:* Increased sedation or respiratory depression

*clozapine:* Risk of respiratory depression or arrest
*digoxin:* Increased risk of elevated blood digoxin level and digitalis toxicity
*flumazenil:* Increased risk of withdrawal symptoms
*levodopa:* Possibly decreased levodopa effects
*oral contraceptives:* Decreased response to temazepam
*phenytoin:* Possibly phenytoin toxicity
*probenecid:* Increased response to temazepam
*zidovudine:* Possibly zidovudine toxicity
**ACTIVITIES**
*alcohol use:* Increased CNS depression and risk of apnea
*smoking:* Increased temazepam clearance

## Adverse Reactions
**CNS:** Aggressiveness, anxiety (in daytime), ataxia, confusion, decreased concentration, depression, dizziness, drowsiness, euphoria, fatigue, headache, insomnia, nightmares, slurred speech, syncope, talkativeness, tremor, vertigo, wakefulness during last third of night
**CV:** Palpitations, tachycardia
**EENT:** Abnormal or blurred vision, increased salivation
**GI:** Abdominal pain, constipation, diarrhea, hepatic dysfunction, nausea, thirst, vomiting
**GU:** Decreased libido
**HEME:** Agranulocytosis, anemia, leukopenia, neutropenia, thrombocytopenia
**MS:** Muscle spasm or weakness
**RESP:** Increased bronchial secretions
**SKIN:** Diaphoresis, flushing, jaundice, pruritus, rash
**Other:** Physical and psychological dependence

## Nursing Considerations
•Use temazepam cautiously in patients with a history of depression or suicidal thoughts.
•**WARNING** Monitor for signs of physical and psychological dependence during therapy.
•Implement safety precautions, according to facility policy, especially in elderly patients, because they're more sensitive to drug's CNS effects.
•Assess patients with respiratory depression, severe COPD, or sleep apnea for signs of ventilatory failure.
•Be aware that temazepam can aggravate acute intermittent porphyria, myasthenia gravis, and severe renal impairment.

T

•Be aware that temazepam may cause worsening psychosis or deterioration of cognition or coordination in patients with late-stage Parkinson's disease.

•Be aware that drug shouldn't be discontinued abruptly, even after only 1 to 2 weeks of therapy, because doing so may cause seizures or withdrawal symptoms, such as insomnia, irritability, and nervousness.

**PATIENT TEACHING**

•Instruct patient to take temazepam exactly as prescribed and not to stop taking it or change dosage without consulting prescriber.

•Explain the risks associated with abrupt cessation, including abdominal cramps, acute sense of hearing, confusion, depression, nausea, numbness, perceptual disturbances, photophobia, sweating, tachycardia, tingling, trembling, and vomiting.

•Advise patient to avoid alcohol because it increases drug's sedative effects.

•Caution patient about possible drowsiness. Advise her to avoid potentially hazardous activities until drug's CNS effects are known.

•Urge patient to notify prescriber immediately about excessive drowsiness, nausea, and known or suspected pregnancy.

# tenecteplase

TNKase

## Class and Category

*Chemical:* Purified glycoprotein
*Therapeutic:* Thrombolytic
*Pregnancy category:* C

## Indications and Dosages

➤ *To reduce mortality associated with acute MI*

**I.V. INJECTION**

**Adults.** Single bolus administered over 5 sec in individualized dosage based on patient's weight, as follows: 30 mg (6 ml) for patients who weigh less than 60 kg; 35 mg (7 ml) for patients who weigh 60 to 69 kg; 40 mg (8 ml) for patients who weigh 70 to 79 kg; 45 mg (9 ml) for patients who weigh 80 to 89 kg; 50 mg (10 ml) for patients who weigh 90 kg or more. Maximum: 50 mg total dose.

## Mechanism of Action

Binds to fibrin and converts plasminogen to plasmin. Plasmin breaks down fibrin, fibrinogen, and other clotting factors, resulting in dissolution of a coronary artery thrombus.

## Incompatibilities

Don't administer tenecteplase through an I.V. line containing dextrose because precipitation may occur.

## Contraindications

Active internal bleeding, aneurysm, arteriovenous malformation, bleeding disorders, brain tumor, history of cerebrovascular accident, hypersensitivity to tenecteplase or its components, intracranial or intraspinal surgery or trauma within past 2 months, severe uncontrolled hypertension

## Interactions

**DRUGS**

*abciximab, aspirin, clopidogrel, dipyridamole, heparin, oral anticoagulants, ticlopidine:* Possibly increased risk of bleeding

## Adverse Reactions

**CNS:** Intracranial hemorrhage
**EENT:** Epistaxis, gingival bleeding, pharyngeal bleeding
**GI:** GI and retroperitoneal bleeding
**GU:** Genitourinary bleeding, prolonged or heavy menstrual bleeding
**HEME:** Hematoma
**RESP:** Hemoptysis
**SKIN:** Bleeding at puncture sites, surgical incision sites, or venous cutdown sites

## Nursing Considerations

•**WARNING** Reconstitute tenecteplase for injection immediately before use because drug contains no antibacterial preservatives. If reconstituted drug isn't used immediately, refrigerate vial at 36° to 46° F (2° to 8° C). Discard solution if not used within 8 hours.

•To reconstitute and administer drug, use supplied 10-ml syringe with dual cannula device. Withdraw 10 ml of supplied (preservative-free) sterile water for injection into syringe, and inject entire contents into vial containing tenecteplase dry powder, directing stream of diluent into powder. Gently swirl—don't shake—vial until contents are completely dissolved. If slight foaming occurs during reconstitution, allow drug to stand undisturbed for a few minutes to allow large bubbles to dissipate. Then withdraw prescribed dose of tenecteplase from reconstituted drug in vial, using supplied syringe. Make sure that reconstituted preparation is a colorless to pale yellow transparent solution. Discard any unused solution.

• Administer drug as a single I.V. bolus over 5 seconds. Although supplied syringe is intended for use with needleless I.V. systems, be aware that it is also compatible with a conventional needle. Follow manufacturer's directions for use with each system. Flush any dextrose-containing I.V. lines with saline solution before and after administering tenecteplase.

• **WARNING** Monitor for signs and symptoms of GI bleeding, including bloody or black, tarry stools; bloody or coffee-ground vomitus; and severe stomach pain. Notify prescriber immediately if any of these signs or symptoms develops.

• Assess tenecteplase injection site for signs and symptoms of hematoma, including deep, dark purple bruises under skin and itching, pain, redness, or swelling. Also monitor for superficial bleeding, delayed bleeding at puncture sites, and bleeding from surgical incisions.

• Assess for signs and symptoms of intracranial bleeding (such as decreased level of consciousness), retroperitoneal bleeding (such as abdominal pain or swelling and back pain), genitourinary bleeding (such as hematuria), or respiratory tract bleeding (such as hemoptysis). Notify prescriber immediately if patient develops any of these signs or symptoms.

• If serious bleeding (not controllable by local pressure) occurs, expect to discontinue concomitant heparin or oral antiplatelet therapy immediately.

• If possible, avoid I.M. injections and nonessential handling of patient for first few hours after drug administration.

• If arterial puncture becomes necessary during first few hours after tenecteplase administration, expect to use an upper extremity that's accessible to manual compression. Apply pressure for at least 30 minutes after procedure, use a pressure dressing, and frequently monitor puncture site for signs of bleeding.

**PATIENT TEACHING**
• Advise patient to immediately report any bleeding, including from nose or gums.
• Instruct patient to limit physical activity during tenecteplase administration to reduce the risk of injury or bleeding.

# terazosin hydrochloride

Hytrin

## Class and Category

*Chemical:* Quinazoline derivative
*Therapeutic:* Antihypertensive, benign prostatic hyperplasia (BPH) treatment
*Pregnancy category:* C

## Indications and Dosages

➤ *To manage hypertension*
**CAPSULES**
**Adults.** *Initial:* 1 mg h.s. *Maintenance:* 1 to 5 mg/day as a single dose or in divided doses q 12 hr. *Maximum:* 20 mg/day.

➤ *To treat symptomatic BPH*
**CAPSULES**
**Adults.** *Initial:* 1 mg h.s., increased in increments to 2 mg, 5 mg, and then 10 mg, as prescribed, based on symptom improvement and urine flow rate. *Maintenance:* 5 to 10 mg/day as a single dose or in divided doses q 12 hr. *Maximum:* 20 mg/day.

| Route | Onset | Peak | Duration |
|-------|-------|------|----------|
| P.O. | 15 min | 2 to 3 hr | 24 hr |

## Mechanism of Action

Blocks postsynaptic alpha$_1$-adrenergic receptors in many tissues, including vascular smooth muscle, the bladder neck, and the prostate. This action promotes vasodilation, which reduces blood pressure and improves urine flow.

## Contraindications

Hypersensitivity to terazosin, other quinazolines, or their components

## Interactions

**DRUGS**
*clonidine:* Possibly decreased clonidine effects
*diuretics, other antihypertensives:* Additive hypotensive effect

T

*dopamine:* Risk of decreased terazosin effects and antagonized vasoconstrictive effect of dopamine (in high doses)

*epinephrine:* Risk of decreased terazosin effects, possibly severe hypotension and tachycardia

*indomethacin, other NSAIDS:* Altered terazosin effects related to sodium and fluid retention

*methoxamine, phenylephrine:* Decreased vasopressor effects, and shortened duration of action of these drugs

*sympathomimetics:* Decreased terazosin effects

## Adverse Reactions

**CNS:** Asthenia, dizziness, headache, lethargy, nervousness, paresthesia, somnolence, syncope, vertigo

**CV:** Chest pain, hypotension, orthostatic hypotension, palpitations, peripheral edema, sinus tachycardia

**EENT:** Blurred vision, dry mouth, nasal congestion, sinusitis

**GI:** Constipation, diarrhea, nausea, vomiting

**MS:** Arthralgia, back pain

**Other:** Flulike symptoms, weight gain

## Nursing Considerations

•Be aware that prostate cancer should be ruled out before terazosin is used to treat BPH.

•Expect prescriber to reduce terazosin dosage if a diuretic or another antihypertensive is added to patient's regimen.

•Monitor blood pressure 2 to 3 hours after initial dose because of possible first-dose hypotension and again after 24 hours to evaluate patient's response.

•If patient requires administration by feeding tube, place capsule in 60 ml of warm tap water. Stir until capsule shell dissolves and liquid contents are released into water (5 to 10 minutes).

•Be aware that elderly patients may have exaggerated hypotension and other adverse reactions.

**PATIENT TEACHING**

•Instruct patient to take terazosin at the same time each night.

•Explain possible first-dose hypotension. Advise patient to change position and rise slowly to prevent syncope early in therapy. Suggest sitting or lying down if dizziness or light-headedness occurs.

•Advise patient to avoid potentially hazardous activities until drug's CNS effects are known.

•Instruct patient to notify prescriber if she misses several doses in a row; caution her against resuming therapy at previous dose.

•Inform patient that drug may take 2 to 6 weeks to improve urinary hesitancy.

•Advise patient to avoid alcohol use, prolonged standing, and excessive exercise or exposure to hot weather because these activities can worsen orthostatic hypotension.

•Stress the importance of regular follow-up visits with prescriber to evaluate patient's response to drug.

# terbinafine hydrochloride

Lamisil

## Class and Category

*Chemical:* Allylamine derivative
*Therapeutic:* Antifungal
*Pregnancy category:* B

## Indications and Dosages

➤ *To treat onychomycosis of fingernails and toenails*

**TABLETS**

**Adults and adolescents.** 125 mg b.i.d. or 250 mg q.d. for 6 to 12 wk.

**DOSAGE ADJUSTMENT** For patients with stable chronic hepatic dysfunction or renal dysfunction (creatinine clearance less than 50 ml/min/1.73 m² or serum creatinine greater than 3.4 mg/dl), dosage reduced by 50%.

---

### Mechanism of Action

Inhibits the conversion of squalene monooxygenase to squalene epoxidase, a key enzyme in fungal biosynthesis. The resulting squalene accumulation weakens cell membranes and creates a deficiency of ergosterol, the fungal membrane component necessary for normal fungal growth.

## Contraindications
Hypersensitivity to terbinafine or its components

## Interactions
**DRUGS**
*beta blockers, MAO inhibitors (type B), selective serotonin reuptake inhibitors, tricyclic antidepressants:* Possibly increased blood levels of these drugs
*cimetidine, other hepatic enzyme inhibitors:* Significantly decreased terbinafine clearance, possibly increased adverse reactions
*hepatotoxic drugs:* Increased risk of hepatotoxicity
*rifampin:* Increased clearance and decreased effectiveness of terbinafine
**FOODS**
*caffeine:* Decreased caffeine clearance
**ACTIVITIES**
*alcohol use:* Increased risk of severe hepatitis

## Adverse Reactions
**CNS:** Headache
**EENT:** Taste perversion
**GI:** Abdominal pain, anorexia, diarrhea, elevated liver function test results, flatulence, hepatic failure, indigestion, nausea, vomiting
**SKIN:** Cutaneous lupus erythematosus, pruritus, rash, urticaria
**OTHER:** Angioedema, systemic lupus erythematosus

## Nursing Considerations
•Because terbinafine has been linked to serious adverse hepatic effects, expect to send nail specimens for laboratory testing to confirm onychomycosis before beginning therapy.
•Be aware that drug shouldn't be given to patients with chronic or active hepatic disease or renal impairment.
•Monitor patient for hepatic failure (anorexia, dark urine, fatigue, jaundice, nausea, pale stools, right upper abdominal pain, and vomiting). Expect to stop drug and obtain liver function tests if these problems develop.
**PATIENT TEACHING**
•Instruct patient to space doses evenly if taking terbinafine more than once a day.
•Stress the need to complete the full course of therapy to prevent relapse of infection.
•Discourage use of alcohol during therapy.
•Tell patient to contact prescriber if onychomycosis doesn't improve in a few weeks.

# terbutaline sulfate
Brethaire, Brethine, Bricanyl, Bricanyl Turbuhaler (CAN)

## Class and Category
*Chemical:* Sympathomimetic amine
*Therapeutic:* Bronchodilator
*Pregnancy category:* B

## Indications and Dosages
➤ *To prevent or reverse bronchospasm from asthma, bronchitis, or emphysema*
**TABLETS (BRETHINE, BRICANYL)**
**Adults and adolescents age 15 and older.** 2.5 to 5 mg t.i.d. at 6-hr intervals while awake. *Maximum:* 15 mg/day.
**Children ages 12 to 15.** 2.5 mg t.i.d. at 6-hr intervals while awake. *Maximum:* 7.5 mg/day.
**Children ages 6 to 11.** 50 to 75 mcg/kg t.i.d. at 6-hr intervals while awake. *Maximum:* 150 mcg/kg/dose or 5 mg/day.
**S.C. INJECTION (BRICANYL)**
**Adults and children age 12 and older.** *Initial:* 0.25 mg, repeated in 15 to 30 min as prescribed. *Maximum:* 0.5 mg/4-hr period.
**Children ages 6 to 12.** 5 to 10 mcg (0.005 to 0.01 mg)/kg q 15 to 20 min, up to 3 doses. *Maximum:* 400 mcg (0.4 mg)/dose.
**INHALATION AEROSOL (BRETHAIRE)**
**Adults and children.** 2 inhalations (400 mcg) q 4 to 6 hr, as needed and as prescribed.
**INHALATION AEROSOL (BRICANYL TURBUHALER)**
**Adults and children.** 1 inhalation (500 mcg), repeated after 5 min, as needed and as prescribed. *Maximum:* 6 inhalations/day.

| Route | Onset | Peak | Duration |
|---|---|---|---|
| P.O. | 30 to 90 min | 2 to 3 hr | 4 to 8 hr |
| S.C. | 15 to 30 min | 30 to 60 min | 1.5 to 4 hr |
| Inhalation | In 5 min | 30 to 90 min | 3 to 6 hr |

## Mechanism of Action
Stimulates beta$_2$-adrenergic receptors in the lungs, which is believed to increase production of cAMP. The increased cAMP level relaxes bronchial smooth muscles, thereby increasing bronchial airflow and relieving bronchospasm.

T

## Contraindications
Hypersensitivity to terbutaline sulfate, other sympathomimetic amines, or their components

## Interactions
**DRUGS**
*antihypertensives, diuretics:* Decreased antihypertensive effect
*beta blockers:* Mutual inhibition of therapeutic effects, increased risk of bronchospasm
*CNS stimulants:* Additive CNS stimulation, possibly resulting in adverse effects
*digoxin:* Increased risk of arrhythmias, possibly digitalis toxicity
*halogenated anesthetics:* Possibly ventricular arrhythmias
*MAO inhibitors:* Possibly potentiated action of terbutaline; headache, hyperpyrexia, hypertension, possibly leading to hypertensive crisis
*maprotiline, tricyclic antidepressants:* Possibly potentiated action of terbutaline
*nitrates:* Decreased effectiveness of nitrates
*ritodrine:* Increased effects of either drug and potential for adverse effects
*sympathomimetics:* Increased CNS stimulation and risk of adverse cardiovascular effects, including prolonged QT interval
*thyroid hormones:* Increased effects of either drug, risk of coronary insufficiency in patients with coronary artery disease
*xanthines (theophylline):* Increased CNS stimulation and other additive toxic effects
**FOODS**
*caffeine:* Increased CNS stimulation and other additive toxic effects

## Adverse Reactions
**CNS:** Anxiety, dizziness, drowsiness, headache, insomnia, light-headedness, nervousness, restlessness, tremor, weakness
**CV:** Chest pain, irregular heartbeat, palpitations, tachycardia
**EENT:** Dry mouth, taste perversion
**ENDO:** Hyperglycemia
**GI:** Heartburn, nausea, vomiting
**MS:** Muscle spasms
**RESP:** Dyspnea
**SKIN:** Diaphoresis, flushing, rash

## Nursing Considerations
• Use terbutaline cautiously in patients with cardiovascular disease because drug can adversely affect cardiovascular function. Monitor patient's heart rate and rhythm and blood pressure and assess for chest pain.
• For S.C. injection, inject into lateral deltoid area.
• Reevaluate patient's respiratory rate, depth, and quality; oxygen saturation; and activity tolerance at regular intervals because continuous use of beta$_2$-agonists for 12 months or longer accelerates the decline in pulmonary function.
**PATIENT TEACHING**
• Teach patient how to use terbutaline aerosol inhaler or administer S.C. injection, as appropriate.
• Instruct patient not to increase dose or frequency without consulting prescriber.
• Urge patient to seek immediate medical attention if symptoms worsen.
• Inform patient that she may experience transient nervousness or tremors during terbutaline therapy.

# teriparatide

Forteo

## Class and Category
*Chemical:* Recombinant human parathyroid hormone (PTH)
*Therapeutic:* Bone growth and density regulator
*Pregnancy category:* C

## Indications and Dosages
➤ *To treat osteoporosis in postmenopausal women and primary or hypogonadal osteoporosis in men at high risk for fracture*
**S.C. INJECTION**
Adults. 20 mcg q.d. for up to 2 yr.

| Route | Onset | Peak | Duration |
|-------|-------|------|----------|
| S.C. | 2 hr | 4 to 6 hr | 16 to 24 hr |

## Contraindications
Hypersensitivity to teriparatide or its components

## Interactions
**DRUGS**
*digitalis glycosides:* Possibly increased risk of digitalis toxicity

## Mechanism of Action

Teriparatide, which contains recombinant PTH, stimulates new bone growth and increases bone density. In a patient with osteoporosis, bone density and mass are diminished by an imbalance between bone destruction and formation. Normally, osteoclasts break down and resorb bone, leaving behind a cavity in a section of bone. Then bone-building cells, called osteoblasts, line the walls of the cavity and stimulate new bone formation. PTH stimulates these actions by attaching to receptors on osteoclasts and osteoblasts, as shown below.

Teriparatide binds to cell-surface receptors on osteoblasts and preferentially stimulates osteoblastic over osteoclastic activity. Also, the drug increases the amount of circulating calcium available for bone formation by increasing the intestinal absorption of calcium and phosphate, thus enhancing the rate of calcium resorption from bone, increasing the reabsorption of calcium, and inhibiting the reabsorption of phosphate in the kidneys. These actions stimulate new bone formation and increase bone density to reduce osteoporotic bone changes.

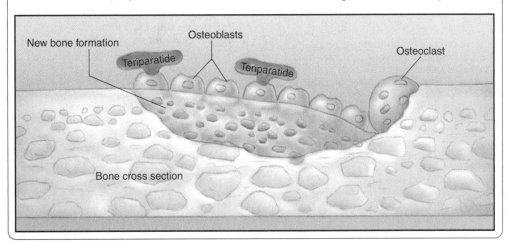

## Adverse Reactions

**CNS:** Asthenia, depression, dizziness, headache, insomnia, paresthesia, syncope, vertigo
**CV:** Angina pectoris, chest pain, hypertension, transient orthostatic hypotension
**EENT:** Pharyngitis, rhinitis, taste perversion, tooth disorder
**ENDO:** Transient hypoparathyroidism
**GI:** Constipation, diarrhea, indigestion, vomiting
**MS:** Arthralgia, leg cramps, neck pain
**RESP:** Cough, dyspnea, pneumonia
**SKIN:** Diaphoresis, pruritus, rash, urticaria
**Other:** Angioedema, generalized pain, injection site reactions (erythema, localized bruising, minor bleeding, pain, pruritus, swelling), transient hypercalcemia or hypocalcemia

## Nursing Considerations

•**WARNING** Be aware that teriparatide shouldn't be used to treat patients at risk for osteosarcoma (such as those with Paget's disease or a metabolic bone disease other than osteoporosis), unexplained elevations of alkaline phosphatase, open epiphyses, or prior skeletal radiation or malignancy.
•**WARNING** Be aware that patients with hypercalcemia shouldn't receive teriparatide because drug may worsen hypercalcemia.
•Use drug cautiously in patients with active or recent urolithiasis because drug could worsen this condition.
•Monitor patient closely for allergic reactions because teriparatide is a peptide agent.
•Monitor patient's blood calcium level, and notify prescriber of any elevation; in persistent

T

hypercalcemia, the drug may need to be stopped.

• Monitor patient's blood pressure during the first several doses of drug therapy because of a risk of transient orthostatic hypotension. If this occurs, place patient in a reclining position and alert prescriber.

**PATIENT TEACHING**

• Teach patient how to administer teriparatide by S.C. injection and how to properly use the delivery pen device and dispose of needles. Advise her not to share pen device with others.

• Inform patient that each delivery pen can be used for up to 28 days after the first injection but then should be discarded even if it still contains solution.

• Instruct patient to store the delivery pen in the refrigerator and to recap it when not in use to protect it from damage and light.

• Tell patient that delivery pen may be used immediately after removal from refrigerator and should be put back in refrigerator as soon as the injection is given.

• Instruct patient to inject drug into thigh or abdominal wall and to rotate injection sites.

• Caution patient to administer drug in a room where she can immediately sit or lie down if light-headedness or palpitations occur. Advise her to notify prescriber if these symptoms persist or worsen.

• Instruct patient to notify prescriber of persistent symptoms of hypercalcemia, such as nausea, vomiting, constipation, lethargy, and muscle weakness.

• Caution patient about potential developing osteosarcoma.

# tetracycline hydrochloride

Achromycin, Achromycin V, Apo-Tetra (CAN), Novo-Tetra (CAN), Nu-Tetra (CAN), Panmycin, Robitet, Sumycin, Tetracap, Tetracyn, Tetracyn 500

## Class and Category

*Chemical:* Chlortetracycline derivative
*Therapeutic:* Antibiotic
*Pregnancy category:* D

## Indications and Dosages

➤ *To treat actinomycosis caused by susceptible organisms*

**CAPSULES, ORAL SUSPENSION, TABLETS**

**Adults and adolescents.** 250 to 500 mg q 6 hr or 500 to 1,000 mg q 12 hr. *Maximum:* 4 g/day.

**Children age 8 and older.** 6.25 to 12.5 mg/kg q 6 hr or 12.5 to 25 mg/kg q 12 hr.

➤ *To treat acne vulgaris*

**CAPSULES, ORAL SUSPENSION, TABLETS**

**Adults and adolescents.** *Initial:* 500 to 2,000 mg/day in divided doses until improvement occurs (usually in 3 wk); then dosage reduced gradually. *Maintenance:* 125 to 1,000 mg/day. *Maximum:* 4 g/day.

➤ *To treat brucellosis caused by susceptible organisms*

**CAPSULES, ORAL SUSPENSION, TABLETS**

**Adults and adolescents.** 500 mg q 6 hr for 3 wk, given concurrently with 1 g of streptomycin I.M. q 12 hr in week 1 and q.d. in week 2. *Maximum:* 4 g/day.

**Children ages 8 to 12.** 6.25 to 12.5 mg/kg q 6 hr, or 12.5 to 25 mg/kg q 12 hr.

➤ *To treat gonorrhea caused by* Neisseria gonorrhoeae

**CAPSULES, ORAL SUSPENSION, TABLETS**

**Adults and adolescents.** 1,500 mg, then 500 mg q 6 hr for 5 days. *Maximum:* 4 g/day.

➤ *To treat syphilis caused by* Treponema pallidum

**CAPSULES, ORAL SUSPENSION, TABLETS**

**Adults and adolescents.** 500 mg q 6 hr for 15 days (for early syphilis) or 30 days (for late syphilis). *Maximum:* 4 g/day.

**Children ages 9 to 12.** 6.25 to 12.5 mg/kg q 6 hr, or 12.5 to 25 mg/kg q 12 hr.

➤ *To treat uncomplicated endocervical, rectal, or urethral infections caused by* Chlamydia trachomatis

**CAPSULES, ORAL SUSPENSION, TABLETS**

**Adults and adolescents.** 500 mg q.i.d. for at least 7 days. *Maximum:* 4 g/day.

**DOSAGE ADJUSTMENT** For patients with renal impairment, dosage possibly reduced because of extended half-life.

## Contraindications

Hypersensitivity to tetracycline or its components

---

### Mechanism of Action

Exerts a bacteriostatic effect against a wide variety of gram-positive and gram-negative organisms by passing through the bacterial lipid bilayer, where it binds reversibly to 30S ribosomal subunits. Bound tetracycline blocks the binding of aminoacyl transfer RNA to messenger RNA, thus inhibiting bacterial protein synthesis.

## Interactions

**DRUGS**

*aluminum-, calcium-, or magnesium-containing antacids; iron supplements (oral); magnesium-containing laxatives; magnesium salicylate; multivitamins (containing manganese or zinc salts); sodium bicarbonate:* Possibly impaired absorption of oral tetracycline and formation of nonabsorbable complexes
*cholestyramine, colestipol:* Possibly impaired absorption of oral tetracycline
*digoxin:* Possibly increased blood digoxin level
*methoxyflurane:* Possibly nephrotoxicity
*oral contraceptives (containing estrogen):* Possibly reduced contraceptive reliability and increased risk of breakthrough bleeding (with long-term tetracycline use)
*penicillins:* Possibly decreased bactericidal effect of penicillins
*vitamin A:* Possibly benign intracranial hypertension

**FOODS**

*dairy products and other foods:* Possibly impaired absorption of oral tetracycline

## Adverse Reactions

**CNS:** Dizziness, light-headedness, unsteadiness
**EENT:** Darkened or discolored tongue, enamel hypoplasia, oral candidiasis, tooth discoloration (in children)
**GI:** Abdominal pain, diarrhea, hepatotoxicity, nausea, rectal candidiasis, vomiting
**GU:** Vaginal candidiasis
**SKIN:** Photosensitivity

## Nursing Considerations

•Avoid giving tetracycline to children under age 8 because drug may cause permanent brown or yellow tooth discoloration and enamel hypoplasia.
•Be aware that tooth discoloration and enamel hypoplasia may occur in breast-feeding infants, along with inhibition of linear skeletal growth, oral and vaginal candidiasis, and photosensitivity.
•To reduce the risk of esophageal irritation or ulceration, avoid bedtime dosing of tetracycline for patient with esophageal obstruction or compression.
•Assess for photosensitivity, which can develop within a few minutes or up to several hours after exposure to sunlight or other ultraviolet (UV) light. Effects may last for 1 to 2 days after discontinuation of drug.

•Be aware that citric acid in tetracycline preparations may accelerate drug deterioration and that using outdated drug may cause Fanconi's syndrome, characterized by multiple defects in renal tubular function. Symptoms include acidosis, bicarbonate wasting, glycosuria, hypokalemia, osteomalacia, and phosphaturia.

**PATIENT TEACHING**

•Instruct patient to take oral tetracycline at least 1 hour before meals or 2 hours after meals because dairy products and some foods may interfere with absorption.
•Advise patient to take each dose with a full glass of water while in an upright position to avoid esophageal or GI irritation.
•Instruct patient taking oral suspension to shake container well before measuring dose and to use a calibrated measuring device.
•Advise patient to avoid taking other drugs, including OTC antacids and other preparations, within 3 hours of oral tetracycline.
•Urge patient to complete the entire course of tetracycline therapy even if she feels better.
•Caution her to avoid direct sunlight or UV light and to wear sunscreen when outdoors.
•Advise women who use oral contraceptives containing estrogen to use another method of contraception while taking tetracycline because contraceptives may be less effective.
•Stress the need to discard outdated tetracycline because of the risk of toxic effects.
•Encourage patient to take safety precautions if she experiences dizziness or other adverse CNS reactions.

# thalidomide

Thalomid

## Class and Category

*Chemical:* Glutamic-acid derivative
*Therapeutic:* Anti-inflammatory, immunomodulator
*Pregnancy category:* X

## Indications and Dosages

➤ *To treat acute cutaneous erythema nodosum leprosum*

**CAPSULES**

**Adults and adolescents.** 100 to 400 mg q.d. h.s. or at least 1 hr after the evening meal. *Usual:* 200 mg.

DOSAGE ADJUSTMENT For those weighing less than 50 kg (110 lb), dosage started at 100 mg.

T

▶ *To prevent or suppress recurrence of cutaneous erythema nodosum leprosum*

**CAPSULES**

**Adults and adolescents.** Minimum dosage necessary to control reaction; dosage tapered q 3 to 6 mo in increments of 50 mg q 2 to 4 wk, as prescribed.

**Mechanism of Action**

Suppresses the production of tumor necrosis factor-alpha, which reduces neutrophils and CD4 T cells in erythema nodosum leprosum lesions, thus preventing or controlling symptoms.

## Contraindications

Hypersensitivity to thalidomide or its components, pregnancy, women of childbearing age who aren't using two reliable contraceptive methods or aren't abstaining from heterosexual intercourse

## Interactions

**DRUGS**

*antihistamines, anxiolytics, barbiturates, chlorpromazine, CNS depressants, hypnotics, opioid analgesics, reserpine, sedatives:* Increased CNS depression

*chloramphenicol, cisplatin, dapsone, didanosine, ethambutol, ethionamide, hydralazine, isoniazid, lithium, metronidazole, nitrofurantoin, nitrous oxide, other drugs associated with peripheral neuropathy, phenytoin, stavudine, vincristine, zalcitabine:* Increased risk of peripheral neuropathy

**ACTIVITIES**

*alcohol use:* Increased CNS depression

## Adverse Reactions

**CNS:** Agitation, asthenia, chills, depression, dizziness, drowsiness, fever, headache, insomnia, lethargy, loss of consciousness, malaise, mood changes, nervousness, paresthesia, peripheral neuropathy, seizures, somnolence, status epilepticus, stupor, syncope, tremor, vertigo

**CV:** Arrhythmias, bradycardia, hyperlipidemia, orthostatic hypotension, peripheral edema, tachycardia

**EENT:** Dry mouth, oral candidiasis, pharyngitis, rhinitis, sinusitis, tooth pain

**ENDO:** Hypothyroidism

**GI:** Abdominal pain, anorexia, constipation, diarrhea, elevated liver function test results, flatulence, hepatic dysfunction, increased appetite, intestinal perforation, nausea

**GU:** Albuminuria, hematuria, impotence

**HEME:** Anemia, leukopenia, neutropenia, prolonged PT

**MS:** Back pain, neck pain or rigidity

**RESP:** Pleural effusion

**SKIN:** Acne, dermatitis, diaphoresis, erythema multiforme, photosensitivity, pruritus, rash

**Other:** Facial edema, hypercalcemia, hyperkalemia, hypocalcemia, hypokalemia, hyponatremia, increased alkaline phosphatase level, lymphadenopathy, pain (generalized), tumor lysis syndrome

## Nursing Considerations

•Be aware that all patients receiving thalidomide must complete an informed consent form and participate in a confidential monitoring registry. Thalidomide may be obtained only through physicians and pharmacies registered in the System for Thalidomide Education and Prescribing Safety (STEPS) Program, a comprehensive safety program designed to prevent fetal exposure to thalidomide. Thalidomide may be dispensed only in original packaging and in no more than a 28-day supply. Prescriptions older than 7 days may not be filled.

•Be aware that female patients of childbearing age must use two contraceptive methods during therapy. Pregnancy testing must be performed 24 hours before starting thalidomide, weekly during first month of therapy, then monthly thereafter in women with regular menstrual cycles or every 2 weeks in women with irregular menstrual cycles.

•**WARNING** Be aware that thalidomide shouldn't be given to pregnant patient. A single dose may cause severe birth defects or fetal death.

•Assess patient's medication history for use of carbamazepine, griseofulvin, HIV-protease inhibitors, modafinil, penicillins, phenytoin, rifabutin, rifampin, and the herbal remedy St. John's wort. These products can decrease the effectiveness of hormonal contraceptives during thalidomide therapy.

•To minimize sedative effect, give thalidomide in divided doses t.i.d. or q.i.d., as prescribed, with larger dose in the evening.

•Assess for early signs of peripheral neuropathy (muscle cramps, numbness and tingling in toes and fingers, pain or superficial sensory loss in feet or hands) in patients receiv-

ing long-term thalidomide therapy. Early detection and drug discontinuation, as prescribed, prevents further damage and increases the chance for reversal.
•Expect to stop thalidomide if absolute neutrophil count is less than 750/mm$^3$. Routine monitoring of WBC count is recommended every other week for first 3 months of treatment in HIV-positive and other immunosuppressed patients and monthly in immunocompetent patients.

**PATIENT TEACHING**
•Instruct patient to have thalidomide prescription filled promptly because prescriptions more than 7 days old may not be filled.
•Urge patient to take drug exactly as prescribed.
•Inform female patient that drug will harm a fetus, and stress the need to avoid pregnancy. Tell her that pregnancy tests will be done before and frequently during therapy.
•Instruct female patient to abstain from sexual intercourse or to use two reliable methods of birth control simultaneously, starting 4 weeks before drug therapy and continuing for up to 4 weeks after therapy has been completed. One contraceptive method must be highly effective, such as an intrauterine device, oral contraceptive, or tubal ligation; the other may be a cervical cap, diaphragm, or latex condom.
•WARNING Inform male patient, even one who has had a vasectomy, that he must use barrier contraception (latex condom) when having sexual intercourse with a woman of childbearing age.
•Caution patient to avoid hazardous activities until drug's CNS effects are known.
•Suggest changing positions slowly to minimize effects of orthostatic hypotension.
•Instruct patient to immediately report signs of peripheral neuropathy, including numbness, pain, or tingling in feet and hands.
•Inform HIV-positive patient of the need for viral-load testing after first and third months of therapy and every 3 months thereafter.
•Urge patient to avoid using alcohol and donating blood or sperm during therapy.

# theophylline

Aerolate, Aerolate III, Aerolate Jr., Aerolate Sr., Apo-Theo LA (CAN), Asmalix, Elixophyllin, Lanophyllin, PMS Theophylline (CAN), Pulmophyllin (CAN), Quibron-T Dividose, Quibron-T/SR Dividose, Respbid, Slo-Bid Gyrocaps, Slo-Phyllin, Theo-24, Theo-SR (CAN), Theobid Duracaps, Theochron, Theoclear, Theoclear LA, Theo-Dur, Theolair, Theolair-SR, Theovent Long-Acting, T-Phyl, Truxophyllin, Uni-Dur, Uniphyl

## Class and Category
*Chemical:* Xanthine derivative
*Therapeutic:* Bronchodilator
*Pregnancy category:* C

## Indications and Dosages
➤ *As loading dose to treat reversible airway obstruction in patients not currently receiving theophylline*
**CAPSULES, ELIXIR, ORAL SOLUTION, SYRUP, TABLETS**
**Adults and children.** 5 mg/kg as a single dose.
**I.V. INFUSION**
**Adults and children.** 5 mg/kg infused over 20 to 30 min.

➤ *As partial loading dose to treat reversible airway obstruction in patients currently receiving theophylline*
**CAPSULES, ELIXIR, ORAL SOLUTION, SYRUP, TABLETS, I.V. INFUSION**
**Adults and children.** Individualized dosage based on blood theophylline level, as prescribed. Loading dose based on principle that 0.5 mg/kg of theophylline will produce a 1-mcg/ml increase in blood theophylline level.

➤ *To provide maintenance treatment of reversible airway obstruction associated with asthma or COPD*
**CAPSULES, TABLETS**
**Adults and children weighing more than 45 kg (99 lb).** *Initial:* 300 mg/day in equally divided doses q 6 to 8 hr; after 3 days, if tolerated, increased to 400 mg/day in divided doses q 6 to 8 hr; after 3 more days, if tolerated, increased to 600 mg/day in divided doses q 6 to 8 hr. Dosages above 600 mg/day are based on blood theophylline level and clinical response.
**Children age 1 and older weighing 45 kg or less.** *Initial:* 12 to 14 mg/kg/day up to maximum of 300 mg/day in equally divided doses q 4 to 6 hr; after 3 days, if tolerated, increased to 16 mg/kg up to maximum of 400

mg/day in equally divided doses q 4 to 6 hr; after 3 more days, if tolerated, 20 mg/kg/day up to maximum of 600 mg/day in equally divided doses q 4 to 6 hr. Dosages above 600 mg/day are based on blood theophylline level and clinical response.

**ELIXIR**

**Adults.** *Initial:* 300 mg/day in equally divided doses q 6 to 8 hr; after 3 days, if tolerated, increased to 400 mg/day in divided doses q 6 to 8 hr; after 3 more days, if tolerated, increased to 600 mg/day in divided doses q 6 to 8 hr. Dosages above 600 mg/day are based on blood theophylline level and clinical response.

**E.R. CAPSULES OR TABLETS**

**Adults and children weighing 45 kg or more.** *Initial:* 300 mg/day in equally divided doses q 8 to 12 hr; after 3 days, if tolerated, increased to 400 mg/day in divided doses q 8 to 12 hr; after 3 more days, if tolerated, increased to 600 mg/day in divided doses q 8 to 12 hr. Dosages above 600 mg/day are based on blood theophylline level and clinical response.

**Children age 1 and older weighing less than 45 kg.** *Initial:* 12 to 14 mg/kg/day up to maximum of 300 mg/day in equally divided doses q 8 to 12 hr; after 3 days, if tolerated, increased to 16 mg/kg up to maximum of 400 mg/day in equally divided doses q 8 to 12 hr; after 3 more days, if tolerated, dosage increased to 20 mg/kg/day up to maximum of 600 mg/day in equally divided doses q 8 to 12 hr. Dosages above 600 mg/day are based on blood theophylline level and clinical response.

**ORAL SOLUTION, SYRUP**

**Adults and children weighing more than 45 kg.** *Initial:* 300 mg/day in equally divided doses q 6 to 8 hr; after 3 days, if tolerated, increased to 400 mg/day in divided doses q 6 to 8 hr; after 3 more days, if tolerated, increased to 600 mg/day in divided doses q 6 to 8 hr. Dosages above 600 mg/day are based on blood theophylline level and clinical response.

**Children age 1 and older weighing 45 kg or less.** *Initial:* 12 to 14 mg/kg/day up to maximum of 300 mg/day in equally divided doses q 4 to 6 hr; after 3 days, if tolerated, increased to 16 mg/kg up to a maximum of 400 mg/day in equally divided doses q 4 to

6 hr; after 3 more days, if tolerated, dosage increased to 20 mg/kg/day up to maximum of 600 mg/day in equally divided doses q 4 to 6 hr. Dosages above 600 mg/day are based on blood theophylline level and clinical response.

**Full-term infants ages 26 to 52 weeks.** Dosage individualized in mg/kg/day, as prescribed, and administered in equally divided doses q 6 hr.

**Full-term infants up to age 26 weeks.** Dosage individualized in mg/kg/day, as prescribed, and administered in equally divided doses q 8 hr.

**Premature infants age 24 days and older.** 1.5 mg/kg q 12 hr.

**Premature infants under age 24 days.** 1 mg/kg q 12 hr.

**I.V. INFUSION**

**Adults and adolescents age 16 and older.** 0.4 mg/kg/hr for nonsmokers, 0.7 mg/kg/hr for smokers.

**DOSAGE ADJUSTMENT** For elderly patients and adults with cardiac decompensation, cor pulmonale, or hepatic impairment, I.V. dosage reduced to 0.2 mg/kg/hr.

**Children ages 9 to 16.** 0.7 mg/kg/hr.

**Children ages 1 to 9.** 0.8 mg/kg/hr.

**Full-term infants up to age 1.** Dosage individualized in mg/kg/day as prescribed.

## Incompatibilities

Don't mix parenteral theophylline solution with any additives. Don't infuse theophylline through same I.V. line as Hetastarch (Hespan), a colloidal plasma volume expander, which is incompatible with theophylline.

## Mechanism of Action

Inhibits phosphodiesterase enzymes, causing bronchodilation. Normally, these enzymes inactivate cAMP and cGMP, which are responsible for bronchial smooth-muscle relaxation. Theophylline also may cause calcium translocation, antagonize prostaglandins and adenosine receptors, stimulate catecholamines, and inhibit cGMP metabolism.

## Contraindications

Hypersensitivity to theophylline or its components, peptic ulcer disease, uncontrolled seizure disorder

## Interactions

**DRUGS**

*adenosine:* Decreased adenosine effectiveness
*allopurinol, cimetidine, ciprofloxacin, cla-rithromycin, disulfiram, enoxacin, erythro-mycin, fluvoxamine, interferon alpha (human recombinant), methotrexate, mexiletine, pen-toxifylline, propafenone, propranolol, tacrine, thiabendazole, ticlopidine, troleandomycin, verapamil:* Increased blood theophylline level and risk of toxicity
*aminoglutethimide, carbamazepine, isopro-terenol (I.V.), moricizine, oral contraceptives (containing estrogen), phenobarbital, pheny-toin, rifampin:* Decreased blood theophylline level and possibly drug effectiveness
*benzodiazepines:* Possibly reversal of benzo-diazepine sedation
*beta blockers:* Possibly decreased bronchodi-lator effect of theophylline
*ephedrine:* Increased adverse effects, includ-ing insomnia, nausea, and nervousness
*halothane anesthetics:* Increased risk of ven-tricular arrhythmias
*ketamine:* Lowered seizure threshold
*lithium:* Decreased lithium effectiveness
*neuromuscular blockers:* Possibly antago-nized neuromuscular blockade
*sucralfate:* Decreased absorption of oral the-ophylline

**FOODS**

*high-carbohydrate, low-protein diet:* Possibly decreased theophylline elimination
*low-carbohydrate, high-protein diet; daily in-take of charbroiled beef:* Possibly increased theophylline elimination

**ACTIVITIES**

*alcohol use:* Increased blood theophylline level and risk of toxicity
*smoking:* Increased drug clearance, decreased drug effectiveness

## Adverse Reactions

**CNS:** Agitation, anxiety (I.V. form), behav-ioral changes, confusion, disorientation, headache, insomnia, nervousness, seizures, tremor
**CV:** Hypotension, tachycardia, ventricular arrhythmias
**ENDO:** Hyperglycemia
**GI:** Abdominal pain, diarrhea, heartburn, nausea, vomiting
**GU:** Increased urine output

## Nursing Considerations

•Be aware that ideal body weight is used to calculate theophylline dosages because drug doesn't bind well in body fat.
•Be aware that E.R. capsules and tablets shouldn't be used for oral loading doses.
•Infuse theophylline loading dose, bolus, or intermittent infusion at a rate that doesn't exceed 25 mg/min.
•Administer continuous theophylline infu-sion with rate-controlled infusion device.
•Monitor blood theophylline level, as or-dered, to gauge therapeutic level and detect toxicity.
•Frequently assess heart rate and rhythm because theophylline can exacerbate existing arrhythmias.
•Be especially alert for signs of toxicity in patient with acute pulmonary edema, hypo-thyroidism, influenza vaccination, prolonged fever, sepsis with multiple organ failure, shock, or viral pulmonary infection because of decreased drug clearance.
•Monitor blood theophylline level in patients with uncorrected acidemia because they have an increased risk of toxicity.
•Expect patient with cystic fibrosis or hy-perthyroidism to experience increased the-ophylline clearance and decreased drug ef-fectiveness. Monitor blood theophylline level, as ordered.
•Suspect toxicity if patient experiences vom-iting, and be prepared to obtain blood the-ophylline level.

**PATIENT TEACHING**

•Instruct patient to swallow theophylline tablets whole and not to chew or crush them, unless scored for breaking.
•Explain that patient may open capsules and mix contents with soft food but that she shouldn't chew or crush granules.
•Instruct patient to take drug with a full glass of water on an empty stomach (30 to 60 minutes before meals or 2 hours after meals). However, suggest that she take drug with food or antacids if GI distress occurs.
•Encourage patient to take drug at the same times every day.
•Advise patient to notify prescriber if she develops a fever, makes a significant dietary change, or starts or stops smoking or taking other drugs because these factors may alter blood theophylline level.

**T**

# thiethylperazine maleate

Torecan

## Class and Category

*Chemical:* Piperazine phenothiazine
*Therapeutic:* Antiemetic
*Pregnancy category:* Not rated

## Indications and Dosages

➤ To treat nausea and vomiting

**TABLETS, I.M. INJECTION, SUPPOSITORIES**
**Adults and adolescents.** 10 mg q.d. to t.i.d.
*Maximum:* 30 mg q.d.

| Route | Onset | Peak | Duration |
|-------|-------|------|----------|
| P.O. | 30 to 60 min | Unknown | 4 hr |

### Mechanism of Action

Relieves nausea and vomiting by centrally blocking dopamine receptors in the medullary chemoreceptor trigger zone.

## Contraindications

Breast-feeding; coma; hypersensitivity to thiethylperazine, sulfites, tartrazine dye, or their components; jaundice; severe CNS depression

## Interactions

**DRUGS**

*aluminum- or magnesium-containing antacids, antidiarrheals (adsorbent):* Decreased absorption of thiethylperazine
*anticonvulsants (including barbiturates):* Lowered seizure threshold
*antihistamines, tricyclic antidepressants:* Additive CNS and GI effects, including ileus and severe constipation
*antihypertensives:* Enhanced hypotensive effect of both drugs
*antimuscarinics (including antiparkinsonian drugs, MAO inhibitors, meperidine, and phenothiazines):* Additive GI effects, including ileus and severe constipation
*appetite suppressants:* Decreased anorectic effect
*barbiturates, benzodiazepines, CNS depressants, general anesthetics, opioid analgesics:* Additive CNS effects
*beta blockers:* Increased blood levels of both drugs; additive hypotensive effects; possibly arrhythmias, irreversible retinopathy, and tardive dyskinesia
*bromocriptine:* Possibly decreased effectiveness of bromocriptine

*hepatotoxic drugs:* Increased risk of hepatotoxicity
*levodopa:* Decreased effectiveness of levodopa
*lithium:* Possibly acute encephalopathy
*methoxsalen, porfimer:* Possibly increased photosensitivity
*metrizamide:* Increased risk of seizures
*ototoxic drugs:* Possibly masked symptoms of ototoxicity (dizziness, tinnitus, and vertigo)
*phenytoin:* Increased risk of phenytoin toxicity
*quinidine:* Possibly adverse cardiac effects
*riboflavin:* Increased requirements for riboflavin
*sympathomimetics:* Reduced vasopressor response and duration of action of sympathomimetics
*tramadol:* Additive CNS effects, increased risk of seizures

**ACTIVITIES**

*alcohol use:* Additive CNS effects

## Adverse Reactions

**CNS:** Confusion, dizziness, EEG abnormalities, extrapyramidal reactions (dystonia, pseudoparkinsonism), sedation
**CV:** ECG changes, hypotension, orthostatic hypotension, tachycardia
**EENT:** Blurred vision, dry mouth
**ENDO:** Gynecomastia
**GI:** Constipation, increased appetite
**GU:** Darkened urine, ejaculation disorders, menstrual irregularities, urine retention
**HEME:** Agranulocytosis, leukopenia (transient)
**SKIN:** Contact dermatitis, photosensitivity
**Other:** Weight gain

## Nursing Considerations

• Avoid using thiethylperazine in patients with neurologic impairment because drug can disrupt central temperature regulation.
• Avoid inadvertent I.V. administration of thiethylperazine; injection is for I.M. administration only.
• Keep patient in recumbent position for 30 to 60 minutes after I.M. injection to minimize the risk of hypotension.
• Be aware that parenteral preparations contain sulfites and that tablets contain tartrazine dye.
• Moisten suppository with water or water-soluble lubricant before insertion. If suppository has softened excessively, chill for 30 minutes or run under cold water before removing wrapper.

•Avoid skin contact with drug to prevent contact dermatitis.

•Because thiethylperazine may cause reactions from anticholinergic effects and adrenergic blockade, assess for blurred vision, constipation, dry mouth, impotence, urine retention (from cholinergic activity) and priapism (from alpha-adrenergic blockade).

•During prolonged therapy, assess for visual disturbances because drug may cause corneal keratopathy and retinal discoloration (pigmentary retinopathy).

•WARNING Be aware that thiethylperazine may cause neuroleptic malignant syndrome, a rare but extremely serious reaction characterized by cardiovascular instability, decreased level of consciousness, extrapyramidal effects, and hyperpyrexia.

•Monitor CBC with differential, as ordered, because drug may worsen existing blood dyscrasias, such as agranulocytosis, neutropenia, and thrombocytopenia, in patients with bone marrow suppression. Be aware that drug may worsen angle-closure glaucoma, encephalopathy, organic or traumatic brain damage, or tardive dyskinesia.

•When possible, avoid combining thiethylperazine with CNS depressants because these drugs may potentiate thiethylperazine's effects.

•Monitor patient with cardiac disease for exaggerated cardiovascular reactions.

•Implement seizure precautions and monitor for seizures in patients with known seizure disorder because drug may lower seizure threshold.

•Implement safety precautions, according to facility policy, for elderly patients. They may be especially sensitive to drug's sedative and extrapyramidal effects.

•Be prepared to discontinue drug 48 hours before myelography and to resume drug 24 to 48 hours afterward to minimize the risk of seizures.

•Be aware that photosensitivity may turn patient's skin yellow-brown, gray, or purple because of hyperpigmentation.

•Be aware that drug shouldn't be given to pregnant patient because it may cause jaundice and extrapyramidal symptoms in her neonate.

PATIENT TEACHING

•Instruct patient to stay recumbent for 1 hour after taking thiethylperazine to minimize effects of orthostatic hypotension.

•Advise patient to notify prescriber immediately about adverse CNS reactions, decreased urine output, or vision changes.

•Urge patient to avoid alcohol use and potentially hazardous activities during therapy.

•Encourage patient to avoid excessive sun exposure and to use sunscreen when she's outdoors.

•Advise patient on long-term therapy to have periodic eye examinations to detect possible eye disorders.

# thiopental sodium

Pentothal

## Class, Category, and Schedule

*Chemical:* Barbiturate
*Therapeutic:* Anticonvulsant, sedative-hypnotic
*Pregnancy category:* C
*Controlled substance:* Schedule III

## Indications and Dosages

➤ *To control seizures from anesthesia or other causes*

I.V. INJECTION

**Adults.** *Initial:* 75 to 125 mg (3 to 5 ml of 2.5% solution) as soon as possible after onset of seizure. *Maximum:* 250 mg given over 10 min.

➤ *To facilitate narcoanalysis*

I.V. INFUSION OR INJECTION

**Adults.** Dosage individualized based on patient's age, condition, sex, and weight; injected at 100 mg/min (4 ml/min of 2.5% solution) with patient counting backwards from 100. Expect to discontinue injection once patient becomes confused with her counting but is still awake. Or, use 0.2% concentration in $D_5W$ for injection and infuse at 50 ml/min.

➤ *To treat cerebral hypertension*

I.V. INFUSION OR INJECTION

**Adults.** 1.5 to 3.5 mg/kg, repeated as required, to reduce elevated intracranial pressure (ICP).

| Route | Onset | Peak | Duration |
|---|---|---|---|
| I.V. | 10 to 40 sec | Unknown | 10 to 30 min |

## Incompatibilities

Don't mix thiopental with acidic I.V. drugs or solutions, succinylcholine, or tubocurarine.

T

## Mechanism of Action

Depresses the CNS and may inhibit the ascending transmission of impulses in the reticular formation. Thiopental possibly enhances or mimics the inhibitory action of gamma-aminobutyric acid, thereby having an anticonvulsant effect and producing sedation and hypnosis. Thiopental may reduce ICP by increasing cerebral vascular resistance, which decreases cerebral blood flow and volume.

## Contraindications

History of porphyria; hypersensitivity to thiopental, its components, or other barbiturates

## Interactions

**DRUGS**

*clonidine, CNS depressants, guanabenz, magnesium sulfate, methyldopa, metyrosine, pargyline, rauwolfia alkaloids:* Additive CNS depressant effects

*diazoxide, diuretics, guanadrel, guanethidine, mecamylamine, trimethaphan:* Possibly additive hypotensive effect

*ketamine:* Increased risk of hypotension or respiratory depression; possibly countered hypnotic effect of thiopental

*phenothiazines:* Possibly increased CNS depression or excitation, increased hypotensive effect

**ACTIVITIES**

*alcohol use:* Additive CNS depressant effects

## Adverse Reactions

**CNS:** Agitation, anxiety, seizures
**CV:** Bradycardia, hypotension, shock, tachycardia, thrombophlebitis
**GI:** Hiccups
**RESP:** Apnea, bronchospasm, cough, laryngospasm, respiratory depression, wheezing
**SKIN:** Hives, itching, rash, redness
**Other:** Angioedema

## Nursing Considerations

•Before administering thiopental, expect to premedicate patient with an anticholinergic, such as atropine or glycopyrrolate, to minimize secretions.
•Be prepared to administer a test dose of 25 to 75 mg (1 to 3 ml of 2.5% solution) to determine tolerance or sensitivity. Expect to observe patient for at least 1 minute after administering test dose.

•Dilute drug with a compatible I.V. solution before administering, such as $D_5W$ for injection, NS for injection, or sterile water for injection. Be aware that sterile water for injection shouldn't be used to prepare 0.2% or 0.4% solution because it would result in a hypotonic solution and cause hemolysis.
•To prepare 0.2% solution, dilute 1 g of thiopental with 500 ml of compatible diluent to produce a final concentration of 2 mg/ml.
•To prepare 0.4% solution, dilute 1 g of thiopental with 250 ml of compatible diluent or 2 g of thiopental with 500 ml of compatible diluent to produce a final concentration of 4 mg/ml.
•To prepare 2.5% solution, dilute 1 g of thiopental with 40 ml of compatible diluent or 5 g of thiopental with 200 ml of compatible diluent to produce a final concentration of 25 mg/ml.
•Inspect solution for particles before administration. Use solution within 24 hours of reconstitution, and discard unused portion after 24 hours.
•Monitor blood and tissue oxygenation and vital signs during I.V. administration. Keep emergency equipment and drugs nearby in case respiratory depression occurs.
•If patient has a history of CV disease or hypotension, monitor her for CV depressant effects, such as bradycardia, hypotension, or shock.
•In patient with a history of seizures, institute seizure precautions according to facility protocol.
•Monitor respiratory rate, rhythm, and quality for signs of respiratory depression in debilitated patient or one with a history of respiratory disease.
•Monitor neurologic status every hour, or as ordered, in patient with increased ICP.

**PATIENT TEACHING**

•Explain the need for frequent hemodynamic monitoring.
•Advise patient to use caution when driving or performing tasks that require alertness for at least 24 hours after thiopental administration.
•Instruct patient not to consume alcohol or other CNS depressants for at least 24 hours after thiopental administration (unless prescribed) because they increase the effects of thiopental.

• Instruct patient to report persistent drowsiness, rash, severe dizziness, or skin lesions to prescriber.

# thioridazine

Mellaril (CAN), Mellaril-S, Novo-Ridazine (CAN)

## thioridazine hydrochloride

Apo-Thioridazine (CAN), Mellaril, Mellaril Concentrate, Novo-Ridazine (CAN), PMS Thioridazine

### Class and Category

*Chemical:* Piperidine phenothiazine
*Therapeutic:* Antipsychotic drug
*Pregnancy category:* Not rated

### Indications and Dosages

➤ *To treat schizophrenia in patients unresponsive to other antipsychotic drugs*

ORAL SOLUTION, ORAL SUSPENSION, TABLETS

**Adults and adolescents.** *Initial:* 50 to 100 mg t.i.d., gradually increased, as needed and tolerated. *Maintenance:* 200 to 800 mg/day in two to four divided doses. *Maximum:* 800 mg/day.
**Children ages 2 to 12.** *Initial:* 0.5 mg/kg/day in divided doses, gradually increased, as needed and tolerated. *Maximum:* 3 mg/kg/day.

| Route | Onset | Peak | Duration |
|-------|-------|------|----------|
| P.O. | Up to several wk | 6 wk to 6 mo | Unknown |

### Mechanism of Action

Depresses areas of the brain that control activity and aggression, including the cerebral cortex, hypothalamus, and limbic system by blocking postsynaptic dopamine$_2$ (D$_2$) receptors. Drug may relieve anxiety by indirectly reducing arousal and increasing filtration of internal stimuli to the brain stem reticular activating system.

### Contraindications

Coma; concurrent use of drugs that inhibit the metabolism of thioridazine, such as fluoxetine, fluvoxamine, paroxetine, pindolol, and propranolol; concurrent use of drugs that prolong the QT interval; concurrent use of high doses of a CNS depressant; history of arrhythmias; hypersensitivity to thioridazine, other phenothiazines, or their components; prolonged QT interval; reduced cytochrome P450 2D6 activity; severe CNS depression; severe hypertensive or hypotensive cardiac disease

### Interactions

DRUGS

*amantadine, antihistamines, antimuscarinics, clozapine, cyclobenzaprine, diphenoxylate, disopyramide, maprotilene:* Additive anticholinergic effects
*amiodarone, bepridil, cisapride, disopyramide, erythromycin, flecainide, grepafloxacin, ibutilide, pimozide, probucol, procainamide, quinidine, sotalol, sparfloxacin, tocainide:* Possibly prolonged QT interval
*amphetamine, chlorpromazine, dextroamphetamine:* Possibly decreased effects of these drugs and thioridazine
*antacids, antidiarrheals (adsorbent), kaolin, rifabutin, rifampin, rifapentine:* Reduced bioavailability of thioridazine
*anxiolytics, benzodiazepines, clonidine, dronabinol, guanabenz, guanfacine, opioid analgesics, phenothiazines, sedative-hypnotics:* Possibly increased CNS effects or hypotension
*barbiturates, fosphenytoin, phenytoin, valproic acid:* Increased CNS depression, lowered seizure threshold
*bromocriptine:* Possibly decreased effectiveness of bromocriptine
*carbamazepine:* Possibly decreased blood thioridazine level
*charcoal:* Reduced thioridazine absorption
*dopamine, droperidol, haloperidol, metoclopramide, metyrosine:* Possibly increased adverse CNS effects
*ephedrine, epinephrine, norepinephrine, phenylephrine:* Possibly severe hypotension, MI, or tachycardia
*fluoxetine, fluvoxamine, other cytochrome P450 2D6 inhibitors, paroxetine, pindolol:* Inhibited metabolism of thioridazine, leading to elevated blood thioridazine level
*general anesthetics:* Possibly potentiated CNS depression
*guanadrel, guanethidine, methyldopa:* Inhibited hypotensive effect of these drugs
*levodopa, pergolide, pramipexole, ropinirole:*

Possibly inhibited antiparkinsonian response
*lithium (high doses):* Risk of encephalopathic
syndrome (characterized by confusion, elevated liver function test results and fasting
blood glucose level, extrapyramidal symptoms,
fever, lethargy, leukocytosis, and weakness)
*MAO inhibitors:* Possibly exaggerated extrapyramidal reactions
*methoxsalen, oral contraceptives, porfimer,
sulfonamides, sulfonylureas, tetracyclines,
thiazide diuretics, vitamin A analogues:* Possibly increased photosensitivity
*propranolol:* Increased blood propranolol and
thioridazine levels, increased CNS effects,
hypotension
*tramadol:* Increased blood tramadol level,
possibly increased risk of seizures
*trazodone:* Possibly additive hypotension
**ACTIVITIES**
*alcohol use:* Additive CNS effects

## Adverse Reactions
**CNS:** Akathisia, altered temperature regulation, depression, dizziness, drowsiness, extrapyramidal reactions (dystonia, laryngospasm, motor restlessness, pseudoparkinsonism), headache, insomnia
**CV:** ECG changes, hypertension, hypotension,
prolonged QT interval, torsades de pointes,
ventricular tachycardia
**EENT:** Blurred vision, change in color perception, dry mouth, impaired night vision,
mydriasis, photophobia
**ENDO:** Breast engorgement, galactorrhea
**GI:** Constipation, ileus, nausea
**GU:** Amenorrhea, decreased libido, ejaculation disorders, impotence, menstrual irregularities, priapism, urine retention
**HEME:** Agranulocytosis, anemia, aplastic
anemia, eosinophilia, leukocytosis, leukopenia, pancytopenia, thrombocytopenia
**SKIN:** Hyperpigmentation, jaundice, photosensitivity
**Other:** Weight gain

## Nursing Considerations
•**WARNING** Expect to give thioridazine only if
patient has failed to respond to therapy with
at least two other antipsychotic drugs because it may prolong the QT interval and
has been associated with torsades de pointes
and sudden death.
•Obtain baseline and serial ECG tracings
and serum potassium levels, as ordered.

Notify prescriber if QT interval is greater
than 500 msec or if potassium level is abnormal, and expect to discontinue drug immediately.
•Frequently monitor blood pressure and assess for chest pain in patients with heart
disease because thioridazine has caused
hypotension and has precipitated angina
on occasion. Also monitor urine output
in patients with benign prostatic hyperplasia because drug can worsen urine retention.
•Be aware that high doses and large dosage
changes in patient with a seizure disorder
may lower seizure threshold. Institute seizure
precautions, as appropriate, according to facility policy.
•Administer drug with food, milk, or a full
glass of water to minimize GI distress.
•Measure oral suspension using calibrated
measuring device. Dilute with 60 to 120 ml
of fruit juice, distilled water, or acidified tap
water immediately before administration.
•Don't administer thioridazine oral suspension with carbamazepine oral suspension; a
rubbery orange precipitate may form in
stool.
•To prevent contact dermatitis, don't let oral
solution come in contact with skin.
•Administer antacid or adsorbent antidiarrheal at least 1 hour before or 2 hours after
thioridazine.
•**WARNING** Be aware that thioridazine can
cause neuroleptic malignant syndrome—most
commonly in males. Signs and symptoms include altered level of consciousness, altered
mental status, autonomic instability (diaphoresis, hypotension or hypertension, sinus
tachycardia), hyperthermia, and severe
extrapyramidal dysfunction. Acute renal
failure, increased serum creatine phosphokinase level, and leukocytosis also have occurred. Notify prescriber immediately if such
symptoms develop, and be prepared to discontinue therapy.
•Be aware that drug shouldn't be discontinued abruptly. Sudden withdrawal of thioridazine may produce transient dizziness, nausea, tremor, and vomiting.
•Assess for eye pain because drug's anticholinergic effects can worsen angle-closure
glaucoma.
•Promptly investigate and report blurred vision, defective color perception, or impaired

night vision because of the risk of pigmentary retinopathy.
• Expect prescriber to discontinue thioridazine and order CBC if patient experiences signs of infection. Also expect drug therapy to be stopped 48 hours before myelography and resumed 24 to 48 hours afterward.
• Monitor patient for signs and symptoms of tardive dyskinesia—such as uncontrollable movements of the arms, face, or legs—even after treatment stops. Notify prescriber if they develop.

**PATIENT TEACHING**
• Instruct patient to take thioridazine exactly as prescribed and not to stop taking drug without consulting prescriber because of the risk of withdrawal symptoms.
• Instruct patient to notify prescriber immediately if she develops unusual symptoms, such as dizziness, palpitations, and syncope, because they may indicate the presence of torsades de pointes.
• Advise patient not to take drug within 2 hours of an antacid.
• Caution patient to avoid alcohol use, which increases drug's sedative effects, and to avoid hazardous activities if drowsiness occurs.
• Urge patient to notify prescriber immediately if she experiences blurred vision, defective color perception, difficulty with nighttime vision, excessive drowsiness, nausea, sore throat, or other signs of infection. Treatment may be discontinued.
• Advise female patient to use effective contraception while taking drug because its fetal effects are unknown. Instruct her to inform prescriber immediately of known or suspected pregnancy.
• Because drug may alter temperature regulation, encourage patient to avoid exposure to extreme temperatures during therapy.
• Advise patient to wear protective dark glasses to minimize the effects of adverse vision reactions.
• If patient requires long-term therapy, explain the risk of tardive dyskinesia, and urge her to notify prescriber immediately if she develops uncontrollable movements of her arms, face, or legs.
• Instruct patient to tell other prescribers that she's taking thioridazine before she takes any new drug.

# thiothixene

Navane

# thiothixene hydrochloride

Navane, Thiothixene HCl Intensol

## Class and Category

*Chemical:* Thioxanthene derivative
*Therapeutic:* Antipsychotic
*Pregnancy category:* Not rated

## Indications and Dosages

➤ *To treat psychotic disorders, such as acute psychosis, psychotic depression, and schizophrenia*

**CAPSULES (THIOTHIXENE), ORAL SOLUTION (THIOTHIXENE HYDROCHLORIDE)**
**Adults and children age 12 and older.** *Initial:* 2 mg t.i.d. (for mild conditions) or 5 mg b.i.d. (for more severe conditions), increased q wk, as needed. *Usual:* 10 to 40 mg/day in divided doses. *Maximum:* 60 mg/day (for severe conditions).

**DOSAGE ADJUSTMENT** For elderly patients, lowest effective dosage used for maintenance therapy; maximum dosage limited to 30 mg/day. For some patients, one daily dose possibly used for maintenance therapy.

**I.M. INJECTION (THIOTHIXENE HYDROCHLORIDE)**
**Adults.** *Initial:* 4 mg b.i.d. to q.i.d. *Optimal:* 4 mg q 6 to 12 hr. *Usual:* 16 to 20 mg/day in divided doses. *Maximum:* 30 mg/day.

---

### Mechanism of Action

Increases dopamine turnover by blocking postsynaptic dopamine receptors in the mesolimbic system. Eventually, dopamine neurotransmission decreases, resulting in antipsychotic effects.

---

## Contraindications

Blood dyscrasias, coma, hypersensitivity to thiothixene or its components, Parkinson's disease, severe CNS depression, shock, use of quinidine

## Interactions

**DRUGS**
*amphetamines:* Decreased effectiveness of either drug
*antacids, antidiarrheals (adsorbent):* Possibly reduced bioavailability of thiothixene

T

*antihistamines, tricyclic antidepressants:* Additive anticholinergic effects, causing severe constipation, ileus, or increased intraocular pressure

*bromocriptine:* Possibly increased serum prolactin level and decreased effectiveness of bromocriptine

*carbamazepine:* Possibly decreased blood thiothixene level

*dopamine:* Decreased vasoconstrictive effect of dopamine (in high doses)

*ephedrine, phenylephrine:* Possibly reduced vasopressor response

*epinephrine:* Possibly epinephrine reversal, leading to severe hypotension, tachycardia, and possibly MI

*erythromycin:* Increased adverse effects of thiothixene

*general anesthetics, opioid analgesics, tramadol:* Additive CNS effects, increased risk of seizures

*guanadrel, guanethidine:* Possibly decreased antihypertensive effect of these drugs

*hypotensive drugs:* Possibly excessive hypotension

*levodopa:* Possibly reduced effectiveness of levodopa

*lithium:* Possibly encephalopathic syndrome (with a blood level that exceeds 12 mEq/L)

*MAO inhibitors:* Possibly exaggerated extrapyramidal reactions

*metaraminol, methoxamine, norepinephrine:* Possibly reduced vasopressor response

*pergolide:* Possibly reduced effectiveness of pergolide

*propranolol:* Possibly seizures and increased hypotension

*quinidine:* Additive orthostatic hypotension, possibly prolonged QT interval

**ACTIVITIES**

*alcohol use:* Additive CNS effects, increased risk of seizures

*smoking:* Possibly decreased blood thiothixene level

## Adverse Reactions

**CNS:** Agitation, akathisia, drowsiness, dystonia, fatigue, insomnia, light-headedness, neuroleptic malignant syndrome, paradoxical exacerbation of psychotic disorder, restlessness, seizures, syncope, tardive dyskinesia, weakness

**CV:** ECG changes, edema, hypotension, peripheral edema, tachycardia

**EENT:** Blurred vision, dry mouth, increased salivation, miosis, mydriasis, nasal congestion, retinopathy

**ENDO:** Breast engorgement, galactorrhea, hyperglycemia, hypoglycemia

**GI:** Anorexia, constipation, diarrhea, elevated liver function test results, ileus, increased appetite, nausea, vomiting

**GU:** Amenorrhea, glycosuria, impotence, priapism

**HEME:** Agranulocytosis, anemia, eosinophilia, hemolytic anemia, leukocytosis, leukopenia, pancytopenia, thrombocytopenia

**SKIN:** Contact dermatitis, decreased sweating, photosensitivity, pruritus, rash

**Other:** Hyperuricemia, weight gain

## Nursing Considerations

• Administer thiothixene capsules with food or milk if needed to minimize GI distress.

• Don't give drug within 1 hr of an antacid.

• Dilute oral solution with 60 to 120 ml of fruit or tomato juice, milk, soup, water, or a carbonated beverage. Measure dose and administer using a calibrated measuring device. Avoid spilling solution on skin because drug may cause contact dermatitis.

• Avoid inadvertent I.V. delivery of thiothixene injection solution. It's intended for I.M. use.

• Be aware that I.M. administration usually is reserved for acute, severe agitation or for patients who can't take oral preparations.

• Maintain patient in recumbent position for 30 minutes after I.M. injection to minimize orthostatic hypotension.

• Assess patient for early signs of potentially irreversible tardive dyskinesia, a syndrome of involuntary rhythmic movements of the face, jaw, mouth, or tongue.

• **WARNING** Be aware that drug can precipitate neuroleptic malignant syndrome, a serious condition characterized by altered mental status, arrhythmias, diaphoresis, hyperpyrexia, muscle rigidity, and tachycardia, especially in patients with hyperthyroidism or thyrotoxicosis. Symptoms may be severe enough to cause life-threatening respiratory depression.

• Monitor patient's serum calcium level because hypocalcemia may lead to dystonic reactions.

• Keep in mind that hypotension from thiothixene may precipitate angina in patients with known cardiac disease.

•**WARNING** Be aware that drug-induced adverse CNS reactions may mimic or suppress neurologic evidence of CNS disorders, such as brain tumor, encephalitis, encephalopathy, meningitis, Reye's syndrome, and tetanus.
•Monitor for extrapyramidal symptoms—particularly dystonias—in children with acute illnesses, including CNS infections, dehydration, gastroenteritis, measles, or varicella-zoster infections.
•Observe for signs of adverse hematologic reactions, such as sore throat and other symptoms of infection. If they occur, be prepared to obtain CBC, as ordered, and discontinue thiothixene, as prescribed.
•Implement seizure precautions in patients with a history of seizures or EEG abnormalities because thiothixene can lower the seizure threshold.
•Assess patient for eye pain because drug's anticholinergic effects may worsen angle-closure glaucoma. Assess patient with benign prostatic hyperplasia for urine retention.

**PATIENT TEACHING**
•Fully inform patient facing long-term thiothixene therapy about risk of developing tardive dyskinesia.
•Advise patient to avoid exposure to sunlight or ultraviolet light, and to apply sunscreen when outdoors.
•Urge patient to avoid smoking or to begin a smoking cessation program while taking thiothixene.
•Encourage patient to avoid extreme temperature changes during drug therapy to prevent hyperthermia or hypothermia caused by decreased sweating.
•Instruct patient to immediately report sore throat or other signs of infection.

# thyroid USP

Armour Thyroid, Thyrar, Thyroid Strong, Westhroid

## Class and Category
*Chemical:* Porcine thyroid gland hormone
*Therapeutic:* Thyroid hormone replacement
*Pregnancy category:* A

## Indications and Dosages
➤ *To treat hypothyroidism without myxedema*

**TABLETS**
**Adults and children.** *Initial:* 60 mg/day, increased by 30 mg/day q mo p.r.n. *Maintenance:* 60 to 120 mg/day.
➤ *To treat hypothyroidism or myxedema in patients with cardiovascular disease*
**TABLETS**
**Adults.** *Initial:* 15 mg/day; daily dosage doubled q 2 wk, as indicated to achieve desired response, up to 180 mg/day. *Maintenance:* 60 to 180 mg/day.
➤ *To treat congenital hypothyroidism (cretinism) or severe hypothyroidism in children and infants*
**TABLETS**
**Children and infants.** *Initial:* 15 mg/day; daily dosage doubled q 2 wk, as indicated to achieve desired response, up to 180 mg/day. If desired response isn't achieved, dosage further increased by 30 to 60 mg/day. *Maintenance:* Individualized.

### Mechanism of Action
Stimulates growth and maturation of tissues, increases energy expenditure, and affects all enzyme actions through several mechanisms. Thyroid hormone:
•regulates cell differentiation and proliferation
•aids in myelination of nerves and development of axonal and dendritic processes in the nervous system
•enhances protein and carbohydrate metabolism by promoting metabolic processes that increase gluconeogenesis and protein synthesis and facilitate the mobilization of glycogen stores.

### Contraindications
Acute MI not associated with hypothyroidism, hypersensitivity to thyroid USP or its components, obesity treatment, untreated thyrotoxicosis

### Interactions
**DRUGS**
*barbiturates, carbamazepine, phenytoin, rifampin:* Possibly increased catabolism of thyroid hormone
*cholestyramine, colestipol:* Decreased effectiveness of thyroid hormone
*corticosteroids:* Decreased metabolism of corticosteroids

*estrogens:* Possibly increased circulating concentrations of thyroxine-binding globulin, decreased effectiveness of thyroid hormone
*insulin, oral antidiabetic drugs:* Possibly altered blood glucose control
*ketamine:* Risk of marked hypertension and tachycardia
*oral anticoagulants:* Altered anticoagulant effect
*sympathomimetics:* Increased adverse cardiovascular effects
*tricyclic antidepressants:* Increased therapeutic and toxic effects of both drugs
**FOODS**
*all foods:* Possibly altered absorption of thyroid hormone

## Adverse Reactions

**CNS:** Headache, insomnia, nervousness, tremor
**CV:** Angina; arrhythmias, including atrial fibrillation and sinus tachycardia; palpitations
**ENDO:** Hyperthyroidism
**GI:** Diarrhea, vomiting
**GU:** Menstrual irregularities
**SKIN:** Alopecia, diaphoresis
**Other:** Heat intolerance, weight loss

## Nursing Considerations

•Avoid giving oral thyroid hormone with food because it may alter drug absorption.
•Don't give thyroid hormone within 5 hours of cholestyramine or colestipol. Giving them together can reduce hormone absorption.
•**WARNING** Be aware that thyroid hormone therapy can unmask or worsen adrenal insufficiency, precipitate adrenal crisis in patients with uncontrolled adrenal insufficiency, and increase the risk of arrhythmias in patients with coronary artery disease.
•Monitor blood glucose level often because thyroid hormone therapy can unmask or exacerbate symptoms of other endocrine disorders and also may alter antidiabetic drug dosage requirements in patients with diabetes mellitus. Be aware that withdrawal of thyroid hormone can precipitate a hypoglycemic response in susceptible patients.
**PATIENT TEACHING**
•Tell patient to take thyroid hormone on an empty stomach at the same time each day.
•Advise her to inform prescriber immediately and seek medical attention if she experiences chest pain, nervousness, or sweating.
•Instruct patient who uses cholestyramine or

colestipol not to take these drugs within 5 hours of thyroid dose.
•Inform patient that full effects may not be evident for 1 to 3 weeks.
•Instruct patient with diabetes mellitus to monitor blood glucose level frequently.

# thyrotropin

## (thyroid-stimulating hormone, TSH)

Thytropar

## thyrotropin alfa

Thyrogen

## Class and Category

*Chemical:* Recombinant glycoprotein of human TSH
*Therapeutic:* Diagnostic aid
*Pregnancy category:* C

## Indications and Dosages

➤ *To provide diagnostic follow-up of patients with well-differentiated thyroid carcinoma*
**I.M. INJECTION (THYROTROPIN ALFA)**
**Adults and adolescents age 16 and older.**
0.9 mg q 24 hr for 2 doses or q 72 hr for 3 doses. Scanning or serum thyroglobulin testing performed 72 hr after last injection.
➤ *To provide differential diagnosis of subclinical hypothyroidism or low thyroid reserve*
**I.M. OR S.C. INJECTION (THYROTROPIN)**
**Adults and adolescents age 16 and older.** 10 IU q.d. for 1 to 3 days, followed by radioactive iodine study 24 hr after last injection. No response indicates thyroid failure; substantial response indicates pituitary failure.
➤ *To determine thyroid status in patients receiving thyroid hormone, to differentiate between primary and secondary hypothyroidism*
**I.M. OR S.C. INJECTION (THYROTROPIN)**
**Adults and adolescents age 16 and older.**
10 IU q.d. for 1 to 3 days.
➤ *To aid in diagnosing thyroid carcinoma remnant after surgery*
**I.M. OR S.C. INJECTION (THYROTROPIN)**
**Adults and adolescents age 16 and older.**
10 IU q.d. for 3 to 7 days.

## Mechanism of Action
Stimulates production of thyroglobulin by active thyroid tissue and enhances uptake of iodine, synthesis of thyroid precursor hormones (monoiodotyrosine, diiodotyrosine, and levothyroxine), and release of triiodothyronine ($T_3$) and thyroxine ($T_4$) from the thyroid gland into systemic circulation. Thyrotropin also binds with thyroid cancer tissue and stimulates iodine uptake in radioactive iodine imaging to detect cancer cells in euthyroid patients after near-total or total thyroidectomy.

## Contraindications
Coronary thrombosis, hypersensitivity to thyrotropin or its components, uncorrected adrenal insufficiency

## Adverse Reactions
**CNS:** Asthenia, fever, headache, paresthesia
**ENDO:** Hyperthyroidism
**GI:** Nausea, vomiting
**RESP:** Respiratory distress
**SKIN:** Rash, urticaria
**Other:** Flulike symptoms; sudden, rapid, painful enlargement of locally recurring papillary carcinoma

## Nursing Considerations
•**WARNING** Be aware that thyrotropin can unmask or worsen adrenal insufficiency, precipitate adrenal crisis in patients with uncontrolled adrenal insufficiency, and increase the risk of arrhythmias in patients with coronary artery disease.
•Reconstitute thyrotropin solution with manufacturer-provided diluent, which contains no preservatives.
•**WARNING** Avoid inadvertent I.V. or intradermal injection of thyrotropin. I.V. administration may result in severe reactions, including diaphoresis, hypotension, nausea, tachycardia, and vomiting. Intradermal injection may damage tissue at injection site.
•Check for chest pain and increased heart rate, especially in patients with cardiac or coronary artery disease, including angina, hypertension, and recent acute MI, and in patients with residual thyroid tissue. Drug may increase serum thyroid hormone level.
**PATIENT TEACHING**
•Advise patient to continue taking any thyroid hormone replacement while receiving injections of thyrotropin alfa unless otherwise directed by prescriber.
•If patient is scheduled for radioactive iodine test, tell her to follow a low-iodine diet.
•Inform patient that testing may take 5 to 12 days to complete.

# tiagabine hydrochloride
Gabitril

## Class and Category
*Chemical:* Nipecotic acid derivative
*Therapeutic:* Anticonvulsant
*Pregnancy category:* C

## Indications and Dosages
➤ *As adjunct to treat partial seizures*
**TABLETS**
**Adults.** *Initial:* 4 mg q.d.; increased by 4 mg/wk up to 16 mg/day, then dosage increased by 4 to 8 mg q wk until desired response occurs. *Usual:* 32 to 56 mg/day. *Maximum:* 56 mg/day in 2 to 4 divided doses.
**Children ages 12 to 18.** *Initial:* 4 mg q.d. for 1 wk, then increased by 4 to 8 mg/wk until desired response occurs. *Maximum:* 32 mg/day in 2 to 4 divided doses.
**DOSAGE ADJUSTMENT** For patients with impaired hepatic function, dosage individualized and reduced, or interval extended if needed, because of reduced drug clearance.

## Mechanism of Action
Appears to inhibit neuronal and glial uptake of gamma-aminobutyric acid (GABA), the major inhibitory neurotransmitter in the CNS. Tiagabine makes more GABA available in the CNS to open chloride channels in postsynaptic membranes, thereby leading to membrane hyperpolarization and preventing transmission of nerve impulses.

## Contraindications
Hypersensitivity to tiagabine or its components

## Interactions
**DRUGS**
*benzodiazepines, CNS depressants:* Possibly additive CNS depression

T

*carbamazepine, phenobarbital, phenytoin:*
Possibly decreased tiagabine effectiveness
**ACTIVITIES**
*alcohol use:* Possibly additive CNS depression

## Adverse Reactions

**CNS:** Amnesia, anxiety, asthenia, ataxia,
confusion, depression, dizziness, drowsiness,
EEG abnormalities, hostility, impaired cog-
nition, insomnia, light-headedness, paresthe-
sia, seizures, status epilepticus, tremor,
weakness
**EENT:** Pharyngitis, stomatitis
**GI:** Abdominal pain, diarrhea, increased ap-
petite, nausea, vomiting
**GU:** UTI
**MS:** Dysarthria
**SKIN:** Ecchymosis, rash

## Nursing Considerations

• Give tiagabine with food.
• **WARNING** Expect to taper dosage gradually,
as prescribed, because stopping drug
abruptly may increase seizure frequency.
• Take seizure precautions because tiagabine
has caused seizures and status epilepticus in
patients with no history of seizures.
**PATIENT TEACHING**
• Instruct patient to take tiagabine with food.
• Advise patient to avoid hazardous activities
until drug's CNS effects are known. Also
urge her to avoid alcoholic beverages during
therapy.
• Caution patient who also takes CNS depressants that drug may increase depressant effect.
• Instruct patient not to stop taking tiagabine
abruptly. Explain that prescriber usually ta-
pers dosage over 4 weeks to reduce the risk
of withdrawal seizures.

# ticarcillin disodium

Ticar

## Class and Category

*Chemical:* Penicillin
*Therapeutic:* Antibiotic
*Pregnancy category:* B

## Indications and Dosages

➤ *To treat moderate to severe infections,
such as bacteremia, diabetic foot ulcers,
empyema, intra-abdominal infections,*
*lower respiratory tract infections (includ-
ing pneumonia), lung abscess, peritonitis,
pulmonary infections due to complications of cystic fibrosis (including bronchiectasis and pneumonia), septicemia, and
skin and soft-tissue infections (including
cellulitis) caused by susceptible organisms*
**I.V. INFUSION**
**Adults and children.** 200 to 300 mg/kg/day in
divided doses q 4 to 6 hr. *Usual:* 3 g q 4 hr or
4 g q 6 hr.
➤ *To treat uncomplicated UTI*
**I.V. INFUSION, I.M. INJECTION**
**Adults and children weighing 40 kg (88 lb)
or more.** 1 g q 6 hr.
**Children over age 1 month and weighing less
than 40 kg.** 50 to 100 mg/kg/day in divided
doses q 6 to 8 hr.
➤ *To treat complicated UTI*
**I.V. INFUSION**
**Adults and children.** 150 to 200 mg/kg in
equally divided doses q 4 to 6 hr. *Usual:* 3 g
q 6 hr.
**DOSAGE ADJUSTMENT** For patients with creatinine clearance of 30 to 60 ml/min/1.73 $m^2$,
2 g I.V. q 4 hr; with creatinine clearance of
10 to 30 ml/min/1.73 $m^2$, 2 g I.V. q 8 hr; with
creatinine clearance of less than 10 ml/min/
1.73 $m^2$, 2 g I.V. q 12 hr or 1 g I.M. q 6 hr.

## Mechanism of Action

Inhibits bacterial cell wall synthesis by
binding to specific penicillin-binding proteins inside the bacterial cell wall. Ultimately, this leads to cell wall lysis and
death.

## Incompatibilities

Don't give ticarcillin through same I.V. line
as amikacin, gentamicin, or tobramycin.
Don't give within 1 hr of aminoglycosides.

## Contraindications

Hypersensitivity to ticarcillin, penicillins, or
their components

## Interactions

**DRUGS**
*aminoglycosides:* Additive or synergistic activity against some bacteria, possibly mutual
inactivation
*anticoagulants:* Possibly interference with
platelet aggregation, prolonged PT

*methotrexate:* Prolonged blood methotrexate level, increased risk of methotrexate toxicity
*probenecid:* Prolonged blood ticarcillin level

## Adverse Reactions

**CV:** Thrombophlebitis, vasculitis
**GI:** Elevated liver function test results, nausea, pseudomembranous colitis, vomiting
**GU:** Proteinuria
**HEME:** Anemia, eosinophilia, hemorrhage, leukopenia, neutropenia, prolonged bleeding time, thrombocytopenia
**SKIN:** Erythema nodosum, exfoliative dermatitis, pruritus, rash, toxic epidermal necrolysis, urticaria
**Other:** Anaphylaxis, hypernatremia, hypokalemia, injection site pain, superinfection

## Nursing Considerations

• Obtain body fluid or tissue samples for culture and sensitivity testing, as ordered. Review test results, if possible, before giving first dose of ticarcillin.
• Don't inject more than 2 g of drug at any one I.M. injection site.
• Reconstitute each gram of ticarcillin with 4 ml of compatible diluent. Further dilute reconstituted I.V. solution to 10 to 100 mg/ml with compatible I.V. solution. To minimize vein irritation, don't exceed concentration of 100 mg/ml. Concentrations of 50 mg/ml or greater are preferred. Infuse appropriate I.V. dose over 30 to 120 minutes.
• Check for local injection site reaction, including thrombophlebitis, during therapy.
• Be aware that ticarcillin may worsen symptoms in patients with a history of GI disease or colitis.
• For patients with renal impairment, take seizure precautions, according to facility policy, because of increased risk of seizures.
• Assess patient for signs of pseudomembranous colitis, such as abdominal cramps and severe watery diarrhea. Also look for other signs of superinfection, such as oral candidiasis and rash in breast-feeding infant.
• Monitor serum electrolyte levels for hypernatremia due to drug's high sodium content and for hypokalemia due to increased urinary potassium loss.
• **WARNING** Monitor patient's platelet count, PT, and APTT because ticarcillin may increase bleeding time and, in rare cases, may induce thrombocytopenia.

**PATIENT TEACHING**
• Stress need to take full course of ticarcillin exactly as prescribed, even if feeling better.
• Urge patient to report past allergies to penicillins and to notify prescriber immediately about adverse reactions, including fever.
• Advise patient to decrease sodium intake to reduce the risk of electrolyte imbalance.

# ticarcillin disodium and clavulanate potassium

Timentin

## Class and Category

*Chemical:* Penicillin
*Therapeutic:* Antibiotic combination
*Pregnancy category:* B

## Indications and Dosages

➤ *To treat moderate to severe infections, such as appendicitis, bacteremia, bone and joint infections (including osteomyelitis), diabetic foot ulcers, diverticulitis, gynecologic infections (including endometritis), infectious arthritis, intra-abdominal infections, lower respiratory tract infections (including pneumonia), peritonitis, septicemia, skin and soft-tissue infections (including cellulitis), and UTIs caused by susceptible organisms; to manage febrile neutropenia*

**I.V. INFUSION**
**Adults and children age 12 and older weighing 60 kg (132 lb) or more.** 3.1 g (3 g of ticarcillin and 100 mg of clavulanic acid) infused over 30 min q 4 to 6 hr.
**Adults and children age 12 and older weighing less than 60 kg.** 200 to 300 mg/kg/day (based on ticarcillin content) in divided doses q 4 to 6 hr.
**Children and infants over age 3 months.** For mild to moderate infections, 200 mg/kg/day (based on ticarcillin content) in divided doses q 6 hr; for severe infections, 300 mg/kg/day (based on ticarcillin content) in divided doses q 4 to 6 hr.

➤ *To treat pulmonary infections caused by complications of cystic fibrosis, such as bronchiectasis or pneumonia*

T

**I.V. INFUSION**
**Children.** 350 to 450 mg/kg/day (based on ticarcillin content) in divided doses.
DOSAGE ADJUSTMENT For patients with renal impairment, loading dose of 3.1 g given, then dosage adjusted based on creatinine clearance.

## Incompatibilities
Don't administer ticarcillin and clavulanate through same I.V. line as amikacin, gentamicin, or tobramycin. Don't administer within 1 hour of aminoglycosides.

## Mechanism of Action
Inhibits bacterial cell wall synthesis by binding to specific penicillin-binding proteins located inside bacterial cell walls. In this way, ticarcillin ultimately leads to cell wall lysis and death. Clavulanic acid, which doesn't alter the action of ticarcillin, binds with bound and extracellular beta-lactamase, preventing beta-lactamase from inactivating ticarcillin.

## Contraindications
Hypersensitivity to ticarcillin, clavulanic acid, or their components

## Interactions
**DRUGS**
*aminoglycosides:* Additive or synergistic activity against some bacteria, possibly mutual inactivation
*anticoagulants:* Possibly interference with platelet aggregation
*methotrexate:* Prolonged blood methotrexate level, increased risk of methotrexate toxicity
*probenecid:* Prolonged blood ticarcillin level

## Adverse Reactions
**CV:** Thrombophlebitis, vasculitis
**GI:** Elevated liver function test results, nausea, pseudomembranous colitis, vomiting
**GU:** Proteinuria
**HEME:** Anemia, eosinophilia, hemorrhage, leukopenia, neutropenia, prolonged bleeding time, thrombocytopenia
**SKIN:** Erythema nodosum, exfoliative dermatitis, pruritus, rash, toxic epidermal necrolysis, urticaria
**Other:** Anaphylaxis, hypernatremia, hypokalemia, infusion site pain

## Nursing Considerations
•Keep in mind that 3.1 g of combination drug ticarcillin and clavulanate corresponds to 3 g of ticarcillin and 100 mg of clavulanic acid.
•Dilute reconstituted I.V. solution to concentration of 10 to 100 mg/ml with compatible I.V. solution. To minimize vein irritation, don't exceed concentration of 100 mg/ml. Concentrations of 50 mg/ml or greater are preferred. Infuse appropriate I.V. dose over 30 to 120 min.
•Know that ticarcillin and clavulanate may exacerbate symptoms in patients with a history of GI disease or colitis.
•For patients with renal impairment, implement seizure precautions, according to facility policy, because they're at increased risk for seizures.
•Assess patient for signs of pseudomembranous colitis, such as abdominal cramps and severe watery diarrhea. Also assess for other signs of superinfection, such as oral candidiasis and rash in breast-feeding infant.
•Monitor serum electrolyte levels for hypernatremia due to drug's high sodium content and for hypokalemia due to increased urinary potassium loss.
•WARNING Monitor patient's platelet count, PT, and APTT because drug may increase bleeding time and, in rare cases, may induce thrombocytopenia.
•Be aware that patient receiving high doses of ticarcillin may develop pseudoproteinuria.
**PATIENT TEACHING**
•Instruct patient taking ticarcillin and clavulanate to report past allergies to penicillins and to notify prescriber immediately about adverse reactions, including fever.
•Advise patient to decrease sodium intake to reduce the risk of electrolyte imbalance.

# ticlopidine hydrochloride
Ticlid

## Class and Category
*Chemical:* Thienopyridine derivative
*Therapeutic:* Antithrombotic, platelet aggregation inhibitor
*Pregnancy category:* B

## Indications and Dosages
➤ *To reduce the risk of initial thrombotic CVA in patients who have experienced transient ischemic attack, to reduce the*

*risk of recurrent CVA in patients who have previously experienced thrombotic CVA*

**TABLETS**

**Adults.** 250 mg b.i.d.

➤ *As adjunct to reduce the risk of sub-acute stent thrombosis after successful coronary stent implantation*

**TABLETS**

**Adults.** 250 mg b.i.d with antiplatelet doses of aspirin for up to 30 days after successful stent implantation.

| Route | Onset | Peak | Duration |
|-------|-------|------|----------|
| P.O. | 2 to 4 days | 8 to 11 days | 1 to 2 wk |

## Contraindications

Coagulopathy, GI bleeding, hematologic disorders related to hematopoiesis (including history of thrombotic thrombocytopenic purpura, neutropenia, and thrombocytopenia), hemophilia, hypersensitivity to ticlopidine or its components, intracranial bleeding, retinal bleeding, severe hepatic disease

## Interactions

**DRUGS**

*aluminum- and magnesium-containing antacids:* Possibly decreased peak blood ticlopidine level

*antineoplastics, antithymocyte globulin, heparin, NSAIDs, oral anticoagulants, platelet aggregation inhibitors, salicylates, strontium-89 chloride, thrombolytics:* Increased risk of bleeding

*cimetidine:* Reduced clearance of ticlopidine, increased risk of adverse reactions

*cyclosporine, digoxin:* Decreased blood level and possibly reduced effectiveness of these drugs

*porfimer:* Decreased effectiveness of porfimer photodynamic therapy

*xanthines (aminophylline, oxytriphylline, theophylline):* Decreased theophylline clearance, increased risk of toxicity

## Mechanism of Action

Normally, platelets don't adhere to blood vessel walls. However, when a thrombotic CVA or other disorder damages blood vessel walls, platelets are activated and adhere within seconds. Once activated, platelets release adenosine diphosphate (ADP). This causes fibrinogen to bind to glycoprotein IIb/IIIa (GP IIb/IIIa) receptors on the surface of activated platelets and connect with other activated platelets. Then a thrombus forms.

Ticlopidine inhibits the release of ADP from activated platelets, which prevents fibrinogen from binding to GP IIb/IIIa receptors on the surface of activated platelets, as shown below. This action prevents platelets from aggregating to form a thrombus, which prevents thrombosis of an implanted stent or recurrence of CVA.

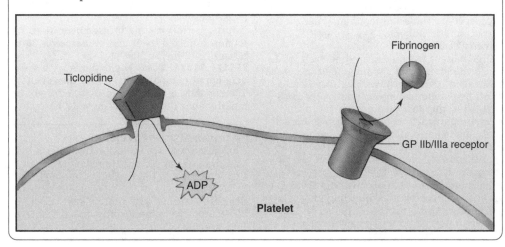

Fibrinogen

Ticlopidine

GP IIb/IIIa receptor

ADP

Platelet

T

## Adverse Reactions
**CNS:** Dizziness
**CV:** Hypercholesterolemia, vasculitis
**EENT:** Tinnitus
**GI:** Abdominal pain, anorexia, diarrhea, elevated liver function test results, flatulence, indigestion, nausea, vomiting
**HEME:** Agranulocytosis, aplastic anemia, hemolysis, hemolytic anemia, neutropenia, pancytopenia, thrombocytopenia, thrombotic thrombocytopenia, thrombotic thrombocytopenic purpura
**SKIN:** Pruritus, purpura, rash
**Other:** Hyponatremia, serum sickness-like reaction

## Nursing Considerations
•Give ticlopidine with food to maximize GI absorption and minimize any GI distress.
•Avoid I.M. injections of other drugs because excessive bleeding, bruising, or hematoma may occur.
•During first 3 months of therapy, monitor CBC every 2 weeks, as ordered (more frequently in patients with depressed neutrophil count).
•Be aware that ticlopidine therapy typically is used for patients with CVA or an increased risk of CVA who can't tolerate aspirin because of the risk of neutropenia or agranulocytosis.
•**WARNING** Be aware that ticlopidine therapy irreversibly affects platelet aggregation. Expect prescriber to discontinue drug 10 to 14 days before surgical procedures to prevent uncontrolled bleeding.
•Monitor serum cholesterol level during first month of ticlopidine therapy for expected increase. Hypercholesterolemia may persist for duration of treatment.

**PATIENT TEACHING**
•Urge patient to take ticlopidine with food.
•Inform patient that she may be at increased risk for infection because drug may decrease WBC or platelet count, especially in first 3 months of therapy.
•Advise patient to notify prescriber immediately if she has chills, fever, or sore throat.
•Encourage patient to keep scheduled appointments for blood tests to detect any abnormalities.
•Instruct patient to apply prolonged pressure to injured areas because bleeding may take longer than usual to stop. Urge her to immediately report to prescriber any unusual bleeding or bruising.

# tigecycline

Tygacil

## Class and Category
*Chemical:* Glycylcycline
*Therapeutic:* Antibiotic
*Pregnancy category:* D

## Indications and Dosages
➤ *To treat complicated skin and skin structure infections caused by* Escherichia coli, Enterococcus faecalis *(vancomycin-susceptible isolates only),* Staphylococcus aureus *(methicillin-susceptible and -resistant isolates),* Streptococcus agalactiae, Streptococcus anginosus *grp. (includes* S. anginosus, S. intermedius, *and* S. constellatus*),* Streptococcus pyogenes, *and* Bacteroides fragilis; *to treat complicated intra-abdominal infections caused by* Citrobacter freundii, Enterobacter cloacae, Escherichia coli, Klebsiella oxytoca, Klebsiella pneumoniae, Enterococcus faecalis *(vancomycin-suseptible isolates only),* Staphylococcus aureus *(methicillin-susceptible isolates only),* Streptococcus anginosus *grp. (includes* S. anginosus, S. intermedius, *and* S. constellatus*),* Bacteroides fragilis, Bacteroides thetaiotaomicron, Bacteroides uniformis, Bacteroides vulgatus, Clostridium perfringens, *and* Peptostreptococcus micros

**I.V. INFUSION**
**Adults.** *Initial:* 100 mg infused over 30 to 60 min followed by 50 mg infused over 30 to 60 min q 12 hr for 5 to 14 days.
**DOSAGE ADJUSTMENT** For patients with severe hepatic impairment, initial dosage of 100 mg should be followed by a reduced maintenance dosage of 25 mg q 12 hr.

---

### Mechanism of Action
Inhibits protein translation in bacteria by binding to the 30S ribosomal subunit, which prevents binding of amino-acyl tRNA molecules to the ribosome complex, thus interfering with protein synthesis. Through this bacteriostatic action, bacteria are weakened.

## Incompatibilities

Don't give amphotericin B, chlorpromazine, methylprednisolone, or voriconazole simultaneously through the same Y-site.

## Contraindications

Hypersensitivity to tigecycline or its components

## Interactions

None known

## Adverse Reactions

**CNS:** Asthenia, chills, dizziness, fever, headache, insomnia, somnolence
**CV:** Bradycardia, hypertension, hypotension, peripheral edema, phlebitis, septic shock, tachycardia, thrombophlebitis, vasodilation
**EENT:** Dry mouth, taste perversion
**ENDO:** Hyperglycemia, hypoglycemia
**GI:** Abdominal pain, acute pancreatitis, anorexia, constipation, diarrhea, dyspepsia, elevated liver enzyme levels, jaundice, nausea, vomiting
**GU:** Elevated BUN and creatinine levels, vaginal candidiasis
**HEME:** Anemia, leukocytosis, thrombocythemia
**MS:** Back pain
**RESP:** Increased cough, dyspnea
**SKIN:** Diaphoresis, photosensitivity, pruritus, rash
**Other:** Hypersensitivity reaction, hypocalcemia; hypokalemia; hyponatremia; hypoproteinemia; injection site reaction, such as edema, phlebitis, inflammation, and pain

## Nursing Considerations

• Obtain body tissue and fluid samples for culture and sensitivity tests as ordered before giving first dose. Expect to begin drug therapy before test results are known.
• Avoid giving tigecycline to children younger than age 8 because drug may cause permanent brown or yellow tooth discoloration and enamel hypoplasia.
• Use tigecycline cautiously in patients hypersensitive to tetracycline class antibiotics because glycylcycline class antibiotics are structurally similar to tetracycline class antibiotics.
• Also use cautiously in patients with complicated intra-abdominal infections secondary to intestinal perforation because of the risk of septic shock.

• Determine whether female patients could be pregnant before starting tigecycline therapy because the drug may cause harm to fetus.
• Reconstitute each vial of tigecycline with 5.3 ml of 0.9% sodium chloride injection or 5% dextrose injection to achieve a concentration of 10 mg/ml. Note that the color will be yellow to orange. If not, the solution should be discarded. Immediately withdraw reconstituted solution from the vial and add to a 100-ml I.V. bag for infusion. Drug may be stored in the I.V. bag at room temperature for up to 6 hours or refrigerated up to 24 hours before use.
• If I.V. line is used to infuse other drugs, flush the line with either 0.9% sodium chloride injection or 5% dextrose injection before and after tigecycline infusion.
• Infuse tigecycline over 30 to 60 minutes.
• Monitor patient closely for diarrhea, which may indicate pseudomembranous colitis, which is known to occur with many antibiotics. If diarrhea occurs during therapy, notify prescriber and expect to withhold drug. Expect to treat psuedomembranous colitis, if confirmed, with fluids, electrolytes, protein, and an antibiotic effective against *Clostridium difficile.*
• Monitor patient for adverse reactions, keeping in mind the similarity between tigecycline and tetracycline.
• Assess patient for superinfection, such as vaginal candiasis, that may result from overgrowth of nonsusceptible organisms, including fungi. If signs of infection are present, notify prescriber and provide supportive care, as prescribed.

**PATIENT TEACHING**
• Instruct patient to report adverse reactions, especially hypersensitivity reactions, such as a rash or itching, as well as diarrhea.
• Tell patient to report discomfort at infusion site because site may need to be changed.

# tiludronate disodium

*(contains 200 mg of tiludronic acid per tablet)*

Skelid

## Class and Category

*Chemical:* Aminobiphosphonate
*Therapeutic:* Bone resorption inhibitor
*Pregnancy category:* C

## Indications and Dosages

➤ *To treat Paget's disease in patients with serum alkaline phosphatase levels at least twice the upper limit of normal, who are symptomatic or at risk for future complications of the disease*

TABLETS

**Adults.** *Initial:* 400 mg of tiludronic acid q.d. 2 hr a.c. or p.c. for 3 mo. *Maximum:* 400 mg of tiludronic acid q.d.

### Mechanism of Action
Reduces the activity of cells that cause bone loss and increases bone mass. Tiludronate may act by inhibiting osteoclast activity on newly formed bone resorption surfaces. This activity reduces the number of sites at which bone is remodeled. When bone formation exceeds bone resorption at these remodeling sites, bone mass increases. Tiludronate may also inhibit bone destruction by binding to hydroxyapatite crystals, which give bone its rigidity.

## Contraindications
Creatinine clearance less than 30 ml/min/ 1.73 m$^2$, esophageal abnormalities that delay esophageal emptying, hypersensitivity to tiludronate or its components

## Interactions
DRUGS
*aluminum- or magnesium-containing antacids, mineral supplements (such as calcium, iron), salicylates, salicylate-containing compounds:* Decreased absorption of tiludronate
*indomethacin:* Possibly increased bioavailability of tiludronate

FOODS
*all foods and beverages (except plain water):* Decreased absorption of tiludronate

## Adverse Reactions
**CNS:** Dizziness, headache
**CV:** Chest pain, edema
**EENT:** Cataracts, conjunctivitis, glaucoma, pharyngitis, rhinitis
**GI:** Diarrhea, esophageal irritation and ulceration, flatulence, indigestion, nausea, vomiting
**MS:** Arthralgia, back pain, myalgia
**RESP:** Cough, upper respiratory tract infection
**SKIN:** Rash
**Other:** Flulike symptoms

## Nursing Considerations
•Be prepared to monitor serum calcium levels before, during, and after tiludronate therapy because drug may exacerbate such conditions as hyperparathyroidism, hypocalcemia, and vitamin D deficiency. Ensure adequate dietary intake of calcium and vitamin D during and after treatment. If hypocalcemia occurs, expect to administer a calcium supplement, as prescribed.
•WARNING Be aware that tiludronate may irritate upper GI mucosa, causing such adverse reactions as esophageal ulcer. To help minimize these reactions, have patient take drug with full glass of plain water and remain upright for at least 30 minutes.

PATIENT TEACHING

•Instruct patient to take tiludronate with 6 to 8 oz of plain water on an empty stomach (at least 2 hours before or after beverages, food, other drugs, or mineral supplements, including mineral water) because food and beverages may severely reduce drug's effect. Also, advise her to remain upright for at least 30 minutes after taking drug.
•Advise patient not to chew or suck on tablet to reduce the risk of esophageal irritation.
•Instruct patient to notify prescriber immediately if she develops signs or symptoms of esophageal irritation, such as trouble swallowing or worsening heartburn; these may indicate a serious esophageal disorder.
•Caution patient not to take salicylate-containing drugs, such as aspirin, during tiludronate therapy.

# timolol maleate

Apo-Timol (CAN), Blocadren, Novo-Timol (CAN)

## Class and Category
*Chemical:* Beta blocker
*Therapeutic:* Antihypertensive, MI prophylactic, vascular headache prophylactic
*Pregnancy category:* C

## Indications and Dosages
➤ *To manage hypertension*
TABLETS
**Adults.** *Initial:* 10 mg b.i.d., increased q wk as prescribed. *Maintenance:* 20 to 40 mg/day in divided doses. *Maximum:* 60 mg/day.

➤ *To provide long-term prophylaxis after MI*
**TABLETS**
**Adults.** 10 mg b.i.d., beginning 1 to 4 wk after MI and continuing for at least 2 yr.

➤ *To prevent migraine headache*
**TABLETS**
**Adults.** *Initial:* 10 mg b.i.d. *Maintenance:* 20 mg/day in divided doses. *Maximum:* 30 mg/day; discontinued after 8 wk, as prescribed, if maximum dose is ineffective.

| Route | Onset | Peak | Duration |
|-------|-------|------|----------|
| P.O. | 30 min | 1 to 2 hr | 4 to 8 hr |

## Mechanism of Action
Selectively blocks $alpha_1$ and $beta_2$ receptors in vascular smooth muscle and $beta_1$ receptors in the heart. This reduces peripheral vascular resistance and blood pressure and relieves migraine headaches. Timolol's potent beta blockade prevents the reflex tachycardia that typically occurs with most alpha blockers, and decreases cardiac excitability, cardiac output, and myocardial oxygen demand, thus preventing MI.

## Contraindications
Acute bronchospasm; asthma; cardiogenic shock; children; COPD (severe); heart failure; hypersensitivity to timolol, other beta blockers, or their components; second- or third-degree AV block; severe sinus bradycardia

## Interactions
**DRUGS**
*allergen immunotherapy, allergenic extracts for skin testing:* Increased risk of serious systemic adverse reactions or anaphylaxis
*amiodarone:* Additive depressant effect on cardiac conduction, negative inotropic effect
*anesthetics (hydrocarbon inhalation):* Increased risk of myocardial depression and hypotension
*beta blockers:* Additive beta blockade effects
*calcium channel blockers, clonidine, diazoxide, guanabenz, reserpine, other hypotension-producing drugs:* Additive hypotensive effect and, possibly, other beta blockade effects
*cimetidine:* Possibly interference with timolol clearance
*estrogens:* Decreased antihypertensive effect of timolol

*fentanyl, fentanyl derivatives:* Possibly increased risk of initial bradycardia after induction doses of fentanyl or derivative (with long-term timolol use)
*glucagon:* Possibly blunted hyperglycemic response
*insulin, oral antidiabetic drugs:* Possibly masking of tachycardia in response to hypoglycemia, impaired glucose control
*lidocaine:* Decreased lidocaine clearance, increased risk of lidocaine toxicity
*MAO inhibitors:* Increased risk of significant hypertension
*neuromuscular blockers:* Possibly potentiated and prolonged action of these drugs
*NSAIDs:* Possibly decreased hypotensive effect
*phenothiazines:* Increased blood levels of both drugs
*phenytoin (parenteral):* Additive cardiac depressant effect
*sympathomimetics, xanthines:* Possibly mutual inhibition of therapeutic effects

## Adverse Reactions
**CNS:** Asthenia, CVA, decreased concentration, depression, dizziness, fatigue, fever, hallucinations, headache, insomnia, nervousness, nightmares, paresthesia, syncope, vertigo
**CV:** Angina, arrhythmias, bradycardia, cardiac arrest, chest pain, edema, palpitations, Raynaud's phenomenon, vasodilation
**EENT:** Diplopia, dry eyes, eye irritation, ptosis, tinnitus, vision changes
**ENDO:** Hyperglycemia, hypoglycemia
**GI:** Abdominal pain, diarrhea, hepatomegaly, indigestion, nausea, vomiting
**GU:** Decreased libido, impotence
**MS:** Arthralgia, decreased tolerance to exercise, extremity pain, muscle weakness
**RESP:** Bronchospasm, cough, crackles, dyspnea
**SKIN:** Alopecia, diaphoresis, hyperpigmentation, pruritus, purpura, rash
**Other:** Anaphylaxis, weight loss

## Nursing Considerations
•**WARNING** Be aware that timolol may mask signs and symptoms of acute hypoglycemia in diabetic patient. The drug also may mask certain signs of hyperthyroidism, such as tachycardia.
•Be aware that timolol may prolong hypoglycemia by interfering with glycogenolysis

**T**

or may promote hyperglycemia by decreasing tissue sensitivity to insulin.
• Monitor blood pressure and cardiac output, as appropriate, for patient with a history of systolic heart failure or left ventricular dysfunction because timolol's negative inotropic effect can depress cardiac output.
• **WARNING** Be aware that timolol shouldn't be discontinued abruptly because this may produce MI, myocardial ischemia, severe hypertension, or ventricular arrhythmias, particularly in patient with known cardiovascular disease.
• Expect varied drug effectiveness in elderly patients; they may be less sensitive to drug's antihypertensive effect or more sensitive because of reduced drug clearance.
• Monitor for impaired circulation in elderly patients with age-related peripheral vascular disease or patients with Raynaud's phenomenon. Such patients may experience exacerbated symptoms from increased alpha stimulation. Elderly patients also are at increased risk for beta blocker–induced hypothermia.
• If timolol exacerbates skin condition, such as psoriasis, notify prescriber.

**PATIENT TEACHING**
• Instruct patient taking timolol to inform prescriber of chest pain, fainting, light-headedness, or shortness of breath, which may indicate the need for dosage change.
• Caution patient not to stop taking drug abruptly. Timolol dosage must be tapered gradually under prescriber's supervision.
• Instruct patient with diabetes mellitus to monitor blood glucose level frequently during therapy.
• Warn patient with psoriasis about possible flare-ups of skin condition.

# tinidazole

Tindamax

## Class and Category
*Chemical:* Synthetic nitroimidazole
*Therapeutic:* Antiprotozoal
*Pregnancy category:* C

## Indications and Dosages
➤ *To treat trichomoniasis caused by* Trichomonas vaginalis

**TABLETS**
**Adults.** 2 g one time with food.
➤ *To treat giardiasis caused by* Giardia duodenalis (G. lamblia)
**TABLETS**
**Adults.** 2 g one time with food.
**Children age 4 and older.** 50 mg/kg (up to 2 g) one time with food.
➤ *To treat intestinal amebiasis caused by* Entamoeba histolytica
**TABLETS**
**Adults.** 2 g q.d. for 3 days with food.
**Children age 4 and older.** 50 mg/kg (up to 2 g) q.d. for 3 days with food.
➤ *To treat amebic liver abscess caused by* Entamoeba histolytica
**TABLETS**
**Adults.** 2 g q.d. for 3 to 5 days with food.
**Children age 4 and older.** 50 mg/kg (up to 2 g) q.d. for 3 to 5 days with food.
**DOSAGE ADJUSTMENT** For patients receiving hemodialysis, an additional dose equivalent to one-half the dose prescribed should be given after the dialysis treatment on the days dialysis is performed.

---

## Mechanism of Action
Tinidazole undergoes intracellular chemical reduction during anaerobic metabolism. After tinidazole is reduced, it damages DNA's helical structure and breaks its strands, which inhibits bacterial nucleic acid synthesis and causes cell death.

---

## Contraindications
Breast-feeding, hypersensitivity to tinidazole or its components, treatment of trichomoniasis during first trimester of pregnancy

## Interactions
**DRUGS**
*cholestyramine:* Possibly decreased bioavailability of tinidazole
*cimetidine, ketoconazole:* Possibly delayed elimination and increased blood level of tinidazole
*cyclosporine, tacrolimus:* Possibly increased serum cyclosporine and tacrolimus levels
*disulfiram:* Possibly combined toxicity, resulting in confusion and psychosis
*fluorouracil:* Possibly decreased fluorouracil clearance

*lithium:* Possibly increased serum lithium levels

*oral anticoagulants:* Possibly increased anticoagulant effect

*oxytetracycline:* Possibly diminished effect of tinidazole

*phenobarbital, phenytoin, rifampin:* Possibly increased metabolism and decreased blood level of tinidazole

**ACTIVITIES**

*alcohol use:* Possibly disulfiram-like effects

## Adverse Reactions

**CNS:** Ataxia, dizziness, coma, confusion, depression, drowsiness, fatigue, fever, headache, insomnia, malaise, peripheral neuropathy, seizures, vertigo, weakness

**CV:** Palpitations

**EENT:** Dry mouth, excessive salivation, furry tongue, metallic or bitter taste, oral candidiasis, pharyngitis, stomatitis, tongue discoloration

**GI:** Abdominal cramps, anorexia, constipation, diarrhea, epigastric discomfort, hepatic abnormalities, indigestion, nausea, thirst, vomiting

**GU:** Candida overgrowth, darkened urine, increased vaginal discharge

**HEME:** Reversible thrombocytopenia, transient leukopenia or neutropenia

**MS:** Arthralgia, arthritis, myalgia

**RESP:** Bronchospasm, dyspnea

**SKIN:** Diaphoresis, flushing, pruritus, rash, urticaria

**Other:** Angioedema

## Nursing Considerations

• Use tinidazole cautiously in patients with CNS disease or blood dyscrasias because tinidazole's adverse effects may worsen these disorders.

• Institute seizure precautions. If a seizure or other abnormal neurological symptoms occur, notify prescriber and expect to discontinue tinidazole.

• Treat a patient diagnosed with trichomoniasis and her sexual partner with the same dose of tinidazole and at the same time, as ordered, because trichomoniasis is a sexually transmitted disease.

• Monitor patient's total WBC count and differential if retreatment with tinidazole is needed because adverse hematological reactions may occur with repeated tinidazole use.

**PATIENT TEACHING**

• Tell patient to take tinidazole with food to minimize gastric discomfort.

• Instruct patient unable to swallow tablets to crush tinidazole and mix in artificial cherry syrup and then take with food.

• Advise patient to avoid alcoholic beverages while taking tinidazole and for 3 days afterward because alcohol can cause intense flushing.

• Tell patient to alert prescriber before taking tinidazole if she thinks or knows she is pregnant because tinidazole crosses the placental barrier during the first trimester and its effects on the fetus are unknown.

# tinzaparin sodium

Innohep

## Class and Category

*Chemical:* Low–molecular-weight heparin
*Therapeutic:* Anticoagulant, antithrombotic
*Pregnancy category:* B

## Indications and Dosages

➤ *As adjunct to treat pulmonary thromboembolism and acute symptomatic deep vein thrombosis*

**S.C. INJECTION**

**Adults.** 175 anti-Xa IU/kg q.d. for at least 6 days. *Maximum:* 18,000 to 21,000 anti-Xa IU/day.

| Route | Onset | Peak | Duration |
|---|---|---|---|
| S.C. | 2 to 3 hr | 4 to 6 hr | 24 hr |

## Mechanism of Action

Potentiates the action of antithrombin III, a coagulation inhibitor. By binding with antithrombin III, tinzaparin rapidly binds with and inactivates clotting factors (primarily fibrin and factor Xa). Without thrombin, fibrinogen can't convert to fibrin and clots can't form.

## Contraindications

Active major bleeding; heparin-induced thrombocytopenia (current or past); hypersensitivity to tinzaparin or its components, other low–molecular-weight heparins, sulfites, benzyl alcohol, or pork products

## Interactions
**DRUGS**
*alteplase, anistreplase, aspirin, dextran, dipyridamole, NSAIDs, oral anticoagulants, streptokinase, sulfinpyrazone, urokinase:* Possibly increased risk of bleeding

## Adverse Reactions
**CNS:** Confusion, dizziness, headache, insomnia, intracranial hemorrhage, paralysis
**CV:** Angina, hypertension, hypotension, tachycardia
**EENT:** Epistaxis, gingival bleeding, pharyngeal bleeding
**GI:** Constipation, elevated liver function test results, GI and retroperitoneal bleeding, hematemesis, nausea, vomiting
**GU:** Hematuria, genitourinary bleeding, prolonged or heavy menstrual bleeding, UTI
**HEME:** Anemia, thrombocytopenia, unusual bruising
**MS:** Back pain
**RESP:** Dyspnea, hemoptysis, pulmonary embolism
**SKIN:** Bleeding at puncture sites, surgical incision sites, or venous cutdown sites; rash
**Other:** Injection site hematoma, including itching, pain, redness, and swelling

## Nursing Considerations
•Expect warfarin therapy to begin within 1 to 3 days of tinzaparin use.
•Monitor patient's international normalized ratio (INR). Expect tinzaparin therapy to be continued until INR reaches 2.0 for 2 consecutive days.
•**WARNING** Monitor patient for signs and symptoms of GI bleeding, including bloody or black, tarry stools; bloody or coffee-ground vomitus; and severe stomach pain. Notify prescriber immediately if patient develops any of these signs or symptoms.
•Assess tinzaparin injection site for signs and symptoms of hematoma, including deep, dark purple bruises under skin and itching, pain, redness, or swelling.
•Assess for signs and symptoms of intracranial bleeding (such as decreased level of consciousness), retroperitoneal bleeding (such as abdominal pain or swelling and back pain), genitourinary bleeding (such as hematuria), or respiratory tract bleeding (such as hemoptysis). Notify prescriber immediately if patient develops any of these signs or symptoms.

•If serious bleeding (not controllable by local pressure) occurs, expect to discontinue any concomitant warfarin or antiplatelet drugs immediately.
•Expect to treat bleeding by administering 1 mg of protamine sulfate 1% solution I.V. per 100 anti-Xa IU of tinzaparin, as prescribed.
•If possible, avoid giving patient I.M. injections while she's receiving tinzaparin. If arterial puncture becomes necessary during tinzaparin therapy, expect to apply pressure after procedure and to monitor puncture site frequently for signs of bleeding.
•Monitor laboratory test results for elevated liver enzyme levels. If significant elevations persist or worsen, notify prescriber immediately.

**PATIENT TEACHING**
•Advise patient who is receiving tinzaparin to immediately report any bleeding, including from nose or gums.
•Instruct patient to limit physical activity during tinzaparin administration to reduce the risk of injury or bleeding.

# tiopronin

Thiola

## Class and Category
*Chemical:* Thiol compound
*Therapeutic:* Antiurolithic
*Pregnancy category:* C

## Indications and Dosages
➤ *To prevent the formation of urinary cystine calculi*
**TABLETS**
**Adults.** 800 mg/day in 3 divided doses.
**Children over age 9.** 15 mg/kg in 3 divided doses.
**DOSAGE ADJUSTMENT** For patients with a history of hypersensitivity to penicillamine, therapy initiated at a reduced dosage; later dosage adjusted as prescribed, according to urine cystine level.

| Route | Onset | Peak | Duration |
|-------|-------|------|----------|
| P.O. | Rapid | Unknown | 8 to 10 hr |

## Contraindications
History of agranulocytosis, aplastic anemia, or thrombocytopenia; hypersensitivity to tiopronin or its components

## Mechanism of Action

Inhibits the formation of urinary cystine calculi by undergoing thiol-disulfide exchange with cystine (cystine-cystine disulfide) to form a water-soluble compound, tiopronin-cystine disulfide.

## Interactions

**DRUGS**

*bone marrow depressants:* Increased risk of adverse hematologic effects
*hepatotoxic drugs:* Increased risk of hepatotoxic effects
*nephrotoxic drugs:* Increased risk of nephrotoxic effects

## Adverse Reactions

**CNS:** Chills, fever
**CV:** Peripheral edema
**EENT:** Laryngeal edema, stomatitis
**GU:** Hematuria, proteinuria
**HEME:** Anemia, eosinophilia, leukopenia, thrombocytopenia
**MS:** Arthralgia
**SKIN:** Ecchymosis, jaundice, pruritus, rash, urticaria

## Nursing Considerations

• Assess for signs of drug fever, which may occur during first month of tiopronin therapy.
• Be aware that drug may be stopped temporarily, then restarted at lower dose.
• Expect to monitor urine cystine level so dosage can be adjusted to keep cystine level below 250 g/ml.

**PATIENT TEACHING**

• Instruct patient to take tiopronin on an empty stomach, 1 hour before or 2 hours after meals, for faster drug absorption.
• Advise patient to drink at least 3 L of fluid daily to maintain a urine output of at least 2 L/day during therapy.
• Encourage the patient to maintain a diet low in methionine, which is an essential amino acid that is found in eggs, cheese, fish, and milk.

# tiotropium bromide

Spiriva HandiHaler

## Class and Category

*Chemical:* Nonane bromide monohydrate

*Therapeutic:* Anticholingeric, bronchodilator
*Pregnancy category:* C

## Indications and Dosages

➤ *To prevent bronchospasm associated with COPD, including chronic bronchitis and emphysema*

**AEROSOL CAPSULES**

**Adults.** 18 mcg (1 capsule) inhaled q.d. using HandiHaler inhalation device

## Mechanism of Action

Prevents acetylcholine from attaching to muscarinic receptors on membranes of smooth-muscle cells. By blocking acetylcholine's effects in the bronchi and bronchioles, tiotropium relaxes smooth muscles and causes bronchodilation.

## Contraindications

Hypersensitivity to atropine or its derivatives, including ipratropium, tiotropium, or their components

## Interactions

**DRUGS**

*anticholinergics:* Possibly increased anticholinergic effects

## Adverse Reactions

**CNS:** Depression, difficulty speaking, paresthesia
**CV:** Angina, atrial fibrillation, chest pain, hypercholesterolemia, palpitations, peripheral edema, supraventricular tachycardia, tachycardia
**EENT:** Blurred vision, cataract, dry mouth, epistaxis, eye pain, glaucoma, laryngitis, pharyngitis, rhinitis, sinusitis, stomatitis, visual halos
**ENDO:** Hyperglycemia
**GI:** Abdominal pain, constipation, gastroesophageal reflux, indigestion, vomiting
**GU:** Urinary difficulty, urine retention, UTI
**MS:** Arthritis, leg or skeletal pain, myalgia
**RESP:** Cough, paradoxical bronchospasm, upper respiratory tract infection
**SKIN:** Pruritus, rash, urticaria
**Other:** Allergic reaction, angioedema, flulike symptpoms, infection, moniliasis

## Nursing Considerations

• Use tiotropium cautiously in patients with angle-closure glaucoma, benign prostatic hyperplasia, or bladder neck obstruction.

T

•Monitor patient closely after giving first dose of tiotropium for immediate hypersensitivity reactions, including angioedema and paradoxical bronchospasm. If any reactions occur, notify prescriber and expect to stop tiotropium.
•Monitor patient's renal function, as ordered, especially in patients with moderate to severe renal impairment, because tiotropium is excreted mainly by the kidneys.
•Monitor patient's pulmonary function, as ordered, to evaluate the effectiveness of tiotropium.

**PATIENT TEACHING**
•Caution patient not to use tiotropium to treat acute bronchospasm.
•Instruct the patient on the proper use of the HandiHaler inhalation device. Tell patient to place the capsule into the center chamber of the inhalation device and then to press and release the button on the side of the inhalation device to pierce the capsule. Then have the patient exhale completely, close her lips around the mouthpiece, inhale slowly and deeply, and hold her breath for as long as is comfortable.
•Alert patient that the HandiHaler device should not be used for taking any other drug and that tiotropium must be taken only using the device and never swallowed.
•Tell patient not to expose capsules to air until ready for use. To remove a capsule from the blister pack, tell patient to open the foil only as far as the stop line to avoid exposing the rest of the capsules in the blister pack to air. Instruct patient to discard capsules if they are inadvertently exposed to air and won't be used immediately.
•Advise patient to keep powder out of her eyes because it may irritate them or blur her vision.
•Instruct patient to rinse her mouth after each treatment to help minimize throat dryness and irritation.
•Advise patient to report decreased response to tiotropium as well as difficulty voiding, eye pain, palpitations, and vision changes.

# tirofiban hydrochloride

Aggrastat

## Class and Category

*Chemical:* Tyrosine derivative
*Therapeutic:* Platelet aggregation inhibitor
*Pregnancy category:* B

## Indications and Dosages

➤ *To treat acute coronary syndrome*
**I.V. INFUSION**
**Adults.** 0.4 mcg/kg/min for 30 min, followed by 0.1 mcg/kg/min.
**DOSAGE ADJUSTMENT** For patients with creatinine clearance of less than 30 ml/min/1.73 m$^2$, infusion rate reduced by one-half.

| Route | Onset | Peak | Duration |
|-------|-------|------|----------|
| I.V. | Immediate | 30 min | 4 to 8 hr |

## Mechanism of Action

Binds to glycoprotein IIb/IIIa receptor sites on the surface of activated platelets. Circulating fibrinogen can bind to these receptor sites and link platelets together, forming a clot that eventually blocks a coronary artery. By binding to receptor sites, tirofiban prevents the normal binding of fibrinogen and other factors and inhibits platelet aggregation.

## Incompatibilities

Don't infuse tirofiban in same I.V. line with any drug other than atropine sulfate, dobutamine, dopamine, epinephrine hydrochloride, furosemide, heparin, lidocaine, midazolam hydrochloride, morphine sulfate, nitroglycerin, potassium chloride, propranolol hydrochloride, or famotidine (Pepcid injection).

## Contraindications

Acute pericarditis; arteriovenous malformation; coagulopathy; CVA that occurred within previous 30 days or a history of hemorrhagic CVA; GI or GU bleeding; hemophilia; history of thrombocytopenia after tirofiban use; hypersensitivity to tirofiban or its components; intracranial aneurysm or mass, intracranial bleeding, retinal bleeding, aortic dissection, or any evidence of active abnormal bleeding within previous 30 days; major surgery or trauma within previous 6 weeks; severe uncontrolled hypertension (systolic blood pressure above 180 mm Hg, diastolic blood pressure above 110 mm Hg)

## Interactions

**DRUGS**
*antineoplastics, antithymocyte globulin, NSAIDs, oral anticoagulants, platelet aggre-*

*gation inhibitors, strontium-89 chloride, thrombolytics:* Increased risk of bleeding
*levothyroxine, omeprazole:* Increased rate of tirofiban clearance
*porfimer:* Decreased effectiveness of porfimer photodynamic therapy
*salicylates:* Increased risk of bleeding, possibly hypoprothrombinemia

## Adverse Reactions
**CNS:** Chills, dizziness, fever, headache, intracranial hemorrhage
**CV:** Edema, hemopericardium, peripheral edema, sinus bradycardia
**GI:** Hematemesis, nausea, retroperitoneal bleeding, vomiting
**GU:** Hematuria, pelvic pain
**HEME:** Severe thrombocytopenia with chills, fever, and possibly fatal bleeding complications
**RESP:** Pulmonary hemorrhage
**SKIN:** Diaphoresis, rash, urticaria
**Other:** Allergic reaction, anaphylaxis, infusion site bleeding

## Nursing Considerations
• **WARNING** Dilute 50-ml vial of tirofiban before use; don't dilute 500-ml container because it holds premixed solution ready for I.V. infusion. Don't use solution unless it's clear and the seal is intact.
• If prescribed, administer tirofiban with heparin for 48 to 108 hours. Expect to continue infusion throughout angiography and for 12 to 24 hours after angioplasty or ather-ectomy.
• **WARNING** If patient is also receiving a heparin infusion, expect to monitor APTT before treatment, 6 hours after heparin infusion starts, and regularly thereafter. Expect to adjust heparin dosage to maintain APTT at about two times the control. Notify prescriber immediately if patient develops an abnormally high APTT. Also, assess patient for signs and symptoms of abnormal bleeding and report them to prescriber immediately because potentially life-threatening bleeding may occur.
• After cardiac catheterization or percutaneous transluminal coronary angioplasty, maintain patient on bed rest and keep head of bed elevated. Ensure percutaneous site hemostasis at least 4 hours before discharge. Minimize invasive procedures, including epidural procedures, to reduce the risk of bleeding.

• Monitor patient's platelet count, hemoglobin level, and hematocrit, as ordered. Expect to discontinue tirofiban if patient's platelet count is less than 90,000/mm$^3$. Expect to administer a platelet transfusion, as prescribed, if patient's platelet count falls below 50,000/mm$^3$.
**PATIENT TEACHING**
• Advise patient to immediately report any bleeding, bruising, headache, pain, or swelling during I.V. infusion of tirofiban.

# tizanidine hydrochloride
Zanaflex

## Class and Category
*Chemical:* Imidazoline
*Therapeutic:* Antispasmodic
*Pregnancy category:* C

## Indications and Dosages
➤ *To manage acute and intermittent increases of muscle tone associated with spasticity*
**TABLETS**
**Adults.** 4 mg q 6 to 8 hr, p.r.n., increased gradually by 2 to 4 mg/dose, as needed and as prescribed. *Maximum:* 36 mg/day or 3 doses/day.

| Route | Onset | Peak | Duration |
|-------|-------|------|----------|
| P.O. | Unknown | 1 to 2 hr | 3 to 6 hr |

### Mechanism of Action
Reduces spasticity by decreasing the release of excitatory amino acids. This alpha$_2$-adrenergic agonist's action increases presynaptic inhibition of spinal motor neurons, with the greatest effects on polysynaptic pathways.

## Contraindications
Hypersensitivity to tizanidine or components

## Interactions
**DRUGS**
*acetaminophen:* Delayed peak effects of acetaminophen
*alpha$_2$-adrenergic agonists:* Possibly significant hypotension
*antihypertensives:* Additive hypotensive effects
*oral contraceptives:* Decreased tizanidine clearance
*rofecoxib:* Possibly increased adverse reactions

T

*alcohol use:* Increased adverse effects of tizanidine, additive CNS depression

## Adverse Reactions
**CNS:** Anxiety, delusions, drowsiness, dyskinesia, fatigue, hallucinations, slurred speech
**CV:** Orthostatic hypotension
**EENT:** Dry mouth, pharyngitis, rhinitis
**GI:** Anorexia, constipation, diarrhea, elevated liver function test results, hepatic failure, hepatomegaly, nausea, vomiting
**GU:** Urinary frequency, UTI
**MS:** Muscle weakness
**SKIN:** Diaphoresis, jaundice, rash, ulceration

## Nursing Considerations
• Monitor hepatic and renal function for first 6 months and periodically thereafter.
• Expect prolonged drug use to inhibit saliva.
• Be aware that tizanidine should be stopped slowly to prevent withdrawal and rebound hypertension, tachycardia, and hypertonia.

PATIENT TEACHING
• Caution patient not to stop taking tizanidine suddenly to prevent adverse effects.
• Advise patient to change positions slowly to minimize effects of orthostatic hypotension.
• Urge patient to avoid alcohol during drug therapy because of its additive CNS effects.
• Advise patient to notify prescriber or a dentist if dry mouth persists for longer than 2 weeks.

# tobramycin sulfate
Tobi

## Class and Category
*Chemical:* Aminoglycoside
*Therapeutic:* Antibiotic
*Pregnancy category:* D

## Indications and Dosages
➤ *To treat bacteremia; bone and joint, gynecologic, intra-abdominal, lower respiratory tract, skin and soft-tissue, and urinary tract infections; endocarditis; meningitis; neonatal sepsis; pyelonephritis; and septicemia caused by susceptible strains of* Acinetobacter *sp.,* Aeromonas *sp.,* Citrobacter *sp.,* Enterobacter *sp.,* Escherichia coli, Haemophilus influenzae *(beta lactamase–negative and –posi-*

*tive),* Klebsiella *sp.,* Morganella morganii, Proteus mirabilis, Proteus vulgaris, Providencia rettgeri, Pseudomonas aeruginosa, Salmonella *sp.,* Serratia *sp.,* Shigella *sp.,* Staphylococcus aureus, *and* Staphylococcus epidermidis; *to treat febrile neutropenia*

I.V. INFUSION, I.M. INJECTION
**Adults.** 3 to 6 mg/kg/day in divided doses q 8 to 12 hr.
**Children over age 5.** 2 to 2.5 mg/kg q 8 hr.
**Children under age 5.** 2.5 mg/kg q 8 to 16 hr.
**Neonates over age 7 days weighing more than 2 kg (4.4 lb).** 2.5 mg/kg q 8 hr.
**Neonates over age 7 days weighing 1.2 to 2 kg (2.6 to 4.4 lb).** 2.5 mg/kg q 8 to 12 hr.
**Neonates age 7 days and under weighing 2 kg or more.** 2.5 mg/kg q 12 hr.
**Neonates age 7 days and under weighing 1.2 to 2 kg.** 2.5 mg/kg q 12 to 18 hr.
**Preterm neonates weighing 1 to 1.2 kg (2.2 to 2.6 lb).** 2.5 mg/kg q 18 to 24 hr.
**Preterm neonates weighing less than 1 kg.** 3.5 mg/kg q 24 hr.
➤ *To treat pulmonary infection caused by* P. aeruginosa *in patients with cystic fibrosis*

I.V. INFUSION
**Adults and children.** 2.5 to 3.3 mg/kg q 8 hr; dosage adjusted to achieve peak blood drug level of 8 to 12 mcg/ml and trough blood drug level below 2 mcg/ml.

INHALATION
**Adults and children over age 6.** 1 ampule (300 mg) b.i.d. in alternating periods of 28 days on and 28 days off.
➤ *To treat meningitis caused by susceptible organisms*

INTRATHECAL INJECTION
**Adults.** 4 to 8 mg q.d. with parenteral therapy.
**Children.** 1 to 2 mg q.d. with parenteral therapy.
➤ *To treat systemic infection*

INTRAPERITONEAL INFUSION
**Adults and children.** 1.5 to 2 mg/kg.
➤ *To treat dialysis-associated peritonitis in patients with end-stage renal disease*

INTRAPERITONEAL INFUSION
**Adults and children.** 4 to 8 mg/L in each dialysate exchange bag, increased, as prescribed, to 6 to 8 mg/L in documented *Pseudomonas* infection or to 20 mg/L administered in one exchange bag q.d.

DOSAGE ADJUSTMENT For patients with renal impairment, dosage possibly reduced.

## Incompatibilities

Don't mix tobramycin in same solution with parenteral aminoglycosides or beta-lactam antibiotics because mutual inactivation may result. Don't dilute or mix inhalation solution in nebulizer with dornase alfa.

## Mechanism of Action

Inhibits bacterial protein synthesis by binding irreversibly to one of two aminoglycoside-binding sites on the 30S ribosomal subunit, resulting in bacteriostatic effects. Bactericidal effects may stem from tobramycin's ability to accumulate within cells so that the intracellular drug level exceeds the extracellular level.

## Contraindications

Concurrent cidofovir therapy; hypersensitivity to tobramycin, aminoglycosides, sodium bisulfite, or their components

## Interactions

**DRUGS**

*acyclovir, aminoglycosides, amphotericin B, carboplatin, cisplatin, NSAIDs, vancomycin:* Additive nephrotoxicity
*carbenicillin, ticarcillin:* Possibly inactivation of tobramycin
*dimenhydrinate:* Possibly masking of symptoms of ototoxicity
*ethacrynic acid, furosemide:* Additive ototoxicity
*general anesthetics, neuromuscular blockers:* Possibly exaggerated neuromuscular blockade

## Adverse Reactions

**CNS:** Confusion, dizziness, headache, lethargy, neurotoxicity, vertigo
**EENT:** Hearing loss, tinnitus
**GI:** Diarrhea, elevated liver function test results, nausea, vomiting
**GU:** Elevated BUN and serum creatinine levels, nephrotoxicity, oliguria, proteinuria, renal failure
**HEME:** Anemia, leukocytosis, leukopenia, neutropenia, thrombocytopenia
**SKIN:** Exfoliative dermatitis, pruritus, rash, urticaria
**Other:** Hypocalcemia, hypokalemia, hypomagnesemia, hyponatremia, injection site pain

## Nursing Considerations

• Obtain body fluid and tissue samples for culture and sensitivity testing before and during tobramycin treatment, as ordered. Review test results, if available, before therapy begins.
• After reconstituting drug with 30 ml of sterile or bacteriostatic water for injection, dilute further with NS or $D_5W$.
• Give each I.V. dose over 20 to 60 minutes.
• WARNING Don't infuse tobramycin over less than 20 minutes because doing so may result in neuromuscular blockade and excessive peak blood drug level.
• Don't expose ampules for inhalation solution to intense light. Refrigerate them at 36° to 46° F (2° to 8° C).
• Because drug can cause bilateral and irreversible hearing loss, assess for early signs of cochlear and vestibular ototoxicity, including high-frequency hearing loss and vertigo.
• Monitor serum calcium, magnesium, potassium, and sodium levels to detect electrolyte imbalances.
• WARNING Be alert for allergic reactions, including anaphylaxis, because some forms of drug contain sodium bisulfite.
• Discontinue tobramycin therapy 7 days before starting cidofovir therapy, as prescribed.
• Assess for signs of nephrotoxicity, such as elevated BUN and serum creatinine levels.
• Expect dehydration to increase the risk of nephrotoxicity.
• WARNING Monitor patient with myasthenia gravis or parkinsonism for increased muscle weakness because of tobramycin's potential curare-like effect.

**PATIENT TEACHING**

• For tobramycin inhalation therapy, instruct patient to inhale over 10 to 15 minutes, using a handheld nebulizer with a compressor.
• Teach patient how to use nebulizer while sitting or standing upright and to breathe normally through its mouthpiece. Nose clips may help patient breathe through her mouth.
• Urge patient to immediately report high-frequency hearing loss and vertigo.
• Instruct female patient to notify prescriber immediately about known or suspected pregnancy because drug poses danger to fetus.

T

# tocainide hydrochloride
Tonocard

## Class and Category
*Chemical:* Lidocaine analogue
*Therapeutic:* Class IB antiarrhythmic
*Pregnancy category:* C

## Indications and Dosages
➤ *To treat life-threatening, sustained ventricular tachycardia*
TABLETS
**Adults.** *Initial:* 400 mg q 8 hr. *Maintenance:* 1.2 to 1.8 g/day in divided doses q 8 hr.
D0SAGE ADJUSTMENT Dosage possibly reduced by 25% if creatinine clearance is 10 to 30 ml/min/1.73 m$^2$ and by 50% if creatinine clearance is less than 10 ml/min/1.73 m$^2$.

| Route | Onset | Peak | Duration |
|-------|-------|------|----------|
| P.O. | Unknown | 0.5 to 2 hr | 8 hr |

## Mechanism of Action
Combines with fast sodium channels in myocardial cell membranes, which inhibits sodium influx into cells and decreases ventricular depolarization, automaticity, and excitability during diastole.

## Contraindications
Hypersensitivity to tocainide or its components, second- or third-degree AV block without ventricular pacemaker

## Interactions
DRUGS
*antiarrhythmics:* Possibly additive cardiac effects, additive toxicity
*beta blockers:* Increased cardiac index, left ventricular pressures, and pulmonary artery wedge pressures
*cimetidine:* Possibly decreased blood tocainide level
*rifampin:* Accelerated hepatic metabolism of tocainide, reduced tocainide effectiveness

## Adverse Reactions
**CNS:** Agitation, anxiety, ataxia, coma, confusion, depression, dizziness, fatigue, hallucinations, headache, mood changes, nervousness, paresthesia, psychosis, seizures, sleep disturbance, syncope, tremor, vertigo
**CV:** AV conduction disorders, bradycardia, chest pain, heart failure, hypertension, hypotension, palpitations, prolonged QT interval, PVCs, tachycardia, ventricular fibrillation
**EENT:** Blurred vision, vision changes
**GI:** Anorexia, diarrhea, nausea, vomiting
**HEME:** Agranulocytosis, anemia, aplastic anemia, bone marrow depression, hemolysis, leukopenia, neutropenia, thrombocytopenia
**RESP:** Pulmonary edema, fibrosis, and hypersensitivity (pneumonitis); respiratory arrest
**SKIN:** Diaphoresis, exfoliative dermatitis, pruritus, rash, skin lesions, urticaria

## Nursing Considerations
• Monitor CBC with differential weekly during first 3 months of tocainide treatment and routinely thereafter to detect blood dyscrasias. Although rare, agranulocytosis, anemia, aplastic anemia, bone marrow depression, hemolysis, leukopenia, neutropenia, or thrombocytopenia may be fatal. Expect findings to normalize about 1 month after therapy stops.
• Maintain continuous cardiac monitoring or obtain periodic ECG tracings, as ordered, to assess drug effectiveness.
• Assess for tremor, a possible sign of maximum dosing.
• Assess for additive adverse cardiac effects, especially if tocainide is used with another antiarrhythmic.
• Be aware that tocainide is secreted in breast milk and has the potential to cause serious adverse reactions in breast-feeding infants.

PATIENT TEACHING
• Inform patient that electrophysiologic studies may be performed before tocainide therapy starts.
• Instruct patient to notify prescriber about tremor because dosage may need to be adjusted.
• Explain that chest X-rays may be needed if adverse pulmonary reactions occur.
• Inform patient that ambulatory monitoring may be needed to verify antiarrhythmic response.
• Stress the importance of keeping all scheduled appointments for follow-up laboratory blood tests.

# tolazamide

Tolinase

## Class and Category

*Chemical:* First-generation sulfonylurea
*Therapeutic:* Antidiabetic
*Pregnancy category:* C

## Indications and Dosages

➤ *As adjunct to treat type 2 diabetes mellitus that's uncontrolled by diet and exercise*

**TABLETS**

**Adults.** *Initial:* 100 mg q.d. with breakfast if fasting blood glucose level is less than 200 mg/dl; 250 mg q.d. if fasting blood glucose level is more than 200 mg/dl. Dose adjusted q wk by 100 to 250 mg, if needed. Doses greater than 500 mg/day are divided and given q 12 hr. *Maximum:* 1,000 mg/day.

**DOSAGE ADJUSTMENT** If patient takes more than 40 U/day of insulin, initial dosage increased to 250 mg q.d. and insulin dosage decreased by 50%.

| Route | Onset | Peak | Duration |
|-------|-------|------|----------|
| P.O. | Unknown | 3 to 4 hr | 10 to 20 hr |

### Mechanism of Action

Stimulates insulin release from beta cells in the pancreas. Tolazamide also increases peripheral tissue sensitivity to insulin either by enhancing insulin binding to cellular receptors or by increasing the number of insulin receptors.

## Contraindications

Diabetic coma; diabetic ketoacidosis; hypersensitivity to tolazamide, sulfonylureas, or their components; pregnancy; sole therapy for type 1 diabetes mellitus

## Interactions

**DRUGS**

*ACE inhibitors, anabolic steroids, androgens, azole antifungals, bromocriptine, chloramphenicol, clofibrate, disopyramide, guanethidine, $H_2$-receptor antagonists, insulin, magnesium salts, MAO inhibitors, methyldopa, octreotide, oxyphenbutazone, phenylbutazone, probenecid, quinidine, salicylates, sulfonamides, tetracycline, theophylline, tricyclic antidepressants, urinary acidifiers:* Increased risk of hypoglycemia
*asparaginase, calcium channel blockers, cholestyramine, clonidine, corticosteroids, danazol, diazoxide, estrogen, glucagon, hydantoins, isoniazid, lithium, morphine, nicotinic acid, oral contraceptives, phenothiazines, rifabutin, rifampin, sympathomimetics, thiazide diuretics, thyroid drugs, urinary alkalizers:* Increased risk of hyperglycemia
*beta blockers:* Possibly hyperglycemia or masking of signs and symptoms of hypoglycemia
*digoxin:* Increased risk of digitalis toxicity
*pentamidine:* Initial hypoglycemia and then hyperglycemia if beta cell damage occurs

**ACTIVITIES**

*alcohol use:* Altered blood glucose control (usually hypoglycemia), possibly disulfiram-like reaction

## Adverse Reactions

**CNS:** Dizziness, fatigue, headache, malaise, paresthesia, vertigo
**ENDO:** Hypoglycemia
**GI:** Anorexia, cholestasis, heartburn, nausea, vomiting
**HEME:** Agranulocytosis, aplastic anemia, hemolysis, hemolytic anemia, leukopenia, thrombocytopenia
**MS:** Muscle weakness
**SKIN:** Erythema, photosensitivity, pruritus, rash, urticaria

## Nursing Considerations

• When switching an insulin-treated patient with type 2 diabetes, expect to start tolazamide at 100 mg q.d. if patient takes less than 20 U/day of insulin, or 250 mg q.d. if patient takes 20 to 40 U/day of insulin.
• Anticipate that patient receiving tolazamide may need temporary insulin treatment during periods of physiologic stress, such as fever, surgery, systemic infection, and trauma.
• For patient over age 65, expect to start tolazamide at 100 mg q.d.
• Assess elderly patients for signs of hypoglycemia because they're more susceptible to drug's hypoglycemic effect. Anticipate that hypoglycemia may be more difficult to detect.
• Assess patient with thyroid disease for altered blood glucose control because thy-

T

roid hormone increases GI absorption of glucose.

• Expect prescriber to stop tolazamide 2 weeks before pregnant patient delivers her neonate to minimize the risk of prolonged hypoglycemia in neonate.

**PATIENT TEACHING**

• Advise patient to avoid alcohol while taking tolazamide.

• Teach patient and family members how to monitor blood glucose level and how to recognize signs of hypoglycemia and hyperglycemia.

• Instruct patient to treat mild hypoglycemia with fruit juice or other simple sugars.

# tolbutamide

Apo-Tolbutamide (CAN), Novo-Butamide (CAN), Orinase

## Class and Category

*Chemical:* First-generation sulfonylurea
*Therapeutic:* Antidiabetic
*Pregnancy category:* C

## Indications and Dosages

➤ *As adjunct to treat type 2 diabetes mellitus that's uncontrolled by diet and exercise*

**TABLETS**

**Adults.** *Initial:* 1 to 2 g/day in divided doses b.i.d. or t.i.d. *Maintenance:* 0.25 to 2 g/day. *Maximum:* 3 g/day.

| Route | Onset | Peak | Duration |
|-------|-------|------|----------|
| P.O. | Unknown | 3 to 4 hr | 6 to 12 hr |

## Mechanism of Action

Stimulates insulin release from beta cells in the pancreas. Tolbutamide also increases peripheral tissue sensitivity to insulin either by enhancing insulin binding to cellular receptors or by increasing the number of insulin receptors.

## Contraindications

Diabetes complicated by pregnancy; diabetic coma; diabetic ketoacidosis; hypersensitivity to tolbutamide, sulfonylureas, or their components; sole therapy for type 1 diabetes mellitus

## Interactions

**DRUGS**

*ACE inhibitors, anabolic steroids, androgens, azole antifungals, bromocriptine, chloramphenicol, clofibrate, disopyramide, guanethidine, $H_2$-receptor antagonists, insulin, magnesium salts, MAO inhibitors, methyldopa, octreotide, oxyphenbutazone, phenylbutazone, probenecid, quinidine, salicylates, sulfonamides, tetracycline, theophylline, tricyclic antidepressants, urinary acidifiers:* Increased risk of hypoglycemia

*asparaginase, calcium channel blockers, cholestyramine, clonidine, corticosteroids, danazol, diazoxide, estrogen, glucagon, hydantoins, isoniazid, lithium, morphine, nicotinic acid, oral contraceptives, phenothiazines, rifabutin, rifampin, sympathomimetics, thiazide diuretics, thyroid drugs, urinary alkalizers:* Increased risk of hyperglycemia

*beta blockers:* Possibly hyperglycemia or masking of signs and symptoms of hypoglycemia

*digoxin:* Increased risk of digitalis toxicity
*pentamidine:* Initial hypoglycemia and then hyperglycemia if beta cell damage occurs

**ACTIVITIES**

*alcohol use:* Altered blood glucose control (usually hypoglycemia), possibly disulfiram-like reaction

## Adverse Reactions

**CNS:** Dizziness, fatigue, headache, malaise, paresthesia, vertigo

**ENDO:** Hypoglycemia

**GI:** Anorexia, cholestasis, heartburn, nausea, vomiting

**HEME:** Agranulocytosis, aplastic anemia, hemolysis, hemolytic anemia, leukopenia, thrombocytopenia

**MS:** Muscle weakness

**SKIN:** Erythema, photosensitivity, pruritus, rash, urticaria

## Nursing Considerations

• If patient takes 20 U or less of insulin/day, expect a possible transfer from insulin to tolbutamide therapy. If patient takes more than 20 U of insulin/day, expect to reduce insulin dosage as tolbutamide therapy starts.

• Anticipate that patient receiving tolbutamide may need temporary insulin treatment during periods of physiologic stress, such as fever, surgery, systemic infection, or trauma.

•Assess elderly patients for signs of hypoglycemia because they're more susceptible to drug's hypoglycemic effect. Anticipate that hypoglycemia may be more difficult to detect.

•Assess patient with thyroid disease for altered blood glucose control because thyroid hormone increases GI absorption of glucose.

•Expect prescriber to stop tolbutamide 2 weeks before pregnant patient delivers her neonate to minimize the risk of prolonged hypoglycemia in neonate.

**PATIENT TEACHING**

•Advise patient to avoid alcohol while taking tolbutamide.

•Teach patient and family members how to monitor blood glucose level and how to recognize signs of hypoglycemia and hyperglycemia.

•Instruct patient to treat mild hypoglycemia with fruit juice or other simple sugars.

# tolcapone

Tasmar

## Class and Category
*Chemical:* Nitrobenzophenone
*Therapeutic:* Antidyskinetic
*Pregnancy category:* C

## Indications and Dosages

➤ *As adjunct (with levodopa and carbidopa) to treat Parkinson's disease*

**TABLETS**

**Adults.** *Initial:* 100 mg t.i.d. *Maximum:* 200 mg t.i.d.

---

## Mechanism of Action

Prolongs plasma half-life of levodopa by inhibiting catechol-*O*-methyltransferase (COMT), an enzyme responsible for metabolizing catecholamines—including dopa, dopamine, epinephrine, norepinephrine, and their hydroxylated metabolites. COMT inhibition reduces the amount of metabolizing enzyme for levodopa, which results in a more sustained plasma levodopa level. This action makes more levodopa available for diffusion into the CNS, where it is converted to dopamine.

---

## Contraindications
Confusion, hyperpyrexia, or rhabdomyolysis with previous use of tolcapone; hepatic dysfunction; hypersensitivity to tolcapone or its components

## Interactions
**DRUGS**
*desipramine:* Possibly increased frequency of adverse effects
*levodopa:* Increased levodopa bioavailability, with increased risk of orthostatic hypotension and syncope
*MAO inhibitors:* Possibly inhibited catecholamine metabolism

## Adverse Reactions
**CNS:** Confusion, dizziness, drowsiness, dyskinesia, fatigue, fever, hallucinations, headache, lethargy, loss of balance
**CV:** Chest pain, orthostatic hypotension
**EENT:** Dry mouth
**GI:** Abdominal pain, anorexia, cholestasis, constipation, diarrhea, elevated liver function test results, vomiting
**GU:** Bright yellow urine, hematuria
**MS:** Muscle cramps, rhabdomyolysis
**RESP:** Dyspnea, upper respiratory tract infection
**SKIN:** Diaphoresis, jaundice

## Nursing Considerations
•Monitor liver function test results, as ordered, during tolcapone therapy to detect hepatic impairment.

•Assess for hallucinations, especially in patient over age 75.

•Anticipate that drug may precipitate or exaggerate preexisting dyskinesia.

•Expect tolcapone to be discontinued if no improvement occurs after 3 weeks of therapy.

**PATIENT TEACHING**

•Inform patient that urine may turn bright yellow during tolcapone therapy.

•Advise patient to avoid potentially hazardous activities until drug's CNS effects are known.

•Urge patient to notify prescriber immediately about darkened urine, decreased appetite, fatigue, jaundice, lethargy, and right-sided abdominal pain.

•Caution patient not to stop taking drug abruptly. Explain that prescriber will supervise tapering of drug dosage.

•Urge patient to have regular follow-up appointments and laboratory tests.

T

# tolmetin

Novo-Tolmetin (CAN), Tolectin DS, Tolectin 200, Tolectin 400 (CAN), Tolectin 600

## Class and Category

*Chemical:* Pyrroleacetic acid derivative
*Therapeutic:* Anti-inflammatory
*Pregnancy category:* C (first trimester), Not rated (later trimesters)

## Indications and Dosages

➤ *To relieve moderate pain from rheumatoid arthritis and osteoarthritis*

CAPSULES, TABLETS

**Adults.** *Initial:* 400 mg t.i.d. *Maintenance:* 600 to 1,800 mg/day in divided doses t.i.d. or q.i.d. *Maximum:* 2,000 mg/day for rheumatoid arthritis, 1,600 mg/day for osteoarthritis.

➤ *To treat juvenile rheumatoid arthritis*

CAPSULES, TABLETS

**Children over age 2.** *Initial:* 20 mg/kg/day in divided doses t.i.d. or q.i.d. *Maintenance:* 15 to 30 mg/kg/day in divided doses. *Maximum:* 30 mg/kg/day.

| Route | Onset | Peak | Duration |
|-------|-------|------|----------|
| P.O. | Unknown | 1 to 2 wk | Unknown |

### Mechanism of Action

Blocks the activity of cyclooxygenase, the enzyme needed to synthesize prostaglandins, which mediate the inflammatory response and cause local vasodilation, swelling, and pain. Prostaglandins also promote pain transmission from the periphery to the spinal cord. By blocking cyclooxygenase and inhibiting prostaglandins, tolmetin reduces inflammatory symptoms and relieves pain.

## Contraindications

Angioedema, asthma, bronchospasm, nasal polyps, rhinitis, or urticaria caused by aspirin, iodides, or other NSAIDs

## Interactions

DRUGS

*ACE inhibitors, beta blockers:* Decreased effectiveness of these drugs, possibly reduced renal function
*alendronate, corticosteroids, other NSAIDs, salicylates:* Increased risk of adverse GI effects
*anticoagulants, platelet aggregation inhibitors, thrombolytics:* Additive inhibition of platelet aggregation; prolonged bleeding time
*antineoplastics, antithymocyte globulin, strontium-89 chloride:* Increased risk of bleeding
*cidofovir:* Possibly nephrotoxicity
*cyclosporine:* Potentiated cyclosporine nephrotoxicity
*digoxin:* Increased blood digoxin level
*lithium:* Possibly lithium toxicity
*methotrexate:* Increased or prolonged blood methotrexate level

ACTIVITIES

*alcohol use:* Increased risk of adverse GI effects

## Adverse Reactions

**CNS:** Aseptic meningitis, cerebral hemorrhage, ischemic CVA, depression, dizziness, drowsiness, fatigue, headache, transient ischemic attack, weakness
**CV:** Chest pain, deep vein thrombosis, edema, hypertension, MI, peripheral edema
**EENT:** Tinnitus
**ENDO:** Hypoglycemia
**GI:** Abdominal pain; constipation; diarrhea; elevated liver function test results; flatulence; gastritis; GI bleeding, perforation, or ulceration; hepatitis; indigestion; jaundice; liver failure; nausea; peptic ulcer disease; vomiting
**GU:** Acute renal failure, dysuria, elevated BUN level, hematuria, interstitial nephritis, nephrotic syndrome, nephrotoxicity, proteinuria, UTI
**HEME:** Agranulocytosis, aplastic anemia, hemolytic anemia, leukopenia, pancytopenia, prolonged bleeding time
**SKIN:** Erythema multiforme, exfoliative dermatitis, maculopapular rash, Stevens-Johnson syndrome, toxic epidermal necrolysis, urticaria
**Other:** Anaphylaxis, angioedema, weight gain or loss

## Nursing Considerations

•Give tolmetin with food or milk to reduce adverse GI reactions.
•Assess patient for improvement within 7 days and progressive improvement over several successive weeks.
•Use tolmetin with extreme caution in patients with a history of ulcer disease or GI bleeding because NSAIDs such as tolmetin increase the risk of GI bleeding and ulcera-

tion. Expect to use tolmetin for the shortest time possible in these patients.

•Be aware that serious GI tract ulceration, bleeding, and perforation may occur without warning symptoms. Elderly patients are at greater risk. To minimize risk, give drug with food. If GI distress occurs, withhold drug and notify prescriber immediately.

•Use tolmetin cautiously in patients with hypertension, and monitor blood pressure closely throughout therapy. Drug may cause hypertension or worsen it.

•WARNING Monitor patient closely for thrombotic events, including MI and stroke, because NSAIDs increase the risk.

•WARNING If patient has bone marrow suppression or is receiving antineoplastic drug therapy, monitor laboratory results (including WBC count), and watch for evidence of infection because anti-inflammatory and antipyretic actions of tolmetin may mask signs and symptoms, such as fever and pain.

•Especially if patient is elderly or taking tolmetin long-term, watch for less common but serious adverse GI reactions, including anorexia, constipation, diverticulitis, dysphagia, esophagitis, gastritis, gastroenteritis, gastroesophageal reflux disease, hemorrhoids, hiatal hernia, melena, stomatitis, and vomiting.

•Monitor liver function test results because, in rare cases, elevated levels may progress to severe hepatic reactions, including fatal hepatitis, liver necrosis, and hepatic failure.

•Monitor BUN and serum creatinine levels in patients with heart failure, impaired renal function, or hepatic dysfunction; those taking diuretics or ACE inhibitors; and elderly patients because drug may cause renal failure.

•Monitor CBC for decreased hemoglobin and hematocrit because drug may worsen anemia.

•Assess patient's skin routinely for rash or other signs of hypersensitivity reaction because tolmetin and other NSAIDs may cause serious skin reactions without warning, even in patients with no history of NSAID hypersensitivity. Stop drug at first sign of reaction, and notify prescriber.

•Assess invasive sites or wounds for bleeding and bruising from drug's effects on platelets.

**PATIENT TEACHING**

•Tell patient to take drug with food or milk.

•Urge patient to limit sodium intake because drug may cause fluid retention.

•Tell patient to avoid alcohol during therapy.

•Teach patient how to perform proper oral hygiene, and advise her to have needed dental work done before tolmetin therapy starts because of the increased risk of bleeding.

•Explain that tolmetin may increase the risk of serious adverse cardiovascular reactions; urge patient to seek immediate medical attention if signs or symptoms arise, such as chest pain, shortness of breath, weakness, and slurring of speech.

•Tell patient that tolmetin also may increase the risk of serious adverse GI reactions; stress the importance of seeking immediate medical attention for such signs and symptoms as epigastric or abdominal pain, indigestion, black or tarry stools, or vomiting blood or material that looks like coffee grounds.

•Alert patient to the possibility of rare but serious skin reactions. Urge her to seek immediate medical attention for rash, blisters, itching, fever, or other indications of hypersensitivity.

# tolterodine tartrate

Detrol, Detrol LA

## Class and Category

*Chemical:* Prodrug of 5-hydroxymethyl-tolterodine
*Therapeutic:* Antispasmodic
*Pregnancy category:* C

## Indications and Dosages

➤ *To treat overactive bladder*

**TABLETS**

**Adults.** 2 mg b.i.d. Reduced to 1 mg b.i.d. based on patient response and tolerance.

DOSAGE ADJUSTMENT Dosage reduced to 1 mg b.i.d. for patients with significant hepatic dysfunction and for patients who are also receiving cytochrome P450 3A4 inhibitors, such as clarithromycin, erythromycin, and the antifungals itraconazole, ketoconazole, and miconazole.

**E.R. TABLETS**

**Adults.** 4 mg q.d. Reduced to 2 mg q.d. based on individual response and tolerance.

## Contraindications

Gastric retention, hypersensitivity to tolterodine tartrate or its components, uncontrolled angle-closure glaucoma, urine retention

**T**

## Mechanism of Action
Exerts antimuscarinic (atropine-like) and potent direct antispasmodic (papaverine-like) actions on smooth muscle in the bladder, which decreases detrusor muscle contractions. This helps reduce urinary frequency and urgency as well as urge-related incontinence.

## Interactions
**DRUGS**
*clarithromycin, erythromycin, itraconazole, ketoconazole, miconazole:* Possibly increased blood tolterodine level
*fluoxetine:* Possibly decreased tolterodine metabolism

## Adverse Reactions
**CNS:** Dizziness, fatigue, hallucinations, headache, somnolence
**CV:** Chest pain, edema, hypertension, palpitations, tachycardia
**EENT:** Abnormal vision, dry eyes, dry mouth
**GI:** Abdominal pain, constipation, diarrhea, flatulence, indigestion, nausea
**GU:** Dysuria, urine retention, UTI
**Other:** Anaphylaxis, angioedema, flulike symptoms

## Nursing Considerations
•**WARNING** Monitor patients with a history of bladder outflow obstruction for decreased urine output or bladder distention because tolterodine poses a risk of urine retention.
•Monitor patients with a history of GI obstructive disorders, such as pyloric stenosis, for abdominal distention or bloating because of increased risk of gastric retention.
•Be aware that drug's antimuscarinic effects may produce blurred vision, dizziness, and drowsiness. If these occur, institute fall precautions according to institution policy.
**PATIENT TEACHING**
•Instruct patient taking tolterodine to immediately report to prescriber difficulty urinating or infrequent urination.
•Advise patient not to drive or perform activities that require high level of alertness until drug's CNS and vision effects are known. Instruct her to notify prescriber if dizziness or blurred vision persists.
•Encourage patient to use sugarless candy, gum, or ice to relieve dry mouth. Advise her to notify prescriber or dentist if dry mouth persists or worsens over 2 weeks.

# topiramate
Topamax

## Class and Category
*Chemical:* Sulfamate-substituted monosaccharide
*Therapeutic:* Anticonvulsant
*Pregnancy category:* C

## Indications and Dosages
➤ *To treat partial-onset or primary generalized tonic-clonic seizures*
**CAPSULES**
**Adults and chidlren age 10 and older.** *Initial:* 25 mg b.i.d. in morning and evening. Increased by 50 mg/day q wk. *Maintenance:* 200 mg b.i.d. in morning and evening.
➤ *As adjunct to treat partial seizures and primary generalized tonic-clonic seizures*
**CAPSULES, TABLETS**
**Adults and adolescents age 17 and older.** *Initial:* 25 to 50 mg/day in divided doses b.i.d. for 1 wk. Increased by 25 to 50 mg/day q wk. *Maintenance:* 200 to 400 mg/day in divided doses b.i.d. *Maximum:* 1,600 mg/day.
**Children ages 2 to 16.** *Initial:* 25 mg or less q h.s. for 1 wk. Increased q 1 to 2 wk by 1 to 3 mg/kg/day in divided doses q 12 hr, as prescribed. *Usual:* 5 to 9 mg/kg/day in divided doses q 12 hr.
➤ *As adjunct to treat seizures associated with Lennox-Gastaut syndrome*
**CAPSULES, TABLETS**
**Children ages 2 to 16.** 25 mg h.s. for 1 wk. Increased q 1 to 2 wk by 1 to 3 mg/kg/day in divided doses q 12 hr, as prescribed. *Usual:* 5 to 9 mg/kg/day in divided doses q 12 hr.
➤ *To prevent migraine headache*
**CAPSULES, TABLETS**
**Adults.** *Initial:* 25 mg q.d. in evening for 1 wk; then 25 mg b.i.d. for 1 wk; then 25 mg in morning and 50 mg in evening for 1 wk. *Maintenance:* 50 mg b.i.d.
**DOSAGE ADJUSTMENT** For patients with moderate to severe renal impairment, dosage possibly reduced by 50%.

## Contraindications
Hypersensitivity to topiramate or its components

## Mechanism of Action

May block the spread of seizures by reducing the length and frequency of excitatory transmission. Topiramate increases the availability of the inhibitory neurotransmitter gamma-aminobutyric acid by blocking voltage-sensitive sodium channels. This action promotes the movement of chloride ions into neurons.

## Interactions

**DRUGS**

*antihistamines, barbiturates, benzodiazepines, CNS depressants, opioid analgesics, skeletal muscle relaxants, tricyclic antidepressants:* Additive CNS depression
*carbamazepine:* Decreased blood topiramate level
*carbonic anhydrase inhibitors:* Increased risk of renal calculus formation
*digoxin:* Possibly decreased blood digoxin level
*ethinyl estradiol:* Increased risk of breakthrough bleeding
*oral contraceptives:* Increased risk of breakthrough bleeding, decreased contraceptive efficacy
*phenobarbital:* Altered blood phenobarbital level
*phenytoin:* Decreased blood level of topiramate
*probenecid:* Possibly blocked renal tubular reabsorption of topiramate and decreased blood topiramate level
*valproic acid:* Decreased blood levels of both drugs

**ACTIVITIES**

*alcohol use:* Additive CNS depression

## Adverse Reactions

**CNS:** Agitation, anxiety, asthenia, ataxia, confusion, decreased concentration, depression, dizziness, fatigue, fever, hallucinations, headache, hyperthermia, hypoesthesia, insomnia, irritability, memory loss, mood changes, nervousness, paresthesia, psychomotor slowing, psychosis, slurred speech, somnolence, suicidal ideology, syncope, tremor
**CV:** Cardiac arrest, chest pain, hot flashes, hypertension, hypotension, palpitations, vasodilation
**EENT:** Diplopia, dry mouth, gingivitis, hearing loss, nystagmus, pharyngitis, rhinitis, secondary angle-closure glaucoma with acute myopia, sinusitis, taste perversion, tinnitus, tongue edema, vision changes
**ENDO:** Breast pain, hyperglycemia
**GI:** Abdominal pain, anorexia, constipation, diarrhea, flatulence, gastroenteritis, gastroesophageal reflux, hepatic failure, hepatitis, indigestion, nausea, pancreatitis, vomiting
**GU:** Cystitis, decreased libido, dysmenorrhea, dysuria, frequent urination, impotence, menstrual irregularities, renal calculi, renal tubular acidosis, UTI, vaginitis
**HEME:** Anemia, leukopenia
**MS:** Arthralgia, back pain, leg cramps or pain, muscle weakness
**RESP:** Bronchitis, cough, dyspnea, pulmonary embolism, upper respiratory tract infection
**SKIN:** Acne, alopecia, decreased sweating, erythema multiforme, pemphigus, pruritus, rash, Stevens-Johnson syndrome, toxic epidermal necrolysis
**Other:** Dehydration, metabolic acidosis, weight gain or loss

## Nursing Considerations

•Obtain baseline serum bicarbonate level before topiramate therapy and monitor periodically throughout therapy, as ordered.
•Give capsule with water and have patient swallow it whole. If needed, open capsules and empty contents onto a spoonful of soft food. Discard unused portion.
•Never store food sprinkled with drug for use at a later time.
•**WARNING** Anticipate an increase in seizures if therapy stops abruptly. Take seizure precautions, as appropriate.
•If patient reports ocular pain or decreased visual acuity, notify prescriber immediately; topiramate may cause increased intraocular pressure and secondary angle-closure glaucoma. Expect to discontinue drug immediately.
•If patient has a history of renal calculi, assess for signs of recurrence.

**PATIENT TEACHING**

•Instruct patient to swallow topiramate tablets whole.
•Urge patient to avoid potentially hazardous activities until drug's CNS effects are known.
•Advise patient to watch for decreased sweating and significantly increased body temperature, especially during hot weather,

and to notify prescriber immediately if they occur.

• Tell patient to maintain adequate fluid intake to minimize the risk of developing kidney stones.

• Advise female patient of possible breakthrough bleeding. If she takes an oral contraceptive, encourage her to use another form of contraception during therapy.

# torsemide

Demadex

## Class and Category

*Chemical:* Anilinopyridine sulfonylurea derivative
*Therapeutic:* Antihypertensive, diuretic
*Pregnancy category:* B

## Indications and Dosages

➤ *To treat edema in heart failure*

TABLETS, I.V. INJECTION

**Adults.** *Initial:* 10 to 20 mg q.d., adjusted by doubling, as prescribed, to achieve desired effect. *Maximum:* 200 mg q.d.

➤ *To treat edema in chronic renal failure*

TABLETS, I.V. INJECTION

**Adults.** *Initial:* 20 mg q.d., adjusted by doubling, as prescribed, to achieve desired effect. *Maximum:* 200 mg q.d.

➤ *To treat ascites, alone or with amiloride or spironolactone*

TABLETS, I.V. INJECTION

**Adults.** *Initial:* 5 to 10 mg q.d. *Maximum:* 40 mg q.d.

➤ *To manage hypertension*

TABLETS

**Adults.** *Initial:* 5 mg q.d., increased to 10 mg q.d. after 4 to 6 wk, as prescribed, if response is inadequate. *Maximum:* 10 mg q.d.

| Route | Onset | Peak | Duration |
|---|---|---|---|
| P.O. | 1 hr | 1 to 2 hr | 6 to 8 hr |
| I.V. | 10 min | 1 hr | 6 to 8 hr |

## Contraindications

Hypersensitivity to torsemide, sulfonamides, or their components

## Interactions

DRUGS

*ACE inhibitors, antihypertensives:* Additive hypotension

*amiloride, spironolactone, triamterene:* Possibly counteracted torsemide-induced hypokalemia

*amphotericin B:* Increased risk of nephrotoxicity and severe, prolonged hypokalemia or hypomagnesemia

*cisplatin:* Increased risk of significant hypokalemia or hypomagnesemia, possibly permanent ototoxicity

*cortisone, fluorocortisone, hydrocortisone:* Increased risk of sodium retention and hypokalemia

*digoxin:* Increased risk of arrhythmias and digitalis toxicity due to hypokalemia or hypomagnesemia

*indomethacin:* Possibly decreased diuretic and antihypertensive effects of torsemide and increased risk of renal failure

*lithium:* Possibly lithium toxicity

*metolazone, thiazide diuretics:* Increased risk of severe fluid and electrolyte loss

*neuromuscular blockers:* Possibly increased neuromuscular blockade due to hypokalemia

*probenecid:* Possibly decreased diuretic effect of torsemide

*quinidine and other ototoxic drugs:* Increased risk of ototoxicity

*salicylates:* Increased risk of salicylate toxicity

ACTIVITIES

*alcohol use:* Additive diuresis and, possibly, dehydration

---

## Mechanism of Action

Blocks active sodium and chloride reabsorption in the ascending loop of Henle by promoting rapid excretion of water, sodium, and chloride. Torsemide also increases the production of renal prostaglandins, increasing the plasma renin level and renal vasodilation. As a result, blood pressure falls, reducing preload and afterload.

---

## Adverse Reactions

**CNS:** Dizziness, drowsiness, fatigue, headache, insomnia, lethargy, nervousness, restlessness, weakness

**CV:** Chest pain, ECG abnormalities, edema, hypotension, tachycardia

**EENT:** Dry mouth, hearing loss, ototoxicity, pharyngitis, rhinitis, tinnitus

**GI:** Constipation, diarrhea, indigestion, nausea, thirst, vomiting

**GU:** Azotemia (prerenal), oliguria, urinary frequency

**MS:** Muscle spasms, myalgia
**RESP:** Cough
**Other:** Hypochloremia, hypokalemia, hypo-magnesemia, hyponatremia, hypovolemia

## Nursing Considerations
•Inject I.V. torsemide slowly over 2 minutes. Flush I.V. line with NS before and afterward.
•Don't exceed 200 mg in a single I.V. dose.
•Monitor serum electrolyte levels and fluid intake and output to detect hypovolemia.
•WARNING Expect torsemide-induced electrolyte imbalances, such as hypokalemia and hypomagnesemia, to increase the risk of toxicity and fatal arrhythmias in a patient who takes a digitalis glycoside. Hypokalemia also potentiates neuromuscular blockade effects of nondepolarizing neuromuscular blockers.

### PATIENT TEACHING
•Advise patient to change position slowly to minimize effects of orthostatic hypotension.
•Instruct patient to notify prescriber at once about drowsiness, dry mouth, hearing changes, lethargy, muscle pain, nausea, restlessness, thirst, vomiting, or weakness.
•Advise diabetic patient to monitor her blood glucose level often because drug may raise it.


# tramadol hydrochloride

Ultram

## Class and Category
*Chemical:* Cyclohexanol
*Therapeutic:* Analgesic
*Pregnancy category:* C

## Indications and Dosages
➤ *To relieve moderate to moderately severe pain*

### TABLETS
**Adults and adolescents over age 16.** 50 to 100 mg q 4 to 6 hr, p.r.n. *Maximum:* 400 mg/day.
DOSAGE ADJUSTMENT If patient has hepatic impairment, dosage reduced to 50 mg q 12 hr. If patient is age 75 or older, maximum dosage reduced to 300 mg/day. If creatinine clearance is 30 ml/min/1.73 m$^2$ or less, interval increased to q 12 hr and maximum dosage limited to 200 mg/day.

| Route | Onset | Peak | Duration |
|-------|-------|------|----------|
| P.O. | 1 hr | 2 to 3 hr | 7 to 14 hr |

## Mechanism of Action
Binds with mu receptors and inhibits the reuptake of norepinephrine and serotonin, which may account for tramadol's analgesic effect.

## Contraindications
Alcohol intoxication; excessive use of central-acting analgesics, hypnotics, opioids, or other psychotropic drugs; hypersensitivity to tramadol or its components; use within 14 days of MAO inhibitor therapy

## Interactions
### DRUGS
*amiodarone, cimetidine, clomipramine, desipramine, fluphenazine, haloperidol, propafenone, quinidine, ritonavir, thioridazine:* Decreased analgesia, increased adverse effects of tramadol
*amphetamines, antipsychotics, bupropion, cyclobenzaprine, dextroamphetamine, MAO inhibitors, naloxone, tricyclic antidepressants:* Increased risk of seizures
*barbiturates, benzodiazepines, opioid analgesics, sedative-hypnotics, tranquilizers:* Additive CNS depression
*carbamazepine:* Increased tramadol metabolism
*general anesthetics:* Increased CNS and respiratory depression
*phenothiazines, rifampin:* Additive CNS depression, increased risk of seizures
*selective serotonin-reuptake inhibitors:* Increased risk of serotonin syndrome and seizures
*warfarin:* Possibly increased INR
### ACTIVITIES
*alcohol use:* Additive CNS depression

## Adverse Reactions
**CNS:** Agitation, dizziness, emotional lability, euphoria, fatigue, hallucinations, headache, hypertonia, nervousness, somnolence, tremor, vertigo, weakness
**CV:** Vasodilation
**EENT:** Dry mouth, vision changes
**GI:** Anorexia, constipation, diarrhea, indigestion, nausea, vomiting
**GU:** Urinary frequency, urine retention
**SKIN:** Diaphoresis, pruritus, rash
**Other:** Physical and psychological dependence

## Nursing Considerations
•Be aware that tramadol shouldn't be given

T

to patients with a history of anaphylactoid reactions to codeine or other opioids.

• Because tramadol may lead to physical and psychological dependence, assess patient for evidence of dependence or abuse. Avoid giving drug to patients with a history of dependence on other opioids.

• Avoid giving tramadol to patients with acute abdominal conditions because it may mask evidence and disrupt assessment of the abdomen.

• After patient receives first dose, watch for allergic reactions, including angioedema, bronchospasm, pruritus, Stevens-Johnson syndrome, toxic epidermal necrolysis, and urticaria. Also watch for evidence of anaphylaxis, such as dyspnea and hypotension.

• If patient has respiratory depression, assess respiratory status often, and expect to give a nonopioid analgesic—not tramadol.

• If patient develops respiratory depression, expect to give naloxone. Watch for seizures because naloxone may increase this risk. Take seizure precautions.

• Assess respiratory status often if patient has increased intracranial pressure or head injury because of possible increased carbon dioxide retention and CSF pressure, either of which may cause respiratory depression. Also, be aware that tramadol may constrict pupils, obscuring evidence of intracranial complications.

• **WARNING** Watch for seizures in patients with epilepsy, a history of seizures, or an increased risk of seizures, such as those with head injury, metabolic disorders, alcohol or drug withdrawal, or CNS infection.

• Expect to taper tramadol rather than stopping it abruptly to avoid such acute withdrawal symptoms as anxiety, diarrhea, insomnia, nausea, pain, panic attacks, paresthesias, piloerection, rigors, sweating, tremor, and upper respiratory symptoms.

**PATIENT TEACHING**

• Urge patient to follow prescribed dose limits and dosing intervals to prevent respiratory depression and seizures.

• Caution patient not to stop drug abruptly.

• Instruct patient to avoid hazardous activities until drug's CNS effects are known.

• Advise patient to avoid alcohol while taking tramadol.

• Urge patient to notify prescriber about known, suspected, or intended pregnancy.

# tramadol hydrochloride and acetaminophen

Ultracet

## Class and Category

*Chemical:* Cyclohexanol (tramadol), aminophenol derivative (acetaminophen)
*Therapeutic:* Opioid analgesic (tramadol), nonnarcotic analgesic (acetaminophen)
*Pregnancy category:* C

## Indications and Dosages

➤ *To provide short-term management of acute pain*

**TABLETS**

**Adults.** *Initial:* 75 mg tramadol and 650 mg acetaminophen q 4 to 6 hr, p.r.n. *Maximum:* 300 mg tramadol and 2,600 mg acetaminophen/day for up to 5 days.

**DOSAGE ADJUSTMENT** Dosing interval increased to 12 hr and maximum dose reduced to 75 mg tramadol and 650 mg acetaminophen/dose in patients with creatinine clearance of less than 30 ml/min/1.73 m².

| Route | Onset | Peak | Duration |
|-------|-------|------|----------|
| P.O. | In 1 hr | Unknown | Unknown |

## Mechanism of Action

Tramadol binds with mu receptors and inhibits the reuptake of norepinephrine and serotonin, which may account for the drug's analgesic effect. Acetaminophen blocks the activity of cyclooxygenase, an enzyme necessary for prostaglandin synthesis. Prostaglandins are important mediators of the inflammatory response that cause local vasodilation, swelling, and pain.

## Contraindications

Acute intoxication with alcohol, centrally acting analgesics, hypnotics, narcotics, opioids, or psychotropic drugs; hypersensitivity to tramadol, other opioids, acetaminophen, or components of these drugs

## Interactions

**DRUGS**

*acetaminophen-containing products:* Increased risk of hepatotoxicity
*carbamazepine:* Increased metabolism of tramadol and increased risk of seizures; possibly

significantly reduced analgesic effect of tramadol

*CNS depressants:* Increased risk of CNS and respiratory depression

*cytochrome P450 2D6 inhibitors, such as amitriptyline, fluoxetine, and paroxetine:* Possibly inhibited tramadol metabolism

*digoxin:* Possibly digitalis toxicity, although rare

*MAO inhibitors, selective serotonin reuptake inhibitors:* Increased risk of seizures and serotonin syndrome

*neuroleptics, opioids, tricyclic antidepressants:* Increased risk of seizures

*quinidine:* Increased blood tramadol level

*warfarin:* Possibly elevated PT and altered effects of warfarin

**FOODS**

*any food:* Possibly delayed peak plasma time

**ACTIVITIES**

*alcohol use:* Increased risk of CNS and respiratory depression

## Adverse Reactions

**CNS:** Dizziness, insomnia, seizures, somnolence

**EENT:** Dry mouth

**GI:** Anorexia, constipation, diarrhea, hepatotoxicity, nausea

**GU:** Prostate disorder

**RESP:** Respiratory depression

**SKIN:** Increased sweating, pruritus

**Other:** Hypersensitivity, physical and psychological dependence

## Nursing Considerations

•Be aware that tramadol and acetaminophen shouldn't be given to patients with a history of anaphylactoid reactions to codeine or other opioid analgesics.

•Avoid giving tramadol and acetaminophen to patients with acute abdominal conditions because drug may mask signs and symptoms and disrupt assessment of the abdomen.

•Monitor liver function test results, as appropriate, and notify prescriber of abnormal results. This drug combination isn't recommended for patients with hepatic impairment.

•After patient receives first dose, watch for allergic reactions, including angioedema, bronchospasm, pruritus, Stevens-Johnson syndrome, toxic epidermal necrolysis, and urticaria. Also watch for evidence of anaphylaxis, such as dyspnea and hypotension.

•If patient has respiratory depression, assess respiratory status often, and expect to give a nonopioid analgesic—not tramadol and acetaminophen.

•If patient develops respiratory depression, expect to give naloxone. Watch for seizures, because naloxone may increase this risk. Take seizure precautions.

•Assess respiratory status often if patient has increased intracranial pressure or head injury because of possible increased carbon dioxide retention and CSF pressure, either of which may cause respiratory depression. Also, be aware that tramadol may constrict pupils, obscuring evidence of intracranial complications.

•**WARNING** Watch for seizures in patients with epilepsy, a history of seizures, or an increased risk of seizures, such as those with head injury, metabolic disorders, alcohol or drug withdrawal, or CNS infection.

•Expect to taper dosage rather than stopping drug abruptly to avoid such acute withdrawal symptoms as anxiety, diarrhea, insomnia, nausea, pain, panic attacks, paresthesia, piloerection, rigors, sweating, tremor, and upper respiratory symptoms.

•Because tramadol and acetaminophen may lead to physical and psychological dependence and abuse, assess patient for evidence of dependence or abuse, such as drug-seeking behavior. Be aware that drug shouldn't be used in patients with a history of dependence on other opioids because dependence may recur.

**PATIENT TEACHING**

•Caution patient that taking more of this drug than prescribed or taking it more often than prescribed can lead to serious adverse reactions, including respiratory depression, seizures, hepatotoxicity, and death.

•Caution patient not to stop drug abruptly.

•Tell patient to avoid potentially hazardous activities until drug's adverse effects are known.

•Warn patient to avoid alcohol while taking tramadol and acetaminophen.

•Warn patient to avoid other drugs that contain tramadol or acetaminophen, including OTC preparations.

•Urge patient to notify prescriber if she becomes pregnant, thinks she might be pregnant, or is trying to become pregnant.

T

# trandolapril

Mavik

## Class and Category

*Chemical:* ACE inhibitor (non-sulfhydryl-containing)
*Therapeutic:* Antihypertensive, vasodilator
*Pregnancy category:* C (first trimester), D (later trimesters)

## Indications and Dosages

➤ *To manage hypertension*

**TABLETS**

**Adults.** *Initial:* 1 mg q.d., increased q wk based on clinical response. Dosage may be given in two daily doses if antihypertensive effect diminishes before 24 hr. *Usual:* 2 to 4 mg/day. *Maximum:* 8 mg/day.

**DOSAGE ADJUSTMENT** Initial dosage increased to 2 mg q.d. for blacks with hypertension. Initial dosage reduced to 0.5 mg for patients also receiving a diuretic, those with a creatinine clearance of less than or equal to 30 ml/min/1.73 m$^2$, and those with cirrhosis.

➤ *To treat heart failure after MI*

**TABLETS**

**Adults.** *Initial:* 1 mg q.d. *Usual:* 4 mg or more q.d. *Maximum:* 8 mg/day.

| Route | Onset | Peak | Duration |
|-------|-------|------|----------|
| P.O. | 2 hr | 8 hr | 24 hr |

## Mechanism of Action

Reduces blood pressure by inhibiting the conversion of angiotensin I to angiotensin II. Angiotensin II is a potent vasoconstrictor that stimulates the renal cortex to secrete aldosterone. Decreased release of aldosterone reduces sodium and water retention and increases their excretion, thereby reducing blood pressure. Trandolapril may also inhibit renal and vascular production of angiotensin II.

## Contraindications

History of angioedema related to previous treatment with ACE inhibitor, hypersensitivity to trandolapril or its components

## Interactions

**DRUGS**

*allopurinol, bone marrow depressants (such as methotrexate), corticosteroids (systemic),*
*cytostatic drugs, procainamide:* Increased risk of potentially fatal neutropenia or agranulocytosis
*antacids:* Decreased blood trandolapril level
*cyclosporine, potassium-containing drugs, potassium-sparing diuretics, potassium supplements:* Increased risk of hyperkalemia
*diuretics, other antihypertensives:* Increased hypotensive effects
*lithium:* Increased blood lithium level and risk of lithium toxicity
*NSAIDs, sympathomimetics:* Possibly reduced antihypertensive effects

**FOODS**

*high-potassium diet, low-sodium milk, potassium-containing salt substitutes:* Increased risk of hyperkalemia

**ACTIVITIES**

*alcohol use:* Possibly increased hypotensive effect

## Adverse Reactions

**CNS:** Dizziness, fatigue, fever, headache
**CV:** Hypotension, orthostatic hypotension
**EENT:** Loss of taste
**GI:** Diarrhea, nausea
**GU:** Decreased libido, impotence
**MS:** Myalgia
**RESP:** Cough, dyspnea, upper respiratory tract infection
**SKIN:** Pruritus, rash
**Other:** Angioedema

## Nursing Considerations

•**WARNING** Closely monitor blood pressure during first 2 weeks of trandolapril therapy and whenever dosage is adjusted, especially in patients with heart failure, hyponatremia, or severe volume or sodium loss. If excessive hypotension occurs, notify prescriber immediately, place patient in supine position, and prepare to infuse I.V. normal saline solution, as prescribed.
•**WARNING** Be alert for signs and symptoms of angioedema. If swelling of tongue, glottis, or larynx causes airway obstruction, notify prescriber and be prepared to discontinue drug and administer emergency measures, including S.C. epinephrine 1:1,000 (0.3 to 0.5 ml).
•Continue to monitor patient's blood pressure to assess drug's long-term effectiveness.

**PATIENT TEACHING**

•Instruct patient to notify prescriber immediately and stop taking trandolapril if she experiences swelling of face, eyes, lips, or tongue or has difficulty breathing.

•Explain that drug may cause dizziness and light-headedness, especially during first few days of therapy. Advise patient to avoid driving and other potentially hazardous activities until drug's CNS effects are known and to notify prescriber immediately if she faints.

•Inform female patient of childbearing age about risks of taking trandolapril during pregnancy, especially during second and third trimesters. Urge her to use effective contraceptive method and to notify prescriber immediately if she becomes or thinks she might be pregnant.

•Advise patient planning to undergo surgery or anesthesia to inform specialist that she's taking trandolapril.

•Instruct patient to consult prescriber before using potassium supplements or salt substitutes containing potassium.

•Inform patient about possible loss of taste, which may result in weight loss. Reassure her that loss of taste is usually reversed after 2 to 3 months.

# trandolapril and verapamil hydrochloride

Tarka

## Class and Category

*Chemical:* ACE inhibitor (non–sulfhydryl-containing) (trandolapril), phenylalkylamine derivative (verapamil)
*Therapeutic:* Antihypertensive
*Pregnancy category:* C (first trimester), D (later trimesters)

## Indications and Dosages

➤ *To manage hypertension*
**E.R. TABLETS**
**Adults.** *Initial:* 1 mg trandolapril and 240 mg verapamil, 2 mg trandolapril and 180 mg verapamil, 2 mg trandolapril and 240 mg verapamil, or 4 mg trandolapril and 240 mg verapamil q.d. *Maximum:* 4 mg trandolapril and 240 mg verapamil.

DOSAGE ADJUSTMENT Patients with hepatic impairment given 30% of normal dosage. Dosage may also be reduced in patients with cirrhosis and those with creatinine clearance less than 30 ml/min/1.73 m².

| Route | Onset | Peak | Duration |
|---|---|---|---|
| P.O. | 1 to 2 hr | Unknown | 24 hr |

## Mechanism of Action

Trandolapril is the prodrug for trandolaprilat, which reduces blood pressure by inhibiting the conversion of angiotensin I to angiotensin II. Angiotensin II is a potent vasoconstrictor that stimulates the renal cortex to secrete aldosterone. Decreased release of aldosterone reduces sodium and water retention and increases their excretion, thereby reducing blood pressure. Trandolapril may also inhibit renal and vascular production of angiotensin II.

Verapamil inhibits calcium entry into coronary and vascular smooth-muscle cells by blocking slow calcium channels in cell membranes. The resulting decrease in the intracellular calcium level inhibits smooth-muscle cell contractions and decreases myocardial oxygen demand by relaxing coronary and vascular smooth muscle, reducing peripheral vascular resistance, and decreasing systolic and diastolic blood pressures.

## Contraindications

Cardiogenic shock; history of angioedema related to previous treatment with ACE inhibitor; hypersensitivity to trandolapril, other ACE inhibitors, verapamil, or their components; hypotension; severe heart failure; severe left ventricular dysfunction; sick sinus syndrome or second- or third-degree AV block (unless artificial pacemaker is in place)

## Interactions
**DRUGS**
*anesthetics (inhaled):* Enhanced cardiodepressive effects of verapamil
*beta blockers:* Increased risk of heart failure, hypotension, and severe bradycardia
*carbamazepine, cyclosporine, theophylline:* Possibly increased blood levels of these drugs and increased risk of toxicity
*cimetidine:* Decreased metabolism and increased blood level of verapamil
*digoxin:* Increased blood level of digoxin and risk of digitalis toxicity
*disopyramide, flecainide:* Possibly additive negative inotropic effects
*diuretics:* Increased risk of hypotension

*lithium:* Increased risk of lithium-induced neurotoxicity
*neuromuscular blockers:* Prolonged recovery from neuromuscular blockade
*phenobarbital:* Increased verapamil clearance
*potassium-sparing diuretics, potassium supplements:* Increased risk of hyperkalemia
*quinidine:* Increased risk of quinidine toxicity, increased QT interval, additive negative inotropic effects
*rifampin:* Decreased bioavailability of oral verapamil

**FOODS**
*all foods:* Decreased verapamil bioavailability
*high-potassium diet, potassium-containing salt substitutes:* Increased risk of hyperkalemia

## Adverse Reactions
**CNS:** Dizziness, fatigue
**CV:** AV block, bradycardia, junctional rhythm, orthostatic hypotension
**EENT:** Dry mouth
**GI:** Constipation
**RESP:** Cough
**Other:** Angioedema

## Nursing Considerations
•Be aware that disopyramide and flecainide should not be given within 48 hours before or 24 hours after trandolapril and verapamil because additive negative inotropic effects can result.
•**WARNING** Closely monitor blood pressure during first 2 weeks of drug therapy and whenever drug dosage or accompanying diuretic dosage is adjusted, especially in patients with heart failure, hyponatremia, or severe volume or sodium loss. If excessive hypotension occurs, notify prescriber immediately, place patient in supine position, and prepare to infuse I.V. normal saline solution, as prescribed.
•**WARNING** Be alert for signs and symptoms of angioedema. If swelling of tongue, glottis, or larynx causes airway obstruction, notify prescriber and be prepared to discontinue drug and administer emergency measures, including S.C. epinephrine 1:1,000 (0.3 to 0.5 ml).
•Assess patient for bradycardia and hypotension, which may indicate AV block, and notify prescriber if heart rate or blood pressure declines significantly.
•Continue to monitor blood pressure to assess drug's long-term effectiveness.

**PATIENT TEACHING**
•Instruct patient not to crush or chew E.R. trandolapril and verapamil tablet, but inform her that she may break tablet in half to aid in swallowing.
•Advise patient to take drug with food.
•Direct patient to monitor pulse rate before taking drug and to notify prescriber if it falls below 50 beats/min or as instructed by prescriber.
•Instruct patient to notify prescriber immediately and stop taking drug if she experiences swelling of face, eyes, lips, or tongue or has difficulty breathing.
•Explain that drug may cause dizziness and light-headedness, especially during first few days of therapy. Urge patient to avoid potentially hazardous activities until drug's adverse CNS effects are known and to notify prescriber immediately if she faints.
•Inform female patient of childbearing age about risks of taking trandolapril and verapamil during pregnancy, especially during second and third trimesters. Urge her to use effective contraception and to notify prescriber immediately if she becomes or thinks she might be pregnant.
•Advise patient planning to undergo surgery or anesthesia to inform specialist that she's taking trandolapril and verapamil.
•Instruct patient to consult prescriber before using potassium supplements or salt substitutes containing potassium.
•Encourage patient to increase dietary fiber intake to prevent constipation. Advise her to notify prescriber if constipation persists.

# tranylcypromine sulfate

Parnate

## Class and Category
*Chemical:* Nonhydrazine derivative
*Therapeutic:* Antidepressant
*Pregnancy category:* Not rated

## Indications and Dosages
➤ *To treat major depressive episodes without melancholia*
**TABLETS**
**Adults and adolescents over age 16.** 30 mg/day in divided doses. After first 2 wk, increased by 10 mg q 1 to 2 wk, as prescribed. *Maintenance:* 10 to 40 mg/day. *Maximum:* 60 mg/day.

DOSAGE ADJUSTMENT For elderly patients, initial dosage possibly reduced to 2.5 to 5 mg/day and increased by 2.5 to 5 mg q 3 to 4 days, as prescribed; maximum dosage 45 mg/day. Alternative therapies should be carefully considered for patients over age 60.

| Route | Onset | Peak | Duration |
|-------|-------|------|----------|
| P.O. | 7 to 10 days | 4 to 8 wk | 10 days |

### Mechanism of Action

Reversibly binds to MAO, reducing its activity and resulting in increased levels of neurotransmitters, including dopamine, epinephrine, and norepinephrine. This regulation of CNS neurotransmitters helps ease depression.

## Contraindications

Cardiovascular disease; cerebrovascular disease; heart failure; hepatic disease; history of headaches; hypersensitivity to tranylcypromine or its components; hypertension; pheochromocytoma; severe renal impairment; use of anesthetics, antihypertensives, bupropion, buspirone, carbamazepine, CNS depressants, cyclobenzaprine, dextromethorphan, meperidine, other MAO inhibitors, selective serotonin-reuptake inhibitors, sympathomimetics, or tricyclic antidepressants

## Interactions

### DRUGS

*amoxapine, bupropion, maprotiline, selective serotonin-reuptake inhibitors, trazodone, tricyclic antidepressants:* Increased risk of severe hypertensive crisis, increased anticholinergic effects
*anticonvulsants:* Additive CNS depression
*antihistamines:* Possibly prolonged anticholinergic and CNS depressant effects
*antipsychotics:* Additive anticholinergic, hypotensive, and sedative effects
*beta blockers:* Possibly worsened bradycardia
*bromocriptine:* Increased blood prolactin level and interference with bromocriptine effects
*buspirone:* Increased blood pressure
*dextroamphetamine, isometheptene, local anesthetics, naphazoline, oxymetazoline, psychostimulants, sympathomimetics, tetrahydrozoline, xylometazoline:* Increased risk of severe hypertensive reaction
*dextromethorphan, tryptophan:* Increased risk of serotonin syndrome

*diuretics:* Additive hypotensive effects
*doxapram:* Increased vasopressor effects
*furazolidone, procarbazine, selegiline:* Increased risk of severe hyperpyretic or hypertensive crisis, seizures, or death
*guanadrel, guanethidine:* Increased risk of moderate to severe hypertension
*insulin, oral antidiabetic drugs:* Possibly prolonged hypoglycemic response
*levodopa:* Increased vasopressor effects, hypertension, adverse cardiovascular effects
*meperidine:* Increased risk of coma, diaphoresis, excitation, hypertension, rigidity, severe respiratory depression, shock, and, possibly, death
*methyldopa:* Increased risk of hallucinations
*metrizamide, tramadol:* Increased risk of seizures
*succinylcholine:* Possibly prolonged succinylcholine effects

### FOODS

*aged cheese; avocadoes; bananas; fava or broad beans; cured sausage (bologna, pepperoni, salami, and summer sausage) or other meat; overripe fruit; pickled fish, meats, or poultry; protein extract; smoked fish, meats, or poultry; soy sauce; yeast extract; and other foods high in pressor amines, such as tyramine:* Increased risk of sudden, severe hypertension
*caffeine-containing beverages and foods:* Increased risk of severe hypertensive crisis and dangerous arrhythmias

### ACTIVITIES

*alcohol-containing products that also may contain tyramine, such as beer (including reduced-alcohol and alcohol-free beer), wine (red and white), sherry, hard liquor, liqueurs:* Increased risk of hypertensive crisis

## Adverse Reactions

**CNS:** Anxiety, chills, dizziness, drowsiness, fever, headache, insomnia, intracranial hemorrhage, paresthesia, restlessness, suicidal ideation, tremor, weakness
**CV:** Bradycardia, chest pain, edema, hypertensive crisis, orthostatic hypotension, palpitations, tachycardia
**EENT:** Blurred vision, dry mouth, mydriasis, photophobia, tinnitus
**GI:** Abdominal pain, anorexia, constipation, diarrhea, nausea, vomiting
**GU:** Ejaculation disorders, impotence, urine retention

T

**HEME:** Agranulocytosis, anemia, leukopenia, thrombocytopenia
**MS:** Muscle spasms, myoclonus, neck stiffness
**SKIN:** Clammy skin, diaphoresis

## Nursing Considerations
•Monitor patient's blood pressure during tranylcypromine therapy to detect hypertensive crisis and to decrease the risk of orthostatic hypotension.
•**WARNING** Notify prescriber immediately if patient has signs of hypertensive crisis, such as chest pain, headache, neck stiffness, and palpitations. Expect to stop drug right away.
•Anticipate that therapeutic response may not occur for up to 4 weeks.
•Expect drug to aggravate symptoms of Parkinson's disease, including muscle spasms, myoclonic movement, and tremor.
•Keep dietary restrictions in place for at least 2 weeks after stopping tranylcypromine because of the slow recovery from drug's enzyme-inhibiting effects.
•Expect to stop drug 10 days before elective surgery, as prescribed, to avoid hypotension.
•Be aware that abrupt cessation of drug can precipitate original symptoms.
•Check diabetic patient's blood glucose level often to detect possible loss of control.
•Anticipate that coadministration with a selective serotonin reuptake inhibitor may cause confusion, seizures, severe hypertension, and other, less severe symptoms.
•Monitor severely depressed patients, including children and teens, for suicidal tendencies. Take safety measures, and notify prescriber immediately.
•Assess patient for sudden insomnia. If it develops, notify prescriber and be prepared to administer drug early in the day.
**PATIENT TEACHING**
•Instruct patient to avoid foods that contain cheese and that are high in tyramine, such as anchovies, avocadoes, bananas, beer, canned figs, caviar, Chianti wine, chocolate, dried fruit, fava beans, liqueurs, meat tenderizers, overripe fruit, pickled herring, raspberries, sauerkraut, sherry, sour cream, soy sauce, yeast extract, and yogurt while taking tranylcypromine.
•Urge patient to continue dietary restrictions for at least 2 weeks after therapy stops.
•Advise patient to notify prescriber immediately about chest pain, dizziness, headache, nausea, neck stiffness, palpitations, rapid heart rate, sweating, and vomiting.

•Urge patient to avoid alcohol and excessive caffeine intake during therapy.
•Suggest changing positions slowly to minimize effects of orthostatic hypotension.
•Advise patient to avoid hazardous activities until drug's CNS effects are known.
•Advise patient not to take other prescribed or OTC drugs without consulting prescriber.
•Caution patient not to stop drug abruptly to avoid recurrence of original symptoms.
•Instruct female patient to use effective contraception during tranylcypromine therapy to prevent fetal abnormalities. Urge her to notify prescriber immediately about known or suspected pregnancy.
•**WARNING** Urge parents to watch their child or adolescent closely for abnormal thinking or behavior or increased aggression or hostility. Stress importance of notifying prescriber about unusual changes.

# trazodone hydrochloride
Desyrel, Trazon, Trialodine

## Class and Category
*Chemical:* Triazolopyridine derivative
*Therapeutic:* Antidepressant, anxiolytic
*Pregnancy category:* C

## Indications and Dosages
➤ *To treat major depression, with or without generalized anxiety*
**TABLETS**
**Adults.** *Initial:* 150 mg/day in divided doses, increased by 50 mg/day q 3 to 4 days, p.r.n., as prescribed. *Maximum:* 400 mg/day for outpatients, 600 mg/day for inpatients.
**Children ages 6 to 18.** *Initial:* 1.5 to 2 mg/kg/day in divided doses, increased q 3 to 4 days, p.r.n., as prescribed. *Maximum:* 6 mg/kg/day in divided doses.

| Route | Onset | Peak | Duration |
|-------|-------|------|----------|
| P.O. | 1 to 2 wk | Unknown | Unknown |

### Mechanism of Action
Blocks serotonin reuptake along the presynaptic neuronal membrane, causing an antidepressant effect. Trazodone exerts an alpha-adrenergic blocking action and produces modest histamine blockade, causing a sedative effect. It also inhibits the vasopressor response to norepinephrine, which reduces blood pressure.

## Contraindications

Hypersensitivity to trazodone or its components, recovery from acute MI

## Interactions

**DRUGS**

*anticonvulsants:* Decreased seizure threshold
*antihypertensives:* Increased risk of excessive hypotension
*anxiolytics, brompheniramine, carbinoxamine, chlorpheniramine, clemastine, dimenhydrinate, diphenhydramine, doxylamine, general anesthetics, methdilazine, opioid analgesics, phenothiazines, sedative-hypnotics, skeletal muscle relaxants:* Increased CNS depression, increased risk of respiratory depression and hypotension
*barbiturates:* Decreased seizure threshold and barbiturate effectiveness, increased drowsiness
*buspirone, selective serotonin-reuptake inhibitors, tricyclic antidepressants:* Possibly excessive serotonergic stimulation
*carbamazepine:* Decreased trazodone level
*clonidine:* Interference with clonidine's antihypertensive effect
*digoxin:* Possibly increased blood digoxin level and risk of digitalis toxicity
*erythromycin, indinavir, itraconazole, ketoconazole, nefazodone, protease inhibitors, ritonavir:* Possibly increased blood trazodone level with increased risk of adverse effects
*MAO inhibitors:* Increased serotonin effects
*warfarin:* Decreased anticoagulation response

**ACTIVITIES**

*alcohol use:* Increased CNS depression, risk of respiratory depression and hypotension

## Adverse Reactions

**CNS:** Dizziness, drowsiness, fatigue, headache, light-headedness, nervousness, suicidal ideation, syncope, tremor
**CV:** Arrhythmias, hypotension, orthostatic hypotension, palpitations
**EENT:** Blurred vision, dry mouth
**GI:** Constipation, indigestion, nausea, vomiting
**GU:** Anorgasmia, ejaculation disorders, increased libido, priapism
**SKIN:** Pruritus, rash

## Nursing Considerations

• Give trazodone shortly after the patient has a meal or light snack to reduce nausea.
• Give larger portion of daily dose at bedtime if drowsiness occurs.

• Because trazodone's mechanism of action is similar to that of selective serotonin reuptake inhibitors, expect high doses (6 to 8 mg/kg) to increase blood serotonin level and low doses (0.05 to 1 mg/kg) to decrease blood serotonin level.
• Expect most patients who respond to trazodone to do so by end of the second week.
• Closely monitor depressed patients, including children and teens, for suicidal thoughts. Notify prescriber if they occur, and take suicide precautions according to facility policy.
• Be aware that adverse CNS reactions usually improve after patient completes a few weeks of therapy.
• **WARNING** Be aware that trazodone therapy may increase the risk of priapism.

**PATIENT TEACHING**

• Urge patient to avoid taking trazodone on an empty stomach because doing so may increase risk of dizziness or light-headedness.
• Caution patient to avoid potentially hazardous activities during therapy.
• Advise patient not to fast during therapy because of possible adverse CNS reactions.
• Instruct male patient to notify prescriber immediately about priapism.
• **WARNING** Urge parents to watch their child or adolescent closely for abnormal thinking or behavior or increased aggression or hostility. Stress importance of notifying prescriber about unusual changes.

# treprostinil sodium

Remodulin

## Class and Category

*Chemical:* Prostaglandin, tricyclic benzidene analog
*Therapeutic:* Vasodilator
*Pregnancy category:* B

## Indications and Dosages

➤ *To treat pulmonary artery hypertension in patients who have New York Heart Association Class II to IV symptoms in order to diminish exercise-induced symptoms*

**I.V. INFUSION, S.C. INFUSION**

**Adults.** *Initial:* 1.25 nanograms/kg/min.
*Maintenance:* Infusion rate increased in increments of no more than 1.25 nanograms/kg/min each wk for first 4 wk, and in increments of no more than 2.5 nanograms/kg/

min each wk thereafter, as needed. *Maximum:* 40 nanograms/kg/min.
**DOSAGE ADJUSTMENT** If initial dosage isn't tolerated or if patient has mild to moderate hepatic insufficiency, decrease initial dose to 0.625 nanogram/kg/min (using ideal body weight).

## Mechanism of Action
Acts directly on pulmonary and systemic arterial vascular beds to produce vasodilation. The vasodilatory effects reduce right and left ventricular afterload and increase cardiac output and stroke volume. These effects improve symptoms of pulmonary hypertension, such as dyspnea, and enable patients with pulmonary hypertension to walk greater distances with less discomfort.

## Contraindications
Hypersensitivity to treprostinil, its components, or structurally related compounds

## Interactions
**DRUGS**
*anticoagulants:* Increased risk of bleeding
*antihypertensives, diuretics, other vasodilators:* Increased risk of hypotension

## Adverse Reactions
**CNS:** Anxiety, dizziness, headache, restlessness
**CV:** Edema, hypotension, vasodilatation
**EENT:** Jaw pain
**GI:** Diarrhea, nausea, vomiting
**SKIN:** Pruritus, rash
**Other:** Infusion site pain or reaction (erythema, induration, rash)

## Nursing Considerations
• Use treprostinil cautiously in patients with hepatic or renal impairment.
• Assess patient's ability to care for an I.V. or S.C. catheter and to use an infusion pump. Discuss findings with prescriber before starting treprostinil therapy.
• Be aware that drug shouldn't be diluted whengiven S.C.
• When drug will be given I.V., dilute with either sterile water for injection or NS according to manufacturer's instructions.
• Calculate infusion rate using the formula provided in the package insert, or refer to charts in package insert to find infusion delivery rate for prescribed dosage and administration route.
• **WARNING** Don't abruptly stop treprostinil infusion or make sudden large reductions in dose because symptoms of pulmonary hypertension may worsen.
• Assess patient frequently for drug effectiveness and for adverse reactions. Know that the goal of chronic dosage adjustments is to find a dose that will improve symptoms of pulmonary hypertension, such as dyspnea and fatigue, while minimizing the drug's adverse effects, such as headache, nausea, vomiting, restlessness, anxiety, and infusion site pain or reaction.
• Monitor patients with mild to moderate hepatic insufficiency closely for adverse reactions, especially after dosage increases, because treprostinil is metabolized primarily by the liver.
• Be aware that patient must be discharged with a backup infusion pump. It should be one that's adjustable to about 0.002 ml/hr and has alarms that indicate occlusion/no delivery, low battery, programming error, and motor malfunction. Also, the pump should have a delivery accuracy of ±6% or better, be positive-pressure driven, and have a reservoir made of polyvinyl chloride, polypropylene, or glass. Make sure patient has additional I.V. or S.C. infusion sets to prevent potential interruptions in drug delivery.

**PATIENT TEACHING**
• Explain to patient that treprostinil is infused continuously through an I.V. or S.C. catheter via an infusion pump.
• Teach patient to operate and maintain the I.V. or S.C. infusion pump and to recognize the drug's adverse effects.
• To reduce the risk of infection, caution patient to always use aseptic technique when preparing and giving drug.
• Tell patient that a single vial of the drug shouldn't be used beyond 14 days after opening and that once the drug is placed in the pump's reservoir, it shouldn't be used after 72 hours.
• Instruct patient to store treprostinil vials at room temperature (about 25° C [77° F]).
• Inform patient that drug will be needed for prolonged periods, possibly years. Stress the importance of not stopping drug abruptly or

making sudden large reductions in dosage without consulting prescriber because symptoms could worsen.
• Make sure patient understands that treprostinil use doesn't preclude the subsequent use of an alternative I.V. prostacyclin therapy such as epoprostenol.
• Make sure patient has emergency contact information for problems or questions about giving treprostinil at home.

# triamcinolone

Aristocort, Aristopak, Atolone, Kenacort, Nasacort AQ

## triamcinolone acetonide

Azmacort, Cenocort A-40, Cinonide-40, Kenaject-40, Kenalog-10, Kenalog-40, Ken-Jec-40, Nasacort, Nasacort HFA, Robalog, Tac-3, Triam-A, Triamonide, Tri-Kort, Trilog

## triamcinolone diacetate

Acetocot, Amcort, Aristocort, Aristocort Forte, Articulose-LA, Cenocort Forte, Cinalone 40, Clinacort, Kenacort Diacetate, Tilone, Tramacort-D, Triam-Forte, Triamolone 40, Tristoject

## triamcinolone hexacetonide

Aristospan

## Class and Category
*Chemical:* Synthetic glucocorticoid
*Therapeutic:* Anti-inflammatory, immunosuppressant
*Pregnancy category:* C (nasal and oral inhalation), Not rated (oral and parenteral)

## Indications and Dosages
➤ *To prevent bronchospasm or provide long-term corticosteroid treatment to control asthma*
**ORAL INHALATION (TRIAMCINOLONE ACETONIDE)**
**Adults and children age 12 and older.** *Initial:* 2 metered sprays (200 mcg) t.i.d. or q.i.d. *Maintenance:* Individualized dosage given b.i.d. *Maximum:* 16 metered sprays/day in divided doses.
**Children ages 6 to 11.** 2 to 4 metered sprays (200 to 400 mcg) b.i.d. to q.i.d. *Maximum:* 12 metered sprays/day.

➤ *To treat acute rheumatic carditis, berylliosis, and Hodgkin's disease; as adjunct to treat fulminating or disseminated pulmonary tuberculosis (with appropriate antituberculosis therapy)*
**SYRUP (TRIAMCINOLONE DIACETATE), TABLETS (TRIAMCINOLONE)**
**Adults and children age 12 and older.** *Initial:* 4 to 48 mg/day as a single dose or in divided doses. Some patients may require an initial dose of 60 mg.
**Children under age 12.** 0.42 to 1.7 mg/kg/day as a single dose or in divided doses.
**I.M. INJECTION (TRIAMCINOLONE ACETONIDE)**
**Adults and children age 12 and older.** 40 to 80 mg q 4 wk, as needed.
**Children ages 6 to 11.** 40 mg q 4 wk, as needed, or 30 to 200 mcg/kg q 1 to 7 days.
**I.M. INJECTION (TRIAMCINOLONE DIACETATE)**
**Adults and children age 12 and older.** 40 mg q wk, or 4 to 7 times the daily P.O. dose as a single injection q 4 days to q 4 wk.
**Children ages 6 to 11.** 40 mg/wk.

➤ *To relieve inflammation caused by acute gouty arthritis, acute nonspecific tenosynovitis, acute or subacute bursitis, epicondylitis, osteoarthritis, posttraumatic osteoarthritis, rheumatoid arthritis, and synovitis*
**SYRUP (TRIAMCINOLONE DIACETATE)**
**Adults and children age 12 and older.** 4 to 48 mg/day as a single dose or in divided doses, adjusted, as prescribed, to lowest effective dose based on clinical response.
**TABLETS (TRIAMCINOLONE)**
**Adults and children age 12 and older.** 8 to 16 mg/day in divided doses t.i.d. or q.i.d., adjusted, as prescribed, to lowest effective dose based on clinical response.
**SYRUP (TRIAMCINOLONE DIACETATE), TABLETS (TRIAMCINOLONE)**
**Children ages 6 to 11.** 0.42 to 1.7 mg/kg/day as a single dose or in divided doses, adjusted, as prescribed, based on clinical response.
**I.M. INJECTION (TRIAMCINOLONE ACETONIDE)**
**Adults and children age 12 and older.** 40 to 80 mg q 4 wk.
**Children ages 6 to 11.** 40 mg q 4 wk.
**I.M. INJECTION (TRIAMCINOLONE DIACETATE)**
**Adults and children age 6 and older.** 40 mg q wk as single injection, repeated q 4 wk if needed.

T

INTRA-ARTICULAR OR INTRABURSAL INJECTION (TRIAM-
CINOLONE ACETONIDE)

**Adults and children age 6 and older.** 2.5 to
15 mg, as needed.

INTRA-ARTICULAR OR INTRASYNOVIAL INJECTION (TRIAM-
CINOLONE DIACETATE)

**Adults.** 5 to 40 mg, repeated as prescribed q
1 to 8 wk, as needed.

INTRA-ARTICULAR INJECTION (TRIAMCINOLONE HEXACE-
TONIDE)

**Adults.** 2 to 20 mg, repeated as prescribed q
3 to 4 wk, as needed.

➤ *To treat primary (Addison's disease) or
secondary adrenocortical insufficiency*

SYRUP (TRIAMCINOLONE DIACETATE)

**Adults and children age 12 and older.** 4 to
12 mg/day as a single dose or in divided
doses.

SYRUP (TRIAMCINOLONE DIACETATE), TABLETS (TRIAM-
CINOLONE)

**Children ages 6 to 11.** 0.12 mg (base)/kg/day
as a single dose or in divided doses.

➤ *To treat inflammatory dermatoses*

TABLETS (TRIAMCINOLONE)

**Adults and children age 12 and older.** 8 to 16
mg/day. *Usual:* 1 to 2 mg/day.

➤ *To treat disseminated lupus erythematosus*

TABLETS (TRIAMCINOLONE)

**Adults and children age 12 and older.** 20 to
30 mg/day. *Usual:* 3 to 30 mg/day.

➤ *To treat nephrotic syndrome*

TABLETS (TRIAMCINOLONE)

**Adults and children age 12 and older.** 16 to
20 mg/day.

➤ *To relieve symptoms of perennial and
seasonal allergic rhinitis*

TABLETS (TRIAMCINOLONE)

**Adults and children age 12 and older.** 8 to
12 mg/day. *Usual:* 2 to 6 mg/day.
**Children ages 6 to 11.** 0.42 to 1.7 mg/kg/day
as a single dose or in divided doses.

NASAL INHALATION (NASACORT)

**Adults and children age 12 and older.** *Initial:*
220 mcg/day in 2 sprays (55 mcg each)/nos-
tril. *Maintenance:* 110 mcg/day in 1 spray (55
mcg)/nostril. *Maximum:* 440 mcg (8
sprays/day).

NASAL INHALATION (NASACORT AQ)

**Adults and children age 12 and older.** *Initial:*
110 mcg/day in 2 sprays (55 mcg each)/nos-
tril. *Maintenance:* 55 mcg/day in 1 spray/
nostril. *Maximum:* 220 mcg or 4 sprays/day.

**Children ages 6 to 11.** 110 mcg/day in 1
spray (55 mcg each)/nostril. *Maximum:* 220
mcg or 4 sprays/day.

NASAL INHALATION (NASACORT HFA)

**Adults and children age 12 and older.** *Initial:*
220 mcg/day in 2 sprays (55 mcg each)/nos-
tril. May be increased to 440 mcg/day in 4
sprays/nostril, as needed.
**Children ages 6 to 11.** 220 mcg/day in 2
sprays (55 mcg each)/nostril.

➤ *To treat chronic idiopathic thrombocytopenic purpura*

TABLETS (TRIAMCINOLONE)

**Adults and children age 12 and older.** 0.8 mg/
kg/day.

| Route | Onset | Peak | Duration |
|---|---|---|---|
| P.O. (tablets) | Unknown | 1 to 2 hr | 2.25 days |
| I.M. (acetonide) | 24 to 48 hr | Unknown | 1 to 6 wk |
| I.M. (diacetate) | Slow | Unknown | 4 days to 4 wk |
| Inhalation | 12 hr | 3 to 4 hr | Unknown |
| Intra-articular, intrabursal (acetonide) | Unknown | Unknown | Several wk |
| Intra-articular, intrasynovial (diacetate) | Unknown | Unknown | 1 to 8 wk |

## Mechanism of Action

Inhibits the release of prostaglandins and
leukotrienes, thus reducing immediate
and late-phase allergic responses in
chronic asthma. Triamcinolone also:
• decreases peribronchial edema and mucus secretion by inhibiting the binding of
allergens to immunoglobulin E antibodies
on the surface of mast cells, thereby inactivating the release of chemotactic substances
• decreases inflammation by interfering
with leukocyte adhesion to capillary walls
• inhibits the release of leukocytic acid
hydrolases, preventing macrophage accumulation at the infection site
• inhibits histamine and kinin release, preventing the formation of scar tissue.

## Incompatibilities

Don't mix triamcinolone hexacetonide with parenteral local anesthetics because precipitation can occur.

## Contraindications

Acute status asthmaticus (inhalation form), hypersensitivity to triamcinolone or its components, live-virus vaccine therapy, systemic fungal infection

## Interactions

### DRUGS

*amphotericin B, ethacrynic acid, furosemide, thiazide diuretics:* Increased potassium-wasting effect, severe hypokalemia
*aspirin:* Increased blood salicylate level, increased risk of salicylate toxicity
*barbiturates, carbamazepine, phenytoin, rifampin:* Increased triamcinolone metabolism
*cholinesterase inhibitors:* Increased risk of severe muscle weakness in patients with myasthenia gravis
*digitalis glycosides:* Increased risk of arrhythmias and digitalis toxicity
*estrogens:* Increased triamcinolone effects
*insulin, oral antidiabetic drugs:* Increased blood glucose level
*isoproterenol:* Increased risk of cardiotoxicity
*live-virus vaccines:* Decreased antibody response, increased risk of neurologic complications
*neuromuscular blockers:* Increased risk of hypokalemia and enhanced neuromuscular blockade
*NSAIDs:* Increased risk of adverse GI effects
*toxoids:* Decreased resistance to toxoids

## Adverse Reactions

**CNS:** Emotional lability, exacerbated psychosis, headache, insomnia, restlessness, seizures, vertigo
**CV:** Edema, heart failure, hypertension
**EENT:** Cataracts, dry mouth, glaucoma, hoarseness, nasal irritation (inhalation form), oropharyngeal candidiasis, pharyngitis, posterior subcapsular cataracts, secondary ocular infection, sinusitis, sneezing
**ENDO:** Cushing's syndrome, diabetes mellitus
**GI:** Abdominal pain, constipation, diarrhea, esophageal ulceration, gastritis, vomiting
**GU:** Cystitis, renal disease, UTI, vaginitis

**MS:** Bursitis, muscle wasting or weakness, myalgia, osteoporosis, tenosynovitis
**RESP:** Bronchospasm (inhalation form), chest congestion
**SKIN:** Ecchymosis, petechiae (parenteral form), photosensitivity, rash, striae, urticaria
**Other:** Anaphylaxis; angioedema; facial edema; herpes infection; impaired wound healing; injection site atrophy, induration, pain, soreness, and sterile abscess; weight gain

## Nursing Considerations

•Give oral form of triamcinolone with meals to minimize GI distress.
•Use calibrated device to measure liquid doses.
•If necessary, crush tablets and mix with food or fluids.
•Shake I.M. suspension thoroughly before drawing it into syringe.
•Be aware that specialized training may be needed to give parenteral triamcinolone.
•Don't administer parenteral forms of triamcinolone I.V.
•Be aware that triamcinolone may reactivate tuberculosis in patients with a history of the disease.
•WARNING Assess patient for signs and symptoms of adrenal insufficiency (fatigue, hypotension, lassitude, nausea, vomiting, and weakness) during times of stress, such as infection, surgery, or trauma. Notify prescriber immediately if you detect these signs and symptoms because adrenal insufficiency may be life-threatening.

### PATIENT TEACHING

•Caution patient not to adjust triamcinolone dosage without consulting prescriber.
•Teach patient how to administer nasal aerosols properly, using manufacturer's instructions, to avoid nasal irritation.
•Instruct patient to dispose of aerosol canister after 240 uses (100 uses for Nasacort HFA) because dosage may not be correct after that time.
•Inform patient that maximum benefit may not occur for up to 2 weeks.
•Advise patient to notify prescriber immediately if asthma fails to respond to inhaled drug because additional systemic therapy may be needed.

T

•Caution patient to avoid exposure to people who have chickenpox or measles throughout triamcinolone therapy and for 12 months afterward.
•Advise patient to have periodic eye examinations during long-term therapy because triamcinolone can cause glaucoma or ocular nerve damage.

# triamterene

Dyrenium

## Class and Category
*Chemical:* Pterdine derivative
*Therapeutic:* Diuretic
*Pregnancy category:* B

## Indications and Dosages
➤ *To treat edema in cirrhosis, heart failure, and nephrotic syndrome*
CAPSULES
**Adults.** *Initial:* 25 to 100 mg/day. *Maximum:* 300 mg/day.

| Route | Onset | Peak | Duration |
|-------|-------|------|----------|
| P.O. | 2 to 4 hr | 1 to several days | 7 to 9 hr |

### Mechanism of Action
Inhibits sodium reabsorption in distal convoluted tubules and cortical collecting ducts, causing sodium and water loss and enhancing potassium retention.

## Contraindications
Anuria, diabetic nephropathy or renal disease linked to renal insufficiency, hyperkalemia (potassium level of 5.5 mEq/L or more), hypersensitivity to triamterene or its components, severe hepatic dysfunction

## Interactions
DRUGS
*ACE inhibitors, amiloride, angiotensin-II receptor antagonists, cyclosporine, heparin, potassium-containing drugs, potassium salts, potassium supplements, spironolactone:* Increased risk of hyperkalemia
*amantadine:* Decreased amantadine clearance, possibly amantadine toxicity

*antihypertensives:* Increased antihypertensive effect
*diuretics:* Increased diuretic effect
*folic acid:* Possibly antagonized action of folic acid
*indomethacin:* Increased risk of renal impairment
*lithium:* Increased risk of lithium toxicity
*NSAIDs:* Decreased diuretic effect of triamterene, increased risk of hyperkalemia
*oral antidiabetic drugs:* Altered blood glucose control

## Adverse Reactions
**CNS:** Dizziness, fatigue, headache, weakness
**EENT:** Dry mouth
**ENDO:** Hyperglycemia, hypoglycemia
**GI:** Diarrhea, nausea, vomiting
**GU:** Azotemia, elevated BUN and serum creatinine levels, renal calculi
**SKIN:** Jaundice, photosensitivity, rash

## Nursing Considerations
•Be aware that triamterene shouldn't be given to patient with creatinine clearance below 10 ml/min/1.73 m² because this condition increases the risk of drug-induced hyperkalemia.
•Monitor serum potassium level during therapy, especially in patient with renal impairment or diabetes mellitus. Also monitor BUN and serum creatinine levels to assess renal function and prevent hyperkalemia.
•Monitor for irregular heartbeat, usually the first sign of hyperkalemia.
•If you suspect hyperkalemia, obtain an ECG tracing, as ordered. A widened QRS complex or an arrhythmia requires prompt additional therapy.
•Monitor laboratory test results and assess for signs of metabolic or respiratory acidosis, which may occur suddenly in patient with cardiac disease or uncontrolled diabetes mellitus.
•Monitor patient's serum uric acid and sodium levels, as ordered, because drug may reduce uric acid clearance and increase the risk of gout and hyperuricemia. It also may worsen preexisting hyponatremia.
•Monitor CBC with differential because drug may increase the risk of megaloblastic anemia in patient with folic acid deficiency.

•Advise patient to take triamterene with food or milk.
•Instruct patient to avoid exposure to excessive heat or sunlight to prevent dehydration and, possibly, photosensitivity.
•Explain to patient with a history of gout that drug may increase the risk of an attack.
•Advise patient to notify prescriber about ineffective diuresis and unexplained weight gain during therapy.

# triazolam

Alti-Triazolam (CAN), Apo-Triazo (CAN), Gen Triazolam (CAN), Halcion, Novo-Triolam (CAN)

## Class, Category, and Schedule
*Chemical:* Benzodiazepine
*Therapeutic:* Sedative-hypnotic
*Pregnancy category:* X
*Controlled substance:* Schedule IV

## Indications and Dosages
➤ *To provide short-term management of insomnia*
TABLETS
**Adults.** 0.125 to 0.25 mg h.s. *Maximum:* 0.5 mg/day (for patients with inadequate response to usual dose).
DOSAGE ADJUSTMENT For elderly or debilitated patients, initial dosage reduced to 0.125 mg h.s. and maximum dosage limited to 0.25 mg/day.

| Route | Onset | Peak | Duration |
|-------|-------|------|----------|
| P.O. | 15 to 30 min | Unknown | Unknown |

### Mechanism of Action
Potentiates the effects of the inhibitory neurotransmitter gamma-aminobutyric acid, which increases the inhibition of the ascending reticular activating system and produces varying levels of CNS depression, including sedation, hypnosis, skeletal muscle relaxation, anticonvulsant activity, and coma.

## Contraindications
Hypersensitivity to triazolam or its components, ketoconazole or itraconazole therapy, pregnancy

## Interactions
DRUGS
*anxiolytics, barbiturates, brompheniramine, carbinoxamine, cetirizine, chlorpheniramine, clemastine, cyproheptadine, dimenhydrinate, diphenhydramine, doxylamine, general anesthetics, methdilazine, opioid analgesics, sedative-hypnotics, phenothiazines, promethazine, tramadol, tricyclic antidepressants, trimeprazine:* Increased sedation, respiratory depression
*cimetidine, diltiazem, disulfiram, erythromycin, probenecid, verapamil:* Increased sedation
*fluconazole:* Increased blood triazolam level and effects
*flumazenil:* Increased risk of withdrawal symptoms
*itraconazole, ketoconazole:* Delayed triazolam elimination
*oral contraceptives:* Increased blood triazolam level
FOODS
*grapefruit juice:* Increased blood triazolam level and sedation
ACTIVITIES
*alcohol use:* Increased sedation, respiratory depression

## Adverse Reactions
**CNS:** Anxiety, ataxia, confusion, depression, dizziness, drowsiness, fatigue, headache, insomnia, nightmares, syncope, talkativeness, tremor, vertigo
**Other:** Physical and psychological dependence

## Nursing Considerations
•Be aware that triazolam shouldn't be discontinued abruptly, even after only 1 to 2 weeks of therapy. Doing so can cause withdrawal symptoms, including abdominal cramps, confusion, depression, diaphoresis, hyperacusis, insomnia, irritability, nausea, nervousness, paresthesia, perceptual disturbances, photophobia, tachycardia, tremor, and vomiting.
•WARNING Assess patient for signs of physical and psychological dependence, and notify prescriber if they occur.
•Monitor respiratory rate and depth and ABG results, as appropriate, because drug may worsen ventilatory failure in patient with pulmonary disease, such as severe COPD, respiratory depression, or sleep apnea. Use drug cautiously in patients with

T

acute intermittent porphyria, myasthenia gravis, and severe renal impairment because it may aggravate these conditions.
• Take safety precautions for elderly patients because drug may impair cognitive and motor function and increase the risk for falls.
• Use triazolam cautiously in patients with advanced Parkinson's disease because drug may worsen cognition, coordination, and psychosis.

**PATIENT TEACHING**
• Instruct patient to take triazolam exactly as prescribed and not to stop taking it abruptly because of the risk of withdrawal symptoms.
• Caution patient about possible drowsiness.
• Urge patient to avoid alcohol because it increases drug's sedative effects.
• Advise patient to notify prescriber about excessive drowsiness, known or suspected pregnancy, or nausea.

# trifluoperazine hydrochloride

Apo-Trifluoperazine (CAN), PMS-Trifluoperazine (CAN)

## Class and Category
*Chemical:* Piperazine phenothiazine
*Therapeutic:* Antianxiety, antipsychotic
*Pregnancy category:* Not rated

## Indications and Dosages
➤ *To treat psychotic disorders*
**SYRUP, TABLETS**
**Adults and adolescents.** *Initial:* 2 to 5 mg b.i.d., increased gradually, as needed. *Maintenance:* 15 to 20 mg/day. *Maximum:* 40 mg/day.
**Children age 6 and older.** *Initial:* 1 mg q.d. or in divided doses b.i.d., increased gradually, as needed.
**I.M. INJECTION**
**Adults and adolescents.** 1 to 2 mg q 4 to 6 hr, as needed. *Maximum:* 10 mg/day.
**Children age 6 and older.** 1 mg q.d. or in divided doses b.i.d., as needed.

➤ *To relieve anxiety*
**SYRUP, TABLETS, I.M. INJECTION**
**Adults and adolescents.** *Initial:* 1 to 2 mg/day, increased gradually, as needed. *Maximum:* 6 mg/day for 12 wk.

## Mechanism of Action
Blocks postsynaptic dopamine receptors, increasing dopamine turnover and decreasing dopamine neurotransmission. This action may depress the areas of the brain that control activity and aggression, including the cerebral cortex, hypothalamus, and limbic system. Trifluoperazine may relieve anxiety by indirectly reducing arousal and increasing the filtering of internal stimuli to the reticular activating system.

## Contraindications
Blood dyscrasias; bone marrow depression; cerebral arteriosclerosis; coma; coronary artery disease; hepatic dysfunction; hypersensitivity to trifluoperazine, other phenothiazines, or their components; myeloproliferative disorders; severe hypertension or hypotension; significant CNS depression; subcortical brain damage; use of high doses of CNS depressants

## Interactions
**DRUGS**
*adsorbent antidiarrheals, aluminum- and magnesium-containing antacids:* Possibly inhibited absorption of oral trifluoperazine
*amantadine, anticholinergics, antidyskinetics, antihistamines:* Possibly intensified adverse anticholinergic effects, increased risk of trifluoperazine-induced hyperpyrexia
*amphetamines:* Decreased stimulant effect of amphetamines, decreased antipsychotic effect of trifluoperazine
*anticonvulsants:* Lowered seizure threshold
*antithyroid drugs:* Increased risk of agranulocytosis
*apomorphine:* Possibly decreased emetic response to apomorphine, additive CNS depression
*appetite suppressants:* Decreased effects of appetite suppressants
*astemizole, cisapride, disopyramide, erythromycin, pimozide, procubol, procainamide, quinidine:* Prolonged QT interval, increased risk of ventricular tachycardia
*beta blockers:* Increased blood levels of both drugs, possibly leading to additive hypotensive effect, arrhythmias, irreversible retinopathy, and tardive dyskinesia

*bromocriptine:* Impaired therapeutic effects of bromocriptine
*CNS depressants:* Additive CNS depression
*ephedrine, metaraminol:* Decreased vasopressor response to ephedrine
*epinephrine:* Blocked alpha-adrenergic effects of epinephrine
*extrapyramidal reaction–causing drugs (droperidol, haloperidol, metoclopramide, metyrosine, risperidone):* Increased severity and frequency of extrapyramidal reactions
*hepatotoxic drugs:* Increased risk of hepatotoxicity
*hypotension-producing drugs:* Possibly severe hypotension with syncope
*levodopa:* Decreased antidyskinetic effect of levodopa
*lithium:* Reduced absorption of oral trifluoperazine, possibly encephalopathy and additive extrapyramidal effects
*MAO inhibitors, maprotiline, tricyclic antidepressants:* Possibly prolonged and intensified sedative and anticholinergic effects, increased blood level of antidepressants, impaired trifluoperazine metabolism, increased risk of neuroleptic malignant syndrome
*mephentermine:* Decreased antipsychotic effect of trifluoperazine and vasopressor effect of mephentermine
*methoxamine, phenylephrine:* Decreased vasopressor effect and shortened duration of action of these drugs
*metrizamide:* Increased risk of seizures
*opioid analgesics:* Increased risk of CNS and respiratory depression, orthostatic hypotension, severe constipation, and urine retention
*ototoxic drugs:* Possibly masking of some symptoms of ototoxicity, such as dizziness, tinnitus, and vertigo
*phenytoin:* Lowered seizure threshold; inhibited phenytoin metabolism, possibly leading to phenytoin toxicity
*photosensitizing drugs:* Possibly additive photosensitivity and intraocular photochemical damage to choroid, lens, or retina
*thiazide diuretics:* Possibly hyponatremia and water intoxication

**ACTIVITIES**
*alcohol use:* Increased CNS and respiratory depression, increased hypotensive effect

## Adverse Reactions

**CNS:** Akathisia, altered temperature regulation, dizziness, drowsiness, extrapyramidal reactions (dystonia, pseudoparkinsonism, tardive dyskinesia)
**CV:** Hypotension, orthostatic hypotension, tachycardia
**EENT:** Blurred vision, dry mouth, nasal congestion, ocular changes (deposits of fine particles in cornea and lens), pigmentary retinopathy
**ENDO:** Galactorrhea, gynecomastia
**GI:** Constipation, epigastric pain, nausea, vomiting
**GU:** Ejaculation disorders, menstrual irregularities, urine retention
**SKIN:** Contact dermatitis, decreased sweating, photosensitivity, pruritus, rash
**Other:** Injection site irritation and sterile abscess, weight gain

## Nursing Considerations

•Use trifluoperazine cautiously in patients with glaucoma because of drug's anticholinergic effect.
•Before administration, observe parenteral solution, which may turn slightly yellow without altering its potency. Don't use solution if discoloration is pronounced or precipitate is present.
•For I.M. administration, inject drug slowly and deep into upper outer quadrant of the buttocks. Keep patient in a supine position for 30 minutes after injection to minimize hypotensive effect.
•Rotate I.M. injection sites to avoid irritation and sterile abscesses.
•**WARNING** Monitor closely for tardive dyskinesia, which may continue after treatment stops. Signs include uncontrolled movements of arms, body, cheeks, jaw, legs, mouth, or tongue. Notify prescriber if such signs occur.
•Closely monitor elderly patients and severely ill or dehydrated children. They're at increased risk for certain adverse CNS reactions.
•To prevent contact dermatitis, avoid skin contact with oral or injection solution.
**PATIENT TEACHING**
•Instruct patient to take trifluoperazine exactly as prescribed and not to stop taking drug abruptly or without consulting prescriber.
•Advise patient to take drug with food or a full glass of milk or water to minimize adverse GI reactions.

•Urge patient to consult prescriber before using other drugs because of possible interactions.

•Instruct patient to notify prescriber immediately if she experiences difficulty swallowing or speaking and tongue protrusion.

•Caution patient to avoid alcohol during therapy.

•Advise patient to avoid potentially hazardous activities until drug's CNS effects are known.

•Instruct patient to change position slowly to minimize effects of orthostatic hypotension.

•Urge patient to avoid exposure to the sun and extreme heat because drug may cause photosensitivity and interfere with thermoregulation. Encourage her to wear sunscreen when outdoors.

# triflupromazine

Vesprin

## Class and Category

*Chemical:* Phenothiazine
*Therapeutic:* Antiemetic, antipsychotic
*Pregnancy category:* Not rated

## Indications and Dosages

➤ *To treat psychotic disorders*
**I.M. INJECTION**
**Adults and adolescents.** 60 mg, as needed. *Maximum:* 150 mg/day.
**Children age 30 months and older.** 0.2 to 0.25 mg/kg, as needed. *Maximum:* 10 mg/day.

➤ *To treat nausea and vomiting*
**I.V. INJECTION**
**Adults.** 1 mg, p.r.n. *Maximum:* 3 mg/day.
**I.M. INJECTION**
**Adults and adolescents.** 5 to 15 mg q 4 hr. *Maximum:* 60 mg/day.
**Children age 30 months and older.** 0.2 to 0.25 mg/kg, p.r.n. *Maximum:* 10 mg/day.

## Contraindications

Blood dyscrasias, bone marrow depression, cerebral arteriosclerosis, coma or severe CNS depression, concurrent use of large amount of CNS depressants, coronary artery disease, hepatic dysfunction, hypersensitivity to phenothiazines, severe hypertension or hypotension, subcortical brain damage

## Mechanism of Action

Blocks postsynaptic dopamine receptors, increasing dopamine turnover and decreasing dopamine neurotransmission. This action may depress the areas of the brain that control activity and aggression, including the cerebral cortex, hypothalamus, and limbic system. Triflupromazine also prevents nausea and vomiting by inhibiting or blocking dopamine receptors in the medullary chemoreceptor trigger zone and, peripherally, by blocking the vagus nerve in the GI tract.

## Interactions

**DRUGS**

*amantadine, anticholinergics, antidyskinetics, antihistamines:* Possibly intensified adverse anticholinergic effects, increased risk of triflupromazine-induced hyperpyrexia

*amphetamines:* Decreased stimulant effect of amphetamines, decreased antipsychotic effect of triflupromazine

*anticonvulsants:* Lowered seizure threshold

*antithyroid drugs:* Increased risk of agranulocytosis

*apomorphine:* Possibly decreased emetic response to apomorphine, additive CNS depression

*appetite suppressants:* Decreased anorectic effect of appetite suppressants

*astemizole, cisapride, disopyramide, erythromycin, pimozide, probucol, procainamide, quinidine:* Prolonged QT interval, increased risk of ventricular tachycardia

*beta blockers:* Increased blood levels of both drugs, possibly leading to additive hypotensive effect, arrhythmias, irreversible retinopathy, and tardive dyskinesia

*bromocriptine:* Impaired therapeutic effects of bromocriptine

*CNS depressants:* Additive CNS depression

*ephedrine:* Decreased vasopressor response to ephedrine

*epinephrine:* Blocked alpha-adrenergic effects of epinephrine

*extrapyramidal reaction–causing drugs (droperidol, haloperidol, metoclopramide, metyrosine, risperidone):* Increased severity and frequency of extrapyramidal reactions

*hepatotoxic drugs:* Increased risk of hepatotoxicity

*hypotension-producing drugs:* Possibly severe hypotension with syncope

*levodopa:* Decreased antidyskinetic effect of levodopa
*lithium:* Possibly encephalopathy and additive extrapyramidal effects
*MAO inhibitors, maprotiline, tricyclic antidepressants:* Increased CNS depression, impaired triflupromazine metabolism, increased risk of neuroleptic malignant syndrome
*mephentermine:* Possibly antagonized antipsychotic effect of triflupromazine and vasopressor effect of mephentermine
*metaraminol:* Decreased vasopressor effect of metaraminol
*methoxamine, phenylephrine:* Decreased vasopressor effect and shortened duration of action of these drugs
*metrizamide:* Increased risk of seizures
*opioid analgesics:* Increased risk of CNS and respiratory depression, orthostatic hypotension, severe constipation, and urine retention
*ototoxic drugs:* Possibly masking of symptoms of ototoxicity, such as dizziness, tinnitus, and vertigo
*phenytoin:* Lowered seizure threshold; inhibited phenytoin metabolism, possibly leading to phenytoin toxicity
*photosensitizing drugs:* Possibly additive photosensitivity and intraocular photochemical damage to choroid, lens, or retina
*thiazide diuretics:* Possibly hyponatremia and water intoxication
**ACTIVITIES**
*alcohol use:* Increased CNS and respiratory depression, increased hypotensive effect

## Adverse Reactions

**CNS:** Akathisia, altered temperature regulation, dizziness, drowsiness, extrapyramidal reactions (dystonia, pseudoparkinsonism, tardive dyskinesia)
**CV:** Hypotension, orthostatic hypotension, tachycardia
**EENT:** Blurred vision, dry mouth, nasal congestion, ocular changes (deposits of fine particles in cornea and lens), pigmentary retinopathy
**ENDO:** Galactorrhea, gynecomastia
**GI:** Constipation, epigastric pain, nausea, vomiting
**GU:** Ejaculation disorders, menstrual irregularities, urine retention
**SKIN:** Decreased sweating, photosensitivity, pruritus, rash
**Other:** Injection site irritation and sterile abscess, weight gain

## Nursing Considerations
•Use triflupromazine cautiously in patients with glaucoma because of drug's anticholinergic effects.
•Before administration, observe parenteral solution, which may turn slightly yellow without altering potency. Don't use solution if discoloration is pronounced or precipitate is present.
•Don't let solution come in contact with your skin because contact dermatitis may occur.
•For I.M. administration, slowly inject drug deep into upper outer quadrant of buttocks. Keep patient supine for 30 minutes afterward to minimize hypotensive effect.
•Rotate I.M. injection sites to avoid irritation and sterile abscesses.
•**WARNING** Monitor closely for tardive dyskinesia, which may continue after treatment stops. Signs include uncontrolled movements of arms, body, cheeks, jaw, legs, mouth, or tongue. Notify prescriber if such signs occur.
•Closely monitor elderly patients and severely ill or dehydrated children. They're at increased risk for certain adverse CNS reactions.
**PATIENT TEACHING**
•Instruct patient to change position slowly to minimize effects of orthostatic hypotension.
•Urge patient to avoid potentially hazardous activities until drug's CNS effects are known.
•Instruct patient to notify prescriber immediately if she experiences difficulty swallowing or speaking and tongue protrusion.
•Caution patient to avoid alcohol during therapy.
•Urge patient to avoid exposure to the sun and extreme heat because drug may cause photosensitivity and interfere with thermoregulation. Encourage her to wear sunscreen when outdoors.

# trihexyphenidyl hydrochloride

Apo-Trihex (CAN), Artane, PMS Trihexyphenidyl (CAN), Trihexane, Trihexy

## Class and Category
*Chemical:* Tertiary amine
*Therapeutic:* Antidyskinetic
*Pregnancy category:* C

## Indications and Dosages

➤ *To treat parkinsonism*

ELIXIR, TABLETS

**Adults.** *Initial:* 1 to 2 mg on day 1, divided into 3 equal doses and given with meals. Total daily dose increased by 2 mg q 3 to 5 days until desired response or maximum dose is reached. *Maximum:* 15 mg/day.

E.R. CAPSULES

**Adults.** 5 mg after breakfast; additional 5 mg 12 hr later, if needed. *Maximum:* 15 mg/day.

➤ *To treat drug-induced extrapyramidal symptoms*

TABLETS

**Adults.** 1 mg/day, increased to 5 to 15 mg/day, as prescribed, to control symptoms.

| Route | Onset | Peak | Duration |
|-------|-------|------|----------|
| P.O. | 1 hr | Unknown | 6 to 12 hr |

### Mechanism of Action

Blocks acetylcholine's action at cholinergic receptor sites, which restores normal dopamine and acetylcholine balance in the brain, relaxing muscle movement and decreasing drooling, rigidity, and tremor. Drug also may inhibit reuptake and storage of dopamine, prolonging its action.

## Contraindications

Achalasia, bladder neck or prostatic obstruction, narrow-angle glaucoma, hypersensitivity to trihexyphenidyl or its components, megacolon, myasthenia gravis, pyloric or duodenal obstruction, stenosing peptic ulcer

## Interactions

DRUGS

*amantadine, anticholinergics, MAO inhibitors, tricyclic antidepressants:* Increased anticholinergic effects
*antidiarrheals (adsorbent):* Possibly decreased therapeutic effects of trihexyphenidyl
*chlorpromazine:* Decreased blood chlorpromazine level
*CNS depressants:* Increased sedative effect
*levodopa:* Increased efficacy of levodopa

ACTIVITIES

*alcohol use:* Increased sedation

## Adverse Reactions

**CNS:** Confusion, dizziness, drowsiness, nervousness
**EENT:** Blurred vision; dry eyes, mouth, nose, or throat; mydriasis
**GI:** Constipation, nausea, vomiting
**GU:** Dysuria, urine retention
**SKIN:** Decreased sweating

## Nursing Considerations

•Use trihexyphenidyl cautiously in patients with cardiovascular, hepatic, or renal disorders. Patients with cardiovascular disorders, such as atherosclerosis, hypertension, and ischemic heart disease, are at risk for tachycardia and coronary ischemia from drug's positive chronotropic effects. Hepatic and renal dysfunction increase the risk of adverse reactions.

•Before therapy begins, assess patient's muscle rigidity and tremor to establish a baseline. During therapy, reassess patient to detect improvement in these signs and evaluate drug effectiveness.

•Obtain patient's intraocular pressure before and periodically during trihexyphenidyl therapy, as ordered, because drug can precipitate incipient glaucoma.

PATIENT TEACHING

•Instruct patient to take trihexyphenidyl after meals.

•Teach patient not to break or chew E.R. capsules.

•Instruct patient to use calibrated device to measure elixir.

•Advise patient to avoid potentially hazardous activities until drug's CNS effects are known.

•Advise patient with dry eyes or increased contact lens awareness to use lubricating drops or stop wearing contact lenses during drug therapy.

•Caution patient being treated for parkinsonism not to stop taking drug suddenly because doing so may worsen symptoms.

•Advise patient to maintain adequate hydration and avoid exercising during hot weather because trihexyphenidyl increases the risk of heatstroke.

# trimethobenzamide hydrochloride

Benzacot, Tebamide, Tigan, Tribenzagan, Trimazide

## Class and Category
*Chemical:* Ethanolamine derivative
*Therapeutic:* Antiemetic
*Pregnancy category:* Not rated

## Indications and Dosages
➤ *To treat nausea and vomiting*
**CAPSULES**
**Adults and adolescents.** 250 mg q 6 to 8 hr, p.r.n.
**Children weighing 15 to 45 kg (33 to 99 lb).** 100 to 200 mg q 6 to 8 hr, p.r.n.
**I.M. INJECTION**
**Adults and adolescents.** 200 mg q 6 to 8 hr, p.r.n.
**RECTAL SUPPOSITORIES**
**Adults and adolescents.** 200 mg q 6 to 8 hr, p.r.n.
**Children weighing 15 to 45 kg.** 100 to 200 mg q 6 to 8 hr, p.r.n.
**Children weighing less than 15 kg.** 100 mg q 6 to 8 hr, p.r.n.

---

### Mechanism of Action
Prevents or stops nausea and vomiting by blocking dopamine receptors and emetic impulses at the chemoreceptor trigger zone in the brain.

---

## Contraindications
Children (I.M.); hypersensitivity to trimethobenzamide, benzocaine, or their components; infants and neonates (suppositories)

## Interactions
**DRUGS**
*apomorphine:* Decreased emetic response to apomorphine, increased CNS effects
*barbiturates, belladonna alkaloids, phenothiazines:* Increased risk of coma, extrapyramidal reactions, opisthotonos, and seizures
*CNS depressants:* Possibly enhanced effects of both drugs
*ototoxic drugs:* Masked signs of ototoxicity

## Adverse Reactions
**CNS:** Dizziness, drowsiness, headache
**EENT:** Blurred vision
**GI:** Diarrhea
**MS:** Muscle cramps
**Other:** Injection site burning, irritation, pain, redness, or swelling

## Nursing Considerations
• Use trimethobenzamide cautiously in patients who are dehydrated and those with an electrolyte imbalance, encephalitis, encephalopathy, gastroenteritis, or high fever.
• Be aware that drug shouldn't be used in children who have viral illnesses because they're at increased risk for Reye's syndrome, characterized by abrupt onset of irrational behavior; lethargy; persistent, severe vomiting; progressive encephalopathy leading to coma, seizures, and possibly death.
• To minimize injection site irritation, inject trimethobenzamide deep into a large muscle mass using the Z-track technique, which blocks solution from escaping along the injection route.
• Moisten rectal suppository with water or water-soluble lubricant before insertion. If suppository is too soft, refrigerate it for 30 minutes or run cold water over it before removing the wrapper.
**PATIENT TEACHING**
• Teach patient how to insert a trimethobenzamide suppository, if necessary.
• Inform patient that drug may cause blurred vision, dizziness, and drowsiness. Advise her to avoid potentially hazardous activities until drug's CNS effects are known.
• Inform patient's parents that drug may cause Reye's syndrome, and urge them to notify prescriber immediately if they notice decreased level of consciousness, irrational behavior, lethargy, or severe vomiting.

# trimethoprim

Proloprim, Trimpex

## Class and Category
*Chemical:* Dihydrofolic acid analogue
*Therapeutic:* Antibiotic
*Pregnancy category:* C

## Indications and Dosages
➤ *To treat UTIs caused by* Enterobacter
   *sp.,* Escherichia coli, Klebsiella pneumo-

niae, Proteus mirabilis, *and coagulase-negative staphylococci, including* Staphylococcus saprophyticus

**TABLETS**

**Adults and children age 12 and older.** 100 mg q 12 hr or 200 mg q.d. for 10 days.

**DOSAGE ADJUSTMENT** For patients with creatinine clearance of 15 to 30 ml/min/1.73 m², dosage usually reduced by 50%.

**Mechanism of Action**

Inhibits formation of tetrahydrofolic acid, the metabolically active form of folic acid, in susceptible bacteria. This depletes folate, an essential component of bacterial development, thereby disrupting production of bacterial nucleic acid and protein.

**Contraindications**

Hypersensitivity to trimethoprim or its components, megaloblastic anemia caused by folate deficiency, severe renal impairment (creatinine clearance of less than 15 ml/min/1.73 m²)

**Interactions**

**DRUGS**

*bone marrow depressants:* Increased risk of leukopenia, thrombocytopenia

*cyclosporine:* Increased risk of nephrotoxicity

*dapsone:* Increased blood levels and risk of adverse effects (especially methemoglobinemia) of both drugs

*folate antagonists:* Increased risk of megaloblastic anemia

*phenytoin:* Decreased phenytoin metabolism, increased risk of phenytoin toxicity

*procainamide:* Increased blood levels of procainamide and its metabolite, *N*-acetylprocainamide

*rifampin:* Increased elimination and decreased effectiveness of trimethoprim

*warfarin:* Increased anticoagulant activity of warfarin

**Adverse Reactions**

**CNS:** Fever, headache

**EENT:** Glossitis

**GI:** Abdominal pain, anorexia, diarrhea, elevated liver function test results, epigastric pain, nausea, vomiting

**GU:** Elevated BUN and serum creatinine levels

**HEME:** Leukopenia, megaloblastic anemia, methemoglobinemia, neutropenia, thrombocytopenia

**SKIN:** Exfoliative dermatitis, pruritus, rash

**Nursing Considerations**

•Obtain urine specimen, as ordered, before trimethoprim therapy starts.

•Give drug on an empty stomach to enhance absorption.

•Evaluate test values for folic acid deficiency and signs of bone marrow depression.

•Monitor serum potassium levels and renal function studies, as ordered, in patients with decreased renal function because they are at increased risk for hyperkalemia and toxic reactions when receiving trimethoprim.

**PATIENT TEACHING**

•Instruct patient to complete entire course of trimethoprim therapy, as prescribed, even if she feels better beforehand.

•Advise patient to take drug with food or milk if GI distress occurs.

•Instruct patient to notify prescriber if she experiences rash, severe fatigue, sore throat, or unusual bleeding or bruising.

# trimipramine maleate

Apo-Trimip (CAN), Novo-Tripramine (CAN), Rhotrimine (CAN), Surmontil

**Class and Category**

*Chemical:* Dibenzazepine derivative

*Therapeutic:* Antidepressant

*Pregnancy category:* C

**Indications and Dosages**

➤ *To treat depression*

**CAPSULES**

**Adults in inpatient settings.** *Initial:* 100 mg/day in divided doses, increased gradually in a few days to 200 mg/day. *Maximum:* 300 mg/day in 2 to 3 wk.

**Adolescents in inpatient settings.** *Initial:* 50 mg/day in divided doses, increased as needed. *Maximum:* 100 mg/day.

**Adults in outpatient settings.** *Initial:* 75 mg/day in divided doses, increased gradually up to 150 mg/day, as needed. *Maintenance:* 50 to 150 mg/day. *Maximum:* 200 mg/day.

**Adolescents in outpatient settings.** *Initial:* 50 mg/day in divided doses, increased as needed. *Maximum:* 100 mg/day.

**DOSAGE ADJUSTMENT** For elderly patients, initial dosage reduced to 50 mg/day in divided doses, and maximum dosage limited to 100 mg/day.

| Route | Onset | Peak | Duration |
|---|---|---|---|
| P.O. | 2 to 3 wk | Unknown | Unknown |

## Mechanism of Action
Inhibits the reuptake of norepinephrine at presynaptic neurons, thus increasing its concentration in synapses. This action may elevate mood and relieve depression.

## Contraindications
Hypersensitivity to trimipramine, other dibenzazepine tricyclic antidepressants, or their components; recovery period after an MI; use within 14 days of therapy with an MAO inhibitor or other tricyclic antidepressant

## Interactions
**DRUGS**
*amantadine, anticholinergics, antidyskinetics, antihistamines:* Increased anticholinergic effects (confusion, hallucinations, nightmares)
*anticonvulsants:* Increased CNS depression, lowered seizure threshold (high trimipramine doses), decreased anticonvulsant effect
*antithyroid drugs:* Risk of agranulocytosis
*barbiturates, carbamazepine:* Decreased blood level and effects of trimipramine
*bupropion, clozapine, cyclobenzaprine, haloperidol, loxapine, maprotiline, molindone, phenothiazines, thioxanthenes:* Increased and prolonged sedative and anticholinergic effects of both drugs, increased risk of seizures
*cimetidine:* Decreased trimipramine metabolism, possibly leading to trimipramine toxicity
*clonidine:* Decreased hypotensive effect and increased CNS depressant effect of clonidine
*CNS depressants:* Increased hypotension and CNS and respiratory depression
*disulfiram, ethchlorvynol:* Transient delirium, risk of CNS depression (ethchlorvynol)
*fluoxetine:* Increased trimipramine level
*guanadrel, guanethidine:* Decreased hypotensive effect
*MAO inhibitors:* Increased risk of death, hyperpyrexia, hypertensive crisis, severe seizures
*methylphenidate:* Decreased methylphenidate effects, increased blood trimipramine level

*metrizamide:* Increased risk of seizures
*naphazoline (ophthalmic), oxymetazoline (nasal or ophthalmic), phenylephrine (nasal or ophthalmic), xylometazoline (nasal):* Increased vasopressor effect of these drugs
*oral anticoagulants:* Increased anticoagulation
*phenothiazines:* Increased blood trimipramine level, decreased phenothiazine metabolism
*pimozide, probucol:* Increased risk of arrhythmias, possibly prolonged QT interval
*sympathomimetics:* Increased risk of arrhythmias, hyperpyrexia, severe hypertension
*thyroid hormones:* Increased therapeutic and toxic effects of both drugs
**ACTIVITIES**
*alcohol use:* Increased hypotension and CNS and respiratory depression

## Adverse Reactions
**CNS:** Anxiety, ataxia, confusion, CVA, delirium, dizziness, drowsiness, excitement, extrapyramidal reactions, hallucinations, headache, insomnia, nervousness, nightmares, parkinsonism, seizures, suicidal ideation, tremor
**CV:** Arrhythmias, orthostatic hypotension
**EENT:** Blurred vision, dry mouth, increased intraocular pressure, taste perversion, tinnitus, tongue swelling
**ENDO:** Gynecomastia, syndrome of inappropriate ADH secretion
**GI:** Constipation, diarrhea, heartburn, ileus, increased appetite, nausea, vomiting
**GU:** Sexual dysfunction, testicular swelling, urine retention
**HEME:** Agranulocytosis, bone marrow depression
**RESP:** Wheezing
**SKIN:** Alopecia, diaphoresis, jaundice, photosensitivity, pruritus, rash, urticaria
**Other:** Facial edema, weight gain

## Nursing Considerations
•Expect to gradually reduce dosage, as prescribed, before electroconvulsive therapy.
**PATIENT TEACHING**
•Instruct patient to take the last dose early in the evening to avoid insomnia.
•Advise patient to avoid hazardous activities until drug's CNS effects are known.
•Advise changing positions slowly to minimize effects of orthostatic hypotension.

T

• Urge patient to avoid alcohol during therapy.
• Advise patient to avoid excessive sunlight and to wear sunscreen when she's outdoors.
• Instruct patient to notify prescriber about unusual bruising and signs of infection.
• Suggest that patient use sugarless gum or hard candy to relieve dry mouth.
•**WARNING** Urge parents to watch their child or adolescent closely for abnormal behavior or increased aggression or hostility. Stress need of notifying prescriber about changes.

# tromethamine

Tham

## Class and Category
*Chemical:* Organic amine
*Therapeutic:* Alkalinizer
*Pregnancy category:* C

## Indications and Dosages
➤ *To treat metabolic acidosis associated with cardiac arrest*
**I.V. INFUSION**
**Adults and children.** 3.6 to 10.8 g (111 to 333 ml) of 0.3 M solution.
**I.V. INJECTION**
**Adults and children.** If chest is opened, 2 to 6 g injected directly into open ventricular cavity.
➤ *To treat metabolic acidosis during cardiac bypass surgery*
**I.V. INFUSION**
**Adults and children.** 9 ml (2.7 mEq or 0.32 g) of 0.3 M solution/kg as a single dose. *Usual:* 500 ml (150 mEq or 18 g) infused over 1 hr. *Maximum:* 500 mg/kg over 1 hr.

## Mechanism of Action
Combines with hydrogen ions and their associated acid anions, including lactic, pyruvic, and carbonic acid, to form salts that are excreted in urine. Tromethamine exerts additional alkalinizing effects by acting as an osmotic diuretic, promoting the excretion of alkaline urine that contains increased amounts of carbon dioxide and electrolytes.

## Contraindications
Anuria, chronic respiratory acidosis, hypersensitivity to tromethamine or its components, uremia

## Interactions
**DRUGS**
*amphetamines, quinidine, other pH-dependent drugs:* Altered excretion of these drugs

## Adverse Reactions
**CNS:** Fever
**CV:** Vasospasm
**ENDO:** Hypoglycemia
**GI:** Hepatic necrosis (hemorrhagic)
**RESP:** Respiratory depression
**Other:** Hypervolemia; infusion site infection, phlebitis, or venous thrombosis; metabolic alkalosis

## Nursing Considerations
• Evaluate blood pH, blood glucose, and serum bicarbonate and electrolyte levels, and partial pressure of arterial carbon dioxide before, during, and after tromethamine therapy, as ordered.
• Be aware that, except in life-threatening situations, tromethamine therapy is limited to 1 day because of the risk of alkalosis.
•**WARNING** Be aware that exceeding the recommended dosage can cause alkalosis, respiratory depression, and reduced carbon dioxide level.
• Expect I.V. administration to increase the risk of hypervolemia and subsequent pulmonary edema.
• Assess infusion site frequently for signs of infiltration, which may cause inflammation, necrosis, thrombosis, tissue sloughing, and vasospasm.
• Be aware that patients with renal failure have an increased risk of developing hyperkalemia. For such patients, be prepared to monitor ECG continuously and assess serum potassium level frequently.
• Monitor blood glucose level frequently during and after therapy because rapid administration can cause hypoglycemia for several hours.
**PATIENT TEACHING**
• Inform family members that patient's vital signs and laboratory test results will be measured frequently to monitor her progress.

# trospium chloride

Sanctura

## Class and Category

*Chemical:* Quaternary ammonium compound
*Therapeutic:* Bladder antispasmodic
*Pregnancy category:* C

## Indications and Dosages

➤ *To treat overactive bladder with symptoms of urge urinary incontinence, urgency, and urinary frequency*

TABLETS

**Adults.** 20 mg b.i.d. 1 hour before meals or on empty stomach.

DOSAGE ADJUSTMENT For patients with severe renal insufficiency (creatinine clearance less than 30 ml/min) and patients age 75 or older, dosage reduced to 20 mg q.d. at bedtime.

| Route | Onset | Peak | Duration |
|-------|-------|------|----------|
| P.O. | Unknown | 5 to 6 hr | Unknown |

### Mechanism of Action

Antagonizes the effect of acetylcholine on muscarinic receptors in the bladder. Trospium's parasympatholytic action reduces the tonus of smooth muscle in the bladder. These actions increase maximum cystometric bladder capacity and volume with the first detrusor contraction, which relieves the sensation of urgency and frequency and enhances bladder control.

## Contraindications

Gastric retention, hypersensitivity to trospium or its components, uncontrolled angle-closure glaucoma, urine retention

## Interactions

DRUGS

*anticholinergics:* Increased frequency or severity of adverse effects; possibly reduced absorption of trospium
*digoxin, metformin, morphine, pancuronium, procainamide:* Possibly increased plasma concentration of trospium, digoxin, metformin, morphine, pancuronium, procainamide

ACTIVITIES

*alcohol use:* Possibly increased drowsiness

## Adverse Reactions

**CNS:** Dizziness, drowsiness, fatigue, headache, light-headedness
**CV:** Palpitations, tachycardia
**EENT:** Blurred vision; dry eyes, mouth, or throat
**GI:** Abdominal distention or pain, constipation, flatulence, indigestion, vomiting
**GU:** Urine retention
**SKIN:** Decreased sweating, dry skin, flushing
**Other:** Angioedema

## Nursing Considerations

• Use trospium cautiously in patients with ulcerative colitis, intestinal atony, or myasthenia gravis because drug may decrease GI motility; patients with significant bladder outflow obstruction because drug may cause urine retention; patients with hepatic impairment because drug's effects on the liver are unknown; and patients with renal impairment because drug excretion may be impaired.
• Monitor elderly patients, especially those age 75 or older, for adverse reactions because elderly patients have an increased risk of trospium-induced adverse reactions.

PATIENT TEACHING

• Instruct patient to take trospium on an empty stomach or at least 1 hour before eating because food delays drug absorption.
• Caution patient to avoid activities in a warm or hot environment because sweating may be delayed, which could cause a sudden increase in body temperature and heatstroke.
• Advise patient to avoid hazardous activities until drug's CNS effects are known.
• Inform patient that alcohol may increase the risk of drowsiness; urge patient to limit or abstain from alcoholic beverages while taking trospium.

# tubocurarine chloride

## Class and Category

*Chemical:* Isoquinoline derivative
*Therapeutic:* Anticonvulsant
*Pregnancy category:* C

## Indications and Dosages

➤ *To manage muscle contractions of seizures associated with electroshock therapy*

T

**I.V. INJECTION**
**Adults.** 157 mcg/kg (0.157 mg/kg) over 30 to 90 sec, given just before electroshock therapy. Expect initial dose to be 3 mg less than calculated total dose.

➤ *To produce skeletal muscle paralysis during anesthesia*

**I.V. OR I.M. INJECTION**
**Adults.** *Initial:* 6 to 9 mg. *Maintenance:* 3 to 4.5 mg in 3 to 5 min. if needed. For prolonged procedures, 3-mg supplemental doses given.
**Infants and children.** 500 mcg/kg I.V.
**Neonates.** *Initial:* 250 to 500 mcg/kg I.V.
*Maintenance:* One-fifth to one-sixth of initial dose if needed.

➤ *To facilitate endotracheal intubation and aid controlled respiration during mechanical ventilation*

**I.V. INJECTION**
**Adults.** *Initial:* 16.5 mcg/kg. *Maintenance:* Dosage individualized based on patient response.

➤ *To aid in the diagnosis of myasthenia gravis*

**I.V. INJECTION**
**Adults.** 4 to 33 mcg/kg. After 2 to 3 min, 1.5 mg of neostigmine is given I.V. to terminate the test.

| Route | Onset | Peak | Duration |
|---|---|---|---|
| I.V. | 1 min | 2 to 5 min | 20 to 40 min |

### Incompatibilities

Don't mix tubocurarine with barbiturates, such as methohexital or thiopental, because a precipitate may form.

## Mechanism of Action

Tubocurarine reduces the intensity of skeletal muscle contractions caused by electrically induced seizures. Normally, when a nerve impulse arrives at a somatic motor nerve terminal, it triggers acetylcholine (ACh) stored in synaptic vesicles to be released into the neuromuscular junction. The released ACh binds with nicotinic receptors embedded in the skeletal muscle motor endplate, as shown below left, triggering muscle cell depolarization and contraction.

Tubocurarine is a nondepolarizing neuromuscular blocker that acts as a competitive antagonist of ACh. By binding to the nicotinic receptors, as shown below right, it prevents transmission of the action potential at the neuromuscular junction, thereby sustaining skeletal muscle relaxation and eliminating the peripheral muscular manifestations of seizures. The drug has no effect on the CNS processes involved with seizures because it doesn't cross the blood-brain barrier.

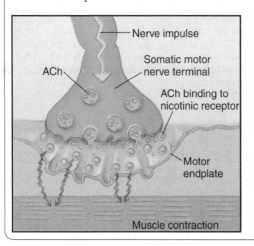

Nerve impulse
ACh
Somatic motor nerve terminal
ACh binding to nicotinic receptor
Motor endplate
Muscle contraction

Tubocurarine binding to nicotinic receptor
Muscle relaxation

## Contraindications
Hypersensitivity to tubocurarine or its components, patients in whom histamine release may be dangerous

## Interactions
**DRUGS**
*alfentanil, fentanyl, sufentanil:* Prevented or reversed muscle rigidity from these drugs
*aminoglycosides, anesthetics, capreomycin, citrate-anticoagulated blood, clindamycin, lidocaine (I.V.), lincomycin, polymyxins, procaine (I.V.), trimethaphan:* Additive neuromuscular blocking effects
*beta blockers, calcium salts:* Prolonged and enhanced effects of tubocurarine
*magnesium salts, procainamide, quinidine:* Enhanced blockade effects
*opioid analgesics:* Additive histamine release effects, additive respiratory depressant effects, worsened bradycardia and hypotension

## Adverse Reactions
**CV:** Arrhythmias, bradycardia, edema, hypotension, shock, tachycardia
**RESP:** Bronchospasm
**SKIN:** Erythema, flushing, itching, rash
**Other:** Anaphylaxis

## Nursing Considerations
•If patient has a history of CV disease or is hypotensive, monitor her for further decrease in blood pressure.
•Monitor patient for bronchospasm and hypotension because tubocurarine may cause increased histamine release.
•Keep emergency equipment and drugs nearby in case respiratory depression occurs.
**PATIENT TEACHING**
•Explain the need for frequent hemodynamic monitoring.

# U·V·W

## urea

### (carbamide)

Ureaphil

### Class and Category

*Chemical:* Carbonic acid diamide salt
*Therapeutic:* Antiglaucoma, diuretic
*Pregnancy category:* C

### Indications and Dosages

➤ *To reduce cerebral edema and intracranial pressure*

**I.V. INFUSION**

**Adults and children age 2 and older.** 500 mg to 1.5 g/kg as 30% solution in $D_5W$, $D_{10}W$, or 10% invert sugar solution infused over 30 min to 2 hr at 4 or 6 ml/min, according to manufacturer's instructions. *Maximum:* 2 g/kg/day.

**Children under age 2.** 100 mg to 1.5 g/kg as 30% solution in $D_5W$, $D_{10}W$, or 10% invert sugar solution infused over 30 min to 2 hr at 4 or 6 ml/min, according to manufacturer's instructions.

➤ *To treat malignant or secondary glaucoma*

**I.V. INFUSION**

**Adults.** 500 mg to 1.5 g/kg as 30% solution in $D_5W$, $D_{10}W$, or 10% invert sugar solution infused over 30 min to 2 hr at 4 or 6 ml/min, according to manufacturer's instructions. *Maximum:* 2 g/kg/day.

**DOSAGE ADJUSTMENT** Dosage reduced or drug withheld for patients with renal impairment if BUN level rises to 75 mg/dl or more or if diuresis fails to occur within 2 hr after administration.

| Route | Onset | Peak | Duration |
|-------|-------|------|----------|
| I.V. | 10 min | 1 to 2 hr | 3 to 10 hr* |

### Contraindications

Active intracranial bleeding, hepatic failure, hypersensitivity to urea or its components, renal impairment, severe dehydration

---

* For diuresis; 5 to 6 hr for reduced intraocular pressure.

### Mechanism of Action

Elevates blood plasma osmolality, creating an osmotic effect that increases the movement of water from the brain, CSF, and anterior portion of the eyes into interstitial fluid and plasma. This action reduces cerebral edema, intracranial pressure, CSF volume, and intraocular pressure. Large doses inhibit the reabsorption of water and solutes in the renal tubules and induce diuresis by affecting the osmotic pressure gradient of the glomerular filtrate.

### Interactions

**DRUGS**

*carbonic anhydrase inhibitors, other diuretics:* Additive diuretic and intraocular pressure–reducing effects
*lithium:* Increased renal excretion of lithium

### Adverse Reactions

**CNS:** Agitation, confusion, fever, headache, hyperthermia, nervousness, subarachnoid hemorrhage, subdural hematoma, syncope
**CV:** Tachycardia
**EENT:** Dry mouth, intraocular hemorrhage
**GI:** Nausea, thirst, vomiting
**GU:** Elevated BUN level
**HEME:** Hemolysis
**SKIN:** Blemishes, extravasation with tissue necrosis and sloughing
**Other:** Dehydration, hypokalemia, hyponatremia, infusion site phlebitis or thrombosis

### Nursing Considerations

• To obtain maximum reduction of intracranial or intraocular pressure, expect to give urea 60 minutes before ocular or intracranial surgery.
• Don't mix urea with invert sugar solution if patient has fructose intolerance from aldolase deficiency.
• Avoid infusing drug into leg veins to reduce risk of phlebitis and thrombosis.
• Discard unused portion of drug after 24 hours.
• Be aware that rapid administration may cause hemolysis, increased capillary bleeding, and, in patients with glaucoma, intraocular hemorrhage.
• Maintain adequate hydration to minimize adverse reactions. Assess for signs of dehydration, including dry mucous membranes or tenting.
• Monitor BUN and serum electrolyte levels as well as fluid intake and output during

urea therapy because prolonged use can cause diuresis.

**PATIENT TEACHING**

•Instruct patient to notify prescriber immediately about difficulty breathing or shortness of breath because drug can cause transient increases in circulatory volume, leading to circulatory overload, exacerbations of heart failure, or pulmonary edema.

•Advise patient to expect increased urine output.

•Encourage patient to remain on bed rest during therapy.

# urokinase

Abbokinase, Abbokinase Open-Cath

## Class and Category

*Chemical:* Renal enzymatic protein
*Therapeutic:* Thrombolytic
*Pregnancy category:* B

## Indications and Dosages

➤ *To treat acute coronary artery thrombosis*

**INTRACORONARY INFUSION**

**Adults.** 6,000 IU/min until artery is maximally opened (up to 2 hr may be required). *Usual:* 500,000 IU.

➤ *To treat acute pulmonary thromboembolism including massive events*

**I.V. INFUSION**

**Adults.** *Initial:* 4,400 IU/kg over 10 min, followed by 4,400 IU/kg/hr for 12 hr.

➤ *To clear I.V. catheter occlusion*

**INSTILLATION**

**Adults and children.** 5,000 IU/ml instilled into occluded line.

| Route | Onset | Peak | Duration |
|---|---|---|---|
| I.V. | Unknown | 20 min to 2 hr | 4 hr |
| Intra-coronary | Unknown | Unknown | 4 hr |

## Incompatibilities

Don't administer I.V. urokinase through the same I.V. line as other drugs or add other drugs to urokinase solution.

## Contraindications

Arteriovenous malformation, bleeding disorder, CVA during previous 2 months, hypersensitivity to urokinase or its components, internal bleeding, intracranial aneurysm, intracranial or intraspinal surgery during previous 2 months, intracranial tumor, recent cardiopulmonary resuscitation, recent trauma, severe uncontrolled hypertension (systolic blood pressure of 200 mm Hg or higher, or diastolic blood pressure of 110 mm Hg or higher)

---

**Mechanism of Action**

Indirectly promotes conversion of plasminogen to plasmin, an enzyme that breaks down fibrin clots, fibrinogen, and other plasma proteins, including procoagulant factors V and VIII.

---

## Interactions

**DRUGS**

*antifibrinolytics (aminocaproic acid, aprotinin):* Mutual antagonism
*antihypertensives:* Increased risk of severe hypotension
*cefamandole, cefoperazone, cefotetan, plicamycin, valproic acid:* Increased risk of hypoprothrombinemia and severe hemorrhage
*corticosteroids, ethacrynic acid, salicylates (nonacetylated):* Increased risk of GI ulceration and bleeding
*enoxaparin, heparin, NSAIDs, oral anticoagulants, platelet-aggregation inhibitors:* Increased risk of hemorrhage
*thiotepa:* Increased therapeutic effects of thiotepa

## Adverse Reactions

**CNS:** Chills, CVA, fever, headache
**CV:** Arrhythmias, including tachycardia; chest pain; cholesterol embolization, hypertension; hypotension
**EENT:** Orolingual edema
**GI:** Nausea, vomiting
**HEME:** Unusual bleeding
**MS:** Back pain, myalgia
**RESP:** Bronchospasm, dyspnea, hypoxemia, wheezing
**SKIN:** Cyanosis, ecchymosis, flushing, pruritus, rash, urticaria
**Other:** Anaphylaxis, infusion site reactions, metabolic acidosis

## Nursing Considerations

•To prevent foaming, don't shake urokinase when reconstituting. Consult with pharmacist about giving drug through 0.45-micron or smaller cellulose membrane filter.

•Assess baseline hematocrit, platelet count, thrombin time, APTT, PT, and INR as ordered.
•Monitor heart rate and rhythm by continuous ECG during therapy, especially during rapid lysis of coronary thrombi, because arrhythmias can occur with reperfusion.
•Monitor blood pressure for hypotension. If hypotension occurs, notify prescriber and expect to reduce infusion rate.
•Check for bleeding at puncture sites and in urine and stool. Check for intracranial bleeding by performing frequent neurologic assessments.
•After arterial puncture is performed, apply pressure for at least 30 minutes and then apply pressure dressing. Check frequently for bleeding during therapy.
•To prevent bleeding and associated complications, avoid venipunctures; use an external blood pressure cuff to measure blood pressure; give acetaminophen (not aspirin), as prescribed, for fever; and handle patient as little as possible.
•**WARNING** If serious bleeding begins and can't be controlled with local pressure, stop infusion immediately and notify prescriber.
**PATIENT TEACHING**
•Instruct patient to remain on bed rest during urokinase therapy.
•Inform patient that minor bleeding may occur at wounds or puncture sites.

# ursodiol
## (ursodeoxycholic acid)
Actigall, Urso Forte, URSO 250, Ursofalk (CAN)

## Class and Category
*Chemical:* Naturally occurring bile acid
*Therapeutic:* Bile salt replenisher, cholelitholytic
*Pregnancy category:* B

## Indications and Dosages
➤ *To prevent gallstone formation in obese patients during rapid weight loss*
**CAPSULES**
**Adults and adolescents.** 300 mg b.i.d. Alternatively, 8 to 10 mg/kg/day in divided doses b.i.d or t.i.d.
➤ *To dissolve gallstones*

**CAPSULES**
**Adults and adolescents.** 8 to 10 mg/kg/day in divided doses b.i.d. or t.i.d.
➤ *To treat primary biliary cirrhosis*
**TABLETS**
**Adults.** 13 to 15 mg/kg/day in two to four divided doses.

## Mechanism of Action
Suppresses hepatic synthesis, biliary secretion, and intestinal reabsorption of cholesterol. Prolonged use promotes dissolution of gallstones.

## Contraindications
Acute cholangiitis; gallstone complications (such as biliary GI fistula; biliary obstruction; calcified, radiopaque, or radiotranslucent bile-pigment gallstones; cholecystitis; pancreatitis); hypersensitivity to ursodiol, other bile acids, or their components

## Interactions
**DRUGS**
*aluminum-containing antacids, cholestyramine, colestipol:* Decreased absorption and therapeutic effects of ursodiol
*clofibrate, estrogens, neomycin, oral contraceptives, progestins:* Interference with ursodiol's therapeutic effects; increased risk of gallstone formation
**FOODS**
*any foods:* Increased dissolution of drug

## Adverse Reactions
**CNS:** Anxiety, asthenia, depression, fatigue, headache, sleep disturbance
**CV:** Chest pain, hypertension, peripheral edema
**ENDO:** Hyperglycemia
**EENT:** Metallic taste, rhinitis, stomatitis
**GI:** Abdominal pain, cholecystitis, constipation, diarrhea, esophagitis, flatulence, indigestion, nausea, peptic ulcer, vomiting
**GU:** Elevated CK level
**HEME:** Leukopenia
**MS:** Arthralgia, back pain, myalgia
**RESP:** Cough
**SKIN:** Alopecia, diaphoresis, dry skin, pruritus, rash, urticaria

## Nursing Considerations
•Administer ursodiol with food to increase drug dissolution.

• Administer aluminum-containing antacids, cholestyramine, and colestipol at least 1 hour before or 4 hours after ursodiol because they may decrease drug's effects.

• Expect drug to be discontinued if gallstones haven't partially dissolved after 12 months of therapy.

• Be aware that if patient inadvertently takes too much ursodiol, diarrhea will most likely result and warrant systemic treatment.

**PATIENT TEACHING**

• Instruct patient to take ursodiol with meals.

• Advise patient to take aluminum-containing antacids at least 1 hour before or 4 hours after ursodiol to avoid impaired absorption.

• Urge patient to notify prescriber immediately if signs of acute cholecystitis develop, such as acute right-upper-quadrant abdominal pain.

• Inform patient that he may need to take ursodiol for a prolonged period before gallstones dissolve.

• Advise diabetic patient to monitor blood glucose levels while taking ursodiol because drug may alter blood glucose control.

# valproic acid

Alti-Valproic (CAN), Depakene, Depakote ER, Deproic (CAN), Dom-Proic (CAN), Med-Valproic (CAN), Novo-Valproic (CAN), Nu-Valproic (CAN), PMS-Valproic Acid (CAN)

## valproate sodium

Depacon

## divalproex sodium

Depakote, Depakote Sprinkle, Epival (CAN)

## Class and Category

*Chemical:* Carboxylic acid derivative
*Therapeutic:* Anticonvulsant
*Pregnancy category:* D

## Indications and Dosages

➤ *To treat simple or complex absence seizures, complex partial seizures, myoclonic seizures, and generalized tonic-clonic seizures as monotherapy*

CAPSULES, DELAYED-RELEASE SPRINKLE CAPSULES, DELAYED-RELEASE TABLETS, SYRUP, I.V. INFUSION

(VALPROIC ACID, VALPROATE SODIUM, DIVALPROEX SODIUM)

**Adults and adolescents.** *Initial:* 10 to 15 mg/kg/day in divided doses b.i.d. or t.i.d., increased

by 5 to 10 mg/kg/day q wk, as needed and as prescribed. *Maximum:* 60 mg/kg/ day.

**Children.** *Initial:* 15 to 45 mg/kg/day in divided doses b.i.d. or t.i.d., increased by 5 to 10 mg/kg/day q wk, as needed and as prescribed.

➤ *As adjunct to treat simple or complex absence seizures, complex partial seizures, myoclonic seizures, and generalized tonic-clonic seizures*

CAPSULES, DELAYED-RELEASE SPRINKLE CAPSULES, DELAYED-RELEASE TABLETS, SYRUP, I.V. INFUSION

(VALPROIC ACID, VALPROATE SODIUM, DIVALPROEX SODIUM)

**Adults and adolescents.** 10 to 30 mg/kg/day in divided doses, increased by 5 to 10 mg/kg/day q wk, as needed and as prescribed.

**Children.** 30 to 100 mg/kg/day in divided doses, as prescribed.

**DOSAGE ADJUSTMENT** For adults being converted from immediate-release divalproex tablets to delayed-release tablets, dosage increased to 8% to 20% more than total daily dose of immediate-release tablets and given once daily.

➤ *To treat acute manic phase of bipolar disorder*

DELAYED-RELEASE TABLETS (DIVALPROEX SODIUM)

**Adults.** *Initial:* 750 mg/day in divided doses. *Maximum:* 60 mg/kg/day.

➤ *To prevent migraine headache*

TABLETS, TABLETS (DIVALPROEX SODIUM)

**Adults.** 250 mg q 12 hr, increased p.r.n. *Maximum:* 1 g/day.

DELAYED-RELEASE TABLETS (DIVALPROEX SODIUM)

**Adults.** 500 mg q.d., increased, as needed and prescribed, up to 1 g/day. *Maximum:* 1 g/day.

## Contraindications

Hepatic dysfunction; hypersensitivity to valproic acid, valproate sodium, divalproex sodium, or their components; urea cycle disorders

---

### Mechanism of Action

May decrease seizure activity by blocking the reuptake of gamma-aminobutyric acid (GABA), the most common inhibitory neurotransmitter in the brain. GABA is known to suppress the rapid firing of neurons by inhibiting voltage-sensitive sodium channels.

## Interactions

### DRUGS

*aspirin, heparin, NSAIDs, oral anticoagulants, thrombolytics:* Increased inhibition of platelet aggregation and risk of bleeding
*barbiturates, primidone:* Increased blood levels of both drugs, additive CNS effects
*carbamazepine:* Possibly decreased valproic acid effectiveness
*cholestyramine:* Decreased bioavailability of valproic acid
*clonazepam:* Increased risk of absence seizures
*CNS depressants:* Increased CNS depression
*diazepam:* Inhibited diazepam metabolism
*ethosuximide:* Unpredictable blood ethosuximide level
*felbamate:* Impaired valproic acid metabolism and increased blood drug level
*haloperidol, loxapine, MAO inhibitors, maprotiline, phenothiazines, thioxanthenes, tricyclic antidepressants:* Increased CNS depression, lowered seizure threshold
*lamotrigine:* Decreased lamotrigine clearance
*mefloquine:* Decreased blood levels of valproic acid, divalproex, and valproate sodium; increased risk of seizures
*phenytoin:* Increased risk of phenytoin toxicity, loss of seizure control

### ACTIVITIES

*alcohol use:* Additive CNS depression

## Adverse Reactions

**CNS:** Agitation, ataxia, confusion, depression, dizziness, drowsiness, euphoria, hallucinations, headache, hyperesthesia, lack of coordination, lethargy, loss of seizure control, paresthesia, psychosis, sedation, tremor, vertigo, weakness
**EENT:** Diplopia, nystagmus, pharyngitis, spots before eyes
**ENDO:** Galactorrhea, hyperglycemia
**GI:** Abdominal pain, anorexia, constipation, diarrhea, elevated liver function test results, hepatotoxicity, increased appetite, indigestion, nausea, pancreatitis, vomiting
**GU:** Menstrual irregularities
**HEME:** Eosinophilia, hematoma, leukopenia, prolonged bleeding time, thrombocytopenia
**MS:** Dysarthria
**SKIN:** Alopecia, diaphoresis, erythema multiforme, jaundice, petechiae, photosensitivity, pruritus, rash, Stevens-Johnson syndrome
**Other:** Facial edema, hyperammonemia, injection site pain, weight gain or loss

## Nursing Considerations

•Give oral valproic acid or divalproex with food to minimize GI irritation, if necessary.
•Administer drug at least 2 hours before or 6 hours after cholestyramine.
•Don't mix syrup with carbonated beverages; doing so may produce an unpleasant-tasting mixture and irritate the mouth and throat.
•Don't break or allow patient to chew delayed-release tablets.
•As needed, sprinkle contents of delayed-release sprinkle capsules on small amount of semisolid food just before administration. Instruct patient not to chew contents of delayed-release sprinkle capsules.
•For I.V. administration, dilute prescribed dose with at least 50 ml of compatible diluent and infuse over 60 minutes.
•Be aware that patient should be switched from I.V. to P.O. form of valproic acid as soon as possible.
•Be aware that patient with hypoalbuminemia or another protein-binding deficiency is at increased risk for valproic acid toxicity.
•Assess for signs and symptoms of decreased hepatic function, including anorexia, facial edema, jaundice, lethargy, loss of seizure control, malaise, vomiting, and weakness.
•Monitor liver function test results, as ordered. Assess for signs and symptoms of hepatotoxicity during first 6 months of treatment, especially in children under age 2. Notify prescriber immediately if you suspect hepatotoxicity.
•Monitor platelet count, as ordered, for signs of thrombocytopenia, and notify prescriber if they appear.
•**WARNING** Be aware that hyperammonemia may occur even if patient's liver function test results are normal. Monitor ammonia levels, as ordered. If patient develops unexplained lethargy, vomiting, or changes in mental status with an increase in ammonia level or if asymptomatic ammonia elevations are detected and persist, expect valproic acid to be discontinued.

### PATIENT TEACHING

•Instruct patient to swallow capsules whole to prevent irritation to mouth and throat. However, delayed-release sprinkle capsules may be opened and contents mixed with food for easier swallowing. Instruct patient not to chew contents of delayed-release sprinkle capsules.

•Advise patient to avoid potentially hazardous activities during therapy because drug may affect mental and motor performance.
•Urge patient to avoid alcohol during therapy.
•Urge female patient to notify prescriber immediately about suspected or known pregnancy.
•Advise patient to notify prescriber if tremor develops during therapy; occurrence of tremor may be dose-related.

# valsartan

Diovan

## Class and Category

*Chemical:* Nonpeptide tetrazole derivative
*Therapeutic:* Antihypertensive
*Pregnancy category:* C (first trimester), D (later trimesters)

## Indications and Dosages

➤ *To manage hypertension, alone or with other antihypertensives*

**CAPSULES**

**Adults.** *Initial:* 80 or 160 mg q.d., increased as needed and prescribed. *Maximum:* 320 mg/day.

➤ *To treat class II to IV heart failure*

**CAPSULES**

**Adults.** *Initial:* 40 mg b.i.d., increased to 80 mg b.i.d. and then 160 mg b.i.d., as needed and prescribed. *Maximum:* 320 mg/day.

➤ *To reduce cardiovascular mortality in stable patients with left ventricular failure or dysfunction following an MI*

**CAPSULES**

**Adults.** *Initial:* 20 mg b.i.d. starting as early as 12 hr after MI, increased to 40 mg b.i.d. within 7 days, followed by subsequent adjustments to 160 mg b.i.d., as tolerated. *Maintenance:* 160 mg b.i.d.

**DOSAGE ADJUSTMENT** If patient develops symptomatic hypotension or renal dysfunction, dosage decreased.

| Route | Onset | Peak | Duration |
|-------|-------|------|----------|
| P.O. | 2 hr | 6 hr | 24 hr |

## Contraindications

Hypersensitivity to valsartan or its components

## Mechanism of Action

Blocks the hormone angiotensin II from binding to the receptor sites in vascular smooth muscle, adrenal glands, and other tissues. This action inhibits angiotensin II's vasoconstrictive and aldosterone-secreting effects, thereby reducing blood pressure.

## Interactions

**DRUGS**

*antihypertensives, diuretics:* Additive hypotensive effect
*potassium salts, potassium-sparing diuretics:* Possibly hyperkalemia

**FOODS**

*potassium-containing salt substitutes:* Possibly hyperkalemia

## Adverse Reactions

**CNS:** Dizziness, fatigue, headache, insomnia
**CV:** Edema
**EENT:** Pharyngitis, rhinitis, sinusitis
**GI:** Abdominal pain, diarrhea, indigestion, nausea, vomiting
**MS:** Arthralgia
**RESP:** Cough, upper respiratory tract infection
**Other:** Hyperkalemia, viral infection

## Nursing Considerations

•Be aware that valsartan shouldn't be given to patients who have hypovolemia or are taking a diuretic because of the increased risk of severe hypotension from volume depletion.
•Use valsartan cautiously during second and third trimesters of pregnancy because of the risk of serious adverse effects on fetus.
•Monitor blood pressure frequently during therapy.
•Be aware that maximal blood pressure reduction typically occurs after 4 weeks.
•Monitor serum potassium level because drug may elevate potassium level by blocking aldosterone secretion.

**PATIENT TEACHING**

•Instruct patient to take valsartan exactly as prescribed at the same time each day to maintain therapeutic effect.
•Advise patient to avoid potentially hazardous activities until drug's CNS effects are known.

•Advise patient to avoid using potassium-containing salt substitutes without consulting prescriber.

•Instruct female patient of childbearing age to use reliable birth control during therapy and to notify prescriber immediately about known or suspected pregnancy.

•Urge patient to keep follow-up appointments with prescriber to monitor progress.

# vancomycin hydrochloride

Vancocin

## Class and Category

*Chemical:* Tricyclic glycopeptide derivative
*Therapeutic:* Antibiotic
*Pregnancy category:* B (oral), C (parenteral)

## Indications and Dosages

➤ *To treat pseudomembranous colitis caused by* Clostridium difficile *and enterocolitis caused by staphylococci*

**CAPSULES, ORAL SOLUTION**
**Adults and adolescents.** 125 to 500 mg q 6 hr for 7 to 10 days. *Maximum:* 2 g/day.
**Children.** 10 mg/kg (up to 125 mg) q 6 hr for 7 to 10 days. *Maximum:* 2 g/day.

➤ *To treat bacterial endocarditis caused by methicillin-resistant* Staphylococcus aureus

**I.V. INFUSION**
**Adults.** 30 mg/kg/day in equally divided doses b.i.d. for 4 to 6 wk. *Maximum:* 2 g/day.

➤ *As adjunct to treat bacterial endocarditis caused by methicillin-resistant* S. aureus *in patients with prosthetic heart valve*

**I.V. INFUSION**
**Adults.** 30 mg/kg/day in equally divided doses b.i.d. to q.i.d. for 6 wk or longer in conjunction with rifampin and gentamicin. *Maximum:* 2 g/day.

➤ *To treat bacterial endocarditis caused by* Streptococcus bovis *or* Streptococcus viridans

**I.V. INFUSION**
**Adults.** 30 mg/kg/day in equally divided doses b.i.d. for 4 wk. *Maximum:* 2 g/day.

➤ *As adjunct to treat bacterial endocarditis caused by enterococci*

**I.V. INFUSION**
**Adults.** 30 mg/kg/day in equally divided doses b.i.d. for 4 to 6 wk in conjunction with gentamicin. *Maximum:* 2 g/day.

➤ *To treat bacterial septicemia, bone and joint infections, pneumonia, and skin and soft-tissue infections caused by* Staphylococcus, *including methicillin-resistant strains, and life-threatening infections*

**I.V. INFUSION**
**Adults and children age 12 and older.** 500 mg q 6 hr or 1 g q 12 hr infused over at least 60 min. *Maximum:* 4 g/day.
**Children ages 1 month to 12 years.** 10 mg/kg q 6 hr or 20 mg/kg q 12 hr infused over at least 60 min.
**Neonates ages 1 week to 1 month.** *Initial:* 15 mg/kg followed by 10 mg/kg q 8 hr infused over at least 60 min.
**Neonates under age 1 week.** *Initial:* 15 mg/kg followed by 10 mg/kg q 12 hr infused over at least 60 min.

## Mechanism of Action

Inhibits bacterial RNA and cell wall synthesis; alters permeability of bacterial membranes, causing cell wall lysis and cell death.

## Incompatibilities

Don't give I.V. vancomycin through the same I.V. line as other drugs. Don't add vancomycin to albumin-containing solutions, alkaline solutions, aminophylline, amobarbital sodium, aztreonam, cefepime, ceftazidime, chloramphenicol sodium succinate, chlorothiazide sodium, dexamethasone sodium phosphate, foscarnet sodium, heparin sodium, methicillin sodium, penicillin G, pentobarbital sodium, phenobarbital sodium, piperacillin sodium and tazobactam sodium, secobarbital sodium, and sodium bicarbonate. Drug may precipitate with heavy metals.

## Contraindications

Hypersensitivity to vancomycin or its components, hypersensitivity to corn or corn products when vancomycin is given with dextrose solutions

## Interactions

**DRUGS**

*aminoglycosides (amikacin, gentamicin, tobramycin), amphotericin B, bacitracin (parenteral), bumetanide, capreomycin, carmustine, cidofovir, cisplatin, cyclosporine, ethacrynic acid, furosemide, paromomycin, pentamidine (parenteral), polymyxins, salicylates (parenteral), streptozocin:* Additive nephrotoxicity or ototoxicity

*antihistamines, buclizine, cyclizine, meclizine, phenothiazines, thioxanthenes, trimethobenzamide:* Masked symptoms of ototoxicity

*cholestyramine, colestipol:* Decreased antibacterial activity of oral vancomycin

*dexamethasone:* Decreased penetration of vancomycin into CSF

*nephrotoxic drugs:* Increased risk of nephrotoxicity

## Adverse Reactions

**CNS:** Chills, dizziness, vertigo
**CV:** Hypotension
**EENT:** Ototoxicity
**GI:** Nausea
**GU:** Nephrotoxicity
**HEME:** Eosinophilia, neutropenia
**RESP:** Dyspnea, wheezing
**SKIN:** Exfoliative dermatitis; extravasation with pain, tenderness, thrombophlebitis, and tissue necrosis; pruritus; rash; toxic epidermal necrolysis; urticaria
**Other:** Anaphylaxis, drug-induced fever, injection site inflammation, superinfection

## Nursing Considerations

• To reconstitute 500-mg vial of vancomycin for I.V. use, add 10 ml of sterile water for injection; further dilute with at least 100 ml of compatible I.V. solution. For 1-g vial of dry, sterile powder, add 20 ml of sterile water for injection; further dilute with at least 200 ml of compatible I.V. solution.

• **WARNING** Infuse over at least 1 hour. Rapid administration may cause hypotension or transient "red man syndrome," characterized by chills; fainting; fever; flushing of face, neck, upper arms, and torso; hypotension; nausea; tachycardia; and vomiting.

• Monitor blood vancomycin levels, as ordered; be aware that therapeutic levels are 10 to 15 mcg/ml trough and 30 to 40 mcg/ml peak.

• Monitor serum vancomycin concentration in patients with renal impairment or colitis because significant increases in blood drug level have occurred in such patients taking multiple oral doses of vancomycin.

• If patient has an inflammatory intestinal disorder, assess him often for adverse reactions because vancomycin absorption may be increased in these conditions.

• Monitor CBC results and serum creatinine and BUN levels during therapy, especially if patient has renal impairment or takes an aminoglycoside.

• Monitor I.V. infusion site for signs and symptoms of extravasation, including necrosis, pain, tenderness, and thrombophlebitis. If extravasation occurs, discontinue infusion immediately and notify prescriber.

• Monitor hearing during therapy. Transient or permanent ototoxicity may occur if patient receives an excessive amount of drug, has an underlying hearing loss, or receives concurrent aminoglycosides.

• Monitor patient receiving prolonged therapy for signs and symptoms of superinfection, such as severe diarrhea and white patches on tongue.

**PATIENT TEACHING**

• Instruct patient to use a calibrated measuring device to accurately measure doses of oral solution.

• Advise patient to notify prescriber if no improvement occurs after a few days.

• Instruct patient to complete full course of vancomycin, as prescribed.

• Caution patient that she should consult prescriber before taking any drug to control diarrhea because that condition may signal superinfection.

• Instruct patient to keep follow-up appointments during and after treatment.

# vardenafil hydrochloride

Levitra

## Class and Category

*Chemical:* Type 5 phosphodiesterase inhibitor
*Therapeutic:* Anti-impotence agent
*Pregnancy category:* B

## Indications and Dosages

➤ *To treat erectile dysfunction*

TABLETS
**Adults.** 10 mg taken 1 hr before sexual activity; increased to 20 mg or decreased to 5 mg, as needed. *Maximum:* 20 mg and taken only once daily regardless of dosage used.

| Route | Onset | Peak | Duration |
|---|---|---|---|
| P.O. | 30 min | 30 min to 2 hr | 4 to 5 hr |

### Mechanism of Action
Enhances effect of nitric oxide (released in the penis by sexual stimulation) and inhibits phosphodiesterase type 5, which increases cGMP level, relaxes smooth muscle, and increases blood flow into the corpus cavernosum, producing an erection.

### Contraindications
Concurrent administration of alpha blockers, concomitant continuous or intermittent nitrate therapy, hypersensitivity to vardenafil or its components

### Interactions
DRUGS
*alpha blockers, nitrates:* Profound hypotension
*erythromycin, indinavir, ketoconazole, ritonavir:* Increased vardenafil effect
*indinavir, ritonavir:* Reduced blood levels of indinavir and ritonavir

### Adverse Reactions
**CNS:** Dizziness, headache
**CV:** Hypotension
**EENT:** Nonarteritic anterior ischemic optic neuropathy, rhinitis, sinusitis
**GI:** Indigestion, nausea
**MS:** Back pain
**SKIN:** Flushing
**Other:** Flulike symptoms, increased creatine kinase level

### Nursing Considerations
• Use vardenafil cautiously in men with renal or hepatic dysfunction, in elderly men, and in men with penile abnormalities that may predispose them to priapism.
• Also use cautiously in patients with left ventricular outflow obstruction, such as aortic stenosis, and those with severely impaired autonomic control of blood pressure because these conditions increase patient's

sensitivity to vasodilators, such as vardenafil.
• Monitor blood pressure and heart rate before and after giving drug, especially if patient is receiving alpha blocker therapy, because of increased risk of symptomatic hypotension.
• Monitor patient's vision, especially if he is older than age 50; has diabetes, hypertension, coronary artery disease, or hyperlipidemia; or smokes, because vardenafil rarely leads to nonarteritic ischemic optic neuropathy and decreased vision, possibly permanent.

PATIENT TEACHING
• Explain that vardenafil should be taken 1 hour before sexual activity is anticipated for best results.
• **WARNING** Instruct patient not to take vardenafil if he also takes an organic nitrate continuously or intermittently, or within 4 hours of taking alpha blockers because profound hypotension and death could result.
• Caution patient not to take vardenafil more than once a day and not to exceed a dosage of 20 mg/day.
• Tell patient to stop taking vardenafil and to notify prescriber if he has sudden loss of vision in one or both eyes.
• Advise patient to seek sexual counseling to enhance drug's effects.
• To avoid possible penile damage and permanent loss of erectile function, urge patient to notify prescriber immediately if erection is painful or lasts longer than 4 hours.

# vasopressin

## (antidiuretic hormone [ADH])
Pitressin, Pressyn (CAN)

### Class and Category
*Chemical:* Polypeptide hormone
*Therapeutic:* Antidiuretic
*Pregnancy category:* C

### Indications and Dosages
➤ *To prevent or control symptoms of central diabetes insipidus caused by insufficient ADH*

## Mechanism of Action

Vasopressin, a synthetic form of antidiuretic hormone, treats diabetes insipidus by decreasing urine output and raising urine osmolality. When vasopressin attaches to vasopressin₂ ($V_2$) receptors on cell membranes in the nephron's collecting duct, it activates the enzyme adenyl cyclase to convert adenosine triphosphate (ATP) to cyclic adenosine monophosphate (cAMP). This action increases the collecting duct's permeability and enhances water reabsorption into the blood.

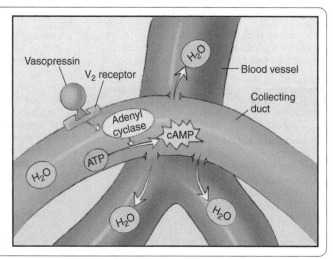

**I.M. OR S.C. INJECTION**
**Adults.** 5 to 10 U b.i.d. or t.i.d., as needed.
**Children.** 2.5 to 10 U t.i.d. or q.i.d., as needed.

➤ *To prevent or treat abdominal distention*
**I.M. INJECTION**
**Adults.** 5 U, increased to 10 U q 3 to 4 hr, as needed.

| Route | Onset | Peak | Duration |
|---|---|---|---|
| I.M., S.C. | Unknown | Unknown | 2 to 8 hr |

## Contraindications

Chronic nephritis with nitrogen retention, hypersensitivity to vasopressin or its components

## Interactions

**DRUGS**
*carbamazepine, chlorpropamide, clofibrate, fludrocortisone, tricyclic antidepressants:* Increased antidiuretic effect
*demeclocycline, lithium, norepinephrine:* Decreased antidiuretic effect

## Adverse Reactions

**CNS:** Dizziness, headache, light-headedness, tremor
**CV:** Angina, MI
**EENT:** Circumoral pallor
**ENDO:** Water intoxication
**GI:** Abdominal cramps, diarrhea, eructation, flatulence, intestinal hypermotility, nausea, vomiting
**SKIN:** Diaphoresis, pallor
**Other:** Allergic reaction

## Nursing Considerations

• Use vasopressin with extreme caution in patients with coronary artery disease because it may cause angina or MI; in those with hypertension because it may increase blood pressure; and in those with asthma, epilepsy, heart failure, or migraine headache because extracellular fluid may increase rapidly.
• Monitor fluid and electrolyte balance during therapy. Monitor intake and output at least every 8 hours, and assess for signs and symptoms of water intoxication and hyponatremia, including anuria, confusion, drowsiness, headache, listlessness, and weight gain.

**PATIENT TEACHING**
• Teach patient how to administer vasopressin; emphasize the need to rotate injection sites.
• Urge patient to notify prescriber immediately if he experiences signs of possible water intoxication, including anuria, confusion, drowsiness, headache, listlessness, and unexplained weight gain.
• Inform patient that abdominal cramps, nausea, and skin blanching will subside after a few minutes and can be minimized by drinking one or two glasses of water.

# venlafaxine hydrochloride

Effexor, Effexor XR

## Class and Category

*Chemical:* Phenylethylamine derivative
*Therapeutic:* Antidepressant
*Pregnancy category:* C

## Indications and Dosages

➤ *To treat and prevent relapse of major depression*

**E.R. CAPSULES**

**Adults.** 75 mg q.d. with a meal same time each day morning or evening (for some patients, 37.5 mg q.d. for 4 to 7 days before increasing to 75 mg/day), then increased by 75 mg/day q 4 days, as prescribed. *Maximum:* 225 mg/day.

**TABLETS**

**Adults.** 75 mg/day in divided doses b.i.d. or t.i.d., increased by 75 mg/day q 4 days, as prescribed. *Maximum:* 375 mg/day (225 mg/ day for outpatients).

➤ *To treat generalized anxiety disorder or social anxiety disorder*

**E.R. CAPSULES**

**Adults.** 75 mg q.d. with a meal at same time each day morning or evening (for some patients, 37.5 mg q.d. for 4 to 7 days before increasing to 75 mg/day), and then increased by 75 mg/day q 4 days, as prescribed. *Maximum:* 225 mg/day.

DOSAGE ADJUSTMENT Initial daily dose decreased by 25% to 50% for patients with mild to moderate renal impairment and by 50% for patients with hepatic impairment.

## Contraindications

Hypersensitivity to venlafaxine or its components, use of an MAO inhibitor within 14 days

---

### Mechanism of Action

Inhibits neuronal reuptake of serotonin and norepinephrine, along with its active metabolite, *O*-desmethylvenlafaxine. These actions raise serotonin and norepinephrine levels at nerve synapses, elevating mood and reducing depression.

---

| Route | Onset | Peak | Duration |
|-------|-------|------|----------|
| P.O. | 2 wk | Unknown | Unknown |

## Interactions

**DRUGS**

*amitriptyline, clomipramine, desipramine, doxepin, haloperidol, imipramine, nortriptyline, protriptyline, trazodone:* Possibly serotonin syndrome
*cimetidine:* Decreased clearance and increased blood level of venlafaxine
*clozapine:* Possibly increased blood clozapine levels and serious adverse reactions, including seizures
*MAO inhibitors:* Increased risk of hypertension; hyperthermia; mental status changes, including coma and delirium; muscle rigidity; and severe myoclonus
*warfarin:* Possibly increased PT, partial thromboplastin time, and INR

## Adverse Reactions

**CNS:** Agitation, anxiety, asthenia, chills, confusion, delusions, depression, dizziness, dream disturbances, drowsiness, dyskinesia, headache, insomnia, mood changes, nervousness, paresthesia, tremor
**CV:** Chest pain, hypertension, palpitations, sinus tachycardia
**EENT:** Blurred vision, dry mouth, pharyngitis, rhinitis, tinnitus
**ENDO:** Syndrome of inappropriate ADH secretion
**GI:** Abdominal pain, anorexia, constipation, diarrhea, flatulence, indigestion, nausea, vomiting
**GU:** Anorgasmia (women), decreased libido, ejaculation disorders, impotence
**MS:** Rhabdomyolysis
**SKIN:** Diaphoresis
**Other:** Hyponatremia, weight loss

## Nursing Considerations

•Monitor blood pressure frequently during venlafaxine therapy because drug may cause dose-related increase in supine diastolic pressure. Expect to reduce or stop drug, as prescribed, if increase develops.
•If patient takes venlafaxine for depression, watch for suicidal tendencies, especially when therapy starts and dosage changes.
•WARNING Be aware that drug shouldn't be discontinued abruptly because doing so may cause asthenia, dizziness, headache, insomnia, and nervousness.

**PATIENT TEACHING**

•Instruct patient not to crush or chew E.R. capsules. However, if she has difficulty swal-

U
V
W

lowing capsules, tell her to open capsule, sprinkle contents on a spoonful of applesauce, and swallow immediately without chewing, followed by a glass of water.
• Advise patient to avoid alcohol during venlafaxine therapy.
• Advise patient not to stop drug abruptly.
• Caution patient to notify prescriber if she becomes pregnant during therapy because she'll need a different antidepressant. Taking venlafaxine during the third trimester of pregnancy increases the risk of complications in the infant after birth.

# verapamil

Apo-Verap (CAN), Calan, Isoptin, Novo-Veramil (CAN), Nu-Verap (CAN)

## verapamil hydrochloride

Calan SR, Isoptin SR, Verelan

## Class and Category

*Chemical:* Phenylalkylamine derivative
*Therapeutic:* Antianginal, antiarrhythmic, antihypertensive
*Pregnancy category:* C

## Indications and Dosages

➤ *To treat chronic angina pectoris*
**TABLETS (VERAPAMIL)**
**Adults and adolescents age 15 and older.** *Initial:* 80 to 120 mg t.i.d., increased q day or wk, as needed and prescribed. *Maximum:* 480 mg/day in divided doses.
**Infants and children up to age 15.** 4 to 8 mg/kg/day in divided doses.
➤ *To manage hypertension*
**E.R. CAPSULES (VERAPAMIL HYDROCHLORIDE)**
**Adults and adolescents.** *Initial:* 240 mg/day, increased q day or wk, as needed and prescribed. *Maximum:* 480 mg/day.
**E.R. TABLETS (VERAPAMIL HYDROCHLORIDE)**
**Adults and adolescents.** *Initial:* 180 mg q.d., increased q day or wk, as needed and prescribed, according to following schedule: 240 mg q.d. in the morning; 180 mg q 12 hr or 240 mg in the morning and 120 mg in the evening; then 240 mg q 12 hr. *Maximum:* 480 mg/day in divided doses.
**TABLETS (VERAPAMIL)**
**Adults and adolescents age 15 and older.** *Initial:* 80 to 120 mg t.i.d., increased q day or

wk, as needed and prescribed. *Maximum:* 480 mg/day in divided doses.
**Infants and children up to age 15.** 4 to 8 mg/kg/day in divided doses.
➤ *To prevent or treat supraventricular tachycardia*
**TABLETS (VERAPAMIL)**
**Adults and adolescents age 15 and older.** *Initial:* 80 to 120 mg t.i.d., increased q day or wk, as needed and prescribed. *Maximum:* 480 mg/day in divided doses.
**DOSAGE ADJUSTMENT** Initial P.O. dosage possibly reduced to 40 mg t.i.d. (120 mg/day for E.R. tablets or capsules) for elderly patients and those with impaired hepatic or left ventricular function.
**I.V. INJECTION (VERAPAMIL HYDROCHLORIDE)**
**Adults and adolescents age 15 and older.** *Initial:* 5 to 10 mg slowly over 2 min; then 10 mg, as prescribed, if response isn't adequate after 30 min.
**Children ages 1 to 15.** *Initial:* 100 to 300 mcg/kg slowly over 2 min, up to maximum of 5 mg; then 10 mg, as prescribed, if response isn't adequate after 30 min.
**Infants up to age 1.** *Initial:* 100 to 200 mcg/kg slowly over 2 min.
**DOSAGE ADJUSTMENT** I.V. drug administered over 3 minutes in elderly patients.

## Incompatibilities

Don't mix I.V. verapamil with albumin, amphotericin B injection, hydralazine hydrochloride injection, nafcillin, or sulfamethoxazole and trimethoprim injection. Solutions with pH above 6.0 cause precipitation.

## Contraindications

Cardiogenic shock, concomitant use of beta blockers (with I.V. verapamil), hypersensitivity to verapamil or its components, hypotension, severe heart failure unless secondary to supraventricular tachycardia that responds to verapamil, severe left ventricular dysfunction, sick sinus syndrome or second- or third-degree heart block unless artificial pacemaker is in place, ventricular tachycardia (with I.V. verapamil)

## Interactions

**DRUGS**
*alpha blockers, antihypertensives, general anesthetics (hydrocarbon), prazosin:* Hypotensive effects
*aspirin:* Increased bleeding time

*beta blockers:* Increased risk of heart failure, hypotension, and severe bradycardia
*calcium supplements:* Decreased response to verapamil
*carbamazepine, cyclosporine, theophylline, valproate:* Increased risk of toxicity from these drugs
*cimetidine:* Decreased metabolism and increased blood level of verapamil
*dantrolene:* Increased risk of hyperkalemia and myocardial depression
*digoxin:* Increased blood digoxin level and risk of digitalis toxicity
*disopyramide, flecainide:* Additive negative inotropic effects
*erythromycin, ritonavir:* Increased blood verapamil level
*lithium:* Increased risk of neurotoxicity
*neuromuscular blockers:* Prolonged recovery from neuromuscular blockade
*NSAIDs, sympathomimetics:* Decreased antihypertensive effect of verapamil
*phenobarbital:* Increased verapamil clearance
*procainamide:* Increased Q-T interval, additive negative inotropic effects
*protein-bound drugs (hydantoins, salicylates, sulfonamides, sulfonylureas, and warfarin and other oral anticoagulants):* Altered blood levels of these drugs
*quinidine:* Increased risk of quinidine toxicity, increased Q-T interval, additive negative inotropic effects
*rifampin:* Decreased bioavailability of oral verapamil

**FOODS**
*grapefruit juice:* Increased concentrations of verapamil

**ACTIVITIES**
*alcohol use:* Increased blood alcohol level and prolonged CNS effects

## Adverse Reactions
**CNS:** Confusion, CVA, disequilibrium, dizziness, extrapyramidal reactions, fatigue, headache, insomnia, paresthesia, psychosis, shakiness, somnolence
**CV:** Angina, AV conduction disorders, bradycardia, claudication, heart failure, hypotension, peripheral edema, tachycardia
**GI:** Constipation, elevated liver function test results, nausea
**GU:** Galactorrhea, menstrual irregularities
**MS:** Muscle spasms
**RESP:** Dyspnea, pulmonary edema, wheezing
**SKIN:** Flushing, rash

| Route | Onset | Peak | Duration |
|---|---|---|---|
| P.O. | 1 to 2 hr | 30 to 90 min | 6 to 8 hr |
| P.O. (E.R.) | 1 to 2 hr | 30 to 90 min | Unknown |
| I.V. | 1 to 5 min | 3 to 5 min | 10 min to 6 hr |

## Mechanism of Action
Inhibits calcium movement into coronary and vascular smooth-muscle cells by blocking slow calcium channels in cell membranes. The resulting decrease in the intracellular calcium level has the following effects:
•inhibits smooth-muscle cell contractions
•decreases myocardial oxygen demand by relaxing coronary and vascular smooth muscle, reducing peripheral vascular resistance, and decreasing systolic and diastolic pressures
•slows AV conduction time and prolongs AV nodal refractoriness
•interrupts reentry circuit in AV nodal reentrant tachycardias.

## Nursing Considerations
•Administer I.V. verapamil with compatible solutions, including Ringer's injection, D₅W, or NS.
•Maintain continuous ECG monitoring and keep emergency resuscitative equipment and drugs readily available during I.V. therapy.
•Assess patient with hypertrophic cardiomyopathy for early development of hypotension and pulmonary edema because second-degree AV block and sinus arrest can result.
•Assess for bradycardia and hypotension, and notify prescriber if heart rate or blood pressure declines significantly.
•Be aware that disopyramide or flecainide shouldn't be given within 48 hours before or 24 hours after verapamil because additive negative inotropic effects can result.
•Institute measures to prevent constipation, including a high-fiber diet and a stool softener, as prescribed.
**PATIENT TEACHING**
•Instruct patient not to crush or chew verapamil E.R. tablets or capsules. Inform her that she may break E.R. tablets in half if necessary to aid swallowing.

- Direct patient to check her pulse rate before taking verapamil and to notify prescriber if it's below 50 beats/minute or as instructed by prescriber.
- Caution patient about possible dizziness and the need to avoid potentially hazardous activities until drug's CNS effects are known.
- Inform patient that adverse skin reactions may subside with continued use. Advise her to notify prescriber if rash persists.
- Encourage patient to increase dietary fiber intake to help prevent constipation. Advise her to notify prescriber if problem becomes persistent or severe.

# voriconazole

Vfend

## Class and Category

*Chemical:* Triazole
*Therapeutic:* Antifungal
*Pregnancy category:* D

## Indications and Dosages

➤ *To treat invasive aspergillosis; to treat serious fungal infections caused by* Scedosporium apiospermum *and* Fusarium *sp., including* Fusarium solani, *in patients intolerant of or refractory to other therapy*

**I.V. INFUSION**

**Adults and children age 12 and older.** *Initial:* 6 mg/kg over 1 to 2 hr at a rate not to exceed 3 mg/kg/hr q 12 hr for 2 doses. *Maintenance:* 4 mg/kg over 1 to 2 hr at a rate not to exceed 3 mg/kg/hr q 12 hr.

**TABLETS**

**Adults and children age 12 and older weighing 40 kg (88 lb) or more.** *Maintenance:* 200 mg q 12 hr, increased to 300 mg q 12 hr, as needed, and taken at least 1 hr before or after a meal.

**Adults and children age 12 and older weighing less than 40 kg.** *Maintenance:* 100 mg q 12 hr, increased to 150 mg q 12 hr, as needed, and taken at least 1 hr before or after a meal.

➤ *To treat candidemia in nonneutropenic patients and other deep-tissue disseminatinated* Candida *infections involving the abdomen, kidney, bladder wall, skin, or a wound*

**I.V. INFUSION**

**Adults.** *Initial:* 6 mg/kg over 1 to 2 hr at a rate not to exceed 3 mg/kg/hr q 12 hr for two doses. *Maintenance:* 3 to 4 mg/kg over 1 to 2 hr at a rate not to exceed 3 mg/kg/hr q 12 hr for at least 14 days after symptoms resolve or last positive culture, whichever takes longer.

**TABLETS**

**Adults.** *Maintenance:* 200 mg q 12 hr taken at least 1 hr before or after a meal.

➤ *To treat esophageal candidiasis*

**TABLETS**

**Adults.** 200 mg q 12 hr taken at least 1 hr before or after a meal for at least 14 days and at least 7 days after symptoms resolve.

**DOSAGE ADJUSTMENT** If patient can't tolerate drug, I.V. maintenance dose may be reduced to 3 mg/kg q 12 hr and oral maintenance dose by 50-mg decrements to at least 200 mg q 12 hr (or to 100 mg q 12 hr for patients weighing less than 40 kg). For use with phenytoin, maintenance dose may be increased to 5 mg/kg I.V. q 12 hr or from 200 mg to 400 mg P.O. q 12 hr (100 mg to 200 mg q 12 hr for patients weighing less than 40 kg). For patients with mild to moderate hepatic cirrhosis, standard loading dose should be used but maintenance dose halved for I.V. or P.O. use. For patients with moderate to severe renal insufficiency (creatinine clearance greater than 50 ml/min), only the oral form should be given, if possible.

## Incompatibilities

Don't infuse into the same line or cannula with other drugs, including parenteral nutrition, to prevent an increase in subvisible particulate matter. Avoid infusion with blood products and any electrolyte supplements. Don't dilute with 4.2% sodium bicarbonate infusion because the mildly alkaline nature of the diluent causes slight degradation of voriconazole after 24 hours of storage at room temperature.

## Mechanism of Action

Prevents fungal ergosterol biosynthesis by inhibiting fungal cytochrome P450–mediated 14 alpha-lanosterol demethylation. The loss of ergosterol in the fungal cell wall renders the fungal cell inactive.

## Contraindications

Coadministration with long-acting barbiturates, carbamazepine, CYP3A4 substrates (astemizole, cisapride, pimozide, quinidine, or terfenadine), efavirenz, ergot alkaloids, rifabutin, rifampin, ritonavir, or sirolimus; hypersensitivity to voriconazole or its components; galactose intolerance, glucose-galactose malabsorption, or Lapp lactase deficiency (oral form only contains lactose)

## Interactions

### DRUGS

*benzodiazepines:* Possibly prolonged sedative effect of benzodiazepines
*calcium channel blockers; HMG-CoA reductase inhibitors, such as lovastatin; omeprazole; sirolimus:* Possibly increased plasma concentrations of these drugs, leading to increased risk of adverse reactions and toxicity
*carbamazepine, long-acting barbiturates, phenytoin, rifampin:* Decreased plasma voriconazole concentration
*coumarin, warfarin:* Possibly increased PTT
*cyclosporine, sirolimus, tacrolimus:* Increased serum concentrations of these drugs and risk of toxicity, especially nephrotoxicity
*CYP3A4 substrates (astemizole, cisapride, pimozide, quinidine, terfenadine):* Increased plasma concentrations of these drugs, which may lead to prolonged QT interval and, rarely, torsades de pointes
*ergot alkaloids (ergotamine, dihydroergotamine):* May increase plasma concentration of ergot alkaloids leading to ergotism
*HIV protease inhibitors (amprenavir, nelfinavir, ritonavir, saquinavir), non-nucleoside reverse transcriptase inhibitors (delavirdine, efavirenz):* Possibly inhibited metabolism of these drugs and voriconazole
*methadone:* Increased plasma concentration of methadone, possibly leading to toxicity, including QT-interval prolongation
*rifabutin:* Increased rifabutin plasma concentration; decreased voriconazole plasma concentrations
*sulfonylureas:* Possibly increased plasma concentrations of sulfonylureas and increased risk of hypoglycemia
*vinca alkaloids:* Possibly increased risk of neurotoxicity

## Adverse Reactions

**CNS:** Chills, dizziness, fever, hallucinations, headache

**CV:** Chest pain, hypertension, hypotension, peripheral edema, tachycardia, vasodilation
**EENT:** Abnormal or blurred vision, altered or enhanced visual perception, change in color perception, chromatopsia, dry mouth, eye hemorrhage, photophobia, visual disturbances
**GI:** Abdominal pain, diarrhea, elevated liver function test results, nausea, vomiting
**GU:** Abnormal kidney function, acute renal failure, elevated serum creatinine level
**HEME:** Anemia, leukopenia, pancytopenia, thrombocytopenia
**RESP:** Respiratory disorders
**SKIN:** Cholestatic jaundice, erythema multiforme, jaundice, maculopapular rash, photosensitivity, pruritus, rash, Stevens-Johnson syndrome, toxic epidermal necrolysis
**Other:** Anaphylaxis (I.V. form), elevated alkaline phosphatase, hypokalemia, hypomagnesemia, sepsis

## Nursing Considerations

• Use voriconazole cautiously in patients with known hypersensitivity to other azoles and in patients at risk for proarrhythmic events (such as those receiving cardiotoxic chemotherapy or those who have cardiomyopathy or hypokalemia) because some azoles may cause prolong QT interval.
• Determine if patient has any problems with galactose intolerance, Lapp lactase deficiency, or glucose-galactose malabsorption before starting therapy because voriconazole tablets contain lactose and shouldn't be given to patients with these conditions.
• Obtain specimens for fungal culture and other relevant laboratory studies (including histopathology), as ordered, before giving first dose. Expect to begin drug before test results are known.
• Assess patient's liver function, including bilirubin, as ordered, at the start of voriconazole therapy and periodically thereafter. Be aware that drug may be discontinued if liver abnormalities occur.
• Check patient's electrolyte levels before start of therapy, as ordered, and correct any imbalances, as prescribed, before administering voriconazole because electrolyte imbalances increase the risk of adverse reactions.
• For I.V. infusion, reconstitute powder with 19 ml of water for injection to obtain 20 ml of concentrate that contains 10 mg/ml of voriconazole. Use a standard 10-ml nonauto-

mated syringe to ensure that exact amount of water is injected into vial. Shake the vial until all powder is dissolved. Further dilute so that final concentration is not less than 0.5 mg/ml nor more than 5 mg/ml. This requires withdrawing and discarding at least an equal volume of diluent from the infusion bag or bottle before instillation of concentrate.

• Discard partially used vials after mixing. If infusion isn't administered immediately, store at 2° to 8° C (37° to 46° F) for no longer than 24 hours.

• Administer I.V. infusion over 1 to 2 hours at a rate that doesn't exceed 3 mg/kg/hr.

• Monitor renal function, especially serum creatinine level, when administering I.V. form of voriconazole because drug may accumulate in body when creatinine clearance is less than 50 ml/min, increasing the risk of adverse reactions.

• **WARNING** Observe patient receiving I.V. voriconazole closely for anaphylactoid-type reactions—such as flushing, fever, sweating, tachycardia, chest tightness, dyspnea, faintness, nausea, pruritus and rash—which may occur immediately after starting the infusion. Stop the infusion if these reactions occur, and notify prescriber immediately.

• Monitor patient closely throughout therapy for skin rash, which may indicate a serious cutaneous reaction, such as Stevens-Johnson syndrome. If a rash occurs, notify prescriber, and expect that drug may be discontinued.

• Monitor cyclosporine, tacrolimus, and warfarin closely for elevated levels when voriconazole is coadministered with any of these drugs.

• Monitor diabetic patients also taking sulfonylureas closely for hypoglycemia, and check blood glucose levels regularly.

• Be aware that voriconazole dosage will need to be adjusted when co-administered with phenytoin. Expect to monitor plasma phenytoin levels and observe patient closely for phenytoin-related adverse reactions.

• Assess patient's visual function, including visual acuity, visual field, and color perception, if voriconazole therapy continues longer than 28 days.

**PATIENT TEACHING**

• Instruct patient taking oral voriconazole to take the tablets at least 1 hour before or 1 hour after a meal.

• Inform female patient of possible fetal risk, and stress the importance of avoiding pregnancy. Tell her to use an effective form of contraception throughout therapy and to notify the prescriber immediately if pregnancy is suspected.

• Caution patient not to drive at night and to avoid potentially hazardous activities because drug may cause visual disturbances, including blurring or photophobia.

• Advise patient to avoid exposure to direct sunlight or UV light and to wear sunscreen when outdoors.

# warfarin sodium

Coumadin

## Class and Category

*Chemical:* Coumarin derivative
*Therapeutic:* Anticoagulant
*Pregnancy category:* X

## Indications and Dosages

➤ *To prevent or treat pulmonary embolism; recurrent MI; thromboembolic complications from atrial fibrillation, heart valve replacement, or MI; and venous thrombosis (and its extension)*

**TABLETS**

**Adults.** *Initial:* 2 to 5 mg/day for 2 to 4 days. *Usual:* 2 to 10 mg/day based on target PT and INR results. *Maximum:* Determined by target PT and INR results, as prescribed.

**I.V. INJECTION**

**Adults.** *Initial:* 2 to 5 mg/day infused over 1 to 2 min. *Usual:* 2 to 10 mg/day infused over 1 to 2 min. *Maximum:* Determined by target PT and INR results, as prescribed.

**DOSAGE ADJUSTMENT** For patients with hepatic dysfunction, dosage reduced to 0.1 mg/kg, as prescribed. For elderly patients, dosage possibly reduced based on PT and INR results.

| Route | Onset | Peak | Duration |
|-------|-------|------|----------|
| P.O | 24 hr | 3 to 4 days | 2 to 5 days |
| I.V. | Unknown | 3 to 4 days | 2 to 5 days |

## Incompatibilities

Don't mix warfarin in solution with amikacin sulfate, epinephrine hydrochloride, metaraminol tartrate, oxytocin, promazine hydrochloride, tetracycline hydrochloride, or vancomycin hydrochloride.

## Mechanism of Action

Interferes with the liver's ability to synthesize vitamin K-dependent clotting factors, depleting clotting factors II (prothrombin), VII, IX, and X. This action, in turn, interferes with the clotting cascade. By depleting vitamin K-dependent clotting factors and interfering with the clotting cascade, warfarin prevents coagulation.

## Contraindications

Bleeding or bleeding tendencies; blood dyscrasias; cerebral or dissecting aneurysm; cerebrovascular hemorrhage; diverticulitis; eclampsia or preeclampsia; history of warfarin-induced necrosis; hypersensitivity to warfarin or its components; malignant or severe uncontrolled hypertension; malnutrition and emaciation; mental state or condition that leads to lack of patient cooperation; pericardial effusion; pericarditis; polyarthritis; pregnancy; prostatectomy; recent or planned neurosurgery, ophthalmic surgery, or spinal puncture; severe hepatic or renal disease

## Interactions

### DRUGS

*acetaminophen, aminoglycosides, amiodarone, androgens, beta blockers, capecitabine, cephalosporins, chloral hydrate, chloramphenicol, chlorpropamide, cimetidine, clofibrate, corticosteroids, cyclophosphamide, dextrothyroxine, diflunisal, disulfiram, erythromycin, fluconazole, gemfibrozil, glucagon, hydantoins, ifosfamide, influenza virus vaccine, isoniazid, ketoconazole, loop diuretics, lovastatin, metronidazole, miconazole, mineral oil, moricizine, nalidixic acid, NSAIDs, omeprazole, penicillins, phenylbutazones, propafenone, propoxyphene, quinidine, quinine, quinolones, salicylates, streptokinase, sulfamethoxazole-trimethoprim, sulfinpyrazone, sulfonamides, tamoxifen, tetracyclines, thyroid hormones, urokinase, vitamin E:* Increased anticoagulant effect of warfarin, increased risk of bleeding
*aminoglutethimide, barbiturates, carbamazepine, cholestyramine, dicloxacillin, estrogens, ethchlorvynol, etretinate, glutethimide, griseofulvin, nafcillin, oral contraceptives, rifampin, spironolactone, sucralfate, thiazide diuretics, trazodone, vitamin C, vitamin K:* Decreased anticoagulant effect of warfarin

*atorvastatin, pravastatin:* Increased or decreased anticoagulant effect of warfarin
*herbal remedies (including bromelains, danshen, dong quai, garlic, ginkgo biloba, and ginseng):* Increased anticoagulant effect of warfarin, increased risk of bleeding
*I.V. lipid emulsion, other medical products that contain soybean oil:* Possibly decreased vitamin K absorption and increased anticoagulant effect of warfarin
*nicotine patch:* Altered response to warfarin

### FOODS

*certain multivitamins, enteral feedings, vitamin–K-rich foods:* Decreased effects of warfarin

### ACTIVITIES

*alcohol use:* Increased risk of hypoprothrombinemia
*smoking, smoking cessation:* Altered response to warfarin

## Adverse Reactions

**CNS:** Intracranial hemorrhage, weakness
**EENT:** Epistaxis, intraocular hemorrhage
**GI:** Abdominal cramps and pain, diarrhea, hepatitis, nausea, vomiting
**GU:** Hematuria, vaginal bleeding (abnormal)
**HEME:** Potentially fatal hemorrhage (from any tissue or organ)
**SKIN:** Alopecia, ecchymosis, jaundice, petechiae, pruritus, purple-toe syndrome, tissue necrosis

## Nursing Considerations

•Reconstitute parenteral warfarin just before administration with 2.7 ml of sterile water for injection to yield 2 mg/ml. Then administer slowly over 1 to 2 minutes through peripheral I.V.
•Expect to administer another parenteral anticoagulant, such as heparin or enoxaparin, with oral warfarin for at least 3 days, or until desired response occurs, before giving warfarin only.
•Avoid I.M. injections during warfarin therapy, if possible, because they can result in bleeding, bruising, and hematoma.
•Monitor INR (daily in acute care setting) and assess for therapeutic effects, as prescribed. Therapeutic INR levels are 2.0 to 3.0 for bioprosthetic heart valve, nonvalvular atrial fibrillation, and venous thromboembolism, and 2.5 to 3.5 after MI and for mechanical heart valve.
•Expect treatment to last up to 12 weeks for bioprosthetic heart valve, 1 to 3 months for nonvalvular atrial fibrillation or venous

thromboembolism, and for rest of life after MI and for mechanical heart valve replacement.

•**WARNING** Be aware of the increased risk for intracranial hemorrhage if patient has cerebral ischemia (such as recent transient ischemic attack or minor ischemic CVA) and INR of 3 to 4.5. As prescribed, withhold next warfarin dose and give vitamin K if INR exceeds 4 because of the risk of bleeding.

•Assess for occult bleeding if patient receives I.V. lipid emulsion or other medical product that contains soybean oil. Such products can decrease vitamin K absorption and increase warfarin's anticoagulant effect.

### PATIENT TEACHING

•Explain that warfarin therapy aims to prevent thrombosis by decreasing clotting ability while avoiding the risk of spontaneous bleeding.

•Instruct patient to take drug exactly as prescribed at the same time each evening.

•Urge patient to keep weekly follow-up appointments for blood tests after discharge until PT and INR levels are stabilized.

•Advise patient to avoid alcohol during warfarin therapy.

•Urge patient to take precautions against bleeding, such as using an electric shaver and a soft-bristled toothbrush. Advise him to continue these precautions for 2 to 5 days after therapy stops, as directed, because anticoagulant effect may persist during this time.

•Caution patient to avoid activities that could cause traumatic injury and bleeding.

•Advise patient to eat consistent amounts of vitamin K–rich foods, such as dark green, leafy vegetables.

•Urge patient to notify prescriber immediately about unusual bleeding and any unexplained symptoms, such as abnormal vaginal bleeding; dizziness; easy bruising; gum bleeding; headache; nosebleeds; prolonged bleeding from cuts; red, black, or tarry stool; red or dark brown urine; swelling; and weakness.

•Advise patient to consult prescriber before taking other drugs—including OTC drugs and herbal remedies—during therapy.

•Instruct female patient of childbearing age to stop taking warfarin and notify prescriber immediately about known or suspected pregnancy.

•Explain that drug may cause reversible purple-toe syndrome and that this syndrome isn't harmful.

•Urge patient to carry medical identification that reveals he's taking warfarin therapy.

# zafirlukast

Accolate

## Class and Category

*Chemical:* Peptide leukotriene receptor antagonist
*Therapeutic:* Antiasthmatic
*Pregnancy category:* B

## Indications and Dosages

➤ *To treat chronic asthma*

**TABLETS**

**Adults and children over age 11.** 20 mg b.i.d.
**Children ages 5 to 11.** 10 mg b.i.d.

| Route | Onset | Peak | Duration |
|-------|-------|------|----------|
| P.O. | 1 wk | Unknown | Unknown |

### Mechanism of Action

Inhibits the selective binding of cysteinyl leukotrienes (arachidonic acid derivatives that usually mediate inflammation in asthma and other inflammatory disorders) by competitively blocking receptor sites. This action causes bronchial relaxation and decreases vascular leakage and edema, mucus secretion, eosinophil movement, and bronchial hyperresponsiveness.

## Contraindications

Hypersensitivity to zafirlukast or its components

## Interactions

**DRUGS**

*alprazolam, amitriptyline, calcium channel blockers, carbamazepine, citalopram, corticosteroids, cyclosporine, diazepam, diclofenac, ibuprofen, imipramine, irbesartan, lidocaine, lovastatin, midazolam, phenytoin, quinidine, simvastatin, tolbutamide, tolterodine, triazolam:* Inhibited metabolism and, possibly, additive adverse effects of these drugs
*aspirin:* Increased blood zafirlukast level
*erythromycin, terfenadine:* Decreased response to zafirlukast
*sildenafil:* Increased adverse effects of sildenafil
*theophylline:* Decreased blood zafirlukast level
*warfarin:* Prolonged PT

**FOODS**

*any food:* Possibly decreased bioavailability of zafirlukast

## Adverse Reactions

**CNS:** Asthenia, dizziness, fever, headache, insomnia, malaise
**GI:** Abdominal pain, diarrhea, elevated liver function test results, hepatic failure, indigestion, nausea, vomiting
**MS:** Back pain, myalgia
**SKIN:** Pruritus
**Other:** Generalized pain

## Nursing Considerations

•Be aware that zafirlukast shouldn't be used to treat bronchospasm during an acute asthma attack or status asthmaticus; it can't relieve symptoms quickly enough.
•Assess respiratory rate, depth, and quality as well as breath sounds before and during treatment to evaluate response to therapy.
•If patient is being weaned from corticosteroids while taking zafirlukast, monitor her for Churg-Strauss syndrome, a rare allergic reaction characterized by eosinophilia, fever, myalgia, and weight loss as well as cardiac complications, neuropathy, and worsening pulmonary symptoms.

**PATIENT TEACHING**

•Instruct patient to take drug exactly as prescribed, in evenly spaced doses, every day. Stress the need to take drug even during symptom-free periods and acute exacerbations.
•Instruct patient to take drug on an empty stomach at least 1 hour before or 2 hours after meals.
•Advise patient to continue using rescue inhalants, as prescribed, for acute attacks.
•Teach patient how to use peak-flow meter to monitor pulmonary function.
•Tell patient to immediately report evidence of liver dysfunction, such as right upperquadrant abdominal pain, nausea, fatigue, lethargy, pruritus, jaundice, flulike symptoms, and anorexia.

# zaleplon

Sonata

## Class, Category, and Schedule

*Chemical:* Imidazopyridine derivative
*Therapeutic:* Sedative-hypnotic
*Pregnancy category:* C
*Controlled substance:* Schedule IV

## Indications and Dosages

➤ *Short-term treatment of insomnia*

**CAPSULES**

**Adults up to age 65.** 10 mg/day h.s., as prescribed, for up to 35 days. *Usual:* 10 mg/day h.s. for 7 to 10 days. *Maximum:* 20 mg/day.

**DOSAGE ADJUSTMENT** For patients who are elderly, have hepatic impairment, or take cimetidine, dosage possibly reduced to 5 mg/day.

| Route | Onset | Peak | Duration |
|-------|-------|------|----------|
| P.O. | 30 min | Unknown | 4 hr |

### Mechanism of Action

Selectively binds with type 1 benzodiazepine (BZ1 or omega$_1$) receptors on the gamma-aminobutyric acid-A receptor complex. This binding produces muscle relaxation and sedation as well as antianxiety and anticonvulsant effects.

## Contraindications

Hypersensitivity to zaleplon or its components

## Interactions

**DRUGS**

*amitriptyline; amoxapine; azatadine; benzodiazepines; brompheniramine; chlorpheniramine; clemastine; clomipramine; clozapine; cyproheptadine; dexchlorpheniramine; diphenhydramine; doxepin; entacapone; haloperidol; hydroxyzine; imipramine; maprotiline; mirtazapine; molindone; nefazodone; nortriptyline; olanzapine; opioid analgesics; other anxiolytics, sedatives, and hypnotics; phenindamine; phenothiazines; pimozide; pramipexole; promethazine; quetiapine; risperidone; ropinirole; thioridazine; trazodone; trimipramine; tripelennamine:* Possibly additive CNS depression

*carbamazepine, phenobarbital, phenytoin, rifampin:* Reduced zaleplon effects

*cimetidine:* Increased blood zaleplon level

*flumazenil:* Reversal of zaleplon's sedation

**FOODS**

*high-fat foods:* Prolonged absorption time and reduced effectiveness of zaleplon

**ACTIVITIES**

*alcohol use:* Increased CNS depression

## Adverse Reactions

**CNS:** Amnesia, anxiety, depression, dizziness, drowsiness, fever, hallucinations, hypertonia, insomnia, paresthesia, seizures, tremor, vertigo

**EENT:** Dry mouth, gingivitis, glossitis, mouth ulcers, stomatitis

**GI:** Anorexia, colitis, constipation, eructation, esophagitis, flatulence, gastritis, gastroenteritis, increased appetite, indigestion, melena, nausea, rectal bleeding, vomiting

**MS:** Back pain

**SKIN:** Photosensitivity, pruritus, rash

**Other:** Physical and psychological dependence

## Nursing Considerations

•Give zaleplon just before bedtime because its onset of action is rapid.

•Avoid giving drug with or after a heavy, high-fat meal because decreased absorption may reduce drug's effects.

•**WARNING** Anticipate an increased risk of suicidal ideation in patient with major depression who takes zaleplon. Take suicide precautions, as needed, according to facility policy.

•Monitor patient for signs of drug abuse because zaleplon has an abuse potential similar to that of benzodiazepines and benzodiazepine-like hypnotics.

**PATIENT TEACHING**

•Inform patient that zaleplon is intended for short-term use. Advise her not to use this drug for any condition other than insomnia.

•Caution patient against exceeding prescribed dosage.

•Instruct patient to take zaleplon immediately before bedtime or right after having trouble falling asleep because of the rapid onset of drug's action.

•Teach patient alternative measures for relaxation and sleep induction.

•Advise patient to consult prescriber before taking other CNS depressants.

•Urge patient to avoid alcohol during therapy.

•Warn patient that zaleplon contains FD & C Yellow No. 5 (tartrazine), which can cause an allergic reaction, especially in those with an aspirin sensitivity. Instruct patient to report any allergic reactions, such as rash or difficulty breathing, to prescriber.

•Instruct patient to notify prescriber if inability to sleep continues. Dosage may need to be adjusted.

# ziconotide

Prialt

## Class and Category

*Chemical:* 25 amino acid polybasic peptide
*Therapeutic:* Analgesic
*Pregnancy category:* C

## Indications and Dosages

➤ *To manage severe chronic pain in patients who are intolerant of or refractory to other pain management measures*

**INTRATHECAL**

**Adults.** *Initial:* 2.4 mcg/day (0.1 mcg/hr), increased as needed by 2.4 mcg/day but no more than 3 times/wk. *Maximum:* 19.2 mcg/day (0.8 mcg/hr) by day 21.

## Contraindications

History of psychosis; hypersensitivity to ziconotide or its components; conditions or treatment that make intrathecal use hazardous (infection at microinfusion site, uncontrolled bleeding diathesis, spinal canal obstruction that impairs circulation of CSF).

## Interactions

**DRUGS**

*CNS depressants:* Increased risk of adverse CNS reactions

## Adverse Reactions

**CNS:** Abnormal gait, agitation, anxiety, aphasia, asthenia, ataxia, chills, confusion, CSF abnormality, CVA, decreased reflexes, depression, difficulty concentrating, dizziness, dysesthesia, emotional lability, fever, hallucinations, headache, hostility, hyperesthesia, hypertonia, incoordination, insomnia, malaise, memory loss, meningitis, nervousness, neuralgia, paranoia, paresthesia, psychosis, somnolence, speech disorder, stupor, syncope, tremor, twitching, unusual dreams, vertigo

**CV:** Atrial fibrillation, bradycardia, chest pain, edema, hypertension, hypotension, orthostatic hypotension, peripheral edema, tachycardia, T-wave changes on ECG, vasodilation

**EENT:** Abnormal vision, diplopia, dry mouth, nystagmus, pharyngitis, photophobia, rhinitis, sinusitis, taste perversion, tinnitus

**GI:** Abdominal pain, anorexia, constipation, diarrhea, indigestion, nausea, vomiting

**GU:** Acute renal failure, dysuria, urinary incontinence, urine retention, UTI

**HEME:** Anemia

**MS:** Arthralgia, arthritis, back pain, leg cramps, myalgia, myasthenia, neck pain or rigidity, rhabdomyolysis

**RESP:** Aspiration pneumonia, bronchitis, cough, dyspnea, lung disorder, pneumonia

**SKIN:** Cellulitis, diaphoresis, dry skin, ecchymosis, pruritus, rash

**Other:** Catheter site infection or pain, dehydration, elevated CK level, flulike symptoms, generalized pain, hypokalemia, sepsis, viral infection, weight loss

## Nursing Considerations

•Determine if patient will receive ziconotide therapy via an implanted variable-rate microinfusion device or an external microinfusion device and catheter. Then, follow manufacturer guidelines for programming the microinfusion devise and doing an initial pump fill, including priming using only undiluted 25-mcg/ml solution and rinsing internal surfaces of pump with 2 ml of drug three times.

•Use strict aseptic technique when preparing the ziconotide solution and filling, refilling, or otherwise handling the microinfusion device.

•Be aware that initial ziconotide dosage shouldn't exceed 2.4 mcg/day.

•Know that refills can use diluted or undiluted ziconotide solutions. If diluting ziconotide, use only NS without preservatives, following manufacturer guidelines. Refrigerate solution up to 24 hours if it isn't used immediately. Expect the device to need refilling about every 40 days if ziconotide is given diluted or about 60 days if given undiluted.

•Assess patient's response to ziconotide regularly. Notify prescriber if pain relief is not adequate, and expect dosage to be increased.

•Check infusion site regularly, and be aware that meningitis can occur within 24 hours after contamination of the delivery system; a disconnected catheter is the most common problem with external devices.

•Monitor patient closely for signs and symptoms of meningitis, such as headache, stiff neck, altered mental status, nausea, vomiting, and occasionally seizures caused by inadvertent contamination of the microinfusion device or catheter tract used to deliver ziconotide. Notify prescriber immediately if you suspect meningitis.

## Mechanism of Action

Pain sensations are transmitted by sensory neurons that travel through N-type calcium channels in the dorsal horn of the spinal cord and ascend to the brain.

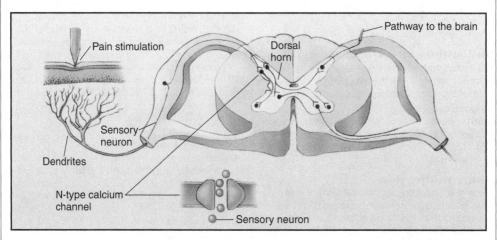

Ziconotide binds to N-type calcium channels on primary nociceptive afferent nerves in superficial layers of the dorsal horn. The channels then become blocked, preventing excitatory neurotransmitter release in the primary afferent nerve terminals and relieving pain.

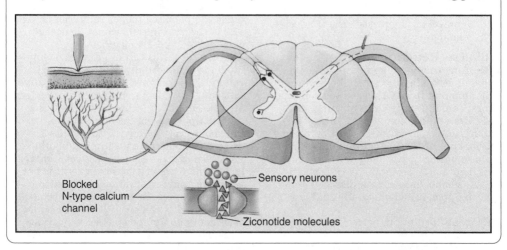

• Monitor patient closely for cognitive impairment, hallucinations, or changes in mood or consciousness because ziconotide may cause severe psychiatric symptoms and neurologic impairment. If present, notify prescriber and expect to decrease dosage or stop ziconotide. Provide appropriate supportive care, as prescribed, to relieve adverse effects. Tell prescriber again if adverse effects are still present after 2 weeks.

• Expect to stop ziconotide temporarily if patient becomes unresponsive or stuporous during therapy; drug may be continued when patient reverts to previous mental status.

•Ziconotide can be stopped abruptly without causing withdrawal symptoms.
•Monitor patient's serum CK level every other week for first month of therapy and monthly thereafter, as ordered. If levels become elevated, notify prescriber and expect to decrease ziconotide dosage or stop drug until levels return to normal.

**PATIENT TEACHING**
•Teach caregiver how to care for external device, if present. Stress need for strict aseptic technique with microinfusion device and connections and importance of checking site often for problems, such as a disconnected catheter, which increase the risk of meningitis.
•Review evidence of meningitis with caregiver, and tell her to contact prescriber immediately if she suspects meningitis.
•Advise patient to notify prescriber if pain relief isn't adequate.
•Tell patient and caregiver to notify prescriber immediately about muscle pain, soreness, and weakness with or without dark urine or a change in mental status or mood, including depression or suicidal ideation.
•Advise patient to avoid hazardous activities that require mental alertness or motor coordination while receiving ziconotide.
•Caution patient to avoid taking OTC preparations that contain CNS depressants because of the risk of adverse CNS effects.

# zileuton

Zyflo

## Class and Category
*Chemical:* Leukotriene inhibitor
*Therapeutic:* Antiasthmatic
*Pregnancy category:* C

## Indications and Dosages
➤ *To treat chronic asthma*
**TABLETS**
Adults and adolescents. 600 mg q.i.d. *Maximum:* 2,400 mg/day.

| Route | Onset | Peak | Duration |
|-------|-------|------|----------|
| P.O. | 2 hr | Unknown | Unknown |

## Contraindications
Hepatic impairment, hypersensitivity to zileuton or its components

## Mechanism of Action
Inhibits the formation of leukotrienes found mainly in neutrophils, eosinophils, monocytes, macrophages, and mast cells. Normally, leukotrienes augment neutrophil and eosinophil migration, neutrophil and monocyte aggregation, leukocyte adhesion, capillary permeability, and smooth-muscle contraction. By inhibiting leukotriene formation, zileuton causes bronchial relaxation and decreases vascular leakage and edema, mucus secretion, eosinophil movement, and bronchial hyperresponsiveness.

## Interactions
**DRUGS**
*propranolol, terfenadine:* Increased effects of these drugs
*theophylline:* Doubled blood theophylline level
*warfarin:* Prolonged PT and INR

## Adverse Reactions
**CNS:** Asthenia, dizziness, fever, headache, hypertonia, insomnia, malaise, nervousness, somnolence
**CV:** Chest pain
**EENT:** Conjunctivitis
**GI:** Abdominal pain, constipation, flatulence, indigestion, nausea, vomiting
**GU:** UTI, vaginitis
**MS:** Arthralgia, myalgia, neck pain or rigidity
**SKIN:** Pruritus
**Other:** Lymphadenopathy

## Nursing Considerations
•Be aware that zileuton shouldn't be used to treat bronchospasm during an acute asthma attack or status asthmaticus; it can't relieve symptoms quickly enough.
•Monitor serum ALT level, as ordered, usually before treatment starts, once a month for 3 months, every 2 to 3 months for remainder of first year, and periodically thereafter during therapy.
•Monitor results of liver and pulmonary function tests and CBC periodically during therapy.

**PATIENT TEACHING**
•Advise patient to take drug exactly as prescribed, in evenly spaced doses, every day. Stress the importance of taking drug even during symptom-free periods and acute exacerbations.

X
Y
Z

•Instruct patient to continue using rescue inhalants, as prescribed, for acute attacks.
•Teach patient how to use peak-flow meter to determine and monitor pulmonary function.

# zinc acetate

*(contains 25 or 50 mg of elemental zinc per capsule)*
Galzin

## zinc chloride

*(contains 1 mg of elemental zinc per ml for I.V. infusion)*

## zinc gluconate

*(contains 1.4 mg of elemental zinc per lozenge; 1.4, 2, 4, 7, 8, 10, 11, 13, 31, 50, or 52 mg of elemental zinc per tablet)*
Orazinc

## zinc sulfate

*(contains 25 or 50 mg of elemental zinc per capsule; 15, 25, 45, or 50 mg of elemental zinc per tablet; 50 mg of elemental zinc per E.R. tablet; and 1 or 5 mg of elemental zinc per ml for I.V. infusion)*
Orazinc, Verazinc, Zinc 15, Zinc-220, Zinca-Pak, Zincate

## Class and Category

*Chemical:* Trace element, mineral
*Therapeutic:* Copper absorption inhibitor, nutritional supplement
*Pregnancy category:* A (oral), C (I.V.)

## Indications and Dosages

➤ *To prevent zinc deficiency based on U.S. and Canadian recommended daily allowances*
**CAPSULES, E.R. TABLETS, LOZENGES, TABLETS**
**Male adults and children age 11 and older.** 15 mg (9 to 12 mg Canadian) of elemental zinc daily.
**Female adults and children age 11 and older.** 12 mg (9 mg Canadian) of elemental zinc daily.
**Pregnant females.** 15 mg (15 mg Canadian) of elemental zinc daily.
**Breast-feeding females.** 16 to 19 mg (15 mg Canadian) of elemental zinc daily.
**Children ages 7 to 10.** 10 mg (7 to 9 mg Canadian) of elemental zinc daily.
**Children ages 4 to 6.** 10 mg (5 mg Canadian) of elemental zinc daily.

**Children from birth to age 3.** 5 to 10 mg (2 to 4 mg Canadian) of elemental zinc daily.
**I.V. INFUSION**
**Adults and children.** 2.5 to 4 mg q.d. added to total parenteral nutrition (TPN) solution. *Maximum:* 12 mg/day.
**Children from birth to age 5.** 100 mcg/kg/day added to TPN solution.
**Premature infants weighing up to 3 kg.** 300 mcg/kg/day added to TPN solution.
➤ *To treat zinc deficiency*
**CAPSULES, E.R. TABLETS, LOZENGES, TABLETS**
**Adults and children.** Dosage individualized based on severity of deficiency.
**I.V. INFUSION**
**Adults and adolescents.** 2.5 to 4 mg q.d. added to TPN solution. *Maximum:* 12 mg/day.
**Children from birth to age 5.** 100 mcg/kg/day added to TPN solution.
**Premature infants weighing up to 3 kg.** 300 mcg/kg/day added to TPN solution.
➤ *As adjunct maintenance therapy for patients previously treated for Wilson's disease*
**CAPSULES**
**Adults.** 50 mg t.i.d.
**Pregnant females.** 25 mg t.i.d., increased to 50 mg t.i.d. if drug effectiveness decreases.
**Children age 10 and older.** 25 mg t.i.d., increased to 50 mg t.i.d. if drug effectiveness decreases.

## Contraindications
Hypersensitivity to zinc or its components

## Interactions
**DRUGS**
*copper supplements:* Impaired copper absorption (with large doses of zinc)
*oral iron supplements, oral phosphate salts, penicillamine, phosphorus-containing drugs:* Decreased zinc absorption
*quinolones, tetracyclines:* Decreased absorption and possibly decreased effectiveness of these antibiotics
*thiazide diuretics:* Increased urinary excretion of zinc
*zinc-containing preparations:* Increased blood zinc level
**FOODS**
*fiber- or phylate-containing foods (such as bran, whole-grain breads, cereal), phosphorus-containing foods (including milk, poultry):* Decreased zinc absorption

## Mechanism of Action

Necessary for proper functioning of more than 200 metalloenzymes (enzymes containing tightly bound zinc atoms as an integral part of their structure), including carbonic anhydrase, carboxypeptidase A, alcohol dehydrogenase, alkaline phosphatase, and RNA polymerase. Zinc also helps maintain nucleic acid, protein, and cell membrane structure and is essential for certain physiologic functions, including cell growth and division, sexual maturation and reproduction, dark adaptation and night vision, wound healing, host immunity, and taste acuity. This mineral also provides cellular antioxidant protection by scavenging free radicals.

In addition, zinc acetate interferes with intestinal absorption of copper and produces a protein that binds with copper, preventing its transfer to the blood. Bound copper is then excreted in stools, thus decreasing copper toxicity in Wilson's disease.

## Adverse Reactions

None with usual dosages

## Nursing Considerations

•**WARNING** Don't administer I.V. zinc preparations that contain benzyl alcohol to neonates or premature infants because this preservative may cause a fatal toxic syndrome characterized by metabolic acidosis and CNS, respiratory, circulatory, and renal function impairment.

•Administer oral zinc supplements 1 hour before or 2 to 3 hours after meals; at least 2 hours after administering oral iron supplements (to prevent decreased zinc absorption) or copper supplements (to prevent decreased copper absorption); and at least 6 hours before or 2 hours after administering quinolone or tetracycline antibiotics (to prevent decreased absorption of these drugs).

•Monitor patient receiving long-term zinc therapy for sideroblastic anemia, which may result from zinc-induced copper deficiency and is characterized by anemia, leukopenia, neutropenia, granulocytopenia, and bone marrow problems. Be aware that these effects are reversible after zinc is discontinued.

•Monitor patient with preexisting copper deficiency for exacerbation of this condition; zinc can decrease serum copper level.

•Assess for signs and symptoms of zinc deficiency, such as growth retardation, hypogonadism, delayed sexual maturation, alopecia, impaired wound healing, skin lesions, immune deficiencies, behavioral disturbances, night blindness, and impaired sense of taste.

•Monitor blood alkaline phosphatase (ALP) level monthly, as ordered; it may increase.

•Be aware that zinc chloride contains aluminum, which may accumulate to the point of toxicity if the patient's kidney function is impaired. Assess kidney function regularly.

**PATIENT TEACHING**

•Explain the need for a zinc supplement.

•Instruct patient to take zinc on an empty stomach, at least 1 hour before or 2 hours after meals. Caution her not to take zinc within 2 hours of iron or copper supplements or phosphorus-containing drugs.

•Instruct patient to let zinc lozenge dissolve in mouth slowly and completely and not to swallow it whole or chew it. Advise her not to take zinc lozenges more often than directed.

# ziprasidone hydrochloride

Geodon

## ziprasidone mesylate

Geodon for Injection

## Class and Category

*Chemical:* Benzisoxazole derivative
*Therapeutic:* Antipsychotic
*Pregnancy category:* C

## Indications and Dosages

➤ *To treat schizophrenia*

**CAPSULES**

**Adults.** *Initial:* 20 mg b.i.d. Dosage increased as indicated q 2 or more days. *Usual:* 20 to 80 mg b.i.d. *Maximum:* 100 mg b.i.d.

**I.M. INJECTION**

**Adults.** *Initial:* 10 to 20 mg. 10 mg dose may be administered q 2 hr up to maximum dose; 20 mg dose may be administered q 4 hr up to maximum dose. *Maximum:* 40 mg/day.

➤ *To treat acute manic or mixed episodes of bipolar disorder*

**CAPSULES**

**Adults.** *Initial:* 40 mg b.i.d. with food on day 1; then increased to 60 or 80 mg on day 2 with further adjustments as needed.

## Incompatibilities

Don't mix injection form with drugs or solvents other than sterile water for injection.

---

## Mechanism of Action

Selectively blocks serotonin and dopamine receptors in the mesocortical tract of the CNS, thereby suppressing psychotic symptoms.

---

## Contraindications

Concomitant use of other drugs that prolong QT interval, history of arrhythmia, hypersensitivity to ziprasidone or its components, known history of QT-interval prolongation, recent acute MI, uncompensated heart failure

## Interactions

**DRUGS**

*antihypertensives:* Additive antihypertensive effects

*carbamazepine:* Possibly decreased blood ziprasidone level

*CNS depressants:* Increased CNS depression

*dopamine agonists, levodopa:* Decreased therapeutic effects of these drugs

*drugs that prolong QT interval (including quinidine, dofetilide, pimozide, sotalol, thioridazine, and sparfloxacin):* Increased risk of prolonged QT or QTc interval, torsades de pointes, and sudden death

*ketoconazole:* Possibly increased blood ziprasidone level

**FOODS**

*all foods:* Increased ziprasidone absorption

## Adverse Reactions

**CNS:** Agitation, akathisia, amnesia, anxiety, asthenia, CVA, depression, dizziness, dystonia, extrapyramidal reactions, headache, hypertonia, insomnia, neuroleptic malignant syndrome, paresthesia, personality or speech disorder, somnolence, tremor

**CV:** Bradycardia, chest pain, hypercholesterolemia, hypertension, orthostatic hypotension, prolonged QT or QTc interval, tachycardia, thrombophlebitis, vasodilation

**EENT:** Abnormal vision, dry mouth, increased salivation, rhinitis, tongue swelling

**ENDO:** Dysmenorrhea, hyperglycemia

**GI:** Abdominal pain, anorexia, constipation, diarrhea, dysphagia, indigestion, nausea, rectal bleeding, vomiting

**MS:** Arthralgia, back pain, dysarthria, myalgia

**RESP:** Cough, pulmonary embolism, upper respiratory tract infection

**SKIN:** Diaphoresis, furunculosis, rash

**Other:** Accidental injury, flulike symptoms, injection site pain, weight gain

## Nursing Considerations

•Protect ziprasidone vials from light. Reconstitute by adding 1.2 ml of sterile water for injection to vial and shaking vigorously until drug is dissolved. Each ml of reconstituted solution contains 20 mg ziprasidone. Discard any unused portion.

•Give only by I.M. route.

•Store reconstituted drug for 24 hours protected from light; if refrigerated, drug may be stored for up to 7 days protected from light.

•Administer I.M. form cautiously to patients with impaired renal function.

•**WARNING** Assess cardiac rhythm in patients with hypokalemia or hypomagnesemia. Be aware that dizziness, palpitations, and syncope may indicate life-threatening torsades de pointes. Be prepared to stop ziprasidone if QTc interval is greater than 500 msec.

•Monitor patient, especially elderly woman, for involuntary movements, which may become irreversible tardive dyskinesia. If symptoms develop, notify prescriber immediately and be prepared to stop drug.

•Immediately report evidence of neuroleptic malignant syndrome, a rare but potentially fatal adverse reaction including hyperpyrexia, muscle rigidity, altered mental status, irregular pulse, blood pressure changes, tachycardia, diaphoresis, arrhythmia, myoglobinuria (rhabdomyolysis), and acute renal failure.

•Monitor patient's blood glucose and lipid levels routinely, as ordered, because drug increases the risk of hyperglycemia and hypercholesterolemia.

**PATIENT TEACHING**

•Instruct patient to take ziprasidone with food to increase drug's absorption.

•Advise patient to avoid hazardous activities until drug's CNS effects are known.

•Tell family to monitor patient closely for suicidal tendencies; patients with psychotic illness or bipolar disorder are at higher risk.
•Urge patient to rise slowly from seated or lying position to minimize orthostatic hypotension.

# zoledronic acid

Zometa

## Class and Category
*Chemical:* Bisphosphonate
*Therapeutic:* Antihypercalcemic, bone resorption inhibitor
*Pregnancy category:* D

## Indications and Dosages
➤ *To treat hypercalcemia caused by cancer*
**I.V. INFUSION**
**Adults.** 4 mg infused over at least 15 min. After 7 days, retreatment with 4 mg if serum calcium level doesn't remain at or return to normal. *Maximum:* 4 mg/dose.
➤ *As adjunct treatment for patients with multiple myeloma or bony metastasis who are receiving standard antineoplastic therapy and have a creatinine clearance above 60 ml/min/1.73 $m^2$*
**I.V. INFUSION**
**Adults.** 4 mg infused over at least 15 min q 3 to 4 wk.
**DOSAGE ADJUSTMENT** If creatinine clearance is 50 to 60 ml/min/1.73 $m^2$, dosage decreased to 3.5 mg; if it's 40 to 49 ml/min/1.73 $m^2$, dosage decreased to 3.3 mg; and if it's 30 to 39 ml/min/1.73 $m^2$, dosage decreased to 3 mg.

## Incompatibilities
Don't mix zoledronic acid with calcium-containing I.V. solutions, such as LR.

## Contraindications
Hypersensitivity to zoledronic acid, other bisphosphonates, or their components

## Interactions
**DRUGS**
*aminoglycosides:* Possibly additive serum calcium–lowering effect
*loop diuretics, such as furosemide:* Possibly increased risk of hypocalcemia

## Adverse Reactions
**CNS:** Chills, fever
**EENT:** Conjunctivitis
**GI:** Nausea, vomiting
**GU:** Elevated serum creatinine level, renal insufficiency or failure
**MS:** Arthralgia, myalgia
**Other:** Hypocalcemia, hypomagnesemia, hypophosphatemia, infusion site redness and swelling

## Nursing Considerations
•Be aware that zoledronic acid isn't indicated for hypercalcemia from hyperparathyroidism or other non–tumor conditions.
•Make sure patient has had a dental checkup before zoledronic acid starts, especially if patient has cancer; is receiving chemotherapy, head or neck radiation, or a corticosteroid; or has poor oral hygiene because the risk of os-

---

> ### Mechanism of Action
> Inhibits resorption of mineralized bone and cartilage by osteoclasts and induces osteoclast breakdown. In cancer-related hypercalcemia, hyperactive osteoclasts cause bone resorption and release of calcium into the blood, which causes polyuria, GI disruption, progressive dehydration, and decreasing GFR. This, in turn, increases renal calcium resorption and worsens hypercalcemia. Zoledronic acid interrupts this process.

---

teonecrosis is increased in these patients, and invasive dental procedures during zoledronic acid therapy may worsen osteonecrosis.
•Expect to aggressively hydrate hypercalcemic patient with I.V. NS before and throughout zoledronic acid therapy, as prescribed, to achieve and maintain a urine output of about 2 L/day.
•**WARNING** During hydration, monitor fluid intake and output often and assess patient, especially one with heart failure, for evidence of life-threatening overhydration.
•Reconstitute zoledronic acid by adding 5 ml of sterile water for injection to drug vial to yield a solution that contains 4 mg of zoledronic acid. Make sure drug is completely dissolved before withdrawing prescribed dose. Further dilute in 100 ml of NS or 5% dextrose injection, and infuse over no less

than 15 minutes.
• Before giving drug, inspect the reconstituted and diluted solution and discard if particles or discoloration are present.
• Refrigerate reconstituted drug at 2° to 8° C (36° to 46° F) and discard it after 24 hours.
• Give drug as a single I.V. solution in a separate I.V. line.
• **WARNING** Be aware that a single dose of zoledronic acid shouldn't exceed 4 mg and shouldn't be infused over less than 15 minutes because this may lead to significant renal function deterioration, which may progress to renal failure.
• **WARNING** Assess patient's renal function, as ordered, before and during zoledronic acid therapy to detect deterioration. For patient with a normal serum creatinine level who develops an increase of 0.5 mg/dl within 2 weeks of receiving drug, expect to withhold next dose until serum creatinine level is within 10% of patient's baseline value. For patient with an abnormal serum creatinine level who develops an increase of 1.0 mg/dl within 2 weeks of receiving drug, expect to withhold next dose until serum creatinine level is within 10% of baseline value.
• Monitor patient's serum calcium, magnesium, and phosphate levels, as ordered, throughout therapy. If hypocalcemia, hypomagnesemia, or hypophosphatemia occurs, expect to give short-term supplemental therapy, as ordered.
• Assess aspirin-sensitive asthma patients for worsening of respiratory symptoms during zoledronic acid therapy because other bisphosphonates have caused bronchoconstriction in these patients.
• Store drug at 25° C (77° F).

**PATIENT TEACHING**
• Teach patient the importance of consuming a nutritious diet, including adequate amounts of calcium and vitamin D.
• Advise patient to alert prescriber about muscle or bone pain.
• Instruct patient on proper oral hygiene and on need to notify prescriber before undergoing invasive dental procedures.

# zolmitriptan

Zomig, Zomig ZMT

## Class and Category

*Chemical:* Selective 5-hydroxytryptamine agonist
*Therapeutic:* Antimigraine
*Pregnancy category:* C

## Indications and Dosages

➤ *To treat acute migraine headache with or without aura*
**DISINTEGRATING TABLETS**
**Adults.** 2.5 mg, repeated q 2 hr p.r.n. *Maximum:* 10 mg in 24 hr or three headaches/mo.
**TABLETS**
**Adults.** 2.5 mg or less, repeated q 2 hr p.r.n. *Maximum:* 10 mg in 24 hr or three headaches/mo.
**NASAL SPRAY**
**Adults.** 5 mg, repeated in 2 hr if needed. *Maximum:* 10 mg/24 hr.
**DOSAGE ADJUSTMENT** Dosage reduced for patients with hepatic impairment.

## Contraindications

Basilar or hemiplegic migraine, cardiovascular disease, concurrent use of ergotamine-containing drugs, hypersensitivity to zolmitriptan or its components, ischemic heart disease, Prinzmetal's angina, symptomatic Wolff-Parkinson-White syndrome or other accessory pathway conduction disorder, use of another 5-hydroxytryptamine agonist within past 24 hours, use of an MAO inhibitor within 14 days

## Interactions
**DRUGS**
*acetaminophen:* Delayed peak effect of acetaminophen (by 1 hour)
*cimetidine:* Prolonged zolmitriptan half-life
*ergot alkaloids:* Prolonged vasoconstriction
*fluoxetine, fluvoxamine, paroxetine, sertraline:* Hyperreflexia, lack of coordination, and weakness
*MAO inhibitors:* Increased zolmitriptan effects
*naratriptan, rizatriptan, sumatriptan:* Prolonged zolmitriptan effects
*oral contraceptives, propranolol:* Increased blood zolmitriptan level

## Adverse Reactions

**CNS:** Asthenia, dizziness, hyperesthesia, paresthesia, somnolence, vertigo
**CV:** Angina, coronary artery vasospasm, hypertension, MI, palpitations, transient myocardial ischemia, ventricular fibrillation or tachycardia
**EENT:** Dry mouth

**GI:** Abdominal pain, bloody diarrhea, dysphagia, GI or splenic infarction, indigestion, ischemic colitis, nausea, vomiting
**MS:** Myalgia; myasthenia; pain, pressure, or tightness in jaw, neck, or throat
**SKIN:** Diaphoresis, flushing
**Other:** Anaphylaxis, anaphylactoid reaction, angioedema

> ### Mechanism of Action
> Constricts inflamed and dilated cranial blood vessels in the carotid circulation and inhibits production of proinflammatory neuropeptides by binding to receptors on intracranial blood vessels and sensory nerves in the trigeminal-vascular system to stimulate negative feedback, which halts the release of serotonin.

## Nursing Considerations
•WARNING Expect an increased risk of vasoconstriction, which may lead to vascular and colonic ischemia with abdominal pain and bloody diarrhea, especially if patient has peripheral vascular disease (including Raynaud's phenomenon) or ischemic bowel disease.
•Monitor elderly patients and those with hepatic impairment for increased blood pressure, and notify prescriber immediately.
### PATIENT TEACHING
•Urge patient to ask prescriber before treating more than three headaches in 30 days.
•Advise patient not to remove disintegrating tablet from blister pack until just before use. Instruct her to peel open pack, let tablet dissolve on her tongue, and then swallow it.

# zolpidem
Ambien, Ambien CR

## Class, Category, and Schedule
*Chemical:* Imidazopyridine derivative
*Therapeutic:* Antianxiety, sedative-hypnotic
*Pregnancy category:* B
*Controlled substance:* Schedule IV

## Indications and Dosages
➤ *To provide short-term treatment of insomnia*
### TABLETS
**Adults.** 10 mg h.s. for 7 to 10 days. *Maximum:* 20 mg/day.

DOSAGE ADJUSTMENT For elderly or debilitated patients and those with hepatic impairment, dosage possibly reduced to 5 mg h.s., with a maximum of 5 mg/day for nursing facility residents
### E.R. TABLETS
**Adults.** 12.5 mg immediately before h.s.
DOSAGE ADJUSTMENT For elderly or debilitated patients and those with hepatic impairment, dosage reduced to 6.25 mg immediately before h.s.

## Contraindications
Hypersensitivity to zolpidem or its components, ritonavir therapy

## Interactions
### DRUGS
*azole antifungals:* Increased CNS activity and additive adverse effects of zolpidem
*barbiturates, chlorpromazine, general anesthetics, opioid agonists, other CNS depressants, phenothiazines, tramadol, tricyclic antidepressants:* Possibly increased CNS depression and reduced psychomotor function
*bupropion:* Increased blood zolpidem level, possibly visual hallucinations, loss of alertness
*desipramine, imipramine:* Increased risk of visual hallucinations and reduced alertness
*flumazenil:* Antagonized sedative effect
*haloperidol:* Increased CNS depression
*nevirapine:* Decreased blood zolpidem level
*rifabutin, rifampin:* Increased zolpidem clearance
*selective serotonin-reuptake inhibitors:* Increased risk of delusions, disorientation, and hallucinations
### FOODS
*all foods:* Increased time to peak blood zolpidem level, decreased effects of zolpidem
### ACTIVITIES
*alcohol use:* Increased CNS depression

## Adverse Reactions
**CNS:** Amnesia, dizziness, drowsiness, headache, lethargy, paradoxical CNS stimulation (including agitation, euphoria, hallucinations, hyperactivity, and nightmares)
**GI:** Constipation, diarrhea, indigestion, nausea, vomiting
**Other:** Withdrawal symptoms

## Mechanism of Action

May potentiate GABA and other inhibitory neurotransmitters. By binding to specific benzodiazepine receptors in limbic and cortical areas of the CNS, zolpidem increases GABA's inhibitory effects, blocks cortical and limbic arousal, and preserves deep sleep (stages 3 and 4).

## Nursing Considerations

• Administer zolpidem just before bedtime because drug has a rapid onset of action.
• Expect patient to receive no more than a 1-month supply of drug for outpatient therapy.
• **WARNING** If zolpidem is withdrawn abruptly (especially after prolonged therapy), monitor for withdrawal symptoms, such as abdominal cramps or discomfort, fatigue, flushing, inconsolable crying, light-headedness, nausea, nervousness, panic attack, rebound insomnia, and vomiting.
• Expect drug to produce anticonvulsant and muscle relaxant effects at high doses.
• If patient takes other CNS depressants, expect to reduce zolpidem dosage, as prescribed.

### PATIENT TEACHING

• Caution patient to take drug exactly as prescribed and not to increase dosage unless directed by prescriber.
• Advise patient taking extended-release form to swallow tablet whole and not to break, crush, or chew it.
• Instruct patient to take zolpidem immediately before bedtime on an empty stomach.
• Advise patient to notify prescriber immediately about abdominal cramps or discomfort, fatigue, flushing, inconsolable crying, light-headedness, nausea, nervousness, panic attack, and vomiting.

# zonisamide

Zonegran

## Class and Category

*Chemical:* Benzisoxazole derivative, sulfonamide
*Therapeutic:* Anticonvulsant
*Pregnancy category:* C

## Indications and Dosages

➤ *As adjunct to treat partial seizures*

### CAPSULES

**Adults.** *Initial:* 100 mg q.d. Dosage increased by 100 mg/day q 2 wk, as needed. *Usual:* 200 to 400 mg/day. *Maximum:* 600 mg/day.

## Contraindications

Hypersensitivity to sulfonamides, zonisamide, or their components

## Interactions

### DRUGS

*carbamazepine, phenobarbital, phenytoin, valproate:* Possibly decreased blood zonisamide level
*CNS depressants:* Additive CNS depressant effects

### FOODS

*grapefruit juice:* Possibly decreased metabolism of zonisamide

## Adverse Reactions

**CNS:** Agitation, ataxia, dizziness, irritability, somnolence
**GI:** Anorexia

## Mechanism of Action

May stop the spread of seizures and suppress their foci by blocking sodium channels and reducing voltage-dependent, inward currents from calcium channels. This action stabilizes neuronal membranes and suppresses synchronized neuronal hyperactivity.

## Nursing Considerations

• **WARNING** Monitor results of CBC and other laboratory tests for signs of blood dyscrasias because zonisamide is a sulfonamide and can be absorbed systemically. Systemic absorption may result in life-threatening reactions, including toxic epidermal necrolysis, Stevens-Johnson syndrome, fulminant hepatic necrosis, agranulocytosis, aplastic anemia, and other blood dyscrasias.
• Be aware that patients receiving doses of 300 mg/day or more are at increased risk for adverse CNS reactions, including decreased concentration, fatigue, drowsiness, and impaired speech.
• Monitor serum creatinine and BUN levels for signs of abnormally decreased glomerular filtration rate (GFR). Expect some decrease in GFR during first 4 weeks of treatment

and a return to baseline within 2 to 3 weeks after drug is discontinued.

•Monitor patient for signs and symptoms of renal calculi.

•Be aware that zonisamide should not be discontinued abruptly because doing so may increase the frequency of seizures.

**PATIENT TEACHING**

•Inform patient that zonisamide is usually prescribed with other anticonvulsants and that she should continue to take all drugs as prescribed.

•Instruct patient to swallow capsules whole, and not to chew them or break them open.

•Inform patient that prescriber may have to adjust dosage over several weeks or months before a stable dose is achieved.

•Advise patient to use caution when driving or performing other activities that require mental alertness because zonisamide commonly causes somnolence, dizziness, and decreased concentration, particularly during first month of therapy.

•Advise patient to wear a medical identification bracelet or necklace with information about her seizure disorder.

•Unless contraindicated, encourage patient to drink 6 to 8 glasses of water each day to prevent kidney stones.

•Advise patient to rise slowly from a lying or seated position to reduce the risk of dizziness.

➤——————————◄

X
Y
Z

# Appendices

# Oral Antidiabetic Combinations

Oral antidiabetic drugs are prescribed, along with life-style changes such as diet and exercise, to manage type 2 diabetes mellitus. A combination of two different types of oral antidiabetic drugs may be prescribed to simplify a patient's drug regimen, enhance drug actions, and, ultimately, provide a patient with better control of his blood glucose level.

The following chart lists the generic and trade names of oral antidiabetic combination drugs, the usual adult dosages for use as monotherapy, and the usual adult dosages for use with patients whose blood glucose levels aren't adequately controlled with one oral antidiabetic drug taken by itself.

Further information about the mechanisms of action, interactions, adverse reactions, and nursing considerations can be found for the specific oral antidiabetic drugs in the alphabetical drug monographs.

| GENERIC AND TRADE NAMES AND CHEMICAL CLASSES | USUAL ADULT DOSAGE AS INITIAL THERAPY | USUAL ADULT DOSAGE WHEN PREVIOUS THERAPY HAS FAILED |
|---|---|---|
| **glipizide and metformin hydrochloride** <br> METAGLIP <br> *Chemical:* Sulfonylurea (glipizide), dimethylbiguanide (metformin) | *Initial:* For blood glucose levels less than 280 mg/dL, 2.5 mg/250 mg tab q.d. with a meal; for blood glucose levels of 280 to 320 mg/dL, 2.5 mg/500 mg tab b.i.d. with meals. Dosage increased by one tab/day q 2 wk, as needed and prescribed. *Maximum:* 10 mg/1000mg or 10 mg/2000 mg daily in divided doses. | *Initial:* 2.5 mg/500 mg or 5 mg/500 mg b.i.d. with morning and evening meals (starting dosage shouldn't exceed daily doses of glipizide or metformin already being taken). Dosage increased in increments of no more than 5 mg/500 mg. *Maximum:* 20 mg/2,000 mg daily. |
| **glyburide and metformin hydrochloride** <br> Glucovance <br> *Chemical:* Sulfonylurea (glyburide), dimethylbiguanide (metformin) | *Initial:* 1.25 mg/250 mg tab q.d. or b.i.d. Dosage increased by 1.25 mg/250 mg/day q 2 wk, as needed. | *Initial:* 2.5 mg/500 mg tab or 5 mg/500 mg tab b.i.d. Dosage increased, as prescribed, by 5 mg/500 mg/day. *Maximum:* 20 mg/2,000 mg daily. |
| **rosiglitazone maleate and metformin hydrochloride** <br> Avandamet <br> *Chemical:* Thiazolidinedione (rosiglitazone), dimethylbiguanide (metformin) | Safety and efficacy as initial therapy hasn't been established. | •If previous metformin dose was 1,000 mg/day, give 1 tab of 2 mg/500 mg b.i.d., as prescribed. <br> •If previous metformin dose was 1,000 to 2,000 mg, dosage must be individualized. <br> •If previous metformin dose was 2,000 mg/day, give 2 tabs of 1 mg/500 mg b.i.d., as prescribed. <br> •If previous rosiglitazone dose was 4 mg/day, give 1 tab of 2 mg/500 mg b.i.d., as prescribed. <br> •If previous rosiglitazone was 8 mg/day, give 1 tab of 4 mg/500 mg b.i.d. <br> •Dosage adjustment required when switching from existing combination therapy.* |

* When switching from combination of rosiglitazone and metformin as separate tablets, usual starting dose is the dose of rosiglitazone and metformin already being taken. For additional blood glucose control, daily dose may be increased in increments of 4 mg rosiglitazone and/or 500 mg metformin, up to maximum daily dose of 8 mg/2,000 mg.

# Insulin Preparations

For each category of insulin, the following chart lists the species; common trade names; onset, peak, and duration; and key nursing considerations.

| CATEGORY, SPECIES, AND TRADE NAMES | KEY NURSING CONSIDERATIONS |
|---|---|
| **Rapid-acting insulin** | |

**Onset:** 15 min  **Peak:** 30 to 90 min  **Duration:** In 6 hr

| | |
|---|---|
| Human<br>•Apidra (insulin glulisine)<br>•Humalog (insulin lispro)<br>•NovoLog (insulin aspart) | •Mix Humalog or NovoLog with other insulin types, but mix Apidra only with NPH insulin, if needed. Administer immediately after mixing.<br>•When mixing rapid-acting insulin with a longer-acting insulin, always draw the rapid-acting insulin into the syringe first to avoid dosage errors.<br>•Give Humalog or NovoLog only by the S.C. route, up to 15 minutes (Humalog) or 5 to 10 minutes (NovoLog) before a meal. Give Apidra by S.C. route up to 15 to 20 minutes before a meal or using an insulin pump. If using a pump, Apidra shouldn't be diluted or mixed with any other insulin.<br>•Be aware that 1 U of rapid-acting insulin has the same glucose-lowering ability as 1 U of short-acting insulin.<br>•Rapid-acting insulin is available as a cartridge. Make sure to use the correct device for brand of insulin prescribed.<br>•Absorption rate of rapid-acting insulin may slow when this type of insulin is mixed in a syringe with human isophane insulin (NPH). Monitor the blood glucose level frequently. |
| **Short-acting insulin** | |

**Onset:** 30 min  **Peak:** 2 to 5 hr  **Duration:** 6 to 8 hr

| | |
|---|---|
| Human<br>•Humulin-R<br>•Novolin ge Toronto (CAN)<br>•Novolin ge Toronto Penfill (CAN)<br>•Novolin R<br>•Novolin R PenFill<br>•Novolin R Prefilled<br>•Velosulin BR<br>•Velosulin Human (CAN)<br>Pork<br>•Regular (concentrated), Iletin II, U-500<br>•Regular Insulin (pork)<br>•Regular Insulin (purified pork) | •Don't use short-acting insulin if it's cloudy, discolored, or unusually viscous.<br>•Use the U-500 strength to treat insulin resistance, as prescribed.<br>•Mix short-acting insulin with other insulin types, if needed. However, don't mix phosphate-buffered insulin with a zinc-containing insulin because the short-acting insulin's effectiveness may be reduced.<br>•Administer by the S.C., I.M., or I.V. route, as prescribed. Use a continuous S.C. infusion pump, if ordered. For an insulin pump, phosphate-buffered insulin is preferred over nonphosphate-buffered insulin. The catheter tubing and reservoir insulin should be changed every 48 hours or as specified by the pump manufacturer.<br>•When administering S.C. or I.M. injections, give the short-acting insulin 15 to 30 minutes before a meal or bedtime snack. |

*(continued)*

# Insulin Preparations (continued)

| CATEGORY, SPECIES, AND TRADE NAMES | KEY NURSING CONSIDERATIONS |
|---|---|

## Intermediate-acting insulin

**Onset:** 1 to 3 hr   **Peak:** 4 to 15 hr   **Duration:** 18 to 24 hr

Human
- Humulin N
- Novolin ge Lente (CAN)
- Novolin ge NPH (CAN)
- Novolin ge NPH Penfill (CAN)
- Novolin N
- Novolin N PenFill
- Novolin N Prefilled

Pork
- Lente
- Lente Iletin II

Beef and pork
- Lente Iletin (CAN)
- NPH Iletin I (CAN)

- Don't use intermediate-acting insulin if it contains precipitate that is clumped or granular or that clings to the sides of the vial.
- Roll the vial gently between your palms to mix; don't shake it. Also gently turn the prefilled syringe up and down several times before using to achieve a uniform mixture.
- Administer by S.C. injection only, 30 minutes before a meal or bedtime snack.
- Be aware that intermediate-acting insulin rarely produces a blood glucose level that's as close to normal as possible. So expect to mix it with a short-acting insulin, as prescribed, for optimum blood glucose control.

## Long-acting insulin

**Onset:** 4 to 6 hr   **Peak:** 8 to 20 hr   **Duration:** 24 to 28 hr

Human
- Humulin-U (CAN)
- Lantus (insulin glargine)
- Levemir (insulin detemir)
- Novolin ge Ultralente (CAN)

- Don't use long-acting insulin if it contains precipitate that is clumped or granular or that clings to the sides of the vial.
- As prescribed, mix Humulin-U or Novolin ge Ultralente with other insulin types—usually a short-acting insulin—if needed. Do not mix Lantus or Levemir with another insulin or solution.
- Roll the vial gently between your palms to obtain a uniform mixture; don't shake it.
- Administer by the S.C. route only. Inject Humulin-U or Novolin ge Ultralente 30 to 60 minutes before a meal or bedtime snack. Inject Lantus once daily at any time, keeping the daily injection time consistent. Inject Levemir prescribed once daily with the evening meal or at bedtime; inject Levemir prescribed twice daily with the morning meal and with the evening meal, at bedtime, or 12 hours after the morning dose.

## Combination insulins

**Onset:** 30 min   **Peak:** 2 to 12 hr   **Duration:** 18 to 24 hr

Human
- Humalog Mix 75/25 Pen
- Humulin 10/90 (CAN)
- Humulin 20/80 (CAN)
- Humulin 30/70 (CAN)
- Humulin 40/60 (CAN)

- Don't use combination insulin if it contains precipitate that is clumped or granular.
- Roll the vial gently between your palms to mix; don't shake it. Also gently turn the prefilled syringe up and down several times before using to achieve a uniform mixture.

## Insulin Preparations (continued)

| CATEGORY, SPECIES, AND TRADE NAMES | KEY NURSING CONSIDERATIONS |
|---|---|

### Combination insulins (continued)

**Onset:** 30 min **Peak:** 2 to 12 hr **Duration:** 18 to 24 hr (continued)

Human (continued)
- Humulin 50/50
- Humulin 70/30
- Novolin 70/30
- Novolin 70/30 PenFill
- Novolin 70/30 Prefilled
- Novolin ge 10/90 Penfill (CAN)
- Novolin ge 20/80 Penfill (CAN)
- Novolin ge 30/70 (CAN)
- Novolin ge 30/70 Penfill (CAN)
- Novolin ge 40/60 Penfill (CAN)
- Novolin ge 50/50 Penfill (CAN)

- Administer combination insulin by the S.C. route only, 30 minutes before a meal.
- Be aware that Canadian and American products contain the same insulin ratio but express it differently. For example, the Canadian Humulin 30/70 and the American Humulin 70/30 both contain 30 units of a short-acting insulin and 70 units of an intermediate-acting insulin. Canadian products list the short-acting insulin first; American products list it second.

## Ophthalmic Drugs

Although less commonly prescribed than oral drugs, drugs instilled into the eyes are frequently brought into the clinical setting by patients with chronic conditions. In most cases, the patient or a family member has administered these preparations at home. Your patient teaching should include a review of proper administration and storage of these drugs. Have the patient or a family member demonstrate proper use of the drug to make sure it will be administered correctly at home. Use this time to reassess the patient's ability to continue self-medication. Also, instruct him to report any changes in the condition being treated, either negative or positive. A properly educated patient not only ensures safe drug administration, but also is more likely to detect adverse reactions that require a dosage reduction or drug discontinuation, thus preventing the development of more serious health problems.

The following chart lists the generic and trade names, FDA-approved indications, and usual adult dosages for those ophthalmic preparations you're most likely to see in your practice setting. The drugs are divided according to therapeutic use.

| GENERIC AND TRADE NAMES | INDICATIONS | USUAL ADULT DOSAGES |
|---|---|---|
| **Ophthalmic antibiotics** | | |
| **bacitracin**<br>AK-Tracin | To treat surface bacterial infections affecting the conjunctiva and cornea | Small amount of ointment applied to conjunctival sac p.r.n. |
| **chloramphenicol**<br>Diochloram, Dioptic (CAN), Pentamycetin (CAN), Sopamycetin (CAN) | To treat surface bacterial infections affecting the conjunctiva and cornea | Apply small amount of ointment to lower conjunctival sac q 3 to 6 hr and p.r.n. for at least 48 hr after eye resumes normal appearance |
| **ciprofloxacin hydrochloride 0.3%**<br>Ciloxan | To treat corneal ulcers due to *Pseudomonas aeruginosa, Staphylococcus aureus, Staphylococcus epidermidis, Streptococcus pneumoniae,* and possibly *Serratia marcescens* and *Streptococcus viridans* | 2 gtt in affected eye q 15 min for first 6 hr, then 2 gtt q 30 min for remainder of first day; on day 2, 2 gtt in affected eye q 1 hr; on days 3 to 14, 2 gtt in affected eye q 4 hr |
| | To treat bacterial conjunctivitis due to *Haemophilus influenzae, S. aureus, S. epidermidis,* and possibly *S. pneumoniae* | 1 or 2 gtt in conjunctival sac of affected eye q 2 hr while awake for first 2 days, then 1 or 2 gtt q 4 hr while awake for next 5 days; or ½-inch strip of ointment applied in affected eye t.i.d. for 2 days, then b.i.d. for next 5 days |
| **erythromycin**<br>Ilotycin | To treat acute or chronic conjunctivitis and other eye infections | 1 cm (0.39 in) of ointment applied in infected eye up to 6 times/day, depending on severity of infection |
| | To treat chlamydial ophthalmic infections (trachoma) | Small amount applied in each eye b.i.d. for 2 mo; or b.i.d. on first 5 days of each month for 6 mo |

## Ophthalmic Drugs (continued)

### Ophthalmic antibiotics (continued)

| GENERIC AND TRADE NAMES | INDICATIONS | USUAL ADULT DOSAGES |
| --- | --- | --- |
| **gatifloxacin 0.3%** Zymar | To treat bacterial conjunctivitis due to *Corynebacterium propinquum, Staphylococcus aureus, Staphylococcus epidermidis, Streptococcus mitis, Streptococcus pneumoniae,* and *Haemophilus influenzae* | 1 gtt q 2 hr while awake, up to 8 times daily on days 1 and 2; then 1 gtt up to q.i.d. while awake on days 3 to 7 |
| **gentamicin sulfate** Garamycin, Genoptic, Gentacidin, Gentak | To treat blepharitis, blepharoconjunctivitis, conjunctivitis, corneal ulcers, dacryocystitis, keratoconjunctivitis, or meibomianitis due to susceptible organisms | 1 or 2 gtt in eye q 4 hr or, for severe infection, up to 2 gtt/hr; alternatively, 1 cm (.39 in) of ointment applied to lower conjunctival sac b.i.d. or t.i.d. |
| **levofloxacin 0.5%** Quixin | To treat bacterial conjunctivitis | On days 1 and 2: 1 or 2 gtt in affected eye q 2 hr while awake, up to 8 times/day; on days 3 to 7: 1 or 2 gtt in affected eye q 4 hr while awake, up to 4 times/day |
| **moxifloxacin 0.5%** Vigamox | To treat bacterial conjunctivitis due to *Staphylococcus aureus, Staphylococcus epidermidis, Staphylococcus haemolyticus, Staphylococcus hominis, Streptococcus pneumoniae,* Streptococcus viridans group, *Haemophilus influenzae, Chlamydia trachomatis* | 1 gtt t.i.d. for 7 days |
| **ofloxacin 0.3%** Ocuflox | To treat conjunctivitis due to *Staphylococcus aureus, Staphylococcus epidermidis, Streptococcus pneumoniae, Enterobacter cloacae, Haemophilus influenzae, Proteus mirabilis, Pseudomonas aeruginosa,* and *Propionibacterium acnes* | 1 or 2 gtt in conjunctival sac q 2 to 4 hr while awake for first 2 days, then 1 gtt q.i.d. for up to 5 more days |
| | To treat bacterial corneal ulcers due to *S. aureus, S. epidermidis, S. pneumoniae, E. cloacae, H. influenzae, P. mirabilis, P. aeruginosa, Serratia marcescens,* and *P. acnes* | 1 or 2 gtt q 30 min while awake and 1 or 2 gtt q 4 to 6 hr after retiring for 2 days; then 1 or 2 gtt/hr while awake for up to 7 more days; then 1 gtt q.i.d. until end of treatment |

(continued)

## Ophthalmic Drugs (continued)

| GENERIC AND TRADE NAMES | INDICATIONS | USUAL ADULT DOSAGES |
|---|---|---|
| **Ophthalmic antibiotics** *(continued)* | | |
| **polymyxin B sulfate** | To treat superficial eye infections involving the conjunctiva or cornea caused by *Pseudomonas* or other gram-negative organisms | 1 to 3 gtt of 0.1% to 0.25% (10,000 to 25,000 U/ml) q 1 hr; or up to 10,000 U in lower conjunctival sac q.d. |
| **sulfacetamide sodium 10%** AK-Sulf, Bleph-10, Ocusulf-10, Sodium Sulamyd 10% (CAN), Sulf-10 **sulfacetamide sodium 15%** Isopto Cetamide **sulfacetamide sodium 30%** | To treat inclusion conjunctivitis, corneal ulcers, and chlamydial infections<br><br><br><br><br><br>To treat trachoma | 1 or 2 gtt solution (10%) in lower conjunctival sac q 2 to 3 hr during day, less often at night; or 1 or 2 gtt (15%) in lower conjunctival sac q 1 to 2 hr; or 1 gtt (30%) in lower conjunctival sac q 2 hr; or 1.25 to 2.5 cm ointment (10%) into conjunctival sac q.i.d. and h.s.<br><br>2 gtt (30%) in lower conjunctival sac q 2 hr in combination with systemic sulfonamide or tetracycline |
| **tobramycin** AKTob, Tobrex | To treat superficial ocular infections involving the conjunctiva or cornea | 1 to 2 gtt q 1 to 4 hr, depending on severity of infection; or 1 cm (.39 in) of ointment applied to lower conjunctival sac q 8 to 12 hr for mild to moderate infections or q 3 to 4 hr for severe infections |
| **tobramycin 0.3% (3 mg) and dexamethasone 0.1% (1 mg)** TobraDex | To treat steroid-responsive inflammatory ocular conditions for which a corticosteroid is indicated and where superficial bacterial ocular infection or a risk of bacterial ocular infection exists | 1 to 2 gtt q 4 to 6 hr; during the initial 24 to 48 hrs, the dosage may be increased to 1 to 2 gtt q 2 hr; or apply 1 cm (.39 inch) of ointment into the conjunctival sac up to q.i.d. |
| **Ophthalmic anti-inflammatory drugs** | | |
| **dexamethasone** Maxidex **dexamethasone sodium phosphate** AK-Dex, Boldex, R.O. Dexasone (CAN) | To treat allergic conjunctivitis; corneal injury from chemical or thermal burns or from penetration of foreign bodies; inflammatory conditions of the anterior segment of globe, conjunctiva, cornea, or eyelids; iridocyclitis; suppression of graft rejection after keratoplasty; and uveitis | 1 or 2 gtt of suspension or solution or 1.25 to 2.5 cm of ointment in conjunctival sac from q 1 hr (in severe disease) to 6 times/day; or ointment may be applied t.i.d. or q.i.d., then tapered to b.i.d., and then q.d. |

## Ophthalmic Drugs (continued)

| GENERIC AND TRADE NAMES | INDICATIONS | USUAL ADULT DOSAGES |
|---|---|---|
| **Ophthalmic anti-inflammatory drugs** *(continued)* | | |
| **diclofenac sodium 0.1%** Voltaren, Voltaren Ophtha (CAN) | To treat postoperative inflammation after removal of cataract | 1 gtt in conjunctival sac q.i.d., beginning 24 hr after surgery and continuing through first 2 wk of postoperative period |
| | To treat photophobia in incisional refractive surgery | 1 or 2 gtt in operative eye 1 hr before surgery; then 1 or 2 gtt 15 min after surgery, followed by 1 gtt q.i.d., beginning 4 to 6 hr after surgery, for up to 3 days p.r.n. |
| **fluorometholone** Fluor-Op, FML Forte, FML Liquifilm, FML S.O.P. **fluorometholone acetate** Eflone, Flarex | To treat inflammatory and allergic conditions of the anterior uvea, conjunctiva, cornea, or sclera | 1 or 2 gtt suspension in conjunctival sac b.i.d. to q.i.d. or, in severe conditions, up to q 2 hr during first 1 to 2 days p.r.n.; or 1 cm (.39 in) of ointment applied to conjunctival sac q.d. to t.i.d. |
| **flurbiprofen sodium** Ocufen | To inhibit intraoperative miosis | 1 gtt in affected eye q 30 min, beginning 2 hr before surgery, up to total of 4 gtt |
| **ketorolac tromethamine** Acular | To relieve ocular itching due to seasonal allergic conjunctivitis | 1 gtt in conjunctival sac of each eye q.i.d. |
| | To treat postoperative inflammation in patients who have undergone cataract extraction | 1 gtt in operative eye q.i.d., beginning 24 hr after cataract surgery and continuing through first 2 wk of postoperative period |
| **loteprednol etabonate** Alrex, Lotemax | To provide temporary relief of seasonal allergic conjunctivitis and to treat steroid-responsive inflammatory conditions of the palpebral and bulbar conjunctiva, cornea, and anterior segment of the globe | 1 gtt of 0.2% suspension in affected eyes q.i.d.; or 1 or 2 gtt of 0.5% suspension in conjunctival sac of affected eye q.i.d. up to 1 gtt/hr |
| | To treat postoperative inflammation following ocular surgery | 1 or 2 gtt in conjunctival sac of operated eye q.i.d., beginning 24 hr after surgery and continuing through first 2 wk of postoperative period |
| **medrysone** HMS Liquifilm | To treat allergic conjunctivitis, episcleritis, ephinephrine sensitivity, and vernal conjunctivitis | 1 gtt into conjunctival sac up to q 4 hr |

*(continued)*

## Ophthalmic Drugs (continued)

| GENERIC AND TRADE NAMES | INDICATIONS | USUAL ADULT DOSAGES |
|---|---|---|
| **Ophthalmic anti-inflammatory drugs _(continued)_** | | |
| **olopatadine hydrochloride 0.1%** Patanol | To treat signs and symptoms of allergic conjunctivitis | 1 gtt b.i.d. at 6- to 8-hr intervals |
| **prednisolone acetate suspension** Econopred Plus, Pred Forte, Pred Mild **prednisolone sodium phosphate solution** AK-Pred, Inflamase Forte, Inflamase Mild | To treat inflammation of the anterior segment of globe, cornea, and palpebral and bulbar conjunctiva | 1 or 2 gtt in conjunctival sac b.i.d. to q.i.d. (suspension) or up to 6 times/day (solution) |
| **rimexolone** Vexol | To treat anterior uveitis | 1 or 2 gtt in conjunctival sac of affected eye q 1 hr while awake in first week; 1 gtt q 2 hr while awake in second week; then tapered until uveitis is resolved |
| | To treat postoperative inflammation after ocular surgery | 1 or 2 gtt in conjunctival sac of affected eye q.i.d., beginning 24 hr after surgery and continuing through first 2 wk of postoperative period |
| **Ophthalmic cycloplegic mydriatics** | | |
| **atropine sulfate** Atropisol, Isopto Atropine, Minims Atropine (CAN) | To treat acute iritis or uveitis | 1 gtt up to q.i.d.; or small strip of ointment applied to conjunctival sac up to b.i.d. |
| | To produce dilation for cycloplegic refraction | 1 or 2 gtt of 1% solution 1 hr before refraction |
| **cyclopentolate hydrochloride** AK-Pentolate, Cyclogyl, Minims Cyclopentolate (CAN), Pentolair | To produce mydriasis and cycloplegia required in specific diagnostic procedures | 1 gtt of 0.5%, 1%, or 2% solution in each eye; then 1 or 2 gtt in 5 to 10 min p.r.n. |
| **homatropine hydrobromide** Isopto Homatropine, Minims Homatropine (CAN) | To dilate pupils for cycloplegic refraction | 1 or 2 gtt in each eye, repeated in 5 to 10 min for 2 or 3 doses p.r.n. |
| | To treat uveitis | 1 or 2 gtt in each eye q 3 to 4 hr |
| **scopolamine hydrobromide** Isopto Hyoscine | To dilate pupils for cycloplegic refraction | 1 or 2 gtt of 0.25% solution 1 hr before refraction |
| | To treat iritis or uveitis | 1 or 2 gtt of 0.25% solution q.d. to q.i.d. |

## Ophthalmic Drugs (continued)

| GENERIC AND TRADE NAMES | INDICATIONS | USUAL ADULT DOSAGES |
|---|---|---|
| **Ophthalmic cycloplegic mydriatics** *(continued)* | | |
| **tropicamide** Mydriacyl, Opticyl, Tropicacyl | To dilate pupils for cycloplegic refraction | 1 gtt of 1% solution, repeated in 5 min; additional 1 gtt in 20 to 30 min p.r.n. |
| **Ophthalmic miotics** | | |
| **acetylcholine chloride** Miochol-E | To produce papillary miosis in anterior segment surgery | 0.5 to 2 ml gently into anterior chamber before or after sutures secured |
| **carbachol 0.01%** Carbastat, Miostat **carbachol 0.75%, 1.5%, 2.25%, 3%** Carboptic, Isopto Carbachol | To produce papillary miosis in ocular surgery<br><br>To treat open-angle glaucoma | 0.5 ml (solution) into anterior chamber before or after sutures secured<br><br>1 or 2 gtt up to t.i.d. |
| **pilocarpine** Ocusert Pilo-20, Ocusert Pilo-40 | To treat primary open-angle glaucoma | 1 or 2 gtt up to q.i.d.; or 1-cm (.39 cm) ribbon of 4% gel applied h.s.; or 1 Ocusert Pilo system (20 or 40 mcg/hr) q 7 days |
| **pilocarpine hydrochloride** Adsorbocarpine, Akarpine, Isopto Carpine, Miocarpine (CAN), Pilocar, Pilopine HS, Pilostat | To treat acute angle-closure glaucoma as emergency therapy | 1 gtt of 2% solution q 5 to 10 min for 3 to 6 doses; then 1 gtt q 1 to 3 hr until pressure is controlled |
| **pilocarpine nitrate** Pilagan, P.V. Carpine Liquifilm (CAN), Minims Pilocarpine (CAN) | To treat mydriasis due to mydriatic or cycloplegic drug therapy | 1 gtt of 1% solution |
| **Ophthalmic vasoconstrictors** | | |
| **naphazoline hydrochloride** Ak-Con, Albalon Liquifilm, Allerest, Clear Eyes, Comfort Eye Drops, Degest 2, Vasocon Regular | To treat ocular congestion, irritation, or itching | 1 gtt of 0.1% solution q 3 to 4 hr; or 1 gtt of 0.012% to 0.03% solution up to q.i.d. for no more than 72 hr |
| **oxymetazoline hydrochloride** OcuClear, Visine L.R. | To provide relief from eye redness due to minor eye irritations | 1 or 2 gtt in conjunctival sac b.i.d. to q.i.d. (at least 6 hr apart) |

*(continued)*

## Ophthalmic Drugs (continued)

| GENERIC AND TRADE NAMES | INDICATIONS | USUAL ADULT DOSAGES |
|---|---|---|
| **Ophthalmic vasoconstrictors** *(continued)* | | |
| **phenylephrine hydrochloride** Ak-Dilate, Ak-Nefrin, Isopto Frin, Mydfrin, Phenoptic, Relief Eye Drops for Red Eyes | To produce mydriasis without cycloplegia | 1 gtt of 2.5% or 10% solution before eye exam, then repeated in 1 hr p.r.n. |
| | To produce mydriasis and vasoconstriction | 1 gtt of 2.5% or 10% solution as single dose |
| | To treat chronic mydriasis | 1 gtt of 2.5% or 10% solution b.i.d. or t.i.d. |
| | To treat posterior adhesion of iris | 1 gtt of 2.5% or 10% solution as single dose |
| **proparacaine hydrochloride** Alcaine, Ophthaine, Ophthetic | To provide deep anesthesia during cataract extraction | 1 gtt q 5 to 10 min for 5 to 7 doses |
| | To provide anesthesia during removal of eye sutures | 1 or 2 gtt 2 to 3 min before procedure |
| | To provide anesthesia during removal of foreign bodies | 1 or 2 gtt in affected eye before surgery |
| | To provide anesthesia during tonometry | 1 or 2 gtt immediately before measurement |
| **tetracaine** Pontocaine | To provide eye anesthesia (short term) | 1 or 2 gtt p.r.n. |
| **tetrahydrozoline hydrochloride** Collyrium Fresh Eye Drops, Eyesine, Murine Plus, Optigene 3, Tetrasine, Visine Moisturizing, Visine Extra | To treat conjunctival congestion, irritation, and allergic conditions | 1 or 2 gtt of 0.05% solution up to q.i.d. or as directed |
| **Miscellaneous ophthalmic drugs** | | |
| **apraclonidine hydrochloride** Iopidine | To prevent or control elevated intraocular pressure (IOP) before and after ocular laser surgery | 1 gtt of 1% solution 1 hr before laser surgery on anterior segment; then 1 drop immediately after surgery |
| **azelastine hydrochloride 0.05%** Optivar | To treat itching of the eye associated with allergic conjunctivitis | 1 gtt in affected eye b.i.d. |
| **betaxolol hydrochloride** Betoptic, Betoptic S | To treat chronic open-angle glaucoma or ocular hypertension | 1 or 2 gtt of 0.5% solution or 0.25% suspension b.i.d. |

## Ophthalmic Drugs (continued)

Miscellaneous ophthalmic drugs (continued)

| GENERIC AND TRADE NAMES | INDICATIONS | USUAL ADULT DOSAGES |
|---|---|---|
| **bimatoprost 0.03%** <br> Lumigan | To reduce elevated IOP in patients with open-angle glaucoma or ocular hypertension who can't tolerate or have insufficiently responded to other IOP-lowering medications | 1 gtt in affected eye q.d. in evening |
| **brimonidine tartrate** <br> Alphagan, Alphagan P | To reduce IOP in open-angle glaucoma or ocular hypertension | 1 gtt in affected eye t.i.d., about 8 hr apart |
| **brinzolamide 1%** <br> Azopt | To reduce IOP in ocular hypertension or open-angle glaucoma | 1 gtt t.i.d. |
| **carteolol hydrochloride** <br> Ocupress | To treat chronic open-angle glaucoma or intraocular hypertension | 1 gtt in conjunctival sac of affected eye b.i.d. |
| **cyclosporine emulsion 0.05%** <br> Restasis | To increase tear production in keratoconjunctivitis sicca | 1 gtt q 12 hr |
| **dipivefrin hydrochloride** <br> Ophto-Dipivefrin (CAN), Propine | To reduce IOP in chronic open-angle glaucoma | 1 drop of 0.1% solution q 12 hr |
| **dorzolamide hydrochloride** <br> Trusopt | To treat increased IOP in ocular hypertension or open-angle glaucoma | 1 gtt in conjunctival sac of affected eye t.i.d. |
| **emedastine difumarate** <br> Emadine | To treat allergic conjunctivitis | 1 gtt in affected eye up to q.i.d. |
| **fluorescein sodium** <br> AK-Fluor, Fluorescite, Fluor-I-Strip, Fluor-I-Strip-A.T., Ful-Glo, Funduscein-10, Funduscein-25, Ophthifluor | To diagnose corneal abrasions and foreign bodies, fit hard contact lenses, determine lacrimal patency, and assist in fundus photography and applanation tonometry | 1 or 2 gtt of 2% solution followed by irrigation; or moisten strip with sterile water, then touch conjunctiva or fornix with moistened tip, and flush with irrigating solution; have patient blink several times after application |
| **ketotifen fumarate** <br> Zaditor | To treat allergic conjunctivitis | 1 gtt in affected eye b.i.d. q 8 to 12 hr |
| **latanoprost** <br> Xalatan | To reduce IOP in ocular hypertension or open-angle glaucoma | 1 gtt in conjunctival sac of affected eye q.d. in evening |

(continued)

## Ophthalmic Drugs (continued)

| GENERIC AND TRADE NAMES | INDICATIONS | USUAL ADULT DOSAGES |
|---|---|---|
| Miscellaneous ophthalmic drugs (continued) | | |
| **levobunolol hydrochloride** AKBeta, Betagan, Novo-Levobunolol (CAN) | To treat chronic open-angle glaucoma or ocular hypertension | 1 or 2 gtt of 0.5% solution q.d. or 0.25% solution b.i.d. |
| **levocabastine hydrochloride 0.05%** Livostin | To treat signs and symptoms of seasonal allergic conjunctivitis | 1 gtt q.i.d. |
| **metipranolol hydrochloride** OptiPranolol | To reduce IOP in ocular hypertension or chronic open-angle glaucoma | 1 gtt in affected eye b.i.d. |
| **nedocromil sodium 2%** Alocril | To treat itching associated with both seasonal and perennial allergic conjunctivitis | 1 or 2 gtt b.i.d. |
| **sodium chloride, hypertonic** Adsorbonac, AK-NaCl, Muro-128, Muroptic-5 | To provide temporary relief from corneal edema | 1 or 2 gtt q 3 to 4 hr; or 6 mm (1/4 in) of ointment applied q 3 to 4 hr |
| **timolol hemihydrate** Betimol **timolol maleate** Apo-Timop (CAN), Timoptic **timolol maleate extended-release solution** Timoptic-XE | To reduce IOP in ocular hypertension or open-angle glaucoma | 1 gtt of 0.25% or 0.5% solution in affected eye b.i.d., then 1 gtt q.d.; or 1 gtt extended-release solution in affected eye q.d. |
| **travoprost 0.004%** Travatan | To reduce elevated IOP in patients with open-angle glaucoma or ocular hypertension who can't tolerate or have insufficiently responded to other IOP-lowering medications | 1 gtt in affected eye q.d. in evening |
| **unoprostone isopropyl 0.15%** Rescula | To reduce elevated IOP in patients with open-angle glaucoma or ocular hypertension who can't tolerate or have insufficiently responded to other IOP-lowering medications | 1 gtt in affected eye b.i.d. |

## Antihistamines

Antihistamines are generally used to relieve immediate hypersensitivity reactions. They're also used as sedatives, antiemetics (especially in motion sickness), antitussives, antidyskinetics, and adjuncts to preoperative or postoperative analgesia.

Antihistamines are contraindicated in patients who are receiving drugs that prolong the QT interval (including some macrolide antibiotics, quinidine, itraconazole, ketoconazole, mibefradil, and zileuton). They're also contraindicated in patients who are hypersensitive to antihistamines or their components.

The chart below includes the trade names; usual dosages; and onset, peak, and duration for the antihistamines your patient is most likely to use daily or intermittently to control the symptoms of allergic rhinitis. When caring for a patient who takes an antihistamine, individualize your plan of care but be sure to include these general interventions:

•Use antihistamines cautiously in patients with a history of glaucoma, peptic ulcer, or urine retention because the drugs' anticholinergic effects may exaggerate these conditions.

•Before antihistamine therapy, assess the patient for hypokalemia and correct the imbalance, as prescribed, to reduce the risk of arrhythmias.

•Before antihistamine therapy, obtain a detailed medication history to help prevent drug interactions.

•Administer antihistamines with food if they cause GI distress.

•Instruct the patient to avoid alcohol and other CNS depressants during antihistamine use because the combination can cause additive CNS depression.

•Monitor blood pressure because the drugs' anticholinergic effects may cause hypertension.

| GENERIC AND TRADE NAMES | USUAL ADULT DOSAGE | ONSET, PEAK, AND DURATION |
|---|---|---|
| **acrivastine**<br>Semprex-D (also includes pseudoephedrine) | 8 mg P.O. q 4 to 6 hr | **Onset:** 30 min<br>**Peak:** Unknown<br>**Duration:** 6 to 8 hr |
| **azatadine**<br>Optimine<br>Trinalin Repetabs (also includes pseudoephedrine) | 1 to 2 mg P.O. q 8 to 12 hr<br>1 tablet P.O. q 12 hr | **Onset:** 15 to 60 min<br>**Peak:** 4 hr<br>**Duration:** 12 hr |
| **azelastine**<br>Astelin | 2 sprays (137 mcg/spray) in each nostril b.i.d. | **Onset:** In 3 hr<br>**Peak:** Unknown<br>**Duration:** 12 hr |
| **cetirizine**<br>Zyrtec<br>Zyrtec D (also includes pseudoephedrine) | 5 to 10 mg P.O. q.d.<br>5 mg/120 mg b.i.d. | **Onset:** 30 to 60 min<br>**Peak:** 1 hr<br>**Duration:** Up to 24 hr |
| **desloratadine**<br>Clarinex<br>Clarinex Reditabs | 5 mg P.O. q.d.<br>5 mg P.O. q.d. | **Onset:** Unknown<br>**Peak:** Unknown (Clarinex);<br>3 hr (Clarinex Reditabs)<br>**Duration:** Unknown |

*(continued)*

## Antihistamines (continued)

| GENERIC AND TRADE NAMES | USUAL ADULT DOSAGE | ONSET, PEAK, AND DURATION |
|---|---|---|
| **fexofenadine**<br>Allegra | 60 mg P.O. b.i.d. or 180 mg P.O. q.d. | **Onset:** 1 hr<br>**Peak:** 2 to 3 hr<br>**Duration:** 12 hr |
| Allegra-D (also includes pseudoephedrine) | 1 tablet P.O. q 12 hr | |
| **loratadine**<br>Claritin | 10 mg P.O. q.d. | **Onset:** 1 to 3 hr<br>**Peak:** 8 to 12 hr<br>**Duration:** At least 24 hr |
| Claritin-D12 (also includes pseudoephedrine) | 1 tablet P.O. q 12 hr | |
| Claritin-D24 (also includes pseudoephedrine) | 1 tablet P.O. q 24 hr | |

# Topical Drugs

Topical preparations consist of an active drug prepared in a specified medium that promotes absorption through the skin. Media are commonly chosen based on drug solubility; rate of drug release; ability to hydrate the outer skin layer; ability to enhance penetration; drug stability; and interactions between the chosen medium, skin, and active ingredient. Topical media include aerosols, creams, gels, lotions, powders, tinctures, and wet dressings. Aerosols, gels, lotions, and tinctures are convenient for applications to the scalp and hairy areas. Acutely inflamed areas are best treated with drying preparations, such as lotions, tinctures, and wet dressings. Chronic inflammations do well with applications of lubricating preparations, including creams and ointments.

Because of its physical properties, the skin can act as a holding area for many drugs, allowing for slow penetration and prolonged duration of action. However, when administering topical or transdermal drugs that aren't prescribed for a specific location, keep in mind that penetration properties may vary in different areas of the skin. For example, the scrotum, face, axillae, and scalp are more permeable than the extremities, and ventral surfaces are generally more permeable than dorsal surfaces.

Topical agents are classified as antibacterials, antifungals (the largest group), antivirals, corticosteroids, retinoids, and other miscellaneous preparations.

•*Antibacterials* may be useful in the early treatment of minor skin infections and wounds. Minor skin infections may respond well to topical drugs applied at the infection site. Minor wounds should be treated at the site and in the immediately surrounding area to prevent other pathogens from colonizing the area.

•*Antifungals* are usually used to treat mucocutaneous infections, such as tineas, primarily ringworm and athlete's foot. Systemic use of antifungals is limited by their potentially toxic adverse effects, most commonly renal damage. Most fungi are completely resistant to conventional antibacterial drugs.

•*Antivirals* are used to inhibit viral replication. They work by targeting any one of the steps involved in viral replication: penetration into susceptible host cells; uncoating of the virus nucleic acid; synthesis of regulatory proteins, RNA and DNA, and structural proteins; assembly of viral particles; and release of the virus from the cell. Topical antivirals such as pencyclovir can shorten the duration of lesions, lessen lesion pain, and minimize viral shedding.

•*Corticosteroids* reduce the signs and symptoms of inflammation. Topical corticosteroids cause vasoconstriction, probably by suppressing cell degranulation. They also cause decreased cell permeability by reducing histamine release from basal and mast cells.

•*Retinoids,* typically derivatives of vitamin A, are very effective in treating acne vulgaris. When applied to the skin, retinoids remain primarily in the dermis; less than 10% of the drug is absorbed into the circulation. Prolonged use of retinoids promotes new dermal growth, new blood vessel formation, and thickening of the epidermis.

•*Miscellaneous topical drugs* are used to treat a variety of topical skin conditions, including dry skin, ichthyosis, parasitic infestations, psoriasis, and unwanted hair growth.

Before you apply a topical preparation, clean the site and let it dry. Use gloves or a finger cot during application to prevent the drug from being absorbed through your own skin. Inform your patient of any expected discomfort, such as temporary stinging or burning. After application, cover the site only if required; some topical drugs shouldn't be covered with an occlusive dressing. Be sure to teach the patient and a family member correct administration technique. Also, review possible adverse reactions, highlighting those that should be reported to the prescriber. Stress the importance of compliance with the drug regimen because some topical drugs require weeks or months of therapy to eradicate the underlying condition.

The following chart includes the generic and trade names of many commonly prescribed topical drugs as well as their FDA-approved indications and usual adult dosage.

*(continued)*

## Topical Drugs (continued)

| GENERIC AND TRADE NAMES | INDICATIONS | USUAL ADULT DOSAGES |
|---|---|---|
| **Antibacterials** | | |
| **azelaic acid cream**<br>Azelex, Finacea, Finevin | To treat mild to moderate inflammatory acne vulgaris | Gently massage thin film into affected area b.i.d., morning and evening. |
| **bacitracin** | To treat topical infections, abrasions, cuts, and minor burns or wounds | Apply thin film to affected area q.d. to t.i.d. up to 3 wk. |
| **benzoyl peroxide**<br>Benzac AC Wash, Clearasil Maximum Strength, Desquam-E 2.5 Gel, Fostex 10 BPO Gel, Triaz | To treat mild to moderate inflammatory acne vulgaris | Apply to affected area q.d., gradually increasing to b.i.d. or t.i.d. |
| **clindamycin phosphate**<br>Cleocin, Cleocin T Gel, Cleocin T Lotion, Clinda-Derm, Dalacin, Dalacin T Topical Solution (CAN) | To treat inflammatory acne vulgaris<br><br>To treat bacterial vaginosis | Apply to affected area b.i.d., morning and evening.<br><br>Insert 1 applicatorful (100 mg) intravaginally q h.s. for 7 days. |
| **clindamycin 1% and benzoyl peroxide 5%**<br>Benzaclin gel<br>DUAC | To treat acne vulgaris | Apply q.d. or b.i.d. (morning and/or evening) to affected areas |
| **erythromycin**<br>Akne-Mycin, A/T/S, Erycette, EryDerm, Erygel, Erymax, Ery-Sol (CAN), Erythrogel, ETS (CAN), Sans-Acne (CAN), Staticin, T-Stat (CAN) | To treat inflammatory acne vulgaris | Apply to affected areas b.i.d., morning and evening. |
| **erythromycin 3% and benzoyl peroxide 5%**<br>Benzamycin | To treat moderate inflammatory acne | Apply to affected areas b.i.d., morning and evening. |
| **gentamicin sulfate**<br>Garamycin, G-myticin | To prevent or treat superficial skin infections due to susceptible bacteria; to treat superficial burns | Rub small amount gently into skin t.i.d. or q.i.d. |
| **mafenide gel 1%**<br>Sulfamylon | As adjunct to treat second- and third-degree burns | Apply 1/16-in layer aseptically to affected areas q.d. or b.i.d. |

## Topical Drugs *(continued)*

| GENERIC AND TRADE NAMES | INDICATIONS | USUAL ADULT DOSAGES |
|---|---|---|
| **Antibacterials** *(continued)* | | |
| **metronidazole** MetroCream, MetroGel, MetroGel-Vaginal | To treat inflammatory papules and pustules of acne rosacea | Apply thin film to affected area b.i.d., morning and evening. |
| | To treat bacterial vaginosis | Insert 1 applicatorful (37.5 mg) intravaginally q h.s. or b.i.d. for 5 days. |
| **mupirocin 2%** Bactroban, Bactroban Cream, Bactroban Nasal | To treat impetigo | Apply to affected areas t.i.d. for 1 to 2 wk. |
| | To treat secondary infections of traumatic skin lesions due to *Staphylococcus aureus* and *Streptococcus pyogenes* | Apply thin film and cover with an occlusive dressing t.i.d. for 10 days. |
| | To eradicate nasal colonization of methicillin-resistant S. aureus | Apply half of the contents of a unit-dose tube to each nostril b.i.d. for 5 days. |
| **neomycin sulfate** Myciguent | To prevent or treat superficial bacterial infections | Rub fingertip-size dose into affected area q.d. to t.i.d. |
| **nitrofurazone** Furacin | As adjunct to treat third-degree burns and to treat infection in skin grafts | Apply directly to lesions or on gauze; repeat p.r.n. |
| **povidone-iodine** Betadine, Betadine Cream, Betadine Spray | To disinfect wounds and burns | Apply or spray to affected area p.r.n. |
| **silver sulfadiazine** Flamazine (CAN), Silvadene, Thermazine | To prevent and treat bacterial and fungal infection in second- and third-degree burns | Apply 1/16-inch layer aseptically q.d. to b.i.d to clean, debrided burns; reapply promptly if removed. |
| **sulfacetamide sodium 10%** Klaron | To treat acne vulgaris | Apply thin film b.i.d. |
| **sulfacetamide sodium 10% and sulfur 5%** Sulfacet-R | To treat acne rosacea, acne vulgaris, and seborrheic dermatitis | Apply thin film, and massage into affected area q.d. to t.i.d. |
| **tetracycline hydrochloride** Achromycin, Topicycline | To treat acne vulgaris | Rub solution into affected area b.i.d. |
| | To prevent or treat superficial skin infections due to susceptible bacteria | Apply to affected area b.i.d. (morning and evening) or t.i.d. |

*(continued)*

## Topical Drugs (continued)

| GENERIC AND TRADE NAMES | INDICATIONS | USUAL ADULT DOSAGES |
|---|---|---|
| **Antifungals** | | |
| **amphotericin B**<br>Fungizone | To treat cutaneous or mucocutaneous candidal infections | Apply liberally and rub in gently b.i.d. to q.i.d. for 1 to 3 wk (interdigital lesions and paronychias), for 2 to 4 wk (perianal candidiasis or glabrous lesions), or for several months (onychomycoses). |
| **butenafine hydrochloride 1%**<br>Lotrimin Ultra, Mentax | To treat tinea corporis, tinea cruris, or tinea versicolor | Apply to affected and immediately surrounding area q.d. for 2 wk. |
| | To treat interdigital tinea pedis due to *Epidermophyton floccosum, Trychophyton mentagrophytes,* or *T. rubrum* | Apply to affected and immediately surrounding area q.d. for 4 wk or b.i.d. for 1 wk. |
| **butoconazole nitrate**<br>Femstat, Femstat One, Mycelex 3 | To treat vulvovaginal mycotic infections caused by *Candida* species | Insert 1 applicatorful (100 mg) intravaginally q h.s. for 3 days; may repeat course for total of 6 days. |
| Gynazole-1 | To treat vulvovaginal infections caused by *Candida albicans* | Insert 1 applicatorful (100 mg) intravaginally once anytime day or night. |
| **ciclopirox olamine 1%**<br>Loprox 0.77% | To treat candidiasis due to *Candida albicans;* tinea corporis, tinea cruris, and tinea pedis due to *E. floccosum, T. mentagrophytes, T. rubrum,* or *Microsporum canis;* tinea versicolor due to *Malassezia furfur;* onychomycosis due to *T. rubrum;* and seborrheic dermatitis | Massage gently into affected and surrounding area b.i.d., morning and evening. |
| **ciclopirox olamine 8%**<br>Penlac | To treat onychomycosis of the fingernails and toenails | Apply evenly to entire nail surface and surrounding 5 mm of skin q h.s. for up to 48 wk. |
| **clotrimazole**<br>Canesten (CAN), Gyne-Lotrimin, Gyne-Lotrimin 3, Lotrimin, Lotrimin Antifungal, Mycelex, Mycelex-7, Mycelex-G, Mycelex OTC, Trivagizole 3 | To treat superficial fungal infections (tinea corporis, tinea cruris, tinea pedis, tinea versicolor, candidiasis) | Apply thin film and massage into affected and surrounding area b.i.d., morning and evening, for 2 to 4 wk. |
| | To treat vulvovaginal candidiasis | Insert 100-mg vaginal tablet q h.s. for 7 days; or 500-mg vaginal tablet q h.s. for 1 day; or 1 applicatorful intravaginally q h.s. for 7 days (or 3 days if using Trivagizole 3). |

## Topical Drugs (continued)

| GENERIC AND TRADE NAMES | INDICATIONS | USUAL ADULT DOSAGES |
|---|---|---|
| **Antifungals** *(continued)* | | |
| **clotrimazole** *(continued)* | To treat oropharyngeal candidiasis | Dissolve oral troche over 15 to 30 min 5 times/day for 14 days. |
| | To prevent oropharyngeal candidiasis | Dissolve oral troche over 15 to 30 min t.i.d. for duration of chemotherapy or until corticosteroid dosage is reduced to maintenance levels. |
| **econazole nitrate** Ecostatin (CAN), Spectazole | To treat tinea corporis, tinea cruris, tinea pedis, tinea versicolor, cutaneous candidiasis | Rub into affected area q.d. or b.i.d for at least 2 wk. |
| | To treat cutaneous candidiasis | Rub into affected area b.i.d. for 2 wk. |
| **gentian violet** Genapax | To treat candidiasis | Insert 1 intravaginal tampon t.i.d. to q.i.d. for 12 days; or apply 1% or 2% solution to affected area q.d. to b.i.d. for 3 days. |
| **haloprogin** Halotex | To treat tinea corporis, tinea cruris, tinea manuum, and tinea pedis due to *E. floccosum, M. canis, T. mentagrophytes, T. rubrum,* or *T. tonsurans;* to treat tinea versicolor due to *M. furfur* | Apply liberally to affected area b.i.d. for 2 to 3 wk or, for intertriginous lesions, up to 4 wk. |
| **ketoconazole 2%** Nizoral | To treat tinea corporis, tinea cruris, and tinea versicolor due to susceptible organisms; to treat cutaneous candidiasis | Apply thin film to affected and immediately surrounding area and cover with an occlusive dressing q.d. for at least 2 wk. |
| | To treat tinea pedis | Apply to affected and immediately surrounding area q.d. for 6 wk; or apply shampoo to wet hair, lather, massage for 1 min, leave drug on scalp for 3 min, then rinse and repeat 2 times/wk for 4 weeks (with at least 3 days between shampoos), then intermittently p.r.n. |
| | To treat seborrheic dermatitis | Apply to affected and immediately surrounding area b.i.d. for 4 wk. |

*(continued)*

## Topical Drugs (continued)

| GENERIC AND TRADE NAMES | INDICATIONS | USUAL ADULT DOSAGES |
|---|---|---|
| **Antifungals** *(continued)* | | |
| **miconazole nitrate** Femizol-M, Fungoid, M-Zole 3, Micatin, Monistat-Derm, Monistat 3, Monistat 7, Ony-Clear Nail | To treat tinea corporis, tinea cruris, tinea pedis; cutaneous candidiasis; and common dermatophyte infections | Apply cream sparingly (or powder or spray liberally) over affected area. b.i.d. for 2 to 4 wk. |
| | To treat tinea versicolor | Apply sparingly to affected area q.d. for 2 wk. |
| | To treat vulvovaginal candidiasis | Insert 1 applicatorful (100 mg) or vaginal suppository (100 mg) h.s. for 7 days, and repeat p.r.n.; or insert vaginal suppository (200 mg) h.s. for 3 days. |
| | To treat onychomycosis | Brush tincture on affected areas of nail surface, beds, and edges and under nail surface b.i.d. for up to several mo; or spray on clean, dry, affected nails, holding actuator down for 1 or 2 sec. |
| **naftifine hydrochloride** Naftin | To treat tinea corporis, tinea cruris, and tinea pedis | Apply cream to affected area q.d.; or apply gel to affected area b.i.d., morning and evening. |
| **nystatin** Mycostatin, Nadostine (CAN), Nilstat | To treat cutaneous and mucocutaneous infections due to *C. albicans* | Apply cream to affected area b.i.d. or as indicated; or apply powder b.i.d. or t.i.d.; or insert 1 or 2 lozenges (200,000 to 400,000 units) 4 to 5 times/day for up to 48 hr after symptoms have subsided or 14 days; or insert 4 to 6 ml (400,000 to 600,000 units) of oral suspension in mouth q.i.d. (one-half of dose in each side of mouth) and retain as long as possible before swallowing. |
| | To treat vulvovaginal candidiasis | Insert 1 intravaginal tablet (100,000 units) or 1 applicatorful (100,000 to 500,000 units) q.d. or b.i.d. for 14 days. |
| **oxiconazole nitrate** Oxistat, Oxizold (CAN) | To treat tinea corporis, tinea cruris, and tinea pedis caused by *E. floccosum, T. mentagrophytes,* or *T. rubrum* | Apply to affected and surrounding area q.d. or b.i.d. for 2 wk (tinea corporis and tinea cruris) or for 4 wk (tinea pedis). |
| | To treat tinea versicolor caused by *M. furfur* | Apply cream to affected and surrounding area q.d. for 2 wk. |

## Topical Drugs (continued)

| GENERIC AND TRADE NAMES | INDICATIONS | USUAL ADULT DOSAGES |
|---|---|---|
| **Antifungals** *(continued)* | | |
| **selenium sulfide**<br>Selsun | To treat tinea versicolor | Apply to scalp, lather with small amount of water, wait 10 min, then rinse, q 7 days. |
| | To treat dandruff and seborrheic scalp dermatitis | Massage into wet scalp, wait 2 to 3 min, rinse, and repeat 2 times/wk for 2 wk, then p.r.n. |
| **sulconazole nitrate**<br>Exelderm | To treat tinea corporis, tinea cruris, and tinea pedis (cream only) caused by *E. floccosum, M. canis, T. mentagrophytes,* or *T. rubrum;* to treat tinea versicolor | Massage small amount gently into affected and surrounding areas q.d. or b.i.d. (tinea pedis) for up to 6 wk. |
| **terbinafine hydrochloride**<br>Lamisil DermGel,<br>Lamisil Solution | To treat tinea versicolor | Apply to affected area b.i.d. for 1 wk. |
| Lamisil AT Cream | To treat tinea corporis, tinea cruris, and tinea pedis | Apply thin film to affected area b.i.d. for 1 wk or 2 wk (plantar tinea pedis). |
| Lamisil AT Solution | To treat interdigital tinea pedis, tinea corporis, and tinea cruris | Apply between the toes b.i.d. for 1 wk (interdigital tinea pedis) or to affected area q.d. for 1 wk (tinea corporis and tinea cruris). |
| **terconazole**<br>Terazol 3, Terazol 7 | To treat vulvovaginal candidiasis | Insert 1 applicatorful (20 mg) intravaginally h.s. for 3 days (0.4%) or 1 applicatorful (40 mg) for 7 days (0.8%); or insert 80-mg vaginal suppository h.s. for 3 consecutive days. |
| **tioconazole**<br>GyneCure Ovules (CAN),<br>Vagistat-1 | To treat vulvovaginal candidiasis | Insert 1 applicatorful (300 mg) or 1 suppository (300 mg) intravaginally h.s. as a single dose. |

*(continued)*

## Topical Drugs (continued)

| GENERIC AND TRADE NAMES | INDICATIONS | USUAL ADULT DOSAGES |
|---|---|---|
| **Antifungals (continued)** | | |
| **tolnaftate** Absorbine Footcare, Aftate for Athlete's Foot, Aftate for Jock Itch, Dr. Scholl's Athlete's Foot, Genaspore, NP-27, Pitrex, Quinsana Plus, Tinactin, Ting, Zeasorb-AF | To treat tinea capitis, corporis, cruris, manuum, pedis, and versicolor | Apply 1% aerosol, cream, gel, powder, or solution to affected and surrounding areas b.i.d.; continue for 2 wk after symptoms subside or up to 6 wk. |
| **Antivirals** | | |
| **acyclovir** Zovirax | To treat mucocutaneous herpes simplex in immunocompromised patients | Apply cream to affected area using finger cot or rubber glove 4 to 6 times a day for 10 days. Apply ointment to affected area using finger cot or rubber glove q 3 hr (6 times/day) for 7 days. |
| **docosanol** Abreva | To treat recurrent oral-facial herpes simplex | Apply cream gently and completely to affected area 5 times daily, starting with first visible sign of lesion and continuing until lesion is healed. |
| **penciclovir** Denavir | To treat recurrent herpes labialis of lips and face | Apply q 2 hr while awake for 4 days. |
| **Corticosteroids** | | |
| **alclometasone dipropionate** Aclovate | To treat corticosteroid-responsive dermatoses | Apply thin film to affected area and massage b.i.d. to t.i.d. |
| **amcinonide** Cyclocort | To treat corticosteroid-responsive dermatoses | Apply thin film to affected area and massage b.i.d. (ointment, lotion) or b.i.d. to t.i.d. (cream). |
| **betamethasone benzoate** Beben (CAN), Uticort | To treat corticosteroid-responsive dermatoses | Apply thin film or a few drops to affected area q.d. to b.i.d. up to 45 g/wk (ointment, cream), 50 g/wk (gel), or 50 ml (lotion). |
| **betamethasone dipropionate** Diprolene, Diprolene AF, Diprosone, Topilene (CAN) | To treat corticosteroid-responsive dermatoses | Apply thin film or a few drops to affected area q.d. to b.i.d. up to 45 g/wk (ointment, cream), 50 g/wk (gel), or 50 ml (lotion). |

## Topical Drugs (continued)

| GENERIC AND TRADE NAMES | INDICATIONS | USUAL ADULT DOSAGES |
|---|---|---|
| **Corticosteroids** (continued) | | |
| **betamethasome valerate** Luxiq | To treat corticosteroid-responsive dermatoses | Apply foam to scalp, and massage until foam disappears, b.i.d. |
| **clobetasol propionate** Dermovate (CAN), Embeline, Temovate | To treat corticosteroid-responsive dermatoses | Apply thin film to affected area and rub in gently b.i.d. to t.i.d., up to 50 g/wk, for 2 wk. |
| Olux | To treat corticosteroid-responsive dermatoses of scalp | Apply to affected area of scalp b.i.d., once in morning and once at night, for 2 wk. |
| **desonide** Desowen, Tridesilon | To treat corticosteroid-responsive dermatoses | Apply thin film to affected area b.i.d. to q.i.d. |
| **diflorasone diacetate** Florone, Maxiflor, Psorcon | To treat corticosteroid-responsive dermatoses | Apply thin film to affected area q.d. to q.i.d. |
| **fluocinolone acetonide** Bio-Syn, Derma Smooth FS, Fluocet, Fluoderm (CAN), Fluolar (CAN), Fluonid (CAN), Fluonide (CAN), Flurosyn, Synalar, Synalar-HP, Synamol (CAN), Synemol | To treat corticosteroid-responsive dermatoses | Apply thin film to affected area b.i.d. to q.i.d. |
| **fluocinonide** Lidemol (CAN), Lidex | To treat corticosteroid-responsive dermatoses | Apply thin film to affected area b.i.d. to q.i.d. |
| **flurandrenolide** Cordran, Cordran Tape, Drenison (CAN) | To treat corticosteroid-responsive dermatoses | Apply thin film to affected area and massage b.i.d. to t.i.d.; or apply tape q 12 to 24 hr. |
| **fluticasone propionate** Cutivate | To treat atopic dermatitis and corticosteroid-responsive dermatoses | Apply thin film q.d. (atopic dermatitis) or b.i.d. (dermatoses). |
| **halcinonide** Halog | To treat corticosteroid-responsive dermatoses | Apply sparingly and massage q.d. to t.i.d. |
| **halobetasol propionate** Ultravate | To treat corticosteroid-responsive dermatoses | Apply thin film to affected area and rub in gently q.d. to b.i.d., up to 50 g/wk, for 2 wk. |

(continued)

## Topical Drugs (continued)

| GENERIC AND TRADE NAMES | INDICATIONS | USUAL ADULT DOSAGES |
|---|---|---|
| **Corticosteroids** *(continued)* | | |
| **hydrocortisone 0.25%** Cetacort, Cort-Dome **hydrocortisone 0.5%** Bactine, Cetacort, Cortate (CAN), Cort-Dome, Cortifair, Delacort, DermiCort, Dermtex HC, Emo-Cort (CAN), Hydro-Tex, Hytone, MyCort, Sential (CAN), S-T Cort **hydrocortisone 1%** Ala-Cort, Allercort, Alphaderm, Acticort 100, Barriere-HC (CAN), Beta-HC, Cetacort, Cort-Dome, Cortifair, Cortril, Dermacort, Emo-Cort (CAN), Gly-Cort, Hi-Cor 1.0, Hydro-Tex, Hytone, LactiCare-HC, Lemoderm, Nutracort, Penecort, Prevex-HC (CAN), Rederm, Sarna HC (CAN), Synacort, Unicort (CAN) **hydrocortisone 2%** Ala-Scalp HP **hydrocortisone 2.5%** Allercort, Anusol-HC, Emo-Cort (CAN), Hi-Cor 2.5, Hytone, LactiCare-HC, Lemoderm, Nutracort, Penecort, Synacort **hydrocortisone acetate 0.1%** Corticreme (CAN) **hydrocortisone acetate 0.5%** 9-1-1, Corticaine, Cortacet (CAN), Cortaid, Cortoderm (CAN), FoilleCort, Gynecort, Hyderm (CAN), Lanacort, Novohydrocort (CAN), Pharma-Cort | To treat corticosteroid-responsive dermatoses | Apply thin film (aerosol foam, cream, lotion, ointment, solution) to affected area q.d. to q.i.d. |

## Topical Drugs *(continued)*

| GENERIC AND TRADE NAMES | INDICATIONS | USUAL ADULT DOSAGES |
|---|---|---|
| **Corticosteroids** *(continued)* | | |
| **hydrocortisone acetate 1%, 2%, 2.5%** Cortaid, Cortef Feminine Itch, Corticreme (CAN), Cortoderm (CAN), Hyderm (CAN), Maximum Strength Cortaid, Micort HC-Lipocream, Novohydrocort (CAN) **hydrocortisone acetate topical aerosol foam** Epifoam | To treat corticosteroid-responsive dermatoses | Apply thin film (aerosol foam, cream, lotion, ointment, solution) to affected area q.d. to q.i.d. |
| **hydrocortisone acetate dental paste** Orabase-HCA | To treat inflamed oral mucosa | Apply to oral mucosa b.i.d. to t.i.d. after meals and h.s. |
| **hydrocortisone butyrate** Locoid **hydrocortisone valerate** Westcort | To treat corticosteroid-responsive dermatoses | Apply to affected area b.i.d. to t.i.d. |
| **hydrocortisone acetate, polymyxin B sulfate, and neomycin sulfate** Cortisporin | To treat corticosteroid-responsive dermatoses (short term) | Apply sparingly and massage b.i.d. to q.i.d. |
| **hydrocortisone and iodoquinol** Vytone | To treat corticosteroid-responsive dermatoses with mild bacterial or fungal infection (short term) | Apply to affected area q.d. to t.i.d. |
| **mometasone furoate** Elocom (CAN), Elocon | To treat corticosteroid-responsive dermatoses | Apply thin film or a few drops to affected area q.d. |
| **prednicarbate** Dermatop | To treat corticosteroid-responsive dermatoses | Apply thin film to affected area b.i.d. |
| **triamcinolone acetonide 0.025%, 0.5%** Aristocort, Aristocort A, Aristocort D (CAN), Flutex, Kenac, Kenalog, Kenonel, Triacet, Triaderm (CAN), Trianide Mild (CAN) | To treat corticosteroid-responsive dermatoses | Apply thin film (cream) to affected area b.i.d. to q.i.d.; 0.025% lotion or ointment q.d. or b.i.d; 0.1% lotion or ointment q.d.; or 0.5% ointment q.d. |

*(continued)*

## Topical Drugs (continued)

| GENERIC AND TRADE NAMES | INDICATIONS | USUAL ADULT DOSAGES |
|---|---|---|
| **Corticosteroids** *(continued)* | | |
| **triamcinolone acetonide 0.1%** Aristocort, Aristocort A, Aristocort R (CAN), Delta-Tritex, Flutex, Kenac, Kenalog, Kenalog-H, Kenonel, Triacet, Triaderm (CAN), Trianide Regular (CAN) **triamcinolone acetonide 0.5%** Aristocort, Aristocort A, Aristocort C (CAN), Flutex, Kenalog, Kenonel, Triacet | To treat corticosteroid-responsive dermatoses | Apply thin film (cream) to affected area b.i.d. to q.i.d.; 0.025% lotion or ointment q.d. or b.i.d; 0.1% lotion or ointment q.d.; or 0.5% ointment q.d. |
| **triamcinolone acetonide dental paste** Kenalog in Orabase, Oracort, Oralone | To treat inflammatory or ulcerative oral lesions | Apply to oral mucosa b.i.d. to t.i.d. after meals and h.s. |
| **triamcinolone acetonide topical aerosol** Kenalog | To treat corticosteroid-responsive dermatoses | Spray affected area t.i.d. to q.i.d. |
| **Retinoids** | | |
| **adapalene** Differin | To treat acne vulgaris | Apply to affected area q h.s. |
| **tazarotene 0.05%, 0.1%** Avage, Tazorac | To treat plaque psoriasis | Apply thin film to affected area q h.s. |
| **tazarotene 0.1%** Avage, Tazorac | To treat facial acne vulgaris or plaque psoriasis | Apply thin film to affected area q h.s. |
| **tretinoin** Avita, Renova, Retin-A, Retin-A Micro, Stieva-A (CAN) | To treat acne vulgaris | Apply sparingly to clean, dry affected area q h.s. |

## Topical Drugs (continued)

| GENERIC AND TRADE NAMES | INDICATIONS | USUAL ADULT DOSAGES |
|---|---|---|
| *Miscellaneous topical drugs* | | |
| **ammonium lactate, 12%** Lac-Hydrin | To treat dry skin and ichthyosis | Apply to affected area, and rub in b.i.d. |
| **anthralin** Anthranol 1 (CAN), Drithocreme, Dritho-Scalp | To treat chronic psoriasis<br><br>To treat chronic scalp psoriasis | Apply sparingly and massage into affected lesions q.d.<br><br>Apply only to lesions q.d. for 1 wk. |
| **becaplermin** Regranex | To treat lower-extremity diabetic neuropathic ulcers that extend into the subcutaneous tissue or beyond and that have an adequate blood supply | Apply to ulcers q.d. |
| **calcipotriene** Dovonex | To treat plaque psoriasis | Apply cream or scalp lotion in a thin layer b.i.d. up to 8 weeks. Apply thin layer of ointment q.d. or b.i.d. up to 8 weeks. |
| **capsaicin** Zostrix Capsin Capzacin-P | To provide temporary pain relief from rheumatoid arthritis and osteoarthritis; to relieve neuralgias from pain following shingles (herpes zoster) infection | Apply to affected area no more than q.i.d. |
| **chlorhexidine** Hibiclens | To clean skin wounds | Rinse area, apply minimal amount to cover, then wash and rinse thoroughly. |
| **chloroxine** Capitrol | To treat dandruff and seborrheic dermatitis | Massage into wet scalp, wait 3 min, rinse, and repeat 2 times/wk. |
| **clotrimazole and betamethasone dipropionate 0.05%, 1%** Lotrisone | To treat symptomatic inflammatory tinea corporis, tinea cruris, and tinea pedis | Massage cream gently into affected and surrounding skin areas b.i.d. for 2 wk (tinea corporis, tinea cruris) or for 4 wk (tinea pedis). |
| **coal tar** Zetar, Zetar Shampoo | To treat psoriasis<br><br>To treat dandruff or scalp seborrhea | Add 15 to 20 ml to lukewarm bath, immerse affected area for 15 to 20 min, and rinse thoroughly 3 to 7 times/wk.<br><br>Massage into wet scalp, rinse, repeat application and wait 5 min, then rinse again. |

*(continued)*

## Topical Drugs (continued)

| GENERIC AND TRADE NAMES | INDICATIONS | USUAL ADULT DOSAGES |
|---|---|---|
| **Miscellaneous topical drugs** *(continued)* | | |
| **crotamiton 10%** Eurax | To treat scabies | Massage into cleansed body from chin to soles of feet, and reapply after 24 hr; change bed linens next day, and bathe 48 hr after second dose; repeat in 7 to 10 days if new lesions appear. |
| **desoximetasone** Topicort | To relieve inflammatory and pruritic manifestations of corticosteroid-responsive dermatoses, including psoriasis, atopic dermatitis, and eczema. | Apply thin film b.i.d. to affected areas; occlusive dressings may be added for severe dermatoses. |
| **diclofenac sodium 3%** Solaraze | To treat actinic keratoses | Massage gel gently onto affected lesion areas b.i.d. for 60 to 90 days. |
| **doxepin hydrochloride** Zonalon | To treat pruritus associated with dermatitis and chronic lichen simplex | Apply thin film to affected area q.i.d. (q 3 to 4 hr) for up to 8 days. |
| **eflornithine** Vaniqa | To retard unwanted hair growth | Apply thin film to affected area of face and chin b.i.d. (at least 8 hr apart); don't wash treated area for at least 4 hr. |
| **fluocinolone acetonide 0.01%, hydroquinone 4%, tretinoin 0.05%** TRI-LUMA Cream | To treat severe facial melasma | Apply a thin film rubbing lightly and uniformly into the hyperpigmented areas of melasma including about 1/2 in of skin surrounding each lesion q.d. at least 30 minutes before bedtime. |
| **fluorouracil cream** Carac, Efudex, Fluoroplex | To treat actinic and solar keratoses | Apply to lesions b.i.d. for 2–6 weeks. |
| **hexachlorophene** pHisoHex | To treat skin preoperatively | Rinse area, apply minimal amount to cover, then wash and rinse thoroughly. |
| **hydrocortisone acetate, polymyxin B sulfate, and neomycin sulfate** Cortisporin | To treat dermatoses associated with secondary bacterial infection | Apply small amount to affected areas b.i.d. to q.i.d. |

## Topical Drugs (continued)

| GENERIC AND TRADE NAMES | INDICATIONS | USUAL ADULT DOSAGES |
|---|---|---|
| **Miscellaneous topical drugs** *(continued)* | | |
| **hydroquinone** Alustra, Claripel, Eldopaque, Eldoquin, Glyquin, Melanex | To treat hyperpigmentation and melanin | Apply b.i.d. to the affected areas for no longer than 2 months |
| **imiquimod 5%** Aldara | To treat external genital and perianal warts | Apply thin layer to affected area and rub in 3 times/wk h.s. for up to 16 wk; remove with soap and water after 6 to 10 hr. |
| **lidocaine and prilocaine** EMLA | For local anesthesia | Apply 1 disk or thick layer of 2.5-g cream occlusively for at least 1 hr. |
| **malathion lotion 0.5%** Ovide | To treat pediculus humanus capitis | Apply to dry hair in amount just sufficient to thoroughly wet the hair and scalp; then allow hair to dry naturally. After 8 to 12 hr, shampoo and rinse hair to remove dead lice and eggs. If lice are still present after 7–9 days, repeat application. |
| **mequinol 2%, retinol 0.01%** Solage | To treat solar lentigines | Apply solution b.i.d. morning and evening at least 8 hours apart. Avoid application to surrounding skin, and do not bathe for 6 hr after application. |
| **minoxidil** Rogaine 2% and 5% | To treat alopecia and androgenetica | Apply 1 ml to affected areas b.i.d. |
| **monobenzone 20%** Benoquin | To treat final depigmentation in extensive vitiligo | Apply b.i.d. to t.i.d. for 1–4 months, then b.i.d. weekly for maintenance |
| **permethrin 1%** Nix | To prevent or treat head lice | Wash and dry hair, saturate scalp with 1% cream, leave on hair for 10 min, then rinse; remove nits with provided comb; repeat in 7 days if living mites are still present. |

*(continued)*

## Topical Drugs (continued)

| GENERIC AND TRADE NAMES | INDICATIONS | USUAL ADULT DOSAGES |
|---|---|---|
| **Miscellaneous topical drugs** (continued) | | |
| **permethrin 5%** Acticin, Elimite | To treat scabies | Massage 5% cream into skin from head to soles of feet, and remove after 8 to 10 hr; repeat in 14 days if living mites are still present. |
| **pimecrolimus 1%** Elidel | To treat mild-to-moderate atopic dermatitis | Apply to affected areas b.i.d. |
| **podofilox** Condylox | To treat anogenital warts (gel); to treat external genital warts (gel or solution) | Apply 0.5% gel to anogenital warts for 3 days, then withhold for 4 days; repeat cycle up to 4 times. Apply 0.5% solution or gel to external genital warts q 12 hr in the morning and evening for 3 days, then withhold for 4 days; repeat cycle up to 4 times |
| **pyrethrum extract and piperonyl butoxide** RID, End Lice, Tegrin-LT | To treat head, pubic, and body lice | Apply to dry hair or affected body area. Massage through all hairy areas until hair is wet. Leave on hair for 10 min; then wash with warm water and soap or shampoo. Repeat in 7 to 10 days. |
| **tacrolimus** Protopic | To treat moderate to severe atopic dermatitis in patients unresponsive to other therapies | Apply thin layer to affected areas b.i.d., rubbing in gently and completely. Continue for 1 wk after signs and symptoms have disappeared. |

# Selected Antivirals

Antivirals are used for viral infections, such as influenza, human immunodeficiency virus (HIV), herpes simplex virus (HSV) I and II, herpes zoster, and cytomegalovirus (CMV) infections.

The following chart lists the generic and trade names, indications, and usual adult dosages for some commonly used antivirals. Although you must individualize your care for a patient who receives an antiviral, be sure to include these general interventions in your plan of care:

•Administer antivirals to patient on an empty stomach, if prescribed, to enhance absorption.

•Avoid administering HIV drugs all at once.

•If patient takes an antacid, administer it 1 hour before or 2 hours after an antiviral because antacids may reduce antiviral absorption.

•Monitor hepatic enzyme levels to detect elevations and help prevent hepatotoxicity.

•Monitor BUN and serum creatinine levels to detect signs of impaired renal function.

•Monitor I.V. injection site for pain or phlebitis, which may result from the high pH of reconstituted solutions.

•Assess immunosuppressed patient for opportunistic infections during antiviral therapy.

•Inform female patient that oral contraceptives may be ineffective when taken with HIV drugs. Suggest alternate contraceptive methods.

| GENERIC AND TRADE NAMES | INDICATIONS | USUAL ADULT DOSAGES |
| --- | --- | --- |
| **Antivirals used for HIV infection** | | |
| **abacavir sulfate** Ziagen | To treat HIV infection | 300 mg P.O. b.i.d. or 600 mg P.O. q.d. |
| **abacavir sulfate and lamivudine** Epzicom | To treat HIV-1 infection | 600 mg abacavir and 300 mg lamivudine (1 tablet) P.O. q.d. |
| **abacavir sulfate, lamivudine, and zidovudine** Trizivir | To treat HIV infection | 300 mg abacavir, 150 mg lamivudine, and 300 mg zidovudine (1 tablet) b.i.d. |
| **amprenavir** Agenerase | To treat HIV infection | 1,200 mg P.O. b.i.d. |
| **atazanavir sulfate** Reyataz | To treat HIV infection in patients not previously treated | 400 mg P.O. q.d. |
| | To treat HIV infection in patients previously treated | 300 mg P.O. q.d. with ritonavir 100 mg P.O. q.d. |
| **delavirdine** Rescriptor | To treat HIV infection | 400 mg P.O. t.i.d. |
| **didanosine** Videx, Videx EC | To treat HIV infection in patients who haven't had success with zidovudine and who weigh 60 kg (132 lb) or more | 200 mg P.O. q 12 hr or 250 mg buffered powder P.O. q 12 hr (Videx); or 400 mg P.O. q.d. (Videx EC). |
| | To treat HIV infection in patients who haven't had success with zidovudine and who weigh less than 60 kg | 125 mg P.O. q 12 hr or 167 mg buffered powder P.O. q 12 hr (Videx); or 250 mg P.O. q.d. (Videx EC). |

*(continued)*

## Selected Antivirals (continued)

| GENERIC AND TRADE NAMES | INDICATIONS | USUAL ADULT DOSAGES |
|---|---|---|
| **Antivirals used for HIV infection** (continued) | | |
| **efavirenz** Sustiva | To treat HIV infection | 600 mg P.O. q.d. |
| **emtricitabine** Emtriva | To treat HIV infection | 200 mg q.d. (capsules) or 240 mg q.d. (oral solution) |
| **enfuvirtide** Fuzeon | To treat HIV infection | 90 mg b.i.d. S.C. |
| **fosamprenavir calcium** Lexiva | To treat HIV infection in patients who don't take ritonavir | 1,400 mg b.i.d. |
| | To treat HIV infection in patients who take ritonavir but don't take a protease inhibitor | 1,400 mg q.d. or 700 mg b.i.d. |
| | To treat HIV infection in patients who take ritonavir and a protease inhibitor | 700 mg b.i.d. |
| **indinavir** Crixivan | To treat HIV infection | 800 mg P.O. q 8 hr. |
| **lamivudine** (3TC, lamivudine triphosphate) Epivir | To treat HIV infection in patients who weigh 50 kg (110 lb) or more | 150 mg P.O. b.i.d. or 300 mg q.d. |
| | To treat HIV infection in patients who weigh less than 50 kg | 2 mg/kg P.O. b.i.d. |
| **lamivudine and zidovudine** (3TC/AZT, 3TC/ZDV) Combivir | To treat HIV infection in patients who weigh 50 kg or more | 150 mg of lamivudine and 300 mg of zidovudine P.O. b.i.d. |
| **lopinavir and ritonavir** Kaletra | To treat HIV infection in patients who weigh more than 40 kg (88 lb) and don't take nevirapine or efavirenz | 400 mg lopinavir and 100 mg ritonavir (2 tablets, 3 capsules, or 5 ml) b.i.d. |
| | As adjunct to treat HIV infection in patients who weigh more than 50 kg and take nevirapine or efavirenz | 533 mg lopinavir and 133 mg ritonavir (4 capsules or 6.5 ml) b.i.d. |
| | To treat HIV infection in patients with no previous treatment | 800 mg lopinavir and 200 mg ritonavir (4 tablets, 6 capsules, or 10 ml) q.d. |
| **nelfinavir** Viracept | To treat HIV infection | 750 mg P.O. t.i.d. |
| **nelfinavir mesylate** Viracept | To treat HIV infection | 1,250 mg b.i.d. or 750 mg t.i.d. |

## Selected Antivirals (continued)

| GENERIC AND TRADE NAMES | INDICATIONS | USUAL ADULT DOSAGES |
|---|---|---|
| **Antivirals used for HIV infection** (continued) | | |
| **nevirapine** Viramune | To treat HIV infection | 200 mg P.O. q.d. for 14 days. |
| **ritonavir** Norvir | To treat HIV infection | 600 mg P.O. b.i.d. |
| **saquinavir** Fortovase, Invirase | To treat HIV infection | 1,200 mg P.O. t.i.d. (Fortovase) or 1,000 mg (Invirase or Fortovase) and 100 mg ritonavir b.i.d. |
| **stavudine** Zerit, Zerit XR | To treat HIV infection in patients who weigh 60 kg or more | 40 mg P.O. q 12 hr (Zerit) or 100 mg P.O. q.d. (Zerit XR). |
| | To treat HIV infection in patients who weigh less than 60 kg | 30 mg P.O. q 12 hr (Zerit) or 75 mg P.O. q.d. (Zerit XR). |
| **tenofovir** Viread | To treat HIV infection | 300 mg P.O. q.d. |
| **tenofovir and emtricitabine** Truvada | To treat HIV-1 infection | 300 mg tenofovir and 200 mg emtricitabine (1 tablet) P.O. q.d. |
| **tipranavir** Aptivus | To treat HIV infection | 500 mg tipranavir and 200 mg ritonavir P.O. b.i.d. |
| **zalcitabine** HIVID | To treat HIV infection | 0.75 mg P.O. q 8 hr. |
| **zidovudine** (AZT, ZDV) Apo-Zidovudine (CAN), Novo-AZT (CAN), Retrovir | To treat HIV infection | 100 mg P.O. q 4 hr while awake, up to 600 mg/day; or 1 to 2 mg/kg I.V. over 1 hr q 4 hr, up to 6 times/day or 6 mg/kg/day. |
| **Antivirals used for herpes virus infection** | | |
| **acyclovir** Zovirax | To treat HSV encephalitis | 10 mg/kg I.V. over 1 hr q 8 hr for 10 days. |
| | To treat HSV genitalis | 200 mg P.O. q 4 hr while awake, up to 5 times/day, for 10 days. |
| | To treat herpes zoster infection | 800 mg P.O. q 4 hr while awake, up to 5 times/day, for 7 to 10 days; or 10 mg/kg I.V. over 1 hr q 8 hr for 7 days. |

*(continued)*

## Selected Antivirals (continued)

| GENERIC AND TRADE NAMES | INDICATIONS | USUAL ADULT DOSAGES |
|---|---|---|
| **Antivirals used for herpes virus infection** (continued) | | |
| **famciclovir** Famvir | To treat HSV genitalis | 125 mg P.O. b.i.d. for 5 days. |
| | To treat herpes zoster infection | 500 mg P.O. q 8 hr for 7 days. |
| **foscarnet** Foscavir | To treat acyclovir-resistant HSV I and II infections | 90 mg/kg I.V. q 12 hr, or 60 mg/kg q 8 hr for 2 to 3 wk. |
| **idoxuridine** Herplex Liquifilm, Stoxil | To treat HSV keratitis | 1 cm applied to conjunctiva q 4 hr while awake, up to 5 times/day; or 1 gtt of 0.1% solution q hr during daytime and q 2 hr during nighttime for 7 to 10 days. |
| **penciclovir** Denavir | To treat HSV labialis | 1% cream applied to lips q 2 hr while awake for 4 days. |
| **valacyclovir** Valtrex | To treat HSV genitalis | 1 g P.O. b.i.d. for 10 days for initial episode; 500 mg P.O. b.i.d. for 3 days for recurrent episodes. |
| | To suppress recurrent HSV genitalis | 1 g P.O. q.d.; alternatively, 500 mg P.O. q.d. for patients with a history of nine or fewer recurrences/year or who have HIV. |
| | To reduce transmisison of genital herpes | 500 mg q.d. for source partner with a history of nine or fewer recurrences/year |
| | To treat herpes zoster infection | 1 g P.O. t.i.d. for 7 days. |
| | To treat herpes labialis (cold sores) | 2 g P.O. b.i.d. for 1 day taken 12 hr apart. |
| **vidarabine** Vira-A | To treat acute viral conjunctivitis and recurrent epithelial keratitis caused by HSV infection | 1.25 cm applied to conjunctiva q 3 hr until re-epithelialized, then 1.25 cm b.i.d. for 7 days. |

## Selected Antivirals (continued)

| GENERIC AND TRADE NAMES | INDICATIONS | USUAL ADULT DOSAGES |
|---|---|---|
| **Antivirals used for CMV infections** | | |
| **cidofovir** Vistide | To treat CMV retinitis | 5 mg/kg I.V. over 1 hr q wk for 2 wk. |
| **foscarnet** Foscavir | To treat CMV infection | 90 mg/kg I.V. q 12 hr, or 60 mg/kg q 8 hr for 2 to 3 wk. |
| **ganciclovir** Cytovene | To treat CMV infection | 5 mg/kg I.V. over 1 hr q 12 hr for 14 to 21 days. *Maintenance:* 1,000 mg P.O. t.i.d. |
| **valganciclovir hydrochloride** Valcyte | To treat CMV retinitis | 900 mg P.O. b.i.d. for 21 days. *Maintenance:* 900 mg P.O. q.d. |
| | To prevent CMV infection in high-risk kidney, heart, and kidney-pancreas transplant patients | 900 mg P.O. q.d., starting within 10 days of transplantation and continuing until 100 days after transplantation |
| **Antivirals used for influenza infections** | | |
| **oseltamivir phosphate** Tamiflu | To treat uncomplicated, acute infections caused by influenza virus A or B in adults who have had symptoms for no more than 2 days | 75 mg P.O. b.i.d. for 5 days, starting within 2 days after symptoms begin. *Maximum:* 75 mg b.i.d. for 5 days. |
| | To prevent influenza following close contact with infected individual | 75 mg P.O. q.d. for 7 days, starting within 2 days of exposure |
| | To prevent influenza during a community outbreak | 75 mg P.O. q.d. during period of potential exposure |
| **rimantadine** Flumadine | To prevent respiratory infections caused by influenza virus A | 100 mg P.O. b.i.d. |
| | To treat respiratory infections caused by influenza virus A | 100 mg P.O. b.i.d. for 5 to 7 days from onset of symptoms. |
| **zanamivir** Relenza | To treat infections caused by influenza virus A or B | 2 inhalations (10 mg) q 12 hr for 5 days. |

*(continued)*

## Selected Antivirals (continued)

| GENERIC AND TRADE NAMES | INDICATIONS | USUAL ADULT DOSAGES |
|---|---|---|
| **Antivirals used for hepatitis B infection** | | |
| **adefovir dipivoxil** <br> Hepsera | To treat chronic hepatitis B | 10 mg P.O. q.d. For patients with creatinine clearance of 20 to 49 ml/min, dosage interval changed to q 48 hr; for 10 to 19 ml/min, dosage interval changed to q 72 hr; for patients receiving hemodialysis, drug given q 7 days following dialysis. |
| **Antivirals used for hepatitis C infection** | | |
| **ribavirin** <br> Copegus, <br> Rebetol, <br> Ribasphere | To treat chronic hepatitis C in combination with interferon alfa-2b in patients who weigh more than 75 kg (165 lb) | 400 mg in the morning and 600 mg in the evening daily |
| | To treat chronic hepatitis C in combination with interferon alfa-2b in patients who weigh 75 kg (165 lb) or less | 600 mg b.i.d. |
| | To treat chronic hepatitis C in combination with peginterferon alfa-2b | 400 mg b.i.d. |
| | To treat chronic hepatitis C in combination with interferon alfa-2a in patients with compensated liver disease who have never received interferon alfa | 400 to 600 mg b.i.d. |

# Antineoplastic Drugs

Antineoplastic drugs have become the standard of treatment for most types of cancer today. Most of these drugs work by inhibiting cell proliferation, thereby leading to cell death. They're most effective at killing cells that are actively dividing. Cell-specific antineoplastics exert their actions during one or more phases of the cell cycle. S-phase antineoplastics interfere with deoxyribonucleic acid (DNA) synthesis; M-phase drugs interfere with the formation of microtubules and disrupt mitosis. Most antineoplastics impair DNA in one of the following four ways:
•preventing separation of DNA strands
•inhibiting DNA repair
•mimicking DNA bases
•disrupting the triplicate codons or producing oxygen free radicals that damage the DNA.

Antineoplastic drugs are cytotoxic, which means that they affect both neoplastic cells and normal cells. As a result, they may cause serious and sometimes life-threatening adverse reactions. Antineoplastics are most harmful to normal cells that exhibit rapid activity and growth, such as bone marrow tissue, the epithelium of the GI mucosa, and hair follicles. When they suppress bone marrow activity, the patient may develop leukopenia, thrombocytopenia, or anemia. When the drugs affect the GI mucosa, the patient may experience nausea, vomiting, anorexia, bowel dysfunction, and mucosal ulcerations. When they affect the hair follicles, the result is hair loss (alopecia), one of the most common adverse reactions; although not life-threatening, hair loss can be emotionally traumatic for patients, especially women.

## Drug Classification
Antineoplastics are classified according to their mechanism of action.
•*Alkylating drugs,* the first drugs developed to fight cancer, are most effective against slow-growing tumors. These agents can damage tissue at the injection site and produce systemic toxicity. They can damage cells during all stages of growth, causing mitotic arrest. Because their actions are not limited to neoplastic cells, they also cause myelosuppression, a predictable adverse reaction. They can also result in secondary tumor development, even years after the initial therapy.
•*Antibiotic antineoplastics* originated from a genus of fungus-like bacteria called *Streptomyces*. Their classification is based on their origin, not on mechanism of action, toxicity, pharmacokinetics, or varying clinical indications. Many of these drugs bind to specific bases and block DNA synthesis to interfere with cell replication.
•*Antimetabolites* are cell-cycle-specific drugs that act by preventing synthesis of nucleotides or inhibiting enzymes by mimicking nucleotides. These drugs are often more effective when used in combination.
•*Antimitotic antineoplastics* disrupt the formation of microtubule structures within the cell during mitosis. This breakdown of microtubule production stops the formation of the mitotic spindle, inhibiting cellular reproduction.
•*Biological response modifiers* alter tumor-host metabolic and immunologic relationships.
•*Antineoplastic enzymes* interfere with the breakdown of extracellular asparagine, an endogenous enzyme that leukemic cells depend on for their survival. The rapid depletion of asparagine eventually kills leukemic cells by fragmenting them into membrane-bound particles that are eliminated by phagocytosis.
•*Hormonal antineoplastics* act as agonists to inhibit tumor cell growth or as antagonists to compete with endogenous growth-promoting hormones. Steroid hormones form specific receptor complexes that bind to certain nuclear proteins necessary for DNA transcription.
•*Miscellaneous antineoplastics* act in a variety of ways, such as by destroying microtubules that are essential for tumor cell structure before mitosis and by inhibiting topoisomerase, the enzyme that affects the degree of supercoiling in DNA by cutting one or both strands. This inhibition causes DNA strands to break and synthesizes toxic compounds that inhibit DNA strand repair.

The following chart lists the generic and common trade names of common antineoplastic drugs, which are grouped according to mechanism of action. It also includes FDA-approved indications and the usual adult dosage for each drug.

## Antineoplastic Drugs (continued)

| GENERIC AND TRADE NAMES | INDICATIONS | USUAL ADULT DOSAGES |
|---|---|---|
| **Alkylating drugs** | | |
| **busulfan** Busulfex, Myleran | To provide palliative treatment of chronic myelocytic leukemia (CML) | *Initial:* 0.06 mg/kg P.O. q.d. until WBC count falls below 15,000/mm$^3$. *Usual:* 4 to 8 mg P.O. q.d. (but may range from 1 to 12 mg P.O. q.d.) *Maintenance:* 1 to 3 mg q.d. During remission, treatment resumed when WBC count reaches 50,000/mm$^3$ |
| | To prepare for hematopoietic progenitor cell transplantation for CML | 0.8 mg/kg I.V. over 2 hr q 6 hr for 4 days for a total of 16 doses as an adjunct with cyclophosphamide |
| **carmustine (BCNU)** BiCNU, Gliadel Wafer | To treat primary brain tumors and glioblastoma multiforme | Up to 8 implants per surgical procedure |
| | To treat primary brain tumors, Hodgkin's disease, non-Hodgkin's lymphoma, and multiple myeloma | 150 to 200 mg/m$^2$ by slow I.V. infusion as a single dose q 6 to 8 wk; or 75 to 100 mg/m$^2$ by slow I.V. infusion q.d. for 2 days q 6 wk |
| **chlorambucil** Leukeran | To provide palliative treatment of chronic lymphocytic leukemia, Hodgkin's disease, malignant lymphomas (including lymphosarcoma and giant follicular lymphoma), and non-Hodgkin's lymphoma | 0.1 to 0.2 mg/kg/day as a single dose or in divided doses for 3 to 6 wk. *Usual:* 4 to 10 mg/day as a single dose or in divided doses for 3 to 6 wk |
| **cyclophosphamide** Cytoxan, Neosar, Procytox (CAN) | To treat acute lymphocytic leukemia, acute nonlymphocytic leukemia, chronic lymphocytic leukemia, chronic myelocytic leukemia, breast cancer, epithelial ovarian cancer, Hodgkin's disease, multiple myeloma, neuroblastoma, non-Hodgkin's lymphoma, and retinoblastoma | 1 to 5 mg/kg P.O. q.d.; or 40 to 50 mg/kg I.V. in divided doses over 2 to 5 days; or 10 to 15 mg/kg I.V. q 7 to 10 days; or 3 to 5 mg/kg I.V. 2 times/wk; or 1.5 to 3 mg/kg I.V. q.d. |
| **ifosfamide** IFEX | To treat germ cell testicular tumors | 1.2 g/m$^2$/day by I.V. infusion for 5 days q 3 wk |
| **lomustine (CCNU)** CeeNU | To treat primary brain tumors and Hodgkin's disease | 100 to 130 mg/m$^2$ P.O. as a single dose q 6 wk |

## Antineoplastic Drugs (continued)

| GENERIC AND TRADE NAMES | INDICATIONS | USUAL ADULT DOSAGES |
|---|---|---|
| **Alkylating drugs** *(continued)* | | |
| **mechlorethamine hydrochloride (nitrogen mustard)** Mustargen | To treat bronchiogenic carcinoma, CML, Hodgkin's disease, lymphosarcoma, and mycosis fungoides | 0.4 mg/kg I.V. as a single dose or in divided doses over 2 to 4 days |
| | To treat malignant pericardial, peritoneal, or pleural effusions | 0.4 mg/kg (peritoneal or pleural effusion); 0.2 mg/kg into affected cavity (pericardial effusion) |
| **melphalan (L-phenylalanine mustard)** Alkeran **melphalan hydrochloride** Alkeran | To treat multiple myeloma | 0.15 mg/kg P.O. q.d. for 7 days, followed by 0.05 mg/kg q.d. after 3-wk period of no drug; or 0.1 to 0.15 mg/kg q.d. for 2 to 3 wk or 0.25 mg/kg for 4 days, followed by 2 to 4 mg q.d. after 2- to 4-wk period of no drug |
| | | 16 mg/m$^2$/I.V. over 15 min q 2 wk for 4 doses, then at 4 wk |
| | To treat epithelial ovarian cancer | 0.2 mg/kg P.O. q.d. for 5 days, repeated q 4 to 5 wk |
| **streptozocin** Zanosar | To treat islet cell or pancreatic carcinoma | 500 mg/m$^2$ I.V. for 5 days q 6 wk, or 1,000 mg/m$^2$ I.V. q wk for 2 wk |
| **temozolomide** Temodar | To treat astrocytoma | 150 mg/m$^2$ P.O. q.d. for first 5 days of 28-day cycle, followed by 200 mg/m$^2$, if tolerated, P.O. q.d. for first 5 days of subsequent 28-day cycles |
| **thiotepa (TESPA, triethylenethio-phosphoramide, TSPA)** Thioplex | To treat malignant pericardial or pleural effusions | 0.6 to 0.8 mg/kg into affected cavity |
| | To treat breast cancer, epithelial ovarian cancer, and Hodgkin's disease | 0.3 to 0.4 mg/kg I.V. q 1 to 4 wk, or 0.2 mg/kg for 4 to 5 days q 2 to 3 wk |
| | To treat bladder tumors | 30 to 60 mg mixed in 30 to 60 ml of normal saline and instilled into bladder q wk for 4 wk |
| **Antibiotic antineoplastics** | | |
| **bleomycin sulfate** Blenoxane | To treat non-Hodgkin's lymphoma, squamous cell carcinoma, and testicular cancer | 0.25 to 0.5 unit/kg or 10 to 20 units/m$^2$ 1 to 2 times/wk I.V., I.M., or S.C.; or 0.25 unit/kg or 15 units/m$^2$ q.d. by I.V. infusion over 24 hr |

*(continued)*

## Antineoplastic Drugs (continued)

| GENERIC AND TRADE NAMES | INDICATIONS | USUAL ADULT DOSAGES |
|---|---|---|
| **Antibiotic antineoplastics** *(continued)* | | |
| **bleomycin sulfate** *(continued)* | To treat Hodgkin's disease | 0.25 to 0.5 unit/kg I.V., I.M., or S.C., or 10 to 20 units/m$^2$ 1 to 2 times/wk |
| | To treat malignant pleural effusions | 60 units intrapleural single bolus dissolved in 50–100 ml of normal saline |
| | To treat squamous cell carcinoma of the cervix, head and neck, penis, or vulva | 30 to 60 units by arterial infusion over 1 to 24 hr |
| **cisplatin** Platinol, Platinol-AQ | To treat bladder cancer | 50 to 70 mg/m$^2$ by I.V. infusion as a single dose q 3 to 4 wk in combination with other agents |
| | To treat advanced ovarian cancer | 75 to 100 mg/m$^2$ by I.V. infusion as a single dose q 21 days in combination with paclitaxel |
| | To treat testicular cancer | 20 mg/m$^2$ by I.V. infusion q.d. for 5 days in combination with bleomycin and etoposide; repeated q 3 wk for two or more cycles |
| **dactinomycin (actinomycin-D)** Cosmegen | To treat Ewing's sarcoma, gestational trophoblastic or Wilms' tumors, rhabdomyosarcoma, sarcoma botryoides, and testicular cancer or tumors | 0.15 to 500 mcg/kg/day I.V. q.d. for 5 days; may repeat after 3 wk |
| | To treat Ewing's sarcoma and sarcoma botryoides | 0.05 mg/kg for lower extremity or pelvis; 0.035 mg/kg for upper extremity as an isolation-perfusion |
| **daunorubicin hydrochloride** Cerubidine | To treat acute lymphocytic leukemia | 45 mg/m$^2$ q.d. for first 3 days of a 32-day course of vincristine, prednisone, and asparaginase combination therapy |
| | To treat acute nonlymphocytic leukemia | 45 mg/m$^2$ q.d. for first 3 days of first course of cytarabine combination therapy and first 2 days of second course of cytarabine combination therapy |
| **daunorubicin, liposomal** DaunoXome | To treat AIDS-related Kaposi's sarcoma | 40 mg/m$^2$ I.V. over 60 min q 2 wk |

## Antineoplastic Drugs (continued)

| GENERIC AND TRADE NAMES | INDICATIONS | USUAL ADULT DOSAGES |
|---|---|---|
| **Antibiotic antineoplastics** *(continued)* | | |
| **doxorubicin hydrochloride** Adriamycin PFS, Adriamycin RDF, Rubex | To treat acute lymphocytic leukemia, acute nonlymphocytic leukemia; bladder, breast, gastric, epithelial ovarian, or thyroid cancer; Hodgkin's disease; neuroblastoma or Wilms' tumor; non-Hodgkin's lymphoma; small-cell lung carcinoma; and soft-tissue sarcoma or osteosarcoma | 60 to 75 mg/m$^2$ I.V. as single dose q 21 days; or 25 to 30 mg/m$^2$ I.V. q.d. for 2 to 3 days q 3 to 4 wk; or 20 mg/m$^2$ q wk; or 40 to 60 mg/m$^2$ q 21 to 28 days in combination with other chemotherapeutic drugs |
| **doxorubicin, liposomal** Caelyx (CAN), Doxil | To treat AIDS-related Kaposi's sarcoma | 20 mg/m$^2$ I.V. over 30 min q 3 wk as tolerated |
| **epirubicin hydrochloride** Ellence | To treat breast cancer | 100 to 120 mg/m$^2$ by I.V. infusion over 3 to 5 min via a free-flowing I.V. solution as a single dose on day 1 or in divided doses on days 1 and 8, repeated q 3 to 4 wk for 6 cycles in combination with other chemotherapy agents |
| **idarubicin hydrochloride** Idamycin | To treat acute nonlymphocytic leukemia | 12 mg/m$^2$/day I.V. over 10 to 15 min for 3 days in combination with cytarabine therapy |
| **mitomycin (mitomycin-C)** Mutamycin | To treat gastric or pancreatic cancer | 20 mg/m$^2$ as a single dose q 6 to 8 wk |
| **pentostatin (2′-deoxycoformycin)** Nipent | To treat hairy cell leukemia | 4 mg/m$^2$ by rapid I.V. injection or diluted for infusion over 20 to 30 min as a single dose q other wk |
| **plicamycin (mithramycin)** Mithracin | To treat testicular cancer | 0.025 to 0.03 mg/kg I.V. q.d. over 4 to 6 hr for 8 to 10 days |
| | To treat hypercalcemia and hypercalciuria | 0.015 to 0.025 mg/kg I.V. q.d. over 4 to 6 hr for 3 to 4 days; may repeat dose q wk as needed |
| **valrubicin** Valstar | To treat bladder cancer | 800 mg q wk for 6 wk into affected cavity |

*(continued)*

## Antineoplastic Drugs (continued)

| GENERIC AND TRADE NAMES | INDICATIONS | USUAL ADULT DOSAGES |
|---|---|---|
| **Antimetabolites** | | |
| **capecitabine** Xeloda | To treat locally advanced or metastatic breast cancer or metastatic colorectal cancer | 1,250 mg/m$^2$ P.O. after a meal b.i.d. (morning and evening) for 2 wk, followed by 1-wk rest period; dose repeated in 3-wk cycles |
| **cladribine (2-CdA, 2-chlorodeoxy-adenosine)** Leustatin | To treat hairy cell leukemia | 0.1 mg/kg/day by continuous I.V. infusion for 7 days |
| **cytarabine (ARA-C, cytosine arabinoside)** Cytosar, Cytosar-U | To treat acute nonlymphocytic leukemia | Initially, 100 mg/m$^2$/day by continuous I.V. infusion for 7 days, alone or in combination with other agents; or 100 mg/m$^2$ I.V. q 12 hr on days 1 to 7, then consult manufacturer's literature for specific dosing; or high-dose therapy of 2 to 3 g/m$^2$ I.V over 1 to 3 hr for 2 to 6 days, then consult manufacturer's literature for specific dosing |
| | To treat meningeal leukemia | 30 mg/m$^2$ intrathecally as a single dose q 4 days |
| | To prevent or treat acute lymphocytic leukemia and chronic myelocytic leukemia | Consult manufacturer's literature for specific dosage. |
| **cytarabine, liposomal** DepoCyt, Depro Tech | To treat lymphomatous meningitis | Initially, 50 mg intrathecally (intraventricular or lumbar puncture) over 1 to 5 min q 14 days for two doses (wk 1 and 3); then 50 mg intrathecally q 14 days for three doses (wk 5, 7, and 9), followed by 1 50-mg dose at wk 13; then 50 mg intrathecally q 28 days for four doses (wk 17, 21, 25, and 29) in combination with dexamethasone 4 mg P.O. or I.V. b.i.d. for 5 days |

## Antineoplastic Drugs *(continued)*

| GENERIC AND TRADE NAMES | INDICATIONS | USUAL ADULT DOSAGES |
|---|---|---|
| **Antimetabolites** *(continued)* | | |
| **floxuridine (fluorodeoxyuridine)** FUDR | To treat colorectal or hepatic cancer | 0.1 to 0.6 mg/kg/day by continuous intra-arterial infusion for 14 to 21 days, followed by 2 wk of no drug; dose repeated in 5-wk cycles |
| **fludarabine phosphate** Fludara | To treat chronic lymphocytic leukemia | 25 mg/m$^2$ I.V. infused over 30 min for 5 days; cycle repeated q 28 days |
| **fluorouracil (5-fluorouracil, 5-FU)** Adrucil, Carac, Efudex, Fluoroplex | To treat colorectal, breast, gastric, or pancreatic cancer | 7 to 12 mg/kg/day I.V. for 4 days, followed by no drug for 3 days, then 7 to 10 mg/kg q 3 to 4 days for total of 2 wk; or 12 mg/kg/day for 4 days, followed by 1 day of no drug, then 6 mg/kg q.o.d. for 4 or 5 days, for total of 12 days; thereafter, 7 to 12 mg/kg/day I.V. q 7 to 10 days |
| | To treat multiple actinic (solar) keratoses | 0.5% cream (face, anterior scalp), 1% cream (head, neck, chest), or 2% to 5% cream (hands) applied to skin q.d. to b.i.d. to cover lesions |
| | To treat superficial basal cell carcinoma | 5% cream applied to skin b.i.d. for up to 12 wk to cover lesions |
| **hydroxyurea** Droxia, Hydrea | To treat epithelial ovarian cancer | 60 to 80 mg/kg P.O. as a single dose q 3 days alone or with radiation therapy; or 20 to 30 mg/kg P.O. q.d. |
| | To treat resistant chronic myelocytic leukemia | 20 to 30 mg/kg P.O. q.d. or in divided doses b.i.d. |
| **mercaptopurine (6-mercaptopurine, 6-MP)** Purinethol | To treat acute lymphocytic leukemia or acute nonlymphocytic leukemia | 2.5 mg/kg/day or 80 to 100 mg/m$^2$/day (rounded off to nearest 25 mg) P.O. as a single dose or in divided doses, followed by 1.5 to 2.5 mg/kg/day P.O. or 50 to 100 mg/m$^2$/day |

*(continued)*

## Antineoplastic Drugs (continued)

| GENERIC AND TRADE NAMES | INDICATIONS | USUAL ADULT DOSAGES |
|---|---|---|
| **Antimetabolites** *(continued)* | | |
| **methotrexate (amethopterin) methotrexate sodium** | To treat chorioadenoma destruens, choriocarcinoma, or hydatidiform mole | 15 to 30 mg/day P.O. or I.M. for 5 days; repeat three to five times with 2 to 3 wk between courses |
| | To treat acute lymphocytic leukemia or meningeal leukemia | Initially, 3.3 mg/m$^2$/day P.O., I.M., or I.V. in combination with prednisone or other drug; as maintenance dose, 30 mg/m$^2$/wk P.O. or I.M. in two divided doses or 2.5 mg/kg I.V. q 14 days |
| | To treat Burkitt's lymphoma (stage I or II) | 10 to 25 mg/day P.O. for 4 to 8 days, followed by no drug for 7 to 10 days; course repeated as needed |
| | To treat Burkitt's lymphoma (stage III) | Same as for stage I or II in combination with other drug |
| | To treat lymphosarcoma (stage III) | 0.625 to 2.5 mg/kg/day P.O. |
| | To treat mycosis fungoides | 2.5 to 10 mg/day P.O. for weeks or months; or 50 mg I.M. q wk or 25 mg I.M. 2 times/wk |
| | To treat osteosarcoma | 12 g/m$^2$ by I.V. infusion over 12 hr, followed by leucovorin rescue on weeks 4, 5, 6, 7, 11, 12, 15, 16, 29, 30, 44, and 45 after surgery in combination with bleomycin, cisplatin, cyclophosphamide, dactinomycin, and doxorubicin |
| | To treat breast or head and neck cancer and non-small-cell or small-cell lung carcinoma | Consult manufacturer's literature for specific dosing. |
| **thioguanine (6-TG, 6-thioguanine)** Lanvis (CAN), Tabloid | To treat acute nonlymphocytic leukemia | 2 mg/kg/day P.O. as a single dose; if no improvement after 4 wk, increase to 3 mg/kg/day |
| **Antimitotic antineoplastics** | | |
| **docetaxel** Taxotere | To treat breast cancer | 60 to 100 mg/m$^2$ by I.V. infusion over 1 hr q 3 wk |
| | To treat non-small-cell lung carcinoma | 75 mg/m$^2$ by I.V. infusion over 1 hr q 3 wk |

## Antineoplastic Drugs (continued)

| GENERIC AND TRADE NAMES | INDICATIONS | USUAL ADULT DOSAGES |
|---|---|---|
| **Antimitotic antineoplastics** *(continued)* | | |
| **paclitaxel**<br>Taxol | To treat ovarian cancer | 135 or 175 mg/m$^2$ by I.V. infusion over 3 or 24 hr q 21 days |
| | To treat breast cancer | 175 mg/m$^2$ by I.V. infusion over 3 or 24 hr q 21 days |
| | To treat AIDS-related Kaposi's sarcoma | 135 mg/m$^2$ by I.V. infusion over 3 or 24 hr q 21 days; or 100 mg/m$^2$ by I.V. infusion over 3 or 24 hr q 14 days |
| | To treat non-small-cell lung carcinoma | 135 mg/m$^2$ by I.V. infusion over 3 or 24 hr, followed by cisplatin 75 mg/m$^2$ I.V. q 21 days |
| **vinblastine sulfate (VLB)**<br>Velban, Velbe (CAN) | To treat breast cancer, Hodgkin's disease, lymphomas, Kaposi's sarcoma, Letterer-Siwe disease, mycosis fungoides, non-Hodgkin's lymphoma, testicular cancer, and trophoblastic gestational tumors | 0.15 to 0.2 mg/kg I.V. q wk |
| **vincristine sulfate (VCR)**<br>Oncovin, Vincasar PFS | To treat acute lymphocytic leukemia, Hodgkin's disease, lymphomas, non-Hodgkin's lymphoma, rhabdomyosarcoma, and Wilms' tumor | 0.01 to 0.03 mg/kg I.V.; or 0.4 to 1.4 mg/m$^2$ I.V. q wk as a single dose (maximum of 2 mg) |
| **vinorelbine tartrate**<br>Navelbine | To treat non-small-cell lung carcinoma | 30 mg/m$^2$ I.V. over 6 to 10 min q wk alone, or 25 mg/m$^2$ I.V. over 6 to 10 min q wk in combination with cisplatin 100 mg/m$^2$ q 4 wk |
| **Biological response modifiers** | | |
| **aldesleukin (IL-2, interleukin-2)**<br>Proleukin | To treat renal cancer and metastatic melanoma | 600,000 IU/kg by I.V. infusion over 15 min q 8 hr for 14 doses, followed by 9 days of no drug; then repeat course of 14 doses for total of 28 doses |
| **alemtuzumab**<br>Campath | To treat B-cell chronic lymphocytic leukemia | *Initial:* 3 mg I.V. over 2 hr daily, then increased to 10 mg I.V. over 2 hr daily. *Maintenance:* 30 mg I.V. over 2 hr 3 times/wk on alternate days for up to 12 wk |

*(continued)*

## Antineoplastic Drugs (continued)

| GENERIC AND TRADE NAMES | INDICATIONS | USUAL ADULT DOSAGES |
|---|---|---|
| **Biological response modifiers** *(continued)* | | |
| **bacillus Calmette-Guérin (BCG) live, Connaught strain** ImmuCyst (CAN), TheraCys | To treat bladder cancer | 81 mg (reconstitute and dilute with 50 ml preservative-free NSS to 53 ml or less) instilled into bladder for 1 to 2 hr q wk for 6 wk, then as a single-dose treatment at 3, 6, 12, 18, and 24 mo |
| **bacillus Calmette-Guérin, Tice strain** TICE BCG | | 50 mg (reconstitute and dilute with 50 ml preservative-free NSS to 50 ml or less) for 1 to 2 hr q 6 wk; may repeat once, followed by single-dose treatment q mo for 6 to 12 mo |
| **denileukin diftitox** Ontak | To treat cutaneous or T-cell lymphomas, including mycosis fungoides | 9 or 18 mcg/kg/day by I.V. infusion over at least 15 min for 5 days; repeated q 21 days |
| **interferon alfa-2a, recombinant** Roferon-A | To treat hairy cell leukemia | 3 million U/day I.M. or S.C. for 16 to 24 wk, followed by 3 million U 3 times/wk |
| | To treat AIDS-related Kaposi's sarcoma | 36 million U/day I.M. or S.C. for 10 to 12 wk; or 3 million U/day I.M. or S.C. on days 1 to 3, 9 million U/day on days 4 to 6, 18 million U/day on days 7 to 9, and 36 million U/day from day 10 until completion of 10- to 12-wk course; maintenance dose, 36 million U 3 times/wk |
| **interferon alfa-2b, recombinant** Intron A | To treat hairy cell leukemia | 2 million $U/m^2$ I.M. or S.C. 3 times/wk |
| | To treat AIDS-related Kaposi's sarcoma | 30 million $U/m^2$ I.M. or S.C. 3 times/wk |
| | To treat malignant melanoma | 20 million $U/m^2$ by I.V. infusion on days 1 to 5 q wk for 4 wk, followed by 10 million $U/m^2$ I.V. 3 times/wk for 48 wk |

## Antineoplastic Drugs (continued)

| GENERIC AND TRADE NAMES | INDICATIONS | USUAL ADULT DOSAGES |
|---|---|---|
| **Biological response modifiers (continued)** | | |
| **levamisole hydrochloride** Ergamisol | To treat colorectal cancer | Beginning 7 to 30 days after surgery, 50 mg P.O. q 8 hr for 3 days, repeated q 2 wk for 1 yr, in combination with fluorouracil 450 mg/m$^2$ by rapid I.V. infusion q.d. for 5 days, starting with first or second course of levamisole |
| | To treat acute lymphocytic | |
| **Antineoplastic enzymes** | | |
| **asparaginase** Colaspase, Elspar, Kidrolase (CAN) | leukemia | 200 IU/kg I.V. q.d. for 28 days |
| **pegaspargase (PEG-L-asparaginase)** Oncaspar | To treat acute lymphoblastic leukemia in adults up to age 21 | 2,500 IU/m$^2$ I.M. or I.V. q 14 days |
| **Hormonal antineoplastics** | | |
| **anastrozole** Arimidex | To treat breast cancer | 1 mg P.O. q.d. |
| **bicalutamide** Casodex | To treat prostate cancer | 50 mg P.O. q.d. in combination with luteinizing hormone-releasing hormone (LHRH) analog or after surgical castration |
| **estramustine phosphate sodium** Emcyt | To treat prostate cancer | 14 mg/kg/day P.O. in three or four divided doses 1 hr a.c. or 2 hr p.c. |
| **exemestane** Aromasin | To treat postmenopausal breast cancer | 25 mg P.O. q.d. p.c. |
| **flutamide** Euflex (CAN), Eulexin | To treat prostate cancer | 250 mg P.O. q 8 hr |
| **goserelin acetate** Zoladex, Zoladex LA, Zoladex 3-Month | To treat breast cancer | 3.6 mg S.C. into upper abdominal wall q 28 days |
| | To treat prostate cancer | 3.6 mg S.C. into upper abdominal wall q 28 days; or 10.8 mg S.C. q 12 wk |
| **letrozole** Femara | To treat breast cancer | 2.5 mg P.O. q.d. |

*(continued)*

## Antineoplastic Drugs (continued)

| GENERIC AND TRADE NAMES | INDICATIONS | USUAL ADULT DOSAGES |
|---|---|---|
| **Hormonal antineoplastics** *(continued)* | | |
| **leuprolide acetate** Lupron, Lupron Depot, Lupron Depot-3 Month, Lupron Depot-4 Month, Viadur | To treat prostate cancer | *Regular:* 1 mg S.C. q.d.; *depot:* 7.5 mg q mo; or 22.5 mg q 3 mo; or 30 mg q 4 mo; *implant:* 1 q 12 mo |
| **medroxyprogesterone acetate** Depo-Provera | To treat endometrial or renal cancer | 400 to 1,000 mg q wk until stable, then 400 mg or more q mo |
| **megestrol acetate** Megace | To treat breast cancer | 160 mg/day P.O. q.d. or in divided doses |
| | To treat endometrial cancer | 40 to 320 mg P.O. q.d. or in divided doses |
| **nilutamide** Anandron (CAN), Nilandron | To treat prostate cancer | 300 mg P.O. q.d. up to 30 days, then 150 mg P.O. q.d. |
| **tamoxifen citrate** Apo-Tamox (CAN), Gen-Tamoxifen (CAN), Nolvadex, Nolvadex-D (CAN), Novo-Tamoxifen (CAN), Tamofen (CAN), Tamone (CAN) | To prevent breast cancer or reduce the risk of invasive breast cancer in women with ductal carcinoma in situ | 20 mg P.O. q.d. for 5 yr |
| | To treat breast cancer (node-negative or node-positive) | 10 mg P.O. b.i.d. or, in metastatic disease, 10 to 20 mg P.O. b.i.d. |
| **testolactone** Teslac | To treat breast cancer | 250 mg P.O. q.i.d. |
| **toremifene citrate** Fareston | To treat breast cancer | 60 mg P.O. q.d. |
| **triptorelin pamoate** Trelstar LA | To provide palliative treatment of advanced prostate cancer | 11.25 mg I.M. q 84 days |
| **Miscellaneous antineoplastics** | | |
| **arsenic trioxide** Trisenox | To treat acute promyelocytic leukemia | *Induction:* 0.15 mg/kg I.V. daily until bone marrow remission occurs. *Maximum:* 60 doses. *Consolidation:* Begun 3 to 6 wk after completion of induction, 0.15 mg/kg I.V. daily for 25 doses over up to 5 wk |

## Antineoplastic Drugs (continued)

| GENERIC AND TRADE NAMES | INDICATIONS | USUAL ADULT DOSAGES |
|---|---|---|
| **Miscellaneous antineoplastics** *(continued)* | | |
| **bexarotene** Targretin | To treat cutaneous manifestations of cutaneous T-cell lymphoma | 300 mg/m$^2$ P.O. q.d. with food; after 8 wk, may increase to 400 mg/m$^2$ P.O. q.d. with food, as needed and tolerated. |
| Targretin Gel | To treat cutaneous lesions of cutaneous T-cell lymphoma (stages IA and IB) | Apply generously to cover only lesions q.o.d. on 1st wk; then increased as tolerated to q.d. on 2nd wk, b.i.d. on 3rd wk, t.i.d on 4th wk and, finally, q.i.d. on 5th wk |
| **dacarbazine** DTIC (CAN), DTIC-Dome | To treat Hodgkin's disease | 150 mg/m$^2$ I.V. q.d. for 5 days in combination with other drugs; may repeat q 28 days; or 375 mg/m$^2$ q 15 days in combination with other drugs |
| | To treat malignant melanoma | 2 to 4.5 mg/kg I.V. q.d. for 10 days and q 28 days thereafter; or 250 mg/m$^2$ I.V. q.d. for 5 days and q 21 days thereafter |
| **etoposide (VP-16)** Toposar, VePesid | To treat germ-cell testicular tumors | 50 to 100 mg/m$^2$/day I.V. on days 1 through 5 up to 100 mg/m$^2$ I.V. on days 1, 3, and 5; course repeated q 3 to 4 wk |
| | To treat small-cell lung carcinoma | 35 mg/m$^2$/day I.V. for 4 days up to 50 mg/m$^2$/day I.V. for 5 days, repeated q 3 to 4 wk; or 70 mg/m$^2$/day P.O. for 4 days to 100 mg/m$^2$/day P.O. for 5 days, repeated q 3 to 4 wk |
| **etoposide phosphate** Etopophos | To treat germ-cell testicular tumors | 50 to 100 mg/m$^2$/day by I.V. infusion on days 1 through 5 to 100 mg/m$^2$/day by I.V. infusion on days 1, 3, and 5; course repeated q 3 to 4 wk |
| | To treat small-cell lung carcinoma | 35 mg/m$^2$/day by I.V. infusion for 4 days to 50 mg/m$^2$/day by I.V. infusion for 5 days, repeated q 3 to 4 wk |

*(continued)*

## Antineoplastic Drugs (continued)

| GENERIC AND TRADE NAMES | INDICATIONS | USUAL ADULT DOSAGES |
|---|---|---|
| Miscellaneous antineoplastics (continued) | | |
| **gemcitabine hydrochloride** Gemzar | To treat non-small-cell lung carcinoma | 1,000 mg/m$^2$ by I.V. infusion over 30 min q.d. on days 1, 8, and 15 q 28 days in combination with cisplatin 100 mg/m$^2$ on day 28; or 1,250 mg/m$^2$ I.V. q.d. on days 1 and 8 q 21 days in combination with cisplatin 100 mg/m$^2$ I.V. on day 21 |
| | To treat pancreatic cancer | 1,000 mg/m$^2$ by I.V. infusion over 30 min q wk for 7 wk, followed by 1 wk of no drug; then q wk for 3 wk, followed by 1 wk of no drug; then repeat 4-wk cycle |
| **gemtuzumab ozogamicin** Mylotarg | To treat first relapse in patients with CD33-positive acute myeloid leukemia who are age 60 or older and who are not candidates for cytotoxic therapy | 9 mg/m$^2$ by I.V. infusion over 2 hr; repeated in 14 days |
| **imatinib mesylate** Gleevec | To treat chronic myeloid leukemia in accelerated phase or blast crisis, or in chronic phase after failure of interferon-alpha therapy | 400 mg P.O. q.d. with food (chronic phase) or 600 mg P.O. q.d. with food (accelerated phase or blast crisis); after 3 mo, dosage may be increased to 600 mg P.O. q.d. (chronic phase) or 800 mg P.O. given in 2 divided doses of 400 mg (accelerated phase or blast crisis), as needed. |
| | To treat gastrointestinal stromal tumor | 400 mg/day P.O. or 600 mg/day P.O. |
| **irinotecan hydrochloride** Camptosar | To treat colorectal cancer | 125 mg/m$^2$ I.V. over 90 min q wk for 4 wk, followed by 2 wk of no drug, then repeat 6-wk cycle; or 350 mg/m$^2$ I.V. over 90 min q 3 wk |
| **iressa** Gefitinib | To treat refractory metastatic nonsmall cell lung cancer | 250 mg P.O. q.d. |
| **mitotane (o,p'-DDD)** Lysodren | To treat adrenocortical carcinoma | 2 to 6 g P.O. q.d. in divided doses t.i.d. or q.i.d. |

## Antineoplastic Drugs (continued)

| GENERIC AND TRADE NAMES | INDICATIONS | USUAL ADULT DOSAGES |
|---|---|---|
| **Miscellaneous antineoplastics** *(continued)* | | |
| **mitoxantrone hydrochloride** Novantrone | To treat hormone-refractory prostate cancer | 12 to 14 mg/m$^2$ I.V. q 21 days |
| | To treat acute nonlymphocytic leukemia | 12 mg/m$^2$ by I.V. infusion through free-flowing NSS or D$_5$W solution over 3 min q.d. on days 1 to 3, in combination with cytarabine 100 mg/m$^2$/day by continuous I.V. infusion on days 1 to 7; if response is inadequate, second course at same dosage may be given |
| **porfimer sodium** Photofrin | To treat esophageal cancer and non-small-cell lung carcinoma | 2 mg/kg I.V. over 3 to 5 min, followed by laser light illumination and debridement of tumor; may repeat course q 30 days three times |
| **procarbazine hydrochloride** Matulane, Natulan (CAN) | To treat Hodgkin's disease | 2 to 4 mg/kg/day (rounded to nearest 50 mg) P.O. as a single dose or in divided doses for 1 wk, followed by 4 to 6 mg/kg/day until leukopenia, thrombocytopenia, or maximal response occurs |
| **rituximab** Rituxan | To treat non-Hodgkin's lymphomas | 375 mg/m$^2$/day by I.V. infusion q wk for 4 or 8 doses |
| **topotecan hydrochloride** Hycamtin | To treat ovarian cancer and small-cell lung carcinoma | 1.5 mg/m$^2$ I.V. over 30 min q.d. for 5 days, repeated q 21 days |
| **trastuzumab** Herceptin | To treat breast cancer | 4 mg/kg I.V. over 90 min, followed by 2 mg/kg I.V. over 30 min q 7 days |
| **velcade** Bortezomib | To treat multiple myeloma | 1.3 mg/m$^2$ I.V. bolus on days 1, 4, 8, and 11 for 2 wk, followed by rest on days 12–21; then repeat 3-wk cycle |

# Selected Antihypertensive Combinations

Antihypertensive drugs are used along with lifestyle changes to manage hypertension. Antihypertensive combinations, which commonly include one or two antihypertensives and a diuretic, are used to simplify patients' drug regimens and, in some cases, to enhance drug actions.

The chart below lists the generic and trade names; functional classes; usual adult dosages;

| ANTIHYPERTENSIVE COMBINATION TRADE NAMES | ANTIHYPERTENSIVE GENERIC NAMES | DIURETIC GENERIC NAMES |
|---|---|---|
| Aldoril-15 | methyldopa 250 mg | hydrochlorothiazide (HCTZ) 15 mg |
| Aldoril-25 | methyldopa 250 mg | HCTZ 25 mg |
| Aldoril D30 | methyldopa 500 mg | HCTZ 30 mg |
| Aldoril D50 | methyldopa 500 mg | HCTZ 50 mg |
| Apresazide 25/25 | hydralazine hydrochloride (HCl) 25 mg | HCTZ 25 mg |
| Apresazide 50/50 | hydralazine HCl 50 mg | HCTZ 50 mg |
| Apresazide 100/50 | hydralazine HCl 100 mg | HCTZ 50 mg |
| Atacand HCT 16/12.5 | candesartan cilexetil 16 mg | HCTZ 12.5 mg |
| Atacand HCT 32/12.5 | candesartan cilexetil 32 mg | HCTZ 12.5 mg |
| Avalide-150 | irbesartan 150 mg | HCTZ 12.5 mg |
| Avalide-300 | irbesartan 300 mg | HCTZ 12.5 mg |
| Benicar HCT 20/12.5 | olmesartan medoxomil 20 mg | HCTZ 12.5 mg |
| Benicar HCT 40/12.5 | olmesartan medoxomil 40 mg | HCTZ 12.5 mg |
| Benicar HCT 40/25 | olmesartan medoxomil 40 mg | HCTZ 25 mg |
| Capozide 25/15 | captopril 25 mg | HCTZ 15 mg |
| Capozide 25/25 | captopril 25 mg | HCTZ 25 mg |
| Capozide 50/15 | captopril 50 mg | HCTZ 15 mg |
| Capozide 50/25 | captopril 50 mg | HCTZ 25 mg |
| Diovan HCT 80/12.5 | valsartan 80 mg | HCTZ 12.5 mg |
| Diovan HCT 160/12.5 | valsartan 160 mg | HCTZ 12.5 mg |
| Diovan HCT 160/25 | valsartan 160 mg | HCTZ 25 mg |
| Dyazide | triamterene 37.5 mg | HCTZ 25 mg |
| Hyzaar 50/12.5 | losartan potassium 50 mg | HCTZ 12.5 mg |
| Hyzaar 100/25 | losartan potassium 100 mg | HCTZ 25 mg |

and onset, peak, and duration for commonly used antihypertensive combinations. For information about the mechanisms of action, interactions, adverse reactions, and nursing considerations related to antihypertensive combinations, review the entries for the specific antihypertensives and diuretics that they contain.

| FUNCTIONAL CLASSES | USUAL ADULT DOSAGES | ONSET, PEAK, AND DURATION |
|---|---|---|
| Centrally acting antiadrenergic and thiazide diuretic | 1 tab b.i.d or t.i.d<br><br>1 tab b.i.d.<br>1 tab q.d.<br>1 tab q.d. | **Onset:** Unknown<br>**Peak:** 4 to 6 hr<br>**Duration:** 12 to 24 hr |
| Peripherally acting arterial dilator and thiazide diuretic | 1 cap q.d. or b.i.d.<br><br>1 cap q.d. or b.i.d.<br>1 cap q.d. or b.i.d. | **Onset:** 20 to 30 min<br>**Peak:** 1 to 2 hr<br>**Duration:** 2 to 4 hr |
| Angiotensin II receptor antagonist and thiazide diuretic | 1 tab q.d. or b.i.d.<br>1 tab q.d. | **Onset:** 1 to 2 wk<br>**Peak:** Within 4 wk<br>**Duration:** Unknown |
| ACE inhibitor and thiazide diuretic | 1 tab q.d.<br>1 tab q.d. | **Onset:** Unknown<br>**Peak:** Unknown<br>**Duration:** Unknown |
| Angiotensin II receptor antagonist and thiazide diuretic | 1 tab q.d.<br>1 tab q.d.<br>1 tab q.d. | **Onset:** Unknown<br>**Peak:** Unknown<br>**Duration:** Unknown |
| ACE inhibitor and thiazide diuretic | 1 tab q.d. to t.i.d.<br>1 tab q.d. or b.i.d.<br>1 tab q.d. to t.i.d.<br>1 tab q.d. or b.i.d. | **Onset:** 15 to 60 min<br>**Peak:** 60 to 90 min<br>**Duration:** 6 to 12 hr |
| ACE inhibitor and thiazide diuretic | 1 or 2 tabs q.d.<br>1 tab q.d.<br>1 tab q.d. | **Onset:** 2 hr<br>**Peak:** 6 hr<br>**Duration:** 24 hr |
| Potassium-sparing diuretic and thiazide diuretic | 1 or 2 caps or tabs q.d. | **Onset:** 2 to 4 hr<br>**Peak:** 1 day<br>**Duration:** 7 to 9 hr |
| ACE inhibitor and thiazide diuretic | 1 or 2 tabs q.d.<br>1 tab q.d. | **Onset:** Unknown<br>**Peak:** 6 hr<br>**Duration:** 24 hr or more |

*(continued)*

## Selected Antihypertensive Combinations (continued)

| ANTIHYPERTENSIVE COMBINATION TRADE NAMES | ANTIHYPERTENSIVE GENERIC NAMES | DIURETIC GENERIC NAMES |
|---|---|---|
| Inderide 80/25 | propranolol HCl 80 mg | HCTZ 25 mg |
| Inderide LA 80/50 | propranolol HCl 80 mg | HCTZ 50 mg |
| Inderide LA 120/50 | propranolol HCl 120 mg | HCTZ 50 mg |
| Inderide LA 160/50 | propranolol HCl 160 mg | HCTZ 50 mg |
| Lopressor HCT 50/25 | metoprolol tartrate 50 mg | HCTZ 25 mg |
| Lopressor HCT 100/25 | metoprolol tartrate 100 mg | HCTZ 25 mg |
| Lopressor HCT 100/50 | metoprolol tartrate 100 mg | HCTZ 50 mg |
| Lotensin HCT 5/6.25 | benazepril HCl 5 mg | HCTZ 6.25 mg |
| Lotensin HCT 10/12.5 | benazepril HCl 10 mg | HCTZ 12.5 mg |
| Lotensin HCT 20/12.5 | benazepril HCl 20 mg | HCTZ 12.5 mg |
| Lotensin HCT 20/25 | benazepril HCl 20 mg | HCTZ 25 mg |
| Lotrel 2.5/10 | amlodipine 2.5 mg, benazepril HCl 10 mg | none |
| Lotrel 5/10 | amlodipine 5 mg, benazepril HCl 10 mg | none |
| Lotrel 5/20 | amlodipine 5 mg, benazepril HCl 10 mg | none |
| Lotrel 10/20 | amlodipine 10 mg, benazepril HCl 20 mg | none |
| Maxzide 37.5/25 | triamterene 37.5 mg | HCTZ 25 mg |
| Maxzide 75/50 | triamterene 75 mg | HCTZ 50 mg |
| Micardis HCT 40/12.5 | telmisartan 40 mg | HCTZ 12.5 mg |
| Micardis HCT 80/12.5 | telmisartan 80 mg | HCTZ 12.5 mg |
| Moduretic | amiloride 5 mg | HCTZ 50 mg |
| Prinzide 10/12.5 | lisinopril 10 mg | HCTZ 12.5 mg |
| Prinzide 20/12.5 | lisinopril 20 mg | HCTZ 12.5 mg |
| Prinzide 20/25 | lisinopril 20 mg | HCTZ 25 mg |
| Timolide 10/25 | timolol maleate 10 mg | HCTZ 25 mg |

| FUNCTIONAL CLASSES | USUAL ADULT DOSAGES | ONSET, PEAK, AND DURATION |
|---|---|---|
| Beta blocker and thiazide diuretic | 1 or 2 tabs b.i.d.<br>1 cap q.d.<br>1 cap q.d.<br>1 cap q.d. | **Onset:** Unknown<br>**Peak:** 1 to 1.5 hr<br>**Duration:** Unknown |
| Beta blocker and thiazide diuretic | 1 or 2 tabs q.d. or 1 tab b.i.d.<br>1 or 2 tabs q.d. or 1 tab b.i.d.<br>1 or 2 tabs q.d. or 1 tab b.i.d. | **Onset:** 1 hr<br>**Peak:** 1 to 2 hr<br>**Duration:** Unknown |
| ACE inhibitor and thiazide diuretic | 1 tab q.d.<br>1 tab q.d.<br>1 tab q.d.<br>1 tab q.d. | **Onset:** 1 hr<br>**Peak:** 2 to 4 hr<br>**Duration:** 24 hr |
| ACE inhibitor and calcium channel blocker | 1 or 2 caps q.d.<br><br>1 cap q.d.<br><br>1 cap q.d.<br><br>1 cap q.d. | **Onset:** Unknown<br>**Peak:** Unknown<br>**Duration:** 24 hr |
| Potassium-sparing diuretic and thiazide diuretic | 1 tab q.d.<br>1 tab q.d. | **Onset:** 2 to 4 hr<br>**Peak:** 1 day<br>**Duration:** 7 to 9 hr |
| Angiotensin II receptor antagonist and thiazide diuretic | 1 tab q.d. or b.i.d.<br>1 tab q.d. or b.i.d. | **Onset:** Within 3 hr<br>**Peak:** In 4 wk<br>**Duration:** Several days to 1 wk |
| Potassium-sparing diuretic and thiazide diuretic | 1 or 2 tabs q.d. | **Onset:** 2 hr<br>**Peak:** 6 to 10 hr<br>**Duration:** 24 hr |
| ACE inhibitor and thiazide diuretic | 1 or 2 tabs q.d.<br>1 or 2 tabs q.d.<br>1 or 2 tabs q.d. | **Onset:** 1 hr<br>**Peak:** 6 hr<br>**Duration:** 24 hr |
| Beta blocker and thiazide diuretic | 1 tab b.i.d. or 2 tabs q.d. | **Onset:** Unknown<br>**Peak:** 1 to 2 hr<br>**Duration:** Unknown |

*(continued)*

## Selected Antihypertensive Combinations (continued)

| ANTIHYPERTENSIVE COMBINATION TRADE NAMES | ANTIHYPERTENSIVE GENERIC NAMES | DIURETIC GENERIC NAMES |
|---|---|---|
| Uniretic 15/25 | moexipril HCl 15 mg | HCTZ 25 mg |
| Vaseretic 5/12.5 | enalapril maleate 5 mg | HCTZ 12.5 mg |
| Vaseretic 10/25 | enalapril maleate 10 mg | HCTZ 25 mg |
| Zestoretic 10/12.5 | lisinopril 10 mg | HCTZ 12.5 mg |
| Zestoretic 20/12.5 | lisinopril 20 mg | HCTZ 12.5 mg |
| Zestoretic 20/25 | lisinopril 20 mg | HCTZ 25 mg |
| Ziac 2.5/6.25 | bisoprolol fumarate 2.5 mg | HCTZ 6.25 mg |
| Ziac 5/6.25 | bisoprolol fumarate 5 mg | HCTZ 6.25 mg |
| Ziac 10/6.25 | bisoprolol fumarate 10 mg | HCTZ 6.25 mg |

| FUNCTIONAL CLASSES | USUAL ADULT DOSAGES | ONSET, PEAK, AND DURATION |
|---|---|---|
| Potassium-sparing diuretic and thiazide diuretic | 1 or 2 tabs q.d. | **Onset:** 1 hr<br>**Peak:** 3 to 6 hr<br>**Duration:** 24 hr |
| ACE inhibitor and thiazide diuretic | 1 tab q.d. or b.i.d.<br>1 tab q.d. or b.i.d. | **Onset:** 1 hr<br>**Peak:** 4 to 6 hr<br>**Duration:** 24 hr |
| ACE inhibitor and thiazide diuretic | 1 or 2 tabs q.d.<br>1 or 2 tabs q.d.<br>1 or 2 tabs q.d. | **Onset:** 1 hr<br>**Peak:** 6 hr<br>**Duration:** 24 hr |
| Beta blocker and thiazide diuretic | 1 or 2 tabs q.d.<br>1 or 2 tabs q.d.<br>1 or 2 tabs q.d. | **Onset:** Unknown<br>**Peak:** Unknown<br>**Duration:** Unknown |

# Vitamins

As you know, an adequate daily intake of vitamins is essential to vital bodily functions, such as embryonic development (vitamin A), regulation of serum calcium and phosphate (vitamin D), and blood clotting (vitamin K).

Vitamins are classified as one of two types: fat soluble (vitamins A, D, E, and K) and water soluble (vitamin C and all forms of vitamin B). Fat-soluble vitamins can accumulate in body tissue over time; when excessive amounts are ingested through diet or sup-

| GENERIC AND TRADE NAMES | RECOMMENDED DAILY INTAKE |
|---|---|
| **vitamin A**<br>**(retinol)**<br>Aquasol A | **Adult men and boys over age 10.** 1,000 mcg/day.<br>**Adult women and girls over age 10.** 800 mcg/day.<br>**Pregnant women.** 800 mcg/day. (900 mcg/day [CAN].)<br>**Breast-feeding women.** 1,200 to 1,300 mcg/day. (1,200 mcg/day [CAN].)<br>**Children ages 7 to 10.** 700 mcg/day. (700 to 800 mcg/day [CAN].)<br>**Children ages 4 to 7.** 500 mcg/day.<br>**Neonates and children to age 4.** 375 to 400 mcg/day. (400 mcg/day [CAN].) |
| **vitamin B₁**<br>**(thiamine hydrochloride)**<br>Betaxin (CAN), Bewon (CAN), Biamine | **Adult men and boys over age 10.** 1.2 to 1.5 mg/day. (0.8 to 1.3 mg/day [CAN].)<br>**Adult women and girls over age 10.** 1 to 1.1 mg/day. (0.8 to 0.9 mg/day [CAN].)<br>**Pregnant women.** 1.5 mg/day. (0.9 to 1 mg/day. [CAN].)<br>**Breast-feeding women.** 1.6 mg/day. (1 to 1.2 mg/day [CAN].) |

plementation, severe and life-threatening toxicity can develop. Water-soluble vitamins don't accumulate in the body; they are excreted daily so that toxicity is not usually a concern with excessive intake.

The following chart lists the generic and trade names of fat-soluble and water-soluble vitamins, the recommended daily intake to prevent vitamin deficiency, dosages when deficiency occurs, other indications and dosages for vitamin therapy, and guidelines for parenteral administration of vitamins.

## OTHER INDICATIONS AND DOSAGES

## PARENTERAL ADMINISTRATION GUIDELINES

*To treat vitamin A deficiency*
CAPSULES, ORAL SOLUTION, TABLETS
**Adults and adolescents.** Dosage individualized based on severity of deficiency, as prescribed.
**I.M. INJECTION**
**Adults and children age 8 and older.** 15,000 to 30,000 retinol equivalent (RE)/day (50,000 to 100,000 IU/day) for 3 days, followed by 15,000 RE/day (50,000 IU/day) for 2 wk.
**Children ages 1 to 8.** 1,500 to 4,500 RE/day (5,000 to 15,000 IU/day) for 10 days; for severe deficiency, 5,250 to 10,500 RE/day (17,500 to 35,000 IU/day) for 10 days.
**Infants to age 1 year.** 1,500 to 3,000 RE/day (5,000 to 10,000 IU/day) for 10 days; for severe deficiency, 2,250 to 4,500 RE/day (7,500 to 15,000 IU/day) for 10 days.
**I.V. INFUSION**
**Adults and children.** Dosage individualized as part of total parenteral nutrition solution, as prescribed.

*To treat xerophthalmia*
CAPSULES, ORAL SOLUTION, TABLETS
**Children age 1 and older.** 60,000 RE (200,000 IU) as a single dose. Dose repeated on day 2 and again in 4 wk.
**Children ages 6 months to 1 year.** 30,000 RE (100,000 IU) as a single dose. Dose repeated on day 2 and again in 4 wk.

*As an adjunct to treat measles*
CAPSULES, ORAL SOLUTION, TABLETS
**Children age 1 and older.** 60,000 RE (200,000 IU) as a single dose when measles are diagnosed.
**Children ages 6 months to 1 year.** 30,000 RE (100,000 IU) as a single dose when measles are diagnosed.

• Be aware that anaphylaxis and death have occurred after I.V. administration of vitamin A; I.V. administration is restricted to special solutions, such as in total parenteral solution. Typically, parenteral administration of vitamin A is by I.M. injection.
• Take precautions to protect vitamin A solution from exposure to light because it's light sensitive.

*To treat vitamin B₁ deficiency (beriberi)*
ELIXIR, TABLETS
**Adults.** 5 to 10 mg t.i.d.
**Children and infants.** 10 mg/day.
**I.V. OR I.M. INJECTION**
**Adults.** *Initial:* 5 to 100 mg q 8 hr, switched to P.O. vitamin B₁ therapy as soon as possible and continued for total of 1 mo.

• Be aware that I.V. administration of vitamin B₁ has caused severe and life-threatening reactions, especially with repeat administration. Monitor patient closely for angioedema, GI bleeding, respiratory distress, throat tightness, urticaria, vascular collapse, and weakness during and after administration.

*(continued)*

## Vitamins (continued)

| GENERIC AND TRADE NAMES | RECOMMENDED DAILY INTAKE |
|---|---|
| **vitamin B$_1$** *(continued)* | **Children ages 7 to 10.** 1 mg/day. (0.8 to 1 mg/day [CAN].) **Children ages 4 to 7.** 0.9 mg/day. (0.7 mg/day [CAN].) **Children ages 1 to 4.** 0.3 to 0.7 mg/day. (0.3 to 0.6 mg/day [CAN].) |
| **vitamin B$_3$** **(niacin)** Endur-Acin, Nia-Bid, Niac, Niacels, Niacor, Nico-400, Nicobid Tempules, Nicolar, Nicotinex Elixir, Novo-Niacin (CAN), Slo-Niacin | **Adult men and boys age 11 and older.** 15 to 20 mg/day. (14 to 23 mg/day [CAN].) **Adult women and girls age 11 and older.** 13 to 15 mg/day. (14 to 16 mg/day [CAN].) **Pregnant women.** 17 mg/day. (14 to 16 mg/day [CAN].) **Breast-feeding women.** 20 mg/day. (14 to 16 mg/day [CAN].) **Children ages 7 to 11.** 13 mg/day. (14 to 18 mg/day [CAN].) **Children ages 4 to 7.** 12 mg/day. (13 mg/day [CAN].) **Neonates and children to age 4.** 5 to 9 mg/day. (4 to 9 mg/day [CAN].) |
| **vitamin B$_6$** **(pyridoxine hydrochloride)** Beesix, Doxine, Nestrex, Pyri, Rodex, Vita-bee 6 | **Adult men and boys age 11 and older.** 1.7 to 2 mg/day. **Adult women and girls age 11 and older.** 1.4 to 1.6 mg/day. **Pregnant women.** 2.2 mg/day. **Breast-feeding women.** 2.1 mg/day. **Children ages 7 to 10.** 1.4 mg/day. **Children ages 4 to 6.** 1.1 mg/day. **Neonates and children to age 3.** 0.3 to 1 mg/day. |

| OTHER INDICATIONS AND DOSAGES | PARENTERAL ADMINISTRATION GUIDELINES |
|---|---|

**OTHER INDICATIONS AND DOSAGES**

*To treat Wernicke's encephalopathy*
**I.V. OR I.M. INJECTION**
**Adults.** *Initial:* 100 mg I.V. *Maintenance:* 50 to 100 mg I.V. or I.M. q.d. until normal recommended daily intake is achieved.

*To treat vitamin B₃ deficiency*
**E.R. CAPSULES, E.R. TABLETS, ORAL SOLUTION, TABLETS**
**Adults and children age 11 and older.** Dosage individualized based on severity of deficiency, as prescribed. *Maximum:* 6 g/day.
**I.V. INJECTION**
**Adults and children age 11 and older.** 25 to 100 mg at least b.i.d.
**Children to age 11.** Up to 300 mg q.d.
**I.M. INJECTION**
**Adults and children age 11 and older.** 50 to 100 mg at least 5 times/day.
**Children to age 11.** Dosage individualized based on severity of deficiency.

*To treat hyperlipidemia (niacin only)*
**E.R. CAPSULES, E.R. TABLETS, ORAL SOLUTION, TABLETS**
**Adults.** *Initial:* 1,000 mg t.i.d. Dosage increased by 500 mg/day q 2 to 4 wk, as needed. *Maintenance:* 1 to 2 g t.i.d. *Maximum:* 6 g/day.
DOSAGE ADJUSTMENT To reduce or prevent facial flushing, initial dosage reduced to 100 mg/day (tab) or 500 mg/day (E.R. tab), and then gradually increased to 3 to 4 g/day.

*To treat vitamin B₆ deficiency*
**E.R. CAPSULES, TABLETS**
**Adults and children.** Dosage individualized based on severity of deficiency, as prescribed.
**E.R. TABLETS**
**Adults.** Dosage individualized based on severity of deficiency, as prescribed.
**I.V. INFUSION**
**Adults and children.** Dosage individualized as part of total parenteral nutrition.

**PARENTERAL ADMINISTRATION GUIDELINES**

•Rotate sites for I.M. administration of vitamin B₁ to help prevent tenderness and induration that may occur following administration.
•I.M. administration may be painful; use the Z-track method of administration
•Because of incompatibilities, don't add parenteral vitamin B₁ to alkaline or neutral solutions; also, don't mix it with oxidizing and reducing agents, including barbiturates, carbonates, citrates, and copper
•Take precautions to protect vitamin B₁ solution from exposure to light because it's light sensitive.

•Be aware that I.V. administration of vitamin B₃ may cause CNS or CV adverse reactions, such as arrhythmias, dizziness, headache, peripheral vasodilation, and syncope. Rate of I.V. administration shouldn't exceed 2 mg/min, regardless of method of I.V. administration.
•Vitamin B₃ must be diluted for I.V. administration. For direct injection, dilute to a concentration of 2 mg/ml; for intermittent or continuous infusion, dilute dose in 500 ml of NS or other compatible solution
•Give I.M. injection following routine I.M. administration guidelines. Vitamin B₃ doesn't need to be diluted for I.M. injection.
•Be aware that parenteral administration shouldn't be used to treat hyperlipidemia.

•Be aware that S.C. or I.M. administration of vitamin B₆ may cause injection site burning or stinging. Before giving injection, alert patient that this adverse effect may occur.
•Know that I.V. administration is given as part of a multivitamin solution; follow the guidelines for administering an I.V. multivitamin solution as recommended for the product being used.

*(continued)*

## Vitamins (continued)

| GENERIC AND TRADE NAMES | RECOMMENDED DAILY INTAKE |
|---|---|
| **vitamin B₆** *(continued)* | **Adult men and boys age 11 and older.** 1.7 to 2 mg/day.<br>**Adult women and girls age 11 and older.** 1.4 to 1.6 mg/day.<br>**Pregnant women.** 2.2 mg/day.<br>**Breast-feeding women.** 2.1 mg/day.<br>**Children ages 7 to 10.** 1.4 mg/day.<br>**Children ages 4 to 6.** 1.1 mg/day.<br>**Neonates and children to age 3.** 0.3 to 1 mg/day. |
| **vitamin B₉**<br>**(folic acid)**<br>Apo-Folic (CAN), Folvite, Novo-Folacid (CAN) | **Adult men and boys age 11 and older.** 150 to 400 mcg/day. (150 to 220 mcg/day [CAN].)<br>**Adult women and girls age 11 and older.** 150 to 400 mcg/day. (145 to 190 mcg/day [CAN].)<br>**Pregnant women.** 400 to 800 mcg/day. (445 to 475 mcg/day [CAN].)<br>**Breast-feeding women.** 260 to 800 mcg/day. (245 to 275 mcg/day [CAN].)<br>**Children ages 7 to 11.** 100 to 400 mcg/day. (125 to 180 mcg/day [CAN].)<br>**Children ages 4 to 7.** 75 to 400 mcg/day. (90 mcg/day [CAN].)<br>**Neonates and children to age 4.** 25 mcg/day. (50 to 80 mcg/day [CAN].) |
| **vitamin B₁₂**<br>**(cyanocobalamin, hydroxycobalamin)** | **Adults age 19 and older.** 2.4 mcg/day.<br>**Pregnant women.** 2.6 mcg/day.<br>**Breast-feeding women.** 2.8 mcg/day.<br>**Adolescents ages 14 to 19.** 2.4 mcg/day.<br>**Children ages 9 to 14.** 1.8 mcg/day.<br>**Children ages 4 to 9.** 1.2 mcg/day.<br>**Children ages 1 to 4.** 0.9 mcg/day.<br>**Infants ages 6 to 12 months.** 0.4 mcg/day.<br>**Neonates and infants to 6 months.** 0.5 mcg/day. |

## OTHER INDICATIONS AND DOSAGES

*To treat pyridoxine dependency syndrome*
**I.V. OR I.M. INJECTION**
**Adults and children age 11 and older.** 30 to 600 mg q.d.
**Infants with seizures.** *Initial:* 10 to 100 mg, then individualized based on severity of deficiency, as prescribed.

*To treat drug-induced pyridoxine deficiency*
**I.V. OR I.M. INJECTION**
**Adults and children age 11 and older.** 50 to 200 mg/day for 3 wk, then 25 to 100 mg/day, as needed.

*To treat vitamin B$_9$ deficiency*
**TABLETS**
**Adults and children.** Dosage individualized based on severity of deficiency, as prescribed.
**I.V. INFUSION, I.M. OR S.C. INJECTION**
**Adults and children.** 0.25 to 1 mg q.d. until hematologic response occurs.

*To treat vitamin B$_{12}$ deficiency caused by nutritional intake imbalance (not for use to treat pernicious anemia)*
**LOZENGES, TABLETS**
**Adults and children.** Dosage individualized based on severity of deficiency, as prescribed.

*To treat vitamin B$_{12}$ deficiency caused by pernicious anemia; malabsorption disorders (tropical or nontropical sprue, partial or total gastrectomy, regional enteritis, gastroenterostomy, ileal resection); or malignancies, granulomas, strictures, or anastomoses involving the ileum.*
**S.C. INJECTION (CYANOCOBALAMIN)**
**Adults.** *Initial:* 30 mcg q.d. for 5 to 10 days, then switched to I.M. administration for maintenance therapy.

## PARENTERAL ADMINISTRATION GUIDELINES

• Vitamin B$_6$ may increase AST (SGOT) levels. Be aware that at least one manufacturer warns against I.V. administration of vitamin B$_6$ to patients with heart disease.
• Take precautions to protect vitamin B$_6$ solution from exposure to light because it's light sensitive.

• Be aware that some vitamin B$_9$ solutions contain benzyl alcohol. Don't administer these solutions to neonates or immature infants because of a risk of fatal toxic syndrome, which may include CNS, respiratory, circulatory, and renal impairment and metabolic acidosis.
• Unless ordered otherwise, dilute 5 mg/ml of vitamin B$_9$ with with 49 ml of sterile water for injection to provide a solution containing 0.1 mg of vitamin/ml.
• Know that parenteral administration may cause anaphylaxis. Parenteral administration should be used only in patients with severe vitamin deficiency or in those with severely impaired GI absorption.
• Be aware that S.C. administration should be injected deeply.
• Take precautions to protect vitamin B$_9$ solution from exposure to light because it's light sensitive.

• Be aware that parenteral vitamin B$_{12}$ solution is incompatible with many drugs, including ascorbic acid, chlorpromazine hydrochloride, dextrose, heavy metals, phytonadione, prochlorperazine edisylate, warfarin sodium, oxidizing or reducing agents, and alkaline or strongly acidic solutions. Do not administer vitamin with other drugs.
• Know that both cyanocobalamin and hydroxycobalamin may be administered by I.M. injection, but only cyanocobalamin may be administered as an S.C. injection. Be alert to which form is being administered to ensure correct route of administration.

*(continued)*

## Vitamins (continued)

| GENERIC AND TRADE NAMES | RECOMMENDED DAILY INTAKE |
|---|---|
| **vitamin B$_{12}$** *(continued)* | **Adults age 19 and older.** 2.4 mcg/day.<br>**Pregnant women.** 2.6 mcg/day.<br>**Breast-feeding women.** 2.8 mcg/day.<br>**Adolescents ages 14 to 19.** 2.4 mcg/day.<br>**Children ages 9 to 14.** 1.8 mcg/day.<br>**Children ages 4 to 9.** 1.2 mcg/day.<br>**Children ages 1 to 4.** 0.9 mcg/day.<br>**Infants ages 6 to 12 months.** 0.4 mcg/day.<br>**Neonates and infants to 6 months.** 0.5 mcg/day. |
| **vitamin C**<br>**(ascorbic acid)**<br>Ascorbic Acid, Cecon Drops, Cenolate, Cevi-Bid, Vicks Vitamin C Drops | **Adult men.** 90 mg/day.<br>**Adult women.** 75 mg/day.<br>**Pregnant women age 19 and older.** 85 mg/day.<br>**Breast-feeding women age 19 and older.** 120 mg/day.<br>**Adolescent boys ages 14 to 19.** 75 mg/day.<br>**Adolescent girls ages 14 to 19.** 65 mg/day.<br>**Pregnant girls ages 14 to 19.** 80 mg/day.<br>**Breast-feeding girls ages 14 to 19.** 115 mg/day.<br>**Children ages 9 to 14.** 45 mg/day.<br>**Children ages 4 to 9.** 25 mg/day.<br>**Children ages 1 to 4.** 15 mg/day.<br>**Infants ages 7 to 12 months.** 50 mg/day.<br>**Neonates and infants to age 7 months.** 40 mg/day.<br>DOSAGE ADJUSTMENT Recommended daily intake for people who smoke is 100 mg/day because of an increased utilization of vitamin C. Recommended daily intake should be increased to promote wound healing and for those with a chronic illness, fever, hemovascular disorder, or infection; the amount of vitamin C increase depends on the severity of the underlying condition. |

## OTHER INDICATIONS AND DOSAGES

## PARENTERAL ADMINISTRATION GUIDELINES

**Children.** *Initial:* 1,000 to 5,000 mcg given in single daily doses of 100 mcg over 2 or more wk. *Maintenance:* 60 or more mcg/mo.

**I.M. INJECTION (CYANOCOBALAMIN OR HYDROXYCOBALAMIN)**

**Adults.** *Initial:* 30 mcg q.d. for 5 to 10 days. *Maintenance:* 100 to 200 mcg q mo.

**Children.** *Initial:* 1,000 to 5,000 mcg, given in single daily doses of 100 mcg over 2 or more wk. *Maintenance:* 60 or more mcg/mo.

**DOSAGE ADJUSTMENT** Dosage adjusted, as needed, to maintain normal hematologic morphology and an erythrocyte count greater than 4.5 million/mm$^3$.

*To treat familial selective B$_{12}$ malabsorption*

**I.M. INJECTION (CYANOCOBALAMIN)**

**Adults.** *Initial.* 1 mg/wk for 3 wk. *Maintenance:* 250 mcg/mo.

*To treat hereditary deficiency of transcobalamin II*

**I.M. INJECTION (CYANOCOBALAMIN)**

**Adults.** 1 to 2 mg/wk.

• Be aware that S.C. administration of cyanocobalamin should be injected deeply.
• Know that vitamin B$_{12}$ is excreted more rapidly after I.V. injection; I.V. administration isn't recommended.
• Take precautions to protect vitamin B$_{12}$ solution from exposure to light because it's light sensitive.

*To treat vitamin C deficiency (scurvy)*

**E.R. CAPSULES; LOZENGES; ORAL SOLUTION; E.R. TABLETS; TABLETS; S.C., I.M., OR I.V. INJECTION**

**Adults.** 100 to 250 mg q.d. or b.i.d. until skeletal changes and signs and symptoms of hemorrhagic disorder are reversed (usually within 2 to 21 days).

**ORAL SOLUTION; TABLETS; S.C., I.M., OR I.V. INJECTION**

**Infants and children.** 100 to 300 mg/day in divided doses until skeletal changes and signs and symptoms of hemorrhagic disorder are reversed (usually within days).

• Be aware that I.M. injection is the preferred parenteral route for administering vitamin C, although it may be administered I.V. or S.C. when necessary.
• Rotate sites for I.M. and S.C. administration to help prevent transient mild soreness that may occur following administration. Inform patient that this adverse effect may occur.
• If giving I.V. vitamin C, avoid rapid administration to prevent faintness or dizziness.
• Administer vitamin C solution by itself because it's incompatible with many drugs.
• Be aware that vitamin C solution rapidly oxidizes in air and in alkaline solutions. Take precautions to protect vitamin solution from exposure to air and light.
• Open vitamin C ampules carefully because increased pressure may develop after prolonged storage.

*(continued)*

## Vitamins (continued)

| GENERIC AND TRADE NAMES | RECOMMENDED DAILY INTAKE |
|---|---|
| **vitamin D$_2$** **(ergocalciferol)** Calciferol, Calciferol Drops, Drisdol, Drisdol Drops, Ostoforte (CAN), Radiostol Forte (CAN) | **Adults and children ages 11 and older.** 200 to 400 IU/day. (100 to 200 IU/day [CAN].) **Pregnant and breast-feeding women.** 400 IU/day. (200 to 300 IU/day [CAN].) **Children ages 7 to 11.** 400 IU/day. (100 to 200 IU/day [CAN].) **Children ages 4 to 7.** 400 IU/day. (200 IU/day [CAN].) **Neonates and children to age 4.** 300 to 400 IU/day. (200 to 400 IU/day [CAN].) |
| **vitamin E** **(alpha tocopherol)** Amino-Opti-E, Aquasol E, E-Complex 600, E-Vitamin succinate, Liqui-E, Pheryl E, Vita-Plus E, Webber Vitamin E (CAN) | **Adult men and adolescent boys.** 16.7 IU/day. (10 to 16.7 IU/day [CAN].) **Adult women and adolescent girls.** 13 IU/day. (8.3 to 11.7 IU/day [CAN].) **Pregnant women.** 16.7 IU/day. (13 to 15 IU/day [CAN].) **Breast-feeding women.** 18 to 20 IU/day. (15 to 16.7 IU/day [CAN].) **Children ages 7 to 10.** 11.7 IU/day. (10 to 13 IU/day [CAN].) **Children ages 4 to 7.** 11.7 IU/day. (8.3 IU/day [CAN].) **Infants and children to age 4.** 5 to 10 IU/day. (5 to 6.7 IU/day [CAN].) |

## OTHER INDICATIONS AND DOSAGES

### PARENTERAL ADMINISTRATION GUIDELINES

*To treat vitamin $D_2$ deficiency*
CAPSULES, ORAL SOLUTION, TABLETS
**Adults and children.** Dosage individualized based on severity of deficiency, as prescribed.

*To treat vitamin D-resistant rickets*
CAPSULES, ORAL SOLUTION, TABLETS
**Adults.** 12,000 to 150,000 IU q.d.

*To treat vitamin D-dependent rickets*
CAPSULES, ORAL SOLUTION, TABLETS
**Adults.** 10,000 to 60,000 IU q.d. *Maximum:* 150,000 IU q.d.
**Children.** 3,000 to 10,000 IU q.d. *Maximum:* 50,000 IU q.d.

*To treat osteomalacia caused by long-term anticonvulsant use*
CAPSULES, ORAL SOLUTION, TABLETS
**Adults.** 1,000 to 4,000 IU q.d.
**Children.** 1,000 IU q.d.

*To treat familial hypophosphatemia*
CAPSULES
**Adults.** 50,000 to 100,000 IU q.d.

*To treat hypoparathyroidism*
CAPSULES
**Adults.** 50,000 to 150,000 IU q.d.
**Children.** 50,000 to 200,000 IU q.d.

*To treat intestinal malabsorption*
I.M. INJECTION
**Adults and children.** 10,000 IU q.d.

•Be aware that vitamin $D_2$ is usually given orally. However, I.M. injection may be required for patients with GI, liver, or biliary disease associated with malabsorption of vitamin D analogs.
Take precautions to protect parenteral vitamin $D_2$ solution from exposure to light because light causes it to decompose.

*To treat vitamin E deficiency*
CAPSULES (ADULTS ONLY), ORAL SOLUTION, TABLETS
**Adults and children.** Dosage individualized based on severity of deficiency, as prescribed.

*Vitamin E isn't administered parenterally.*

*(continued)*

## Vitamins (continued)

| GENERIC AND TRADE NAMES | RECOMMENDED DAILY INTAKE |
|---|---|
| **vitamin K$_1$**<br>**(phytonadione)**<br>AquaMEPHYTON, Mephyton | *Recommended daily intake hasn't been established for vitamin K$_1$. However, adequate intake is suggested as follows:*<br>**Adult men age 19 and older.** 120 mcg/day.<br>**Adult women age 19 and older, pregnant and breast-feeding women.** 90 mcg/day.<br>**Adolescents ages 14 to 19.** 75 mcg/day.<br>**Children ages 9 to 14.** 60 mcg/day.<br>**Children ages 4 to 9.** 55 mcg/day.<br>**Children ages 1 to 4.** 30 mcg/day.<br>**Infants ages 7 to 12 months.** 2.5 mcg/day.<br>**Neonates and infants to age 7 months.** 2 mcg/day. |

## OTHER INDICATIONS AND DOSAGES

*To prevent hypoprothrombinemia during prolonged use of total parenteral nutrition*
**I.M. INJECTION**
**Adults.** 5 to 10 mg/wk.
**Children.** 2 to 5 mg/wk.

*To prevent hypoprothrombinemia in infants with diets deficient in vitamin K (less than 100 mcg/L)*
**I.M. INJECTION**
**Infants.** 1 mg/mo.

*To treat anticoagulant-induced hypoprothrombinemia*
**TABLETS, I.M. OR S.C. INJECTION**
**Adults.** 2.5 to 25 mg, repeated 12 to 48 hr after P.O. dose or 6 to 8 hr after S.C. or I.M. dose, as prescribed. *Maximum:* 50 mg/dose.
**Children.** 2.5 to 10 mg S.C. or I.M., repeated in 6 to 8 hr, as prescribed.
**Infants.** 1 to 2 mg S.C. or I.M., repeated in 4 to 8 hr, as prescribed.

*To treat hypoprothrombinemia from other causes*
**TABLETS, I.M. OR S.C. INJECTION**
**Adults.** 2 to 25 mg. *Usual:* 25 mg. *Maximum:* 50 mg/dose.
**Children.** 5 to 10 mg S.C. or I.M.
**Infants.** 2 mg S.C. or I.M.

*To prevent hemorrhagic disease in neonates*
**I.M. OR S.C. INJECTION**
**Neonates.** 0.5 to 1 mg within 1 hr after birth, repeated in 6 to 8 hr, as prescribed.

*To treat hemorrhagic disease in neonates*
**I.M. OR S.C. INJECTION**
**Neonates.** 1 mg (or higher dose if mother took an oral anticoagulant or anticonvulsant during pregnancy).

## PARENTERAL ADMINISTRATION GUIDELINES

• Be aware that severe adverse reactions, including anaphylaxis, cardiac and respiratory arrest, hypersensitivity, and shock, may occur during or immediately after I.M. or I.V. administration of vitamin $K_1$, even if it's diluted to avoid rapid infusion. Administer vitamin by S.C. route whenever possible.
• If vitamin $K_1$ must be administered I.V., do not exceed rate of 1 mg/min, as prescribed.
• Be aware that some vitamin $K_1$ solutions contain benzyl alcohol. Don't administer these solutions to neonates or immature infants because of a risk of fatal toxic syndrome, which may include CNS, respiratory, circulatory, and renal impairment and metabolic acidosis.
• Take precautions to protect vitamin $K_1$ solution from exposure to light because it's light sensitive.

## Interferons

Interferons are classified as biological response modifiers or antineoplastics. They fall into three major categories—alpha, beta, and gamma—which are described below.

The chart on the following pages lists the trade names, indications, usual adult dosages, adverse reactions, and nursing considerations for these interferons.

### Interferon alpha

Highly purified proteins produced by a recombinant DNA process, drugs in this category exhibit antiviral and antitumor activity. Antiviral activity depends on their inhibition of viral protein synthesis. Antitumor activity results from their ability to exert a cytostatic effect, reducing the rate of cell proliferation by delaying RNA and protein production. This delay induces cells to enter a resting stage. These drugs also increase the activity of human natural killer (NK) cells, which have the ability to lyse certain tumor cells and normal targets. They also selectively increase the number of cytotoxic T-cells, thereby affecting tumor growth. Phagocytic activity of macrophages also is increased.

INTERFERON ALFACON

This specific form of interferon is produced by fermentation of genetically engineered *Escherichia coli*. It's structurally and functionally related to interferon beta and has greater biological activity than other interferon alfas.

### Interferon beta

Produced by fibroblasts and epithelial cells, drugs in this category neutralize the activity of endoge-

| GENERIC AND TRADE NAMES | INDICATIONS AND USUAL ADULT DOSAGES |
| --- | --- |
| **Interferon alpha drugs** | |
| **peginterferon alfa-2a** PEGASYS | *As monotherapy to treat patients with chronic heptatitis C who have compensated liver disease and have never received an interferon alpha:* 180 mcg/wk S.C. for 48 wk. |
| | *As adjunct to treat patients with chronic hepatitis C who have compensated liver disease and have never received an interferon alpha:* 180 mcg/wk S.C. with ribavirin (Copegus) 800 to 1,200 mg/day P.O. in 2 divided doses with food for 48 wk. |
| **peginterferon alfa-2b** PEG-Intron | *As monotherapy to treat patients with chronic hepatitis C who have compensated liver disease and have never received an interferon alpha:* 1 mcg/kg/wk S.C. for 1 year. |
| | *As adjunct to treat patients with chronic hepatitis C who have compensated liver disease and have never received an interferon alpha:* 1.5 mcg/kg/wk S.C. with ribavirin 800 mg/day P.O. in 2 divided doses. |
| **recombinant interferon alfa-2a** Roferon-A | *To treat hairy cell leukemia:* 3 million U/day I.M. or S.C. for 16 to 24 wk, followed by 3 million U 3 times/wk for maintenance. |
| | *To treat AIDS-associated Kaposi's sarcoma:* 36 million U/day I.M. or S.C. for 10 to 12 wk; alternatively, 3 million U/day I.M. or S.C. on days 1 to 3, 9 million U/day on days 4 to 6, 18 million U/day on days 7 to 9, and 36 million U/day for remainder of 10- to 12-wk induction period, followed by 36 million U 3 times/wk for maintenance. |
| **recombinant interferon alfa-2b** Intron A | *To treat hairy cell leukemia:* 2 million U/m$^2$ I.M. or S.C. 3 times/wk. |

nous interferon gamma (IFNG), the substance believed to be responsible for triggering the autoimmune process that leads to multiple sclerosis. In multiple sclerosis, an initial viral infection may stimulate IFNG production by T-lymphocytes. Then IFNG induces macrophages to produce proteinases that degrade the myelin sheath around the spinal cord. Cytotoxic T-cells then move to the site of inflammation, recognizing antigens as receptor sites, where they attack the tissue affected by IFNG, resulting in progressive neurologic dysfunction. Interferon beta drugs interfere with IFNG production by lymphocytes and the mRNA transcription caused by IFNG. As a result, cytotoxic T-cells can't locate receptor sites and cause further damage in the CNS.

## Interferon gamma

Produced from genetically engineered *Escherichia coli,* this type of interferon is chemically and therapeutically distinct from interferon alpha. Drugs in this category have potent phagocyte-activating properties. By enhancing oxidative metabolism, they produce toxic oxygen metabolites in phagocytes, which permits more efficient killing of certain fungi, bacteria, and protozoal microbes. Enhanced antibody-dependent cellular cytotoxicity and NK-cell activity reduce the risk of developing a serious infection in patients with chronic disease. These drugs also stimulate production of cytokines, such as interleukin-1-beta, and regulate the immune system by suppressing the IgE level and inhibiting collagen production.

| ADVERSE REACTIONS | NURSING CONSIDERATIONS |
|---|---|
| **CNS:** Dizziness, fatigue, headache<br>**CV:** Hypotension<br>**EENT:** Dry mouth<br>**GI:** Anorexia, diarrhea, hepatotoxicity, nausea, vomiting<br>**HEME:** Anemia, leukopenia, thrombocytopenia<br>**SKIN:** Alopecia, rash<br>**Other:** Flulike symptoms | •Use interferon alpha drugs cautiously in patients with renal impairment and in elderly patients.<br>•Be aware that cross-sensitivity may occur among interferon alpha drugs.<br>•Be aware that interferon alpha drugs aren't interchangeable.<br>•Be aware that patients who are sensitive to mouse immunoglobulin also may be sensitive to recombinant interferon alfa-2a.<br>•Unless contraindicated, ensure that patient is well hydrated at the start of and throughout therapy to reduce the risk of hypotension.<br>•Reconstitute by adding 3 ml of diluent provided by manufacturer and swirling gently to dissolve.<br>•Be aware that reconstitution of peginterferon alfa-2a and interferon alfa-n3 is not necessary.<br>•Don't shake vial.<br>•Be aware that cross-sensitivity with interferon alfa-n3 to mouse immunoglobulin, egg protein, or neomycin may occur.<br>•WARNING Because interferon alpha drugs may cause or aggravate fatal or life-threatening autoimmune, ischemic, infectious, or neuropsychiatric disorders, monitor patient periodically with clinical and laboratory evaluations and expect drug to be discontinued if he develops severe or worsening signs and symptoms of these conditions.<br>•Obtain CBC before and regularly during treatment, as ordered, because interferon alpha drugs may cause bone marrow suppression. Expect drug to be discontinued if patient develops severe decreases in platelet or neutrophil count.<br>•Implement bleeding and infection-control measures, according to facility policy. |

*(continued)*

## Interferons (continued)

| GENERIC AND TRADE NAMES | INDICATIONS AND USUAL ADULT DOSAGES |
|---|---|
| **Interferon alpha drugs** (continued) | |
| **recombinant interferon alfa-2b**<br>Intron A<br>(continued) | *To treat condyloma acuminatum:* 1 million U (using only the 10-million U/ml strength) intralesionally at base of wart (up to 5 warts/course) 3 times/wk on alternate days for 3 wk. If response is inadequate 12 to 16 wk after initial treatment, repeat course, as prescribed.<br><br>*To treat AIDS-associated Kaposi's sarcoma:* 30 million U/$m^2$ (using 50 million-U/ml strength) I.M. or S.C. 3 times/wk.<br><br>*To treat chronic, active hepatitis B and C:* 3 million U I.M. or S.C. 3 times/wk. *To treat chronic hepatitis B:* 5 million U/day or 10 million U 3 times/wk I.M. or S.C. for 16 wk.<br><br>*To treat malignant melanoma:* 20 million U/$m^2$ as I.V. infusion for 5 consecutive days/wk for 4 wk, followed by 10 million U/$m^2$ S.C. 3 times/wk for 48 wk. |
| **interferon alfa-n3**<br>Alferon N | *To treat condyloma acuminatum:* 250,000 U intralesionally at base of wart 2 times/wk for up to 8 wk. |
| **Interferon alfacon drugs** | |
| **interferon alfacon-1**<br>Infergen | *To treat chronic, active hepatitis C:* 9 mcg S.C. 3 times/wk, at intervals of at least 48 hours, for 24 wk. If inadequate response or relapse occurs, 15 mcg 3 times/wk for 6 mo. |
| **Interferon beta drugs** | |
| **interferon beta-1a**<br>Avonex | *To treat initial attack or relapsing forms of multiple sclerosis:* 30 mcg I.M. once/wk. |
| Rebif | *To treat relapsing forms of multiple sclerosis:* 44 mcg S.C. 3 times/wk. |
| **interferon beta-1b**<br>Betaseron | *To treat relapsing forms of multiple sclerosis:* 0.25 mg S.C. q.o.d. |

| ADVERSE REACTIONS | NURSING CONSIDERATIONS |
|---|---|
| **CNS:** Fatigue, headache<br>**GI:** Diarrhea, nausea, vomiting<br>**HEME:** Leukopenia<br>**SKIN:** Rash<br>**Other:** Flulike symptoms | •Use gamma interferon cautiously in patients previously exposed to cytotoxic drugs or radiation therapy.<br>•Be aware that cross-sensitivity may occur with *Escherichia coli–*derived products.<br>•Discard vial if left at room temperature for more than 12 hours.<br>•Implement bleeding and infection-control measures, according to facility policy.<br>•Administer acetaminophen, as prescribed, to prevent or treat headache and fever. |
| **CNS:** Anxiety, confusion, decreased concentration, depression, insomnia, nervousness<br>**EENT:** Abnormal vision<br>**HEME:** Leukopenia, thrombocytopenia | •Be aware that use of interferon alfacon-1 isn't recommended for patients with autoimmune hepatitis or psychiatric disorders.<br>•Be aware that cross-sensitivity may occur with other interferon alfa drugs or *Escherichia coli–*derived products.<br>•Don't shake vial.<br>•Implement bleeding and infection-control measures, according to facility policy.<br>•Monitor patient for signs and symptoms of vision abnormalities. |
| **CNS:** Fatigue, headache, weakness<br>**GI:** Diarrhea, nausea<br>**HEME:** Anemia, unusual bleeding or bruising<br>**Other:** Flulike symptoms, infection | •Use beta interferons with extreme caution in patients with depression or seizure disorder.<br>•Be aware that cross-sensitivity may occur with natural or recombinant interferon beta or human albumin.<br>•Reconstitute following manufacturer's directions and refrigerate. Use interferon beta-1a within 6 hours of reconstitution. Use interferon beta-1b within 3 hours of reconstitution.<br>•Implement bleeding and infection-control measures, according to facility policy. |

*(continued)*

## Interferons (continued)

| GENERIC AND TRADE NAMES | INDICATIONS AND USUAL ADULT DOSAGES |
|---|---|
| **Interferon gamma drugs** | |
| **interferon gamma-1b**<br>Actimmune | *To treat chronic granulomatous disease or to delay progression of severe, malignant osteopetrosis in patients with body surface area greater than 0.5 m²:* 50 mcg/m² (1 million IU/m²) S.C. 3 times/wk.<br><br>*To treat chronic granulomatous disease or to delay progression of severe, malignant osteopetrosis in patients with body surface area of 0.5 m² or less:* 1.5 mcg/kg/dose S.C. 3 times/wk. |

| ADVERSE REACTIONS | NURSING CONSIDERATIONS |
|---|---|
| **CNS:** Fatigue, headache<br>**GI:** Diarrhea, nausea, vomiting<br>**HEME:** Leukopenia<br>**SKIN:** Rash<br>**Other:** Flulike symptoms | •Use gamma interferon cautiously in patients previously exposed to cytotoxic drugs or radiation therapy.<br>•Be aware that cross-sensitivity may occur with *Escherichia coli*–derived products.<br>•Discard vial if left at room temperature for more than 12 hours.<br>•Implement bleeding and infection-control measures, according to facility policy.<br>•Administer acetaminophen, as prescribed, to prevent or treat headache and fever. |

# Compatible Drugs in a Syringe

The chart below lets you know at a glance whether particular drugs are compatible for at least 15 minutes when mixed together in a syringe for immediate administration. However, keep in mind that drugs listed as compatible when mixed in a syringe may not be compatible when prepared for other routes of administration. Drug combinations prepared for immediate administration usually require a more concentrated solution than those prepared for infusion.

(**Key:** C = Compatible; I = Incompatible; n/a = Compatibility information not available; no recommendations can be given.)

| | atropine | chlorpromazine | dexamethasone | diazepam | diphenhydramine | droperidol | furosemide | glycopyrrolate | haloperidol | heparin | hydromorphone |
|---|---|---|---|---|---|---|---|---|---|---|---|
| atropine | | C | n/a | n/a | C | C | n/a | C | I | n/a | C |
| chlorpromazine | C | | n/a | n/a | C | C | n/a | C | n/a | I | C |
| dexamethasone | n/a | n/a | | n/a | I | n/a | n/a | n/a | n/a | n/a | C |
| diazepam | n/a | n/a | n/a | | n/a | n/a | n/a | I | n/a | I | n/a |
| diphenhydramine | C | C | I | n/a | | C | n/a | C | I | n/a | C |
| droperidol | C | C | n/a | n/a | C | | I | C | n/a | I | n/a |
| furosemide | n/a | n/a | n/a | n/a | n/a | I | | n/a | n/a | C | n/a |
| glycopyrrolate | C | C | I | C | C | C | n/a | | C | n/a | C |
| haloperidol | n/a | n/a | n/a | n/a | C | n/a | n/a | n/a | | I | C |
| heparin | C | I | n/a | I | n/a | I | C | n/a | I | | n/a |
| hydromorphone | C | C | n/a | n/a | C | n/a | n/a | C | C | n/a | |
| hydroxyzine | C | C | n/a | n/a | C | C | n/a | C | I | n/a | C |
| ketorolac | n/a | n/a | n/a | I | n/a | n/a | n/a | n/a | I | n/a | I |
| lidocaine | n/a | n/a | n/a | n/a | n/a | n/a | n/a | C | n/a | C | n/a |
| lorazepam | n/a | n/a | n/a | n/a | n/a | n/a | n/a | n/a | n/a | n/a | C |
| meperidine | C | C | n/a | C | C | C | n/a | C | n/a | I | n/a |
| metoclopramide | C | C | n/a | n/a | C | C | I | n/a | n/a | C | C |
| midazolam | C | C | n/a | n/a | C | n/a | n/a | C | C | n/a | C |
| morphine | C | C | n/a | n/a | C | C | n/a | C | I | C* | n/a |
| pentobarbital | C | I | n/a | n/a | I | I | n/a | I | n/a | n/a | C |
| prochlorperazine | C | n/a | n/a | n/a | C | C | n/a | C | n/a | n/a | I |
| ranitidine | C | I | C | n/a | C | n/a | n/a | C | n/a | n/a | C |
| scopolamine | C | C | n/a | n/a | C | C | n/a | C | n/a | n/a | C |

* Compatible only with morphine doses of 1 mg, 2 mg, and 5 mg.

| hydroxyzine | ketorolac | lidocaine | lorazepam | meperidine | metoclopramide | midazolam | morphine | pentobarbital | prochlorperazine | ranitidine | scopolamine |
|---|---|---|---|---|---|---|---|---|---|---|---|
| C | n/a | n/a | n/a | C | C | C | C | C | C | C | C |
| C | n/a | n/a | n/a | C | C | C | I | I | C | C | C |
| n/a | n/a | n/a | n/a | n/a | C | n/a | n/a | n/a | n/a | C | n/a |
| n/a | I | n/a | n/a | n/a | n/a | n/a | n/a | n/a | n/a | I | n/a |
| C | n/a | n/a | n/a | C | C | C | C | I | C | C | C |
| C | n/a | n/a | n/a | C | C | C | C | I | C | n/a | C |
| n/a | n/a | n/a | n/a | n/a | I | n/a | n/a | n/a | n/a | n | n/a |
| C | n/a | C | n/a | C | n/a | C | C | I | C | C | C |
| I | I | n/a | n/a | n/a | n/a | n/a | I | n/a | n/a | n/a | n/a |
| n/a | n/a | C | n/a | I | C | n/a | C | n/a | n/a | n | n/a |
| C | I | n/a | C | n/a | n/a | C | n/a | C | I | C | C |
|  | I | C | n/a | C | C | C | C | I | C | C | C |
| I |  | n/a | n/a | n/a | n/a | n/a | n/a | n/a | I | n/a | n/a |
| C | n/a |  | n/a | n/a | C | n/a | n/a | n/a | n/a | n/a | n/a |
| n/a | n/a | n/a |  | n/a | n/a | n/a | n/a | n/a | n/a | I | n/a |
| C | n/a | n/a | n/a |  | C | C | I | I | C | C | C |
| n/a | n/a | C | n/a | C |  | C | C | n/a | C | C | C |
| C | n/a | n/a | n/a | C | C |  | C | I | I | I | C |
| C | n/a | n/a | n/a | n/a | C | C |  | I | C | C | C |
| I | n/a | n/a | n/a | I | I | I | I |  | I | I | C |
| C | I | n/a | n/a | C | C | I | C | I |  | C | C |
| I | n/a | n/a | I | C | C | I | C | I | C |  | C |
| C | n/a | n/a | n/a | C | C | C | C | C | C | C |  |

# Drug Formulas and Calculations

When administering drugs, you must be familiar with drug formulas and calculation methods to ensure that your patient receives the prescribed drug in the correct dosage, strength, or flow rate. This appendix will provide you with a quick review of how to calculate the strength of a solution, drug dosages, and I.V. flow rates.

## Calculating the Strength of a Solution

Most solutions come prepared in the required strength by the pharmacy or medical supply source. But sometimes only the concentrated form is available, and you'll need to dilute the solution or solid to administer the prescribed strength.

When a solid form of a drug is used to prepare a solution, the drug must be completely dissolved. Solid drug forms, such as tablets, crystals, and powders, are considered 100% strength. (An exception to this is boric acid, which is only 5% at full strength.) The final diluted solution is stated in terms of liquid measurement. To prepare a solution, you'll need to add the prescribed solid or liquid form of the drug (the solute) to the prescribed amount of diluent (the solvent). Two of the most common diluents used in the clinical setting are normal saline solution and sterile water.

You can use two formulas to calculate the strength of a solution, as shown in the examples below.

### Method 1: Calculating percentage and volume
Use the following formula:

$$\frac{\text{Weaker solution}}{\text{Stronger solution}} = \frac{\text{Solute}}{\text{Solvent}}$$

*Example:* You need to dilute a stock solution of 100% strength to a 5% solution. How much solute will you need to add to obtain 500 ml of the 5% solution?

Calculate as follows:

$$\frac{5\ (\%)\ \text{(weaker solution)}}{100\ (\%)\ \text{(stronger solution)}} = \frac{X\ (g)\ \text{(solute)}}{500\ \text{ml (solvent)}}$$

$$100\ X = (500)(5)\ \text{or}\ 2{,}500$$

$$X = 25\ g$$

*Answer:* You'll need to add 25 g of solute to each 500 ml of solvent to prepare a 5% solution.

### Method 2: Calculating percentage and volume
Use the following formula:

$$\frac{\text{(Desired strength)}}{\text{(Available strength)}} \times \frac{\text{Total amount of}}{\text{desired solution}} = X\ \frac{\text{(amount of undiluted drug}}{\text{needed to make solution)}}$$

*Example:* You need to make 100 ml of a 20% solution, using an 80% solution. How much of the 80% solution must you add to the sterile water to yield a final volume of 100 ml of a 20% solution?

Calculate as follows:

$$\frac{20\ (\%)\ \text{(Desired strength)}}{80\ (\%)\ \text{(Available strength)}} \times \frac{100\ \text{ml (Total amount}}{\text{of desired solution)}} = X$$

$$\frac{0.20}{0.80} = 0.25$$

$$0.25 \times 100\ \text{(ml)} = X$$

$$X = 25\ \text{ml of 80\% solution}$$

*Answer:* You'll need to add 25 ml of the 80% solution to the water to make a final volume of 100 ml of a 20% solution.

## Drug Formulas and Calculations (continued)

## Calculating Drug Dosages

You may be required to calculate drug dosages when you need to administer a drug that's available only in one measure, but prescribed in another. You should also be prepared to convert various units of measure, such as milligrams (mg) to grains (gr), and dry measurements to liquid. You can use three common methods of ratio and proportion to calculate drug dosages, as shown in the examples below.

### CALCULATING ORAL DRUG DOSAGES

*Example:* You need to give a patient 0.25 mg of digoxin, which comes only in 0.125-mg tablets. How many tablets will you need to give him to attain the proper dosage?

### Method 1: Using labeled amount of drug

In this method, true proportions between the drug label and the prescribed dose are used to determine ratio and proportion. The drug label, which states the amount of drug in one unit of measurement—in this case, 0.125-mg in each tablet of digoxin—is the first ratio, expressed as follows:

$$\text{milligrams : tablets} = \text{milligrams : tablets}$$

$$0.125 \text{ mg (amount of drug) : 1 tablet (unit of measure)}$$

The prescribed dose—in this case, 0.25-mg—is the second ratio; it must be stated in the same order and units of measure as the first, as follows:

$$0.125 \text{ mg : 1 tablet} = 0.25 \text{ mg : X (tablets)}$$

Calculate as follows:

$$0.125 \text{ X} = 0.25$$

$$X = \frac{0.25}{0.125}$$

$$X = 2$$

*Answer:* You'll need to give the patient 2 tablets of digoxin 0.125 mg.

Be sure to use critical thinking to assess whether your answer is correct. Because the amount of drug prescribed is greater than the amount of drug in one tablet, it's reasonable to expect the required number of tablets to be greater than one.

### Method 2: Using an established formula

To determine the correct number of digoxin tablets to give using this method, use the following formula:

$$\frac{\text{Prescribed dose}}{\text{Dose available}} \times \text{Quantity (unit of measure)} = \text{X (unknown quantity to be given)}$$

Calculate as follows:

$$\frac{0.25 \text{ mg}}{0.125 \text{ mg}} \times 1 \text{ tablet} = \text{X (number of 0.125-mg tablets)}$$

$$\frac{0.25}{0.125} = 2\text{X}$$

$$2 = \text{X}$$

*Answer:* You'll need to give the patient 2 tablets of digoxin 0.125 mg.

*(continued)*

## Drug Formulas and Calculations (continued)

### Method 3: Calculating according to proportion size

This method uses the same components as method #1, but the ratio is based on proportions according to size. To determine the correct number of digoxin tablets to give using this method, use the following formula:

$$\frac{\text{smaller}}{\text{larger}} = \frac{\text{smaller}}{\text{larger}}$$

Substitute 0.125 into the smaller part and 0.25 into the greater part of the first ratio. Critical thinking leads us to believe that you'll need more than 1 tablet of the weaker 0.125-mg strength to equal the stronger 0.25 mg. Set up the proportion as follows:

$$\frac{0.125 \text{ mg}}{0.25 \text{ mg}} = \frac{1 \text{ (tablet)}}{X \text{ (tablets)}}$$

Calculate as follows:

$$0.125\ X = 0.25$$

$$X = \frac{0.25}{0.125}$$

$$X = 2 \text{ tablets}$$

*Answer:* You'll need to give the patient 2 tablets of digoxin 0.125 mg.

---

### CALCULATING PARENTERAL DRUG DOSAGES

The same methods used for calculating oral drugs and solutions can be used for preparing parenteral injections.

*Example:* You need to administer a prescribed dose of 1 mg morphine sulfate from a unit-dose cartridge containing 4 mg per 2 ml. How many milliliters will you need to give to equal the prescribed dose of 1 mg?

### Method 1: Using labeled amount of drug

Using the same ratio as for oral drugs, the drug label—in this case, 4 mg—is the first ratio, and the prescribed dose—in this case, 1 mg—is the second ratio, expressed as follows:

$$4 \text{ mg (the amount of drug)} : 2 \text{ ml (the unit of measure)}$$

Calculate as follows:

$$4 \text{ mg} : 2 \text{ ml} = 1 \text{ mg} : X \text{ ml}$$

$$4X = 2$$

$$X = \frac{2}{4}$$

$$X = 0.5 \text{ ml}$$

*Answer:* You'll need to give 0.5 ml of morphine sulfate to equal the prescribed dose of 1 mg.

### Method 2: Using an established formula

Use this formula:

$$\frac{\text{Prescribed dose}}{\text{Dose available}} \times \text{Quantity (unit of measure)} = X \text{ (unknown quantity to be given)}$$

## Drug Formulas and Calculations (continued)

Calculate as follows:

$$\frac{1 \text{ mg}}{4 \text{ mg}} \times 2 \text{ ml} = X \text{ (number of ml)}$$

$$\frac{4}{2} = 0.5$$

*Answer:* You'll need to give 0.5 ml of morphine sulfate to equal the prescribed dose of 1 mg.

### Method 3: Calculating according to proportion size
To determine the correct amount of morphine sulfate to give using this method, use the following formula:

$$\text{smaller : greater} = \text{smaller : greater}$$

$$\text{milligrams : milligrams} = \text{milliliters : milliliters}$$

Critical thinking leads us to believe that 1 mg is less than 4 mg and that you'll need less than 2 ml to give 1 mg of the drug; therefore, 1 mg goes into the smaller part of the first ratio, and X goes into the smaller part of the second ratio. Set up the proportion as follows:

$$1 \text{ mg} : 4 \text{ mg} = X \text{ (ml)} : 2 \text{ ml}$$

$$4X = 2$$

$$X = \frac{2}{4}$$

$$X = 0.5$$

*Answer:* You'll need to give 0.5 ml of morphine sulfate to equal the prescribed dose of 1 mg.

## Calculating I.V. Flow Rates
When an I.V. solution is delivered by gravity, you must calculate the number of drops needed per minute for proper infusion. To calculate I.V. flow rates, you need to know three things:
- the drip factor—or the number of drops contained in 1 ml for the type of I.V. set you'll be using. This information is provided on the individual package label.
- the amount and type of fluid that you'll infuse as prescribed on the physician's order sheet
- the infusion duration time in minutes.

Once you've gathered this information, you can calculate the I.V. flow rate using the following equation:

$$\frac{\text{Total number of ml}}{\text{Total number of minutes}} \times \text{drip factor (gtt/ml)} = \text{flow rate (gtt/min)}$$

*Example 1:* If the physician prescribes 1,000 ml of $D_5W$ to infuse over 10 hours, and the drip rate for your administration set delivers 15 drops (gtt) per ml, calculate as follows:

$$\frac{1,000 \text{ ml}}{10 \text{ hours} \times 60 \text{ minutes}} \times 15 \text{ gtt/ml} = X \text{ gtt/minute}$$

$$\frac{1,000 \text{ ml}}{600 \text{ minutes}} \times 15 \text{ gtt/ml} = X \text{ gtt/minute}$$

*(continued)*

## Drug Formulas and Calculations (continued)

1.67 ml/minute $\times$ 15 gtt/ml = X gtt/minute

25.05 gtt/minute = X

*Answer:* To infuse, round off 25.05 to 25 gtt/minute or according to your institution's policy.

*Example 2:* If the physician prescribes 500 ml of 0.45% NS to infuse over 2 hours, and the drip rate for your administration set delivers 10 gtt/ml, calculate as follows:

$$\frac{500 \text{ ml}}{2 \text{ hours} \times 60 \text{ minutes}} \times 10 \text{ gtt/ml} = X \text{ gtt/minute}$$

$$\frac{500 \text{ ml}}{120 \text{ minutes}} \times 10 \text{ gtt/ml} = X \text{ gtt/minute}$$

4.17 ml/minute $\times$ 10 gtt/ml = X gtt/minute

41.7 gtt/minute = X

*Answer:* To infuse, round off 41.7 to 42 gtt/minute or according to your institution's policy.

*Note:* When preparing for I.V. administration using a controlled infusion device, the electronic flow-regulator will either count drops using an electronic eye or use a controlled pumping action to deliver the fluid in milliliters. Your final calculation will be based on the unit of measure used by the device: drops per minute, or ml per hour.

# Weights and Equivalents

The following three tables show approximate equivalents among the various systems of measurement.

## Table 1: Liquid Equivalents Among Household, Apothecaries', and Metric Systems

| HOUSEHOLD | APOTHECARIES' | METRIC |
|---|---|---|
| 1 teaspoon (tsp) | 1 fluid dram ($f\mathbf{3}$) | 5 milliliters (ml) |
| 1 tablespoon (tbs) | 0.5 fluid ounce ($f\mathbf{3}$) | 15 ml |
| 2 tbs (1 ounce [oz]) | 1 fluid ounce | 30 ml |
| 1 cupful | 8 fluid ounces | 240 ml |
| 1 pint (pt) | 16 fluid ounces | 473 ml |
| 1 quart (qt) | 32 fluid ounces | 946 ml (1 liter) |

## Table 2: Solid Equivalents Among Apothecaries' and Metric Systems

| APOTHECARIES' | METRIC |
|---|---|
| 15 grains (gr) | 1 gram (g) (1,000 milligrams [mg]) |
| 10 gr | 0.6 g (600 mg) |
| 7.5 gr | 0.5 g (500 mg) |
| 5 gr | 0.3 g (300 mg) |
| 3 gr | 0.2 g (200 mg) |
| 1.5 gr | 0.1 g (100 mg) |
| 1 gr | 0.06 g (60 mg) or 0.065 g (65 mg) |
| 0.75 gr | 0.05 g (50 mg) |
| 0.5 gr | 0.03 g (30 mg) |
| 0.25 gr | 0.015 g (15 mg) |
| 1/60 gr | 0.001 g (1 mg) |
| 1/100 gr | 0.6 mg |
| 1/120 gr | 0.5 mg |
| 1/150 gr | 0.4 mg |

(continued)

## Weights and Equivalents (continued)

### Table 3: Solid Equivalents Among Avoirdupois, Apothecaries', and Metric Systems

| AVOIRDUPOIS | APOTHECARIES' | METRIC |
|---|---|---|
| 1 gr | 1 gr | 0.065 g |
| 15.4 gr | 15 gr | 1 g |
| 1 ounce (1 oz) | 480 gr | 28.35 g |
| 437.5 gr | 1 oz | 31 g |
| 1 pound (lb) | 1.33 lb | 454 g |
| 0.75 lb | 1 lb | 373 g |
| 2.2 lb | 2.7 lb | 1 kilogram (kg) |

# Equianalgesic Doses for Opioid Agonists

An equianalgesic dose of a synthetic opioid agonist is the dose that produces the same level of analgesia as 10 mg of I.M. or S.C. morphine, the prinicipal opioid obtained from opium poppies. If your patient is switched from one opioid to another, expect to use the equianalgesic dose to decrease the risk of adverse reactions while increasing the likelihood of adequate pain relief. The chart below compares equianalgesic doses (oral and parenteral) for adults and children who weigh 50 kg (110 lb) or more.

| OPIOID | ORAL DOSE | PARENTERAL DOSE |
|---|---|---|
| codeine | 200 mg (Not recommended dose) | 120 to 130 mg |
| hydrocodone | 30 mg | Not applicable |
| hydromorphone | 7.5 mg | 1.5 mg |
| levorphanol | 4 mg | 2 mg |
| meperidine | 300 mg | 75 to 100 mg |
| morphine (around-the-clock dosing) | 30 mg | 10 mg |
| morphine (single or intermittent dosing) | 60 mg | 10 mg |
| oxycodone | 30 mg | Not applicable |

## Abbreviations

The following abbreviations, which are common to nursing practice, are used throughout the book.

| | | | | |
|---|---|---|---|---|
| ABG | arterial blood gas | | EEG | electroencephalogram |
| a.c. | before meals | | EENT | eyes, ears, nose, and throat |
| ACE | angiotensin-converting enzyme | | ENDO | endocrine |
| ADH | antidiuretic hormone | | E.R. | extended-release |
| AIDS | acquired immunodeficiency syndrome | | °F | degrees Fahrenheit |
| ALT | alanine aminotransferase | | FDA | Food and Drug Administration |
| ANA | antinuclear antibodies | | g | gram |
| APTT | activated partial thromboplastin time | | GFR | glomerular filtration rate |
| AST | aspartate aminotransferase | | GI | gastrointestinal |
| ATP | adenosine triphosphate | | gtt | drop |
| AV | atrioventricular | | GU | genitourinary |
| b.i.d. | twice a day | | $H_1$ | histamine$_1$ |
| BUN | blood urea nitrogen | | $H_2$ | histamine$_2$ |
| °C | degrees Celsius | | HDL | high-density lipoprotein |
| cAMP | cyclic adenosine monophosphate | | HEME | hematologic |
| (CAN) | Canadian drug trade name | | HIV | human immunodeficiency virus |
| cap | capsule | | HPV | human papilloma virus |
| CBC | complete blood count | | hr | hour |
| cGMP | cyclic guanosine monophosphate | | h.s. | at bedtime |
| CK | creatine kinase | | HSV | herpes simplex virus |
| Cl | chloride | | HZV | herpes zoster virus |
| cm | centimeter | | ICP | intracranial pressure |
| CMV | cytomegalovirus | | I.D. | intradermal |
| CNS | central nervous system | | IgA | immunoglobulin A |
| COPD | chronic obstructive pulmonary disease | | IgE | immunoglobulin E |
| C.R. | controlled-release | | I.M. | intramuscular |
| CSF | cerebrospinal fluid | | INR | international normalized ratio |
| CV | cardiovascular | | IU | international unit |
| CVA | cerebrovascular accident | | I.V. | intravenous |
| $D_5LR$ | dextrose 5% in lactated Ringer's solution | | IVPB | intravenous piggyback |
| $D_5NS$ | dextrose 5% in normal saline solution | | kg | kilogram |
| $D_5/0.2NS$ | dextrose 5% in quarter-normal saline solution | | KIU | kallikrein inactivator units |
| $D_5/0.45NS$ | dextrose 5% in half-normal saline solution | | L | liter |
| $D_5W$ | dextrose 5% in water | | LA | long-acting |
| $D_{10}W$ | dextrose 10% in water | | LD | lactate dehydrogenase |
| $D_{50}W$ | dextrose 50% in water | | LDL | low-density lipoprotein |
| dl | deciliter | | LOC | level of consciousness |
| DNA | deoxyribonucleic acid | | LR | lactated Ringer's solution |
| DS | double-strength | | M | molar |
| EC | enteric-coated | | $m^2$ | square meter |
| ECG | electrocardiogram | | MAO | monoamine oxidase |
| | | | mcg | microgram |
| | | | mEq | milliequivalent |
| | | | mg | milligram |
| | | | MI | myocardial infarction |
| | | | min | minute |
| | | | ml | milliliter |

## Abbreviations (continued)

| | | | | |
|---|---|---|---|---|
| **mm** | millimeter | | **q** | every |
| **mm³** | cubic millimeter | | **q.d.** | every day |
| **mmol** | millimole | | **q.i.d.** | four times a day |
| **mo** | month | | **q.o.d.** | every other day |
| **MS** | musculoskeletal | | **RBC** | red blood cell |
| **Na** | sodium | | **REM** | rapid eye movement |
| **NaCl** | sodium chloride | | **RESP** | respiratory |
| **NG** | nasogastric | | **RNA** | ribonucleic acid |
| **NPH** | human isophane insulin | | **RSV** | respiratory syncytial virus |
| **NPO** | nothing by mouth | | **SA** | sinoatrial |
| **NS** | normal saline solution | | **S.C.** | subcutaneous |
| **0.225NS** | quarter-normal saline (0.225%) solution | | **sec** | second |
| **0.45NS** | half-normal saline (0.45%) solution | | **S.L.** | sublingual |
| **NSAID** | nonsteroidal anti-inflammatory drug | | **S.R.** | sustained-release |
| | | | **stat** | immediately |
| **OTC** | over the counter | | **supp** | suppository |
| **p.c.** | after meals | | **tab** | tablet |
| **PCA** | patient-controlled analgesia | | **T₃** | triiodothyronine |
| **P.O.** | by mouth | | **T₄** | thyroxine |
| **P.R.** | by rectum | | **t.i.d.** | three times a day |
| **p.r.n.** | as needed | | **U** | units |
| **PSVT** | paroxysmal supraventricular tachycardia | | **USP** | United States Pharmacopeia |
| **PT** | prothrombin time | | **UTI** | urinary tract infection |
| **PTCA** | percutaneous transluminal coronary angioplasty | | **VLDL** | very low-density lipoprotein |
| | | | **WBC** | white blood cell |
| **PVC** | premature ventricular contraction | | **wk** | week |

# Index

- **Generic and alternate names:** lowercase initial letter
- **Trade names:** uppercase initial letter
- **Illustrations:** *i* after page number
- **Tables:** *t* after page number

# NOTES

# NOTES